OPTUM360°®

MW00356262

Current Procedural Coding Expert

CPT® codes with Medicare essentials for enhanced accuracy

2021

optum360coding.com

Notice

The *2021 Current Procedural Coding Expert* is designed to be an accurate and authoritative source of information about the CPT® coding system. Every effort has been made to verify the accuracy of the listings, and all information is believed reliable at the time of publication. Absolute accuracy cannot be guaranteed, however. This publication is made available with the understanding that the publisher is not engaged in rendering legal or other services that require a professional license.

American Medical Association Notice

Fee schedules, relative value units, conversion factors and/or related components are not assigned by the AMA, are not part of CPT, and the AMA is not recommending their use. The AMA does not directly or indirectly practice medicine or dispense medical services. The AMA assumes no liability for data contained or not contained herein.

CPT is a registered trademark of the American Medical Association.

Our Commitment to Accuracy

Optum360 is committed to producing accurate and reliable materials.

To report corrections, please email accuracy@optum.com. You can also reach customer service by calling 1.800.464.3649, option 1.

Copyright

Made in the USA

ISBN 978-1-62254-551-3

Acknowledgments

Gregory A. Kemp, MA, *Product Manager*
Stacy Perry, *Manager, Desktop Publishing*
Elizabeth Leibold, RHIT, *Subject Matter Expert*
Anita Schmidt, BS, RHIA, AHIMA-approved ICD-10-CM/PCS Trainer, *Subject Matter Expert*
LaJuana Green, RHIA, CCS, *Subject Matter Expert*
Tracy Betzler, *Senior Desktop Publishing Specialist*
Hope M. Dunn, *Senior Desktop Publishing Specialist*
Katie Russell, *Desktop Publishing Specialist*
Kate Holden, *Editor*

About the Contributors

Elizabeth Leibold, RHIT

Ms. Leibold has more than 25 years of experience in the health care profession. She has served in a variety of roles, ranging from patient registration to billing and collections, and has an extensive background in both physician and hospital outpatient coding and compliance. She has worked for large health care systems and health information management services companies, and has wide-ranging experience in facility and professional component coding, along with CPT expertise in interventional procedures, infusion services, emergency department, observation, and ambulatory surgery coding. Her areas of expertise include chart-to-claim coding audits and providing staff education to both tenured and new coding staff. She is an active member of the American Health Information Management Association (AHIMA) and West Tennessee Health Information Management Association (WTHIMA).

Anita Schmidt, BS, RHIA, AHIMA-approved ICD-10-CM/PCS Trainer

Ms. Schmidt has expertise in ICD-10-CM/PCS, DRG, and CPT with more than 15 years' experience in coding in multiple settings, including inpatient, observation, and same-day surgery. Her experience includes analysis of medical record documentation, assignment of ICD-10-CM and PCS codes, and DRG validation. She has conducted training for ICD-10-CM/PCS and electronic health record. She has also collaborated with clinical documentation specialists to identify documentation needs and potential areas for physician education. Most recently she has been developing content for resource and educational products related to ICD-10-CM, ICD-10-PCS, DRG, and CPT. Ms. Schmidt is an AHIMA-approved ICD-10-CM/PCS trainer and is an active member of the American Health Information Management Association (AHIMA) and the Minnesota Health Information Management Association.

LaJuana Green, RHIA, CCS

Ms. Green is a Registered Health Information Administrator with over 35 years of experience in multiple areas of information management. She has proven expertise in the analysis of medical record documentation, assignment of ICD-10-CM and PCS codes, DRG validation, and CPT code assignment in ambulatory surgery units and the hospital outpatient setting. Her experience includes serving as a director of a health information management department, clinical technical editing, new technology research and writing, medical record management, utilization review activities, quality assurance, tumor registry, medical library services, and chargemaster maintenance. Ms. Green is an active member of the American Health Information Management Association (AHIMA).

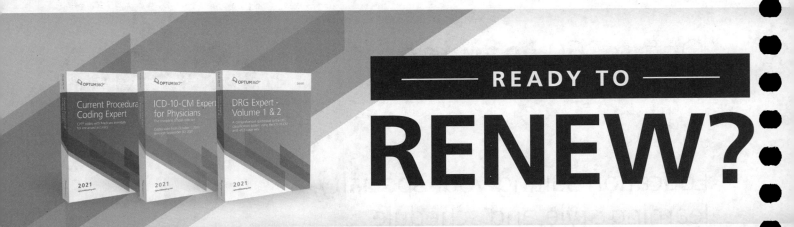

Contents

Introduction

Welcome to Optum360's *Current Procedural Coding Expert*, an exciting Medicare coding and reimbursement tool and definitive procedure coding source that combines the work of the Centers for Medicare and Medicaid Services, American Medical Association, and Optum360 experts with the technical components you need for proper reimbursement and coding accuracy. Handy snap in tabs are included to indicate those sections used most often for easy reference.

This approach to CPT® Medicare coding utilizes innovative and intuitive ways of communicating the information you need to code claims accurately and efficiently. *Includes* and *Excludes* notes, similar to those found in the ICD-10-CM manual, help determine what services are related to the codes you are reporting. Icons help you crosswalk the code you are reporting to laboratory and radiology procedures necessary for proper reimbursement. CMS-mandated icons and relative value units (RVUs) help you determine which codes are most appropriate for the service you are reporting. Add to that additional information identifying age and sex edits, ambulatory surgery center (ASC) and ambulatory payment classification (APC) indicators, and Medicare coverage and payment rule citations, and *Current Procedural Coding Expert* provides the best in Medicare procedure reporting.

Current Procedural Coding Expert includes the information needed to submit claims to federal contractors and most commercial payers, and is correct at the time of printing. However, CMS, federal contractors, and commercial payers may change payment rules at any time throughout the year. *Current Procedural Coding Expert* includes effective codes that will not be published in the AMA's Current Procedural Terminology (CPT) book until the following year. Commercial payers will announce changes through monthly news or information posted on their websites. CMS will post changes in policy on its website at http://www.cms.gov/transmittals. National and local coverage determinations (NCDs and LCDs) provide universal and individual contractor guidelines for specific services. The existence of a procedure code does not imply coverage under any given insurance plan.

Current Procedural Coding Expert is based on the AMA's Current Procedural Terminology coding system, which is copyrighted and owned by the physician organization. The CPT codes are the nation's official, Health Information Portability and Accountability Act (HIPAA) compliant code set for procedures and services provided by physicians, ambulatory surgery centers (ASCs), and hospital outpatient services, as well as laboratories, imaging centers, physical therapy clinics, urgent care centers, and others.

Getting Started with *Current Procedural Coding Expert*

Current Procedural Coding Expert is an exciting tool combining the most current material at the time of our publication from the AMA's CPT 2021, CMS's online manual system, the Correct Coding initiative, CMS fee schedules, official Medicare guidelines for reimbursement and coverage, the Integrated Outpatient Code Editor (I/OCE), and Optum360's own coding expertise.

These coding rules and guidelines are incorporated into more specific section notes and code notes. Section notes are listed under a range of codes and apply to all codes in that range. Code notes are found under individual codes and apply to the single code.

Material is presented in a logical fashion for those billing Medicare, Medicaid, and many private payers. The format, based on customer comments, better addresses what customers tell us they need in a comprehensive Medicare procedure coding guide.

Designed to be easy to use and full of information, this product is an excellent companion to your AMA CPT manual, and other Optum360 and Medicare resources.

For mid-year code updates, official errata changes, correction notices, and any other changes pertinent to the information in *Current Procedural Coding Expert*, see our product update page at https://www.optum360coding.com/ProductUpdates/. The password for 2021 is PROCEDURE2021.

Note: The AMA releases code changes quarterly as well as errata or corrections to CPT codes and guidelines and posts them on their web site. Some of these changes may not appear in the AMA's CPT book until the following year. *Current Procedural Coding Expert* incorporates the most recent errata or release notes found on the AMA's web site at our publication time, including new, revised and deleted codes. *Current Procedural Coding Expert* identifies these new or revised codes from the AMA website errata or release notes with an icon similar to the AMA's current new ● and revised ▲ icons. For purposes of this publication, new CPT codes and revisions that won't be in the AMA book until the next edition are indicated with a ● and a ▲ icon. For the next year's edition of *Current Procedural Coding Expert*, these codes will appear with standard black new or revised icons, as appropriate, to correspond with those changes as indicated in the AMA's CPT book. CPT codes that were new for 2020 and appeared in the 2020 *Current Procedural Coding Expert* but did not appear in the AMA's CPT code book until 2021 are identified in appendix B as "Web Release New and Revised Codes."

General Conventions

Many of the sources of information in this book can be determined by color.

- All CPT codes and descriptions and the Evaluation and Management guidelines from the American Medical Association are in **black text**.
- Includes, Excludes, and other notes appear in **blue text**. The resources used for this information are a variety of Medicare policy manuals, the *National Correct Coding Initiative Policy Manual* (NCCI), AMA resources and guidelines, and specialty association resources and our Optum360 clinical experts.

Resequencing of CPT Codes

The American Medical Association (AMA) uses a numbering methodology of resequencing, which is the practice of displaying codes outside of their numerical order according to the description relationship. According to the AMA, there are instances in which a new code is needed within an existing grouping of codes but an unused code number is not available. In these situations, the AMA will resequence the codes. In other words, it will assign a code that is not in numeric sequence with the related codes. However, the code and description will appear in the CPT manual with the other related codes.

An example of resequencing from *Current Procedural Coding Expert* follows:

	21555	**Excision, tumor, soft tissue of neck or anterior thorax, subcutaneous; less than 3 cm**
#	**21552**	**3 cm or greater**
	21556	**Excision, tumor, soft tissue of neck or anterior thorax, subfascial (eg, intramuscular); less than 5 cm**
#	**21554**	**5 cm or greater**

In *Current Procedural Coding Expert* the resequenced codes are listed twice. They appear in their resequenced position as shown above as well as in their original numeric position with a note indicating that the code is out of numerical sequence and where it can be found. (See example below.)

21554 **Resequenced code. See code following 21556.**

This differs from the AMA CPT book, in which the coder is directed to a code range that contains the resequenced code and description, rather than to a specific location.

Resequenced codes will appear in brackets in the headers, section notes, and code ranges. For example:

27327-27339 [27337, 27339] Excision Soft Tissue Tumors Femur/Knee. Codes [27337, 27339] are included in section 27327-27339 in their resequenced positions.

Code also toxoid/vaccine (90476-90749 [90620, 90621, 90625, 90630, 90644, 90672, 90673, 90674, 90750, 90756])

This shows codes 90620, 90621, 90625, 90630, 90644, 90672, 90673, 90674, 90750, and 90756 are resequenced in this range of codes.

Code Ranges for Medicare Billing

Appendix E identifies all resequenced CPT codes. Optum360 will display the resequenced coding as assigned by the AMA in its CPT products so that the user may understand the code description relationships.

Each particular group of CPT codes in *Current Procedural Coding Expert* is organized in a more intuitive fashion for Medicare billing, being grouped by the Medicare rules and regulations as found in the official CMS online manuals that govern payment of these particular procedures and services, as in this example:

99221-99233 Inpatient Hospital Visits: Initial and Subsequent
CMS: 100-4,11,40.1.3 Independent Attending Physician Services; 100-4,12,100.1.1 Teaching Physicians E/M Services; 100-4,12,30.6.10 Consultation Services; 100-4,12,30.6.15.1 Prolonged Services With Direct Face-to-Face Patient Contact; 100-4,12,30.6.4 Services Furnished Incident to Physician's Service; 100-4,12,30.6.9 Hospital Visit and Critical Care on Same Day

Icons

● **New Codes**
Codes that have been added since the last edition of the AMA CPT book was printed.

▲ **Revised Codes**
Codes that have been revised since the last edition of the AMA CPT book was printed.

● **New Web Release**
Codes that are new for the current year but will not be in the AMA CPT book until 2022.

▲ **Revised Web Release**
Codes that have been revised for the current year, but will not be in the AMA CPT book until 2022.

Resequenced Codes
Codes that are out of numeric order but apply to the appropriate category.

★ **Telemedicine Services**
Codes that may be reported for telemedicine services. Modifier 95 must be appended to code.

❍ **Reinstated Code**
Codes that have been reinstated since the last edition of the book was printed.

Pink Color Bar—Not Covered by Medicare
Services and procedures identified by this color bar are never covered benefits under Medicare. Services and procedures that are not covered may be billed directly to the patient at the time of the service.

Gray Color Bar—Unlisted Procedure
Unlisted CPT codes report procedures that have not been assigned a specific code number. An unlisted code delays payment due to the extra time necessary for review.

Green Color Bar—Resequenced Codes
Resequenced codes are codes that are out of numeric sequence—they are indicated with a green color bar. They are listed twice, in their resequenced position as well as in their original numeric position with a note that the code is out of numerical sequence and where the resequenced code and description can be found.

INCLUDES **Includes notes**
Includes notes identify procedures and services that would be bundled in the procedure code. These are derived from AMA, CMS, NCCI, and Optum360 coding guidelines. This is not meant to be an all-inclusive list.

EXCLUDES **Excludes notes**
Excludes notes may lead the user to other codes. They may identify services that are not bundled and may be separately reported, OR may lead the user to another more appropriate code. These are derived from AMA, CMS, NCCI, and Optum360 coding guidelines. This is not meant to be an all-inclusive list.

Code Also This note identifies an additional code that should be reported with the service and may relate to another CPT code or an appropriate HCPCS code(s) that should be reported along with the CPT code when appropriate.

Code First Found under add-on codes, this note identifies codes for primary procedures that should be reported first, with the add-on code reported as a secondary code.

Laboratory/Pathology Crosswalk
This icon denotes CPT codes in the laboratory and pathology section of CPT that may be reported separately with the primary CPT code.

Radiology Crosswalk
This icon denotes codes in the radiology section that may be used with the primary CPT code being reported.

TC **Technical Component Only**
Codes with this icon represent only the technical component (staff and equipment costs) of a procedure or service. Do not use either modifier 26 (professional component) or TC (technical component) with these codes.

26 **Professional Component**
Only codes with this icon represent the physician's work or professional component of a procedure or service. Do not use either modifier 26 (professional component) or TC (technical component) with these codes.

50 **Bilateral Procedure**
This icon identifies codes that can be reported bilaterally when the same surgeon provides the service for the same patient on the same date. Medicare allows payment for both procedures at 150 percent of the usual amount for one procedure. The modifier does not apply to bilateral procedures inclusive to one code.

80 **Assist-at-Surgery Allowed**
Services noted by this icon are allowed an assistant at surgery with a Medicare payment equal to 16 percent of the allowed amount for the global surgery for that procedure. No documentation is required.

80 **Assist-at-Surgery Allowed with Documentation**
Services noted by this icon are allowed an assistant at surgery with a Medicare payment equal to 16 percent of the allowed amount for the global surgery for that procedure. Documentation is required.

\+ **Add-on Codes**
This icon identifies procedures reported in addition to the primary procedure. The icon "+" denotes add-on codes. An add-on code is neither a stand-alone code nor subject to multiple procedure rules since it describes work in addition to the primary procedure.

According to Medicare guidelines, add-on codes may be identified in the following ways:

- The code is found on Change Request (CR) 7501 or successive CRs as a Type I, Type II, or Type III add-on code.

- The add-on code most often has a global period of "ZZZ" in the Medicare Physician Fee Schedule Database.
- The code is found in the CPT book with the icon "+" appended. Add-on code descriptors typically include the phrases "each additional" or "(List separately in addition to primary procedure)."

(50) **Optum Modifier 50 Exempt**
Codes identified by this icon indicate that the procedure should not be reported with modifier 50 (Bilateral procedures).

⊘ **Modifier 51 Exempt**
Codes identified by this icon indicate that the procedure should not be reported with modifier 51 (Multiple procedures).

(51) **Optum Modifier 51 Exempt**
Codes identified by this Optum360 icon indicate that the procedure should not be reported with modifier 51 (Multiple procedures). Any code with this icon is backed by official AMA guidelines but was not identified by the AMA with their modifier 51 exempt icon.

Correct Coding Initiative (CCI)
Current Procedural Coding Expert identifies those codes with corresponding CCI edits. The CCI edits define correct coding practices that serve as the basis of the national Medicare policy for paying claims. The code noted is the major service/procedure. The code may represent a column 1 code within the column 1/column 2 correct coding edits table or a code pair that is mutually exclusive of each other.

CLIA Waived Test
This symbol is used to distinguish those laboratory tests that can be performed using test systems that are waived from regulatory oversight established by the Clinical Laboratory Improvement Amendments of 1988 (CLIA). The applicable CPT code for a CLIA waived test may be reported by providers who perform the testing but do not hold a CLIA license.

(63) **Modifier 63 Exempt**
This icon identifies procedures performed on infants that weigh less than 4 kg. Due to the complexity of performing procedures on infants less than 4 kg, modifier 63 may be added to the surgery codes to inform the payers of the special circumstances involved.

A2–Z3 **ASC Payment Indicators**
This icon identifies ASC status payment indicators. They indicate how the ASC payment rate was derived and/or how the procedure, item, or service is treated under the revised ASC payment system. For more information about these indicators and how they affect billing, consult Optum360's *Revenue Cycle Pro*.

- A2 Surgical procedure on ASC list in 2007; payment based on OPPS relative payment weight.
- B5 Alternative code may be available; no payment made.
- Deleted/discontinued code; no payment made.
- F4 Corneal tissue acquisition; hepatitis B vaccine; paid at reasonable cost.
- G2 Non-office-based surgical procedure added in CY 2008 or later; payment based on OPPS relative payment weight.
- H2 Brachytherapy source paid separately when provided integral to a surgical procedure on ASC list; payment based on OPPS rate.
- J7 OPPS pass-through device paid separately when provided integral to a surgical procedure on ASC list; payment contractor-priced.
- J8 Device-intensive procedure; paid at adjusted rate.
- K2 Drugs and biologicals paid separately when provided integral to a surgical procedure on ASC list; payment based on OPPS rate.
- K7 Unclassified drugs and biologicals; payment contractor-priced.
- L1 Influenza vaccine; pneumococcal vaccine. Packaged item/service; no separate payment made.
- L6 New technology intraocular lens (NTIOL); special payment.
- N1 Packaged service/item; no separate payment made.
- P2 Office-based surgical procedure added to ASC list in CY 2008 or later with MPFS nonfacility practice expense (PE) RVUs; payment based on OPPS relative payment weight.
- P3 Office-based surgical procedure added to ASC list in CY 2008 or later with MPFS nonfacility PE RVUs; payment based on MPFS nonfacility PE RVUs.
- R2 Office-based surgical procedure added to ASC list in CY 2008 or later without MPFS nonfacility PE RVUs; payment based on OPPS relative payment weight.
- Z2 Radiology or diagnostic service paid separately when provided integral to a surgical procedure on ASC list; payment based on OPPS relative payment weight.
- Z3 Radiology or diagnostic service paid separately when provided integral to a surgical procedure on ASC list; payment based on MPFS nonfacility PE RVUs.

A **Age Edit**
This icon denotes codes intended for use with a specific age group, such as neonate, newborn, pediatric, and adult. This edit is based on age specifications in the CPT code descriptors, the product/service represented by the code *may* have age restrictions, and/or updates from the Integrated Outpatient Code Editor (I/OCE). Carefully review the code description to ensure the code you report most appropriately reflects the patient's age.

M **Maternity**
This icon identifies procedures that by definition should be used only for maternity patients generally between 9 and 64 years of age based on CMS I/OCE designations.

♀ **Female Only**
This icon identifies procedures designated by CMS for females only based on CMS I/OCE designations.

♂ **Male Only**
This icon identifies procedures designated by CMS for males only based on CMS I/OCE designations.

Facility RVU
This icon precedes the facility RVU from CMS's 2018 physician fee schedule (PFS). It can be found under the code description.

New codes include no RVU information.

Nonfacility RVU
This icon precedes the nonfacility RVU from CMS's 2018 PFS. It can be found under the code description.

New codes include no RVU information.

FUD: Global days are sometimes referred to as "follow-up days" or FUDs. The global period is the time following surgery during which routine care by the physician is considered postoperative and included in the surgical fee. Office visits or other routine care related to the original surgery cannot be separately reported if provided during the global period. The statuses are:

000	No follow-up care included in this procedure
010	Normal postoperative care is included in this procedure for ten days
090	Normal postoperative care is included in the procedure for 90 days
MMM	Maternity codes; usual global period does not apply
XXX	The global concept does not apply to the code

YYY The carrier is to determine whether the global concept applies and establishes postoperative period, if appropriate, at time of pricing

ZZZ The code is related to another service and is always included in the global period of the other service

CMS: This notation indicates that there is a specific CMS guideline pertaining to this code in the CMS Online Manual System which includes the internet-only manual (IOM) *National Coverage Determinations Manual* (NCD). These CMS sources present the rules for submitting these services to the federal government or its contractors and a link to the IOMs is included in appendix G of this book.

AMA: This indicates discussion of the code in the American Medical Association's *CPT Assistant* newsletter. Use the citation to find the correct issue. This includes citations for the current year and the preceding six years. In the event no citations can be found during this time period, the most recent citations that can be found are used.

Drug Not Approved by FDA
The AMA CPT Editorial Panel is publishing new vaccine product codes prior to Food and Drug Administration approval. This symbol indicates which of these codes are pending FDA approval at press time.

[A]–[Y] **OPPS Status Indicators (OPSI)**
Status indicators identify how individual CPT codes are paid or not paid under the latest available hospital outpatient prospective payment system (OPPS). The same status indicator is assigned to all the codes within an ambulatory payment classification (APC). Consult your payer or other resource to learn which CPT codes fall within various APCs.

[A] Services furnished to a hospital outpatient that are paid under a fee schedule or payment system other than OPPS. For example:
- Ambulance services
- Separately payable clinical diagnostic laboratory services
- Separately payable non-implantable prosthetics and orthotics
- Physical, occupational, and speech therapy
- Diagnostic mammography
- Screening mammography

[B] Codes that are not recognized by OPPS when submitted on an outpatient hospital Part B bill type (12x and 13x)

[C] Inpatient procedures

[D] Discontinued codes

[E] Items, codes, and services:
- Not covered by any Medicare outpatient benefit category
- Statutorily excluded by Medicare
- Not reasonable and necessary

[NC] Items, codes, and services for which pricing information and claims data are not available

[F] Corneal tissue acquisition; certain CRNA services and hepatitis B vaccines

[G] Pass-through drugs and biologicals

[H] Pass-through device categories

[J1] Hospital Part B services paid through a comprehensive APC

[L1] Hospital Part B services that may be paid through a comprehensive APC

[K] Nonpass-through drugs and nonimplantable biologicals, including therapeutic radiopharmaceuticals

[L] Influenza vaccine; pneumococcal pneumonia vaccine

[M] Items and services not billable to the MAC

[N] Items and services packaged into APC rates

[P] Partial hospitalization

[Q1] STV-packaged codes

[Q2] T-packaged codes

[Q3] Codes that may be paid through a composite APC

[NI] Conditionally packaged laboratory tests

[R] Blood and blood products

[S] Procedure or service, not discounted when multiple

[T] Procedure or service, multiple procedure reduction applies

[U] Brachytherapy sources

[V] Clinic or emergency department visit

[Y] Nonimplantable durable medical equipment

Appendixes

Appendix A: Modifiers—This appendix identifies modifiers. A modifier is a two-position alpha or numeric code that is appended to a CPT or HCPCS code to clarify the services being billed. Modifiers provide a means by which a service can be altered without changing the procedure code. They add more information, such as anatomical site, to the code. In addition, they help eliminate the appearance of duplicate billing and unbundling. Modifiers are used to increase the accuracy in reimbursement and coding consistency, ease editing, and capture payment data.

Appendix B: New, Revised, and Deleted Codes—This is a list of new, revised, and deleted CPT codes for the current year. This appendix also includes a list of web release new and revised codes, which indicate official code changes in *Current Procedural Coding Expert* that will not be in the CPT code book until the following year.

Appendix C: Evaluation and Management Extended Guidelines—This appendix presents an overview of evaluation and management (E/M) services that augment the official AMA CPT E/M services. It includes tables that distinguish documentation components of each E/M code and the federal documentation guidelines (1995 and 1997) currently in use by the Centers for Medicare and Medicaid Services (CMS).

Appendix D: Crosswalk of Deleted Codes—This appendix is a cross-reference from a deleted CPT code to an active code when one is available. The deleted code cross-reference will also appear under the deleted code description in the tabular section of the book.

Appendix E: Resequenced Codes—This appendix contains a list of codes that are not in numeric order in the book. AMA resequenced some of the code numbers to relocate codes in the same category but not in numeric sequence. In addition to the list of codes, this appendix provides the page number where the resequenced code may be found.

Appendix F: Add-on, Optum Modifier 50 Exempt, Modifier 51 Exempt, Optum Modifier 51 Exempt, Modifier 63 Exempt, and Modifier 95 Telemedicine Services—This list includes add-on codes that cannot be reported alone, codes that are exempt from modifiers 50 and 51, codes that should not be reported with modifier 63, and codes identified by the ★ icon to which modifier 95 may be appended when the service is provided as a synchronous telemedicine service.

Appendix G: Medicare Internet-only Manual (IOMs)—Previously, this appendix contained a verbatim printout of the Medicare Internet-only Manual references pertaining to specific codes. This appendix now contains a link to the IOMs on the Centers for Medicare and Medicaid Services website. The IOM references applicable to specific codes can still be found at the code level. For example:

93784-93790 Ambulatory Blood Pressure Monitoring

CMS: 100-3,20.19 Ambulatory Blood Pressure Monitoring (20.19); 100-4,32,10.1 Ambulatory Blood Pressure Monitoring Billing Requirements

Appendix H: Quality Payment Program (QPP)—Previously, this appendix contained lists of the numerators and denominators applicable to the Medicare PQRS. However, with the implementation of the Quality Payment Program (QPP) mandated by passage of the Medicare Access and Chip Reauthorization Act (MACRA) of 2015, the PQRS system will be obsolete. This appendix now contains information pertinent to that legislation as well as a brief overview of the proposed changes for the following year.

Appendix I: Medically Unlikely Edits—This appendix contains the published medically unlikely edits (MUEs). These edits establish maximum daily allowable units of service. The edits will be applied to the services provided to the same patient, for the same CPT code, on the same date of service when billed by the same provider. Included are the physician and facility edits.

Appendix J: Inpatient-Only Procedures—This appendix identifies services with the status indicator "C." Medicare will not pay an OPPS hospital or ASC when these procedures are performed on a Medicare patient as an outpatient. Physicians should refer to this list when scheduling Medicare patients for surgical procedures. CMS updates this list quarterly.

Appendix K: Place of Service and Type of Service—This appendix contains lists of place-of-service codes that should be used on professional claims and type-of-service codes used by the Medicare Common Working File.

Appendix L: Multianalyte Assays with Algorithmic Analyses —This appendix lists the administrative codes for multianalyte assays with algorithmic analyses. The AMA updates this list three times a year.

Appendix M: Glossary—This appendix contains general terms and definitions as well as those that would apply to or be helpful for billing and reimbursement.

Appendix N: Listing of Sensory, Motor, and Mixed Nerves—This appendix lists a summary of each sensory, motor, and mixed nerve with its appropriate nerve conduction study code.

Appendix O: Vascular Families—Appendix O contains a table of vascular families starting with the aorta. Additional information can be found in the interventional radiology illustrations located behind the index.

Appendix P: Interventional Radiology Illustrations—This appendix contains illustrations specific to interventional radiology procedures.

Note: All data current as of November 12, 2020.

Anatomical Illustrations

Body Planes and Movements

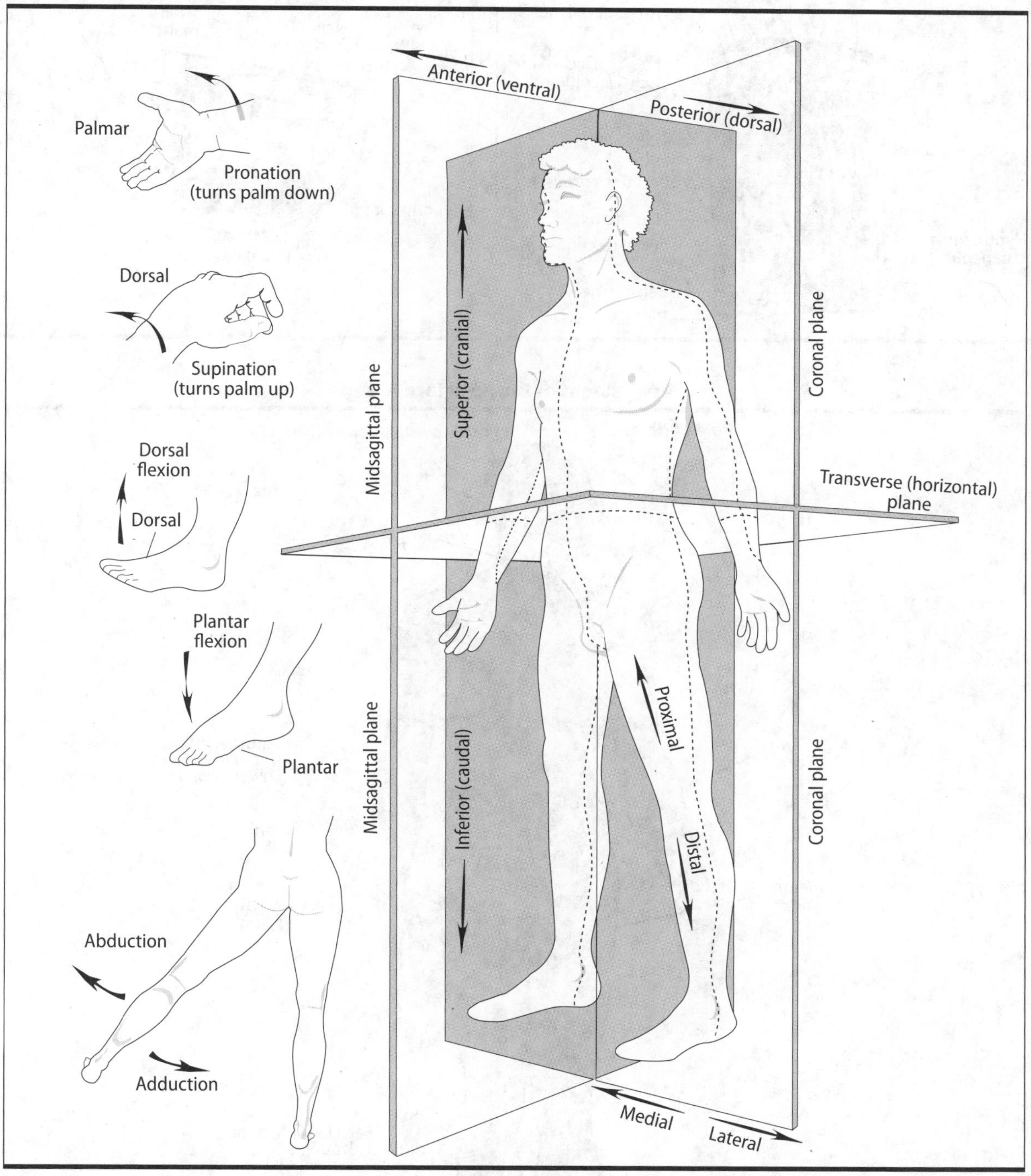

Integumentary System

Skin and Subcutaneous Tissue

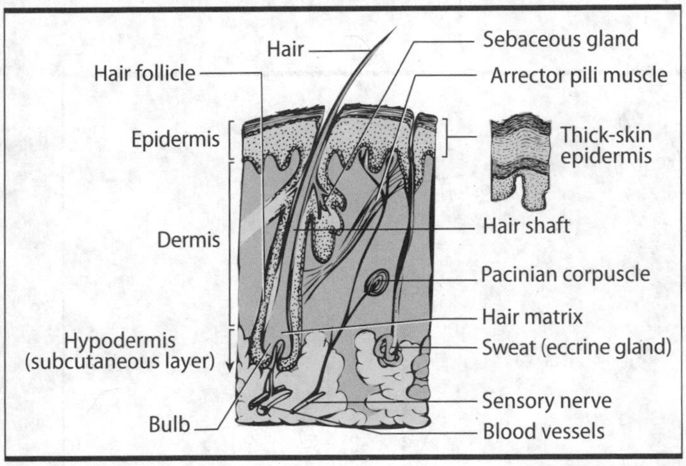

Nail Anatomy

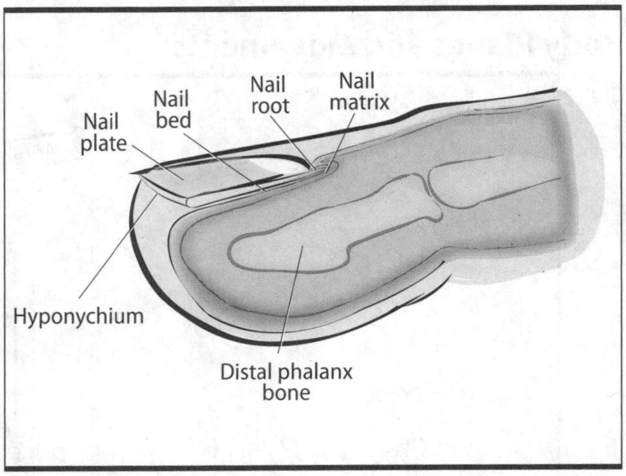

Assessment of Burn Surface Area

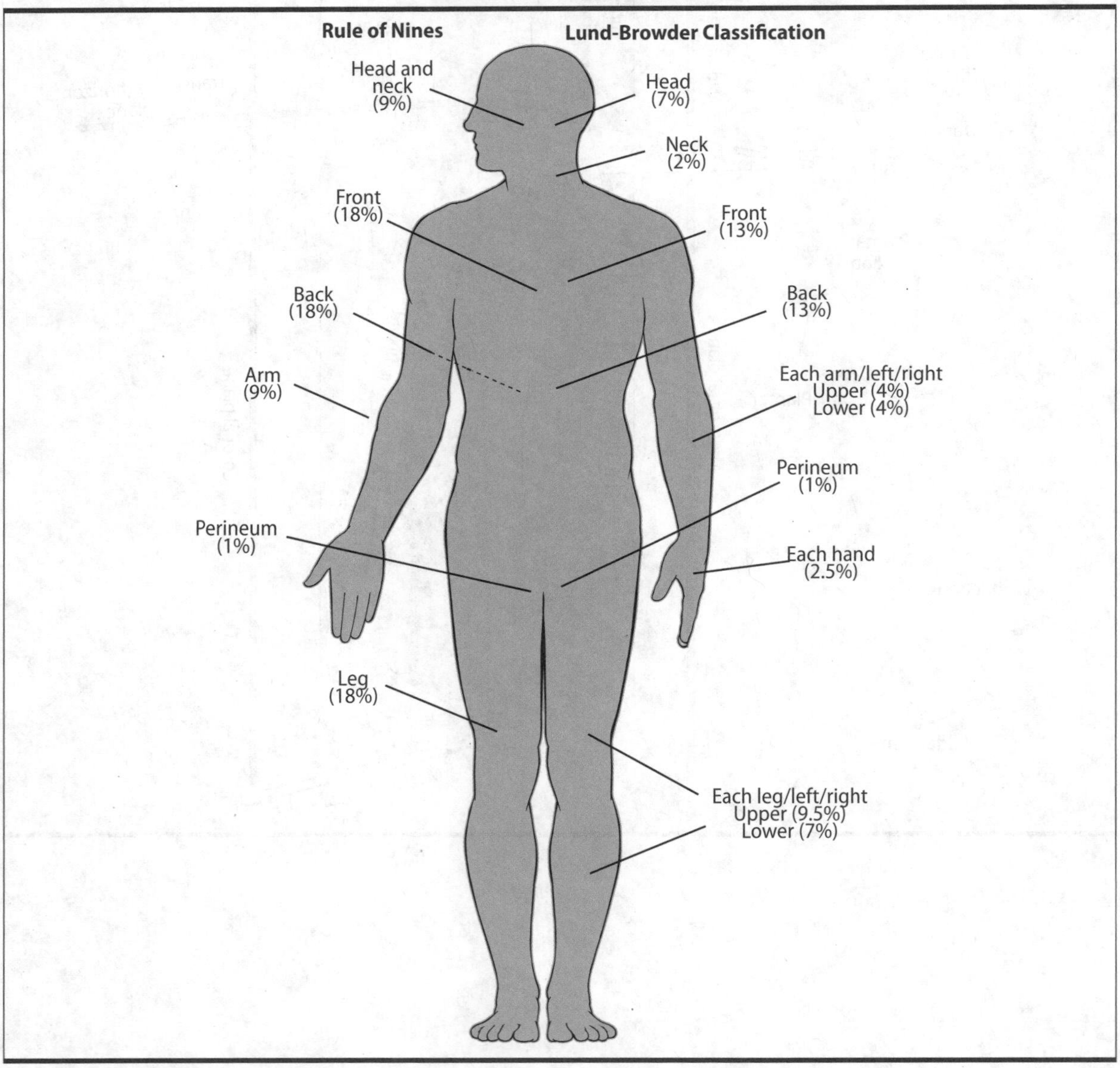

Musculoskeletal System

Bones and Joints

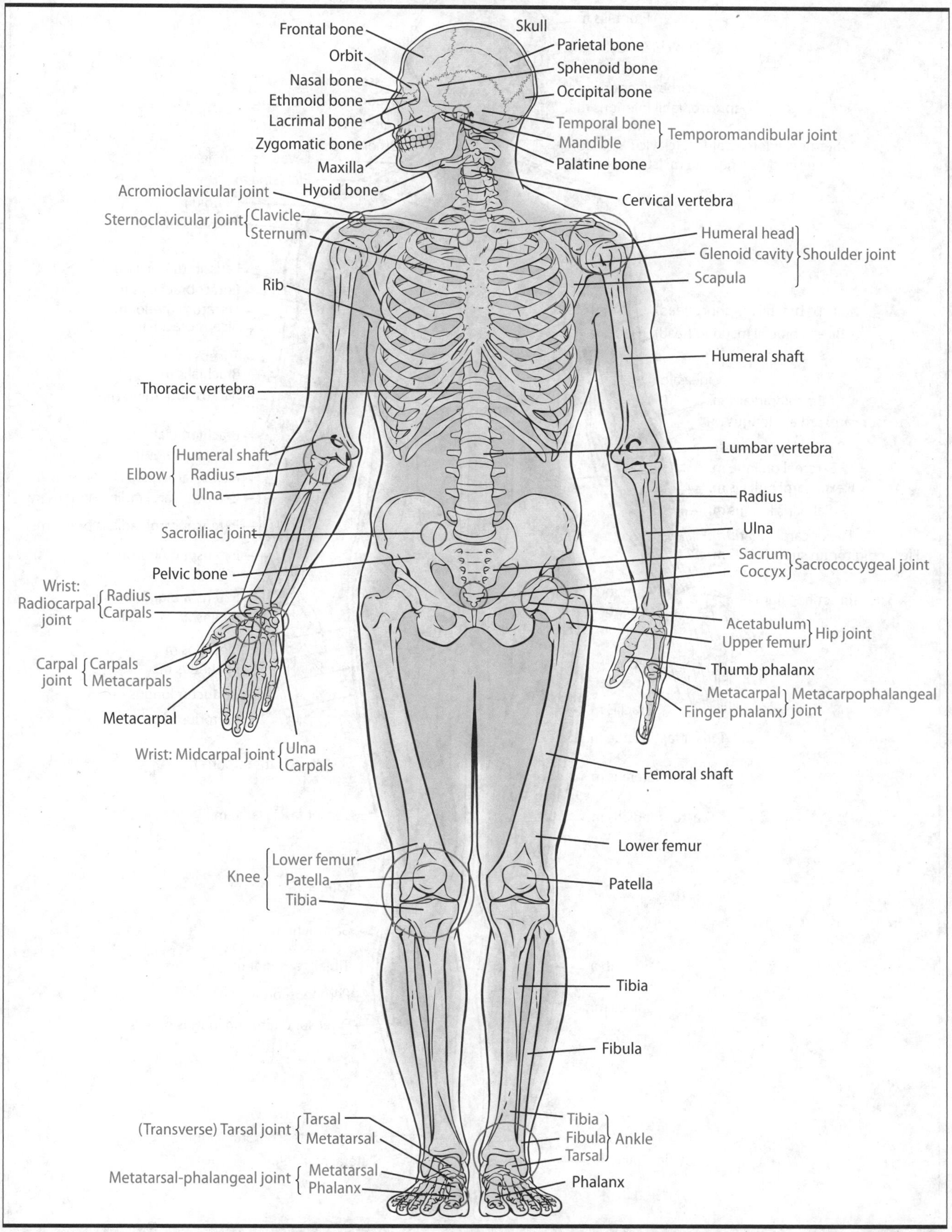

Muscles

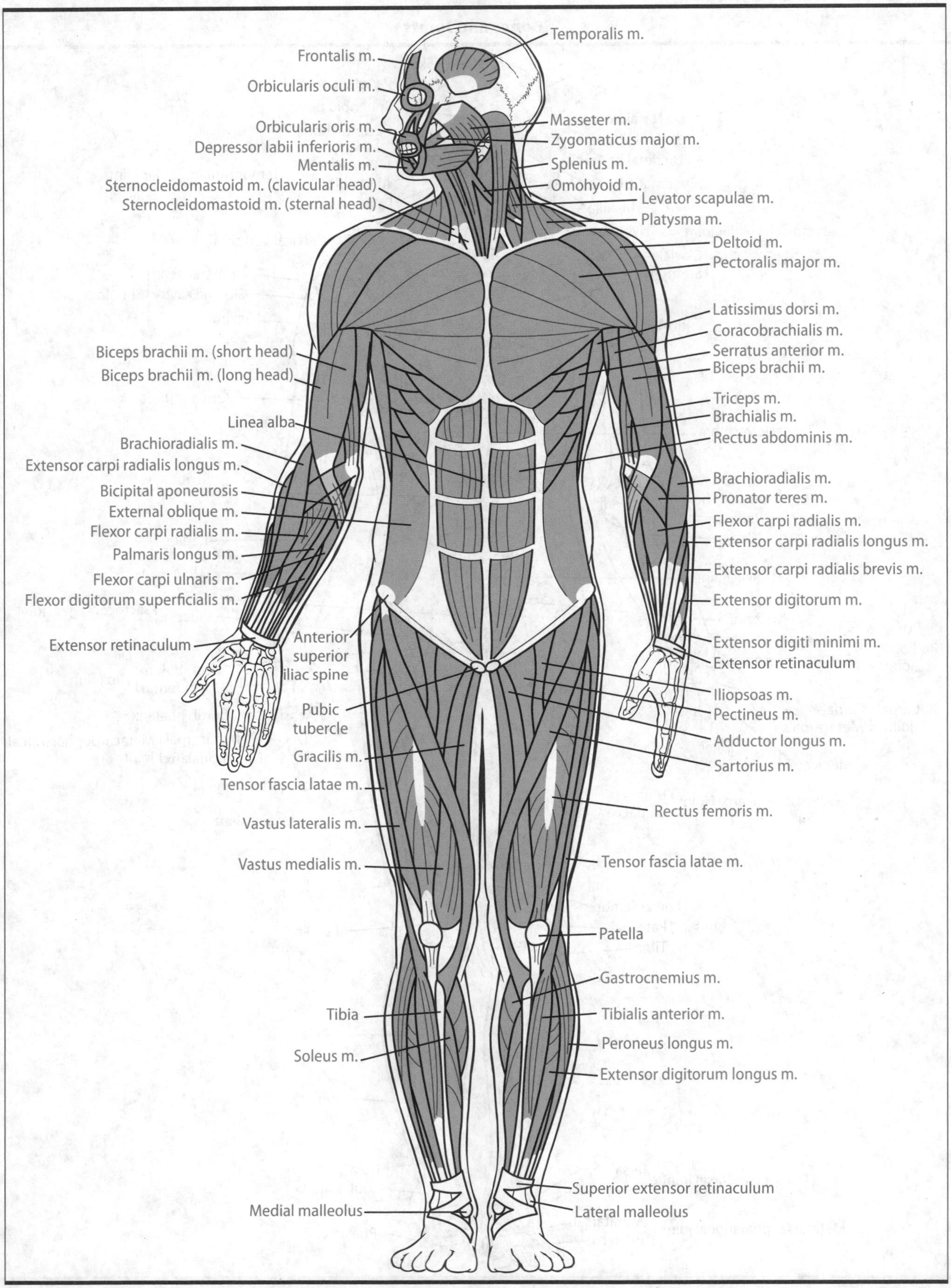
Temporalis m.
Frontalis m.
Orbicularis oculi m.
Orbicularis oris m.
Depressor labii inferioris m.
Mentalis m.
Sternocleidomastoid m. (clavicular head)
Sternocleidomastoid m. (sternal head)
Masseter m.
Zygomaticus major m.
Splenius m.
Omohyoid m.
Levator scapulae m.
Platysma m.
Deltoid m.
Pectoralis major m.
Latissimus dorsi m.
Coracobrachialis m.
Serratus anterior m.
Biceps brachii m.
Biceps brachii m. (short head)
Biceps brachii m. (long head)
Triceps m.
Brachialis m.
Rectus abdominis m.
Linea alba
Brachioradialis m.
Extensor carpi radialis longus m.
Bicipital aponeurosis
External oblique m.
Flexor carpi radialis m.
Palmaris longus m.
Flexor carpi ulnaris m.
Flexor digitorum superficialis m.
Brachioradialis m.
Pronator teres m.
Flexor carpi radialis m.
Extensor carpi radialis longus m.
Extensor carpi radialis brevis m.
Extensor digitorum m.
Extensor retinaculum
Anterior superior iliac spine
Extensor digiti minimi m.
Extensor retinaculum
Pubic tubercle
Iliopsoas m.
Pectineus m.
Adductor longus m.
Sartorius m.
Gracilis m.
Tensor fascia latae m.
Rectus femoris m.
Vastus lateralis m.
Vastus medialis m.
Tensor fascia latae m.
Patella
Gastrocnemius m.
Tibia
Tibialis anterior m.
Peroneus longus m.
Soleus m.
Extensor digitorum longus m.
Superior extensor retinaculum
Medial malleolus
Lateral malleolus

Head and Facial Bones

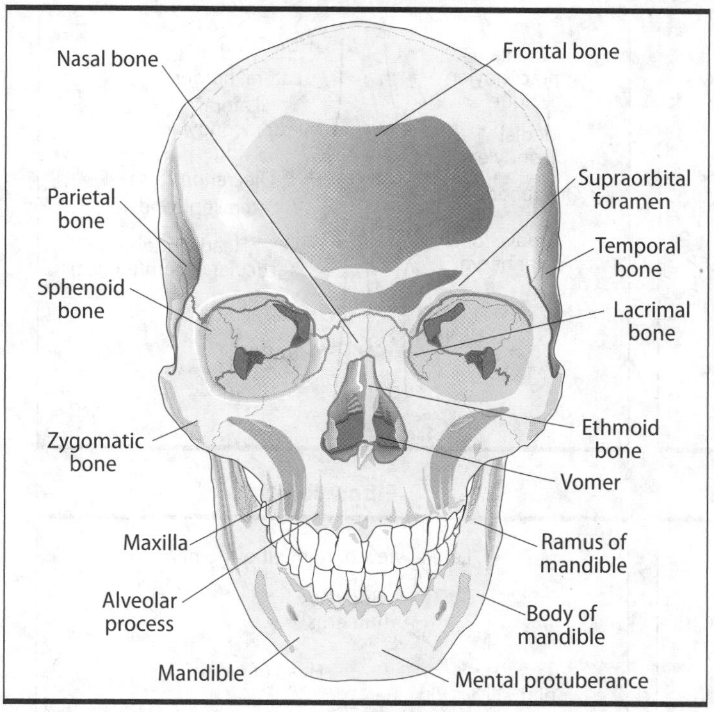
Nasal bone
Frontal bone
Parietal bone
Supraorbital foramen
Temporal bone
Sphenoid bone
Lacrimal bone
Ethmoid bone
Zygomatic bone
Vomer
Maxilla
Ramus of mandible
Alveolar process
Body of mandible
Mandible
Mental protuberance

Nose

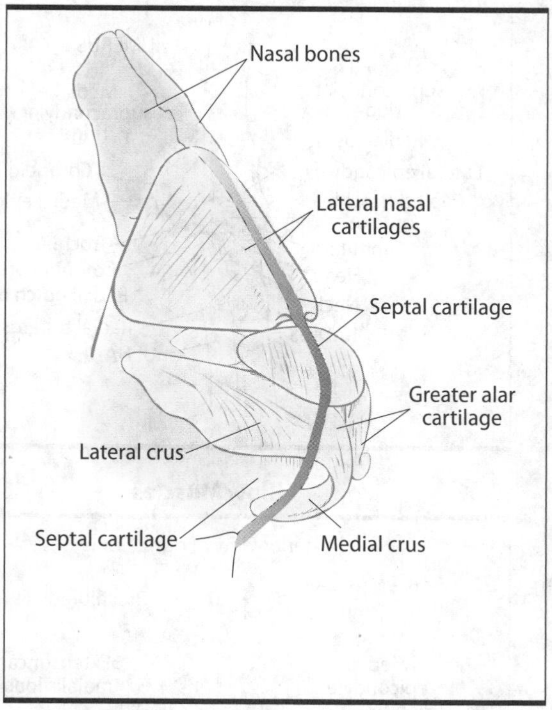
Nasal bones
Lateral nasal cartilages
Septal cartilage
Greater alar cartilage
Lateral crus
Septal cartilage
Medial crus

Shoulder (Anterior View)

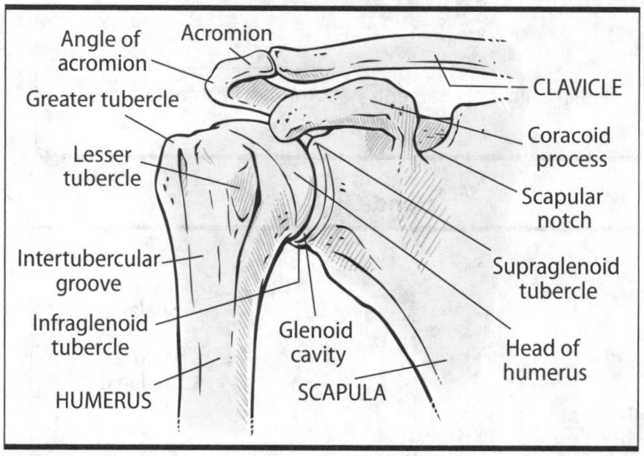
Angle of acromion
Acromion
CLAVICLE
Greater tubercle
Coracoid process
Lesser tubercle
Scapular notch
Intertubercular groove
Supraglenoid tubercle
Infraglenoid tubercle
Glenoid cavity
Head of humerus
HUMERUS
SCAPULA

Shoulder (Posterior View)

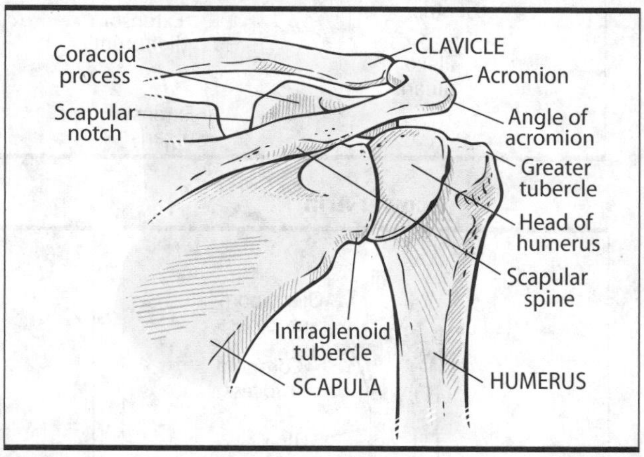
Coracoid process
CLAVICLE
Acromion
Scapular notch
Angle of acromion
Greater tubercle
Head of humerus
Scapular spine
Infraglenoid tubercle
SCAPULA
HUMERUS

Shoulder Muscles

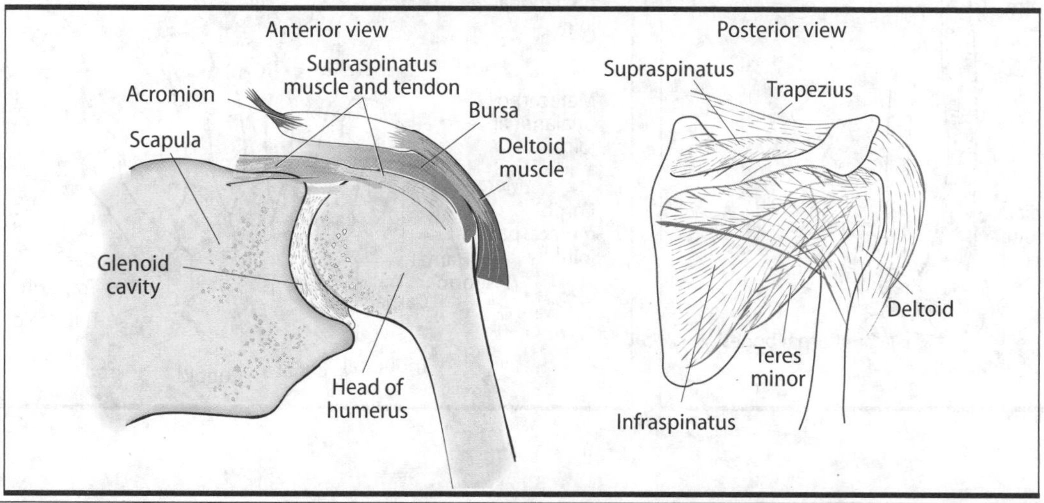
Anterior view
Supraspinatus muscle and tendon
Acromion
Bursa
Scapula
Deltoid muscle
Glenoid cavity
Head of humerus
Posterior view
Supraspinatus
Trapezius
Deltoid
Teres minor
Infraspinatus

Elbow (Anterior View)

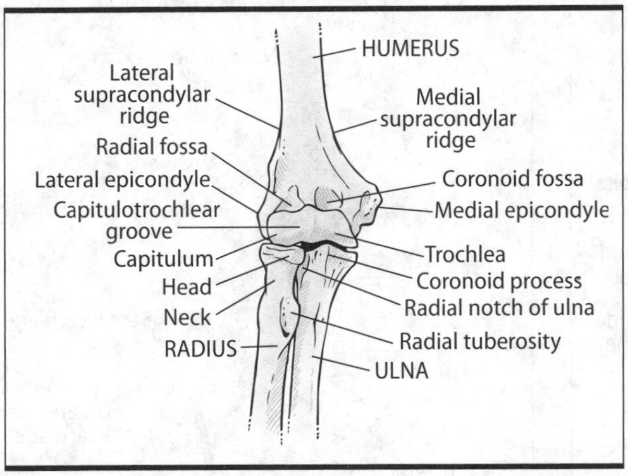
HUMERUS
Lateral supracondylar ridge
Medial supracondylar ridge
Radial fossa
Lateral epicondyle
Capitulotrochlear groove
Coronoid fossa
Medial epicondyle
Capitulum
Trochlea
Head
Coronoid process
Neck
Radial notch of ulna
RADIUS
Radial tuberosity
ULNA

Elbow (Posterior View)

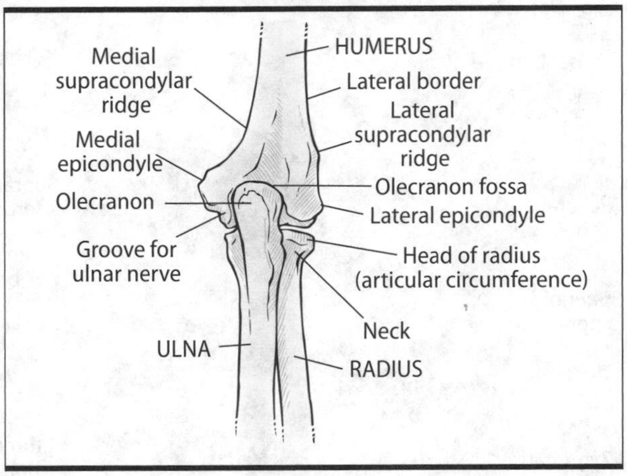
HUMERUS
Medial supracondylar ridge
Lateral border
Lateral supracondylar ridge
Medial epicondyle
Olecranon fossa
Olecranon
Lateral epicondyle
Groove for ulnar nerve
Head of radius (articular circumference)
Neck
ULNA
RADIUS

Elbow Muscles

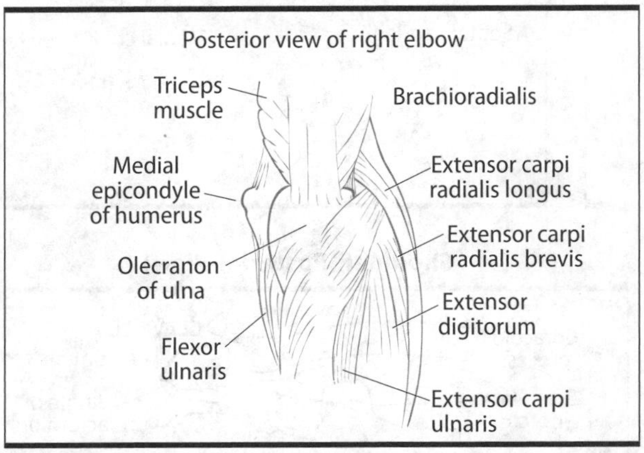
Posterior view of right elbow
Triceps muscle
Brachioradialis
Medial epicondyle of humerus
Extensor carpi radialis longus
Extensor carpi radialis brevis
Olecranon of ulna
Extensor digitorum
Flexor ulnaris
Extensor carpi ulnaris

Elbow Joint

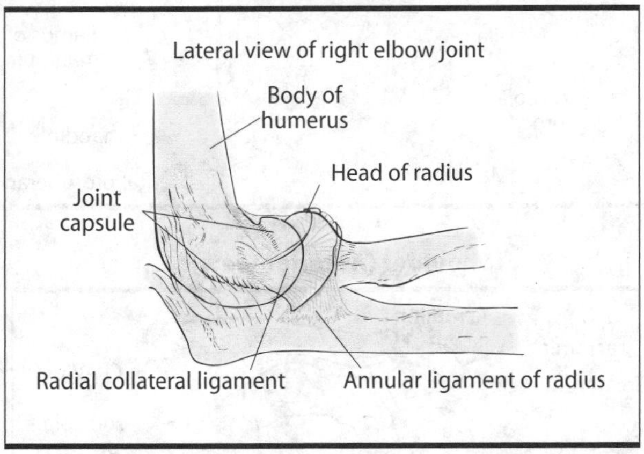
Lateral view of right elbow joint
Body of humerus
Head of radius
Joint capsule
Radial collateral ligament
Annular ligament of radius

Lower Arm

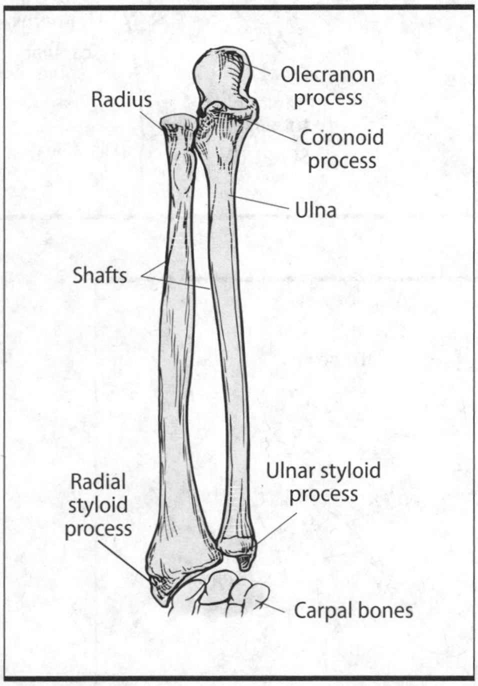
Radius
Olecranon process
Coronoid process
Ulna
Shafts
Radial styloid process
Ulnar styloid process
Carpal bones

Hand

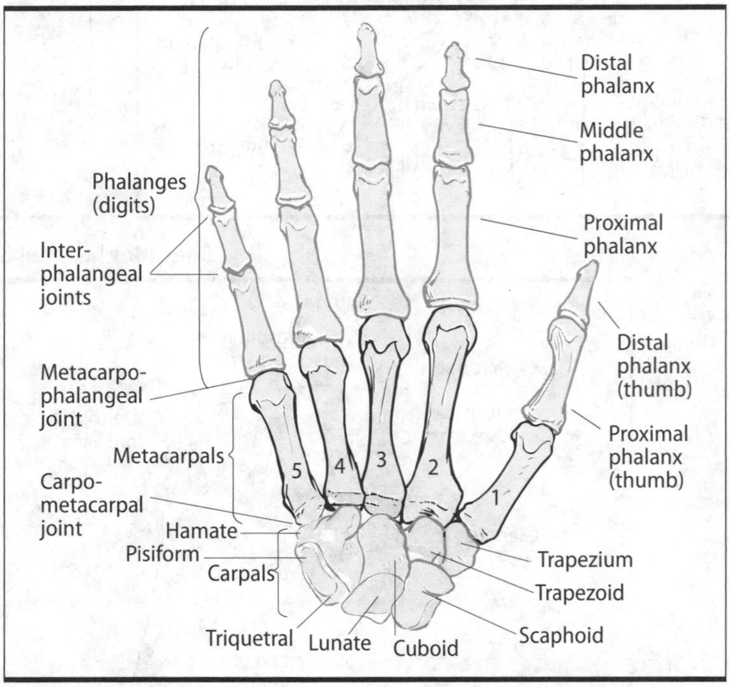
Distal phalanx
Middle phalanx
Phalanges (digits)
Proximal phalanx
Inter-phalangeal joints
Distal phalanx (thumb)
Metacarpo-phalangeal joint
Proximal phalanx (thumb)
Metacarpals
5
4
3
2
1
Carpo-metacarpal joint
Hamate
Pisiform
Carpals
Trapezium
Trapezoid
Triquetral
Lunate
Cuboid
Scaphoid

Hip (Anterior View)

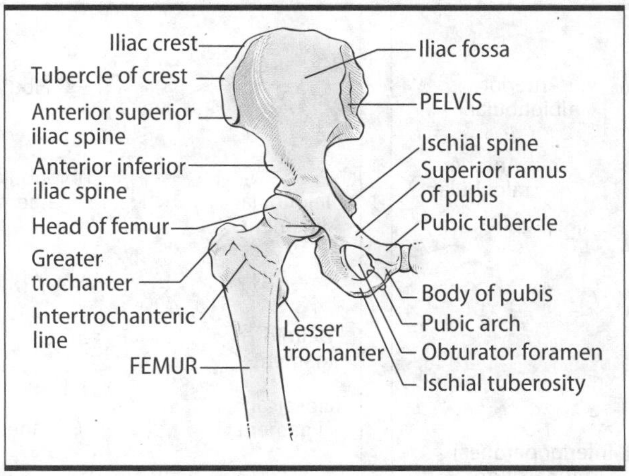
Iliac crest
Tubercle of crest
Anterior superior iliac spine
Anterior inferior iliac spine
Head of femur
Greater trochanter
Intertrochanteric line
FEMUR
Lesser trochanter
Iliac fossa
PELVIS
Ischial spine
Superior ramus of pubis
Pubic tubercle
Body of pubis
Pubic arch
Obturator foramen
Ischial tuberosity

Hip (Posterior View)

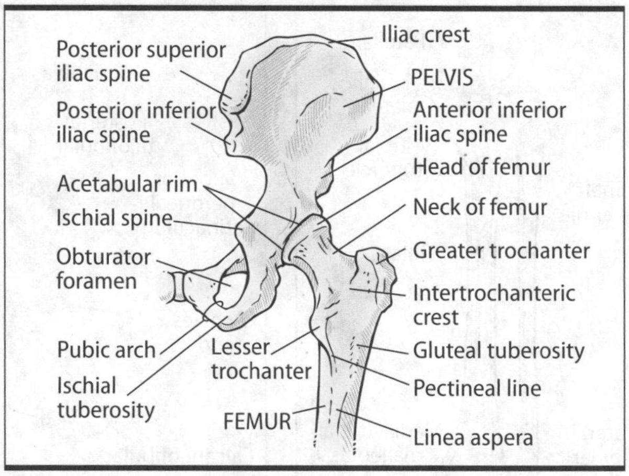
Posterior superior iliac spine
Posterior inferior iliac spine
Acetabular rim
Ischial spine
Obturator foramen
Pubic arch
Ischial tuberosity
Lesser trochanter
FEMUR
Iliac crest
PELVIS
Anterior inferior iliac spine
Head of femur
Neck of femur
Greater trochanter
Intertrochanteric crest
Gluteal tuberosity
Pectineal line
Linea aspera

Knee (Anterior View)

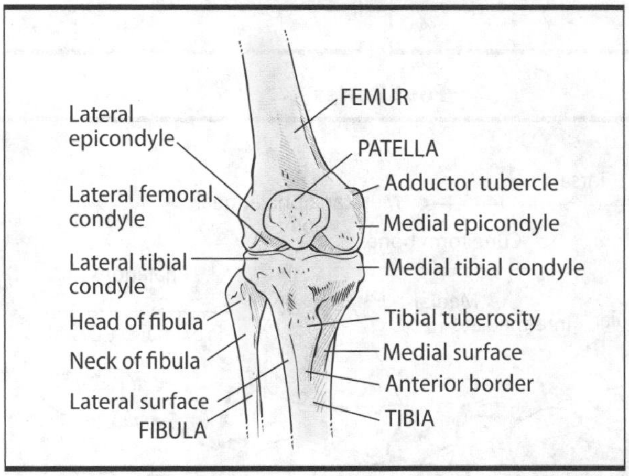
Lateral epicondyle
Lateral femoral condyle
Lateral tibial condyle
Head of fibula
Neck of fibula
Lateral surface
FIBULA
FEMUR
PATELLA
Adductor tubercle
Medial epicondyle
Medial tibial condyle
Tibial tuberosity
Medial surface
Anterior border
TIBIA

Knee (Posterior View)

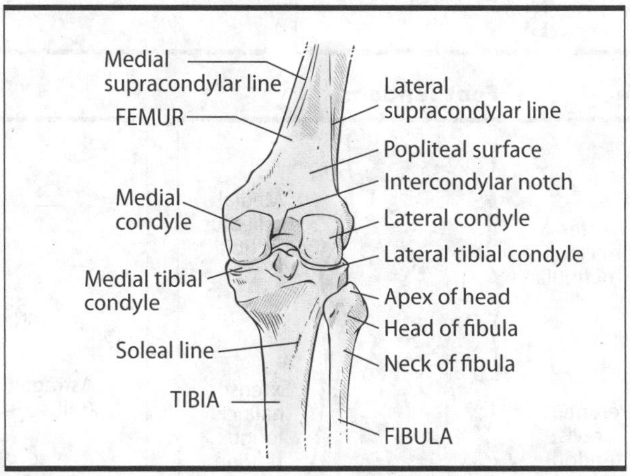
Medial supracondylar line
FEMUR
Medial condyle
Medial tibial condyle
Soleal line
TIBIA
Lateral supracondylar line
Popliteal surface
Intercondylar notch
Lateral condyle
Lateral tibial condyle
Apex of head
Head of fibula
Neck of fibula
FIBULA

Knee Joint (Anterior View)

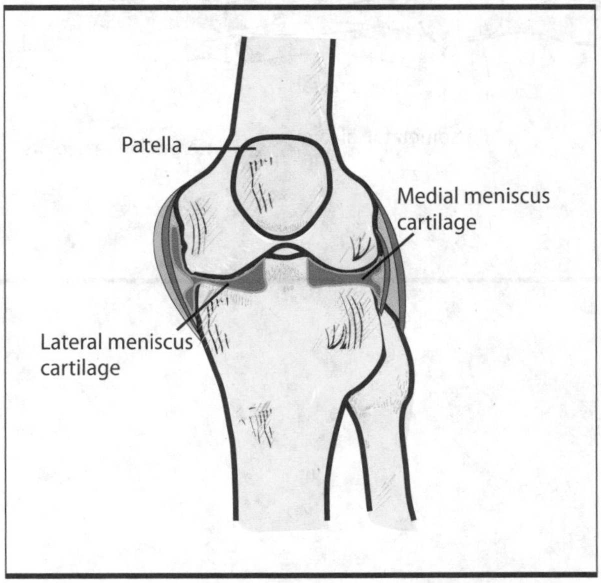
Patella
Medial meniscus cartilage
Lateral meniscus cartilage

Knee Joint (Lateral View)

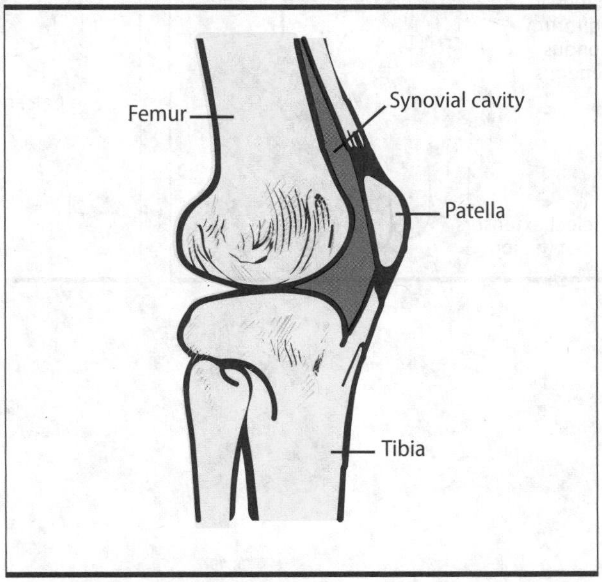
Femur
Synovial cavity
Patella
Tibia

Lower Leg

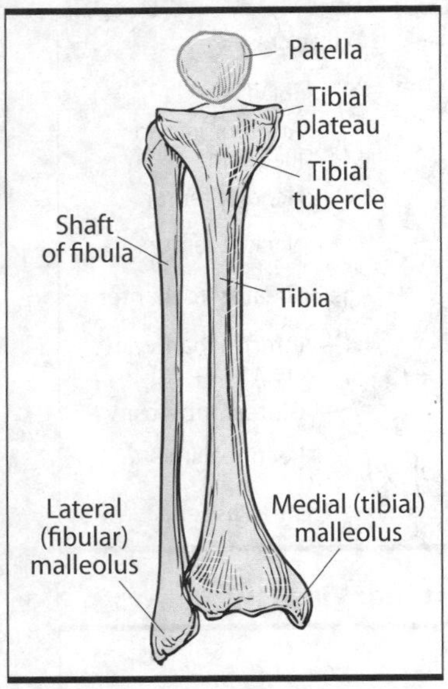
Patella
Tibial plateau
Tibial tubercle
Shaft of fibula
Tibia
Lateral (fibular) malleolus
Medial (tibial) malleolus

Ankle Ligament (Lateral View)

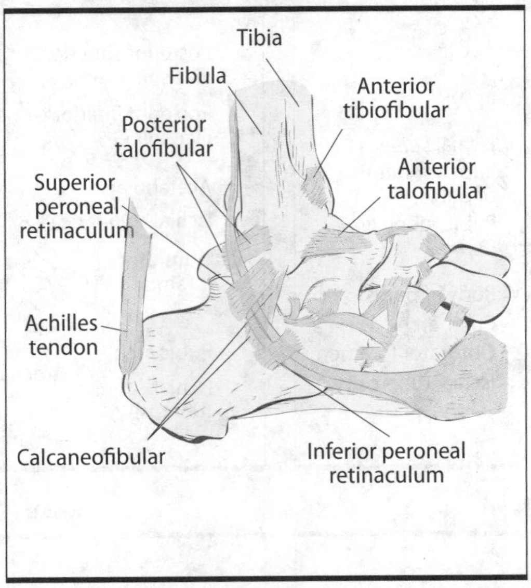
Tibia
Fibula
Anterior tibiofibular
Posterior talofibular
Anterior talofibular
Superior peroneal retinaculum
Achilles tendon
Calcaneofibular
Inferior peroneal retinaculum

Ankle Ligament (Posterior View)

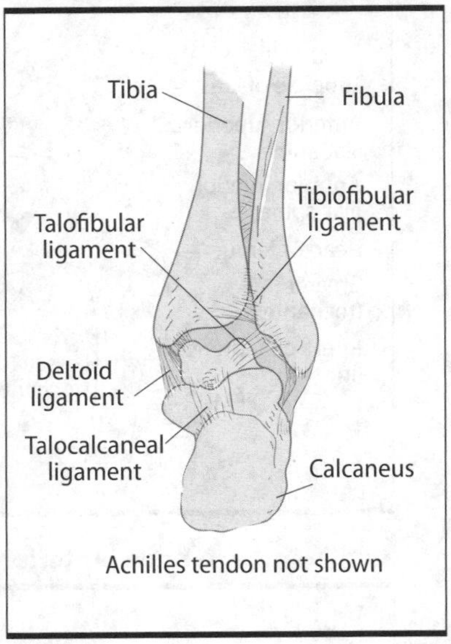
Tibia
Fibula
Tibiofibular ligament
Talofibular ligament
Deltoid ligament
Talocalcaneal ligament
Calcaneus
Achilles tendon not shown

Foot Tendons

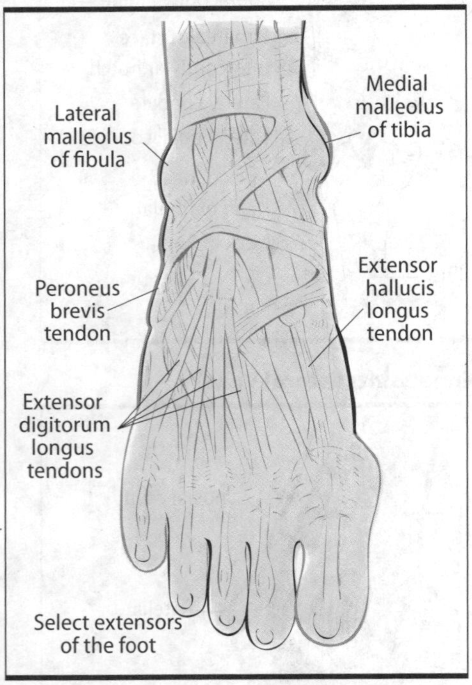
Medial malleolus of tibia
Lateral malleolus of fibula
Extensor hallucis longus tendon
Peroneus brevis tendon
Extensor digitorum longus tendons
Select extensors of the foot

Foot Bones

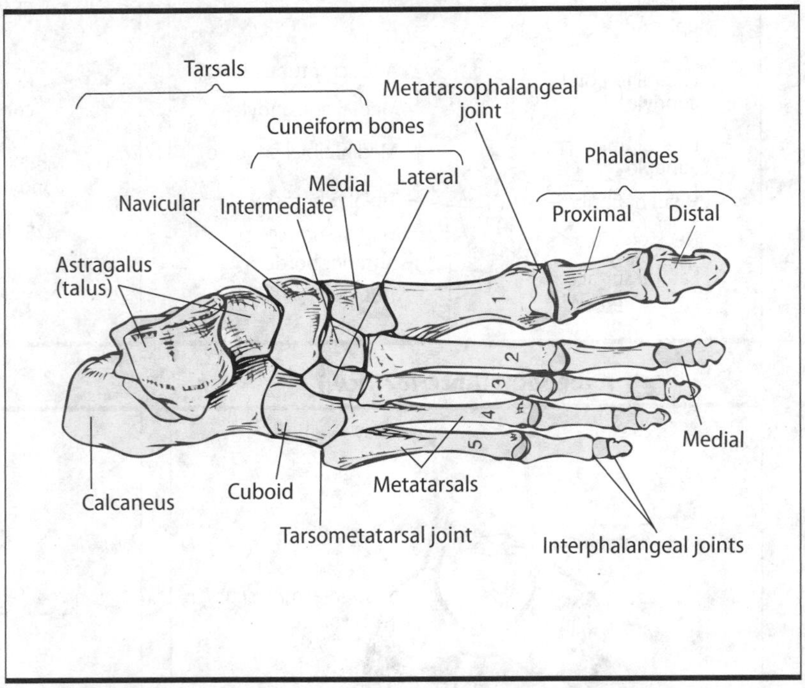
Tarsals
Metatarsophalangeal joint
Cuneiform bones
Phalanges
Medial
Lateral
Navicular
Intermediate
Proximal
Distal
Astragalus (talus)
1
2
3
4
5
Medial
Calcaneus
Cuboid
Metatarsals
Tarsometatarsal joint
Interphalangeal joints

Respiratory System

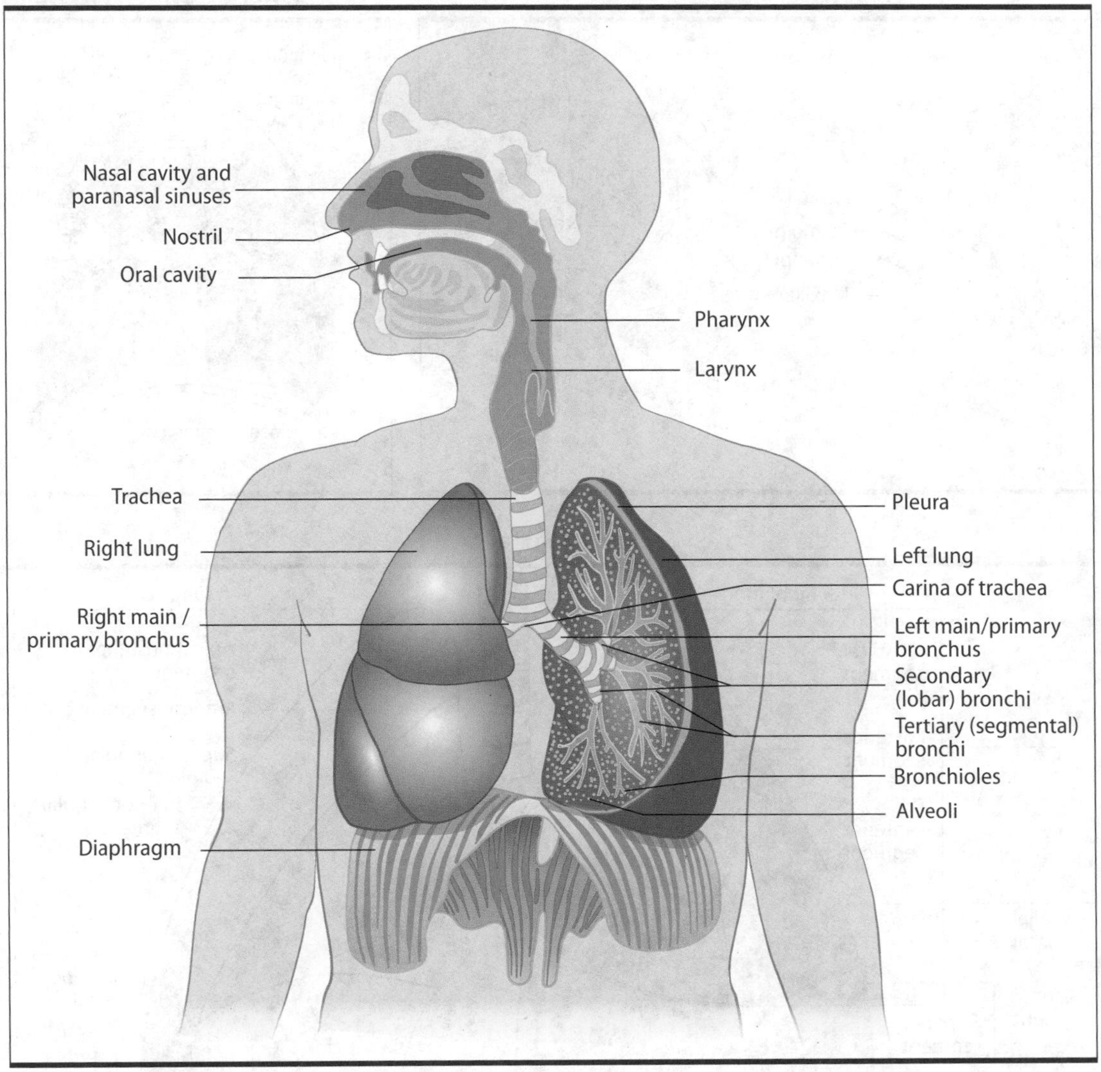
Nasal cavity and paranasal sinuses
Nostril
Oral cavity
Pharynx
Larynx
Trachea
Right lung
Right main / primary bronchus
Diaphragm
Pleura
Left lung
Carina of trachea
Left main/primary bronchus
Secondary (lobar) bronchi
Tertiary (segmental) bronchi
Bronchioles
Alveoli

Upper Respiratory System

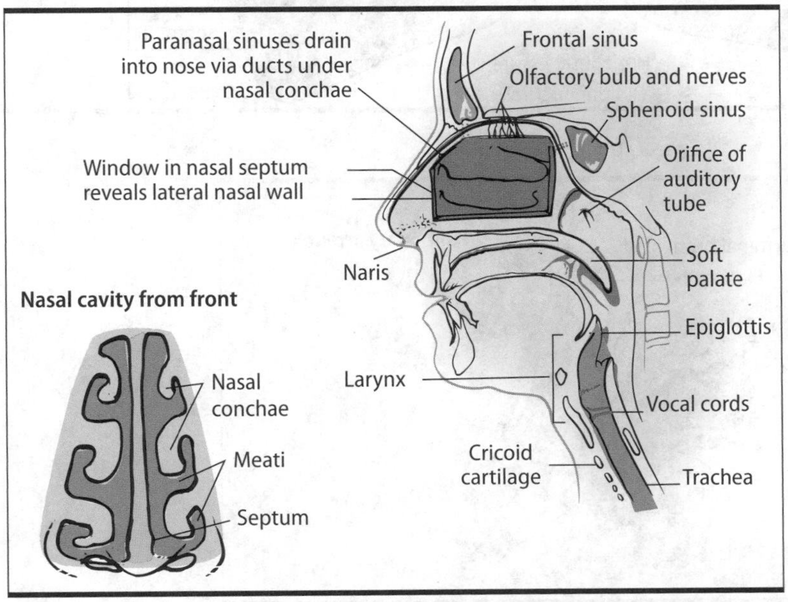
Paranasal sinuses drain into nose via ducts under nasal conchae
Window in nasal septum reveals lateral nasal wall
Naris
Larynx
Frontal sinus
Olfactory bulb and nerves
Sphenoid sinus
Orifice of auditory tube
Soft palate
Epiglottis
Vocal cords
Cricoid cartilage
Trachea
Nasal cavity from front
Nasal conchae
Meati
Septum

Nasal Turbinates

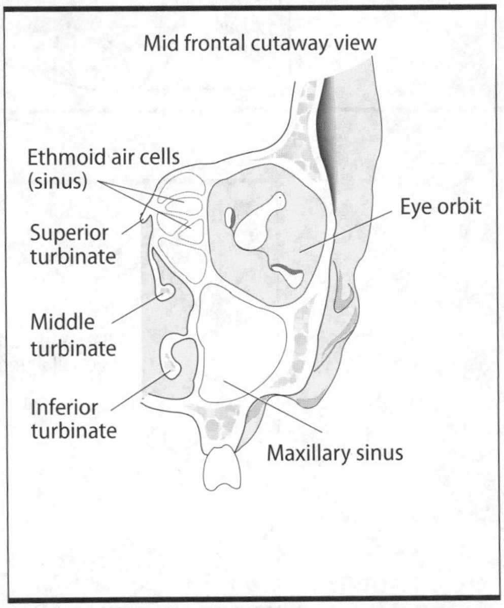
Mid frontal cutaway view
Ethmoid air cells (sinus)
Superior turbinate
Middle turbinate
Inferior turbinate
Eye orbit
Maxillary sinus

Paranasal Sinuses

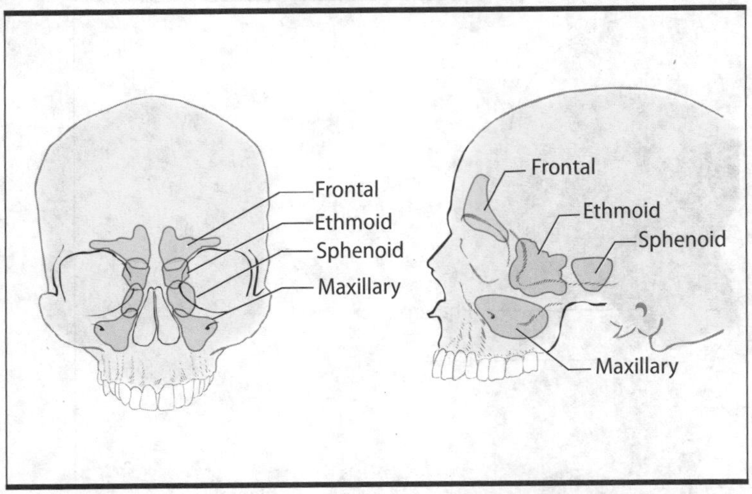
Frontal
Ethmoid
Sphenoid
Maxillary
Frontal
Ethmoid
Sphenoid
Maxillary

Lower Respiratory System

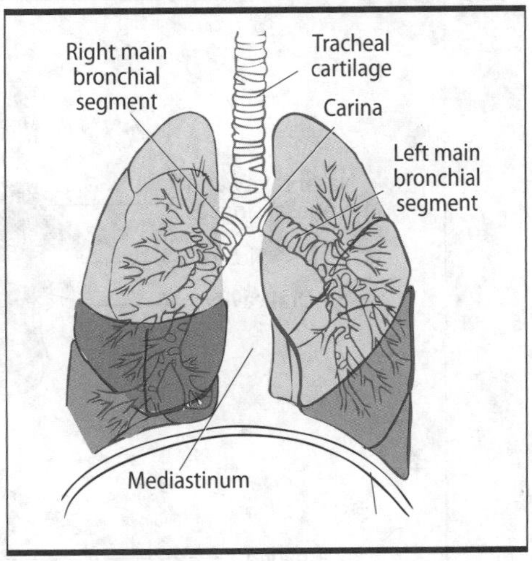
Right main bronchial segment
Tracheal cartilage
Carina
Left main bronchial segment
Mediastinum

Lung Segments

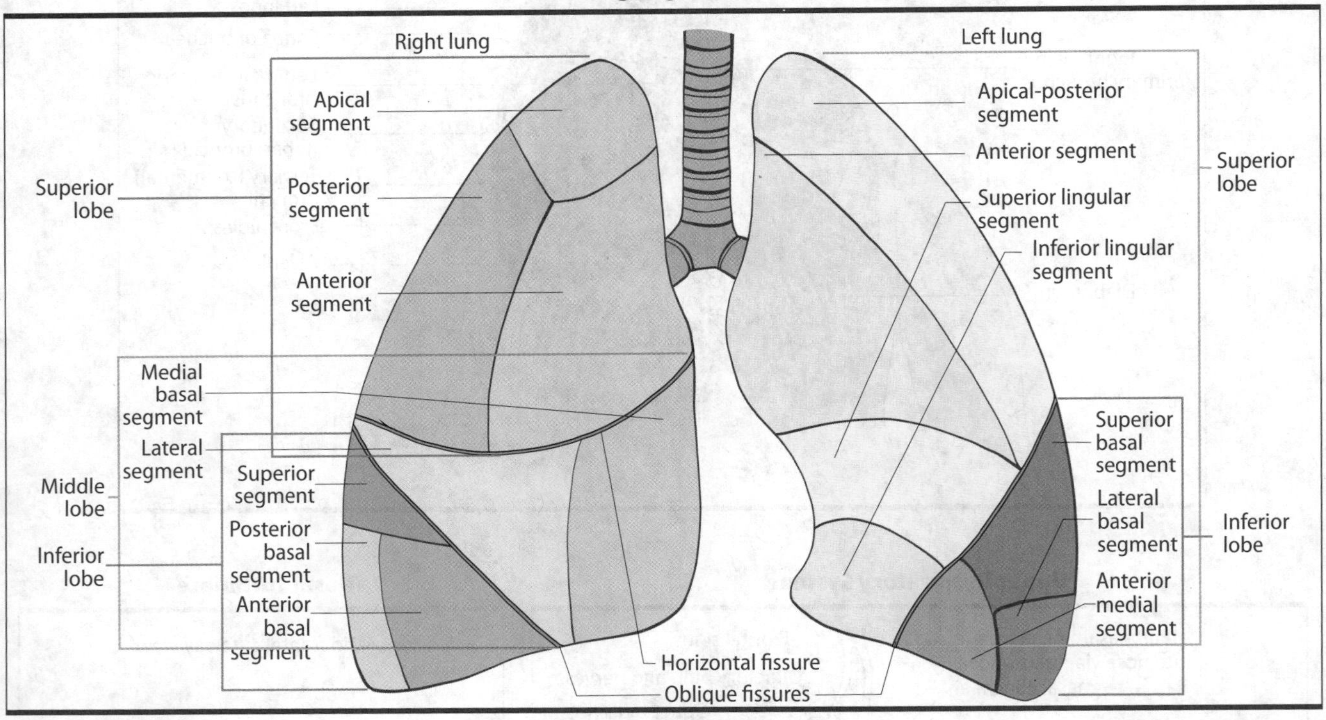
Right lung
Left lung
Apical segment
Posterior segment
Anterior segment
Superior lobe
Medial basal segment
Lateral segment
Middle lobe
Superior segment
Posterior basal segment
Inferior lobe
Anterior basal segment
Apical-posterior segment
Anterior segment
Superior lingular segment
Inferior lingular segment
Superior lobe
Superior basal segment
Lateral basal segment
Inferior lobe
Anterior medial segment
Horizontal fissure
Oblique fissures

Alveoli

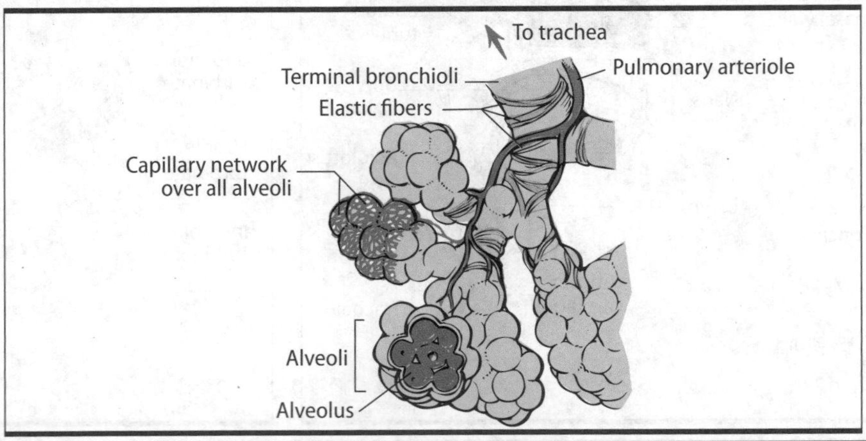
To trachea
Terminal bronchioli
Pulmonary arteriole
Elastic fibers
Capillary network over all alveoli
Alveoli
Alveolus

Arterial System

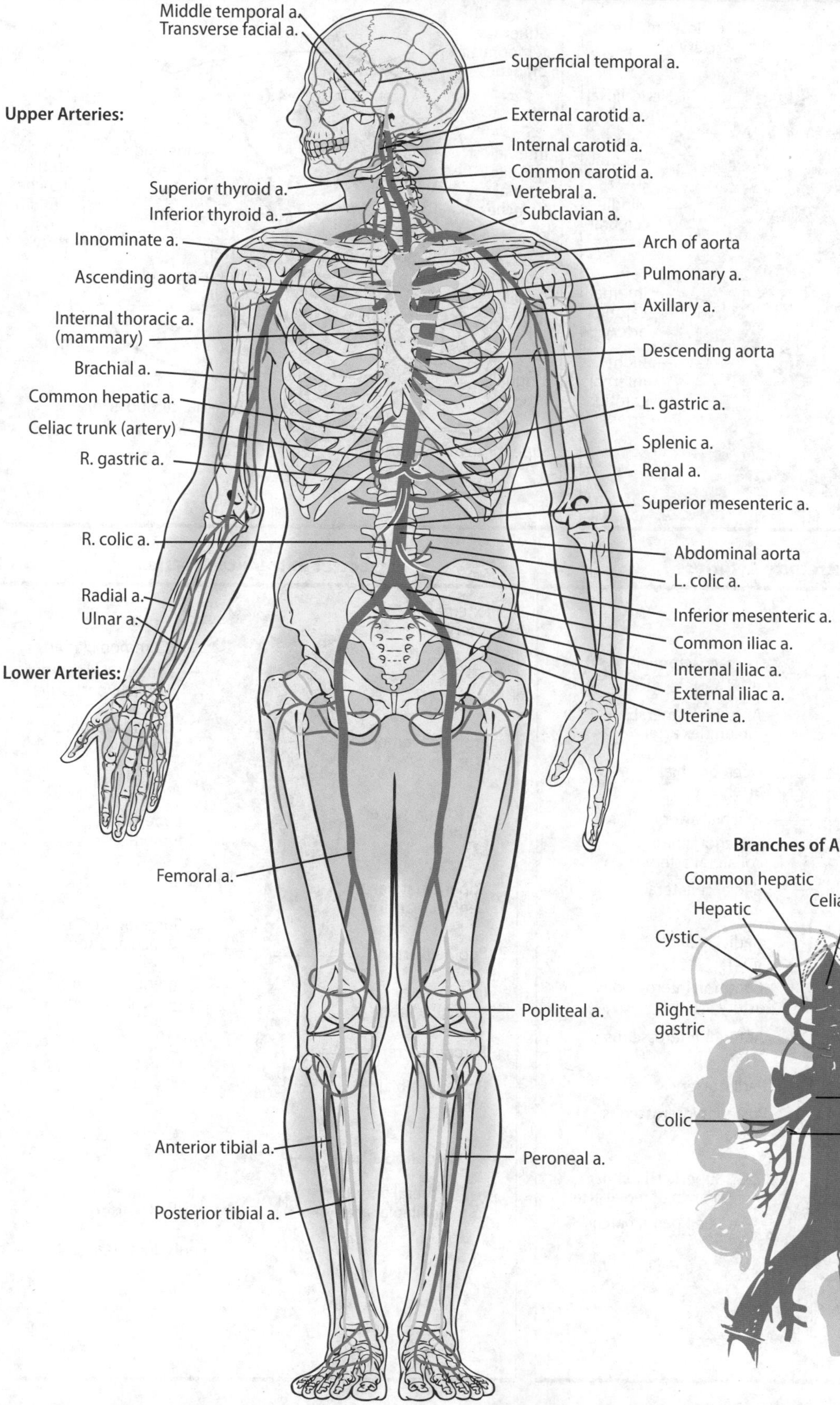
Middle temporal a.
Transverse facial a.
Superficial temporal a.
Upper Arteries:
External carotid a.
Internal carotid a.
Common carotid a.
Superior thyroid a.
Vertebral a.
Inferior thyroid a.
Subclavian a.
Innominate a.
Arch of aorta
Ascending aorta
Pulmonary a.
Axillary a.
Internal thoracic a. (mammary)
Descending aorta
Brachial a.
Common hepatic a.
L. gastric a.
Celiac trunk (artery)
Splenic a.
R. gastric a.
Renal a.
Superior mesenteric a.
R. colic a.
Abdominal aorta
L. colic a.
Radial a.
Ulnar a.
Inferior mesenteric a.
Common iliac a.
Lower Arteries:
Internal iliac a.
External iliac a.
Uterine a.
Femoral a.
Popliteal a.
Anterior tibial a.
Peroneal a.
Posterior tibial a.

Branches of Abdominal Aorta

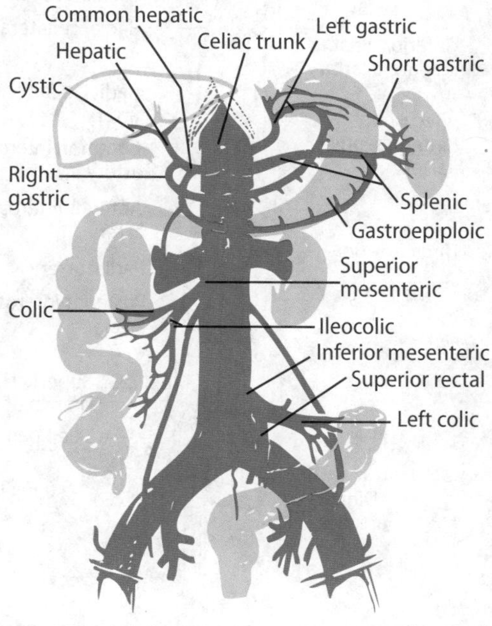
Common hepatic
Celiac trunk
Left gastric
Hepatic
Short gastric
Cystic
Right gastric
Splenic
Gastroepiploic
Superior mesenteric
Colic
Ileocolic
Inferior mesenteric
Superior rectal
Left colic

Internal Carotid and Arteries and Branches

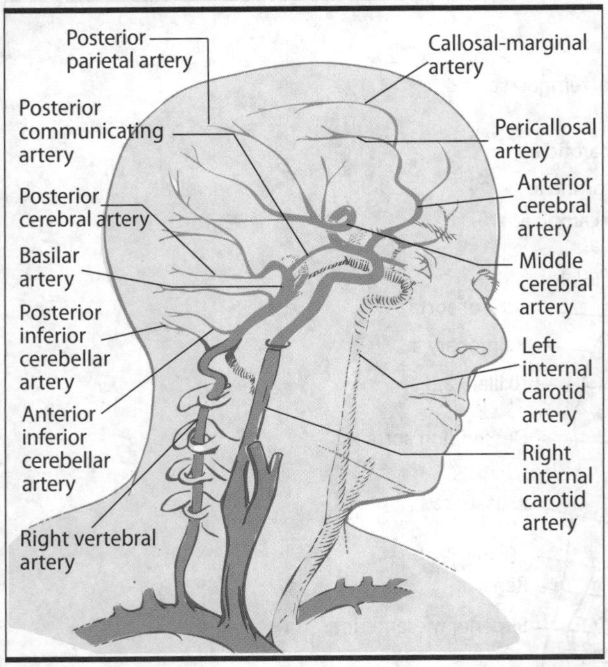
Posterior parietal artery
Callosal-marginal artery
Posterior communicating artery
Pericallosal artery
Anterior cerebral artery
Posterior cerebral artery
Basilar artery
Middle cerebral artery
Posterior inferior cerebellar artery
Left internal carotid artery
Anterior inferior cerebellar artery
Right internal carotid artery
Right vertebral artery

External Carotid Arteries and Branches

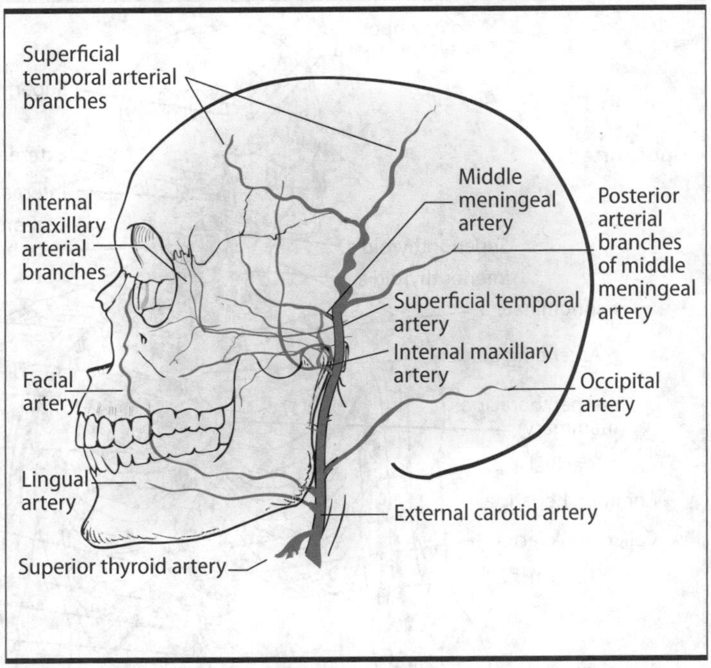
Superficial temporal arterial branches
Internal maxillary arterial branches
Middle meningeal artery
Posterior arterial branches of middle meningeal artery
Superficial temporal artery
Internal maxillary artery
Facial artery
Occipital artery
Lingual artery
External carotid artery
Superior thyroid artery

Upper Extremity Arteries

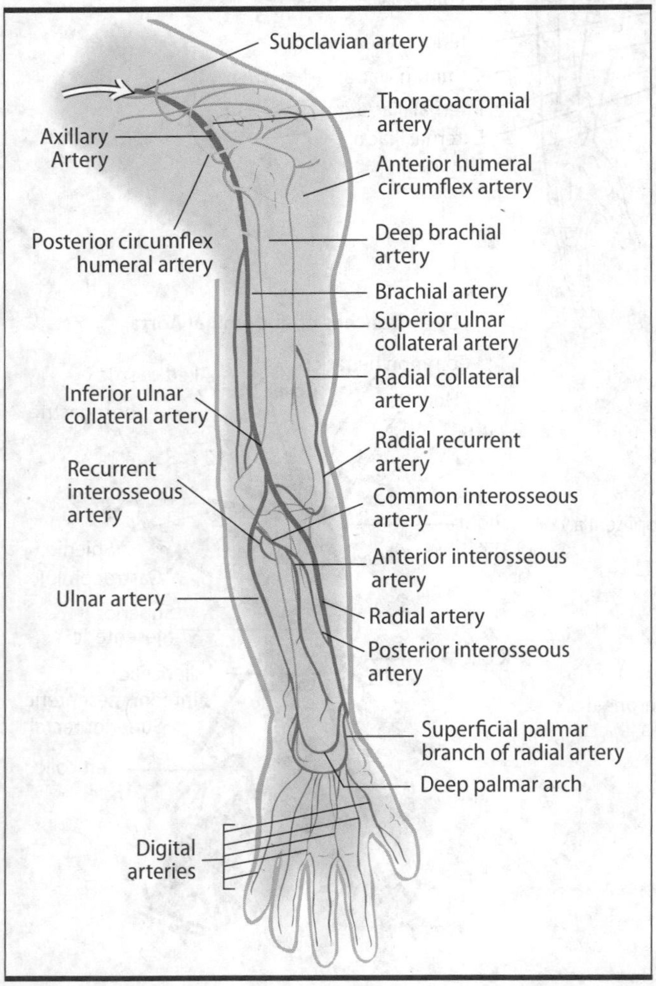
Subclavian artery
Thoracoacromial artery
Axillary Artery
Anterior humeral circumflex artery
Posterior circumflex humeral artery
Deep brachial artery
Brachial artery
Superior ulnar collateral artery
Radial collateral artery
Inferior ulnar collateral artery
Radial recurrent artery
Recurrent interosseous artery
Common interosseous artery
Anterior interosseous artery
Ulnar artery
Radial artery
Posterior interosseous artery
Superficial palmar branch of radial artery
Deep palmar arch
Digital arteries

Lower Extremity Arteries

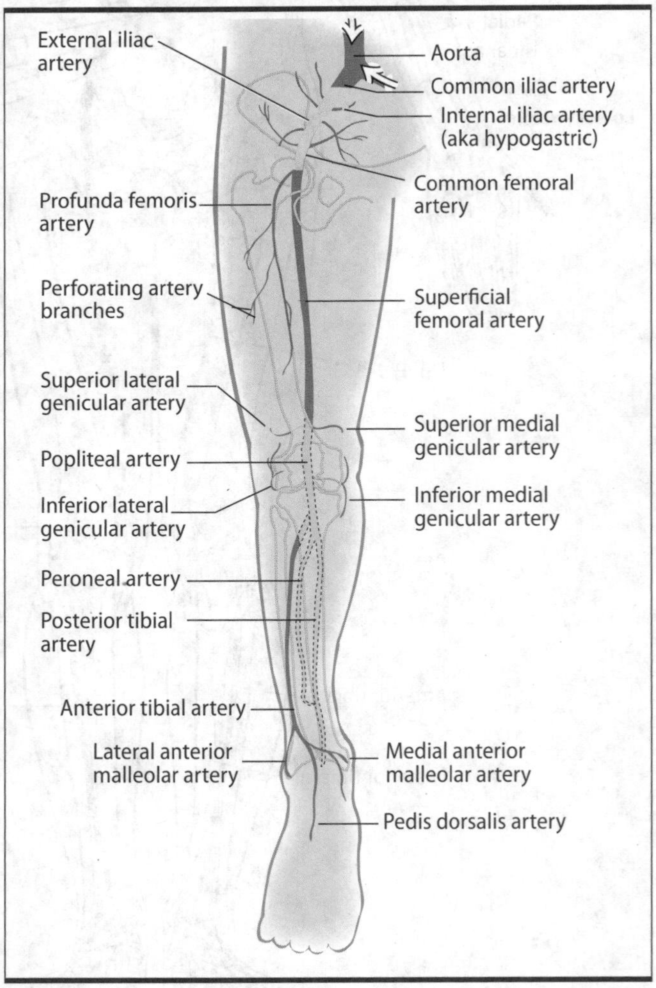
External iliac artery
Aorta
Common iliac artery
Internal iliac artery (aka hypogastric)
Common femoral artery
Profunda femoris artery
Perforating artery branches
Superficial femoral artery
Superior lateral genicular artery
Superior medial genicular artery
Popliteal artery
Inferior medial genicular artery
Inferior lateral genicular artery
Peroneal artery
Posterior tibial artery
Anterior tibial artery
Lateral anterior malleolar artery
Medial anterior malleolar artery
Pedis dorsalis artery

Venous System

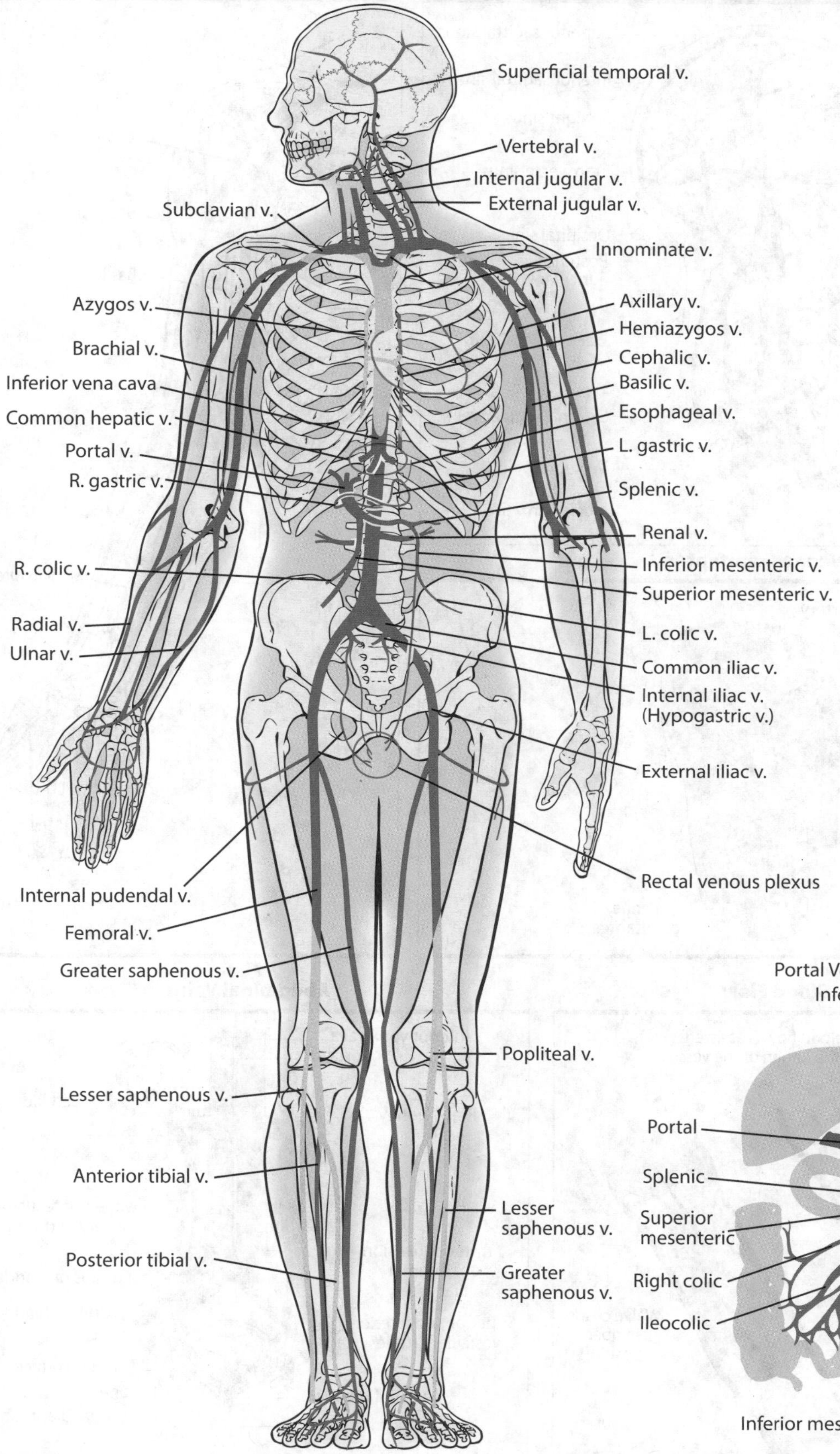
Superficial temporal v.
Vertebral v.
Internal jugular v.
External jugular v.
Subclavian v.
Innominate v.
Azygos v.
Axillary v.
Hemiazygos v.
Brachial v.
Cephalic v.
Inferior vena cava
Basilic v.
Common hepatic v.
Esophageal v.
Portal v.
L. gastric v.
R. gastric v.
Splenic v.
Renal v.
R. colic v.
Inferior mesenteric v.
Superior mesenteric v.
Radial v.
L. colic v.
Ulnar v.
Common iliac v.
Internal iliac v.
(Hypogastric v.)
External iliac v.
Rectal venous plexus
Internal pudendal v.
Femoral v.
Greater saphenous v.
Popliteal v.
Lesser saphenous v.
Anterior tibial v.
Lesser
saphenous v.
Posterior tibial v.
Greater
saphenous v.

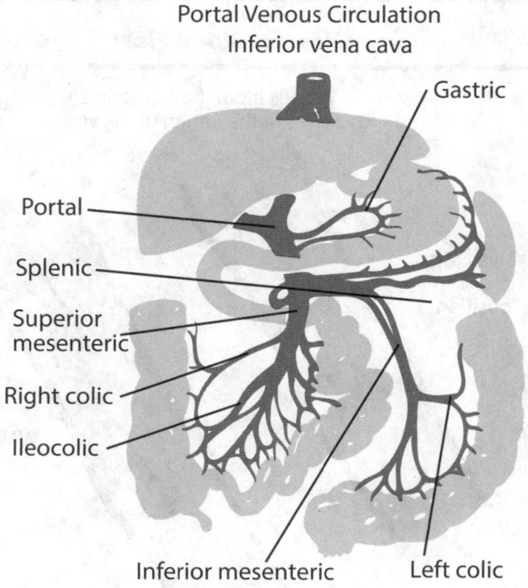
Portal Venous Circulation
Inferior vena cava
Gastric
Portal
Splenic
Superior
mesenteric
Right colic
Ileocolic
Inferior mesenteric
Left colic

Head and Neck Veins

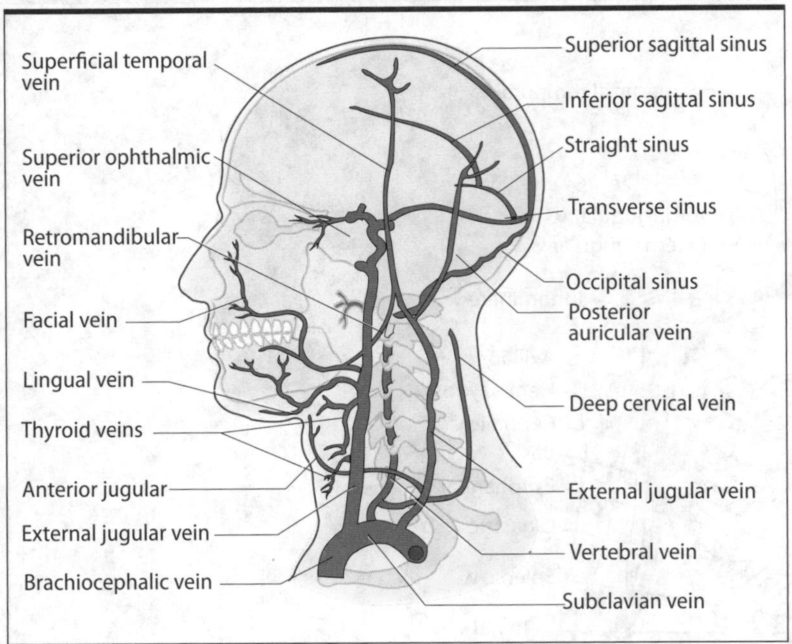
Superficial temporal vein
Superior ophthalmic vein
Retromandibular vein
Facial vein
Lingual vein
Thyroid veins
Anterior jugular
External jugular vein
Brachiocephalic vein
Superior sagittal sinus
Inferior sagittal sinus
Straight sinus
Transverse sinus
Occipital sinus
Posterior auricular vein
Deep cervical vein
External jugular vein
Vertebral vein
Subclavian vein

Upper Extremity Veins

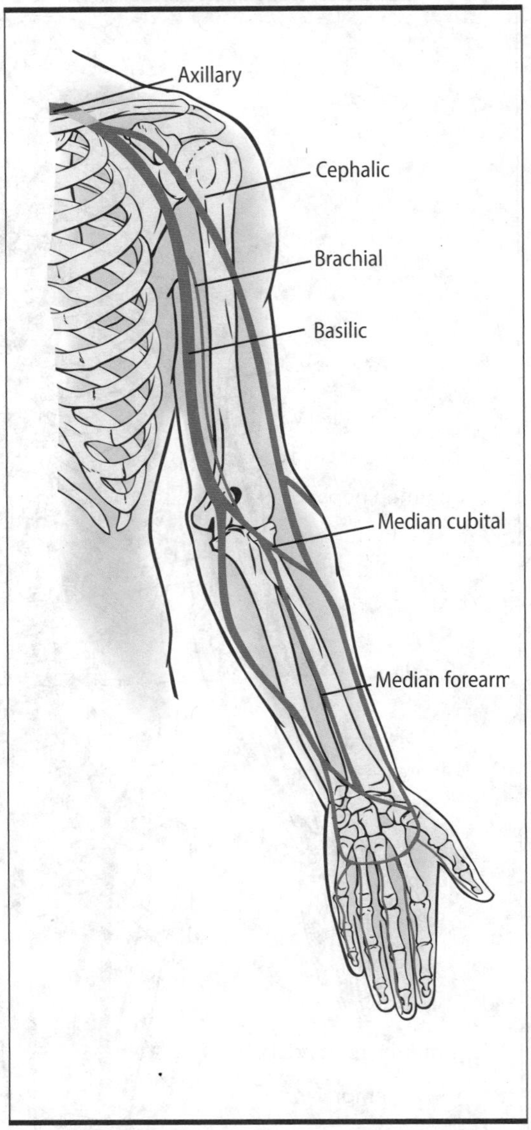
Axillary
Cephalic
Brachial
Basilic
Median cubital
Median forearm

Venae Comitantes

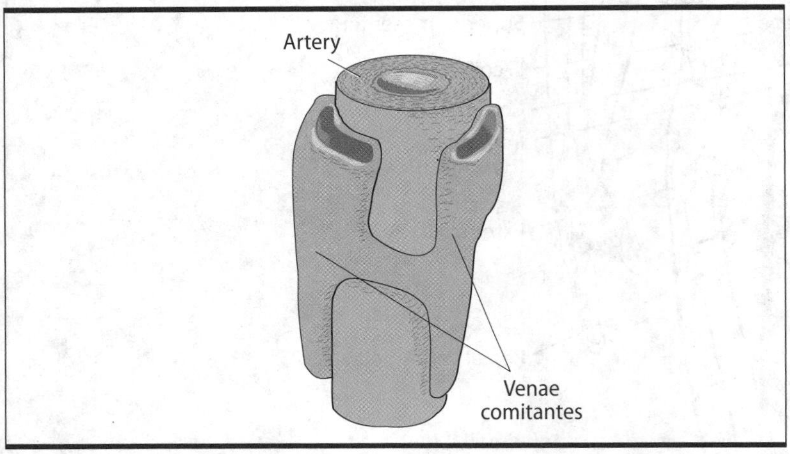
Artery
Venae comitantes

Venous Blood Flow

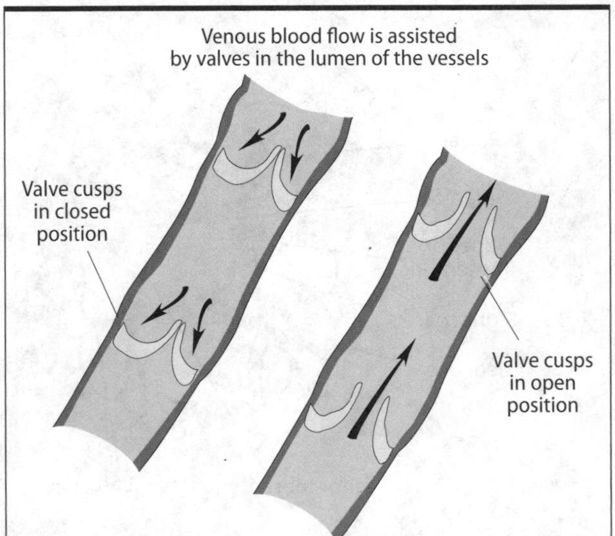
Venous blood flow is assisted by valves in the lumen of the vessels
Valve cusps in closed position
Valve cusps in open position

Abdominal Veins

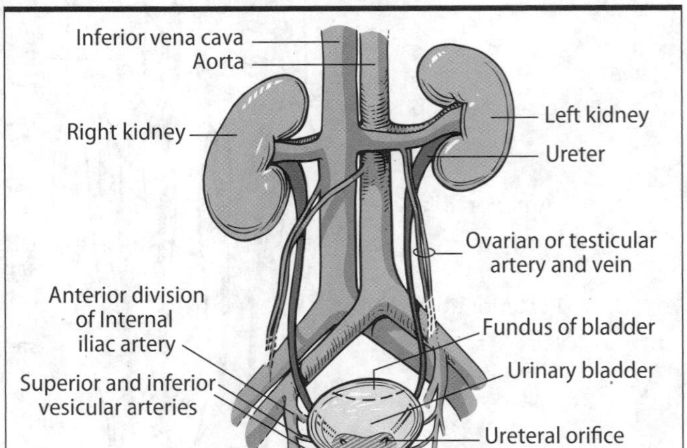
Inferior vena cava
Aorta
Right kidney
Left kidney
Ureter
Ovarian or testicular artery and vein
Anterior division of Internal iliac artery
Fundus of bladder
Urinary bladder
Superior and inferior vesicular arteries
Ureteral orifice
Trigone
Uvula of bladder
Urogenital diaphragm
Urethra

Cardiovascular System

Coronary Veins

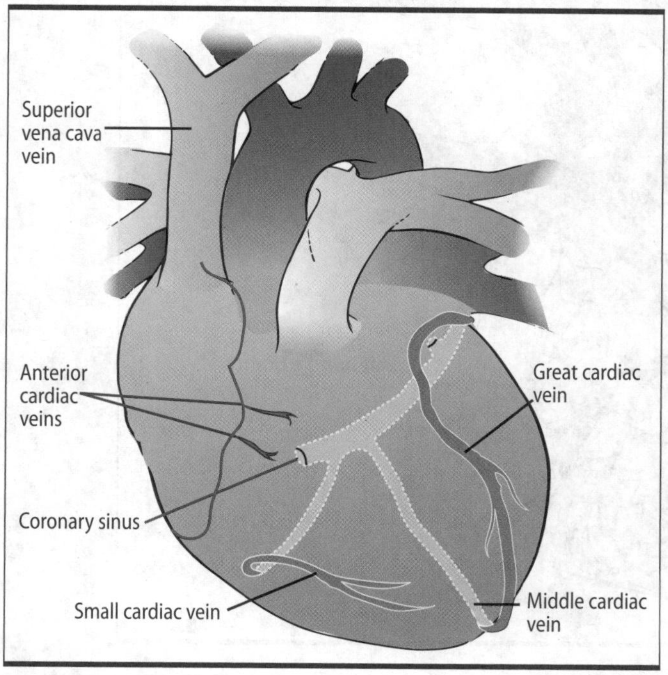

Anatomy of the Heart

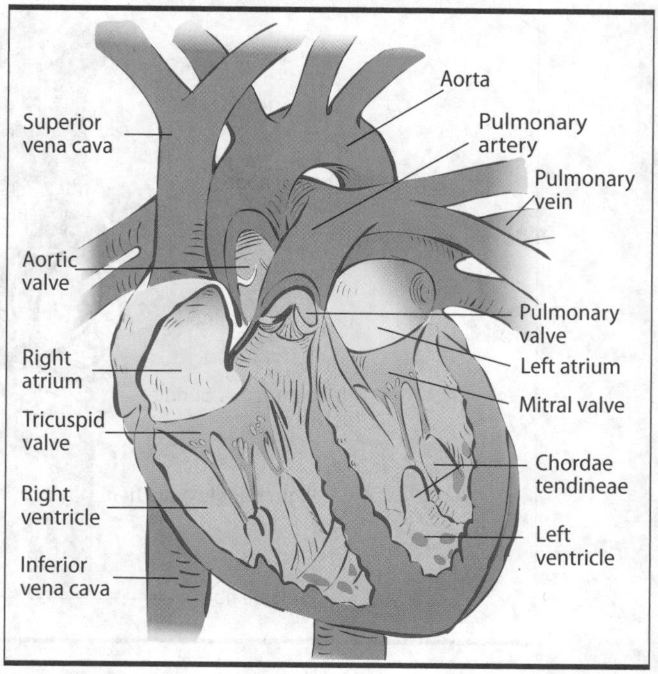

Heart Cross Section

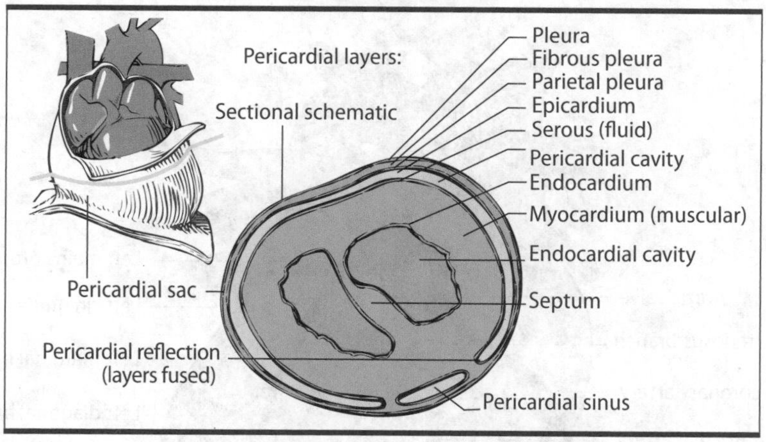

Heart Valves

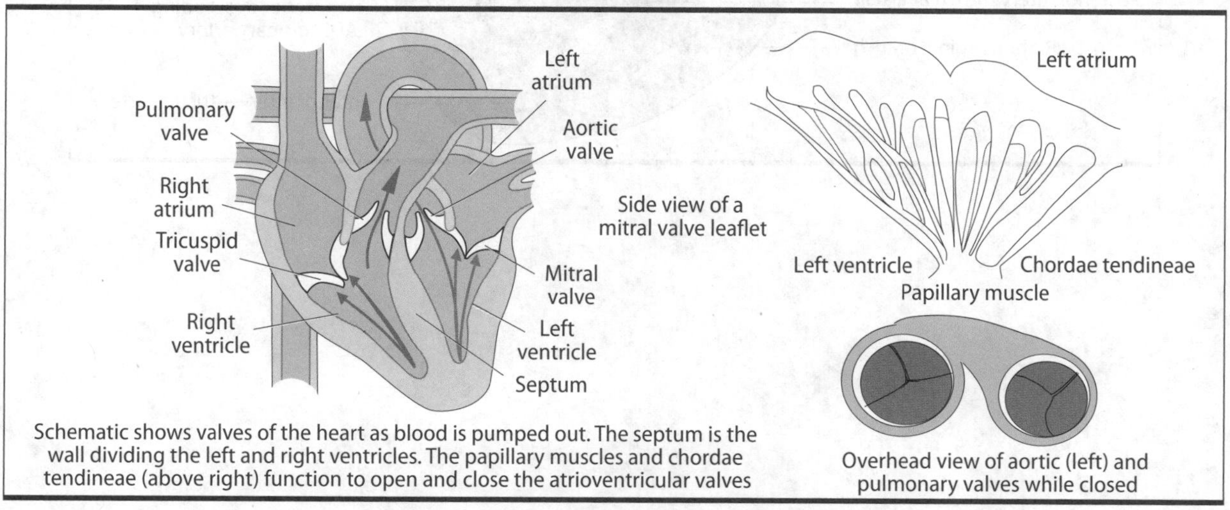

Schematic shows valves of the heart as blood is pumped out. The septum is the wall dividing the left and right ventricles. The papillary muscles and chordae tendineae (above right) function to open and close the atrioventricular valves

Overhead view of aortic (left) and pulmonary valves while closed

Heart Conduction System

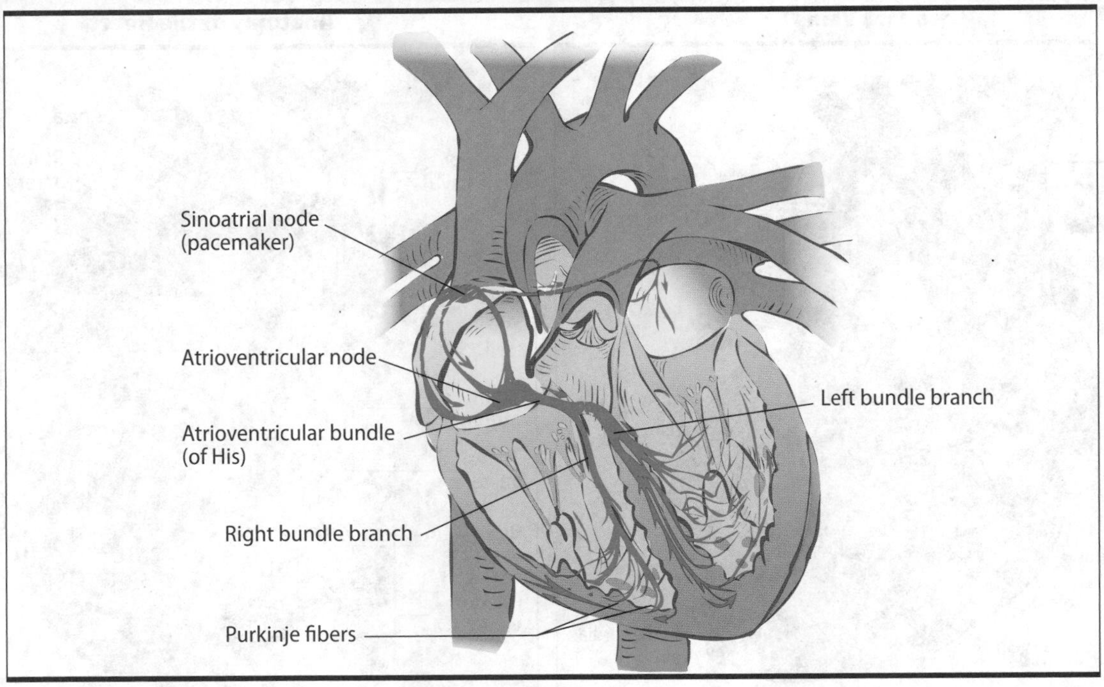
Sinoatrial node
(pacemaker)
Atrioventricular node
Left bundle branch
Atrioventricular bundle
(of His)
Right bundle branch
Purkinje fibers

Coronary Arteries

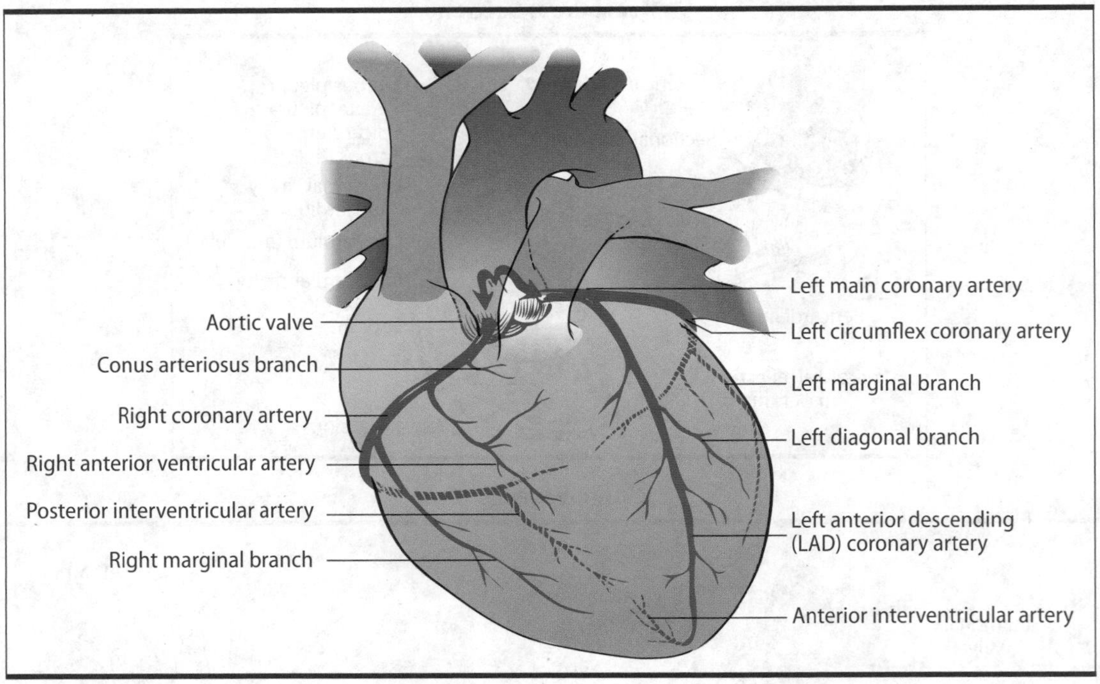
Left main coronary artery
Aortic valve
Left circumflex coronary artery
Conus arteriosus branch
Left marginal branch
Right coronary artery
Left diagonal branch
Right anterior ventricular artery
Posterior interventricular artery
Left anterior descending
(LAD) coronary artery
Right marginal branch
Anterior interventricular artery

Lymphatic System

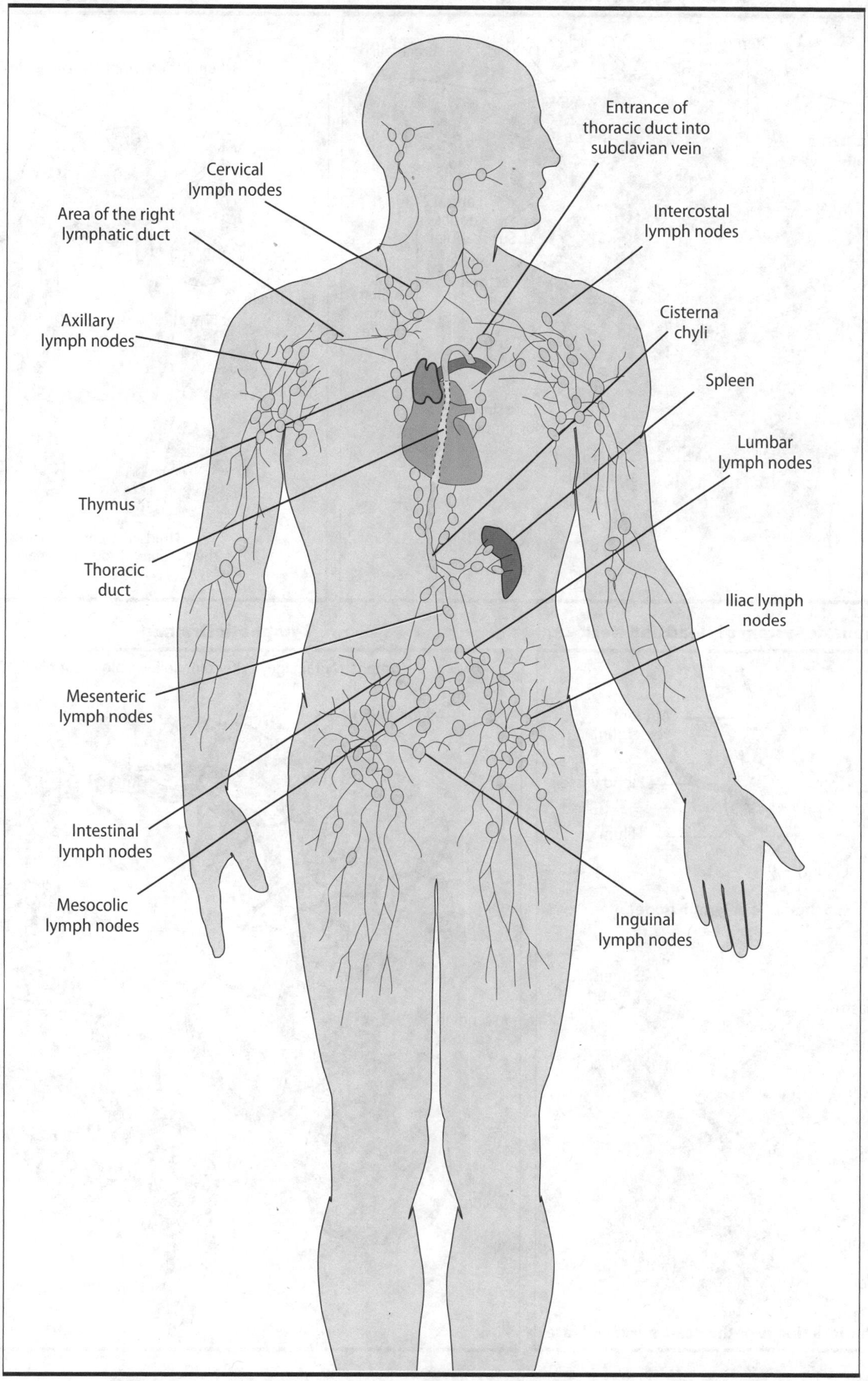

Axillary Lymph Nodes

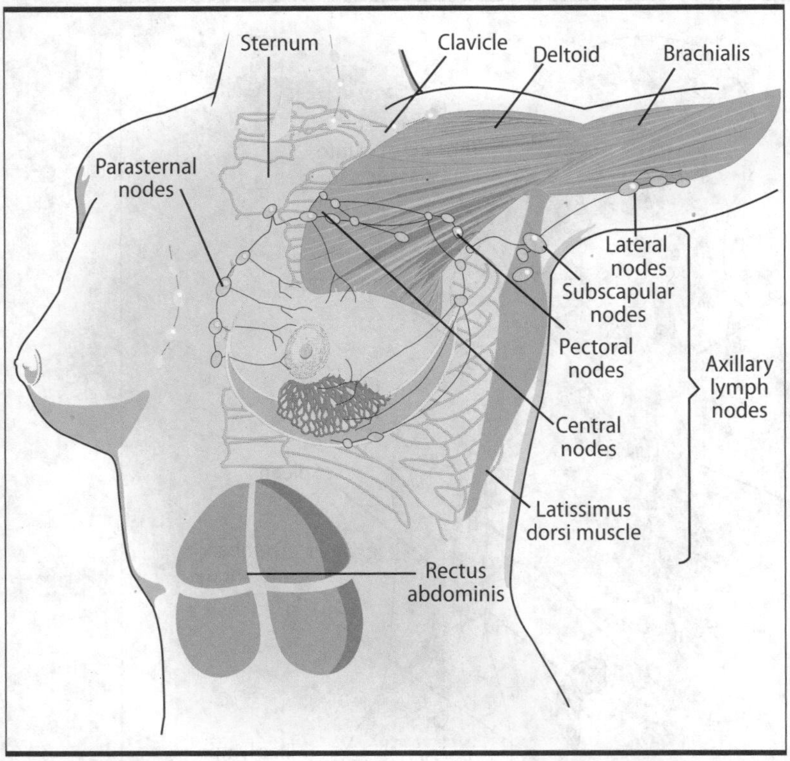

Lymphatic Capillaries

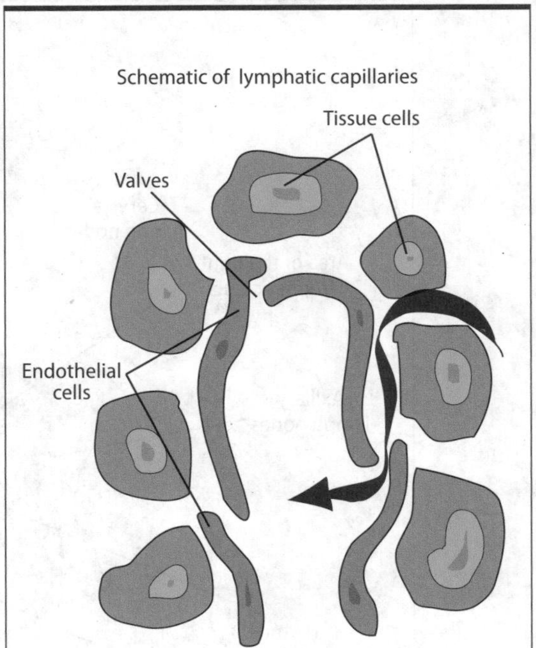

Fluids and particles can enter the capillary through overlapping valves

Lymphatic System of Head and Neck

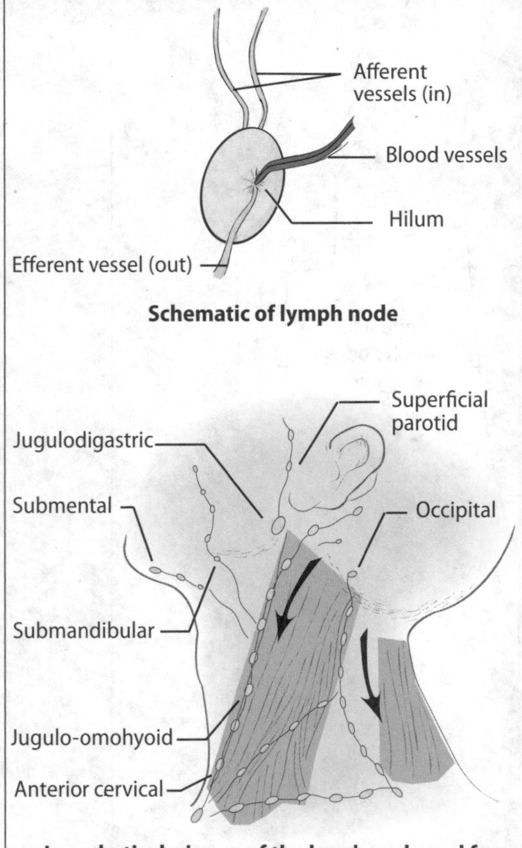

Lymphatic drainage of the head, neck, and face

Lymphatic Drainage

Lymphatic drainage of the colon follows blood supply

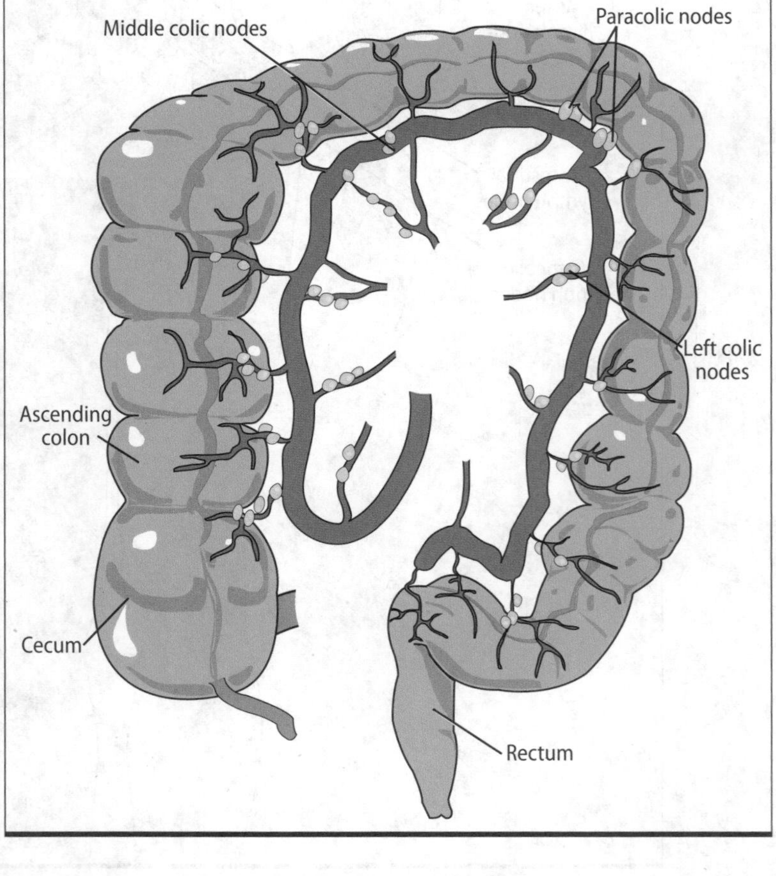

Spleen Internal Structures

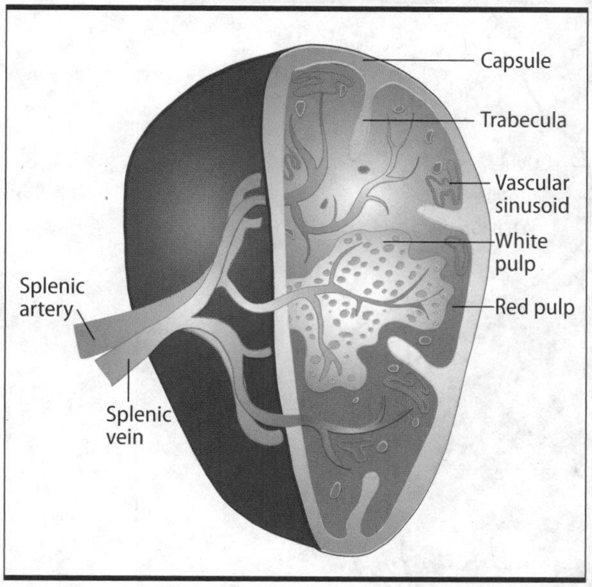

Spleen External Structures

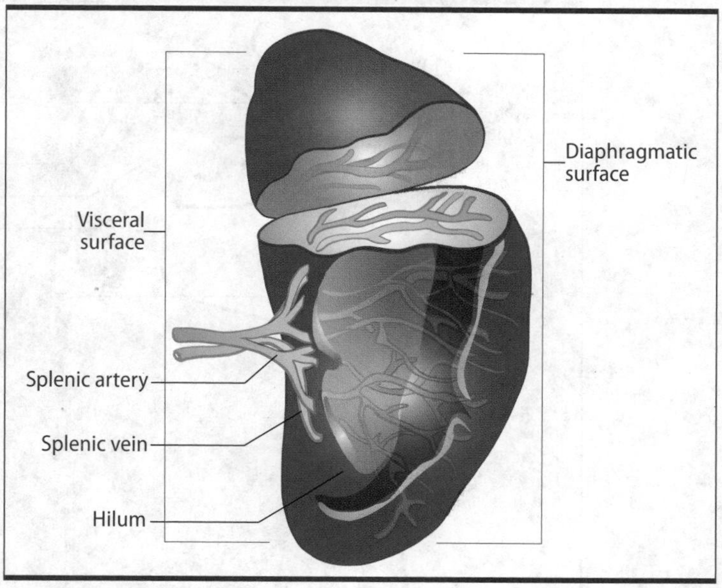

Anatomical Illustrations—Lymphatic System

Digestive System

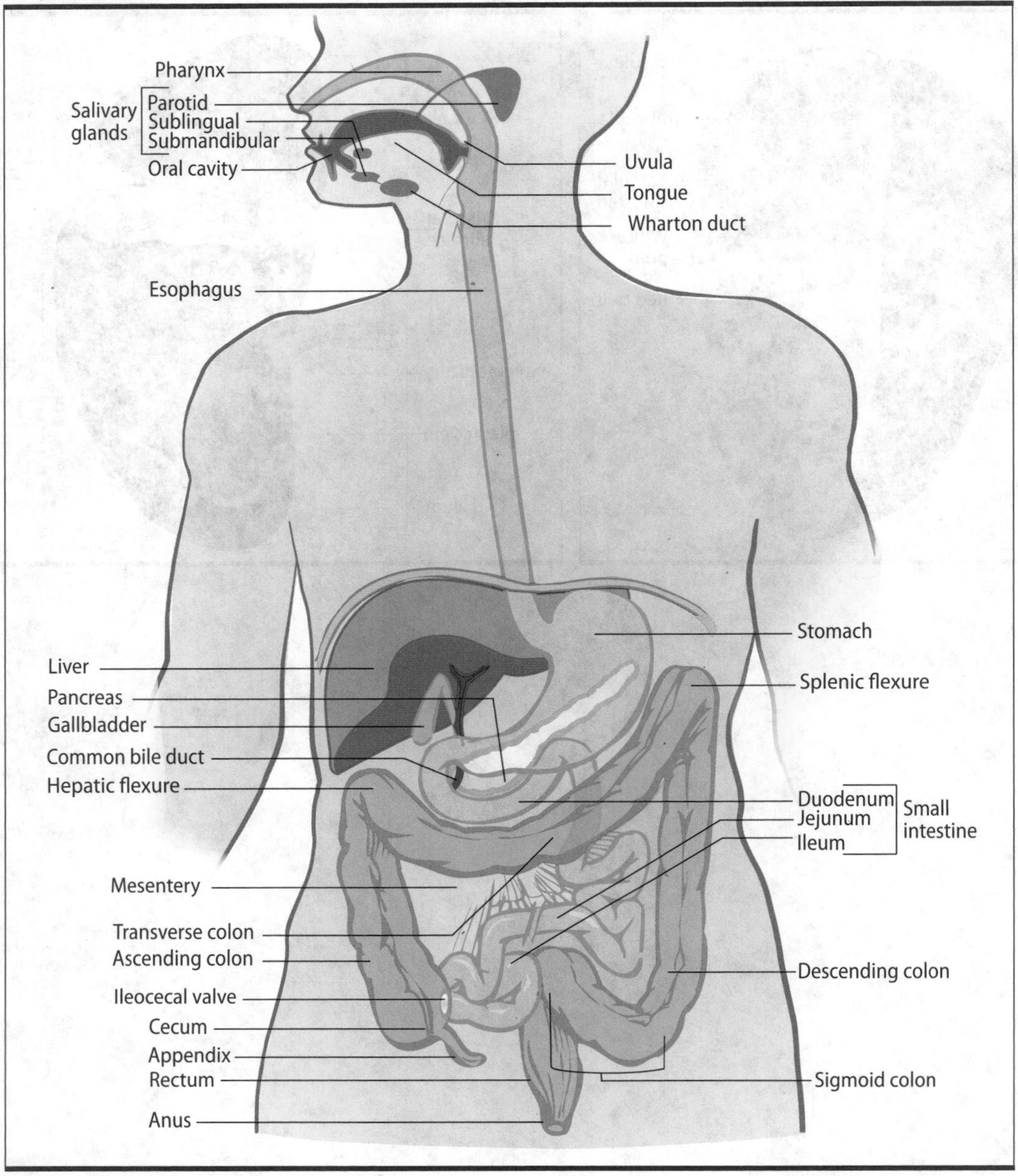
Pharynx
Salivary glands
Parotid
Sublingual
Submandibular
Oral cavity
Uvula
Tongue
Wharton duct
Esophagus
Stomach
Liver
Pancreas
Gallbladder
Common bile duct
Hepatic flexure
Splenic flexure
Duodenum
Jejunum
Ileum
Small intestine
Mesentery
Transverse colon
Ascending colon
Descending colon
Ileocecal valve
Cecum
Appendix
Rectum
Anus
Sigmoid colon

Gallbladder

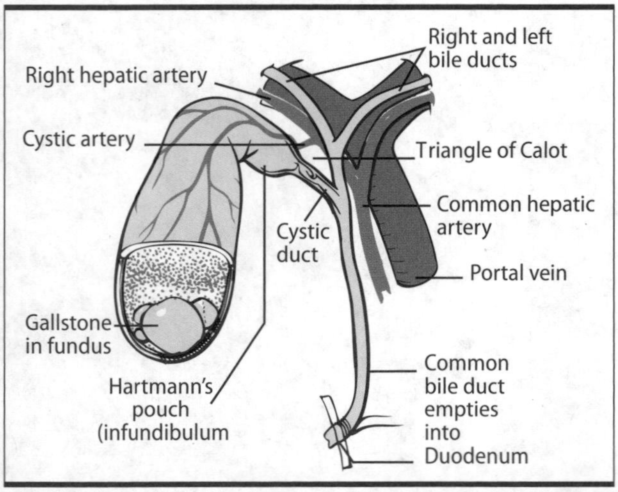
Right and left bile ducts
Right hepatic artery
Cystic artery
Triangle of Calot
Common hepatic artery
Cystic duct
Portal vein
Gallstone in fundus
Hartmann's pouch (infundibulum
Common bile duct empties into Duodenum

Stomach

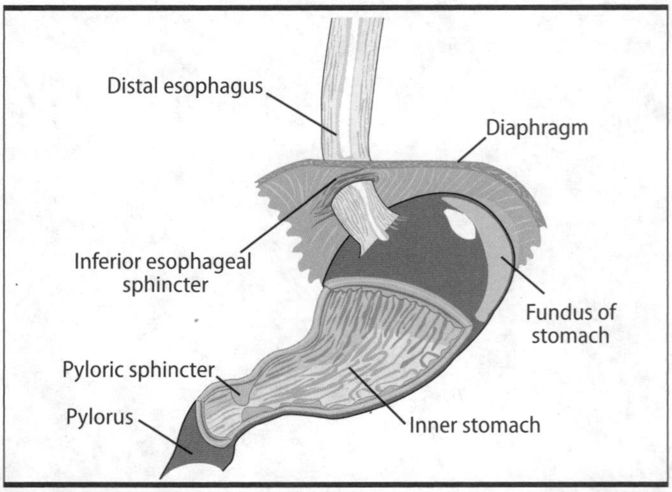
Distal esophagus
Diaphragm
Inferior esophageal sphincter
Fundus of stomach
Pyloric sphincter
Pylorus
Inner stomach

Anatomical Illustrations—Digestive System

Mouth (Upper)

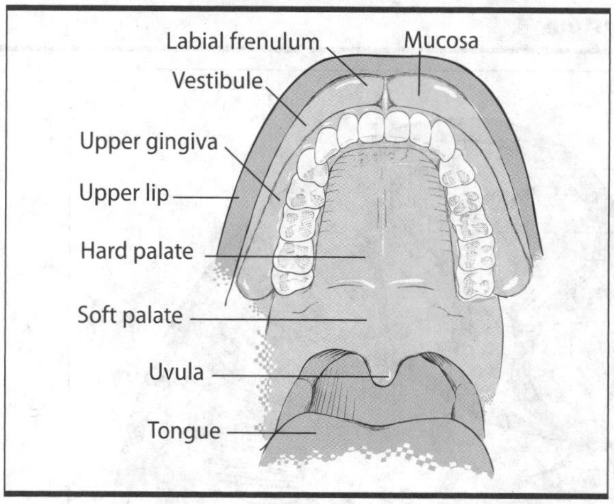

- Labial frenulum
- Mucosa
- Vestibule
- Upper gingiva
- Upper lip
- Hard palate
- Soft palate
- Uvula
- Tongue

Mouth (Lower)

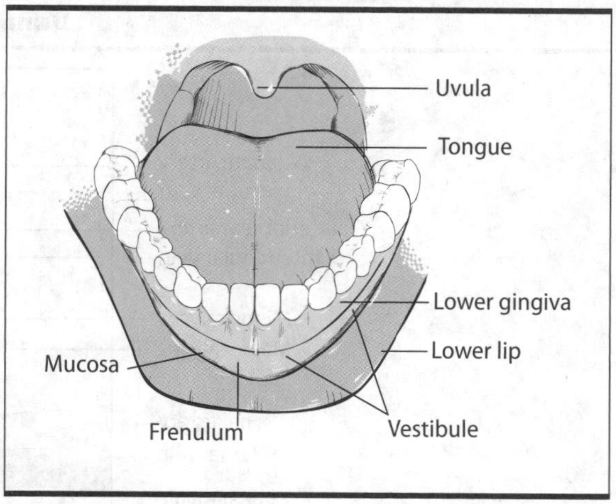

- Uvula
- Tongue
- Lower gingiva
- Lower lip
- Mucosa
- Vestibule
- Frenulum

Pancreas

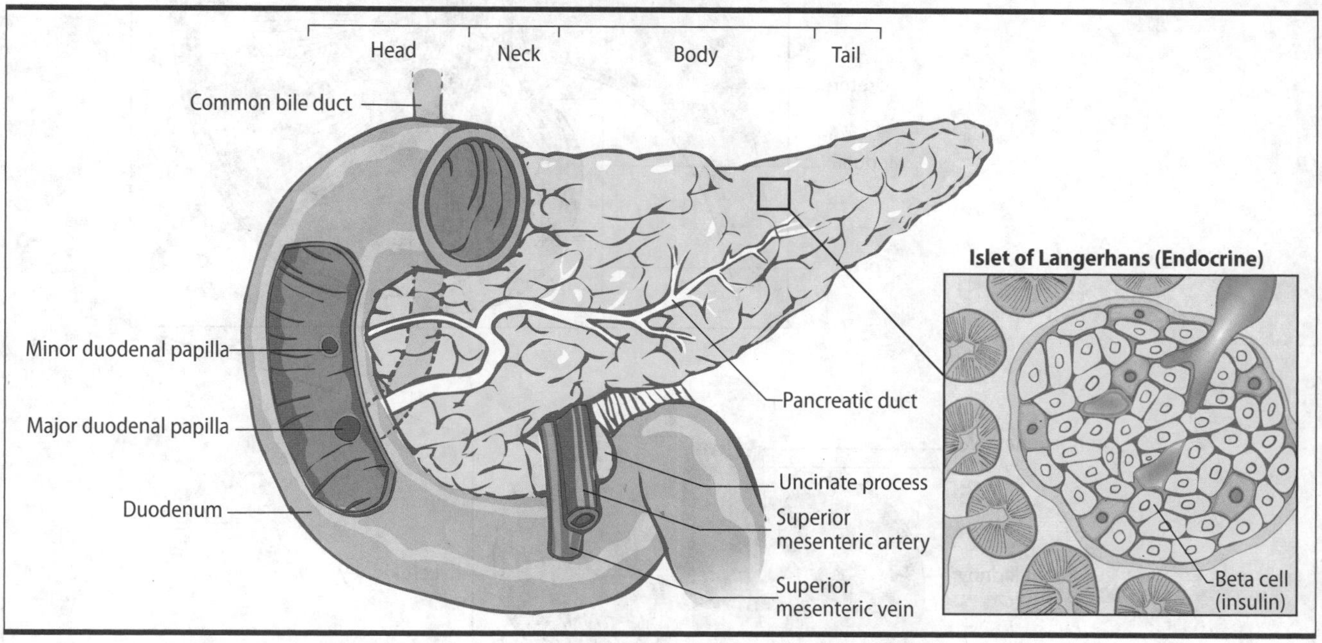

- Head
- Neck
- Body
- Tail
- Common bile duct
- Minor duodenal papilla
- Major duodenal papilla
- Duodenum
- Pancreatic duct
- Uncinate process
- Superior mesenteric artery
- Superior mesenteric vein

Islet of Langerhans (Endocrine)

- Beta cell (insulin)

Liver

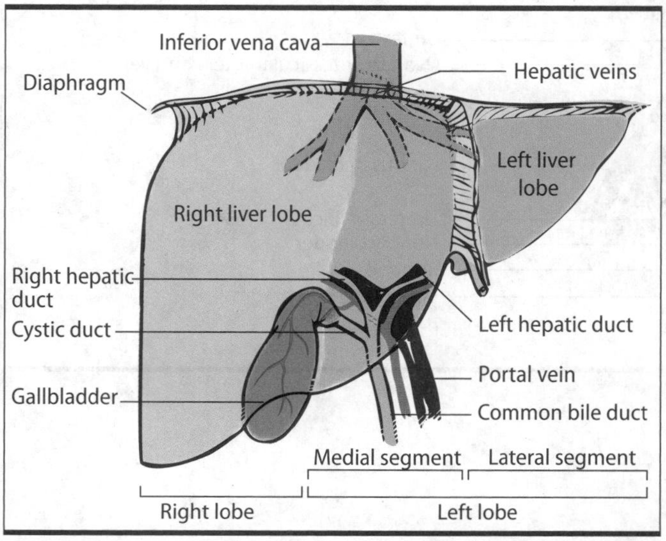

- Inferior vena cava
- Hepatic veins
- Diaphragm
- Left liver lobe
- Right liver lobe
- Right hepatic duct
- Cystic duct
- Left hepatic duct
- Gallbladder
- Portal vein
- Common bile duct
- Medial segment
- Lateral segment
- Right lobe
- Left lobe

Anus

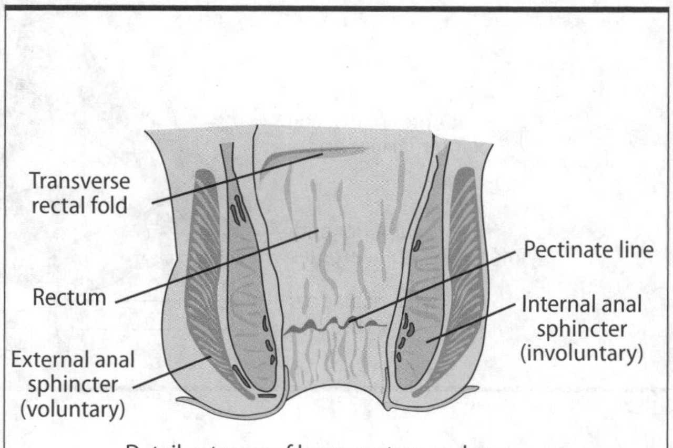

- Transverse rectal fold
- Pectinate line
- Rectum
- Internal anal sphincter (involuntary)
- External anal sphincter (voluntary)

Detail cutaway of lower rectum and anus

Genitourinary System

Urinary System

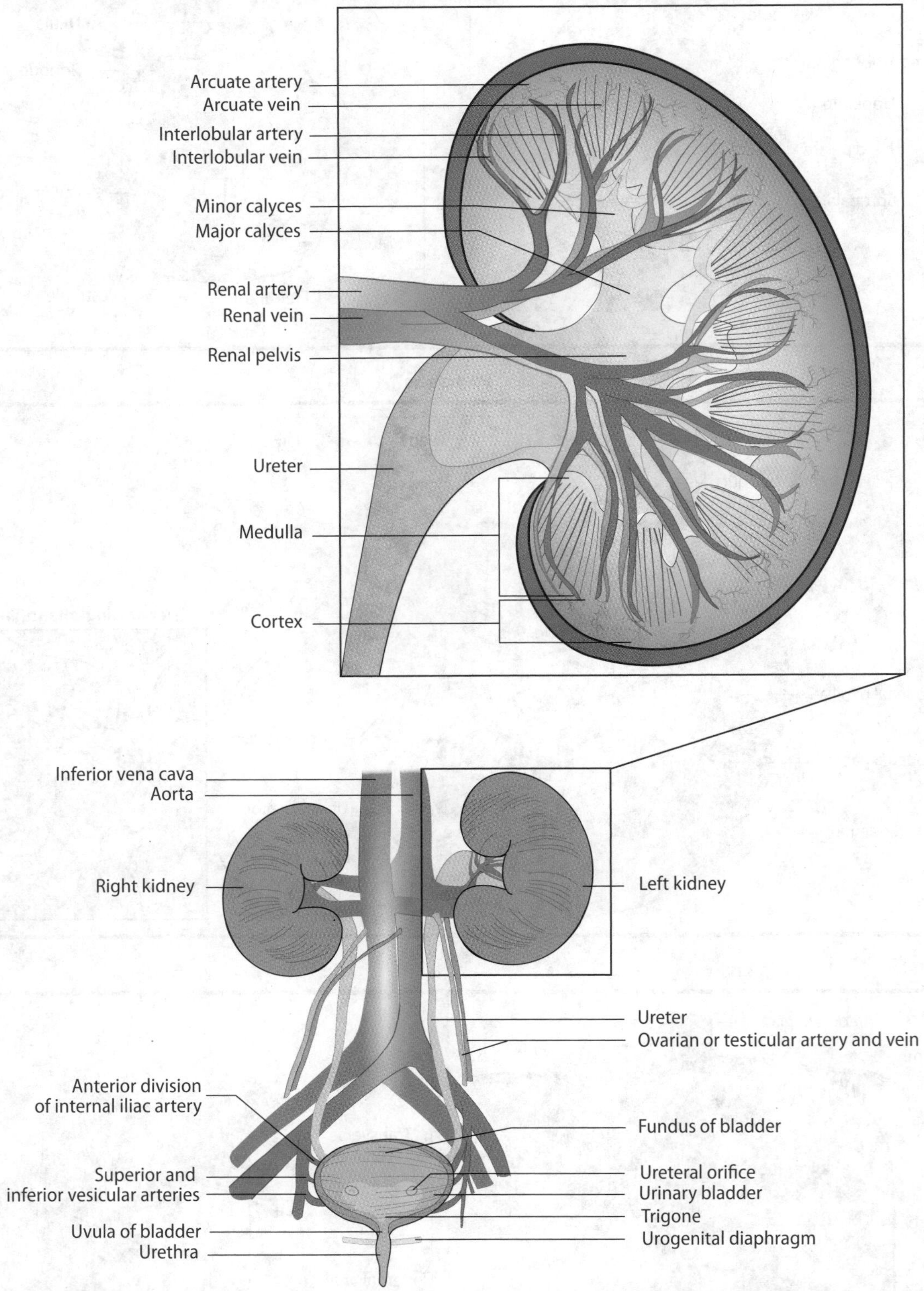
Arcuate artery
Arcuate vein
Interlobular artery
Interlobular vein
Minor calyces
Major calyces
Renal artery
Renal vein
Renal pelvis
Ureter
Medulla
Cortex
Inferior vena cava
Aorta
Right kidney
Left kidney
Ureter
Ovarian or testicular artery and vein
Anterior division of internal iliac artery
Fundus of bladder
Superior and inferior vesicular arteries
Ureteral orifice
Urinary bladder
Trigone
Uvula of bladder
Urogenital diaphragm
Urethra

Nephron

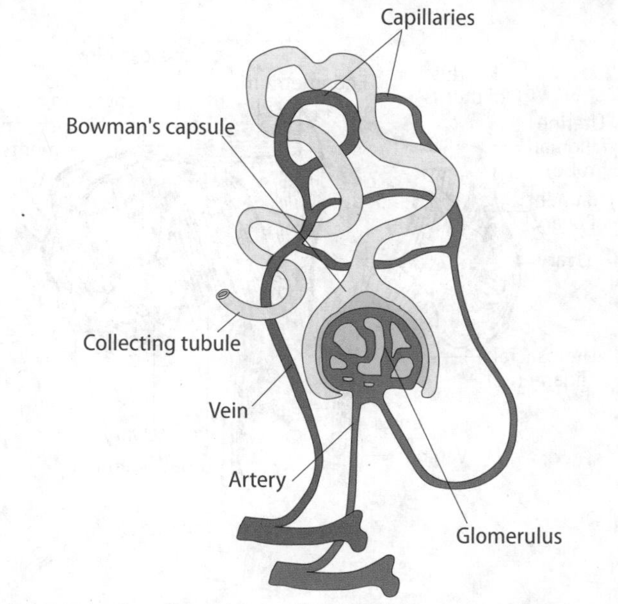

Schematic of nephron, the tiny filtering mechanism of the kidney

Male Genitourinary

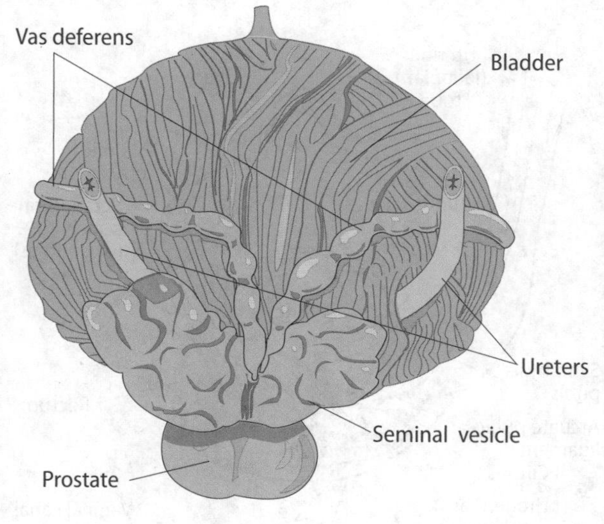

Posterior view of male bladder and prostate

Testis and Associate Structures

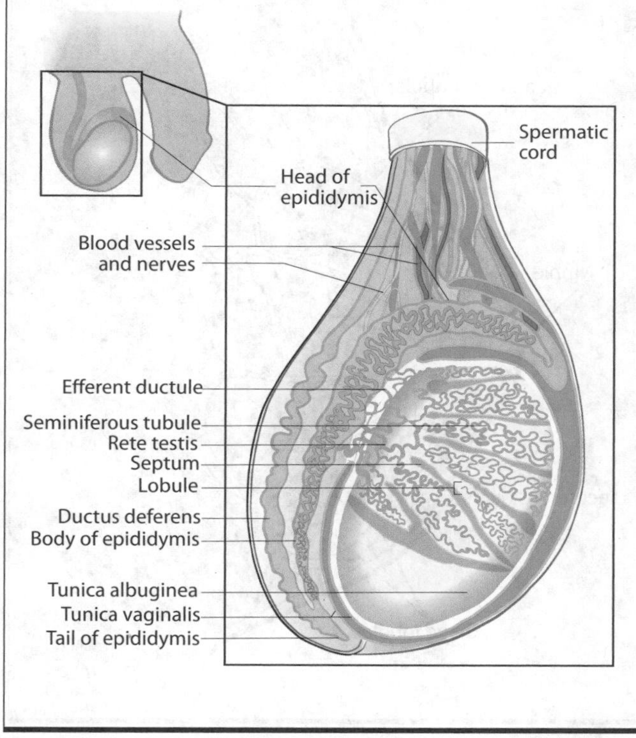

Male Genitourinary System

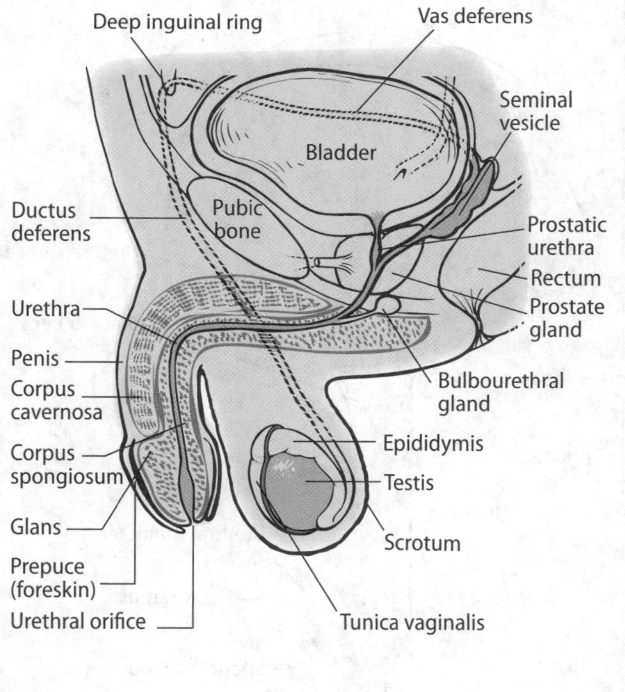

Female Genitourinary

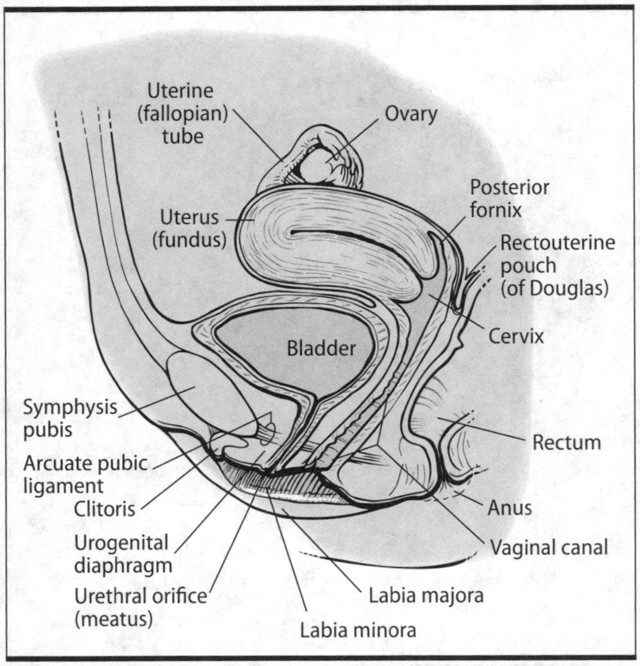

Female Reproductive System

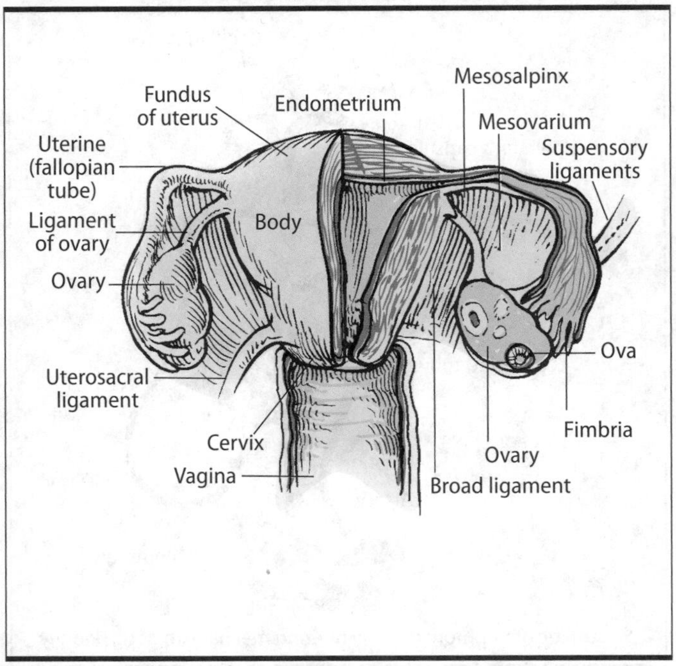

Female Bladder

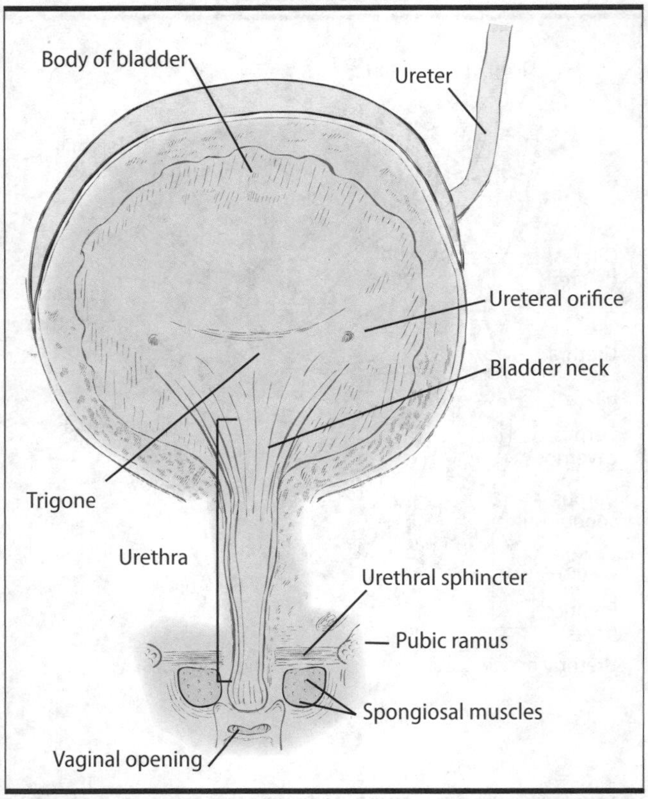

Female Breast

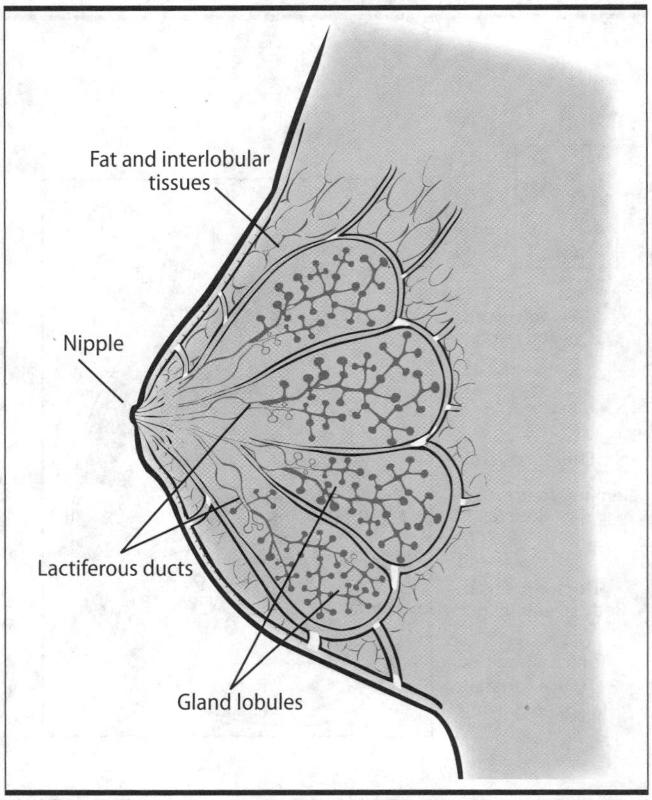

Endocrine System

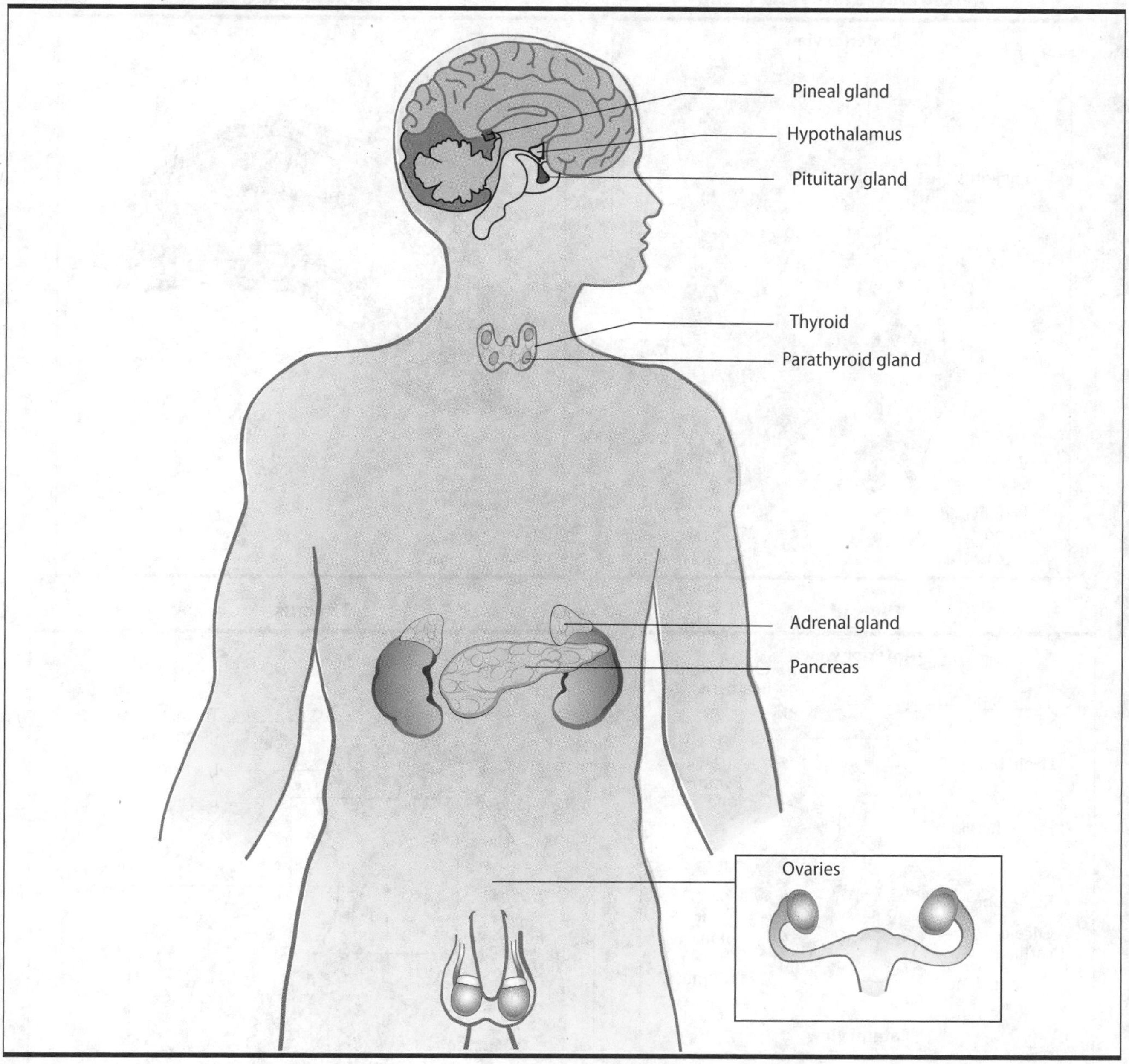

Structure of an Ovary

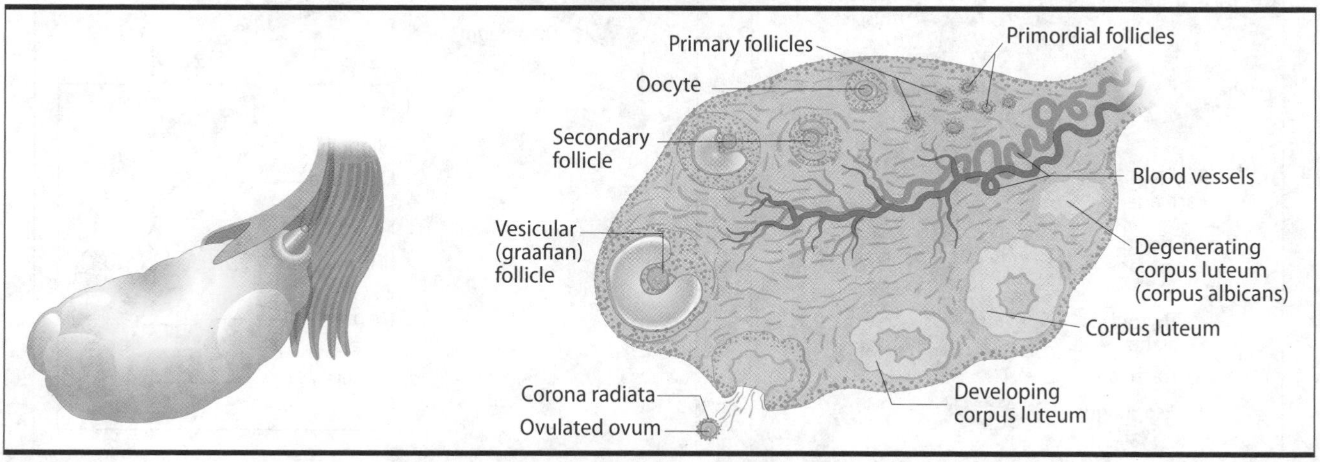

Thyroid and Parathyroid Glands

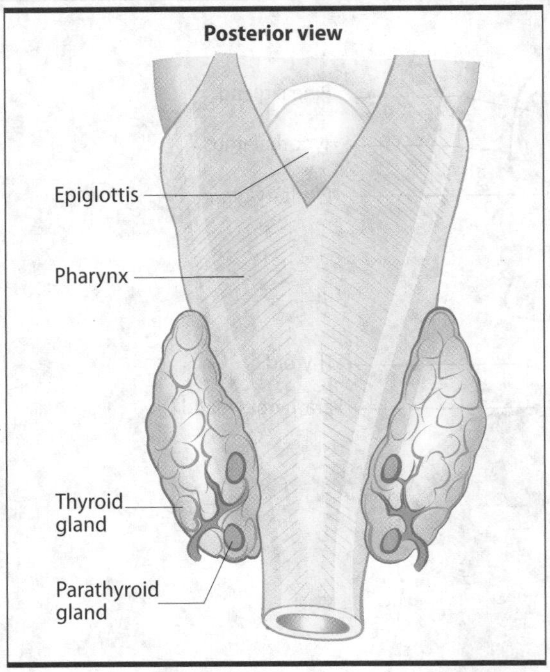

Adrenal Gland

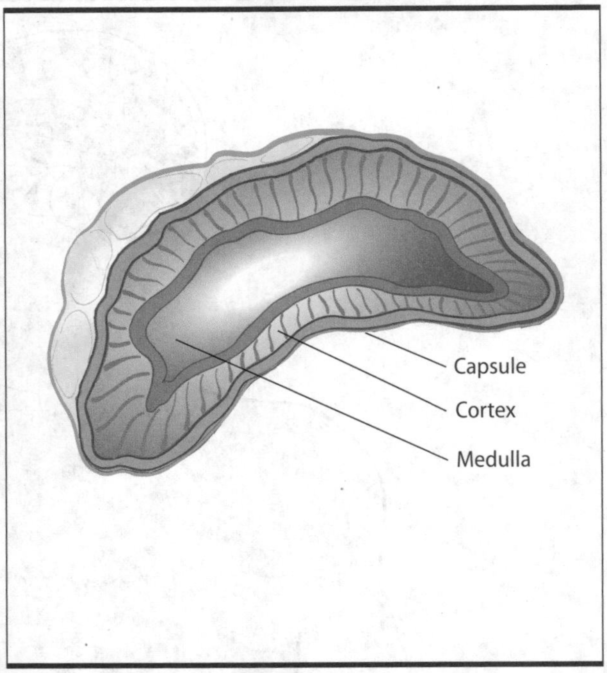

Thyroid

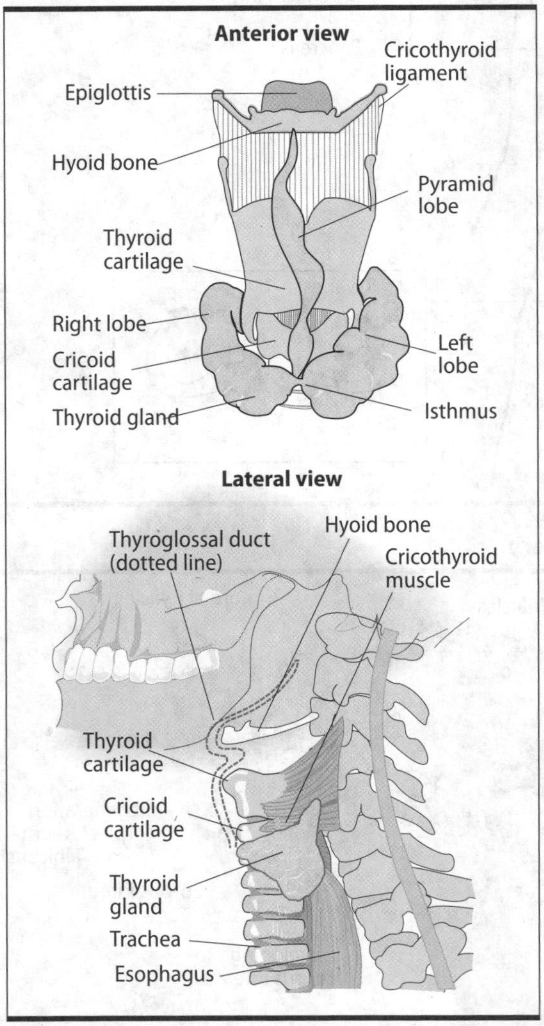

Thymus

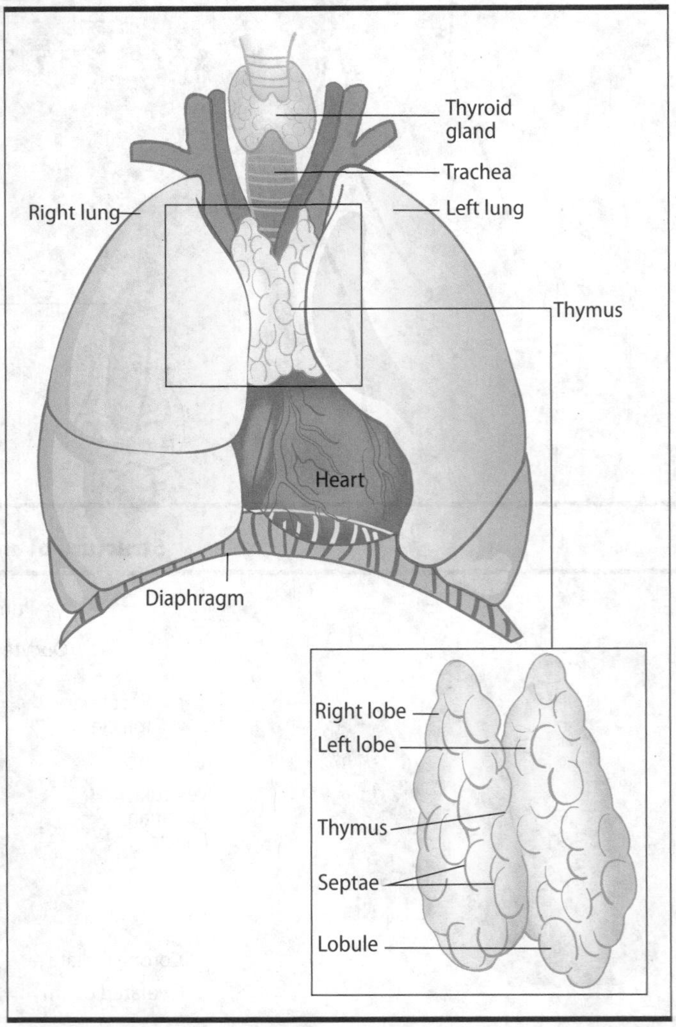

Nervous System

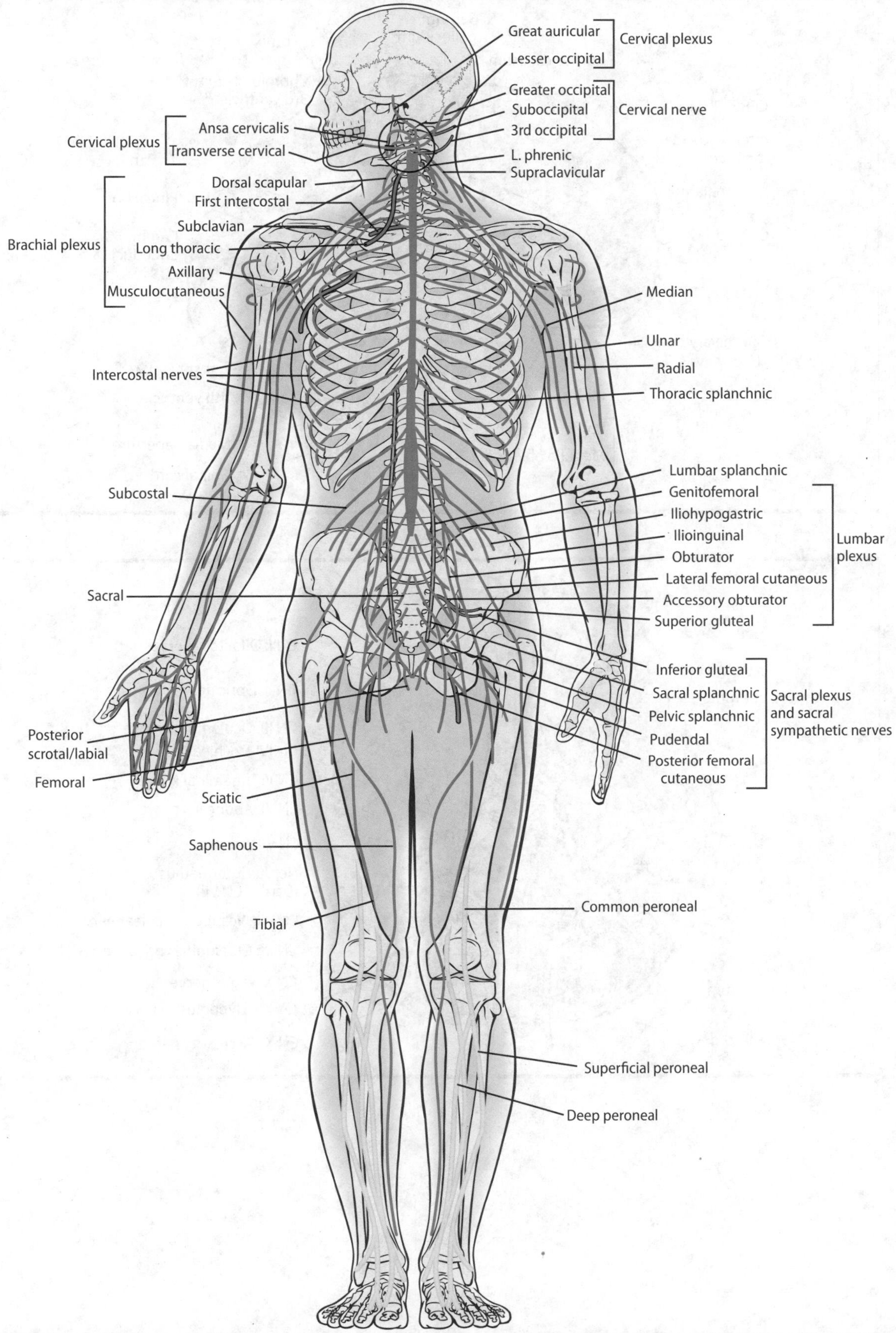

Brain

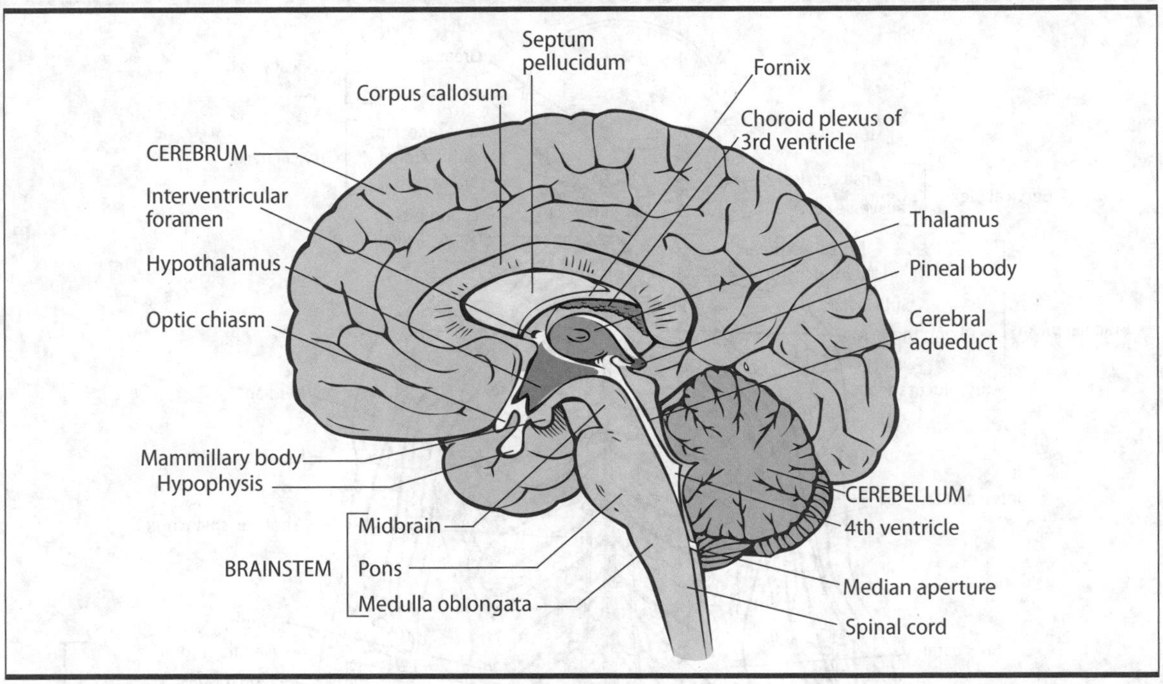
Septum pellucidum
Corpus callosum
Fornix
Choroid plexus of 3rd ventricle
CEREBRUM
Interventricular foramen
Thalamus
Hypothalamus
Pineal body
Optic chiasm
Cerebral aqueduct
Mammillary body
Hypophysis
CEREBELLUM
Midbrain
4th ventricle
BRAINSTEM
Pons
Medulla oblongata
Median aperture
Spinal cord

Cranial Nerves

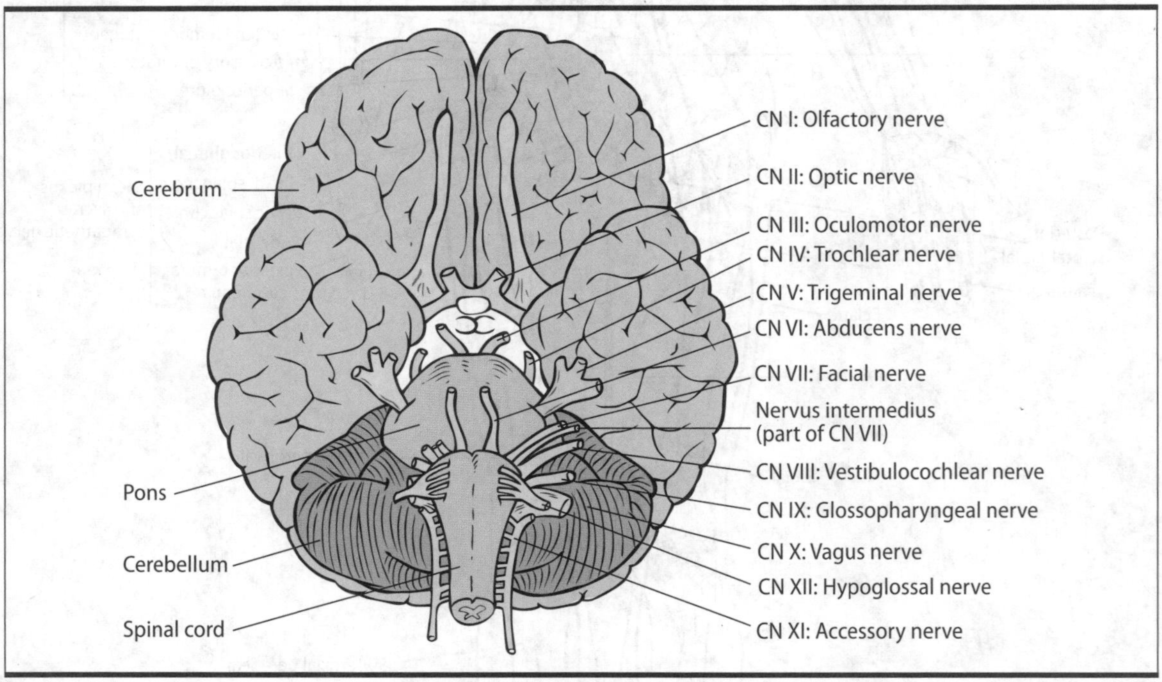
CN I: Olfactory nerve
Cerebrum
CN II: Optic nerve
CN III: Oculomotor nerve
CN IV: Trochlear nerve
CN V: Trigeminal nerve
CN VI: Abducens nerve
CN VII: Facial nerve
Nervus intermedius (part of CN VII)
CN VIII: Vestibulocochlear nerve
Pons
CN IX: Glossopharyngeal nerve
Cerebellum
CN X: Vagus nerve
CN XII: Hypoglossal nerve
Spinal cord
CN XI: Accessory nerve

Spinal Cord and Spinal Nerves

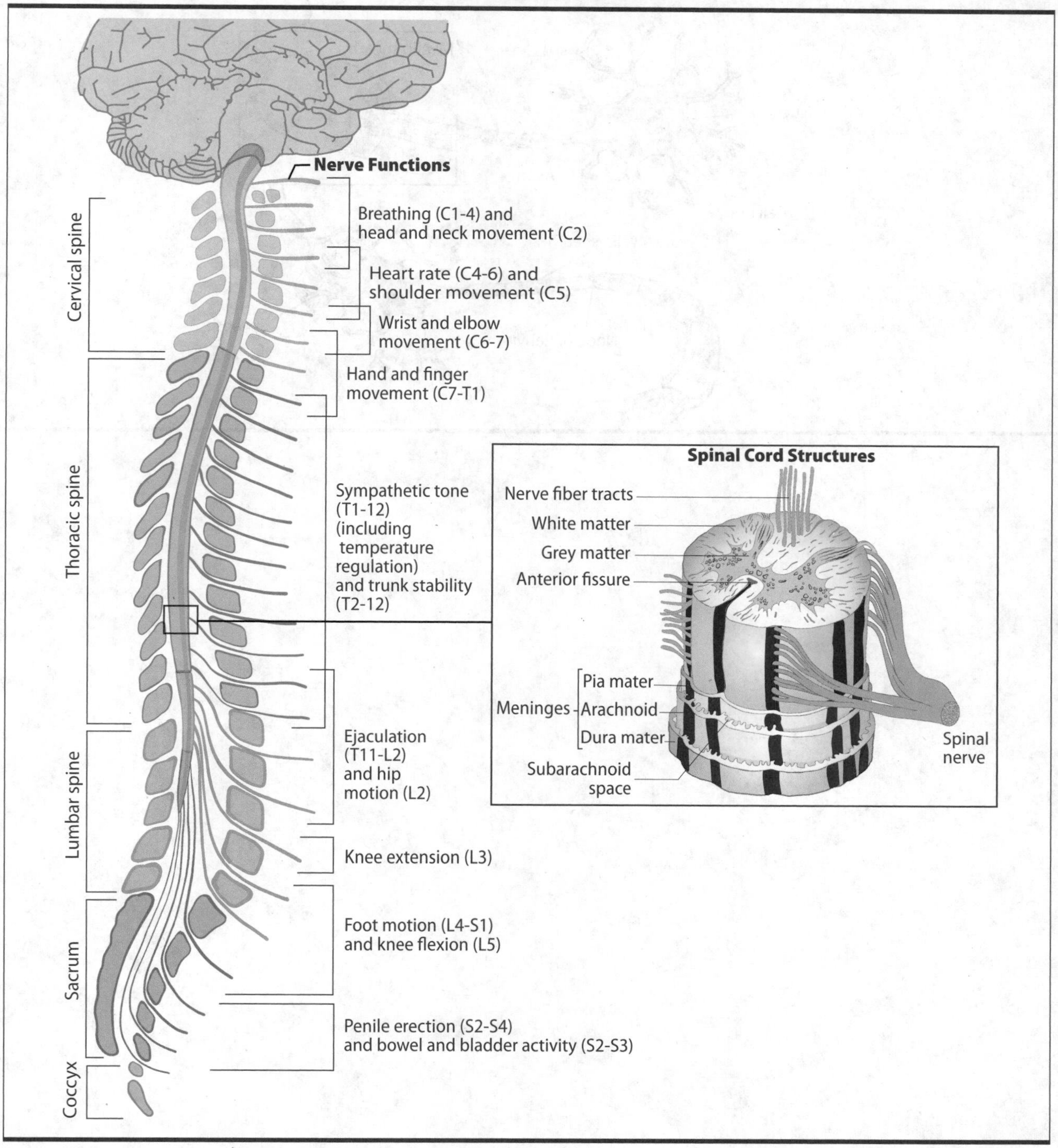
Nerve Functions
Breathing (C1-4) and
head and neck movement (C2)
Heart rate (C4-6) and
shoulder movement (C5)
Wrist and elbow
movement (C6-7)
Hand and finger
movement (C7-T1)
Sympathetic tone
(T1-12)
(including
temperature
regulation)
and trunk stability
(T2-12)
Ejaculation
(T11-L2)
and hip
motion (L2)
Knee extension (L3)
Foot motion (L4-S1)
and knee flexion (L5)
Penile erection (S2-S4)
and bowel and bladder activity (S2-S3)
Cervical spine
Thoracic spine
Lumbar spine
Sacrum
Coccyx
Spinal Cord Structures
Nerve fiber tracts
White matter
Grey matter
Anterior fissure
Meninges
Pia mater
Arachnoid
Dura mater
Subarachnoid
space
Spinal
nerve

Nerve Cell

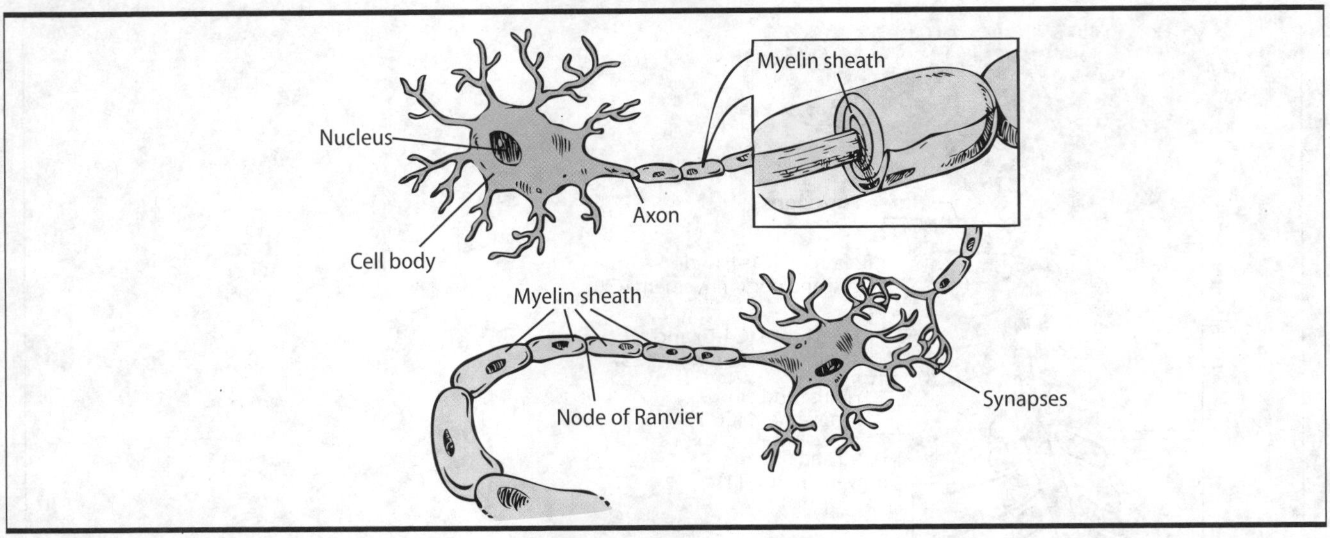
Myelin sheath
Nucleus
Axon
Cell body
Myelin sheath
Synapses
Node of Ranvier

Eye

Eye Structure

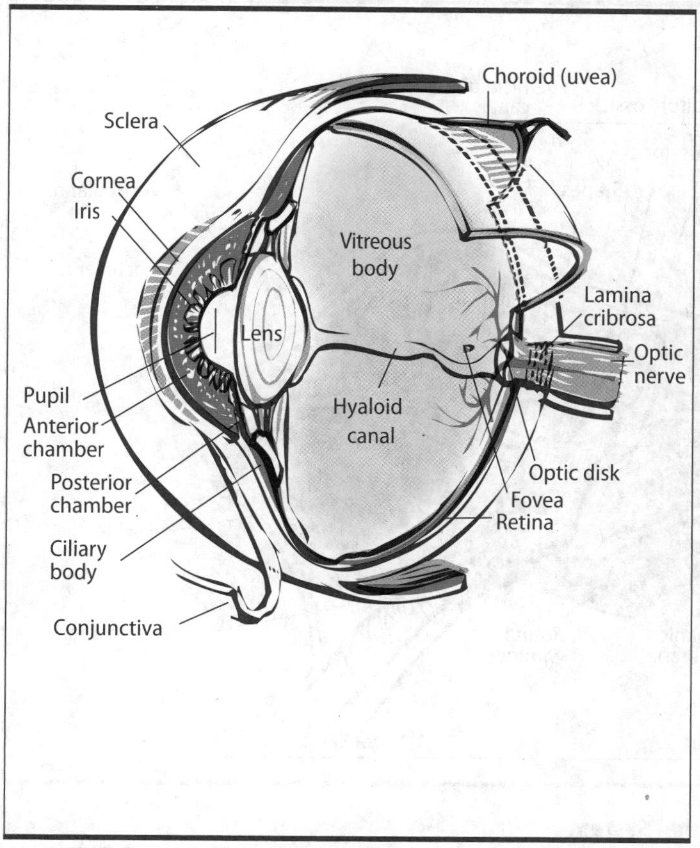

Posterior Pole of Globe/Flow of Aqueous Humor

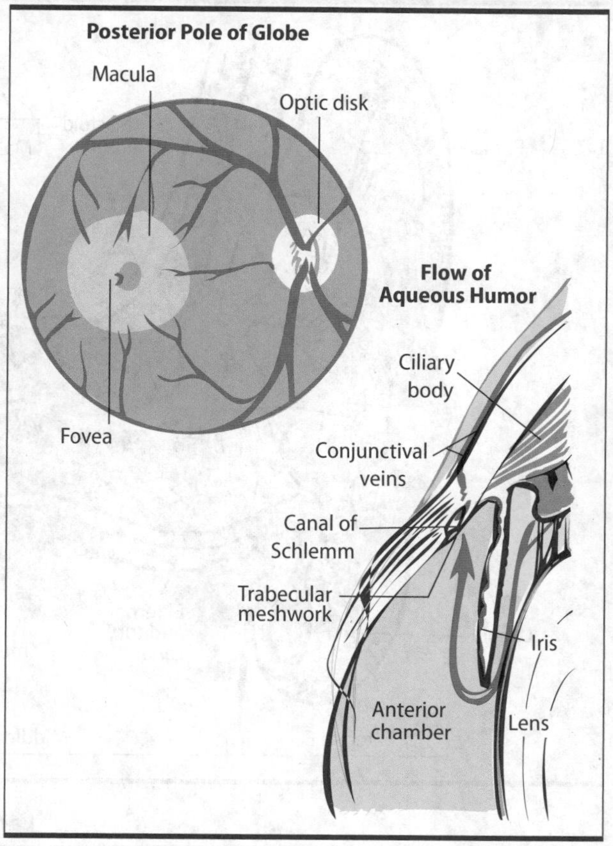

Eye Musculature

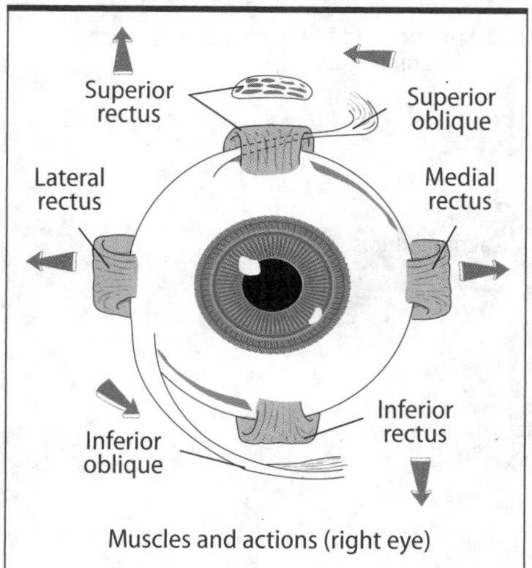

Muscles and actions (right eye)

Eyelid Structures

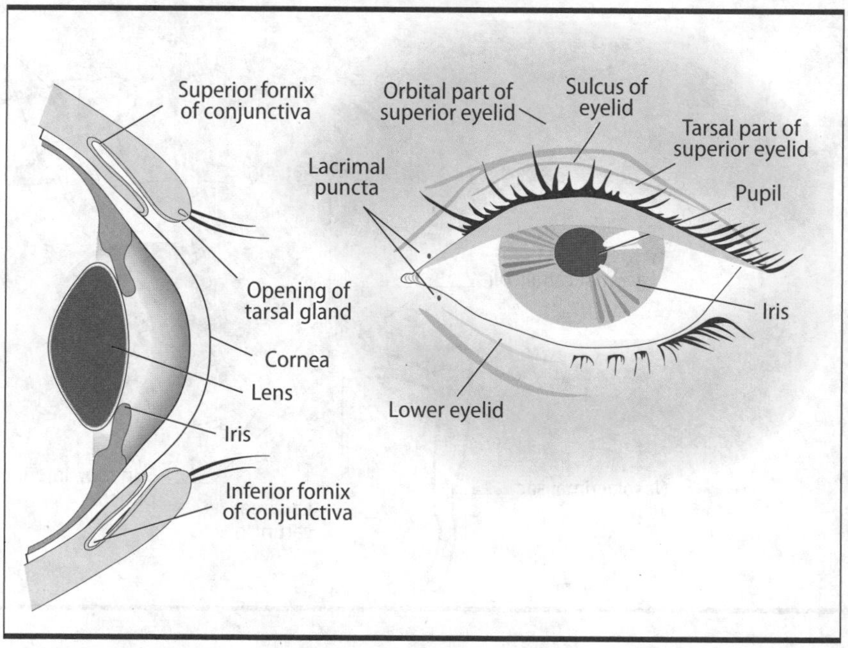

Ear and Lacrimal System

Ear Anatomy

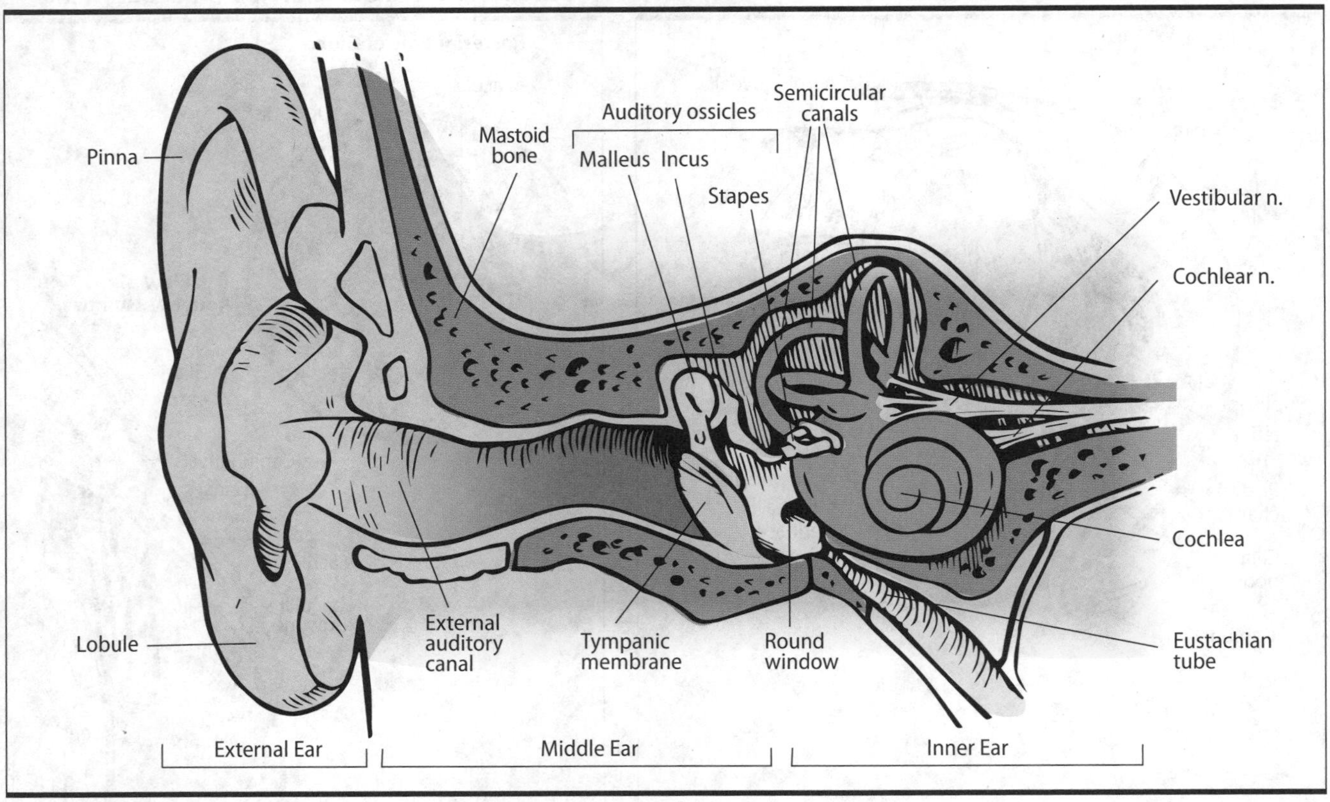

Lacrimal System

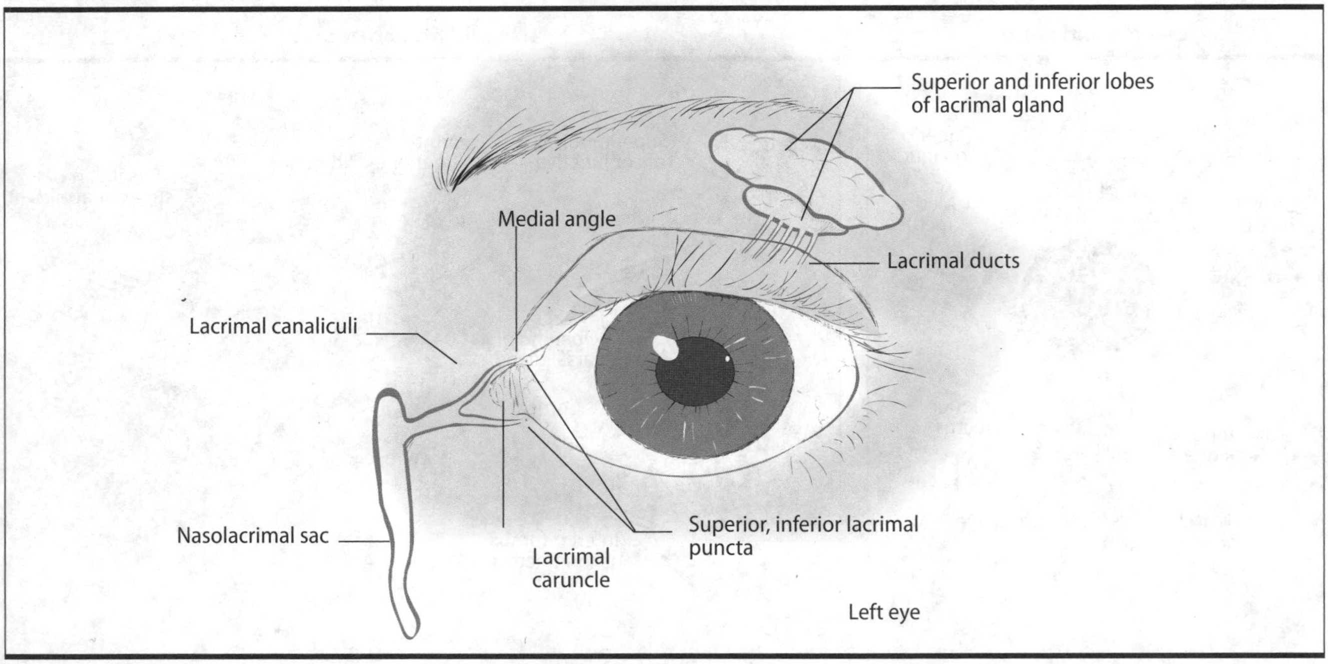

0-Numeric

A

[Resequenced]

 [Resequenced]

 [Resequenced]

 [Resequenced]

[Resequenced]

[Resequenced]

 [Resequenced]

 [Resequenced]

 [Resequenced]

[Resequenced]

 [Resequenced]

D

 [Resequenced]

E

Index

Ear — Education

[Resequenced]

 [Resequenced]

 [Resequenced]

 [Resequenced]

 [Resequenced]

[Resequenced]

 [Resequenced]

[Resequenced]

 [Resequenced]

L

[Resequenced]

M

 [Resequenced]

[Resequenced]

 [Resequenced]

[Resequenced]

[Resequenced]

 [Resequenced]

Q

Index

 [Resequenced]

 [Resequenced]

 [Resequenced]

S

[Resequenced]

 [Resequenced]

 [Resequenced]

 [Resequenced]

[Resequenced]

 [Resequenced]

 [Resequenced]

X

 [Resequenced]

Y

Z

00100-00126 Anesthesia for Cleft Lip, Ear, ECT, Eyelid, and Salivary Gland Procedures

CMS: 100-04,12,140.1 Qualified Nonphysician Anesthetists; 100-04,12,140.3 Payment for Qualified Nonphysician Anesthetists; 100-04,12,140.3.3 Billing Modifiers; 100-04,12,140.3.4 General Billing Instructions; 100-04,12,140.4.1 Anesthesiologist/Qualified Nonphysican Anesthetist; 100-04,12,140.4.2 Anesthetist and Anesthesiologist in a Single Procedure; 100-04,12,140.4.3 Payment for Medical /Surgical Services by CRNAs; 100-04,12,140.4.4 Conversion Factors for Anesthesia Services; 100-04,12,140.5 Payment for Anesthesia Services Furnished by a Teaching CRNA; 100-04,4,250.3.2 Anesthesia in a Hospital Outpatient Setting

00100 **Anesthesia for procedures on salivary glands, including biopsy**

 0.00   0.00   **FUD** XXX   N ▢

AMA: 2019,Oct,10; 2018,Jan,8; 2017,Dec,8; 2017,Jan,8; 2016,Jan,13; 2015,Jan,16

00102 **Anesthesia for procedures involving plastic repair of cleft lip**

 0.00   0.00   **FUD** XXX   N ▢

AMA: 2019,Oct,10; 2018,Jan,8; 2017,Dec,8; 2017,Jan,8; 2016,Jan,13; 2015,Jan,16

00103 **Anesthesia for reconstructive procedures of eyelid (eg, blepharoplasty, ptosis surgery)**

 0.00   0.00   **FUD** XXX   N ▢

AMA: 2019,Oct,10; 2018,Jan,8; 2017,Dec,8; 2017,Jan,8; 2016,Jan,13; 2015,Jan,16

00104 **Anesthesia for electroconvulsive therapy**

 0.00   0.00   **FUD** XXX   N ▢

AMA: 2019,Oct,10; 2018,Jan,8; 2017,Dec,8; 2017,Jan,8; 2016,Jan,13; 2015,Jan,16

00120 **Anesthesia for procedures on external, middle, and inner ear including biopsy; not otherwise specified**

 0.00   0.00   **FUD** XXX   N ▢

AMA: 2019,Oct,10; 2018,Jan,8; 2017,Dec,8; 2017,Jan,8; 2016,Jan,13; 2015,Jan,16

00124 **otoscopy**

 0.00   0.00   **FUD** XXX   N ▢

AMA: 2019,Oct,10; 2018,Jan,8; 2017,Dec,8; 2017,Jan,8; 2016,Jan,13; 2015,Jan,16

00126 **tympanotomy**

 0.00   0.00   **FUD** XXX   N ▢

AMA: 2019,Oct,10; 2018,Jan,8; 2017,Dec,8; 2017,Jan,8; 2016,Jan,13; 2015,Jan,16

00140-00148 Anesthesia for Eye Procedures

CMS: 100-04,12,140.1 Qualified Nonphysician Anesthetists; 100-04,12,140.3 Payment for Qualified Nonphysician Anesthetists; 100-04,12,140.3.3 Billing Modifiers; 100-04,12,140.3.4 General Billing Instructions; 100-04,12,140.4.1 Anesthesiologist/Qualified Nonphysican Anesthetist; 100-04,12,140.4.2 Anesthetist and Anesthesiologist in a Single Procedure; 100-04,12,140.4.3 Payment for Medical /Surgical Services by CRNAs; 100-04,12,140.4.4 Conversion Factors for Anesthesia Services; 100-04,12,140.5 Payment for Anesthesia Services Furnished by a Teaching CRNA; 100-04,4,250.3.2 Anesthesia in a Hospital Outpatient Setting

00140 **Anesthesia for procedures on eye; not otherwise specified**

 0.00   0.00   **FUD** XXX   N ▢

AMA: 2019,Oct,10; 2018,Jan,8; 2017,Dec,8; 2017,Jan,8; 2016,Jan,13; 2015,Jan,16

00142 **lens surgery**

 0.00   0.00   **FUD** XXX   N ▢

AMA: 2019,Oct,10; 2018,Jan,8; 2017,Dec,8; 2017,Jan,8; 2016,Jan,13; 2015,Jan,16

00144 **corneal transplant**

 0.00   0.00   **FUD** XXX   N ▢

AMA: 2019,Oct,10; 2018,Jan,8; 2017,Dec,8; 2017,Jan,8; 2016,Jan,13; 2015,Jan,16

00145 **vitreoretinal surgery**

 0.00   0.00   **FUD** XXX   N ▢

AMA: 2019,Oct,10; 2018,Jan,8; 2017,Dec,8; 2017,Jan,8; 2016,Jan,13; 2015,Jan,16

00147 **iridectomy**

 0.00   0.00   **FUD** XXX   N ▢

AMA: 2019,Oct,10; 2018,Jan,8; 2017,Dec,8; 2017,Jan,8; 2016,Jan,13; 2015,Jan,16

00148 **ophthalmoscopy**

 0.00   0.00   **FUD** XXX   N ▢

AMA: 2019,Oct,10; 2018,Jan,8; 2017,Dec,8; 2017,Jan,8; 2016,Jan,13; 2015,Jan,16

00160-00326 Anesthesia for Face and Head Procedures

CMS: 100-04,12,140.1 Qualified Nonphysician Anesthetists; 100-04,12,140.3 Payment for Qualified Nonphysician Anesthetists; 100-04,12,140.3.3 Billing Modifiers; 100-04,12,140.3.4 General Billing Instructions; 100-04,12,140.4.1 Anesthesiologist/Qualified Nonphysican Anesthetist; 100-04,12,140.4.2 Anesthetist and Anesthesiologist in a Single Procedure; 100-04,12,140.4.4 Conversion Factors for Anesthesia Services; 100-04,12,140.5 Payment for Anesthesia Services Furnished by a Teaching CRNA; 100-04,4,250.3.2 Anesthesia in a Hospital Outpatient Setting

00160 **Anesthesia for procedures on nose and accessory sinuses; not otherwise specified**

 0.00   0.00   **FUD** XXX   N ▢

AMA: 2019,Oct,10; 2018,Jan,8; 2017,Dec,8; 2017,Jan,8; 2016,Jan,13; 2015,Jan,16

00162 **radical surgery**

 0.00   0.00   **FUD** XXX   N ▢

AMA: 2019,Oct,10; 2018,Jan,8; 2017,Dec,8; 2017,Jan,8; 2016,Jan,13; 2015,Jan,16

00164 **biopsy, soft tissue**

 0.00   0.00   **FUD** XXX   N ▢

AMA: 2019,Oct,10; 2018,Jan,8; 2017,Dec,8; 2017,Jan,8; 2016,Jan,13; 2015,Jan,16

00170 **Anesthesia for intraoral procedures, including biopsy; not otherwise specified**

 0.00   0.00   **FUD** XXX   N ▢

AMA: 2019,Oct,10; 2018,Jan,8; 2017,Dec,8; 2017,Jan,8; 2016,Jan,13; 2015,Jan,16

00172 **repair of cleft palate**

 0.00   0.00   **FUD** XXX   N ▢

AMA: 2019,Oct,10; 2018,Jan,8; 2017,Dec,8; 2017,Jan,8; 2016,Jan,13; 2015,Jan,16

00174 **excision of retropharyngeal tumor**

 0.00   0.00   **FUD** XXX   N ▢

AMA: 2019,Oct,10; 2018,Jan,8; 2017,Dec,8; 2017,Jan,8; 2016,Jan,13; 2015,Jan,16

00176 **radical surgery**

 0.00   0.00   **FUD** XXX   C ▢

AMA: 2019,Oct,10; 2018,Jan,8; 2017,Dec,8; 2017,Jan,8; 2016,Jan,13; 2015,Jan,16

00190 **Anesthesia for procedures on facial bones or skull; not otherwise specified**

 0.00   0.00   **FUD** XXX   N ▢

AMA: 2019,Oct,10; 2018,Jan,8; 2017,Dec,8; 2017,Jan,8; 2016,Jan,13; 2015,Jan,16

00192 **radical surgery (including prognathism)**

 0.00   0.00   **FUD** XXX   C ▢

AMA: 2019,Oct,10; 2018,Jan,8; 2017,Dec,8; 2017,Jan,8; 2016,Jan,13; 2015,Jan,16

00210 **Anesthesia for intracranial procedures; not otherwise specified**

 0.00   0.00   **FUD** XXX   N ▢

AMA: 2019,Oct,10; 2018,Jan,8; 2017,Dec,8; 2017,Jan,8; 2016,Jan,13; 2015,Jan,16

00211 **craniotomy or craniectomy for evacuation of hematoma**

 0.00   0.00   **FUD** XXX   C ▢

AMA: 2019,Oct,10; 2018,Jan,8; 2017,Dec,8; 2017,Jan,8; 2016,Jan,13; 2015,Jan,16

00212 **subdural taps**

 0.00   0.00   **FUD** XXX   N ▢

AMA: 2019,Oct,10; 2018,Jan,8; 2017,Dec,8; 2017,Jan,8; 2016,Jan,13; 2015,Jan,16

00214 **burr holes, including ventriculography**

 0.00   0.00   **FUD** XXX   C ▢

AMA: 2019,Oct,10; 2018,Jan,8; 2017,Dec,8; 2017,Jan,8; 2016,Jan,13; 2015,Jan,16

● New Code   ▲ Revised Code   ○ Reinstated   ● New Web Release   ▲ Revised Web Release   + Add-on   Unlisted   Not Covered   # Resequenced
50 Optum Mod 50 Exempt   ⊘ AMA Mod 51 Exempt   51 Optum Mod 51 Exempt   63 Mod 63 Exempt   ✗ Non-FDA Drug   ★ Telemedicine   M Maternity   A Age Edit

CPT © 2020 American Medical Association. All Rights Reserved.

00215 **cranioplasty or elevation of depressed skull fracture, extradural (simple or compound)**
0.00 0.00 FUD XXX C
AMA: 2019,Oct,10; 2018,Jan,8; 2017,Dec,8; 2017,Jan,8; 2016,Jan,13; 2015,Jan,16

00216 **vascular procedures**
0.00 0.00 FUD XXX N
AMA: 2019,Oct,10; 2018,Jan,8; 2017,Dec,8; 2017,Jan,8; 2016,Jan,13; 2015,Jan,16

00218 **procedures in sitting position**
0.00 0.00 FUD XXX N
AMA: 2019,Oct,10; 2018,Jan,8; 2017,Dec,8; 2017,Jan,8; 2016,Jan,13; 2015,Jan,16

00220 **cerebrospinal fluid shunting procedures**
0.00 0.00 FUD XXX N
AMA: 2019,Oct,10; 2018,Jan,8; 2017,Dec,8; 2017,Jan,8; 2016,Jan,13; 2015,Jan,16

00222 **electrocoagulation of intracranial nerve**
0.00 0.00 FUD XXX N
AMA: 2019,Oct,10; 2018,Jan,8; 2017,Dec,8; 2017,Jan,8; 2016,Jan,13; 2015,Jan,16

00300 **Anesthesia for all procedures on the integumentary system, muscles and nerves of head, neck, and posterior trunk, not otherwise specified**
0.00 0.00 FUD XXX N
AMA: 2019,Oct,10; 2018,Jan,8; 2017,Dec,8; 2017,Jan,8; 2016,Jan,13; 2015,Jan,16

00320 **Anesthesia for all procedures on esophagus, thyroid, larynx, trachea and lymphatic system of neck; not otherwise specified, age 1 year or older**
0.00 0.00 FUD XXX N
AMA: 2019,Oct,10; 2018,Jan,8; 2017,Dec,8; 2017,Jan,8; 2016,Jan,13; 2015,Jan,16

00322 **needle biopsy of thyroid**
EXCLUDES *Cervical spine and spinal cord procedures (00600, 00604, 00670)*
0.00 0.00 FUD XXX N
AMA: 2019,Oct,10; 2018,Jan,8; 2017,Dec,8; 2017,Jan,8; 2016,Jan,13; 2015,Jan,16

00326 **Anesthesia for all procedures on the larynx and trachea in children younger than 1 year of age** A
INCLUDES Anesthesia for patient of extreme age, younger than 1 year and older than 70 (99100)
0.00 0.00 FUD XXX N
AMA: 2019,Oct,10; 2018,Jan,8; 2017,Dec,8; 2017,Jan,8; 2016,Jan,13; 2015,Jan,16

00350-00352 Anesthesia for Neck Vessel Procedures

CMS: 100-04,12,140.1 Qualified Nonphysician Anesthetists; 100-04,12,140.3 Payment for Qualified Nonphysician Anesthetists; 100-04,12,140.3.3 Billing Modifiers; 100-04,12,140.3.4 General Billing Instructions; 100-04,12,140.4.1 Anesthesiologist/Qualified Nonphysican Anesthetist; 100-04,12,140.4.2 Anesthetist and Anesthesiologist in a Single Procedure; 100-04,12,140.4.3 Payment for Medical /Surgical Services by CRNAs; 100-04,12,140.4.4 Conversion Factors for Anesthesia Services; 100-04,12,140.5 Payment for Anesthesia Services Furnished by a Teaching CRNA; 100-04,4,250.3.2 Anesthesia in a Hospital Outpatient Setting

EXCLUDES *Arteriography (01916)*

00350 **Anesthesia for procedures on major vessels of neck; not otherwise specified**
0.00 0.00 FUD XXX N
AMA: 2019,Oct,10; 2018,Jan,8; 2017,Dec,8; 2017,Jan,8; 2016,Jan,13; 2015,Jan,16

00352 **simple ligation**
0.00 0.00 FUD XXX N
AMA: 2019,Oct,10; 2018,Jan,8; 2017,Dec,8; 2017,Jan,8; 2016,Jan,13; 2015,Jan,16

00400-00529 Anesthesia for Chest/Pectoral Girdle Procedures

CMS: 100-04,12,140.1 Qualified Nonphysician Anesthetists; 100-04,12,140.3 Payment for Qualified Nonphysician Anesthetists; 100-04,12,140.3.3 Billing Modifiers; 100-04,12,140.3.4 General Billing Instructions; 100-04,12,140.4.1 Anesthesiologist/Qualified Nonphysican Anesthetist; 100-04,12,140.4.2 Anesthetist and Anesthesiologist in a Single Procedure; 100-04,12,140.4.3 Payment for Medical /Surgical Services by CRNAs; 100-04,12,140.4.4 Conversion Factors for Anesthesia Services; 100-04,12,140.5 Payment for Anesthesia Services Furnished by a Teaching CRNA; 100-04,4,250.3.2 Anesthesia in a Hospital Outpatient Setting

00400 **Anesthesia for procedures on the integumentary system on the extremities, anterior trunk and perineum; not otherwise specified**
0.00 0.00 FUD XXX N
AMA: 2019,Oct,10; 2018,Jan,8; 2017,Dec,8; 2017,Jan,8; 2016,Jan,13; 2015,Jan,16

00402 **reconstructive procedures on breast (eg, reduction or augmentation mammoplasty, muscle flaps)**
0.00 0.00 FUD XXX N
AMA: 2019,Oct,10; 2018,Jan,8; 2017,Dec,8; 2017,Jan,8; 2016,Jan,13; 2015,Jan,16

00404 **radical or modified radical procedures on breast**
0.00 0.00 FUD XXX N
AMA: 2019,Oct,10; 2018,Jan,8; 2017,Dec,8; 2017,Jan,8; 2016,Jan,13; 2015,Jan,16

00406 **radical or modified radical procedures on breast with internal mammary node dissection**
0.00 0.00 FUD XXX N
AMA: 2019,Oct,10; 2018,Jan,8; 2017,Dec,8; 2017,Jan,8; 2016,Jan,13; 2015,Jan,16

00410 **electrical conversion of arrhythmias**
0.00 0.00 FUD XXX N
AMA: 2019,Oct,10; 2018,Jan,8; 2017,Dec,8; 2017,Jan,8; 2016,Jan,13; 2015,Jan,16

00450 **Anesthesia for procedures on clavicle and scapula; not otherwise specified**
0.00 0.00 FUD XXX N
AMA: 2019,Oct,10; 2018,Jan,8; 2017,Dec,8; 2017,Jan,8; 2016,Jan,13; 2015,Jan,16

00454 **biopsy of clavicle**
0.00 0.00 FUD XXX N
AMA: 2019,Oct,10; 2018,Jan,8; 2017,Dec,8; 2017,Jan,8; 2016,Jan,13; 2015,Jan,16

00470 **Anesthesia for partial rib resection; not otherwise specified**
0.00 0.00 FUD XXX N
AMA: 2019,Oct,10; 2018,Jan,8; 2017,Dec,8; 2017,Jan,8; 2016,Jan,13; 2015,Jan,16

00472 **thoracoplasty (any type)**
0.00 0.00 FUD XXX N
AMA: 2019,Oct,10; 2018,Jan,8; 2017,Dec,8; 2017,Jan,8; 2016,Jan,13; 2015,Jan,16

00474 **radical procedures (eg, pectus excavatum)**
0.00 0.00 FUD XXX C
AMA: 2019,Oct,10; 2018,Jan,8; 2017,Dec,8; 2017,Jan,8; 2016,Jan,13; 2015,Jan,16

00500 **Anesthesia for all procedures on esophagus**
0.00 0.00 FUD XXX N
AMA: 2019,Oct,10; 2018,Jan,8; 2017,Dec,8; 2017,Jan,8; 2016,Jan,13; 2015,Jan,16

00520 **Anesthesia for closed chest procedures; (including bronchoscopy) not otherwise specified**
0.00 0.00 FUD XXX N
AMA: 2019,Oct,10; 2018,Jan,8; 2017,Dec,8; 2017,Jan,8; 2016,Jan,13; 2015,Jan,16

00522 **needle biopsy of pleura**
0.00 0.00 FUD XXX N
AMA: 2019,Oct,10; 2018,Jan,8; 2017,Dec,8; 2017,Jan,8; 2016,Jan,13; 2015,Jan,16

00524 **pneumocentesis**

0.00 0.00 **FUD** XXX C

AMA: 2019,Oct,10; 2018,Jan,8; 2017,Dec,8; 2017,Jan,8; 2016,Jan,13; 2015,Jan,16

00528 **mediastinoscopy and diagnostic thoracoscopy not utilizing 1 lung ventilation**

EXCLUDES *Tracheobronchial reconstruction (00539)*

0.00 0.00 **FUD** XXX N

AMA: 2019,Oct,10; 2018,Jan,8; 2017,Dec,8; 2017,Jan,8; 2016,Jan,13; 2015,Jan,16

00529 **mediastinoscopy and diagnostic thoracoscopy utilizing 1 lung ventilation**

0.00 0.00 **FUD** XXX N

AMA: 2019,Oct,10; 2018,Jan,8; 2017,Dec,8; 2017,Jan,8; 2016,Jan,13; 2015,Jan,16

00530 Anesthesia for Cardiac Pacemaker Procedure

CMS: 100-03,10.6 Anesthesia in Cardiac Pacemaker Surgery; 100-04,12,140.1 Qualified Nonphysician Anesthetists; 100-04,12,140.3 Payment for Qualified Nonphysician Anesthetists; 100-04,12,140.3.3 Billing Modifiers; 100-04,12,140.3.4 General Billing Instructions; 100-04,12,140.4.1 Anesthesiologist/Qualified Nonphysican Anesthetist; 100-04,12,140.4.2 Anesthetist and Anesthesiologist in a Single Procedure; 100-04,12,140.4.3 Payment for Medical /Surgical Services by CRNAs; 100-04,12,140.4.4 Conversion Factors for Anesthesia Services; 100-04,12,140.5 Payment for Anesthesia Services Furnished by a Teaching CRNA; 100-04,4,250.3.2 Anesthesia in a Hospital Outpatient Setting

00530 **Anesthesia for permanent transvenous pacemaker insertion**

0.00 0.00 **FUD** XXX N

AMA: 2019,Oct,10; 2018,Jan,8; 2017,Dec,8; 2017,Jan,8; 2016,Jan,13; 2015,Jan,16

00532-00550 Anesthesia for Heart and Lung Procedures

CMS: 100-04,12,140.1 Qualified Nonphysician Anesthetists; 100-04,12,140.3 Payment for Qualified Nonphysician Anesthetists; 100-04,12,140.3.3 Billing Modifiers; 100-04,12,140.3.4 General Billing Instructions; 100-04,12,140.4.1 Anesthesiologist/Qualified Nonphysican Anesthetist; 100-04,12,140.4.2 Anesthetist and Anesthesiologist in a Single Procedure; 100-04,12,140.4.3 Payment for Medical /Surgical Services by CRNAs; 100-04,12,140.4.4 Conversion Factors for Anesthesia Services; 100-04,12,140.5 Payment for Anesthesia Services Furnished by a Teaching CRNA; 100-04,4,250.3.2 Anesthesia in a Hospital Outpatient Setting

00532 **Anesthesia for access to central venous circulation**

0.00 0.00 **FUD** XXX N

AMA: 2019,Oct,10; 2018,Jan,8; 2017,Dec,8; 2017,Jan,8; 2016,Jan,13; 2015,Jan,16

00534 **Anesthesia for transvenous insertion or replacement of pacing cardioverter-defibrillator**

EXCLUDES *Transthoracic approach (00560)*

0.00 0.00 **FUD** XXX N

AMA: 2019,Oct,10; 2018,Jan,8; 2017,Dec,8; 2017,Jan,8; 2016,Jan,13; 2015,Jan,16

00537 **Anesthesia for cardiac electrophysiologic procedures including radiofrequency ablation**

0.00 0.00 **FUD** XXX N

AMA: 2019,Oct,10; 2018,Jan,8; 2017,Dec,8; 2017,Jan,8; 2016,Jan,13; 2015,Jan,16

00539 **Anesthesia for tracheobronchial reconstruction**

0.00 0.00 **FUD** XXX N

AMA: 2019,Oct,10; 2018,Jan,8; 2017,Dec,8; 2017,Jan,8; 2016,Jan,13; 2015,Jan,16

00540 **Anesthesia for thoracotomy procedures involving lungs, pleura, diaphragm, and mediastinum (including surgical thoracoscopy); not otherwise specified**

EXCLUDES *Thoracic spine and spinal cord procedures via anterior transthoracic approach (00625-00626)*

0.00 0.00 **FUD** XXX C

AMA: 2019,Oct,10; 2018,Jan,8; 2017,Dec,8; 2017,Jan,8; 2016,Jan,13; 2015,Jan,16

00541 **utilizing 1 lung ventilation**

EXCLUDES *Thoracic spine and spinal cord procedures via anterior transthoracic approach (00625-00626)*

0.00 0.00 **FUD** XXX N

AMA: 2019,Oct,10; 2018,Jan,8; 2017,Dec,8; 2017,Jan,8; 2016,Jan,13; 2015,Jan,16

00542 **decortication**

0.00 0.00 **FUD** XXX C

AMA: 2019,Oct,10; 2018,Jan,8; 2017,Dec,8; 2017,Jan,8; 2016,Jan,13; 2015,Jan,16

00546 **pulmonary resection with thoracoplasty**

0.00 0.00 **FUD** XXX C

AMA: 2019,Oct,10; 2018,Jan,8; 2017,Dec,8; 2017,Jan,8; 2016,Jan,13; 2015,Jan,16

00548 **intrathoracic procedures on the trachea and bronchi**

0.00 0.00 **FUD** XXX N

AMA: 2019,Oct,10; 2018,Jan,8; 2017,Dec,8; 2017,Jan,8; 2016,Jan,13; 2015,Jan,16

00550 **Anesthesia for sternal debridement**

0.00 0.00 **FUD** XXX N

AMA: 2019,Oct,10; 2018,Jan,8; 2017,Dec,8; 2017,Jan,8; 2016,Jan,13; 2015,Jan,16

00560-00580 Anesthesia for Open Heart Procedures

CMS: 100-04,12,140.1 Qualified Nonphysician Anesthetists; 100-04,12,140.3 Payment for Qualified Nonphysician Anesthetists; 100-04,12,140.3.3 Billing Modifiers; 100-04,12,140.3.4 General Billing Instructions; 100-04,12,140.4.1 Anesthesiologist/Qualified Nonphysican Anesthetist; 100-04,12,140.4.2 Anesthetist and Anesthesiologist in a Single Procedure; 100-04,12,140.4.3 Payment for Medical /Surgical Services by CRNAs; 100-04,12,140.4.4 Conversion Factors for Anesthesia Services; 100-04,12,140.5 Payment for Anesthesia Services Furnished by a Teaching CRNA; 100-04,4,250.3.2 Anesthesia in a Hospital Outpatient Setting

00560 **Anesthesia for procedures on heart, pericardial sac, and great vessels of chest; without pump oxygenator**

0.00 0.00 **FUD** XXX C

AMA: 2019,Oct,10; 2018,Jan,8; 2017,Dec,8; 2017,Jan,8; 2016,Jan,13; 2015,Jan,16

00561 **with pump oxygenator, younger than 1 year of age** A

INCLUDES Anesthesia complicated by utilization of controlled hypotension (99135)

Anesthesia complicated by utilization of total body hypothermia (99116)

Anesthesia for patient of extreme age, younger than 1 year and older than 70 (99100)

0.00 0.00 **FUD** XXX C

AMA: 2019,Oct,10; 2018,Jan,8; 2017,Dec,8; 2017,Jan,8; 2016,Jan,13; 2015,Jan,16

00562 **with pump oxygenator, age 1 year or older, for all noncoronary bypass procedures (eg, valve procedures) or for re-operation for coronary bypass more than 1 month after original operation** A

0.00 0.00 **FUD** XXX C

AMA: 2019,Oct,10; 2018,Jan,8; 2017,Dec,8; 2017,Jan,8; 2016,Jan,13; 2015,Jan,16

00563 **with pump oxygenator with hypothermic circulatory arrest**

0.00 0.00 **FUD** XXX N

AMA: 2019,Oct,10; 2018,Jan,8; 2017,Dec,8; 2017,Jan,8; 2016,Jan,13; 2015,Jan,16

00566 **Anesthesia for direct coronary artery bypass grafting; without pump oxygenator**

0.00 0.00 **FUD** XXX N

AMA: 2019,Oct,10; 2018,Jan,8; 2017,Dec,8; 2017,Jan,8; 2016,Jan,13; 2015,Jan,16

00567 **with pump oxygenator**

0.00 0.00 **FUD** XXX C

AMA: 2019,Oct,10; 2018,Jan,8; 2017,Dec,8; 2017,Jan,8; 2016,Jan,13; 2015,Jan,16

00580 **Anesthesia for heart transplant or heart/lung transplant**

0.00 0.00 **FUD** XXX C

AMA: 2019,Oct,10; 2018,Jan,8; 2017,Dec,8; 2017,Jan,8; 2016,Jan,13; 2015,Jan,16

00600-00670 Anesthesia for Spinal Procedures

CMS: 100-04,12,140.1 Qualified Nonphysician Anesthetists; 100-04,12,140.3 Payment for Qualified Nonphysician Anesthetists; 100-04,12,140.3.3 Billing Modifiers; 100-04,12,140.3.4 General Billing Instructions; 100-04,12,140.4.1 Anesthesiologist/Qualified Nonphysican Anesthetist; 100-04,12,140.4.2 Anesthetist and Anesthesiologist in a Single Procedure; 100-04,12,140.4.3 Payment for Medical /Surgical Services by CRNAs; 100-04,12,140.4.4 Conversion Factors for Anesthesia Services; 100-04,12,140.5 Payment for Anesthesia Services Furnished by a Teaching CRNA; 100-04,4,250.3.2 Anesthesia in a Hospital Outpatient Setting

00600 **Anesthesia for procedures on cervical spine and cord; not otherwise specified**

EXCLUDES *Percutaneous image-guided spine and spinal cord anesthesia services (01935-01936)*

0.00 0.00 **FUD** XXX N

AMA: 2019,Oct,10; 2018,Jan,8; 2017,Dec,8; 2017,Jan,8; 2016,Jan,13; 2015,Jan,16

00604 **procedures with patient in the sitting position**

0.00 0.00 **FUD** XXX C

AMA: 2019,Oct,10; 2018,Jan,8; 2017,Dec,8; 2017,Jan,8; 2016,Jan,13; 2015,Jan,16

00620 **Anesthesia for procedures on thoracic spine and cord, not otherwise specified**

0.00 0.00 **FUD** XXX N

AMA: 2019,Oct,10; 2018,Jan,8; 2017,Dec,8; 2017,Jan,8; 2016,Jan,13; 2015,Jan,16

00625 **Anesthesia for procedures on the thoracic spine and cord, via an anterior transthoracic approach; not utilizing 1 lung ventilation**

EXCLUDES *Anesthesia services for thoracotomy procedures other than spine (00540-00541)*

0.00 0.00 **FUD** XXX N

AMA: 2019,Oct,10; 2018,Jan,8; 2017,Dec,8; 2017,Jan,8; 2016,Jan,13; 2015,Jan,16

00626 **utilizing 1 lung ventilation**

EXCLUDES *Anesthesia services for thoracotomy procedures other than spine (00540-00541)*

0.00 0.00 **FUD** XXX N

AMA: 2019,Oct,10; 2018,Jan,8; 2017,Dec,8; 2017,Jan,8; 2016,Jan,13; 2015,Jan,16

00630 **Anesthesia for procedures in lumbar region; not otherwise specified**

0.00 0.00 **FUD** XXX N

AMA: 2019,Oct,10; 2018,Jan,8; 2017,Dec,8; 2017,Jan,8; 2016,Jan,13; 2015,Jan,16

00632 **lumbar sympathectomy**

0.00 0.00 **FUD** XXX C

AMA: 2019,Oct,10; 2018,Jan,8; 2017,Dec,8; 2017,Jan,8; 2016,Jan,13; 2015,Jan,16

00635 **diagnostic or therapeutic lumbar puncture**

0.00 0.00 **FUD** XXX N

AMA: 2019,Oct,10; 2018,Jan,8; 2017,Dec,8; 2017,Jan,8; 2016,Jan,13; 2015,Jan,16

00640 **Anesthesia for manipulation of the spine or for closed procedures on the cervical, thoracic or lumbar spine**

0.00 0.00 **FUD** XXX N

AMA: 2019,Oct,10; 2018,Jan,8; 2017,Dec,8; 2017,Jan,8; 2016,Jan,13; 2015,Jan,16

00670 **Anesthesia for extensive spine and spinal cord procedures (eg, spinal instrumentation or vascular procedures)**

0.00 0.00 **FUD** XXX C

AMA: 2019,Oct,10; 2018,Jan,8; 2017,Dec,8; 2017,Jan,8; 2016,Jan,13; 2015,Jan,16

00700-00882 Anesthesia for Abdominal Procedures

CMS: 100-04,12,140.1 Qualified Nonphysician Anesthetists; 100-04,12,140.3 Payment for Qualified Nonphysician Anesthetists; 100-04,12,140.3.3 Billing Modifiers; 100-04,12,140.3.4 General Billing Instructions; 100-04,12,140.4.1 Anesthesiologist/Qualified Nonphysican Anesthetist; 100-04,12,140.4.2 Anesthetist and Anesthesiologist in a Single Procedure; 100-04,12,140.4.3 Payment for Medical /Surgical Services by CRNAs; 100-04,12,140.4.4 Conversion Factors for Anesthesia Services; 100-04,12,140.5 Payment for Anesthesia Services Furnished by a Teaching CRNA; 100-04,4,250.3.2 Anesthesia in a Hospital Outpatient Setting

00700 **Anesthesia for procedures on upper anterior abdominal wall; not otherwise specified**

0.00 0.00 **FUD** XXX N

AMA: 2019,Oct,10; 2018,Jan,8; 2017,Dec,8; 2017,Jan,8; 2016,Jan,13; 2015,Jan,16

00702 **percutaneous liver biopsy**

0.00 0.00 **FUD** XXX N

AMA: 2019,Oct,10; 2018,Jan,8; 2017,Dec,8; 2017,Jan,8; 2016,Jan,13; 2015,Jan,16

00730 **Anesthesia for procedures on upper posterior abdominal wall**

0.00 0.00 **FUD** XXX N

AMA: 2019,Oct,10; 2018,Jan,8; 2017,Dec,8; 2017,Jan,8; 2016,Jan,13; 2015,Jan,16

00731 **Anesthesia for upper gastrointestinal endoscopic procedures, endoscope introduced proximal to duodenum; not otherwise specified**

EXCLUDES *Combination of upper and lower endoscopic gastrointestinal procedures (00813)*

0.00 0.00 **FUD** XXX N

AMA: 2019,Oct,10; 2018,Jan,8; 2017,Dec,8

00732 **endoscopic retrograde cholangiopancreatography (ERCP)**

EXCLUDES *Combination of upper and lower endoscopic gastrointestinal procedures (00813)*

0.00 0.00 **FUD** XXX N

AMA: 2019,Oct,10; 2018,Jan,8; 2017,Dec,8

00750 **Anesthesia for hernia repairs in upper abdomen; not otherwise specified**

0.00 0.00 **FUD** XXX N

AMA: 2019,Oct,10; 2018,Jan,8; 2017,Dec,8; 2017,Jan,8; 2016,Jan,13; 2015,Jan,16

00752 **lumbar and ventral (incisional) hernias and/or wound dehiscence**

0.00 0.00 **FUD** XXX N

AMA: 2019,Oct,10; 2018,Jan,8; 2017,Dec,8; 2017,Jan,8; 2016,Jan,13; 2015,Jan,16

00754 **omphalocele**

0.00 0.00 **FUD** XXX N

AMA: 2019,Oct,10; 2018,Jan,8; 2017,Dec,8; 2017,Jan,8; 2016,Jan,13; 2015,Jan,16

00756 **transabdominal repair of diaphragmatic hernia**

0.00 0.00 **FUD** XXX N

AMA: 2019,Oct,10; 2018,Jan,8; 2017,Dec,8; 2017,Jan,8; 2016,Jan,13; 2015,Jan,16

00770 **Anesthesia for all procedures on major abdominal blood vessels**

0.00 0.00 **FUD** XXX N

AMA: 2019,Oct,10; 2018,Jan,8; 2017,Dec,8; 2017,Jan,8; 2016,Jan,13; 2015,Jan,16

00790 **Anesthesia for intraperitoneal procedures in upper abdomen including laparoscopy; not otherwise specified**

0.00 0.00 **FUD** XXX N

AMA: 2019,Oct,10; 2018,Jan,8; 2017,Dec,8; 2017,Jan,8; 2016,Jan,13; 2015,Jan,16

00792 **partial hepatectomy or management of liver hemorrhage (excluding liver biopsy)**

0.00 0.00 **FUD** XXX C

AMA: 2019,Oct,10; 2018,Jan,8; 2017,Dec,8; 2017,Jan,8; 2016,Jan,13; 2015,Jan,16

00794 pancreatectomy, partial or total (eg, Whipple procedure)
    🚑 0.00   👤 0.00   **FUD** XXX   C 🖵
    AMA: 2019,Oct,10; 2018,Jan,8; 2017,Dec,8; 2017,Jan,8; 2016,Jan,13; 2015,Jan,16

00796 liver transplant (recipient)
    EXCLUDES *Physiological support during liver harvest (01990)*
    🚑 0.00   👤 0.00   **FUD** XXX   C 🖵
    AMA: 2019,Oct,10; 2018,Jan,8; 2017,Dec,8; 2017,Jan,8; 2016,Jan,13; 2015,Jan,16

00797 gastric restrictive procedure for morbid obesity
    🚑 0.00   👤 0.00   **FUD** XXX   N 🖵
    AMA: 2019,Oct,10; 2018,Jan,8; 2017,Dec,8; 2017,Jan,8; 2016,Jan,13; 2015,Jan,16

00800 Anesthesia for procedures on lower anterior abdominal wall; not otherwise specified
    🚑 0.00   👤 0.00   **FUD** XXX   N 🖵
    AMA: 2019,Oct,10; 2018,Jan,8; 2017,Dec,8; 2017,Jan,8; 2016,Jan,13; 2015,Jan,16

00802 panniculectomy
    🚑 0.00   👤 0.00   **FUD** XXX   C 🖵
    AMA: 2019,Oct,10; 2018,Jan,8; 2017,Dec,8; 2017,Jan,8; 2016,Jan,13; 2015,Jan,16

00811 Anesthesia for lower intestinal endoscopic procedures, endoscope introduced distal to duodenum; not otherwise specified
    🚑 0.00   👤 0.00   **FUD** XXX   N 🖵
    AMA: 2019,Oct,10; 2018,Jan,8; 2017,Dec,8

00812 screening colonoscopy
    INCLUDES Anesthesia services for all screening colonoscopy irrespective of findings
    🚑 0.00   👤 0.00   **FUD** XXX   N 🖵
    AMA: 2019,Oct,10; 2018,Jan,8; 2017,Dec,8

00813 Anesthesia for combined upper and lower gastrointestinal endoscopic procedures, endoscope introduced both proximal to and distal to the duodenum
    🚑 0.00   👤 0.00   **FUD** XXX   N 🖵
    AMA: 2019,Oct,10; 2018,Jan,8; 2017,Dec,8

00820 Anesthesia for procedures on lower posterior abdominal wall
    🚑 0.00   👤 0.00   **FUD** XXX   N 🖵
    AMA: 2019,Oct,10; 2018,Jan,8; 2017,Dec,8; 2017,Jan,8; 2016,Jan,13; 2015,Jan,16

00830 Anesthesia for hernia repairs in lower abdomen; not otherwise specified
    EXCLUDES *Anesthesia for hernia repairs on infants one year old or less (00834, 00836)*
    🚑 0.00   👤 0.00   **FUD** XXX   N 🖵
    AMA: 2019,Oct,10; 2018,Jan,8; 2017,Dec,8; 2017,Jan,8; 2016,Jan,13; 2015,Jan,16

00832 ventral and incisional hernias
    EXCLUDES *Anesthesia for hernia repairs on infants one year old or less (00834, 00836)*
    🚑 0.00   👤 0.00   **FUD** XXX   N 🖵
    AMA: 2019,Oct,10; 2018,Jan,8; 2017,Dec,8; 2017,Jan,8; 2016,Jan,13; 2015,Jan,16

00834 Anesthesia for hernia repairs in the lower abdomen not otherwise specified, younger than 1 year of age   A
    INCLUDES Anesthesia for patient of extreme age, younger than 1 year and older than 70 (99100)
    🚑 0.00   👤 0.00   **FUD** XXX   N 🖵
    AMA: 2019,Oct,10; 2018,Jan,8; 2017,Dec,8; 2017,Jan,8; 2016,Jan,13; 2015,Jan,16

00836 Anesthesia for hernia repairs in the lower abdomen not otherwise specified, infants younger than 37 weeks gestational age at birth and younger than 50 weeks gestational age at time of surgery   A
    INCLUDES Anesthesia for patient of extreme age, younger than 1 year and older than 70 (99100)
    🚑 0.00   👤 0.00   **FUD** XXX   N 🖵
    AMA: 2019,Oct,10; 2018,Jan,8; 2017,Dec,8; 2017,Jan,8; 2016,Jan,13; 2015,Jan,16

00840 Anesthesia for intraperitoneal procedures in lower abdomen including laparoscopy; not otherwise specified
    🚑 0.00   👤 0.00   **FUD** XXX   N 🖵
    AMA: 2019,Oct,10; 2018,Jan,8; 2017,Dec,8; 2017,Jan,8; 2016,Jan,13; 2015,Jan,16

00842 amniocentesis   M ♀
    🚑 0.00   👤 0.00   **FUD** XXX   N 🖵
    AMA: 2019,Oct,10; 2018,Jan,8; 2017,Dec,8; 2017,Jan,8; 2016,Jan,13; 2015,Jan,16

00844 abdominoperineal resection
    🚑 0.00   👤 0.00   **FUD** XXX   C 🖵
    AMA: 2019,Oct,10; 2018,Jan,8; 2017,Dec,8; 2017,Jan,8; 2016,Jan,13; 2015,Jan,16

00846 radical hysterectomy   ♀
    🚑 0.00   👤 0.00   **FUD** XXX   C 🖵
    AMA: 2019,Oct,10; 2018,Jan,8; 2017,Dec,8; 2017,Jan,8; 2016,Jan,13; 2015,Jan,16

00848 pelvic exenteration
    🚑 0.00   👤 0.00   **FUD** XXX   C 🖵
    AMA: 2019,Oct,10; 2018,Jan,8; 2017,Dec,8; 2017,Jan,8; 2016,Jan,13; 2015,Jan,16

00851 tubal ligation/transection   ♀
    🚑 0.00   👤 0.00   **FUD** XXX   N 🖵
    AMA: 2019,Oct,10; 2018,Jan,8; 2017,Dec,8; 2017,Jan,8; 2016,Jan,13; 2015,Jan,16

00860 Anesthesia for extraperitoneal procedures in lower abdomen, including urinary tract; not otherwise specified
    🚑 0.00   👤 0.00   **FUD** XXX   N 🖵
    AMA: 2019,Oct,10; 2018,Jan,8; 2017,Dec,8; 2017,Jan,8; 2016,Jan,13; 2015,Jan,16

00862 renal procedures, including upper one-third of ureter, or donor nephrectomy
    🚑 0.00   👤 0.00   **FUD** XXX   N 🖵
    AMA: 2019,Oct,10; 2018,Jan,8; 2017,Dec,8; 2017,Jan,8; 2016,Jan,13; 2015,Jan,16

00864 total cystectomy
    🚑 0.00   👤 0.00   **FUD** XXX   C 🖵
    AMA: 2019,Oct,10; 2018,Jan,8; 2017,Dec,8; 2017,Jan,8; 2016,Jan,13; 2015,Jan,16

00865 radical prostatectomy (suprapubic, retropubic)   ♂
    🚑 0.00   👤 0.00   **FUD** XXX   C 🖵
    AMA: 2019,Oct,10; 2018,Jan,8; 2017,Dec,8; 2017,Jan,8; 2016,Jan,13; 2015,Jan,16

00866 adrenalectomy
    🚑 0.00   👤 0.00   **FUD** XXX   C 🖵
    AMA: 2019,Oct,10; 2018,Jan,8; 2017,Dec,8; 2017,Jan,8; 2016,Jan,13; 2015,Jan,16

00868 renal transplant (recipient)
    EXCLUDES *Anesthesia for donor nephrectomy (00862)*
    Physiological support during kidney harvest (01990)
    🚑 0.00   👤 0.00   **FUD** XXX   C 🖵
    AMA: 2019,Oct,10; 2018,Jan,8; 2017,Dec,8; 2017,Jan,8; 2016,Jan,13; 2015,Jan,16

00870 cystolithotomy
    🚑 0.00   👤 0.00   **FUD** XXX   N 🖵
    AMA: 2019,Oct,10; 2018,Jan,8; 2017,Dec,8; 2017,Jan,8; 2016,Jan,13; 2015,Jan,16

● New Code   ▲ Revised Code   ○ Reinstated   ● New Web Release   ▲ Revised Web Release   + Add-on   Unlisted   Not Covered   # Resequenced
50 Optum Mod 50 Exempt   ⊘ AMA Mod 51 Exempt   51 Optum Mod 51 Exempt   63 Mod 63 Exempt   ✗ Non-FDA Drug   ★ Telemedicine   M Maternity   A Age Edit

00872 **Anesthesia for lithotripsy, extracorporeal shock wave; with water bath**
0.00 0.00 FUD XXX N
AMA: 2019,Oct,10; 2018,Jan,8; 2017,Dec,8; 2017,Jan,8; 2016,Jan,13; 2015,Jan,16

00873 **without water bath**
0.00 0.00 FUD XXX N
AMA: 2019,Oct,10; 2018,Jan,8; 2017,Dec,8; 2017,Jan,8; 2016,Jan,13; 2015,Jan,16

00880 **Anesthesia for procedures on major lower abdominal vessels; not otherwise specified**
0.00 0.00 FUD XXX N
AMA: 2019,Oct,10; 2018,Jan,8; 2017,Dec,8; 2017,Jan,8; 2016,Jan,13; 2015,Jan,16

00882 **inferior vena cava ligation**
0.00 0.00 FUD XXX C
AMA: 2019,Oct,10; 2018,Jan,8; 2017,Dec,8; 2017,Jan,8; 2016,Jan,13; 2015,Jan,16

00902-00952 Anesthesia for Genitourinary Procedures

CMS: 100-04,12,140.1 Qualified Nonphysician Anesthetists; 100-04,12,140.3 Payment for Qualified Nonphysician Anesthetists; 100-04,12,140.3.3 Billing Modifiers; 100-04,12,140.3.4 General Billing Instructions; 100-04,12,140.4.1 Anesthesiologist/Qualified Nonphysician Anesthetist; 100-04,12,140.4.2 Anesthetist and Anesthesiologist in a Single Procedure; 100-04,12,140.4.3 Payment for Medical /Surgical Services by CRNAs; 100-04,12,140.4.4 Conversion Factors for Anesthesia Services; 100-04,12,140.5 Payment for Anesthesia Services Furnished by a Teaching CRNA; 100-04,4,250.3.2 Anesthesia in a Hospital Outpatient Setting

EXCLUDES *Procedures on perineal skin, muscles, and nerves (00300, 00400)*

00902 **Anesthesia for; anorectal procedure**
0.00 0.00 FUD XXX N
AMA: 2019,Oct,10; 2018,Jan,8; 2017,Dec,8; 2017,Jan,8; 2016,Jan,13; 2015,Jan,16

00904 **radical perineal procedure**
0.00 0.00 FUD XXX C
AMA: 2019,Oct,10; 2018,Jan,8; 2017,Dec,8; 2017,Jan,8; 2016,Jan,13; 2015,Jan,16

00906 **vulvectomy** ♀
0.00 0.00 FUD XXX N
AMA: 2019,Oct,10; 2018,Jan,8; 2017,Dec,8; 2017,Jan,8; 2016,Jan,13; 2015,Jan,16

00908 **perineal prostatectomy** ♂
0.00 0.00 FUD XXX C
AMA: 2019,Oct,10; 2018,Jan,8; 2017,Dec,8; 2017,Jan,8; 2016,Jan,13; 2015,Jan,16

00910 **Anesthesia for transurethral procedures (including urethrocystoscopy); not otherwise specified**
0.00 0.00 FUD XXX N
AMA: 2019,Oct,10; 2018,Jan,8; 2017,Dec,8; 2017,Jan,8; 2016,Jan,13; 2015,Jan,16

00912 **transurethral resection of bladder tumor(s)**
0.00 0.00 FUD XXX N
AMA: 2019,Oct,10; 2018,Jan,8; 2017,Dec,8; 2017,Jan,8; 2016,Jan,13; 2015,Jan,16

00914 **transurethral resection of prostate** ♂
0.00 0.00 FUD XXX N
AMA: 2019,Oct,10; 2018,Jan,8; 2017,Dec,8; 2017,Jan,8; 2016,Jan,13; 2015,Jan,16

00916 **post-transurethral resection bleeding**
0.00 0.00 FUD XXX N
AMA: 2019,Oct,10; 2018,Jan,8; 2017,Dec,8; 2017,Jan,8; 2016,Jan,13; 2015,Jan,16

00918 **with fragmentation, manipulation and/or removal of ureteral calculus**
0.00 0.00 FUD XXX N
AMA: 2019,Oct,10; 2018,Jan,8; 2017,Dec,8; 2017,Jan,8; 2016,Jan,13; 2015,Jan,16

00920 **Anesthesia for procedures on male genitalia (including open urethral procedures); not otherwise specified** ♂
0.00 0.00 FUD XXX N
AMA: 2019,Oct,10; 2018,Jan,8; 2017,Dec,8; 2017,Jan,8; 2016,Jan,13; 2015,Jan,16

00921 **vasectomy, unilateral or bilateral** ♂
0.00 0.00 FUD XXX N
AMA: 2019,Oct,10; 2018,Jan,8; 2017,Dec,8; 2017,Jan,8; 2016,Jan,13; 2015,Jan,16

00922 **seminal vesicles** ♂
0.00 0.00 FUD XXX N
AMA: 2019,Oct,10; 2018,Jan,8; 2017,Dec,8; 2017,Jan,8; 2016,Jan,13; 2015,Jan,16

00924 **undescended testis, unilateral or bilateral** ♂
0.00 0.00 FUD XXX N
AMA: 2019,Oct,10; 2018,Jan,8; 2017,Dec,8; 2017,Jan,8; 2016,Jan,13; 2015,Jan,16

00926 **radical orchiectomy, inguinal** ♂
0.00 0.00 FUD XXX N
AMA: 2019,Oct,10; 2018,Jan,8; 2017,Dec,8; 2017,Jan,8; 2016,Jan,13; 2015,Jan,16

00928 **radical orchiectomy, abdominal** ♂
0.00 0.00 FUD XXX N
AMA: 2019,Oct,10; 2018,Jan,8; 2017,Dec,8; 2017,Jan,8; 2016,Jan,13; 2015,Jan,16

00930 **orchiopexy, unilateral or bilateral** ♂
0.00 0.00 FUD XXX N
AMA: 2019,Oct,10; 2018,Jan,8; 2017,Dec,8; 2017,Jan,8; 2016,Jan,13; 2015,Jan,16

00932 **complete amputation of penis** ♂
0.00 0.00 FUD XXX C
AMA: 2019,Oct,10; 2018,Jan,8; 2017,Dec,8; 2017,Jan,8; 2016,Jan,13; 2015,Jan,16

00934 **radical amputation of penis with bilateral inguinal lymphadenectomy** ♂
0.00 0.00 FUD XXX C
AMA: 2019,Oct,10; 2018,Jan,8; 2017,Dec,8; 2017,Jan,8; 2016,Jan,13; 2015,Jan,16

00936 **radical amputation of penis with bilateral inguinal and iliac lymphadenectomy** ♂
0.00 0.00 FUD XXX C
AMA: 2019,Oct,10; 2018,Jan,8; 2017,Dec,8; 2017,Jan,8; 2016,Jan,13; 2015,Jan,16

00938 **insertion of penile prosthesis (perineal approach)** ♂
0.00 0.00 FUD XXX N
AMA: 2019,Oct,10; 2018,Jan,8; 2017,Dec,8; 2017,Jan,8; 2016,Jan,13; 2015,Jan,16

00940 **Anesthesia for vaginal procedures (including biopsy of labia, vagina, cervix or endometrium); not otherwise specified** ♀
0.00 0.00 FUD XXX N
AMA: 2019,Oct,10; 2018,Jan,8; 2017,Dec,8; 2017,Jan,8; 2016,Jan,13; 2015,Jan,16

00942 **colpotomy, vaginectomy, colporrhaphy, and open urethral procedures** ♀
0.00 0.00 FUD XXX N
AMA: 2019,Oct,10; 2018,Jan,8; 2017,Dec,8; 2017,Jan,8; 2016,Jan,13; 2015,Jan,16

00944 **vaginal hysterectomy** ♀
0.00 0.00 FUD XXX C
AMA: 2019,Oct,10; 2018,Jan,8; 2017,Dec,8; 2017,Jan,8; 2016,Jan,13; 2015,Jan,16

00948 **cervical cerclage** ♀
0.00 0.00 FUD XXX N
AMA: 2019,Oct,10; 2018,Jan,8; 2017,Dec,8; 2017,Jan,8; 2016,Jan,13; 2015,Jan,16

00950 **culdoscopy** ♀
0.00 0.00 **FUD** XXX N
AMA: 2019,Oct,10; 2018,Jan,8; 2017,Dec,8; 2017,Jan,8; 2016,Jan,13; 2015,Jan,16

00952 **hysteroscopy and/or hysterosalpingography** ♀
0.00 0.00 **FUD** XXX N
AMA: 2019,Oct,10; 2018,Jan,8; 2017,Dec,8; 2017,Jan,8; 2016,Jan,13; 2015,Jan,16

01112-01522 Anesthesia for Lower Extremity Procedures

CMS: 100-04,12,140.1 Qualified Nonphysician Anesthetists; 100-04,12,140.3 Payment for Qualified Nonphysician Anesthetists; 100-04,12,140.3.3 Billing Modifiers; 100-04,12,140.3.4 General Billing Instructions; 100-04,12,140.4.1 Anesthesiologist/Qualified Nonphysican Anesthetist; 100-04,12,140.4.2 Anesthetist and Anesthesiologist in a Single Procedure; 100-04,12,140.4.3 Payment for Medical /Surgical Services by CRNAs; 100-04,12,140.4.4 Conversion Factors for Anesthesia Services; 100-04,12,140.5 Payment for Anesthesia Services Furnished by a Teaching CRNA; 100-04,4,250.3.2 Anesthesia in a Hospital Outpatient Setting

01112 **Anesthesia for bone marrow aspiration and/or biopsy, anterior or posterior iliac crest**
0.00 0.00 **FUD** XXX N
AMA: 2019,Oct,10; 2018,Jan,8; 2017,Dec,8; 2017,Jan,8; 2016,Jan,13; 2015,Jan,16

01120 **Anesthesia for procedures on bony pelvis**
0.00 0.00 **FUD** XXX N
AMA: 2019,Oct,10; 2018,Jan,8; 2017,Dec,8; 2017,Jan,8; 2016,Jan,13; 2015,Jan,16

01130 **Anesthesia for body cast application or revision**
0.00 0.00 **FUD** XXX N
AMA: 2019,Oct,10; 2018,Jan,8; 2017,Dec,8; 2017,Jan,8; 2016,Jan,13; 2015,Jan,16

01140 **Anesthesia for interpelviabdominal (hindquarter) amputation**
0.00 0.00 **FUD** XXX C
AMA: 2019,Oct,10; 2018,Jan,8; 2017,Dec,8; 2017,Jan,8; 2016,Jan,13; 2015,Jan,16

01150 **Anesthesia for radical procedures for tumor of pelvis, except hindquarter amputation**
0.00 0.00 **FUD** XXX C
AMA: 2019,Oct,10; 2018,Jan,8; 2017,Dec,8; 2017,Jan,8; 2016,Jan,13; 2015,Jan,16

01160 **Anesthesia for closed procedures involving symphysis pubis or sacroiliac joint**
0.00 0.00 **FUD** XXX N
AMA: 2019,Oct,10; 2018,Jan,8; 2017,Dec,8; 2017,Jan,8; 2016,Jan,13; 2015,Jan,16

01170 **Anesthesia for open procedures involving symphysis pubis or sacroiliac joint**
0.00 0.00 **FUD** XXX N
AMA: 2019,Oct,10; 2018,Jan,8; 2017,Dec,8; 2017,Jan,8; 2016,Jan,13; 2015,Jan,16

01173 **Anesthesia for open repair of fracture disruption of pelvis or column fracture involving acetabulum**
0.00 0.00 **FUD** XXX N
AMA: 2019,Oct,10; 2018,Jan,8; 2017,Dec,8; 2017,Jan,8; 2016,Jan,13; 2015,Jan,16

01200 **Anesthesia for all closed procedures involving hip joint**
0.00 0.00 **FUD** XXX N
AMA: 2019,Oct,10; 2018,Jan,8; 2017,Dec,8; 2017,Jan,8; 2016,Jan,13; 2015,Jan,16

01202 **Anesthesia for arthroscopic procedures of hip joint**
0.00 0.00 **FUD** XXX N
AMA: 2019,Oct,10; 2018,Jan,8; 2017,Dec,8; 2017,Jan,8; 2016,Jan,13; 2015,Jan,16

01210 **Anesthesia for open procedures involving hip joint; not otherwise specified**
0.00 0.00 **FUD** XXX N
AMA: 2019,Oct,10; 2018,Jan,8; 2017,Dec,8; 2017,Jan,8; 2016,Jan,13; 2015,Jan,16

01212 **hip disarticulation**
0.00 0.00 **FUD** XXX C
AMA: 2019,Oct,10; 2018,Jan,8; 2017,Dec,8; 2017,Jan,8; 2016,Jan,13; 2015,Jan,16

01214 **total hip arthroplasty**
0.00 0.00 **FUD** XXX C
AMA: 2019,Oct,10; 2018,Jan,8; 2017,Dec,8; 2017,Jan,8; 2016,Jan,13; 2015,Jan,16

01215 **revision of total hip arthroplasty**
0.00 0.00 **FUD** XXX N
AMA: 2019,Oct,10; 2018,Jan,8; 2017,Dec,8; 2017,Jan,8; 2016,Jan,13; 2015,Jan,16

01220 **Anesthesia for all closed procedures involving upper two-thirds of femur**
0.00 0.00 **FUD** XXX N
AMA: 2019,Oct,10; 2018,Jan,8; 2017,Dec,8; 2017,Jan,8; 2016,Jan,13; 2015,Jan,16

01230 **Anesthesia for open procedures involving upper two-thirds of femur; not otherwise specified**
0.00 0.00 **FUD** XXX N
AMA: 2019,Oct,10; 2018,Jan,8; 2017,Dec,8; 2017,Jan,8; 2016,Jan,13; 2015,Jan,16

01232 **amputation**
0.00 0.00 **FUD** XXX C
AMA: 2019,Oct,10; 2018,Jan,8; 2017,Dec,8; 2017,Jan,8; 2016,Jan,13; 2015,Jan,16

01234 **radical resection**
0.00 0.00 **FUD** XXX C
AMA: 2019,Oct,10; 2018,Jan,8; 2017,Dec,8; 2017,Jan,8; 2016,Jan,13; 2015,Jan,16

01250 **Anesthesia for all procedures on nerves, muscles, tendons, fascia, and bursae of upper leg**
0.00 0.00 **FUD** XXX N
AMA: 2019,Oct,10; 2018,Jan,8; 2017,Dec,8; 2017,Jan,8; 2016,Jan,13; 2015,Jan,16

01260 **Anesthesia for all procedures involving veins of upper leg, including exploration**
0.00 0.00 **FUD** XXX N
AMA: 2019,Oct,10; 2018,Jan,8; 2017,Dec,8; 2017,Jan,8; 2016,Jan,13; 2015,Jan,16

01270 **Anesthesia for procedures involving arteries of upper leg, including bypass graft; not otherwise specified**
0.00 0.00 **FUD** XXX N
AMA: 2019,Oct,10; 2018,Jan,8; 2017,Dec,8; 2017,Jan,8; 2016,Jan,13; 2015,Jan,16

01272 **femoral artery ligation**
0.00 0.00 **FUD** XXX C
AMA: 2019,Oct,10; 2018,Jan,8; 2017,Dec,8; 2017,Jan,8; 2016,Jan,13; 2015,Jan,16

01274 **femoral artery embolectomy**
0.00 0.00 **FUD** XXX C
AMA: 2019,Oct,10; 2018,Jan,8; 2017,Dec,8; 2017,Jan,8; 2016,Jan,13; 2015,Jan,16

01320 **Anesthesia for all procedures on nerves, muscles, tendons, fascia, and bursae of knee and/or popliteal area**
0.00 0.00 **FUD** XXX N
AMA: 2019,Oct,10; 2018,Jan,8; 2017,Dec,8; 2017,Jan,8; 2016,Jan,13; 2015,Jan,16

01340 **Anesthesia for all closed procedures on lower one-third of femur**
0.00 0.00 **FUD** XXX N
AMA: 2019,Oct,10; 2018,Jan,8; 2017,Dec,8; 2017,Jan,8; 2016,Jan,13; 2015,Jan,16

01360 **Anesthesia for all open procedures on lower one-third of femur**
0.00 0.00 **FUD** XXX N
AMA: 2019,Oct,10; 2018,Jan,8; 2017,Dec,8; 2017,Jan,8; 2016,Jan,13; 2015,Jan,16

01380 **Anesthesia for all closed procedures on knee joint**
0.00 0.00 FUD XXX N
AMA: 2019,Oct,10; 2018,Jan,8; 2017,Dec,8; 2017,Jan,8; 2016,Jan,13; 2015,Jan,16

01382 **Anesthesia for diagnostic arthroscopic procedures of knee joint**
0.00 0.00 FUD XXX N
AMA: 2019,Oct,10; 2018,Jan,8; 2017,Dec,8; 2017,Jan,8; 2016,Jan,13; 2015,Jan,16

01390 **Anesthesia for all closed procedures on upper ends of tibia, fibula, and/or patella**
0.00 0.00 FUD XXX N
AMA: 2019,Oct,10; 2018,Jan,8; 2017,Dec,8; 2017,Jan,8; 2016,Jan,13; 2015,Jan,16

01392 **Anesthesia for all open procedures on upper ends of tibia, fibula, and/or patella**
0.00 0.00 FUD XXX N
AMA: 2019,Oct,10; 2018,Jan,8; 2017,Dec,8; 2017,Jan,8; 2016,Jan,13; 2015,Jan,16

01400 **Anesthesia for open or surgical arthroscopic procedures on knee joint; not otherwise specified**
0.00 0.00 FUD XXX N
AMA: 2019,Oct,10; 2018,Jan,8; 2017,Dec,8; 2017,Jan,8; 2016,Jan,13; 2015,Jan,16

01402 **total knee arthroplasty**
0.00 0.00 FUD XXX C
AMA: 2019,Oct,10; 2018,Jan,8; 2017,Dec,8; 2017,Jan,8; 2016,Jan,13; 2015,Jan,16

01404 **disarticulation at knee**
0.00 0.00 FUD XXX C
AMA: 2019,Oct,10; 2018,Jan,8; 2017,Dec,8; 2017,Jan,8; 2016,Jan,13; 2015,Jan,16

01420 **Anesthesia for all cast applications, removal, or repair involving knee joint**
0.00 0.00 FUD XXX N
AMA: 2019,Oct,10; 2018,Jan,8; 2017,Dec,8; 2017,Jan,8; 2016,Jan,13; 2015,Jan,16

01430 **Anesthesia for procedures on veins of knee and popliteal area; not otherwise specified**
0.00 0.00 FUD XXX N
AMA: 2019,Oct,10; 2018,Jan,8; 2017,Dec,8; 2017,Jan,8; 2016,Jan,13; 2015,Jan,16

01432 **arteriovenous fistula**
0.00 0.00 FUD XXX N
AMA: 2019,Oct,10; 2018,Jan,8; 2017,Dec,8; 2017,Jan,8; 2016,Jan,13; 2015,Jan,16

01440 **Anesthesia for procedures on arteries of knee and popliteal area; not otherwise specified**
0.00 0.00 FUD XXX N
AMA: 2019,Oct,10; 2018,Jan,8; 2017,Dec,8; 2017,Jan,8; 2016,Jan,13; 2015,Jan,16

01442 **popliteal thromboendarterectomy, with or without patch graft**
0.00 0.00 FUD XXX C
AMA: 2019,Oct,10; 2018,Jan,8; 2017,Dec,8; 2017,Jan,8; 2016,Jan,13; 2015,Jan,16

01444 **popliteal excision and graft or repair for occlusion or aneurysm**
0.00 0.00 FUD XXX C
AMA: 2019,Oct,10; 2018,Jan,8; 2017,Dec,8; 2017,Jan,8; 2016,Jan,13; 2015,Jan,16

01462 **Anesthesia for all closed procedures on lower leg, ankle, and foot**
0.00 0.00 FUD XXX N
AMA: 2019,Oct,10; 2018,Jan,8; 2017,Dec,8; 2017,Jan,8; 2016,Jan,13; 2015,Jan,16

01464 **Anesthesia for arthroscopic procedures of ankle and/or foot**
0.00 0.00 FUD XXX N
AMA: 2019,Oct,10; 2018,Jan,8; 2017,Dec,8; 2017,Jan,8; 2016,Jan,13; 2015,Jan,16

01470 **Anesthesia for procedures on nerves, muscles, tendons, and fascia of lower leg, ankle, and foot; not otherwise specified**
0.00 0.00 FUD XXX N
AMA: 2019,Oct,10; 2018,Jan,8; 2017,Dec,8; 2017,Jan,8; 2016,Jan,13; 2015,Jan,16

01472 **repair of ruptured Achilles tendon, with or without graft**
0.00 0.00 FUD XXX N
AMA: 2019,Oct,10; 2018,Jan,8; 2017,Dec,8; 2017,Jan,8; 2016,Jan,13; 2015,Jan,16

01474 **gastrocnemius recession (eg, Strayer procedure)**
0.00 0.00 FUD XXX N
AMA: 2019,Oct,10; 2018,Jan,8; 2017,Dec,8; 2017,Jan,8; 2016,Jan,13; 2015,Jan,16

01480 **Anesthesia for open procedures on bones of lower leg, ankle, and foot; not otherwise specified**
0.00 0.00 FUD XXX N
AMA: 2019,Oct,10; 2018,Jan,8; 2017,Dec,8; 2017,Jan,8; 2016,Jan,13; 2015,Jan,16

01482 **radical resection (including below knee amputation)**
0.00 0.00 FUD XXX N
AMA: 2019,Oct,10; 2018,Jan,8; 2017,Dec,8; 2017,Jan,8; 2016,Jan,13; 2015,Jan,16

01484 **osteotomy or osteoplasty of tibia and/or fibula**
0.00 0.00 FUD XXX N
AMA: 2019,Oct,10; 2018,Jan,8; 2017,Dec,8; 2017,Jan,8; 2016,Jan,13; 2015,Jan,16

01486 **total ankle replacement**
0.00 0.00 FUD XXX C
AMA: 2019,Oct,10; 2018,Jan,8; 2017,Dec,8; 2017,Jan,8; 2016,Jan,13; 2015,Jan,16

01490 **Anesthesia for lower leg cast application, removal, or repair**
0.00 0.00 FUD XXX N
AMA: 2019,Oct,10; 2018,Jan,8; 2017,Dec,8; 2017,Jan,8; 2016,Jan,13; 2015,Jan,16

01500 **Anesthesia for procedures on arteries of lower leg, including bypass graft; not otherwise specified**
0.00 0.00 FUD XXX N
AMA: 2019,Oct,10; 2018,Jan,8; 2017,Dec,8; 2017,Jan,8; 2016,Jan,13; 2015,Jan,16

01502 **embolectomy, direct or with catheter**
0.00 0.00 FUD XXX C
AMA: 2019,Oct,10; 2018,Jan,8; 2017,Dec,8; 2017,Jan,8; 2016,Jan,13; 2015,Jan,16

01520 **Anesthesia for procedures on veins of lower leg; not otherwise specified**
0.00 0.00 FUD XXX N
AMA: 2019,Oct,10; 2018,Jan,8; 2017,Dec,8; 2017,Jan,8; 2016,Jan,13; 2015,Jan,16

01522 **venous thrombectomy, direct or with catheter**
0.00 0.00 FUD XXX N
AMA: 2019,Oct,10; 2018,Jan,8; 2017,Dec,8; 2017,Jan,8; 2016,Jan,13; 2015,Jan,16

01610-01680 Anesthesia for Shoulder Procedures

CMS: 100-04,12,140.1 Qualified Nonphysician Anesthetists; 100-04,12,140.3 Payment for Qualified Nonphysician Anesthetists; 100-04,12,140.3.3 Billing Modifiers; 100-04,12,140.3.4 General Billing Instructions; 100-04,12,140.4.1 Anesthesiologist/Qualified Nonphysican Anesthetist; 100-04,12,140.4.2 Anesthetist and Anesthesiologist in a Single Procedure; 100-04,12,140.4.3 Payment for Medical /Surgical Services by CRNAs; 100-04,12,140.4.4 Conversion Factors for Anesthesia Services; 100-04,12,140.5 Payment for Anesthesia Services Furnished by a Teaching CRNA; 100-04,4,250.3.2 Anesthesia in a Hospital Outpatient Setting

INCLUDES Acromioclavicular joint
Humeral head and neck
Shoulder joint
Sternoclavicular joint

01610 **Anesthesia for all procedures on nerves, muscles, tendons, fascia, and bursae of shoulder and axilla**
0.00 0.00 **FUD** XXX N
AMA: 2019,Oct,10; 2018,Jan,8; 2017,Dec,8; 2017,Jan,8; 2016,Jan,13; 2015,Jan,16

01620 **Anesthesia for all closed procedures on humeral head and neck, sternoclavicular joint, acromioclavicular joint, and shoulder joint**
0.00 0.00 **FUD** XXX N
AMA: 2019,Oct,10; 2018,Jan,8; 2017,Dec,8; 2017,Jan,8; 2016,Jan,13; 2015,Jan,16

01622 **Anesthesia for diagnostic arthroscopic procedures of shoulder joint**
0.00 0.00 **FUD** XXX N
AMA: 2019,Oct,10; 2018,Jan,8; 2017,Dec,8; 2017,Jan,8; 2016,Jan,13; 2015,Jan,16

01630 **Anesthesia for open or surgical arthroscopic procedures on humeral head and neck, sternoclavicular joint, acromioclavicular joint, and shoulder joint; not otherwise specified**
0.00 0.00 **FUD** XXX N
AMA: 2019,Oct,10; 2018,Jan,8; 2017,Dec,8; 2017,Jan,8; 2016,Jan,13; 2015,Jan,16

01634 **shoulder disarticulation**
0.00 0.00 **FUD** XXX C
AMA: 2019,Oct,10; 2018,Jan,8; 2017,Dec,8; 2017,Jan,8; 2016,Jan,13; 2015,Jan,16

01636 **interthoracoscapular (forequarter) amputation**
0.00 0.00 **FUD** XXX C
AMA: 2019,Oct,10; 2018,Jan,8; 2017,Dec,8; 2017,Jan,8; 2016,Jan,13; 2015,Jan,16

01638 **total shoulder replacement**
0.00 0.00 **FUD** XXX C
AMA: 2019,Oct,10; 2018,Jan,8; 2017,Dec,8; 2017,Jan,8; 2016,Jan,13; 2015,Jan,16

01650 **Anesthesia for procedures on arteries of shoulder and axilla; not otherwise specified**
0.00 0.00 **FUD** XXX N
AMA: 2019,Oct,10; 2018,Jan,8; 2017,Dec,8; 2017,Jan,8; 2016,Jan,13; 2015,Jan,16

01652 **axillary-brachial aneurysm**
0.00 0.00 **FUD** XXX C
AMA: 2019,Oct,10; 2018,Jan,8; 2017,Dec,8; 2017,Jan,8; 2016,Jan,13; 2015,Jan,16

01654 **bypass graft**
0.00 0.00 **FUD** XXX C
AMA: 2019,Oct,10; 2018,Jan,8; 2017,Dec,8; 2017,Jan,8; 2016,Jan,13; 2015,Jan,16

01656 **axillary-femoral bypass graft**
0.00 0.00 **FUD** XXX C
AMA: 2019,Oct,10; 2018,Jan,8; 2017,Dec,8; 2017,Jan,8; 2016,Jan,13; 2015,Jan,16

01670 **Anesthesia for all procedures on veins of shoulder and axilla**
0.00 0.00 **FUD** XXX N
AMA: 2019,Oct,10; 2018,Jan,8; 2017,Dec,8; 2017,Jan,8; 2016,Jan,13; 2015,Jan,16

01680 **Anesthesia for shoulder cast application, removal or repair, not otherwise specified**
0.00 0.00 **FUD** XXX N
AMA: 2019,Oct,10; 2018,Jan,8; 2017,Dec,8; 2017,Jan,8; 2016,Jan,13; 2015,Jan,16

01710-01860 Anesthesia for Upper Extremity Procedures

CMS: 100-04,12,140.1 Qualified Nonphysician Anesthetists; 100-04,12,140.3 Payment for Qualified Nonphysician Anesthetists; 100-04,12,140.3.3 Billing Modifiers; 100-04,12,140.3.4 General Billing Instructions; 100-04,12,140.4.1 Anesthesiologist/Qualified Nonphysican Anesthetist; 100-04,12,140.4.2 Anesthetist and Anesthesiologist in a Single Procedure; 100-04,12,140.4.3 Payment for Medical /Surgical Services by CRNAs; 100-04,12,140.4.4 Conversion Factors for Anesthesia Services; 100-04,12,140.5 Payment for Anesthesia Services Furnished by a Teaching CRNA; 100-04,4,250.3.2 Anesthesia in a Hospital Outpatient Setting

01710 **Anesthesia for procedures on nerves, muscles, tendons, fascia, and bursae of upper arm and elbow; not otherwise specified**
0.00 0.00 **FUD** XXX N
AMA: 2019,Oct,10; 2018,Jan,8; 2017,Dec,8; 2017,Jan,8; 2016,Jan,13; 2015,Jan,16

01712 **tenotomy, elbow to shoulder, open**
0.00 0.00 **FUD** XXX N
AMA: 2019,Oct,10; 2018,Jan,8; 2017,Dec,8; 2017,Jan,8; 2016,Jan,13; 2015,Jan,16

01714 **tenoplasty, elbow to shoulder**
0.00 0.00 **FUD** XXX N
AMA: 2019,Oct,10; 2018,Jan,8; 2017,Dec,8; 2017,Jan,8; 2016,Jan,13; 2015,Jan,16

01716 **tenodesis, rupture of long tendon of biceps**
0.00 0.00 **FUD** XXX N
AMA: 2019,Oct,10; 2018,Jan,8; 2017,Dec,8; 2017,Jan,8; 2016,Jan,13; 2015,Jan,16

01730 **Anesthesia for all closed procedures on humerus and elbow**
0.00 0.00 **FUD** XXX N
AMA: 2019,Oct,10; 2018,Jan,8; 2017,Dec,8; 2017,Jan,8; 2016,Jan,13; 2015,Jan,16

01732 **Anesthesia for diagnostic arthroscopic procedures of elbow joint**
0.00 0.00 **FUD** XXX N
AMA: 2019,Oct,10; 2018,Jan,8; 2017,Dec,8; 2017,Jan,8; 2016,Jan,13; 2015,Jan,16

01740 **Anesthesia for open or surgical arthroscopic procedures of the elbow; not otherwise specified**
0.00 0.00 **FUD** XXX N
AMA: 2019,Oct,10; 2018,Jan,8; 2017,Dec,8; 2017,Jan,8; 2016,Jan,13; 2015,Jan,16

01742 **osteotomy of humerus**
0.00 0.00 **FUD** XXX N
AMA: 2019,Oct,10; 2018,Jan,8; 2017,Dec,8; 2017,Jan,8; 2016,Jan,13; 2015,Jan,16

01744 **repair of nonunion or malunion of humerus**
0.00 0.00 **FUD** XXX N
AMA: 2019,Oct,10; 2018,Jan,8; 2017,Dec,8; 2017,Jan,8; 2016,Jan,13; 2015,Jan,16

01756 **radical procedures**
0.00 0.00 **FUD** XXX C
AMA: 2019,Oct,10; 2018,Jan,8; 2017,Dec,8; 2017,Jan,8; 2016,Jan,13; 2015,Jan,16

01758 **excision of cyst or tumor of humerus**
0.00 0.00 **FUD** XXX N
AMA: 2019,Oct,10; 2018,Jan,8; 2017,Dec,8; 2017,Jan,8; 2016,Jan,13; 2015,Jan,16

01760 **total elbow replacement**
0.00 0.00 **FUD** XXX N
AMA: 2019,Oct,10; 2018,Jan,8; 2017,Dec,8; 2017,Jan,8; 2016,Jan,13; 2015,Jan,16

01770 **Anesthesia for procedures on arteries of upper arm and elbow; not otherwise specified**
0.00 0.00 FUD XXX N
AMA: 2019,Oct,10; 2018,Jan,8; 2017,Dec,8; 2017,Jan,8; 2016,Jan,13; 2015,Jan,16

01772 **embolectomy**
0.00 0.00 FUD XXX N
AMA: 2019,Oct,10; 2018,Jan,8; 2017,Dec,8; 2017,Jan,8; 2016,Jan,13; 2015,Jan,16

01780 **Anesthesia for procedures on veins of upper arm and elbow; not otherwise specified**
0.00 0.00 FUD XXX N
AMA: 2019,Oct,10; 2018,Jan,8; 2017,Dec,8; 2017,Jan,8; 2016,Jan,13; 2015,Jan,16

01782 **phleborrhaphy**
0.00 0.00 FUD XXX N
AMA: 2019,Oct,10; 2018,Jan,8; 2017,Dec,8; 2017,Jan,8; 2016,Jan,13; 2015,Jan,16

01810 **Anesthesia for all procedures on nerves, muscles, tendons, fascia, and bursae of forearm, wrist, and hand**
0.00 0.00 FUD XXX N
AMA: 2019,Oct,10; 2018,Jan,8; 2017,Dec,8; 2017,Jan,8; 2016,Jan,13; 2015,Jan,16

01820 **Anesthesia for all closed procedures on radius, ulna, wrist, or hand bones**
0.00 0.00 FUD XXX N
AMA: 2019,Oct,10; 2018,Jan,8; 2017,Dec,8; 2017,Jan,8; 2016,Jan,13; 2015,Jan,16

01829 **Anesthesia for diagnostic arthroscopic procedures on the wrist**
0.00 0.00 FUD XXX N
AMA: 2019,Oct,10; 2018,Jan,8; 2017,Dec,8; 2017,Jan,8; 2016,Jan,13; 2015,Jan,16

01830 **Anesthesia for open or surgical arthroscopic/endoscopic procedures on distal radius, distal ulna, wrist, or hand joints; not otherwise specified**
0.00 0.00 FUD XXX N
AMA: 2019,Oct,10; 2018,Jan,8; 2017,Dec,8; 2017,Jan,8; 2016,Jan,13; 2015,Jan,16

01832 **total wrist replacement**
0.00 0.00 FUD XXX N
AMA: 2019,Oct,10; 2018,Jan,8; 2017,Dec,8; 2017,Jan,8; 2016,Jan,13; 2015,Jan,16

01840 **Anesthesia for procedures on arteries of forearm, wrist, and hand; not otherwise specified**
0.00 0.00 FUD XXX N
AMA: 2019,Oct,10; 2018,Jan,8; 2017,Dec,8; 2017,Jan,8; 2016,Jan,13; 2015,Jan,16

01842 **embolectomy**
0.00 0.00 FUD XXX N
AMA: 2019,Oct,10; 2018,Jan,8; 2017,Dec,8; 2017,Jan,8; 2016,Jan,13; 2015,Jan,16

01844 **Anesthesia for vascular shunt, or shunt revision, any type (eg, dialysis)**
0.00 0.00 FUD XXX N
AMA: 2019,Oct,10; 2018,Jan,8; 2017,Dec,8; 2017,Jan,8; 2016,Jan,13; 2015,Jan,16

01850 **Anesthesia for procedures on veins of forearm, wrist, and hand; not otherwise specified**
0.00 0.00 FUD XXX N
AMA: 2019,Oct,10; 2018,Jan,8; 2017,Dec,8; 2017,Jan,8; 2016,Jan,13; 2015,Jan,16

01852 **phleborrhaphy**
0.00 0.00 FUD XXX N
AMA: 2019,Oct,10; 2018,Jan,8; 2017,Dec,8; 2017,Jan,8; 2016,Jan,13; 2015,Jan,16

01860 **Anesthesia for forearm, wrist, or hand cast application, removal, or repair**
0.00 0.00 FUD XXX N
AMA: 2019,Oct,10; 2018,Jan,8; 2017,Dec,8; 2017,Jan,8; 2016,Jan,13; 2015,Jan,16

01916-01936 Anesthesia for Interventional Radiology Procedures

CMS: 100-04,12,140.1 Qualified Nonphysician Anesthetists; 100-04,12,140.3 Payment for Qualified Nonphysician Anesthetists; 100-04,12,140.3.3 Billing Modifiers; 100-04,12,140.3.4 General Billing Instructions; 100-04,12,140.4.1 Anesthesiologist/Qualified Nonphysican Anesthetist; 100-04,12,140.4.2 Anesthetist and Anesthesiologist in a Single Procedure; 100-04,12,140.4.3 Payment for Medical /Surgical Services by CRNAs; 100-04,12,140.4.4 Conversion Factors for Anesthesia Services; 100-04,12,140.5 Payment for Anesthesia Services Furnished by a Teaching CRNA; 100-04,4,250.3.2 Anesthesia in a Hospital Outpatient Setting

01916 **Anesthesia for diagnostic arteriography/venography**
EXCLUDES *Anesthesia for therapeutic interventional radiological procedures involving the arterial system (01924-01926)*
Anesthesia for therapeutic interventional radiological procedures involving the venous/lymphatic system (01930-01933)
0.00 0.00 FUD XXX N
AMA: 2019,Oct,10; 2018,Jan,8; 2017,Dec,8; 2017,Jan,8; 2016,Jan,13; 2015,Jan,16

01920 **Anesthesia for cardiac catheterization including coronary angiography and ventriculography (not to include Swan-Ganz catheter)**
0.00 0.00 FUD XXX N
AMA: 2019,Oct,10; 2018,Jan,8; 2017,Dec,8; 2017,Jan,8; 2016,Jan,13; 2015,Jan,16

01922 **Anesthesia for non-invasive imaging or radiation therapy**
0.00 0.00 FUD XXX N
AMA: 2019,Oct,10; 2018,Jan,8; 2017,Dec,8; 2017,Jan,8; 2016,Jan,13; 2015,Jan,16

01924 **Anesthesia for therapeutic interventional radiological procedures involving the arterial system; not otherwise specified**
0.00 0.00 FUD XXX N
AMA: 2019,Oct,10; 2018,Jan,8; 2017,Dec,8; 2017,Jan,8; 2016,Jan,13; 2015,Jan,16

01925 **carotid or coronary**
0.00 0.00 FUD XXX N
AMA: 2019,Oct,10; 2018,Jan,8; 2017,Dec,8; 2017,Jan,8; 2016,Jan,13; 2015,Jan,16

01926 **intracranial, intracardiac, or aortic**
0.00 0.00 FUD XXX N
AMA: 2019,Oct,10; 2018,Jan,8; 2017,Dec,8; 2017,Jan,8; 2016,Jan,13; 2015,Jan,16

01930 **Anesthesia for therapeutic interventional radiological procedures involving the venous/lymphatic system (not to include access to the central circulation); not otherwise specified**
0.00 0.00 FUD XXX N
AMA: 2019,Oct,10; 2018,Jan,8; 2017,Dec,8; 2017,Jan,8; 2016,Jan,13; 2015,Jan,16

01931 **intrahepatic or portal circulation (eg, transvenous intrahepatic portosystemic shunt[s] [TIPS])**
0.00 0.00 FUD XXX N
AMA: 2019,Oct,10; 2018,Jan,8; 2017,Dec,8; 2017,Jan,8; 2016,Jan,13; 2015,Jan,16

01932 **intrathoracic or jugular**
0.00 0.00 FUD XXX N
AMA: 2019,Oct,10; 2018,Jan,8; 2017,Dec,8; 2017,Jan,8; 2016,Jan,13; 2015,Jan,16

01933 **intracranial**
0.00 0.00 FUD XXX N
AMA: 2019,Oct,10; 2018,Jan,8; 2017,Dec,8; 2017,Jan,8; 2016,Jan,13; 2015,Jan,16

01935 **Anesthesia for percutaneous image guided procedures on the spine and spinal cord; diagnostic**
0.00 0.00 FUD XXX N
AMA: 2019,Oct,10; 2018,Jan,8; 2017,Dec,8; 2017,Jan,8; 2016,Jan,13; 2015,Jan,16

01936 **therapeutic**
0.00 0.00 FUD XXX N
AMA: 2019,Oct,10; 2018,Jan,8; 2017,Dec,8; 2017,Jan,8; 2016,Jan,13; 2015,Jan,16

01951-01953 Anesthesia for Burn Procedures

CMS: 100-04,12,140.1 Qualified Nonphysician Anesthetists; 100-04,12,140.3 Payment for Qualified Nonphysician Anesthetists; 100-04,12,140.3.3 Billing Modifiers; 100-04,12,140.3.4 General Billing Instructions; 100-04,12,140.4.1 Anesthesiologist/Qualified Nonphysican Anesthetist; 100-04,12,140.4.2 Anesthetist and Anesthesiologist in a Single Procedure; 100-04,12,140.4.3 Payment for Medical /Surgical Services by CRNAs; 100-04,12,140.4.4 Conversion Factors for Anesthesia Services; 100-04,12,140.5 Payment for Anesthesia Services Furnished by a Teaching CRNA; 100-04,4,250.3.2 Anesthesia in a Hospital Outpatient Setting

01951 **Anesthesia for second- and third-degree burn excision or debridement with or without skin grafting, any site, for total body surface area (TBSA) treated during anesthesia and surgery; less than 4% total body surface area**
0.00 0.00 FUD XXX N
AMA: 2019,Oct,10; 2018,Jan,8; 2017,Dec,8; 2017,Jan,8; 2016,Jan,13; 2015,Jan,16

01952 **between 4% and 9% of total body surface area**
0.00 0.00 FUD XXX N
AMA: 2019,Oct,10; 2018,Jan,8; 2017,Dec,8; 2017,Jan,8; 2016,Jan,13; 2015,Jan,16

+ 01953 **each additional 9% total body surface area or part thereof (List separately in addition to code for primary procedure)**
Code first (01952)
0.00 0.00 FUD XXX N
AMA: 2019,Oct,10; 2018,Jan,8; 2017,Dec,8; 2017,Jan,8; 2016,Jan,13; 2015,Jan,16

01958-01969 Anesthesia for Obstetric Procedures

CMS: 100-04,12,140.1 Qualified Nonphysician Anesthetists; 100-04,12,140.3 Payment for Qualified Nonphysician Anesthetists; 100-04,12,140.3.3 Billing Modifiers; 100-04,12,140.3.4 General Billing Instructions; 100-04,12,140.4.1 Anesthesiologist/Qualified Nonphysican Anesthetist; 100-04,12,140.4.2 Anesthetist and Anesthesiologist in a Single Procedure; 100-04,12,140.4.3 Payment for Medical /Surgical Services by CRNAs; 100-04,12,140.4.4 Conversion Factors for Anesthesia Services; 100-04,12,140.5 Payment for Anesthesia Services Furnished by a Teaching CRNA; 100-04,4,250.3.2 Anesthesia in a Hospital Outpatient Setting

01958 **Anesthesia for external cephalic version procedure** M
0.00 0.00 FUD XXX N
AMA: 2019,Oct,10; 2018,Jan,8; 2017,Dec,8; 2017,Jan,8; 2016,Jan,13; 2015,Jan,16

01960 **Anesthesia for vaginal delivery only** M ♀
0.00 0.00 FUD XXX N
AMA: 2019,Oct,10; 2018,Jan,8; 2017,Dec,8; 2017,Jan,8; 2016,Jan,13; 2015,Jan,16

01961 **Anesthesia for cesarean delivery only** M ♀
0.00 0.00 FUD XXX N
AMA: 2019,Oct,10; 2018,Jan,8; 2017,Dec,8; 2017,Jan,8; 2016,Jan,13; 2015,Jan,16

01962 **Anesthesia for urgent hysterectomy following delivery** M ♀
0.00 0.00 FUD XXX N
AMA: 2019,Oct,10; 2018,Jan,8; 2017,Dec,8; 2017,Jan,8; 2016,Jan,13; 2015,Jan,16

01963 **Anesthesia for cesarean hysterectomy without any labor analgesia/anesthesia care** M ♀
0.00 0.00 FUD XXX N
AMA: 2019,Oct,10; 2018,Jan,8; 2017,Dec,8; 2017,Jan,8; 2016,Jan,13; 2015,Jan,16

01965 **Anesthesia for incomplete or missed abortion procedures** M ♀
0.00 0.00 FUD XXX N
AMA: 2019,Oct,10; 2018,Jan,8; 2017,Dec,8; 2017,Jan,8; 2016,Jan,13; 2015,Jan,16

01966 **Anesthesia for induced abortion procedures** M ♀
0.00 0.00 FUD XXX N
AMA: 2019,Oct,10; 2018,Jan,8; 2017,Dec,8; 2017,Jan,8; 2016,Jan,13; 2015,Jan,16

01967 **Neuraxial labor analgesia/anesthesia for planned vaginal delivery (this includes any repeat subarachnoid needle placement and drug injection and/or any necessary replacement of an epidural catheter during labor)** M ♀
0.00 0.00 FUD XXX N
AMA: 2019,Oct,10; 2018,Jan,8; 2017,Dec,8; 2017,Jan,8; 2016,Jan,13; 2015,Jan,16

+ 01968 **Anesthesia for cesarean delivery following neuraxial labor analgesia/anesthesia (List separately in addition to code for primary procedure performed)** M ♀
Code first (01967)
0.00 0.00 FUD XXX N
AMA: 2019,Oct,10; 2018,Jan,8; 2017,Dec,8; 2017,Jan,8; 2016,Jan,13; 2015,Jan,16

+ 01969 **Anesthesia for cesarean hysterectomy following neuraxial labor analgesia/anesthesia (List separately in addition to code for primary procedure performed)** M ♀
Code first (01967)
0.00 0.00 FUD XXX N
AMA: 2019,Oct,10; 2018,Jan,8; 2017,Dec,8; 2017,Jan,8; 2016,Jan,13; 2015,Jan,16

01990-01999 Anesthesia Miscellaneous

CMS: 100-04,12,140.1 Qualified Nonphysician Anesthetists; 100-04,12,140.3 Payment for Qualified Nonphysician Anesthetists; 100-04,12,140.3.3 Billing Modifiers; 100-04,12,140.3.4 General Billing Instructions; 100-04,12,140.4.1 Anesthesiologist/Qualified Nonphysican Anesthetist; 100-04,12,140.4.2 Anesthetist and Anesthesiologist in a Single Procedure; 100-04,12,140.4.3 Payment for Medical /Surgical Services by CRNAs; 100-04,12,140.4.4 Conversion Factors for Anesthesia Services; 100-04,12,140.5 Payment for Anesthesia Services Furnished by a Teaching CRNA; 100-04,4,250.3.2 Anesthesia in a Hospital Outpatient Setting

01990 **Physiological support for harvesting of organ(s) from brain-dead patient**
0.00 0.00 FUD XXX C
AMA: 2019,Oct,10; 2018,Jan,8; 2017,Dec,8; 2017,Jan,8; 2016,Jan,13; 2015,Jan,16

01991 **Anesthesia for diagnostic or therapeutic nerve blocks and injections (when block or injection is performed by a different physician or other qualified health care professional); other than the prone position**
EXCLUDES *Bier block for pain management (64999)*
Moderate Sedation (99151-99153, 99155-99157)
Pain management via intra-arterial or IV therapy (96373-96374)
Regional or local anesthesia of arms or legs for surgical procedure
0.00 0.00 FUD XXX N
AMA: 2019,Oct,10; 2018,Jan,8; 2017,Dec,8; 2017,Jan,8; 2016,Jan,13; 2015,Jan,16

01992 **prone position**
EXCLUDES *Bier block for pain management (64999)*
Moderate sedation (99151-99153, 99155-99157)
Pain management via intra-arterial or IV therapy (96373-96374)
Regional or local anesthesia of arms or legs for surgical procedure
0.00 0.00 FUD XXX N
AMA: 2019,Oct,10; 2018,Jan,8; 2017,Dec,8; 2017,Jan,8; 2016,Jan,13; 2015,Jan,16

01996 Daily hospital management of epidural or subarachnoid continuous drug administration

INCLUDES Continuous epidural or subarachnoid drug services performed after insertion of an epidural or subarachnoid catheter

0.00 0.00 FUD XXX N

AMA: 2019,Oct,10; 2018,Jan,8; 2017,Dec,8; 2017,Sep,6; 2017,Jan,8; 2016,Jan,13; 2015,May,10; 2015,Jan,16

01999 Unlisted anesthesia procedure(s)

0.00 0.00 FUD XXX N

AMA: 2019,Oct,10; 2018,Jan,8; 2017,Dec,8; 2017,Jan,8; 2016,Jan,13; 2015,May,10; 2015,Jan,16

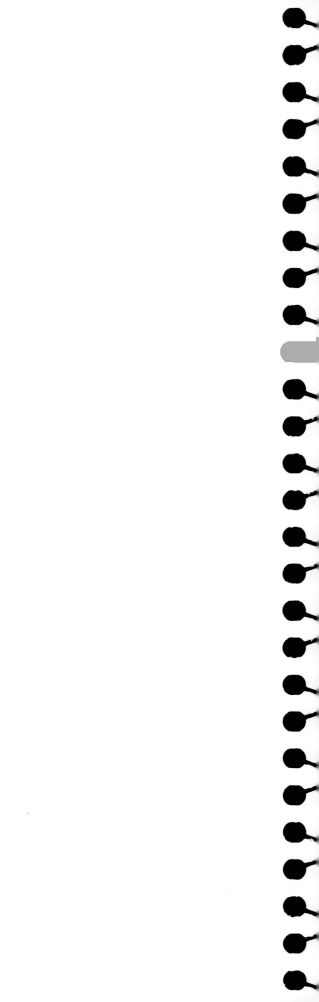

10004-10012 [10004, 10005, 10006, 10007, 10008, 10009, 10010, 10011, 10012] Fine Needle Aspiration

EXCLUDES *Core needle biopsy, lung or mediastinum (32408)*
Percutaneous localization clip placement during breast biopsy (19081-19086)
Percutaneous needle biopsy:
Abdominal or retroperitoneal mass (49180)
Epididymis (54800)
Kidney (50200)
Liver (47000-47001)
Lymph node (38505)
Muscle (20206)
Nucleus pulposus, paravertebral tissue, intervertebral disc (62267)
Pancreas (48102)
Pleura (32400)
Prostate (55700, 55706)
Salivary gland (42400)
Spinal cord (62269)
Testis (54500)
Thyroid (60100)
Soft tissue percutaneous fluid drainage by catheter using image guidance (10030)
Thyroid cyst (60300)

Code also multiple biopsies on same service date:
FNA biopsies using same imaging guidance: report imaging add-on code for second and successive procedures
FNA biopsies separate lesions, different imaging guidance: append modifier 59 to codes for additional imaging modality used
FNA and core needle biopsy same lesion, same imaging guidance, procedure includes imaging guidance for core needle procedure
FNA and core needle biopsies separate lesions, same or different imaging guidance, append modifier 59 to code for core needle biopsy and imaging guidance

10004 **Resequenced code. See code following 10021.**
10005 **Resequenced code. See code following 10021.**
10006 **Resequenced code. See code following 10021.**
10007 **Resequenced code. See code following 10021.**
10008 **Resequenced code. See code following 10021.**
10009 **Resequenced code. See code following 10021.**
10010 **Resequenced code. See code following 10021.**
10011 **Resequenced code. See code following 10021.**
10012 **Resequenced code. See code following 10021.**

10021 **Fine needle aspiration biopsy, without imaging guidance; first lesion**
(88172-88173, [88177])
1.60 2.80 FUD XXX T P3 80
AMA: 2019,May,10; 2019,Apr,4; 2019,Feb,8; 2018,Jan,8; 2017,Jan,8; 2016,Jan,13; 2015,Jan,16

+ # **10004** **each additional lesion (List separately in addition to code for primary procedure)**
EXCLUDES *Fine needle biopsy using other imaging methods for same lesion ([10005, 10006, 10007, 10008, 10009, 10010, 10011, 10012])*
Imaging guidance (76942)
(88172-88173, [88177])
Code first (10021)
1.25 1.48 FUD ZZZ N1 80
AMA: 2019,Apr,4; 2019,Feb,8

10005 **Fine needle aspiration biopsy, including ultrasound guidance; first lesion**
INCLUDES Imaging guidance (76942)
(88172-88173, [88177])
2.10 3.59 FUD XXX P3 80
AMA: 2019,May,10; 2019,Feb,8; 2019,Apr,4

+ # **10006** **each additional lesion (List separately in addition to code for primary procedure)**
INCLUDES Imaging guidance (76942)
(88172-88173, [88177])
Code first ([10005])
1.42 1.70 FUD ZZZ N1 80
AMA: 2019,Apr,4; 2019,Feb,8

10007 **Fine needle aspiration biopsy, including fluoroscopic guidance; first lesion**
INCLUDES Imaging guidance (77002)
(88172-88173, [88177])
2.70 8.09 FUD XXX P3 80
AMA: 2019,Apr,4; 2019,Feb,8

+ # **10008** **each additional lesion (List separately in addition to code for primary procedure)**
INCLUDES Imaging guidance (77002)
(88172-88173, [88177])
Code first ([10007])
1.76 4.79 FUD ZZZ N1 80
AMA: 2019,Apr,4; 2019,Feb,8

10009 **Fine needle aspiration biopsy, including CT guidance; first lesion**
INCLUDES Imaging guidance (77012)
(88172-88173, [88177])
3.28 13.3 FUD XXX P2 80
AMA: 2019,Apr,4; 2019,Feb,8

+ # **10010** **each additional lesion (List separately in addition to code for primary procedure)**
INCLUDES Imaging guidance (77012)
(88172-88173, [88177])
Code first ([10009])
2.38 8.02 FUD ZZZ N1 80
AMA: 2019,Apr,4; 2019,Feb,8

10011 **Fine needle aspiration biopsy, including MR guidance; first lesion**
INCLUDES Imaging guidance (77021)
(88172-88173, [88177])
0.00 0.00 FUD XXX R2 80
AMA: 2019,Apr,4; 2019,Feb,8

+ # **10012** **each additional lesion (List separately in addition to code for primary procedure)**
INCLUDES Imaging guidance (77021)
(88172-88173, [88177])
Code first ([10011])
0.00 0.00 FUD ZZZ N1 80
AMA: 2019,Apr,4; 2019,Feb,8

10030-10180 Treatment of Lesions: Skin and Subcutaneous Tissues

EXCLUDES *Excision benign lesion (11400-11471)*

10030 **Image-guided fluid collection drainage by catheter (eg, abscess, hematoma, seroma, lymphocele, cyst), soft tissue (eg, extremity, abdominal wall, neck), percutaneous**
INCLUDES Radiologic guidance (75989, 76942, 77002-77003, 77012, 77021)
EXCLUDES *Percutaneous drainage with imaging guidance:*
Peritoneal or retroperitoneal collections (49406)
Visceral collections (49405)
Transvaginal or transrectal drainage with imaging guidance peritoneal or retroperitoneal collections (49407)
Code also every instance of fluid collection drained using a separate catheter (10030)
3.98 17.5 FUD 000 T G2 80
AMA: 2019,Apr,4; 2018,Jan,8; 2017,Aug,9; 2017,Jan,8; 2016,Jan,13; 2015,Jan,16

Integumentary System

10004 — 10030

10035 Placement of soft tissue localization device(s) (eg, clip, metallic pellet, wire/needle, radioactive seeds), percutaneous, including imaging guidance; first lesion

INCLUDES Radiologic guidance (76942, 77002, 77012, 77021)

EXCLUDES *Sites with more specific code descriptor, such as breast*

Reporting code more than one time per site, regardless number markers used

Code also each additional target on same or opposite side (10036)

2.46 12.8 **FUD** 000 T N1 80 50

AMA: 2018,Jan,8; 2017,Jan,8; 2016,Jun,3

\+ **10036 each additional lesion (List separately in addition to code for primary procedure)**

INCLUDES Radiologic guidance (76942, 77002, 77012, 77021)

EXCLUDES *Sites with more specific code descriptor, such as breast*

Reporting code more than one time per site, regardless number markers used

Code first (10035)

1.25 11.7 **FUD** ZZZ N N1 80

AMA: 2018,Jan,8; 2017,Jan,8; 2016,Jun,3

10040 Acne surgery (eg, marsupialization, opening or removal of multiple milia, comedones, cysts, pustules)

1.53 3.11 **FUD** 010 Q1 N1

AMA: 2018,Jan,8; 2017,Jan,8; 2016,Jan,13; 2015,Jan,16

10060 Incision and drainage of abscess (eg, carbuncle, suppurative hidradenitis, cutaneous or subcutaneous abscess, cyst, furuncle, or paronychia); simple or single

2.87 3.44 **FUD** 010 T P3

AMA: 2018,Jan,8; 2017,Jan,8; 2016,Jan,13; 2015,Jan,16

10061 complicated or multiple

5.16 5.87 **FUD** 010 T P3

AMA: 2018,Jan,8; 2017,Jan,8; 2016,Jan,13; 2015,Jan,16

10080 Incision and drainage of pilonidal cyst; simple

2.95 5.99 **FUD** 010 T P3

AMA: 2018,Jan,8; 2017,Jan,8; 2016,Jan,13; 2015,Jan,16

10081 complicated

EXCLUDES *Excision pilonidal cyst (11770-11772)*

4.93 8.67 **FUD** 010 T P3

AMA: 2018,Jan,8; 2017,Jan,8; 2016,Jan,13; 2015,Jan,16

10120 Incision and removal of foreign body, subcutaneous tissues; simple

2.94 4.31 **FUD** 010 T P3

AMA: 2018,Jan,8; 2017,Jan,8; 2016,Jan,13; 2015,Jan,16

10121 complicated

EXCLUDES *Debridement associated with fracture or dislocation (11010-11012)*

Exploration penetrating wound (20100-20103)

5.33 7.76 **FUD** 010 J A2

AMA: 2018,Jan,8; 2017,Jan,8; 2016,Jan,13; 2015,Jan,16

10140 Incision and drainage of hematoma, seroma or fluid collection

(76942, 77002, 77012, 77021)

3.40 4.77 **FUD** 010 J P3

AMA: 2018,Jan,8; 2017,Jan,8; 2016,Jan,13; 2015,Jan,16

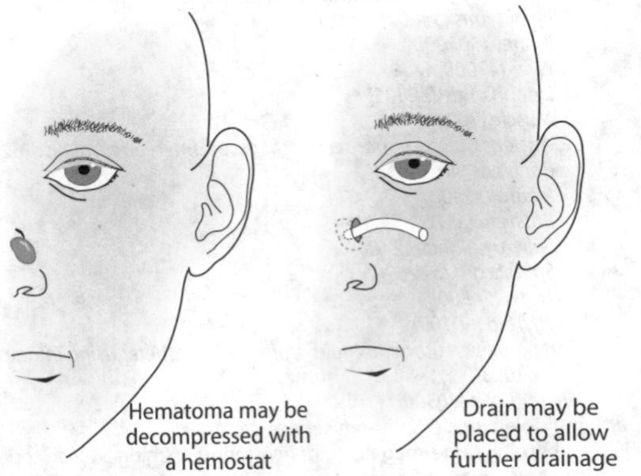

Hematoma may be decompressed with a hemostat
Drain may be placed to allow further drainage

10160 Puncture aspiration of abscess, hematoma, bulla, or cyst

(76942, 77002, 77012, 77021)

2.71 3.71 **FUD** 010 T P3

AMA: 2018,Jan,8; 2017,Aug,9; 2017,Jan,8; 2016,Jan,13; 2015,Jan,16

10180 Incision and drainage, complex, postoperative wound infection

EXCLUDES *Wound dehiscence (12020-12021, 13160)*

5.10 7.12 **FUD** 010 J A2

AMA: 2018,Jan,8; 2017,Jan,8; 2016,Jan,13; 2015,Jan,16

11000-11012 Removal of Foreign Substances and Infected/Devitalized Tissue

EXCLUDES *Debridement:*

Burns (16000-16030)

Deeper tissue (11042-11047 [11045, 11046])

Nails (11720-11721)

Nonelective debridement/active care management (97597-97598)

Wounds (11042-11047 [11045, 11046])

Dermabrasions (15780-15783)

Pressure ulcer excision (15920-15999)

11000 Debridement of extensive eczematous or infected skin; up to 10% of body surface

EXCLUDES *Necrotizing soft tissue infection:*

Abdominal wall (11005-11006)

External genitalia and perineum (11004, 11006)

0.82 1.61 **FUD** 000 T P3

AMA: 2018,Feb,10; 2018,Jan,8; 2017,Jan,8; 2016,Jan,13; 2015,Jan,16

\+ **11001 each additional 10% of the body surface, or part thereof (List separately in addition to code for primary procedure)**

EXCLUDES *Necrotizing soft tissue infection:*

Abdominal wall (11005-11006)

External genitalia and perineum (11004, 11006)

Code first (11000)

0.41 0.62 **FUD** ZZZ N N1

AMA: 2018,Feb,10; 2018,Jan,8; 2017,Jan,8; 2016,Jan,13; 2015,Jan,16

11004 Debridement of skin, subcutaneous tissue, muscle and fascia for necrotizing soft tissue infection; external genitalia and perineum

Code also skin grafts or flaps, when performed (14000-14350, 15040-15770 [15769], 15771-15776)

16.6 16.6 **FUD** 000 C

AMA: 2019,Nov,14; 2018,Feb,10; 2018,Jan,8; 2017,Jan,8; 2016,Jan,13; 2015,Jan,16

11005 **abdominal wall, with or without fascial closure**

Code also skin grafts or flaps, when performed (14000-14350, 15040-15770 [15769], 15771-15776)

22.6 22.6 **FUD** 000 C 80

AMA: 2019,Nov,14; 2018,Feb,10; 2018,Jan,8; 2017,Jan,8; 2016,Jan,13; 2015,Jan,16

11006 **external genitalia, perineum and abdominal wall, with or without fascial closure**

EXCLUDES *Orchiectomy (54520)*

Testicular transplant (54680)

Code also skin grafts or flaps, when performed (14000-14350, 15040-15770 [15769], 15771-15776)

20.4 20.4 **FUD** 000 C

AMA: 2019,Nov,14; 2018,Jan,8; 2017,Jan,8; 2016,Jan,13; 2015,Jan,16

\+ **11008** **Removal of prosthetic material or mesh, abdominal wall for infection (eg, for chronic or recurrent mesh infection or necrotizing soft tissue infection) (List separately in addition to code for primary procedure)**

EXCLUDES *Debridement (11000-11001, 11010-11044 [11045, 11046])*

Insertion mesh (49568)

Code also skin grafts or flaps, when performed (14000-14350, 15040-15770 [15769], 15771-15776)

Code first (10180, 11004-11006)

7.99 7.99 **FUD** ZZZ C 80

AMA: 2019,Jan,14; 2018,Jan,8; 2017,Jan,8; 2016,Jan,13; 2015,Jan,16

11010 **Debridement including removal of foreign material at the site of an open fracture and/or an open dislocation (eg, excisional debridement); skin and subcutaneous tissues**

7.96 13.5 **FUD** 010 T A2

AMA: 2018,Jan,8; 2017,Jan,8; 2016,Jan,13; 2015,Jan,16

11011 **skin, subcutaneous tissue, muscle fascia, and muscle**

8.68 15.2 **FUD** 000 T A2

AMA: 2018,Jan,8; 2017,Jan,8; 2016,Jan,13; 2015,Jan,16

11012 **skin, subcutaneous tissue, muscle fascia, muscle, and bone**

12.0 19.3 **FUD** 000 J A2

AMA: 2018,Jan,8; 2017,Jan,8; 2016,Jan,13; 2015,Jan,16

11042-11047 [11045, 11046] Removal of Infected/Devitalized Tissue

INCLUDES Debridement reported by size and depth

Debridement reported for multiple wounds by adding total surface area wounds with same depth

Injuries, wounds, chronic ulcers, infections

EXCLUDES *Debridement:*

Burn (16020-16030)

Eczematous or infected skin (11000-11001)

Nails (11720-11721)

Necrotizing soft tissue infection external genitalia, perineum, or abdominal wall (11004-11006)

Non-elective debridement/active care management same wound (97597-97602)

Dermabrasions (15780-15783)

Excision pressure ulcers (15920-15999)

Code also each additional single wound with different depths

Code also modifier 59 for additional wound debridement

Code also multiple wound groups with different depths

11042 **Debridement, subcutaneous tissue (includes epidermis and dermis, if performed); first 20 sq cm or less**

1.75 3.57 **FUD** 000 T A2

AMA: 2018,Jan,8; 2017,Jan,8; 2016,Oct,3; 2016,Aug,9; 2016,Feb,13; 2016,Jan,13; 2015,Jan,16

\+ # **11045** **each additional 20 sq cm, or part thereof (List separately in addition to code for primary procedure)**

Code first (11042)

0.77 1.19 **FUD** ZZZ N N1 80

AMA: 2018,Jan,8; 2017,Jan,8; 2016,Oct,3; 2016,Aug,9; 2016,Jan,13; 2015,Jan,16

11043 **Debridement, muscle and/or fascia (includes epidermis, dermis, and subcutaneous tissue, if performed); first 20 sq cm or less**

4.47 6.64 **FUD** 000 T A2

AMA: 2020,Apr,8; 2018,Jan,8; 2017,Jan,8; 2016,Oct,3; 2016,Aug,9; 2016,Jan,13; 2015,Jan,16

\+ # **11046** **each additional 20 sq cm, or part thereof (List separately in addition to code for primary procedure)**

Code first (11043)

1.62 2.12 **FUD** ZZZ N N1 80

AMA: 2018,Jan,8; 2017,Jan,8; 2016,Oct,3; 2016,Aug,9; 2016,Jan,13; 2015,Jan,16

11044 **Debridement, bone (includes epidermis, dermis, subcutaneous tissue, muscle and/or fascia, if performed); first 20 sq cm or less**

6.58 8.93 **FUD** 000 J A2

AMA: 2018,Jan,8; 2017,Jan,8; 2016,Oct,3; 2016,Aug,9; 2016,Jan,13; 2015,Jan,16

11045 **Resequenced code. See code following 11042.**

11046 **Resequenced code. See code following 11043.**

\+ **11047** **each additional 20 sq cm, or part thereof (List separately in addition to code for primary procedure)**

Code first (11044)

2.86 3.53 **FUD** ZZZ N N1 80

AMA: 2018,Jan,8; 2017,Jan,8; 2016,Oct,3; 2016,Aug,9; 2016,Jan,13; 2015,Jan,16

11055-11057 Excision Benign Hypertrophic Skin Lesions

CMS: 100-04,32,80.8 CSF Edits: Routine Foot Care

EXCLUDES *Destruction benign lesions other than cutaneous vascular proliferative lesions or skin tags (17110-17111)*

11055 **Paring or cutting of benign hyperkeratotic lesion (eg, corn or callus); single lesion**

0.46 1.78 **FUD** 000 Q1 N1

AMA: 2018,Jan,8; 2017,Jan,8; 2016,Jan,13; 2015,Jan,16

11056 **2 to 4 lesions**

0.65 1.90 **FUD** 000 Q1 N1

AMA: 2018,Jan,8; 2017,Jan,8; 2016,Jan,13; 2015,Jan,16

11057 **more than 4 lesions**

0.85 2.31 **FUD** 000 T P3

AMA: 2018,Jan,8; 2017,Jan,8; 2016,Jan,13; 2015,Jan,16

11102-11107 Surgical Biopsy Skin and Mucous Membranes

INCLUDES Attaining tissue for pathologic exam

EXCLUDES *Biopsies performed during related procedures*

Biopsy:

Anterior 2/3 tongue (41100)

Conjunctiva (68100)

Ear (69100)

Eyelid ([67810])

Floor of mouth (41108)

Intranasal (30100)

Lip (40490)

Nail (11755)

Penis (54100)

Perineum/vulva (56605-56606)

Vestibule of mouth (40808)

11102 **Tangential biopsy of skin (eg, shave, scoop, saucerize, curette); single lesion**

1.12 2.84 **FUD** 000 P3

AMA: 2020,May,13; 2019,Dec,9; 2019,Jan,9

\+ **11103** **each separate/additional lesion (List separately in addition to code for primary procedure)**

Code first different biopsy techniques used for additional separate lesions, when performed (11102, 11104, 11106)

0.66 1.51 **FUD** ZZZ N1

AMA: 2020,May,13; 2019,Dec,9; 2019,Jan,9

11104 **Punch biopsy of skin (including simple closure, when performed); single lesion**

1.40 3.57 **FUD** 000 P2

AMA: 2019,Dec,9; 2019,Jan,9

Integumentary System

11005 — 11104

\+ **11105** **each separate/additional lesion (List separately in addition to code for primary procedure)**

Code first different biopsy techniques used for additional separate lesions, when performed (11104, 11106)

0.76 | 1.72 | FUD ZZZ | N1

AMA: 2019,Dec,9; 2019,Jan,9

11106 **Incisional biopsy of skin (eg, wedge) (including simple closure, when performed); single lesion**

1.74 | 4.26 | FUD 000 | P3

AMA: 2019,Dec,9; 2019,Jan,9

\+ **11107** **each separate/additional lesion (List separately in addition to code for primary procedure)**

Code first (11106)

0.93 | 2.04 | FUD ZZZ | N1

AMA: 2019,Dec,9; 2019,Jan,9

11200-11201 Skin Tag Removal - All Techniques

INCLUDES Chemical destruction
Electrocauterization
Electrosurgical destruction
Ligature strangulation
Removal with or without local anesthesia
Sharp excision or scissoring

11200 **Removal of skin tags, multiple fibrocutaneous tags, any area; up to and including 15 lesions**

2.10 | 2.52 | FUD 010 | Q1 N1

AMA: 2018,Jan,8; 2017,Jan,8; 2016,Jan,13; 2015,Jan,16

\+ **11201** **each additional 10 lesions, or part thereof (List separately in addition to code for primary procedure)**

Code first (11200)

0.48 | 0.54 | FUD ZZZ | N N1

AMA: 2018,Jan,8; 2017,Jan,8; 2016,Jan,13; 2015,Jan,16

11300-11313 Skin Lesion Removal: Shaving

INCLUDES Local anesthesia
Partial thickness excision by horizontal slicing
Wound cauterization

11300 **Shaving of epidermal or dermal lesion, single lesion, trunk, arms or legs; lesion diameter 0.5 cm or less**

0.99 | 2.84 | FUD 000 | Q1 N1 80

AMA: 2019,Jan,9; 2018,Feb,10; 2018,Jan,8; 2017,Dec,14; 2017,Jan,8; 2016,Jan,13; 2015,Jan,16

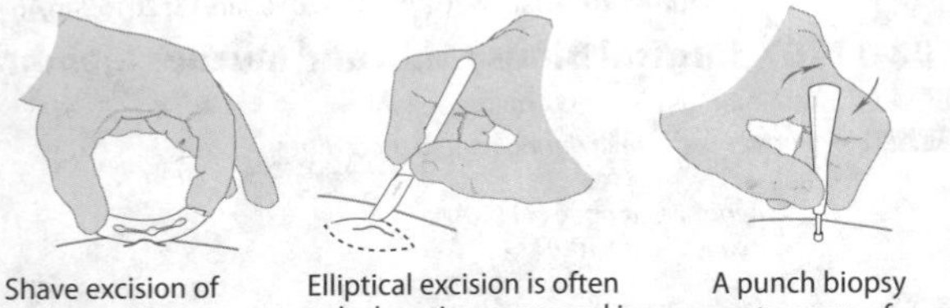

Shave excision of an elevated lesion; technique also used to biopsy

Elliptical excision is often used when tissue removal is larger than 4 mm or when deep pathology is suspected

A punch biopsy cuts a core of tissue as the tool is twisted downward

11301 **lesion diameter 0.6 to 1.0 cm**

1.50 | 3.45 | FUD 000 | Q1 N1 80

AMA: 2019,Jan,9; 2018,Feb,10; 2018,Jan,8; 2017,Dec,14; 2017,Jan,8; 2016,Jan,13; 2015,Jan,16

11302 **lesion diameter 1.1 to 2.0 cm**

1.76 | 3.99 | FUD 000 | Q1 N1 80

AMA: 2019,Jan,9; 2018,Feb,10; 2018,Jan,8; 2017,Dec,14; 2017,Jan,8; 2016,Jan,13; 2015,Jan,16

11303 **lesion diameter over 2.0 cm**

2.07 | 4.39 | FUD 000 | Q1 N1 80

AMA: 2019,Jan,9; 2018,Feb,10; 2018,Jan,8; 2017,Dec,14; 2017,Jan,8; 2016,Jan,13; 2015,Jan,16

11305 **Shaving of epidermal or dermal lesion, single lesion, scalp, neck, hands, feet, genitalia; lesion diameter 0.5 cm or less**

1.12 | 2.90 | FUD 000 | Q1 N1 80

AMA: 2019,Jan,9; 2018,Feb,10; 2018,Jan,8; 2017,Dec,14; 2017,Jan,8; 2016,Jan,13; 2015,Jan,16

11306 **lesion diameter 0.6 to 1.0 cm**

1.45 | 3.50 | FUD 000 | Q1 N1 80

AMA: 2019,Jan,9; 2018,Feb,10; 2018,Jan,8; 2017,Dec,14; 2017,Jan,8; 2016,Jan,13; 2015,Jan,16

11307 **lesion diameter 1.1 to 2.0 cm**

1.87 | 4.09 | FUD 000 | T P2 80

AMA: 2019,Jan,9; 2018,Feb,10; 2018,Jan,8; 2017,Dec,14; 2017,Jan,8; 2016,Jan,13; 2015,Jan,16

11308 **lesion diameter over 2.0 cm**

2.11 | 4.37 | FUD 000 | Q1 N1 80

AMA: 2019,Jan,9; 2018,Feb,10; 2018,Jan,8; 2017,Dec,14; 2017,Jan,8; 2016,Jan,13; 2015,Jan,16

11310 **Shaving of epidermal or dermal lesion, single lesion, face, ears, eyelids, nose, lips, mucous membrane; lesion diameter 0.5 cm or less**

1.34 | 3.29 | FUD 000 | T P3 80

AMA: 2019,Jan,9; 2018,Feb,10; 2018,Jan,8; 2017,Dec,14; 2017,Jan,8; 2016,Jan,13; 2015,Jan,16

11311 **lesion diameter 0.6 to 1.0 cm**

1.88 | 3.86 | FUD 000 | T P2 80

AMA: 2019,Jan,9; 2018,Feb,10; 2018,Jan,8; 2017,Dec,14; 2017,Jan,8; 2016,Jan,13; 2015,Jan,16

11312 **lesion diameter 1.1 to 2.0 cm**

2.17 | 4.51 | FUD 000 | T P3 80

AMA: 2019,Jan,9; 2018,Feb,10; 2018,Jan,8; 2017,Dec,14; 2017,Jan,8; 2016,Jan,13; 2015,Jan,16

11313 **lesion diameter over 2.0 cm**

2.82 | 5.27 | FUD 000 | T P3 80

AMA: 2019,Jan,9; 2018,Feb,10; 2018,Jan,8; 2017,Dec,14; 2017,Jan,8; 2016,Jan,13; 2015,Jan,16

11400-11446 Skin Lesion Removal: Benign

INCLUDES Biopsy on same lesion
Cicatricial lesion excision
Full thickness removal including margins
Lesion measurement before excision at largest diameter plus margin
Local anesthesia
Simple, nonlayered closure

EXCLUDES *Adjacent tissue transfer: report only adjacent tissue transfer (14000-14302)*
Biopsy eyelid ([67810])
Destruction:
Benign lesions, any method (17110-17111)
Cutaneous vascular proliferative lesions (17106-17108)
Destruction of eyelid lesion (67850)
Malignant lesions (17260-17286)
Premalignant lesions (17000, 17003-17004)
Escharotomy (16035-16036)
Excision and reconstruction eyelid (67961-67975)
Excision chalazion (67800-67808)
Eyelid procedures involving more than skin (67800 and subsequent codes)
Laser fenestration for scars (0479T-0480T)
Shave removal (11300-11313)

Code also complex closure (13100-13153)
Code also each separate lesion
Code also intermediate closure (12031-12057)
Code also modifier 22 when excision complicated or unusual
Code also reconstruction (15002-15261, 15570-15770)

11400 **Excision, benign lesion including margins, except skin tag (unless listed elsewhere), trunk, arms or legs; excised diameter 0.5 cm or less**

2.33 | 3.57 | FUD 010 | T P3

AMA: 2019,Nov,3; 2018,Sep,7; 2018,Feb,10; 2018,Jan,8; 2017,Jan,8; 2016,Apr,3; 2016,Jan,13; 2015,Jan,16

11401 **excised diameter 0.6 to 1.0 cm**

2.96 | 4.35 | FUD 010 | T P3

AMA: 2019,Nov,3; 2018,Sep,7; 2018,Feb,10; 2018,Jan,8; 2017,Jan,8; 2016,Apr,3; 2016,Jan,13; 2015,Jan,16

11402 **excised diameter 1.1 to 2.0 cm**

3.29 | 4.78 | FUD 010 | T P3

AMA: 2019,Nov,3; 2018,Sep,7; 2018,Feb,10; 2018,Jan,8; 2017,Jan,8; 2016,Apr,3; 2016,Jan,13; 2015,Jan,16

26/TC PC/TC Only | A2-Z3 ASC Payment | 50 Bilateral | ♂ Male Only | ♀ Female Only | Facility RVU | Non-Facility RVU | CCI | CLIA
FUD Follow-up Days | CMS: IOM | AMA: CPT Asst | A-Y OPPSI | 80/80 Surg Assist Allowed / w/Doc | Lab Crosswalk | Radiology Crosswalk
16

11403   excised diameter 2.1 to 3.0 cm
    🔲 4.23   5.58   **FUD** 010   T P3 ▣
    AMA: 2019,Nov,3; 2018,Sep,7; 2018,Feb,10; 2018,Jan,8; 2017,Jan,8; 2016,Apr,3; 2016,Jan,13; 2015,Jan,16

11404   excised diameter 3.1 to 4.0 cm
    🔲 4.66   6.34   **FUD** 010   J A2 ▣
    AMA: 2019,Nov,3; 2018,Sep,7; 2018,Feb,10; 2018,Jan,8; 2017,Jan,8; 2016,Apr,3; 2016,Jan,13; 2015,Jan,16

11406   excised diameter over 4.0 cm
    🔲 7.09   9.07   **FUD** 010   J A2 ▣
    AMA: 2019,Nov,3; 2018,Sep,7; 2018,Feb,10; 2018,Jan,8; 2017,Jan,8; 2016,Apr,3; 2016,Jan,13; 2015,Jan,16

11420   **Excision, benign lesion including margins, except skin tag (unless listed elsewhere), scalp, neck, hands, feet, genitalia; excised diameter 0.5 cm or less**
    🔲 2.34   3.60   **FUD** 010   J P3 ▣
    AMA: 2019,Nov,3; 2018,Sep,7; 2018,Feb,10; 2018,Jan,8; 2017,Jan,8; 2016,Apr,3; 2016,Jan,13; 2015,Jan,16

11421   excised diameter 0.6 to 1.0 cm
    🔲 3.15   4.49   **FUD** 010   T P3 ▣
    AMA: 2019,Nov,3; 2018,Sep,7; 2018,Feb,10; 2018,Jan,8; 2017,Jan,8; 2016,Apr,3; 2016,Jan,13; 2015,Jan,16

11422   excised diameter 1.1 to 2.0 cm
    🔲 3.88   5.11   **FUD** 010   J P3 ▣
    AMA: 2019,Nov,3; 2018,Sep,7; 2018,Feb,10; 2018,Jan,8; 2017,Jan,8; 2016,Apr,3; 2016,Jan,13; 2015,Jan,16

11423   excised diameter 2.1 to 3.0 cm
    🔲 4.45   5.81   **FUD** 010   J P3 ▣
    AMA: 2019,Nov,3; 2018,Sep,7; 2018,Feb,10; 2018,Jan,8; 2017,Jan,8; 2016,Apr,3; 2016,Jan,13; 2015,Jan,16

11424   excised diameter 3.1 to 4.0 cm
    🔲 5.11   6.71   **FUD** 010   J A2 ▣
    AMA: 2019,Nov,3; 2018,Sep,7; 2018,Feb,10; 2018,Jan,8; 2017,Jan,8; 2016,Apr,3; 2016,Jan,13; 2015,Jan,16

11426   excised diameter over 4.0 cm
    🔲 7.89   9.63   **FUD** 010   J A2 ▣
    AMA: 2019,Nov,3; 2018,Sep,7; 2018,Feb,10; 2018,Jan,8; 2017,Jan,8; 2016,Apr,3; 2016,Jan,13; 2015,Jan,16

11440   **Excision, other benign lesion including margins, except skin tag (unless listed elsewhere), face, ears, eyelids, nose, lips, mucous membrane; excised diameter 0.5 cm or less**
    🔲 2.96   3.91   **FUD** 010   T P3 ▣
    AMA: 2019,Nov,3; 2019,Jan,14; 2018,Sep,7; 2018,Feb,10; 2018,Jan,8; 2017,Jan,8; 2016,Apr,3; 2016,Jan,13; 2015,Jan,16

The physician removes a benign lesion from the external ear, nose, or mucous membranes

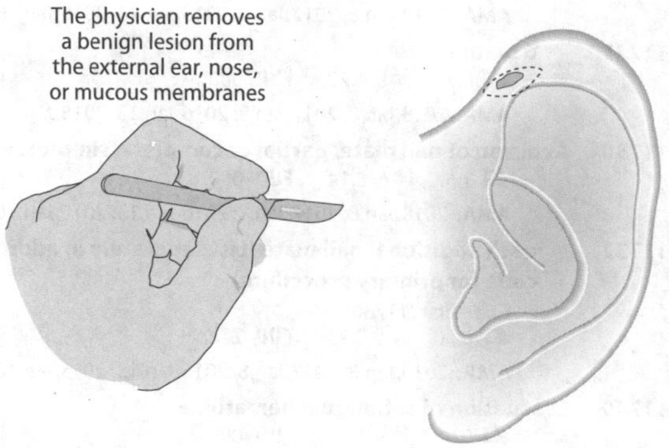

11441   excised diameter 0.6 to 1.0 cm
    🔲 3.73   4.88   **FUD** 010   T P3 ▣
    AMA: 2019,Nov,3; 2019,Jan,14; 2018,Sep,7; 2018,Feb,10; 2018,Jan,8; 2017,Jan,8; 2016,Apr,3; 2016,Jan,13; 2015,Jan,16

11442   excised diameter 1.1 to 2.0 cm
    🔲 4.14   5.43   **FUD** 010   T P3 ▣
    AMA: 2019,Nov,3; 2019,Jan,14; 2018,Sep,7; 2018,Feb,10; 2018,Jan,8; 2017,Jan,8; 2016,Apr,3; 2016,Jan,13; 2015,Jan,16

11443   excised diameter 2.1 to 3.0 cm
    🔲 5.08   6.45   **FUD** 010   J P3 ▣
    AMA: 2019,Nov,3; 2019,Jan,14; 2018,Sep,7; 2018,Feb,10; 2018,Jan,8; 2017,Jan,8; 2016,Apr,3; 2016,Jan,13; 2015,Jan,16

11444   excised diameter 3.1 to 4.0 cm
    🔲 6.49   8.09   **FUD** 010   J A2 ▣
    AMA: 2019,Nov,3; 2019,Jan,14; 2018,Sep,7; 2018,Feb,10; 2018,Jan,8; 2017,Jan,8; 2016,Apr,3; 2016,Jan,13; 2015,Jan,16

11446   excised diameter over 4.0 cm
    🔲 9.33   11.1   **FUD** 010   J A2 ▣
    AMA: 2019,Nov,3; 2019,Jan,14; 2018,Sep,7; 2018,Feb,10; 2018,Jan,8; 2017,Jan,8; 2016,Apr,3; 2016,Jan,13; 2015,Jan,16

11450-11471 Treatment of Hidradenitis: Excision and Repair

Code also closure by skin graft or flap (14000-14350, 15040-15770 [15769], 15771-15776)

11450   **Excision of skin and subcutaneous tissue for hidradenitis, axillary; with simple or intermediate repair**
    🔲 7.36   11.6   **FUD** 090   J A2 50 ▣
    AMA: 2019,Nov,3; 2018,Sep,7; 2018,Feb,10; 2018,Jan,8; 2017,Jan,8; 2016,Aug,9; 2016,Jan,13; 2015,Jan,16

Hidradenitis is a disease process stemming from clogged specialized sweat glands, principally located in the axilla and groin areas

Hair shaft

Hidradenitis of the axilla

Hair matrix

Sweat (eccrine gland)

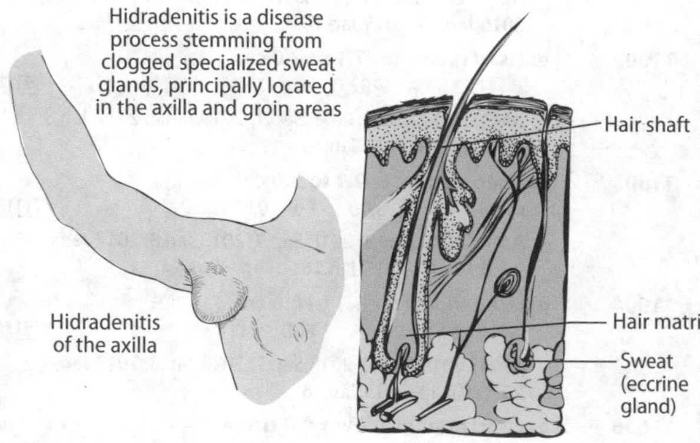

11451   **with complex repair**
    🔲 9.41   14.5   **FUD** 090   J A2 80 50 ▣
    AMA: 2019,Nov,3; 2018,Sep,7; 2018,Feb,10;.2018,Jan,8; 2017,Jan,8; 2016,Aug,9; 2016,Jan,13; 2015,Jan,16

11462   **Excision of skin and subcutaneous tissue for hidradenitis, inguinal; with simple or intermediate repair**
    🔲 7.01   11.3   **FUD** 090   J A2 80 50 ▣
    AMA: 2019,Nov,3; 2018,Sep,7; 2018,Feb,10; 2018,Jan,8; 2017,Jan,8; 2016,Aug,9; 2016,Jan,13; 2015,Jan,16

11463   **with complex repair**
    🔲 9.42   14.3   **FUD** 090   J A2 80 50 ▣
    AMA: 2019,Nov,3; 2018,Sep,7; 2018,Feb,10; 2018,Jan,8; 2017,Jan,8; 2016,Aug,9; 2016,Jan,13; 2015,Jan,16

11470   **Excision of skin and subcutaneous tissue for hidradenitis, perianal, perineal, or umbilical; with simple or intermediate repair**
    🔲 8.08   12.0   **FUD** 090   J A2 ▣
    AMA: 2019,Nov,3; 2018,Sep,7; 2018,Feb,10; 2018,Jan,8; 2017,Jan,8; 2016,Aug,9; 2016,Jan,13; 2015,Jan,16

11471   **with complex repair**
    🔲 10.0   15.0   **FUD** 090   J A2 80 ▣
    AMA: 2019,Nov,3; 2018,Sep,7; 2018,Feb,10; 2018,Jan,8; 2017,Jan,8; 2016,Aug,9; 2016,Jan,13; 2015,Jan,16

● New Code   ▲ Revised Code   ○ Reinstated   ● New Web Release   ▲ Revised Web Release   + Add-on   Unlisted   Not Covered   # Resequenced
50 Optum Mod 50 Exempt   ⊘ AMA Mod 51 Exempt   51 Optum Mod 51 Exempt   63 Mod 63 Exempt   ✔ Non-FDA Drug   ★ Telemedicine   M Maternity   A Age Edit

11600-11646 Skin Lesion Removal: Malignant

INCLUDES Biopsy on same lesion
Excision additional margin at same operative session
Full thickness removal including margins
Lesion measurement before excision at largest diameter plus margin
Local anesthesia
Simple, nonlayered closure

EXCLUDES *Adjacent tissue transfer. Report only adjacent tissue transfer (14000-14302)*
Destruction (17260-17286)
Excision additional margin at subsequent operative session (11600-11646)

Code also complex closure (13100-13153)
Code also each separate lesion
Code also intermediate closure (12031-12057)
Code also modifier 58 when re-excision performed during postoperative period
Code also reconstruction (15002-15261, 15570-15770)

11600 **Excision, malignant lesion including margins, trunk, arms, or legs; excised diameter 0.5 cm or less**
3.46 5.61 FUD 010 T P3
AMA: 2019,Nov,3; 2018,Sep,7; 2018,Jan,8; 2017,Jan,8; 2016,Jan,13; 2015,Jan,16

11601 **excised diameter 0.6 to 1.0 cm**
4.29 6.52 FUD 010 T P3
AMA: 2019,Nov,3; 2018,Sep,7; 2018,Jan,8; 2017,Jan,8; 2016,Jan,13; 2015,Jan,16

11602 **excised diameter 1.1 to 2.0 cm**
4.63 7.02 FUD 010 T P2
AMA: 2019,Nov,3; 2018,Sep,7; 2018,Jan,8; 2017,Jan,8; 2016,Jan,13; 2015,Jan,16

11603 **excised diameter 2.1 to 3.0 cm**
5.54 8.00 FUD 010 T P3
AMA: 2019,Nov,3; 2018,Sep,7; 2018,Jan,8; 2017,Jan,8; 2016,Jan,13; 2015,Jan,16

11604 **excised diameter 3.1 to 4.0 cm**
6.12 8.93 FUD 010 T A2
AMA: 2019,Nov,3; 2018,Sep,7; 2018,Jan,8; 2017,Jan,8; 2016,Jan,13; 2015,Jan,16

11606 **excised diameter over 4.0 cm**
9.24 12.8 FUD 010 J A2
AMA: 2019,Nov,3; 2018,Sep,7; 2018,Jan,8; 2017,Jan,8; 2016,Jan,13; 2015,Jan,16

11620 **Excision, malignant lesion including margins, scalp, neck, hands, feet, genitalia; excised diameter 0.5 cm or less**
3.50 5.64 FUD 010 J P3
AMA: 2019,Nov,3; 2018,Sep,7; 2018,Jan,8; 2017,Jan,8; 2016,Jan,13; 2015,Jan,16

11621 **excised diameter 0.6 to 1.0 cm**
4.27 6.55 FUD 010 T P3
AMA: 2019,Nov,3; 2018,Sep,7; 2018,Jan,8; 2017,Jan,8; 2016,Jan,13; 2015,Jan,16

11622 **excised diameter 1.1 to 2.0 cm**
4.93 7.30 FUD 010 T P3
AMA: 2019,Nov,3; 2018,Sep,7; 2018,Jan,8; 2017,Jan,8; 2016,Jan,13; 2015,Jan,16

11623 **excised diameter 2.1 to 3.0 cm**
6.03 8.52 FUD 010 J P3
AMA: 2019,Nov,3; 2018,Sep,7; 2018,Jan,8; 2017,Jan,8; 2016,Jan,13; 2015,Jan,16

11624 **excised diameter 3.1 to 4.0 cm**
6.85 9.65 FUD 010 J A2
AMA: 2019,Nov,3; 2018,Sep,7; 2018,Jan,8; 2017,Jan,8; 2016,Jan,13; 2015,Jan,16

11626 **excised diameter over 4.0 cm**
8.44 11.6 FUD 010 J A2
AMA: 2019,Nov,3; 2018,Sep,7; 2018,Jan,8; 2017,Jan,8; 2016,Jan,13; 2015,Jan,16

11640 **Excision, malignant lesion including margins, face, ears, eyelids, nose, lips; excised diameter 0.5 cm or less**
EXCLUDES *Eyelid excision involving more than skin (67800-67808, 67840-67850, 67961-67966)*
3.59 5.77 FUD 010 T P3
AMA: 2019,Nov,3; 2018,Sep,7; 2018,Jan,8; 2017,Jan,8; 2016,Jan,13; 2015,Jan,16

11641 **excised diameter 0.6 to 1.0 cm**
EXCLUDES *Eyelid excision involving more than skin (67800-67808, 67840-67850, 67961-67966)*
4.45 6.78 FUD 010 T P3
AMA: 2019,Nov,3; 2018,Sep,7; 2018,Jan,8; 2017,Jan,8; 2016,Jan,13; 2015,Jan,16

11642 **excised diameter 1.1 to 2.0 cm**
EXCLUDES *Eyelid excision involving more than skin (67800-67808, 67840-67850, 67961-67966)*
5.30 7.73 FUD 010 T P3
AMA: 2019,Nov,3; 2018,Sep,7; 2018,Jan,8; 2017,Jan,8; 2016,Jan,13; 2015,Jan,16

11643 **excised diameter 2.1 to 3.0 cm**
EXCLUDES *Eyelid excision involving more than skin (67800-67808, 67840-67850, 67961-67966)*
6.55 9.06 FUD 010 J P3
AMA: 2019,Nov,3; 2018,Sep,7; 2018,Jan,8; 2017,Jan,8; 2016,Jan,13; 2015,Jan,16

11644 **excised diameter 3.1 to 4.0 cm**
EXCLUDES *Eyelid excision involving more than skin (67800-67808, 67840-67850, 67961-67966)*
8.14 11.1 FUD 010 J A2
AMA: 2019,Nov,3; 2018,Sep,7; 2018,Jan,8; 2017,Jan,8; 2016,Jan,13; 2015,Jan,16

11646 **excised diameter over 4.0 cm**
EXCLUDES *Eyelid excision involving more than skin (67800-67808, 67840-67850, 67961-67966)*
11.2 14.5 FUD 010 J A2
AMA: 2019,Nov,3; 2018,Sep,7; 2018,Jan,8; 2017,Jan,8; 2016,Jan,13; 2015,Jan,16

11719-11765 Nails and Supporting Structures

CMS: 100-02,15,290 Foot Care

EXCLUDES *Drainage paronychia or onychia (10060-10061)*

11719 **Trimming of nondystrophic nails, any number**
0.22 0.41 FUD 000 Q1 N1
AMA: 2018,Jan,8; 2017,Jan,8; 2016,Jan,13; 2015,Jan,16

11720 **Debridement of nail(s) by any method(s); 1 to 5**
0.42 0.93 FUD 000 Q1 N1
AMA: 2018,Jan,8; 2017,Jan,8; 2016,Jan,13; 2015,Jan,16

11721 **6 or more**
0.72 1.29 FUD 000 Q1 N1
AMA: 2018,Jan,8; 2017,Jan,8; 2016,Jan,13; 2015,Jan,16

11730 **Avulsion of nail plate, partial or complete, simple; single**
1.57 3.14 FUD 000 Q1 N1
AMA: 2018,Jan,8; 2017,Jan,8; 2016,Jan,13; 2015,Jan,16

\+ **11732** **each additional nail plate (List separately in addition to code for primary procedure)**
Code first (11730)
0.50 0.95 FUD ZZZ N N1
AMA: 2018,Jan,8; 2017,Jan,8; 2016,Jan,13; 2015,Jan,16

11740 **Evacuation of subungual hematoma**
0.90 1.52 FUD 000 Q1 N1
AMA: 2018,Jan,8; 2017,Jan,8; 2016,Jan,13; 2015,Jan,16

11750 **Excision of nail and nail matrix, partial or complete (eg, ingrown or deformed nail), for permanent removal;**
EXCLUDES *Pinch graft (15050)*
2.92 4.41 FUD 010 T P3
AMA: 2018,Jan,8; 2017,Jan,8; 2016,Jan,13; 2015,Jan,16

11755 **Biopsy of nail unit (eg, plate, bed, matrix, hyponychium, proximal and lateral nail folds) (separate procedure)**
1.79 3.47 FUD 000 T P3 80
AMA: 2019,Jan,9; 2018,Jan,8; 2017,Jan,8; 2016,Jan,13; 2015,Jan,16

11760 **Repair of nail bed**
3.27 5.46 FUD 010 T G2
AMA: 2018,Jan,8; 2017,Jan,8; 2016,Jan,13; 2015,Jan,16

11762 **Reconstruction of nail bed with graft**
5.33 8.15 FUD 010 T P3
AMA: 2018,Jan,8; 2017,Jan,8; 2016,Jan,13; 2015,Jan,16

11765 **Wedge excision of skin of nail fold (eg, for ingrown toenail)**
INCLUDES Cotting's operation
2.64 4.80 FUD 010 Q1 N1
AMA: 2018,Jan,8; 2017,Jan,8; 2016,Jan,13; 2015,Jan,16

11770-11772 Treatment Pilonidal Cyst: Excision

EXCLUDES *Incision of pilonidal cyst (10080-10081)*

11770 **Excision of pilonidal cyst or sinus; simple**
5.34 8.92 FUD 010 J A2

11771 **extensive**
12.7 17.2 FUD 090 J A2

11772 **complicated**
16.6 20.9 FUD 090 J A2
AMA: 2018,Jan,8; 2017,Jan,8; 2016,Jan,13; 2015,Sep,12

11900-11901 Treatment of Lesions: Injection

EXCLUDES *Injection local anesthesia performed preoperatively*
Injection veins (36470-36471)
Intralesional chemotherapy (96405-96406)

11900 **Injection, intralesional; up to and including 7 lesions**
0.90 1.54 FUD 000 Q1 N1
AMA: 2018,Jan,8; 2017,Jan,8; 2016,Jan,13; 2015,Jan,16

11901 **more than 7 lesions**
1.36 1.97 FUD 000 Q1 N1
AMA: 2018,Jan,8; 2017,Jan,8; 2016,Jan,13; 2015,Jan,16

11920-11971 Tattoos, Tissue Expanders, and Dermal Fillers

CMS: 100-02,16,10 Exclusions from Coverage; 100-02,16,120 Cosmetic Procedures; 100-02,16,180 Services Related to Noncovered Procedures

11920 **Tattooing, intradermal introduction of insoluble opaque pigments to correct color defects of skin, including micropigmentation; 6.0 sq cm or less**
3.23 5.33 FUD 000 T P3 80
AMA: 2018,Jan,8; 2017,Jan,8; 2016,Aug,9

11921 **6.1 to 20.0 sq cm**
3.81 6.08 FUD 000 T P3 80
AMA: 2018,Jan,8; 2017,Jan,8; 2016,Aug,9

\+ 11922 **each additional 20.0 sq cm, or part thereof (List separately in addition to code for primary procedure)**
Code first (11921)
0.86 1.71 FUD ZZZ N N1 80

11950 **Subcutaneous injection of filling material (eg, collagen); 1 cc or less**
1.51 2.26 FUD 000 T P3 80
AMA: 2019,Aug,10; 2018,Jan,8; 2017,Jan,8; 2016,Jan,13; 2015,Jan,16

11951 **1.1 to 5.0 cc**
1.98 2.80 FUD 000 T P3 80
AMA: 2019,Aug,10; 2018,Jan,8; 2017,Jan,8; 2016,Jan,13; 2015,Jan,16

11952 **5.1 to 10.0 cc**
3.03 4.13 FUD 000 T P3 80
AMA: 2019,Aug,10; 2018,Jan,8; 2017,Jan,8; 2016,Jan,13; 2015,Jan,16

11954 **over 10.0 cc**
3.21 4.41 FUD 000 T P3 80
AMA: 2019,Aug,10; 2018,Jan,8; 2017,Jan,8; 2016,Jan,13; 2015,Jan,16

11960 **Insertion of tissue expander(s) for other than breast, including subsequent expansion**
EXCLUDES *Breast reconstruction with tissue expander(s) (19357)*
Decompression, nerve (64722-64726)
Endoscopic release transverse carpal ligament (29848)
Neuroplasty (64702-64721)
Removal tissue expander without implant insertion (11971)
Secondary closure, surgical wound or dehiscence (13160)
28.1 28.1 FUD 090 T A2
AMA: 1991,Win,1

▲ 11970 **Replacement of tissue expander with permanent implant**
17.6 17.6 FUD 090 J A2 50
AMA: 2018,Jan,8; 2017,Jan,8; 2016,Jan,13; 2015,Jan,16

▲ 11971 **Removal of tissue expander without insertion of implant**
EXCLUDES *Insertion/replacement tissue expander (11960, 11970)*
9.31 13.7 FUD 090 Q2 A2 80 50
AMA: 2018,Jan,8; 2017,Jan,8; 2016,Jan,13; 2015,Jan,16

11976-11983 Drug Implantation

11976 **Removal, implantable contraceptive capsules** ♀
2.73 4.15 FUD 000 Q2 P3 80
AMA: 1992,Win,1; 1991,Win,1

11980 **Subcutaneous hormone pellet implantation (implantation of estradiol and/or testosterone pellets beneath the skin)**
1.61 2.69 FUD 000 Q1 N1
AMA: 2018,Jan,8; 2017,Jan,8; 2016,Jan,13; 2015,Jan,16

11981 **Insertion, non-biodegradable drug delivery implant**
EXCLUDES *Insertion deep drug-delivery device:*
Intra-articular (20704)
Intramedullary (20702)
Subfascial (20700)
1.86 2.96 FUD 000 Q1 N1 80
AMA: 2018,Jan,8; 2017,Jan,8; 2016,Jan,13; 2015,Jan,16

11982 **Removal, non-biodegradable drug delivery implant**
EXCLUDES *Removal deep drug-delivery device:*
Intra-articular (20705)
Intramedullary (20703)
Subfascial (20701)
2.87 4.49 FUD XXX Q1 N1 80

11983 **Removal with reinsertion, non-biodegradable drug delivery implant**
3.01 4.15 FUD 000 Q1 N1 80

Integumentary System
11755 — 11983

12001-12021 Suturing of Superficial Wounds

INCLUDES Administration local anesthesia
Cauterization without closure
Simple:
- Exploration nerves, blood vessels, tendons
- Vessel ligation, in wound

Simple repair that involves:
- Routine debridement and decontamination
- Simple one layer closure
- Superficial tissues
- Sutures, staples, tissue adhesives
- Total length several repairs in same code category

EXCLUDES *Adhesive strips only, see appropriate E/M service*
Complex repair nerves, blood vessels, tendons (see appropriate anatomical section)
Debridement requiring:
- *Comprehensive cleaning*
- *Removal significant tissue*
- *Removal soft tissue and/or bone, no fracture/dislocation, performed separately (11042-11047 [11045, 11046])*
- *Removal soft tissue and/or bone with open fracture/dislocation (11010-11012)*

Deep tissue repair (12031-13153)
Major exploration (20100-20103)
Repair nerves, blood vessels, tendons (See appropriate anatomical section. These repairs include simple and intermediate closure. Report complex closure with modifier 59.)
Secondary closure/dehiscence (13160)

Code also modifier 59 added to less complicated procedure code when reporting more than one wound repair classification

12001 **Simple repair of superficial wounds of scalp, neck, axillae, external genitalia, trunk and/or extremities (including hands and feet); 2.5 cm or less**
1.30 2.58 **FUD** 000 Q1 N1
AMA: 2018,Sep,7; 2018,Jan,8; 2017,Dec,14; 2017,Jan,8; 2016,Jan,13; 2015,Jan,16

12002 **2.6 cm to 7.5 cm**
1.67 3.08 **FUD** 000 Q1 N1
AMA: 2018,Sep,7; 2018,Jan,8; 2017,Jan,8; 2016,Jan,13; 2015,Jan,16

12004 **7.6 cm to 12.5 cm**
2.15 3.69 **FUD** 000 Q1 N1
AMA: 2018,Sep,7; 2018,Jan,8; 2017,Jan,8; 2016,Jan,13; 2015,Jan,16

12005 **12.6 cm to 20.0 cm**
2.71 4.69 **FUD** 000 Q1 A2
AMA: 2018,Sep,7; 2018,Jan,8; 2017,Jan,8; 2016,Jan,13; 2015,Jan,16

12006 **20.1 cm to 30.0 cm**
3.43 5.76 **FUD** 000 Q2 A2
AMA: 2018,Sep,7; 2018,Jan,8; 2017,Jan,8; 2016,Jan,13; 2015,Jan,16

12007 **over 30.0 cm**
4.23 6.58 **FUD** 000 T A2
AMA: 2018,Sep,7; 2018,Jan,8; 2017,Jan,8; 2016,Jan,13; 2015,Jan,16

12011 **Simple repair of superficial wounds of face, ears, eyelids, nose, lips and/or mucous membranes; 2.5 cm or less**
1.57 3.09 **FUD** 000 Q1 N1
AMA: 2018,Sep,7; 2018,Jan,8; 2017,Jan,8; 2016,Nov,7; 2016,Jan,13; 2015,Jan,16

12013 **2.6 cm to 5.0 cm**
1.72 3.29 **FUD** 000 Q1 N1
AMA: 2018,Sep,7; 2018,Jan,8; 2017,Jan,8; 2016,Jan,13; 2015,Jan,16

12014 **5.1 cm to 7.5 cm**
2.20 4.00 **FUD** 000 Q1 N1
AMA: 2018,Sep,7; 2018,Jan,8; 2017,Jan,8; 2016,Jan,13; 2015,Jan,16

12015 **7.6 cm to 12.5 cm**
2.78 4.84 **FUD** 000 Q1 G2
AMA: 2018,Sep,7; 2018,Jan,8; 2017,Jan,8; 2016,Jan,13; 2015,Jan,16

12016 **12.6 cm to 20.0 cm**
3.77 6.16 **FUD** 000 Q1 A2
AMA: 2018,Sep,7; 2018,Jan,8; 2017,Jan,8; 2016,Jan,13; 2015,Jan,16

12017 **20.1 cm to 30.0 cm**
4.48 4.48 **FUD** 000 Q1 A2 80
AMA: 2018,Sep,7; 2018,Jan,8; 2017,Jan,8; 2016,Jan,13; 2015,Jan,16

12018 **over 30.0 cm**
5.08 5.08 **FUD** 000 Q1 A2 80
AMA: 2018,Sep,7; 2018,Jan,8; 2017,Jan,8; 2016,Jan,13; 2015,Jan,16

12020 **Treatment of superficial wound dehiscence; simple closure**
EXCLUDES *Secondary closure major/complex wound or dehiscence (13160)*
5.43 8.41 **FUD** 010 T A2
AMA: 2019,Nov,3; 2018,Jan,8; 2017,Jan,8; 2016,Jan,13; 2015,Jan,16

12021 **with packing**
EXCLUDES *Secondary closure major/complex wound or dehiscence (13160)*
4.01 4.90 **FUD** 010 T A2
AMA: 2019,Nov,3; 2018,Jan,8; 2017,Jan,8; 2016,Jan,13; 2015,Jan,16

12031-12057 Suturing of Intermediate Wounds

INCLUDES Administration local anesthesia
Repair that involves:
- Closure contaminated single layer wound
- Layered closure (e.g., subcutaneous tissue, superficial fascia)
- Limited undermining
- Removal foreign material (e.g., gravel, glass)
- Routine debridement and decontamination

Simple:
- Exploration nerves, blood vessels, tendons in wound
- Vessel ligation, in wound

Total length several repairs in same code category

EXCLUDES *Debridement requiring:*
- *Removal soft tissue and/or bone, no fracture/dislocation, performed separately (11042-11047 [11045, 11046])*
- *Removal soft tissue/bone due to open fracture/dislocation (11010-11012)*

Major exploration (20100-20103)
Repair nerves, blood vessels, tendons (See appropriate anatomical section. These repairs include simple and intermediate closure. Report complex closure with modifier 59.)
Secondary closure major/complex wound or dehiscence (13160)
Wound repair involving more than layered closure

Code also modifier 59 added to less complicated procedure code when reporting more than one wound repair classification

12031 **Repair, intermediate, wounds of scalp, axillae, trunk and/or extremities (excluding hands and feet); 2.5 cm or less**
4.36 7.17 **FUD** 010 T P2
AMA: 2019,Nov,3; 2018,Sep,7; 2018,Jan,8; 2017,Jan,8; 2016,Jan,13; 2015,Jan,16

12032 **2.6 cm to 7.5 cm**
5.46 8.59 **FUD** 010 T P2
AMA: 2019,Nov,3; 2018,Sep,7; 2018,Jan,8; 2017,Jan,8; 2016,Jan,13; 2015,Jan,16

12034 **7.6 cm to 12.5 cm**
5.96 9.07 **FUD** 010 T A2
AMA: 2019,Nov,3; 2018,Sep,7; 2018,Jan,8; 2017,Jan,8; 2016,Jan,13; 2015,Jan,16

12035 **12.6 cm to 20.0 cm**
6.94 11.0 **FUD** 010 T A2
AMA: 2019,Nov,3; 2018,Sep,7; 2018,Jan,8; 2017,Jan,8; 2016,Jan,13; 2015,Jan,16

12036 **20.1 cm to 30.0 cm**
8.15 12.3 **FUD** 010 T A2
AMA: 2019,Nov,3; 2018,Sep,7; 2018,Jan,8; 2017,Jan,8; 2016,Jan,13; 2015,Jan,16

12037 **over 30.0 cm**
9.53 14.0 **FUD** 010 T A2 80
AMA: 2019,Nov,3; 2018,Sep,7; 2018,Jan,8; 2017,Jan,8; 2016,Jan,13; 2015,Jan,16

12041 **Repair, intermediate, wounds of neck, hands, feet and/or external genitalia; 2.5 cm or less**
4.22 7.19 **FUD** 010 Q2 P2
AMA: 2019,Nov,3; 2018,Sep,7; 2018,Jan,8; 2017,Jan,8; 2016,Jan,13; 2015,Jan,16

12042 **2.6 cm to 7.5 cm**
5.75 8.41 **FUD** 010 T P2
AMA: 2019,Nov,3; 2018,Sep,7; 2018,Jan,8; 2017,Jan,8; 2016,Jan,13; 2015,Jan,16

12044 **7.6 cm to 12.5 cm**
6.16 10.6 **FUD** 010 T A2
AMA: 2019,Nov,3; 2018,Sep,7; 2018,Jan,8; 2017,Jan,8; 2016,Jan,13; 2015,Jan,16

12045 **12.6 cm to 20.0 cm**
7.71 11.4 **FUD** 010 T A2
AMA: 2019,Nov,3; 2018,Sep,7; 2018,Jan,8; 2017,Jan,8; 2016,Jan,13; 2015,Jan,16

12046 **20.1 cm to 30.0 cm**
9.01 13.8 **FUD** 010 T A2 80
AMA: 2019,Nov,3; 2018,Sep,7; 2018,Jan,8; 2017,Jan,8; 2016,Jan,13; 2015,Jan,16

12047 **over 30.0 cm**
10.1 15.4 **FUD** 010 T A2 80
AMA: 2019,Nov,3; 2018,Sep,7; 2018,Jan,8; 2017,Jan,8; 2016,Jan,13; 2015,Jan,16

12051 **Repair, intermediate, wounds of face, ears, eyelids, nose, lips and/or mucous membranes; 2.5 cm or less**
4.85 7.73 **FUD** 010 T P2
AMA: 2019,Nov,3; 2018,Sep,7; 2018,Jan,8; 2017,Jan,8; 2016,Jan,13; 2015,Jan,16

12052 **2.6 cm to 5.0 cm**
5.74 8.67 **FUD** 010 T P2
AMA: 2019,Nov,3; 2018,Sep,7; 2018,Jan,8; 2017,Jan,8; 2016,Jan,13; 2015,Jan,16

12053 **5.1 cm to 7.5 cm**
6.20 10.1 **FUD** 010 T P2
AMA: 2019,Nov,3; 2018,Sep,7; 2018,Jan,8; 2017,Jan,8; 2016,Jan,13; 2015,Jan,16

12054 **7.6 cm to 12.5 cm**
6.35 10.7 **FUD** 010 Q2 A2
AMA: 2019,Nov,3; 2018,Sep,7; 2018,Jan,8; 2017,Jan,8; 2016,Jan,13; 2015,Jan,16

12055 **12.6 cm to 20.0 cm**
8.66 13.9 **FUD** 010 T A2
AMA: 2019,Nov,3; 2018,Sep,7; 2018,Jan,8; 2017,Jan,8; 2016,Jan,13; 2015,Jan,16

12056 **20.1 cm to 30.0 cm**
11.0 15.9 **FUD** 010 Q2 A2 80
AMA: 2019,Nov,3; 2018,Sep,7; 2018,Jan,8; 2017,Jan,8; 2016,Jan,13; 2015,Jan,16

12057 **over 30.0 cm**
12.2 16.9 **FUD** 010 T A2 80
AMA: 2019,Nov,3; 2018,Sep,7; 2018,Jan,8; 2017,Jan,8; 2016,Jan,13; 2015,Jan,16

13100-13160 Suturing of Complicated Wounds

INCLUDES Creation limited defect for repair
Debridement complicated wounds/avulsions
Repair with layered closure that involves at least one of the following:
- Debridement wound edges
- Exposure underlying structures, such as bone, cartilage, tendon, or named neovascular structure
- Extensive undermining
- Free margin involvement helical or nostril rim or vermillion border
- Retention suture placement

Simple:
- Exploration nerves, vessels, tendons in wound
- Vessel ligation in wound

Total length several repairs in same code category

EXCLUDES *Excision:*
- *Benign lesions (11400-11446)*
- *Extensive debridement open fracture/dislocation (11010-11012)*
- *Extensive debridement penetrating or blunt trauma not associated with open fracture/dislocation (11042-11047 [11045, 11046])*
- *Malignant lesions (11600-11646)*
- *Surgical preparation wound bed (15002-15005)*

Extensive exploration (20100-20103)
Repair nerves, blood vessel, tendons (See appropriate anatomical section. These repairs include simple and intermediate closure. Report complex closure with modifier 59.)

Code also modifier 59 added to less complicated procedure code when reporting more than one wound repair classification

13100 **Repair, complex, trunk; 1.1 cm to 2.5 cm**
EXCLUDES *Complex repair 1.0 cm or less (12001, 12031)*
5.81 9.72 **FUD** 010 T A2
AMA: 2019,Nov,14; 2019,Nov,3; 2018,Sep,7; 2018,Jan,8; 2017,Apr,9; 2017,Jan,8; 2016,Jan,13; 2015,Jan,16

13101 **2.6 cm to 7.5 cm**
7.14 11.4 **FUD** 010 T A2
AMA: 2019,Dec,14; 2019,Nov,3; 2018,Sep,7; 2018,Jan,8; 2017,Apr,9; 2017,Jan,8; 2016,Jan,13; 2015,Jan,16

+ **13102** **each additional 5 cm or less (List separately in addition to code for primary procedure)**
Code first (13101)
2.14 3.46 **FUD** ZZZ N N1
AMA: 2019,Nov,14; 2019,Nov,3; 2018,Sep,7; 2018,Jan,8; 2017,Apr,9; 2017,Jan,8; 2016,Jan,13; 2015,Jan,16

13120 **Repair, complex, scalp, arms, and/or legs; 1.1 cm to 2.5 cm**
EXCLUDES *Complex repair 1.0 cm or less (12001, 12031)*
6.68 10.1 **FUD** 010 T A2
AMA: 2019,Nov,3; 2018,Sep,7; 2018,Jan,8; 2017,Jan,8; 2016,Jan,13; 2015,Jan,16

13121 **2.6 cm to 7.5 cm**
7.67 12.2 **FUD** 010 T A2
AMA: 2019,Nov,3; 2018,Sep,7; 2018,Jan,8; 2017,Jan,8; 2016,Jan,13; 2015,Jan,16

+ **13122** **each additional 5 cm or less (List separately in addition to code for primary procedure)**
Code first (13121)
2.42 3.74 **FUD** ZZZ N N1
AMA: 2019,Nov,3; 2018,Sep,7; 2018,Jan,8; 2017,Jan,8; 2016,Jan,13; 2015,Jan,16

13131 **Repair, complex, forehead, cheeks, chin, mouth, neck, axillae, genitalia, hands and/or feet; 1.1 cm to 2.5 cm**
EXCLUDES *Complex repair 1.0 cm or less (12001, 12011, 12031, 12041, 12051)*
7.04 11.1 **FUD** 010 T A2
AMA: 2019,Nov,3; 2018,Sep,7; 2018,Jan,8; 2017,Apr,9; 2017,Jan,8; 2016,Jan,13; 2015,Jan,16

13132 **2.6 cm to 7.5 cm**
8.81 13.5 **FUD** 010 T A2
AMA: 2019,Nov,3; 2018,Sep,7; 2018,Jan,8; 2017,Apr,9; 2017,Jan,8; 2016,Jan,13; 2015,Jan,16

+ **13133** **each additional 5 cm or less (List separately in addition to code for primary procedure)**

Code first (13132)

3.69 4.98 **FUD** ZZZ N N1

AMA: 2019,Nov,3; 2018,Sep,7; 2018,Jan,8; 2017,Apr,9; 2017,Jan,8; 2016,Jan,13; 2015,Jan,16

13151 **Repair, complex, eyelids, nose, ears and/or lips; 1.1 cm to 2.5 cm**

EXCLUDES *Complex repair 1.0 cm or less (12011, 12051)*

8.25 12.1 **FUD** 010 T A2

AMA: 2019,Nov,3; 2018,Sep,7; 2018,Jan,8; 2017,Jan,8; 2016,Jan,13; 2015,Jan,16

13152 **2.6 cm to 7.5 cm**

9.74 14.3 **FUD** 010 T A2

AMA: 2019,Nov,3; 2018,Sep,7; 2018,Jan,8; 2017,Jan,8; 2016,Jan,13; 2015,Jan,16

+ **13153** **each additional 5 cm or less (List separately in addition to code for primary procedure)**

Code first (13152)

4.02 5.45 **FUD** ZZZ N N1

AMA: 2019,Nov,3; 2018,Sep,7; 2018,Jan,8; 2017,Jan,8; 2016,Jan,13; 2015,Jan,16

13160 **Secondary closure of surgical wound or dehiscence, extensive or complicated**

EXCLUDES *Insertion tissue expander, other than breast (11960)*
Packing or simple secondary wound closure (12020-12021)

22.9 22.9 **FUD** 090 T A2

AMA: 2019,Nov,3; 2018,Jan,8; 2017,Jan,8; 2016,Jan,13; 2015,Jan,16

14000-14350 Reposition Contiguous Tissue

INCLUDES Excision (with or without lesion) with repair by adjacent tissue transfer or tissue rearrangement
Size includes primary (due to excision) and secondary (due to flap design)
Z-plasty, W-plasty, VY-plasty, rotation flap, advancement flap, double pedicle flap, random island flap

EXCLUDES *Closure wounds by undermining surrounding tissue without additional incisions (13100-13160)*
Full thickness closure:
Eyelid (67930-67935, 67961-67975)
Lip (40650-40654)

Code also skin graft necessary to repair secondary defect (15040-15731)

14000 **Adjacent tissue transfer or rearrangement, trunk; defect 10 sq cm or less**

INCLUDES Burrow's operation

EXCLUDES *Excision lesion with repair by adjacent tissue transfer or tissue rearrangement (11400-11446, 11600-11646)*

14.3 17.8 **FUD** 090 T A2

AMA: 2018,Jan,8; 2017,Oct,9; 2017,Jan,8; 2016,Jan,13; 2015,Sep,12; 2015,Feb,10; 2015,Jan,16

Example of common Z-plasty. Lesion is removed with oval-shaped incision

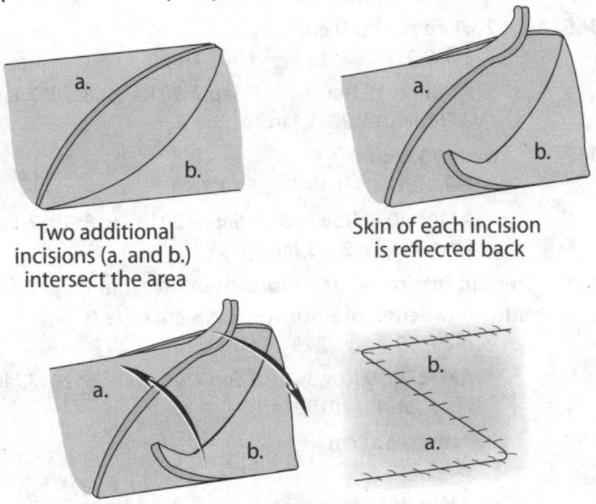
a.
b.
Two additional incisions (a. and b.) intersect the area
a.
b.
Skin of each incision is reflected back
a.
b.
b.
a.
The flaps are then transposed and the repair is closed

An adjacent flap, or other rearrangement flap, is performed to repair a defect

14001 **defect 10.1 sq cm to 30.0 sq cm**

EXCLUDES *Excision lesion with repair by adjacent tissue transfer or tissue rearrangement (11400-11446, 11600-11646)*

18.7 22.8 **FUD** 090 T A2

AMA: 2018,Jan,8; 2017,Oct,9; 2017,Jan,8; 2016,Jan,13; 2015,Feb,10; 2015,Jan,16

14020 **Adjacent tissue transfer or rearrangement, scalp, arms and/or legs; defect 10 sq cm or less**

EXCLUDES *Excision lesion with repair by adjacent tissue transfer or tissue rearrangement (11400-11446, 11600-11646)*

16.0 19.8 **FUD** 090 T A2

AMA: 2018,Jan,8; 2017,Jan,8; 2016,Jan,13; 2015,Jan,16

14021 **defect 10.1 sq cm to 30.0 sq cm**

EXCLUDES *Excision lesion with repair by adjacent tissue transfer or tissue rearrangement (11400-11446, 11600-11646)*

20.5 24.7 **FUD** 090 T A2

AMA: 2018,Jan,8; 2017,Jan,8; 2016,Jan,13; 2015,Jan,16

14040 **Adjacent tissue transfer or rearrangement, forehead, cheeks, chin, mouth, neck, axillae, genitalia, hands and/or feet; defect 10 sq cm or less**

INCLUDES Krimer's palatoplasty

EXCLUDES *Excision lesion with repair by adjacent tissue transfer or tissue rearrangement (11400-11446, 11600-11646)*

18.1 21.7 **FUD** 090 T A2

AMA: 2018,Jan,8; 2017,Nov,6; 2017,Jan,8; 2016,Jan,13; 2015,Jan,16

14041 **defect 10.1 sq cm to 30.0 sq cm**

EXCLUDES *Excision lesion with repair by adjacent tissue transfer or tissue rearrangement (11400-11446, 11600-11646)*

22.3 26.7 **FUD** 090 T A2

AMA: 2018,Jan,8; 2017,Nov,6; 2017,Jan,8; 2016,Jan,13; 2015,Jan,16

14060 **Adjacent tissue transfer or rearrangement, eyelids, nose, ears and/or lips; defect 10 sq cm or less**

INCLUDES Denonvillier's operation

EXCLUDES *Excision lesion with repair by adjacent tissue transfer or tissue rearrangement (11400-11446, 11600-11646)*
Eyelid, full thickness (67961-67966)

19.0 21.9 **FUD** 090 T A2

AMA: 2018,Jan,8; 2017,Nov,6; 2017,Jan,8; 2016,Jan,13; 2015,Jan,16

14061 **defect 10.1 sq cm to 30.0 sq cm**

EXCLUDES *Excision lesion with repair by adjacent tissue transfer or tissue rearrangement (11400-11446, 11600-11646)*
Eyelid, full thickness (67961 and subsequent codes)

23.4 28.3 **FUD** 090 T A2

AMA: 2018,Jan,8; 2017,Nov,6; 2017,Jan,8; 2016,Jan,13; 2015,Jan,16

14301 **Adjacent tissue transfer or rearrangement, any area; defect 30.1 sq cm to 60.0 sq cm**

EXCLUDES *Excision lesion with repair by adjacent tissue transfer or tissue rearrangement (11400-11446, 11600-11646)*

25.0 30.8 **FUD** 090 T G2 80

AMA: 2018,Jan,8; 2017,Nov,6; 2017,Apr,9; 2017,Jan,8; 2016,Jan,13; 2015,Jan,16

+ **14302** **each additional 30.0 sq cm, or part thereof (List separately in addition to code for primary procedure)**

EXCLUDES *Excision lesion with repair by adjacent tissue transfer or tissue rearrangement (11400-11446, 11600-11646)*

Code first (14301)

6.31 6.31 **FUD** ZZZ N N1 80

AMA: 2018,Jan,8; 2017,Nov,6; 2017,Jan,8; 2016,Jan,13; 2015,Jan,16

14350 **Filleted finger or toe flap, including preparation of recipient site**

19.7 19.7 **FUD** 090 T A2 80

AMA: 2018,Jan,8; 2017,Jan,8; 2016,Jan,13; 2015,Jan,16

15002-15005 Development of Base for Tissue Grafting

INCLUDES Add together surface area multiple wounds in same anatomical locations as indicated in code descriptor groups, such as face and scalp. Do not add together multiple wounds at different anatomical site groups such as trunk and face
Ankle or wrist when code description describes leg or arm
Cleaning and preparing viable wound surface for grafting or negative pressure wound therapy used to heal wound primarily
Code selection based on defect size and location
Percentage applies to children younger than age 10
Removal nonviable tissue in nonchronic wounds for primary healing
Square centimeters applies to children and adults age 10 or older

EXCLUDES *Chronic wound management on wounds left to heal by secondary intention (11042-11047 [11045, 11046], 97597-97598)*
Necrotizing soft tissue infections for specific anatomical locations (11004-11008)

15002 **Surgical preparation or creation of recipient site by excision of open wounds, burn eschar, or scar (including subcutaneous tissues), or incisional release of scar contracture, trunk, arms, legs; first 100 sq cm or 1% of body area of infants and children**

EXCLUDES *Linear scar revision (13100-13153)*

6.45 10.0 **FUD** 000 T A2 80

AMA: 2019,Nov,3; 2018,Jan,8; 2017,Jan,8; 2016,Jan,13; 2015,Jan,16

+ **15003** **each additional 100 sq cm, or part thereof, or each additional 1% of body area of infants and children (List separately in addition to code for primary procedure)**

Code first (15002)

1.32 2.11 **FUD** ZZZ N N1 80

AMA: 2019,Nov,3; 2018,Jan,8; 2017,Jan,8; 2016,Jan,13; 2015,Jan,16

15004 **Surgical preparation or creation of recipient site by excision of open wounds, burn eschar, or scar (including subcutaneous tissues), or incisional release of scar contracture, face, scalp, eyelids, mouth, neck, ears, orbits, genitalia, hands, feet and/or multiple digits; first 100 sq cm or 1% of body area of infants and children**

7.65 11.4 **FUD** 000 T A2 80

AMA: 2019,Nov,3; 2018,Jan,8; 2017,Jan,8; 2016,Jan,13; 2015,Jan,16

+ **15005** **each additional 100 sq cm, or part thereof, or each additional 1% of body area of infants and children (List separately in addition to code for primary procedure)**

Code first (15004)

2.66 3.50 **FUD** ZZZ N N1 80

AMA: 2019,Nov,3; 2018,Jan,8; 2017,Jan,8; 2016,Jan,13; 2015,Jan,16

15040 Obtain Autograft

INCLUDES Ankle or wrist when code description describes leg or arm
Percentage applies to children younger than age 10
Square centimeters applies to children and adults age 10 or older

15040 **Harvest of skin for tissue cultured skin autograft, 100 sq cm or less**

3.60 7.47 **FUD** 000 T A2

AMA: 2018,Jan,8; 2017,Jan,8; 2016,Jan,13; 2015,Jan,16

15050 Pinch Graft

INCLUDES Autologous skin graft harvest and application
Current graft removal
Fixation and anchoring skin graft
Simple cleaning

EXCLUDES *Removal devitalized tissue from wound(s), non-selective debridement, without anesthesia (97602)*

Code also graft or flap necessary to repair donor site

15050 **Pinch graft, single or multiple, to cover small ulcer, tip of digit, or other minimal open area (except on face), up to defect size 2 cm diameter**

13.0 16.7 **FUD** 090 T A2

AMA: 2018,Jan,8; 2017,Jan,8; 2016,Jun,8; 2016,Jan,13; 2015,Jan,16

15100-15261 Skin Grafts and Replacements

INCLUDES Add together surface area multiple wounds in same anatomical locations as indicated in code descriptor groups, such as face and scalp. Do not add together multiple wounds at different anatomical site groups such as trunk and face
Ankle or wrist when code description describes leg or arm
Autologous skin graft harvest and application
Code selection based on recipient site location and graft size and type
Current graft removal
Fixation and anchoring skin graft
Percentage applies to children younger than age 10
Simple cleaning
Simple tissue debridement
Square centimeters applies to children and adults age 10 or older

EXCLUDES *Debridement without immediate primary closure, when wound grossly contaminated and extensive cleaning needed, or when necrotic or contaminated tissue removed (11042-11047 [11045, 11046], 97597-97598)*
Removal devitalized tissue from wound(s), non-selective debridement, without anesthesia (97602)

Code also graft or flap necessary to repair donor site
Code also primary procedure requiring skin graft for definitive closure

15100 **Split-thickness autograft, trunk, arms, legs; first 100 sq cm or less, or 1% of body area of infants and children (except 15050)**
20.5 24.5 FUD 090 T A2
AMA: 2018,Jan,8; 2017,Jan,8; 2016,Jun,8; 2016,Jan,13; 2015,Jan,16

+ **15101** **each additional 100 sq cm, or each additional 1% of body area of infants and children, or part thereof (List separately in addition to code for primary procedure)**
Code first (15100)
3.24 5.40 FUD ZZZ N N1
AMA: 2018,Jan,8; 2017,Jan,8; 2016,Jun,8; 2016,Jan,13; 2015,Jan,16

15110 **Epidermal autograft, trunk, arms, legs; first 100 sq cm or less, or 1% of body area of infants and children**
19.9 23.1 FUD 090 T A2
AMA: 2018,Jan,8; 2017,Jan,8; 2016,Jan,13; 2015,Jan,16

+ **15111** **each additional 100 sq cm, or each additional 1% of body area of infants and children, or part thereof (List separately in addition to code for primary procedure)**
Code first (15110)
3.02 3.33 FUD ZZZ N N1
AMA: 2018,Jan,8; 2017,Jan,8; 2016,Jan,13; 2015,Jan,16

15115 **Epidermal autograft, face, scalp, eyelids, mouth, neck, ears, orbits, genitalia, hands, feet, and/or multiple digits; first 100 sq cm or less, or 1% of body area of infants and children**
19.6 22.8 FUD 090 T A2
AMA: 2018,Jan,8; 2017,Jan,8; 2016,Jan,13; 2015,Jan,16

+ **15116** **each additional 100 sq cm, or each additional 1% of body area of infants and children, or part thereof (List separately in addition to code for primary procedure)**
Code first (15115)
4.39 4.81 FUD ZZZ N N1
AMA: 2018,Jan,8; 2017,Jan,8; 2016,Jan,13; 2015,Jan,16

15120 **Split-thickness autograft, face, scalp, eyelids, mouth, neck, ears, orbits, genitalia, hands, feet, and/or multiple digits; first 100 sq cm or less, or 1% of body area of infants and children (except 15050)**
EXCLUDES *Other eyelid repair (67961-67975)*
19.9 24.3 FUD 090 T A2
AMA: 2018,Jan,8; 2017,Jan,8; 2016,Jun,8; 2016,Jan,13; 2015,Jan,16

+ **15121** **each additional 100 sq cm, or each additional 1% of body area of infants and children, or part thereof (List separately in addition to code for primary procedure)**
EXCLUDES *Other eyelid repair (67961-67975)*
Code first (15120)
3.86 5.95 FUD ZZZ N N1
AMA: 2018,Jan,8; 2017,Jan,8; 2016,Jun,8; 2016,Jan,13; 2015,Jan,16

15130 **Dermal autograft, trunk, arms, legs; first 100 sq cm or less, or 1% of body area of infants and children**
17.1 20.6 FUD 090 T A2
AMA: 2018,Jan,8; 2017,Jan,8; 2016,Jan,13; 2015,Jan,16

+ **15131** **each additional 100 sq cm, or each additional 1% of body area of infants and children, or part thereof (List separately in addition to code for primary procedure)**
Code first (15130)
2.65 2.86 FUD ZZZ N N1
AMA: 2018,Jan,8; 2017,Jan,8; 2016,Jan,13; 2015,Jan,16

15135 **Dermal autograft, face, scalp, eyelids, mouth, neck, ears, orbits, genitalia, hands, feet, and/or multiple digits; first 100 sq cm or less, or 1% of body area of infants and children**
21.4 24.5 FUD 090 T A2
AMA: 2018,Jan,8; 2017,Jan,8; 2016,Jan,13; 2015,Jan,16

+ **15136** **each additional 100 sq cm, or each additional 1% of body area of infants and children, or part thereof (List separately in addition to code for primary procedure)**
Code first (15135)
2.65 2.83 FUD ZZZ N N1
AMA: 2018,Jan,8; 2017,Jan,8; 2016,Jan,13; 2015,Jan,16

15150 **Tissue cultured skin autograft, trunk, arms, legs; first 25 sq cm or less**
18.4 20.3 FUD 090 T A2
AMA: 2018,Jan,8; 2017,Jan,8; 2016,Jan,13; 2015,Jan,16

+ **15151** **additional 1 sq cm to 75 sq cm (List separately in addition to code for primary procedure)**
EXCLUDES *Grafts over 75 sq cm (15152)*
Reporting code more than one time per session
Code first (15150)
3.19 3.45 FUD ZZZ N N1
AMA: 2018,Jan,8; 2017,Jan,8; 2016,Jan,13; 2015,Jan,16

+ **15152** **each additional 100 sq cm, or each additional 1% of body area of infants and children, or part thereof (List separately in addition to code for primary procedure)**
Code first (15151)
4.22 4.47 FUD ZZZ N N1
AMA: 2018,Jan,8; 2017,Jan,8; 2016,Jan,13; 2015,Jan,16

15155 **Tissue cultured skin autograft, face, scalp, eyelids, mouth, neck, ears, orbits, genitalia, hands, feet, and/or multiple digits; first 25 sq cm or less**
21.1 23.0 FUD 090 T A2
AMA: 2018,Jan,8; 2017,Jan,8; 2016,Jan,13; 2015,Jan,16

+ **15156** **additional 1 sq cm to 75 sq cm (List separately in addition to code for primary procedure)**
EXCLUDES *Grafts over 75 sq cm (15157)*
Reporting code more than one time per session
Code first (15155)
4.39 4.64 FUD ZZZ N N1
AMA: 2018,Jan,8; 2017,Jan,8; 2016,Jan,13; 2015,Jan,16

+ **15157** **each additional 100 sq cm, or each additional 1% of body area of infants and children, or part thereof (List separately in addition to code for primary procedure)**
Code first (15156)
4.78 5.17 FUD ZZZ N N1
AMA: 2018,Jan,8; 2017,Jan,8; 2016,Jan,13; 2015,Jan,16

15200 **Full thickness graft, free, including direct closure of donor site, trunk; 20 sq cm or less**
19.2 23.9 **FUD** 090 T A2
AMA: 2018,Jan,8; 2017,Jan,8; 2016,Jun,8; 2016,Jan,13; 2015,Jan,16

\+ **15201** **each additional 20 sq cm, or part thereof (List separately in addition to code for primary procedure)**
Code first (15200)
2.26 4.20 **FUD** ZZZ N N1
AMA: 2018,Jan,8; 2017,Jan,8; 2016,Jun,8; 2016,Jan,13; 2015,Jan,16

15220 **Full thickness graft, free, including direct closure of donor site, scalp, arms, and/or legs; 20 sq cm or less**
17.4 21.9 **FUD** 090 T A2
AMA: 2018,Jan,8; 2017,Jan,8; 2016,Jun,8; 2016,Jan,13; 2015,Jan,16

\+ **15221** **each additional 20 sq cm, or part thereof (List separately in addition to code for primary procedure)**
Code first (15220)
2.03 3.86 **FUD** ZZZ N N1
AMA: 2018,Jan,8; 2017,Jan,8; 2016,Jun,8; 2016,Jan,13; 2015,Jan,16

15240 **Full thickness graft, free, including direct closure of donor site, forehead, cheeks, chin, mouth, neck, axillae, genitalia, hands, and/or feet; 20 sq cm or less**
EXCLUDES *Fingertip graft (15050)*
Syndactyly repair fingers (26560-26562)
23.0 26.6 **FUD** 090 T A2
AMA: 2018,Jan,8; 2017,Jan,8; 2016,Jun,8; 2016,Jan,13; 2015,Jan,16

\+ **15241** **each additional 20 sq cm, or part thereof (List separately in addition to code for primary procedure)**
Code first (15240)
3.18 5.22 **FUD** ZZZ N N1
AMA: 2018,Jan,8; 2017,Jan,8; 2016,Jun,8; 2016,Jan,13; 2015,Jan,16

15260 **Full thickness graft, free, including direct closure of donor site, nose, ears, eyelids, and/or lips; 20 sq cm or less**
EXCLUDES *Other eyelid repair (67961-67975)*
24.1 28.5 **FUD** 090 T A2
AMA: 2018,Jan,8; 2017,Jan,8; 2016,Jun,8; 2016,Jan,13; 2015,Jan,16

\+ **15261** **each additional 20 sq cm, or part thereof (List separately in addition to code for primary procedure)**
EXCLUDES *Other eyelid repair (67961-67975)*
Code first (15260)
3.96 5.99 **FUD** ZZZ N N1
AMA: 2018,Jan,8; 2017,Jan,8; 2016,Jun,8; 2016,Jan,13; 2015,Jan,16

15271-15278 Skin Substitute Graft Application

INCLUDES Add together surface area multiple wounds in same anatomical locations as indicated in code descriptor groups, such as face and scalp. Do not add together multiple wounds at different anatomical site groups such as trunk and face
Ankle or wrist when code description describes leg or arm
Code selection based on defect site location and size
Fixation and anchoring skin graft
Graft types include:
- Biological material used for tissue engineering (e.g., scaffold) for growing skin
- Nonautologous human skin such as:
  - Acellular
  - Allograft
  - Cellular
  - Dermal
  - Epidermal
  - Homograft
- Nonhuman grafts

Percentage applies to children younger than age 10
Removing current graft
Simple cleaning
Simple tissue debridement
Square centimeters applies to children and adults age 10 or older

EXCLUDES *Application nongraft dressing*
Injected skin substitutes
Removal devitalized tissue from wound(s), non-selective debridement, without anesthesia (97602)
Skin application procedures, low cost (C5271-C5278)

Code also biologic implant for soft tissue reinforcement (15777)
Code also primary procedure requiring skin graft for definitive closure
Code also supply high-cost skin substitute product (C1849, C9363, Q4101, Q4103-Q4110, Q4116, Q4121-Q4123, Q4126-Q4128, Q4132-Q4133, Q4137-Q4138, Q4140-Q4141, Q4143, Q4146-Q4148, Q4150-Q4161, Q4163-Q4164, Q4169, Q4173, Q4175, Q4176, Q4178, Q4179, Q4180, Q4181, Q4183, Q4184, Q4186-Q4187, Q4194, Q4195, Q4196, Q4197, Q4203, Q4205, Q4208, Q4226, Q4234)

15271 **Application of skin substitute graft to trunk, arms, legs, total wound surface area up to 100 sq cm; first 25 sq cm or less wound surface area**
EXCLUDES *Total wound area greater than or equal to 100 sq cm (15273-15274)*
2.42 4.14 **FUD** 000 T G2
AMA: 2018,Jan,8; 2017,Oct,9; 2017,Jan,8; 2016,Jan,13; 2015,Jan,16

\+ **15272** **each additional 25 sq cm wound surface area, or part thereof (List separately in addition to code for primary procedure)**
EXCLUDES *Total wound area greater than or equal to 100 sq cm (15273-15274)*
Code first (15271)
0.50 0.76 **FUD** ZZZ N N1
AMA: 2018,Jan,8; 2017,Jan,8; 2016,Jan,13; 2015,Jan,16

15273 **Application of skin substitute graft to trunk, arms, legs, total wound surface area greater than or equal to 100 sq cm; first 100 sq cm wound surface area, or 1% of body area of infants and children**
EXCLUDES *Total wound surface area up to 100 cm (15271-15272)*
5.84 8.73 **FUD** 000 T G2
AMA: 2018,Jan,8; 2017,Jan,8; 2016,Jan,13; 2015,Jan,16

\+ **15274** **each additional 100 sq cm wound surface area, or part thereof, or each additional 1% of body area of infants and children, or part thereof (List separately in addition to code for primary procedure)**
EXCLUDES *Total wound surface area up to 100 cm (15271-15272)*
Code first (15273)
1.33 2.15 **FUD** ZZZ N N1
AMA: 2018,Jan,8; 2017,Jan,8; 2016,Jan,13; 2015,Jan,16

15275 **Application of skin substitute graft to face, scalp, eyelids, mouth, neck, ears, orbits, genitalia, hands, feet, and/or multiple digits, total wound surface area up to 100 sq cm; first 25 sq cm or less wound surface area**

EXCLUDES *Total wound area greater than or equal to 100 sq cm (15277-15278)*

2.74 4.37 **FUD** 000 T G2

AMA: 2018,Jan,8; 2017,Jan,8; 2016,Jan,13; 2015,Jan,16

\+ **15276** **each additional 25 sq cm wound surface area, or part thereof (List separately in addition to code for primary procedure)**

EXCLUDES *Total wound area greater than or equal to 100 sq cm (15277-15278)*

Code first (15275)

0.73 0.98 **FUD** ZZZ N N1

AMA: 2018,Jan,8; 2017,Jan,8; 2016,Jan,13; 2015,Jan,16

15277 **Application of skin substitute graft to face, scalp, eyelids, mouth, neck, ears, orbits, genitalia, hands, feet, and/or multiple digits, total wound surface area greater than or equal to 100 sq cm; first 100 sq cm wound surface area, or 1% of body area of infants and children**

EXCLUDES *Total surface area up to 100 sq cm (15275-15276)*

6.60 9.55 **FUD** 000 T G2

AMA: 2018,Jan,8; 2017,Jan,8; 2016,Jan,13; 2015,Jan,16

\+ **15278** **each additional 100 sq cm wound surface area, or part thereof, or each additional 1% of body area of infants and children, or part thereof (List separately in addition to code for primary procedure)**

EXCLUDES *Total surface area up to 100 sq cm (15275-15276)*

Code first (15277)

1.66 2.54 **FUD** ZZZ N N1

AMA: 2018,Jan,8; 2017,Jan,8; 2016,Jan,13; 2015,Jan,16

15570-15731 Wound Reconstruction: Skin Flaps

INCLUDES Ankle or wrist when code description describes leg or arm
Code selection based on recipient site when flap attached in transfer or to final site and based on donor site when tube created for transfer later or when flap delayed prior to transfer
Fixation and anchoring skin graft
Simple tissue debridement
Tube formation for later transfer

EXCLUDES *Contiguous tissue transfer flaps (14040-14041, 14060-14061, 14301-14302)*
Debridement without immediate primary closure (11042-11047 [11045, 11046], 97597-97598)
Excision:
Benign lesion (11400-11471)
Burn eschar or scar (15002-15005)
Malignant lesion (11600-11646)
Microvascular repair (15756-15758)
Primary procedure--see appropriate anatomical site

Code also application extensive immobilization apparatus
Code also repair donor site with skin grafts or flaps

15570 **Formation of direct or tubed pedicle, with or without transfer; trunk**

INCLUDES Flaps without vascular pedicle

21.1 26.2 **FUD** 090 T A2

AMA: 2018,Jan,8; 2017,Jan,8; 2016,Jan,13; 2015,Jan,16

Pedicle flap

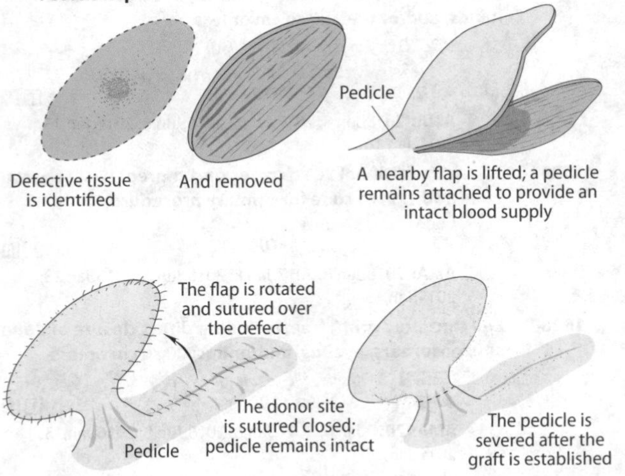
Defective tissue is identified
And removed
Pedicle
A nearby flap is lifted; a pedicle remains attached to provide an intact blood supply
The flap is rotated and sutured over the defect
The donor site is sutured closed; pedicle remains intact
Pedicle
The pedicle is severed after the graft is established

15572 **scalp, arms, or legs**

INCLUDES Flaps without vascular pedicle

21.2 25.3 **FUD** 090 T A2

AMA: 2018,Jan,8; 2017,Jan,8; 2016,Jan,13; 2015,Jan,16

15574 **forehead, cheeks, chin, mouth, neck, axillae, genitalia, hands or feet**

INCLUDES Flaps without vascular pedicle

21.6 25.7 **FUD** 090 T A2

AMA: 2018,Jan,8; 2017,Jan,8; 2016,Jan,13; 2015,Jan,16

15576 **eyelids, nose, ears, lips, or intraoral**

INCLUDES Flaps without vascular pedicle

19.1 22.9 **FUD** 090 T A2

AMA: 2018,Jan,8; 2017,Jan,8; 2016,Jan,13; 2015,Jan,16

15600 **Delay of flap or sectioning of flap (division and inset); at trunk**

5.96 9.47 **FUD** 090 T A2 80

AMA: 2019,Jun,14; 2018,Jan,8; 2017,Jan,8; 2016,Jan,13; 2015,Jan,16

15610 **at scalp, arms, or legs**

6.89 10.2 **FUD** 090 T A2 80

AMA: 2018,Jan,8; 2017,Jan,8; 2016,Jan,13; 2015,Jan,16

15620 at forehead, cheeks, chin, neck, axillae, genitalia, hands, or feet

🚑 9.26   ⚕ 12.6   **FUD** 090   T A2 ▱

AMA: 2018,Jan,8; 2017,Jan,8; 2016,Jan,13; 2015,Jan,16

15630 at eyelids, nose, ears, or lips

🚑 9.77   ⚕ 13.0   **FUD** 090   T A2 ▱

AMA: 2018,Jan,8; 2017,Jan,8; 2016,Jan,13; 2015,Jan,16

15650 Transfer, intermediate, of any pedicle flap (eg, abdomen to wrist, Walking tube), any location

EXCLUDES Defatting, revision, or rearranging transferred pedicle flap or skin graft (13100-14302)

Eyelids, ears, lips, and nose - refer to anatomical area

🚑 11.0   ⚕ 14.5   **FUD** 090   T A2 80 ▱

AMA: 2018,Jan,8; 2017,Jan,8; 2016,Jan,13; 2015,Jan,16

15730 Midface flap (ie, zygomaticofacial flap) with preservation of vascular pedicle(s)

🚑 26.3   ⚕ 42.9   **FUD** 090   T G2 ▱

AMA: 2018,Apr,10; 2018,Jan,8; 2017,Nov,6

15731 Forehead flap with preservation of vascular pedicle (eg, axial pattern flap, paramedian forehead flap)

EXCLUDES Muscle, myocutaneous, or fasciocutaneous flap head or neck (15733)

🚑 28.6   ⚕ 32.0   **FUD** 090   T A2 80 ▱

AMA: 2018,Jan,8; 2017,Nov,6; 2017,Jan,8; 2016,Jan,13; 2015,Jan,16

15733-15738 Wound Reconstruction: Muscle Flaps

INCLUDES Code based on donor site

EXCLUDES Contiguous tissue transfer flaps (14040-14041, 14060-14061, 14301-14302)

Microvascular repair (15756-15758)

Code also application extensive immobilization apparatus

Code also repair donor site with skin grafts or flaps

15733 Muscle, myocutaneous, or fasciocutaneous flap; head and neck with named vascular pedicle (ie, buccinators, genioglossus, temporalis, masseter, sternocleidomastoid, levator scapulae)

INCLUDES Repair extracranial defect by anterior pericranial flap on vascular pedicle (15731)

🚑 29.9   ⚕ 29.9   **FUD** 090   T A2 ▱

AMA: 2018,Apr,10; 2018,Jan,8; 2017,Nov,6

15734 trunk

🚑 43.6   ⚕ 43.6   **FUD** 090   T A2 80 ▱

AMA: 2018,Aug,10; 2018,Jan,8; 2017,Nov,6; 2017,Jan,8; 2016,Jan,13; 2015,Jan,16

15736 upper extremity

🚑 35.3   ⚕ 35.3   **FUD** 090   T A2 ▱

AMA: 2018,Jan,8; 2017,Nov,6; 2017,Jan,8; 2016,Jan,13; 2015,Jan,16

15738 lower extremity

🚑 37.4   ⚕ 37.4   **FUD** 090   T A2 80 ▱

AMA: 2018,Jan,8; 2017,Nov,6; 2017,Jan,8; 2016,Jan,13; 2015,Jan,16

15740-15758 Wound Reconstruction: Other

INCLUDES Fixation and anchoring skin graft

Routine dressing

Simple tissue debridement

EXCLUDES Adjacent tissue transfer (14000-14302)

Excision:

Benign lesion (11400-11471)

Burn eschar or scar (15002-15005)

Malignant lesion (11600-11646)

Flaps without vascular pedicle addition (15570-15576)

Primary procedure--see appropriate anatomical section

Skin graft for repair donor site (15050-15278)

Code also repair donor site with skin grafts or flaps (14000-14350, 15050-15278)

15740 Flap; island pedicle requiring identification and dissection of an anatomically named axial vessel

EXCLUDES V-Y subcutaneous flaps, random island flaps, and other flaps from adjacent areas (14000-14302)

🚑 24.2   ⚕ 28.8   **FUD** 090   T A2 ▱

AMA: 2018,Jan,8; 2017,Dec,14; 2017,Jan,8; 2016,Jan,13; 2015,Jan,16

15750 neurovascular pedicle

EXCLUDES V-Y subcutaneous flaps, random island flaps, and other flaps from adjacent areas (14000-14302)

🚑 26.4   ⚕ 26.4   **FUD** 090   T A2 80 ▱

AMA: 2018,Jan,8; 2017,Dec,14

15756 Free muscle or myocutaneous flap with microvascular anastomosis

INCLUDES Operating microscope (69990)

🚑 66.0   ⚕ 66.0   **FUD** 090   C 80 ▱

AMA: 2019,Dec,5; 2018,Jan,8; 2017,Jan,8; 2016,Feb,12; 2016,Jan,13; 2015,Jan,16

15757 Free skin flap with microvascular anastomosis

INCLUDES Operating microscope (69990)

🚑 65.5   ⚕ 65.5   **FUD** 090   C 80 ▱

AMA: 2019,Dec,5; 2018,Jan,8; 2017,Jan,8; 2016,Apr,8; 2016,Feb,12; 2016,Jan,13; 2015,Jan,16

15758 Free fascial flap with microvascular anastomosis

INCLUDES Operating microscope (69990)

🚑 66.0   ⚕ 66.0   **FUD** 090   C 80 ▱

AMA: 2019,Dec,5; 2018,Jan,8; 2017,Jan,8; 2016,Feb,12; 2016,Jan,13; 2015,Jan,16

15760-15774 [15769] Other Grafts

EXCLUDES Adjacent tissue transfer (14000-14302)

Excision:

Benign lesion (11400-11471)

Burn eschar or scar (15002-15005)

Malignant lesion (11600-11646)

Flaps without vascular pedicle addition (15570-15576)

Microvascular repair (15756-15758)

Primary procedure (see appropriate anatomical site)

Repair donor site with skin grafts or flaps (14000-14350, 15050-15278)

15760 Graft; composite (eg, full thickness of external ear or nasal ala), including primary closure, donor area

INCLUDES Fixation and anchoring skin graft

Routine dressing

Simple tissue debridement

🚑 20.2   ⚕ 24.2   **FUD** 090   T A2 ▱

AMA: 2018,Jan,8; 2017,Jan,8; 2016,Jan,13; 2015,Jan,16

15769 Resequenced code. See code following 15770.

15770 derma-fat-fascia

INCLUDES Fixation and anchoring skin graft

Routine dressing

Simple tissue debridement

🚑 19.0   ⚕ 19.0   **FUD** 090   T A2 80 ▱

AMA: 2019,Oct,5; 2018,Jan,8; 2017,Jan,8; 2016,Jan,13; 2015,Jan,16

● New Code   ▲ Revised Code   ○ Reinstated   ● New Web Release   ▲ Revised Web Release   + Add-on   Unlisted   Not Covered   # Resequenced

50 Optum Mod 50 Exempt   ⊘ AMA Mod 51 Exempt   51 Optum Mod 51 Exempt   63 Mod 63 Exempt   ✗ Non-FDA Drug   ★ Telemedicine   M Maternity   A Age Edit

15769 **Grafting of autologous soft tissue, other, harvested by direct excision (eg, fat, dermis, fascia)**

INCLUDES Excisional graft harvest and recipient site placement

EXCLUDES *Autologous grafts specific tissue types, such as skin, bone, nerve, tendon, fascia lata, or vessels*
Autologous white blood cell concentrate injection (0481T)
Harvesting adipose tissue for adipose-derived regenerative cell therapy (0489T-0490T)
Platelet-rich plasma injection (0232T)
Suction assisted lipectomy (15876-15879)

Facility RVU 13.8 | Non-Facility RVU 13.8 | FUD 090 | G2

15771 **Grafting of autologous fat harvested by liposuction technique to trunk, breasts, scalp, arms, and/or legs; 50 cc or less injectate**

INCLUDES Add together injectate volume harvested from each anatomical area indicated in code description, such as face and neck, to report total volume. Do not add together injectate harvested from different anatomical site groups, such as trunk and face
Code based on recipient site

EXCLUDES *Autologous white blood cell concentrate injection (0481T)*
Liposuction not for grafting purposes (15876-15879)
Obtaining tissue for adipose-derived regenerative cell therapy (0489T-0490T)
Platelet-rich plasma injection (0232T)
Subcutaneous injection filling material, at same anatomical site (11950-11954)
Reporting code more than one time per session

Facility RVU 13.7 | Non-Facility RVU 16.5 | FUD 090 | G2

AMA: 2020,Apr,10

+ 15772 **each additional 50 cc injectate, or part thereof (List separately in addition to code for primary procedure)**

Code first (15771)

Facility RVU 4.07 | Non-Facility RVU 5.22 | FUD ZZZ

AMA: 2020,Apr,10

15773 **Grafting of autologous fat harvested by liposuction technique to face, eyelids, mouth, neck, ears, orbits, genitalia, hands, and/or feet; 25 cc or less injectate**

INCLUDES Add together injectate volume harvested from each anatomical area indicated in code description, such as face and neck, to report total volume. Do not add together injectate harvested from different anatomical site groups, such as trunk and face
Code based on recipient site

EXCLUDES *Autologous white blood cell concentrate injection (0481T)*
Liposuction not for grafting purposes (15876-15879)
Obtaining tissue for adipose-derived regenerative cell therapy (0489T-0490T)
Platelet-rich plasma injection (0232T)
Subcutaneous injection filling material, at same anatomical site (11950-11954)
Reporting code more than one time per session

Facility RVU 13.9 | Non-Facility RVU 16.7 | FUD 090 | G2

+ 15774 **each additional 25 cc injectate, or part thereof (List separately in addition to code for primary procedure)**

Code first (15773)

Facility RVU 3.91 | Non-Facility RVU 5.06 | FUD ZZZ

15775-15839 Plastic, Reconstructive, and Aesthetic Surgery

CMS: 100-02,16,10 Exclusions from Coverage; 100-02,16,120 Cosmetic Procedures; 100-02,16,180 Services Related to Noncovered Procedures

15775 **Punch graft for hair transplant; 1 to 15 punch grafts**

EXCLUDES *Strip transplant (15220)*

Facility RVU 6.42 | Non-Facility RVU 8.74 | FUD 000 | T A2 80

AMA: 2018,Jan,8; 2017,Jan,8; 2016,Jan,13; 2015,Jan,16

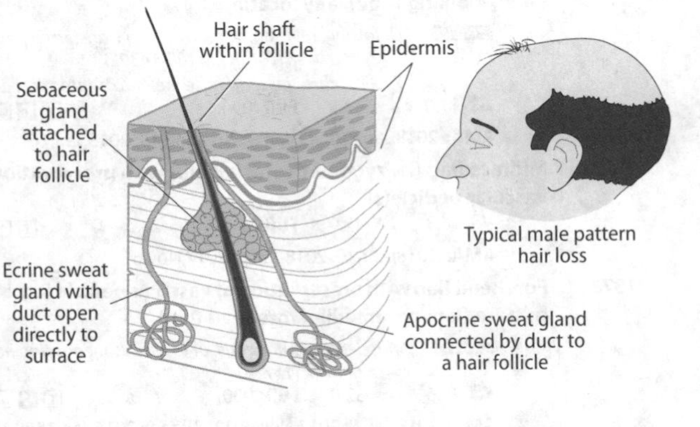

15776 **more than 15 punch grafts**

EXCLUDES *Strip transplant (15220)*

Facility RVU 10.2 | Non-Facility RVU 14.5 | FUD 000 | T A2 80

AMA: 2018,Jan,8; 2017,Jan,8; 2016,Jan,13; 2015,Jan,16

+ 15777 **Implantation of biologic implant (eg, acellular dermal matrix) for soft tissue reinforcement (ie, breast, trunk) (List separately in addition to code for primary procedure)**

EXCLUDES *Application high cost skin substitute to external wound (15271-15278)*
Application low cost skin substitute to external wound (C5271-C5278)
Mesh implantation for:
Open repair ventral or incisional hernia (49560-49566) and (49568)
Repair devitalized soft tissue infection (11004-11006) and (49568)
Repair pelvic floor (57267)
Repair anorectal fistula with plug (46707)
Soft tissue reinforcement with biologic implants other than in the breast or trunk (17999)
Reporting modifier 50 for bilateral breast procedure. Report once for each side when performed bilaterally

Code also supply biologic implant
Code also synthetic or non-biological implant to reinforce abdominal wall (0437T)
Code first primary procedure

Facility RVU 6.25 | Non-Facility RVU 6.25 | FUD ZZZ | N N1 50

AMA: 2019,Nov,14; 2019,Jan,14; 2018,Jan,8; 2017,Jan,8; 2016,Jan,13; 2015,Jan,16

15780 **Dermabrasion; total face (eg, for acne scarring, fine wrinkling, rhytids, general keratosis)**

Facility RVU 19.3 | Non-Facility RVU 25.2 | FUD 090 | J P3 80

AMA: 2018,Jan,8; 2017,Jan,8; 2016,Jan,13; 2015,Jan,16

15781 **segmental, face**

Facility RVU 12.3 | Non-Facility RVU 15.6 | FUD 090 | T P2

AMA: 1997,Nov,1

15782 **regional, other than face**

Facility RVU 11.2 | Non-Facility RVU 15.3 | FUD 090 | J P3 80

AMA: 1997,Nov,1

15783 **superficial, any site (eg, tattoo removal)**

Facility RVU 10.6 | Non-Facility RVU 13.6 | FUD 090 | T P2 80

AMA: 2018,Jan,8; 2017,Jan,8; 2016,Jan,13; 2015,Jan,16

15786 **Abrasion; single lesion (eg, keratosis, scar)**

Facility RVU 3.85 | Non-Facility RVU 6.87 | FUD 010 | Q1 N1

AMA: 1997,Nov,1

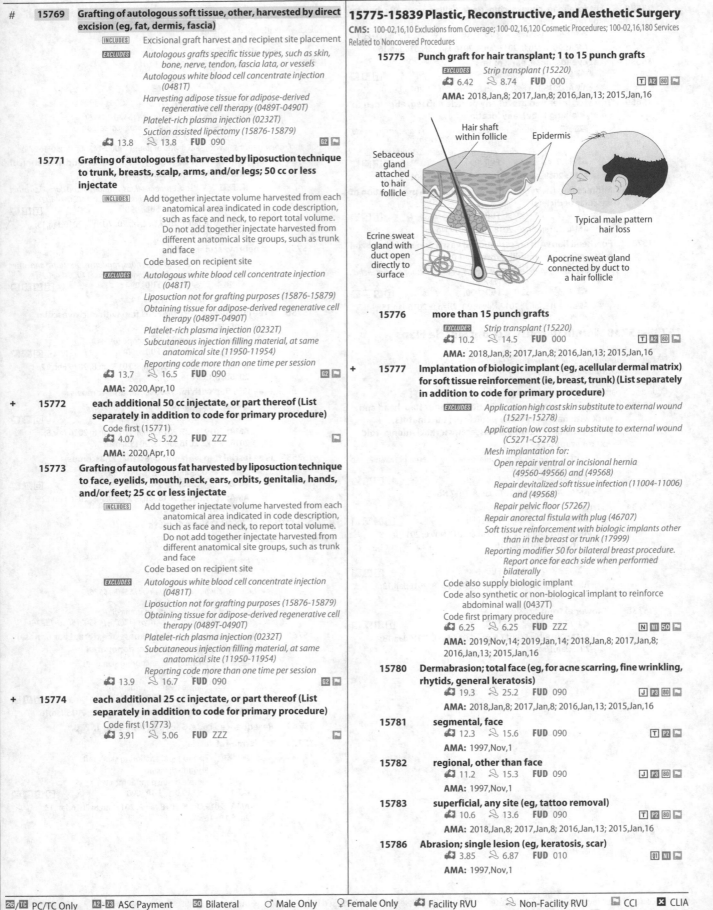

\+ **15787** **each additional 4 lesions or less (List separately in addition to code for primary procedure)**
Code first (15786)
0.50 | 1.27 | FUD ZZZ | N NI
AMA: 1997,Nov,1

15788 **Chemical peel, facial; epidermal**
6.55 | 12.2 | FUD 090 | Q1 NI
AMA: 1997,Nov,1; 1993,Win,1

15789 **dermal**
11.6 | 15.3 | FUD 090 | T P2
AMA: 1997,Nov,1; 1993,Win,1

15792 **Chemical peel, nonfacial; epidermal**
6.61 | 10.9 | FUD 090 | Q1 NI 80
AMA: 1997,Nov,1; 1993,Win,1

15793 **dermal**
10.0 | 13.6 | FUD 090 | Q1 NI 80
AMA: 1997,Nov,1; 1993,Win,1

15819 **Cervicoplasty**
22.7 | 22.7 | FUD 090 | T G2 80
AMA: 1997,Nov,1

15820 **Blepharoplasty, lower eyelid;**
14.5 | 16.2 | FUD 090 | T A2 80 50
AMA: 2018,Jan,8; 2017,Jan,8; 2016,Jan,13; 2015,Jan,16

15821 **with extensive herniated fat pad**
15.5 | 17.4 | FUD 090 | T A2 80 50
AMA: 2018,Jan,8; 2017,Jan,8; 2016,Jan,13; 2015,Jan,16

15822 **Blepharoplasty, upper eyelid;**
11.2 | 12.9 | FUD 090 | T A2 50
AMA: 2018,Jan,8; 2017,Jan,8; 2016,Jan,13; 2015,Jan,16

15823 **with excessive skin weighting down lid**
15.5 | 17.4 | FUD 090 | T A2 50
AMA: 2018,Jan,8; 2017,Jan,8; 2016,Jan,13; 2015,Jan,16

15824 **Rhytidectomy; forehead**
EXCLUDES *Repair brow ptosis (67900)*
0.00 | 0.00 | FUD 000 | T A2 80 50
AMA: 2018,Jan,8; 2017,Apr,9

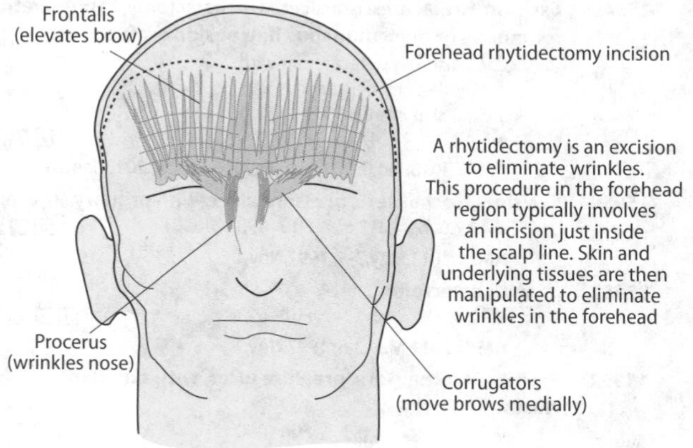

Frontalis
(elevates brow)
Forehead rhytidectomy incision
A rhytidectomy is an excision to eliminate wrinkles. This procedure in the forehead region typically involves an incision just inside the scalp line. Skin and underlying tissues are then manipulated to eliminate wrinkles in the forehead
Procerus
(wrinkles nose)
Corrugators
(move brows medially)

15825 **neck with platysmal tightening (platysmal flap, P-flap)**
0.00 | 0.00 | FUD 000 | T A2 80 50
AMA: 2018,Jan,8; 2017,Apr,9

15826 **glabellar frown lines**
0.00 | 0.00 | FUD 000 | T A2 80 50
AMA: 1997,Nov,1

15828 **cheek, chin, and neck**
0.00 | 0.00 | FUD 000 | T A2 80 50
AMA: 1997,Nov,1

15829 **superficial musculoaponeurotic system (SMAS) flap**
0.00 | 0.00 | FUD 000 | T A2 80 50
AMA: 1997,Nov,1

15830 **Excision, excessive skin and subcutaneous tissue (includes lipectomy); abdomen, infraumbilical panniculectomy**
EXCLUDES *For same wound:*
Adjacent tissue transfer, trunk (14000-14001, 14302)
Complex wound repair, trunk (13100-13102)
Intermediate wound repair, trunk (12031-12032, 12034-12037)
Other abdominoplasty (17999)
Code also, when performed (15847)
33.9 | 33.9 | FUD 090 | J A2 80

15832 **thigh**
26.5 | 26.5 | FUD 090 | J A2 80 50
AMA: 1997,Nov,1

15833 **leg**
25.2 | 25.2 | FUD 090 | J A2 80 50
AMA: 1997,Nov,1

15834 **hip**
25.7 | 25.7 | FUD 090 | J A2 80 50
AMA: 1997,Nov,1

15835 **buttock**
26.9 | 26.9 | FUD 090 | J A2 80
AMA: 1997,Nov,1

15836 **arm**
22.6 | 22.6 | FUD 090 | J A2 80 50
AMA: 1997,Nov,1

15837 **forearm or hand**
20.6 | 24.7 | FUD 090 | J G2 80
AMA: 1997,Nov,1

15838 **submental fat pad**
18.5 | 18.5 | FUD 090 | J G2 80
AMA: 1998,Feb,1; 1997,Nov,1

15839 **other area**
21.2 | 25.4 | FUD 090 | J A2 80
AMA: 1997,Nov,1

15840-15845 Reanimation of the Paralyzed Face

INCLUDES Routine dressing and supplies
EXCLUDES *Intravenous fluorescein evaluation blood flow in graft or flap (15860)*
Nerve:
Decompression (69720, 69725, 69955)
Pedicle transfer (64905, 64907)
Suture (64831-64876, 69740, 69745)
Code also repair donor site with skin grafts or flaps

15840 **Graft for facial nerve paralysis; free fascia graft (including obtaining fascia)**
28.9 | 28.9 | FUD 090 | T A2
AMA: 1997,Nov,1

15841 **free muscle graft (including obtaining graft)**
51.2 | 51.2 | FUD 090 | T A2 80
AMA: 1997,Nov,1

15842 **free muscle flap by microsurgical technique**
INCLUDES Operating microscope (69990)
78.5 | 78.5 | FUD 090 | T G2 80
AMA: 2016,Feb,12

15845 **regional muscle transfer**
28.8 | 28.8 | FUD 090 | T A2 80
AMA: 1998,Feb,1; 1997,Nov,1

15847 Removal of Excess Abdominal Tissue Add-on

CMS: 100-02,16,10 Exclusions from Coverage; 100-02,16,120 Cosmetic Procedures; 100-02,16,180 Services Related to Noncovered Procedures

\+ **15847** **Excision, excessive skin and subcutaneous tissue (includes lipectomy), abdomen (eg, abdominoplasty) (includes umbilical transposition and fascial plication) (List separately in addition to code for primary procedure)**
EXCLUDES *Abdominal wall hernia repair (49491-49587)*
Other abdominoplasty (17999)
Code first (15830)
0.00 | 0.00 | FUD YYY | N NI 80

15850-15852 Suture Removal/Dressing Change: Anesthesia Required

15850 **Removal of sutures under anesthesia (other than local), same surgeon**
Facility RVU 1.14 Non-Facility RVU 2.57 **FUD** XXX T G2 CCI
AMA: 2018,Jan,8; 2017,Jan,8; 2016,Jan,13; 2015,Jan,16

15851 **Removal of sutures under anesthesia (other than local), other surgeon**
Facility RVU 1.31 Non-Facility RVU 2.85 **FUD** 000 T P3 CCI
AMA: 2018,Jan,8; 2017,Jan,8; 2016,Jan,13; 2015,Jan,16

15852 **Dressing change (for other than burns) under anesthesia (other than local)**
EXCLUDES *Dressing change for burns (16020-16030)*
Facility RVU 1.34 Non-Facility RVU 1.34 **FUD** 000 Q1 N1 CCI
AMA: 1997,Nov,1

15860 Injection for Vascular Flow Determination

15860 **Intravenous injection of agent (eg, fluorescein) to test vascular flow in flap or graft**
Facility RVU 3.13 Non-Facility RVU 3.13 **FUD** 000 Q1 N1 80 CCI
AMA: 2002,May,7; 1997,Nov,1

15876-15879 Liposuction

CMS: 100-02,16,10 Exclusions from Coverage; 100-02,16,120 Cosmetic Procedures; 100-02,16,180 Services Related to Noncovered Procedures

EXCLUDES *Liposuction for autologous fat grafting (15771-15774)*
Obtaining tissue for adipose-derived regenerative cell therapy (0489T-0490T)

15876 **Suction assisted lipectomy; head and neck**
Facility RVU 0.00 Non-Facility RVU 0.00 **FUD** 000 T A2 80 CCI
AMA: 2019,Oct,5; 2019,Aug,10; 2018,Sep,12

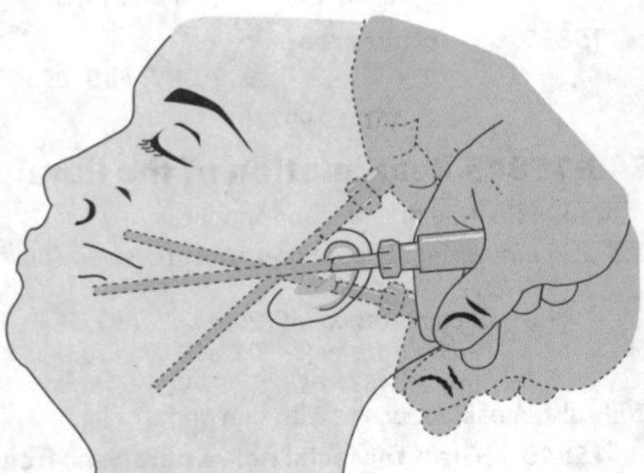

Cannula typically inserted through incision in front of ear

15877 **trunk**
Facility RVU 0.00 Non-Facility RVU 0.00 **FUD** 000 T A2 80 CCI
AMA: 2019,Oct,5; 2019,Aug,10; 2018,Sep,12; 2018,Jan,8; 2017,Jan,8; 2016,Jan,13; 2015,Jan,16

15878 **upper extremity**
Facility RVU 0.00 Non-Facility RVU 0.00 **FUD** 000 T A2 80 50 CCI
AMA: 2019,Oct,5; 2019,Aug,10; 2018,Sep,12

15879 **lower extremity**
Facility RVU 0.00 Non-Facility RVU 0.00 **FUD** 000 T A2 80 50 CCI
AMA: 2019,Oct,5; 2019,Aug,10; 2018,Sep,12

15920-15999 Treatment of Decubitus Ulcers

Code also free skin graft to repair ulcer or donor site

15920 **Excision, coccygeal pressure ulcer, with coccygectomy; with primary suture**
Facility RVU 17.8 Non-Facility RVU 17.8 **FUD** 090 J A2 80 CCI
AMA: 2011,May,3-5; 1997,Nov,1

15922 **with flap closure**
Facility RVU 22.8 Non-Facility RVU 22.8 **FUD** 090 T A2 80 CCI
AMA: 2011,May,3-5; 1997,Nov,1

15931 **Excision, sacral pressure ulcer, with primary suture;**
Facility RVU 20.1 Non-Facility RVU 20.1 **FUD** 090 J A2 CCI
AMA: 2011,May,3-5; 1997,Nov,1

15933 **with ostectomy**
Facility RVU 24.5 Non-Facility RVU 24.5 **FUD** 090 J A2 80 CCI
AMA: 2011,May,3-5; 1997,Nov,1

15934 **Excision, sacral pressure ulcer, with skin flap closure;**
Facility RVU 27.3 Non-Facility RVU 27.3 **FUD** 090 T A2 CCI
AMA: 2011,May,3-5; 1997,Nov,1

15935 **with ostectomy**
Facility RVU 31.6 Non-Facility RVU 31.6 **FUD** 090 T A2 80 CCI
AMA: 2011,May,3-5; 1997,Nov,1

15936 **Excision, sacral pressure ulcer, in preparation for muscle or myocutaneous flap or skin graft closure;**
Code also any defect repair with:
Muscle or myocutaneous flap (15734, 15738)
Split skin graft (15100-15101)
Facility RVU 26.0 Non-Facility RVU 26.0 **FUD** 090 T A2 CCI
AMA: 2011,May,3-5; 1998,Nov,1

15937 **with ostectomy**
Code also any defect repair with:
Muscle or myocutaneous flap (15734, 15738)
Split skin graft (15100-15101)
Facility RVU 30.1 Non-Facility RVU 30.1 **FUD** 090 T A2 CCI
AMA: 2011,May,3-5; 1998,Nov,1

15940 **Excision, ischial pressure ulcer, with primary suture;**
Facility RVU 20.1 Non-Facility RVU 20.1 **FUD** 090 J A2 CCI
AMA: 2011,May,3-5; 1997,Nov,1

15941 **with ostectomy (ischiectomy)**
Facility RVU 26.4 Non-Facility RVU 26.4 **FUD** 090 J A2 80 CCI
AMA: 2011,May,3-5; 1997,Nov,1

15944 **Excision, ischial pressure ulcer, with skin flap closure;**
Facility RVU 26.2 Non-Facility RVU 26.2 **FUD** 090 T A2 80 CCI
AMA: 2011,May,3-5; 1997,Nov,1

15945 **with ostectomy**
Facility RVU 29.3 Non-Facility RVU 29.3 **FUD** 090 T A2 80 CCI
AMA: 2011,May,3-5; 1997,Nov,1

15946 **Excision, ischial pressure ulcer, with ostectomy, in preparation for muscle or myocutaneous flap or skin graft closure**
Code also any defect repair with:
Muscle or myocutaneous flap (15734, 15738)
Split skin graft (15100-15101)
Facility RVU 47.0 Non-Facility RVU 47.0 **FUD** 090 T A2 CCI
AMA: 2018,Jan,8; 2017,Jan,8; 2016,Jan,13; 2015,Jan,16

15950 **Excision, trochanteric pressure ulcer, with primary suture;**
Facility RVU 17.6 Non-Facility RVU 17.6 **FUD** 090 J A2 CCI
AMA: 2011,May,3-5; 1997,Nov,1

15951 **with ostectomy**
Facility RVU 25.2 Non-Facility RVU 25.2 **FUD** 090 J A2 80 CCI
AMA: 2011,May,3-5; 1997,Nov,1

15952 **Excision, trochanteric pressure ulcer, with skin flap closure;**
Facility RVU 26.3 Non-Facility RVU 26.3 **FUD** 090 T A2 80 CCI
AMA: 2011,May,3-5; 1997,Nov,1

15953 **with ostectomy**
Facility RVU 28.9 Non-Facility RVU 28.9 **FUD** 090 T A2 CCI
AMA: 2011,May,3-5; 1997,Nov,1

15956 **Excision, trochanteric pressure ulcer, in preparation for muscle or myocutaneous flap or skin graft closure;**
Code also any defect repair with:
Muscle or myocutaneous flap (15734, 15738)
Split skin graft (15100-15101)
Facility RVU 33.3 Non-Facility RVU 33.3 **FUD** 090 T A2 CCI
AMA: 2011,May,3-5; 1998,Nov,1

15958 **with ostectomy**

Code also any defect repair with:

Muscle or myocutaneous flap (15734-15738)

Split skin graft (15100-15101)

34.0 34.0 **FUD** 090 T A2

AMA: 2011,May,3-5; 1998,Nov,1

15999 **Unlisted procedure, excision pressure ulcer**

0.00 0.00 **FUD** YYY T 80

AMA: 2011,May,3-5; 1997,Nov,1

16000-16036 Burn Care

INCLUDES Local care burn surface only

EXCLUDES *Application skin grafts and flaps including all services described in:(15100-15777)*

E/M services

Laser fenestration for scars (0479T-0480T)

16000 **Initial treatment, first degree burn, when no more than local treatment is required**

1.33 2.09 **FUD** 000 Q1 N1

AMA: 2018,Jan,8; 2017,Jan,8; 2016,Jan,13; 2015,Jan,16

16020 **Dressings and/or debridement of partial-thickness burns, initial or subsequent; small (less than 5% total body surface area)**

INCLUDES Wound coverage other than skin graft

1.56 2.35 **FUD** 000 Q1 N1

AMA: 2018,Jan,8; 2017,Jan,8; 2016,Jan,13; 2015,Jan,16

16025 **medium (eg, whole face or whole extremity, or 5% to 10% total body surface area)**

INCLUDES Wound coverage other than skin graft

3.16 4.26 **FUD** 000 T A2

AMA: 2018,Jan,8; 2017,Jan,8; 2016,Jan,13; 2015,Jan,16

16030 **large (eg, more than 1 extremity, or greater than 10% total body surface area)**

INCLUDES Wound coverage other than skin graft

3.84 5.54 **FUD** 000 T A2

AMA: 2018,Jan,8; 2017,Jan,8; 2016,Jan,13; 2015,Jan,16

16035 **Escharotomy; initial incision**

EXCLUDES *Debridement scraping of burn (16020-16030)*

5.71 5.71 **FUD** 000 T G2

AMA: 2018,Jan,8; 2017,Jan,8; 2016,Jan,13; 2015,Jan,16

+ **16036** **each additional incision (List separately in addition to code for primary procedure)**

EXCLUDES *Debridement or scraping burn (16020-16030)*

Code first (16035)

2.37 2.37 **FUD** ZZZ C

AMA: 2018,Jan,8; 2017,Jan,8; 2016,Jan,13; 2015,Jan,16

17000-17004 Destruction Any Method: Premalignant Lesion

CMS: 100-03,140.5 Laser Procedures

EXCLUDES *Cryotherapy acne (17340)*

Destruction, skin:

Benign lesions other than cutaneous vascular proliferative lesions (17110-17111)

Cutaneous vascular proliferative lesions (17106-17108)

Malignant lesions (17260-17286)

Destruction lesion:

Anus (46900-46917, 46924)

Conjunctiva (68135)

Eyelid (67850)

Penis (54050-54057, 54065)

Vagina (57061, 57065)

Vestibule of mouth (40820)

Vulva (56501, 56515)

Destruction or excision skin tags (11200-11201)

Escharotomy (16035-16036)

Excision benign lesion (11400-11446)

Laser fenestration for scars (0479T-0480T)

Localized chemotherapy treatment see appropriate office visit service code

Paring or excision benign hyperkeratotic lesion (11055-11057)

Shaving skin lesions (11300-11313)

Treatment inflammatory skin disease via laser (96920-96922)

17000 **Destruction (eg, laser surgery, electrosurgery, cryosurgery, chemosurgery, surgical curettement), premalignant lesions (eg, actinic keratoses); first lesion**

1.53 1.85 **FUD** 010 Q1 N1

AMA: 2018,Jan,8; 2017,Dec,14; 2017,Jan,8; 2016,Apr,3; 2016,Jan,13; 2015,Jan,16

+ **17003** **second through 14 lesions, each (List separately in addition to code for first lesion)**

Code first (17000)

0.06 0.17 **FUD** ZZZ N N1

AMA: 2018,Jan,8; 2017,Dec,14; 2017,Jan,8; 2016,Apr,3; 2016,Jan,13; 2015,Jan,16

17004 **Destruction (eg, laser surgery, electrosurgery, cryosurgery, chemosurgery, surgical curettement), premalignant lesions (eg, actinic keratoses), 15 or more lesions**

EXCLUDES *Reporting code for destruction less than 15 lesions (17000-17003)*

2.79 4.48 **FUD** 010 T P3

AMA: 2018,Jan,8; 2017,Dec,14; 2017,Jan,8; 2016,Apr,3; 2016,Jan,13; 2015,Jan,16

17106-17250 Destruction Any Method: Vascular Proliferative Lesion

CMS: 100-02,16,10 Exclusions from Coverage; 100-02,16,120 Cosmetic Procedures

EXCLUDES *Cryotherapy acne (17340)*

Destruction, skin:

Malignant lesions (17260-17286)

Premalignant lesions (17000-17004)

Destruction lesion:

Anus (46900-46917, 46924)

Conjunctiva (68135)

Eyelid (67850)

Penis (54050-54057, 54065)

Vagina (57061, 57065)

Vestibule of mouth (40820)

Vulva (56501, 56515)

Destruction or excision skin tags (11200-11201)

Escharotomy (16035-16036)

Excision benign lesion (11400-11446)

Laser fenestration for scars (0479T-0480T)

Localized chemotherapy treatment see appropriate office visit service code

Paring or excision benign hyperkeratotic lesion (11055-11057)

Shaving skin lesions (11300-11313)

Treatment inflammatory skin disease via laser (96920-96922)

17106 **Destruction of cutaneous vascular proliferative lesions (eg, laser technique); less than 10 sq cm**

7.84 9.72 **FUD** 090 T P2

AMA: 2019,Sep,10; 2018,Jan,8; 2017,Dec,14; 2017,Jan,8; 2016,Apr,3; 2016,Jan,13; 2015,Jan,16

17107 **10.0 to 50.0 sq cm**
10.1 12.7 FUD 090 T P2
AMA: 2018,Jan,8; 2017,Dec,14; 2017,Jan,8; 2016,Apr,3; 2016,Jan,13; 2015,Jan,16

17108 **over 50.0 sq cm**
15.0 18.1 FUD 090 T P3 80
AMA: 2018,Jan,8; 2017,Dec,14; 2017,Jan,8; 2016,Apr,3; 2016,Jan,13; 2015,Jan,16

17110 **Destruction (eg, laser surgery, electrosurgery, cryosurgery, chemosurgery, surgical curettement), of benign lesions other than skin tags or cutaneous vascular proliferative lesions; up to 14 lesions**
1.91 3.17 FUD 010 Q1 N1
AMA: 2020,Apr,10; 2018,Jan,8; 2017,Dec,14; 2017,Jan,8; 2016,Apr,3; 2016,Jan,13; 2015,Jan,16

17111 **15 or more lesions**
EXCLUDES *Destruction neurofibromas, 50-100 lesions (0419T-0420T)*
2.34 3.72 FUD 010 Q1 N1
AMA: 2018,Jan,8; 2017,Dec,14; 2017,Jan,8; 2016,Apr,3; 2016,Jan,13; 2015,Jan,16

17250 **Chemical cauterization of granulation tissue (ie, proud flesh)**
EXCLUDES *Excision/removal codes for same lesion*
Chemical cauterization when applied for wound hemostasis
Wound care management (97597-97598, 97602)
1.05 2.31 FUD 000 Q1 N1
AMA: 2018,Jan,8; 2017,Dec,14; 2017,Jan,8; 2016,Jan,13; 2015,Jan,16

17260-17286 Destruction, Any Method: Malignant Lesion

CMS: 100-03,140.5 Laser Procedures

EXCLUDES *Cryotherapy acne (17340)*
Destruction, skin:
Benign lesions other than cutaneous vascular proliferative lesions (17110-17111)
Cutaneous vascular proliferative lesions (17106-17108)
Premalignant lesions (17000-17004)
Destruction lesion:
Anus (46900-46917, 46924)
Conjunctiva (68135)
Eyelid (67850)
Penis (54050-54057, 54065)
Vestibule of mouth (40820)
Vulva (56501-56515)
Destruction or excision skin tags (11200-11201)
Escharotomy (16035-16036)
Excision benign lesion (11400-11446)
Laser fenestration for scars (0479T-0480T)
Localized chemotherapy treatment see appropriate office visit service code
Paring or excision benign hyperkeratotic lesion (11055-11057)
Shaving skin lesion (11300-11313)
Treatment inflammatory skin disease via laser (96920-96922)

17260 **Destruction, malignant lesion (eg, laser surgery, electrosurgery, cryosurgery, chemosurgery, surgical curettement), trunk, arms or legs; lesion diameter 0.5 cm or less**
2.03 2.71 FUD 010 Q1 N1
AMA: 2018,Jan,8; 2017,Dec,14; 2017,Jan,8; 2016,Jan,13; 2015,Jan,16

17261 **lesion diameter 0.6 to 1.0 cm**
2.58 4.11 FUD 010 Q1 N1
AMA: 2018,Jan,8; 2017,Dec,14; 2017,Jan,8; 2016,Jan,13; 2015,Jan,16

17262 **lesion diameter 1.1 to 2.0 cm**
3.30 5.01 FUD 010 Q1 N1
AMA: 2018,Jan,8; 2017,Dec,14; 2017,Jan,8; 2016,Jan,13; 2015,Jan,16

17263 **lesion diameter 2.1 to 3.0 cm**
3.55 5.45 FUD 010 Q1 N1
AMA: 2018,Jan,8; 2017,Dec,14; 2017,Jan,8; 2016,Jan,13; 2015,Jan,16

17264 **lesion diameter 3.1 to 4.0 cm**
3.79 5.84 FUD 010 T P3
AMA: 2018,Jan,8; 2017,Dec,14; 2017,Jan,8; 2016,Jan,13; 2015,Jan,16

17266 **lesion diameter over 4.0 cm**
4.47 6.66 FUD 010 T P3
AMA: 2018,Jan,8; 2017,Dec,14; 2017,Jan,8; 2016,Jan,13; 2015,Jan,16

17270 **Destruction, malignant lesion (eg, laser surgery, electrosurgery, cryosurgery, chemosurgery, surgical curettement), scalp, neck, hands, feet, genitalia; lesion diameter 0.5 cm or less**
2.74 4.22 FUD 010 T P2
AMA: 2018,Jan,8; 2017,Dec,14; 2017,Jan,8; 2016,Jan,13; 2015,Jan,16

17271 **lesion diameter 0.6 to 1.0 cm**
3.14 4.67 FUD 010 T P2
AMA: 2018,Jan,8; 2017,Dec,14; 2017,Jan,8; 2016,Jan,13; 2015,Jan,16

17272 **lesion diameter 1.1 to 2.0 cm**
3.52 5.32 FUD 010 Q1 N1
AMA: 2018,Jan,8; 2017,Dec,14; 2017,Jan,8; 2016,Jan,13; 2015,Jan,16

17273 **lesion diameter 2.1 to 3.0 cm**
4.11 5.94 FUD 010 T P3
AMA: 2018,Jan,8; 2017,Dec,14; 2017,Jan,8; 2016,Jan,13; 2015,Jan,16

17274 **lesion diameter 3.1 to 4.0 cm**
4.88 6.97 FUD 010 T P3
AMA: 2018,Jan,8; 2017,Dec,14; 2017,Jan,8; 2016,Jan,13; 2015,Jan,16

17276 **lesion diameter over 4.0 cm**
5.86 8.07 FUD 010 T P2
AMA: 2018,Jan,8; 2017,Dec,14; 2017,Jan,8; 2016,Jan,13; 2015,Jan,16

17280 **Destruction, malignant lesion (eg, laser surgery, electrosurgery, cryosurgery, chemosurgery, surgical curettement), face, ears, eyelids, nose, lips, mucous membrane; lesion diameter 0.5 cm or less**
2.48 3.94 FUD 010 Q1 N1
AMA: 2018,Jan,8; 2017,Dec,14; 2017,Jan,8; 2016,Jan,13; 2015,Jan,16

17281 **lesion diameter 0.6 to 1.0 cm**
3.54 5.09 FUD 010 T P3
AMA: 2018,Jan,8; 2017,Dec,14; 2017,Jan,8; 2016,Jan,13; 2015,Jan,16

17282 **lesion diameter 1.1 to 2.0 cm**
3.97 5.82 FUD 010 T P3
AMA: 2018,Jan,8; 2017,Dec,14; 2017,Jan,8; 2016,Jan,13; 2015,Jan,16

17283 **lesion diameter 2.1 to 3.0 cm**
4.97 6.94 FUD 010 T P3
AMA: 2018,Jan,8; 2017,Dec,14; 2017,Jan,8; 2016,Jan,13; 2015,Jan,16

17284 **lesion diameter 3.1 to 4.0 cm**
5.80 7.90 FUD 010 T P3
AMA: 2018,Jan,8; 2017,Dec,14; 2017,Jan,8; 2016,Jan,13; 2015,Jan,16

17286 **lesion diameter over 4.0 cm**
7.86 10.1 FUD 010 T P3
AMA: 2018,Jan,8; 2017,Dec,14; 2017,Jan,8; 2016,Jan,13; 2015,Jan,16

17311-17315 Mohs Surgery

INCLUDES Surgical/pathology services performed by same physician or other qualified health care provider:
- Evaluation skin margins by surgeon
- Pathology exam on Mohs surgery specimen (by Mohs surgeon) (88302-88309)
- Routine frozen section stain (88314)
- Tumor removal, mapping, preparation, and examination lesion

EXCLUDES *Frozen section if no prior diagnosis determination has been performed (88331)*

Code also any special histochemical stain on frozen section, nonroutine (with modifier 59) (88311-88314, 88342)
Code also biopsy (with modifier 59) when no prior diagnosis determination has been performed, biopsy indeterminate, or performed more than 90 days preoperatively (11102, 11104, 11106)
Code also complex repair (13100-13160)
Code also flaps or grafts (14000-14350, 15050-15770)
Code also intermediate repair (12031-12057)
Code also simple repair (12001-12021)

17311 Mohs micrographic technique, including removal of all gross tumor, surgical excision of tissue specimens, mapping, color coding of specimens, microscopic examination of specimens by the surgeon, and histopathologic preparation including routine stain(s) (eg, hematoxylin and eosin, toluidine blue), head, neck, hands, feet, genitalia, or any location with surgery directly involving muscle, cartilage, bone, tendon, major nerves, or vessels; first stage, up to 5 tissue blocks
10.4 18.8 FUD 000 T P2
AMA: 2018,Jan,8; 2017,Jan,8; 2016,Jan,13; 2015,Jan,16

+ **17312 each additional stage after the first stage, up to 5 tissue blocks (List separately in addition to code for primary procedure)**
Code first (17311)
5.76 11.2 FUD ZZZ N N1
AMA: 2018,Jan,8; 2017,Jan,8; 2016,Jan,13; 2015,Jan,16

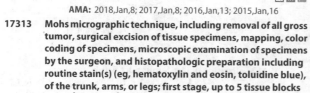

17313 Mohs micrographic technique, including removal of all gross tumor, surgical excision of tissue specimens, mapping, color coding of specimens, microscopic examination of specimens by the surgeon, and histopathologic preparation including routine stain(s) (eg, hematoxylin and eosin, toluidine blue), of the trunk, arms, or legs; first stage, up to 5 tissue blocks
9.34 17.6 FUD 000 T P2
AMA: 2018,Jan,8; 2017,Jan,8; 2016,Jan,13; 2015,Jan,16

+ **17314 each additional stage after the first stage, up to 5 tissue blocks (List separately in addition to code for primary procedure)**
Code first (17313)
5.14 10.8 FUD ZZZ N N1
AMA: 2018,Jan,8; 2017,Jan,8; 2016,Jan,13; 2015,Jan,16

+ **17315 Mohs micrographic technique, including removal of all gross tumor, surgical excision of tissue specimens, mapping, color coding of specimens, microscopic examination of specimens by the surgeon, and histopathologic preparation including routine stain(s) (eg, hematoxylin and eosin, toluidine blue), each additional block after the first 5 tissue blocks, any stage (List separately in addition to code for primary procedure)**
Code first (17311-17314)
1.47 2.22 FUD ZZZ N N1
AMA: 2018,Jan,8; 2017,Jan,8; 2016,Jan,13; 2015,Jan,16

17340-17999 Treatment for Active Acne and Permanent Hair Removal

CMS: 100-02,16,10 Exclusions from Coverage; 100-02,16,120 Cosmetic Procedures

17340 Cryotherapy (CO2 slush, liquid N2) for acne
1.40 1.49 FUD 010 Q1 N1
AMA: 2018,Jan,8; 2017,Jan,8; 2016,Jan,13; 2015,Jan,16

17360 Chemical exfoliation for acne (eg, acne paste, acid)
2.77 3.61 FUD 010 Q1 N1
AMA: 2018,Jan,8; 2017,Jan,8; 2016,Jan,13; 2015,Jan,16

17380 Electrolysis epilation, each 30 minutes
EXCLUDES *Actinotherapy (96900)*
0.00 0.00 FUD 000 T R2 80
AMA: 2018,Jan,8; 2017,Jan,8; 2016,Jan,13; 2015,Jan,16

17999 Unlisted procedure, skin, mucous membrane and subcutaneous tissue
0.00 0.00 FUD YYY Q1 80
AMA: 2019,Sep,10; 2019,Mar,10; 2019,Jan,14; 2018,Jan,8; 2017,Dec,13; 2017,Jan,8; 2016,May,13; 2016,Jan,13; 2015,Jan,16

19000-19030 Treatment of Breast Abscess and Cyst with Injection, Aspiration, Incision

19000 Puncture aspiration of cyst of breast;
(76942, 77021)
1.26 3.11 FUD 000 T P3
AMA: 2018,Jan,8; 2017,Jan,8; 2016,Jan,13; 2015,Jan,16

+ **19001 each additional cyst (List separately in addition to code for primary procedure)**
Code first (19000)
(76942, 77021)
0.62 0.77 FUD ZZZ N N1
AMA: 2018,Jan,8; 2017,Jan,8; 2016,Jan,13; 2015,Jan,16

19020 Mastotomy with exploration or drainage of abscess, deep
8.93 13.5 FUD 090 J A2 50
AMA: 2018,Jan,8; 2017,Jan,8; 2016,Jan,13; 2015,Jan,16

19030 Injection procedure only for mammary ductogram or galactogram
(77053-77054)
2.23 4.74 FUD 000 N N1 50
AMA: 2018,Jan,8; 2017,Jan,8; 2016,Jan,13; 2015,Jan,16

19081-19086 Breast Biopsy with Imaging Guidance

CMS: 100-03,220.13 Percutaneous Image-guided Breast Biopsy; 100-04,12,40.7 Bilateral Procedures; 100-04,13,80.1 Physician Presence; 100-04,13,80.2 S&I Multiple Procedure Reduction

INCLUDES Breast biopsy with placement localization devices
- Fluoroscopic guidance for needle placement (77002)
- Magnetic resonance guidance for needle placement (77021)
- Radiological examination, surgical specimen (76098)
- Ultrasonic guidance for needle placement (76942)

EXCLUDES *Biopsy breast without imaging guidance (19100-19101)*
- *Lesion removal without concentration on surgical margins (19110-19126)*
- *Open biopsy after placement localization device (19101)*
- *Partial mastectomy (19301-19302)*
- *Placement localization devices only (19281-19288)*
- *Total mastectomy (19303-19307)*

Code also additional biopsies performed with different imaging modalities

19081 Biopsy, breast, with placement of breast localization device(s) (eg, clip, metallic pellet), when performed, and imaging of the biopsy specimen, when performed, percutaneous; first lesion, including stereotactic guidance
4.82 17.3 FUD 000 J G2 80 50
AMA: 2019,Apr,4; 2018,Jan,8; 2017,Jan,8; 2016,Jun,3; 2016,Jan,13; 2015,May,8; 2015,Mar,5; 2015,Jan,16

+ **19082 each additional lesion, including stereotactic guidance (List separately in addition to code for primary procedure)**
Code first (19081)
2.42 13.9 FUD ZZZ N N1 80
AMA: 2019,Apr,4; 2018,Jan,8; 2017,Jan,8; 2016,Jun,3; 2016,Jan,13; 2015,May,8; 2015,Mar,5; 2015,Jan,16

19083 Biopsy, breast, with placement of breast localization device(s) (eg, clip, metallic pellet), when performed, and imaging of the biopsy specimen, when performed, percutaneous; first lesion, including ultrasound guidance
4.56 17.1 FUD 000 J G2 80 50
AMA: 2019,Apr,4; 2018,Jan,8; 2017,Jan,8; 2016,Jun,3; 2016,Jan,13; 2015,May,8; 2015,Mar,5; 2015,Jan,16

+ **19084** **each additional lesion, including ultrasound guidance (List separately in addition to code for primary procedure)**
Code first (19083)
2.25 13.6 FUD ZZZ N N1 80
AMA: 2019,Apr,4; 2018,Jan,8; 2017,Jan,8; 2016,Jun,3; 2016,Jan,13; 2015,May,8; 2015,Mar,5; 2015,Jan,16

19085 **Biopsy, breast, with placement of breast localization device(s) (eg, clip, metallic pellet), when performed, and imaging of the biopsy specimen, when performed, percutaneous; first lesion, including magnetic resonance guidance**
5.28 26.1 FUD 000 J G2 80 50
AMA: 2019,Apr,4; 2018,Jan,8; 2017,Jan,8; 2016,Jun,3; 2016,Jan,13; 2015,May,8; 2015,Mar,5; 2015,Jan,16

+ **19086** **each additional lesion, including magnetic resonance guidance (List separately in addition to code for primary procedure)**
Code first (19085)
2.65 21.9 FUD ZZZ N N1 80
AMA: 2019,Apr,4; 2018,Jan,8; 2017,Jan,8; 2016,Jun,3; 2016,Jan,13; 2015,May,8; 2015,Mar,5; 2015,Jan,16

19100-19101 Breast Biopsy Without Imaging Guidance

EXCLUDES *Biopsy breast with imaging guidance (19081-19086)*
Lesion removal without concentration on surgical margins (19110-19126)
Partial mastectomy (19301-19302)
Total mastectomy (19303-19307)

19100 **Biopsy of breast; percutaneous, needle core, not using imaging guidance (separate procedure)**
EXCLUDES *Fine needle aspiration:*
With imaging guidance ([10005, 10006, 10007, 10008, 10009, 10010, 10011, 10012])
Without imaging guidance (10021, [10004])
2.03 4.32 FUD 000 J A2 50
AMA: 2018,Jan,8; 2017,Jan,8; 2016,Jan,13; 2015,Jan,16

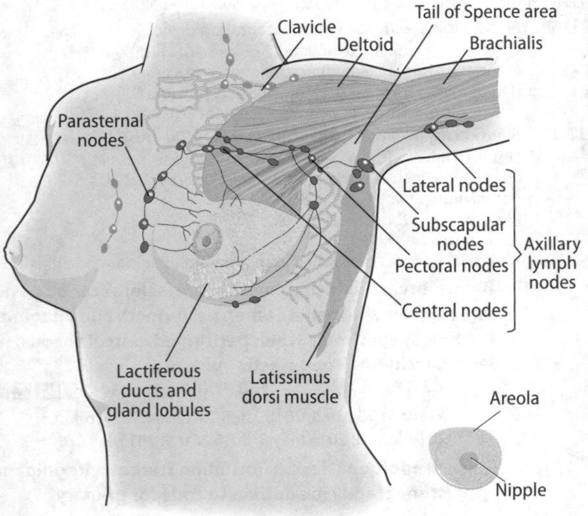

19101 **open, incisional**
Code also placement localization device with imaging guidance (19281-19288)
6.45 9.62 FUD 010 J A2 50
AMA: 2018,Jan,8; 2017,Jan,8; 2016,Jan,13; 2015,Jan,16

19105 Treatment of Fibroadenoma: Cryoablation

CMS: 100-04,13,80.1 Physician Presence; 100-04,13,80.2 S&I Multiple Procedure Reduction

INCLUDES Adjacent lesions treated with one cryoprobe
Ultrasound guidance (76940, 76942)

EXCLUDES *Cryoablation malignant breast tumors (0581T)*

19105 **Ablation, cryosurgical, of fibroadenoma, including ultrasound guidance, each fibroadenoma**
6.14 77.6 FUD 000 J G2 50
AMA: 2007,Mar,7-8

19110-19126 Excisional Procedures: Breast

INCLUDES Open removal breast mass without concentration on surgical margins
Code also placement localization device with imaging guidance (19281-19288)

19110 **Nipple exploration, with or without excision of a solitary lactiferous duct or a papilloma lactiferous duct**
9.94 13.9 FUD 090 J A2 50
AMA: 2018,Jan,8; 2017,Jan,8; 2016,Jan,13; 2015,Jan,16

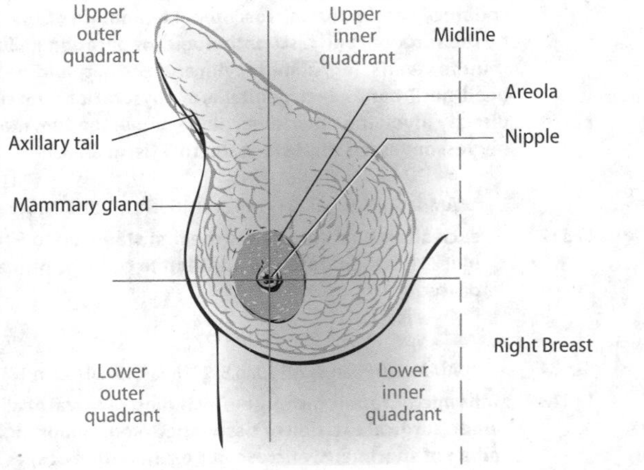

19112 **Excision of lactiferous duct fistula**
9.12 13.2 FUD 090 J A2 80 50
AMA: 2018,Jan,8; 2017,Jan,8; 2016,Jan,13; 2015,Jan,16

19120 **Excision of cyst, fibroadenoma, or other benign or malignant tumor, aberrant breast tissue, duct lesion, nipple or areolar lesion (except 19300), open, male or female, 1 or more lesions**
12.0 14.5 FUD 090 J A2 50
AMA: 2018,Jan,8; 2017,Jan,8; 2016,Jan,13; 2015,Mar,5; 2015,Jan,16

19125 **Excision of breast lesion identified by preoperative placement of radiological marker, open; single lesion**
INCLUDES Intraoperative clip placement
13.2 15.8 FUD 090 J A2 50
AMA: 2018,Jan,8; 2017,Jan,8; 2016,Jan,13; 2015,Mar,5; 2015,Jan,16

+ **19126** **each additional lesion separately identified by a preoperative radiological marker (List separately in addition to code for primary procedure)**
INCLUDES Intraoperative clip placement
Code first (19125)
4.68 4.68 FUD ZZZ N N1
AMA: 2018,Jan,8; 2017,Jan,8; 2016,Jan,13; 2015,Jan,16

19281-19288 Placement of Localization Markers

INCLUDES Placement localization devices only

EXCLUDES *Biopsy breast without imaging guidance (19100-19101)*
When performed on same lesion:
Fluoroscopic guidance for needle placement (77002)
Localization device placement with biopsy breast (19081-19086)
Magnetic resonance guidance for needle placement (77021)
Ultrasonic guidance for needle placement (76942)

Code also open excision of breast lesion when performed after localization device placement (19110-19126)
Code also open incisional breast biopsy when performed after localization device placement (19101)
Code also radiography surgical specimen (76098)

19281 **Placement of breast localization device(s) (eg, clip, metallic pellet, wire/needle, radioactive seeds), percutaneous; first lesion, including mammographic guidance**
2.91 6.90 **FUD** 000 Q1 N1 80 50
AMA: 2018,Jan,8; 2017,Jan,8; 2016,Jun,3; 2016,Jan,13; 2015,May,8; 2015,Jan,16

\+ **19282** **each additional lesion, including mammographic guidance (List separately in addition to code for primary procedure)**
Code first (19281)
1.46 4.92 **FUD** ZZZ N N1 80
AMA: 2018,Jan,8; 2017,Jan,8; 2016,Jun,3; 2016,Jan,13; 2015,May,8; 2015,Jan,16

19283 **Placement of breast localization device(s) (eg, clip, metallic pellet, wire/needle, radioactive seeds), percutaneous; first lesion, including stereotactic guidance**
2.93 7.74 **FUD** 000 Q1 N1 80 50
AMA: 2018,Jan,8; 2017,Jan,8; 2016,Jun,3; 2016,May,13; 2016,Jan,13; 2015,May,8; 2015,Jan,16

\+ **19284** **each additional lesion, including stereotactic guidance (List separately in addition to code for primary procedure)**
Code first (19283)
1.49 5.90 **FUD** ZZZ N N1 80
AMA: 2018,Jan,8; 2017,Jan,8; 2016,Jun,3; 2016,May,13; 2016,Jan,13; 2015,May,8; 2015,Jan,16

19285 **Placement of breast localization device(s) (eg, clip, metallic pellet, wire/needle, radioactive seeds), percutaneous; first lesion, including ultrasound guidance**
2.49 12.9 **FUD** 000 Q1 N1 80 50
AMA: 2018,Jan,8; 2017,Jan,8; 2016,Jun,3; 2016,May,13; 2016,Jan,13; 2015,May,8; 2015,Jan,16

\+ **19286** **each additional lesion, including ultrasound guidance (List separately in addition to code for primary procedure)**
Code first (19285)
1.25 11.9 **FUD** ZZZ N N1 80
AMA: 2018,Jan,8; 2017,Jan,8; 2016,Jun,3; 2016,May,13; 2016,Jan,13; 2015,May,8; 2015,Jan,16

19287 **Placement of breast localization device(s) (eg clip, metallic pellet, wire/needle, radioactive seeds), percutaneous; first lesion, including magnetic resonance guidance**
3.72 22.1 **FUD** 000 Q1 N1 80 50
AMA: 2018,Jan,8; 2017,Jan,8; 2016,Jun,3; 2016,May,13; 2016,Jan,13; 2015,Jan,16

\+ **19288** **each additional lesion, including magnetic resonance guidance (List separately in addition to code for primary procedure)**
Code first (19287)
1.87 18.6 **FUD** ZZZ N N1 80
AMA: 2018,Jan,8; 2017,Jan,8; 2016,Jun,3; 2016,May,13; 2016,Jan,13; 2015,Jan,16

19294-19298 Radioelement Application

\+ **19294** **Preparation of tumor cavity, with placement of a radiation therapy applicator for intraoperative radiation therapy (IORT) concurrent with partial mastectomy (List separately in addition to code for primary procedure)**
Code first (19301-19302)
4.71 4.71 **FUD** ZZZ N N1 80
AMA: 2020,May,9

19296 **Placement of radiotherapy afterloading expandable catheter (single or multichannel) into the breast for interstitial radioelement application following partial mastectomy, includes imaging guidance; on date separate from partial mastectomy**
6.11 114. **FUD** 000 J J8 80 50
AMA: 2020,May,9; 2018,Jan,8; 2017,Jan,8; 2016,Jan,13; 2015,Jan,16

\+ **19297** **concurrent with partial mastectomy (List separately in addition to code for primary procedure)**
Code first (19301-19302)
2.75 2.75 **FUD** ZZZ N N1 80
AMA: 2020,May,9; 2019,Apr,10; 2018,Jan,8; 2017,Jan,8; 2016,Jan,13; 2015,Jan,16

19298 **Placement of radiotherapy after loading brachytherapy catheters (multiple tube and button type) into the breast for interstitial radioelement application following (at the time of or subsequent to) partial mastectomy, includes imaging guidance**
9.22 28.4 **FUD** 000 J G2 80 50
AMA: 2020,May,9; 2018,Jan,8; 2017,Jan,8; 2016,Jan,13; 2015,Jan,16

19300-19307 Mastectomies: Partial, Simple, Radical

CMS: 100-04,12,40.7 Bilateral Procedures

INCLUDES Intraoperative clip placement

EXCLUDES *Insertion prosthesis (19340, 19342)*

19300 **Mastectomy for gynecomastia** ♂
EXCLUDES *Removal breast tissue for:*
Other than gynecomastia (19318)
Treatment or prevention breast cancer (19301-19307)
12.1 15.8 **FUD** 090 J A2 50
AMA: 2020,May,9; 2018,Jan,8; 2017,Jan,8; 2016,Jan,13; 2015,Jan,16

19301 **Mastectomy, partial (eg, lumpectomy, tylectomy, quadrantectomy, segmentectomy);**
EXCLUDES *Insertion radiotherapy afterloading balloon during separate encounter (19296)*
Code also intraoperative radiofrequency spectroscopy margin assessment and report (0546T)
Code also insertion radiotherapy afterloading balloon catheter, when performed at same time (19297)
Code also insertion radiotherapy afterloading brachytherapy catheter, when performed at same time (19298)
Code also tumor cavity preparation with intraoperative radiation therapy applicator, when performed (19294)
19.0 19.0 **FUD** 090 J A2 80 50
AMA: 2020,May,9; 2018,Jan,8; 2017,Oct,9; 2017,Jan,8; 2016,Jan,13; 2015,Mar,5; 2015,Jan,16

19302 **with axillary lymphadenectomy**
EXCLUDES *Insertion radiotherapy afterloading balloon during separate encounter (19296)*
Code also intraoperative radiofrequency spectroscopy margin assessment and report (0546T)
Code also insertion radiotherapy afterloading balloon catheter, when performed at same time (19297)
Code also insertion radiotherapy afterloading brachytherapy catheter, when performed at same time (19298)
Code also tumor cavity preparation with intraoperative radiation therapy applicator, when performed (19294)
25.9 25.9 **FUD** 090 J A2 80 50
AMA: 2020,May,9; 2019,Feb,8; 2018,Jan,8; 2017,Jan,8; 2016,Jan,13; 2015,Mar,5; 2015,Jan,16

19303 Mastectomy, simple, complete

EXCLUDES *Excision pectoral muscles and axillary or internal mammary lymph nodes*
Removal breast tissue for:
Gynecomastia (19300)
Other than gynecomastia (19318)

27.6 27.6 FUD 090 J A2 80 50

AMA: 2020,May,9; 2019,Dec,4; 2018,Jan,8; 2017,Jan,8; 2016,Jan,13; 2015,Mar,5; 2015,Jan,16

19305 Mastectomy, radical, including pectoral muscles, axillary lymph nodes

33.0 33.0 FUD 090 C 80 50

AMA: 2020,May,9; 2018,Jan,8; 2017,Jan,8; 2016,Jan,13; 2015,Jan,16

19306 Mastectomy, radical, including pectoral muscles, axillary and internal mammary lymph nodes (Urban type operation)

34.7 34.7 FUD 090 C 80 50

AMA: 2020,May,9; 2018,Jan,8; 2017,Jan,8; 2016,Jan,13; 2015,Jan,16

19307 Mastectomy, modified radical, including axillary lymph nodes, with or without pectoralis minor muscle, but excluding pectoralis major muscle

34.6 34.6 FUD 090 J 80 50

AMA: 2020,May,9; 2019,Feb,8; 2018,Jan,8; 2017,Jan,8; 2016,Jan,13; 2015,Mar,5; 2015,Jan,16

19316-19499 Plastic, Reconstructive, and Aesthetic Breast Procedures

CMS: 100-03,140.2 Breast Reconstruction Following Mastectomy; 100-04,12,40.7 Bilateral Procedures

Code also biologic implant for tissue reinforcement (15777)

19316 Mastopexy

22.3 22.3 FUD 090 J A2 80 50

AMA: 2018,Jan,8; 2017,Jan,8; 2016,Jan,13; 2015,Jan,16

▲ **19318 Breast reduction**

INCLUDES Aries-Pitanguy mammaplasty
Biesenberger mammaplasty

31.5 31.5 FUD 090 J A2 80 50

AMA: 2020,May,9; 2018,Jan,8; 2017,Jan,8; 2016,Jan,13; 2015,Jan,16

19324 ~~**Mammaplasty, augmentation; without prosthetic implant**~~

To report, see (15771-15772)

▲ **19325 Breast augmentation with implant**

EXCLUDES *Flap or graft (15100-15650)*

Code also fat grafting, when performed (15771-15772)

18.6 18.6 FUD 090 J G2 80 50

AMA: 2018,Jan,8; 2017,Jan,8; 2016,Jan,13; 2015,Jan,16

▲ **19328 Removal of intact breast implant**

EXCLUDES *Removal tissue expander (11970-11971)*
Revision peri-implant capsule, breast (19370)

14.4 14.4 FUD 090 Q2 A2 50

AMA: 2018,Jan,8; 2017,Jan,8; 2016,Jan,13; 2015,Jan,16

▲ **19330 Removal of ruptured breast implant, including implant contents (eg, saline, silicone gel)**

EXCLUDES *Insertion new breast implant during same operative session (19342)*
Removal ruptured tissue expander (11970-11971)

18.3 18.3 FUD 090 Q2 A2 50

AMA: 2018,Jan,8; 2017,Jan,8; 2016,Jan,13; 2015,Jan,16

▲ **19340 Insertion of breast implant on same day of mastectomy (ie, immediate)**

EXCLUDES *Preparation moulage for custom breast implant (19396)*
Supply prosthetic implant (99070, C1789, L8600)

28.6 28.6 FUD 090 J A2 50

AMA: 2020,May,9; 2018,Jan,8; 2017,Jan,8; 2016,Jan,13; 2015,Dec,18; 2015,Jan,16

▲ **19342 Insertion or replacement of breast implant on separate day from mastectomy**

EXCLUDES *Preparation moulage for custom breast implant (19396)*
Removal intact breast implant (19328)
Removal tissue expander with insertion breast implant (11970)
Supply prosthetic implant (99070, C1789, L8600)

26.7 26.7 FUD 090 J A2 80 50

AMA: 2020,May,9; 2018,Jan,8; 2017,Jan,8; 2016,Jan,13; 2015,Nov,10; 2015,Jan,16

19350 Nipple/areola reconstruction

INCLUDES Adjacent tissue transfer, trunk (14000-14001)
Full-thickness graft, trunk (15200-15201)
Split-thickness autograft, trunk, arms, legs (15100)
Tattooing to correct skin color defects (11920-11922)

19.4 23.8 FUD 090 J A2 50

AMA: 2018,Jan,8; 2017,Jan,8; 2016,Aug,9; 2016,Jan,13; 2015,Jan,16

19355 Correction of inverted nipples

17.8 21.7 FUD 090 J A2 80 50

AMA: 2018,Jan,8; 2017,Jan,8; 2016,Jan,13; 2015,Jan,16

▲ **19357 Tissue expander placement in breast reconstruction, including subsequent expansion(s)**

43.1 43.1 FUD 090 J J8 80 50

AMA: 2018,Jan,8; 2017,Jan,8; 2016,Jan,13; 2015,Feb,10; 2015,Jan,16

▲ **19361 Breast reconstruction; with latissimus dorsi flap**

INCLUDES Closure donor site
Harvesting skin graft
Inset shaping flap into breast

EXCLUDES *Implant prosthesis with latissimus dorsi implant:*
performed different day than mastectomy (19342)
performed same day as mastectomy (19340)
Insertion tissue expander with latissimus dorsi flap (19357)

45.4 45.4 FUD 090 C 80 50

AMA: 2019,Nov,14; 2018,Jan,8; 2017,Jan,8; 2016,Jan,13; 2015,Feb,10; 2015,Jan,16

▲ **19364 with free flap (eg, fTRAM, DIEP, SIEA, GAP flap)**

INCLUDES Closure donor site
Harvesting skin graft
Inset shaping flap into breast
Microvascular repair
Operating microscope (69990)

79.7 79.7 FUD 090 C 80 50

AMA: 2019,Nov,14; 2018,Jan,8; 2017,Jan,8; 2016,Feb,12; 2016,Jan,13; 2015,Feb,10; 2015,Jan,16

19366 ~~**Breast reconstruction with other technique**~~

▲ **19367 with single-pedicled transverse rectus abdominis myocutaneous (TRAM) flap**

INCLUDES Closure donor site
Harvesting skin graft
Inset shaping flap into breast

51.5 51.5 FUD 090 C 80 50

AMA: 2019,Nov,14; 2018,Jan,8; 2017,Jan,8; 2016,Jan,13; 2015,Feb,10; 2015,Jan,16

▲ **19368 with single-pedicled transverse rectus abdominis myocutaneous (TRAM) flap, requiring separate microvascular anastomosis (supercharging)**

INCLUDES Closure donor site
Harvesting skin graft
Inset shaping flap into breast
Operating microscope (69990)

63.2 63.2 FUD 090 C 80 50

AMA: 2019,Nov,14; 2018,Jan,8; 2017,Jan,8; 2016,Feb,12; 2016,Jan,13; 2015,Feb,10; 2015,Jan,16

▲ **19369 with bipedicled transverse rectus abdominis myocutaneous (TRAM) flap**

INCLUDES Closure donor site
Harvesting skin graft
Inset shaping flap into breast

59.0 59.0 **FUD** 090 C 80 50

AMA: 2019,Nov,14; 2018,Jan,8; 2017,Jan,8; 2016,Jan,13; 2015,Feb,10; 2015,Jan,16

▲ **19370 Revision of peri-implant capsule, breast, including capsulotomy, capsulorrhaphy, and/or partial capsulectomy**

EXCLUDES *Removal and replacement with new implant (19342)*
Removal intact breast implant (19328)

19.9 19.9 **FUD** 090 J A2 50

AMA: 2018,Jan,8; 2017,Jan,8; 2016,Jan,13; 2015,Dec,18; 2015,Jan,16

▲ **19371 Peri-implant capsulectomy, breast, complete, including removal of all intracapsular contents**

EXCLUDES *Removal and replacement with new implant (19342)*
Removal intact breast implant (19328)
Removal ruptured breast implant (19330)
Revision peri-implant capsule on same breast (19370)

22.5 22.5 **FUD** 090 J A2 50

AMA: 2018,Jan,8; 2017,Jan,8; 2016,Jan,13; 2015,Jan,16

▲ **19380 Revision of reconstructed breast (eg, significant removal of tissue, re-advancement and/or re-inset of flaps in autologous reconstruction or significant capsular revision combined with soft tissue excision in implant-based reconstruction)**

INCLUDES Removal portion or reshaping flap
Revision flap position on chest wall
Revision scar(s)
When performed on same breast:
Breast reduction (19318)
Mastopexy (19316)
Repair complex, trunk (13100-13102)
Repair intermediate, trunk (12031-12037)
Revision peri-implant capsule, breast (19370)
Suction assisted lipectomy; trunk (15877)

EXCLUDES *Autologuous fat graft (15771-15772)*
Implant replacement (19342)

22.4 22.4 **FUD** 090 J A2 50

AMA: 2019,Nov,14; 2018,Jan,8; 2017,Dec,13; 2017,Jan,8; 2016,Jan,13; 2015,Dec,18; 2015,Jan,16

19396 Preparation of moulage for custom breast implant

4.17 8.23 **FUD** 000 J G2 80 50

AMA: 2018,Jan,8; 2017,Jan,8; 2016,Jan,13; 2015,Jan,16

19499 Unlisted procedure, breast

0.00 0.00 **FUD** YYY J 80 50

AMA: 2019,Aug,10; 2019,Apr,10; 2018,Jan,8; 2017,Jan,8; 2016,Dec,16; 2016,Jan,13; 2015,Mar,5; 2015,Jan,16

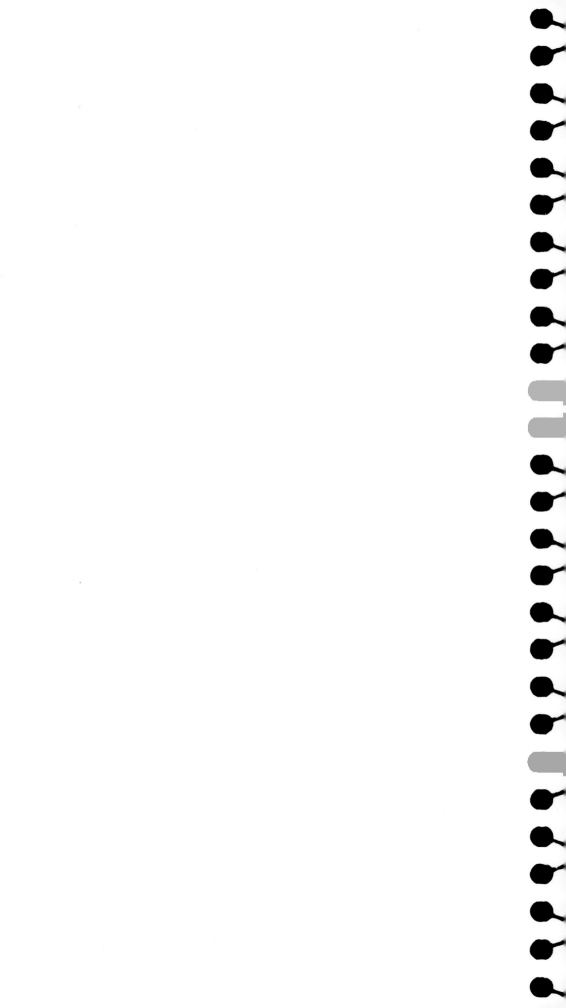

20100-20103 Exploratory Surgery of Traumatic Wound

INCLUDES Debridement
Expanded dissection wound for exploration
Extraction foreign material
Open examination
Tying or coagulation small vessels

EXCLUDES *Cutaneous/subcutaneous incision and drainage procedures (10060-10061)*
Laparotomy (49000-49010)
Repair major vessels:
Abdomen (35221, 35251, 35281)
Chest (35211, 35216, 35241, 35246, 35271, 35276)
Extremity (35206-35207, 35226, 35236, 35256, 35266, 35286)
Neck (35201, 35231, 35261)
Thoracotomy (32100-32160)

20100 Exploration of penetrating wound (separate procedure); neck
17.4 17.4 FUD 010 T 80 50
AMA: 2018,Jan,8; 2017,Jan,8; 2016,Jan,13; 2015,Jan,16

20101 chest
6.10 13.7 FUD 010 T
AMA: 2018,Jan,8; 2017,Jan,8; 2016,Jan,13; 2015,Jan,16

20102 abdomen/flank/back
7.39 14.0 FUD 010 T
AMA: 2020,Jan,6; 2018,Jan,8; 2017,Jan,8; 2016,Jan,13; 2015,Jan,16

20103 extremity
10.0 16.5 FUD 010 T G2 80
AMA: 2018,Jan,8; 2017,Jan,8; 2016,Jan,13; 2015,Jan,16

20150 Epiphyseal Bar Resection

20150 Excision of epiphyseal bar, with or without autogenous soft tissue graft obtained through same fascial incision
29.0 29.0 FUD 090 J G2 80 50
AMA: 1996,Nov,1

20200-20206 Muscle Biopsy

EXCLUDES *Removal of muscle tumor (see appropriate anatomic section)*

20200 Biopsy, muscle; superficial
2.73 6.07 FUD 000 J A2

20205 deep
4.44 8.47 FUD 000 J A2

20206 Biopsy, muscle, percutaneous needle
EXCLUDES *Fine needle aspiration (10021, [10004, 10005, 10006, 10007, 10008, 10009, 10010, 10011, 10012])*
(76942, 77002, 77012, 77021)
(88172-88173)
1.67 6.76 FUD 000 J A2
AMA: 2019,Apr,4

20220-20225 Percutaneous Bone Biopsy

EXCLUDES *Bone marrow aspiration(s) or biopsy(ies) (38220-38222)*

20220 Biopsy, bone, trocar, or needle; superficial (eg, ilium, sternum, spinous process, ribs)
(77002, 77012, 77021)
2.55 7.04 FUD 000 J A2
AMA: 2018,Jan,8; 2017,Jan,8; 2016,Jan,13; 2015,Jan,16

20225 deep (eg, vertebral body, femur)
EXCLUDES *When performed at same level:*
Percutaneous vertebroplasty (22510-22515)
Percutaneous sacral augmentation (sacroplasty) (0200T-0201T)
(77002, 77012, 77021)
3.07 14.7 FUD 000 J A2
AMA: 2018,Jan,8; 2017,Jan,8; 2016,Jan,13; 2015,Jan,8; 2015,Jan,16

20240-20251 Open Bone Biopsy

EXCLUDES *Sequestrectomy or incision and drainage of bone abscess of:*
Calcaneus (28120)
Carpal bone (25145)
Clavicle (23170)
Humeral head (23174)
Humerus (24134)
Olecranon process (24138)
Radius (24136, 25145)
Scapula (23172)
Skull (61501)
Talus (28120)
Ulna (24138, 24145)

20240 Biopsy, bone, open; superficial (eg, sternum, spinous process, rib, patella, olecranon process, calcaneus, tarsal, metatarsal, carpal, metacarpal, phalanx)
4.21 4.21 FUD 000 J A2
AMA: 2018,Jan,8; 2017,Jan,8; 2016,Jan,13; 2015,Jan,16

20245 deep (eg, humeral shaft, ischium, femoral shaft)
10.1 10.1 FUD 000 J A2
AMA: 2018,Jan,8; 2017,Jan,8; 2016,Jan,13; 2015,Jan,16

20250 Biopsy, vertebral body, open; thoracic
11.3 11.3 FUD 010 J A2
AMA: 2018,Jan,8; 2017,Jan,8; 2016,Jan,13; 2015,Jan,16

20251 lumbar or cervical
12.4 12.4 FUD 010 J A2 80
AMA: 2018,Jan,8; 2017,Jan,8; 2016,Jan,13; 2015,Jan,16

20500-20501 Injection Fistula/Sinus Tract

EXCLUDES *Arthrography injection of:*
Ankle (27648)
Elbow (24220)
Hip (27093, 27095)
Sacroiliac joint (27096)
Shoulder (23350)
Temporomandibular joint (TMJ) (21116)
Wrist (25246)
Autologous adipose-derived regenerative cells injection (0489T-0490T)

20500 Injection of sinus tract; therapeutic (separate procedure)
(76080)
2.49 3.25 FUD 010 T P3

20501 diagnostic (sinogram)
EXCLUDES *Contrast injection or injections for radiological evaluation existing gastrostomy, duodenostomy, jejunostomy, gastro-jejunostomy, or cecostomy (or other colonic) tube from percutaneous approach (49465)*
(76080)
1.09 3.62 FUD 000 N N1

20520-20525 Foreign Body Removal

20520 Removal of foreign body in muscle or tendon sheath; simple
4.22 6.03 FUD 010 J P3

20525 deep or complicated
7.11 13.6 FUD 010 J A2

20526-20561 [20560, 20561] Therapeutic Injections: Tendons, Trigger Points

20526 Injection, therapeutic (eg, local anesthetic, corticosteroid), carpal tunnel
1.66 2.20 FUD 000 T P3 50
AMA: 2018,Jan,8; 2017,Jan,8; 2016,Jan,13; 2015,Jan,16

20527 Injection, enzyme (eg, collagenase), palmar fascial cord (ie, Dupuytren's contracture)
EXCLUDES *Post injection palmar fascial cord manipulation (26341)*
1.90 2.39 FUD 000 T P3 50
AMA: 2018,Jan,8; 2017,Jan,8; 2016,Jan,13; 2015,Jan,16

20550 **Injection(s); single tendon sheath, or ligament, aponeurosis (eg, plantar "fascia")**

EXCLUDES *Autologous WBC injection (0481T)*
Morton's neuroma (64455, 64632)
Platelet rich plasma injection (0232T)

(76942, 77002, 77021)

1.13 1.51 FUD 000 T P3 50

AMA: 2018,Jan,8; 2017,Jan,8; 2016,Jan,13; 2015,Jan,16

20551 **single tendon origin/insertion**

EXCLUDES *Autologous WBC injection (0481T)*
Platelet rich plasma injection (0232T)

(76942, 77002, 77021)

1.15 1.60 FUD 000 T P3

AMA: 2018,Jan,8; 2017,Dec,13; 2017,Jan,8; 2016,Jan,13; 2015,Jan,16

20552 **Injection(s); single or multiple trigger point(s), 1 or 2 muscle(s)**

EXCLUDES *Autologous WBC injection (0481T)*
Needle insertion(s) without injection(s) for same muscle(s) ([20560, 20561])
Platelet rich plasma injection (0232T)

(76942, 77002, 77021)

1.11 1.59 FUD 000 T P3

AMA: 2020,Feb,9; 2018,Jan,8; 2017,Dec,13; 2017,Jun,10; 2017,Jan,8; 2016,Jan,13; 2015,Jan,16

20553 **single or multiple trigger point(s), 3 or more muscles**

EXCLUDES *Needle insertion(s) without injection(s) for same muscle(s) ([20560, 20561])*

(76942, 77002, 77021)

1.25 1.82 FUD 000 T P3

AMA: 2020,Feb,9; 2018,Dec,8; 2018,Dec,8; 2018,Jan,8; 2017,Jun,10; 2017,Jan,8; 2016,Jan,13; 2015,Jan,16

20560 **Needle insertion(s) without injection(s); 1 or 2 muscle(s)**

INCLUDES Dry needling and trigger-point acupuncture

0.47 0.74 FUD XXX

AMA: 2020,Feb,9

20561 **3 or more muscles**

INCLUDES Dry needling and trigger-point acupuncture

0.71 1.10 FUD XXX

AMA: 2020,Feb,9

20555-20561 [20560, 20561] Placement of Catheters/Needles for Brachytherapy

Code also interstitial radioelement application (77770-77772, 77778)

20555 **Placement of needles or catheters into muscle and/or soft tissue for subsequent interstitial radioelement application (at the time of or subsequent to the procedure)**

EXCLUDES *Interstitial radioelement:*
Devices placed into breast (19296-19298)
Placement needle, catheters, or devices into muscle or soft tissue head and neck (41019)
Placement needles or catheters into pelvic organs or genitalia (55920)
Placement needles or catheters into prostate (55875)

(76942, 77002, 77012, 77021)

9.49 9.49 FUD 000 J R2 80

AMA: 2018,Jan,8; 2017,Jan,8; 2016,Jan,13; 2015,Jan,16

20560 **Resequenced code. See code following 20553.**

20561 **Resequenced code. See code before 20555.**

20600-20611 Aspiration and/or Injection of Joint

CMS: 100-03,150.7 Prolotherapy, Joint Sclerotherapy, and Ligamentous Injections with Sclerosing Agents

20600 **Arthrocentesis, aspiration and/or injection, small joint or bursa (eg, fingers, toes); without ultrasound guidance**

EXCLUDES *Autologous adipose-derived regenerative cells injection (0489T-0490T)*
Platelet rich plasma (PRP) injections (0232T)
Ultrasound guidance (76942)

(77002, 77012, 77021)

1.04 1.44 FUD 000 T P3 50

AMA: 2018,Sep,12; 2018,Jan,8; 2017,Aug,9; 2017,Jan,8; 2016,Jan,13; 2015,Nov,10; 2015,Feb,6; 2015,Jan,16

20604 **with ultrasound guidance, with permanent recording and reporting**

INCLUDES Ultrasound guidance (76942)

EXCLUDES *Autologous adipose-derived regenerative cells injection (0489T-0490T)*
Platelet rich plasma (PRP) injections (0232T)

(77002, 77012, 77021)

1.32 2.17 FUD 000 T P3 50

AMA: 2018,Sep,12; 2018,Jan,8; 2017,Jan,8; 2016,Jan,13; 2015,Jul,10; 2015,Feb,6

20605 **Arthrocentesis, aspiration and/or injection, intermediate joint or bursa (eg, temporomandibular, acromioclavicular, wrist, elbow or ankle, olecranon bursa); without ultrasound guidance**

EXCLUDES *Ultrasound guidance (76942)*

(77002, 77012, 77021)

1.08 1.49 FUD 000 T P3 50

AMA: 2018,Jan,8; 2017,Aug,9; 2017,Jan,8; 2016,Jan,13; 2015,Nov,10; 2015,Feb,6; 2015,Jan,16

20606 **with ultrasound guidance, with permanent recording and reporting**

INCLUDES Ultrasound guidance (76942)

EXCLUDES *Platelet rich plasma (PRP) injections (0232T)*

(77002, 77012, 77021)

1.53 2.32 FUD 000 T P3 50

AMA: 2018,Jan,8; 2017,Jan,8; 2016,Jan,13; 2015,Jul,10; 2015,Feb,6

20610 **Arthrocentesis, aspiration and/or injection, major joint or bursa (eg, shoulder, hip, knee, subacromial bursa); without ultrasound guidance**

EXCLUDES *Injection contrast for knee arthrography (27369)*
Platelet rich plasma (PRP) injections (0232T)
Ultrasound guidance (76942)

(77002, 77012, 77021)

1.32 1.77 FUD 000 T P3 50

AMA: 2019,Aug,7; 2018,Jan,8; 2017,Apr,9; 2017,Jan,8; 2016,Jan,13; 2015,Nov,10; 2015,Aug,6; 2015,Feb,6; 2015,Jan,16

20611 **with ultrasound guidance, with permanent recording and reporting**

INCLUDES Ultrasound guidance (76942)

EXCLUDES *Injection contrast for knee arthrography (27369)*
Platelet rich plasma (PRP) injections (0232T)

(77002, 77012, 77021)

1.75 2.61 FUD 000 T P3 50

AMA: 2019,Aug,7; 2018,Jan,8; 2017,Jan,8; 2016,Jan,13; 2015,Nov,10; 2015,Aug,6; 2015,Jul,10; 2015,Feb,6

20612-20615 Aspiration and/or Injection of Cyst

20612 **Aspiration and/or injection of ganglion cyst(s) any location**

Code also modifier 59 for multiple ganglion aspirations or injections

1.19 1.76 FUD 000 T P3

20615 **Aspiration and injection for treatment of bone cyst**

4.60 7.10 FUD 010 T P3

26/TC PC/TC Only A2-Z3 ASC Payment 50 Bilateral ♂ Male Only ♀ Female Only Facility RVU Non-Facility RVU CCI CLIA
FUD Follow-up Days CMS: IOM AMA: CPT Asst A-Y OPPSI 80/80 Surg Assist Allowed / w/Doc Lab Crosswalk Radiology Crosswalk

40

20650-20697 Procedures Related to Bony Fixation

20650 **Insertion of wire or pin with application of skeletal traction, including removal (separate procedure)**
4.54 6.08 FUD 010 J A2

20660 **Application of cranial tongs, caliper, or stereotactic frame, including removal (separate procedure)**
7.00 7.00 FUD 000 Q2
AMA: 2018,Jan,8; 2017,Jan,8; 2016,Jan,13; 2015,Jan,16

20661 **Application of halo, including removal; cranial**
14.4 14.4 FUD 090 C
AMA: 2018,Jan,8; 2017,Jan,8; 2016,Jan,13; 2015,Jan,16

20662 **pelvic**
14.8 14.8 FUD 090 J R2 80

20663 **femoral**
13.6 13.6 FUD 090 J R2 80 50

20664 **Application of halo, including removal, cranial, 6 or more pins placed, for thin skull osteology (eg, pediatric patients, hydrocephalus, osteogenesis imperfecta)**
25.0 25.0 FUD 090 C
AMA: 2018,Jan,8; 2017,Jan,8; 2016,Jan,13; 2015,Jan,16

20665 **Removal of tongs or halo applied by another individual**
2.65 3.13 FUD 010 Q1 G2 80
AMA: 2018,Jan,8; 2017,Jan,8; 2016,Jan,13; 2015,Jan,16

20670 **Removal of implant; superficial (eg, buried wire, pin or rod) (separate procedure)**
4.18 10.5 FUD 010 Q2 A2
AMA: 2018,Jan,3; 2018,Jan,8; 2017,Jan,8; 2016,Jan,13; 2015,Jan,16

20680 **deep (eg, buried wire, pin, screw, metal band, nail, rod or plate)**
EXCLUDES *Removal and reinsertion sinus tarsi implant ([0511T])*
Removal sinus tarsi implant ([0510T])
12.1 17.6 FUD 090 Q2 A2 80
AMA: 2018,Jan,3; 2018,Jan,8; 2017,Jan,8; 2016,Nov,9; 2016,Jan,13; 2015,Nov,10; 2015,Jan,16

20690 **Application of a uniplane (pins or wires in 1 plane), unilateral, external fixation system**
17.2 17.2 FUD 090 J J8
AMA: 2018,Jan,3; 2018,Jan,8; 2017,Jan,8; 2016,Jan,13; 2015,Jan,16

20692 **Application of a multiplane (pins or wires in more than 1 plane), unilateral, external fixation system (eg, Ilizarov, Monticelli type)**
32.2 32.2 FUD 090 J J8 80
AMA: 2019,May,10; 2018,Jan,8; 2018,Jan,3; 2017,Jan,8; 2016,Jan,13; 2015,Jan,16

20693 **Adjustment or revision of external fixation system requiring anesthesia (eg, new pin[s] or wire[s] and/or new ring[s] or bar[s])**
12.7 12.7 FUD 090 J A2
AMA: 2018,Jan,3; 2018,Jan,8; 2017,Jan,8; 2016,Jan,13; 2015,Jan,16

20694 **Removal, under anesthesia, of external fixation system**
9.72 12.2 FUD 090 Q2 A2
AMA: 2018,Jan,3; 2018,Jan,8; 2017,Jan,8; 2016,Jan,13; 2015,Jan,16

20696 **Application of multiplane (pins or wires in more than 1 plane), unilateral, external fixation with stereotactic computer-assisted adjustment (eg, spatial frame), including imaging; initial and subsequent alignment(s), assessment(s), and computation(s) of adjustment schedule(s)**
EXCLUDES *Application multiplane external fixation system (20692)*
Osteotomy with insertion intramedullary lengthening device, humerus (0594T)
Removal and replacement each strut (20697)
34.4 34.4 FUD 090 J J8 80
AMA: 2018,Jan,3; 2018,Jan,8; 2017,Jan,8; 2016,Jan,13; 2015,Jan,16

20697 **exchange (ie, removal and replacement) of strut, each**
EXCLUDES *Application multiplane external fixation system (20692)*
Exchange strut for multiplane external fixation system (20697)
58.9 58.9 FUD 000 ⊘ J P2 80 TC
AMA: 2018,Jan,3; 2018,Jan,8; 2017,Jan,8; 2016,Jan,13; 2015,Jan,16

20700-20705 Drug Delivery Device

\+ **20700** **Manual preparation and insertion of drug-delivery device(s), deep (eg, subfascial) (List separately in addition to code for primary procedure)**
INCLUDES Combining therapeutic agents, including antibiotics, with carrier substance during operative episode
Forming resulting mixture into drug delivery devices (beads, nails, spacers)
Insertion therapeutic device/agent once per anatomic location
EXCLUDES *Insertion drug delivery implant, non-biodegradable (11981)*
Insertion prefabricated drug device
Code first (11010-11012, 11043, [11046], 11044, 11047, 20240-20251, 21010, 21025-21026, 21501-21510, 21627-21630, 22010-22015, 23030-23044, 23170-23184, 23334-23335, 23930-24000, 24134-24140, 24147, 24160, 25031-25040, 25145-25151, 26070, 26230-26236, 26990-26992, 27030, 27070-27071, 27090, 27301-27303, 27310, 27360, 27603-27604, 27610, 27640-27641, 28001-28003, 28020, 28120-28122)
2.44 2.44 FUD ZZZ 80

\+ **20701** **Removal of drug-delivery device(s), deep (eg, subfascial) (List separately in addition to code for primary procedure)**
INCLUDES Removal therapeutic device/agent once per anatomic location from subfascial tissues
EXCLUDES *Removal drug delivery device, performed alone (20680)*
Removal drug delivery implant, non-biodegradable (11982)
Code first (11010-11012, 11043, [11046], 11044, 11047, 20240-20251, 21010, 21025-21026, 21501-21510, 21627-21630, 22010-22015, 23030-23044, 23170-23184, 23334-23335, 23930-24000, 24134-24140, 24147, 24160, 25031-25040, 25145-25151, 26070, 26230-26236, 26990-26992, 27030, 27070-27071, 27090, 27301-27303, 27310, 27360, 27603-27604, 27610, 27640-27641, 28001-28003, 28020, 28120-28122)
1.82 1.82 FUD ZZZ 80

+ **20702 Manual preparation and insertion of drug-delivery device(s), intramedullary (List separately in addition to code for primary procedure)**

INCLUDES Combining therapeutic agents, including antibiotics, with carrier substance during operative episode
Forming resulting mixture into drug delivery devices (beads, nails, spacers)
Insertion therapeutic device/agent once per anatomic location into intramedullary spaces

EXCLUDES *Insertion drug delivery implant, non-biodegradable (11981)*
Insertion prefabricated drug device

Code first (20680-20692, 20694, 20802-20805, 20838, 21510, 23035, 23170, 23180, 23184, 23515, 23615, 23935, 24134, 24138-24140, 24147, 24430, 24516, 25035, 25145-25151, 25400, 25515, 25525-25526, 25545, 25574-25575, 27245, 27259, 27360, 27470, 27506, 27640, 27720)

4.06 4.06 FUD ZZZ 80

+ **20703 Removal of drug-delivery device(s), intramedullary (List separately in addition to code for primary procedure)**

INCLUDES Removal therapeutic device/agent once per anatomic location from intramedullary spaces

EXCLUDES *Removal drug delivery device, performed alone (20680)*
Removal drug delivery implant, non-biodegradable (11982)

Code first (20690-20692, 20694, 20802-20805, 20838, 21510, 23035, 23170, 23180, 23184, 23515, 23615, 23935, 24134, 24138-24140, 24147, 24430, 24516, 25035, 25145-25151, 25400, 25515, 25525-25526, 25545, 25574-25575, 27245, 27259, 27360, 27470, 27506, 27640, 27720)

2.91 2.91 FUD ZZZ 80

+ **20704 Manual preparation and insertion of drug-delivery device(s), intra-articular (List separately in addition to code for primary procedure)**

INCLUDES Combining therapeutic agents, including antibiotics, with carrier substance during operative episode
Forming resulting mixture into drug delivery devices (beads, nails, spacers)
Insertion therapeutic device/agent once per anatomic location into intra-articular spaces

EXCLUDES *Insertion drug delivery implant, non-biodegradable (11981)*
Insertion prefabricated drug device
Removal hip prosthesis (27091)
Removal knee prosthesis (27488)

Code first (22864-22865, 23040-23044, 23334, 24000, 24160, 25040, 25250-25251, 26070-26080, 26990, 27030, 27090, 27301, 27310, 27603, 27610, 28020)

4.23 4.23 FUD ZZZ 80

+ **20705 Removal of drug-delivery device(s), intra-articular (List separately in addition to code for primary procedure)**

INCLUDES Removal therapeutic device/agent once per anatomic location from intra-articular space(s)

EXCLUDES *Open treatment femoral neck fracture/internal fixation or prosthetic replacement (27236)*
Partial knee replacement (27446)
Partial or total hip replacement (27125-27130)
Patella arthroplasty with prosthesis (27438)
Removal drug delivery device, performed alone (20680)
Removal drug delivery implant, non-biodegradable (11982)
Removal hip prosthesis (27091)
Removal knee prosthesis (27488)
Removal shoulder prosthesis (23335)
Revision hip arthroplasty (27134-27138)
Revision knee arthroplasty (27486-27487)

Code first (22864-22865, 23040-23044, 23334, 24000, 24160, 25040, 25250-25251, 26070-26080, 26990, 27030, 27090, 27301, 27310, 27603, 27610, 28020)

3.48 3.48 FUD ZZZ 80

20802-20838 Reimplantation Procedures

EXCLUDES *Repair incomplete amputation (see individual repair codes for bone(s), ligament(s), tendon(s), nerve(s), or blood vessel(s) and append modifier 52)*

20802 Replantation, arm (includes surgical neck of humerus through elbow joint), complete amputation
79.5 79.5 FUD 090 C 80 50
AMA: 1997,Apr,4

20805 Replantation, forearm (includes radius and ulna to radial carpal joint), complete amputation
94.7 94.7 FUD 090 C 80 50
AMA: 1997,Apr,4

20808 Replantation, hand (includes hand through metacarpophalangeal joints), complete amputation
114. 114. FUD 090 C 80 50
AMA: 1997,Apr,4

20816 Replantation, digit, excluding thumb (includes metacarpophalangeal joint to insertion of flexor sublimis tendon), complete amputation
59.5 59.5 FUD 090 C 80
AMA: 2018,Jan,8; 2017,Jan,8; 2016,Jan,13; 2015,Jan,16

20822 Replantation, digit, excluding thumb (includes distal tip to sublimis tendon insertion), complete amputation
51.2 51.2 FUD 090 J G2 80
AMA: 1997,Apr,4

20824 Replantation, thumb (includes carpometacarpal joint to MP joint), complete amputation
59.7 59.7 FUD 090 C 80 50
AMA: 1997,Apr,4

20827 Replantation, thumb (includes distal tip to MP joint), complete amputation
52.6 52.6 FUD 090 C 80 50
AMA: 1997,Apr,4

20838 Replantation, foot, complete amputation
80.6 80.6 FUD 090 C 80 50
AMA: 1997,Apr,4

20900-20924 Bone and Tissue Autografts

EXCLUDES *Acquisition autogenous bone, bone marrow, cartilage, tendon, fascia lata or other grafts through distinct incision unless included in code description*
Autologous fat graft obtained by liposuction (15771-15774)
Bone graft procedures on spine (20930-20938)
Other autologous soft tissue grafts (fat, dermis, fascia) harvested by direct excision ([15769])

20900 Bone graft, any donor area; minor or small (eg, dowel or button)
5.33 11.6 FUD 000 J A2 80
AMA: 2020,May,13; 2018,Jul,14; 2018,Jan,8; 2017,Jan,8; 2016,Jan,13; 2015,Jan,16

20902 major or large
8.20 8.20 FUD 000 J A2 80
AMA: 2020,May,13; 2018,Jul,14; 2018,Jan,8; 2017,Jan,8; 2016,Jan,13; 2015,Jan,16

20910 Cartilage graft; costochondral
EXCLUDES *Graft with ear cartilage (21235)*
13.5 13.5 FUD 090 T A2 80
AMA: 2020,May,13; 2018,Jul,14; 2018,Jan,8; 2017,Jan,8; 2016,Jan,13; 2015,Jan,16

20912 nasal septum
EXCLUDES *Graft with ear cartilage (21235)*
13.6 13.6 FUD 090 T A2 80
AMA: 2020,May,13; 2018,Jul,14

20920 Fascia lata graft; by stripper
11.3 11.3 FUD 090 T A2
AMA: 2020,May,13; 2018,Jul,14; 2018,Jan,8; 2017,Jan,8; 2016,Jan,13; 2015,Jan,16

20922 **by incision and area exposure, complex or sheet**
13.9 17.0 FUD 090 T A2 80
AMA: 2020,May,13; 2018,Jul,14; 2018,Jan,8; 2017,Jan,8; 2016,Jan,13; 2015,Jan,16

20924 **Tendon graft, from a distance (eg, palmaris, toe extensor, plantaris)**
14.6 14.6 FUD 090 J A2 80
AMA: 2020,May,13; 2018,Jul,14

20930-20939 Bone Allograft and Autograft of Spine

EXCLUDES *Acquisition autogenous bone, bone marrow, cartilage, tendon, fascia lata, or other grafts through distinct incision unless included in code description*
Autologous fat graft obtained by liposuction (15771-15774)
Other autologous soft tissue grafts (fat, dermis, fascia) harvested by direct excision ([15769])

+ 20930 **Allograft, morselized, or placement of osteopromotive material, for spine surgery only (List separately in addition to code for primary procedure)**
Code first (22319, 22532-22533, 22548-22558, 22590-22612, 22630, 22633-22634, 22800-22812)
0.00 0.00 FUD XXX N N1
AMA: 2020,May,13; 2019,May,7; 2018,Jul,14; 2018,Jan,8; 2017,Mar,7; 2017,Jan,8; 2016,Jan,13; 2015,Jan,16

+ 20931 **Allograft, structural, for spine surgery only (List separately in addition to code for primary procedure)**
Code first (22319, 22532-22533, 22548-22558, 22590-22612, 22630, 22633-22634, 22800-22812)
3.26 3.26 FUD ZZZ N N1
AMA: 2020,May,13; 2019,May,7; 2018,Jul,14; 2018,Jan,8; 2017,Mar,7; 2017,Jan,8; 2016,Jan,13; 2015,Jan,16

+ 20932 **Allograft, includes templating, cutting, placement and internal fixation, when performed; osteoarticular, including articular surface and contiguous bone (List separately in addition to code for primary procedure)**
EXCLUDES *Allograft, intercalary (20933-20934)*
Injection contrast for ankle arthrography (27648)
Osteotomy, femur (27448)
Radical resection tumor:
Clavicle (23200)
Fibula (27646)
Ischial tuberosity/greater trochanter femur (27078)
Radial head or neck (24152)
Talus or calcaneus (27647)
Removal hip prosthesis (27090-27091)
Code also insertion joint prosthesis
Code first (23210, 23220, 24150, 25170, 27075-27077, 27365, 27645, 27704)
20.6 20.6 FUD ZZZ N1 80
AMA: 2020,May,13; 2019,May,7

+ 20933 **hemicortical intercalary, partial (ie, hemicylindrical) (List separately in addition to code for primary procedure)**
EXCLUDES *Allograft, intercalary, complete (20934)*
Allograft, osteoarticular (20932)
Arthroplasty procedures, hip (27130, 27132, 27134, 27138)
Bone graft (20955-20957, 20962)
Excision cyst with allograft (23146, 23156, 24116, 24126, 25126, 25136, 27356, 27638, 28103, 28107)
Injection contrast for ankle arthrography (27648)
Open treatment femoral fractures (27236, 27244)
Osteotomy, femur (27448)
Radical resection tumor:
Clavicle (23200)
Fibula (27646)
Ischial tuberosity/greater trochanter femur (27078)
Radial head or neck (24152)
Talus or calcaneus (27647)
Removal hip prosthesis (27090-27091)
Code also insertion joint prosthesis
Code first (23210, 23220, 24150, 25170, 27075-27077, 27365, 27645, 27704)
18.9 18.9 FUD ZZZ N1 80
AMA: 2020,May,13; 2019,May,7

+ 20934 **intercalary, complete (ie, cylindrical) (List separately in addition to code for primary procedure)**
Allograft, intercalary, partial (20933)
Allograft, osteoarticular (20932)
Excision cyst with allograft (23146, 23156)
Injection contrast for ankle arthrography (27648)
Osteotomy, femur (27448)
Radical resection tumor:
Clavicle (23200)
Fibula (27646)
Ischial tuberosity/greater trochanter femur (27078)
Radial head or neck (24152)
Talus or calcaneus (27647)
Removal hip prosthesis (27090-27091)
Code also insertion joint prosthesis
Code first (23210, 23220, 24150, 25170, 27075-27077, 27365, 27645, 27704)
20.6 20.6 FUD ZZZ N1 80
AMA: 2020,May,13; 2019,May,7

+ 20936 **Autograft for spine surgery only (includes harvesting the graft); local (eg, ribs, spinous process, or laminar fragments) obtained from same incision (List separately in addition to code for primary procedure)**
Code first (22319, 22532-22533, 22548-22558, 22590-22612, 22630, 22633-22634, 22800-22812)
0.00 0.00 FUD XXX N N1
AMA: 2020,May,13; 2018,Jul,14; 2018,Jan,8; 2017,Mar,7; 2017,Jan,8; 2016,Jan,13; 2015,Jan,16

+ 20937 **morselized (through separate skin or fascial incision) (List separately in addition to code for primary procedure)**
Code first (22319, 22532-22533, 22548-22558, 22590-22612, 22630, 22633-22634, 22800-22812)
4.85 4.85 FUD ZZZ N N1 80
AMA: 2020,May,13; 2018,Jul,14; 2018,Jan,8; 2017,Mar,7; 2017,Jan,8; 2016,Jan,13; 2015,Jan,16

+ 20938 **structural, bicortical or tricortical (through separate skin or fascial incision) (List separately in addition to code for primary procedure)**
EXCLUDES *Bone marrow for bone grafting in spinal surgery (20939)*
Code first (22319, 22532-22533, 22548-22558, 22590-22612, 22630, 22633-22634, 22800-22812)
5.34 5.34 FUD ZZZ N N1 80
AMA: 2020,May,13; 2018,Jul,14; 2018,Jan,8; 2017,Mar,7; 2017,Jan,8; 2016,Jan,13; 2015,Jan,16

+ **20939 Bone marrow aspiration for bone grafting, spine surgery only, through separate skin or fascial incision (List separately in addition to code for primary procedure)**

EXCLUDES *Bone marrow aspiration for other than bone grafting in spinal surgery (20999)*
Diagnostic bone marrow aspiration (38220, 38222)
Platelet rich plasma injection (0232T)
Reporting with modifier 50. Report once for each side when performed bilaterally

Code first (22319, 22532-22534, 22548, 22551-22552, 22554, 22556, 22558, 22590, 22595, 22600, 22610, 22612, 22630, 22633-22634, 22800, 22802, 22804, 22808, 22810, 22812)

2.03 2.03 FUD ZZZ N N1 80 50

AMA: 2018,May,3

20950 Measurement of Intracompartmental Pressure

20950 Monitoring of interstitial fluid pressure (includes insertion of device, eg, wick catheter technique, needle manometer technique) in detection of muscle compartment syndrome

2.56 7.43 FUD 000 T G2 80

AMA: 2018,Jan,8; 2017,Jan,8; 2016,Jan,13; 2015,Jan,16

20955-20973 Bone and Osteocutaneous Grafts

INCLUDES Operating microscope (69990)

20955 Bone graft with microvascular anastomosis; fibula

70.9 70.9 FUD 090 C 80

AMA: 2019,Dec,5; 2019,May,7; 2018,Jan,8; 2017,Jan,8; 2016,Feb,12; 2016,Jan,13; 2015,Jan,16

20956 iliac crest

76.6 76.6 FUD 090 C 80

AMA: 2019,Dec,5; 2019,May,7; 2018,Jan,8; 2017,Jan,8; 2016,Feb,12; 2016,Jan,13; 2015,Jan,16

20957 metatarsal

79.6 79.6 FUD 090 C 80

AMA: 2019,Dec,5; 2019,May,7; 2018,Jan,8; 2017,Jan,8; 2016,Feb,12; 2016,Jan,13; 2015,Jan,16

20962 other than fibula, iliac crest, or metatarsal

76.9 76.9 FUD 090 C 80

AMA: 2019,Dec,5; 2019,May,7; 2016,Feb,12

20969 Free osteocutaneous flap with microvascular anastomosis; other than iliac crest, metatarsal, or great toe

78.6 78.6 FUD 090 C 80

AMA: 2019,Dec,5; 2019,Oct,10; 2018,Jan,8; 2017,Jan,8; 2016,Feb,12; 2016,Jan,13; 2015,Jan,16

20970 iliac crest

82.6 82.6 FUD 090 C 80

AMA: 2019,Dec,5; 2018,Jan,8; 2017,Jan,8; 2016,Feb,12; 2016,Jan,13; 2015,Jan,16

20972 metatarsal

82.4 82.4 FUD 090 J G2 80

AMA: 2019,Dec,5; 2018,Jan,8; 2017,Jan,8; 2016,Feb,12; 2016,Jan,13; 2015,Jan,16

20973 great toe with web space

EXCLUDES *Great toe wrap-around with bone graft (26551)*

87.0 87.0 FUD 090 J R2 80 50

AMA: 2019,Dec,5; 2018,Jan,8; 2017,Jan,8; 2016,Feb,12; 2016,Jan,13; 2015,Jan,16

20974-20979 Osteogenic Stimulation

CMS: 100-03,150.2 Osteogenic Stimulation

20974 Electrical stimulation to aid bone healing; noninvasive (nonoperative)

1.45 2.26 FUD 000 ⊘ A

AMA: 2018,Jan,8; 2017,Jan,8; 2016,Jan,13; 2015,Jan,16

20975 invasive (operative)

5.18 5.18 FUD 000 ⊘ N N1 80

AMA: 2002,Apr,13; 2000,Nov,8

20979 Low intensity ultrasound stimulation to aid bone healing, noninvasive (nonoperative)

0.93 1.53 FUD 000 Q1 N1

AMA: 2018,Jan,8; 2017,Jan,8; 2016,Jan,13; 2015,Jan,16

20982-20999 General Musculoskeletal Procedures

20982 Ablation therapy for reduction or eradication of 1 or more bone tumors (eg, metastasis) including adjacent soft tissue when involved by tumor extension, percutaneous, including imaging guidance when performed; radiofrequency

EXCLUDES *Radiologic guidance (76940, 77002, 77013, 77022)*

10.5 110. FUD 000 J G2 50

AMA: 2018,Jan,8; 2017,Jan,8; 2016,Jan,13; 2015,Sep,12; 2015,Jul,8

20983 cryoablation

EXCLUDES *Radiologic guidance (76940, 77002, 77013, 77022)*

10.1 163. FUD 000 J J8 50

AMA: 2018,Jan,8; 2017,Jan,8; 2016,Jan,13; 2015,Jul,8

+ **20985 Computer-assisted surgical navigational procedure for musculoskeletal procedures, image-less (List separately in addition to code for primary procedure)**

EXCLUDES *Image guidance derived from intraoperative and preoperative obtained images (0054T-0055T)*
Stereotactic computer-assisted navigational procedure; cranial or intradural (61781-61783)

Code first primary procedure

4.24 4.24 FUD ZZZ N N1 80

AMA: 2018,Jan,8; 2017,Jan,8; 2016,Jan,13; 2015,Jan,16

20999 Unlisted procedure, musculoskeletal system, general

0.00 0.00 FUD YYY T 80

AMA: 2018,May,3; 2018,Jan,8; 2017,Jan,8; 2016,Jan,13; 2015,Jul,8; 2015,Jan,16

21010 Temporomandibular Joint Arthrotomy

21010 Arthrotomy, temporomandibular joint

EXCLUDES *Cutaneous/subcutaneous abscess and hematoma drainage (10060-10061)*
Excision foreign body from dentoalveolar site (41805-41806)

22.0 22.0 FUD 090 J A2 80 50

AMA: 2002,Apr,13

21011-21016 Excision Soft Tissue Tumors Face and Scalp

INCLUDES Any necessary elevation tissue planes or dissection
Measurement tumor and necessary margin at greatest diameter prior to excision
Simple and intermediate repairs
Excision types:
- Fascial or subfascial soft tissue tumors: simple and marginal resection tumors found either in or below deep fascia, not including bone or excision substantial amount normal tissue; primarily benign and intramuscular tumors
- Radical resection soft tissue tumor: wide resection tumor involving substantial margins normal tissue and may include tissue removal from one or more layers; most often malignant or aggressive benign
- Subcutaneous: simple and marginal resection tumors in subcutaneous tissue above deep fascia; most often benign

EXCLUDES *Complex repair*
Excision benign cutaneous lesions (eg, sebaceous cyst) (11420-11426)
Radical resection cutaneous tumors (eg, melanoma) (11620-11646)
Significant vessel exploration or neuroplasty

21011 Excision, tumor, soft tissue of face or scalp, subcutaneous; less than 2 cm

7.38 10.3 FUD 090 J P3 80

AMA: 2018,Sep,7; 2018,Jan,8; 2017,Jan,8; 2016,Jan,13; 2015,Jan,16

21012 2 cm or greater

9.72 9.72 FUD 090 J R2 80

AMA: 2018,Sep,7; 2018,Jan,8; 2017,Jan,8; 2016,Jan,13; 2015,Jan,16

26/TC PC/TC Only A2-Z3 ASC Payment 50 Bilateral ♂ Male Only ♀ Female Only Facility RVU Non-Facility RVU CCI CLIA
FUD Follow-up Days CMS: IOM AMA: CPT Asst A-Y OPPSI 80/80 Surg Assist Allowed / w/Doc Lab Crosswalk Radiology Crosswalk

21013 **Excision, tumor, soft tissue of face and scalp, subfascial (eg, subgaleal, intramuscular); less than 2 cm**
11.5 | 15.1 | FUD 090 | J P3 80
AMA: 2018,Sep,7; 2018,Jan,8; 2017,Jan,8; 2016,Jan,13; 2015,Jan,16

21014 **2 cm or greater**
15.0 | 15.0 | FUD 090 | J R2 80
AMA: 2018,Sep,7; 2018,Jan,8; 2017,Jan,8; 2016,Jan,13; 2015,Jan,16

21015 **Radical resection of tumor (eg, sarcoma), soft tissue of face or scalp; less than 2 cm**
EXCLUDES *Removal of cranial tumor for osteomyelitis (61501)*
20.3 | 20.3 | FUD 090 | J G2
AMA: 2018,Sep,7; 2018,Jan,8; 2017,Jan,8; 2016,Jan,13; 2015,Jan,16

21016 **2 cm or greater**
29.0 | 29.0 | FUD 090 | J G2 80
AMA: 2018,Sep,7; 2018,Jan,8; 2017,Jan,8; 2016,Jan,13; 2015,Jan,16

21025-21070 Procedures of Cranial and Facial Bones

INCLUDES
Any necessary elevation tissue planes or dissection
Measurement tumor and necessary margins prior to excision
Radical resection bone tumor involves resection tumor (may include entire bone) and wide margins normal tissue primarily for malignant or aggressive benign tumors
Simple and intermediate repairs

EXCLUDES
Complex repair
Excision soft tissue tumors, face and scalp (21011-21016)
Radical resection cutaneous tumors (e.g., melanoma) (11620-11646)
Significant vessel exploration, neuroplasty, reconstruction, or complex bone repair

21025 **Excision of bone (eg, for osteomyelitis or bone abscess); mandible**
19.9 | 23.6 | FUD 090 | J A2
AMA: 2018,Sep,7; 2018,Jan,8; 2017,Jan,8; 2016,Jan,13; 2015,Jan,16

21026 **facial bone(s)**
12.9 | 16.0 | FUD 090 | J A2
AMA: 2018,Sep,7

21029 **Removal by contouring of benign tumor of facial bone (eg, fibrous dysplasia)**
17.9 | 21.8 | FUD 090 | J A2 80
AMA: 2018,Sep,7

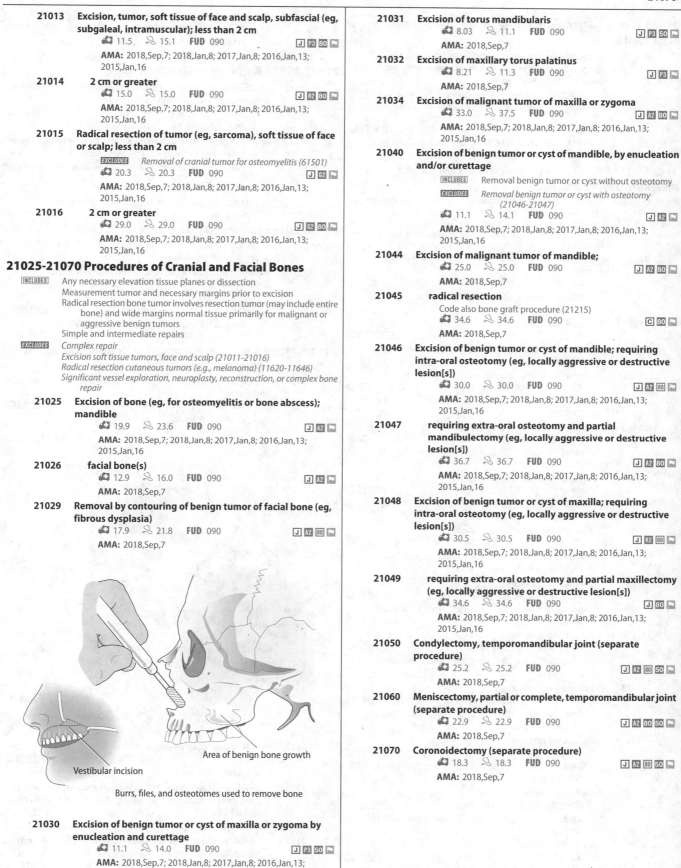

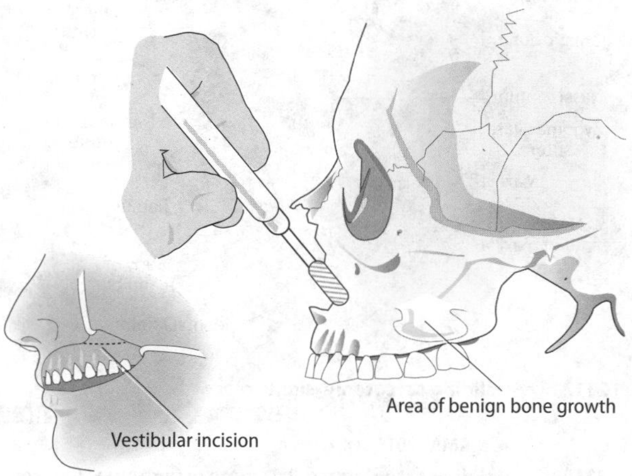

21030 **Excision of benign tumor or cyst of maxilla or zygoma by enucleation and curettage**
11.1 | 14.0 | FUD 090 | J P3 50
AMA: 2018,Sep,7; 2018,Jan,8; 2017,Jan,8; 2016,Jan,13; 2015,Jan,16

21031 **Excision of torus mandibularis**
8.03 | 11.1 | FUD 090 | J P3 50
AMA: 2018,Sep,7

21032 **Excision of maxillary torus palatinus**
8.21 | 11.3 | FUD 090 | J P3
AMA: 2018,Sep,7

21034 **Excision of malignant tumor of maxilla or zygoma**
33.0 | 37.5 | FUD 090 | J A2 80
AMA: 2018,Sep,7; 2018,Jan,8; 2017,Jan,8; 2016,Jan,13; 2015,Jan,16

21040 **Excision of benign tumor or cyst of mandible, by enucleation and/or curettage**
INCLUDES Removal benign tumor or cyst without osteotomy
EXCLUDES *Removal benign tumor or cyst with osteotomy (21046-21047)*
11.1 | 14.1 | FUD 090 | J A2
AMA: 2018,Sep,7; 2018,Jan,8; 2017,Jan,8; 2016,Jan,13; 2015,Jan,16

21044 **Excision of malignant tumor of mandible;**
25.0 | 25.0 | FUD 090 | J A2 80
AMA: 2018,Sep,7

21045 **radical resection**
Code also bone graft procedure (21215)
34.6 | 34.6 | FUD 090 | C 80
AMA: 2018,Sep,7

21046 **Excision of benign tumor or cyst of mandible; requiring intra-oral osteotomy (eg, locally aggressive or destructive lesion[s])**
30.0 | 30.0 | FUD 090 | J A2 80
AMA: 2018,Sep,7; 2018,Jan,8; 2017,Jan,8; 2016,Jan,13; 2015,Jan,16

21047 **requiring extra-oral osteotomy and partial mandibulectomy (eg, locally aggressive or destructive lesion[s])**
36.7 | 36.7 | FUD 090 | J A2 80
AMA: 2018,Sep,7; 2018,Jan,8; 2017,Jan,8; 2016,Jan,13; 2015,Jan,16

21048 **Excision of benign tumor or cyst of maxilla; requiring intra-oral osteotomy (eg, locally aggressive or destructive lesion[s])**
30.5 | 30.5 | FUD 090 | J R2 80
AMA: 2018,Sep,7; 2018,Jan,8; 2017,Jan,8; 2016,Jan,13; 2015,Jan,16

21049 **requiring extra-oral osteotomy and partial maxillectomy (eg, locally aggressive or destructive lesion[s])**
34.6 | 34.6 | FUD 090 | J 80
AMA: 2018,Sep,7; 2018,Jan,8; 2017,Jan,8; 2016,Jan,13; 2015,Jan,16

21050 **Condylectomy, temporomandibular joint (separate procedure)**
25.2 | 25.2 | FUD 090 | J A2 80 50
AMA: 2018,Sep,7

21060 **Meniscectomy, partial or complete, temporomandibular joint (separate procedure)**
22.9 | 22.9 | FUD 090 | J A2 80 50
AMA: 2018,Sep,7

21070 **Coronoidectomy (separate procedure)**
18.3 | 18.3 | FUD 090 | J A2 80 50
AMA: 2018,Sep,7

Musculoskeletal System
21013 — 21070

21073 Temporomandibular Joint Manipulation with Anesthesia

21073 **Manipulation of temporomandibular joint(s) (TMJ), therapeutic, requiring an anesthesia service (ie, general or monitored anesthesia care)**

EXCLUDES *Closed treatment TMJ dislocation (21480, 21485)*
Manipulation TMJ without general or MAC anesthesia (97140, 98925-98929, 98943)

7.19 10.9 **FUD** 090 T P3 80 50

AMA: 2018,Sep,7; 2018,Jan,8; 2018,Jan,3; 2017,Jan,8; 2016,Jan,13; 2015,Jan,16

21076-21089 Medical Impressions for Fabrication Maxillofacial Prosthesis

INCLUDES Design, preparation, and professional services rendered by physician or other qualified health care professional

EXCLUDES *Application or removal caliper or tongs (20660, 20665)*
Professional services rendered for outside laboratory designed and prepared prosthesis

21076 **Impression and custom preparation; surgical obturator prosthesis**
23.1 27.6 **FUD** 010 T P3 80
AMA: 2018,Sep,7; 2018,Jan,8; 2017,Jan,8; 2016,Jan,13; 2015,Jan,16

21077 **orbital prosthesis**
53.4 64.0 **FUD** 090 J P3 80 50
AMA: 2018,Sep,7; 2018,Jan,8; 2017,Jan,8; 2016,Jan,13; 2015,Jan,16

21079 **interim obturator prosthesis**
35.8 43.5 **FUD** 090 J P3
AMA: 2018,Sep,7; 2018,Jan,8; 2017,Jan,8; 2016,Jan,13; 2015,Jan,16

21080 **definitive obturator prosthesis**
40.4 49.8 **FUD** 090 J P3
AMA: 2018,Sep,7; 2018,Jan,8; 2017,Jan,8; 2016,Jan,13; 2015,Jan,16

21081 **mandibular resection prosthesis**
37.0 45.7 **FUD** 090 J P3 80
AMA: 2018,Sep,7; 2018,Jan,8; 2017,Jan,8; 2016,Jan,13; 2015,Jan,16

21082 **palatal augmentation prosthesis**
34.0 42.4 **FUD** 090 J P3 80
AMA: 2018,Sep,7; 2018,Jan,8; 2017,Jan,8; 2016,Jan,13; 2015,Jan,16

21083 **palatal lift prosthesis**
31.6 40.4 **FUD** 090 J P3 80
AMA: 2018,Sep,7; 2018,Jan,8; 2017,Jan,8; 2016,Jan,13; 2015,Jan,16

21084 **speech aid prosthesis**
36.5 46.2 **FUD** 090 J P3 80
AMA: 2018,Sep,7; 2018,Jan,8; 2017,Jan,8; 2016,Jan,13; 2015,Jan,16

21085 **oral surgical splint**
15.7 21.0 **FUD** 010 T P2 80
AMA: 2018,Sep,7; 2018,Jan,8; 2017,Sep,14; 2017,Jan,8; 2016,Jan,13; 2015,Jan,16

21086 **auricular prosthesis**
39.4 47.6 **FUD** 090 J P3 80 50
AMA: 2018,Sep,7; 2018,Jan,8; 2017,Jan,8; 2016,Jan,13; 2015,Jan,16

21087 **nasal prosthesis**
42.7 51.1 **FUD** 090 J P3 80
AMA: 2018,Sep,7; 2018,Jan,8; 2017,Jan,8; 2016,Jan,13; 2015,Jan,16

21088 **facial prosthesis**
0.00 0.00 **FUD** 090 J R2 80
AMA: 2018,Sep,7; 2018,Jan,8; 2017,Jan,8; 2016,Jan,13; 2015,Jan,16

21089 **Unlisted maxillofacial prosthetic procedure**
0.00 0.00 **FUD** YYY T
AMA: 2018,Sep,7; 2018,Jan,8; 2017,Jan,8; 2016,Jan,13; 2015,Jan,16

21100-21110 Application Fixation Device

21100 **Application of halo type appliance for maxillofacial fixation, includes removal (separate procedure)**
10.6 18.9 **FUD** 090 J A2 80
AMA: 2018,Sep,7

21110 **Application of interdental fixation device for conditions other than fracture or dislocation, includes removal**

EXCLUDES *Interdental fixation device removal by different provider (20670-20680)*

19.5 23.3 **FUD** 090 Q2 P2
AMA: 2018,Sep,7; 2018,Jan,8; 2017,Jan,8; 2016,Jan,13; 2015,Jan,16

21116 Injection for TMJ Arthrogram

CMS: 100-02,15,150.1 Treatment of Temporomandibular Joint (TMJ) Syndrome; 100-04,13,80.1 Physician Presence; 100-04,13,80.2 S&I Multiple Procedure Reduction

21116 **Injection procedure for temporomandibular joint arthrography**
(70332)
1.34 5.62 **FUD** 000 N N1 50
AMA: 2018,Sep,7; 2018,Jan,8; 2017,Jan,8; 2016,May,13; 2016,Jan,13; 2015,Aug,6

21120-21299 Repair/Reconstruction Craniofacial Bones

EXCLUDES *Cranioplasty (21179-21180, 62120, 62140-62147)*

21120 **Genioplasty; augmentation (autograft, allograft, prosthetic material)**
15.0 19.2 **FUD** 090 J G2
AMA: 2018,Sep,7

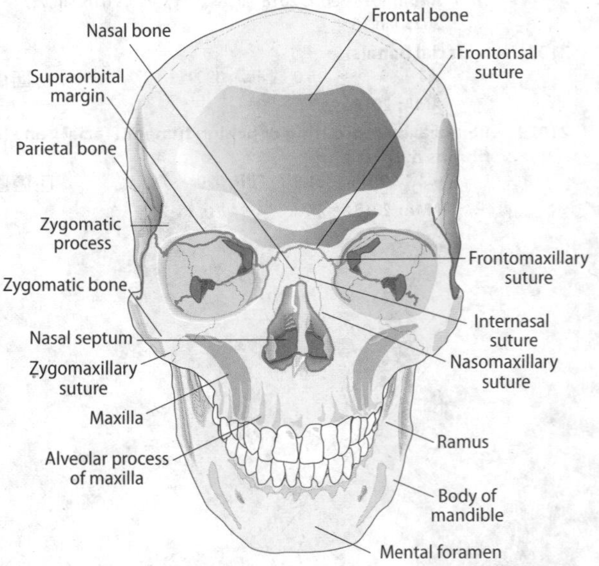

21121 **sliding osteotomy, single piece**
17.8 20.9 **FUD** 090 J A2 80
AMA: 2018,Sep,7

21122 **sliding osteotomies, 2 or more osteotomies (eg, wedge excision or bone wedge reversal for asymmetrical chin)**
22.1 22.1 **FUD** 090 J A2 80
AMA: 2018,Sep,7

21123 **sliding, augmentation with interpositional bone grafts (includes obtaining autografts)**
26.1 26.1 **FUD** 090 J A2 80
AMA: 2018,Sep,7

21125 Augmentation, mandibular body or angle; prosthetic material
🚗 19.8   ⚕ 80.8   **FUD** 090   J A2 80 ▨
AMA: 2018,Sep,7

21127 with bone graft, onlay or interpositional (includes obtaining autograft)
🚗 24.6   ⚕ 112.   **FUD** 090   J A2 80 ▨
AMA: 2018,Sep,7

21137 Reduction forehead; contouring only
🚗 21.7   ⚕ 21.7   **FUD** 090   J G2 80 ▨
AMA: 2018,Sep,7

21138 contouring and application of prosthetic material or bone graft (includes obtaining autograft)
🚗 26.5   ⚕ 26.5   **FUD** 090   J G2 80 ▨
AMA: 2018,Sep,7

21139 contouring and setback of anterior frontal sinus wall
🚗 32.0   ⚕ 32.0   **FUD** 090   J G2 80 ▨
AMA: 2018,Sep,7

21141 Reconstruction midface, LeFort I; single piece, segment movement in any direction (eg, for Long Face Syndrome), without bone graft
🚗 39.4   ⚕ 39.4   **FUD** 090   C 80 ▨
AMA: 2018,Sep,7

21142 2 pieces, segment movement in any direction, without bone graft
🚗 40.5   ⚕ 40.5   **FUD** 090   C 80 ▨
AMA: 2018,Sep,7

21143 3 or more pieces, segment movement in any direction, without bone graft
🚗 41.0   ⚕ 41.0   **FUD** 090   C 80 ▨
AMA: 2018,Sep,7

21145 single piece, segment movement in any direction, requiring bone grafts (includes obtaining autografts)
🚗 46.2   ⚕ 46.2   **FUD** 090   C 80 ▨
AMA: 2018,Sep,7

21146 2 pieces, segment movement in any direction, requiring bone grafts (includes obtaining autografts) (eg, ungrafted unilateral alveolar cleft)
🚗 46.8   ⚕ 46.8   **FUD** 090   C 80 ▨
AMA: 2018,Sep,7

21147 3 or more pieces, segment movement in any direction, requiring bone grafts (includes obtaining autografts) (eg, ungrafted bilateral alveolar cleft or multiple osteotomies)
🚗 50.8   ⚕ 50.8   **FUD** 090   C 80 ▨
AMA: 2018,Sep,7

21150 Reconstruction midface, LeFort II; anterior intrusion (eg, Treacher-Collins Syndrome)
🚗 47.3   ⚕ 47.3   **FUD** 090   J G2 80 ▨
AMA: 2018,Sep,7

21151 any direction, requiring bone grafts (includes obtaining autografts)
🚗 52.0   ⚕ 52.0   **FUD** 090   C 80 ▨
AMA: 2018,Sep,7

21154 Reconstruction midface, LeFort III (extracranial), any type, requiring bone grafts (includes obtaining autografts); without LeFort I
🚗 56.0   ⚕ 56.0   **FUD** 090   C 80 ▨
AMA: 2018,Sep,7

21155 with LeFort I
🚗 62.2   ⚕ 62.2   **FUD** 090   C 80 ▨
AMA: 2018,Sep,7

Bicoronal scalp flap
Lower eyelid
Circum-vestibular

Typical transcutaneous and transoral incisions

LeFort III with LeFort I down-fracture

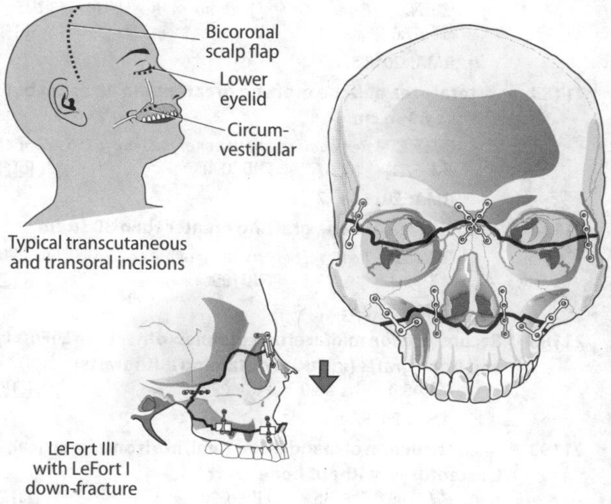

21159 Reconstruction midface, LeFort III (extra and intracranial) with forehead advancement (eg, mono bloc), requiring bone grafts (includes obtaining autografts); without LeFort I
🚗 74.5   ⚕ 74.5   **FUD** 090   C 80 ▨
AMA: 2018,Sep,7

21160 with LeFort I
🚗 81.4   ⚕ 81.4   **FUD** 090   C 80 ▨
AMA: 2018,Sep,7

21172 Reconstruction superior-lateral orbital rim and lower forehead, advancement or alteration, with or without grafts (includes obtaining autografts)
EXCLUDES   *Frontal or parietal craniotomy for craniosynostosis (61556)*
🚗 60.2   ⚕ 60.2   **FUD** 090   J 80 ▨
AMA: 2018,Sep,7

21175 Reconstruction, bifrontal, superior-lateral orbital rims and lower forehead, advancement or alteration (eg, plagiocephaly, trigonocephaly, brachycephaly), with or without grafts (includes obtaining autografts)
EXCLUDES   *Bifrontal craniotomy for craniosynostosis (61557)*
🚗 64.3   ⚕ 64.3   **FUD** 090   J 80 ▨
AMA: 2018,Sep,7

21179 Reconstruction, entire or majority of forehead and/or supraorbital rims; with grafts (allograft or prosthetic material)
EXCLUDES   *Extensive craniotomy for numerous suture craniosynostosis (61558-61559)*
🚗 44.2   ⚕ 44.2   **FUD** 090   C 80 ▨
AMA: 2018,Sep,7

21180 with autograft (includes obtaining grafts)
EXCLUDES   *Extensive craniotomy for numerous suture craniosynostosis (61558-61559)*
🚗 49.4   ⚕ 49.4   **FUD** 090   C 80 ▨
AMA: 2018,Sep,7

21181 Reconstruction by contouring of benign tumor of cranial bones (eg, fibrous dysplasia), extracranial
🚗 21.4   ⚕ 21.4   **FUD** 090   J A2 80 ▨
AMA: 2018,Sep,7

● New Code   ▲ Revised Code   ○ Reinstated   ● New Web Release   ▲ Revised Web Release   + Add-on   Unlisted   Not Covered   # Resequenced
⑤⓪ Optum Mod 50 Exempt   ⊘ AMA Mod 51 Exempt   ⑤① Optum Mod 51 Exempt   ⑥③ Mod 63 Exempt   ✗ Non-FDA Drug   ★ Telemedicine   M Maternity   A Age Edit

21182 **Reconstruction of orbital walls, rims, forehead, nasoethmoid complex following intra- and extracranial excision of benign tumor of cranial bone (eg, fibrous dysplasia), with multiple autografts (includes obtaining graft); total area of bone grafting less than 40 sq cm**
EXCLUDES *Removal obenign tumor of the skull (61563-61564)*
61.6 61.6 FUD 090 C 80
AMA: 2018,Sep,7

21183 **total area of bone grafting greater than 40 sq cm but less than 80 sq cm**
EXCLUDES *Removal benign tumor of the skull (61563-61564)*
67.1 67.1 FUD 090 C 80
AMA: 2018,Sep,7

21184 **total area of bone grafting greater than 80 sq cm**
EXCLUDES *Removal benign tumor of the skull (61563-61564)*
72.3 72.3 FUD 090 C 80
AMA: 2018,Sep,7

21188 **Reconstruction midface, osteotomies (other than LeFort type) and bone grafts (includes obtaining autografts)**
48.0 48.0 FUD 090 C 80
AMA: 2018,Sep,7

21193 **Reconstruction of mandibular rami, horizontal, vertical, C, or L osteotomy; without bone graft**
36.8 36.8 FUD 090 J 80
AMA: 2018,Sep,7; 2018,Jan,8; 2017,Jan,8; 2016,Jan,13; 2015,Jan,16

21194 **with bone graft (includes obtaining graft)**
41.2 41.2 FUD 090 C 80
AMA: 2018,Sep,7; 2018,Jan,8; 2017,Jan,8; 2016,Jan,13; 2015,Jan,16

21195 **Reconstruction of mandibular rami and/or body, sagittal split; without internal rigid fixation**
39.5 39.5 FUD 090 J 80
AMA: 2018,Sep,7; 2018,Jan,8; 2017,Jan,8; 2016,Jan,13; 2015,Jan,16

21196 **with internal rigid fixation**
40.9 40.9 FUD 090 C 80
AMA: 2018,Sep,7; 2018,Jan,8; 2017,Jan,8; 2016,Jan,13; 2015,Jan,16

21198 **Osteotomy, mandible, segmental;**
EXCLUDES *Total maxillary osteotomy (21141-21160)*
33.0 33.0 FUD 090 J G2 80
AMA: 2018,Sep,7; 2018,Jan,8; 2017,Jan,8; 2016,Jan,13; 2015,Jan,16

21199 **with genioglossus advancement**
EXCLUDES *Total maxillary osteotomy (21141-21160)*
31.0 31.0 FUD 090 J G2 80
AMA: 2018,Sep,7; 2018,Jan,8; 2017,Jan,8; 2016,Jan,13; 2015,Jan,16

21206 **Osteotomy, maxilla, segmental (eg, Wassmund or Schuchard)**
34.1 34.1 FUD 090 J A2 80
AMA: 2018,Sep,7

21208 **Osteoplasty, facial bones; augmentation (autograft, allograft, or prosthetic implant)**
23.2 49.9 FUD 090 J J8 80
AMA: 2018,Sep,7

21209 **reduction**
17.4 22.9 FUD 090 J A2 80
AMA: 2018,Sep,7

21210 **Graft, bone; nasal, maxillary or malar areas (includes obtaining graft)**
EXCLUDES *Cleft palate procedures (42200-42225)*
22.3 56.5 FUD 090 J A2
AMA: 2018,Sep,7

21215 **mandible (includes obtaining graft)**
24.9 114. FUD 090 J A2
AMA: 2018,Sep,7

21230 **Graft; rib cartilage, autogenous, to face, chin, nose or ear (includes obtaining graft)**
EXCLUDES *Augmentation facial bones (21208)*
21.3 21.3 FUD 090 J A2 80
AMA: 2018,Sep,7

21235 **ear cartilage, autogenous, to nose or ear (includes obtaining graft)**
EXCLUDES *Augmentation facial bones (21208)*
16.2 20.7 FUD 090 J A2
AMA: 2018,Sep,7; 2018,Jan,8; 2017,Jan,8; 2016,Jan,13; 2015,Jan,16

21240 **Arthroplasty, temporomandibular joint, with or without autograft (includes obtaining graft)**
30.8 30.8 FUD 090 J A2 80 50
AMA: 2018,Sep,7

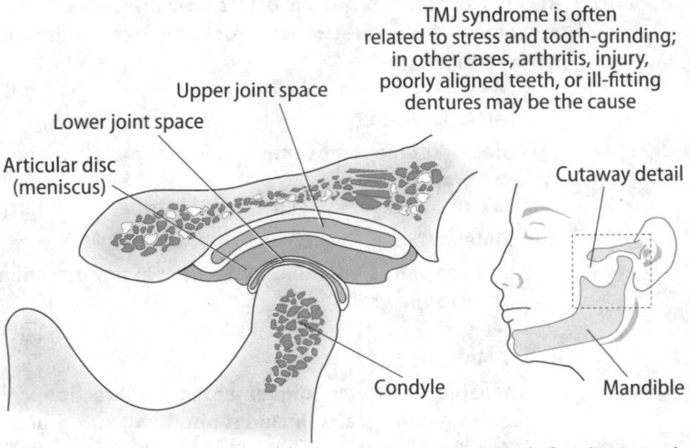
TMJ syndrome is often related to stress and tooth-grinding; in other cases, arthritis, injury, poorly aligned teeth, or ill-fitting dentures may be the cause
Upper joint space
Lower joint space
Articular disc (meniscus)
Cutaway detail
Condyle
Mandible
Symptoms include facial pain and chewing problems; TMJ syndrome occurs more frequently in women

Cutaway view of temporomandibular joint (TMJ)

21242 **Arthroplasty, temporomandibular joint, with allograft**
29.2 29.2 FUD 090 J A2 80 50
AMA: 2018,Sep,7

21243 **Arthroplasty, temporomandibular joint, with prosthetic joint replacement**
48.9 48.9 FUD 090 J J8 80 50
AMA: 2018,Sep,7

21244 **Reconstruction of mandible, extraoral, with transosteal bone plate (eg, mandibular staple bone plate)**
29.3 29.3 FUD 090 J G2 80
AMA: 2018,Sep,7

21245 **Reconstruction of mandible or maxilla, subperiosteal implant; partial**
26.8 34.5 FUD 090 J A2 80
AMA: 2018,Sep,7

21246 **complete**
25.4 25.4 FUD 090 J A2 80
AMA: 2018,Sep,7

21247 **Reconstruction of mandibular condyle with bone and cartilage autografts (includes obtaining grafts) (eg, for hemifacial microsomia)**
45.9 45.9 FUD 090 C 80 50
AMA: 2018,Sep,7

21248 **Reconstruction of mandible or maxilla, endosteal implant (eg, blade, cylinder); partial**
EXCLUDES *Midface reconstruction (21141-21160)*
25.3 31.1 FUD 090 J A2
AMA: 2018,Sep,7

21249 **complete**

EXCLUDES *Midface reconstruction (21141-21160)*

33.4 40.1 FUD 090 J A2 80

AMA: 2018,Sep,7

21255 **Reconstruction of zygomatic arch and glenoid fossa with bone and cartilage (includes obtaining autografts)**

40.6 40.6 FUD 090 C 80 50

AMA: 2018,Sep,7

21256 **Reconstruction of orbit with osteotomies (extracranial) and with bone grafts (includes obtaining autografts) (eg, micro-ophthalmia)**

35.9 35.9 FUD 090 J 80 50

AMA: 2018,Sep,7

21260 **Periorbital osteotomies for orbital hypertelorism, with bone grafts; extracranial approach**

40.1 40.1 FUD 090 J G2 80

AMA: 2018,Sep,7

21261 **combined intra- and extracranial approach**

71.1 71.1 FUD 090 J 80

AMA: 2018,Sep,7

21263 **with forehead advancement**

65.7 65.7 FUD 090 J 80

AMA: 2018,Sep,7

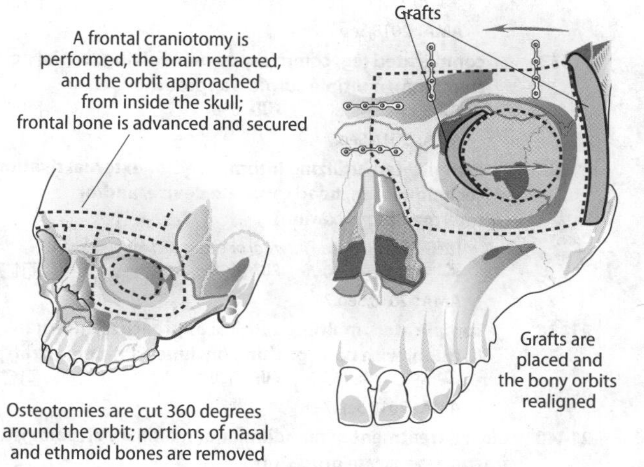
Grafts
A frontal craniotomy is performed, the brain retracted, and the orbit approached from inside the skull; frontal bone is advanced and secured
Grafts are placed and the bony orbits realigned
Osteotomies are cut 360 degrees around the orbit; portions of nasal and ethmoid bones are removed

21267 **Orbital repositioning, periorbital osteotomies, unilateral, with bone grafts; extracranial approach**

46.8 46.8 FUD 090 J A2 80 50

AMA: 2018,Sep,7

21268 **combined intra- and extracranial approach**

58.8 58.8 FUD 090 C 80 50

AMA: 2018,Sep,7

21270 **Malar augmentation, prosthetic material**

EXCLUDES *Augmentation procedure with bone graft (21210)*

21.7 29.1 FUD 090 J A2 80 50

AMA: 2018,Sep,7

21275 **Secondary revision of orbitocraniofacial reconstruction**

24.1 24.1 FUD 090 J G2 80

AMA: 2018,Sep,7

21280 **Medial canthopexy (separate procedure)**

EXCLUDES *Reconstruction canthus (67950)*

16.4 16.4 FUD 090 J A2 80 50

AMA: 2018,Sep,7

21282 **Lateral canthopexy**

11.0 11.0 FUD 090 J A2 50

AMA: 2018,Sep,7

21295 **Reduction of masseter muscle and bone (eg, for treatment of benign masseteric hypertrophy); extraoral approach**

5.39 5.39 FUD 090 T A2 80 50

AMA: 2018,Sep,7

21296 **intraoral approach**

11.7 11.7 FUD 090 J A2 80 50

AMA: 2018,Sep,7

21299 **Unlisted craniofacial and maxillofacial procedure**

0.00 0.00 FUD YYY T 80

AMA: 2018,Sep,7

21310-21499 Care of Fractures/Dislocations of the Cranial and Facial Bones

EXCLUDES *Closed treatment skull fracture, report with appropriate E/M service*
Open treatment skull fracture (62000-62010)

21310 **Closed treatment of nasal bone fracture without manipulation**

0.78 3.76 FUD 000 T A2

AMA: 2019,Nov,12; 2019,Sep,3; 2018,Sep,7; 2018,Jan,3

21315 **Closed treatment of nasal bone fracture; without stabilization**

4.31 7.80 FUD 010 T A2

AMA: 2019,Nov,12; 2019,Sep,3; 2018,Sep,7; 2018,Jan,3

21320 **with stabilization**

3.83 7.23 FUD 010 J A2

AMA: 2019,Sep,3; 2018,Sep,7

21325 **Open treatment of nasal fracture; uncomplicated**

12.4 12.4 FUD 090 J A2 80

AMA: 2018,Sep,7

21330 **complicated, with internal and/or external skeletal fixation**

16.0 16.0 FUD 090 J A2 80

AMA: 2018,Sep,7

21335 **with concomitant open treatment of fractured septum**

20.3 20.3 FUD 090 J A2

AMA: 2018,Sep,7

21336 **Open treatment of nasal septal fracture, with or without stabilization**

18.2 18.2 FUD 090 J A2 80

AMA: 2018,Sep,7

21337 **Closed treatment of nasal septal fracture, with or without stabilization**

8.41 11.7 FUD 090 J A2 80

AMA: 2019,Sep,3; 2018,Sep,7

21338 **Open treatment of nasoethmoid fracture; without external fixation**

18.8 18.8 FUD 090 J J8 80

AMA: 2018,Sep,7

21339 **with external fixation**

21.3 21.3 FUD 090 J A2 80

AMA: 2018,Sep,7

21340 **Percutaneous treatment of nasoethmoid complex fracture, with splint, wire or headcap fixation, including repair of canthal ligaments and/or the nasolacrimal apparatus**

21.3 21.3 FUD 090 J A2 80

AMA: 2018,Sep,7

21343 **Open treatment of depressed frontal sinus fracture**

30.7 30.7 FUD 090 C 80

AMA: 2018,Sep,7

21344 **Open treatment of complicated (eg, comminuted or involving posterior wall) frontal sinus fracture, via coronal or multiple approaches**

39.7 39.7 FUD 090 C 80

AMA: 2018,Sep,7

21345 **Closed treatment of nasomaxillary complex fracture (LeFort II type), with interdental wire fixation or fixation of denture or splint**
17.9 22.2 **FUD** 090 T A2 80
AMA: 2018,Sep,7

21346 **Open treatment of nasomaxillary complex fracture (LeFort II type); with wiring and/or local fixation**
27.4 27.4 **FUD** 090 J
AMA: 2018,Sep,7

21347 **requiring multiple open approaches**
29.0 29.0 **FUD** 090 C 80
AMA: 2018,Sep,7

21348 **with bone grafting (includes obtaining graft)**
31.0 31.0 **FUD** 090 C 80
AMA: 2018,Sep,7

21355 **Percutaneous treatment of fracture of malar area, including zygomatic arch and malar tripod, with manipulation**
9.18 12.2 **FUD** 010 J A2 80 50
AMA: 2018,Sep,7

21356 **Open treatment of depressed zygomatic arch fracture (eg, Gillies approach)**
10.7 14.2 **FUD** 010 J A2 80 50
AMA: 2018,Sep,7

21360 **Open treatment of depressed malar fracture, including zygomatic arch and malar tripod**
14.6 14.6 **FUD** 090 J G2 80 50
AMA: 2018,Sep,7

21365 **Open treatment of complicated (eg, comminuted or involving cranial nerve foramina) fracture(s) of malar area, including zygomatic arch and malar tripod; with internal fixation and multiple surgical approaches**
31.6 31.6 **FUD** 090 J 80 50
AMA: 2018,Sep,7

21366 **with bone grafting (includes obtaining graft)**
36.5 36.5 **FUD** 090 C 80 50
AMA: 2018,Sep,7

21385 **Open treatment of orbital floor blowout fracture; transantral approach (Caldwell-Luc type operation)**
21.5 21.5 **FUD** 090 J 80 50
AMA: 2018,Sep,7

21386 **periorbital approach**
18.7 18.7 **FUD** 090 J 80 50
AMA: 2018,Sep,7

21387 **combined approach**
22.5 22.5 **FUD** 090 J 80 50
AMA: 2018,Sep,7

21390 **periorbital approach, with alloplastic or other implant**
22.9 22.9 **FUD** 090 J G2 80 50
AMA: 2018,Sep,7

21395 **periorbital approach with bone graft (includes obtaining graft)**
29.0 29.0 **FUD** 090 J 80 50
AMA: 2018,Sep,7

21400 **Closed treatment of fracture of orbit, except blowout; without manipulation**
4.59 5.77 **FUD** 090 T A2 80 50
AMA: 2018,Sep,7

21401 **with manipulation**
9.23 14.7 **FUD** 090 T A2 80 50
AMA: 2018,Sep,7

21406 **Open treatment of fracture of orbit, except blowout; without implant**
16.7 16.7 **FUD** 090 J G2 80 50
AMA: 2018,Sep,7

21407 **with implant**
18.4 18.4 **FUD** 090 J G2 80 50
AMA: 2018,Sep,7

21408 **with bone grafting (includes obtaining graft)**
26.1 26.1 **FUD** 090 J 80 50
AMA: 2018,Sep,7

21421 **Closed treatment of palatal or maxillary fracture (LeFort I type), with interdental wire fixation or fixation of denture or splint**
17.2 20.3 **FUD** 090 J A2 80
AMA: 2018,Sep,7

21422 **Open treatment of palatal or maxillary fracture (LeFort I type);**
18.4 18.4 **FUD** 090 C 80
AMA: 2018,Sep,7

21423 **complicated (comminuted or involving cranial nerve foramina), multiple approaches**
22.0 22.0 **FUD** 090 C 80
AMA: 2018,Sep,7

21431 **Closed treatment of craniofacial separation (LeFort III type) using interdental wire fixation of denture or splint**
19.9 19.9 **FUD** 090 C 80
AMA: 2018,Sep,7

21432 **Open treatment of craniofacial separation (LeFort III type); with wiring and/or internal fixation**
20.7 20.7 **FUD** 090 C 80
AMA: 2018,Sep,7

21433 **complicated (eg, comminuted or involving cranial nerve foramina), multiple surgical approaches**
50.1 50.1 **FUD** 090 C 80
AMA: 2018,Sep,7

21435 **complicated, utilizing internal and/or external fixation techniques (eg, head cap, halo device, and/or intermaxillary fixation)**
EXCLUDES *Removal internal or external fixation (20670)*
40.7 40.7 **FUD** 090 C 80
AMA: 2018,Sep,7

21436 **complicated, multiple surgical approaches, internal fixation, with bone grafting (includes obtaining graft)**
59.2 59.2 **FUD** 090 C 80
AMA: 2018,Sep,7

21440 **Closed treatment of mandibular or maxillary alveolar ridge fracture (separate procedure)**
14.0 17.3 **FUD** 090 J P3 80
AMA: 2018,Sep,7

21445 **Open treatment of mandibular or maxillary alveolar ridge fracture (separate procedure)**
17.9 22.2 **FUD** 090 J A2 80
AMA: 2018,Sep,7

21450 **Closed treatment of mandibular fracture; without manipulation**
13.4 16.4 **FUD** 090 T A2 80
AMA: 2018,Sep,7

21451 **with manipulation**
18.0 21.5 **FUD** 090 T A2 80
AMA: 2018,Sep,7

21452 **Percutaneous treatment of mandibular fracture, with external fixation**
12.0 20.1 FUD 090 J A2 80
AMA: 2018,Sep,7

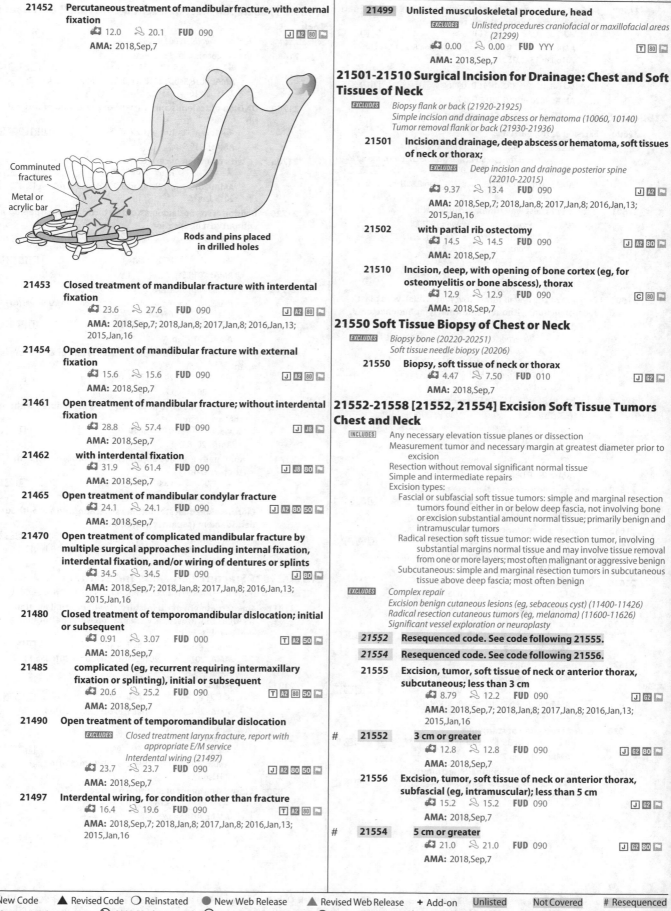

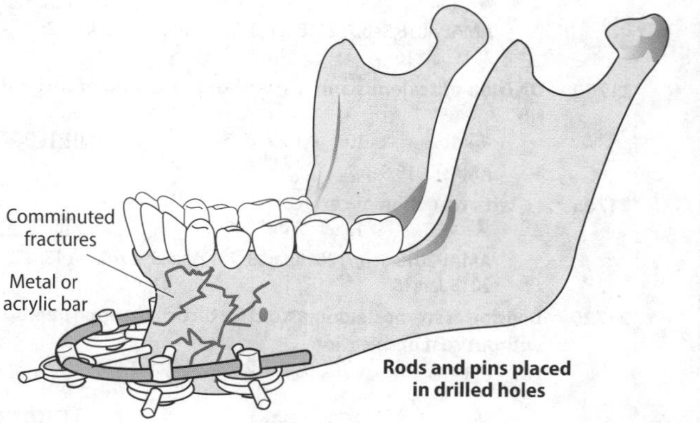

21453 **Closed treatment of mandibular fracture with interdental fixation**
23.6 27.6 FUD 090 J A2 80
AMA: 2018,Sep,7; 2018,Jan,8; 2017,Jan,8; 2016,Jan,13; 2015,Jan,16

21454 **Open treatment of mandibular fracture with external fixation**
15.6 15.6 FUD 090 J A2 80
AMA: 2018,Sep,7

21461 **Open treatment of mandibular fracture; without interdental fixation**
28.8 57.4 FUD 090 J J8
AMA: 2018,Sep,7

21462 **with interdental fixation**
31.9 61.4 FUD 090 J J8 80
AMA: 2018,Sep,7

21465 **Open treatment of mandibular condylar fracture**
24.1 24.1 FUD 090 J A2 80 50
AMA: 2018,Sep,7

21470 **Open treatment of complicated mandibular fracture by multiple surgical approaches including internal fixation, interdental fixation, and/or wiring of dentures or splints**
34.5 34.5 FUD 090 J 80
AMA: 2018,Sep,7; 2018,Jan,8; 2017,Jan,8; 2016,Jan,13; 2015,Jan,16

21480 **Closed treatment of temporomandibular dislocation; initial or subsequent**
0.91 3.07 FUD 000 T A2 50
AMA: 2018,Sep,7

21485 **complicated (eg, recurrent requiring intermaxillary fixation or splinting), initial or subsequent**
20.6 25.2 FUD 090 T A2 80 50
AMA: 2018,Sep,7

21490 **Open treatment of temporomandibular dislocation**
EXCLUDES *Closed treatment larynx fracture, report with appropriate E/M service*
Interdental wiring (21497)
23.7 23.7 FUD 090 J A2 80 50
AMA: 2018,Sep,7

21497 **Interdental wiring, for condition other than fracture**
16.4 19.6 FUD 090 T A2 80
AMA: 2018,Sep,7; 2018,Jan,8; 2017,Jan,8; 2016,Jan,13; 2015,Jan,16

21499 **Unlisted musculoskeletal procedure, head**
EXCLUDES *Unlisted procedures craniofacial or maxillofacial areas (21299)*
0.00 0.00 FUD YYY T 80
AMA: 2018,Sep,7

21501-21510 Surgical Incision for Drainage: Chest and Soft Tissues of Neck

EXCLUDES *Biopsy flank or back (21920-21925)*
Simple incision and drainage abscess or hematoma (10060, 10140)
Tumor removal flank or back (21930-21936)

21501 **Incision and drainage, deep abscess or hematoma, soft tissues of neck or thorax;**
EXCLUDES *Deep incision and drainage posterior spine (22010-22015)*
9.37 13.4 FUD 090 J A2
AMA: 2018,Sep,7; 2018,Jan,8; 2017,Jan,8; 2016,Jan,13; 2015,Jan,16

21502 **with partial rib ostectomy**
14.5 14.5 FUD 090 J A2 80
AMA: 2018,Sep,7

21510 **Incision, deep, with opening of bone cortex (eg, for osteomyelitis or bone abscess), thorax**
12.9 12.9 FUD 090 C 80
AMA: 2018,Sep,7

21550 Soft Tissue Biopsy of Chest or Neck

EXCLUDES *Biopsy bone (20220-20251)*
Soft tissue needle biopsy (20206)

21550 **Biopsy, soft tissue of neck or thorax**
4.47 7.50 FUD 010 J G2
AMA: 2018,Sep,7

21552-21558 [21552, 21554] Excision Soft Tissue Tumors Chest and Neck

INCLUDES Any necessary elevation tissue planes or dissection
Measurement tumor and necessary margin at greatest diameter prior to excision
Resection without removal significant normal tissue
Simple and intermediate repairs
Excision types:
Fascial or subfascial soft tissue tumors: simple and marginal resection tumors found either in or below deep fascia, not involving bone or excision substantial amount normal tissue; primarily benign and intramuscular tumors
Radical resection soft tissue tumor: wide resection tumor, involving substantial margins normal tissue and may involve tissue removal from one or more layers; most often malignant or aggressive benign
Subcutaneous: simple and marginal resection tumors in subcutaneous tissue above deep fascia; most often benign

EXCLUDES *Complex repair*
Excision benign cutaneous lesions (eg, sebaceous cyst) (11400-11426)
Radical resection cutaneous tumors (eg, melanoma) (11600-11626)
Significant vessel exploration or neuroplasty

21552 **Resequenced code. See code following 21555.**

21554 **Resequenced code. See code following 21556.**

21555 **Excision, tumor, soft tissue of neck or anterior thorax, subcutaneous; less than 3 cm**
8.79 12.2 FUD 090 J G2
AMA: 2018,Sep,7; 2018,Jan,8; 2017,Jan,8; 2016,Jan,13; 2015,Jan,16

\# **21552** **3 cm or greater**
12.8 12.8 FUD 090 J G2 80
AMA: 2018,Sep,7

21556 **Excision, tumor, soft tissue of neck or anterior thorax, subfascial (eg, intramuscular); less than 5 cm**
15.2 15.2 FUD 090 J G2
AMA: 2018,Sep,7

\# **21554** **5 cm or greater**
21.0 21.0 FUD 090 J G2 80
AMA: 2018,Sep,7

21557 **Radical resection of tumor (eg, sarcoma), soft tissue of neck or anterior thorax; less than 5 cm**
27.5 27.5 **FUD** 090 J G2 80
AMA: 2020,Apr,10; 2018,Sep,7; 2018,Jan,8; 2017,Jan,8; 2016,Jan,13; 2015,Jan,16

21558 **5 cm or greater**
38.8 38.8 **FUD** 090 J G2 80
AMA: 2020,Apr,10; 2018,Sep,7

21600-21632 Bony Resection Chest and Neck

21600 **Excision of rib, partial**
EXCLUDES *Extensive debridement (11044, 11047)*
Radical resection, chest wall/rib cage for tumor (21601)
15.9 15.9 **FUD** 090 J A2 80
AMA: 2018,Sep,7; 2018,Jan,8; 2017,Jan,8; 2016,Jan,13; 2015,Jan,16

21601 **Excision of chest wall tumor including rib(s)**
EXCLUDES *Exploratory thoracotomy (32100)*
Resection apical lung tumor (32503-32504)
Thoracentesis (32554-32555)
Tube thoracostomy (32551)
34.1 34.1 **FUD** 090 80
AMA: 2019,Dec,4

21602 **Excision of chest wall tumor involving rib(s), with plastic reconstruction; without mediastinal lymphadenectomy**
EXCLUDES *Exploratory thoracotomy (32100)*
Resection apical lung tumor (32503-32504)
Thoracentesis (32554-32555)
Tube thoracostomy (32551)
45.8 45.8 **FUD** 090 80
AMA: 2019,Dec,4

21603 **with mediastinal lymphadenectomy**
EXCLUDES *Exploratory thoracotomy (32100)*
Resection apical lung tumor (32503-32504)
Thoracentesis (32554-32555)
Tube thoracostomy (32551)
50.7 50.7 **FUD** 090 80
AMA: 2019,Dec,4

21610 **Costotransversectomy (separate procedure)**
34.5 34.5 **FUD** 090 J A2 80
AMA: 2018,Sep,7

21615 **Excision first and/or cervical rib;**
17.8 17.8 **FUD** 090 C 80 50
AMA: 2018,Sep,7; 2018,Jan,8; 2017,Jan,8; 2016,Jan,13; 2015,Jan,16

21616 **with sympathectomy**
20.7 20.7 **FUD** 090 C 80 50
AMA: 2018,Sep,7

21620 **Ostectomy of sternum, partial**
14.6 14.6 **FUD** 090 C 80
AMA: 2018,Sep,7

21627 **Sternal debridement**
EXCLUDES *Debridement with sternotomy closure (21750)*
15.5 15.5 **FUD** 090 C 80
AMA: 2018,Sep,7; 2018,Jan,8; 2017,Jan,8; 2016,Jan,13; 2015,Jan,16

21630 **Radical resection of sternum;**
35.1 35.1 **FUD** 090 C 80
AMA: 2018,Sep,7

21632 **with mediastinal lymphadenectomy**
34.9 34.9 **FUD** 090 C 80
AMA: 2018,Sep,7

21685-21750 Repair/Reconstruction Chest and Soft Tissues Neck

EXCLUDES *Repair simple wounds (12001-12007)*

21685 **Hyoid myotomy and suspension**
28.2 28.2 **FUD** 090 J G2 80
AMA: 2018,Sep,7; 2018,Jan,8; 2017,Jan,8; 2016,Jan,13; 2015,Jan,16

21700 **Division of scalenus anticus; without resection of cervical rib**
10.3 10.3 **FUD** 090 J A2 80 50
AMA: 2018,Sep,7

21705 **with resection of cervical rib**
15.5 15.5 **FUD** 090 C 80 50
AMA: 2018,Sep,7; 2018,Jan,8; 2017,Jan,8; 2016,Jan,13; 2015,Jan,16

21720 **Division of sternocleidomastoid for torticollis, open operation; without cast application**
EXCLUDES *Transection spinal accessory and cervical nerves (63191, 64722)*
15.0 15.0 **FUD** 090 J A2 80
AMA: 2018,Sep,7

21725 **with cast application**
EXCLUDES *Transection spinal accessory and cervical nerves (63191, 64722)*
15.5 15.5 **FUD** 090 T A2 80
AMA: 2018,Sep,7

21740 **Reconstructive repair of pectus excavatum or carinatum; open**
29.7 29.7 **FUD** 090 C 80
AMA: 2018,Sep,7

21742 **minimally invasive approach (Nuss procedure), without thoracoscopy**
0.00 0.00 **FUD** 090 J 80
AMA: 2018,Sep,7

21743 **minimally invasive approach (Nuss procedure), with thoracoscopy**
0.00 0.00 **FUD** 090 J 80
AMA: 2019,Nov,14; 2018,Sep,7

21750 **Closure of median sternotomy separation with or without debridement (separate procedure)**
19.7 19.7 **FUD** 090 C 80
AMA: 2018,Sep,7; 2018,Jan,8; 2017,Jan,8; 2016,Jan,13; 2015,Jan,16

21811-21825 Fracture Care: Ribs and Sternum

EXCLUDES *Closed treatment uncomplicated rib fractures, report appropriate E/M services*

21811 **Open treatment of rib fracture(s) with internal fixation, includes thoracoscopic visualization when performed, unilateral; 1-3 ribs**
17.2 17.2 **FUD** 000 J 80 50
AMA: 2018,Sep,7; 2018,Jan,8; 2017,Jan,8; 2016,Jan,13; 2015,Aug,3

21812 **4-6 ribs**
21.0 21.0 **FUD** 000 J 80 50
AMA: 2018,Sep,7; 2018,Jan,8; 2017,Jan,8; 2016,Jan,13; 2015,Aug,3

21813 **7 or more ribs**
28.7 28.7 **FUD** 000 J 80 50
AMA: 2018,Sep,7; 2018,Jan,8; 2017,Jan,8; 2016,Jan,13; 2015,Aug,3

21820 **Closed treatment of sternum fracture**
4.15 4.18 **FUD** 090 T A2
AMA: 2018,Sep,7

21825 **Open treatment of sternum fracture with or without skeletal fixation**

EXCLUDES *Treatment sternoclavicular dislocation (23520-23532)*

15.6 15.6 FUD 090 C 80

AMA: 2018,Sep,7

21899 Unlisted Procedures of Chest or Neck

CMS: 100-04,4,180.3 Unlisted Service or Procedure

21899 **Unlisted procedure, neck or thorax**

0.00 0.00 FUD YYY T 80

AMA: 2018,Sep,7; 2018,Jan,8; 2017,Jan,8; 2016,Jan,13; 2015,Aug,3

21920-21925 Biopsy Soft Tissue of Back and Flank

EXCLUDES *Soft tissue needle biopsy (20206)*

21920 **Biopsy, soft tissue of back or flank; superficial**

4.55 7.30 FUD 010 J P3

AMA: 2018,Sep,7

21925 **deep**

10.4 13.4 FUD 090 J A2

AMA: 2018,Sep,7

21930-21936 Excision Soft Tissue Tumors Back or Flank

INCLUDES Any necessary elevation tissue planes or dissection
Measurement tumor and necessary margin at greatest diameter prior to excision
Simple and intermediate repairs
Excision types:
Fascial or subfascial soft tissue tumors: simple and marginal resection tumors found either in or below deep fascia, not involving bone or excision substantial amount normal tissue; most often benign and intramuscular tumors
Radical resection soft tissue tumor: wide resection of tumor, involving substantial margins normal tissue and may include tissue removal from one or more layers; most often malignant or aggressive benign
Subcutaneous: simple and marginal resection tumors in subcutaneous tissue above deep fascia; most often benign

EXCLUDES *Complex repair*
Excision benign cutaneous lesions (eg, sebaceous cyst) (11400-11406)
Radical resection cutaneous tumors (eg, melanoma) (11600-11606)
Significant vessel exploration or neuroplasty

21930 **Excision, tumor, soft tissue of back or flank, subcutaneous; less than 3 cm**

10.4 14.1 FUD 090 J G2

AMA: 2018,Sep,7; 2018,Jan,8; 2017,Jan,8; 2016,Jan,13; 2015,Jan,16

21931 **3 cm or greater**

13.6 13.6 FUD 090 J G2 80

AMA: 2018,Sep,7

21932 **Excision, tumor, soft tissue of back or flank, subfascial (eg, intramuscular); less than 5 cm**

19.0 19.0 FUD 090 J G2 80

AMA: 2018,Sep,7

21933 **5 cm or greater**

21.3 21.3 FUD 090 J G2 80

AMA: 2018,Sep,7

21935 **Radical resection of tumor (eg, sarcoma), soft tissue of back or flank; less than 5 cm**

29.7 29.7 FUD 090 J G2

AMA: 2018,Sep,7

21936 **5 cm or greater**

40.9 40.9 FUD 090 J G2 80

AMA: 2018,Sep,7

22010-22015 Incision for Drainage of Deep Spinal Abscess

EXCLUDES *Incision and drainage hematoma (10060, 10140)*
Injection:
Chemonucleolysis (62292)
Discography (62290-62291)
Facet joint (64490-64495, [64633, 64634, 64635, 64636])
Myelography (62284)
Needle/trocar biopsy (20220-20225)

22010 **Incision and drainage, open, of deep abscess (subfascial), posterior spine; cervical, thoracic, or cervicothoracic**

27.7 27.7 FUD 090 C 80

AMA: 2018,Sep,7

22015 **lumbar, sacral, or lumbosacral**

EXCLUDES *Incision and drainage, complex, postoperative wound infection (10180)*
Incision and drainage, open, deep abscess (subfascial), posterior spine; cervical, thoracic, or cervicothoracic (22010)
Removal posterior nonsegmental instrumentation (eg, Harrington rod) (22850)
Removal posterior segmental instrumentation (22852)

27.2 27.2 FUD 090 C

AMA: 2018,Sep,7

22100-22103 Partial Resection Vertebral Component

EXCLUDES *Back or flank biopsy (21920-21925)*
Bone biopsy (20220-20251)
Bone grafting procedures (20930-20938)
Harvest bone graft (20931, 20938)
Injection:
Chemonucleolysis (62292)
Discography (62290-62291)
Facet joint (64490-64495, [64633, 64634, 64635, 64636])
Myelography (62284)
Osteotomy (22210-22226)
Reconstruction after vertebral body resection (22585, 63082, 63086, 63088, 63091)
Removal tumor flank or back (21930)
Soft tissue needle biopsy (20206)
Spinal reconstruction with bone graft or vertebral body prosthesis:
Cervical (20931, 20938, 22554, 63081)
Lumbar (20931, 20938, 22558, 63087, 63090)
Thoracic (20931, 20938, 22556, 63085, 63087)
Vertebral corpectomy (63081-63091)

22100 **Partial excision of posterior vertebral component (eg, spinous process, lamina or facet) for intrinsic bony lesion, single vertebral segment; cervical**

24.8 24.8 FUD 090 J 80

AMA: 2018,Sep,7; 2018,Jan,8; 2017,Mar,7; 2017,Jan,8; 2016,Jan,13; 2015,Jan,16

22101 **thoracic**

25.1 25.1 FUD 090 J 80

AMA: 2018,Sep,7; 2018,Jan,8; 2017,Mar,7; 2017,Jan,8; 2016,Jan,13; 2015,Jan,16

22102 **lumbar**

Code also posterior spinous process distraction device insertion, when applicable (22867-22870)

23.6 23.6 FUD 090 J G2 80

AMA: 2018,Sep,7; 2018,Jan,8; 2017,Mar,7; 2017,Jan,8; 2016,Jan,13; 2015,Jan,16

+ 22103 **each additional segment (List separately in addition to code for primary procedure)**

Code first (22100-22102)

4.09 4.09 FUD ZZZ N N1 80

AMA: 2018,Sep,7

22110-22116 Partial Resection Vertebral Component without Decompression

EXCLUDES *Back or flank biopsy (21920-21925)*
Bone biopsy (20220-20251)
Bone grafting procedures (20930-20938)
Harvest bone graft (20931, 20938)
Injection:
Chemonucleolysis (62292)
Discography (62290-62291)
Facet joint (64490-64495, [64633, 64634, 64635, 64636])
Myelography (62284)
Osteotomy (22210-22226)
Reconstruction after vertebral body resection (22585, 63082, 63086, 63088, 63091)
Removal tumor flank or back (21930)
Soft tissue needle biopsy (20206)
Spinal reconstruction with bone graft or vertebral body prosthesis:
Cervical (20931, 20938, 22554, 22853-22854 [22859], 63081)
Lumbar (20931, 20938, 22558, 22853-22854 [22859], 63087, 63090)
Thoracic (20931, 20938, 22556, 22853-22854 [22859], 63085, 63087)
Vertebral corpectomy (63081-63091)

22110 **Partial excision of vertebral body, for intrinsic bony lesion, without decompression of spinal cord or nerve root(s), single vertebral segment; cervical**
30.1 30.1 **FUD** 090 C 80
AMA: 2018,Sep,7; 2018,Jan,8; 2017,Mar,7; 2017,Jan,8; 2016,Jan,13; 2015,Jan,16

22112 **thoracic**
32.7 32.7 **FUD** 090 C 80
AMA: 2018,Sep,7; 2018,Jan,8; 2017,Mar,7; 2017,Jan,8; 2016,Jan,13; 2015,Jan,16

22114 **lumbar**
32.4 32.4 **FUD** 090 C 80
AMA: 2018,Sep,7; 2018,Jan,8; 2017,Mar,7; 2017,Jan,8; 2016,Jan,13; 2015,Jan,16

\+ **22116** **each additional vertebral segment (List separately in addition to code for primary procedure)**
Code first (22110-22114)
4.12 4.12 **FUD** ZZZ C 80
AMA: 2018,Sep,7

22206-22216 Spinal Osteotomy: Posterior/Posterolateral Approach

EXCLUDES *Decompression spinal cord and/or nerve roots (63001-63308)*
Injection:
Chemonucleolysis (62292)
Discography (62290-62292)
Facet joint (64490-64495, [64633, 64634, 64635, 64636])
Myelography (62284)
Vertebral corpectomy (63081-63091)
Code also arthrodesis (22590-22632)
Code also bone grafting procedures (20930-20938)
Code also spinal instrumentation (22840-22855 [22859])

22206 **Osteotomy of spine, posterior or posterolateral approach, 3 columns, 1 vertebral segment (eg, pedicle/vertebral body subtraction); thoracic**
EXCLUDES *Osteotomy spine, posterior or posterolateral approach, lumbar (22207)*
Procedures performed at same level (22210-22226, 22830, 63001-63048, 63055-63066, 63075-63091, 63101-63103)
71.3 71.3 **FUD** 090 C 80
AMA: 2018,Sep,7; 2018,Jan,8; 2017,Mar,7; 2017,Jan,8; 2016,Jan,13; 2015,Jan,16

22207 **lumbar**
EXCLUDES *Osteotomy spine, posterior or posterolateral approach, thoracic (22206)*
Procedures performed at same level (22210-22226, 22830, 63001-63048, 63055-63066, 63075-63091, 63101-63103)
69.8 69.8 **FUD** 090 C 80
AMA: 2018,Sep,7; 2018,Jan,8; 2017,Mar,7; 2017,Jan,8; 2016,Jan,13; 2015,Jan,16

\+ **22208** **each additional vertebral segment (List separately in addition to code for primary procedure)**
EXCLUDES *Procedures performed at same level (22210-22226, 22830, 63001-63048, 63055-63066, 63075-63091, 63101-63103)*
Code first (22206, 22207)
17.1 17.1 **FUD** ZZZ C 80
AMA: 2018,Sep,7; 2018,Jan,8; 2017,Jan,8; 2016,Jan,13; 2015,Jan,16

22210 **Osteotomy of spine, posterior or posterolateral approach, 1 vertebral segment; cervical**
51.7 51.7 **FUD** 090 C 80
AMA: 2018,Sep,7; 2018,Jan,8; 2017,Mar,7; 2017,Jan,8; 2016,Jan,13; 2015,Jan,16

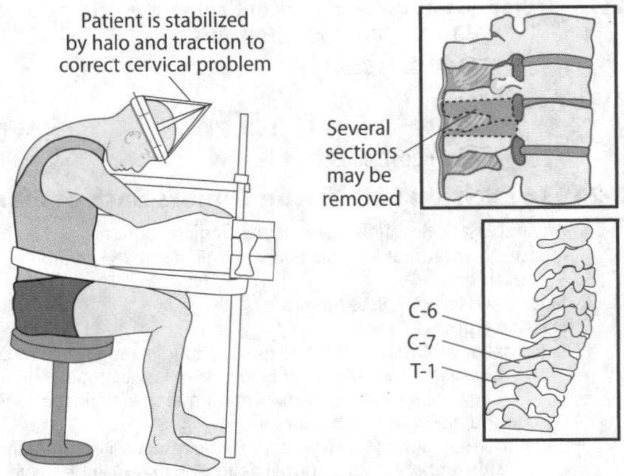
Patient is stabilized by halo and traction to correct cervical problem
Several sections may be removed
C-6
C-7
T-1
Physician removes spinous processes, lamina

22212 **thoracic**
43.2 43.2 **FUD** 090 C 80
AMA: 2018,Sep,7; 2018,Jan,8; 2017,Mar,7; 2017,Jan,8; 2016,Jan,13; 2015,Jan,16

22214 **lumbar**
43.4 43.4 **FUD** 090 C 80
AMA: 2018,Sep,7; 2018,Jan,8; 2017,Mar,7; 2017,Jan,8; 2016,Jan,13; 2015,Jan,16

\+ **22216** **each additional vertebral segment (List separately in addition to primary procedure)**
Code first (22210-22214)
10.5 10.5 **FUD** ZZZ C 80
AMA: 2018,Sep,7; 2018,Jan,8; 2017,Jan,8; 2016,Jan,13; 2015,Jan,16

22220-22226 Spinal Osteotomy: Anterior Approach

EXCLUDES *Decompression spinal cord and/or nerve roots (63001-63308)*
Injection:
Chemonucleolysis (62292)
Discography (62290-62291)
Facet joint (64490-64495, [64633, 64634, 64635, 64636])
Myelography (62284)
Needle/trocar biopsy (20220-20225)
Vertebral corpectomy (63081-63091)
Code also arthrodesis (22590-22632)
Code also bone grafting procedures (20930-20938)
Code also spinal instrumentation (22840-22855 [22859])

22220 **Osteotomy of spine, including discectomy, anterior approach, single vertebral segment; cervical**
47.0 47.0 **FUD** 090 C 80
AMA: 2018,Sep,7; 2018,Jan,8; 2017,Mar,7; 2017,Jan,8; 2016,Jan,13; 2015,Jan,16

22222 **thoracic**
51.1 51.1 **FUD** 090 C 80
AMA: 2018,Sep,7; 2018,Jan,8; 2017,Mar,7; 2017,Jan,8; 2016,Jan,13; 2015,Jan,16

22224 **lumbar**
46.1 46.1 **FUD** 090 C 80
AMA: 2018,Sep,7; 2018,Jan,8; 2017,Mar,7; 2017,Jan,8; 2016,Jan,13; 2015,Jan,16

\+ 22226 **each additional vertebral segment (List separately in addition to code for primary procedure)**
Code first (22220-22224)
10.5 10.5 **FUD** ZZZ C 80
AMA: 2018,Sep,7

22310-22315 Closed Treatment Vertebral Fractures

EXCLUDES *Injection:*
Chemonucleolysis (62292)
Discography (62290-62291)
Facet joint (64490-64495, [64633, 64634, 64635, 64636])
Myelography (62284)
Percutaneous vertebroplasty at same level (22510-22515)
Code also arthrodesis (22590-22632)
Code also bone grafting procedures (20930-20938)
Code also spinal instrumentation (22840-22855 [22859])

22310 **Closed treatment of vertebral body fracture(s), without manipulation, requiring and including casting or bracing**
8.38 8.70 **FUD** 090 T A2
AMA: 2018,Sep,7; 2018,Jan,8; 2017,Mar,7; 2017,Jan,8; 2016,Jan,13; 2015,Jan,16; 2015,Jan,8

22315 **Closed treatment of vertebral fracture(s) and/or dislocation(s) requiring casting or bracing, with and including casting and/or bracing by manipulation or traction**
EXCLUDES *Spinal manipulation (97140)*
22.2 25.3 **FUD** 090 J A2
AMA: 2018,Sep,7; 2018,Jan,8; 2017,Mar,7; 2017,Jan,8; 2016,Jan,13; 2015,Jan,8; 2015,Jan,16

22318-22319 Open Treatment Odontoid Fracture: Anterior Approach

EXCLUDES *Injection:*
Chemonucleolysis (62292)
Discography (62290-62291)
Facet joint (64490-64495, [64633, 64634, 64635, 64636])
Myelography (62284)
Needle/trocar biopsy (20220-20225)
Code also arthrodesis (22590-22632)
Code also bone grafting procedures (20930-20938)
Code also spinal instrumentation (22840-22855 [22859])

22318 **Open treatment and/or reduction of odontoid fracture(s) and or dislocation(s) (including os odontoideum), anterior approach, including placement of internal fixation; without grafting**
47.6 47.6 **FUD** 090 C 80
AMA: 2018,Sep,7; 2018,Jan,8; 2017,Mar,7; 2017,Jan,8; 2016,Jan,13; 2015,Jan,16

22319 **with grafting**
53.6 53.6 **FUD** 090 C 80
AMA: 2018,Sep,7; 2018,May,3; 2018,Jan,8; 2017,Mar,7; 2017,Jan,8; 2016,Jan,13; 2015,Jan,16

22325-22328 Open Treatment Vertebral Fractures: Posterior Approach

EXCLUDES *Injection:*
Chemonucleolysis (62292)
Discography (62290-62291)
Facet joint (64490-64495, [64633, 64634, 64635, 64636])
Myelography (62284)
Needle/trocar biopsy (20220-20225)
Spine decompression (63001-63091)
Vertebral corpectomy (63081-63091)
Vertebral fracture care by arthrodesis (22548-22632)
Code also arthrodesis (22548-22632)
Code also bone grafting procedures (20930-20938)
Code also spinal instrumentation (22840-22855 [22859])

22325 **Open treatment and/or reduction of vertebral fracture(s) and/or dislocation(s), posterior approach, 1 fractured vertebra or dislocated segment; lumbar**
EXCLUDES *Percutaneous vertebral augmentation performed at same level (22514-22515)*
Percutaneous vertebroplasty performed at same level (22511-22512)
41.9 41.9 **FUD** 090 C 80
AMA: 2018,Sep,7; 2018,Jan,8; 2017,Aug,9; 2017,Mar,7; 2017,Jan,8; 2016,Jan,13; 2015,Jan,16; 2015,Jan,8

22326 **cervical**
EXCLUDES *Percutaneous vertebroplasty performed at same level (22510, 22512)*
43.4 43.4 **FUD** 090 C 80
AMA: 2018,Sep,7; 2018,Jan,8; 2017,Mar,7; 2017,Jan,8; 2016,Jan,13; 2015,Jan,16

22327 **thoracic**
EXCLUDES *Percutaneous vertebral augmentation performed at same level (22515)*
Percutaneous vertebroplasty performed at same level (22510, 22512-22513)
43.7 43.7 **FUD** 090 C 80
AMA: 2018,Sep,7; 2018,Jan,8; 2017,Mar,7; 2017,Jan,8; 2016,Jan,13; 2015,Jan,8; 2015,Jan,16

\+ 22328 **each additional fractured vertebra or dislocated segment (List separately in addition to code for primary procedure)**
Code first (22325-22327)
8.25 8.25 **FUD** ZZZ C 80
AMA: 2018,Sep,7

22505 Spinal Manipulation with Anesthesia

EXCLUDES *Manipulation not requiring anesthesia (97140)*

22505 **Manipulation of spine requiring anesthesia, any region**
3.76 3.76 **FUD** 010 J A2
AMA: 2018,Sep,7; 2018,Jan,8; 2017,Jan,8; 2016,Jan,13; 2015,Jan,16

22510-22515 Percutaneous Vertebroplasty/Kyphoplasty

INCLUDES Radiological guidance
When performed at same level:
Bone biopsy (20225)
Closed treatment vertebral fractures (22310, 22315)
Open treatment/reduction vertebral fractures (22325, 22327)
EXCLUDES *Sacroplasty/augmentation (0200T-0201T)*

22510 **Percutaneous vertebroplasty (bone biopsy included when performed), 1 vertebral body, unilateral or bilateral injection, inclusive of all imaging guidance; cervicothoracic**
12.5 49.8 **FUD** 010 J G2
AMA: 2018,Sep,7; 2018,Jan,8; 2017,Jan,8; 2016,Jan,13; 2015,Jan,8

22511 **lumbosacral**
11.7 49.3 **FUD** 010 J G2
AMA: 2018,Sep,7; 2018,Jan,8; 2017,Jan,8; 2016,Jan,13; 2015,Apr,8; 2015,Jan,8

+ **22512** **each additional cervicothoracic or lumbosacral vertebral body (List separately in addition to code for primary procedure)**
Code first (22510-22511)
5.96 24.4 **FUD** ZZZ N N1
AMA: 2018,Sep,7; 2018,Jan,8; 2017,Jan,8; 2016,Jan,13; 2015,Jan,8

22513 **Percutaneous vertebral augmentation, including cavity creation (fracture reduction and bone biopsy included when performed) using mechanical device (eg, kyphoplasty), 1 vertebral body, unilateral or bilateral cannulation, inclusive of all imaging guidance; thoracic**
14.9 195. **FUD** 010 J G2
AMA: 2018,Sep,7; 2018,Jan,8; 2017,Jan,8; 2016,Jan,13; 2015,Jan,8

22514 **lumbar**
13.9 194. **FUD** 010 J G2
AMA: 2018,Sep,7; 2018,Jan,8; 2017,Jan,8; 2016,Jan,13; 2015,Jan,8

+ **22515** **each additional thoracic or lumbar vertebral body (List separately in addition to code for primary procedure)**
Code first (22513-22514)
6.39 105. **FUD** ZZZ N N1
AMA: 2018,Sep,7; 2018,Jan,8; 2017,Jan,8; 2016,Jan,13; 2015,Jan,8

22526-22527 Percutaneous Annuloplasty

CMS: 100-04,32,220.1 Thermal Intradiscal Procedures (TIPS)

INCLUDES Fluoroscopic guidance (77002, 77003)
EXCLUDES *Needle/trocar biopsy (20220-20225)*
Injection:
Chemonucleolysis (62292)
Discography (62290-62291)
Facet joint (64490-64495, [64633, 64634, 64635, 64636])
Myelography (62284)
Procedure performed by other methods (22899)

22526 **Percutaneous intradiscal electrothermal annuloplasty, unilateral or bilateral including fluoroscopic guidance; single level**
9.76 65.0 **FUD** 010 E
AMA: 2018,Sep,7; 2018,Jan,8; 2017,Jan,8; 2016,Jan,13; 2015,Jan,8; 2015,Jan,16

+ **22527** **1 or more additional levels (List separately in addition to code for primary procedure)**
Code first (22526)
4.44 53.1 **FUD** ZZZ E
AMA: 2018,Sep,7; 2018,Jan,8; 2017,Jan,8; 2016,Jan,13; 2015,Jan,8; 2015,Jan,16

22532-22534 Spinal Fusion: Lateral Extracavitary Approach

EXCLUDES *Corpectomy (63101-63103)*
Exploration spinal fusion (22830)
Fracture care (22310-22328)
Injection:
Chemonucleolysis (62292)
Discography (62290-62291)
Facet joint (64490-64495, [64633, 64634, 64635, 64636])
Myelography (62284)
Laminectomy (63001-63017)
Needle/trocar biopsy (20220-20225)
Osteotomy (22206-22226)
Code also bone grafting procedures (20930-20938)
Code also spinal instrumentation (22840-22855 [22859])

22532 **Arthrodesis, lateral extracavitary technique, including minimal discectomy to prepare interspace (other than for decompression); thoracic**
52.1 52.1 **FUD** 090 C 80
AMA: 2020,May,13; 2018,Sep,7; 2018,May,3; 2018,Jan,8; 2017,Mar,7; 2017,Feb,9; 2017,Jan,8; 2016,Jan,13; 2015,Jan,16

22533 **lumbar**
48.0 48.0 **FUD** 090 C 80
AMA: 2020,May,13; 2018,Sep,7; 2018,May,3; 2018,Jan,8; 2017,Mar,7; 2017,Feb,9; 2017,Jan,8; 2016,Jan,13; 2015,Jan,16

+ **22534** **thoracic or lumbar, each additional vertebral segment (List separately in addition to code for primary procedure)**
Code first (22532-22533)
10.5 10.5 **FUD** ZZZ C 80
AMA: 2020,May,13; 2018,Sep,7; 2018,May,3; 2017,Feb,9

22548-22634 Spinal Fusion: Anterior and Posterior Approach

EXCLUDES *Corpectomy (63081-63091)*
Exploration spinal fusion (22830)
Fracture care (22310-22328)
Injection:
Chemonucleolysis (62292)
Discography (62290-62291)
Facet joint (64490-64495, [64633, 64634, 64635, 64636])
Myelography (62284)
Laminectomy (63001-63017)
Needle/trocar biopsy (20220-20225)
Osteotomy (22206-22226)
Code also bone grafting procedures (20930-20938)
Code also spinal instrumentation (22840-22855 [22859])

22548 **Arthrodesis, anterior transoral or extraoral technique, clivus-C1-C2 (atlas-axis), with or without excision of odontoid process**
EXCLUDES *Laminectomy or laminotomy with disc removal (63020-63042)*
56.4 56.4 **FUD** 090 C 80
AMA: 2020,May,13; 2018,Sep,7; 2018,May,3; 2018,Jan,8; 2017,Mar,7; 2017,Jan,8; 2016,Jan,13; 2015,Jan,16

22551 **Arthrodesis, anterior interbody, including disc space preparation, discectomy, osteophytectomy and decompression of spinal cord and/or nerve roots; cervical below C2**
INCLUDES Operating microscope (69990)
49.3 49.3 **FUD** 090 J J8 80
AMA: 2020,May,13; 2018,Sep,7; 2018,Aug,10; 2018,May,3; 2018,Jan,8; 2017,Mar,7; 2017,Jan,8; 2016,May,13; 2016,Feb,12; 2016,Jan,13; 2015,Jan,16; 2015,Jan,13

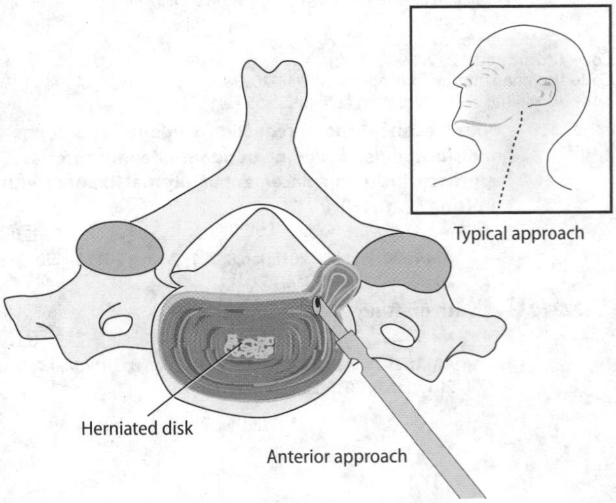

+ **22552** **cervical below C2, each additional interspace (List separately in addition to code for separate procedure)**
INCLUDES Operating microscope (69990)
Code first (22551)
11.6 11.6 **FUD** ZZZ N N1 80
AMA: 2020,May,13; 2018,Sep,7; 2018,Aug,10; 2018,May,3; 2018,Jan,8; 2017,Mar,7; 2017,Jan,8; 2016,Feb,12; 2016,Jan,13; 2015,Jan,16

22554 **Arthrodesis, anterior interbody technique, including minimal discectomy to prepare interspace (other than for decompression); cervical below C2**

EXCLUDES *Anterior discectomy and interbody fusion during same operative session (regardless if performed by multiple surgeons) (22551)*

Discectomy, anterior, with decompression spinal cord and/or nerve root(s), cervical (even by separate individual) (63075-63076)

36.3 36.3 **FUD** 090 J J8 80

AMA: 2020,May,13; 2018,Sep,7; 2018,May,3; 2018,Jan,8; 2017,Mar,7; 2017,Jan,8; 2016,Jan,13; 2015,Apr,7; 2015,Jan,16

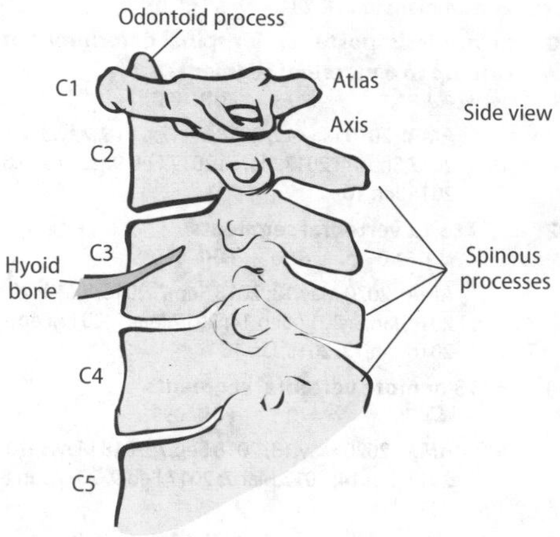

22556 **thoracic**

48.1 48.1 **FUD** 090 C 80

AMA: 2020,May,13; 2018,Sep,7; 2018,May,3; 2018,Jan,8; 2017,Mar,7; 2017,Jan,8; 2016,Jan,13; 2015,Jan,16

22558 **lumbar**

EXCLUDES *Arthrodesis using pre-sacral interbody technique (22586)*

44.3 44.3 **FUD** 090 C 80

AMA: 2020,May,13; 2018,Sep,7; 2018,May,3; 2018,Jan,8; 2017,Mar,7; 2017,Feb,9; 2017,Jan,8; 2016,Jan,13; 2015,Mar,9; 2015,Jan,16

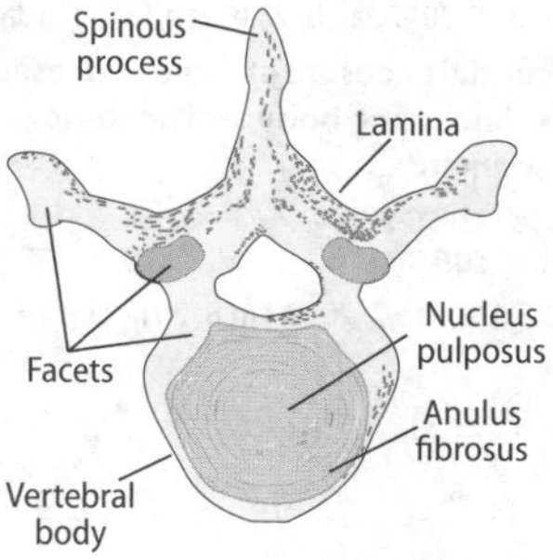

Thoracic vertebra (superior views)

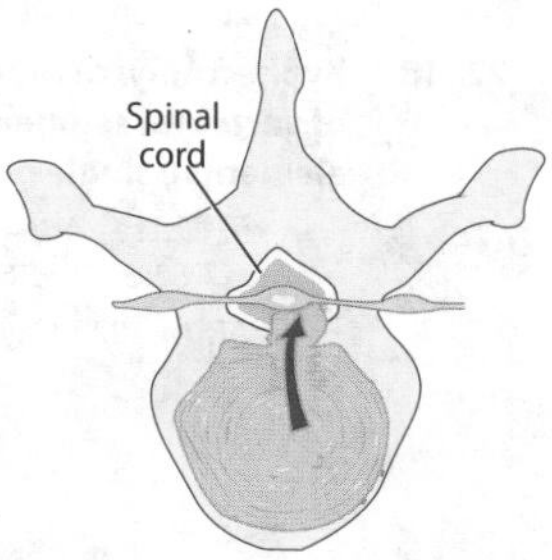

Depiction of nucleus herniating through anulus and pressuring spinal nerve

\+ **22585** **each additional interspace (List separately in addition to code for primary procedure)**

EXCLUDES *Anterior discectomy and interbody fusion during same operative session (regardless if performed by multiple surgeons) (22552)*

Discectomy, anterior, with decompression spinal cord and/or nerve root(s), cervical (even by separate individual) (63075)

Code first (22554-22558)

9.51 9.51 **FUD** ZZZ N N1 80

AMA: 2020,May,13; 2018,Sep,7; 2018,Jan,8; 2017,Jan,8; 2016,Jan,13; 2015,Jan,16

22586 **Arthrodesis, pre-sacral interbody technique, including disc space preparation, discectomy, with posterior instrumentation, with image guidance, includes bone graft when performed, L5-S1 interspace**

INCLUDES Radiologic guidance (77002-77003, 77011-77012)

EXCLUDES *Allograft and autograft spinal bone (20930-20938)*

Epidurography, radiological supervision and interpretation (72275)

Pelvic fixation, other than sacrum (22848)

Posterior non-segmental instrumentation (22840)

59.6 59.6 **FUD** 090 C 80

AMA: 2020,May,13; 2018,Sep,7

22590 **Arthrodesis, posterior technique, craniocervical (occiput-C2)**

EXCLUDES *Posterior intrafacet implant insertion (0219T-0222T)*

45.6 45.6 **FUD** 090 C 80

AMA: 2020,May,13; 2018,Sep,7; 2018,May,3; 2018,Jan,8; 2017,Mar,7; 2017,Jan,8; 2016,Jan,13; 2015,Jan,16

Skull and cervical vertebrae; posterior view

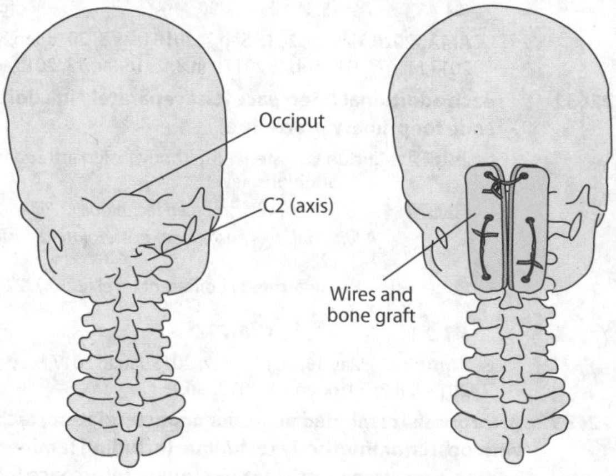

The physician fuses skull to C2 (axis) to stabilize cervical vertebrae; anchor holes are drilled in the occiput of the skull

22595 **Arthrodesis, posterior technique, atlas-axis (C1-C2)**

EXCLUDES *Posterior intrafacet implant insertion (0219T-0222T)*

43.8 43.8 **FUD** 090 C 80

AMA: 2020,May,13; 2018,Sep,7; 2018,May,3; 2018,Jan,8; 2017,Mar,7; 2017,Jan,8; 2016,Jan,13; 2015,Jan,16

22600 **Arthrodesis, posterior or posterolateral technique, single level; cervical below C2 segment**

EXCLUDES *Posterior intrafacet implant insertion (0219T-0222T)*

37.4 37.4 **FUD** 090 C 80

AMA: 2020,May,13; 2018,Sep,7; 2018,May,3; 2018,Jan,8; 2017,Mar,7; 2017,Jan,8; 2016,Jan,13; 2015,Jan,16

22610 **thoracic (with lateral transverse technique, when performed)**

EXCLUDES *Posterior intrafacet implant insertion (0219T-0222T)*

36.7 36.7 **FUD** 090 C 80

AMA: 2020,May,13; 2018,Sep,7; 2018,May,3; 2018,Jan,8; 2017,Mar,7; 2017,Jan,8; 2016,Jan,13; 2015,Jan,16

22612 **lumbar (with lateral transverse technique, when performed)**

EXCLUDES *Arthrodesis performed at same interspace and segment (22630)*

Combined technique at same interspace and segment (22633)

Posterior intrafacet implant insertion (0219T-0222T)

46.0 46.0 **FUD** 090 J J8 80

AMA: 2020,May,13; 2018,Sep,7; 2018,May,3; 2018,Jan,8; 2017,Mar,7; 2017,Feb,9; 2017,Jan,8; 2016,Jan,13; 2015,Jan,16

+ **22614** **each additional vertebral segment (List separately in addition to code for primary procedure)**

INCLUDES Additional level fusion arthrodesis posterior or posterolateral interbody

EXCLUDES *Additional level interbody arthrodesis combined posterolateral or posterior with posterior interbody arthrodesis (22634)*

Additional level posterior interbody arthrodesis (22632)

Posterior intrafacet implant insertion (0219T-0222T)

Code first when performed at different level (22600, 22610, 22612, 22630, 22633)

11.4 11.4 **FUD** ZZZ N N1 80

AMA: 2020,May,13; 2018,Sep,7; 2018,Jan,8; 2017,Feb,9; 2017,Jan,8; 2016,Jan,13; 2015,Jan,16

22630 **Arthrodesis, posterior interbody technique, including laminectomy and/or discectomy to prepare interspace (other than for decompression), single interspace; lumbar**

EXCLUDES *Arthrodesis performed at same interspace and segment (22612)*

Combined technique (22612 and 22630) for same interspace and segment (22633)

45.5 45.5 **FUD** 090 C 80

AMA: 2020,May,13; 2018,Sep,7; 2018,May,3; 2018,Jan,8; 2017,Mar,7; 2017,Feb,9; 2017,Jan,8; 2016,Jan,13; 2015,Jan,16

+ **22632** **each additional interspace (List separately in addition to code for primary procedure)**

INCLUDES Includes posterior interbody fusion arthrodesis, additional level

EXCLUDES *Additional level combined technique (22634)*

Additional level posterior or posterolateral fusion (22614)

Code first when performed at different level (22612, 22630, 22633)

9.36 9.36 **FUD** ZZZ C 80

AMA: 2020,May,13; 2018,Sep,7; 2018,Jan,8; 2017,Feb,9; 2017,Jan,8; 2016,Jan,13; 2015,Jan,16

22633 **Arthrodesis, combined posterior or posterolateral technique with posterior interbody technique including laminectomy and/or discectomy sufficient to prepare interspace (other than for decompression), single interspace and segment; lumbar**

EXCLUDES *Arthrodesis performed at same interspace and segment (22612, 22630)*

53.8 53.8 **FUD** 090 C 80

AMA: 2020,May,13; 2018,Sep,7; 2018,Jul,14; 2018,May,9; 2018,May,3; 2018,Jan,8; 2017,Mar,7; 2017,Feb,9; 2017,Jan,8; 2016,Oct,11; 2016,Jan,13; 2015,Jan,16

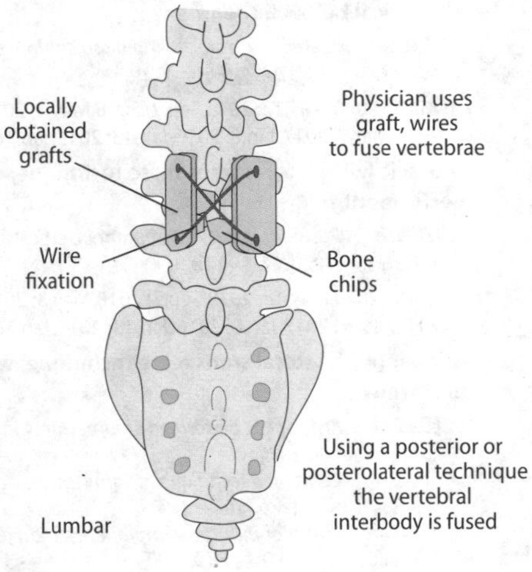
Locally obtained grafts
Physician uses graft, wires to fuse vertebrae
Wire fixation
Bone chips
Using a posterior or posterolateral technique the vertebral interbody is fused
Lumbar

+ **22634** **each additional interspace and segment (List separately in addition to code for primary procedure)**

Code first (22633)

14.4 14.4 **FUD** ZZZ C 80

AMA: 2020,May,13; 2018,Sep,7; 2018,Jul,14; 2018,May,3; 2018,Jan,8; 2017,Mar,7; 2017,Feb,9; 2017,Jan,8; 2016,Jan,13; 2015,Jan,16

22800-22819 Procedures to Correct Anomalous Spinal Vertebrae

CMS: 100-03,150.2 Osteogenic Stimulation

EXCLUDES *Facet injection (64490-64495, [64633, 64634, 64635, 64636])*

Code also bone grafting procedures (20930-20938)

Code also spinal instrumentation (22840-22855 [22859])

22800 **Arthrodesis, posterior, for spinal deformity, with or without cast; up to 6 vertebral segments**

39.3 39.3 **FUD** 090 C 80

AMA: 2020,May,13; 2018,Sep,7; 2018,May,3; 2018,Jan,8; 2017,Sep,14; 2017,Mar,7; 2017,Feb,9; 2017,Jan,8; 2016,Jan,13; 2015,Jan,16

22802 **7 to 12 vertebral segments**

61.0 61.0 **FUD** 090 C 80

AMA: 2020,May,13; 2018,Sep,7; 2018,Jul,14; 2018,May,3; 2018,Jan,8; 2017,Sep,14; 2017,Mar,7; 2017,Feb,9; 2017,Jan,8; 2016,Jan,13; 2015,Jan,16

22804 **13 or more vertebral segments**

70.3 70.3 **FUD** 090 C 80

AMA: 2020,May,13; 2018,Sep,7; 2018,May,3; 2018,Jan,8; 2017,Sep,14; 2017,Mar,7; 2017,Feb,9; 2017,Jan,8; 2016,Jan,13; 2015,Jan,16

22808 **Arthrodesis, anterior, for spinal deformity, with or without cast; 2 to 3 vertebral segments**

INCLUDES Smith-Robinson arthrodesis

53.1 53.1 **FUD** 090 C 80

AMA: 2020,May,13; 2018,Sep,7; 2018,May,3; 2018,Jan,8; 2017,Sep,14; 2017,Mar,7; 2017,Jan,8; 2016,Jan,13; 2015,Jan,16

22810 **4 to 7 vertebral segments**

60.2 60.2 **FUD** 090 C 80

AMA: 2020,May,13; 2018,Sep,7; 2018,May,3; 2018,Jan,8; 2017,Sep,14; 2017,Mar,7; 2017,Jan,8; 2016,Jan,13; 2015,Jan,16

22812 **8 or more vertebral segments**

63.9 63.9 **FUD** 090 C 80

AMA: 2020,May,13; 2018,Sep,7; 2018,May,3; 2018,Jan,8; 2017,Sep,14; 2017,Mar,7; 2017,Jan,8; 2016,Jan,13; 2015,Jan,16

22818 **Kyphectomy, circumferential exposure of spine and resection of vertebral segment(s) (including body and posterior elements); single or 2 segments**

EXCLUDES *Arthrodesis (22800-22804)*

62.6 62.6 **FUD** 090 C 80

AMA: 2020,May,13; 2018,Sep,7; 2018,Jan,8; 2017,Sep,14

22819 **3 or more segments**

> EXCLUDES *Arthrodesis (22800-22804)*
>
> 🚑 72.2   👤 72.2   **FUD** 090   C 80 ▣
>
> **AMA:** 2020,May,13; 2018,Sep,7; 2018,Jan,8; 2017,Sep,14

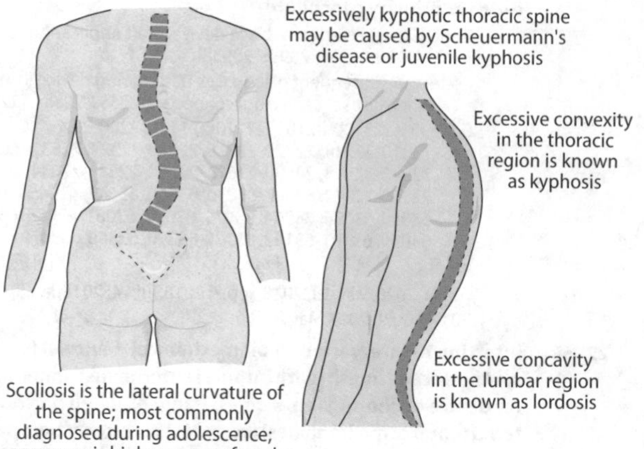

Excessively kyphotic thoracic spine may be caused by Scheuermann's disease or juvenile kyphosis

Excessive convexity in the thoracic region is known as kyphosis

Excessive concavity in the lumbar region is known as lordosis

Scoliosis is the lateral curvature of the spine; most commonly diagnosed during adolescence; occurrence is higher among females

22830 Surgical Exploration Previous Spinal Fusion

CMS: 100-03,150.2 Osteogenic Stimulation

> EXCLUDES *Arthrodesis (22532-22819)*
> *Bone grafting procedures (20930-20938)*
> *Instrumentation removal (22850, 22852, 22855)*
> *Spinal decompression (63001-63103)*
> Code also spinal instrumentation (22840-22855 [22859])

22830 **Exploration of spinal fusion**

> 🚑 23.6   👤 23.6   **FUD** 090   C 80 ▣
>
> **AMA:** 2018,Sep,7; 2018,Jan,8; 2017,Jan,8; 2016,Jan,13; 2015,Jan,16

22840-22848 Posterior, Anterior, Pelvic Spinal Instrumentation

> INCLUDES Removal or revision previously placed spinal instrumentation during same session as insertion new instrumentation at levels including all or part of previously instrumented segments (22849, 22850, 22852, 22855)
>
> EXCLUDES *Arthrodesis (22532-22534, 22548-22812)*
> *Bone grafting procedures (20930-20938)*
> *Exploration spinal fusion (22830)*
> *Fracture treatment (22325-22328)*
> *Reporting more than one instrumentation code per incision*

+ **22840** **Posterior non-segmental instrumentation (eg, Harrington rod technique, pedicle fixation across 1 interspace, atlantoaxial transarticular screw fixation, sublaminar wiring at C1, facet screw fixation) (List separately in addition to code for primary procedure)**

> Code first (22100-22102, 22110-22114, 22206-22207, 22210-22214, 22220-22224, 22310-22327, 22532-22533, 22548-22558, 22590-22612, 22630, 22633-22634, 22800-22812, 63001-63030, 63040-63042, 63045-63047, 63050-63056, 63064, 63075, 63077, 63081, 63085, 63087, 63090, 63101-63102, 63170-63290, 63300-63307)
>
> 🚑 22.2   👤 22.2   **FUD** ZZZ   N N1 80 ▣
>
> **AMA:** 2020,May,13; 2018,Sep,7; 2018,Jan,8; 2017,Jun,10; 2017,Feb,9; 2017,Jan,8; 2016,Jan,13; 2015,Jan,16

+ **22841** **Internal spinal fixation by wiring of spinous processes (List separately in addition to code for primary procedure)**

> Code first (22100-22102, 22110-22114, 22206-22207, 22210-22214, 22220-22224, 22310-22327, 22532-22533, 22548-22558, 22590-22612, 22630, 22633-22634, 22800-22812, 63001-63030, 63040-63042, 63045-63047, 63050-63056, 63064, 63075, 63077, 63081, 63085, 63087, 63090, 63101-63102, 63170-63290, 63300-63307)
>
> 🚑 0.00   👤 0.00   **FUD** XXX   C ▣
>
> **AMA:** 2020,May,13; 2018,Sep,7; 2018,Jan,8; 2017,Feb,9; 2017,Jan,8; 2016,Jan,13; 2015,Jan,16

+ **22842** **Posterior segmental instrumentation (eg, pedicle fixation, dual rods with multiple hooks and sublaminar wires); 3 to 6 vertebral segments (List separately in addition to code for primary procedure)**

> Code first (22100-22102, 22110-22114, 22206-22207, 22210-22214, 22220-22224, 22310-22327, 22532-22533, 22548-22558, 22590-22612, 22630, 22633-22634, 22800-22812, 63001-63030, 63040-63042, 63045-63047, 63050-63056, 63064, 63075, 63077, 63081, 63085, 63087, 63090, 63101-63102, 63170-63290, 63300-63307)
>
> 🚑 22.1   👤 22.1   **FUD** ZZZ   N N1 80 ▣
>
> **AMA:** 2020,May,13; 2018,Sep,7; 2018,Jan,8; 2017,Feb,9; 2017,Jan,8; 2016,Jan,13; 2015,Jan,16

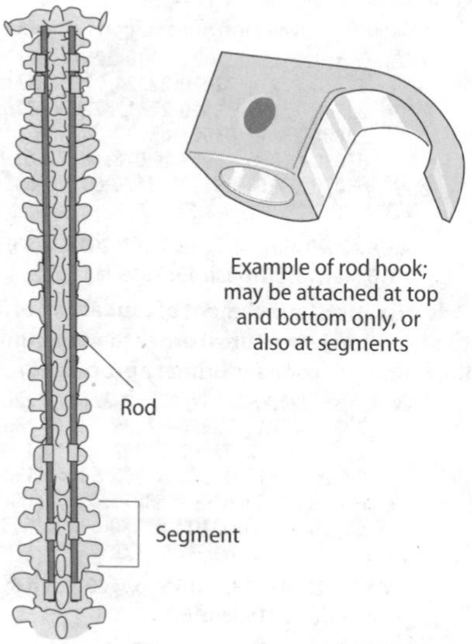

Example of rod hook; may be attached at top and bottom only, or also at segments

Rod

Segment

+ **22843** **7 to 12 vertebral segments (List separately in addition to code for primary procedure)**

> Code first (22100-22102, 22110-22114, 22206-22207, 22210-22214, 22220-22224, 22310-22327, 22532-22533, 22548-22558, 22590-22612, 22630, 22633-22634, 22800-22812, 63001-63030, 63040-63042, 63045-63047, 63050-63056, 63064, 63075, 63077, 63081, 63085, 63087, 63090, 63101-63102, 63170-63290, 63300-63307)
>
> 🚑 23.8   👤 23.8   **FUD** ZZZ   C 80 ▣
>
> **AMA:** 2020,May,13; 2018,Sep,7; 2018,Jul,14; 2018,Jan,8; 2017,Jan,8; 2016,Jan,13; 2015,Jan,16

+ **22844** **13 or more vertebral segments (List separately in addition to code for primary procedure)**

> Code first (22100-22102, 22110-22114, 22206-22207, 22210-22214, 22220-22224, 22310-22327, 22532-22533, 22548-22558, 22590-22612, 22630, 22633-22634, 22800-22812, 63001-63030, 63040-63042, 63045-63047, 63050-63056, 63064, 63075, 63077, 63081, 63085, 63087, 63090, 63101-63102, 63170-63290, 63300-63307)
>
> 🚑 28.6   👤 28.6   **FUD** ZZZ   C 80 ▣
>
> **AMA:** 2020,May,13; 2018,Sep,7; 2018,Jan,8; 2017,Jan,8; 2016,Jan,13; 2015,Jan,16

+ **22845** **Anterior instrumentation; 2 to 3 vertebral segments (List separately in addition to code for primary procedure)**

> INCLUDES Dwyer instrumentation technique
>
> Code first (22100-22102, 22110-22114, 22206-22207, 22210-22214, 22220-22224, 22310-22327, 22532-22533, 22548-22558, 22590-22612, 22630, 22633-22634, 22800-22812, 63001-63030, 63040-63042, 63045-63047, 63050-63056, 63064, 63075, 63077, 63081, 63085, 63087, 63090, 63101-63102, 63170-63290, 63300-63307)
>
> 🚑 21.1   👤 21.1   **FUD** ZZZ   N N1 80 ▣
>
> **AMA:** 2020,May,13; 2018,Sep,7; 2018,Jan,8; 2017,Mar,7; 2017,Jan,8; 2016,May,13; 2016,Jan,13; 2015,Apr,7; 2015,Mar,9; 2015,Jan,13; 2015,Jan,16

● New Code   ▲ Revised Code   ○ Reinstated   ● New Web Release   ▲ Revised Web Release   + Add-on   Unlisted   Not Covered   # Resequenced
50 Optum Mod 50 Exempt   ⊘ AMA Mod 51 Exempt   51 Optum Mod 51 Exempt   63 Mod 63 Exempt   ⚹ Non-FDA Drug   ★ Telemedicine   M Maternity   A Age Edit

+ 22846 4 to 7 vertebral segments (List separately in addition to code for primary procedure)

INCLUDES Dwyer instrumentation technique

Code first (22100-22102, 22110-22114, 22206-22207, 22210-22214, 22220-22224, 22310-22327, 22532-22533, 22548-22558, 22590-22612, 22630, 22633-22634, 22800-22812, 63001-63030, 63040-63042, 63045-63047, 63050-63056, 63064, 63075, 63077, 63081, 63085, 63087, 63090, 63101-63102, 63170-63290, 63300-63307)

22.0 22.0 FUD ZZZ C 80

AMA: 2020,May,13; 2018,Sep,7; 2018,Jan,8; 2017,Jan,8; 2016,May,13; 2016,Jan,13; 2015,Jan,16

+ 22847 8 or more vertebral segments (List separately in addition to code for primary procedure)

INCLUDES Dwyer instrumentation technique

Code first (22100-22102, 22110-22114, 22206-22207, 22210-22214, 22220-22224, 22310-22327, 22532-22533, 22548-22558, 22590-22612, 22630, 22633-22634, 22800-22812, 63001-63030, 63040-63042, 63045-63047, 63050-63056, 63064, 63075, 63077, 63081, 63085, 63087, 63090, 63101-63102, 63170-63290, 63300-63307)

23.4 23.4 FUD ZZZ C 80

AMA: 2020,May,13; 2018,Sep,7; 2018,Jan,8; 2017,Jan,8; 2016,May,13; 2016,Jan,13; 2015,Jan,16

+ 22848 Pelvic fixation (attachment of caudal end of instrumentation to pelvic bony structures) other than sacrum (List separately in addition to code for primary procedure)

Code first (22100-22102, 22110-22114, 22206-22207, 22210-22214, 22220-22224, 22310-22327, 22532-22533, 22548-22558, 22590-22612, 22630, 22633-22634, 22800-22812, 63001-63030, 63040-63042, 63045-63047, 63050-63056, 63064, 63075, 63077, 63081, 63085, 63087, 63090, 63101-63102, 63170-63290, 63300-63307)

10.4 10.4 FUD ZZZ C 80

AMA: 2020,May,13; 2018,Sep,7; 2018,Jan,8; 2017,Jan,8; 2016,Jan,13; 2015,Jan,16

22849-22855 [22859] Miscellaneous Spinal Instrumentation

EXCLUDES *Arthrodesis (22532-22534, 22548-22812)*
Bone grafting procedures (20930-20938)
Exploration spinal fusion (22830)
Facet injection (64490-64495, [64633, 64634, 64635, 64636])
Fracture treatment (22325-22328)

22849 Reinsertion of spinal fixation device

INCLUDES Removal of instrumentation at the same level (22850, 22852, 22855)

37.7 37.7 FUD 090 C 80

AMA: 2020,May,13; 2018,Sep,7; 2018,Jan,8; 2017,Jun,10; 2017,Jan,8; 2016,May,13; 2016,Jan,13; 2015,Jan,16

22850 Removal of posterior nonsegmental instrumentation (eg, Harrington rod)

21.0 21.0 FUD 090 C 80

AMA: 2020,May,13; 2018,Sep,7; 2018,Jan,8; 2017,Jun,10; 2017,Jan,8; 2016,May,13; 2016,Jan,13; 2015,Jan,16

22852 Removal of posterior segmental instrumentation

20.2 20.2 FUD 090 C 80

AMA: 2020,May,13; 2018,Sep,7; 2018,Jan,8; 2017,Jun,10; 2017,Jan,8; 2016,Jan,13; 2015,Jan,16

+ 22853 Insertion of interbody biomechanical device(s) (eg, synthetic cage, mesh) with integral anterior instrumentation for device anchoring (eg, screws, flanges), when performed, to intervertebral disc space in conjunction with interbody arthrodesis, each interspace (List separately in addition to code for primary procedure)

Code also intervertebral bone device/graft application (20930-20931, 20936-20938)

Code also subsequent disc spaces undergoing device insertion when disc spaces are not connected (22853-22854, [22859])

Code first (22100-22102, 22110-22114, 22206-22207, 22210-22214, 22220-22224, 22310-22327, 22532-22533, 22548-22558, 22590-22612, 22630, 22633-22634, 22800-22812, 63001-63030, 63040, 63042, 63045-63047, 63050-63056, 63064, 63075, 63077, 63081, 63085, 63087, 63090, 63101-63102, 63170-63290, 63300-63307)

7.52 7.52 FUD ZZZ N N1 80

AMA: 2020,May,13; 2018,Sep,7; 2018,Jul,14; 2018,Jan,8; 2017,Aug,9; 2017,Mar,7

+ 22854 Insertion of intervertebral biomechanical device(s) (eg, synthetic cage, mesh) with integral anterior instrumentation for device anchoring (eg, screws, flanges), when performed, to vertebral corpectomy(ies) (vertebral body resection, partial or complete) defect, in conjunction with interbody arthrodesis, each contiguous defect (List separately in addition to code for primary procedure)

Code also intervertebral bone device/graft application (20930-20931, 20936-20938)

Code also subsequent disc spaces undergoing device insertion when disc spaces are not connected (22853-22854, [22859])

Code first (22100-22102, 22110-22114, 22206-22207, 22210-22214, 22220-22224, 22310-22327, 22532-22533, 22548-22558, 22590-22612, 22630, 22633-22634, 22800-22812, 63001-63030, 63040, 63042, 63045-63047, 63050-63056, 63064, 63075, 63077, 63081, 63085, 63087, 63090, 63101-63102, 63170-63290, 63300-63307)

9.74 9.74 FUD ZZZ N N1 80

AMA: 2020,May,13; 2018,Sep,7; 2018,Jan,8; 2017,Mar,7

+ # 22859 Insertion of intervertebral biomechanical device(s) (eg, synthetic cage, mesh, methylmethacrylate) to intervertebral disc space or vertebral body defect without interbody arthrodesis, each contiguous defect (List separately in addition to code for primary procedure)

Code also intervertebral bone device/graft application (20930-20931, 20936-20938)

Code also subsequent disc spaces undergoing device insertion when disc spaces are not connected (22853-22854, 22854)

Code first (22100-22102, 22110-22114, 22206-22207, 22210-22214, 22220-22224, 22310-22327, 22532-22533, 22548-22558, 22590-22612, 22630, 22633-22634, 22800-22812, 63001-63030, 63040-63042, 63045-63047, 63050-63056, 63064, 63075, 63077, 63081, 63085, 63087, 63090, 63101-63102, 63170-63290, 63300-63307)

9.74 9.74 FUD ZZZ N N1 80

AMA: 2020,May,13; 2018,Sep,7; 2018,Jan,8; 2017,Mar,7

22855 Removal of anterior instrumentation

32.1 32.1 FUD 090 C 80

AMA: 2020,May,13; 2018,Sep,7; 2018,Jan,8; 2017,Jun,10; 2017,Jan,8; 2016,Jan,13; 2015,Jan,16

22856-22865 [22858, 22859] Artificial Disc Replacement

EXCLUDES *Fluoroscopy*
Spinal decompression (63001-63048)

22856 **Total disc arthroplasty (artificial disc), anterior approach, including discectomy with end plate preparation (includes osteophytectomy for nerve root or spinal cord decompression and microdissection); single interspace, cervical**

INCLUDES Operating microscope (69990)

EXCLUDES *Application intervertebral biomechanical device(s) at same level (22853-22854, [22859])*
Arthrodesis at same level (22554)
Discectomy at same level (63075)
Insertion instrumentation at same level (22845)

Code also arthroplasty more than one interspace, when performed ([22858])

47.3 47.3 FUD 090 J J8 80

AMA: 2020,May,13; 2018,Sep,7; 2018,Jan,8; 2017,Jan,8; 2016,Feb,12; 2016,Jan,13; 2015,Apr,7

+ # **22858** **second level, cervical (List separately in addition to code for primary procedure)**

Code first (22856)

14.8 14.8 FUD ZZZ N N1 80

AMA: 2020,May,13; 2018,Sep,7; 2018,Jan,8; 2017,Jan,8; 2016,Feb,12; 2016,Jan,13; 2015,Apr,7

22857 **Total disc arthroplasty (artificial disc), anterior approach, including discectomy to prepare interspace (other than for decompression), single interspace, lumbar**

INCLUDES Operating microscope (69990)

EXCLUDES *Application intervertebral biomechanical device(s) at same level (22853-22854, [22859])*
Arthrodesis at same level (22558)
Insertion instrumentation at same level (22845)
Retroperitoneal exploration (49010)

Code also arthroplasty more than one interspace, when performed (0163T)

50.8 50.8 FUD 090 C 80

AMA: 2020,May,13; 2018,Sep,7; 2016,Feb,12

22858 **Resequenced code. See code following 22856.**

22859 **Resequenced code. See code following 22854.**

22861 **Revision including replacement of total disc arthroplasty (artificial disc), anterior approach, single interspace; cervical**

INCLUDES Operating microscope (69990)

EXCLUDES *Procedures performed at same level (22845, 22853-22854, [22859], 22864, 63075)*
Revision additional cervical arthroplasty (0098T)

66.9 66.9 FUD 090 C 80

AMA: 2020,May,13; 2018,Sep,7; 2016,Feb,12

22862 **lumbar**

EXCLUDES *Arthroplasty revision more than one interspace (0165T)*
Procedures performed at same level (22558, 22845, 22853-22854, [22859], 22865, 49010)

66.8 66.8 FUD 090 C 80

AMA: 2020,May,13; 2018,Sep,7; 2018,Jan,8; 2017,Jan,8; 2016,Jan,13; 2015,Jan,16

22864 **Removal of total disc arthroplasty (artificial disc), anterior approach, single interspace; cervical**

INCLUDES Operating microscope (69990)

EXCLUDES *Cervical total disc arthroplasty with additional interspace removal (0095T)*
Revision total disc arthroplasty (22861)

59.7 59.7 FUD 090 C 80

AMA: 2020,May,13; 2018,Sep,7

22865 **lumbar**

EXCLUDES *Arthroplasty more than one level (0164T)*
Exploration, retroperitoneal area with or without biopsy(s) (49010)

65.1 65.1 FUD 090 C 80

AMA: 2020,May,13; 2018,Sep,7; 2018,Jan,8; 2017,Jan,8; 2016,Jan,13; 2015,Jan,16

22867-22899 Spinal Distraction/Stabilization Device

22867 **Insertion of interlaminar/interspinous process stabilization/distraction device, without fusion, including image guidance when performed, with open decompression, lumbar; single level**

EXCLUDES *Interlaminar/interspinous stabilization/distraction device insertion (22869, 22870)*
Procedures at same level (22532-22534, 22558, 22612, 22614, 22630, 22632-22634, 22800, 22802, 22804, 22840-22842, 22869-22870, 63005, 63012, 63017, 63030, 63035, 63042, 63044, 63047-63048, 77003)

28.2 28.2 FUD 090 J J8 80

AMA: 2020,May,13; 2018,Sep,7; 2018,Jan,8; 2017,Feb,9

+ **22868** **second level (List separately in addition to code for primary procedure)**

EXCLUDES *Interlaminar/interspinous stabilization/distraction device insertion (22869-22870)*
Procedures at same level (22532-22534, 22558, 22612, 22614, 22630, 22632-22634, 22800, 22802, 22804, 22840-22842, 22869-22870, 63005, 63012, 63017, 63030, 63035, 63042, 63044, 63047-63048, 77003)

Code first (22867)

7.08 7.08 FUD ZZZ N N1 80

AMA: 2020,May,13; 2018,Sep,7; 2018,Jan,8; 2017,Feb,9

22869 **Insertion of interlaminar/interspinous process stabilization/distraction device, without open decompression or fusion, including image guidance when performed, lumbar; single level**

EXCLUDES *Procedures at the same level (22532-22534, 22558, 22612, 22614, 22630, 22632-22634, 22800, 22802, 22804, 22840-22842, 63005, 63012, 63017, 63030, 63035, 63042, 63044, 63047-63048, 77003)*

12.8 12.8 FUD 090 J J8 80

AMA: 2020,May,13; 2018,Sep,7; 2018,Jan,8; 2017,Feb,9

+ **22870** **second level (List separately in addition to code for primary procedure)**

EXCLUDES *Procedures at the same level (22532-22534, 22558, 22612, 22614, 22630, 22632-22634, 22800, 22802, 22804, 22840-22842, 63005, 63012, 63017, 63030, 63035, 63042, 63044, 63047-63048, 77003)*

Code first (22869)

3.96 3.96 FUD ZZZ N N1 80

AMA: 2020,May,13; 2018,Sep,7; 2018,Jan,8; 2017,Feb,9

22899 **Unlisted procedure, spine**

0.00 0.00 FUD YYY T 80

AMA: 2020,Jun,14; 2018,Sep,7; 2018,May,10; 2018,Jan,8; 2017,Feb,9; 2017,Jan,8; 2016,Jan,13; 2015,Jan,8; 2015,Jan,16

22900-22999 Musculoskeletal Procedures of Abdomen

INCLUDES Any necessary elevation tissue planes or dissection
Measurement tumor and necessary margin at greatest diameter prior to excision
Simple and intermediate repairs
Excision types:
Fascial or subfascial soft tissue tumors: simple and marginal resection tumors found either in or below deep fascia, not involving bone or excision substantial amount normal tissue; primarily benign and intramuscular tumors
Radical resection soft tissue tumor: wide resection tumor involving substantial margins normal tissue and may include tissue removal from one or more layers; most often malignant or aggressive benign
Subcutaneous: simple and marginal resection tumors in subcutaneous tissue above deep fascia; most often benign

EXCLUDES *Complex repair*
Excision benign cutaneous lesions (eg, sebaceous cyst) (11400-11406)
Radical resection cutaneous tumors (eg, melanoma) (11600-11606)
Significant vessel exploration or neuroplasty

22900 **Excision, tumor, soft tissue of abdominal wall, subfascial (eg, intramuscular); less than 5 cm**
16.3 16.3 FUD 090 J G2 80
AMA: 2018,Sep,7

22901 **5 cm or greater**
19.3 19.3 FUD 090 J G2 80
AMA: 2018,Sep,7

22902 **Excision, tumor, soft tissue of abdominal wall, subcutaneous; less than 3 cm**
9.57 13.1 FUD 090 J G2 80
AMA: 2018,Sep,7

22903 **3 cm or greater**
12.6 12.6 FUD 090 J G2 80
AMA: 2018,Sep,7

22904 **Radical resection of tumor (eg, sarcoma), soft tissue of abdominal wall; less than 5 cm**
30.5 30.5 FUD 090 J G2 80
AMA: 2018,Sep,7

22905 **5 cm or greater**
38.5 38.5 FUD 090 J G2 80
AMA: 2018,Sep,7

22999 **Unlisted procedure, abdomen, musculoskeletal system**
0.00 0.00 FUD YYY T 80
AMA: 2018,Sep,7

23000-23044 Surgical Incision Shoulder: Drainage, Foreign Body Removal, Contracture Release

23000 **Removal of subdeltoid calcareous deposits, open**
EXCLUDES *Arthroscopic removal calcium deposits bursa (29999)*
10.5 16.4 FUD 090 J A2 80 50
AMA: 2018,Sep,7

23020 **Capsular contracture release (eg, Sever type procedure)**
EXCLUDES *Simple incision and drainage (10040-10160)*
19.9 19.9 FUD 090 J A2 80 50
AMA: 2018,Sep,7

23030 **Incision and drainage, shoulder area; deep abscess or hematoma**
7.20 12.4 FUD 010 J A2
AMA: 2018,Sep,7

23031 **infected bursa**
6.01 11.5 FUD 010 J A2 50
AMA: 2018,Sep,7

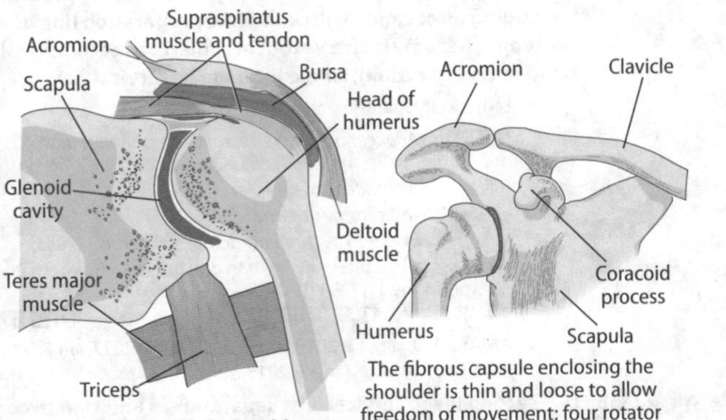

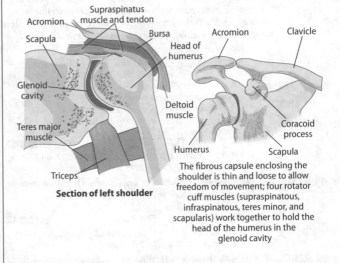

Section of left shoulder

The fibrous capsule enclosing the shoulder is thin and loose to allow freedom of movement; four rotator cuff muscles (supraspinatous, infraspinatous, teres minor, and scapularis) work together to hold the head of the humerus in the glenoid cavity

23035 **Incision, bone cortex (eg, osteomyelitis or bone abscess), shoulder area**
19.6 19.6 FUD 090 J A2 80 50
AMA: 2018,Sep,7

23040 **Arthrotomy, glenohumeral joint, including exploration, drainage, or removal of foreign body**
20.7 20.7 FUD 090 J A2 80 50
AMA: 2018,Sep,7

23044 **Arthrotomy, acromioclavicular, sternoclavicular joint, including exploration, drainage, or removal of foreign body**
16.3 16.3 FUD 090 J A2 50
AMA: 2018,Sep,7

23065-23066 Shoulder Biopsy

EXCLUDES *Soft tissue needle biopsy (20206)*

23065 **Biopsy, soft tissue of shoulder area; superficial**
4.81 6.34 FUD 010 J P3 50
AMA: 2018,Sep,7

23066 **deep**
10.4 16.2 FUD 090 J A2 50
AMA: 2018,Sep,7

23071-23078 [23071, 23073] Excision Soft Tissue Tumors of Shoulder

INCLUDES Any necessary elevation tissue planes or dissection
Measurement tumor and necessary margin at greatest diameter prior to excision
Simple and intermediate repairs
Excision types:
Fascial or subfascial soft tissue tumors: simple and marginal resection tumors found either in or below deep fascia, not involving bone or excision substantial amount normal tissue; primarily benign and intramuscular tumors
Radical resection soft tissue tumor: wide resection tumor, involving substantial margins normal tissue and may involve tissue removal from one or more layers; most often malignant or aggressive benign
Subcutaneous: simple and marginal resection tumors in subcutaneous tissue above deep fascia; most often benign

EXCLUDES *Complex repair*
Excision benign cutaneous lesions (eg, sebaceous cyst) (11400-11406)
Radical resection cutaneous tumors (eg, melanoma) (11600-11606)
Significant vessel exploration or neuroplasty

23071 **Resequenced code. See code following 23075.**

23073 **Resequenced code. See code following 23076.**

23075 **Excision, tumor, soft tissue of shoulder area, subcutaneous; less than 3 cm**
9.44 14.3 **FUD** 090 J G2 50
AMA: 2018,Sep,7; 2018,Jan,8; 2017,Jan,8; 2016,Jan,13; 2015,Jan,16

\# **23071** **3 cm or greater**
12.1 12.1 **FUD** 090 J G2 80 50
AMA: 2018,Sep,7

23076 **Excision, tumor, soft tissue of shoulder area, subfascial (eg, intramuscular); less than 5 cm**
15.6 15.6 **FUD** 090 J G2 50
AMA: 2018,Sep,7; 2018,Jan,8; 2017,Jan,8; 2016,Jan,13; 2015,Jan,16

\# **23073** **5 cm or greater**
20.1 20.1 **FUD** 090 J G2 80 50
AMA: 2018,Sep,7

23077 **Radical resection of tumor (eg, sarcoma), soft tissue of shoulder area; less than 5 cm**
32.7 32.7 **FUD** 090 J G2 80 50
AMA: 2018,Sep,7

23078 **5 cm or greater**
41.4 41.4 **FUD** 090 J G2 80 50
AMA: 2018,Sep,7

23100-23195 Bone and Joint Procedures of Shoulder

INCLUDES Acromioclavicular joint
Clavicle
Head and neck of humerus
Scapula
Shoulder joint
Sternoclavicular joint

23100 **Arthrotomy, glenohumeral joint, including biopsy**
14.5 14.5 **FUD** 090 J A2 80 50
AMA: 2018,Sep,7

23101 **Arthrotomy, acromioclavicular joint or sternoclavicular joint, including biopsy and/or excision of torn cartilage**
13.1 13.1 **FUD** 090 J A2 50
AMA: 2018,Sep,7

23105 **Arthrotomy; glenohumeral joint, with synovectomy, with or without biopsy**
18.3 18.3 **FUD** 090 J A2 80 50
AMA: 2018,Sep,7

23106 **sternoclavicular joint, with synovectomy, with or without biopsy**
14.3 14.3 **FUD** 090 J A2 50
AMA: 2018,Sep,7

23107 **Arthrotomy, glenohumeral joint, with joint exploration, with or without removal of loose or foreign body**
19.0 19.0 **FUD** 090 J A2 80 50
AMA: 2018,Sep,7

23120 **Claviculectomy; partial**
INCLUDES Mumford operation
EXCLUDES *Arthroscopic claviculectomy (29824)*
16.8 16.8 **FUD** 090 J A2 80 50
AMA: 2018,Sep,7; 2018,Jan,8; 2017,Jan,8; 2016,Jan,13; 2015,Jan,16

23125 **total**
20.4 20.4 **FUD** 090 J A2 80 50
AMA: 2018,Sep,7

23130 **Acromioplasty or acromionectomy, partial, with or without coracoacromial ligament release**
17.6 17.6 **FUD** 090 J A2 50
AMA: 2018,Sep,7; 2018,Jan,8; 2017,Jan,8; 2016,Jan,13; 2015,Mar,7; 2015,Feb,10; 2015,Jan,16

23140 **Excision or curettage of bone cyst or benign tumor of clavicle or scapula;**
15.9 15.9 **FUD** 090 J A2 50
AMA: 2018,Sep,7

23145 **with autograft (includes obtaining graft)**
20.0 20.0 **FUD** 090 J A2 80 50
AMA: 2018,Sep,7

23146 **with allograft**
17.9 17.9 **FUD** 090 J A2 80 50
AMA: 2019,May,7; 2018,Sep,7

23150 **Excision or curettage of bone cyst or benign tumor of proximal humerus;**
19.2 19.2 **FUD** 090 J A2 80 50
AMA: 2018,Sep,7

23155 **with autograft (includes obtaining graft)**
22.9 22.9 **FUD** 090 J A2 80 50
AMA: 2018,Sep,7

23156 **with allograft**
19.4 19.4 **FUD** 090 J J8 80 50
AMA: 2019,May,7; 2018,Sep,7

23170 **Sequestrectomy (eg, for osteomyelitis or bone abscess), clavicle**
16.2 16.2 **FUD** 090 J A2 50
AMA: 2018,Sep,7

23172 **Sequestrectomy (eg, for osteomyelitis or bone abscess), scapula**
16.3 16.3 **FUD** 090 J A2 80 50
AMA: 2018,Sep,7

23174 **Sequestrectomy (eg, for osteomyelitis or bone abscess), humeral head to surgical neck**
21.9 21.9 **FUD** 090 J A2 80 50
AMA: 2018,Sep,7

23180 **Partial excision (craterization, saucerization, or diaphysectomy) bone (eg, osteomyelitis), clavicle**
19.1 19.1 **FUD** 090 J A2 50
AMA: 2018,Sep,7

23182 **Partial excision (craterization, saucerization, or diaphysectomy) bone (eg, osteomyelitis), scapula**
19.0 19.0 **FUD** 090 J A2 80 50
AMA: 2018,Sep,7

23184 **Partial excision (craterization, saucerization, or diaphysectomy) bone (eg, osteomyelitis), proximal humerus**
21.1 21.1 **FUD** 090 J A2 80 50
AMA: 2018,Sep,7

23190 **Ostectomy of scapula, partial (eg, superior medial angle)**
16.5 16.5 **FUD** 090 J A2 80 50
AMA: 2018,Sep,7

23195 **Resection, humeral head**
EXCLUDES *Arthroplasty with replacement with implant (23470)*
21.5 21.5 **FUD** 090 J A2 80 50
AMA: 2018,Sep,7

23200-23220 Radical Resection of Bone Tumors of Shoulder

INCLUDES Any necessary elevation tissue planes or dissection
Excision adjacent soft tissue during bone tumor resection (23071-23078 [23071, 23073])
Measurement tumor and necessary margin at greatest diameter prior to excision
Radical resection cutaneous tumors (e.g., melanoma)
Resection tumor (may include entire bone) and wide margins normal tissues primarily for malignant or aggressive benign tumors
Simple and intermediate repairs

EXCLUDES *Complex repair*
Significant vessel exploration, neuroplasty, reconstruction, or complex bone repair

23200 **Radical resection of tumor; clavicle**
43.6 43.6 **FUD** 090 C 80 50
AMA: 2019,May,7; 2018,Sep,7

23210 **scapula**
51.2 51.2 **FUD** 090 C 80 50
AMA: 2019,May,7; 2018,Sep,7

23220 **Radical resection of tumor, proximal humerus**
56.3 56.3 FUD 090 C 80 50
AMA: 2019,May,7; 2018,Sep,7

23330-23335 Removal Implant/Foreign Body from Shoulder

EXCLUDES *Bursal arthrocentesis or needling (20610)*
K-wire or pin insertion (20650)
K-wire or pin removal (20670, 20680)

23330 **Removal of foreign body, shoulder; subcutaneous**
4.79 8.03 FUD 010 T A2 80 50
AMA: 2018,Sep,7; 2018,Jan,8; 2017,Jan,8; 2016,Jan,13; 2015,Jan,16

23333 **deep (subfascial or intramuscular)**
13.2 13.2 FUD 090 J G2 80 50
AMA: 2018,Sep,7; 2018,Jan,8; 2017,Jan,8; 2016,Jan,13; 2015,Jan,16

23334 **Removal of prosthesis, includes debridement and synovectomy when performed; humeral or glenoid component**
EXCLUDES *Foreign body removal (23330, 23333)*
Prosthesis removal and replacement in same shoulder (eg, glenoid and/or humeral components) (23473-23474)
30.8 30.8 FUD 090 J G2 50
AMA: 2018,Sep,7; 2018,Jan,8; 2017,Jan,8; 2016,Jan,13; 2015,Jan,16

23335 **humeral and glenoid components (eg, total shoulder)**
EXCLUDES *Foreign body removal (23330, 23333)*
Prosthesis removal and replacement in same shoulder (eg, glenoid and/or humeral components) (23473-23474)
36.7 36.7 FUD 090 C 50
AMA: 2018,Sep,7; 2018,Jan,8; 2017,Jan,8; 2016,Jan,13; 2015,Jan,16

23350 Injection for Shoulder Arthrogram

23350 **Injection procedure for shoulder arthrography or enhanced CT/MRI shoulder arthrography**
EXCLUDES *Shoulder biopsy (29805-29826)*
(73040, 73201-73202, 73222-73223, 77002)
1.47 3.97 FUD 000 N N1 50
AMA: 2018,Sep,7; 2018,Jan,8; 2017,Jan,8; 2016,May,13; 2016,Jan,13; 2015,Aug,6; 2015,Jan,16

23395-23491 Repair/Reconstruction of Shoulder

23395 **Muscle transfer, any type, shoulder or upper arm; single**
37.0 37.0 FUD 090 J A2 80
AMA: 2018,Sep,7

23397 **multiple**
32.9 32.9 FUD 090 J A2 80
AMA: 2018,Sep,7

23400 **Scapulopexy (eg, Sprengels deformity or for paralysis)**
28.0 28.0 FUD 090 J A2 80 50
AMA: 2018,Sep,7

23405 **Tenotomy, shoulder area; single tendon**
17.8 17.8 FUD 090 J A2 80
AMA: 2018,Sep,7

23406 **multiple tendons through same incision**
22.2 22.2 FUD 090 J J8 80
AMA: 2018,Sep,7

23410 **Repair of ruptured musculotendinous cuff (eg, rotator cuff) open; acute**
EXCLUDES *Arthroscopic repair (29827)*
23.6 23.6 FUD 090 J A2 80 50
AMA: 2018,Sep,7; 2018,Jan,8; 2017,Jan,8; 2016,Jan,13; 2015,Jan,16

23412 **chronic**
EXCLUDES *Arthroscopic repair (29827)*
24.5 24.5 FUD 090 J A2 80 50
AMA: 2018,Sep,7; 2018,Jan,8; 2017,Jan,8; 2016,Jan,13; 2015,Jun,10; 2015,Feb,10; 2015,Jan,16

23415 **Coracoacromial ligament release, with or without acromioplasty**
EXCLUDES *Arthroscopic repair (29826)*
20.1 20.1 FUD 090 J A2 50
AMA: 2018,Sep,7; 2018,Jan,8; 2017,Jan,8; 2016,Jan,13; 2015,Mar,7

23420 **Reconstruction of complete shoulder (rotator) cuff avulsion, chronic (includes acromioplasty)**
28.0 28.0 FUD 090 J A2 80 50
AMA: 2018,Sep,7; 2018,Jan,8; 2017,Jan,8; 2016,Jan,13; 2015,Jan,16

23430 **Tenodesis of long tendon of biceps**
EXCLUDES *Arthroscopic biceps tenodesis (29828)*
21.4 21.4 FUD 090 J A2 80 50
AMA: 2018,Sep,7

23440 **Resection or transplantation of long tendon of biceps**
21.7 21.7 FUD 090 J A2 80 50
AMA: 2018,Sep,7

23450 **Capsulorrhaphy, anterior; Putti-Platt procedure or Magnuson type operation**
EXCLUDES *Arthroscopic thermal capsulorrhaphy (29999)*
27.3 27.3 FUD 090 J A2 80 50
AMA: 2018,Sep,7

23455 **with labral repair (eg, Bankart procedure)**
EXCLUDES *Arthroscopic repair (29806)*
28.7 28.7 FUD 090 J A2 80 50
AMA: 2018,Sep,7

23460 **Capsulorrhaphy, anterior, any type; with bone block**
INCLUDES Bristow procedure
31.4 31.4 FUD 090 J A2 80 50
AMA: 2018,Sep,7

23462 **with coracoid process transfer**
EXCLUDES *Open thermal capsulorrhaphy (23929)*
30.9 30.9 FUD 090 J A2 80 50
AMA: 2018,Sep,7

23465 **Capsulorrhaphy, glenohumeral joint, posterior, with or without bone block**
EXCLUDES *Sternoclavicular and acromioclavicular joint repair (23530, 23550)*
32.3 32.3 FUD 090 J G2 80 50
AMA: 2018,Sep,7

23466 **Capsulorrhaphy, glenohumeral joint, any type multi-directional instability**
32.0 32.0 FUD 090 J A2 80 50
AMA: 2018,Sep,7

23470 **Arthroplasty, glenohumeral joint; hemiarthroplasty**
34.7 34.7 FUD 090 J 80 50
AMA: 2018,Sep,7; 2018,Jan,8; 2017,Jan,8; 2016,Jan,13; 2015,Jan,16

23472 **total shoulder (glenoid and proximal humeral replacement (eg, total shoulder))**
EXCLUDES *Proximal humerus osteotomy (24400)*
Removal total shoulder components (23334-23335)
41.9 41.9 FUD 090 C 80 50
AMA: 2018,Sep,7; 2018,Jan,8; 2017,Jan,8; 2016,Jan,13; 2015,Jan,16

23473 Revision of total shoulder arthroplasty, including allograft when performed; humeral or glenoid component

EXCLUDES Removal prosthesis only (glenoid and/or humeral component) same shoulder/same operative sessions (23334-23335)

46.7 46.7 **FUD** 090   J 80 50

AMA: 2018,Sep,7; 2018,Jan,8; 2017,Jan,8; 2016,Jan,13; 2015,Jan,16

23474 humeral and glenoid component

EXCLUDES Removal prosthesis only (glenoid and/or humeral component) same shoulder/same operative sessions (23334-23335)

50.5 50.5 **FUD** 090   C 80 50

AMA: 2018,Sep,7; 2018,Jan,8; 2017,Jan,8; 2016,Jan,13; 2015,Jan,16

23480 Osteotomy, clavicle, with or without internal fixation;

23.7 23.7 **FUD** 090   J A2 50

AMA: 2018,Sep,7

23485 with bone graft for nonunion or malunion (includes obtaining graft and/or necessary fixation)

27.6 27.6 **FUD** 090   J J8 80 50

AMA: 2018,Sep,7

23490 Prophylactic treatment (nailing, pinning, plating or wiring) with or without methylmethacrylate; clavicle

24.6 24.6 **FUD** 090   J A2 80 50

AMA: 2018,Sep,7

23491 proximal humerus

29.3 29.3 **FUD** 090   J J8 80 50

AMA: 2018,Sep,7

23500-23680 Treatment of Shoulder Fracture/Dislocation

23500 Closed treatment of clavicular fracture; without manipulation

6.37 6.24 **FUD** 090   T A2 50

AMA: 2018,Sep,7

23505 with manipulation

9.61 10.2 **FUD** 090   J A2 50

AMA: 2018,Sep,7

23515 Open treatment of clavicular fracture, includes internal fixation, when performed

20.7 20.7 **FUD** 090   J J8 80 50

AMA: 2018,Sep,7; 2018,Jan,8; 2017,Jan,8; 2016,Jan,13; 2015,Jan,16

23520 Closed treatment of sternoclavicular dislocation; without manipulation

6.73 6.72 **FUD** 090   J A2 80 50

AMA: 2018,Sep,7

23525 with manipulation

10.2 11.1 **FUD** 090   T A2 80 50

AMA: 2018,Sep,7

23530 Open treatment of sternoclavicular dislocation, acute or chronic;

16.5 16.5 **FUD** 090   J A2 80 50

AMA: 2018,Sep,7

23532 with fascial graft (includes obtaining graft)

18.0 18.0 **FUD** 090   J A2 80 50

AMA: 2018,Sep,7

23540 Closed treatment of acromioclavicular dislocation; without manipulation

6.64 6.67 **FUD** 090   T A2 50

AMA: 2018,Sep,7

23545 with manipulation

8.93 9.91 **FUD** 090   T A2 80 50

AMA: 2018,Sep,7

23550 Open treatment of acromioclavicular dislocation, acute or chronic;

16.3 16.3 **FUD** 090   J A2 80 50

AMA: 2018,Sep,7

23552 with fascial graft (includes obtaining graft)

18.8 18.8 **FUD** 090   J J8 80 50

AMA: 2019,Nov,14; 2018,Sep,7

23570 Closed treatment of scapular fracture; without manipulation

6.89 6.69 **FUD** 090   T A2 50

AMA: 2018,Sep,7

23575 with manipulation, with or without skeletal traction (with or without shoulder joint involvement)

10.8 11.6 **FUD** 090   J A2 80 50

AMA: 2018,Sep,7

23585 Open treatment of scapular fracture (body, glenoid or acromion) includes internal fixation, when performed

28.2 28.2 **FUD** 090   J A2 80 50

AMA: 2018,Sep,7; 2018,Jan,8; 2017,Jan,8; 2016,Jan,13; 2015,Jan,16

23600 Closed treatment of proximal humeral (surgical or anatomical neck) fracture; without manipulation

8.92 9.45 **FUD** 090   T P2 50

AMA: 2018,Sep,7

23605 with manipulation, with or without skeletal traction

12.2 13.4 **FUD** 090   J A2 50

AMA: 2018,Sep,7

23615 Open treatment of proximal humeral (surgical or anatomical neck) fracture, includes internal fixation, when performed, includes repair of tuberosity(s), when performed;

25.5 25.5 **FUD** 090   J J8 80 50

AMA: 2018,Sep,7; 2018,Jan,8; 2017,Jan,8; 2016,Jan,13; 2015,Jan,16

23616 with proximal humeral prosthetic replacement

35.7 35.7 **FUD** 090   J J8 80 50

AMA: 2018,Sep,7

23620 Closed treatment of greater humeral tuberosity fracture; without manipulation

7.32 7.65 **FUD** 090   T P2 50

AMA: 2018,Sep,7

23625 with manipulation

10.1 10.9 **FUD** 090   J A2 50

AMA: 2018,Sep,7

23630 Open treatment of greater humeral tuberosity fracture, includes internal fixation, when performed

22.4 22.4 **FUD** 090   J J8 80 50

AMA: 2018,Sep,7

23650 Closed treatment of shoulder dislocation, with manipulation; without anesthesia

8.36 9.18 **FUD** 090   T A2 50

AMA: 2018,Sep,7

23655 requiring anesthesia

11.5 11.5 **FUD** 090   J A2 50

AMA: 2018,Sep,7

23660 Open treatment of acute shoulder dislocation

EXCLUDES Chronic dislocation repair (23450-23466)

16.8 16.8 **FUD** 090   J A2 80 50

AMA: 2018,Sep,7; 2018,Jan,8; 2017,Jan,8; 2016,Jan,13; 2015,Jan,16

23665 Closed treatment of shoulder dislocation, with fracture of greater humeral tuberosity, with manipulation

11.4 12.3 **FUD** 090   J A2 50

AMA: 2019,Feb,10; 2018,Sep,7

23670 Open treatment of shoulder dislocation, with fracture of greater humeral tuberosity, includes internal fixation, when performed

25.2 25.2 **FUD** 090   J A2 80 50

AMA: 2018,Sep,7

● New Code ▲ Revised Code ○ Reinstated ● New Web Release ▲ Revised Web Release + Add-on Unlisted Not Covered # Resequenced
50 Optum Mod 50 Exempt ⊘ AMA Mod 51 Exempt 51 Optum Mod 51 Exempt 63 Mod 63 Exempt ✗ Non-FDA Drug ★ Telemedicine M Maternity A Age Edit

23675 **Closed treatment of shoulder dislocation, with surgical or anatomical neck fracture, with manipulation**
14.4 15.9 FUD 090 J A2 50
AMA: 2018,Sep,7

23680 **Open treatment of shoulder dislocation, with surgical or anatomical neck fracture, includes internal fixation, when performed**
26.8 26.8 FUD 090 J J8 80 50
AMA: 2018,Sep,7

23700-23929 Other/Unlisted Shoulder Procedures

23700 **Manipulation under anesthesia, shoulder joint, including application of fixation apparatus (dislocation excluded)**
5.63 5.63 FUD 010 J A2 50
AMA: 2018,Sep,7; 2018,Jan,8; 2017,Jan,8; 2016,Jan,13; 2015,Jun,10; 2015,Jan,16

23800 **Arthrodesis, glenohumeral joint;**
29.6 29.6 FUD 090 J G2 80 50
AMA: 2020,May,13; 2018,Sep,7

23802 **with autogenous graft (includes obtaining graft)**
37.0 37.0 FUD 090 J G2 80 50
AMA: 2020,May,13; 2018,Sep,7

23900 **Interthoracoscapular amputation (forequarter)**
40.0 40.0 FUD 090 C 80
AMA: 2018,Sep,7

23920 **Disarticulation of shoulder;**
32.4 32.4 FUD 090 C 80 50
AMA: 2018,Sep,7

23921 **secondary closure or scar revision**
13.5 13.5 FUD 090 T A2 50
AMA: 2018,Sep,7

23929 **Unlisted procedure, shoulder**
0.00 0.00 FUD YYY T 80
AMA: 2018,Sep,7

23930-24006 Surgical Incision Elbow/Upper Arm

EXCLUDES *Simple incision and drainage procedures (10040-10160)*

23930 **Incision and drainage, upper arm or elbow area; deep abscess or hematoma**
6.12 10.2 FUD 010 J A2 50
AMA: 2018,Sep,7

23931 **bursa**
4.48 8.19 FUD 010 J A2 50
AMA: 2018,Sep,7

23935 **Incision, deep, with opening of bone cortex (eg, for osteomyelitis or bone abscess), humerus or elbow**
14.7 14.7 FUD 090 J A2 80 50
AMA: 2018,Sep,7

24000 **Arthrotomy, elbow, including exploration, drainage, or removal of foreign body**
13.7 13.7 FUD 090 J A2 80 50
AMA: 2018,Sep,7

24006 **Arthrotomy of the elbow, with capsular excision for capsular release (separate procedure)**
20.5 20.5 FUD 090 J A2 80 50
AMA: 2018,Sep,7

24065-24066 Biopsy of Elbow/Upper Arm

EXCLUDES *Soft tissue needle biopsy (20206)*

24065 **Biopsy, soft tissue of upper arm or elbow area; superficial**
4.71 7.41 FUD 010 J P3 50
AMA: 2018,Sep,7

24066 **deep (subfascial or intramuscular)**
12.0 18.0 FUD 090 J A2 50
AMA: 2018,Sep,7

24071-24079 [24071, 24073] Excision Soft Tissue Tumors Elbow/Upper Arm

INCLUDES Any necessary elevation tissue planes or dissection
Measurement tumor and necessary margin at greatest diameter prior to excision
Excision types:
- Fascial or subfascial soft tissue tumors: simple and marginal resection tumors found either in or below deep fascia, not involving bone or excision substantial amount normal tissue; primarily benign and intramuscular tumors
- Radical resection soft tissue tumor: wide resection tumor involving substantial margins normal tissue and may involve tissue removal from one or more layers; most often malignant or aggressive benign
- Subcutaneous: simple and marginal resection tumors found in subcutaneous tissue above deep fascia; most often benign

EXCLUDES *Complex repair*
Excision benign cutaneous lesion (eg, sebaceous cyst) (11400-11406)
Radical resection cutaneous tumors (eg, melanoma) (11600-11606)
Significant vessel exploration or neuroplasty

24071 **Resequenced code. See code following 24075.**

24073 **Resequenced code. See code following 24076.**

24075 **Excision, tumor, soft tissue of upper arm or elbow area, subcutaneous; less than 3 cm**
9.47 14.8 FUD 090 J G2 50
AMA: 2018,Sep,7

\# **24071** **3 cm or greater**
11.7 11.7 FUD 090 J G2 80 50
AMA: 2018,Sep,7

24076 **Excision, tumor, soft tissue of upper arm or elbow area, subfascial (eg, intramuscular); less than 5 cm**
15.6 15.6 FUD 090 J G2 50
AMA: 2018,Sep,7

\# **24073** **5 cm or greater**
19.9 19.9 FUD 090 J G2 80 50
AMA: 2018,Sep,7

24077 **Radical resection of tumor (eg, sarcoma), soft tissue of upper arm or elbow area; less than 5 cm**
29.9 29.9 FUD 090 J G2 50
AMA: 2018,Sep,7

24079 **5 cm or greater**
38.3 38.3 FUD 090 J G2 80 50
AMA: 2018,Sep,7

24100-24149 Bone/Joint Procedures Upper Arm/Elbow

24100 **Arthrotomy, elbow; with synovial biopsy only**
12.0 12.0 FUD 090 J A2 80 50
AMA: 2018,Sep,7

24101 **with joint exploration, with or without biopsy, with or without removal of loose or foreign body**
14.4 14.4 FUD 090 J A2 80 50
AMA: 2018,Sep,7

24102 **with synovectomy**
17.7 17.7 FUD 090 J A2 80 50
AMA: 2018,Sep,7

24105 **Excision, olecranon bursa**
10.1 10.1 FUD 090 J A2 50
AMA: 2018,Sep,7

24110 **Excision or curettage of bone cyst or benign tumor, humerus;**
16.8 16.8 FUD 090 J A2 50
AMA: 2018,Sep,7

24115 **with autograft (includes obtaining graft)**
21.2 21.2 FUD 090 J A2 80 50
AMA: 2018,Sep,7

24116 **with allograft**
24.8 24.8 FUD 090 J A2 80 50
AMA: 2019,May,7; 2018,Sep,7

24120 **Excision or curettage of bone cyst or benign tumor of head or neck of radius or olecranon process;**
15.3 15.3 FUD 090 J A2 80 50
AMA: 2018,Sep,7

24125 **with autograft (includes obtaining graft)**
17.9 17.9 FUD 090 J A2 80 50
AMA: 2018,Sep,7

24126 **with allograft**
18.7 18.7 FUD 090 J J8 80 50
AMA: 2019,May,7; 2018,Sep,7

24130 **Excision, radial head**
EXCLUDES *Radial head arthroplasty with implant (24366)*
14.6 14.6 FUD 090 J A2 50
AMA: 2018,Sep,7

24134 **Sequestrectomy (eg, for osteomyelitis or bone abscess), shaft or distal humerus**
21.4 21.4 FUD 090 J A2 80 50
AMA: 2018,Sep,7

24136 **Sequestrectomy (eg, for osteomyelitis or bone abscess), radial head or neck**
18.2 18.2 FUD 090 J A2 50
AMA: 2018,Sep,7

24138 **Sequestrectomy (eg, for osteomyelitis or bone abscess), olecranon process**
19.6 19.6 FUD 090 J A2 80 50
AMA: 2018,Sep,7

24140 **Partial excision (craterization, saucerization, or diaphysectomy) bone (eg, osteomyelitis), humerus**
20.2 20.2 FUD 090 J A2 80 50
AMA: 2018,Sep,7

24145 **Partial excision (craterization, saucerization, or diaphysectomy) bone (eg, osteomyelitis), radial head or neck**
17.1 17.1 FUD 090 J A2 50
AMA: 2018,Sep,7

24147 **Partial excision (craterization, saucerization, or diaphysectomy) bone (eg, osteomyelitis), olecranon process**
17.9 17.9 FUD 090 J A2 50
AMA: 2018,Sep,7

24149 **Radical resection of capsule, soft tissue, and heterotopic bone, elbow, with contracture release (separate procedure)**
EXCLUDES *Capsular and soft tissue release (24006)*
33.8 33.8 FUD 090 J G2 80 50
AMA: 2018,Sep,7

24150-24152 Radical Resection Bone Tumor Upper Arm

INCLUDES Any necessary elevation tissue planes or dissection
Excision adjacent soft tissue during bone tumor resection (24071-24079 [24071, 24073])
Measurement tumor and necessary margin at greatest diameter prior to excision
Resection tumor (may include entire bone) and wide margins normal tissue primarily for malignant or aggressive benign tumors
Simple and intermediate repairs

EXCLUDES *Complex repair*
Significant vessel exploration, neuroplasty, reconstruction, or complex bone repair

24150 **Radical resection of tumor, shaft or distal humerus**
44.9 44.9 FUD 090 J 80 50
AMA: 2019,May,7; 2018,Sep,7

24152 **Radical resection of tumor, radial head or neck**
38.9 38.9 FUD 090 J G2 80 50
AMA: 2019,May,7; 2018,Sep,7

24155 Elbow Arthrectomy

24155 **Resection of elbow joint (arthrectomy)**
24.6 24.6 FUD 090 J A2 80 50
AMA: 2018,Sep,7

24160-24201 Removal Implant/Foreign Body from Elbow/Upper Arm

EXCLUDES *Bursal or joint arthrocentesis or needling (20605)*
K-wire or pin insertion (20650)
K-wire or pin removal (20670, 20680)

24160 **Removal of prosthesis, includes debridement and synovectomy when performed; humeral and ulnar components**
INCLUDES Prosthesis removal and replacement in same elbow (eg, humeral and/or ulnar component(s)) (24370-24371)
EXCLUDES *Foreign body removal (24200-24201)*
Hardware removal other than prosthesis (20680)
36.3 36.3 FUD 090 02 A2 50
AMA: 2018,Sep,7; 2018,Jan,8; 2017,Jan,8; 2016,Jan,13; 2015,Jan,16

24164 **radial head**
EXCLUDES *Foreign body removal (24200-24201)*
Hardware removal other than prosthesis (20680)
20.8 20.8 FUD 090 02 A2 50
AMA: 2018,Sep,7; 2018,Jan,8; 2017,Jan,8; 2016,Jan,13; 2015,Jan,16

24200 **Removal of foreign body, upper arm or elbow area; subcutaneous**
4.05 6.20 FUD 010 J P3 80 50
AMA: 2018,Sep,7; 2018,Jan,8; 2017,Jan,8; 2016,Jan,13; 2015,Jan,16

24201 **deep (subfascial or intramuscular)**
10.4 15.7 FUD 090 J A2 50
AMA: 2018,Sep,7; 2018,Jan,8; 2017,Jan,8; 2016,Jan,13; 2015,Jan,16

24220 Injection for Elbow Arthrogram

24220 **Injection procedure for elbow arthrography**
EXCLUDES *Injection tennis elbow (20550)*
(73085)
1.95 4.71 FUD 000 N N1 80 50
AMA: 2018,Sep,7; 2018,Jan,8; 2017,Jan,8; 2016,May,13; 2016,Jan,13; 2015,Aug,6

24300-24498 Repair/Reconstruction of Elbow/Upper Arm

24300 **Manipulation, elbow, under anesthesia**
EXCLUDES *External fixation (20690, 20692)*
12.2 12.2 FUD 090 J G2 50
AMA: 2018,Sep,7

24301 **Muscle or tendon transfer, any type, upper arm or elbow, single (excluding 24320-24331)**
21.6 21.6 FUD 090 J A2 80
AMA: 2018,Sep,7

24305 **Tendon lengthening, upper arm or elbow, each tendon**
16.7 16.7 FUD 090 J A2 80
AMA: 2018,Sep,7

24310 **Tenotomy, open, elbow to shoulder, each tendon**
13.5 13.5 FUD 090 J A2 80
AMA: 2018,Sep,7

24320 **Tenoplasty, with muscle transfer, with or without free graft, elbow to shoulder, single (Seddon-Brookes type procedure)**
22.5 22.5 FUD 090 J A2 80
AMA: 2018,Sep,7

24330 **Flexor-plasty, elbow (eg, Steindler type advancement);**
20.6 20.6 FUD 090 J A2 80 50
AMA: 2018,Sep,7

24331 **with extensor advancement**
22.7 22.7 FUD 090 J A2 80 50
AMA: 2018,Sep,7

24332 Tenolysis, triceps
17.6 17.6 FUD 090 J G2 50
AMA: 2018,Sep,7

24340 Tenodesis of biceps tendon at elbow (separate procedure)
17.7 17.7 FUD 090 J A2 80 50
AMA: 2018,Sep,7

24341 Repair, tendon or muscle, upper arm or elbow, each tendon or muscle, primary or secondary (excludes rotator cuff)
21.4 21.4 FUD 090 J A2 80 50
AMA: 2018,Sep,7

24342 Reinsertion of ruptured biceps or triceps tendon, distal, with or without tendon graft
22.3 22.3 FUD 090 J A2 80 50
AMA: 2018,Sep,7; 2018,Jan,8; 2017,Apr,9

24343 Repair lateral collateral ligament, elbow, with local tissue
20.4 20.4 FUD 090 J G2 80 50
AMA: 2018,Sep,7

24344 Reconstruction lateral collateral ligament, elbow, with tendon graft (includes harvesting of graft)
31.5 31.5 FUD 090 J G2 80 50
AMA: 2018,Sep,7

24345 Repair medial collateral ligament, elbow, with local tissue
20.2 20.2 FUD 090 J A2 80 50
AMA: 2018,Sep,7

24346 Reconstruction medial collateral ligament, elbow, with tendon graft (includes harvesting of graft)
31.7 31.7 FUD 090 J G2 80 50
AMA: 2018,Sep,7

24357 Tenotomy, elbow, lateral or medial (eg, epicondylitis, tennis elbow, golfer's elbow); percutaneous
EXCLUDES *Arthroscopy, elbow, surgical; debridement (29837-29838)*
11.9 11.9 FUD 090 J G2 80 50
AMA: 2018,Sep,7; 2018,Jan,8; 2017,Jan,8; 2016,Jan,13; 2015,Jan,16

24358 debridement, soft tissue and/or bone, open
EXCLUDES *Arthroscopy, elbow, surgical; debridement (29837-29838)*
15.1 15.1 FUD 090 J G2 80 50
AMA: 2018,Sep,7; 2018,Jan,8; 2017,Jan,8; 2016,Jan,13; 2015,Jan,16

24359 debridement, soft tissue and/or bone, open with tendon repair or reattachment
EXCLUDES *Arthroscopy, elbow, surgical; debridement (29837-29838)*
19.0 19.0 FUD 090 J G2 80 50
AMA: 2018,Sep,7; 2018,Jan,8; 2017,Jan,8; 2016,Jan,13; 2015,Jan,16

24360 Arthroplasty, elbow; with membrane (eg, fascial)
26.0 26.0 FUD 090 J A2 80 50
AMA: 2018,Sep,7

24361 with distal humeral prosthetic replacement
29.0 29.0 FUD 090 J J8 80 50
AMA: 2018,Sep,7

24362 with implant and fascia lata ligament reconstruction
30.6 30.6 FUD 090 J A2 80 50
AMA: 2018,Sep,7

24363 with distal humerus and proximal ulnar prosthetic replacement (eg, total elbow)
EXCLUDES *Total elbow implant revision (24370-24371)*
41.9 41.9 FUD 090 J J8 80 50
AMA: 2018,Sep,7; 2018,Jan,8; 2017,Jan,8; 2016,Jan,13; 2015,Jan,16

24365 Arthroplasty, radial head;
18.4 18.4 FUD 090 J J8 80 50
AMA: 2018,Sep,7

24366 with implant
19.7 19.7 FUD 090 J J8 80 50
AMA: 2018,Sep,7

24370 Revision of total elbow arthroplasty, including allograft when performed; humeral or ulnar component
EXCLUDES *Prosthesis removal without replacement in same elbow (eg, humeral and/or ulnar component/s) (24160)*
44.7 44.7 FUD 090 J J8 80 50
AMA: 2018,Sep,7; 2018,Jan,8; 2017,Jan,8; 2016,Jan,13; 2015,Jan,16

24371 humeral and ulnar component
EXCLUDES *Prosthesis removal without replacement in same elbow (eg, humeral and/or ulnar component/s) (24160)*
51.3 51.3 FUD 090 J J8 80 50
AMA: 2018,Sep,7; 2018,Jan,8; 2017,Jan,8; 2016,Jan,13; 2015,Jan,16

24400 Osteotomy, humerus, with or without internal fixation
EXCLUDES *Osteotomy with insertion intramedullary lengthening device, humerus (0594T)*
23.7 23.7 FUD 090 J A2 80 50
AMA: 2018,Sep,7; 2018,Jan,8; 2017,Jan,8; 2016,Jan,13; 2015,Jan,16

24410 Multiple osteotomies with realignment on intramedullary rod, humeral shaft (Sofield type procedure)
EXCLUDES *Osteotomy with insertion intramedullary lengthening device, humerus (0594T)*
30.5 30.5 FUD 090 J G2 80 50
AMA: 2018,Sep,7

24420 Osteoplasty, humerus (eg, shortening or lengthening) (excluding 64876)
EXCLUDES *Osteotomy with insertion intramedullary lengthening device, humerus (0594T)*
29.5 29.5 FUD 090 J A2 80 50
AMA: 2018,Sep,7

24430 Repair of nonunion or malunion, humerus; without graft (eg, compression technique)
EXCLUDES *Repair proximal radius and/or ulna (25400-25420)*
30.5 30.5 FUD 090 J J8 80 50
AMA: 2018,Sep,7

24435 with iliac or other autograft (includes obtaining graft)
EXCLUDES *Repair proximal radius and/or ulna (25400-25420)*
31.0 31.0 FUD 090 J J8 80 50
AMA: 2018,Sep,7

24470 Hemiepiphyseal arrest (eg, cubitus varus or valgus, distal humerus)
19.3 19.3 FUD 090 J A2 80 50
AMA: 2018,Sep,7

24495 Decompression fasciotomy, forearm, with brachial artery exploration
23.4 23.4 FUD 090 J A2 80 50
AMA: 2018,Sep,7

24498 Prophylactic treatment (nailing, pinning, plating or wiring), with or without methylmethacrylate, humeral shaft
24.9 24.9 FUD 090 J J8 80 50
AMA: 2018,Sep,7

24500-24685 Treatment of Fracture/Dislocation of Elbow/Upper Arm

INCLUDES Treatment for either closed or open fractures or dislocations

24500 Closed treatment of humeral shaft fracture; without manipulation
9.46 10.2 FUD 090 T A2 50
AMA: 2018,Sep,7

24505 with manipulation, with or without skeletal traction
12.9 14.3 FUD 090 J A2 50
AMA: 2018,Sep,7

24515 **Open treatment of humeral shaft fracture with plate/screws, with or without cerclage**
25.3 25.3 **FUD** 090 J J8 80 50
AMA: 2018,Sep,7

24516 **Treatment of humeral shaft fracture, with insertion of intramedullary implant, with or without cerclage and/or locking screws**
EXCLUDES *Osteotomy with insertion intramedullary lengthening device, humerus (0594T)*
24.7 24.7 **FUD** 090 J J8 80 50
AMA: 2018,Sep,7; 2018,Jan,8; 2018,Jan,3; 2017,Jan,8; 2016,Jan,13; 2015,Jan,16

24530 **Closed treatment of supracondylar or transcondylar humeral fracture, with or without intercondylar extension; without manipulation**
9.96 10.9 **FUD** 090 T A2 50
AMA: 2018,Sep,7

24535 **with manipulation, with or without skin or skeletal traction**
16.3 17.7 **FUD** 090 J A2 50
AMA: 2018,Sep,7

24538 **Percutaneous skeletal fixation of supracondylar or transcondylar humeral fracture, with or without intercondylar extension**
21.5 21.5 **FUD** 090 J A2 50
AMA: 2018,Sep,7; 2018,Jan,8; 2017,Jan,8; 2016,Jan,13; 2015,Jan,16

24545 **Open treatment of humeral supracondylar or transcondylar fracture, includes internal fixation, when performed; without intercondylar extension**
26.8 26.8 **FUD** 090 J J8 80 50
AMA: 2018,Sep,7

24546 **with intercondylar extension**
29.9 29.9 **FUD** 090 J J8 80 50
AMA: 2018,Sep,7

24560 **Closed treatment of humeral epicondylar fracture, medial or lateral; without manipulation**
8.41 9.43 **FUD** 090 T A2 50
AMA: 2018,Sep,7

24565 **with manipulation**
14.1 15.3 **FUD** 090 J A2 50
AMA: 2018,Sep,7

24566 **Percutaneous skeletal fixation of humeral epicondylar fracture, medial or lateral, with manipulation**
20.6 20.6 **FUD** 090 J A2 50
AMA: 2018,Sep,7

24575 **Open treatment of humeral epicondylar fracture, medial or lateral, includes internal fixation, when performed**
21.0 21.0 **FUD** 090 J J8 80 50
AMA: 2018,Sep,7

24576 **Closed treatment of humeral condylar fracture, medial or lateral; without manipulation**
8.75 9.80 **FUD** 090 T A2 50
AMA: 2018,Sep,7

24577 **with manipulation**
14.4 15.8 **FUD** 090 J A2 50
AMA: 2018,Sep,7

24579 **Open treatment of humeral condylar fracture, medial or lateral, includes internal fixation, when performed**
EXCLUDES *Closed treatment without manipulation (24530, 24560, 24576, 24650, 24670)*
Repair with manipulation (24535, 24565, 24577, 24675)
24.0 24.0 **FUD** 090 J J8 80 50
AMA: 2018,Sep,7

24582 **Percutaneous skeletal fixation of humeral condylar fracture, medial or lateral, with manipulation**
23.3 23.3 **FUD** 090 J A2 50
AMA: 2018,Sep,7

24586 **Open treatment of periarticular fracture and/or dislocation of the elbow (fracture distal humerus and proximal ulna and/or proximal radius);**
31.2 31.2 **FUD** 090 J G2 80 50
AMA: 2018,Sep,7

24587 **with implant arthroplasty**
EXCLUDES *Distal humerus arthroplasty with implant (24361)*
31.4 31.4 **FUD** 090 J J8 80 50
AMA: 2018,Sep,7

24600 **Treatment of closed elbow dislocation; without anesthesia**
9.71 10.6 **FUD** 090 T A2 50
AMA: 2018,Sep,7

24605 **requiring anesthesia**
13.6 13.6 **FUD** 090 J A2 50
AMA: 2018,Sep,7

24615 **Open treatment of acute or chronic elbow dislocation**
20.6 20.6 **FUD** 090 J A2 80 50
AMA: 2018,Sep,7

24620 **Closed treatment of Monteggia type of fracture dislocation at elbow (fracture proximal end of ulna with dislocation of radial head), with manipulation**
15.8 15.8 **FUD** 090 J A2 80 50
AMA: 2018,Sep,7

24635 **Open treatment of Monteggia type of fracture dislocation at elbow (fracture proximal end of ulna with dislocation of radial head), includes internal fixation, when performed**
19.3 19.3 **FUD** 090 J J8 80 50
AMA: 2018,Sep,7

24640 **Closed treatment of radial head subluxation in child, nursemaid elbow, with manipulation** A
2.26 2.89 **FUD** 010 T P3 80 50
AMA: 2018,Sep,7

24650 **Closed treatment of radial head or neck fracture; without manipulation**
6.96 7.51 **FUD** 090 T P2 50
AMA: 2018,Sep,7

24655 **with manipulation**
11.4 12.6 **FUD** 090 J A2 50
AMA: 2018,Sep,7

24665 **Open treatment of radial head or neck fracture, includes internal fixation or radial head excision, when performed;**
18.8 18.8 **FUD** 090 J A2 80 50
AMA: 2018,Sep,7

24666 **with radial head prosthetic replacement**
21.1 21.1 **FUD** 090 J J8 80 50
AMA: 2018,Sep,7

24670 **Closed treatment of ulnar fracture, proximal end (eg, olecranon or coronoid process[es]); without manipulation**
7.53 8.28 **FUD** 090 T A2 50
AMA: 2018,Sep,7

24675 **with manipulation**
11.9 13.1 **FUD** 090 J A2 50
AMA: 2018,Sep,7

24685 **Open treatment of ulnar fracture, proximal end (eg, olecranon or coronoid process[es]), includes internal fixation, when performed**
EXCLUDES *Arthrotomy, elbow (24100-24102)*
18.8 18.8 **FUD** 090 J J8 80 50
AMA: 2018,Sep,7; 2018,Jan,3

24800-24999 Other/Unlisted Elbow/Upper Arm Procedures

24800 **Arthrodesis, elbow joint; local**
23.9 23.9 FUD 090 J A2 80 50
AMA: 2020,May,13; 2018,Sep,7

24802 **with autogenous graft (includes obtaining graft)**
28.9 28.9 FUD 090 J G2 80 50
AMA: 2020,May,13; 2018,Sep,7

24900 **Amputation, arm through humerus; with primary closure**
21.3 21.3 FUD 090 C 80 50
AMA: 2018,Sep,7

24920 **open, circular (guillotine)**
21.1 21.1 FUD 090 C 80 50
AMA: 2018,Sep,7

24925 **secondary closure or scar revision**
16.3 16.3 FUD 090 J A2 80 50
AMA: 2018,Sep,7

24930 **re-amputation**
22.3 22.3 FUD 090 C 80 50
AMA: 2018,Sep,7

24931 **with implant**
26.9 26.9 FUD 090 C 80 50
AMA: 2018,Sep,7

24935 **Stump elongation, upper extremity**
33.6 33.6 FUD 090 J 80 50
AMA: 2018,Sep,7

24940 **Cineplasty, upper extremity, complete procedure**
0.00 0.00 FUD 090 C 80 50
AMA: 2018,Sep,7

24999 **Unlisted procedure, humerus or elbow**
0.00 0.00 FUD YYY T 80 50
AMA: 2018,Sep,7

25000-25001 Incision Tendon Sheath of Wrist

25000 **Incision, extensor tendon sheath, wrist (eg, deQuervains disease)**
EXCLUDES *Carpal tunnel release (64721)*
9.70 9.70 FUD 090 J A2 50
AMA: 2018,Sep,7

25001 **Incision, flexor tendon sheath, wrist (eg, flexor carpi radialis)**
9.88 9.88 FUD 090 J G2 50
AMA: 2018,Sep,7

25020-25025 Decompression Fasciotomy Forearm/Wrist

25020 **Decompression fasciotomy, forearm and/or wrist, flexor OR extensor compartment; without debridement of nonviable muscle and/or nerve**
EXCLUDES *Brachial artery exploration (24495)*
Superficial incision and drainage (10060-10160)
16.4 16.4 FUD 090 J A2 50
AMA: 2018,Sep,7

25023 **with debridement of nonviable muscle and/or nerve**
EXCLUDES *Debridement (11000-11044 [11045, 11046])*
Decompression fasciotomy with exploration brachial artery exploration (24495)
Superficial incision and drainage (10060-10160)
34.4 34.4 FUD 090 J A2 80 50
AMA: 2018,Sep,7

25024 **Decompression fasciotomy, forearm and/or wrist, flexor AND extensor compartment; without debridement of nonviable muscle and/or nerve**
22.5 22.5 FUD 090 J A2 50
AMA: 2018,Sep,7

25025 **with debridement of nonviable muscle and/or nerve**
34.8 34.8 FUD 090 J A2 80 50
AMA: 2018,Sep,7

25028-25040 Incision for Drainage/Foreign Body Removal

25028 **Incision and drainage, forearm and/or wrist; deep abscess or hematoma**
17.0 17.0 FUD 090 J A2 50
AMA: 2018,Sep,7

25031 **bursa**
10.0 10.0 FUD 090 J A2 80 50
AMA: 2018,Sep,7

25035 **Incision, deep, bone cortex, forearm and/or wrist (eg, osteomyelitis or bone abscess)**
16.8 16.8 FUD 090 J A2 80 50
AMA: 2018,Sep,7

25040 **Arthrotomy, radiocarpal or midcarpal joint, with exploration, drainage, or removal of foreign body**
16.1 16.1 FUD 090 J A2 80 50
AMA: 2018,Sep,7

25065-25066 Biopsy Forearm/Wrist

EXCLUDES *Soft tissue needle biopsy (20206)*

25065 **Biopsy, soft tissue of forearm and/or wrist; superficial**
4.59 7.37 FUD 010 J P3 50
AMA: 2018,Sep,7

25066 **deep (subfascial or intramuscular)**
10.3 10.3 FUD 090 J A2 50
AMA: 2018,Sep,7

25071-25078 [25071, 25073] Excision Soft Tissue Tumors Forearm/Wrist

INCLUDES Any necessary elevation tissue planes or dissection
Measurement tumor and necessary margin at greatest diameter prior to excision
Simple and intermediate repairs
Excision types:
Fascial or subfascial soft tissue tumors: simple and marginal resection tumors found either in or below deep fascia, not involving bone or excision substantial amount normal tissue; primarily benign and intramuscular tumors
Radical resection soft tissue tumor: wide resection tumor involving substantial margins normal tissue and may include tissue removal from one or more layers; most often malignant or aggressive benign
Subcutaneous: simple and marginal resection tumors in subcutaneous tissue above deep fascia; most often benign

EXCLUDES *Complex repair*
Excision benign cutaneous lesions (eg, sebaceous cyst) (11400-11406)
Radical resection cutaneous tumors (eg, melanoma) (11600-11606)
Significant vessel exploration or neuroplasty

25071 **Resequenced code. See code following 25075.**

25073 **Resequenced code. See code following 25076.**

25075 **Excision, tumor, soft tissue of forearm and/or wrist area, subcutaneous; less than 3 cm**
9.09 14.5 FUD 090 J G2 50
AMA: 2018,Sep,7

\# **25071** **3 cm or greater**
12.2 12.2 FUD 090 J G2 80 50
AMA: 2018,Sep,7

25076 **Excision, tumor, soft tissue of forearm and/or wrist area, subfascial (eg, intramuscular); less than 3 cm**
14.9 14.9 FUD 090 J G2 50
AMA: 2018,Sep,7

\# **25073** **3 cm or greater**
15.4 15.4 FUD 090 J G2 80 50
AMA: 2018,Sep,7

25077 **Radical resection of tumor (eg, sarcoma), soft tissue of forearm and/or wrist area; less than 3 cm**
25.6 25.6 FUD 090 J G2 50
AMA: 2018,Sep,7

25078 **3 cm or greater**
33.6 33.6 FUD 090 J G2 80 50
AMA: 2018,Sep,7

26/TC PC/TC Only A2-Z3 ASC Payment 50 Bilateral ♂ Male Only ♀ Female Only Facility RVU Non-Facility RVU CCI CLIA
FUD Follow-up Days CMS: IOM AMA: CPT Asst A-Y OPPSI 80/80 Surg Assist Allowed / w/Doc Lab Crosswalk Radiology Crosswalk

25085-25240 Procedures of Bones/Joints Lower Arm/Wrist

25085 **Capsulotomy, wrist (eg, contracture)**
12.9 12.9 **FUD** 090 J A2 80 50
AMA: 2018,Sep,7

25100 **Arthrotomy, wrist joint; with biopsy**
10.0 10.0 **FUD** 090 J A2 80 50
AMA: 2018,Sep,7

25101 **with joint exploration, with or without biopsy, with or without removal of loose or foreign body**
11.6 11.6 **FUD** 090 J A2 80 50
AMA: 2018,Sep,7

25105 **with synovectomy**
13.9 13.9 **FUD** 090 J A2 80 50
AMA: 2018,Sep,7

25107 **Arthrotomy, distal radioulnar joint including repair of triangular cartilage, complex**
17.7 17.7 **FUD** 090 J A2 80 50
AMA: 2018,Sep,7

25109 **Excision of tendon, forearm and/or wrist, flexor or extensor, each**
15.4 15.4 **FUD** 090 J G2 50
AMA: 2018,Sep,7

25110 **Excision, lesion of tendon sheath, forearm and/or wrist**
9.84 9.84 **FUD** 090 J A2 50
AMA: 2018,Sep,7

25111 **Excision of ganglion, wrist (dorsal or volar); primary**
EXCLUDES *Excision ganglion hand or finger (26160)*
9.24 9.24 **FUD** 090 J A2 50
AMA: 2018,Sep,7

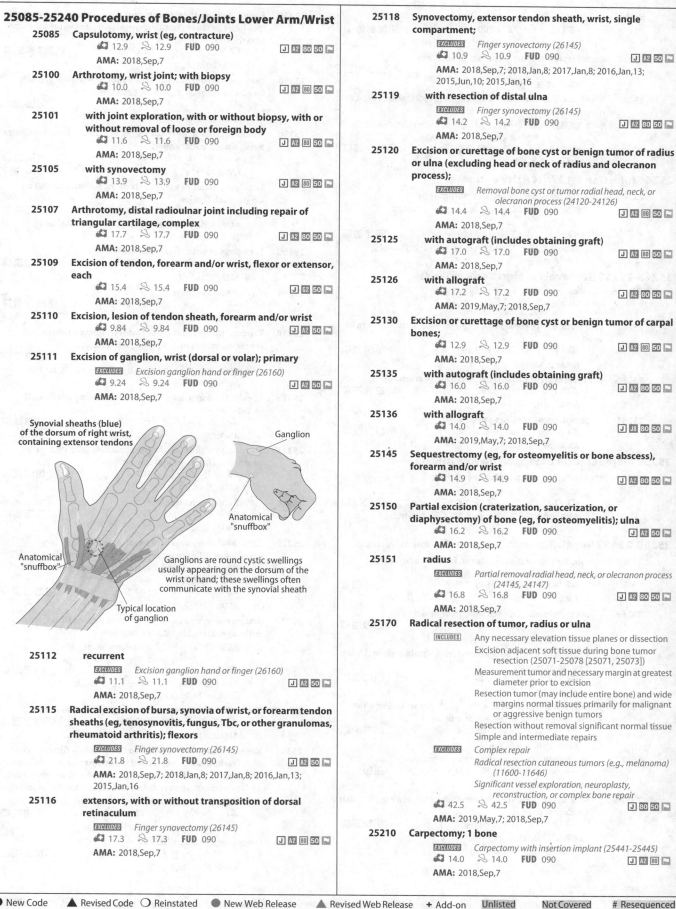

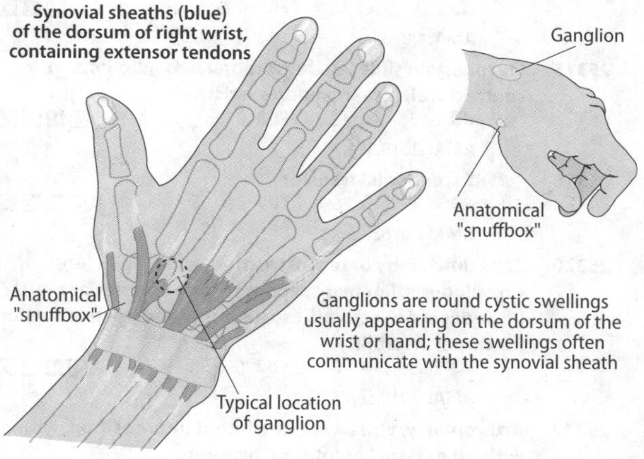
Synovial sheaths (blue) of the dorsum of right wrist, containing extensor tendons
Ganglion
Anatomical "snuffbox"
Anatomical "snuffbox"
Ganglions are round cystic swellings usually appearing on the dorsum of the wrist or hand; these swellings often communicate with the synovial sheath
Typical location of ganglion

25112 **recurrent**
EXCLUDES *Excision ganglion hand or finger (26160)*
11.1 11.1 **FUD** 090 J A2 50
AMA: 2018,Sep,7

25115 **Radical excision of bursa, synovia of wrist, or forearm tendon sheaths (eg, tenosynovitis, fungus, Tbc, or other granulomas, rheumatoid arthritis); flexors**
EXCLUDES *Finger synovectomy (26145)*
21.8 21.8 **FUD** 090 J A2 50
AMA: 2018,Sep,7; 2018,Jan,8; 2017,Jan,8; 2016,Jan,13; 2015,Jan,16

25116 **extensors, with or without transposition of dorsal retinaculum**
EXCLUDES *Finger synovectomy (26145)*
17.3 17.3 **FUD** 090 J A2 80 50
AMA: 2018,Sep,7

25118 **Synovectomy, extensor tendon sheath, wrist, single compartment;**
EXCLUDES *Finger synovectomy (26145)*
10.9 10.9 **FUD** 090 J A2 50
AMA: 2018,Sep,7; 2018,Jan,8; 2017,Jan,8; 2016,Jan,13; 2015,Jun,10; 2015,Jan,16

25119 **with resection of distal ulna**
EXCLUDES *Finger synovectomy (26145)*
14.2 14.2 **FUD** 090 J A2 80 50
AMA: 2018,Sep,7

25120 **Excision or curettage of bone cyst or benign tumor of radius or ulna (excluding head or neck of radius and olecranon process);**
EXCLUDES *Removal bone cyst or tumor radial head, neck, or olecranon process (24120-24126)*
14.4 14.4 **FUD** 090 J A2 80 50
AMA: 2018,Sep,7

25125 **with autograft (includes obtaining graft)**
17.0 17.0 **FUD** 090 J A2 80 50
AMA: 2018,Sep,7

25126 **with allograft**
17.2 17.2 **FUD** 090 J A2 80 50
AMA: 2019,May,7; 2018,Sep,7

25130 **Excision or curettage of bone cyst or benign tumor of carpal bones;**
12.9 12.9 **FUD** 090 J A2 80 50
AMA: 2018,Sep,7

25135 **with autograft (includes obtaining graft)**
16.0 16.0 **FUD** 090 J A2 80 50
AMA: 2018,Sep,7

25136 **with allograft**
14.0 14.0 **FUD** 090 J J8 80 50
AMA: 2019,May,7; 2018,Sep,7

25145 **Sequestrectomy (eg, for osteomyelitis or bone abscess), forearm and/or wrist**
14.9 14.9 **FUD** 090 J A2 80 50
AMA: 2018,Sep,7

25150 **Partial excision (craterization, saucerization, or diaphysectomy) of bone (eg, for osteomyelitis); ulna**
16.2 16.2 **FUD** 090 J A2 50
AMA: 2018,Sep,7

25151 **radius**
EXCLUDES *Partial removal radial head, neck, or olecranon process (24145, 24147)*
16.8 16.8 **FUD** 090 J A2 80 50
AMA: 2018,Sep,7

25170 **Radical resection of tumor, radius or ulna**
INCLUDES Any necessary elevation tissue planes or dissection
Excision adjacent soft tissue during bone tumor resection (25071-25078 [25071, 25073])
Measurement tumor and necessary margin at greatest diameter prior to excision
Resection tumor (may include entire bone) and wide margins normal tissues primarily for malignant or aggressive benign tumors
Resection without removal significant normal tissue
Simple and intermediate repairs
EXCLUDES *Complex repair*
Radical resection cutaneous tumors (e.g., melanoma) (11600-11646)
Significant vessel exploration, neuroplasty, reconstruction, or complex bone repair
42.5 42.5 **FUD** 090 J 80 50
AMA: 2019,May,7; 2018,Sep,7

25210 **Carpectomy; 1 bone**
EXCLUDES *Carpectomy with insertion implant (25441-25445)*
14.0 14.0 **FUD** 090 J A2 80
AMA: 2018,Sep,7

25215 **all bones of proximal row**
17.8 17.8 FUD 090 J A2 80 50
AMA: 2019,Dec,14; 2019,Feb,10; 2018,Sep,7

25230 **Radial styloidectomy (separate procedure)**
12.4 12.4 FUD 090 J A2 50
AMA: 2018,Sep,7

25240 **Excision distal ulna partial or complete (eg, Darrach type or matched resection)**
EXCLUDES *Acquisition fascia for interposition (20920, 20922)*
Implant replacement (25442)
12.3 12.3 FUD 090 J A2 80 50
AMA: 2018,Sep,7

25246 Injection for Wrist Arthrogram

25246 **Injection procedure for wrist arthrography**
EXCLUDES *Excision superficial foreign body (20520)*
(73115)
2.14 5.25 FUD 000 N N1 50
AMA: 2018,Sep,7; 2018,Jan,8; 2017,Jan,8; 2016,Jan,13; 2015,Aug,6

25248-25251 Removal Foreign Body of Wrist

EXCLUDES *Excision superficial foreign body (20520)*
K-wire, pin, or rod insertion (20650)
K-wire, pin, or rod removal (20670, 20680)

25248 **Exploration with removal of deep foreign body, forearm or wrist**
11.8 11.8 FUD 090 J A2 50
AMA: 2018,Sep,7

25250 **Removal of wrist prosthesis; (separate procedure)**
15.3 15.3 FUD 090 Q2 A2 80 50
AMA: 2018,Sep,7

25251 **complicated, including total wrist**
20.7 20.7 FUD 090 Q2 A2 80 50
AMA: 2018,Sep,7

25259 Manipulation of Wrist with Anesthesia

25259 **Manipulation, wrist, under anesthesia**
EXCLUDES *Application external fixation (20690, 20692)*
12.1 12.1 FUD 090 J G2 50
AMA: 2018,Sep,7; 2018,Jan,8; 2017,Jan,8; 2016,Jan,13; 2015,Jan,16

25260-25492 Repair/Reconstruction of Forearm/Wrist

25260 **Repair, tendon or muscle, flexor, forearm and/or wrist; primary, single, each tendon or muscle**
18.1 18.1 FUD 090 J A2
AMA: 2018,Sep,7

25263 **secondary, single, each tendon or muscle**
18.1 18.1 FUD 090 J A2 80
AMA: 2018,Sep,7

25265 **secondary, with free graft (includes obtaining graft), each tendon or muscle**
21.4 21.4 FUD 090 J A2 80
AMA: 2018,Sep,7

25270 **Repair, tendon or muscle, extensor, forearm and/or wrist; primary, single, each tendon or muscle**
14.1 14.1 FUD 090 J A2 80
AMA: 2018,Sep,7

25272 **secondary, single, each tendon or muscle**
15.9 15.9 FUD 090 J A2 80
AMA: 2018,Sep,7

25274 **secondary, with free graft (includes obtaining graft), each tendon or muscle**
19.1 19.1 FUD 090 J A2 80
AMA: 2018,Sep,7

25275 **Repair, tendon sheath, extensor, forearm and/or wrist, with free graft (includes obtaining graft) (eg, for extensor carpi ulnaris subluxation)**
19.3 19.3 FUD 090 J A2 80 50
AMA: 2018,Sep,7

25280 **Lengthening or shortening of flexor or extensor tendon, forearm and/or wrist, single, each tendon**
16.3 16.3 FUD 090 J A2 80
AMA: 2018,Sep,7

25290 **Tenotomy, open, flexor or extensor tendon, forearm and/or wrist, single, each tendon**
12.5 12.5 FUD 090 J A2
AMA: 2018,Sep,7

25295 **Tenolysis, flexor or extensor tendon, forearm and/or wrist, single, each tendon**
15.1 15.1 FUD 090 J A2
AMA: 2018,Sep,7; 2018,Jan,8; 2017,Jan,8; 2016,Jan,13; 2015,Jan,16

25300 **Tenodesis at wrist; flexors of fingers**
19.5 19.5 FUD 090 J A2 80 50
AMA: 2018,Sep,7

25301 **extensors of fingers**
18.5 18.5 FUD 090 J A2 80 50
AMA: 2018,Sep,7

25310 **Tendon transplantation or transfer, flexor or extensor, forearm and/or wrist, single; each tendon**
17.8 17.8 FUD 090 J A2 80
AMA: 2018,Sep,7; 2018,Jan,8; 2017,Jan,8; 2016,Jan,13; 2015,Jan,16

25312 **with tendon graft(s) (includes obtaining graft), each tendon**
20.7 20.7 FUD 090 J A2 80
AMA: 2018,Sep,7

25315 **Flexor origin slide (eg, for cerebral palsy, Volkmann contracture), forearm and/or wrist;**
22.2 22.2 FUD 090 J A2 80 50
AMA: 2018,Sep,7

25316 **with tendon(s) transfer**
26.4 26.4 FUD 090 J A2 80 50
AMA: 2018,Sep,7

25320 **Capsulorrhaphy or reconstruction, wrist, open (eg, capsulodesis, ligament repair, tendon transfer or graft) (includes synovectomy, capsulotomy and open reduction) for carpal instability**
28.3 28.3 FUD 090 J A2 80 50
AMA: 2018,Sep,7

25332 **Arthroplasty, wrist, with or without interposition, with or without external or internal fixation**
EXCLUDES *Acquiring fascia for interposition (20920, 20922)*
Arthroplasty with prosthesis (25441-25446)
24.2 24.2 FUD 090 J A2 80 50
AMA: 2019,Feb,10; 2018,Sep,7; 2018,Jan,8; 2017,Jan,8; 2016,Jan,13; 2015,Jan,16

25335 **Centralization of wrist on ulna (eg, radial club hand)**
27.2 27.2 FUD 090 J A2 80 50
AMA: 2018,Sep,7; 2018,May,10

25337 **Reconstruction for stabilization of unstable distal ulna or distal radioulnar joint, secondary by soft tissue stabilization (eg, tendon transfer, tendon graft or weave, or tenodesis) with or without open reduction of distal radioulnar joint**
EXCLUDES *Acquiring fascia lata graft (20920, 20922)*
25.5 25.5 FUD 090 J A2 50
AMA: 2018,Sep,7

25350 **Osteotomy, radius; distal third**
19.4 19.4 FUD 090 J J8 80 50
AMA: 2018,Sep,7

25355 **middle or proximal third**
22.0 22.0 FUD 090 J A2 80 50
AMA: 2018,Sep,7

25360 **Osteotomy; ulna**
18.8 18.8 FUD 090 J A2 80 50
AMA: 2018,Sep,7

25365 **radius AND ulna**
26.4 26.4 FUD 090 J A2 80 50
AMA: 2018,Sep,7

25370 **Multiple osteotomies, with realignment on intramedullary rod (Sofield type procedure); radius OR ulna**
29.0 29.0 FUD 090 J A2 80 50
AMA: 2018,Sep,7

25375 **radius AND ulna**
27.5 27.5 FUD 090 J A2 80 50
AMA: 2018,Sep,7

25390 **Osteoplasty, radius OR ulna; shortening**
22.1 22.1 FUD 090 J J8 80 50
AMA: 2018,Sep,7

25391 **lengthening with autograft**
28.7 28.7 FUD 090 J J8 80 50
AMA: 2018,Sep,7

25392 **Osteoplasty, radius AND ulna; shortening (excluding 64876)**
29.3 29.3 FUD 090 J A2 80 50
AMA: 2018,Sep,7

25393 **lengthening with autograft**
32.6 32.6 FUD 090 J A2 80 50
AMA: 2018,Sep,7

25394 **Osteoplasty, carpal bone, shortening**
22.6 22.6 FUD 090 J G2 80 50
AMA: 2018,Sep,7

25400 **Repair of nonunion or malunion, radius OR ulna; without graft (eg, compression technique)**
23.1 23.1 FUD 090 J J8 80 50
AMA: 2018,Sep,7

25405 **with autograft (includes obtaining graft)**
29.9 29.9 FUD 090 J J8 80 50
AMA: 2018,Sep,7

25415 **Repair of nonunion or malunion, radius AND ulna; without graft (eg, compression technique)**
27.8 27.8 FUD 090 J J8 80 50
AMA: 2018,Sep,7

25420 **with autograft (includes obtaining graft)**
33.5 33.5 FUD 090 J G2 80 50
AMA: 2018,Sep,7

25425 **Repair of defect with autograft; radius OR ulna**
27.6 27.6 FUD 090 J A2 80 50
AMA: 2018,Sep,7

25426 **radius AND ulna**
32.4 32.4 FUD 090 J G2 80 50
AMA: 2018,Sep,7

25430 **Insertion of vascular pedicle into carpal bone (eg, Hori procedure)**
21.0 21.0 FUD 090 J G2 50
AMA: 2018,Sep,7

25431 **Repair of nonunion of carpal bone (excluding carpal scaphoid (navicular)) (includes obtaining graft and necessary fixation), each bone**
22.7 22.7 FUD 090 J G2 80 50
AMA: 2018,Sep,7

25440 **Repair of nonunion, scaphoid carpal (navicular) bone, with or without radial styloidectomy (includes obtaining graft and necessary fixation)**
22.1 22.1 FUD 090 J A2 80 50
AMA: 2018,Sep,7

25441 **Arthroplasty with prosthetic replacement; distal radius**
27.0 27.0 FUD 090 J J8 80 50
AMA: 2018,Sep,7; 2018,Jan,8; 2017,Aug,9; 2017,Jan,8; 2016,Jan,13; 2015,Jan,16

25442 **distal ulna**
23.2 23.2 FUD 090 J J8 80 50
AMA: 2018,Sep,7; 2018,Jan,8; 2017,Aug,9; 2017,Jan,8; 2016,Jan,13; 2015,Jan,16

25443 **scaphoid carpal (navicular)**
22.6 22.6 FUD 090 J J8 80 50
AMA: 2018,Sep,7; 2018,Jan,8; 2017,Jan,8; 2016,Jan,13; 2015,Jan,16

25444 **lunate**
23.7 23.7 FUD 090 J J8 80 50
AMA: 2018,Sep,7; 2018,Jan,8; 2017,Jan,8; 2016,Jan,13; 2015,Jan,16

25445 **trapezium**
20.8 20.8 FUD 090 J J8 50
AMA: 2018,Sep,7; 2018,Jan,8; 2017,Jan,8; 2016,Jan,13; 2015,Jan,16

25446 **distal radius and partial or entire carpus (total wrist)**
33.8 33.8 FUD 090 J J8 80 50
AMA: 2018,Sep,7; 2018,Jan,8; 2017,Jan,8; 2016,Jan,13; 2015,Jan,16

25447 **Arthroplasty, interposition, intercarpal or carpometacarpal joints**
EXCLUDES *Wrist arthroplasty (25332)*
23.8 23.8 FUD 090 J A2 80 50
AMA: 2018,Sep,7; 2018,Jan,8; 2017,Jan,8; 2016,Jan,13; 2015,Jan,16

25449 **Revision of arthroplasty, including removal of implant, wrist joint**
29.8 29.8 FUD 090 J A2 80 50
AMA: 2018,Sep,7

25450 **Epiphyseal arrest by epiphysiodesis or stapling; distal radius OR ulna**
17.7 17.7 FUD 090 J A2 50
AMA: 2018,Sep,7

25455 **distal radius AND ulna**
21.0 21.0 FUD 090 J A2 50
AMA: 2018,Sep,7

25490 **Prophylactic treatment (nailing, pinning, plating or wiring) with or without methylmethacrylate; radius**
20.7 20.7 FUD 090 J A2 80 50
AMA: 2018,Sep,7

25491 **ulna**
21.3 21.3 FUD 090 J A2 80 50
AMA: 2018,Sep,7

25492 **radius AND ulna**
26.1 26.1 FUD 090 J A2 80 50
AMA: 2018,Sep,7

25500-25695 Treatment of Fracture/Dislocation of Forearm/Wrist

Code also external fixation, when performed (20690, 20692)

25500 **Closed treatment of radial shaft fracture; without manipulation**
7.25 7.98 FUD 090 T P2 50
AMA: 2018,Sep,7

25505 **with manipulation**
13.2 14.4 FUD 090 J A2 50
AMA: 2018,Sep,7

25515 **Open treatment of radial shaft fracture, includes internal fixation, when performed**
19.2 19.2 FUD 090 J J8 80 50
AMA: 2018,Sep,7

25520 **Closed treatment of radial shaft fracture and closed treatment of dislocation of distal radioulnar joint (Galeazzi fracture/dislocation)**
15.5 16.4 FUD 090 J A2 50
AMA: 2018,Sep,7

25525 **Open treatment of radial shaft fracture, includes internal fixation, when performed, and closed treatment of distal radioulnar joint dislocation (Galeazzi fracture/ dislocation), includes percutaneous skeletal fixation, when performed**
22.6 22.6 FUD 090 J A2 80 50
AMA: 2018,Sep,7

25526 **Open treatment of radial shaft fracture, includes internal fixation, when performed, and open treatment of distal radioulnar joint dislocation (Galeazzi fracture/ dislocation), includes internal fixation, when performed, includes repair of triangular fibrocartilage complex**
27.5 27.5 FUD 090 J J8 80 50
AMA: 2018,Sep,7

25530 **Closed treatment of ulnar shaft fracture; without manipulation**
6.88 7.52 FUD 090 T P2 50
AMA: 2018,Sep,7

25535 **with manipulation**
13.0 14.0 FUD 090 T A2 50
AMA: 2018,Sep,7

25545 **Open treatment of ulnar shaft fracture, includes internal fixation, when performed**
17.9 17.9 FUD 090 J J8 80 50
AMA: 2018,Sep,7; 2018,Jan,8; 2017,Jan,8; 2016,Jan,13; 2015,Jan,16

25560 **Closed treatment of radial and ulnar shaft fractures; without manipulation**
7.31 8.15 FUD 090 T P2 50
AMA: 2018,Sep,7

25565 **with manipulation**
13.2 14.7 FUD 090 J A2 50
AMA: 2018,Sep,7

25574 **Open treatment of radial AND ulnar shaft fractures, with internal fixation, when performed; of radius OR ulna**
19.4 19.4 FUD 090 J J8 80 50
AMA: 2018,Sep,7; 2018,Jan,8; 2017,Jan,8; 2016,Jan,13; 2015,Jan,16

25575 **of radius AND ulna**
25.9 25.9 FUD 090 J J8 80 50
AMA: 2018,Sep,7

25600 **Closed treatment of distal radial fracture (eg, Colles or Smith type) or epiphyseal separation, includes closed treatment of fracture of ulnar styloid, when performed; without manipulation**
INCLUDES Closed treatment ulnar styloid fracture (25650)
9.06 9.51 FUD 090 T P2 50
AMA: 2018,Sep,7; 2018,Jan,8; 2017,Jan,8; 2016,Jan,13; 2015,Jan,16

25605 **with manipulation**
INCLUDES Closed treatment ulnar styloid fracture (25650)
14.7 15.5 FUD 090 J A2 50
AMA: 2018,Sep,7; 2018,Jan,8; 2017,Jan,8; 2016,Jan,13; 2015,Jan,16

25606 **Percutaneous skeletal fixation of distal radial fracture or epiphyseal separation**
EXCLUDES *Closed treatment ulnar styloid fracture (25650)*
Open repair ulnar styloid fracture (25652)
Percutaneous repair ulnar styloid fracture (25651)
19.1 19.1 FUD 090 J A2 50
AMA: 2018,Sep,7

25607 **Open treatment of distal radial extra-articular fracture or epiphyseal separation, with internal fixation**
EXCLUDES *Closed treatment ulnar styloid fracture (25650)*
Open repair ulnar styloid fracture (25652)
Percutaneous repair ulnar styloid fracture (25651)
21.1 21.1 FUD 090 J J8 80 50
AMA: 2018,Sep,7; 2018,Jan,8; 2017,Jan,8; 2016,Jan,13; 2015,Jan,16

25608 **Open treatment of distal radial intra-articular fracture or epiphyseal separation; with internal fixation of 2 fragments**
EXCLUDES *Closed treatment ulnar styloid fracture (25650)*
Open repair ulnar styloid fracture (25652)
Open treatment distal radial intra-articular fracture or epiphyseal separation; with internal fixation of 3 or more fragments (25609)
Percutaneous repair ulnar styloid fracture (25651)
23.7 23.7 FUD 090 J J8 80 50
AMA: 2018,Sep,7; 2018,Jan,8; 2017,Jan,8; 2016,Jan,13; 2015,Jan,16

25609 **with internal fixation of 3 or more fragments**
EXCLUDES *Closed treatment ulnar styloid fracture (25650)*
Open repair ulnar styloid fracture (25652)
Percutaneous repair ulnar styloid fracture (25651)
30.2 30.2 FUD 090 J J8 80 50
AMA: 2018,Sep,7; 2018,Jan,8; 2017,Jan,8; 2016,Jan,13; 2015,Jan,16

25622 **Closed treatment of carpal scaphoid (navicular) fracture; without manipulation**
8.07 8.76 FUD 090 T P2 50
AMA: 2018,Sep,7

25624 **with manipulation**
12.6 13.8 FUD 090 J A2 80 50
AMA: 2018,Sep,7

25628 **Open treatment of carpal scaphoid (navicular) fracture, includes internal fixation, when performed**
20.7 20.7 FUD 090 J A2 80 50
AMA: 2018,Sep,7

25630 **Closed treatment of carpal bone fracture (excluding carpal scaphoid [navicular]); without manipulation, each bone**
8.13 8.77 FUD 090 T P2 50
AMA: 2018,Sep,7

25635 **with manipulation, each bone**
11.9 13.1 FUD 090 J A2 80 50
AMA: 2018,Sep,7

25645 **Open treatment of carpal bone fracture (other than carpal scaphoid [navicular]), each bone**
16.4 16.4 FUD 090 J A2 80 50
AMA: 2018,Sep,7

25650 **Closed treatment of ulnar styloid fracture**
EXCLUDES *Closed treatment distal radial fracture (25600, 25605)*
Open treatment distal radial extra-articular fracture or epiphyseal separation, with internal fixation (25607-25609)
8.70 9.35 FUD 090 T P2 50
AMA: 2018,Sep,7; 2018,Jan,8; 2017,Jan,8; 2016,Jan,13; 2015,Jan,16

25651 **Percutaneous skeletal fixation of ulnar styloid fracture**
14.0 14.0 FUD 090 J G2 80 50
AMA: 2018,Sep,7

25652 **Open treatment of ulnar styloid fracture**
17.9 17.9 FUD 090 J G2 50
AMA: 2018,Sep,7; 2018,Jan,8; 2017,Jan,8; 2016,Jan,13; 2015,Jan,16

25660 **Closed treatment of radiocarpal or intercarpal dislocation, 1 or more bones, with manipulation**
11.9 11.9 FUD 090 T A2 80 50
AMA: 2018,Sep,7

25670 **Open treatment of radiocarpal or intercarpal dislocation, 1 or more bones**
17.5 17.5 **FUD** 090 J A2 80 50
AMA: 2018,Sep,7

25671 **Percutaneous skeletal fixation of distal radioulnar dislocation**
15.3 15.3 **FUD** 090 J A2 50
AMA: 2018,Sep,7

25675 **Closed treatment of distal radioulnar dislocation with manipulation**
11.2 12.4 **FUD** 090 T A2 80 50
AMA: 2018,Sep,7

25676 **Open treatment of distal radioulnar dislocation, acute or chronic**
18.0 18.0 **FUD** 090 J A2 80 50
AMA: 2018,Sep,7

25680 **Closed treatment of trans-scaphoperilunar type of fracture dislocation, with manipulation**
15.1 15.1 **FUD** 090 T A2 80 50
AMA: 2018,Sep,7

25685 **Open treatment of trans-scaphoperilunar type of fracture dislocation**
21.2 21.2 **FUD** 090 J A2 80 50
AMA: 2018,Sep,7

25690 **Closed treatment of lunate dislocation, with manipulation**
14.0 14.0 **FUD** 090 J A2 80 50
AMA: 2018,Sep,7

25695 **Open treatment of lunate dislocation**
18.2 18.2 **FUD** 090 J A2 80 50
AMA: 2018,Sep,7

25800-25830 Wrist Fusion

25800 **Arthrodesis, wrist; complete, without bone graft (includes radiocarpal and/or intercarpal and/or carpometacarpal joints)**
21.0 21.0 **FUD** 090 J J8 80 50
AMA: 2020,May,13; 2018,Sep,7

25805 **with sliding graft**
24.4 24.4 **FUD** 090 J J8 80 50
AMA: 2020,May,13; 2018,Sep,7

25810 **with iliac or other autograft (includes obtaining graft)**
24.9 24.9 **FUD** 090 J J8 80 50
AMA: 2020,May,13; 2018,Sep,7

25820 **Arthrodesis, wrist; limited, without bone graft (eg, intercarpal or radiocarpal)**
18.1 18.1 **FUD** 090 J J8 80 50
AMA: 2020,May,13; 2018,Sep,7

25825 **with autograft (includes obtaining graft)**
22.3 22.3 **FUD** 090 J J8 80 50
AMA: 2020,May,13; 2018,Sep,7; 2018,Jan,8; 2017,Jan,8; 2016,Jan,13; 2015,Jan,16

25830 **Arthrodesis, distal radioulnar joint with segmental resection of ulna, with or without bone graft (eg, Sauve-Kapandji procedure)**
27.0 27.0 **FUD** 090 J J8 80 50
AMA: 2020,May,13; 2018,Sep,7

25900-25999 Amputation Through Forearm/Wrist

25900 **Amputation, forearm, through radius and ulna;**
20.5 20.5 **FUD** 090 C 80 50
AMA: 2018,Sep,7

25905 **open, circular (guillotine)**
20.2 20.2 **FUD** 090 C 80 50
AMA: 2018,Sep,7

25907 **secondary closure or scar revision**
17.6 17.6 **FUD** 090 J A2 80 50
AMA: 2018,Sep,7

25909 **re-amputation**
19.7 19.7 **FUD** 090 J 80 50
AMA: 2018,Sep,7

25915 **Krukenberg procedure**
33.7 33.7 **FUD** 090 C 80 50
AMA: 2018,Sep,7

25920 **Disarticulation through wrist;**
20.5 20.5 **FUD** 090 C 80 50
AMA: 2018,Sep,7

25922 **secondary closure or scar revision**
17.7 17.7 **FUD** 090 J A2 80 50
AMA: 2018,Sep,7

25924 **re-amputation**
20.0 20.0 **FUD** 090 C 80 50
AMA: 2018,Sep,7

25927 **Transmetacarpal amputation;**
24.0 24.0 **FUD** 090 C 80 50
AMA: 2018,Sep,7

25929 **secondary closure or scar revision**
17.2 17.2 **FUD** 090 T A2 80 50
AMA: 2018,Sep,7

25931 **re-amputation**
22.1 22.1 **FUD** 090 J G2 50
AMA: 2018,Sep,7

25999 **Unlisted procedure, forearm or wrist**
0.00 0.00 **FUD** YYY T 80 50
AMA: 2019,Feb,10; 2018,Sep,7

26010-26037 Incision Hand/Fingers

26010 **Drainage of finger abscess; simple**
3.97 8.62 **FUD** 010 T P2
AMA: 2018,Sep,7

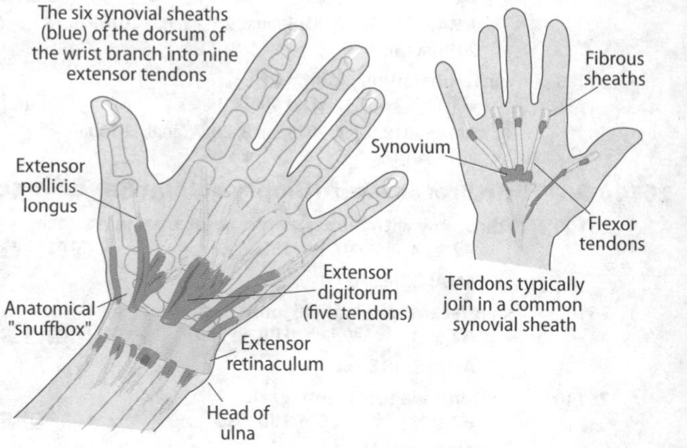

26011 **complicated (eg, felon)**
5.32 12.4 **FUD** 010 J A2
AMA: 2018,Sep,7

26020 **Drainage of tendon sheath, digit and/or palm, each**
15.9 15.9 **FUD** 090 J A2
AMA: 2018,Sep,7

26025 **Drainage of palmar bursa; single, bursa**
12.1 12.1 **FUD** 090 J A2 80 50
AMA: 2018,Sep,7

26030 **multiple bursa**
14.0 14.0 **FUD** 090 J A2 80 50
AMA: 2018,Sep,7

26034 **Incision, bone cortex, hand or finger (eg, osteomyelitis or bone abscess)**
15.7 15.7 **FUD** 090 J A2
AMA: 2018,Sep,7

Musculoskeletal System

26035 — 26123

26035 **Decompression fingers and/or hand, injection injury (eg, grease gun)**
24.7 24.7 FUD 090 J G2 80
AMA: 2018,Sep,7

26037 **Decompressive fasciotomy, hand (excludes 26035)**
EXCLUDES *Injection injury (26035)*
16.3 16.3 FUD 090 J G2 80 50
AMA: 2018,Sep,7

26040-26045 Incision Palmar Fascia

EXCLUDES *Enzyme injection fasciotomy (20527, 26341)*
Fasciectomy (26121, 26123, 26125)

26040 **Fasciotomy, palmar (eg, Dupuytren's contracture); percutaneous**
9.00 9.00 FUD 090 J A2 50
AMA: 2018,Sep,7; 2018,Jan,8; 2017,Jan,8; 2016,Jan,13; 2015,Jan,16

26045 **open, partial**
13.5 13.5 FUD 090 J A2 50
AMA: 2018,Sep,7; 2018,Jan,8; 2017,Jan,8; 2016,Jan,13; 2015,Jan,16

26055-26080 Incision Tendon/Joint of Fingers/Hand

26055 **Tendon sheath incision (eg, for trigger finger)**
8.91 16.1 FUD 090 J A2
AMA: 2018,Sep,7

26060 **Tenotomy, percutaneous, single, each digit**
7.41 7.41 FUD 090 J A2 80
AMA: 2018,Sep,7

26070 **Arthrotomy, with exploration, drainage, or removal of loose or foreign body; carpometacarpal joint**
9.23 9.23 FUD 090 J A2 50
AMA: 2018,Sep,7

26075 **metacarpophalangeal joint, each**
9.64 9.64 FUD 090 J A2 50
AMA: 2018,Sep,7; 2018,Jan,8; 2017,Jan,8; 2016,Jan,13; 2015,Jan,16

26080 **interphalangeal joint, each**
11.3 11.3 FUD 090 J A2
AMA: 2018,Sep,7; 2018,Jan,8; 2017,Jan,8; 2016,Jan,13; 2015,Jan,16

26100-26110 Arthrotomy with Biopsy of Joint Hand/Fingers

26100 **Arthrotomy with biopsy; carpometacarpal joint, each**
9.64 9.64 FUD 090 J A2 80 50
AMA: 2018,Sep,7

26105 **metacarpophalangeal joint, each**
9.71 9.71 FUD 090 J A2 80 50
AMA: 2018,Sep,7

26110 **interphalangeal joint, each**
9.28 9.28 FUD 090 J A2
AMA: 2018,Sep,7

26111-26118 [26111, 26113] Excision Soft Tissue Tumors Fingers and Hand

INCLUDES Any necessary elevation tissue planes or dissection
Measurement tumor and necessary margin at greatest diameter prior to excision
Simple and intermediate repairs
Excision types:
- Fascial or subfascial soft tissue tumors: simple and marginal resection tumors found either in or below deep fascia, not involving bone or excision substantial amount normal tissue; primarily benign and intramuscular tumors
  - Tumors fingers and toes involving joint capsules, tendons and tendon sheaths
- Radical resection soft tissue tumor: wide resection tumor, involving substantial margins normal tissue and may include tissue removal from one or more layers; most often malignant or aggressive benign
  - Tumors fingers and toes adjacent to joints, tendons and tendon sheaths
- Subcutaneous: simple and marginal resection tumors found in subcutaneous tissue above deep fascia; most often benign

EXCLUDES *Complex repair*
Excision benign cutaneous lesions (eg, sebaceous cyst) (11420-11426)
Radical resection cutaneous tumors (eg, melanoma) (11620-11626)
Significant vessel exploration or neuroplasty

26111 **Resequenced code. See code following 26115.**

26113 **Resequenced code. See code following 26116.**

26115 **Excision, tumor or vascular malformation, soft tissue of hand or finger, subcutaneous; less than 1.5 cm**
9.51 15.2 FUD 090 J G2
AMA: 2018,Sep,7

\# **26111** **1.5 cm or greater**
11.9 11.9 FUD 090 J G2 80
AMA: 2018,Sep,7

26116 **Excision, tumor, soft tissue, or vascular malformation, of hand or finger, subfascial (eg, intramuscular); less than 1.5 cm**
15.1 15.1 FUD 090 J G2
AMA: 2018,Sep,7; 2018,Jan,8; 2017,Jan,8; 2016,Jan,13; 2015,Jan,16

\# **26113** **1.5 cm or greater**
15.7 15.7 FUD 090 J G2 80
AMA: 2018,Sep,7

26117 **Radical resection of tumor (eg, sarcoma), soft tissue of hand or finger; less than 3 cm**
21.4 21.4 FUD 090 J G2
AMA: 2018,Sep,7

26118 **3 cm or greater**
30.3 30.3 FUD 090 J G2 80
AMA: 2018,Sep,7

26121-26236 Procedures of Bones, Fascia, Joints and Tendons Hands and Fingers

26121 **Fasciectomy, palm only, with or without Z-plasty, other local tissue rearrangement, or skin grafting (includes obtaining graft)**
EXCLUDES *Enzyme injection fasciotomy (20527, 26341)*
Fasciotomy (26040, 26045)
17.2 17.2 FUD 090 J A2 50
AMA: 2018,Sep,7; 2018,Jan,8; 2017,Jan,8; 2016,Jan,13; 2015,Jan,16

26123 **Fasciectomy, partial palmar with release of single digit including proximal interphalangeal joint, with or without Z-plasty, other local tissue rearrangement, or skin grafting (includes obtaining graft);**
EXCLUDES *Enzyme injection fasciotomy (20527, 26341)*
Fasciotomy (26040, 26045)
24.0 24.0 FUD 090 J A2 50
AMA: 2018,Sep,7; 2018,Jan,8; 2017,Jan,8; 2016,Jan,13; 2015,Jan,16

\+ **26125** **each additional digit (List separately in addition to code for primary procedure)**

EXCLUDES *Enzyme injection fasciotomy (20527, 26341)*
Fasciotomy (26040, 26045)

Code first (26123)

7.87 | 7.87 | FUD ZZZ | N N1

AMA: 2018,Sep,7; 2018,Jan,8; 2017,Jan,8; 2016,Jan,13; 2015,Jan,16

26130 **Synovectomy, carpometacarpal joint**

13.4 | 13.4 | FUD 090 | J A2 50

AMA: 2018,Sep,7

26135 **Synovectomy, metacarpophalangeal joint including intrinsic release and extensor hood reconstruction, each digit**

15.9 | 15.9 | FUD 090 | J A2 80

AMA: 2018,Sep,7

26140 **Synovectomy, proximal interphalangeal joint, including extensor reconstruction, each interphalangeal joint**

14.5 | 14.5 | FUD 090 | J A2

AMA: 2018,Sep,7

26145 **Synovectomy, tendon sheath, radical (tenosynovectomy), flexor tendon, palm and/or finger, each tendon**

EXCLUDES *Wrist synovectomy (25115-25116)*

14.7 | 14.7 | FUD 090 | J A2

AMA: 2018,Sep,7

26160 **Excision of lesion of tendon sheath or joint capsule (eg, cyst, mucous cyst, or ganglion), hand or finger**

EXCLUDES *Trigger finger (26055)*
Wrist ganglion removal (25111-25112)

9.04 | 16.3 | FUD 090 | J A2

AMA: 2019,Jul,10; 2018,Sep,7

26170 **Excision of tendon, palm, flexor or extensor, single, each tendon**

EXCLUDES *Excision extensor tendon, with implantation synthetic rod for delayed tendon graft, hand or finger, each rod (26415)*
Excision flexor tendon, with implantation synthetic rod for delayed tendon graft, hand or finger, each rod (26390)

11.7 | 11.7 | FUD 090 | J A2 80

AMA: 2018,Sep,7; 2018,Jan,8; 2017,Jan,8; 2016,Jan,13; 2015,Jan,16

26180 **Excision of tendon, finger, flexor or extensor, each tendon**

EXCLUDES *Excision extensor tendon, with implantation synthetic rod for delayed tendon graft, hand or finger, each rod (26415)*
Excision flexor tendon, with implantation synthetic rod for delayed tendon graft, hand or finger, each rod (26390)

12.8 | 12.8 | FUD 090 | J A2 80

AMA: 2018,Sep,7

26185 **Sesamoidectomy, thumb or finger (separate procedure)**

15.8 | 15.8 | FUD 090 | J A2 80 50

AMA: 2018,Sep,7

26200 **Excision or curettage of bone cyst or benign tumor of metacarpal;**

13.0 | 13.0 | FUD 090 | J A2 80

AMA: 2018,Sep,7

26205 **with autograft (includes obtaining graft)**

17.3 | 17.3 | FUD 090 | J A2

AMA: 2018,Sep,7

26210 **Excision or curettage of bone cyst or benign tumor of proximal, middle, or distal phalanx of finger;**

12.7 | 12.7 | FUD 090 | J A2

AMA: 2018,Sep,7

26215 **with autograft (includes obtaining graft)**

16.2 | 16.2 | FUD 090 | J A2

AMA: 2018,Sep,7

26230 **Partial excision (craterization, saucerization, or diaphysectomy) bone (eg, osteomyelitis); metacarpal**

14.4 | 14.4 | FUD 090 | J A2 80

AMA: 2018,Sep,7

26235 **proximal or middle phalanx of finger**

14.1 | 14.1 | FUD 090 | J A2 80

AMA: 2019,Jul,10; 2018,Sep,7

26236 **distal phalanx of finger**

12.6 | 12.6 | FUD 090 | J A2

AMA: 2019,Jul,10; 2018,Sep,7

26250-26262 Radical Resection Bone Tumor of Hand/Finger

INCLUDES Any necessary elevation tissue planes or dissection
Excision adjacent soft tissue during bone tumor resection (26111-26118 [26111, 26113])
Measurement tumor and necessary margin at greatest diameter prior to excision
Resection tumor (may include entire bone) and wide margins normal tissue primarily for malignant or aggressive benign tumors
Simple and intermediate repairs

EXCLUDES *Complex repair*
Significant vessel exploration, neuroplasty, reconstruction, or complex bone repair

26250 **Radical resection of tumor, metacarpal**

30.8 | 30.8 | FUD 090 | J A2 80

AMA: 2018,Sep,7

26260 **Radical resection of tumor, proximal or middle phalanx of finger**

23.0 | 23.0 | FUD 090 | J A2 80

AMA: 2018,Sep,7

26262 **Radical resection of tumor, distal phalanx of finger**

18.1 | 18.1 | FUD 090 | J A2 80

AMA: 2018,Sep,7

26320 Implant Removal Hand/Finger

26320 **Removal of implant from finger or hand**

EXCLUDES *Excision foreign body (20520, 20525)*

9.98 | 9.98 | FUD 090 | Q2 A2

AMA: 2018,Sep,7

26340-26548 Repair/Reconstruction of Fingers and Hand

26340 **Manipulation, finger joint, under anesthesia, each joint**

EXCLUDES *Application external fixation (20690, 20692)*

9.67 | 9.67 | FUD 090 | J G2 50

AMA: 2018,Sep,7; 2018,Jan,8; 2017,Jan,8; 2016,Jan,13; 2015,Jan,16

26341 **Manipulation, palmar fascial cord (ie, Dupuytren's cord), post enzyme injection (eg, collagenase), single cord**

EXCLUDES *Enzyme injection fasciotomy (20527)*

Code also custom orthotic fabrication and/or fitting

2.17 | 2.90 | FUD 010 | T P3 50

AMA: 2018,Sep,7; 2018,Jan,8; 2017,Jan,8; 2016,Jan,13; 2015,Jan,16

26350 **Repair or advancement, flexor tendon, not in zone 2 digital flexor tendon sheath (eg, no man's land); primary or secondary without free graft, each tendon**

20.8 | 20.8 | FUD 090 | J A2

AMA: 2018,Sep,7

26352 **secondary with free graft (includes obtaining graft), each tendon**

23.3 | 23.3 | FUD 090 | J A2 80

AMA: 2018,Sep,7

26356 **Repair or advancement, flexor tendon, in zone 2 digital flexor tendon sheath (eg, no man's land); primary, without free graft, each tendon**

22.8 | 22.8 | FUD 090 | J A2

AMA: 2018,Sep,7; 2018,Jan,8; 2017,Dec,14; 2017,Jan,8; 2016,Jan,13; 2015,Jan,16

26357 secondary, without free graft, each tendon
25.6 25.6 FUD 090 J A2 80
AMA: 2018,Sep,7

26358 secondary, with free graft (includes obtaining graft), each tendon
28.3 28.3 FUD 090 J A2 80
AMA: 2018,Sep,7

26370 Repair or advancement of profundus tendon, with intact superficialis tendon; primary, each tendon
21.9 21.9 FUD 090 J A2 80
AMA: 2018,Sep,7; 2018,Jan,8; 2017,Jan,8; 2016,Jan,13; 2015,Jan,16

26372 secondary with free graft (includes obtaining graft), each tendon
25.7 25.7 FUD 090 J A2 80
AMA: 2018,Sep,7

26373 secondary without free graft, each tendon
24.7 24.7 FUD 090 J A2 80
AMA: 2018,Sep,7

26390 Excision flexor tendon, with implantation of synthetic rod for delayed tendon graft, hand or finger, each rod
23.6 23.6 FUD 090 J J8 80
AMA: 2018,Sep,7

26392 Removal of synthetic rod and insertion of flexor tendon graft, hand or finger (includes obtaining graft), each rod
27.4 27.4 FUD 090 J A2 80
AMA: 2018,Sep,7

26410 Repair, extensor tendon, hand, primary or secondary; without free graft, each tendon
16.5 16.5 FUD 090 J A2
AMA: 2018,Sep,7

26412 with free graft (includes obtaining graft), each tendon
19.7 19.7 FUD 090 J A2 80
AMA: 2018,Sep,7

26415 Excision of extensor tendon, with implantation of synthetic rod for delayed tendon graft, hand or finger, each rod
23.7 23.7 FUD 090 J A2 80
AMA: 2018,Sep,7

26416 Removal of synthetic rod and insertion of extensor tendon graft (includes obtaining graft), hand or finger, each rod
25.7 25.7 FUD 090 J A2
AMA: 2018,Sep,7; 2018,Jan,8; 2017,Jan,8; 2016,Jan,13; 2015,Jan,16

26418 Repair, extensor tendon, finger, primary or secondary; without free graft, each tendon
16.2 16.2 FUD 090 J A2
AMA: 2018,Sep,7; 2018,Jan,8; 2017,Jan,8; 2016,Jan,13; 2015,Jan,16

26420 with free graft (includes obtaining graft) each tendon
20.6 20.6 FUD 090 J A2 80
AMA: 2018,Sep,7

26426 Repair of extensor tendon, central slip, secondary (eg, boutonniere deformity); using local tissue(s), including lateral band(s), each finger
14.4 14.4 FUD 090 J A2
AMA: 2018,Sep,7

26428 with free graft (includes obtaining graft), each finger
21.3 21.3 FUD 090 J A2 80
AMA: 2018,Sep,7

26432 Closed treatment of distal extensor tendon insertion, with or without percutaneous pinning (eg, mallet finger)
13.9 13.9 FUD 090 J A2
AMA: 2018,Sep,7

26433 Repair of extensor tendon, distal insertion, primary or secondary; without graft (eg, mallet finger)
EXCLUDES *Trigger finger (26055)*
15.6 15.6 FUD 090 J A2
AMA: 2018,Sep,7

26434 with free graft (includes obtaining graft)
EXCLUDES *Trigger finger (26055)*
18.2 18.2 FUD 090 J A2 80
AMA: 2018,Sep,7

26437 Realignment of extensor tendon, hand, each tendon
17.5 17.5 FUD 090 J A2
AMA: 2018,Sep,7

26440 Tenolysis, flexor tendon; palm OR finger, each tendon
18.0 18.0 FUD 090 J A2
AMA: 2018,Sep,7; 2018,Jan,8; 2017,Jan,8; 2016,Jan,13; 2015,Jun,10; 2015,Jan,16

26442 palm AND finger, each tendon
27.1 27.1 FUD 090 J A2
AMA: 2018,Sep,7

26445 Tenolysis, extensor tendon, hand OR finger, each tendon
16.8 16.8 FUD 090 J A2
AMA: 2018,Sep,7; 2018,Jan,8; 2017,Jan,8; 2016,Jan,13; 2015,Jan,16

26449 Tenolysis, complex, extensor tendon, finger, including forearm, each tendon
19.9 19.9 FUD 090 J A2 80
AMA: 2018,Sep,7

26450 Tenotomy, flexor, palm, open, each tendon
11.4 11.4 FUD 090 J A2 80
AMA: 2018,Sep,7

26455 Tenotomy, flexor, finger, open, each tendon
12.1 12.1 FUD 090 J A2 80
AMA: 2018,Sep,7

26460 Tenotomy, extensor, hand or finger, open, each tendon
11.8 11.8 FUD 090 J A2
AMA: 2018,Sep,7

26471 Tenodesis; of proximal interphalangeal joint, each joint
18.0 18.0 FUD 090 J A2 80
AMA: 2018,Sep,7

26474 of distal joint, each joint
17.7 17.7 FUD 090 J A2 80
AMA: 2018,Sep,7

26476 Lengthening of tendon, extensor, hand or finger, each tendon
17.5 17.5 FUD 090 J A2
AMA: 2018,Sep,7

26477 Shortening of tendon, extensor, hand or finger, each tendon
16.3 16.3 FUD 090 J A2
AMA: 2018,Sep,7

26478 Lengthening of tendon, flexor, hand or finger, each tendon
18.2 18.2 FUD 090 J A2 80
AMA: 2018,Sep,7; 2018,Jan,8; 2017,Jan,8; 2016,Jan,13; 2015,Jan,16

26479 Shortening of tendon, flexor, hand or finger, each tendon
17.6 17.6 FUD 090 J A2 80
AMA: 2018,Sep,7

26480 Transfer or transplant of tendon, carpometacarpal area or dorsum of hand; without free graft, each tendon
21.1 21.1 FUD 090 J A2 80
AMA: 2018,Sep,7; 2018,Jan,8; 2017,Jan,8; 2016,Jan,13; 2015,Jan,16

26483 **with free tendon graft (includes obtaining graft), each tendon**
24.4 24.4 FUD 090 J A2 80
AMA: 2018,Sep,7

26485 **Transfer or transplant of tendon, palmar; without free tendon graft, each tendon**
22.7 22.7 FUD 090 J A2 80
AMA: 2018,Sep,7

26489 **with free tendon graft (includes obtaining graft), each tendon**
27.1 27.1 FUD 090 J A2 80
AMA: 2018,Sep,7

26490 **Opponensplasty; superficialis tendon transfer type, each tendon**
EXCLUDES *Thumb fusion (26820)*
22.5 22.5 FUD 090 J A2 80
AMA: 2018,Sep,7

26492 **tendon transfer with graft (includes obtaining graft), each tendon**
EXCLUDES *Thumb fusion (26820)*
25.0 25.0 FUD 090 J A2 80
AMA: 2018,Sep,7

26494 **hypothenar muscle transfer**
EXCLUDES *Thumb fusion (26820)*
23.3 23.3 FUD 090 J A2 80
AMA: 2018,Sep,7

26496 **other methods**
EXCLUDES *Thumb fusion (26820)*
24.9 24.9 FUD 090 J A2 80
AMA: 2018,Sep,7

26497 **Transfer of tendon to restore intrinsic function; ring and small finger**
25.2 25.2 FUD 090 J A2 80
AMA: 2018,Sep,7

26498 **all 4 fingers**
33.2 33.2 FUD 090 J A2 80
AMA: 2018,Sep,7

26499 **Correction claw finger, other methods**
24.2 24.2 FUD 090 J A2 80
AMA: 2018,Sep,7

26500 **Reconstruction of tendon pulley, each tendon; with local tissues (separate procedure)**
18.2 18.2 FUD 090 J A2 80
AMA: 2018,Sep,7

26502 **with tendon or fascial graft (includes obtaining graft) (separate procedure)**
20.8 20.8 FUD 090 J A2 80
AMA: 2018,Sep,7

26508 **Release of thenar muscle(s) (eg, thumb contracture)**
18.6 18.6 FUD 090 J A2 80 50
AMA: 2018,Sep,7

26510 **Cross intrinsic transfer, each tendon**
17.6 17.6 FUD 090 J A2 80
AMA: 2018,Sep,7

26516 **Capsulodesis, metacarpophalangeal joint; single digit**
20.5 20.5 FUD 090 J A2 80 50
AMA: 2018,Sep,7

26517 **2 digits**
24.1 24.1 FUD 090 J A2 80 50
AMA: 2018,Sep,7

26518 **3 or 4 digits**
24.4 24.4 FUD 090 J A2 80 50
AMA: 2018,Sep,7

26520 **Capsulectomy or capsulotomy; metacarpophalangeal joint, each joint**
EXCLUDES *Carpometacarpal joint arthroplasty (25447)*
18.2 18.2 FUD 090 J A2
AMA: 2018,Sep,7

26525 **interphalangeal joint, each joint**
EXCLUDES *Carpometacarpal joint arthroplasty (25447)*
18.9 18.9 FUD 090 J A2
AMA: 2018,Sep,7; 2018,Jan,8; 2017,Jan,8; 2016,Jan,13; 2015,Jun,10; 2015,Jan,16

26530 **Arthroplasty, metacarpophalangeal joint; each joint**
EXCLUDES *Carpometacarpal joint arthroplasty (25447)*
15.4 15.4 FUD 090 J A2 80
AMA: 2018,Sep,7

26531 **with prosthetic implant, each joint**
EXCLUDES *Carpometacarpal joint arthroplasty (25447)*
18.0 18.0 FUD 090 J J8 80
AMA: 2018,Sep,7; 2018,Jan,8; 2017,Jan,8; 2016,Jan,13; 2015,Jan,16

26535 **Arthroplasty, interphalangeal joint; each joint**
EXCLUDES *Carpometacarpal joint arthroplasty (25447)*
12.3 12.3 FUD 090 J A2
AMA: 2018,Sep,7

26536 **with prosthetic implant, each joint**
EXCLUDES *Carpometacarpal joint arthroplasty (25447)*
20.8 20.8 FUD 090 J J8 80
AMA: 2018,Sep,7

26540 **Repair of collateral ligament, metacarpophalangeal or interphalangeal joint**
19.3 19.3 FUD 090 J A2 80
AMA: 2018,Sep,7

26541 **Reconstruction, collateral ligament, metacarpophalangeal joint, single; with tendon or fascial graft (includes obtaining graft)**
22.5 22.5 FUD 090 J A2 80
AMA: 2018,Sep,7; 2018,Jan,8; 2017,Jan,8; 2016,Jan,13; 2015,Jan,16

26542 **with local tissue (eg, adductor advancement)**
19.9 19.9 FUD 090 J A2 80
AMA: 2018,Sep,7; 2018,Jan,8; 2017,Jan,8; 2016,Jan,13; 2015,Jan,16

26545 **Reconstruction, collateral ligament, interphalangeal joint, single, including graft, each joint**
20.7 20.7 FUD 090 J A2 80
AMA: 2018,Sep,7

26546 **Repair non-union, metacarpal or phalanx (includes obtaining bone graft with or without external or internal fixation)**
28.9 28.9 FUD 090 J A2 80 50
AMA: 2018,Sep,7

26548 **Repair and reconstruction, finger, volar plate, interphalangeal joint**
22.2 22.2 FUD 090 J A2 80
AMA: 2018,Sep,7

26550-26556 Reconstruction Procedures with Finger and Toe Transplants

26550 **Pollicization of a digit**
46.8 46.8 FUD 090 J A2 80 50
AMA: 2018,Sep,7

26551 **Transfer, toe-to-hand with microvascular anastomosis; great toe wrap-around with bone graft**
INCLUDES Operating microscope (69990)
EXCLUDES *Big toe with web space (20973)*
95.1 95.1 FUD 090 C 80 50
AMA: 2018,Sep,7; 2018,Jan,8; 2017,Jan,8; 2016,Feb,12; 2016,Jan,13; 2015,Jan,16

26553 **other than great toe, single**
INCLUDES Operating microscope (69990)
94.5 94.5 FUD 090 C 80 50
AMA: 2018,Sep,7; 2018,Jan,8; 2017,Jan,8; 2016,Feb,12; 2016,Jan,13; 2015,Jan,16

26554 **other than great toe, double**
INCLUDES Operating microscope (69990)
109. 109. FUD 090 C 80 50
AMA: 2018,Sep,7; 2018,Jan,8; 2017,Jan,8; 2016,Feb,12; 2016,Jan,13; 2015,Jan,16

26555 **Transfer, finger to another position without microvascular anastomosis**
39.6 39.6 FUD 090 J A2 80
AMA: 2018,Sep,7

26556 **Transfer, free toe joint, with microvascular anastomosis**
INCLUDES Operating microscope (69990)
EXCLUDES *Big toe to hand transfer (20973)*
98.2 98.2 FUD 090 C 80
AMA: 2018,Sep,7; 2018,Jan,8; 2017,Jan,8; 2016,Feb,12; 2016,Jan,13; 2015,Jan,16

26560-26596 Repair of Other Deformities of the Fingers/Hand

26560 **Repair of syndactyly (web finger) each web space; with skin flaps**
16.5 16.5 FUD 090 J A2 80
AMA: 2018,Sep,7

26561 **with skin flaps and grafts**
27.5 27.5 FUD 090 J A2 80
AMA: 2018,Sep,7

26562 **complex (eg, involving bone, nails)**
38.8 38.8 FUD 090 J A2 80
AMA: 2018,Sep,7

26565 **Osteotomy; metacarpal, each**
19.0 19.0 FUD 090 J A2 80
AMA: 2018,Sep,7

26567 **phalanx of finger, each**
19.9 19.9 FUD 090 J A2 80
AMA: 2018,Sep,7; 2018,Jan,8; 2017,Jan,8; 2016,Jan,13; 2015,Jan,16

26568 **Osteoplasty, lengthening, metacarpal or phalanx**
26.1 26.1 FUD 090 J A2 80
AMA: 2018,Sep,7

26580 **Repair cleft hand**
INCLUDES Barsky's procedure
43.7 43.7 FUD 090 J A2 80 50
AMA: 2018,Sep,7

26587 **Reconstruction of polydactylous digit, soft tissue and bone**
EXCLUDES *Soft tissue removal only (11200)*
30.0 30.0 FUD 090 J A2 80
AMA: 2018,Sep,7; 2018,Jan,8; 2017,Jan,8; 2016,Jan,13; 2015,Jan,16

26590 **Repair macrodactylia, each digit**
40.7 40.7 FUD 090 J A2 80
AMA: 2018,Sep,7; 2018,Jan,8; 2017,Jan,8; 2016,Jan,13; 2015,Jan,16

26591 **Repair, intrinsic muscles of hand, each muscle**
13.0 13.0 FUD 090 J A2 80
AMA: 2018,Sep,7; 2018,Jan,8; 2017,Jan,8; 2016,Jan,13; 2015,Jan,16

26593 **Release, intrinsic muscles of hand, each muscle**
17.6 17.6 FUD 090 J A2
AMA: 2018,Sep,7

26596 **Excision of constricting ring of finger, with multiple Z-plasties**
EXCLUDES *Graft repair or scar contracture release (11042, 14040-14041, 15120, 15240)*
22.5 22.5 FUD 090 J A2 80
AMA: 2018,Sep,7

26600-26785 Treatment of Fracture/Dislocation of Fingers and Hand

INCLUDES Closed, percutaneous, and open treatment fractures or dislocations

26600 **Closed treatment of metacarpal fracture, single; without manipulation, each bone**
8.06 8.50 FUD 090 T P2
AMA: 2018,Sep,7

26605 **with manipulation, each bone**
8.45 9.33 FUD 090 T A2
AMA: 2018,Sep,7

26607 **Closed treatment of metacarpal fracture, with manipulation, with external fixation, each bone**
13.9 13.9 FUD 090 J A2 80
AMA: 2018,Sep,7

26608 **Percutaneous skeletal fixation of metacarpal fracture, each bone**
13.7 13.7 FUD 090 J A2 80
AMA: 2018,Sep,7

26615 **Open treatment of metacarpal fracture, single, includes internal fixation, when performed, each bone**
16.5 16.5 FUD 090 J A2
AMA: 2018,Sep,7

26641 **Closed treatment of carpometacarpal dislocation, thumb, with manipulation**
9.97 11.0 FUD 090 T P2 80 50
AMA: 2018,Sep,7

26645 **Closed treatment of carpometacarpal fracture dislocation, thumb (Bennett fracture), with manipulation**
11.3 12.3 FUD 090 J A2 80 50
AMA: 2018,Sep,7

26650 **Percutaneous skeletal fixation of carpometacarpal fracture dislocation, thumb (Bennett fracture), with manipulation**
13.7 13.7 FUD 090 J A2 50
AMA: 2018,Sep,7

26665 **Open treatment of carpometacarpal fracture dislocation, thumb (Bennett fracture), includes internal fixation, when performed**
18.0 18.0 FUD 090 J A2 50
AMA: 2018,Sep,7

26670 **Closed treatment of carpometacarpal dislocation, other than thumb, with manipulation, each joint; without anesthesia**
8.87 9.86 FUD 090 T P2 80
AMA: 2018,Sep,7

26675 **requiring anesthesia**
12.0 13.1 FUD 090 J A2 80
AMA: 2018,Sep,7

26676 **Percutaneous skeletal fixation of carpometacarpal dislocation, other than thumb, with manipulation, each joint**
14.5 14.5 FUD 090 J A2
AMA: 2018,Sep,7

26685 **Open treatment of carpometacarpal dislocation, other than thumb; includes internal fixation, when performed, each joint**
16.5 16.5 FUD 090 J A2
AMA: 2018,Sep,7

26686 **complex, multiple, or delayed reduction**
18.0 18.0 FUD 090 J A2 80
AMA: 2018,Sep,7

26700 **Closed treatment of metacarpophalangeal dislocation, single, with manipulation; without anesthesia**
8.73 9.38 **FUD** 090 T P2
AMA: 2018,Sep,7

26705 **requiring anesthesia**
10.9 11.9 **FUD** 090 J A2 80
AMA: 2018,Sep,7

26706 **Percutaneous skeletal fixation of metacarpophalangeal dislocation, single, with manipulation**
12.6 12.6 **FUD** 090 J A2
AMA: 2018,Sep,7

26715 **Open treatment of metacarpophalangeal dislocation, single, includes internal fixation, when performed**
16.4 16.4 **FUD** 090 J A2 80
AMA: 2018,Sep,7

26720 **Closed treatment of phalangeal shaft fracture, proximal or middle phalanx, finger or thumb; without manipulation, each**
5.26 5.62 **FUD** 090 T P2
AMA: 2018,Sep,7

26725 **with manipulation, with or without skin or skeletal traction, each**
8.73 9.75 **FUD** 090 T P2
AMA: 2018,Sep,7

26727 **Percutaneous skeletal fixation of unstable phalangeal shaft fracture, proximal or middle phalanx, finger or thumb, with manipulation, each**
13.5 13.5 **FUD** 090 J A2
AMA: 2018,Sep,7

26735 **Open treatment of phalangeal shaft fracture, proximal or middle phalanx, finger or thumb, includes internal fixation, when performed, each**
17.1 17.1 **FUD** 090 J A2
AMA: 2018,Sep,7

26740 **Closed treatment of articular fracture, involving metacarpophalangeal or interphalangeal joint; without manipulation, each**
6.25 6.60 **FUD** 090 T P2
AMA: 2018,Sep,7

26742 **with manipulation, each**
9.64 10.6 **FUD** 090 J A2
AMA: 2018,Sep,7

26746 **Open treatment of articular fracture, involving metacarpophalangeal or interphalangeal joint, includes internal fixation, when performed, each**
21.3 21.3 **FUD** 090 J A2
AMA: 2018,Sep,7

26750 **Closed treatment of distal phalangeal fracture, finger or thumb; without manipulation, each**
5.35 5.32 **FUD** 090 T P2
AMA: 2018,Sep,7

26755 **with manipulation, each**
7.77 8.99 **FUD** 090 T G2
AMA: 2018,Sep,7

26756 **Percutaneous skeletal fixation of distal phalangeal fracture, finger or thumb, each**
12.1 12.1 **FUD** 090 J A2 80
AMA: 2018,Sep,7

26765 **Open treatment of distal phalangeal fracture, finger or thumb, includes internal fixation, when performed, each**
14.3 14.3 **FUD** 090 J A2
AMA: 2018,Sep,7

26770 **Closed treatment of interphalangeal joint dislocation, single, with manipulation; without anesthesia**
7.41 8.08 **FUD** 090 T G2
AMA: 2018,Sep,7

26775 **requiring anesthesia**
9.96 11.0 **FUD** 090 T P2
AMA: 2018,Sep,7

26776 **Percutaneous skeletal fixation of interphalangeal joint dislocation, single, with manipulation**
12.8 12.8 **FUD** 090 J A2
AMA: 2018,Sep,7

26785 **Open treatment of interphalangeal joint dislocation, includes internal fixation, when performed, single**
15.7 15.7 **FUD** 090 J A2
AMA: 2018,Sep,7

26820-26863 Fusion of Joint(s) of Fingers or Hand

26820 **Fusion in opposition, thumb, with autogenous graft (includes obtaining graft)**
22.2 22.2 **FUD** 090 J J8 80 50
AMA: 2020,May,13; 2018,Sep,7

26841 **Arthrodesis, carpometacarpal joint, thumb, with or without internal fixation;**
21.2 21.2 **FUD** 090 J A2 80 50
AMA: 2020,May,13; 2018,Sep,7

26842 **with autograft (includes obtaining graft)**
22.8 22.8 **FUD** 090 J A2 80 50
AMA: 2020,May,13; 2018,Sep,7

26843 **Arthrodesis, carpometacarpal joint, digit, other than thumb, each;**
21.6 21.6 **FUD** 090 J A2 80
AMA: 2020,May,13; 2018,Sep,7; 2018,Jan,8; 2017,Jan,8; 2016,Jan,13; 2015,Jan,16

26844 **with autograft (includes obtaining graft)**
23.9 23.9 **FUD** 090 J A2 80
AMA: 2020,May,13; 2018,Sep,7

26850 **Arthrodesis, metacarpophalangeal joint, with or without internal fixation;**
20.2 20.2 **FUD** 090 J A2 80
AMA: 2020,May,13; 2018,Sep,7

26852 **with autograft (includes obtaining graft)**
23.2 23.2 **FUD** 090 J A2 80
AMA: 2020,May,13; 2018,Sep,7

26860 **Arthrodesis, interphalangeal joint, with or without internal fixation;**
15.9 15.9 **FUD** 090 J A2
AMA: 2020,May,13; 2018,Sep,7; 2018,Jan,8; 2017,Jan,8; 2016,Jan,13; 2015,Jan,16

\+ **26861** **each additional interphalangeal joint (List separately in addition to code for primary procedure)**
Code first (26860)
2.98 2.98 **FUD** ZZZ N N1
AMA: 2020,May,13; 2018,Sep,7; 2018,Jan,8; 2017,Jan,8; 2016,Jan,13; 2015,Jan,16

26862 **with autograft (includes obtaining graft)**
21.1 21.1 **FUD** 090 J A2 80
AMA: 2020,May,13; 2018,Sep,7

\+ **26863** **with autograft (includes obtaining graft), each additional joint (List separately in addition to code for primary procedure)**
Code first (26862)
6.62 6.62 **FUD** ZZZ N N1 80
AMA: 2020,May,13; 2018,Sep,7

26910-26989 Amputations and Unlisted Procedures Finger/Hand

26910 **Amputation, metacarpal, with finger or thumb (ray amputation), single, with or without interosseous transfer**
EXCLUDES *Repositioning (26550, 26555)*
Transmetacarpal amputation hand (25927)
20.4 20.4 **FUD** 090 J A2
AMA: 2018,Sep,7

26951 **Amputation, finger or thumb, primary or secondary, any joint or phalanx, single, including neurectomies; with direct closure**

EXCLUDES *Repair necessitating flaps or grafts (15050-15758)*
Transmetacarpal amputation hand (25927)

19.1 19.1 FUD 090 J A2

AMA: 2018,Sep,7

26952 **with local advancement flaps (V-Y, hood)**

EXCLUDES *Repair necessitating flaps or grafts (15050-15758)*
Transmetacarpal amputation hand (25927)

18.9 18.9 FUD 090 J A2

AMA: 2018,Sep,7

26989 **Unlisted procedure, hands or fingers**

0.00 0.00 FUD YYY T

AMA: 2018,Sep,7

26990-26992 Incision for Drainage of Pelvis or Hip

EXCLUDES *Simple incision and drainage procedures (10040-10160)*

26990 **Incision and drainage, pelvis or hip joint area; deep abscess or hematoma**

18.8 18.8 FUD 090 J A2

AMA: 2018,Sep,7

26991 **infected bursa**

15.1 20.4 FUD 090 J A2 80

AMA: 2018,Sep,7

26992 **Incision, bone cortex, pelvis and/or hip joint (eg, osteomyelitis or bone abscess)**

28.5 28.5 FUD 090 C 80

AMA: 2018,Sep,7; 2018,Jan,8; 2017,Jan,8; 2016,Jan,13; 2015,Jan,16

27000-27006 Tenotomy Procedures of Hip

27000 **Tenotomy, adductor of hip, percutaneous (separate procedure)**

11.6 11.6 FUD 090 J A2 50

AMA: 2018,Sep,7

27001 **Tenotomy, adductor of hip, open**

15.6 15.6 FUD 090 J A2 80 50

AMA: 2018,Sep,7

27003 **Tenotomy, adductor, subcutaneous, open, with obturator neurectomy**

17.1 17.1 FUD 090 J A2 80 50

AMA: 2018,Sep,7

27005 **Tenotomy, hip flexor(s), open (separate procedure)**

20.8 20.8 FUD 090 C 80 50

AMA: 2018,Sep,7

27006 **Tenotomy, abductors and/or extensor(s) of hip, open (separate procedure)**

20.7 20.7 FUD 090 J 80 50

AMA: 2018,Sep,7

27025-27036 Surgical Incision of Hip

27025 **Fasciotomy, hip or thigh, any type**

26.5 26.5 FUD 090 C 80 50

AMA: 2018,Sep,7

27027 **Decompression fasciotomy(ies), pelvic (buttock) compartment(s) (eg, gluteus medius-minimus, gluteus maximus, iliopsoas, and/or tensor fascia lata muscle), unilateral**

25.8 25.8 FUD 090 J 80 50

AMA: 2018,Sep,7

27030 **Arthrotomy, hip, with drainage (eg, infection)**

27.1 27.1 FUD 090 C 80 50

AMA: 2018,Sep,7

27033 **Arthrotomy, hip, including exploration or removal of loose or foreign body**

28.1 28.1 FUD 090 J A2 80 50

AMA: 2018,Sep,7; 2018,Jan,8; 2017,Jan,8; 2016,Jan,13; 2015,Jan,16

27035 **Denervation, hip joint, intrapelvic or extrapelvic intra-articular branches of sciatic, femoral, or obturator nerves**

EXCLUDES *Transection obturator nerve (64763, 64766)*

32.8 32.8 FUD 090 J A2 80 50

AMA: 2018,Sep,7; 2018,Jan,8; 2017,Jan,8; 2016,Jan,13; 2015,Jan,16

27036 **Capsulectomy or capsulotomy, hip, with or without excision of heterotopic bone, with release of hip flexor muscles (ie, gluteus medius, gluteus minimus, tensor fascia latae, rectus femoris, sartorius, iliopsoas)**

29.1 29.1 FUD 090 C 80 50

AMA: 2018,Sep,7

27040-27041 Biopsy of Hip/Pelvis

EXCLUDES *Soft tissue needle biopsy (20206)*

27040 **Biopsy, soft tissue of pelvis and hip area; superficial**

5.70 9.83 FUD 010 J A2 50

AMA: 2018,Sep,7

27041 **deep, subfascial or intramuscular**

20.1 20.1 FUD 090 J A2 50

AMA: 2018,Sep,7

27043-27059 [27043, 27045, 27059] Excision Soft Tissue Tumors Hip/ Pelvis

INCLUDES Any necessary elevation tissue planes or dissection
Measurement tumor and necessary margin at greatest diameter prior to excision
Simple and intermediate repairs
Excision types:
Fascial or subfascial soft tissue tumors: simple and marginal resection tumors found either in or below deep fascia, not involving bone or excision substantial amount normal tissue; primarily benign and intramuscular tumors
Radical resection soft tissue tumor: wide resection tumor involving substantial margins normal tissue and may involve tissue removal from one or more layers; mostly malignant or aggressive benign,
Subcutaneous: simple and marginal resection tumors found in subcutaneous tissue above deep fascia; most often benign

EXCLUDES *Complex repair*
Excision benign cutaneous lesions (eg, sebaceous cyst) (11400-11406)
Radical resection cutaneous tumors (eg, melanoma) (11600-11606)
Significant vessel exploration, neuroplasty, reconstruction, or complex bone repair

27043 **Resequenced code. See code following 27047.**

27045 **Resequenced code. See code following 27048.**

27047 **Excision, tumor, soft tissue of pelvis and hip area, subcutaneous; less than 3 cm**

10.4 13.6 FUD 090 J G2 50

AMA: 2018,Sep,7

\# **27043** **3 cm or greater**

13.5 13.5 FUD 090 J G2 50

AMA: 2018,Sep,7

27048 **Excision, tumor, soft tissue of pelvis and hip area, subfascial (eg, intramuscular); less than 5 cm**

17.6 17.6 FUD 090 J G2 80 50

AMA: 2018,Sep,7

\# **27045** **5 cm or greater**

21.3 21.3 FUD 090 J G2 80 50

AMA: 2018,Sep,7

27049 **Radical resection of tumor (eg, sarcoma), soft tissue of pelvis and hip area; less than 5 cm**

38.6 38.6 FUD 090 J G2 80 50

AMA: 2018,Sep,7

\# **27059** **5 cm or greater**
52.6 52.6 **FUD** 090 J G2 80 50
AMA: 2018,Sep,7

27050-27071 [27059] Procedures of Bones and Joints of Hip and Pelvis

27050 **Arthrotomy, with biopsy; sacroiliac joint**
11.5 11.5 **FUD** 090 J A2 80 50
AMA: 2018,Sep,7

27052 **hip joint**
16.6 16.6 **FUD** 090 J A2 80 50
AMA: 2018,Sep,7

27054 **Arthrotomy with synovectomy, hip joint**
19.8 19.8 **FUD** 090 C 80 50
AMA: 2018,Sep,7

27057 **Decompression fasciotomy(ies), pelvic (buttock) compartment(s) (eg, gluteus medius-minimus, gluteus maximus, iliopsoas, and/or tensor fascia lata muscle) with debridement of nonviable muscle, unilateral**
29.2 29.2 **FUD** 090 J 80 50
AMA: 2018,Sep,7

27059 **Resequenced code. See code following 27049.**

27060 **Excision; ischial bursa**
13.4 13.4 **FUD** 090 J A2 50
AMA: 2018,Sep,7

27062 **trochanteric bursa or calcification**
EXCLUDES *Arthrocentesis (20610)*
13.1 13.1 **FUD** 090 J A2 50
AMA: 2018,Sep,7

27065 **Excision of bone cyst or benign tumor, wing of ilium, symphysis pubis, or greater trochanter of femur; superficial, includes autograft, when performed**
15.0 15.0 **FUD** 090 J A2 80 50
AMA: 2018,Sep,7

27066 **deep (subfascial), includes autograft, when performed**
23.1 23.1 **FUD** 090 J A2 80 50
AMA: 2018,Sep,7

27067 **with autograft requiring separate incision**
29.8 29.8 **FUD** 090 J A2 80 50
AMA: 2018,Sep,7

27070 **Partial excision, wing of ilium, symphysis pubis, or greater trochanter of femur, (craterization, saucerization) (eg, osteomyelitis or bone abscess); superficial**
25.3 25.3 **FUD** 090 C 80 50
AMA: 2018,Sep,7

27071 **deep (subfascial or intramuscular)**
27.2 27.2 **FUD** 090 C 80 50
AMA: 2018,Sep,7

27075-27078 Radical Resection Bone Tumor of Hip/Pelvis

INCLUDES Any necessary elevation tissue planes or dissection
Excision adjacent soft tissue during bone tumor resection (27043-27049 [27043, 27045, 27059])
Measurement tumor and necessary margin at greatest diameter prior to excision
Resection tumor (may include entire bone) and wide margins normal tissue primarily for malignant or aggressive benign tumors
Simple and intermediate repairs

EXCLUDES *Complex repair*
Significant vessel exploration, neuroplasty, reconstruction, or complex bone repair

27075 **Radical resection of tumor; wing of ilium, 1 pubic or ischial ramus or symphysis pubis**
60.5 60.5 **FUD** 090 C 80
AMA: 2019,May,7; 2018,Sep,7

27076 **ilium, including acetabulum, both pubic rami, or ischium and acetabulum**
73.5 73.5 **FUD** 090 C 80
AMA: 2019,May,7; 2018,Sep,7

27077 **innominate bone, total**
81.8 81.8 **FUD** 090 C 80
AMA: 2019,May,7; 2018,Sep,7

27078 **ischial tuberosity and greater trochanter of femur**
59.6 59.6 **FUD** 090 C 80 50
AMA: 2019,May,7; 2018,Sep,7

27080 Excision of Coccyx

EXCLUDES *Surgical excision decubitus ulcers (15920, 15922, 15931-15958)*

27080 **Coccygectomy, primary**
14.7 14.7 **FUD** 090 J A2 80
AMA: 2018,Sep,7

27086-27091 Removal Foreign Body or Hip Prosthesis

27086 **Removal of foreign body, pelvis or hip; subcutaneous tissue**
4.82 8.78 **FUD** 010 J A2 80 50
AMA: 2018,Sep,7; 2018,Jan,8; 2017,Jan,8; 2016,Jan,13; 2015,Jan,16

27087 **deep (subfascial or intramuscular)**
17.7 17.7 **FUD** 090 J A2 80 50
AMA: 2018,Sep,7

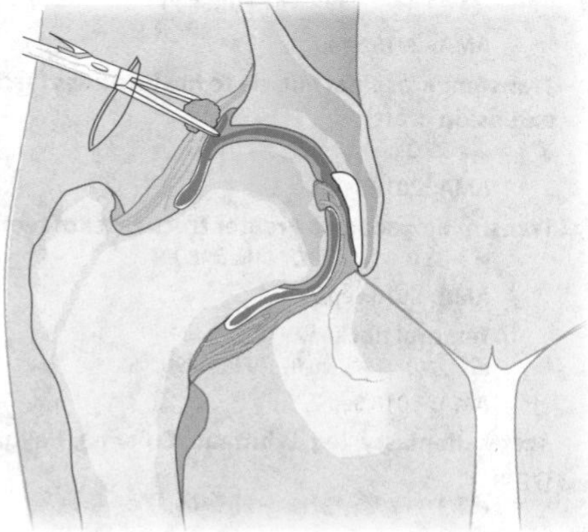

A foreign body is removed from the pelvis or hip

27090 **Removal of hip prosthesis; (separate procedure)**
24.0 24.0 **FUD** 090 C 80 50
AMA: 2019,May,7; 2018,Sep,7

27091 **complicated, including total hip prosthesis, methylmethacrylate with or without insertion of spacer**
46.0 46.0 **FUD** 090 C 80 50
AMA: 2019,May,7; 2018,Sep,7; 2018,Jan,8; 2017,Jan,8; 2016,Jan,13; 2015,Jan,16

27093-27096 Injection for Arthrogram Hip/Sacroiliac Joint

27093 **Injection procedure for hip arthrography; without anesthesia**
(73525)
2.01 5.72 **FUD** 000 N N1 50
AMA: 2018,Sep,7; 2018,Jan,8; 2017,Jan,8; 2016,Jan,13; 2015,Aug,6; 2015,Jan,16

27095 **with anesthesia**
(73525)
2.43 8.36 **FUD** 000 N N1 50
AMA: 2018,Sep,7; 2018,Jan,8; 2017,Jan,8; 2016,Jan,13; 2016,Jan,11; 2015,Aug,6; 2015,Jan,16

27096 **Injection procedure for sacroiliac joint, anesthetic/steroid, with image guidance (fluoroscopy or CT) including arthrography when performed**

INCLUDES Confirmation intra-articular needle placement with CT or fluoroscopy
Fluoroscopic guidance (77002-77003)

EXCLUDES *Procedure performed without fluoroscopy or CT guidance (20552)*

2.39 4.61 **FUD** 000 B 50

AMA: 2018,Sep,7; 2018,Jan,8; 2017,Jan,8; 2016,Jan,13; 2015,Aug,6; 2015,Jan,16

27097-27187 Revision/Reconstruction Hip and Pelvis

INCLUDES Closed, open and percutaneous treatment fractures and dislocations

27097 **Release or recession, hamstring, proximal**

19.7 19.7 **FUD** 090 J A2 80 50

AMA: 2018,Sep,7

27098 **Transfer, adductor to ischium**

20.0 20.0 **FUD** 090 J A2 80 50

AMA: 2018,Sep,7

27100 **Transfer external oblique muscle to greater trochanter including fascial or tendon extension (graft)**

INCLUDES Eggers procedure

23.6 23.6 **FUD** 090 J A2 80 50

AMA: 2018,Sep,7

27105 **Transfer paraspinal muscle to hip (includes fascial or tendon extension graft)**

25.0 25.0 **FUD** 090 J A2 80 50

AMA: 2018,Sep,7

27110 **Transfer iliopsoas; to greater trochanter of femur**

28.0 28.0 **FUD** 090 J A2 80 50

AMA: 2018,Sep,7

27111 **to femoral neck**

26.0 26.0 **FUD** 090 J A2 80 50

AMA: 2018,Sep,7

27120 **Acetabuloplasty; (eg, Whitman, Colonna, Haygroves, or cup type)**

37.5 37.5 **FUD** 090 C 80 50

AMA: 2018,Sep,7

27122 **resection, femoral head (eg, Girdlestone procedure)**

31.7 31.7 **FUD** 090 C 80 50

AMA: 2018,Sep,7

27125 **Hemiarthroplasty, hip, partial (eg, femoral stem prosthesis, bipolar arthroplasty)**

EXCLUDES *Hip replacement following hip fracture (27236)*

32.7 32.7 **FUD** 090 C 80 50

AMA: 2018,Sep,7; 2018,Jan,8; 2017,Jan,8; 2016,Jan,13; 2015,Jan,16

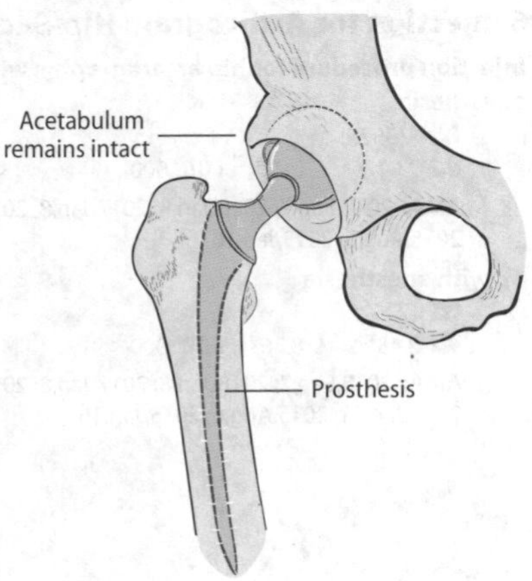

27130 **Arthroplasty, acetabular and proximal femoral prosthetic replacement (total hip arthroplasty), with or without autograft or allograft**

39.2 39.2 **FUD** 090 C 80 50

AMA: 2019,May,7; 2018,Sep,7; 2018,Jan,8; 2017,Jan,8; 2016,Jan,13; 2015,Jan,16

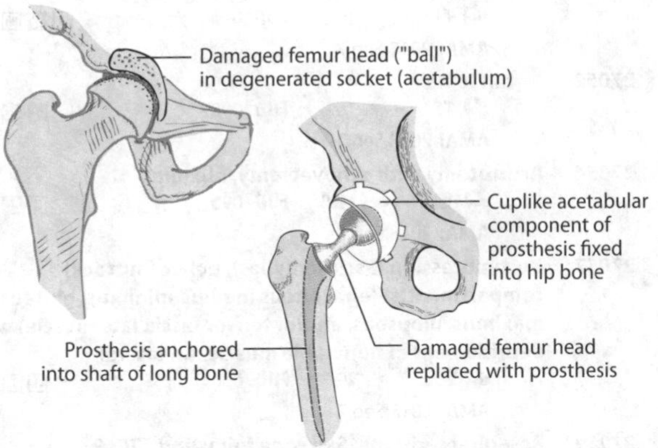

27132 **Conversion of previous hip surgery to total hip arthroplasty, with or without autograft or allograft**

48.3 48.3 **FUD** 090 C 80 50

AMA: 2019,May,7; 2018,Sep,7; 2018,Jan,8; 2017,Sep,14; 2017,Jan,8; 2016,Jan,13; 2015,Jan,16

27134 **Revision of total hip arthroplasty; both components, with or without autograft or allograft**

55.3 55.3 **FUD** 090 C 80 50

AMA: 2019,May,7; 2018,Sep,7; 2018,Jan,8; 2017,Jan,8; 2016,Jan,13; 2015,Jan,16

27137 **acetabular component only, with or without autograft or allograft**

42.5 42.5 **FUD** 090 C 80 50

AMA: 2018,Sep,7; 2018,Jan,8; 2017,Jan,8; 2016,Jan,13; 2015,Jan,16

27138 **femoral component only, with or without allograft**

44.1 44.1 **FUD** 090 C 80 50

AMA: 2019,May,7; 2018,Sep,7; 2018,Jan,8; 2017,Jan,8; 2016,Jan,13; 2015,Jan,16

27140 **Osteotomy and transfer of greater trochanter of femur (separate procedure)**

25.8 25.8 **FUD** 090 C 80 50

AMA: 2018,Sep,7

27146 **Osteotomy, iliac, acetabular or innominate bone;**

INCLUDES Salter osteotomy

36.9 36.9 **FUD** 090 C 80 50

AMA: 2018,Sep,7; 2018,Jan,8; 2017,Jan,8; 2016,Jan,13; 2015,Jan,16

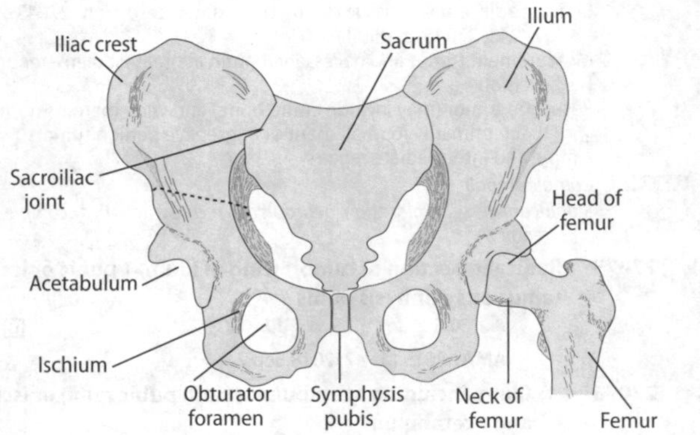

27147 **with open reduction of hip**
INCLUDES Pemberton osteotomy
42.4 42.4 **FUD** 090 C 80 50
AMA: 2018,Sep,7

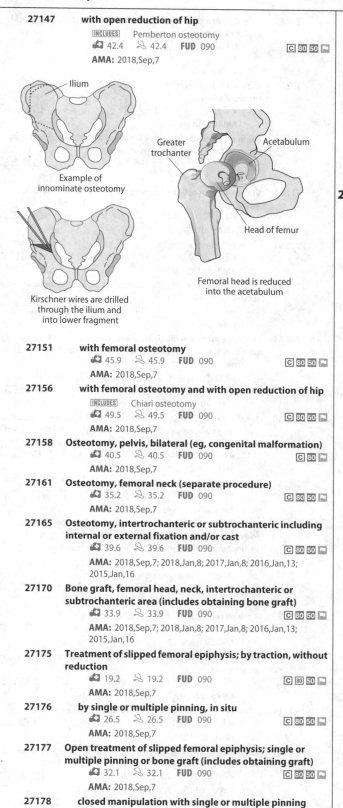

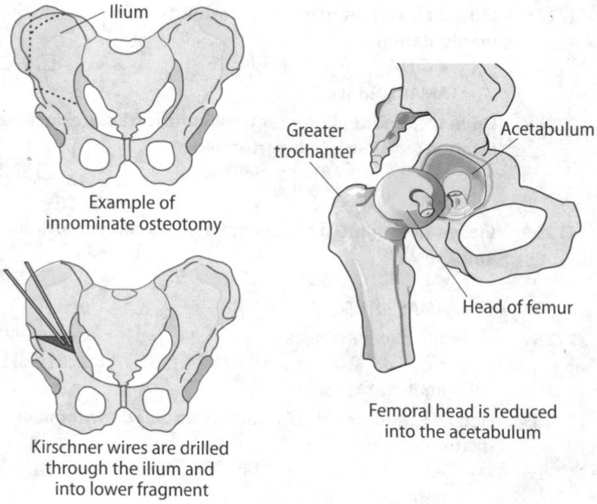

27151 **with femoral osteotomy**
45.9 45.9 **FUD** 090 C 80 50
AMA: 2018,Sep,7

27156 **with femoral osteotomy and with open reduction of hip**
INCLUDES Chiari osteotomy
49.5 49.5 **FUD** 090 C 80 50
AMA: 2018,Sep,7

27158 **Osteotomy, pelvis, bilateral (eg, congenital malformation)**
40.5 40.5 **FUD** 090 C 80
AMA: 2018,Sep,7

27161 **Osteotomy, femoral neck (separate procedure)**
35.2 35.2 **FUD** 090 C 80 50
AMA: 2018,Sep,7

27165 **Osteotomy, intertrochanteric or subtrochanteric including internal or external fixation and/or cast**
39.6 39.6 **FUD** 090 C 80 50
AMA: 2018,Sep,7; 2018,Jan,8; 2017,Jan,8; 2016,Jan,13; 2015,Jan,16

27170 **Bone graft, femoral head, neck, intertrochanteric or subtrochanteric area (includes obtaining bone graft)**
33.9 33.9 **FUD** 090 C 80 50
AMA: 2018,Sep,7; 2018,Jan,8; 2017,Jan,8; 2016,Jan,13; 2015,Jan,16

27175 **Treatment of slipped femoral epiphysis; by traction, without reduction**
19.2 19.2 **FUD** 090 C 80 50
AMA: 2018,Sep,7

27176 **by single or multiple pinning, in situ**
26.5 26.5 **FUD** 090 C 80 50
AMA: 2018,Sep,7

27177 **Open treatment of slipped femoral epiphysis; single or multiple pinning or bone graft (includes obtaining graft)**
32.1 32.1 **FUD** 090 C 80 50
AMA: 2018,Sep,7

27178 **closed manipulation with single or multiple pinning**
26.5 26.5 **FUD** 090 C 80 50
AMA: 2018,Sep,7

27179 **osteoplasty of femoral neck (Heyman type procedure)**
28.2 28.2 **FUD** 090 J 80 50
AMA: 2018,Sep,7

27181 **osteotomy and internal fixation**
32.3 32.3 **FUD** 090 C 80 50
AMA: 2018,Sep,7

27185 **Epiphyseal arrest by epiphysiodesis or stapling, greater trochanter of femur**
20.7 20.7 **FUD** 090 C 50
AMA: 2018,Sep,7

27187 **Prophylactic treatment (nailing, pinning, plating or wiring) with or without methylmethacrylate, femoral neck and proximal femur**
28.7 28.7 **FUD** 090 C 80 50
AMA: 2018,Sep,7; 2018,Jan,8; 2017,Jan,8; 2016,Jan,13; 2015,Jan,16

27197-27269 Treatment of Fracture/Dislocation Hip/Pelvis

27197 **Closed treatment of posterior pelvic ring fracture(s), dislocation(s), diastasis or subluxation of the ilium, sacroiliac joint, and/or sacrum, with or without anterior pelvic ring fracture(s) and/or dislocation(s) of the pubic symphysis and/or superior/inferior rami, unilateral or bilateral; without manipulation**
3.68 3.68 **FUD** 000 T G2
AMA: 2018,Sep,7; 2018,Jan,8; 2017,Jun,9

27198 **with manipulation, requiring more than local anesthesia (ie, general anesthesia, moderate sedation, spinal/epidural)**
EXCLUDES *Closed treatment anterior pelvic ring, pubic symphysis, inferior rami fracture/dislocation--see appropriate E/M codes*
8.84 8.84 **FUD** 000 T G2 80
AMA: 2018,Sep,7; 2018,Jan,3; 2018,Jan,8; 2017,Jun,9

27200 **Closed treatment of coccygeal fracture**
5.40 5.32 **FUD** 090 T P2
AMA: 2018,Sep,7

27202 **Open treatment of coccygeal fracture**
15.2 15.2 **FUD** 090 J A2 80
AMA: 2018,Sep,7

27215 **Open treatment of iliac spine(s), tuberosity avulsion, or iliac wing fracture(s), unilateral, for pelvic bone fracture patterns that do not disrupt the pelvic ring, includes internal fixation, when performed**
17.4 17.4 **FUD** 090 E
AMA: 2018,Sep,7

27216 **Percutaneous skeletal fixation of posterior pelvic bone fracture and/or dislocation, for fracture patterns that disrupt the pelvic ring, unilateral (includes ipsilateral ilium, sacroiliac joint and/or sacrum)**
EXCLUDES *Sacroiliac joint arthrodesis without fracture and/or dislocation, percutaneous or minimally invasive (27279)*
26.7 26.7 **FUD** 090 E
AMA: 2018,Sep,7; 2018,Jan,8; 2017,Jan,8; 2016,Jan,13; 2015,Jan,16

27217 **Open treatment of anterior pelvic bone fracture and/or dislocation for fracture patterns that disrupt the pelvic ring, unilateral, includes internal fixation, when performed (includes pubic symphysis and/or ipsilateral superior/inferior rami)**
25.0 25.0 **FUD** 090 E
AMA: 2018,Sep,7

27218 **Open treatment of posterior pelvic bone fracture and/or dislocation, for fracture patterns that disrupt the pelvic ring, unilateral, includes internal fixation, when performed (includes ipsilateral ilium, sacroiliac joint and/or sacrum)**

EXCLUDES *Sacroiliac joint arthrodesis without fracture and/or dislocation, percutaneous or minimally invasive (27279)*

34.6 34.6 FUD 090 E

AMA: 2018,Sep,7; 2018,Jan,8; 2017,Jan,8; 2016,Jan,13; 2015,Jan,16

27220 **Closed treatment of acetabulum (hip socket) fracture(s); without manipulation**

12.2 12.4 FUD 090 T G2 50

AMA: 2018,Sep,7

27222 **with manipulation, with or without skeletal traction**

28.1 28.1 FUD 090 C 50

AMA: 2018,Sep,7

27226 **Open treatment of posterior or anterior acetabular wall fracture, with internal fixation**

30.4 30.4 FUD 090 C 80 50

AMA: 2018,Sep,7

27227 **Open treatment of acetabular fracture(s) involving anterior or posterior (one) column, or a fracture running transversely across the acetabulum, with internal fixation**

47.9 47.9 FUD 090 C 80 50

AMA: 2018,Sep,7

27228 **Open treatment of acetabular fracture(s) involving anterior and posterior (two) columns, includes T-fracture and both column fracture with complete articular detachment, or single column or transverse fracture with associated acetabular wall fracture, with internal fixation**

54.3 54.3 FUD 090 C 80 50

AMA: 2018,Sep,7

27230 **Closed treatment of femoral fracture, proximal end, neck; without manipulation**

13.6 13.8 FUD 090 T A2 50

AMA: 2018,Sep,7

27232 **with manipulation, with or without skeletal traction**

21.6 21.6 FUD 090 C 50

AMA: 2018,Sep,7

27235 **Percutaneous skeletal fixation of femoral fracture, proximal end, neck**

26.2 26.2 FUD 090 J 50

AMA: 2018,Sep,7; 2018,Jan,8; 2017,Jan,8; 2016,Jan,13; 2015,Jan,16

27236 **Open treatment of femoral fracture, proximal end, neck, internal fixation or prosthetic replacement**

34.4 34.4 FUD 090 C 80 50

AMA: 2019,May,7; 2018,Sep,7; 2018,Jan,8; 2017,Jan,8; 2016,Nov,9; 2016,Jan,13; 2015,Jan,16

27238 **Closed treatment of intertrochanteric, peritrochanteric, or subtrochanteric femoral fracture; without manipulation**

13.3 13.3 FUD 090 J A2 50

AMA: 2018,Sep,7; 2018,Jan,8; 2017,Jan,8; 2016,Jan,13; 2015,Jan,16

27240 **with manipulation, with or without skin or skeletal traction**

27.5 27.5 FUD 090 C 50

AMA: 2018,Sep,7; 2018,Jan,8; 2017,Jan,8; 2016,Jan,13; 2015,Jan,16

27244 **Treatment of intertrochanteric, peritrochanteric, or subtrochanteric femoral fracture; with plate/screw type implant, with or without cerclage**

35.5 35.5 FUD 090 C 80 50

AMA: 2019,May,7; 2018,Sep,7; 2018,Jan,8; 2017,Jan,8; 2016,Jan,13; 2015,Jan,16

27245 **with intramedullary implant, with or without interlocking screws and/or cerclage**

35.5 35.5 FUD 090 C 80 50

AMA: 2018,Sep,7; 2018,Jan,8; 2017,Jan,8; 2016,Jan,13; 2015,Jan,16

27246 **Closed treatment of greater trochanteric fracture, without manipulation**

11.1 11.1 FUD 090 T A2 50

AMA: 2018,Sep,7

27248 **Open treatment of greater trochanteric fracture, includes internal fixation, when performed**

21.5 21.5 FUD 090 C 80 50

AMA: 2018,Sep,7

27250 **Closed treatment of hip dislocation, traumatic; without anesthesia**

5.33 5.33 FUD 000 T A2 50

AMA: 2018,Sep,7

27252 **requiring anesthesia**

21.8 21.8 FUD 090 J A2 50

AMA: 2018,Sep,7

27253 **Open treatment of hip dislocation, traumatic, without internal fixation**

27.2 27.2 FUD 090 C 80 50

AMA: 2018,Sep,7

27254 **Open treatment of hip dislocation, traumatic, with acetabular wall and femoral head fracture, with or without internal or external fixation**

EXCLUDES *Acetabular fracture treatment (27226-27227)*

36.4 36.4 FUD 090 C 80 50

AMA: 2018,Sep,7

27256 **Treatment of spontaneous hip dislocation (developmental, including congenital or pathological), by abduction, splint or traction; without anesthesia, without manipulation**

6.78 8.73 FUD 010 T G2 80 50

AMA: 2018,Sep,7

27257 **with manipulation, requiring anesthesia**

10.4 10.4 FUD 010 J A2 80 50

AMA: 2018,Sep,7

27258 **Open treatment of spontaneous hip dislocation (developmental, including congenital or pathological), replacement of femoral head in acetabulum (including tenotomy, etc);**

INCLUDES Lorenz's operation

32.1 32.1 FUD 090 C 80 50

AMA: 2018,Sep,7

27259 **with femoral shaft shortening**

44.7 44.7 FUD 090 C 80 50

AMA: 2018,Sep,7

27265 **Closed treatment of post hip arthroplasty dislocation; without anesthesia**

11.6 11.6 FUD 090 T A2 50

AMA: 2018,Sep,7

27266 **requiring regional or general anesthesia**

16.8 16.8 FUD 090 J A2 50

AMA: 2018,Sep,7

27267 **Closed treatment of femoral fracture, proximal end, head; without manipulation**

12.5 12.5 FUD 090 J G2 80 50

AMA: 2018,Sep,7; 2018,Jan,8; 2017,Jan,8; 2016,Jan,13; 2015,Jan,16

27268 **with manipulation**

15.6 15.6 FUD 090 C 80 50

AMA: 2018,Sep,7; 2018,Jan,8; 2017,Jan,8; 2016,Jan,13; 2015,Jan,16

26/TC PC/TC Only A2-Z3 ASC Payment 50 Bilateral ♂ Male Only ♀ Female Only Facility RVU Non-Facility RVU CCI CLIA
FUD Follow-up Days CMS: IOM AMA: CPT Asst A-Y OPPSI 80/80 Surg Assist Allowed / w/Doc Lab Crosswalk Radiology Crosswalk

86

27269 **Open treatment of femoral fracture, proximal end, head, includes internal fixation, when performed**

EXCLUDES *Arthrotomy, hip (27033)*
Open treatment hip dislocation, traumatic, without internal fixation (27253)

35.9 35.9 FUD 090 C 80 50

AMA: 2018,Sep,7; 2018,Jan,8; 2017,Jan,8; 2016,Jan,13; 2015,Jan,16

27275 Hip Manipulation with Anesthesia

27275 **Manipulation, hip joint, requiring general anesthesia**

5.26 5.26 FUD 010 J A2

AMA: 2018,Sep,7; 2018,Jan,8; 2017,Jan,8; 2016,May,13; 2016,Jan,11; 2016,Jan,13; 2015,Jan,16

27279-27286 Arthrodesis of Hip and Pelvis

27279 **Arthrodesis, sacroiliac joint, percutaneous or minimally invasive (indirect visualization), with image guidance, includes obtaining bone graft when performed, and placement of transfixing device**

25.3 25.3 FUD 090 J J8 80 50

AMA: 2020,May,13; 2018,Sep,7

27280 **Arthrodesis, open, sacroiliac joint, including obtaining bone graft, including instrumentation, when performed**

EXCLUDES *Sacroiliac joint arthrodesis without fracture and/or dislocation, percutaneous or minimally invasive (27279)*

39.2 39.2 FUD 090 C 80 50

AMA: 2020,May,13; 2018,Sep,7; 2018,Jan,8; 2017,Jan,8; 2016,Jan,13; 2015,Jan,16

27282 **Artnrodesis, symphysis pubis (including obtaining graft)**

24.7 24.7 FUD 090 C 80

AMA: 2020,May,13; 2018,Sep,7

27284 **Arthrodesis, hip joint (including obtaining graft);**

46.6 46.6 FUD 090 C 80 50

AMA: 2020,May,13; 2018,Sep,7

27286 **with subtrochanteric osteotomy**

47.6 47.6 FUD 090 C 80 50

AMA: 2020,May,13; 2018,Sep,7; 2018,Jan,8; 2017,Jan,8; 2016,Jan,13; 2015,Jan,16

27290-27299 Amputations and Unlisted Procedures of Hip and Pelvis

27290 **Interpelviabdominal amputation (hindquarter amputation)**

46.9 46.9 FUD 090 C 80

AMA: 2018,Sep,7; 2018,Jan,8; 2017,Jan,8; 2016,Jan,13; 2015,Jan,16

27295 **Disarticulation of hip**

36.4 36.4 FUD 090 C 80 50

AMA: 2018,Sep,7; 2018,Jan,8; 2017,Jan,8; 2016,Jan,13; 2015,Jan,16

27299 **Unlisted procedure, pelvis or hip joint**

0.00 0.00 FUD YYY T 80 50

AMA: 2018,Sep,7; 2018,Jan,8; 2017,Jan,8; 2016,Jun,8; 2016,Jan,13; 2015,Jan,16

27301-27310 Incisional Procedures Femur or Knee

EXCLUDES *Superficial incision and drainage (10040-10160)*

27301 **Incision and drainage, deep abscess, bursa, or hematoma, thigh or knee region**

14.5 19.4 FUD 090 J A2 50

AMA: 2018,Sep,7; 2018,Jan,8; 2017,Jan,8; 2016,Jan,13; 2015,Jan,16

27303 **Incision, deep, with opening of bone cortex, femur or knee (eg, osteomyelitis or bone abscess)**

18.5 18.5 FUD 090 C 80 50

AMA: 2018,Sep,7

27305 **Fasciotomy, iliotibial (tenotomy), open**

EXCLUDES *Ober-Yount (gluteal-iliotibial) fasciotomy (27025)*

13.8 13.8 FUD 090 J A2 80 50

AMA: 2018,Sep,7

27306 **Tenotomy, percutaneous, adductor or hamstring; single tendon (separate procedure)**

9.89 9.89 FUD 090 J A2 80 50

AMA: 2018,Sep,7; 2018,Jan,8; 2017,Aug,9

27307 **multiple tendons**

13.8 13.8 FUD 090 J A2 80 50

AMA: 2018,Sep,7; 2018,Jan,8; 2017,Aug,9

27310 **Arthrotomy, knee, with exploration, drainage, or removal of foreign body (eg, infection)**

21.1 21.1 FUD 090 J A2 80 50

AMA: 2018,Sep,7; 2018,Jan,8; 2017,Jan,8; 2016,Jan,13; 2015,Jan,16

27323-27324 Biopsy Femur or Knee

EXCLUDES *Soft tissue needle biopsy (20206)*

27323 **Biopsy, soft tissue of thigh or knee area; superficial**

5.08 7.91 FUD 010 J A2 50

AMA: 2018,Sep,7; 2018,Jan,8; 2017,Jan,8; 2016,Jan,13; 2015,Jan,16

27324 **deep (subfascial or intramuscular)**

11.6 11.6 FUD 090 J A2 50

AMA: 2018,Sep,7; 2018,Jan,8; 2017,Jan,8; 2016,Jan,13; 2015,Jan,16

27325-27326 Neurectomy

27325 **Neurectomy, hamstring muscle**

16.1 16.1 FUD 090 J A2 80 50

AMA: 2018,Sep,7

27326 **Neurectomy, popliteal (gastrocnemius)**

14.9 14.9 FUD 090 J A2 80 50

AMA: 2018,Sep,7

27327-27339 [27329, 27337, 27339] Excision Soft Tissue Tumors Femur/ Knee

INCLUDES Any necessary elevation tissue planes or dissection
Measurement tumor and necessary margin at greatest diameter prior to excision
Simple and intermediate repairs
Excision types:
Fascial or subfascial soft tissue tumors: simple and marginal resection tumors found either in or below deep fascia, not including bone or excision substantial amount normal tissue; primarily benign and intramuscular tumors
Radical resection soft tissue tumor: wide resection tumor involving substantial margins normal tissue and may involve tissue removal from one or more layers; most often malignant or aggressive benign
Subcutaneous: simple and marginal resection tumors in subcutaneous tissue above deep fascia; most often benign

EXCLUDES *Complex repair*
Excision benign cutaneous lesions (eg, sebaceous cyst) (11400-11406)
Radical resection cutaneous tumors (eg, melanoma) (11600-11606)
Significant vessel exploration or neuroplasty

27327 **Excision, tumor, soft tissue of thigh or knee area, subcutaneous; less than 3 cm**

9.00 13.5 FUD 090 J G2 50

AMA: 2018,Sep,7

\# **27337** **3 cm or greater**

12.1 12.1 FUD 090 J G2 80 50

AMA: 2018,Sep,7

27328 **Excision, tumor, soft tissue of thigh or knee area, subfascial (eg, intramuscular); less than 5 cm**

18.0 18.0 FUD 090 J G2 50

AMA: 2018,Sep,7; 2018,Jan,8; 2017,Jan,8; 2016,Nov,9

27329 **Resequenced code. See code following 27360.**

\# **27339** **5 cm or greater**

21.7 21.7 FUD 090 J G2 80 50

AMA: 2018,Sep,7

27330-27360 [27337, 27339] Resection Procedures Thigh/Knee

27330 **Arthrotomy, knee; with synovial biopsy only**
11.9 11.9 **FUD** 090 J A2 50
AMA: 2018,Sep,7; 2018,Jan,8; 2017,Jan,8; 2016,Jan,13; 2015,Jan,16

27331 **including joint exploration, biopsy, or removal of loose or foreign bodies**
13.6 13.6 **FUD** 090 J A2 80 50
AMA: 2018,Sep,7; 2018,Jan,8; 2017,Jan,8; 2016,Jan,13; 2015,Jan,16

27332 **Arthrotomy, with excision of semilunar cartilage (meniscectomy) knee; medial OR lateral**
18.5 18.5 **FUD** 090 J A2 80 50
AMA: 2018,Sep,7

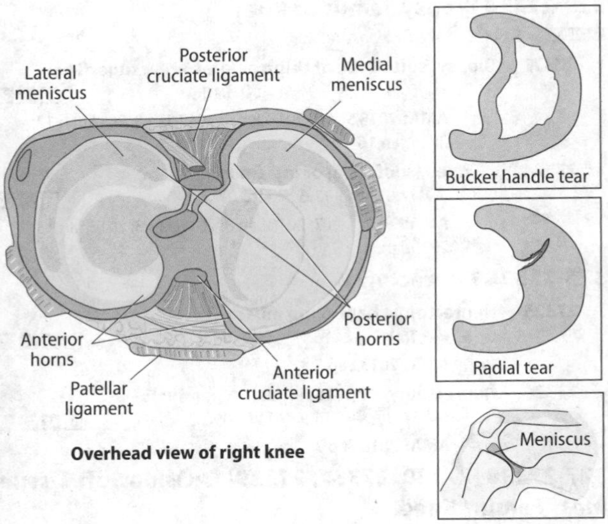

Overhead view of right knee

27333 **medial AND lateral**
16.9 16.9 **FUD** 090 J A2 80 50
AMA: 2018,Sep,7; 2018,Jan,8; 2017,Jan,8; 2016,Jan,13; 2015,Jan,16

27334 **Arthrotomy, with synovectomy, knee; anterior OR posterior**
19.7 19.7 **FUD** 090 J A2 80 50
AMA: 2018,Sep,7

27335 **anterior AND posterior including popliteal area**
22.0 22.0 **FUD** 090 J A2 80 50
AMA: 2018,Sep,7

27337 **Resequenced code. See code following 27327.**

27339 **Resequenced code. See code before 27330.**

27340 **Excision, prepatellar bursa**
10.6 10.6 **FUD** 090 J A2 50
AMA: 2018,Sep,7

27345 **Excision of synovial cyst of popliteal space (eg, Baker's cyst)**
13.9 13.9 **FUD** 090 J A2 80 50
AMA: 2018,Sep,7

27347 **Excision of lesion of meniscus or capsule (eg, cyst, ganglion), knee**
15.1 15.1 **FUD** 090 J A2 80 50
AMA: 2018,Sep,7

27350 **Patellectomy or hemipatellectomy**
18.8 18.8 **FUD** 090 J A2 80 50
AMA: 2018,Sep,7

27355 **Excision or curettage of bone cyst or benign tumor of femur;**
17.4 17.4 **FUD** 090 J A2 80 50
AMA: 2018,Sep,7

27356 **with allograft**
21.3 21.3 **FUD** 090 J G2 80 50
AMA: 2019,May,7; 2018,Sep,7

27357 **with autograft (includes obtaining graft)**
23.5 23.5 **FUD** 090 J A2 80 50
AMA: 2018,Sep,7; 2018,Jan,8; 2017,Jan,8; 2016,Jan,13; 2015,Jan,16

\+ **27358** **with internal fixation (List in addition to code for primary procedure)**
Code first (27355-27357)
8.03 8.03 **FUD** ZZZ N N1 80
AMA: 2018,Sep,7

27360 **Partial excision (craterization, saucerization, or diaphysectomy) bone, femur, proximal tibia and/or fibula (eg, osteomyelitis or bone abscess)**
24.7 24.7 **FUD** 090 J A2 80 50
AMA: 2018,Sep,7

27329-27365 [27329] Radical Resection Tumor Knee/Thigh

INCLUDES Any necessary elevation tissue planes or dissection
Excision adjacent soft tissue during bone tumor resection
Measurement tumor and necessary margin at greatest diameter prior to excision
Radical resection bone tumor: resection tumor (may include entire bone) and wide margins normal tissue primarily for malignant or aggressive benign tumors
Radical resection soft tissue tumor: wide resection tumor involving substantial margins normal tissue that may include tissue removal from one or more layers; most often malignant or aggressive benign
Simple and intermediate repairs

EXCLUDES *Complex repair*
Radical resection cutaneous tumors (eg, melanoma) (11600-11606)
Significant vessel exploration, neuroplasty, reconstruction, or complex bone repair

\# **27329** **Radical resection of tumor (eg, sarcoma), soft tissue of thigh or knee area; less than 5 cm**
30.1 30.1 **FUD** 090 J G2 80 50
AMA: 2018,Sep,7

27364 **5 cm or greater**
45.2 45.2 **FUD** 090 J G2 80 50
AMA: 2018,Sep,7

27365 **Radical resection of tumor, femur or knee**
EXCLUDES *Soft tissue tumor excision thigh or knee area (27329, 27364)*
59.6 59.6 **FUD** 090 C 80 50
AMA: 2019,May,7; 2018,Sep,7

27369 Injection for Arthrogram of Knee

EXCLUDES *Arthrocentesis, aspiration and/or injection, knee (20610-20611)*
Arthroscopy, knee (29871)

27369 **Injection procedure for contrast knee arthrography or contrast enhanced CT/MRI knee arthrography**
Code also fluoroscopic guidance, when performed for CT/MRI arthrography (73701-73702, 73722-73723, 77002)
(73580, 73701-73702, 73722-73723)
1.17 4.06 **FUD** 000 N1 50
AMA: 2019,Aug,7

27372 Foreign Body Removal Femur or Knee

EXCLUDES *Arthroscopic procedures (29870-29887)*
Removal knee prosthesis (27488)

27372 **Removal of foreign body, deep, thigh region or knee area**
11.4 17.0 **FUD** 090 J A2 80 50
AMA: 2018,Sep,7

27380-27499 Repair/Reconstruction of Femur or Knee

27380 **Suture of infrapatellar tendon; primary**
17.5 17.5 **FUD** 090 J A2 80 50
AMA: 2018,Sep,7

27381 **secondary reconstruction, including fascial or tendon graft**
23.0 23.0 **FUD** 090 J A2 80 50
AMA: 2018,Sep,7

27385 **Suture of quadriceps or hamstring muscle rupture; primary**
16.9 16.9 **FUD** 090 J A2 80 50
AMA: 2018,Sep,7; 2018,Jan,8; 2017,Aug,9

27386 **secondary reconstruction, including fascial or tendon graft**
24.3 24.3 **FUD** 090 J A2 80 50
AMA: 2020,Apr,10; 2018,Sep,7

27390 **Tenotomy, open, hamstring, knee to hip; single tendon**
12.9 12.9 **FUD** 090 J A2 80 50
AMA: 2018,Sep,7

27391 **multiple tendons, 1 leg**
16.2 16.2 **FUD** 090 J A2 80
AMA: 2018,Sep,7

27392 **multiple tendons, bilateral**
20.4 20.4 **FUD** 090 J A2 80
AMA: 2018,Sep,7

27393 **Lengthening of hamstring tendon; single tendon**
14.6 14.6 **FUD** 090 J A2 80 50
AMA: 2018,Sep,7

27394 **multiple tendons, 1 leg**
18.8 18.8 **FUD** 090 J A2 80
AMA: 2018,Sep,7

27395 **multiple tendons, bilateral**
25.4 25.4 **FUD** 090 J A2 80
AMA: 2018,Sep,7

27396 **Transplant or transfer (with muscle redirection or rerouting), thigh (eg, extensor to flexor); single tendon**
17.7 17.7 **FUD** 090 J A2 80 50
AMA: 2018,Sep,7

27397 **multiple tendons**
26.3 26.3 **FUD** 090 J G2 80 50
AMA: 2018,Sep,7

27400 **Transfer, tendon or muscle, hamstrings to femur (eg, Egger's type procedure)**
20.0 20.0 **FUD** 090 J A2 80 50
AMA: 2018,Sep,7

27403 **Arthrotomy with meniscus repair, knee**
EXCLUDES *Arthroscopic treatment (29882)*
18.5 18.5 **FUD** 090 J J8 80 50
AMA: 2019,May,10; 2018,Sep,7

27405 **Repair, primary, torn ligament and/or capsule, knee; collateral**
19.5 19.5 **FUD** 090 J A2 80 50
AMA: 2018,Sep,7; 2018,Jan,8; 2017,Jan,8; 2016,Jan,13; 2015,Jan,16

27407 **cruciate**
EXCLUDES *Reconstruction (27427)*
22.9 22.9 **FUD** 090 J A2 80 50
AMA: 2018,Sep,7

27409 **collateral and cruciate ligaments**
EXCLUDES *Reconstruction (27427-27429)*
27.9 27.9 **FUD** 090 J A2 80 50
AMA: 2018,Sep,7

27412 **Autologous chondrocyte implantation, knee**
EXCLUDES *Arthrotomy, knee (27331)*
Autologous fat graft obtained by liposuction (15771-15774)
Manipulation knee joint under general anesthesia (27570)
Obtaining chondrocytes (29870)
Other autologous soft tissue grafts (fat, dermis, fascia) harvested by direct excision ([15769])
47.1 47.1 **FUD** 090 J 80 50
AMA: 2018,Sep,7

27415 **Osteochondral allograft, knee, open**
EXCLUDES *Arthroscopic procedure (29867)*
Osteochondral autograft knee (27416)
39.6 39.6 **FUD** 090 J J8 80 50
AMA: 2019,Apr,10; 2018,Sep,7; 2018,Jan,8; 2017,Jan,8; 2016,Jan,13; 2015,Jan,16

27416 **Osteochondral autograft(s), knee, open (eg, mosaicplasty) (includes harvesting of autograft[s])**
EXCLUDES *Procedures in same compartment (29874, 29877, 29879, 29885-29887)*
Procedures performed at same surgical session (27415, 29870-29871, 29875, 29884)
Surgical arthroscopy knee with osteochondral autograft(s) (29866)
28.3 28.3 **FUD** 090 J G2 80 50
AMA: 2018,Sep,7; 2018,Jan,8; 2017,Jan,8; 2016,Jan,13; 2015,Jan,16

27418 **Anterior tibial tubercleplasty (eg, Maquet type procedure)**
23.8 23.8 **FUD** 090 J A2 80 50
AMA: 2018,Sep,7; 2018,Jan,8; 2017,Jan,8; 2016,Jan,13; 2015,Jan,16

27420 **Reconstruction of dislocating patella; (eg, Hauser type procedure)**
21.4 21.4 **FUD** 090 J A2 80 50
AMA: 2018,Sep,7; 2018,Jan,8; 2017,Jan,8; 2016,Jan,13; 2015,Jan,16

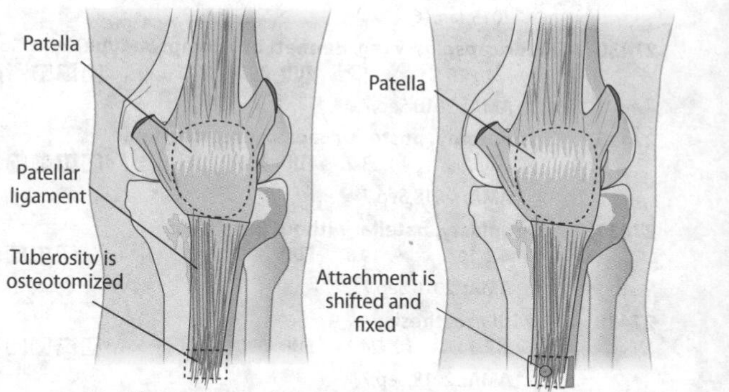

Patellar tendon insertion point is resected and shifted

27422 **with extensor realignment and/or muscle advancement or release (eg, Campbell, Goldwaite type procedure)**
21.4 21.4 **FUD** 090 J A2 80 50
AMA: 2018,Sep,7; 2018,Jan,8; 2017,Jan,8; 2016,Jan,13; 2015,Jan,16

27424 **with patellectomy**
21.5 21.5 **FUD** 090 J A2 80 50
AMA: 2018,Sep,7

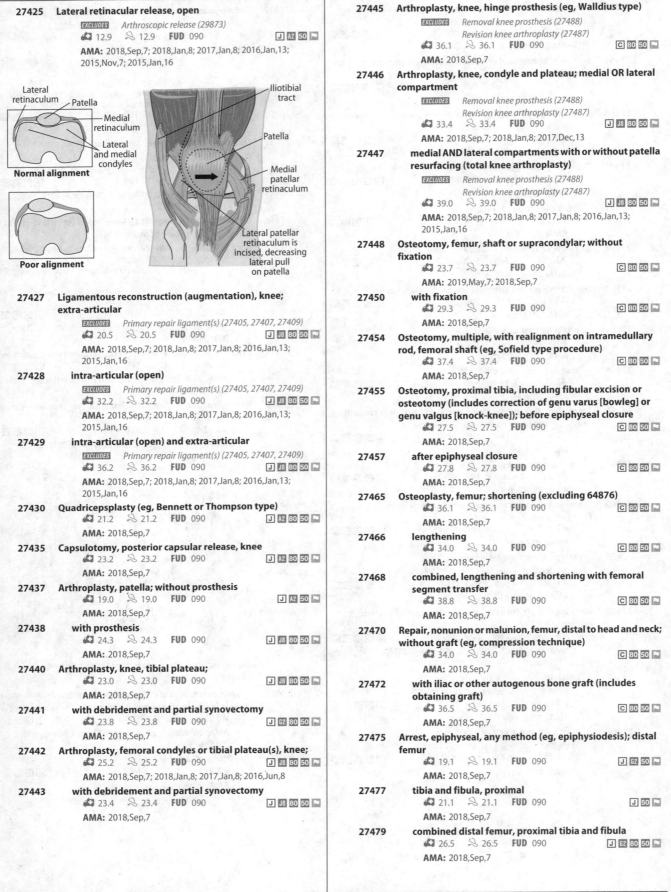

27425 Lateral retinacular release, open

EXCLUDES *Arthroscopic release (29873)*

Facility RVU 12.9 Non-Facility RVU 12.9 FUD 090 J A2 50

AMA: 2018,Sep,7; 2018,Jan,8; 2017,Jan,8; 2016,Jan,13; 2015,Nov,7; 2015,Jan,16

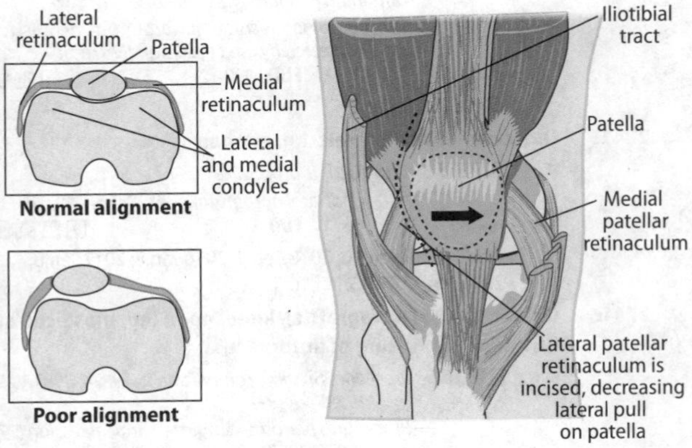

27427 Ligamentous reconstruction (augmentation), knee; extra-articular

EXCLUDES *Primary repair ligament(s) (27405, 27407, 27409)*

Facility RVU 20.5 Non-Facility RVU 20.5 FUD 090 J J8 80 50

AMA: 2018,Sep,7; 2018,Jan,8; 2017,Jan,8; 2016,Jan,13; 2015,Jan,16

27428 intra-articular (open)

EXCLUDES *Primary repair ligament(s) (27405, 27407, 27409)*

Facility RVU 32.2 Non-Facility RVU 32.2 FUD 090 J J8 80 50

AMA: 2018,Sep,7; 2018,Jan,8; 2017,Jan,8; 2016,Jan,13; 2015,Jan,16

27429 intra-articular (open) and extra-articular

EXCLUDES *Primary repair ligament(s) (27405, 27407, 27409)*

Facility RVU 36.2 Non-Facility RVU 36.2 FUD 090 J J8 80 50

AMA: 2018,Sep,7; 2018,Jan,8; 2017,Jan,8; 2016,Jan,13; 2015,Jan,16

27430 Quadricepsplasty (eg, Bennett or Thompson type)

Facility RVU 21.2 Non-Facility RVU 21.2 FUD 090 J A2 80 50

AMA: 2018,Sep,7

27435 Capsulotomy, posterior capsular release, knee

Facility RVU 23.2 Non-Facility RVU 23.2 FUD 090 J A2 80 50

AMA: 2018,Sep,7

27437 Arthroplasty, patella; without prosthesis

Facility RVU 19.0 Non-Facility RVU 19.0 FUD 090 J A2 50

AMA: 2018,Sep,7

27438 with prosthesis

Facility RVU 24.3 Non-Facility RVU 24.3 FUD 090 J J8 80 50

AMA: 2018,Sep,7

27440 Arthroplasty, knee, tibial plateau;

Facility RVU 23.0 Non-Facility RVU 23.0 FUD 090 J J8 80 50

AMA: 2018,Sep,7

27441 with debridement and partial synovectomy

Facility RVU 23.8 Non-Facility RVU 23.8 FUD 090 J G2 80 50

AMA: 2018,Sep,7

27442 Arthroplasty, femoral condyles or tibial plateau(s), knee;

Facility RVU 25.2 Non-Facility RVU 25.2 FUD 090 J J8 80 50

AMA: 2018,Sep,7; 2018,Jan,8; 2017,Jan,8; 2016,Jun,8

27443 with debridement and partial synovectomy

Facility RVU 23.4 Non-Facility RVU 23.4 FUD 090 J J8 80 50

AMA: 2018,Sep,7

27445 Arthroplasty, knee, hinge prosthesis (eg, Walldius type)

EXCLUDES *Removal knee prosthesis (27488)*
Revision knee arthroplasty (27487)

Facility RVU 36.1 Non-Facility RVU 36.1 FUD 090 C 80 50

AMA: 2018,Sep,7

27446 Arthroplasty, knee, condyle and plateau; medial OR lateral compartment

EXCLUDES *Removal knee prosthesis (27488)*
Revision knee arthroplasty (27487)

Facility RVU 33.4 Non-Facility RVU 33.4 FUD 090 J J8 80 50

AMA: 2018,Sep,7; 2018,Jan,8; 2017,Dec,13

27447 medial AND lateral compartments with or without patella resurfacing (total knee arthroplasty)

EXCLUDES *Removal knee prosthesis (27488)*
Revision knee arthroplasty (27487)

Facility RVU 39.0 Non-Facility RVU 39.0 FUD 090 J J8 80 50

AMA: 2018,Sep,7; 2018,Jan,8; 2017,Jan,8; 2016,Jan,13; 2015,Jan,16

27448 Osteotomy, femur, shaft or supracondylar; without fixation

Facility RVU 23.7 Non-Facility RVU 23.7 FUD 090 C 80 50

AMA: 2019,May,7; 2018,Sep,7

27450 with fixation

Facility RVU 29.3 Non-Facility RVU 29.3 FUD 090 C 80 50

AMA: 2018,Sep,7

27454 Osteotomy, multiple, with realignment on intramedullary rod, femoral shaft (eg, Sofield type procedure)

Facility RVU 37.4 Non-Facility RVU 37.4 FUD 090 C 80 50

AMA: 2018,Sep,7

27455 Osteotomy, proximal tibia, including fibular excision or osteotomy (includes correction of genu varus [bowleg] or genu valgus [knock-knee]); before epiphyseal closure

Facility RVU 27.5 Non-Facility RVU 27.5 FUD 090 C 80 50

AMA: 2018,Sep,7

27457 after epiphyseal closure

Facility RVU 27.8 Non-Facility RVU 27.8 FUD 090 C 80 50

AMA: 2018,Sep,7

27465 Osteoplasty, femur; shortening (excluding 64876)

Facility RVU 36.1 Non-Facility RVU 36.1 FUD 090 C 80 50

AMA: 2018,Sep,7

27466 lengthening

Facility RVU 34.0 Non-Facility RVU 34.0 FUD 090 C 80 50

AMA: 2018,Sep,7

27468 combined, lengthening and shortening with femoral segment transfer

Facility RVU 38.8 Non-Facility RVU 38.8 FUD 090 C 80 50

AMA: 2018,Sep,7

27470 Repair, nonunion or malunion, femur, distal to head and neck; without graft (eg, compression technique)

Facility RVU 34.0 Non-Facility RVU 34.0 FUD 090 C 80 50

AMA: 2018,Sep,7

27472 with iliac or other autogenous bone graft (includes obtaining graft)

Facility RVU 36.5 Non-Facility RVU 36.5 FUD 090 C 80 50

AMA: 2018,Sep,7

27475 Arrest, epiphyseal, any method (eg, epiphysiodesis); distal femur

Facility RVU 19.1 Non-Facility RVU 19.1 FUD 090 J G2 50

AMA: 2018,Sep,7

27477 tibia and fibula, proximal

Facility RVU 21.1 Non-Facility RVU 21.1 FUD 090 J 50

AMA: 2018,Sep,7

27479 combined distal femur, proximal tibia and fibula

Facility RVU 26.5 Non-Facility RVU 26.5 FUD 090 J G2 80 50

AMA: 2018,Sep,7

27485 **Arrest, hemiepiphyseal, distal femur or proximal tibia or fibula (eg, genu varus or valgus)**
19.3 19.3 FUD 090 J 50
AMA: 2018,Sep,7

27486 **Revision of total knee arthroplasty, with or without allograft; 1 component**
40.6 40.6 FUD 090 C 80 50
AMA: 2018,Sep,7; 2018,Apr,10; 2018,Jan,8; 2017,Jan,8; 2016,Jan,13; 2015,Jul,10; 2015,Jan,16

27487 **femoral and entire tibial component**
50.8 50.8 FUD 090 C 80 50
AMA: 2018,Sep,7; 2018,Jan,8; 2017,Jan,8; 2016,Jan,13; 2015,Jan,16

27488 **Removal of prosthesis, including total knee prosthesis, methylmethacrylate with or without insertion of spacer, knee**
34.7 34.7 FUD 090 C 80 50
AMA: 2018,Sep,7; 2018,Jan,8; 2017,Jan,8; 2016,Jan,13; 2015,Jan,16

27495 **Prophylactic treatment (nailing, pinning, plating, or wiring) with or without methylmethacrylate, femur**
32.5 32.5 FUD 090 C 80 50
AMA: 2018,Sep,7

27496 **Decompression fasciotomy, thigh and/or knee, 1 compartment (flexor or extensor or adductor);**
15.7 15.7 FUD 090 J A2 50
AMA: 2018,Sep,7

27497 **with debridement of nonviable muscle and/or nerve**
16.7 16.7 FUD 090 J A2 80 50
AMA: 2018,Sep,7

27498 **Decompression fasciotomy, thigh and/or knee, multiple compartments;**
18.8 18.8 FUD 090 J A2 80 50
AMA: 2018,Sep,7

27499 **with debridement of nonviable muscle and/or nerve**
20.2 20.2 FUD 090 J A2 80 50
AMA: 2018,Sep,7

27500-27566 Treatment of Fracture/Dislocation of Femur/Knee

INCLUDES Closed, percutaneous, and open treatment fractures and dislocations

27500 **Closed treatment of femoral shaft fracture, without manipulation**
13.8 15.0 FUD 090 T A2 50
AMA: 2018,Sep,7

27501 **Closed treatment of supracondylar or transcondylar femoral fracture with or without intercondylar extension, without manipulation**
14.3 14.5 FUD 090 T A2 80 50
AMA: 2018,Sep,7

27502 **Closed treatment of femoral shaft fracture, with manipulation, with or without skin or skeletal traction**
21.9 21.9 FUD 090 J A2 50
AMA: 2018,Sep,7; 2018,Jan,8; 2017,Jan,8; 2016,Jan,13; 2015,Jan,16

27503 **Closed treatment of supracondylar or transcondylar femoral fracture with or without intercondylar extension, with manipulation, with or without skin or skeletal traction**
23.1 23.1 FUD 090 J A2 80 50
AMA: 2018,Sep,7

27506 **Open treatment of femoral shaft fracture, with or without external fixation, with insertion of intramedullary implant, with or without cerclage and/or locking screws**
38.6 38.6 FUD 090 C 80 50
AMA: 2018,Sep,7; 2018,Jan,8; 2017,Jan,8; 2016,Jan,13; 2015,Jan,16

27507 **Open treatment of femoral shaft fracture with plate/screws, with or without cerclage**
28.0 28.0 FUD 090 C 80 50
AMA: 2018,Sep,7

27508 **Closed treatment of femoral fracture, distal end, medial or lateral condyle, without manipulation**
14.3 15.0 FUD 090 T A2 50
AMA: 2018,Sep,7

27509 **Percutaneous skeletal fixation of femoral fracture, distal end, medial or lateral condyle, or supracondylar or transcondylar, with or without intercondylar extension, or distal femoral epiphyseal separation**
18.6 18.6 FUD 090 J A2 80 50
AMA: 2018,Dec,10; 2018,Dec,10; 2018,Sep,7

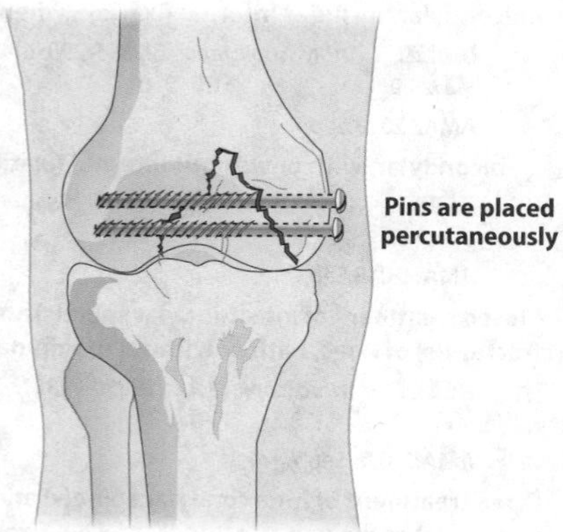

27510 **Closed treatment of femoral fracture, distal end, medial or lateral condyle, with manipulation**
19.6 19.6 FUD 090 J A2 50
AMA: 2018,Sep,7

27511 **Open treatment of femoral supracondylar or transcondylar fracture without intercondylar extension, includes internal fixation, when performed**
28.8 28.8 FUD 090 C 80 50
AMA: 2018,Sep,7

27513 **Open treatment of femoral supracondylar or transcondylar fracture with intercondylar extension, includes internal fixation, when performed**
35.9 35.9 FUD 090 C 80 50
AMA: 2018,Sep,7

27514 **Open treatment of femoral fracture, distal end, medial or lateral condyle, includes internal fixation, when performed**
27.9 27.9 FUD 090 C 80 50
AMA: 2018,Sep,7

27516 **Closed treatment of distal femoral epiphyseal separation; without manipulation**
13.8 14.7 FUD 090 T A2 50
AMA: 2018,Sep,7

27517 **with manipulation, with or without skin or skeletal traction**
19.6 19.6 FUD 090 J A2 80 50
AMA: 2018,Sep,7

27519 **Open treatment of distal femoral epiphyseal separation, includes internal fixation, when performed**
25.7 25.7 FUD 090 C 80 50
AMA: 2018,Sep,7

27520 **Closed treatment of patellar fracture, without manipulation**
8.54 9.25 FUD 090 T A2 50
AMA: 2018,Sep,7

27524 **Open treatment of patellar fracture, with internal fixation and/or partial or complete patellectomy and soft tissue repair**
21.7 21.7 **FUD** 090 J 62 80 50
AMA: 2018,Sep,7

27530 **Closed treatment of tibial fracture, proximal (plateau); without manipulation**
EXCLUDES *Arthroscopic repair (29855-29856)*
8.05 8.63 **FUD** 090 T A2 50
AMA: 2018,Sep,7

27532 **with or without manipulation, with skeletal traction**
EXCLUDES *Arthroscopic repair (29855-29856)*
16.5 17.7 **FUD** 090 J A2 50
AMA: 2018,Sep,7

27535 **Open treatment of tibial fracture, proximal (plateau); unicondylar, includes internal fixation, when performed**
EXCLUDES *Arthroscopic repair (29855-29856)*
25.9 25.9 **FUD** 090 C 80 50
AMA: 2018,Sep,7

27536 **bicondylar, with or without internal fixation**
EXCLUDES *Arthroscopic repair (29855-29856)*
34.3 34.3 **FUD** 090 C 80 50
AMA: 2018,Sep,7

27538 **Closed treatment of intercondylar spine(s) and/or tuberosity fracture(s) of knee, with or without manipulation**
EXCLUDES *Arthroscopic repair (29850-29851)*
12.7 13.6 **FUD** 090 T A2 80 50
AMA: 2018,Sep,7

27540 **Open treatment of intercondylar spine(s) and/or tuberosity fracture(s) of the knee, includes internal fixation, when performed**
23.4 23.4 **FUD** 090 C 80 50
AMA: 2018,Sep,7

27550 **Closed treatment of knee dislocation; without anesthesia**
13.8 14.9 **FUD** 090 T A2 80 50
AMA: 2018,Sep,7

27552 **requiring anesthesia**
18.0 18.0 **FUD** 090 J A2 80 50
AMA: 2018,Sep,7

27556 **Open treatment of knee dislocation, includes internal fixation, when performed; without primary ligamentous repair or augmentation/reconstruction**
25.3 25.3 **FUD** 090 C 80 50
AMA: 2018,Sep,7

27557 **with primary ligamentous repair**
30.2 30.2 **FUD** 090 C 80 50
AMA: 2018,Sep,7

27558 **with primary ligamentous repair, with augmentation/reconstruction**
34.5 34.5 **FUD** 090 C 80 50
AMA: 2018,Sep,7

27560 **Closed treatment of patellar dislocation; without anesthesia**
EXCLUDES *Recurrent dislocation (27420-27424)*
9.66 10.5 **FUD** 090 T A2 50
AMA: 2018,Sep,7

27562 **requiring anesthesia**
EXCLUDES *Recurrent dislocation (27420-27424)*
13.9 13.9 **FUD** 090 T A2 80 50
AMA: 2018,Sep,7

27566 **Open treatment of patellar dislocation, with or without partial or total patellectomy**
EXCLUDES *Recurrent dislocation (27420-27424)*
25.8 25.8 **FUD** 090 J A2 80 50
AMA: 2018,Sep,7

27570 Knee Manipulation with Anesthesia

27570 **Manipulation of knee joint under general anesthesia (includes application of traction or other fixation devices)**
4.34 4.34 **FUD** 010 J A2 50
AMA: 2018,Sep,7; 2018,Jan,8; 2017,Jan,8; 2016,Jan,13; 2015,Jan,16

27580 Knee Arthrodesis

27580 **Arthrodesis, knee, any technique**
42.1 42.1 **FUD** 090 C 80 50
AMA: 2020,May,13; 2018,Sep,7

27590-27599 Amputations and Unlisted Procedures at Femur or Knee

27590 **Amputation, thigh, through femur, any level;**
23.0 23.0 **FUD** 090 C 80 50
AMA: 2018,Sep,7; 2018,Jan,8; 2017,Dec,13

27591 **immediate fitting technique including first cast**
27.9 27.9 **FUD** 090 C 80 50
AMA: 2018,Sep,7

27592 **open, circular (guillotine)**
19.5 19.5 **FUD** 090 C 80 50
AMA: 2018,Sep,7

27594 **secondary closure or scar revision**
14.6 14.6 **FUD** 090 J A2 50
AMA: 2018,Sep,7

27596 **re-amputation**
20.6 20.6 **FUD** 090 C 50
AMA: 2018,Sep,7

27598 **Disarticulation at knee**
INCLUDES Batch-Spittler-McFaddin operation
Callander knee disarticulation
Gritti amputation
20.6 20.6 **FUD** 090 C 80 50
AMA: 2018,Sep,7

27599 **Unlisted procedure, femur or knee**
0.00 0.00 **FUD** YYY T 80 50
AMA: 2019,Apr,10; 2018,Dec,10; 2018,Dec,10; 2018,Sep,7; 2018,Apr,10; 2018,Jan,8; 2017,Aug,9; 2017,Mar,10; 2017,Jan,8; 2016,Nov,9; 2016,Jun,8; 2016,Jan,13; 2015,Jan,13; 2015,Jan,16

27600-27602 Decompression Fasciotomy of Leg

EXCLUDES *Fasciotomy with debridement (27892-27894)*
Simple incision and drainage (10140-10160)

27600 **Decompression fasciotomy, leg; anterior and/or lateral compartments only**
11.7 11.7 **FUD** 090 J A2 50
AMA: 2018,Sep,7

27601 **posterior compartment(s) only**
12.8 12.8 **FUD** 090 J A2 50
AMA: 2018,Sep,7

27602 **anterior and/or lateral, and posterior compartment(s)**
14.0 14.0 **FUD** 090 J A2 80 50
AMA: 2018,Sep,7

27603-27612 Incisional Procedures Lower Leg and Ankle

27603 **Incision and drainage, leg or ankle; deep abscess or hematoma**
11.1 15.2 **FUD** 090 J A2 50
AMA: 2018,Sep,7

27604 **infected bursa**
9.61 13.6 **FUD** 090 J A2 80 50
AMA: 2018,Sep,7

27605 **Tenotomy, percutaneous, Achilles tendon (separate procedure); local anesthesia**
5.34 9.83 **FUD** 010 J A2 80 50
AMA: 2018,Sep,14; 2018,Sep,7

27606 general anesthesia
7.99 7.99 FUD 010 J A2 50
AMA: 2018,Sep,7; 2018,Sep,14

27607 Incision (eg, osteomyelitis or bone abscess), leg or ankle
17.5 17.5 FUD 090 J A2 50
AMA: 2018,Sep,7

27610 Arthrotomy, ankle, including exploration, drainage, or removal of foreign body
18.7 18.7 FUD 090 J A2 50
AMA: 2018,Sep,7

27612 Arthrotomy, posterior capsular release, ankle, with or without Achilles tendon lengthening
EXCLUDES *Lengthening or shortening tendon (27685)*
16.0 16.0 FUD 090 J A2 80 50
AMA: 2018,Sep,7

27613-27614 Biopsy Lower Leg and Ankle

EXCLUDES *Needle biopsy (20206)*

27613 Biopsy, soft tissue of leg or ankle area; superficial
4.60 7.22 FUD 010 J P3 50
AMA: 2018,Sep,7

27614 deep (subfascial or intramuscular)
11.7 16.6 FUD 090 J A2 50
AMA: 2018,Sep,7

27615-27634 [27632, 27634] Excision Soft Tissue Tumors Lower Leg/Ankle

INCLUDES Any necessary elevation tissue planes or dissection
Measurement tumor and necessary margin at greatest diameter prior to excision
Resection without removal significant normal tissue
Simple and intermediate repairs
Excision types:
Fascial or subfascial soft tissue tumors: simple and marginal resection most often benign and intramuscular tumors found either in or below deep fascia, not involving bone
Resection tumor (may include entire bone) and wide margins normal tissue primarily for malignant or aggressive benign tumors
Subcutaneous: simple and marginal resection most often benign tumors found in subcutaneous tissue above deep fascia

EXCLUDES *Complex repair*
Excision benign cutaneous lesions (eg, sebaceous cyst) (11400-11406)
Radical resection cutaneous tumors (eg, melanoma) (11600-11606)
Significant vessel exploration or neuroplasty

27615 Radical resection of tumor (eg, sarcoma), soft tissue of leg or ankle area; less than 5 cm
29.6 29.6 FUD 090 J G2 80 50
AMA: 2018,Sep,7

27616 5 cm or greater
36.6 36.6 FUD 090 J G2 80 50
AMA: 2018,Sep,7

27618 Excision, tumor, soft tissue of leg or ankle area, subcutaneous; less than 3 cm
8.83 13.2 FUD 090 J G2 50
AMA: 2018,Sep,7; 2018,Jan,8; 2017,Jan,8; 2016,Jan,13; 2015,Jan,16

27632 3 cm or greater
11.9 11.9 FUD 090 J G2 80 50
AMA: 2018,Sep,7

27619 Excision, tumor, soft tissue of leg or ankle area, subfascial (eg, intramuscular); less than 5 cm
13.3 13.3 FUD 090 J G2 50
AMA: 2018,Sep,7

27634 5 cm or greater
19.7 19.7 FUD 090 J G2 80 50
AMA: 2018,Sep,7

27620-27641 [27632, 27634] Bone and Joint Procedures Ankle/Leg

27620 Arthrotomy, ankle, with joint exploration, with or without biopsy, with or without removal of loose or foreign body
12.9 12.9 FUD 090 J A2 80 50
AMA: 2018,Sep,7

27625 Arthrotomy, with synovectomy, ankle;
16.4 16.4 FUD 090 J A2 80 50
AMA: 2018,Sep,7

27626 including tenosynovectomy
17.4 17.4 FUD 090 J A2 80 50
AMA: 2018,Sep,7

27630 Excision of lesion of tendon sheath or capsule (eg, cyst or ganglion), leg and/or ankle
10.4 15.9 FUD 090 J A2 50
AMA: 2018,Sep,7

27632 Resequenced code. See code following 27618.

27634 Resequenced code. See code following 27619.

27635 Excision or curettage of bone cyst or benign tumor, tibia or fibula;
16.7 16.7 FUD 090 J A2 50
AMA: 2018,Sep,7; 2018,Jan,8; 2017,Jan,8; 2016,Jan,13; 2015,Jan,16

27637 with autograft (includes obtaining graft)
21.5 21.5 FUD 090 J A2 80 50
AMA: 2018,Sep,7

27638 with allograft
22.0 22.0 FUD 090 J A2 80 50
AMA: 2019,May,7; 2018,Sep,7

27640 Partial excision (craterization, saucerization, or diaphysectomy), bone (eg, osteomyelitis); tibia
EXCLUDES *Excision exostosis (27635)*
23.9 23.9 FUD 090 J A2 50
AMA: 2018,Sep,7; 2018,Jan,8; 2017,Jan,8; 2016,Jan,13; 2015,Jan,16

27641 fibula
EXCLUDES *Excision exostosis (27635)*
19.0 19.0 FUD 090 J A2 50
AMA: 2018,Sep,7

27645-27647 Radical Resection Bone Tumor Ankle/Leg

INCLUDES Any necessary elevation tissue planes or dissection
Excision adjacent soft tissue during bone tumor resection (27615-27619 [27632, 27634])
Measurement tumor and necessary margin at greatest diameter prior to excision
Resection tumor (may include entire bone) and wide margins normal tissue primarily for malignant or aggressive benign tumors
Simple and intermediate repairs

EXCLUDES *Complex repair*
Significant vessel exploration, neuroplasty, reconstruction, or complex bone repair

27645 Radical resection of tumor; tibia
51.2 51.2 FUD 090 C 80 50
AMA: 2019,May,7; 2018,Sep,7

27646 fibula
44.5 44.5 FUD 090 C 80 50
AMA: 2019,May,7; 2018,Sep,7

27647 talus or calcaneus
29.3 29.3 FUD 090 J A2 80 50
AMA: 2019,May,7; 2018,Sep,7

27648 Injection for Ankle Arthrogram

EXCLUDES *Arthroscopy (29894-29898)*

27648 **Injection procedure for ankle arthrography**
(73615)
1.52 5.22 FUD 000 N N1 80 50
AMA: 2019,May,7; 2018,Sep,7; 2018,Jan,8; 2017,Jan,8; 2016,Jan,13; 2015,Aug,6

27650-27745 Repair/Reconstruction Lower Leg/Ankle

27650 **Repair, primary, open or percutaneous, ruptured Achilles tendon;**
18.9 18.9 FUD 090 J A2 80 50
AMA: 2020,Jun,14; 2018,Sep,7; 2018,Jan,8; 2017,Jan,8; 2016,Jan,13; 2015,Jan,16

27652 **with graft (includes obtaining graft)**
19.1 19.1 FUD 090 J A2 50
AMA: 2018,Sep,7; 2018,Jan,8; 2017,Jan,8; 2016,Jan,13; 2015,Jan,16

27654 **Repair, secondary, Achilles tendon, with or without graft**
20.4 20.4 FUD 090 J A2 80 50
AMA: 2020,Jun,14; 2020,Apr,8; 2018,Sep,7; 2018,Jan,8; 2017,Jan,8; 2016,Dec,16; 2016,Jan,13; 2015,Jan,16

27656 **Repair, fascial defect of leg**
11.4 18.2 FUD 090 J A2 80 50
AMA: 2018,Sep,7

27658 **Repair, flexor tendon, leg; primary, without graft, each tendon**
10.6 10.6 FUD 090 J A2 80
AMA: 2018,Sep,7

27659 **secondary, with or without graft, each tendon**
13.5 13.5 FUD 090 J A2 80
AMA: 2018,Sep,7; 2018,Jan,8; 2017,Jan,8; 2016,Jan,13; 2015,Jan,13

27664 **Repair, extensor tendon, leg; primary, without graft, each tendon**
10.3 10.3 FUD 090 J A2 80
AMA: 2018,Sep,7; 2018,Jan,8; 2017,Jan,8; 2016,Jan,13; 2015,Jan,13

27665 **secondary, with or without graft, each tendon**
11.9 11.9 FUD 090 J A2 80
AMA: 2018,Sep,7

27675 **Repair, dislocating peroneal tendons; without fibular osteotomy**
14.1 14.1 FUD 090 J A2 80 50
AMA: 2018,Sep,7

27676 **with fibular osteotomy**
17.2 17.2 FUD 090 J A2 80 50
AMA: 2018,Sep,7

27680 **Tenolysis, flexor or extensor tendon, leg and/or ankle; single, each tendon**
12.2 12.2 FUD 090 J A2
AMA: 2018,Sep,7; 2018,Jan,8; 2017,Jan,8; 2016,Jan,13; 2015,Jan,16

27681 **multiple tendons (through separate incision[s])**
15.7 15.7 FUD 090 J A2 50
AMA: 2018,Sep,7

27685 **Lengthening or shortening of tendon, leg or ankle; single tendon (separate procedure)**
13.3 19.0 FUD 090 J A2 80 50
AMA: 2018,Sep,7; 2018,Sep,14; 2018,Jan,8; 2017,Jan,8; 2016,Jan,13; 2015,Jan,16

27686 **multiple tendons (through same incision), each**
15.6 15.6 FUD 090 J A2 50
AMA: 2018,Sep,7; 2018,Jan,8; 2017,Jan,8; 2016,Jan,13; 2015,Jan,16

27687 **Gastrocnemius recession (eg, Strayer procedure)**
13.0 13.0 FUD 090 J A2 80 50
AMA: 2018,Sep,7

27690 **Transfer or transplant of single tendon (with muscle redirection or rerouting); superficial (eg, anterior tibial extensors into midfoot)**
INCLUDES Toe extensors considered single tendon with transplant into midfoot
18.3 18.3 FUD 090 J A2 80 50
AMA: 2018,Sep,7

27691 **deep (eg, anterior tibial or posterior tibial through interosseous space, flexor digitorum longus, flexor hallucis longus, or peroneal tendon to midfoot or hindfoot)**
INCLUDES Barr procedure
Toe extensors considered single tendon with transplant into midfoot
21.4 21.4 FUD 090 J A2 80 50
AMA: 2018,Sep,7

\+ **27692** **each additional tendon (List separately in addition to code for primary procedure)**
INCLUDES Toe extensors considered single tendon with transplant into midfoot
Code first (27690-27691)
3.01 3.01 FUD ZZZ N N1 80
AMA: 2018,Sep,7

27695 **Repair, primary, disrupted ligament, ankle; collateral**
13.6 13.6 FUD 090 J A2 50
AMA: 2018,Nov,11; 2018,Sep,7; 2018,Jan,8; 2017,Jan,8; 2016,Jan,13; 2015,Jan,16

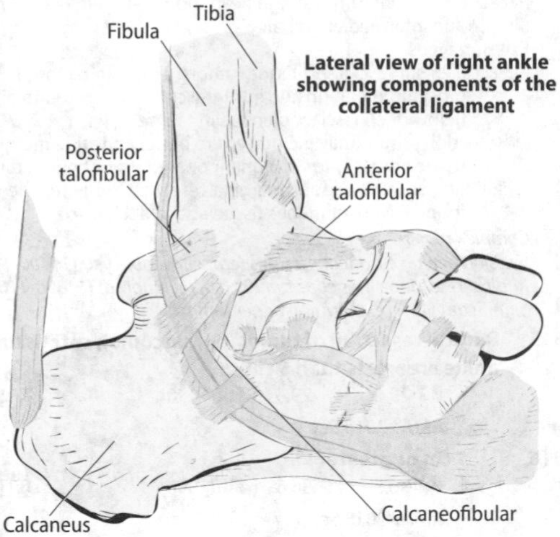

Lateral view of right ankle showing components of the collateral ligament

27696 **both collateral ligaments**
16.0 16.0 FUD 090 J A2 50
AMA: 2018,Nov,11; 2018,Sep,7; 2018,Jan,8; 2017,Jan,8; 2016,Jan,13; 2015,Jan,16

27698 **Repair, secondary, disrupted ligament, ankle, collateral (eg, Watson-Jones procedure)**
18.3 18.3 FUD 090 J A2 80 50
AMA: 2018,Sep,7; 2018,Jan,8; 2017,Jan,8; 2016,Jan,13; 2015,Jan,16

27700 **Arthroplasty, ankle;**
17.6 17.6 FUD 090 J A2 80 50
AMA: 2018,Sep,7

27702 **with implant (total ankle)**
27.7 27.7 FUD 090 C 80 50
AMA: 2018,Sep,7

27703 **revision, total ankle**
32.2 32.2 FUD 090 C 80 50
AMA: 2018,Sep,7

27704 Removal of ankle implant
16.5 16.5 FUD 090 Q2 A2 50
AMA: 2019,May,7; 2018,Sep,7

27705 Osteotomy; tibia
EXCLUDES *Genu varus or genu valgus repair (27455-27457)*
21.8 21.8 FUD 090 J J8 80 50
AMA: 2018,Sep,7

27707 fibula
EXCLUDES *Genu varus or genu valgus repair (27455-27457)*
11.4 11.4 FUD 090 J A2 50
AMA: 2018,Sep,7

27709 tibia and fibula
EXCLUDES *Genu varus or genu valgus repair (27455-27457)*
33.6 33.6 FUD 090 J A2 80 50
AMA: 2018,Sep,7

27712 multiple, with realignment on intramedullary rod (eg, Sofield type procedure)
EXCLUDES *Genu varus or genu valgus repair (27455-27457)*
31.8 31.8 FUD 090 C 80 50
AMA: 2018,Sep,7

27715 Osteoplasty, tibia and fibula, lengthening or shortening
INCLUDES Anderson tibial lengthening
30.9 30.9 FUD 090 C 80 50
AMA: 2018,Sep,7

27720 Repair of nonunion or malunion, tibia; without graft, (eg, compression technique)
25.1 25.1 FUD 090 J J8 80 50
AMA: 2018,Sep,7

27722 with sliding graft
25.7 25.7 FUD 090 J 80 50
AMA: 2018,Sep,7

27724 with iliac or other autograft (includes obtaining graft)
36.4 36.4 FUD 090 C 80 50
AMA: 2018,Sep,7; 2018,Jan,8; 2017,Jan,8; 2016,Jan,13; 2015,Jan,16

27725 by synostosis, with fibula, any method
35.1 35.1 FUD 090 C 80 50
AMA: 2018,Sep,7

27726 Repair of fibula nonunion and/or malunion with internal fixation
INCLUDES Osteotomy; fibula (27707)
27.6 27.6 FUD 090 J J8 50
AMA: 2018,Sep,7; 2018,Jan,8; 2017,Jan,8; 2016,Jan,13; 2015,Jan,16

27727 Repair of congenital pseudarthrosis, tibia
29.9 29.9 FUD 090 C 80 50
AMA: 2018,Sep,7

27730 Arrest, epiphyseal (epiphysiodesis), open; distal tibia
16.9 16.9 FUD 090 J A2 50
AMA: 2018,Sep,7

27732 distal fibula
12.9 12.9 FUD 090 J A2 50
AMA: 2018,Sep,7

27734 distal tibia and fibula
18.9 18.9 FUD 090 J A2 50
AMA: 2018,Sep,7

27740 Arrest, epiphyseal (epiphysiodesis), any method, combined, proximal and distal tibia and fibula;
EXCLUDES *Epiphyseal arrest proximal tibia and fibula (27477)*
20.4 20.4 FUD 090 J G2 80 50
AMA: 2018,Sep,7

27742 and distal femur
EXCLUDES *Epiphyseal arrest proximal tibia and fibula (27477)*
22.4 22.4 FUD 090 J A2 80 50
AMA: 2018,Sep,7

27745 Prophylactic treatment (nailing, pinning, plating or wiring) with or without methylmethacrylate, tibia
21.7 21.7 FUD 090 J J8 80 50
AMA: 2018,Sep,7

27750-27848 Treatment of Fracture/Dislocation Lower Leg/Ankle

INCLUDES Treatment open or closed fracture or dislocation

27750 Closed treatment of tibial shaft fracture (with or without fibular fracture); without manipulation
9.18 9.91 FUD 090 T A2 50
AMA: 2018,Sep,7; 2018,Jan,8; 2017,Jan,8; 2016,Jan,13; 2015,Jan,16

27752 with manipulation, with or without skeletal traction
14.1 15.4 FUD 090 J A2 50
AMA: 2018,Sep,7; 2018,Jan,8; 2018,Jan,3; 2017,Jan,8; 2016,Jan,13; 2015,Jan,16

27756 Percutaneous skeletal fixation of tibial shaft fracture (with or without fibular fracture) (eg, pins or screws)
16.6 16.6 FUD 090 J J8 80 50
AMA: 2018,Sep,7; 2018,Jan,8; 2017,Jan,8; 2016,Jan,13; 2015,Jan,16

27758 Open treatment of tibial shaft fracture (with or without fibular fracture), with plate/screws, with or without cerclage
25.8 25.8 FUD 090 J J8 80 50
AMA: 2018,Sep,7; 2018,Jan,8; 2017,Jan,8; 2016,Jan,13; 2015,Jan,16

27759 Treatment of tibial shaft fracture (with or without fibular fracture) by intramedullary implant, with or without interlocking screws and/or cerclage
28.8 28.8 FUD 090 J J8 80 50
AMA: 2018,Sep,7; 2018,Jan,8; 2017,Jan,8; 2016,Jan,13; 2015,Jan,16

27760 Closed treatment of medial malleolus fracture; without manipulation
8.81 9.56 FUD 090 T A2 50
AMA: 2018,Sep,7

27762 with manipulation, with or without skin or skeletal traction
12.4 13.7 FUD 090 J A2 50
AMA: 2018,Sep,7

27766 Open treatment of medial malleolus fracture, includes internal fixation, when performed
17.4 17.4 FUD 090 J A2 50
AMA: 2018,Sep,7

27767 Closed treatment of posterior malleolus fracture; without manipulation
EXCLUDES *Treatment bimalleolar ankle fracture (27808-27814)*
Treatment trimalleolar ankle fracture (27816-27823)
8.20 8.24 FUD 090 T P2 50
AMA: 2018,Sep,7

27768 with manipulation
EXCLUDES *Treatment bimalleolar ankle fracture (27808-27814)*
Treatment trimalleolar ankle fracture (27816-27823)
12.7 12.7 FUD 090 J G2 50
AMA: 2018,Sep,7

27769 Open treatment of posterior malleolus fracture, includes internal fixation, when performed
EXCLUDES *Treatment bimalleolar ankle fracture (27808-27814)*
Treatment trimalleolar ankle fracture (27816-27823)
21.0 21.0 FUD 090 J G2 50
AMA: 2018,Sep,7

27780 Closed treatment of proximal fibula or shaft fracture; without manipulation
8.08 8.80 FUD 090 T A2 50
AMA: 2018,Sep,7; 2018,Jan,8; 2017,Jan,8; 2016,Jan,13; 2015,Jan,16

Musculoskeletal System

27704 — 27780

● New Code ▲ Revised Code ○ Reinstated ● New Web Release ▲ Revised Web Release + Add-on Unlisted Not Covered # Resequenced
Optum Mod 50 Exempt AMA Mod 51 Exempt Optum Mod 51 Exempt Mod 63 Exempt Non-FDA Drug ★ Telemedicine Maternity Age Edit

27781 **with manipulation**
11.3 | 12.3 | FUD 090 | J A2 50
AMA: 2018,Sep,7

27784 **Open treatment of proximal fibula or shaft fracture, includes internal fixation, when performed**
20.6 | 20.6 | FUD 090 | J A2 50
AMA: 2018,Sep,7; 2018,Jan,8; 2017,Jan,8; 2016,Jan,13; 2015,Jan,16

27786 **Closed treatment of distal fibular fracture (lateral malleolus); without manipulation**
8.25 | 9.01 | FUD 090 | T A2 50
AMA: 2018,Sep,7

27788 **with manipulation**
11.1 | 12.2 | FUD 090 | T A2 50
AMA: 2018,Sep,7

27792 **Open treatment of distal fibular fracture (lateral malleolus), includes internal fixation, when performed**
EXCLUDES *Repair tibia and fibula shaft fracture (27750-27759)*
18.6 | 18.6 | FUD 090 | J J8 50
AMA: 2018,Sep,7; 2018,Jan,8; 2017,Jan,8; 2016,Jan,13; 2015,Jan,16

27808 **Closed treatment of bimalleolar ankle fracture (eg, lateral and medial malleoli, or lateral and posterior malleoli or medial and posterior malleoli); without manipulation**
8.70 | 9.57 | FUD 090 | T A2 50
AMA: 2018,Sep,7

27810 **with manipulation**
12.1 | 13.3 | FUD 090 | J A2 50
AMA: 2018,Sep,7

27814 **Open treatment of bimalleolar ankle fracture (eg, lateral and medial malleoli, or lateral and posterior malleoli, or medial and posterior malleoli), includes internal fixation, when performed**
22.1 | 22.1 | FUD 090 | J J8 80 50
AMA: 2018,Sep,7; 2018,Jan,8; 2017,Jan,8; 2016,Feb,13

27816 **Closed treatment of trimalleolar ankle fracture; without manipulation**
8.36 | 9.36 | FUD 090 | T A2 50
AMA: 2018,Sep,7

27818 **with manipulation**
12.4 | 13.9 | FUD 090 | J A2 50
AMA: 2018,Sep,7

27822 **Open treatment of trimalleolar ankle fracture, includes internal fixation, when performed, medial and/or lateral malleolus; without fixation of posterior lip**
24.9 | 24.9 | FUD 090 | J J8 80 50
AMA: 2018,Sep,7

27823 **with fixation of posterior lip**
28.0 | 28.0 | FUD 090 | J J8 80 50
AMA: 2018,Sep,7

27824 **Closed treatment of fracture of weight bearing articular portion of distal tibia (eg, pilon or tibial plafond), with or without anesthesia; without manipulation**
8.71 | 9.02 | FUD 090 | T A2 50
AMA: 2018,Sep,7

27825 **with skeletal traction and/or requiring manipulation**
14.2 | 15.7 | FUD 090 | J A2 80 50
AMA: 2018,Sep,7

27826 **Open treatment of fracture of weight bearing articular surface/portion of distal tibia (eg, pilon or tibial plafond), with internal fixation, when performed; of fibula only**
24.2 | 24.2 | FUD 090 | J J8 80 50
AMA: 2018,Sep,7

27827 **of tibia only**
32.0 | 32.0 | FUD 090 | J J8 80 50
AMA: 2018,Sep,7

27828 **of both tibia and fibula**
38.1 | 38.1 | FUD 090 | J J8 80 50
AMA: 2018,Sep,7; 2018,Jan,8; 2017,Jan,8; 2016,Jan,13; 2015,Jan,16

27829 **Open treatment of distal tibiofibular joint (syndesmosis) disruption, includes internal fixation, when performed**
20.0 | 20.0 | FUD 090 | J A2 80 50
AMA: 2018,Sep,7; 2018,Jan,8; 2017,Jan,8; 2016,Feb,13; 2016,Jan,13; 2015,Jan,16

27830 **Closed treatment of proximal tibiofibular joint dislocation; without anesthesia**
10.2 | 11.1 | FUD 090 | T A2 80 50
AMA: 2018,Sep,7

27831 **requiring anesthesia**
11.6 | 11.6 | FUD 090 | J A2 80 50
AMA: 2018,Sep,7

27832 **Open treatment of proximal tibiofibular joint dislocation, includes internal fixation, when performed, or with excision of proximal fibula**
21.8 | 21.8 | FUD 090 | J A2 80 50
AMA: 2018,Sep,7

27840 **Closed treatment of ankle dislocation; without anesthesia**
10.7 | 10.7 | FUD 090 | T A2 50
AMA: 2018,Sep,7

27842 **requiring anesthesia, with or without percutaneous skeletal fixation**
14.2 | 14.2 | FUD 090 | J A2 50
AMA: 2018,Sep,7

27846 **Open treatment of ankle dislocation, with or without percutaneous skeletal fixation; without repair or internal fixation**
EXCLUDES *Arthroscopy (29894-29898)*
20.6 | 20.6 | FUD 090 | J A2 80 50
AMA: 2018,Sep,7

27848 **with repair or internal or external fixation**
EXCLUDES *Arthroscopy (29894-29898)*
23.0 | 23.0 | FUD 090 | J J8 80 50
AMA: 2018,Sep,7

27860 Ankle Manipulation with Anesthesia

27860 **Manipulation of ankle under general anesthesia (includes application of traction or other fixation apparatus)**
4.91 | 4.91 | FUD 010 | J A2 80 50
AMA: 2018,Sep,7

27870-27871 Arthrodesis Lower Leg/Ankle

27870 **Arthrodesis, ankle, open**
EXCLUDES *Arthroscopic arthrodesis ankle (29899)*
29.5 | 29.5 | FUD 090 | J J8 80 50
AMA: 2020,May,13; 2018,Sep,7

27871 **Arthrodesis, tibiofibular joint, proximal or distal**
19.8 | 19.8 | FUD 090 | J J8 80 50
AMA: 2020,May,13; 2018,Sep,7

27880-27889 Amputations of Lower Leg/Ankle

27880 **Amputation, leg, through tibia and fibula;**
INCLUDES Burgess amputation
26.3 | 26.3 | FUD 090 | C 80 50
AMA: 2018,Sep,7

27881 **with immediate fitting technique including application of first cast**
24.8 | 24.8 | FUD 090 | C 80 50
AMA: 2018,Sep,7

27882 **open, circular (guillotine)**
17.3 | 17.3 | FUD 090 | C 80 50
AMA: 2018,Sep,7

27884 secondary closure or scar revision
16.5 16.5 FUD 090 J A2 50
AMA: 2018,Sep,7

27886 re-amputation
18.9 18.9 FUD 090 C 50
AMA: 2018,Sep,7

27888 **Amputation, ankle, through malleoli of tibia and fibula (eg, Syme, Pirogoff type procedures), with plastic closure and resection of nerves**
18.9 18.9 FUD 090 C 80 50
AMA: 2018,Sep,7

27889 **Ankle disarticulation**
18.6 18.6 FUD 090 J A2 50
AMA: 2018,Sep,7

27892-27899 Decompression Fasciotomy Lower Leg

EXCLUDES *Decompression fasciotomy without debridement (27600-27602)*

27892 **Decompression fasciotomy, leg; anterior and/or lateral compartments only, with debridement of nonviable muscle and/or nerve**
15.8 15.8 FUD 090 J A2 80 50
AMA: 2018,Sep,7

27893 posterior compartment(s) only, with debridement of nonviable muscle and/or nerve
17.5 17.5 FUD 090 J A2 80 50
AMA: 2018,Sep,7

27894 anterior and/or lateral, and posterior compartment(s), with debridement of nonviable muscle and/or nerve
24.3 24.3 FUD 090 J A2 80 50
AMA: 2018,Sep,7

27899 **Unlisted procedure, leg or ankle**
0.00 0.00 FUD YYY T 80 50
AMA: 2020,Apr,8; 2018,Sep,7; 2018,Jan,8; 2017,Jan,8; 2016,Dec,16; 2016,Jan,13; 2015,Jan,16

28001-28008 Surgical Incision Foot/Toe

EXCLUDES *Simple incision and drainage (10060-10160)*

28001 **Incision and drainage, bursa, foot**
4.90 8.03 FUD 010 J P3
AMA: 2018,Sep,7

28002 **Incision and drainage below fascia, with or without tendon sheath involvement, foot; single bursal space**
9.20 12.7 FUD 010 J A2
AMA: 2018,Sep,7

28003 multiple areas
16.0 20.1 FUD 090 J A2
AMA: 2018,Sep,7

28005 **Incision, bone cortex (eg, osteomyelitis or bone abscess), foot**
16.6 16.6 FUD 090 J A2
AMA: 2018,Sep,7

28008 **Fasciotomy, foot and/or toe**
EXCLUDES *Plantar fascia division (28250)*
Plantar fasciectomy (28060, 28062)
8.46 12.5 FUD 090 J A2 50
AMA: 2018,Sep,7

28010-28011 Tenotomy/Toe

EXCLUDES *Open tenotomy (28230-28234)*
Simple incision and drainage (10140-10160)

28010 **Tenotomy, percutaneous, toe; single tendon**
5.99 6.69 FUD 090 J P3
AMA: 2018,Sep,7

28011 multiple tendons
8.10 9.09 FUD 090 J A2
AMA: 2018,Sep,7

28020-28024 Arthrotomy Foot/Toe

EXCLUDES *Simple incision and drainage (10140-10160)*

28020 **Arthrotomy, including exploration, drainage, or removal of loose or foreign body; intertarsal or tarsometatarsal joint**
10.3 15.5 FUD 090 J A2
AMA: 2018,Sep,7

28022 metatarsophalangeal joint
9.36 14.0 FUD 090 J A2
AMA: 2018,Sep,7

28024 interphalangeal joint
8.71 13.1 FUD 090 J A2
AMA: 2018,Sep,7

28035 Tarsal Tunnel Release

EXCLUDES *Other nerve decompression (64722)*
Other neuroplasty (64704)

28035 **Release, tarsal tunnel (posterior tibial nerve decompression)**
10.2 15.2 FUD 090 J A2 50
AMA: 2018,Sep,7

28039-28047 [28039, 28041] Excision Soft Tissue Tumors Foot/Toe

INCLUDES Any necessary elevation tissue planes or dissection
Measurement tumor and necessary margin at greatest diameter prior to excision
Simple and intermediate repairs
Excision types:
- Fascial or subfascial soft tissue tumors: simple and marginal resection tumors found either in or below deep fascia, not involving bone or excision substantial amount normal tissue; primarily benign and intramuscular tumors
  - Tumors fingers and toes involving joint capsules, tendons and tendon sheaths
- Radical resection soft tissue tumor: wide resection tumor, involving substantial margins normal tissue and may involve tissue removal from one or more layers; most often malignant or aggressive benign
  - Tumors fingers and toes adjacent to joints, tendons and tendon sheaths
- Subcutaneous: simple and marginal resection tumors in subcutaneous tissue above deep fascia; most often benign

EXCLUDES *Complex repair*
Excision benign cutaneous lesions (eg, sebaceous cyst) (11420-11426)
Radical resection cutaneous tumors (eg, melanoma) (11620-11626)
Significant vessel exploration, neuroplasty, or reconstruction

28039 **Resequenced code. See code following 28043.**

28041 **Resequenced code. See code following 28045.**

28043 **Excision, tumor, soft tissue of foot or toe, subcutaneous; less than 1.5 cm**
7.52 11.3 FUD 090 J G2 50
AMA: 2018,Sep,7

28039 1.5 cm or greater
9.94 14.3 FUD 090 J G2 80 50
AMA: 2018,Sep,7

28045 **Excision, tumor, soft tissue of foot or toe, subfascial (eg, intramuscular); less than 1.5 cm**
9.97 14.0 FUD 090 J G2 80 50
AMA: 2018,Sep,7

28041 1.5 cm or greater
13.0 13.0 FUD 090 J G2 80 50
AMA: 2018,Sep,7

28046 **Radical resection of tumor (eg, sarcoma), soft tissue of foot or toe; less than 3 cm**
20.6 20.6 FUD 090 J G2 50
AMA: 2018,Sep,7

28047 3 cm or greater
30.1 30.1 FUD 090 J G2 80 50
AMA: 2018,Sep,7

28050-28160 Resection Procedures Foot/Toes

28050 **Arthrotomy with biopsy; intertarsal or tarsometatarsal joint**
8.03 | 12.1 | FUD 090 | J A2 50
AMA: 2002,Apr,13; 1998,Nov,1

28052 **metatarsophalangeal joint**
8.15 | 12.8 | FUD 090 | J A2 50
AMA: 2002,Apr,13

28054 **interphalangeal joint**
6.77 | 10.8 | FUD 090 | J A2 80 50
AMA: 2002,Apr,13

28055 **Neurectomy, intrinsic musculature of foot**
11.1 | 11.1 | FUD 090 | J A2 80 50
AMA: 2002,Apr,13

28060 **Fasciectomy, plantar fascia; partial (separate procedure)**
EXCLUDES *Plantar fasciotomy (28008, 28250)*
10.3 | 15.0 | FUD 090 | J A2 50
AMA: 2018,Jan,8; 2017,Jan,8; 2016,Jan,13; 2015,Jan,16

28062 **radical (separate procedure)**
EXCLUDES *Plantar fasciotomy (28008, 28250)*
11.7 | 16.7 | FUD 090 | J A2 50
AMA: 2002,Apr,13

28070 **Synovectomy; intertarsal or tarsometatarsal joint, each**
10.1 | 15.2 | FUD 090 | J A2
AMA: 2002,Apr,13

28072 **metatarsophalangeal joint, each**
9.23 | 14.0 | FUD 090 | J A2
AMA: 2002,Apr,13

28080 **Excision, interdigital (Morton) neuroma, single, each**
10.6 | 15.1 | FUD 090 | J A2 80
AMA: 2018,Jan,8; 2017,Jan,8; 2016,Jan,13; 2015,Jan,16

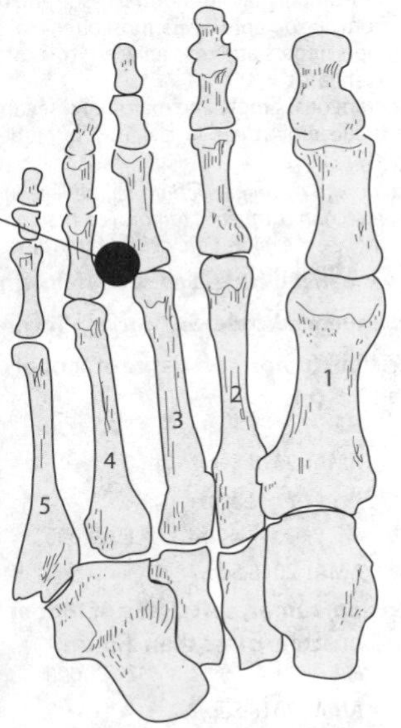

Morton neuroma is a chronic inflammation or irritation of the nerves in the web space between the heads of the metatarsals and phalanges

28086 **Synovectomy, tendon sheath, foot; flexor**
10.2 | 15.4 | FUD 090 | J A2 80 50
AMA: 2002,Apr,13

28088 **extensor**
7.92 | 12.5 | FUD 090 | J A2 80 50
AMA: 2002,Apr,13

28090 **Excision of lesion, tendon, tendon sheath, or capsule (including synovectomy) (eg, cyst or ganglion); foot**
8.86 | 13.5 | FUD 090 | J A2 50
AMA: 2002,Apr,13; 1998,Nov,1

28092 **toe(s), each**
7.75 | 12.2 | FUD 090 | J A2
AMA: 2002,Apr,13; 1998,Nov,1

28100 **Excision or curettage of bone cyst or benign tumor, talus or calcaneus;**
11.9 | 17.6 | FUD 090 | J A2 80 50
AMA: 2002,Apr,13

28102 **with iliac or other autograft (includes obtaining graft)**
17.5 | 17.5 | FUD 090 | J A2 80 50
AMA: 2002,Apr,13

28103 **with allograft**
11.2 | 11.2 | FUD 090 | J A2 80 50
AMA: 2019,May,7

28104 **Excision or curettage of bone cyst or benign tumor, tarsal or metatarsal, except talus or calcaneus;**
10.2 | 15.2 | FUD 090 | J A2 80
AMA: 2002,May,7; 2002,Apr,13

28106 **with iliac or other autograft (includes obtaining graft)**
12.3 | 12.3 | FUD 090 | J A2 80
AMA: 2002,May,7; 2002,Apr,13

28107 **with allograft**
10.0 | 14.7 | FUD 090 | J A2 80
AMA: 2019,May,7

28108 **Excision or curettage of bone cyst or benign tumor, phalanges of foot**
EXCLUDES *Partial excision bone, toe (28124)*
8.30 | 12.7 | FUD 090 | J A2
AMA: 2002,Apr,13

28110 **Ostectomy, partial excision, fifth metatarsal head (bunionette) (separate procedure)**
8.35 | 13.3 | FUD 090 | J A2 50
AMA: 2018,Jan,8; 2017,Jan,8; 2016,Jan,13; 2015,Jan,16

28111 **Ostectomy, complete excision; first metatarsal head**
9.33 | 14.0 | FUD 090 | J A2 50
AMA: 2002,Apr,13

28112 **other metatarsal head (second, third or fourth)**
9.00 | 14.0 | FUD 090 | J A2 50
AMA: 2002,Apr,13

28113 **fifth metatarsal head**
12.1 | 16.9 | FUD 090 | J A2 80 50
AMA: 2002,Apr,13

28114 **all metatarsal heads, with partial proximal phalangectomy, excluding first metatarsal (eg, Clayton type procedure)**
23.9 | 30.7 | FUD 090 | J A2 80 50
AMA: 2002,Apr,13; 1998,Nov,1

28116 **Ostectomy, excision of tarsal coalition**
16.6 | 22.0 | FUD 090 | J A2 50
AMA: 2002,Apr,13

28118 **Ostectomy, calcaneus;**
11.9 | 17.2 | FUD 090 | J A2 80 50
AMA: 2018,Jan,8; 2017,Jan,8; 2016,Jan,13; 2015,Jan,13; 2015,Jan,16

28119 **for spur, with or without plantar fascial release**
10.3 | 15.1 | FUD 090 | J A2 50
AMA: 2018,Jan,8; 2017,Jan,8; 2016,Jan,13; 2015,Jan,16

28120 **Partial excision (craterization, saucerization, sequestrectomy, or diaphysectomy) bone (eg, osteomyelitis or bossing); talus or calcaneus**
INCLUDES Barker operation
14.3 | 19.5 | FUD 090 | J A2 50
AMA: 2018,Jan,8; 2017,Jan,8; 2016,Jan,13; 2015,Jan,16

28122 **tarsal or metatarsal bone, except talus or calcaneus**
EXCLUDES *Hallux rigidus cheilectomy (28289)*
Partial removal talus or calcaneus (28120)
12.6 17.2 FUD 090 J A2 80 50
AMA: 2020,Aug,14

28124 **phalanx of toe**
9.55 13.8 FUD 090 J P3 50
AMA: 2002,Apr,13

28126 **Resection, partial or complete, phalangeal base, each toe**
7.11 11.3 FUD 090 J A2
AMA: 2018,Jan,8; 2017,Jan,8; 2016,Jan,13; 2015,Mar,9

28130 **Talectomy (astragalectomy)**
INCLUDES Whitman astragalectomy
EXCLUDES *Calcanectomy (28118)*
18.2 18.2 FUD 090 J J8 80 50
AMA: 2002,Apr,13

28140 **Metatarsectomy**
12.5 16.9 FUD 090 J A2
AMA: 2002,Apr,13

28150 **Phalangectomy, toe, each toe**
8.04 12.2 FUD 090 J A2
AMA: 2002,Apr,13; 1998,Nov,1

28153 **Resection, condyle(s), distal end of phalanx, each toe**
7.63 11.9 FUD 090 J A2
AMA: 2018,Jan,8; 2017,Jan,8; 2016,Jan,13; 2015,Jan,16

28160 **Hemiphalangectomy or interphalangeal joint excision, toe, proximal end of phalanx, each**
7.69 11.9 FUD 090 J A2
AMA: 2002,Apr,13; 1998,Nov,1

28171-28175 Radical Resection Bone Tumor Foot/Toes

INCLUDES Any necessary elevation tissue planes or dissection
Excision adjacent soft tissue during bone tumor resection (28039-28047 [28039, 28041])
Measurement tumor and necessary margin at greatest diameter prior to excision
Resection tumor (may include entire bone) and wide margins normal tissue primarily for malignant or aggressive benign tumors
Simple and intermediate repairs
EXCLUDES *Complex repair*
Radical tumor resection calcaneus or talus (27647)
Significant vessel exploration, neuroplasty, reconstruction, or complex bone repair

28171 **Radical resection of tumor; tarsal (except talus or calcaneus)**
32.1 32.1 FUD 090 J A2 80
AMA: 2002,Apr,13; 1994,Win,1

28173 **metatarsal**
21.3 21.3 FUD 090 J A2
AMA: 2002,Apr,13; 1994,Win,1

28175 **phalanx of toe**
13.6 13.6 FUD 090 J A2
AMA: 2002,Apr,13

28190-28193 Foreign Body Removal: Foot

28190 **Removal of foreign body, foot; subcutaneous**
3.85 7.35 FUD 010 T P3 50
AMA: 2018,Jan,8; 2017,Jan,8; 2016,Jan,13; 2015,Jan,16

28192 **deep**
9.01 13.5 FUD 090 J A2 50
AMA: 2018,Jan,8; 2017,Jan,8; 2016,Jan,13; 2015,Jan,16

28193 **complicated**
10.6 15.2 FUD 090 J A2 50
AMA: 2002,Apr,13

28200-28360 [28295] Repair/Reconstruction of Foot/Toe

INCLUDES Closed, open, and percutaneous treatment fractures and dislocations

28200 **Repair, tendon, flexor, foot; primary or secondary, without free graft, each tendon**
9.33 14.2 FUD 090 J A2
AMA: 2018,Jan,8; 2017,Jan,8; 2016,Feb,15; 2016,Jan,13; 2015,Jan,16

28202 **secondary with free graft, each tendon (includes obtaining graft)**
12.4 17.4 FUD 090 J A2 80
AMA: 2002,Apr,13

28208 **Repair, tendon, extensor, foot; primary or secondary, each tendon**
9.11 13.9 FUD 090 J A2
AMA: 2002,Apr,13; 1998,Nov,1

28210 **secondary with free graft, each tendon (includes obtaining graft)**
12.0 16.9 FUD 090 J A2 80
AMA: 2002,Apr,13

28220 **Tenolysis, flexor, foot; single tendon**
8.72 13.0 FUD 090 J P3 50
AMA: 2002,Apr,13; 1998,Nov,1

28222 **multiple tendons**
10.2 14.9 FUD 090 J A2 50
AMA: 2002,Apr,13; 1998,Nov,1

28225 **Tenolysis, extensor, foot; single tendon**
7.59 12.0 FUD 090 J A2 50
AMA: 2002,Apr,13; 1998,Nov,1

28226 **multiple tendons**
11.3 17.6 FUD 090 J A2 50
AMA: 2002,Apr,13; 1998,Nov,1

28230 **Tenotomy, open, tendon flexor; foot, single or multiple tendon(s) (separate procedure)**
8.16 12.5 FUD 090 J P3 50
AMA: 2002,Apr,13; 1998,Nov,1

28232 **toe, single tendon (separate procedure)**
6.95 11.1 FUD 090 J P3
AMA: 2020,Apr,10; 2018,Jan,8; 2017,Jan,8; 2016,Jan,13; 2015,Mar,9

28234 **Tenotomy, open, extensor, foot or toe, each tendon**
EXCLUDES *Tendon transfer (27690-27691)*
7.59 11.8 FUD 090 J A2
AMA: 2018,Jan,8; 2017,Jan,8; 2016,Jan,13; 2015,Jan,16

28238 **Reconstruction (advancement), posterior tibial tendon with excision of accessory tarsal navicular bone (eg, Kidner type procedure)**
EXCLUDES *Extensor hallucis longus transfer with big toe fusion (Jones procedure) (28760)*
Subcutaneous tenotomy (28010-28011)
Transfer or transplant tendon with muscle redirection or rerouting (27690-27692)
13.9 19.2 FUD 090 J A2 80 50
AMA: 2002,Apr,13; 2002,May,7

28240 **Tenotomy, lengthening, or release, abductor hallucis muscle**
8.46 12.9 FUD 090 J A2 50
AMA: 2002,Apr,13

28250 **Division of plantar fascia and muscle (eg, Steindler stripping) (separate procedure)**
11.6 16.7 FUD 090 J A2 80 50
AMA: 2002,Apr,13; 1998,Nov,1

28260 **Capsulotomy, midfoot; medial release only (separate procedure)**
14.9 20.2 FUD 090 J A2 80 50
AMA: 2002,Apr,13

28261 **with tendon lengthening**
27.0 34.6 **FUD** 090 J A2 80 50
AMA: 2002,Apr,13

28262 **extensive, including posterior talotibial capsulotomy and tendon(s) lengthening (eg, resistant clubfoot deformity)**
32.5 40.4 **FUD** 090 J J8 80 50
AMA: 2002,Apr,13; 1998,Nov,1

28264 **Capsulotomy, midtarsal (eg, Heyman type procedure)**
22.2 29.1 **FUD** 090 J A2 80 50
AMA: 2002,Apr,13; 1998,Nov,1

28270 **Capsulotomy; metatarsophalangeal joint, with or without tenorrhaphy, each joint (separate procedure)**
9.64 14.2 **FUD** 090 J A2 50
AMA: 2018,Jan,8; 2017,Jan,8; 2016,Jan,13; 2015,Jan,16

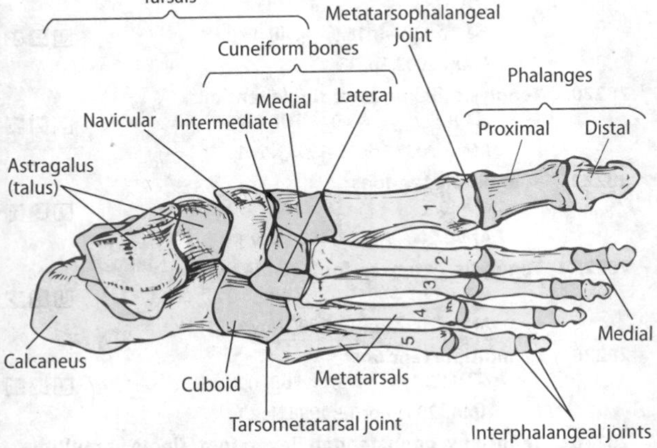

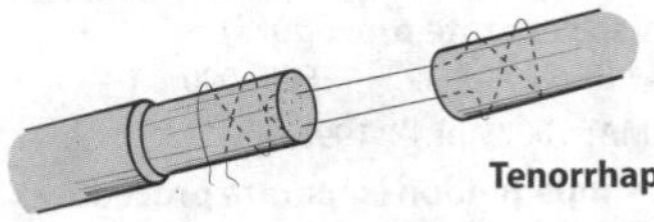
Tenorrhaphy

28272 **interphalangeal joint, each joint (separate procedure)**
7.27 11.3 **FUD** 090 J P3 50
AMA: 2018,Jan,8; 2017,Jan,8; 2016,Jan,13; 2015,Jan,16

28280 **Syndactylization, toes (eg, webbing or Kelikian type procedure)**
10.0 14.8 **FUD** 090 J A2 80 50
AMA: 2002,Apr,13; 1998,Nov,1

28285 **Correction, hammertoe (eg, interphalangeal fusion, partial or total phalangectomy)**
10.9 15.5 **FUD** 090 J A2 50
AMA: 2018,Jan,8; 2017,Jan,8; 2016,Jun,8; 2016,Jan,13; 2015,Mar,9; 2015,Jan,16

28286 **Correction, cock-up fifth toe, with plastic skin closure (eg, Ruiz-Mora type procedure)**
8.56 12.8 **FUD** 090 J A2 50
AMA: 2002,Apr,13; 1998,Nov,1

28288 **Ostectomy, partial, exostectomy or condylectomy, metatarsal head, each metatarsal head**
12.4 17.5 **FUD** 090 J A2
AMA: 2002,Apr,13; 1998,Nov,1

28289 **Hallux rigidus correction with cheilectomy, debridement and capsular release of the first metatarsophalangeal joint; without implant**
13.2 20.5 **FUD** 090 J A2 80 50
AMA: 2020,Aug,14; 2020,Jul,13; 2018,Jan,8; 2017,Jan,8; 2016,Dec,3; 2016,Jan,13; 2015,Sep,12; 2015,Jan,16

28291 **with implant**
14.1 21.0 **FUD** 090 J J8 80 50
AMA: 2020,Aug,14; 2018,Jan,8; 2017,Nov,10; 2017,Jan,8; 2016,Dec,3

28292 **Correction, hallux valgus (bunionectomy), with sesamoidectomy, when performed; with resection of proximal phalanx base, when performed, any method**
13.9 21.3 **FUD** 090 J A2 80 50
AMA: 2018,Jan,8; 2017,Jan,8; 2016,Dec,3; 2016,Jan,13; 2015,Jan,16

28295 **Resequenced code. See code following 28296.**

28296 **with distal metatarsal osteotomy, any method**
14.8 26.3 **FUD** 090 J A2 80 50
AMA: 2020,Jul,13; 2018,Sep,14; 2018,Jan,8; 2017,Jan,8; 2016,Dec,3; 2016,Jan,13; 2015,Jan,16

28295 **with proximal metatarsal osteotomy, any method**
16.1 28.5 **FUD** 090 J G2 80 50
AMA: 2018,Jan,8; 2017,Jan,8; 2016,Dec,3

28297 **with first metatarsal and medial cuneiform joint arthrodesis, any method**
17.4 30.2 **FUD** 090 J J8 80 50
AMA: 2018,Jan,8; 2017,Jan,8; 2016,Dec,3; 2016,Jan,13; 2015,Jan,16

28298 **with proximal phalanx osteotomy, any method**
INCLUDES Akin procedure
14.3 24.3 **FUD** 090 J A2 80 50
AMA: 2018,Jan,8; 2017,Jan,8; 2016,Dec,3; 2016,Jan,13; 2015,Jan,16

28299 **with double osteotomy, any method**
16.8 29.1 **FUD** 090 J A2 80 50
AMA: 2018,Jan,8; 2017,Jan,8; 2016,Dec,3; 2016,Apr,8; 2016,Jan,13; 2015,Jan,16

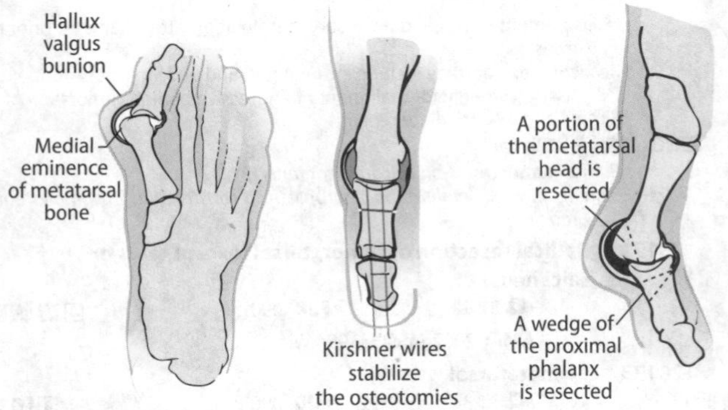

28300 **Osteotomy; calcaneus (eg, Dwyer or Chambers type procedure), with or without internal fixation**
18.7 18.7 **FUD** 090 J J8 80 50
AMA: 2002,Apr,13; 1998,Nov,1

28302 **talus**
20.6 20.6 **FUD** 090 J A2 80 50
AMA: 2002,Apr,13

28304 **Osteotomy, tarsal bones, other than calcaneus or talus;**
17.3 23.6 **FUD** 090 J A2 80 50
AMA: 2002,Apr,13; 1998,Nov,1

28305 **with autograft (includes obtaining graft) (eg, Fowler type)**
19.3 19.3 **FUD** 090 J J8 80 50
AMA: 2002,Apr,13; 1998,Nov,1

28306 **Osteotomy, with or without lengthening, shortening or angular correction, metatarsal; first metatarsal**
11.6 17.6 **FUD** 090 J A2 80 50
AMA: 2018,Jan,8; 2017,Jan,8; 2016,Jan,13; 2015,Jan,16

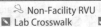

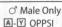

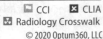

28307 **first metatarsal with autograft (other than first toe)**
11.9 17.9 **FUD** 090 J A2 80 50
AMA: 2002,Apr,13; 1998,Nov,1

28308 **other than first metatarsal, each**
10.9 16.4 **FUD** 090 J A2 80 50
AMA: 2002,Apr,13; 1998,Nov,1

28309 **multiple (eg, Swanson type cavus foot procedure)**
25.5 25.5 **FUD** 090 J A2 80 50
AMA: 2018,Jan,8; 2017,Jan,8; 2016,Jan,13; 2015,Jan,16

28310 **Osteotomy, shortening, angular or rotational correction; proximal phalanx, first toe (separate procedure)**
10.3 15.7 **FUD** 090 J A2 50
AMA: 2018,Jan,8; 2017,Jan,8; 2016,Jan,13; 2015,Jan,16

28312 **other phalanges, any toe**
9.12 14.4 **FUD** 090 J A2
AMA: 2002,Apr,13

28313 **Reconstruction, angular deformity of toe, soft tissue procedures only (eg, overlapping second toe, fifth toe, curly toes)**
10.2 15.1 **FUD** 090 J A2
AMA: 2002,Apr,13; 1998,Nov,1

28315 **Sesamoidectomy, first toe (separate procedure)**
9.38 13.9 **FUD** 090 J A2 50
AMA: 2002,Apr,13

28320 **Repair, nonunion or malunion; tarsal bones**
17.5 17.5 **FUD** 090 J J8 80 50
AMA: 2002,Apr,13; 1998,Nov,1

28322 **metatarsal, with or without bone graft (includes obtaining graft)**
16.5 22.5 **FUD** 090 J J8 80
AMA: 2002,Apr,13

28340 **Reconstruction, toe, macrodactyly; soft tissue resection**
11.8 16.5 **FUD** 090 J A2
AMA: 2002,Apr,13

28341 **requiring bone resection**
14.1 19.3 **FUD** 090 J A2
AMA: 2002,Apr,13

28344 **Reconstruction, toe(s); polydactyly**
8.04 12.2 **FUD** 090 J A2 50
AMA: 2002,Apr,13

28345 **syndactyly, with or without skin graft(s), each web**
10.5 14.9 **FUD** 090 J A2 80
AMA: 2002,Apr,13

28360 **Reconstruction, cleft foot**
31.4 31.4 **FUD** 090 J 80 50
AMA: 2002,Apr,13

28400-28675 Treatment of Fracture/Dislocation of Foot/Toe

28400 **Closed treatment of calcaneal fracture; without manipulation**
6.55 7.09 **FUD** 090 T A2 50
AMA: 2002,Apr,13

28405 **with manipulation**
INCLUDES Bohler reduction
10.0 11.1 **FUD** 090 T A2 80 50
AMA: 2002,Apr,13

28406 **Percutaneous skeletal fixation of calcaneal fracture, with manipulation**
15.1 15.1 **FUD** 090 J A2 80 50
AMA: 2002,Apr,13

28415 **Open treatment of calcaneal fracture, includes internal fixation, when performed;**
32.2 32.2 **FUD** 090 J J8 80 50
AMA: 2002,Apr,13

28420 **with primary iliac or other autogenous bone graft (includes obtaining graft)**
37.1 37.1 **FUD** 090 J J8 80 50
AMA: 2002,Apr,13

28430 **Closed treatment of talus fracture; without manipulation**
6.03 6.85 **FUD** 090 T P2 50
AMA: 2002,Apr,13

28435 **with manipulation**
9.31 10.4 **FUD** 090 J A2 80 50
AMA: 2002,Apr,13

28436 **Percutaneous skeletal fixation of talus fracture, with manipulation**
12.9 12.9 **FUD** 090 J G2 50
AMA: 2002,Apr,13

28445 **Open treatment of talus fracture, includes internal fixation, when performed**
29.9 29.9 **FUD** 090 J J8 80 50
AMA: 2002,Apr,13

28446 **Open osteochondral autograft, talus (includes obtaining graft[s])**
INCLUDES Osteotomy; fibula (27707)
Osteotomy; tibia (27705)
EXCLUDES *Arthroscopically aided osteochondral talus graft (29892)*
Open osteochondral allograft or repairs with industrial grafts (28899)
35.3 35.3 **FUD** 090 J G2 80 50
AMA: 2018,Jan,8; 2017,Jan,8; 2016,Jan,13; 2015,Jan,16

28450 **Treatment of tarsal bone fracture (except talus and calcaneus); without manipulation, each**
5.47 6.07 **FUD** 090 T P2
AMA: 2018,Jan,8; 2017,Jan,8; 2016,Jan,13; 2015,Jan,16

28455 **with manipulation, each**
7.40 8.27 **FUD** 090 J P3 80
AMA: 2002,Apr,13

28456 **Percutaneous skeletal fixation of tarsal bone fracture (except talus and calcaneus), with manipulation, each**
9.74 9.74 **FUD** 090 J A2
AMA: 2002,Apr,13

28465 **Open treatment of tarsal bone fracture (except talus and calcaneus), includes internal fixation, when performed, each**
18.1 18.1 **FUD** 090 J J8
AMA: 2019,Aug,10

28470 **Closed treatment of metatarsal fracture; without manipulation, each**
5.85 6.26 **FUD** 090 T P2
AMA: 2002,Apr,13

28475 **with manipulation, each**
6.52 7.37 **FUD** 090 T P2
AMA: 2002,Apr,13

28476 **Percutaneous skeletal fixation of metatarsal fracture, with manipulation, each**
10.5 10.5 **FUD** 090 J A2 80
AMA: 2002,Apr,13

28485 **Open treatment of metatarsal fracture, includes internal fixation, when performed, each**
15.8 15.8 **FUD** 090 J J8
AMA: 2019,Aug,10

28490 **Closed treatment of fracture great toe, phalanx or phalanges; without manipulation**
3.57 4.12 **FUD** 090 T P3 50
AMA: 2002,Apr,13

28495 **with manipulation**
4.25 5.10 **FUD** 090 T P2 50
AMA: 2002,Apr,13

28496 **Percutaneous skeletal fixation of fracture great toe, phalanx or phalanges, with manipulation**
6.93 12.9 FUD 090 J A2 50
AMA: 2002,Apr,13

28505 **Open treatment of fracture, great toe, phalanx or phalanges, includes internal fixation, when performed**
14.3 19.1 FUD 090 J A2 50
AMA: 2002,Apr,13

28510 **Closed treatment of fracture, phalanx or phalanges, other than great toe; without manipulation, each**
3.41 3.47 FUD 090 T P3
AMA: 2002,Apr,13

28515 **with manipulation, each**
4.08 4.67 FUD 090 T P3
AMA: 2002,Apr,13

28525 **Open treatment of fracture, phalanx or phalanges, other than great toe, includes internal fixation, when performed, each**
11.6 16.5 FUD 090 J A2 80
AMA: 2002,Apr,13

28530 **Closed treatment of sesamoid fracture**
2.88 3.30 FUD 090 T P3 80 50
AMA: 2002,Apr,13

28531 **Open treatment of sesamoid fracture, with or without internal fixation**
5.22 9.73 FUD 090 J A2 50
AMA: 2002,Apr,13

28540 **Closed treatment of tarsal bone dislocation, other than talotarsal; without anesthesia**
5.01 5.57 FUD 090 T P2 80 50
AMA: 2002,Apr,13

28545 **requiring anesthesia**
7.62 8.67 FUD 090 J G2 80 50
AMA: 2002,Apr,13

28546 **Percutaneous skeletal fixation of tarsal bone dislocation, other than talotarsal, with manipulation**
9.85 16.7 FUD 090 J A2 80 50
AMA: 2002,Apr,13

28555 **Open treatment of tarsal bone dislocation, includes internal fixation, when performed**
18.7 24.6 FUD 090 J A2 80 50
AMA: 2002,Apr,13

28570 **Closed treatment of talotarsal joint dislocation; without anesthesia**
5.52 6.57 FUD 090 T P2 80 50
AMA: 2002,Apr,13

28575 **requiring anesthesia**
9.57 10.6 FUD 090 J A2 80 50
AMA: 2002,Apr,13

28576 **Percutaneous skeletal fixation of talotarsal joint dislocation, with manipulation**
11.1 11.1 FUD 090 J A2 80 50
AMA: 2002,Apr,13

28585 **Open treatment of talotarsal joint dislocation, includes internal fixation, when performed**
19.6 25.0 FUD 090 J J8 80 50
AMA: 2018,Jan,8; 2017,Jan,8; 2016,Jan,13; 2015,Jan,16

28600 **Closed treatment of tarsometatarsal joint dislocation; without anesthesia**
5.35 6.26 FUD 090 T P2 80
AMA: 2002,Apr,13

28605 **requiring anesthesia**
8.57 9.58 FUD 090 T A2 80
AMA: 2002,Apr,13

28606 **Percutaneous skeletal fixation of tarsometatarsal joint dislocation, with manipulation**
11.1 11.1 FUD 090 J A2
AMA: 2002,Apr,13

28615 **Open treatment of tarsometatarsal joint dislocation, includes internal fixation, when performed**
23.4 23.4 FUD 090 J J8 80
AMA: 2002,Apr,13

28630 **Closed treatment of metatarsophalangeal joint dislocation; without anesthesia**
3.15 4.49 FUD 010 T P3 80
AMA: 2002,Apr,13

28635 **requiring anesthesia**
3.81 5.04 FUD 010 J A2 80
AMA: 2002,Apr,13

28636 **Percutaneous skeletal fixation of metatarsophalangeal joint dislocation, with manipulation**
5.74 8.98 FUD 010 J A2
AMA: 2002,Apr,13

28645 **Open treatment of metatarsophalangeal joint dislocation, includes internal fixation, when performed**
14.0 18.9 FUD 090 J A2
AMA: 2018,Jan,8; 2017,Jan,8; 2016,Jan,13; 2015,Jan,16

28660 **Closed treatment of interphalangeal joint dislocation; without anesthesia**
2.56 3.38 FUD 010 T P3
AMA: 2002,Apr,13

28665 **requiring anesthesia**
3.72 4.41 FUD 010 T A2 80
AMA: 2002,Apr,13

28666 **Percutaneous skeletal fixation of interphalangeal joint dislocation, with manipulation**
4.79 4.79 FUD 010 J A2
AMA: 2002,Apr,13

28675 **Open treatment of interphalangeal joint dislocation, includes internal fixation, when performed**
11.6 16.4 FUD 090 J A2
AMA: 2002,Apr,13

28705-28760 Arthrodesis of Foot/Toe

28705 **Arthrodesis; pantalar**
35.4 35.4 FUD 090 J J8 80 50
AMA: 2020,May,13

28715 **triple**
27.1 27.1 FUD 090 J J8 80 50
AMA: 2020,May,13

28725 **subtalar**
INCLUDES Dunn arthrodesis
Grice arthrodesis
22.4 22.4 FUD 090 J J8 80 50
AMA: 2020,May,13; 2018,Jan,8; 2017,Jan,8; 2016,Jan,13; 2015,Jan,16

28730 **Arthrodesis, midtarsal or tarsometatarsal, multiple or transverse;**
INCLUDES Lambrinudi arthrodesis
21.2 21.2 FUD 090 J J8 80 50
AMA: 2020,May,13

28735 **with osteotomy (eg, flatfoot correction)**
22.4 22.4 FUD 090 J J8 80 50
AMA: 2020,May,13; 2019,May,10

28737 **Arthrodesis, with tendon lengthening and advancement, midtarsal, tarsal navicular-cuneiform (eg, Miller type procedure)**
19.8 19.8 FUD 090 J J8 80 50
AMA: 2020,May,13

28740 **Arthrodesis, midtarsal or tarsometatarsal, single joint**
17.9 24.3 FUD 090 J J8 80 50
AMA: 2020,May,13; 2018,Jan,8; 2017,Jan,8; 2016,Jan,13; 2015,Jan,16

28750 **Arthrodesis, great toe; metatarsophalangeal joint**
16.8 22.9 FUD 090 J J8 80 50
AMA: 2020,May,13; 2018,Jan,8; 2017,Jan,8; 2016,Dec,3; 2016,Jan,13; 2015,Jan,16

28755 **interphalangeal joint**
9.56 14.7 FUD 090 J A2 50
AMA: 2020,May,13

28760 **Arthrodesis, with extensor hallucis longus transfer to first metatarsal neck, great toe, interphalangeal joint (eg, Jones type procedure)**
INCLUDES Jones procedure
EXCLUDES *Hammer toe repair or interphalangeal fusion (28285)*
16.6 22.5 FUD 090 J A2 80 50
AMA: 2020,May,13

28800-28825 Amputation Foot/Toe

28800 **Amputation, foot; midtarsal (eg, Chopart type procedure)**
15.4 15.4 FUD 090 C 80 50
AMA: 2002,Apr,13; 1998,Nov,1

28805 **transmetatarsal**
20.9 20.9 FUD 090 J 80 50
AMA: 2002,Apr,13; 1997,May,4

28810 **Amputation, metatarsal, with toe, single**
12.3 12.3 FUD 090 J A2 80
AMA: 2002,Apr,13

28820 **Amputation, toe; metatarsophalangeal joint**
11.3 16.1 FUD 090 J A2
AMA: 2002,Apr,13; 1997,May,4

28825 **interphalangeal joint**
10.6 15.4 FUD 090 J A2
AMA: 2002,Apr,13

28890-28899 Other/Unlisted Procedures Foot/Toe

28890 **Extracorporeal shock wave, high energy, performed by a physician or other qualified health care professional, requiring anesthesia other than local, including ultrasound guidance, involving the plantar fascia**
EXCLUDES *Extracorporeal shock wave therapy integumentary system not otherwise specified, when performed on same treatment area ([0512T, 0513T])*
Extracorporeal shock wave therapy musculoskeletal system not otherwise specified (0101T-0102T)
6.38 9.18 FUD 090 J P3 50
AMA: 2018,Dec,5; 2018,Dec,5; 2018,Jan,8; 2017,Jan,8; 2016,Jan,13; 2015,Jan,16

28899 **Unlisted procedure, foot or toes**
0.00 0.00 FUD YYY T 80
AMA: 2018,Oct,11; 2018,Jan,8; 2017,Nov,10; 2017,Sep,14; 2017,Jan,8; 2016,Dec,3; 2016,Jun,8; 2016,Jan,13; 2015,Nov,10; 2015,Jan,16

29000-29086 Casting: Arm/Shoulder/Torso

INCLUDES Application cast or strapping when provided as:
- Initial service to stabilize fracture or injury without restorative treatment
- Replacement procedure

Removal cast

EXCLUDES *Cast or splint material*
E/M services provided as initial service when restorative treatment not provided
Orthotic supervision and training (97760-97763)

29000 **Application of halo type body cast (see 20661-20663 for insertion)**
5.57 9.69 FUD 000 T G2 80
AMA: 2018,Jan,8; 2018,Jan,3; 2017,Jan,8; 2016,Jan,13; 2015,Jan,16

29010 **Application of Risser jacket, localizer, body; only**
4.58 7.63 FUD 000 T P2 80
AMA: 2018,Jan,8; 2018,Jan,3; 2017,Jan,8; 2016,Jan,13; 2015,Jan,16

29015 **including head**
5.18 8.22 FUD 000 T P2 80
AMA: 2018,Jan,8; 2018,Jan,3; 2017,Jan,8; 2016,Jan,13; 2015,Jan,16

29035 **Application of body cast, shoulder to hips;**
4.08 7.13 FUD 000 T P2 80
AMA: 2018,Jan,8; 2018,Jan,3; 2017,Jan,8; 2016,Jan,13; 2015,Jan,16

29040 **including head, Minerva type**
4.95 8.17 FUD 000 T G2 80
AMA: 2018,Jan,8; 2018,Jan,3; 2017,Jan,8; 2016,Jan,13; 2015,Jan,16

29044 **including 1 thigh**
4.78 8.01 FUD 000 T P2 80
AMA: 2018,Jan,8; 2018,Jan,3; 2017,Jan,8; 2016,Jan,13; 2015,Jan,16

29046 **including both thighs**
5.37 8.78 FUD 000 T G2 80
AMA: 2018,Jan,8; 2018,Jan,3; 2017,Jan,8; 2016,Jan,13; 2015,Jan,16

29049 **Application, cast; figure-of-eight**
2.00 2.79 FUD 000 T P3 80
AMA: 2018,Jan,3; 2018,Jan,8; 2017,Jan,8; 2016,Jan,13; 2015,Jan,16

29055 **shoulder spica**
3.93 6.22 FUD 000 T P2 80
AMA: 2018,Jan,8; 2018,Jan,3; 2017,Jan,8; 2016,Jan,13; 2015,Jan,16

29058 **plaster Velpeau**
2.71 3.51 FUD 000 T P3 80
AMA: 2018,Jan,8; 2018,Jan,3; 2017,Jan,8; 2016,Jan,13; 2015,Jan,16

29065 **shoulder to hand (long arm)**
1.95 2.70 FUD 000 T P3 50
AMA: 2018,Jan,8; 2018,Jan,3; 2017,Jan,8; 2016,Jan,13; 2015,Jan,16

29075 **elbow to finger (short arm)**
1.76 2.43 FUD 000 T P3 50
AMA: 2018,Jan,8; 2018,Jan,3; 2017,Jan,8; 2016,Jan,13; 2015,Jan,16

29085 **hand and lower forearm (gauntlet)**
1.92 2.68 FUD 000 T P3 50
AMA: 2018,Jan,3; 2018,Jan,8; 2017,Jan,8; 2016,Jan,13; 2015,Jan,16

29086 **finger (eg, contracture)**
1.47 2.22 FUD 000 T P3 50
AMA: 2018,Jan,8; 2018,Jan,3; 2017,Jan,8; 2016,Jan,13; 2015,Jan,16

29105-29280 Splinting and Strapping: Torso/Upper Extremities

INCLUDES Application splint or strapping when provided as:
- Initial service to stabilize fracture or dislocation
- Replacement procedure

EXCLUDES *E/M services provided as initial service when restorative treatment not provided*
Orthotic supervision and training (97760-97763)
Splinting and strapping material

29105 **Application of long arm splint (shoulder to hand)**
1.38 2.33 FUD 000 T P3 50
AMA: 2018,Jan,3; 2018,Jan,8; 2017,Jan,8; 2016,Jan,13; 2015,Jan,16

29125 **Application of short arm splint (forearm to hand); static**
1.13 1.82 FUD 000 01 N1 50
AMA: 2018,Jan,8; 2018,Jan,3; 2017,Jan,8; 2016,Jan,13; 2015,Jan,16

29126 **dynamic**
1.40 | 2.18 | FUD 000 | Q1 N1 50
AMA: 2018,Jan,8; 2018,Jan,3; 2017,Jan,8; 2016,Jan,13; 2015,Jan,16

29130 **Application of finger splint; static**
0.85 | 1.18 | FUD 000 | Q1 N1 50
AMA: 2018,Jan,8; 2018,Jan,3; 2017,Jan,8; 2016,Jan,13; 2015,Jan,16

29131 **dynamic**
0.98 | 1.48 | FUD 000 | Q1 N1 50
AMA: 2018,Jan,8; 2018,Jan,3; 2017,Jan,8; 2016,Jan,13; 2015,Jan,16

29200 **Strapping; thorax**
EXCLUDES *Strapping of low back (29799)*
0.54 | 0.93 | FUD 000 | T P3
AMA: 2018,Jan,8; 2018,Jan,3; 2017,Jan,8; 2016,Jan,13; 2015,Jan,16

29240 **shoulder (eg, Velpeau)**
0.54 | 0.87 | FUD 000 | Q1 N1 50
AMA: 2018,Jan,3; 2018,Jan,8; 2017,Jan,8; 2016,Jan,13; 2015,Jan,16

29260 **elbow or wrist**
0.56 | 0.86 | FUD 000 | Q1 N1 50
AMA: 2018,Jan,8; 2018,Jan,3; 2017,Jan,8; 2016,Jan,13; 2015,Jan,16

29280 **hand or finger**
0.60 | 0.88 | FUD 000 | Q1 N1 50
AMA: 2018,Jan,8; 2018,Jan,3; 2017,Jan,8; 2016,Jan,13; 2015,Jan,16

29305-29450 Casting: Legs

INCLUDES Application cast when provided as:
- Initial service to stabilize fracture or injury without restorative treatment
- Replacement procedure

Removal cast

EXCLUDES *Cast or splint materials*
E/M services provided as part initial service when restorative treatment is not provided
Orthotic supervision and training (97760-97763)

29305 **Application of hip spica cast; 1 leg**
EXCLUDES *Hip spica cast thighs only (29046)*
4.57 | 7.02 | FUD 000 | T P2 80
AMA: 2018,Jan,8; 2018,Jan,3; 2017,Jan,8; 2016,Jan,13; 2015,Jan,16

29325 **1 and one-half spica or both legs**
EXCLUDES *Hip spica cast thighs only (29046)*
5.11 | 7.75 | FUD 000 | T P2 80
AMA: 2018,Jan,8; 2018,Jan,3; 2017,Jan,8; 2016,Jan,13; 2015,Jan,16

29345 **Application of long leg cast (thigh to toes);**
2.87 | 3.85 | FUD 000 | T P3 50
AMA: 2018,Jan,3; 2018,Jan,8; 2017,Jan,8; 2016,Jan,13; 2015,Jan,16

29355 **walker or ambulatory type**
3.07 | 4.03 | FUD 000 | T P3 50
AMA: 2018,Jan,3; 2018,Jan,8; 2017,Jan,8; 2016,Jan,13; 2015,Jan,16

29358 **Application of long leg cast brace**
2.96 | 4.51 | FUD 000 | T P3 50
AMA: 2018,Jan,3; 2018,Jan,8; 2017,Jan,8; 2016,Jan,13; 2015,Jan,16

29365 **Application of cylinder cast (thigh to ankle)**
2.51 | 3.49 | FUD 000 | T P3 50
AMA: 2018,Jan,3; 2018,Jan,8; 2017,Jan,8; 2016,Jan,13; 2015,Jan,16

29405 **Application of short leg cast (below knee to toes);**
1.69 | 2.26 | FUD 000 | T P3 50
AMA: 2018,Jan,3; 2018,Jan,8; 2017,Jan,8; 2016,Jan,13; 2015,Jan,16

29425 **walking or ambulatory type**
1.59 | 2.17 | FUD 000 | T P3 50
AMA: 2018,Jan,3; 2018,Jan,8; 2017,Jan,8; 2016,Jan,13; 2015,Jan,16

29435 **Application of patellar tendon bearing (PTB) cast**
2.35 | 3.25 | FUD 000 | T P3 50
AMA: 2018,Jan,3; 2018,Jan,8; 2017,Jan,8; 2016,Jan,13; 2015,Jan,16

29440 **Adding walker to previously applied cast**
0.83 | 1.23 | FUD 000 | T P3 50
AMA: 2018,Jan,8; 2018,Jan,3; 2017,Jan,8; 2016,Jan,13; 2015,Jan,16

29445 **Application of rigid total contact leg cast**
2.94 | 3.73 | FUD 000 | T P3 50
AMA: 2018,Jan,3; 2018,Jan,8; 2017,Jan,8; 2016,Jan,13; 2015,Jan,16

29450 **Application of clubfoot cast with molding or manipulation, long or short leg**
3.26 | 4.11 | FUD 000 | T P3 50
AMA: 2018,Jan,8; 2018,Jan,3; 2017,Jan,8; 2016,Jan,13; 2015,Jan,16

29505-29584 Splinting and Strapping Ankle/Foot/Leg/Toes

INCLUDES Application splinting and strapping when provided as:
- Initial service to stabilize fracture or injury without restorative treatment
- Replacement procedure

EXCLUDES *E/M services provided as part initial service when restorative treatment not provided*
Orthotic supervision and training (97760-97763)

29505 **Application of long leg splint (thigh to ankle or toes)**
1.45 | 2.41 | FUD 000 | T P3 50
AMA: 2018,Jan,3; 2018,Jan,8; 2017,Jan,8; 2016,Jan,13; 2015,Jan,16

29515 **Application of short leg splint (calf to foot)**
1.42 | 2.01 | FUD 000 | T P3 50
AMA: 2019,Oct,10; 2018,Jan,8; 2018,Jan,3; 2017,Jan,8; 2016,Jan,13; 2015,Jan,16

29520 **Strapping; hip**
EXCLUDES *For treatment in same extremity:*
Endovenous ablation therapy incompetent vein (36473-36479, [36482], [36483])
Sclerosal injection for incompetent vein(s) ([36465], [36466], 36468-36471)
0.55 | 1.00 | FUD 000 | Q1 N1 80 50
AMA: 2018,Jan,8; 2018,Jan,3; 2017,Jan,8; 2016,Jan,13; 2015,Jan,16

29530 **knee**
EXCLUDES *For treatment in same extremity:*
Endovenous ablation therapy incompetent vein (36473-36479, [36482], [36483])
Sclerosal injection for incompetent vein(s) ([36465], [36466], 36468-36471)
0.54 | 0.87 | FUD 000 | Q1 N1 50
AMA: 2018,Jan,3; 2018,Jan,8; 2017,Jan,8; 2016,Jan,13; 2015,Jan,16

29540 **ankle and/or foot**
EXCLUDES *For treatment in same extremity:*
Endovenous ablation therapy incompetent vein (36473-36479, [36482, 36483])
Multi-layer compression system (29581)
Sclerosal injection for incompetent vein(s) ([36465], [36466], 36468-36471)
Unna boot (29580)
0.51 | 0.81 | FUD 000 | T P3 50
AMA: 2018,Jan,3; 2018,Jan,8; 2017,Jan,8; 2016,Aug,3; 2016,Jan,13; 2015,Jan,16

29550 **toes**

EXCLUDES *For treatment in same extremity:*
Endovenous ablation therapy incompetent vein (36473-36479, [36482, 36483])
Sclerosal injection for incompetent vein(s) ([36465], [36466], 36468-36471)

0.33 0.54 FUD 000 Q1 N1 50

AMA: 2018,Jan,8; 2018,Jan,3; 2017,Jan,8; 2016,Jan,13; 2015,Jan,16

29580 **Unna boot**

EXCLUDES *Application multilayer compression system (29581)*
For treatment in same extremity:
Endovenous ablation therapy incompetent vein (36473-36479, [36482, 36483])
Sclerosal injection for incompetent vein(s) ([36465], [36466], 36468-36471)
Strapping ankle or foot (29540)

0.79 1.80 FUD 000 T P3 50

AMA: 2018,Jan,3; 2018,Jan,8; 2017,Jan,8; 2016,Aug,3; 2016,Jan,13; 2015,Jan,16

29581 **Application of multi-layer compression system; leg (below knee), including ankle and foot**

EXCLUDES *For treatment in same extremity:*
Endovenous ablation therapy incompetent vein (36473-36479, [36482, 36483])
Sclerosal injection for incompetent vein(s) ([36465], [36466], 36468-36471)
Strapping (29540, 29580)

0.80 2.47 FUD 000 T P2 80 50

AMA: 2018,Mar,3; 2018,Jan,8; 2018,Jan,3; 2017,Jan,8; 2016,Nov,3; 2016,Aug,3; 2016,Jan,13; 2015,Mar,9; 2015,Jan,16

29584 **upper arm, forearm, hand, and fingers**

EXCLUDES *For treatment in same extremity:*
Endovenous ablation therapy incompetent vein (36473-36479, [36482], [36483])
Sclerosal injection for incompetent vein(s) ([36465], [36466], 36468-36471)

0.47 2.29 FUD 000 T P2 80 50

AMA: 2018,Jan,3; 2018,Jan,8; 2017,Jan,8; 2016,Aug,3; 2016,Jan,13; 2015,Mar,9

29700-29799 Casting Services Other Than Application

INCLUDES Casts applied by treating individual
Removal casts applied by treating individual

29700 **Removal or bivalving; gauntlet, boot or body cast**

0.96 1.78 FUD 000 T P3

AMA: 2018,Jan,3; 2018,Jan,8; 2017,Jan,8; 2016,Jan,13; 2015,Jan,16

29705 **full arm or full leg cast**

1.31 1.82 FUD 000 T P3 50

AMA: 2018,Jan,3; 2018,Jan,8; 2017,Jan,8; 2016,Jan,13; 2015,Jan,16

29710 **shoulder or hip spica, Minerva, or Risser jacket, etc.**

2.41 3.48 FUD 000 T P3 80 50

AMA: 2018,Jan,3; 2018,Jan,8; 2017,Jan,8; 2016,Jan,13; 2015,Jan,16

29720 **Repair of spica, body cast or jacket**

1.26 2.38 FUD 000 T P3

AMA: 2018,Jan,3; 2018,Jan,8; 2017,Jan,8; 2016,Jan,13; 2015,Jan,16

29730 **Windowing of cast**

1.25 1.76 FUD 000 T P3

AMA: 2018,Jan,3; 2018,Jan,8; 2017,Jan,8; 2016,Jan,13; 2015,Jan,16

29740 **Wedging of cast (except clubfoot casts)**

2.02 2.82 FUD 000 T P3

AMA: 2018,Jan,3; 2018,Jan,8; 2017,Jan,8; 2016,Jan,13; 2015,Jan,16

29750 **Wedging of clubfoot cast**

2.26 3.07 FUD 000 T P3 80 50

AMA: 2018,Jan,3; 2018,Jan,8; 2017,Jan,8; 2016,Jan,13; 2015,Jan,16

29799 **Unlisted procedure, casting or strapping**

0.00 0.00 FUD YYY T 80

AMA: 2018,Jan,3; 2018,Jan,8; 2017,Jan,8; 2016,Aug,3; 2016,Jan,13; 2015,Jan,16

29800-29999 [29914, 29915, 29916] Arthroscopic Procedures

INCLUDES Diagnostic arthroscopy with surgical arthroscopy
EXCLUDES *Reporting removal foreign or loose body(ies) smaller than arthroscopic cannula diameter utilized for procedure*
Code also modifier 51 when arthroscopy performed with arthrotomy

29800 **Arthroscopy, temporomandibular joint, diagnostic, with or without synovial biopsy (separate procedure)**

15.2 15.2 FUD 090 J A2 80 50

AMA: 2018,Jan,8; 2017,Jan,8; 2016,Jan,13; 2015,Jan,16

29804 **Arthroscopy, temporomandibular joint, surgical**

EXCLUDES *Open surgery (21010)*

17.7 17.7 FUD 090 J A2 80 50

AMA: 2018,Jan,8; 2017,Jan,8; 2016,Jan,13; 2015,Jan,16

29805 **Arthroscopy, shoulder, diagnostic, with or without synovial biopsy (separate procedure)**

EXCLUDES *Open surgery (23065-23066, 23100-23101)*

13.5 13.5 FUD 090 J A2 50

AMA: 2018,Jan,8; 2017,Jan,8; 2016,Jan,13; 2015,Jun,10; 2015,Jan,16

29806 **Arthroscopy, shoulder, surgical; capsulorrhaphy**

EXCLUDES *Open surgery (23450-23466)*
Thermal capsulorrhaphy (29999)

30.5 30.5 FUD 090 J A2 50

AMA: 2018,Jun,11; 2018,Jan,8; 2017,Jan,8; 2016,Jan,13; 2015,Jul,10; 2015,Mar,7; 2015,Jan,16

29807 **repair of SLAP lesion**

29.8 29.8 FUD 090 J A2 50

AMA: 2018,Jan,8; 2017,Jan,8; 2016,Jan,13; 2015,Mar,7; 2015,Jan,16

29819 **with removal of loose body or foreign body**

EXCLUDES *Open surgery (23040-23044, 23107)*

16.9 16.9 FUD 090 J A2 50

AMA: 2018,Jun,11; 2018,Jan,8; 2017,Jan,8; 2016,Jan,13; 2015,Mar,7; 2015,Jan,16

29820 **synovectomy, partial**

EXCLUDES *Open surgery (23105)*

15.3 15.3 FUD 090 J A2 80 50

AMA: 2018,Jan,8; 2017,Jan,8; 2016,Jan,13; 2015,Mar,7; 2015,Jan,16

29821 **synovectomy, complete**

EXCLUDES *Open surgery (23105)*

17.1 17.1 FUD 090 J A2 80 50

AMA: 2018,Jan,8; 2017,Jan,8; 2016,Jan,13; 2015,Mar,7; 2015,Jan,16

▲ **29822** **debridement, limited, 1 or 2 discrete structures (eg, humeral bone, humeral articular cartilage, glenoid bone, glenoid articular cartilage, biceps tendon, biceps anchor complex, labrum, articular capsule, articular side of the rotator cuff, bursal side of the rotator cuff, subacromial bursa, foreign body[ies])**

EXCLUDES *Open surgery (see specific shoulder section)*

16.6 16.6 FUD 090 J A2 80 50

AMA: 2018,Jan,7; 2018,Jan,8; 2017,Jan,8; 2016,Jan,13; 2015,Mar,7; 2015,Jan,16

▲ **29823** **debridement, extensive, 3 or more discrete structures (eg, humeral bone, humeral articular cartilage, glenoid bone, glenoid articular cartilage, biceps tendon, biceps anchor complex, labrum, articular capsule, articular side of the rotator cuff, bursal side of the rotator cuff, subacromial bursa, foreign body[ies])**

EXCLUDES *Open surgery (see specific shoulder section)*

18.1 18.1 **FUD** 090 J A2 80 50

AMA: 2018,Jan,7; 2018,Jan,8; 2017,Jan,8; 2016,Dec,16; 2016,Jan,13; 2015,Mar,7; 2015,Jan,16

29824 **distal claviculectomy including distal articular surface (Mumford procedure)**

EXCLUDES *Open surgery (23120)*

19.1 19.1 **FUD** 090 J A2 80 50

AMA: 2018,Jan,8; 2017,Jan,8; 2016,Jan,13; 2015,Mar,7; 2015,Jan,16

29825 **with lysis and resection of adhesions, with or without manipulation**

EXCLUDES *Open surgery (see specific shoulder section)*

16.9 16.9 **FUD** 090 J A2 80 50

AMA: 2018,Jan,8; 2017,Jan,8; 2016,Jan,13; 2015,Mar,7; 2015,Jan,16

+ **29826** **decompression of subacromial space with partial acromioplasty, with coracoacromial ligament (ie, arch) release, when performed (List separately in addition to code for primary procedure)**

EXCLUDES *Open surgery (23130, 23415)*

Code first (29806-29825, 29827-29828)

5.07 5.07 **FUD** ZZZ N N1 80 50

AMA: 2018,Jan,8; 2017,Jan,8; 2016,Jan,13; 2015,Mar,7; 2015,Jan,16

29827 **with rotator cuff repair**

EXCLUDES *Distal clavicle excision (29824)*
Open surgery or mini open repair (23412)
Subacromial decompression (29826)

30.9 30.9 **FUD** 090 J A2 80 50

AMA: 2018,Jan,8; 2017,Jan,8; 2016,Jul,8; 2016,Jan,13; 2015,Mar,7; 2015,Jan,16

29828 **biceps tenodesis**

EXCLUDES *Arthroscopy, shoulder, diagnostic, with or without synovial biopsy (29805)*
Arthroscopy, shoulder, surgical; debridement, limited (29822)
Arthroscopy, shoulder, surgical; synovectomy, partial (29820)
Tenodesis long tendon biceps (23430)

26.5 26.5 **FUD** 090 J G2 80 50

AMA: 2018,Jan,8; 2017,Jan,8; 2016,Jul,8; 2016,Jan,13; 2015,Mar,7; 2015,Jan,16

29830 **Arthroscopy, elbow, diagnostic, with or without synovial biopsy (separate procedure)**

13.1 13.1 **FUD** 090 J A2 50

AMA: 2018,Jan,8; 2017,Jan,8; 2016,Jan,13; 2015,Jan,16

29834 **Arthroscopy, elbow, surgical; with removal of loose body or foreign body**

13.9 13.9 **FUD** 090 J A2 80 50

AMA: 2018,Jan,8; 2017,Jan,8; 2016,Jan,13; 2015,Jan,16

29835 **synovectomy, partial**

14.4 14.4 **FUD** 090 J A2 80 50

AMA: 2018,Jan,8; 2017,Jan,8; 2016,Jan,13; 2015,Jan,16

29836 **synovectomy, complete**

16.8 16.8 **FUD** 090 J A2 80 50

AMA: 2018,Jan,8; 2017,Jan,8; 2016,Jan,13; 2015,Jan,16

29837 **debridement, limited**

15.2 15.2 **FUD** 090 J A2 80 50

AMA: 2018,Jan,8; 2017,Jan,8; 2016,Jan,13; 2015,Jan,16

29838 **debridement, extensive**

17.0 17.0 **FUD** 090 J A2 80 50

AMA: 2018,Jan,8; 2017,Jan,8; 2016,Jan,13; 2015,Jan,16

29840 **Arthroscopy, wrist, diagnostic, with or without synovial biopsy (separate procedure)**

12.9 12.9 **FUD** 090 J A2 80 50

AMA: 2018,Jan,8; 2017,Jan,8; 2016,Jan,13; 2015,Jan,16

29843 **Arthroscopy, wrist, surgical; for infection, lavage and drainage**

14.0 14.0 **FUD** 090 J A2 80 50

AMA: 2018,Jan,8; 2017,Jan,8; 2016,Jan,13; 2015,Jan,16

29844 **synovectomy, partial**

14.2 14.2 **FUD** 090 J A2 80 50

AMA: 2018,Jan,8; 2017,Jan,8; 2016,Jan,13; 2015,Jan,16

29845 **synovectomy, complete**

16.8 16.8 **FUD** 090 J A2 80 50

AMA: 2018,Jan,8; 2017,Jan,8; 2016,Jan,13; 2015,Jan,16

29846 **excision and/or repair of triangular fibrocartilage and/or joint debridement**

15.0 15.0 **FUD** 090 J A2 80 50

AMA: 2018,Jan,8; 2017,Jan,8; 2016,Jan,13; 2015,Jan,16

29847 **internal fixation for fracture or instability**

15.6 15.6 **FUD** 090 J A2 80 50

AMA: 2018,Jan,8; 2017,Jan,8; 2016,Jan,13; 2015,Jan,16

29848 **Endoscopy, wrist, surgical, with release of transverse carpal ligament**

EXCLUDES *Open surgery (64721)*
Tissue expander, other than breast (11960)

14.7 14.7 **FUD** 090 J A2 50

AMA: 2018,Apr,10; 2018,Jan,8; 2017,Jan,8; 2017,Jan,6; 2016,Jan,13; 2015,Jul,10; 2015,Jan,16

29850 **Arthroscopically aided treatment of intercondylar spine(s) and/or tuberosity fracture(s) of the knee, with or without manipulation; without internal or external fixation (includes arthroscopy)**

17.9 17.9 **FUD** 090 J A2 80 50

AMA: 2018,Jan,8; 2017,Jan,8; 2016,Jan,13; 2015,Jan,16

29851 **with internal or external fixation (includes arthroscopy)**

EXCLUDES *Bone graft (20900, 20902)*

26.8 26.8 **FUD** 090 J A2 80 50

AMA: 2018,Jan,8; 2017,Jan,8; 2016,Jan,13; 2015,Jan,16

29855 **Arthroscopically aided treatment of tibial fracture, proximal (plateau); unicondylar, includes internal fixation, when performed (includes arthroscopy)**

EXCLUDES *Bone graft (20900, 20902)*

22.5 22.5 **FUD** 090 J J8 80 50

AMA: 2019,Nov,13; 2018,Sep,14; 2018,Jan,8; 2017,Jan,8; 2016,Jan,13; 2015,Jan,16

29856 **bicondylar, includes internal fixation, when performed (includes arthroscopy)**

EXCLUDES *Bone graft (20900, 20902)*

28.6 28.6 **FUD** 090 J J8 80 50

AMA: 2018,Jan,8; 2017,Jan,8; 2016,Jan,13; 2015,Jan,16

29860 **Arthroscopy, hip, diagnostic with or without synovial biopsy (separate procedure)**

19.2 19.2 **FUD** 090 J A2 80 50

AMA: 2018,Jan,8; 2017,Jan,8; 2016,Jan,13; 2015,Jan,16

29861 **Arthroscopy, hip, surgical; with removal of loose body or foreign body**

20.8 20.8 **FUD** 090 J A2 80 50

AMA: 2018,Jan,8; 2017,Jan,8; 2016,Jan,13; 2015,Jan,16

29862 **with debridement/shaving of articular cartilage (chondroplasty), abrasion arthroplasty, and/or resection of labrum**

23.4 23.4 **FUD** 090 J A2 80 50

AMA: 2018,Jan,8; 2017,Jan,8; 2016,Jan,13; 2015,Jan,16

29863 **with synovectomy**
23.2 23.2 FUD 090 J A2 80 50
AMA: 2018,Jan,8; 2017,Jan,8; 2016,Jan,13; 2015,Jan,16

29914 **with femoroplasty (ie, treatment of cam lesion)**
INCLUDES Chondroplasty (29862)
Synovectomy (29863)
28.7 28.7 FUD 090 J G2 80 50
AMA: 2018,Jan,8; 2017,Jan,8; 2016,Jan,13; 2015,Jan,16

29915 **with acetabuloplasty (ie, treatment of pincer lesion)**
INCLUDES Chondroplasty (29862)
Synovectomy (29863)
29.5 29.5 FUD 090 J G2 80 50
AMA: 2018,Jan,8; 2017,Jan,8; 2016,Jan,13; 2015,Jan,16

29916 **with labral repair**
INCLUDES Acetabuloplasty ([29915])
Chondroplasty (29862)
Synovectomy (29863)
29.5 29.5 FUD 090 J G2 80 50
AMA: 2018,Jan,8; 2017,Jan,8; 2016,Jan,13; 2015,Jan,16

29866 **Arthroscopy, knee, surgical; osteochondral autograft(s) (eg, mosaicplasty) (includes harvesting of the autograft[s])**
EXCLUDES *Open osteochondral autograft knee (27416)*
Procedures performed at same surgical session (29870-29871, 29875, 29884)
Procedures performed in same compartment (29874, 29877, 29879, 29885-29887)
30.3 30.3 FUD 090 J G2 80 50
AMA: 2018,Jan,8; 2017,Jan,8; 2016,Jan,13; 2015,Jan,16

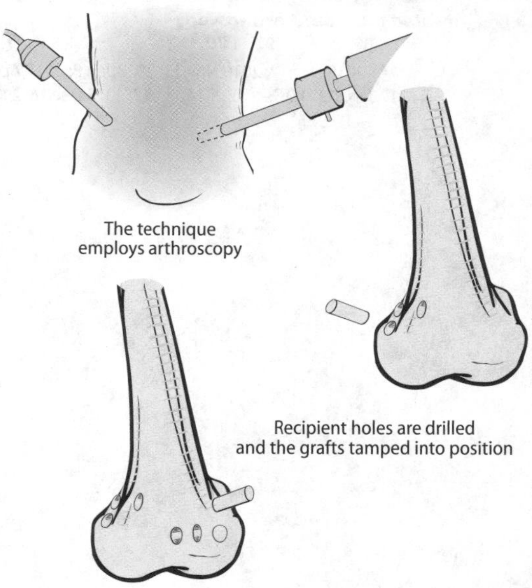
Cylindrical plugs of healthy bone are harvested, usually from a non-weight bearing area of the femur
The technique employs arthroscopy
Recipient holes are drilled and the grafts tamped into position

29867 **osteochondral allograft (eg, mosaicplasty)**
EXCLUDES *Procedures performed at same surgical session (27415, 27570, 29870-29871, 29875, 29884)*
Procedures performed in same compartment (29874, 29877, 29879, 29885-29887)
36.9 36.9 FUD 090 J J8 80 50
AMA: 2018,Jan,8; 2017,Jan,8; 2016,Jan,13; 2015,Jan,16

29868 **meniscal transplantation (includes arthrotomy for meniscal insertion), medial or lateral**
EXCLUDES *Procedures performed at same surgical session (29870-29871, 29875, 29880, 29883-29884)*
Procedures performed in same compartment (29874, 29877, 29881-29882)
48.4 48.4 FUD 090 J 80 50
AMA: 2018,Jan,8; 2017,Jan,8; 2016,Jan,13; 2015,Jan,16

29870 **Arthroscopy, knee, diagnostic, with or without synovial biopsy (separate procedure)**
EXCLUDES *Open procedure (27412)*
11.7 16.4 FUD 090 J A2 50
AMA: 2019,Nov,14; 2018,Jan,8; 2017,Jan,8; 2016,Jan,13; 2015,Jan,16

29871 **Arthroscopy, knee, surgical; for infection, lavage and drainage**
EXCLUDES *Injection contrast for knee arthrography (27369)*
Osteochondral graft (27412, 27415, 29866-29867)
14.8 14.8 FUD 090 J A2 50
AMA: 2019,Aug,7; 2018,Jan,8; 2017,Jan,8; 2016,Jan,13; 2015,Aug,6; 2015,Jan,16

29873 **with lateral release**
EXCLUDES *Open procedure (27425)*
15.2 15.2 FUD 090 J A2 50
AMA: 2018,Jan,8; 2017,Jan,8; 2016,Jan,13; 2015,Nov,7; 2015,Jan,16

29874 **for removal of loose body or foreign body (eg, osteochondritis dissecans fragmentation, chondral fragmentation)**
15.5 15.5 FUD 090 J A2 80 50
AMA: 2018,Jan,8; 2017,Jan,8; 2016,Jan,13; 2015,Jan,16

29875 **synovectomy, limited (eg, plica or shelf resection) (separate procedure)**
14.3 14.3 FUD 090 J A2 80 50
AMA: 2018,Jan,8; 2017,Jan,8; 2016,Jan,13; 2016,Jan,11; 2015,Jan,16

29876 **synovectomy, major, 2 or more compartments (eg, medial or lateral)**
18.8 18.8 FUD 090 J A2 50
AMA: 2018,Jan,8; 2017,Jan,8; 2016,Jan,13; 2015,Jan,16

29877 **debridement/shaving of articular cartilage (chondroplasty)**
EXCLUDES *Arthroscopy, knee, surgical; with meniscectomy (29880-29881)*
17.9 17.9 FUD 090 J A2 80 50
AMA: 2020,May,13; 2018,Jan,8; 2017,Jan,8; 2016,Jan,13; 2015,Jan,16

29879 **abrasion arthroplasty (includes chondroplasty where necessary) or multiple drilling or microfracture**
19.0 19.0 FUD 090 J A2 80 50
AMA: 2018,Jan,8; 2017,Jan,8; 2016,Jan,13; 2015,Jan,16

29880 **with meniscectomy (medial AND lateral, including any meniscal shaving) including debridement/shaving of articular cartilage (chondroplasty), same or separate compartment(s), when performed**
16.1 16.1 FUD 090 J A2 80 50
AMA: 2018,Jan,8; 2017,Jan,8; 2016,Jan,13; 2015,Jan,16

29881 **with meniscectomy (medial OR lateral, including any meniscal shaving) including debridement/shaving of articular cartilage (chondroplasty), same or separate compartment(s), when performed**
15.5 15.5 FUD 090 J A2 80 50
AMA: 2020,Sep,14; 2020,May,13; 2019,Nov,14; 2018,Jan,8; 2017,Jan,8; 2016,Jan,13; 2016,Jan,11; 2015,Jan,16

29882 **with meniscus repair (medial OR lateral)**
EXCLUDES *Meniscus transplant (29868)*
19.9 19.9 **FUD** 090 J A2 50
AMA: 2019,May,10; 2018,Jan,8; 2017,Jan,8; 2016,Jan,13; 2015,Jan,16

29883 **with meniscus repair (medial AND lateral)**
EXCLUDES *Meniscus transplant (29868)*
24.2 24.2 **FUD** 090 J A2 80 50
AMA: 2018,Jan,8; 2017,Jan,8; 2016,Jan,13; 2015,Jan,16

29884 **with lysis of adhesions, with or without manipulation (separate procedure)**
17.8 17.8 **FUD** 090 J A2 80 50
AMA: 2018,Jan,8; 2017,Jan,8; 2016,Jan,13; 2015,Jan,16

29885 **drilling for osteochondritis dissecans with bone grafting, with or without internal fixation (including debridement of base of lesion)**
21.7 21.7 **FUD** 090 J A2 80 50
AMA: 2018,Jan,8; 2017,Jan,8; 2016,Jan,13; 2015,Jan,16

29886 **drilling for intact osteochondritis dissecans lesion**
18.3 18.3 **FUD** 090 J A2 50
AMA: 2018,Jan,8; 2017,Jan,8; 2016,Jan,13; 2015,Jan,16

29887 **drilling for intact osteochondritis dissecans lesion with internal fixation**
21.5 21.5 **FUD** 090 J A2 80 50
AMA: 2018,Jan,8; 2017,Jan,8; 2016,Jan,13; 2015,Jan,16

29888 **Arthroscopically aided anterior cruciate ligament repair/augmentation or reconstruction**
28.3 28.3 **FUD** 090 J J8 80 50
AMA: 2018,Jan,8; 2017,Jan,8; 2016,Nov,9; 2016,Jan,13; 2015,Jan,16

29889 **Arthroscopically aided posterior cruciate ligament repair/augmentation or reconstruction**
35.3 35.3 **FUD** 090 J J8 80 50
AMA: 2018,Jan,8; 2017,Jan,8; 2016,Jan,13; 2015,Jan,16

29891 **Arthroscopy, ankle, surgical, excision of osteochondral defect of talus and/or tibia, including drilling of the defect**
19.3 19.3 **FUD** 090 J A2 80 50
AMA: 2018,Jan,8; 2017,Jan,8; 2016,Jan,13; 2015,Jan,16

29892 **Arthroscopically aided repair of large osteochondritis dissecans lesion, talar dome fracture, or tibial plafond fracture, with or without internal fixation (includes arthroscopy)**
18.7 18.7 **FUD** 090 J A2 80 50
AMA: 2018,Jan,8; 2017,Jan,8; 2016,Jan,13; 2015,Jan,16

29893 **Endoscopic plantar fasciotomy**
12.3 17.8 **FUD** 090 J A2 50
AMA: 2018,Jan,8; 2017,Jan,8; 2016,Jan,13; 2015,Jan,16

29894 **Arthroscopy, ankle (tibiotalar and fibulotalar joints), surgical; with removal of loose body or foreign body**
14.2 14.2 **FUD** 090 J A2 80 50
AMA: 2018,Jan,8; 2017,Jan,8; 2016,Jan,13; 2015,Jan,16

29895 **synovectomy, partial**
13.4 13.4 **FUD** 090 J A2 80 50
AMA: 2018,Jan,8; 2017,Jan,8; 2016,Jan,13; 2015,Jan,16

29897 **debridement, limited**
14.4 14.4 **FUD** 090 J A2 80 50
AMA: 2018,Jan,8; 2017,Jan,8; 2016,Jan,13; 2015,Jan,16

29898 **debridement, extensive**
16.1 16.1 **FUD** 090 J A2 80 50
AMA: 2018,Jan,8; 2017,Jan,8; 2016,Jan,13; 2015,Jan,16

29899 **with ankle arthrodesis**
EXCLUDES *Open procedure (27870)*
29.7 29.7 **FUD** 090 J J8 80 50
AMA: 2018,Jan,8; 2017,Jan,8; 2016,Jan,13; 2015,Jan,16

29900 **Arthroscopy, metacarpophalangeal joint, diagnostic, includes synovial biopsy**
EXCLUDES *Arthroscopy, metacarpophalangeal joint, surgical (29901-29902)*
14.3 14.3 **FUD** 090 J A2 80 50
AMA: 2018,Jan,8; 2017,Jan,8; 2016,Jan,13; 2015,Jan,16

29901 **Arthroscopy, metacarpophalangeal joint, surgical; with debridement**
15.4 15.4 **FUD** 090 J A2 80 50
AMA: 2018,Jan,8; 2017,Jan,8; 2016,Jan,13; 2015,Jan,16

29902 **with reduction of displaced ulnar collateral ligament (eg, Stenar lesion)**
16.4 16.4 **FUD** 090 J A2 80 50
AMA: 2018,Jan,8; 2017,Jan,8; 2016,Jan,13; 2015,Jan,16

29904 **Arthroscopy, subtalar joint, surgical; with removal of loose body or foreign body**
18.3 18.3 **FUD** 090 J G2 80 50
AMA: 2018,Jan,8; 2017,Jan,8; 2016,Jan,13; 2015,Jan,16

29905 **with synovectomy**
14.9 14.9 **FUD** 090 J G2 80 50
AMA: 2018,Jan,8; 2017,Jan,8; 2016,Jan,13; 2015,Jan,16

29906 **with debridement**
19.5 19.5 **FUD** 090 J G2 80 50
AMA: 2018,Jan,8; 2017,Jan,8; 2016,Jan,13; 2015,Jan,16

29907 **with subtalar arthrodesis**
25.3 25.3 **FUD** 090 J J8 80 50
AMA: 2018,Jan,8; 2017,Jan,8; 2016,Jan,13; 2015,Jan,16

29914 **Resequenced code. See code following 29863.**

29915 **Resequenced code. See code following 29863.**

29916 **Resequenced code. See code before 29866.**

29999 **Unlisted procedure, arthroscopy**
0.00 0.00 **FUD** YYY T 80 50
AMA: 2019,Dec,12; 2019,Nov,13; 2018,Jan,8; 2017,Apr,9; 2017,Jan,8; 2016,Dec,16; 2016,Jan,13; 2015,Dec,16; 2015,Jan,16

30000-30115 I&D, Biopsy, Excision Procedures of the Nose

30000 **Drainage abscess or hematoma, nasal, internal approach**

EXCLUDES *Incision and drainage (10060, 10140)*

3.38 7.18 FUD 010 T P2 80

AMA: 2005,May,13-14; 1994,Spr,24

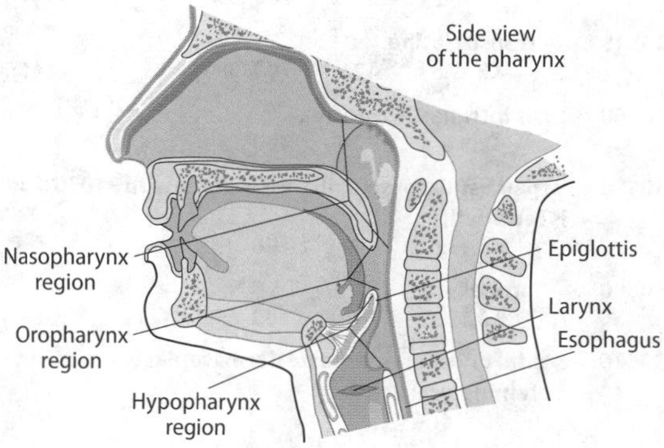

The nasopharynx is the membranous passage above the level of the soft palate; the oropharynx is the region between the soft palate and the upper edge of the epiglottis; the hypopharynx is the region of the epiglottis to the juncture of the larynx and esophagus; the three regions are collectively known as the pharynx

30020 **Drainage abscess or hematoma, nasal septum**

EXCLUDES *Lateral rhinotomy incision (30118, 30320)*

3.37 6.90 FUD 010 T P3

30100 **Biopsy, intranasal**

EXCLUDES *Superficial biopsy nose (11102-11107)*

1.91 4.03 FUD 000 T P3

AMA: 2019,Jan,9

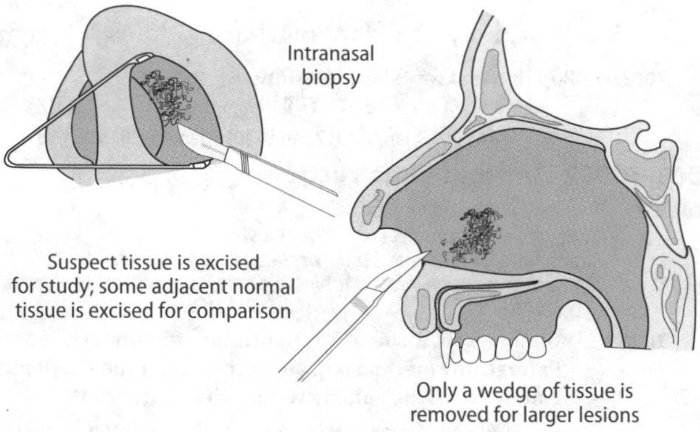

30110 **Excision, nasal polyp(s), simple**

3.70 6.82 FUD 010 T P3 50

30115 **Excision, nasal polyp(s), extensive**

12.7 12.7 FUD 090 J A2 50

30117-30118 Destruction Procedures Nose

CMS: 100-03,140.5 Laser Procedures

30117 **Excision or destruction (eg, laser), intranasal lesion; internal approach**

9.47 26.4 FUD 090 J A2

AMA: 2020,Sep,14; 2019,Nov,14; 2019,Jul,10

30118 **external approach (lateral rhinotomy)**

22.0 22.0 FUD 090 J A2

30120-30140 Excision Procedures Nose, Turbinate

30120 **Excision or surgical planing of skin of nose for rhinophyma**

12.3 14.6 FUD 090 J A2

AMA: 2018,Jan,8; 2017,Jan,8; 2016,Jan,13; 2015,Jan,16

30124 **Excision dermoid cyst, nose; simple, skin, subcutaneous**

8.33 8.33 FUD 090 T R2

30125 **complex, under bone or cartilage**

17.5 17.5 FUD 090 J A2 80

30130 **Excision inferior turbinate, partial or complete, any method**

EXCLUDES *Ablation, soft tissue inferior turbinates, unilateral or bilateral, any method (30801-30802)*
Excision middle/superior turbinate(s) (30999)
Fracture nasal inferior turbinate(s), therapeutic (30930)

11.2 11.2 FUD 090 J A2 50

AMA: 2018,Jan,8; 2017,Jan,8; 2016,Jan,13; 2015,Jan,16

30140 **Submucous resection inferior turbinate, partial or complete, any method**

EXCLUDES *Ablation, soft tissue inferior turbinates, unilateral or bilateral, any method (30801-30802)*
Endoscopic resection concha bullosa middle turbinate (31240)
Fracture nasal inferior turbinate(s), therapeutic (30930)
Submucous resection:
Nasal septum (30520)
Superior or middle turbinate (30999)

5.12 7.92 FUD 000 J A2 50

AMA: 2020,Jan,12; 2018,Jan,8; 2017,Jan,8; 2016,Jan,13; 2015,Jan,16

30150-30160 Surgical Removal: Nose

EXCLUDES *Reconstruction and/or closure (primary or delayed primary intention) (13151-13160, 14060-14302, 15120-15121, 15260-15261, 15760, 20900-20912)*

30150 **Rhinectomy; partial**

22.4 22.4 FUD 090 J A2

30160 **total**

22.6 22.6 FUD 090 J A2 80

30200-30320 Turbinate Injection, Removal Foreign Substance in the Nose

30200 **Injection into turbinate(s), therapeutic**

1.66 3.18 FUD 000 T P3

AMA: 2018,Jan,8; 2017,Jan,8; 2016,Jan,13; 2015,Jan,16

30210 **Displacement therapy (Proetz type)**

2.82 4.24 FUD 010 T P3

AMA: 2018,Jan,8; 2017,Jan,8; 2016,Jan,13; 2015,Jan,16

30220 **Insertion, nasal septal prosthesis (button)**

3.57 8.70 FUD 010 T A2

30300 **Removal foreign body, intranasal; office type procedure**

3.23 5.40 FUD 010 Q1 N1

AMA: 2018,Jan,8; 2017,Jan,8; 2016,Jan,13; 2015,Jan,16

30310 **requiring general anesthesia**

5.80 5.80 FUD 010 J A2 80

30320 **by lateral rhinotomy**

13.2 13.2 FUD 090 T A2 80

30400-30630 Reconstruction or Repair of Nose

EXCLUDES *Harvesting bone/tissue/fat grafts ([15769], 15773-15774, 20900-20924, 21210)*
Liposuction for autologous fat grafting (15773-15774)

30400 **Rhinoplasty, primary; lateral and alar cartilages and/or elevation of nasal tip**

INCLUDES Carpue's operation

EXCLUDES *Reconstruction columella (13151-13153)*

34.3 34.3 FUD 090 J A2 80

30410 **complete, external parts including bony pyramid, lateral and alar cartilages, and/or elevation of nasal tip**

39.8 39.8 FUD 090 J A2 80

30420 **including major septal repair**
40.3 40.3 **FUD** 090 J A2
AMA: 2018,Jan,8; 2017,Nov,11; 2017,Jan,8; 2016,Jul,8

30430 **Rhinoplasty, secondary; minor revision (small amount of nasal tip work)**
29.7 29.7 **FUD** 090 J A2 80

30435 **intermediate revision (bony work with osteotomies)**
37.6 37.6 **FUD** 090 J A2 80

30450 **major revision (nasal tip work and osteotomies)**
49.8 49.8 **FUD** 090 J A2 80

30460 **Rhinoplasty for nasal deformity secondary to congenital cleft lip and/or palate, including columellar lengthening; tip only**
23.5 23.5 **FUD** 090 J A2 80
AMA: 2018,Jan,8; 2017,Jan,8; 2016,Jan,13; 2015,Jan,16

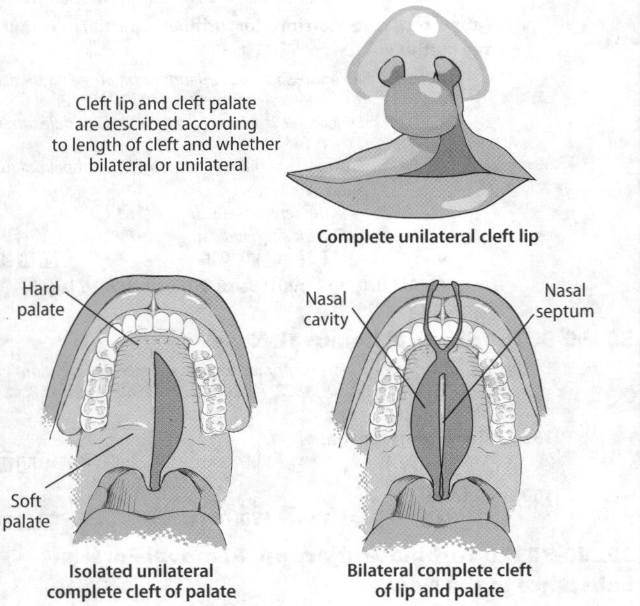

30462 **tip, septum, osteotomies**
45.1 45.1 **FUD** 090 J A2 80
AMA: 2018,Jan,8; 2017,Jan,8; 2016,Jan,13; 2015,Jan,16

30465 **Repair of nasal vestibular stenosis (eg, spreader grafting, lateral nasal wall reconstruction)**
INCLUDES Bilateral procedure
EXCLUDES *Harvesting ear cartilage graft, autogenous (21235)*
Repair nasal valve or vestibular lateral wall collapse with implants same side during same operative session (30468)
Repair nasal vestibular stenosis without graft, implant, or reconstruction lateral wall (30999)
Code also modifier 52 for unilateral procedure
28.5 28.5 **FUD** 090 J A2 80
AMA: 2020,Sep,14

● **30468** **Repair of nasal valve collapse with subcutaneous/submucosal lateral wall implant(s)**
INCLUDES Bilateral procedure
EXCLUDES *Repair nasal vestibular stenosis same side during same operative session (30465)*
Repair nasal vestibular stenosis without graft, implant, or reconstruction lateral wall (30999)
Code also modifier 52 for unilateral procedure

30520 **Septoplasty or submucous resection, with or without cartilage scoring, contouring or replacement with graft**
EXCLUDES *Turbinate resection (30140)*
18.0 18.0 **FUD** 090 J A2
AMA: 2019,Jul,10; 2018,Jan,8; 2017,Jan,8; 2016,Jan,13; 2015,Jul,10; 2015,Jan,16

30540 **Repair choanal atresia; intranasal**
20.2 20.2 **FUD** 090 63 J A2 80

30545 **transpalatine**
27.6 27.6 **FUD** 090 63 J A2 80

30560 **Lysis intranasal synechia**
3.95 7.96 **FUD** 010 T A2

30580 **Repair fistula; oromaxillary (combine with 31030 if antrotomy is included)**
13.6 17.8 **FUD** 090 J A2

30600 **oronasal**
12.3 16.8 **FUD** 090 J A2 80

30620 **Septal or other intranasal dermatoplasty (does not include obtaining graft)**

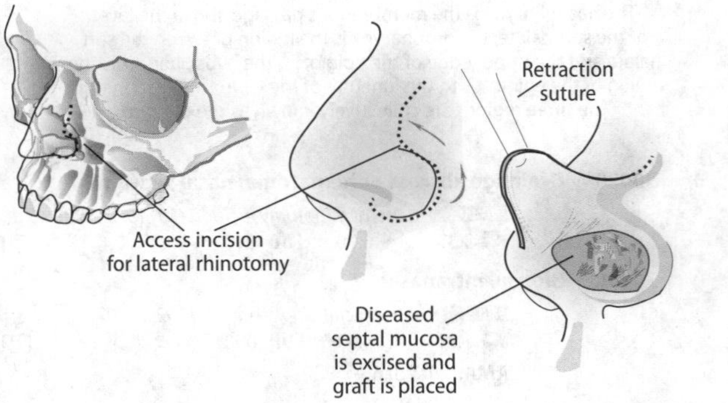

18.2 18.2 **FUD** 090 J A2

30630 **Repair nasal septal perforations**
18.0 18.0 **FUD** 090 J A2 80
AMA: 2018,Jan,8; 2017,Jan,8; 2016,Jan,13; 2015,Jan,16

30801-30802 Turbinate Destruction

EXCLUDES *Ablation middle/superior turbinates (30999)*
Cautery to stop nasal bleeding (30901-30906)
Excision inferior turbinate, partial or complete, any method (30130)
Submucous resection inferior turbinate, partial or complete, any method (30140)

30801 **Ablation, soft tissue of inferior turbinates, unilateral or bilateral, any method (eg, electrocautery, radiofrequency ablation, or tissue volume reduction); superficial**
EXCLUDES *Submucosal ablation inferior turbinates (30802)*
4.10 6.18 **FUD** 010 T A2
AMA: 2019,Jul,10

30802 **intramural (ie, submucosal)**
EXCLUDES *Superficial ablation inferior turbinates (30801)*
5.58 7.86 **FUD** 010 T A2
AMA: 2019,Jul,10; 2018,Jan,8; 2017,Jan,8; 2016,Jan,13; 2015,Jan,16

30901-30920 Control Nose Bleed

30901 **Control nasal hemorrhage, anterior, simple (limited cautery and/or packing) any method**
1.64 4.09 **FUD** 000 01 N1 50
AMA: 2020,Jul,13

30903 **Control nasal hemorrhage, anterior, complex (extensive cautery and/or packing) any method**
2.28 6.49 **FUD** 000 T A2 50
AMA: 1990,Win,4

30905 **Control nasal hemorrhage, posterior, with posterior nasal packs and/or cautery, any method; initial**
3.07 9.64 FUD 000 T A2
AMA: 2018,Jan,8; 2017,Jan,8; 2016,Jan,13; 2015,Jan,16

30906 **subsequent**
3.92 10.0 FUD 000 T A2
AMA: 2002,May,7

30915 **Ligation arteries; ethmoidal**
EXCLUDES *External carotid artery (37600)*
16.7 16.7 FUD 090 T A2

30920 **internal maxillary artery, transantral**
EXCLUDES *External carotid artery (37600)*
24.3 24.3 FUD 090 T A2

30930-30999 Other and Unlisted Procedures of Nose

30930 **Fracture nasal inferior turbinate(s), therapeutic**
EXCLUDES *Excision inferior turbinate, partial or complete, any method (30130)*
Fracture superior or middle turbinate(s) (30999)
Submucous resection inferior turbinate, partial or complete, any method (30140)
3.43 3.43 FUD 010 J A2
AMA: 2018,Jan,8; 2017,Nov,11; 2017,Jan,8; 2016,Jul,8; 2016,Jan,13; 2015,Jan,16

30999 **Unlisted procedure, nose**
0.00 0.00 FUD YYY T 80
AMA: 2020,Sep,14; 2019,Nov,14; 2018,Jan,8; 2017,Jan,8; 2016,Jan,13; 2015,Jan,16

31000-31230 Opening Sinuses

31000 **Lavage by cannulation; maxillary sinus (antrum puncture or natural ostium)**
3.02 5.17 FUD 010 T P2 50
AMA: 2018,Jan,8; 2017,Jan,8; 2016,Jan,13; 2015,Jan,16

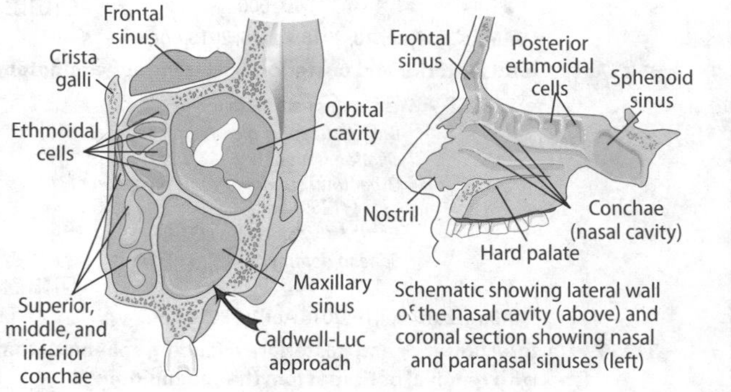

Schematic showing lateral wall of the nasal cavity (above) and coronal section showing nasal and paranasal sinuses (left)

31002 **sphenoid sinus**
5.39 5.39 FUD 010 T R2 80 50

31020 **Sinusotomy, maxillary (antrotomy); intranasal**
10.4 13.6 FUD 090 J A2 50

31030 **radical (Caldwell-Luc) without removal of antrochoanal polyps**
14.7 18.4 FUD 090 J A2 50

31032 **radical (Caldwell-Luc) with removal of antrochoanal polyps**
16.5 16.5 FUD 090 J A2 50

31040 **Pterygomaxillary fossa surgery, any approach**
EXCLUDES *Transantral ligation internal maxillary artery (30920)*
22.0 22.0 FUD 090 J R2 50

31050 **Sinusotomy, sphenoid, with or without biopsy;**
14.1 14.1 FUD 090 J A2 50

31051 **with mucosal stripping or removal of polyp(s)**
19.0 19.0 FUD 090 J A2 50

31070 **Sinusotomy frontal; external, simple (trephine operation)**
INCLUDES Killian operation
EXCLUDES *Intranasal frontal sinusotomy (31276)*
12.9 12.9 FUD 090 J A2 50

31075 **transorbital, unilateral (for mucocele or osteoma, Lynch type)**
22.8 22.8 FUD 090 J A2 80 50

31080 **obliterative without osteoplastic flap, brow incision (includes ablation)**
INCLUDES Ridell sinusotomy
30.0 30.0 FUD 090 J A2 80 50

31081 **obliterative, without osteoplastic flap, coronal incision (includes ablation)**
32.3 32.3 FUD 090 J A2 80 50

31084 **obliterative, with osteoplastic flap, brow incision**
33.5 33.5 FUD 090 J A2 80 50

31085 **obliterative, with osteoplastic flap, coronal incision**
34.6 34.6 FUD 090 J A2 80 50

31086 **nonobliterative, with osteoplastic flap, brow incision**
32.6 32.6 FUD 090 J A2 80 50

31087 **nonobliterative, with osteoplastic flap, coronal incision**
31.2 31.2 FUD 090 J A2 80 50

31090 **Sinusotomy, unilateral, 3 or more paranasal sinuses (frontal, maxillary, ethmoid, sphenoid)**
30.3 30.3 FUD 090 J A2 50
AMA: 1998,Nov,1; 1997,Nov,1

31200 **Ethmoidectomy; intranasal, anterior**
16.7 16.7 FUD 090 J A2 50
AMA: 2018,Jan,8; 2017,Jan,8; 2016,Feb,10

31201 **intranasal, total**
21.9 21.9 FUD 090 J A2 50
AMA: 2018,Jan,8; 2017,Jan,8; 2016,Feb,10

31205 **extranasal, total**
26.3 26.3 FUD 090 J A2 80 50
AMA: 2018,Jan,8; 2017,Jan,8; 2016,Feb,10

31225 **Maxillectomy; without orbital exenteration**
52.1 52.1 FUD 090 C 80 50

31230 **with orbital exenteration (en bloc)**
EXCLUDES *Orbital exenteration without maxillectomy (65110-65114)*
Skin grafts (15120-15121)
58.3 58.3 FUD 090 C 80 50

31231-31235 Nasal Endoscopy, Diagnostic

INCLUDES Complete sinus exam (e.g., nasal cavity, turbinates, sphenoethmoidal recess)
Code also stereotactic navigation, when performed (61782)

31231 **Nasal endoscopy, diagnostic, unilateral or bilateral (separate procedure)**
1.82 5.48 FUD 000 T P2
AMA: 2018,Apr,3; 2018,Jan,8; 2017,Jul,7; 2017,Jan,8; 2017,Jan,6; 2016,Dec,13; 2016,Feb,10; 2016,Jan,13; 2015,Jan,16

31233 **Nasal/sinus endoscopy, diagnostic; with maxillary sinusoscopy (via inferior meatus or canine fossa puncture)**
EXCLUDES *When performed on same side:*
Dilation of maxillary sinus ostium (31295)
Maxillary antrostomy (31256, 31267)
3.87 7.41 FUD 000 T A2 80 50
AMA: 2018,Apr,3; 2018,Jan,8; 2017,Jan,8; 2016,Jan,13; 2015,Jan,16

31235 **with sphenoid sinusoscopy (via puncture of sphenoidal face or cannulation of ostium)**

EXCLUDES *Insertion drug-eluting implant performed with biopsy, debridement, or polypectomy (31237)*
Insertion drug-eluting implant without other nasal/sinus endoscopic procedure (31299)
When performed on same side:
Sinus dilation (31297-31298)
Sphenoidotomy (31287-31288)
Total ethmoidectomy with sphenoidotomy ([31257, 31259])

4.54 8.49 FUD 000 J A2 80 50

AMA: 2018,Apr,3; 2018,Jan,8; 2017,Jan,8; 2016,Jan,13; 2015,Jan,16

31237-31253 [31253] Nasal Endoscopy, Surgical

INCLUDES Diagnostic nasal/sinus endoscopy

Code also stereotactic navigation, when performed (61782)

31237 **Nasal/sinus endoscopy, surgical; with biopsy, polypectomy or debridement (separate procedure)**

EXCLUDES *When performed on same side:*
Frontal sinus exploration (31276)
Maxillary antrostomy (31256, 31267)
Nasal hemorrhage control (31238)
Optic nerve decompression (31294)
Orbital wall decompression, medial and/or inferior (31292-31293)
Other total ethmoidectomy procedures ([31253], 31255, [31257], [31259])
Partial ethmoidectomy (31254)
Repair CSF leak (31290-31291)
Sphenoidotomy (31287-31288)

4.54 7.21 FUD 000 J A2 50

AMA: 2020,Jan,12; 2019,Jul,7; 2019,Apr,10; 2018,Apr,3; 2018,Jan,8; 2017,Jan,8; 2016,Feb,10; 2016,Jan,13; 2015,Jan,16; 2015,Jan,13

31238 **with control of nasal hemorrhage**

EXCLUDES *When performed on same side:*
Biopsy, polypectomy, or debridement (31237)
Sphenopalatine artery ligation (31241)

4.80 7.17 FUD 000 J A2 80 50

AMA: 2018,Apr,3; 2018,Jan,8; 2017,Jan,8; 2016,Jan,13; 2015,Jan,16

31239 **with dacryocystorhinostomy**

17.4 17.4 FUD 010 J A2 80 50

AMA: 2018,Apr,3; 2018,Jan,8; 2017,Jan,8; 2016,Jan,13; 2015,Jan,16

31240 **with concha bullosa resection**

4.52 4.52 FUD 000 J A2 80 50

AMA: 2018,Apr,3; 2018,Jan,8; 2017,Jan,8; 2016,Feb,10; 2016,Jan,13; 2015,Jan,16

31241 **with ligation of sphenopalatine artery**

EXCLUDES *When performed on same side:*
Nasal hemorrhage control (31238)

12.7 12.7 FUD 000 C 80 50

AMA: 2018,Apr,3

31253 **Resequenced code. See code following 31255.**

31254-31259 [31253, 31257, 31259] Nasal Endoscopy with Ethmoid Removal

INCLUDES Diagnostic nasal/sinus endoscopy
Sinusotomy, when applicable

EXCLUDES *When performed on same side:*
Biopsy, polypectomy, or debridement (31237)
Optic nerve decompression (31294)
Orbital wall decompression, medial, and/or inferior (31292-31293)
Repair CSF leak (31290-31291)

Code also stereotactic navigation, when performed (61782)

31254 **Nasal/sinus endoscopy, surgical with ethmoidectomy; partial (anterior)**

EXCLUDES *When performed on same side:*
Other total ethmoidectomy procedures (31253, 31255, [31257], [31259])

7.01 11.7 FUD 000 J A2 50

AMA: 2019,Apr,10; 2018,Apr,3; 2018,Jan,8; 2017,Jan,8; 2016,Feb,10; 2016,Jan,13; 2015,Jan,16

31255 **with ethmoidectomy, total (anterior and posterior)**

EXCLUDES *When performed on same side:*
Frontal sinus exploration (31276)
Other total ethmoidectomy procedures (31253, [31257], [31259])
Partial ethmoidectomy (31254)
Sphenoidotomy (31287-31288)

9.31 9.31 FUD 000 J A2 50

AMA: 2019,Apr,10; 2018,Apr,3; 2018,Apr,10; 2018,Jan,8; 2017,Jan,8; 2016,Feb,10; 2016,Jan,13; 2015,Jan,16

\# **31253** **total (anterior and posterior), including frontal sinus exploration, with removal of tissue from frontal sinus, when performed**

EXCLUDES *When performed on same side:*
Dilation sinus (31296, 31298)
Frontal sinus exploration (31276)
Partial ethmoidectomy (31254)
Total ethmoidectomy (31255)

14.4 14.4 FUD 000 J G2 50

AMA: 2019,Apr,10; 2018,Apr,10; 2018,Apr,3

\# **31257** **total (anterior and posterior), including sphenoidotomy**

EXCLUDES *When performed on same side:*
Diagnostic sphenoid sinusoscopy (31235)
Dilation sinus (31297-31298)
Other total ethmoidectomy procedures (31255, [31259])
Partial ethmoidectomy (31254)
Sphenoidotomy (31287-31288)

12.8 12.8 FUD 000 J G2 50

AMA: 2019,Apr,10; 2018,Apr,10; 2018,Apr,3

\# **31259** **total (anterior and posterior), including sphenoidotomy, with removal of tissue from the sphenoid sinus**

EXCLUDES *When performed on same side:*
Diagnostic sphenoid sinusoscopy (31235)
Dilation sinus (31297-31298)
Other total ethmoidectomy procedures (31255, [31257])
Partial ethmoidectomy (31254)
Sphenoidotomy (31287-31288)

13.6 13.6 FUD 000 J G2 50

AMA: 2019,Apr,10; 2018,Apr,3

31256-31267 [31257, 31259] Nasal Endoscopy with Maxillary Procedures

INCLUDES Diagnostic nasal/sinus endoscopy
Sinusotomy, when applicable

EXCLUDES *When performed on same side:*
Biopsy, polypectomy, or debridement (31237)
Dilation maxillary sinus ostium (31295)
Maxillary sinusoscopy (31233)

Code also stereotactic navigation, when performed (61782)

31256 **Nasal/sinus endoscopy, surgical, with maxillary antrostomy;**

EXCLUDES *When performed on the same side:*
Maxillary antrostomy with removal of tissue from maxillary sinus (31267)

5.19 5.19 **FUD** 000 J A2 50

AMA: 2019,Apr,10; 2018,Apr,3; 2018,Apr,10; 2018,Jan,8; 2017,Jan,8; 2016,Jan,13; 2015,Jan,16

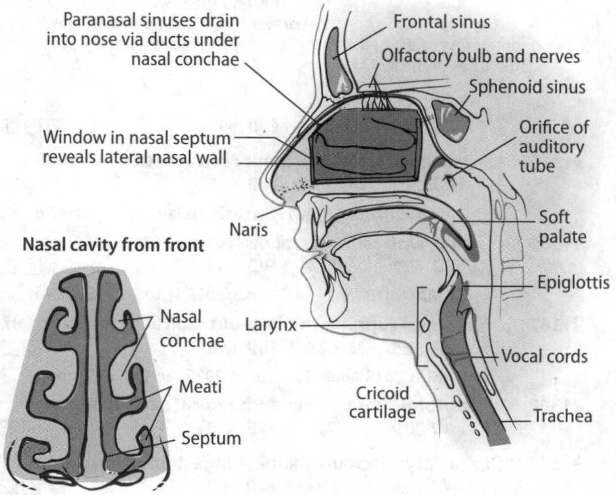

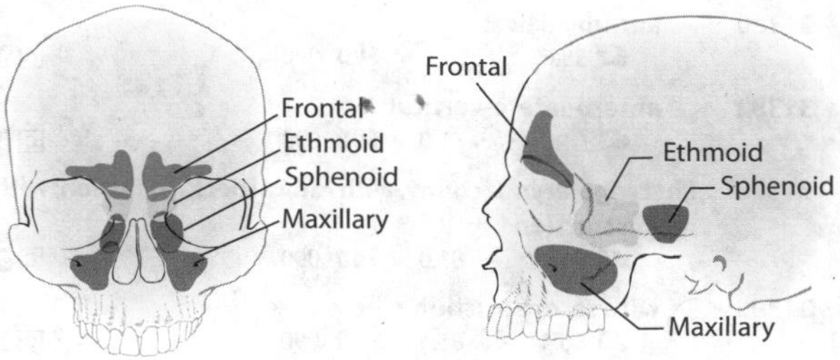

31257 **Resequenced code. See code following 31255.**

31259 **Resequenced code. See code following 31255.**

31267 **with removal of tissue from maxillary sinus**

EXCLUDES *When performed on same side:*
Maxillary antrostomy without removal tissue (31256)

7.61 7.61 **FUD** 000 J A2 50

AMA: 2019,Apr,10; 2018,Apr,3; 2018,Jan,8; 2017,Jan,8; 2016,Jan,13; 2015,Jan,16

31276 Nasal Endoscopy with Frontal Sinus Examination

INCLUDES Diagnostic nasal/sinus endoscopy
Sinusotomy, when applicable

EXCLUDES *When performed on same side:*
Biopsy, polypectomy, or debridement (31237)
Dilation frontal or frontal and sphenoid sinus (31296, 31298)
Other total ethmoidectomy procedures (31253, 31255)

Code also stereotactic navigation, when performed (61782)

31276 **Nasal/sinus endoscopy, surgical, with frontal sinus exploration, including removal of tissue from frontal si[nus], when performed**

10.9 10.9 **FUD** 000 J A2

AMA: 2019,Apr,10; 2018,Apr,3; 2018,Apr,10; 2018,Jan,8; 2017,Jan,8; 2016,Jan,13; 2015,Jan,16

31287-31288 Nasal Endoscopy with Sphenoid Procedur[es]

EXCLUDES *Sinus dilation (31297-31298)*
When performed on same side:
Biopsy, polypectomy, or debridement (31237)
Diagnostic sphenoid sinusoscopy (31235)
Optic nerve decompression (31294)
Other total ethmoidectomy procedures (31255, [31257], [31259])
Repair CSF leak (31291)

Code also stereotactic navigation, when performed (61782)

31287 **Nasal/sinus endoscopy, surgical, with sphenoidotomy;**

EXCLUDES *When performed on same side:*
Sphenoidotomy with removal tissue (31288)

5.78 5.78 **FUD** 000 J A2 80 50

AMA: 2019,Apr,10; 2018,Apr,3; 2018,Jan,8; 2017,Jan,8; 2016,Jan,13; 2015,Jan,16

31288 **with removal of tissue from the sphenoid sinus**

EXCLUDES *When performed on same side:*
Sphenoidotomy without removal tissue (31287)

6.71 6.71 **FUD** 000 J A2 80 50

AMA: 2019,Apr,10; 2018,Apr,3; 2018,Jan,8; 2017,Jan,8; 2016,Feb,10; 2016,Jan,13; 2015,Jan,16

31290-31294 Nasal Endoscopy with Repair and Decompression

INCLUDES Diagnostic nasal/sinus endoscopy
Sinusotomy, when applicable

EXCLUDES *When performed on same side:*
Biopsy, polypectomy, or debridement (31237)
Other total ethmoidectomy procedures ([31253], 31255, [31257], [31259])
Partial ethmoidectomy (31254)

Code also stereotactic navigation, when performed (61782)

31290 **Nasal/sinus endoscopy, surgical, with repair of cerebrospinal fluid leak; ethmoid region**

32.7 32.7 **FUD** 010 C 80 50

AMA: 2018,Apr,3; 2018,Jan,8; 2017,Jan,8; 2016,Feb,10; 2016,Jan,13; 2015,Jan,16

31291 **sphenoid region**

EXCLUDES *When performed on same side:*
Sphenoidotomy (31287-31288)

34.9 34.9 **FUD** 010 C 80 50

AMA: 2018,Apr,3; 2018,Jan,8; 2017,Jan,8; 2016,Jan,13; 2015,Jan,16

31292 **Nasal/sinus endoscopy, surgical, with orbital decompression; medial or inferior wall**

EXCLUDES *When performed on same side:*
Dilation frontal sinus only (31296)
Orbital wall decompression, medial and inferior (31293)

28.4 28.4 **FUD** 010 J 80 50

AMA: 2018,Apr,3; 2018,Jan,8; 2017,Jan,8; 2016,Jan,13; 2015,Jan,16

31293 **medial and inferior wall**

EXCLUDES *When performed on same side:*
Orbital wall decompression, medial or inferior (31292)

30.7 30.7 **FUD** 010 J 80 50

AMA: 2018,Apr,3; 2018,Jan,8; 2017,Jan,8; 2016,Jan,13; 2015,Jan,16

31294 **Nasal/sinus endoscopy, surgical, with optic nerve decompression**

EXCLUDES *When performed on same side:*
Sphenoidotomy (31287-31288)

35.2 | 35.2 | FUD 010 | J 80 50

AMA: 2018,Apr,3; 2018,Jan,8; 2017,Jan,8; 2016,Jan,13; 2015,Jan,16

31295-31298 Nasal Endoscopy with Sinus Ostia Dilation

INCLUDES Any method tissue displacement
Fluoroscopy, when performed

Code also stereotactic navigation, when performed (61782)

31295 **Nasal/sinus endoscopy, surgical, with dilation (eg, balloon dilation); maxillary sinus ostium, transnasal or via canine fossa**

EXCLUDES *When performed on same side:*
Maxillary antrostomy (31256-31267)
Maxillary sinusoscopy (31233)

4.55 | 55.6 | FUD 000 | J P3 80 50

AMA: 2020,Jun,14; 2018,Apr,3; 2018,Jan,8; 2017,Jan,8; 2016,Jan,13; 2015,Jan,16

31296 **frontal sinus ostium**

EXCLUDES *When performed on same side:*
Frontal sinus exploration (31276)
Dilation frontal and sphenoid sinus (31298)
Dilation sphenoid sinus only (31297)
Total ethmoidectomy (31253)

5.15 | 54.2 | FUD 000 | J P3 80 50

AMA: 2020,Jun,14; 2018,Apr,3; 2018,Jan,8; 2017,Jan,8; 2016,Jan,13; 2015,Jan,16

31297 **sphenoid sinus ostium**

EXCLUDES *When performed on same side:*
Diagnostic sphenoid sinusoscopy (31235)
Dilation frontal and sphenoid sinus (31298)
Dilation frontal sinus only (31296)
Sphenoidotomy (31287-31288)
Total ethmoidectomy procedures ([31257], [31259])

4.12 | 53.1 | FUD 000 | J P3 80 50

AMA: 2020,Jun,14; 2018,Apr,3; 2018,Jan,8; 2017,Jan,8; 2016,Jan,13; 2015,Jan,16

31298 **frontal and sphenoid sinus ostia**

EXCLUDES *When performed on same side:*
Diagnostic sphenoid sinusoscopy (31235)
Dilation frontal sinus only (31296)
Dilation sphenoid sinus only (31297)
Frontal sinus exploration (31276)
Other total ethmoidectomy procedures (31253, [31257], [31259])
Sphenoidotomy (31287-31288)

7.34 | 102. | FUD 000 | J P2 80 50

AMA: 2020,Jun,14; 2018,Apr,3

31299 Unlisted Procedures of Accessory Sinuses

CMS: 100-04,4,180.3 Unlisted Service or Procedure

EXCLUDES *Hypophysectomy (61546, 61548)*

31299 **Unlisted procedure, accessory sinuses**

0.00 | 0.00 | FUD YYY | T 80

AMA: 2019,Jul,7; 2019,Apr,10; 2018,Jan,8; 2017,Nov,11; 2017,Jan,8; 2016,Feb,10; 2016,Jan,13; 2015,Jul,10; 2015,Jan,16

31300-31502 Procedures of the Larynx

31300 **Laryngotomy (thyrotomy, laryngofissure), with removal of tumor or laryngocele, cordectomy**

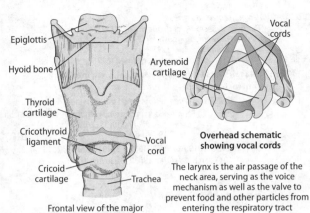

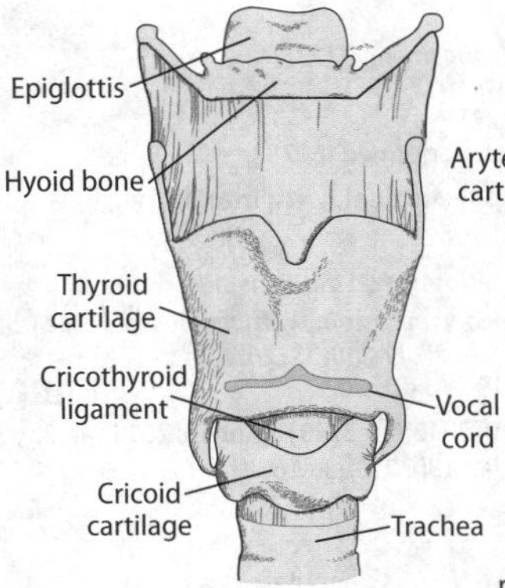

Frontal view of the major structures of the larynx

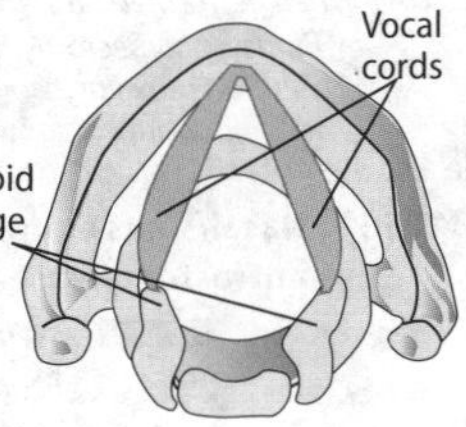

Overhead schematic showing vocal cords

The larynx is the air passage of the neck area, serving as the voice mechanism as well as the valve to prevent food and other particles from entering the respiratory tract

36.6 | 36.6 | FUD 090 | J A2 80

31360 **Laryngectomy; total, without radical neck dissection**

59.2 | 59.2 | FUD 090 | C 80

AMA: 2018,Jan,8; 2017,Jan,8; 2016,Jan,13; 2015,Jan,16

31365 **total, with radical neck dissection**

73.2 | 73.2 | FUD 090 | C 80

AMA: 2018,Jan,8; 2017,Jan,8; 2016,Jan,13; 2015,Jan,16

31367 **subtotal supraglottic, without radical neck dissection**

62.6 | 62.6 | FUD 090 | C 80

AMA: 2018,Jan,8; 2017,Jan,8; 2016,Jan,13; 2015,Jan,16

31368 **subtotal supraglottic, with radical neck dissection**

70.2 | 70.2 | FUD 090 | C 80

31370 **Partial laryngectomy (hemilaryngectomy); horizontal**

59.4 | 59.4 | FUD 090 | C 80

31375 **laterovertical**

55.8 | 55.8 | FUD 090 | C 80

31380 **anterovertical**

55.6 | 55.6 | FUD 090 | C 80

31382 **antero-latero-vertical**

61.0 | 61.0 | FUD 090 | C 80

31390 **Pharyngolaryngectomy, with radical neck dissection; without reconstruction**

81.0 | 81.0 | FUD 090 | C 80

31395 **with reconstruction**

86.4 | 86.4 | FUD 090 | C 80

31400 **Arytenoidectomy or arytenoidopexy, external approach**

EXCLUDES *Endoscopic arytenoidectomy (31560)*

28.0 | 28.0 | FUD 090 | J A2 80

31420 **Epiglottidectomy**

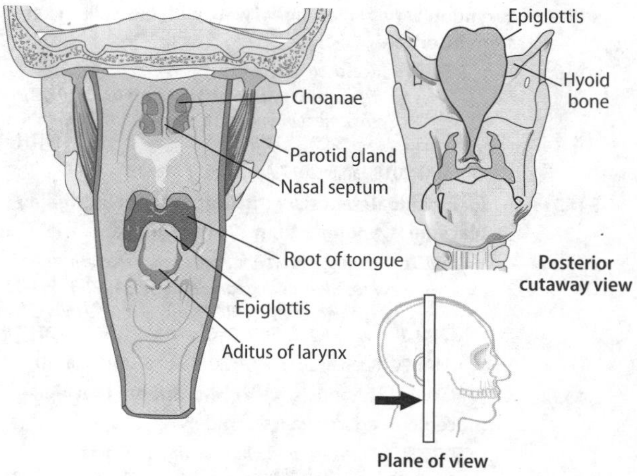

23.4 23.4 FUD 090 J A2 80

31500 **Intubation, endotracheal, emergency procedure**

EXCLUDES *Chest x-ray performed to confirm endotracheal tube position*

4.14 4.14 FUD 000 T G2

AMA: 2018,Jan,8; 2017,Jan,8; 2016,Oct,8; 2016,May,3; 2016,Jan,13; 2015,Jan,16

31502 **Tracheotomy tube change prior to establishment of fistula tract**

1.01 1.01 FUD 000 T G2

AMA: 1990,Win,4

31505-31541 Endoscopy of the Larynx

31505 **Laryngoscopy, indirect; diagnostic (separate procedure)**

1.39 2.48 FUD 000 T P3

AMA: 2018,Jan,8; 2017,Jan,8; 2016,Jan,13; 2015,Jan,16

31510 **with biopsy**

3.46 6.01 FUD 000 J A2 80

AMA: 2018,Jan,8; 2017,Jan,8; 2016,Jan,13; 2015,Jan,16

31511 **with removal of foreign body**

3.79 6.04 FUD 000 T A2

AMA: 2018,Jan,8; 2017,Jan,8; 2016,Jan,13; 2015,Jan,16

31512 **with removal of lesion**

3.70 5.92 FUD 000 J A2 80

AMA: 2018,Jan,8; 2017,Jan,8; 2016,Jan,13; 2015,Jan,16

31513 **with vocal cord injection**

3.76 3.76 FUD 000 T A2 80

AMA: 2018,Jan,8; 2017,Jan,8; 2016,Jan,13; 2015,Jan,16

31515 **Laryngoscopy direct, with or without tracheoscopy; for aspiration**

3.12 5.79 FUD 000 T A2

AMA: 1998,Nov,1; 1997,Nov,1

31520 **diagnostic, newborn** A

4.48 4.48 FUD 000 63 T G2 80

AMA: 1998,Nov,1; 1997,Nov,1

31525 **diagnostic, except newborn**

4.56 7.15 FUD 000 J A2

AMA: 2018,Jan,8; 2017,Jan,8; 2016,Jan,13; 2015,Jan,16

31526 **diagnostic, with operating microscope or telescope**

INCLUDES Operating microscope (69990)

4.49 4.49 FUD 000 J A2

AMA: 2018,Jan,8; 2017,Jun,10; 2016,Feb,12

31527 **with insertion of obturator**

5.55 5.55 FUD 000 J A2 80

AMA: 1998,Nov,1; 1997,Nov,1

31528 **with dilation, initial**

4.09 4.09 FUD 000 J A2 80

AMA: 2002,May,7; 1998,Nov,1

31529 **with dilation, subsequent**

4.59 4.59 FUD 000 J A2 80

AMA: 2002,May,7; 1998,Nov,1

31530 **Laryngoscopy, direct, operative, with foreign body removal;**

5.70 5.70 FUD 000 J A2

AMA: 1998,Nov,1; 1997,Nov,1

31531 **with operating microscope or telescope**

INCLUDES Operating microscope (69990)

6.08 6.08 FUD 000 J A2 80

AMA: 2018,Jan,8; 2017,Jun,10; 2016,Feb,12

31535 **Laryngoscopy, direct, operative, with biopsy;**

5.39 5.39 FUD 000 J A2

AMA: 1998,Nov,1; 1997,Nov,1

31536 **with operating microscope or telescope**

INCLUDES Operating microscope (69990)

6.00 6.00 FUD 000 J A2

AMA: 2018,Jan,8; 2017,Jun,10; 2016,Feb,12

31540 **Laryngoscopy, direct, operative, with excision of tumor and/or stripping of vocal cords or epiglottis;**

6.89 6.89 FUD 000 J A2

AMA: 1998,Nov,1; 1997,Nov,1

31541 **with operating microscope or telescope**

INCLUDES Operating microscope (69990)

7.52 7.52 FUD 000 J A2

AMA: 2019,Sep,10; 2019,Jul,10; 2018,Jan,8; 2017,Jun,10; 2016,Feb,12

31545-31554 [31551, 31552, 31553, 31554] Endoscopy of Larynx with Reconstruction

INCLUDES Operating microscope (69990)

EXCLUDES *Laryngoscopy, direct, operative, with excision tumor and/or vocal cord or epiglottis stripping (31540-31541)*

Vocal cord reconstruction with allograft (31599)

31545 **Laryngoscopy, direct, operative, with operating microscope or telescope, with submucosal removal of non-neoplastic lesion(s) of vocal cord; reconstruction with local tissue flap(s)**

10.3 10.3 FUD 000 J A2 50

AMA: 2016,Feb,12

31546 **reconstruction with graft(s) (includes obtaining autograft)**

EXCLUDES *Autologous fat graft obtained by liposuction (15771-15774)*

Autologous soft tissue grafts obtained by direct excision ([15769])

15.7 15.7 FUD 000 J A2 50

AMA: 2018,Jan,8; 2017,Jan,8; 2016,Feb,12; 2016,Jan,13; 2015,Jan,16

31551 **Resequenced code. See code following 31580.**

31552 **Resequenced code. See code following 31580.**

31553 **Resequenced code. See code following 31580.**

31554 **Resequenced code. See code following 31580.**

31560-31571 Endoscopy of Larynx with Arytenoid Removal, Vocal Cord Injection

31560 **Laryngoscopy, direct, operative, with arytenoidectomy;**

8.97 8.97 FUD 000 J A2 80

AMA: 1998,Nov,1; 1997,Nov,1

31561 **with operating microscope or telescope**

INCLUDES Operating microscope (69990)

9.82 9.82 FUD 000 J A2 80

AMA: 2018,Jan,8; 2017,Jun,10; 2016,Feb,12

31570 **Laryngoscopy, direct, with injection into vocal cord(s), therapeutic;**

6.53 9.68 FUD 000 J A2

AMA: 2018,Jan,8; 2017,Jan,8; 2017,Jan,6; 2016,Jan,13; 2015,Jan,16

31571 **with operating microscope or telescope**

INCLUDES *Operating microscope (69990)*

7.14 7.14 FUD 000 J A2

AMA: 2018,Jan,8; 2017,Jun,10; 2017,Jan,8; 2017,Jan,6; 2016,Feb,12; 2016,Jan,13; 2015,Jan,16

31572-31579 [31572, 31573, 31574] Endoscopy of Larynx, Flexible Fiberoptic

EXCLUDES *Evaluation by flexible fiberoptic endoscope:*
Sensory assessment (92614-92615)
Swallowing (92612-92613)
Swallowing and sensory assessment (92616-92617)
Flexible fiberoptic endoscopic examination/testing by cine or video recording (92612-92617)

31572 **Resequenced code. See code following 31578.**

31573 **Resequenced code. See code following 31578.**

31574 **Resequenced code. See code following 31578.**

31575 **Laryngoscopy, flexible; diagnostic**

EXCLUDES *Diagnostic nasal endoscopy not through additional endoscope (31231)*
Procedures during same session (31572-31574, 31576-31578, 43197-43198, 92511, 92612, 92614, 92616)

1.90 3.49 FUD 000 T P2

AMA: 2018,Jan,8; 2017,Jul,7; 2017,Apr,8; 2017,Jan,8; 2016,Dec,13

31576 **with biopsy(ies)**

EXCLUDES *Destruction or excision lesion (31572, 31578)*

3.38 7.63 FUD 000 J A2

AMA: 2018,Jan,8; 2017,Jul,7; 2017,Apr,8; 2017,Jan,8; 2016,Dec,13

31577 **with removal of foreign body(s)**

3.82 7.93 FUD 000 T A2 80

AMA: 2018,Jan,8; 2017,Jul,7; 2017,Apr,8; 2017,Jan,8; 2016,Dec,13

31578 **with removal of lesion(s), non-laser**

4.27 8.59 FUD 000 J A2 80

AMA: 2018,Jan,8; 2017,Jul,7; 2017,Apr,8; 2017,Jan,8; 2016,Dec,13

\# **31572** **with ablation or destruction of lesion(s) with laser, unilateral**

EXCLUDES *Biopsy or excision lesion (31576, 31578)*

5.15 14.7 FUD 000 J G2 80 50

AMA: 2019,Sep,10; 2018,Jan,8; 2017,Jul,7; 2017,Apr,8; 2017,Jan,8; 2016,Dec,13

\# **31573** **with therapeutic injection(s) (eg, chemodenervation agent or corticosteroid, injected percutaneous, transoral, or via endoscope channel), unilateral**

4.27 7.61 FUD 000 J P3 80 50

AMA: 2018,May,7; 2018,Jan,8; 2017,Jul,7; 2017,Apr,8; 2017,Jan,8; 2016,Dec,13

\# **31574** **with injection(s) for augmentation (eg, percutaneous, transoral), unilateral**

4.27 28.7 FUD 000 J G2 80 50

AMA: 2018,May,7; 2018,Jan,8; 2017,Jul,7; 2017,Apr,8; 2017,Jan,8; 2016,Dec,13

31579 **Laryngoscopy, flexible or rigid telescopic, with stroboscopy**

3.41 5.46 FUD 000 T P3

AMA: 2018,Jan,8; 2017,Jul,7; 2017,Apr,8; 2017,Jan,8; 2016,Dec,13

31580-31599 [31551, 31552, 31553, 31554] Larynx Reconstruction

31580 **Laryngoplasty; for laryngeal web, with indwelling keel or stent insertion**

EXCLUDES *Keel or stent removal (31599)*
Tracheostomy (31600-31601, 31603, 31605, 31610)
Treatment laryngeal stenosis (31551-31554)

35.7 35.7 FUD 090 J A2 80

AMA: 2018,Jan,8; 2017,Apr,5; 2017,Mar,10

\# **31551** **for laryngeal stenosis, with graft, without indwelling stent placement, younger than 12 years of age** A

EXCLUDES *Cartilage graft obtained through same incision*
Procedure during same session (31552-31554, 31580)
Tracheostomy (31600-31601, 31603, 31605, 31610)

41.2 41.2 FUD 090 J G2 80

AMA: 2018,Jan,8; 2017,Jul,7; 2017,Apr,5; 2017,Mar,10

\# **31552** **for laryngeal stenosis, with graft, without indwelling stent placement, age 12 years or older** A

EXCLUDES *Cartilage graft obtained through same incision*
Procedure during same session (31551, 31553-31554, 31580)
Tracheostomy (31600-31601, 31603, 31605, 31610)

42.0 42.0 FUD 090 J G2 80

AMA: 2018,Jan,8; 2017,Jul,7; 2017,Apr,5; 2017,Mar,10

\# **31553** **for laryngeal stenosis, with graft, with indwelling stent placement, younger than 12 years of age** A

EXCLUDES *Cartilage graft obtained through same incision*
Procedure during same session (31551-31552, 31554, 31580)
Stent removal (31599)
Tracheostomy (31600-31601, 31603, 31605, 31610)

47.8 47.8 FUD 090 J G2 80

AMA: 2018,Jan,8; 2017,Jul,7; 2017,Apr,5; 2017,Mar,10

\# **31554** **for laryngeal stenosis, with graft, with indwelling stent placement, age 12 years or older** A

EXCLUDES *Cartilage graft obtained through same incision*
Procedure during same session (31551-31553, 31580)
Stent removal (31599)
Tracheostomy (31600-31601, 31603, 31605, 31610)

47.8 47.8 FUD 090 J G2 80

AMA: 2018,Jan,8; 2017,Jul,7; 2017,Apr,5; 2017,Mar,10

31584 **with open reduction and fixation of (eg, plating) fracture, includes tracheostomy, if performed**

EXCLUDES *Cartilage graft obtained through same incision*

39.6 39.6 FUD 090 J 80

AMA: 2018,Jan,8; 2017,Apr,5; 2017,Mar,10

31587 **Laryngoplasty, cricoid split, without graft placement**

EXCLUDES *Tracheostomy (31600-31601, 31603, 31605, 31610)*

33.2 33.2 FUD 090 J 80

AMA: 2018,Jan,8; 2017,Apr,5; 2017,Mar,10

31590 **Laryngeal reinnervation by neuromuscular pedicle**

24.9 24.9 FUD 090 J A2 80

AMA: 2018,Jan,8; 2017,Mar,10

31591 **Laryngoplasty, medialization, unilateral**

30.7 30.7 FUD 090 J G2 80

AMA: 2018,Jan,8; 2017,Jul,7; 2017,Apr,5; 2017,Mar,10

31592 **Cricotracheal resection**

EXCLUDES *Advancement or rotational flaps performed not requiring additional incision*
Cartilage graft obtained through same incision
Tracheal stenosis excision/anastomosis (31780-31781)
Tracheostomy (31600-31601, 31603, 31605, 31610)

49.2 49.2 FUD 090 J G2 80

AMA: 2018,Jan,8; 2017,Jul,7; 2017,Apr,5; 2017,Mar,10; 2017,Feb,14

31599 **Unlisted procedure, larynx**
0.00 0.00 FUD YYY — T 80
AMA: 2018,Jan,8; 2017,Apr,5; 2017,Mar,10; 2017,Jan,8; 2017,Jan,6; 2016,Dec,13; 2016,Jan,13; 2015,Jan,16

31600-31610 Stoma Creation: Trachea

EXCLUDES *Aspiration trachea, direct vision (31515)*
Endotracheal intubation (31500)

31600 **Tracheostomy, planned (separate procedure);**
8.91 8.91 FUD 000 — J
AMA: 2019,Sep,10; 2017,Apr,5

31601 **younger than 2 years** — A
12.9 12.9 FUD 000 — J 80
AMA: 2017,Apr,5

31603 **Tracheostomy, emergency procedure; transtracheal**
9.30 9.30 FUD 000 — T A2
AMA: 2017,Apr,5

31605 **cricothyroid membrane**
9.70 9.70 FUD 000 — T G2
AMA: 2017,Apr,5

31610 **Tracheostomy, fenestration procedure with skin flaps**
27.2 27.2 FUD 090 — J
AMA: 2017,Apr,5

31611-31614 Procedures of the Trachea

31611 **Construction of tracheoesophageal fistula and subsequent insertion of an alaryngeal speech prosthesis (eg, voice button, Blom-Singer prosthesis)**
15.1 15.1 FUD 090 — J A2 80

31612 **Tracheal puncture, percutaneous with transtracheal aspiration and/or injection**
EXCLUDES *Tracheal aspiration under direct vision (31515)*
1.37 2.46 FUD 000 — J A2 80
AMA: 1994,Win,1

31613 **Tracheostoma revision; simple, without flap rotation**
12.6 12.6 FUD 090 — J A2

31614 **complex, with flap rotation**
20.7 20.7 FUD 090 — J A2

31615 Endoscopy Through Tracheostomy

INCLUDES Diagnostic bronchoscopy
EXCLUDES *Endobronchial ultrasound [EBUS] guided biopsies mediastinal or hilar lymph nodes (31652-31653)*
Tracheoscopy (31515-31578)
Code also endobronchial ultrasound [EBUS] during diagnostic/therapeutic peripheral lesion intervention (31654)

31615 **Tracheobronchoscopy through established tracheostomy incision**
3.29 4.83 FUD 000 — T A2
AMA: 2018,Jan,8; 2017,Jan,8; 2016,Jan,13; 2015,Jan,16

31622-31654 [31651] Endoscopy of Lung

INCLUDES Diagnostic bronchoscopy with surgical bronchoscopy procedures
Fluoroscopic imaging guidance, when performed

31622 **Bronchoscopy, rigid or flexible, including fluoroscopic guidance, when performed; diagnostic, with cell washing, when performed (separate procedure)**
3.78 6.84 FUD 000 — J A2
AMA: 2018,Jan,8; 2017,Jan,8; 2016,Apr,5; 2016,Jan,13; 2015,Jan,16

31623 **with brushing or protected brushings**
3.82 7.66 FUD 000 — J A2
AMA: 2018,Jan,8; 2017,Jan,8; 2016,Apr,5; 2016,Jan,13; 2015,Jan,16

31624 **with bronchial alveolar lavage**
3.87 7.16 FUD 000 — J A2
AMA: 2018,Jan,8; 2017,Jun,10; 2017,Jan,8; 2016,Apr,5; 2016,Jan,13; 2015,Jan,16

31625 **with bronchial or endobronchial biopsy(s), single or multiple sites**
4.50 9.80 FUD 000 — J A2
AMA: 2018,Jan,8; 2017,Jan,8; 2016,Apr,5; 2016,Jan,13; 2015,Jan,16

31626 **with placement of fiducial markers, single or multiple**
Code also device
5.72 23.9 FUD 000 — J G2 80
AMA: 2018,Jan,8; 2017,Jun,10; 2017,Jan,8; 2016,Apr,5; 2016,Jan,13; 2015,Jun,6; 2015,Jan,16

\+ **31627** **with computer-assisted, image-guided navigation (List separately in addition to code for primary procedure[s])**
INCLUDES 3D reconstruction (76376-76377)
Code first (31615, 31622-31626, 31628-31631, 31635-31636, 31638-31643)
2.78 36.3 FUD ZZZ — N N1 80
AMA: 2018,Jan,8; 2017,Jan,8; 2016,Jan,13; 2015,Jan,16

31628 **with transbronchial lung biopsy(s), single lobe**
INCLUDES All biopsies taken from lobe
EXCLUDES *Transbronchial biopsies by needle aspiration (31629, 31633)*
Code also transbronchial biopsies additional lobe(s) (31632)
5.06 10.4 FUD 000 — J A2
AMA: 2018,Jan,8; 2017,Jun,10; 2017,Jan,8; 2016,Apr,5; 2016,Jan,13; 2015,Jan,16

31629 **with transbronchial needle aspiration biopsy(s), trachea, main stem and/or lobar bronchus(i)**
INCLUDES All biopsies from same lobe or upper airway
EXCLUDES *Transbronchial biopsies lung (31628, 31632)*
Code also transbronchial needle biopsies additional lobe(s) (31633)
5.37 12.8 FUD 000 — J A2
AMA: 2018,Jan,8; 2017,Jan,8; 2016,Apr,5; 2016,Jan,13; 2015,Jan,16

31630 **with tracheal/bronchial dilation or closed reduction of fracture**
5.72 5.72 FUD 000 — J A2
AMA: 2018,Jan,8; 2017,Jan,8; 2016,Jan,13; 2015,Jan,16

31631 **with placement of tracheal stent(s) (includes tracheal/bronchial dilation as required)**
EXCLUDES *Bronchial stent placement (31636-31637)*
Revision bronchial or tracheal stent (31638)
6.58 6.58 FUD 000 — J A2
AMA: 2018,Jan,8; 2017,Jan,8; 2016,Jan,13; 2015,Jan,16

\+ **31632** **with transbronchial lung biopsy(s), each additional lobe (List separately in addition to code for primary procedure)**
INCLUDES All biopsies taken from additional lobe lung
Code first (31628)
1.43 1.82 FUD ZZZ — N N1
AMA: 2018,Jan,8; 2017,Jan,8; 2016,Jan,13; 2015,Jan,16

\+ **31633** **with transbronchial needle aspiration biopsy(s), each additional lobe (List separately in addition to code for primary procedure)**
INCLUDES All needle biopsies from another lobe or from trachea
Code first (31629)
1.82 2.26 FUD ZZZ — N N1
AMA: 2018,Jan,8; 2017,Jan,8; 2016,Jan,13; 2015,Jan,16

31634 **with balloon occlusion, with assessment of air leak, with administration of occlusive substance (eg, fibrin glue), if performed**
EXCLUDES *When performed during same operative session:*
Bronchoscopy, rigid or flexible, including fluoroscopic guidance; with balloon occlusio, assessment air leak, airway sizing, and insertion bronchial valve(s), initial lobe (31647, [31651])
5.53 49.4 FUD 000 — J G2 80
AMA: 2018,Jan,8; 2017,Jan,8; 2016,Jan,13; 2015,Jan,16

31635 **with removal of foreign body**
EXCLUDES *Removal implanted bronchial valves (31648-31649)*
5.06 8.03 FUD 000 J A2
AMA: 2018,Jan,8; 2017,Jan,8; 2016,Jan,13; 2015,Jan,16

31636 **with placement of bronchial stent(s) (includes tracheal/bronchial dilation as required), initial bronchus**
6.33 6.33 FUD 000 J J8
AMA: 2018,Jan,8; 2017,Jan,8; 2016,Jan,13; 2015,Jan,16

+ **31637** **each additional major bronchus stented (List separately in addition to code for primary procedure)**
Code first (31636)
2.22 2.22 FUD ZZZ N N1
AMA: 2018,Jan,8; 2017,Jan,8; 2016,Jan,13; 2015,Jan,16

31638 **with revision of tracheal or bronchial stent inserted at previous session (includes tracheal/bronchial dilation as required)**
7.21 7.21 FUD 000 J A2
AMA: 2018,Jan,8; 2017,Jan,8; 2016,Jan,13; 2015,Jan,16

31640 **with excision of tumor**
7.21 7.21 FUD 000 J A2
AMA: 2018,Jan,8; 2017,Jan,8; 2016,Apr,5; 2016,Jan,13; 2015,Jan,16

31641 **with destruction of tumor or relief of stenosis by any method other than excision (eg, laser therapy, cryotherapy)**
Code also any photodynamic therapy via bronchoscopy (96570-96571)
7.39 7.39 FUD 000 J A2
AMA: 2018,Jan,8; 2017,Jan,8; 2016,Jan,13; 2015,Jan,16

31643 **with placement of catheter(s) for intracavitary radioelement application**
Code also when appropriate (77761-77763, 77770-77772)
5.04 5.04 FUD 000 J A2
AMA: 2018,Jan,8; 2017,Jan,8; 2016,Apr,5; 2016,Jan,13; 2015,Jan,16

31645 **with therapeutic aspiration of tracheobronchial tree, initial (eg, drainage of lung abscess)**
EXCLUDES *Bedside aspiration trachea, bronchi (31725)*
4.21 7.42 FUD 000 J A2
AMA: 2018,Jan,8; 2017,Jan,8; 2016,Apr,5; 2016,Jan,13; 2015,Jan,16

31646 **with therapeutic aspiration of tracheobronchial tree, subsequent**
EXCLUDES *Bedside aspiration trachea, bronchi (31725)*
4.08 4.08 FUD 000 T A2
AMA: 2018,Sep,3; 2018,Jan,8; 2017,Jan,8; 2016,Apr,5; 2016,Jan,13; 2015,Jan,16

31647 **with balloon occlusion, when performed, assessment of air leak, airway sizing, and insertion of bronchial valve(s), initial lobe**
6.10 6.10 FUD 000 J J8
AMA: 2018,Sep,3; 2018,Jan,8; 2017,Jan,8; 2016,Jan,13; 2015,Jan,16

+ # **31651** **with balloon occlusion, when performed, assessment of air leak, airway sizing, and insertion of bronchial valve(s), each additional lobe (List separately in addition to code for primary procedure[s])**
Code first (31647)
2.13 2.13 FUD ZZZ N N1
AMA: 2018,Sep,3; 2018,Jan,8; 2017,Jan,8; 2016,Jan,13; 2015,Jan,16

31648 **with removal of bronchial valve(s), initial lobe**
EXCLUDES *Removal with reinsertion bronchial valve during same session (31647 and 31648) and ([31651])*
5.80 5.80 FUD 000 J G2
AMA: 2018,Sep,3; 2018,Jan,8; 2017,Jan,8; 2016,Jan,13; 2015,Jan,16

+ **31649** **with removal of bronchial valve(s), each additional lobe (List separately in addition to code for primary procedure)**
Code first (31648)
1.94 1.94 FUD ZZZ Q2 G2
AMA: 2018,Sep,3; 2018,Jan,8; 2017,Jan,8; 2016,Jan,13; 2015,Jan,16

31651 **Resequenced code. See code following 31647.**

31652 **with endobronchial ultrasound (EBUS) guided transtracheal and/or transbronchial sampling (eg, aspiration[s]/biopsy[ies]), one or two mediastinal and/or hilar lymph node stations or structures**
EXCLUDES *Procedures performed more than one time per session*
6.38 31.2 FUD 000 J G2
AMA: 2018,Jan,8; 2017,Jan,8; 2016,Apr,5

31653 **with endobronchial ultrasound (EBUS) guided transtracheal and/or transbronchial sampling (eg, aspiration[s]/biopsy[ies]), 3 or more mediastinal and/or hilar lymph node stations or structures**
EXCLUDES *Procedures performed more than one time per session*
7.08 28.7 FUD 000 J G2
AMA: 2018,Jan,8; 2017,Jan,8; 2016,Apr,5

+ **31654** **with transendoscopic endobronchial ultrasound (EBUS) during bronchoscopic diagnostic or therapeutic intervention(s) for peripheral lesion(s) (List separately in addition to code for primary procedure[s])**
EXCLUDES *Endobronchial ultrasound [EBUS] for mediastinal/hilar lymph node station/adjacent structure access (31652-31653)*
Procedures performed more than one time per session
Code first (31622-31626, 31628-31629, 31640, 31643-31646)
1.94 3.48 FUD ZZZ N N1
AMA: 2018,Jan,8; 2017,Jan,8; 2016,Apr,5

31660-31661 Bronchial Thermoplasty

INCLUDES Fluoroscopic imaging guidance, when performed

31660 **Bronchoscopy, rigid or flexible, including fluoroscopic guidance, when performed; with bronchial thermoplasty, 1 lobe**
5.62 5.62 FUD 000 J
AMA: 2018,Jan,8; 2017,Jan,8; 2016,Jan,13; 2015,Jan,16

31661 **with bronchial thermoplasty, 2 or more lobes**
5.93 5.93 FUD 000 J
AMA: 2018,Jan,8; 2017,Jan,8; 2016,Jan,13; 2015,Jan,16

31717-31899 Respiratory Procedures

EXCLUDES *Endotracheal intubation (31500)*
Tracheal aspiration under direct vision (31515)

31717 **Catheterization with bronchial brush biopsy**
3.18 7.98 FUD 000 T A2
AMA: 2018,Jan,8; 2017,Jan,8; 2016,Jan,13; 2015,Jan,16

31720 **Catheter aspiration (separate procedure); nasotracheal**
1.59 1.59 FUD 000 Q1 N1
AMA: 1994,Win,1

31725 **tracheobronchial with fiberscope, bedside**
2.27 2.27 FUD 000 C

31730 **Transtracheal (percutaneous) introduction of needle wire dilator/stent or indwelling tube for oxygen therapy**
4.33 33.8 FUD 000 J A2
AMA: 1992,Win,1

31750 **Tracheoplasty; cervical**
39.1 39.1 FUD 090 J A2 80

31755 **tracheopharyngeal fistulization, each stage**
49.1 49.1 FUD 090 J A2 80

31760 **intrathoracic**
39.6 39.6 FUD 090 C 80

31766 **Carinal reconstruction**
51.3 51.3 FUD 090 C 80

31770 Bronchoplasty; graft repair

EXCLUDES *Bronchoplasty done with lobectomy (32501)*

38.4 38.4 FUD 090 C 80

31775 excision stenosis and anastomosis

EXCLUDES *Bronchoplasty done with lobectomy (32501)*

40.4 40.4 FUD 090 C 80

31780 Excision tracheal stenosis and anastomosis; cervical

34.2 34.2 FUD 090 C 80

AMA: 2018,Jan,8; 2017,Apr,5; 2017,Feb,14

31781 cervicothoracic

39.8 39.8 FUD 090 C 80

AMA: 2018,Jan,8; 2017,Apr,5; 2017,Feb,14

31785 Excision of tracheal tumor or carcinoma; cervical

30.8 30.8 FUD 090 J 80

AMA: 2003,Jan,1

31786 thoracic

41.6 41.6 FUD 090 C 80

31800 Suture of tracheal wound or injury; cervical

20.3 20.3 FUD 090 C 80

AMA: 1994,Win,1

31805 intrathoracic

23.5 23.5 FUD 090 C 80

31820 Surgical closure tracheostomy or fistula; without plastic repair

EXCLUDES *Tracheoesophageal fistula repair (43305, 43312)*

9.35 12.3 FUD 090 J A2 80

31825 with plastic repair

EXCLUDES *Tracheoesophageal fistula repair (43305, 43312)*

13.6 17.1 FUD 090 J A2 80

31830 Revision of tracheostomy scar

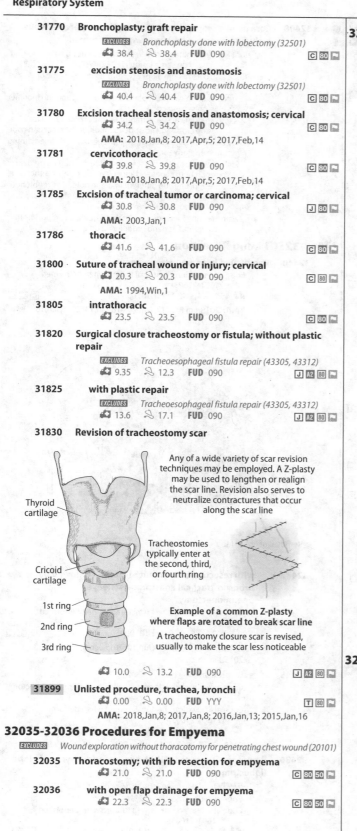

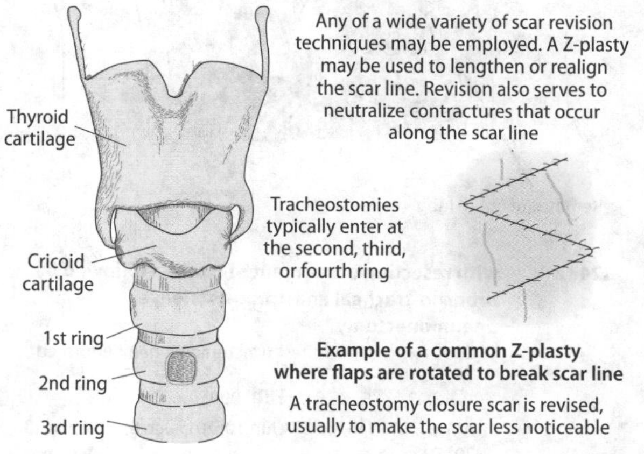

Any of a wide variety of scar revision techniques may be employed. A Z-plasty may be used to lengthen or realign the scar line. Revision also serves to neutralize contractures that occur along the scar line
Thyroid cartilage
Tracheostomies typically enter at the second, third, or fourth ring
Cricoid cartilage
1st ring
2nd ring
3rd ring
Example of a common Z-plasty where flaps are rotated to break scar line
A tracheostomy closure scar is revised, usually to make the scar less noticeable

10.0 13.2 FUD 090 J A2 80

31899 Unlisted procedure, trachea, bronchi

0.00 0.00 FUD YYY T 80

AMA: 2018,Jan,8; 2017,Jan,8; 2016,Jan,13; 2015,Jan,16

32035-32036 Procedures for Empyema

EXCLUDES *Wound exploration without thoracotomy for penetrating chest wound (20101)*

32035 Thoracostomy; with rib resection for empyema

21.0 21.0 FUD 090 C 80 50

32036 with open flap drainage for empyema

22.3 22.3 FUD 090 C 80 50

32096-32098 Open Biopsy of Chest and Pleura

INCLUDES Varying amounts of lung tissue excised for analysis
Wedge technique with tissue obtained without precise consideration of margins

EXCLUDES *Core needle biopsy, lung or mediastinum (32408)*
Percutaneous needle biopsy pleura (32400)
Thoracoscopy:
with biopsy (32607-32609)
with diagnostic wedge resection resulting in anatomic lung resection (32668)
with diagnostic wedge resection resulting in anatomic lung resection (32507)

32096 Thoracotomy, with diagnostic biopsy(ies) of lung infiltrate(s) (eg, wedge, incisional), unilateral

EXCLUDES *Procedure performed more than one time per lung*
Removal lung (32440-32445, 32488)

Code also appropriate add-on code for the more extensive procedure at the same location if diagnostic wedge resection results in the need for further surgery (32507, 32668)

23.2 23.2 FUD 090 C 80

AMA: 2018,Jan,8; 2017,Jan,8; 2016,Jan,13; 2015,Jan,16

32097 Thoracotomy, with diagnostic biopsy(ies) of lung nodule(s) or mass(es) (eg, wedge, incisional), unilateral

EXCLUDES *Procedure performed more than one time per lung*
Removal lung (32440-32445, 32488)

Code also appropriate add-on code for the more extensive procedure in the same location if diagnostic wedge resection results in the need for further surgery (32507, 32668)

23.1 23.1 FUD 090 C 80

AMA: 2018,Jan,8; 2017,Jan,8; 2016,Jan,13; 2015,Jan,16

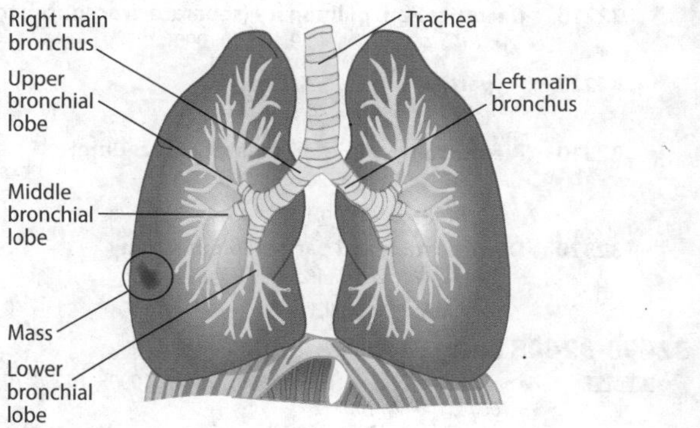

32098 Thoracotomy, with biopsy(ies) of pleura

21.9 21.9 FUD 090 C 80

AMA: 2018,Jan,8; 2017,Jan,8; 2016,Jan,13; 2015,Jan,16

32100-32160 Open Procedures: Chest

INCLUDES Exploration penetrating chest wound

EXCLUDES *Lung resection (32480-32504)*
Wound exploration without thoracotomy for penetrating chest wound (20101)

32100 Thoracotomy; with exploration

EXCLUDES *Excision chest wall tumor, when performed (21601-21603)*
Extracorporeal membrane oxygenation (ECMO)/extracorporeal life support (ECLS) (33955-33957, [33963, 33964])
Resection apical lung tumor (32503-32504)

23.3 23.3 FUD 090 C 80

AMA: 2019,Dec,5; 2019,Dec,4; 2018,Jan,8; 2017,Jan,8; 2016,Jan,13; 2015,Jul,3; 2015,Jan,16

32110 with control of traumatic hemorrhage and/or repair of lung tear

42.4 42.4 FUD 090 C 80

AMA: 2018,Jan,8; 2017,Jan,8; 2016,Jan,13; 2015,Jan,16

32120 for postoperative complications

25.2 25.2 FUD 090 C 80

32124 **with open intrapleural pneumonolysis**
26.7 26.7 **FUD** 090
AMA: 2018,Jan,8; 2017,Jan,8; 2016,Jan,13; 2015,Jan,16

32140 **with cyst(s) removal, includes pleural procedure when performed**
28.5 28.5 **FUD** 090
AMA: 2018,Jan,8; 2017,Jan,8; 2016,Jan,13; 2015,Jan,16

32141 **with resection-plication of bullae, includes any pleural procedure when performed**
EXCLUDES *Lung volume reduction (32491)*
44.0 44.0 **FUD** 090
AMA: 2018,Jan,8; 2017,Jan,8; 2016,Jan,13; 2015,Jan,16

32150 **with removal of intrapleural foreign body or fibrin deposit**
28.9 28.9 **FUD** 090
AMA: 2018,Jan,8; 2017,Jan,8; 2016,Jan,13; 2015,Jan,16

32151 **with removal of intrapulmonary foreign body**
29.0 29.0 **FUD** 090

32160 **with cardiac massage**
22.9 22.9 **FUD** 090

32200-32320 Open Procedures: Lung

32200 **Pneumonostomy, with open drainage of abscess or cyst**
EXCLUDES *Image-guided, percutaneous drainage (eg, abscess, cyst) of lungs/mediastinum via catheter (49405)*
(75989)
32.7 32.7 **FUD** 090
AMA: 2013,Nov,9; 1997,Nov,1

32215 **Pleural scarification for repeat pneumothorax**
23.0 23.0 **FUD** 090

32220 **Decortication, pulmonary (separate procedure); total**
45.9 45.9 **FUD** 090

32225 **partial**
28.7 28.7 **FUD** 090

32310 **Pleurectomy, parietal (separate procedure)**
26.3 26.3 **FUD** 090
AMA: 1994,Win,1

32320 **Decortication and parietal pleurectomy**
46.1 46.1 **FUD** 090
AMA: 1994,Fall,1

32400-32408 Lung Biopsy

EXCLUDES *Fine needle aspiration ([10004, 10005, 10006, 10007, 10008, 10009, 10010, 10011, 10012], 10021)*
Open lung biopsy (32096-32097)
Open mediastinal biopsy (39000-39010)
Thoracoscopic (VATS) biopsy lung, pericardium, pleural, or mediastinal space (32604-32609)

32400 **Biopsy, pleura, percutaneous needle**
(76942, 77002, 77012, 77021)
2.48 4.56 **FUD** 000
AMA: 2019,Apr,4; 2018,Jan,8; 2017,Jan,8; 2016,Jan,13; 2015,Jan,16

32405 ~~**Biopsy, lung or mediastinum, percutaneous needle**~~
To report, see ([32408])

● **32408** **Core needle biopsy, lung or mediastinum, percutaneous, including imaging guidance, when performed**
INCLUDES Imaging guidance performed during tsame session on same lesion (76942, 77002, 77012, 77021)
Code also core needle biopsy performed during same operative session:
other anatomical site; report both codes and append modifier 59 on second code
same anatomical site, different lesion; report 32408 for each lesion biopsied and append modifier 59 on second code
Code also FNA biopsy and core needle biopsy performed during same operative session:
different lesion, utilizing same or different imaging guidance; report both codes and append modifier 59 on either code
same lesion, utilizing different imaging guidance; report both image-guided biopsy codes and append modifier 59 on either code
same lesion, utilizing same imaging guidance; report both codes and append modifier 52 on either code

32440-32501 Lung Resection

32440 **Removal of lung, pneumonectomy;**
Code also excision chest wall tumor, when performed (21601-21603)
45.1 45.1 **FUD** 090
AMA: 2018,Jan,8; 2017,Jan,8; 2016,Jan,13; 2015,Jan,16

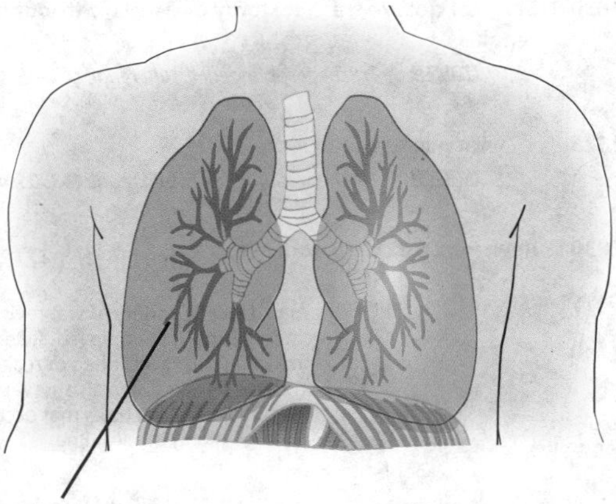

Removal of entire lung

32442 **with resection of segment of trachea followed by broncho-tracheal anastomosis (sleeve pneumonectomy)**
Code also excision chest wall tumor, when performed (21601-21603)
88.9 88.9 **FUD** 090
AMA: 2018,Jan,8; 2017,Jun,10; 2017,Jan,8; 2016,Jan,13; 2015,Jan,16

32445 **extrapleural**
Code also empyemectomy with extrapleural pneumonectomy (32540)
Code also excision chest wall tumor, when performed (21601-21603)
102. 102. **FUD** 090
AMA: 2018,Jan,8; 2017,Jan,8; 2016,Jan,13; 2015,Jan,16

32480 **Removal of lung, other than pneumonectomy; single lobe (lobectomy)**
EXCLUDES *Lung removal with bronchoplasty (32501)*
Code also decortication (32320)
Code also excision chest wall tumor, when performed (21601-21603)
42.6 42.6 **FUD** 090
AMA: 2018,Jan,8; 2017,Jan,8; 2016,Jan,13; 2015,Jan,16

32482 **2 lobes (bilobectomy)**

EXCLUDES *Lung removal with bronchoplasty (32501)*

Code also decortication (32320)

Code also excision chest wall tumor, when performed (21601-21603)

45.8 45.8 **FUD** 090 C 80

AMA: 2018,Jan,8; 2017,Jan,8; 2016,Jan,13; 2015,Jan,16

32484 **single segment (segmentectomy)**

EXCLUDES *Lung removal with bronchoplasty (32501)*

Code also decortication (32320)

Code also excision chest wall tumor, when performed (21601-21603)

41.3 41.3 **FUD** 090 C 80

AMA: 2018,Jan,8; 2017,Jan,8; 2016,Jan,13; 2015,Jan,16

32486 **with circumferential resection of segment of bronchus followed by broncho-bronchial anastomosis (sleeve lobectomy)**

Code also decortication (32320)

Code also excision chest wall tumor, when performed (21601-21603)

68.1 68.1 **FUD** 090 C 80

AMA: 2018,Jan,8; 2017,Jun,10; 2017,Jan,8; 2016,Jan,13; 2015,Jan,16

32488 **with all remaining lung following previous removal of a portion of lung (completion pneumonectomy)**

Code also decortication (32320)

Code also excision chest wall tumor, when performed (21601-21603)

69.1 69.1 **FUD** 090 C 80

AMA: 2018,Jan,8; 2017,Jan,8; 2016,Jan,13; 2015,Jan,16

32491 **with resection-plication of emphysematous lung(s) (bullous or non-bullous) for lung volume reduction, sternal split or transthoracic approach, includes any pleural procedure, when performed**

Code also decortication (32320)

Code also excision chest wall tumor, when performed (21601-21603)

42.4 42.4 **FUD** 090 C 80 50

AMA: 2018,Jan,8; 2017,Jan,8; 2016,Jan,13; 2015,Jan,16

+ **32501** **Resection and repair of portion of bronchus (bronchoplasty) when performed at time of lobectomy or segmentectomy (List separately in addition to code for primary procedure)**

INCLUDES Plastic closure bronchus, not closure resected bronchus

Code first (32480-32484)

7.04 7.04 **FUD** ZZZ C 80

AMA: 1995,Win,1

32503-32504 Excision of Lung Neoplasm

EXCLUDES *Excision chest wall tumor (21601-21603)*
Thoracentesis, needle or catheter, aspiration pleural space (32554-32555)
Thoracotomy; with exploration (32100)
Tube thoracostomy (32551)

32503 **Resection of apical lung tumor (eg, Pancoast tumor), including chest wall resection, rib(s) resection(s), neurovascular dissection, when performed; without chest wall reconstruction(s)**

51.9 51.9 **FUD** 090 C 80

AMA: 2019,Dec,4

32504 **with chest wall reconstruction**

59.1 59.1 **FUD** 090 C 80

AMA: 2019,Dec,4

32505-32507 Thoracotomy with Wedge Resection

INCLUDES Wedge technique with tissue obtained with precise consideration margins and complete resection

Code also resection chest wall tumor with lung resection, when performed (21601-21603)

32505 **Thoracotomy; with therapeutic wedge resection (eg, mass, nodule), initial**

EXCLUDES *Removal lung (32440, 32442, 32445, 32488)*

Code also more extensive procedure lung when performed on contralateral lung or different lobe with modifier 59 despite intraoperative pathology consultation

26.8 26.8 **FUD** 090 C 80

AMA: 2018,Jan,8; 2017,Jan,8; 2016,Jan,13; 2015,Jan,16

+ **32506** **with therapeutic wedge resection (eg, mass or nodule), each additional resection, ipsilateral (List separately in addition to code for primary procedure)**

Code also more extensive procedure lung when performed on contralateral lung or different lobe with modifier 59 despite intraoperative pathology consultation

Code first (32505)

4.53 4.53 **FUD** ZZZ C 80

AMA: 2018,Jan,8; 2017,Jan,8; 2016,Jan,13; 2015,Jan,16

+ **32507** **with diagnostic wedge resection followed by anatomic lung resection (List separately in addition to code for primary procedure)**

INCLUDES Classification as diagnostic wedge resection when intraoperative pathology consultation dictates more extensive resection in same anatomical area

EXCLUDES *Diagnostic wedge resection by thoracoscopy (32668)*
Therapeutic wedge resection (32505-32506, 32666-32667)

Code first (32440, 32442, 32445, 32480-32488, 32503-32504)

4.52 4.52 **FUD** ZZZ C 80

AMA: 2018,Jan,8; 2017,Jan,8; 2016,Jan,13; 2015,Jan,16

32540 Removal of Empyema

32540 **Extrapleural enucleation of empyema (empyemectomy)**

Code also appropriate removal lung code when done with lobectomy (32480-32488)

50.1 50.1 **FUD** 090 C 80

AMA: 1994,Fall,1

32550-32552 Chest Tube/Catheter

32550 **Insertion of indwelling tunneled pleural catheter with cuff**

EXCLUDES *Procedures performed on same side chest with (32554-32557)*

(75989)

5.98 21.2 **FUD** 000 J G2

AMA: 2018,Jan,8; 2017,Jan,8; 2016,Jan,13; 2015,Jan,16

32551 **Tube thoracostomy, includes connection to drainage system (eg, water seal), when performed, open (separate procedure)**

EXCLUDES *Procedures performed on same side chest with (33020, 33025)*

4.56 4.56 **FUD** 000 T 50

AMA: 2019,Dec,4; 2018,Jul,7; 2018,Jan,8; 2017,Jun,10; 2017,Jan,8; 2016,Jan,13; 2015,Jan,16

32552 **Removal of indwelling tunneled pleural catheter with cuff**

4.55 5.28 **FUD** 010 Q2 G2 80

AMA: 2018,Jan,8; 2017,Jan,8; 2016,Jan,13; 2015,Jan,16

32553 Intrathoracic Placement Radiation Therapy Devices

EXCLUDES *Percutaneous placement interstitial device(s) for radiation therapy guidance: intra-abdominal, intrapelvic, and/or retroperitoneal (49411)*

Code also device

32553 Placement of interstitial device(s) for radiation therapy guidance (eg, fiducial markers, dosimeter), percutaneous, intra-thoracic, single or multiple

(76942, 77002, 77012, 77021)

5.17 15.1 FUD 000 S G2 80

AMA: 2018,Jan,8; 2017,Jan,8; 2016,Jun,3; 2016,Jan,13; 2015,Jun,6; 2015,Jan,16

32554-32557 Pleural Aspiration and Drainage

EXCLUDES *Chest x-ray performed to confirm chest tube position, complications, procedure adequacy*
Open tube thoracostomy (32551)
Placement indwelling tunneled pleural drainage catheter (cuffed) (32550)

32554 Thoracentesis, needle or catheter, aspiration of the pleural space; without imaging guidance

EXCLUDES *Radiologic guidance (75989, 76942, 77002, 77012, 77021)*

2.58 6.01 FUD 000 T G2 50

AMA: 2019,Dec,4; 2018,Jan,8; 2017,Jan,8; 2016,Jan,13; 2015,Jan,16

32555 with imaging guidance

INCLUDES Radiologic guidance (75989, 76942, 77002, 77012, 77021)

3.22 8.51 FUD 000 T G2 50

AMA: 2019,Dec,4; 2018,Jan,8; 2017,Jan,8; 2016,Jan,13; 2015,Jan,16

32556 Pleural drainage, percutaneous, with insertion of indwelling catheter; without imaging guidance

EXCLUDES *Radiologic guidance (75989, 76942, 77002, 77012, 77021)*

3.55 17.4 FUD 000 J G2 50

AMA: 2018,Jan,8; 2017,Jan,8; 2016,Jan,13; 2015,Jan,16

32557 with imaging guidance

INCLUDES Radiologic guidance (75989, 76942, 77002, 77012, 77021)

4.39 16.0 FUD 000 T G2 50

AMA: 2018,Jan,8; 2017,Jan,8; 2016,Jan,13; 2015,Jan,16

32560-32562 Instillation Drug/Chemical by Chest Tube

EXCLUDES *Insertion chest tube (32551)*

32560 Instillation, via chest tube/catheter, agent for pleurodesis (eg, talc for recurrent or persistent pneumothorax)

2.25 7.38 FUD 000 T

AMA: 2018,Jan,8; 2017,Jan,8; 2016,Jan,13; 2015,Jan,16

32561 Instillation(s), via chest tube/catheter, agent for fibrinolysis (eg, fibrinolytic agent for break up of multiloculated effusion); initial day

EXCLUDES *Reporting code more than one time on initial treatment date*

1.95 2.66 FUD 000 T 80

AMA: 2018,Jan,8; 2017,Jan,8; 2016,Jan,13; 2015,Jan,16

32562 subsequent day

EXCLUDES *Reporting code more than one time on each day subsequent treatment*

1.75 2.40 FUD 000 T 80

AMA: 2018,Jan,8; 2017,Jan,8; 2016,Jan,13; 2015,Jan,16

32601-32674 Thoracic Surgery: Video-Assisted (VATS)

INCLUDES Diagnostic thoracoscopy in surgical thoracoscopy

32601 Thoracoscopy, diagnostic (separate procedure); lungs, pericardial sac, mediastinal or pleural space, without biopsy

8.90 8.90 FUD 000 J 80

AMA: 2018,Jan,8; 2017,Jan,8; 2016,Jan,13; 2015,Jan,16

32604 pericardial sac, with biopsy

EXCLUDES *Open biopsy pericardium (39010)*

13.8 13.8 FUD 000 J 80

AMA: 2018,Jan,8; 2017,Jan,8; 2016,Jan,13; 2015,Jan,16

32606 mediastinal space, with biopsy

13.3 13.3 FUD 000 J 80

AMA: 2018,Jan,8; 2017,Jan,8; 2016,Jan,13; 2015,Jan,16

32607 Thoracoscopy; with diagnostic biopsy(ies) of lung infiltrate(s) (eg, wedge, incisional), unilateral

EXCLUDES *Removal lung (32440-32445, 32488)*
Thoracoscopy, surgical; with removal lung (32671)
Reporting code more than one time per lung

8.89 8.89 FUD 000 J 80

AMA: 2018,Jan,8; 2017,Jan,8; 2016,Jan,13; 2015,Jan,16

32608 with diagnostic biopsy(ies) of lung nodule(s) or mass(es) (eg, wedge, incisional), unilateral

EXCLUDES *Removal lung (32440-32445, 32488)*
Thoracoscopy, surgical; with removal lung (32671)
Reporting code more than one time per lung

10.9 10.9 FUD 000 J 80

AMA: 2018,Jan,8; 2017,Jan,8; 2016,Jan,13; 2015,Jan,16

32609 with biopsy(ies) of pleura

7.45 7.45 FUD 000 J 80

AMA: 2018,Jan,8; 2017,Jan,8; 2016,Jan,13; 2015,Jan,16

32650 Thoracoscopy, surgical; with pleurodesis (eg, mechanical or chemical)

19.1 19.1 FUD 090 C 80 50

AMA: 2018,Jan,8; 2017,Jan,8; 2016,Jan,13; 2015,Jan,16

32651 with partial pulmonary decortication

31.6 31.6 FUD 090 C 80 50

AMA: 2018,Jan,8; 2017,Jan,8; 2016,Jan,13; 2015,Jan,16

32652 with total pulmonary decortication, including intrapleural pneumonolysis

47.9 47.9 FUD 090 C 80 50

AMA: 2018,Jan,8; 2017,Jan,8; 2016,Jan,13; 2015,Jan,16

32653 with removal of intrapleural foreign body or fibrin deposit

30.6 30.6 FUD 090 C 80

AMA: 2018,Jan,8; 2017,Jan,8; 2016,Jan,13; 2015,Jan,16

32654 with control of traumatic hemorrhage

33.5 33.5 FUD 090 C 80 50

AMA: 2018,Jan,8; 2017,Jan,8; 2016,Jan,13; 2015,Jan,16

32655 with resection-plication of bullae, includes any pleural procedure when performed

EXCLUDES *Thoracoscopic lung volume reduction surgery (32672)*

27.5 27.5 FUD 090 C 80 50

AMA: 2018,Jan,8; 2017,Jan,8; 2016,Jan,13; 2015,Jan,16

32656 with parietal pleurectomy

23.0 23.0 FUD 090 C 80 50

AMA: 2018,Jan,8; 2017,Jan,8; 2016,Jan,13; 2015,Jan,16

32658 with removal of clot or foreign body from pericardial sac

20.6 20.6 FUD 090 C 80

AMA: 2018,Jan,8; 2017,Jan,8; 2016,Jan,13; 2015,Jan,16

32659 with creation of pericardial window or partial resection of pericardial sac for drainage

21.1 21.1 FUD 090 C 80

AMA: 2018,Jan,8; 2017,Jan,8; 2016,Jan,13; 2015,Jan,16

32661 with excision of pericardial cyst, tumor, or mass

23.0 23.0 FUD 090 C 80

AMA: 2018,Jan,8; 2017,Jan,8; 2016,Jan,13; 2015,Jan,16

32662 with excision of mediastinal cyst, tumor, or mass

25.7 25.7 FUD 090 C 80

AMA: 2018,Jan,8; 2017,Jan,8; 2016,Jan,13; 2015,Jan,16

32663 **with lobectomy (single lobe)**

EXCLUDES *Thoracoscopic segmentectomy (32669)*

40.4 40.4 FUD 090 C 80

AMA: 2018,Jan,8; 2017,Jan,8; 2016,Jan,13; 2015,Jan,16

32664 **with thoracic sympathectomy**

24.4 24.4 FUD 090 C 80 50

AMA: 2018,Jan,8; 2017,Jan,8; 2016,Jan,13; 2015,Dec,16; 2015,Jan,16

32665 **with esophagomyotomy (Heller type)**

EXCLUDES *Exploratory thoracoscopy with and without biopsy (32601-32609)*

35.6 35.6 FUD 090 C 80

AMA: 2018,Jan,8; 2017,Jan,8; 2016,Jan,13; 2015,Jan,16

32666 **with therapeutic wedge resection (eg, mass, nodule), initial unilateral**

EXCLUDES *Removal lung (32440-32445, 32488)*
Thoracoscopy, surgical; with removal lung (32671)

Code also more extensive procedure lung when performed on contralateral lung or different lobe with modifier 59 despite pathology consultation

25.1 25.1 FUD 090 C 80 50

AMA: 2018,Jan,8; 2017,Jan,8; 2016,Jan,13; 2015,Jan,16

\+ **32667** **with therapeutic wedge resection (eg, mass or nodule), each additional resection, ipsilateral (List separately in addition to code for primary procedure)**

EXCLUDES *Removal lung (32440-32445, 32488)*
Thoracoscopy, surgical; with removal lung (32671)

Code also more extensive procedure lung when performed on contralateral lung or different lobe with modifier 59 despite intraoperative pathology consultation

Code first (32666)

4.54 4.54 FUD ZZZ C 80

AMA: 2018,Jan,8; 2017,Jan,8; 2016,Jan,13; 2015,Jan,16

\+ **32668** **with diagnostic wedge resection followed by anatomic lung resection (List separately in addition to code for primary procedure)**

INCLUDES Classification as diagnostic wedge resection when intraoperative pathology consultation dictates more extensive resection in same anatomical area

Code first (32440-32488, 32503-32504, 32663, 32669-32671)

4.54 4.54 FUD ZZZ C 80

AMA: 2018,Jan,8; 2017,Jan,8; 2016,Jan,13; 2015,Jan,16

32669 **with removal of a single lung segment (segmentectomy)**

38.7 38.7 FUD 090 C 80

AMA: 2018,Jan,8; 2017,Jan,8; 2016,Jan,13; 2015,Jan,16

32670 **with removal of two lobes (bilobectomy)**

46.2 46.2 FUD 090 C 80

AMA: 2018,Jan,8; 2017,Jan,8; 2016,Jan,13; 2015,Jan,16

32671 **with removal of lung (pneumonectomy)**

51.5 51.5 FUD 090 C 80

AMA: 2018,Jan,8; 2017,Jan,8; 2016,Jan,13; 2015,Jan,16

32672 **with resection-plication for emphysematous lung (bullous or non-bullous) for lung volume reduction (LVRS), unilateral includes any pleural procedure, when performed**

44.0 44.0 FUD 090 C 80

AMA: 2018,Jan,8; 2017,Jan,8; 2016,Jan,13; 2015,Jan,16

32673 **with resection of thymus, unilateral or bilateral**

EXCLUDES *Exploratory thoracoscopy with and without biopsy (32601-32609)*
Open excision mediastinal cyst (39200)
Open excision mediastinal tumor (39220)
Open thymectomy (60520-60522)

35.0 35.0 FUD 090 C 80

AMA: 2018,Jan,8; 2017,Jan,8; 2016,Jan,13; 2015,Jan,16

\+ **32674** **with mediastinal and regional lymphadenectomy (List separately in addition to code for primary procedure)**

INCLUDES Mediastinal lymph nodes:
- Left side:
  - Aortopulmonary window
  - Inferior pulmonary ligament
  - Paraesophageal
  - Subcarinal
- Right side:
  - Inferior pulmonary ligament
  - Paraesophageal
  - Paratracheal
  - Subcarinal

EXCLUDES *Mediastinal and regional lymphadenectomy by thoracotomy (38746)*

Code first (21601, 31760, 31766, 31786, 32096-32200, 32220-32320, 32440-32491, 32503-32505, 32601-32663, 32666, 32669-32673, 32815, 33025, 33030, 33050-33130, 39200-39220, 39560-39561, 43101, 43112, 43117-43118, 43122-43123, 43287-43288, 43351, 60270, 60505)

6.24 6.24 FUD ZZZ C 80

AMA: 2018,Jan,8; 2017,Jan,8; 2016,Jan,13; 2015,Jan,16

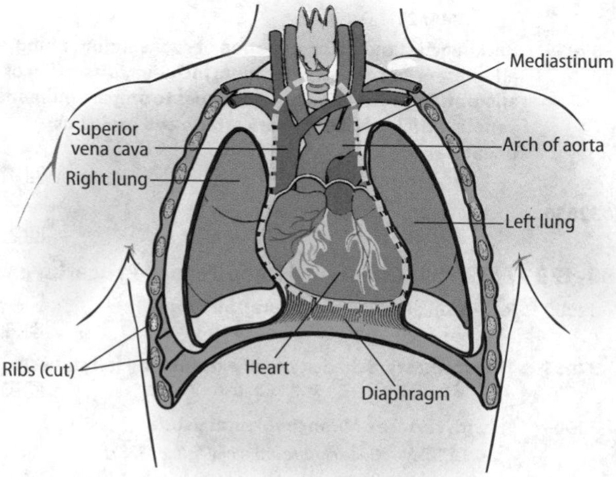

32701 Target Delineation for Stereotactic Radiation Therapy

INCLUDES Collaboration between radiation oncologist and surgeon
Correlation tumor and contiguous body structures
Determination borders and volume of tumor
Identification fiducial markers
Verification target when fiducial markers not used

EXCLUDES *Fiducial marker insertion (31626, 32553)*
Procedure performed by same physician as radiation treatment management (77427-77499)
Radiation oncology services (77295, 77331, 77370, 77373, 77435)
Therapeutic radiology (77261-77799 [77295, 77385, 77386, 77387, 77424, 77425])

32701 **Thoracic target(s) delineation for stereotactic body radiation therapy (SRS/SBRT), (photon or particle beam), entire course of treatment**

6.21 6.21 FUD XXX B 80 26

AMA: 2018,Jan,8; 2017,Jan,8; 2016,Jan,13; 2015,Jun,6

32800-32820 Chest Repair and Reconstruction Procedures

32800 **Repair lung hernia through chest wall**

27.0 27.0 FUD 090 C 80

32810 **Closure of chest wall following open flap drainage for empyema (Clagett type procedure)**

26.0 26.0 FUD 090 C 80

32815 **Open closure of major bronchial fistula**

81.0 81.0 FUD 090 C 80

32820 **Major reconstruction, chest wall (posttraumatic)**

38.3 38.3 FUD 090 C 80

32850-32856 Lung Transplant Procedures

INCLUDES Harvesting donor lung(s), cold preservation, preparation donor lung(s), transplantation into recipient

EXCLUDES *Assessment marginal cadaver donor lungs (0494T-0496T)*
Repairs or resection donor lung(s) (32491, 32505-32507, 35216, 35276)

32850 Donor pneumonectomy(s) (including cold preservation), from cadaver donor
0.00 0.00 FUD XXX C
AMA: 1993,Win,1

32851 Lung transplant, single; without cardiopulmonary bypass
94.8 94.8 FUD 090 C 80
AMA: 1993,Win,1

32852 with cardiopulmonary bypass
103. 103. FUD 090 C 80
AMA: 2017,Dec,3

32853 Lung transplant, double (bilateral sequential or en bloc); without cardiopulmonary bypass
133. 133. FUD 090 C 80
AMA: 1993,Win,1

32854 with cardiopulmonary bypass
141. 141. FUD 090 C 80
AMA: 2017,Dec,3

32855 Backbench standard preparation of cadaver donor lung allograft prior to transplantation, including dissection of allograft from surrounding soft tissues to prepare pulmonary venous/atrial cuff, pulmonary artery, and bronchus; unilateral
0.00 0.00 FUD XXX C 80

32856 bilateral
0.00 0.00 FUD XXX C 80

32900-32997 [32994] Chest and Respiratory Procedures

32900 Resection of ribs, extrapleural, all stages
41.0 41.0 FUD 090 C 80

32905 Thoracoplasty, Schede type or extrapleural (all stages);
38.5 38.5 FUD 090 C 80

32906 with closure of bronchopleural fistula
EXCLUDES *Open closure bronchial fistula (32815)*
Resection first rib for thoracic compression (21615-21616)
47.6 47.6 FUD 090 C 80

32940 Pneumonolysis, extraperiosteal, including filling or packing procedures
35.7 35.7 FUD 090 C 80

32960 Pneumothorax, therapeutic, intrapleural injection of air
2.62 3.61 FUD 000 T G2

32994 Resequenced code. See code following 32998.

32997 Total lung lavage (unilateral)
EXCLUDES *Broncho-alveolar lavage by bronchoscopy (31624)*
9.84 9.84 FUD 000 C 50
AMA: 2018,Jan,8; 2017,Jan,8; 2016,Jan,13; 2015,Jan,16

32998-32999 [32994] Destruction of Lung Neoplasm

32998 Ablation therapy for reduction or eradication of 1 or more pulmonary tumor(s) including pleura or chest wall when involved by tumor extension, percutaneous, including imaging guidance when performed, unilateral; radiofrequency
12.7 99.5 FUD 000 J G2 80 50
AMA: 2018,Jan,8; 2017,Nov,8

\# **32994 cryoablation**
12.8 155. FUD 000 J G2 80 50
AMA: 2018,Jan,8; 2017,Nov,8

32999 Unlisted procedure, lungs and pleura
0.00 0.00 FUD YYY T
AMA: 2018,Jan,8; 2017,Jan,8; 2016,Jan,13; 2015,Dec,16; 2015,Jun,6; 2015,Jan,16

33016-33050 Procedures of the Pericardial Sac

EXCLUDES *Surgical thoracoscopy (video-assisted thoracic surgery [VATS]) procedures pericardium (32601, 32604, 32658-32659, 32661)*

33016 **Pericardiocentesis, including imaging guidance, when performed**

INCLUDES Imaging guidance for needle placement:
- Computed tomography (77012)
- Fluoroscopy (77002)
- Magnetic resonance (77021)
- Ultrasound (76942)

EXCLUDES *Echocardiography for pericardiocentesis guidance (93303-93325)*

6.85 6.85 FUD 000 G2

AMA: 2020,Jan,7

33017 **Pericardial drainage with insertion of indwelling catheter, percutaneous, including fluoroscopy and/or ultrasound guidance, when performed; 6 years and older without congenital cardiac anomaly**

INCLUDES Catheters that remain in patient at procedure conclusion

Imaging guidance for needle placement:
- Fluoroscopy (77002)
- Magnetic resonance (77021)
- Ultrasound (76942)

EXCLUDES *CT guided pericardial drainage (33019)*

Echocardiography for pericardiocentesis guidance (93303-93325)

Pericardial drainage for patients:
- *Any age with congenital cardiac anomaly (33018)*
- *Younger than 6 years of age (33018)*

Radiologically guided catheter placement for percutaneous drainage (75989)

7.10 7.10 FUD 000

AMA: 2020,Jan,7

33018 **birth through 5 years of age or any age with congenital cardiac anomaly**

INCLUDES Catheters that remain in patient at procedure conclusion

Imaging guidance for needle placement:
- Fluoroscopy (77002)
- Magnetic resonance (77021)
- Ultrasound (76942)

Patient age birth to 5 years without congenital cardiac anomaly

Patient any age with congenital cardiac anomaly, such as heterotaxy, dextrocardia, mesocardia, or single ventricle anomaly, or 90 days following repair congenital cardiac anomaly

EXCLUDES *CT guided pericardial drainage (33019)*

Echocardiography for pericardiocentesis guidance (93303-93325)

Radiologically guided catheter placement for percutaneous drainage (75989)

8.09 8.09 FUD 000

AMA: 2020,Jan,7

33019 **Pericardial drainage with insertion of indwelling catheter, percutaneous, including CT guidance**

INCLUDES Catheters that remain in patient at procedure conclusion

Imaging guidance for needle placement:
- Computed tomography (77012)
- Fluoroscopy (77002)
- Magnetic resonance (77021)
- Ultrasound (76942)

EXCLUDES *Radiologically guided catheter placement for percutaneous drainage (75989)*

6.57 6.57 FUD 000

AMA: 2020,Jan,7

33020 **Pericardiotomy for removal of clot or foreign body (primary procedure)**

INCLUDES Tube thoracostomy when chest tube or pleural drain placed on same side (32551)

23.8 23.8 FUD 090 C 80

AMA: 1997,Nov,1

33025 **Creation of pericardial window or partial resection for drainage**

INCLUDES Tube thoracostomy when chest tube or pleural drain placed on same side (32551)

EXCLUDES *Surgical thoracoscopy (video-assisted thoracic surgery [VATS]) creation of pericardial window (32659)*

22.2 22.2 FUD 090 C 80

AMA: 1997,Nov,1

33030 **Pericardiectomy, subtotal or complete; without cardiopulmonary bypass**

INCLUDES Delorme pericardiectomy

57.8 57.8 FUD 090 C 80

AMA: 1997,Nov,1; 1994,Win,1

33031 **with cardiopulmonary bypass**

71.7 71.7 FUD 090 C 80

AMA: 2017,Dec,3

33050 **Resection of pericardial cyst or tumor**

EXCLUDES *Open biopsy pericardium (39010)*

Surgical thoracoscopy (video-assisted thoracic surgery [VATS]) resection of cyst, mass, or tumor pericardium (32661)

28.9 28.9 FUD 090 C 80

AMA: 1997,Nov,1

33120-33130 Neoplasms of Heart

Code also removal thrombus through separate heart incision, when performed (33310-33315); append modifier 59 to (33315)

33120 **Excision of intracardiac tumor, resection with cardiopulmonary bypass**

60.6 60.6 FUD 090 C 80

AMA: 2018,Jan,8; 2017,Dec,3; 2017,Jan,8; 2016,Jan,13; 2015,Jan,16

33130 **Resection of external cardiac tumor**

39.5 39.5 FUD 090 C 80

AMA: 2018,Jan,8; 2017,Jan,8; 2016,Jan,13; 2015,Jan,16

33140-33141 Transmyocardial Revascularization

33140 **Transmyocardial laser revascularization, by thoracotomy; (separate procedure)**

45.5 45.5 FUD 090 C 80

AMA: 2018,Jan,8; 2017,Jan,8; 2016,Jan,13; 2015,Jan,16

\+ **33141** **performed at the time of other open cardiac procedure(s) (List separately in addition to code for primary procedure)**

Code first (33390-33391, 33404-33496, 33510-33536, 33542)

3.80 3.80 FUD ZZZ C 80

AMA: 2018,Jan,8; 2017,Jan,8; 2016,Jan,13; 2015,Jan,16

33202-33203 Placement Epicardial Leads

INCLUDES Imaging guidance:
Fluoroscopy (76000)
Ultrasound (76942, 76998, 93318)
Temporary pacemaker (33210-33211)

Code also insertion pulse generator when performed by same physician/same surgical session (33212-33213, [33221], 33230-33231, 33240)

33202 **Insertion of epicardial electrode(s); open incision (eg, thoracotomy, median sternotomy, subxiphoid approach)**
Facility RVU 22.3 Non-Facility RVU 22.3 **FUD** 090 C
AMA: 2019,Mar,6; 2018,Jan,8; 2017,Jan,8; 2016,Aug,5; 2016,May,5; 2016,Jan,13; 2015,May,3; 2015,Jan,16

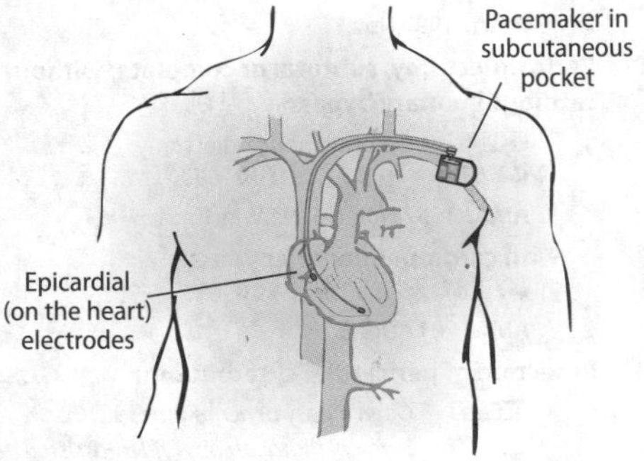

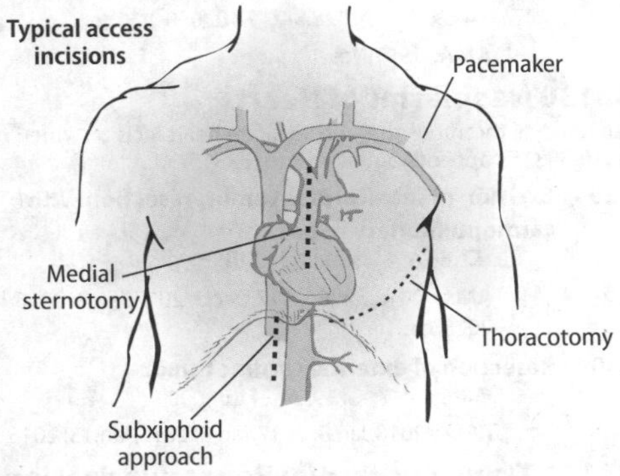

33203 **endoscopic approach (eg, thoracoscopy, pericardioscopy)**
Facility RVU 23.3 Non-Facility RVU 23.3 **FUD** 090 C
AMA: 2019,Mar,6; 2018,Jan,8; 2017,Jan,8; 2016,Aug,5; 2016,May,5; 2016,Jan,13; 2015,May,3; 2015,Jan,16

33206-33214 [33221] Pacemakers

INCLUDES Device evaluation (93279-93298 [93260, 93261])
Dual lead: device that paces and senses in two heart chambers
Imaging guidance:
Fluoroscopy (76000)
Ultrasound (76942, 76998, 93318)
Multiple lead: device that paces and senses in three or more heart chambers
Radiological supervision and interpretation for pacemaker procedure
Single lead: device that paces and senses in one heart chamber
Skin pocket revision, when performed
Temporary pacemaker (33210-33211)

EXCLUDES *Electrode repositioning:*
Left ventricle (33226)
Pacemaker (33215)
Insertion lead for left ventricular (biventricular) pacing (33224-33225)
Leadless pacemaker systems ([33274, 33275])

Code also wound infection or hematoma incision/drainage, when performed (10140, 10180, 11042-11047 [11045, 11046])

33206 **Insertion of new or replacement of permanent pacemaker with transvenous electrode(s); atrial**
INCLUDES Pulse generator insertion/single transvenous electrode placement
EXCLUDES *Insertion transvenous electrode only (33216-33217)*
Removal with immediate replacement pacemaker pulse generator only, single lead system ([33227])
Code also removal old pacemaker pulse generator and electrode, when replacement entire system performed:
Electrode (33234)
Pulse generator (33233)
Facility RVU 13.1 Non-Facility RVU 13.1 **FUD** 090 J J8
AMA: 2019,Oct,3; 2019,Mar,6; 2018,Jan,8; 2017,Jan,8; 2016,Aug,5; 2016,May,5; 2016,Jan,13; 2015,May,3; 2015,Jan,16

33207 **ventricular**
INCLUDES Pulse generator insertion/single transvenous electrode placement
EXCLUDES *Insertion transvenous electrode only (33216-33217)*
Removal with immediate replacement pacemaker pulse generator only, single lead system ([33227])
Code also removal old pacemaker pulse generator and electrode, when replacement entire system performed:
Electrode (33234)
Pulse generator (33233)
Facility RVU 13.9 Non-Facility RVU 13.9 **FUD** 090 J J8
AMA: 2019,Oct,3; 2019,Mar,6; 2018,Jan,8; 2017,Jan,8; 2016,Aug,5; 2016,May,5; 2016,Jan,13; 2015,May,3; 2015,Jan,16

33208 **atrial and ventricular**
INCLUDES Pulse generator insertion/dual transvenous electrode placement
EXCLUDES *Insertion transvenous electrode(s) only (33216-33217)*
Removal with immediate replacement pacemaker pulse generator only, dual or multiple lead system ([33228, 33229])
Code also removal old pacemaker pulse generator and electrode, when replacement entire system performed:
Electrodes (33235)
Pulse generator (33233)
Facility RVU 15.1 Non-Facility RVU 15.1 **FUD** 090 J J8
AMA: 2019,Oct,3; 2019,Mar,6; 2018,Jan,8; 2017,Jan,8; 2016,Aug,5; 2016,May,5; 2016,Jan,13; 2015,May,3; 2015,Jan,16

33210 **Insertion or replacement of temporary transvenous single chamber cardiac electrode or pacemaker catheter (separate procedure)**
Facility RVU 4.74 Non-Facility RVU 4.74 **FUD** 000 J G2
AMA: 2019,Oct,3; 2019,Mar,6; 2018,Jan,8; 2017,Jan,8; 2016,Aug,5; 2016,May,5; 2016,Jan,13; 2015,May,3; 2015,Jan,16

33211 **Insertion or replacement of temporary transvenous dual chamber pacing electrodes (separate procedure)**
Facility RVU 4.90 Non-Facility RVU 4.90 **FUD** 000 J J8
AMA: 2019,Oct,3; 2019,Mar,6; 2018,Jan,8; 2017,Jan,8; 2016,Aug,5; 2016,May,5; 2016,Jan,13; 2015,May,3; 2015,Jan,16

33212 Insertion of pacemaker pulse generator only; with existing single lead

EXCLUDES *Insertion for replacement single lead pacemaker pulse generator ([33227])*

Insertion transvenous electrode(s) (33216-33217)

Removal permanent pacemaker pulse generator only (33233)

Code also placement epicardial leads by same physician/same surgical session (33202-33203)

🚑 9.31 ⚕ 9.31 **FUD** 090   J J8 ▭

AMA: 2019,Oct,3; 2019,Mar,6; 2018,Jan,8; 2017,Jan,8; 2016,Aug,5; 2016,May,5; 2016,Jan,13; 2015,May,3; 2015,Jan,16

33213 with existing dual leads

EXCLUDES *Insertion for replacement dual lead pacemaker pulse generator ([33228])*

Insertion transvenous electrode(s) (33216-33217)

Removal permanent pacemaker pulse generator only (33233)

Code also placement epicardial leads by same physician/same surgical session (33202-33203)

🚑 9.73 ⚕ 9.73 **FUD** 090   J J8 ▭

AMA: 2019,Oct,3; 2019,Mar,6; 2018,Jan,8; 2017,Jan,8; 2016,Aug,5; 2016,May,5; 2016,Jan,13; 2015,May,3; 2015,Jan,16

\# **33221** with existing multiple leads

EXCLUDES *Insertion for replacement multiple lead pacemaker pulse generator ([33229])*

Insertion transvenous electrode(s) (33216-33217)

Removal permanent pacemaker pulse generator only (33233)

Code also placement epicardial leads by same physician/same surgical session (33202-33203)

🚑 10.4 ⚕ 10.4 **FUD** 090   J J8 ▭

AMA: 2019,Oct,3; 2019,Mar,6; 2018,Jan,8; 2017,Jan,8; 2016,Aug,5; 2016,May,5; 2016,Jan,13; 2015,May,3; 2015,Jan,16

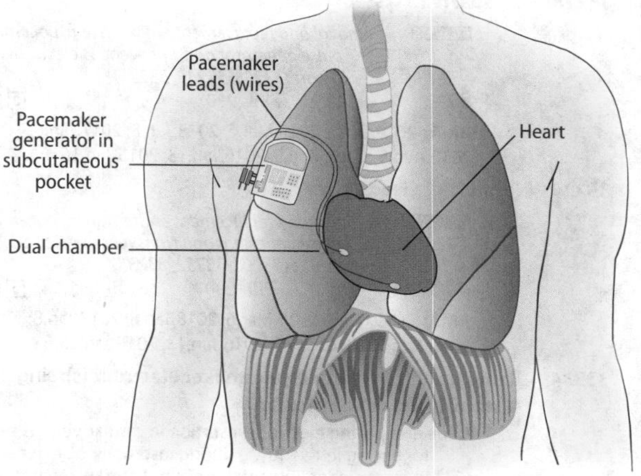

Pacemaker leads (wires)

Pacemaker generator in subcutaneous pocket

Heart

Dual chamber

33214 Upgrade of implanted pacemaker system, conversion of single chamber system to dual chamber system (includes removal of previously placed pulse generator, testing of existing lead, insertion of new lead, insertion of new pulse generator)

EXCLUDES *Insertion transvenous electrode(s) (33216-33217)*

Removal and replacement pacemaker pulse generator (33227-33229)

🚑 13.8 ⚕ 13.8 **FUD** 090   J J8 80 ▭

AMA: 2019,Oct,3; 2019,Mar,6; 2018,Jan,8; 2017,Jan,8; 2016,Aug,5; 2016,May,5; 2016,Jan,13; 2015,May,3; 2015,Jan,16

33215-33249 [33221, 33227, 33228, 33229, 33230, 33231, 33262, 33263, 33264] Pacemakers/Implantable Defibrillator/Electrode Insertion/Replacement/Revision/Repair

INCLUDES Device evaluation (93279-93298 [93260, 93261])

Dual lead: device that paces and senses in two heart chambers

Imaging guidance:
  Fluoroscopy (76000)
  Ultrasound (76942, 76998, 93318)

Multiple lead: device that paces and senses in three or more heart chambers

Radiological supervision and interpretation for pacemaker or pacing cardioverter-defibrillator procedure

Single lead: device that paces and senses in one heart chamber

Skin pocket revision, when performed

Temporary pacemaker (33210-33211)

EXCLUDES *Electrode repositioning:*
  Left ventricle (33226)
  Pacemaker or implantable defibrillator (33215)

Insertion lead for left ventricular (biventricular) pacing (33224-33225)

Removal leadless pacemaker system ([33275])

Removal subcutaneous implantable defibrillator electrode ([33272])

Testing defibrillator threshold (DFT) during follow-up evaluation (93642-93644)

Testing defibrillator threshold (DFT) during insertion/replacement (93640-93641)

Code also wound infection or hematoma incision/drainage, when performed (10140, 10180, 11042-11047 [11045, 11046])

33215 Repositioning of previously implanted transvenous pacemaker or implantable defibrillator (right atrial or right ventricular) electrode

🚑 9.01 ⚕ 9.01 **FUD** 090   T 62 ▭

AMA: 2019,Oct,3; 2019,Mar,6; 2018,Jan,8; 2017,Jan,8; 2016,Aug,5; 2016,May,5; 2016,Jan,13; 2015,May,3; 2015,Jan,16

33216 Insertion of a single transvenous electrode, permanent pacemaker or implantable defibrillator

EXCLUDES *Insertion or replacement lead for cardiac venous system (33224-33225)*

Insertion or replacement permanent implantable defibrillator generator or system (33249)

Removal and replacement permanent pacemaker or implantable defibrillator (33206-33208, 33212-33213, [33221], 33227-33229, 33230-33231, 33240, [33262, 33263, 33264])

🚑 10.7 ⚕ 10.7 **FUD** 090   J J8 ▭

AMA: 2019,Oct,3; 2019,Mar,6; 2018,Jan,8; 2017,Jan,8; 2016,Aug,5; 2016,May,5; 2016,Jan,13; 2015,May,3; 2015,Jan,16

33217 Insertion of 2 transvenous electrodes, permanent pacemaker or implantable defibrillator

EXCLUDES *Insertion or replacement lead for cardiac venous system (33224-33225)*

Insertion or replacement permanent implantable defibrillator generator or system (33249)

Removal and replacement permanent pacemaker or implantable defibrillator (33206-33208, 33212-33213, [33221], 33227-33229, 33230-33231, 33240, [33262, 33263, 33264])

🚑 10.6 ⚕ 10.6 **FUD** 090   J J8 ▭

AMA: 2019,Oct,3; 2019,Mar,6; 2018,Jan,8; 2017,Jan,8; 2016,Aug,5; 2016,May,5; 2016,Jan,13; 2015,May,3; 2015,Jan,16

33218 Repair of single transvenous electrode, permanent pacemaker or implantable defibrillator

Code also removal old generator with insertion new generator replacement, when performed:
  Implantable defibrillator ([33262, 33263, 33264])
  Pacemaker ([33227, 33228, 33229])

🚑 11.2 ⚕ 11.2 **FUD** 090   T 62 ▭

AMA: 2019,Oct,3; 2019,Mar,6; 2018,Jan,8; 2017,Jan,8; 2016,Aug,5; 2016,May,5; 2016,Jan,13; 2015,May,3; 2015,Jan,16

● New Code   ▲ Revised Code   ○ Reinstated   ● New Web Release   ▲ Revised Web Release   + Add-on   Unlisted   Not Covered   # Resequenced

50 Optum Mod 50 Exempt   ⊘ AMA Mod 51 Exempt   51 Optum Mod 51 Exempt   63 Mod 63 Exempt   ✗ Non-FDA Drug   ★ Telemedicine   M Maternity   A Age Edit

33220 **Repair of 2 transvenous electrodes for permanent pacemaker or implantable defibrillator**

Code also modifier 52 Reduced services, when one electrode in two-chamber system repaired

Code also removal old generator with insertion new generator replacement, when performed:

Implantable defibrillator ([33263, 33264])

Pacemaker ([33228, 33229])

10.9 10.9 FUD 090 T J8

AMA: 2019,Oct,3; 2019,Mar,6; 2018,Jan,8; 2017,Jan,8; 2016,Aug,5; 2016,May,5; 2016,Jan,13; 2015,May,3; 2015,Jan,16

33221 **Resequenced code. See code following 33213.**

33222 **Relocation of skin pocket for pacemaker**

INCLUDES Formation new pocket

Procedures related to existing pocket:

Accessing pocket

Incision/drainage abscess or hematoma (10140, 10180)

Pocket closure (13100-13102)

EXCLUDES *Debridement, subcutaneous tissue (11042-11047 [11045, 11046])*

Code also removal and replacement existing generator

9.84 9.84 FUD 090 T A2

AMA: 2019,Oct,3; 2019,Mar,6; 2018,Jan,8; 2017,Jan,8; 2016,Aug,5; 2016,May,5; 2016,Jan,13; 2015,May,3; 2015,Jan,16

33223 **Relocation of skin pocket for implantable defibrillator**

INCLUDES Formation new pocket

Procedures related to existing pocket:

Accessing pocket

Incision/drainage abscess or hematoma (10140, 10180)

Pocket closure (13100-13102)

EXCLUDES *Debridement, subcutaneous tissue (11042-11047 [11045, 11046])*

Code also removal and replacement existing generator

11.8 11.8 FUD 090 T A2 80

AMA: 2019,Oct,3; 2019,Mar,6; 2018,Jan,8; 2017,Jan,8; 2016,Aug,5; 2016,Jan,13; 2015,Jan,16

33224 **Insertion of pacing electrode, cardiac venous system, for left ventricular pacing, with attachment to previously placed pacemaker or implantable defibrillator pulse generator (including revision of pocket, removal, insertion, and/or replacement of existing generator)**

Code also placement epicardial electrode when appropriate (33202-33203)

14.9 14.9 FUD 000 J J8

AMA: 2019,Oct,3; 2019,Mar,6; 2018,Jan,8; 2017,Jan,8; 2016,Aug,5; 2016,May,5; 2016,Jan,13; 2015,May,3; 2015,Jan,16

\+ **33225** **Insertion of pacing electrode, cardiac venous system, for left ventricular pacing, at time of insertion of implantable defibrillator or pacemaker pulse generator (eg, for upgrade to dual chamber system) (List separately in addition to code for primary procedure)**

Code also placement epicardial electrode when appropriate (33202-33203)

Code first (33206-33208, 33212-33213, [33221], 33214, 33216-33217, 33223, 33228-33229, 33230-33231, 33233, 33234-33235, 33240, [33263, 33264], 33249)

Code first (33223) for relocation pocket for implantable defibrillator

Code first (33222) for relocation pocket for pacemaker pulse generator

13.6 13.6 FUD ZZZ N N1

AMA: 2019,Oct,3; 2019,Mar,6; 2018,Jan,8; 2017,Jan,8; 2016,Aug,5; 2016,May,5; 2016,Jan,13; 2015,May,3; 2015,Jan,16

33226 **Repositioning of previously implanted cardiac venous system (left ventricular) electrode (including removal, insertion and/or replacement of existing generator)**

14.4 14.4 FUD 000 T G2

AMA: 2019,Oct,3; 2019,Mar,6; 2018,Jan,8; 2017,Jan,8; 2016,Aug,5; 2016,May,5; 2016,Jan,13; 2015,May,3; 2015,Jan,16

33227 **Resequenced code. See code following 33233.**

33228 **Resequenced code. See code following 33233.**

33229 **Resequenced code. See code before 33234.**

33230 **Resequenced code. See code following 33240.**

33231 **Resequenced code. See code before 33241.**

33233 **Removal of permanent pacemaker pulse generator only**

EXCLUDES *Removal with immediate replacement pacemaker pulse generator, without replacement electrode(s):*

Dual lead system ([33228])

Multiple lead system ([33229])

Single lead system ([33227])

Code also insertion replacement pacemaker pulse generator with transvenous electrode(s) (total system), when performed:

Pacemaker and dual leads (33208)

Pacemaker and single atrial lead (33206)

Pacemaker and single ventricular lead (33207)

Code also removal electrode(s), when removal total system without replacement performed:

Dual leads (atrial and ventricular) (33235)

Single lead (atrial or ventricular) (33234)

6.68 6.68 FUD 090 Q2 J8

AMA: 2019,Oct,3; 2019,Mar,6; 2018,Jan,8; 2017,Jan,8; 2016,Aug,5; 2016,May,5; 2016,Jan,13; 2015,Jan,16

\# **33227** **Removal of permanent pacemaker pulse generator with replacement of pacemaker pulse generator; single lead system**

EXCLUDES *Removal and replacement entire system, pacemaker pulse generator and transvenous electrode, report (33206-33207, 33233, 33234)*

Removal and replacement for conversion from single chamber to dual chamber system (33214)

9.82 9.82 FUD 090 J J8

AMA: 2019,Oct,3; 2019,Mar,6; 2018,Jan,8; 2017,Jan,8; 2016,Aug,5; 2016,May,5; 2016,Jan,13; 2015,Jan,16

\# **33228** **dual lead system**

EXCLUDES *Removal and replacement entire system, pacemaker pulse generator and transvenous electrode(s), report (33208, 33233, 33235)*

10.2 10.2 FUD 090 J J8

AMA: 2019,Oct,3; 2019,Mar,6; 2018,Jan,8; 2017,Jan,8; 2016,Aug,5; 2016,May,5; 2016,Jan,13; 2015,Jan,16

\# **33229** **multiple lead system**

EXCLUDES *Removal and replacement entire system, pacemaker pulse generator and transvenous electrode(s), report (33208, 33233, 33235)*

10.8 10.8 FUD 090 J J8

AMA: 2019,Oct,3; 2019,Mar,6; 2018,Jan,8; 2017,Jan,8; 2016,Aug,5; 2016,May,5; 2016,Jan,13; 2015,Jan,16

33234 **Removal of transvenous pacemaker electrode(s); single lead system, atrial or ventricular**

Code also pacing electrode insertion in cardiac venous system for pacing left ventricle during insertion pulse generator (pacemaker or implantable defibrillator) when performed (33225)

Code also removal old pacemaker pulse generator and insertion replacement pacemaker pulse generator with transvenous electrode (total system), when performed:

Insertion pacemaker and atrial lead (33206) OR

Insertion pacemaker and ventricular lead (33207) AND

Removal generator (33233)

Code also thoracotomy to remove electrode, when performed, for unsuccessful transvenous removal (33238)

14.0 14.0 FUD 090 Q2 G2

AMA: 2019,Oct,3; 2019,Mar,6; 2018,Jan,8; 2017,Jan,8; 2016,Aug,5; 2016,May,5; 2016,Jan,13; 2015,Jan,16

33235 **dual lead system**

Code also pacing electrode insertion in cardiac venous system for pacing left ventricle during insertion pulse generator (pacemaker or implantable defibrillator) when performed (33225)

Code also removal old pacemaker pulse generator and insertion replacement pacemaker pulse generator with transvenous electrodes (total system), when performed:

Insertion generator and dual leads (33208) AND

Insertion pacemaker and atrial lead (33206) OR

Insertion pacemaker and ventricular lead (33207) AND

Removal generator (33233)

Code also thoracotomy to remove electrode, when performed, for unsuccessful transvenous removal (33238)

18.5 18.5 **FUD** 090 Q2 J8

AMA: 2019,Oct,3; 2019,Mar,6; 2018,Jan,8; 2017,Jan,8; 2016,Aug,5; 2016,May,5; 2016,Jan,13; 2015,Jan,16

33236 **Removal of permanent epicardial pacemaker and electrodes by thoracotomy; single lead system, atrial or ventricular**

EXCLUDES *Removal implantable defibrillator electrode(s) by thoracotomy (33243)*

Removal transvenous electrodes by thoracotomy (33238)

Removal transvenous pacemaker electrodes, single or dual lead system; without thoracotomy (33234, 33235)

22.5 22.5 **FUD** 090 C 80

AMA: 2019,Oct,3; 2019,Mar,6; 2018,Jan,8; 2017,Jan,8; 2016,Aug,5; 2016,May,5; 2016,Jan,13; 2015,Jan,16

33237 **dual lead system**

EXCLUDES *Removal implantable defibrillator electrode(s) by thoracotomy (33243)*

Removal transvenous electrodes by thoracotomy (33238)

Removal transvenous pacemaker electrodes, single or dual lead system; without thoracotomy (33234, 33235)

24.1 24.1 **FUD** 090 C 80

AMA: 2019,Oct,3; 2019,Mar,6; 2018,Jan,8; 2017,Jan,8; 2016,Aug,5; 2016,May,5; 2016,Jan,13; 2015,Jan,16

33238 **Removal of permanent transvenous electrode(s) by thoracotomy**

EXCLUDES *Removal implantable defibrillator electrode(s) by thoracotomy (33243)*

Removal transvenous pacemaker electrodes, single or dual lead system; without thoracotomy (33234, 33235)

27.0 27.0 **FUD** 090 C 80

AMA: 2019,Oct,3; 2018,Jan,8; 2017,Jan,8; 2016,Aug,5; 2016,May,5; 2016,Jan,13; 2015,Jan,16

33240 **Insertion of implantable defibrillator pulse generator only; with existing single lead**

EXCLUDES *Insertion electrode(s) (33216-33217, [33271])*

Removal and replacement implantable defibrillator pulse generator only ([33262, 33263, 33264])

Code also placement epicardial leads by same physician/same surgical session as generator insertion (33202-33203)

10.5 10.5 **FUD** 090 J J8

AMA: 2019,Oct,3; 2018,Jan,8; 2017,Jan,8; 2016,Aug,5; 2016,Jan,13; 2015,Jan,16

33230 **with existing dual leads**

EXCLUDES *Insertion single transvenous electrode, permanent pacemaker or implantable defibrillator (33216-33217)*

Removal and replacement implantable defibrillator pulse generator only ([33262, 33263, 33264])

Code also placement epicardial leads by same physician/same surgical session as generator insertion (33202-33203)

11.0 11.0 **FUD** 090 J J8

AMA: 2019,Oct,3; 2019,Mar,6; 2018,Jan,8; 2017,Jan,8; 2016,Aug,5; 2016,Jan,13; 2015,Jan,16

33231 **with existing multiple leads**

EXCLUDES *Insertion single transvenous electrode, permanent pacemaker or implantable defibrillator (33216-33217)*

Removal and replacement implantable defibrillator pulse generator only ([33262, 33263, 33264])

Code also placement epicardial leads by same physician/same surgical session as generator placement (33202-33203)

11.6 11.6 **FUD** 090 J J8

AMA: 2019,Oct,3; 2019,Mar,6; 2018,Jan,8; 2017,Jan,8; 2016,Aug,5; 2016,Jan,13; 2015,Jan,16

33241 **Removal of implantable defibrillator pulse generator only**

EXCLUDES *Removal substernal implantable defibrillator pulse generator only (0580T)*

Removal with immediate replacement implantable defibrillator pulse generator only ([33262, 33263, 33264])

Code also removal electrode(s) and insertion replacement defibrillator with electrode(s) (total system), when performed:

Removal electrode(s) (33243-33244) AND

Insertion defibrillator system, single or dual (33249) OR

Removal subcutaneous electrode ([33272]) AND

Insertion subcutaneous defibrillator system ([33270])

Code also removal electrode(s), when total system removed without replacement:

Subcutaneous electrode ([33272])

Transvenous electrode(s) (33243)

6.20 6.20 **FUD** 090 Q2 G2

AMA: 2019,Oct,3; 2018,Jan,8; 2017,Jan,8; 2016,Aug,5; 2016,Jan,13; 2015,Jan,16

33262 **Removal of implantable defibrillator pulse generator with replacement of implantable defibrillator pulse generator; single lead system**

EXCLUDES *Insertion electrode(s) (33216-33217, [33271])*

Removal and replacement implantable defibrillator pulse generator and electrode(s) (total system) (33241, 33243-33244, 33249)

Removal and replacement subcutaneous defibrillator pulse generator and electrode(s) (total system) (33241, [33270], [33272])

Removal and replacement substernal implantable defibrillator pulse generator ([0614T])

Removal implantable defibrillator pulse generator only (33241)

Repair implantable defibrillator pulse generator and/or leads (33218, 33220)

Code also electrode(s) removal by thoracotomy (33243)

Code also subcutaneous electrode removal ([33272])

Code also transvenous removal of electrode(s) (33244)

10.8 10.8 **FUD** 090 J J8

AMA: 2019,Oct,3; 2018,Jan,8; 2017,Jan,8; 2016,Aug,5; 2016,Jan,13; 2015,Jan,16

\# **33263** **dual lead system**

EXCLUDES *Insertion single transvenous electrode, permanent pacemaker or implantable defibrillator (33216-33217)*
Removal and replacement implantable defibrillator pulse generator and electrode(s) (total system) (33241, 33243-33244, 33249)
Removal and replacement subcutaneous defibrillator pulse generator and electrode (total system) (33241, [33270], [33272])
Removal implantable defibrillator pulse generator only (33241)
Repair implantable defibrillator pulse generator and/or leads (33218, 33220)

Code also removal electrodes by thoracotomy (33243)
Code also transvenous removal electrodes (33244)

11.2 11.2 **FUD** 090 J J8

AMA: 2019,Oct,3; 2018,Jan,8; 2017,Jan,8; 2016,Aug,5; 2016,Jan,13; 2015,Jan,16

\# **33264** **multiple lead system**

EXCLUDES *Insertion single transvenous electrode, permanent pacemaker or implantable defibrillator (33216-33217)*
Removal and replacement implantable defibrillator pulse generator and electrode(s) (total system) (33241, 33243-33244, 33249)
Removal and replacement subcutaneous defibrillator pulse generator and electrode(s) (total system) (33241, [33270], [33272])
Removal implantable defibrillator pulse generator only (33241)
Repair implantable defibrillator pulse generator and/or leads (33218, 33220)

Code also removal electrodes by thoracotomy (33243)
Code also transvenous removal electrodes (33244)

11.7 11.7 **FUD** 090 J J8

AMA: 2019,Oct,3; 2018,Jan,8; 2017,Jan,8; 2016,Aug,5; 2016,Jan,13; 2015,Jan,16

33243 **Removal of single or dual chamber implantable defibrillator electrode(s); by thoracotomy**

EXCLUDES *Transvenous removal defibrillator electrode(s) (33244)*

Code also removal implantable defibrillator pulse generator and insertion replacement defibrillator with electrodes (total system), when entire system replaced:
Insertion defibrillator system, single or dual (33249)
Removal generator (33241)
Code also removal implantable defibrillator pulse generator, when entire system removed without replacement (33241)
Code also replacement implantable defibrillator pulse generator, when performed:
Dual lead system ([33263])
Multiple lead system ([33264])
Single lead system ([33262])

39.6 39.6 **FUD** 090 C 80

AMA: 2019,Oct,3; 2018,Jan,8; 2017,Jan,8; 2016,Aug,5; 2016,Jan,13; 2015,Jan,16

33244 **by transvenous extraction**

Code also removal implantable defibrillator pulse generator and insertion replacement defibrillator with electrodes (total system), when entire system replaced:
Insertion defibrillator system, single or dual (33249)
Removal generator (33241)
Code also removal implantable defibrillator pulse generator, when entire system removed without replacement (33241)
Code also replacement implantable defibrillator pulse generator, when performed:
Dual lead system ([33263])
Multiple lead system ([33264])
Single lead system ([33262])
Code also thoracotomy to remove electrode, when performed, if transvenous removal unsuccessful (33238, 33243)

25.1 25.1 **FUD** 090 Q2

AMA: 2019,Oct,3; 2018,Jan,8; 2017,Jan,8; 2016,Aug,5; 2016,Jan,13; 2015,Jan,16

33249 **Insertion or replacement of permanent implantable defibrillator system, with transvenous lead(s), single or dual chamber**

EXCLUDES *Insertion single transvenous electrode, permanent pacemaker or implantable defibrillator (33216-33217)*

Code also removal defibrillator generator when upgrading from single to dual-chamber system (33241)
Code also removal implantable defibrillator pulse generator and removal electrode(s), when entire system replaced:
Removal electrode(s) (33243-33244)
Removal generator (33241)

26.6 26.6 **FUD** 090 J J8

AMA: 2019,Oct,3; 2018,Jan,8; 2017,Jan,8; 2016,Aug,5; 2016,Jan,13; 2015,Jan,16

33270-33275 [33270, 33271, 33272, 33273, 33274, 33275] Subcutaneous Implantable Defibrillator

INCLUDES Programming and interrogation of:
Leadless pacemaker (93279, 93286, 93288, 93294, 93296)
Subcutaneous implantable defibrillator ([93260, 93261])

\# **33270** **Insertion or replacement of permanent subcutaneous implantable defibrillator system, with subcutaneous electrode, including defibrillation threshold evaluation, induction of arrhythmia, evaluation of sensing for arrhythmia termination, and programming or reprogramming of sensing or therapeutic parameters, when performed**

INCLUDES Electrophysiologic evaluation at initial insertion (93644)

EXCLUDES *Insertion subcutaneous implantable defibrillator electrode only ([33271])*
Insertion/replacement permanent implantable defibrillator system with substernal electrode (0571T)

Code also electrophysiologic evaluation following replacement subcutaneous implantable defibrillator, when performed (93644)
Code also removal subcutaneous implantable defibrillator and removal subcutaneous electrode, when entire system is being replaced:
Defibrillator (33241)
Electrode ([33272])

16.4 16.4 **FUD** 090 J J8

AMA: 2019,Oct,3; 2018,Jan,8; 2017,Jan,8; 2016,Aug,5; 2016,Jan,13; 2015,Jan,16

\# **33271** **Insertion of subcutaneous implantable defibrillator electrode**

EXCLUDES *Insertion implantable defibrillator pulse generator only, other than subcutaneous:*
Initial insertion (33240)
Removal/replacement ([33262])
Insertion subcutaneous implantable defibrillator and electrode (total system) ([33270])
Insertion substernal defibrillator electrode (0572T)

13.1 13.1 **FUD** 090 J J8

AMA: 2019,Oct,3; 2018,Jan,8; 2017,Jan,8; 2016,Aug,5; 2016,Jan,13; 2015,Jan,16

\# **33272** **Removal of subcutaneous implantable defibrillator electrode**

EXCLUDES *Removal substernal defibrillator electrode (0573T)*

Code also removal implantable defibrillator, when performed:
Removal with replacement ([33262])
Removal without replacement (33241)
Code also removal subcutaneous implantable defibrillator and insertion replacement implantable subcutaneous defibrillator with electrode (total system), when entire system is being replaced:
Insertion total system ([33270])
Removal defibrillator (33241)

10.0 10.0 **FUD** 090 Q2

AMA: 2019,Oct,3; 2018,Jan,8; 2017,Jan,8; 2016,Aug,5; 2016,Jan,13; 2015,Jan,16

33273 **Repositioning of previously implanted subcutaneous implantable defibrillator electrode**

EXCLUDES *Repositioning substernal defibrillator electrode (0574T)*

11.5 11.5 FUD 090 T G2

AMA: 2019,Oct,3; 2018,Jan,8; 2017,Jan,8; 2016,Aug,5; 2016,Jan,13; 2015,Jan,16

33274 **Transcatheter insertion or replacement of permanent leadless pacemaker, right ventricular, including imaging guidance (eg, fluoroscopy, venous ultrasound, ventriculography, femoral venography) and device evaluation (eg, interrogation or programming), when performed**

INCLUDES Cardiac catheterization for insertion leadless pacemaker (93451, 93453, 93456-93457, 93460-93461, 93530-93533)
Femoral venography (75820)
Imaging guidance (76000, 76937, 77002)
Right ventriculography (93566)

EXCLUDES *Removal permanent leadless pacemaker ([33275])*
Services for pacemakers with leads (33202-33203, 33206-33208, 33212-33214 [33221], 33215-33218, 33220, 33233-33237 [33227, 33228, 33229])

14.2 14.2 FUD 090 J8

AMA: 2019,Mar,6

33275 **Transcatheter removal of permanent leadless pacemaker, right ventricular, including imaging guidance (eg, fluoroscopy, venous ultrasound, ventriculography, femoral venography), when performed**

INCLUDES Cardiac catheterization for insertion leadless pacemaker (93451, 93453, 93456-93457, 93460-93461, 93530-93533)
Femoral venography (75820)
Imaging guidance (76000, 76937, 77002)
Right ventriculography (93566)

EXCLUDES *Insertion/replacement leadless pacemaker ([33274])*
Services for pacemakers with leads (33202-33203, 33206-33208, 33212-33214 [33221], 33215-33218, 33220, 33233-33237 [33227, 33228, 33229])

15.4 15.4 FUD 090 G2

AMA: 2019,Mar,6

33250-33251 Surgical Ablation Arrhythmogenic Foci, Supraventricular

INCLUDES Procedures using cryotherapy, laser, microwave, radiofrequency, and ultrasound

33250 **Operative ablation of supraventricular arrhythmogenic focus or pathway (eg, Wolff-Parkinson-White, atrioventricular node re-entry), tract(s) and/or focus (foci); without cardiopulmonary bypass**

EXCLUDES *Pacing and mapping during surgery by other provider (93631)*

41.7 41.7 FUD 090 C 80

AMA: 2018,Jan,8; 2017,Jan,8; 2016,Jan,13; 2015,Jan,16

33251 **with cardiopulmonary bypass**

47.0 47.0 FUD 090 C 80

AMA: 2018,Jan,8; 2017,Dec,3; 2017,Jan,8; 2016,Jan,13; 2015,Jan,16

33254-33256 Surgical Ablation Arrhythmogenic Foci, Atrial (e.g., Maze)

INCLUDES Excision or isolation left atrial appendage
Procedures using cryotherapy, laser, microwave, radiofrequency, and ultrasound

EXCLUDES *Any procedure involving median sternotomy or cardiopulmonary bypass*
Aortic valve procedures (33390-33391, 33404-33415)
Aortoplasty (33417)
Ascending aorta graft (33858-33859, 33863-33864)
Coronary artery bypass (33510-33516, 33517-33523, 33533-33536)
Excision intracardiac tumor, resection (33120)
Mitral valve procedures (33418-33430)
Outflow tract augmentation (33478)
Prosthetic valve repair (33496)
Pulmonary artery embolectomy (33910-33920)
Pulmonary valve procedures (33470-33477)
Repair aberrant coronary artery anatomy (33500-33507)
Repair aberrant heart anatomy (33600-33853)
Resection external cardiac tumor (33130)
Temporary pacemaker (33210-33211)
Thoracotomy; with exploration (32100)
Tricuspid valve procedures (33460-33468)
Tube thoracostomy, includes connection to drainage system (32551)
Ventricular reconstruction (33542-33548)
Ventriculomyotomy (33416)

33254 **Operative tissue ablation and reconstruction of atria, limited (eg, modified maze procedure)**

39.0 39.0 FUD 090 C 80

AMA: 2018,Jan,8; 2017,Jan,8; 2016,Jan,13; 2015,Jan,16

33255 **Operative tissue ablation and reconstruction of atria, extensive (eg, maze procedure); without cardiopulmonary bypass**

47.4 47.4 FUD 090 C 80

AMA: 2018,Jan,8; 2017,Jan,8; 2016,Jan,13; 2015,Jan,16

33256 **with cardiopulmonary bypass**

56.1 56.1 FUD 090 C 80

AMA: 2018,Jan,8; 2017,Dec,3; 2017,Jan,8; 2016,Jan,13; 2015,Jan,16

33257-33259 Surgical Ablation Arrhythmogenic Foci, Atrial, with Other Heart Procedure(s)

EXCLUDES *Operative tissue ablation and reconstruction atria (without other cardiac procedure), limited or extensive:*
Endoscopic (33265-33266)
Open (33254-33256)
Temporary pacemaker (33210-33211)
Tube thoracostomy, includes connection to drainage system (32551)

+ 33257 **Operative tissue ablation and reconstruction of atria, performed at the time of other cardiac procedure(s), limited (eg, modified maze procedure) (List separately in addition to code for primary procedure)**

Code first (33120-33130, 33250-33251, 33261, 33300-33335, 33365, 33390-33391, 33404-33417 [33440], 33420-33430, 33460-33476, 33478, 33496, 33500-33507, 33510-33516, 33533-33548, 33600-33619, 33641-33697, 33702-33732, 33735-33767, 33770-33877, 33910-33922, 33925-33926, 33975-33983)

16.8 16.8 FUD ZZZ C 80

+ 33258 **Operative tissue ablation and reconstruction of atria, performed at the time of other cardiac procedure(s), extensive (eg, maze procedure), without cardiopulmonary bypass (List separately in addition to code for primary procedure)**

Code first, when performed without cardiopulmonary bypass (33130, 33250, 33300, 33310, 33320-33321, 33330, 33365, 33420, 33470-33471, 33501-33503, 33510-33516, 33533-33536, 33690, 33735, 33737, 33750-33766, 33800-33813, 33820-33824, 33840-33852, 33875, 33877, 33915, 33925, 33981, 33982)

18.7 18.7 FUD ZZZ C 80

Cardiovascular, Hemic, and Lymphatic

33273 — 33258

\+ **33259** **Operative tissue ablation and reconstruction of atria, performed at the time of other cardiac procedure(s), extensive (eg, maze procedure), with cardiopulmonary bypass (List separately in addition to code for primary procedure)**

Code first, when performed with cardiopulmonary bypass (33120, 33251, 33261, 33305, 33315, 33322, 33335, 33390-33391, 33404-33410, 33411-33417, 33422-33430, 33460-33468, 33474-33478, 33496, 33500, 33504-33507, 33510-33516, 33533-33548, 33600-33688, 33692-33726, 33730, 33732, 33736, 33767, 33770, 33783, 33786-33788, 33814, 33853, 33858-33877, 33910, 33916-33922, 33926, 33975-33980, 33983)

24.3 24.3 FUD ZZZ C 80

AMA: 2017,Dec,3

33261-33264 [33262, 33263, 33264] Surgical Ablation Arrhythmogenic Foci, Ventricular

33261 **Operative ablation of ventricular arrhythmogenic focus with cardiopulmonary bypass**

47.0 47.0 FUD 090 C 80

AMA: 2018,Jan,8; 2017,Dec,3; 2017,Jan,8; 2016,Jan,13; 2015,Jan,16

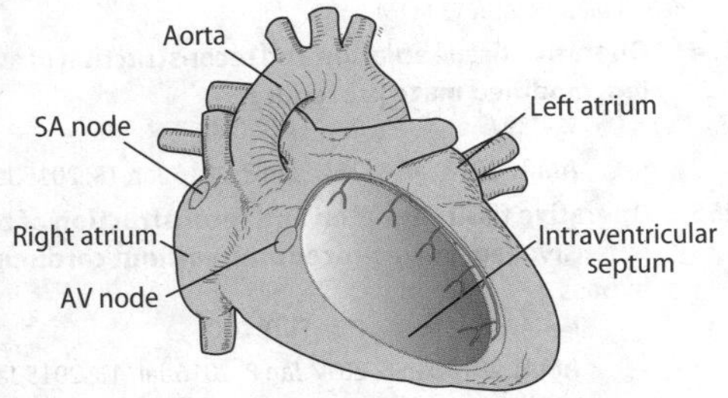

Impulse centers that are causing arrhythmia are treated with ablation

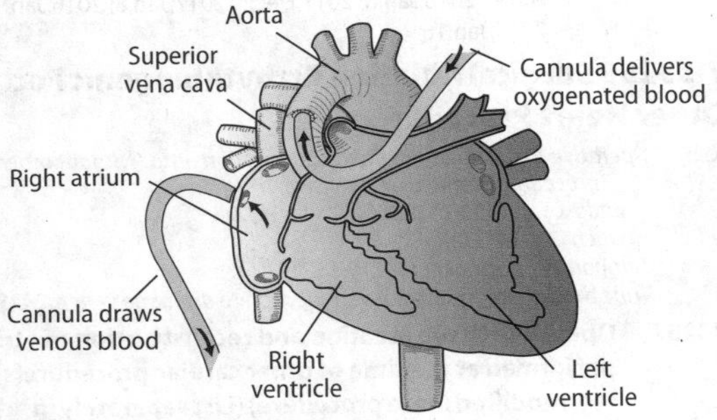

Bypass schematic

33262 **Resequenced code. See code following 33241.**

33263 **Resequenced code. See code following 33241.**

33264 **Resequenced code. See code before 33243.**

33265-33275 [33270, 33271, 33272, 33273, 33274, 33275] Surgical Ablation Arrhythmogenic Foci, Endoscopic

EXCLUDES *Insertion or replacement temporary transvenous single chamber cardiac electrode or pacemaker catheter (separate procedure) (33210-33211)*
Tube thoracostomy, includes connection to drainage system (32551)

33265 **Endoscopy, surgical; operative tissue ablation and reconstruction of atria, limited (eg, modified maze procedure), without cardiopulmonary bypass**

39.3 39.3 FUD 090 C 80

AMA: 2018,Jan,8; 2017,Jan,8; 2016,Jan,13; 2015,Jan,16

33266 **operative tissue ablation and reconstruction of atria, extensive (eg, maze procedure), without cardiopulmonary bypass**

53.4 53.4 FUD 090 C 80

AMA: 2018,Jan,8; 2017,Jan,8; 2016,Jan,13; 2015,Jan,16

33270 **Resequenced code. See code following 33249.**

33271 **Resequenced code. See code following 33249.**

33272 **Resequenced code. See code following 33249.**

33273 **Resequenced code. See code following 33249.**

33274 **Resequenced code. See code following 33249.**

33275 **Resequenced code. See code following 33249.**

33285-33289 Cardiac Rhythm Monitor System

33285 **Insertion, subcutaneous cardiac rhythm monitor, including programming**

INCLUDES Implantation device into subcutaneous prepectoral pocket
Initial programming

EXCLUDES *Successive analysis and/or reprogramming (93285, 93291, 93298)*

2.57 142. FUD 000 J8

AMA: 2019,Oct,3; 2019,Apr,3

33286 **Removal, subcutaneous cardiac rhythm monitor**

2.54 3.80 FUD 000 G2

AMA: 2019,Apr,3

33289 **Transcatheter implantation of wireless pulmonary artery pressure sensor for long-term hemodynamic monitoring, including deployment and calibration of the sensor, right heart catheterization, selective pulmonary catheterization, radiological supervision and interpretation, and pulmonary artery angiography, when performed**

INCLUDES Device implantation into subcutaneous pocket
Fluoroscopy (76000)
Pulmonary artery angiography/injection (75741, 75743, 75746, 93568)
Pulmonary artery catheterization (36013-36015)
Radiologic supervision and interpretation
Remote monitoring (93264)
Right heart catheterization (93451, 93453, 93456-93457, 93460-93461, 93530-93533)
Sensor deployment and calibration

9.55 9.55 FUD 000 80

AMA: 2019,Jun,3

33300-33315 Procedures for Injury of the Heart

INCLUDES Procedures with and without cardiopulmonary bypass

Code also transvascular ventricular support, when performed:
Balloon pump (33967, 33968, 33970-33974)
Extracorporeal membrane oxygenation (ECMO)/extracorporeal life support (ECLS) (33946-33949)
Ventricular assist device (33975-33983, [33995], 33990-33993 [33997])

33300 **Repair of cardiac wound; without bypass**

71.0 71.0 FUD 090 C 80

AMA: 1997,Nov,1

33305 **with cardiopulmonary bypass**

118. 118. FUD 090 C 80

AMA: 2017,Dec,3

33310 **Cardiotomy, exploratory (includes removal of foreign body, atrial or ventricular thrombus); without bypass**

EXCLUDES *Other cardiac procedures unless separate incision into heart necessary to remove thrombus*

33.7 33.7 FUD 090 C 80

AMA: 1997,Nov,1

33315 **with cardiopulmonary bypass**

EXCLUDES *Other cardiac procedures unless separate incision into heart necessary to remove thrombus*

Code also excision thrombus with cardiopulmonary bypass and append modifier 59 when separate incision required with (33120, 33130, 33420-33430, 33460-33468, 33496, 33542, 33545, 33641-33647, 33670, 33681, 33975-33980)

55.3 55.3 FUD 090 C 80

AMA: 2018,Jan,8; 2017,Dec,3; 2017,Jan,8; 2016,Jan,13; 2015,Jan,16

33320-33335 Procedures for Injury of the Aorta/Great Vessels

Code also transvascular ventricular support, when performed:
- Balloon pump (33967, 33968, 33970-33974)
- Extracorporeal membrane oxygenation (ECMO)/extracorporeal life support (ECLS) (33946-33949)
- Ventricular assist device (33975-33983, [33995], 33990-33993 [33997])

33320 **Suture repair of aorta or great vessels; without shunt or cardiopulmonary bypass**
30.5 30.5 **FUD** 090 C 80
AMA: 2018,Jun,11; 2018,Jan,8; 2017,Jan,8; 2016,Jan,13; 2015,Jan,16

33321 **with shunt bypass**
34.3 34.3 **FUD** 090 C 80
AMA: 2018,Jun,11

33322 **with cardiopulmonary bypass**
40.2 40.2 **FUD** 090 C 80
AMA: 2018,Jun,11; 2018,Jan,8; 2017,Dec,3; 2017,Jan,8; 2016,Jan,13; 2015,Jan,16

33330 **Insertion of graft, aorta or great vessels; without shunt, or cardiopulmonary bypass**
41.2 41.2 **FUD** 090 C 80
AMA: 2018,Jun,11

33335 **with cardiopulmonary bypass**
54.6 54.6 **FUD** 090 C 80
AMA: 2018,Jun,11; 2017,Dec,3

33340 Closure Left Atrial Appendage

EXCLUDES *Cardiac catheterization except for reasons other than closure left atrial appendage (93451-93453, 93456, 93458-93461, 93462, 93530-93533)*

Code also transvascular ventricular support, when performed:
- Balloon pump (33967, 33968, 33970-33974)
- Extracorporeal membrane oxygenation (ECMO)/extracorporeal life support (ECLS) (33946-33949)
- Ventricular assist device (33975-33983, [33995], 33990-33993 [33997])

33340 **Percutaneous transcatheter closure of the left atrial appendage with endocardial implant, including fluoroscopy, transseptal puncture, catheter placement(s), left atrial angiography, left atrial appendage angiography, when performed, and radiological supervision and interpretation**
22.9 22.9 **FUD** 000 C 80
AMA: 2018,Jan,8; 2017,Jul,3

33361-33369 Transcatheter Aortic Valve Replacement

CMS: 100-03,20.32 Transcatheter Aortic Valve Replacement (TAVR); 100-04,32,290.3 Claims Processing TAVR Inpatient; 100-04,32,290.4 Payment of TAVR for MA Plan Participants

INCLUDES
- Access and implantation aortic valve (33361-33366)
- Access sheath placement
- Advancement valve delivery system
- Arteriotomy closure
- Balloon aortic valvuloplasty
- Cardiac or open arterial approach
- Deployment of valve
- Percutaneous access
- Radiology procedures:
  - Angiography during and after procedure
  - Assessment access site for closure
  - Documentation intervention completion
  - Guidance for valve placement
  - Supervision and interpretation
- Temporary pacemaker
- Valve repositioning when necessary

EXCLUDES
- *Cardiac catheterization procedures included in TAVR/TAVI service (93452-93453, 93458-93461, 93567)*
- *Percutaneous coronary interventional procedures*

Code also cardiac catheterization services for purposes other than TAVR/TAVI

Code also diagnostic coronary angiography at different session from interventional procedure

Code also diagnostic coronary angiography same time as TAVR/TAVI when:
- Previous study available, but documentation states patient's condition has changed since previous study, visualization anatomy/pathology inadequate, or change occurs during procedure warranting additional evaluation outside current target area
- No previous catheter-based coronary angiography study available, and full diagnostic study performed, with decision to perform intervention based on that study

Code also modifier 59 when diagnostic coronary angiography procedures performed as separate and distinct procedural services on same day or session as TAVR/TAVI

Code also modifier 62 as all TAVI/TAVR procedures require work two physicians

Code also transvascular ventricular support, when performed:
- Balloon pump (33967, 33970, 33973)
- Ventricular assist device (33975-33976, [33995], 33990-33993 [33997])

33361 **Transcatheter aortic valve replacement (TAVR/TAVI) with prosthetic valve; percutaneous femoral artery approach**
Code also cardiopulmonary bypass when performed (33367-33369)
39.4 39.4 **FUD** 000 C 80
AMA: 2018,Jan,8; 2017,Jan,8; 2016,Jan,13; 2015,Mar,9; 2015,Jan,16

33362 **open femoral artery approach**
Code also cardiopulmonary bypass when performed (33367-33369)
43.1 43.1 **FUD** 000 C 80
AMA: 2018,Jan,8; 2017,Dec,3; 2017,Jan,8; 2016,Jan,13; 2015,Mar,9; 2015,Jan,16

33363 **open axillary artery approach**
Code also cardiopulmonary bypass when performed (33367-33369)
44.6 44.6 **FUD** 000 C 80
AMA: 2018,Jan,8; 2017,Dec,3; 2017,Jan,8; 2016,Jan,13; 2015,Mar,9; 2015,Jan,16

33364 **open iliac artery approach**
Code also cardiopulmonary bypass when performed (33367-33369)
46.1 46.1 **FUD** 000 C 80
AMA: 2018,Jan,8; 2017,Dec,3; 2017,Jan,8; 2016,Jan,13; 2015,Mar,9; 2015,Jan,16

33365 **transaortic approach (eg, median sternotomy, mediastinotomy)**
Code also cardiopulmonary bypass when performed (33367-33369)
51.8 51.8 **FUD** 000 C 80
AMA: 2018,Jan,8; 2017,Jan,8; 2016,Jan,13; 2015,Mar,9; 2015,Jan,16

33366 **transapical exposure (eg, left thoracotomy)**
Code also cardiopulmonary bypass when performed (33367-33369)
45.7 45.7 FUD 000 C 80
AMA: 2018,Jan,8; 2017,Jan,8; 2016,Jan,13; 2015,Mar,9; 2015,Jan,16

\+ **33367** **cardiopulmonary bypass support with percutaneous peripheral arterial and venous cannulation (eg, femoral vessels) (List separately in addition to code for primary procedure)**
EXCLUDES *Cardiopulmonary bypass support with open or central arterial and venous cannulation (33368-33369)*
Code first (33361-33366, 33418, 33477, 0483T-0484T, 0544T, 0545T, 0569T-0570T)
18.2 18.2 FUD ZZZ C 80
AMA: 2018,Jan,8; 2017,Jan,8; 2016,Mar,5; 2016,Jan,13; 2015,Sep,3; 2015,Jan,16

\+ **33368** **cardiopulmonary bypass support with open peripheral arterial and venous cannulation (eg, femoral, iliac, axillary vessels) (List separately in addition to code for primary procedure)**
EXCLUDES *Cardiopulmonary bypass support with percutaneous or central arterial and venous cannulation (33367, 33369)*
Code first (33361-33366, 33418, 33477, 0483T-0484T, 0544T, 0545T, 0569T-0570T)
21.7 21.7 FUD ZZZ C 80
AMA: 2018,Jan,8; 2017,Jan,8; 2016,Mar,5; 2016,Jan,13; 2015,Sep,3; 2015,Jan,16

\+ **33369** **cardiopulmonary bypass support with central arterial and venous cannulation (eg, aorta, right atrium, pulmonary artery) (List separately in addition to code for primary procedure)**
EXCLUDES *Cardiopulmonary bypass support with percutaneous or open arterial and venous cannulation (33367-33368)*
Code first (33361-33366, 33418, 33477, 0483T-0484T, 0544T, 0545T, 0569T-0570T)
28.6 28.6 FUD ZZZ C 80
AMA: 2018,Jan,8; 2017,Jan,8; 2016,Mar,5; 2016,Jan,13; 2015,Sep,3; 2015,Jan,16

33390-33415 [33440] Aortic Valve Procedures

Code also transvascular ventricular support, when performed:
Balloon pump (33967, 33968, 33970-33974)
Extracorporeal membrane oxygenation (ECMO)/extracorporeal life support (ECLS) (33946-33949)
Ventricular assist device (33975-33983, [33995], 33990-33993 [33997])

33390 **Valvuloplasty, aortic valve, open, with cardiopulmonary bypass; simple (ie, valvotomy, debridement, debulking, and/or simple commissural resuspension)**
54.9 54.9 FUD 090 C 80
AMA: 2018,Jan,8; 2017,Dec,3

33391 **complex (eg, leaflet extension, leaflet resection, leaflet reconstruction, or annuloplasty)**
INCLUDES Simple aortic valvuloplasty (33390)
66.4 66.4 FUD 090 C 80
AMA: 2018,Jan,8; 2017,Dec,3

33404 **Construction of apical-aortic conduit**
50.6 50.6 FUD 090 C 80
AMA: 2018,Jan,8; 2017,Dec,3; 2017,Jan,8; 2016,Jan,13; 2015,Jan,16

33405 **Replacement, aortic valve, open, with cardiopulmonary bypass; with prosthetic valve other than homograft or stentless valve**
65.7 65.7 FUD 090 C 80
AMA: 2019,Nov,9; 2019,Apr,6; 2018,Jan,8; 2017,Dec,3; 2017,Jan,8; 2016,Jan,13; 2015,Jan,16

33406 **with allograft valve (freehand)**
83.4 83.4 FUD 090 C 80
AMA: 2019,Nov,9; 2019,Apr,6; 2018,Jan,8; 2017,Dec,3; 2017,Jan,8; 2016,Jan,13; 2015,Jan,16

33410 **with stentless tissue valve**
73.6 73.6 FUD 090 C 80
AMA: 2019,Nov,9; 2019,Apr,6; 2018,Jan,8; 2017,Dec,3; 2017,Jan,8; 2016,Jan,13; 2015,Jan,16

\# **33440** **Replacement, aortic valve; by translocation of autologous pulmonary valve and transventricular aortic annulus enlargement of the left ventricular outflow tract with valved conduit replacement of pulmonary valve (Ross-Konno procedure)**
INCLUDES Open replacement aortic valve with aortic annulus enlargement (33411-33412)
Open replacement aortic valve with translocation pulmonary valve (33413)
EXCLUDES *Aortoplasty for supravalvular stenosis (33417)*
Open replacement aortic valve (33405-33406, 33410)
Repair complex cardiac anomaly (except pulmonary atresia) (33608)
Repair left ventricular outlet obstruction (33414)
Repair pulmonary atresia (33920)
Replacement pulmonary valve (33475)
Resection/incision subvalvular tissue for aortic stenosis (33416)
98.1 98.1 FUD 090 80
AMA: 2019,Apr,6

33411 **with aortic annulus enlargement, noncoronary sinus**
97.4 97.4 FUD 090 C 80
AMA: 2019,Nov,9; 2019,Apr,6; 2018,Jan,8; 2017,Dec,3; 2017,Jan,8; 2016,Jan,13; 2015,Jan,16

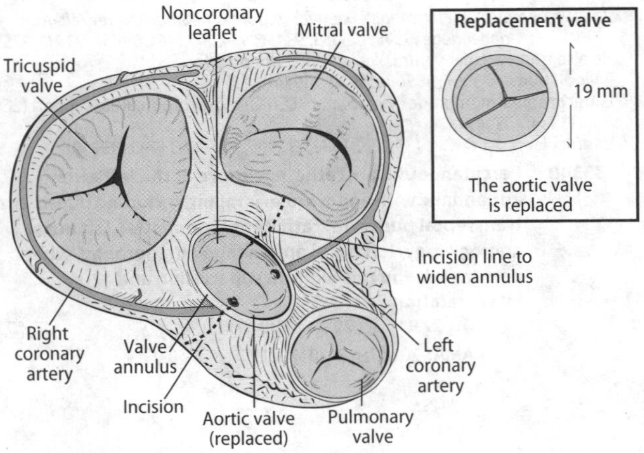

Overhead schematic of major heart valves

33412 **with transventricular aortic annulus enlargement (Konno procedure)**
EXCLUDES *Replacement aortic valve by translocation pulmonary valve, aortic annulus enlargement, valved conduit pulmonary valve replacement ([33440])*
Replacement aortic valve with translocation pulmonary valve (33413)
91.4 91.4 FUD 090 C 80
AMA: 2019,Nov,9; 2019,Apr,6; 2018,Jan,8; 2017,Dec,3; 2017,Jan,8; 2016,Jan,13; 2015,Jan,16

33413 **by translocation of autologous pulmonary valve with allograft replacement of pulmonary valve (Ross procedure)**
EXCLUDES *Replacement aortic valve by translocation pulmonary valve, aortic annulus enlargement, valved conduit pulmonary valve replacement ([33440])*
Replacement aortic valve with transventricular aortic annulus enlargement (33412)
94.3 94.3 FUD 090 C 80
AMA: 2019,Nov,9; 2019,Apr,6; 2018,Jan,8; 2017,Dec,3; 2017,Jan,8; 2016,Jan,13; 2015,Jan,16

33414 **Repair of left ventricular outflow tract obstruction by patch enlargement of the outflow tract**
62.2 62.2 FUD 090 C 80
AMA: 2019,Apr,6; 2018,Jan,8; 2017,Dec,3; 2017,Jan,8; 2016,Jan,13; 2015,Jan,16

33415 **Resection or incision of subvalvular tissue for discrete subvalvular aortic stenosis**
58.7 58.7 FUD 090 C 80
AMA: 2018,Jan,8; 2017,Dec,3; 2017,Jan,8; 2016,Jan,13; 2015,Jan,16

33416 Ventriculectomy

CMS: 100-03,20.26 Partial Ventriculectomy

EXCLUDES *Percutaneous transcatheter septal reduction therapy (93583)*

Code also transvascular ventricular support, when performed:
- Balloon pump (33967, 33968, 33970-33974)
- Extracorporeal membrane oxygenation (ECMO)/extracorporeal life support (ECLS) (33946-33949)
- Ventricular assist device (33975-33983, [33995], 33990-33993 [33997])

33416 **Ventriculomyotomy (-myectomy) for idiopathic hypertrophic subaortic stenosis (eg, asymmetric septal hypertrophy)**
58.5 58.5 FUD 090 C 80
AMA: 2019,Apr,6; 2018,Jan,8; 2017,Dec,3; 2017,Jan,8; 2016,Jan,13; 2015,Jan,16

33417 Repair of Supravalvular Stenosis by Aortoplasty

Code also transvascular ventricular support, when performed:
- Balloon pump (33967, 33968, 33970-33974)
- Extracorporeal membrane oxygenation (ECMO)/extracorporeal life support (ECLS) (33946-33949)
- Ventricular assist device (33975-33983, [33995], 33990-33993 [33997])

33417 **Aortoplasty (gusset) for supravalvular stenosis**
48.2 48.2 FUD 090 C 80
AMA: 2019,Apr,6; 2018,Jan,8; 2017,Dec,3; 2017,Jan,8; 2016,Jan,13; 2015,Jan,16

33418-33419 Transcatheter Mitral Valve Procedures

INCLUDES
- Access sheath placement
- Advancement valve delivery system
- Deployment valve
- Radiology procedures:
  - Angiography during and after procedure
  - Documentation intervention completion
  - Guidance for valve placement
  - Supervision and interpretation
- Valve repositioning when necessary

EXCLUDES
- *Cardiac catheterization services for purposes other than TMVR*
- *Diagnostic angiography different session from interventional procedure*
- *Percutaneous approach through the coronary sinus for TMVR (0345T)*
- *Percutaneous coronary interventional procedures*
- *Transcatheter mitral valve annulus reconstruction (0544T)*
- *Transcatheter TMVI by percutaneous or transthoracic approach (0483T-0484T)*

Code also cardiopulmonary bypass:
- Central (33369)
- Open peripheral (33368)
- Percutaneous peripheral (33367)

Code also diagnostic coronary angiography and cardiac catheterization procedures when:
- No previous study available and full diagnostic study performed
- Previous study inadequate or patient's clinical indication for study changed prior to or during procedure
- Report modifier 59 with cardiac catheterization procedures when on same day or same session as TMVR

Code also transvascular ventricular support, when performed:
- Balloon pump (33967, 33970, 33973)
- Ventricular assist device ([33995], 33990-33993 [33997])

33418 **Transcatheter mitral valve repair, percutaneous approach, including transseptal puncture when performed; initial prosthesis**
Code also left heart catheterization when performed by transapical puncture (93462)
52.1 52.1 FUD 090 C 80
AMA: 2018,Jan,8; 2017,Jan,8; 2016,Jan,13; 2015,Sep,3

\+ **33419** **additional prosthesis(es) during same session (List separately in addition to code for primary procedure)**
EXCLUDES *Procedures performed more than one time per session*
Code first (33418)
12.3 12.3 FUD ZZZ N N1 80
AMA: 2018,Jan,8; 2017,Jan,8; 2016,Jan,13; 2015,Sep,3

33420-33440 [33440] Mitral Valve Procedures

Code also thrombus removal through separate heart incision, when performed (33310-33315); append modifier 59 to (33315)

Code also transvascular ventricular support, when performed:
- Balloon pump (33967, 33968, 33970-33974)
- Extracorporeal membrane oxygenation (ECMO)/extracorporeal life support (ECLS) (33946-33949)
- Ventricular assist device (33975-33983, [33995], 33990-33993 [33997])

33420 **Valvotomy, mitral valve; closed heart**
42.3 42.3 FUD 090 C
AMA: 2018,Jan,8; 2017,Jan,8; 2016,Jan,13; 2015,Sep,3; 2015,Jan,16

33422 **open heart, with cardiopulmonary bypass**
48.1 48.1 FUD 090 C 80
AMA: 2018,Jan,8; 2017,Dec,3; 2017,Jan,8; 2016,Jan,13; 2015,Sep,3; 2015,Jan,16

33425 **Valvuloplasty, mitral valve, with cardiopulmonary bypass;**
79.1 79.1 FUD 090 C 80
AMA: 2018,Jan,8; 2017,Dec,3; 2017,Jan,8; 2016,Jan,13; 2015,Sep,3; 2015,Jan,16

33426 **with prosthetic ring**
69.0 69.0 FUD 090 C 80
AMA: 2018,Jan,8; 2017,Dec,3; 2017,Jan,8; 2016,Jan,13; 2015,Sep,3; 2015,Jan,16

33427 **radical reconstruction, with or without ring**
70.7 70.7 FUD 090 C 80
AMA: 2018,Jan,8; 2017,Dec,3; 2017,Jan,8; 2016,Jan,13; 2015,Sep,3; 2015,Jan,16

33430 **Replacement, mitral valve, with cardiopulmonary bypass**
81.1 81.1 FUD 090 C 80
AMA: 2018,Jan,8; 2017,Dec,3; 2017,Jan,8; 2016,Jan,13; 2015,Sep,3; 2015,Jan,16

33440 **Resequenced code. See code following 33410.**

33460-33468 Tricuspid Valve Procedures

EXCLUDES
- *Transcatheter tricuspid valve annulus reconstruction (0545T)*
- *Transcatheter tricuspid valve repair (0569T-0570T)*

Code also thrombus removal through separate heart incision, when performed (33310-33315); append modifier 59 to (33315)

Code also transvascular ventricular support, when performed:
- Balloon pump (33967, 33968, 33970-33974)
- Extracorporeal membrane oxygenation (ECMO)/extracorporeal life support (ECLS) (33946-33949)
- Ventricular assist device (33975-33983, [33995], 33990-33993 [33997])

33460 **Valvectomy, tricuspid valve, with cardiopulmonary bypass**
69.6 69.6 FUD 090 C 80
AMA: 2018,Jan,8; 2017,Dec,3; 2017,Jan,8; 2016,Jan,13; 2015,Jan,16

33463 **Valvuloplasty, tricuspid valve; without ring insertion**
89.5 89.5 FUD 090 C 80
AMA: 2018,Jan,8; 2017,Dec,3; 2017,Jan,8; 2016,Jan,13; 2015,Jan,16

33464 **with ring insertion**
70.7 70.7 FUD 090 C 80
AMA: 2018,Jan,8; 2017,Dec,3; 2017,Jan,8; 2016,Jan,13; 2015,Jan,16

33465 **Replacement, tricuspid valve, with cardiopulmonary bypass**
79.9 79.9 FUD 090 C 80
AMA: 2018,Jan,8; 2017,Dec,3; 2017,Jan,8; 2016,Jan,13; 2015,Jan,16

33468 **Tricuspid valve repositioning and plication for Ebstein anomaly**
71.0 71.0 FUD 090 C 80
AMA: 2018,Jan,8; 2017,Dec,3; 2017,Jan,8; 2016,Jan,13; 2015,Jan,16

33470-33474 Pulmonary Valvotomy

INCLUDES Brock's operation

Code also concurrent systemic-to-pulmonary artery shunt ligation/takedown (33924)
Code also transvascular ventricular support, when performed:
Balloon pump (33967, 33968, 33970-33974)
Extracorporeal membrane oxygenation (ECMO)/extracorporeal life support (ECLS) (33946-33949)
Ventricular assist device (33975-33983, [33995], 33990-33993 [33997])

33470 **Valvotomy, pulmonary valve, closed heart; transventricular**
35.8 35.8 FUD 090 63 C 80
AMA: 2018,Jan,8; 2017,Jan,8; 2016,Jan,13; 2015,Jan,16

33471 **via pulmonary artery**
EXCLUDES *Percutaneous valvuloplasty pulmonary valve (92990)*
38.3 38.3 FUD 090 C 80
AMA: 2018,Jan,8; 2017,Jan,8; 2016,Jan,13; 2015,Jan,16

33474 **Valvotomy, pulmonary valve, open heart, with cardiopulmonary bypass**
63.0 63.0 FUD 090 C 80
AMA: 2017,Dec,3

33475-33476 Other Procedures Pulmonary Valve

Code also concurrent systemic-to-pulmonary artery shunt ligation/takedown (33924)
Code also transvascular ventricular support, when performed:
Balloon pump (33967, 33968, 33970-33974)
Extracorporeal membrane oxygenation (ECMO)/extracorporeal life support (ECLS) (33946-33949)
Ventricular assist device (33975-33983, [33995], 33990-33993 [33997])

33475 **Replacement, pulmonary valve**
67.5 67.5 FUD 090 C 80
AMA: 2019,Apr,6; 2018,Jan,8; 2017,Dec,3; 2017,Jan,8; 2016,Jan,13; 2015,Jan,16

33476 **Right ventricular resection for infundibular stenosis, with or without commissurotomy**
INCLUDES Brock's operation
44.0 44.0 FUD 090 C 80
AMA: 2018,Jan,8; 2017,Dec,3; 2017,Jan,8; 2016,Jan,13; 2015,Jan,16

33477 Transcatheter Pulmonary Valve Implantation

INCLUDES Cardiac catheterization, contrast injection, angiography, fluoroscopic guidance and supervision and interpretation for device placement
Percutaneous balloon angioplasty within treatment area
Pre-, intra-, and postoperative hemodynamic measurements
Valvuloplasty or stent insertion in pulmonary valve conduit (37236-37237, 92997-92998)

EXCLUDES *Fluoroscopy (76000)*
Injection procedure during cardiac catheterization (93563, 93566-93568)
Percutaneous cardiac intervention procedures, when performed
Procedures performed more than one time per session
Right heart catheterization (93451, 93453-93461, 93530-93533)

Code also concurrent systemic-to-pulmonary artery shunt ligation/takedown (33924)
Code also transvascular ventricular support, when performed:
Balloon pump (33967, 33970, 33973)
Extracorporeal membrane oxygenation (ECMO)/extracorporeal life support (ECLS) (33946-33959, [33962], [33963], [33964], [33965], [33966], [33969], [33984], [33985], [33986], [33987], [33988], [33989])
Ventricular assist device ([33995], 33990-33993 [33997])

33477 **Transcatheter pulmonary valve implantation, percutaneous approach, including pre-stenting of the valve delivery site, when performed**
39.4 39.4 FUD 000 C 80
AMA: 2018,Jan,8; 2017,Jan,8; 2016,Aug,9; 2016,Mar,5

33478 Outflow Tract Augmentation

Code also for cavopulmonary anastomosis to second superior vena cava (33768)
Code also concurrent ligation/takedown systemic-to-pulmonary artery shunt (33924)
Code also transvascular ventricular support, when performed:
Balloon pump (33967, 33968, 33970-33974)
Extracorporeal membrane oxygenation (ECMO)/extracorporeal life support (ECLS) (33946-33949)
Ventricular assist device (33975-33983, [33995], 33990-33993 [33997])

33478 **Outflow tract augmentation (gusset), with or without commissurotomy or infundibular resection**
45.4 45.4 FUD 090 C 80
AMA: 2018,Jan,8; 2017,Dec,3; 2017,Jan,8; 2016,Jan,13; 2015,Jan,16

33496 Prosthetic Valve Repair

Code also thrombus removal through separate heart incision, when performed (33310-33315); append modifier 59 to (33315)
Code also reoperation if performed (33530)

33496 **Repair of non-structural prosthetic valve dysfunction with cardiopulmonary bypass (separate procedure)**
48.5 48.5 FUD 090 C 80
AMA: 2018,Jan,8; 2017,Dec,3; 2017,Jan,8; 2016,Jan,13; 2015,Jan,16

33500-33507 Repair Aberrant Coronary Artery Anatomy

INCLUDES Angioplasty and/or endarterectomy

33500 **Repair of coronary arteriovenous or arteriocardiac chamber fistula; with cardiopulmonary bypass**
45.5 45.5 FUD 090 C 80
AMA: 2017,Dec,3

33501 **without cardiopulmonary bypass**
32.2 32.2 FUD 090 C 80
AMA: 2007,Mar,1-3; 1997,Nov,1

33502 **Repair of anomalous coronary artery from pulmonary artery origin; by ligation**
36.9 36.9 FUD 090 63 C 80
AMA: 2017,Dec,3

33503 **by graft, without cardiopulmonary bypass**
38.3 38.3 FUD 090 63 C 80
AMA: 2007,Mar,1-3; 1997,Nov,1

33504 **by graft, with cardiopulmonary bypass**
42.3 42.3 FUD 090 C 80
AMA: 2017,Dec,3

33505 **with construction of intrapulmonary artery tunnel (Takeuchi procedure)**
59.8 59.8 FUD 090 63 C 80
AMA: 2017,Dec,3

33506 **by translocation from pulmonary artery to aorta**
59.7 59.7 FUD 090 63 C 80
AMA: 2017,Dec,3

33507 **Repair of anomalous (eg, intramural) aortic origin of coronary artery by unroofing or translocation**
49.8 49.8 FUD 090 C 80
AMA: 2018,Jan,8; 2017,Dec,3; 2017,Jan,8; 2016,Jan,13; 2015,Jan,16

33508 Endoscopic Harvesting of Venous Graft

INCLUDES Diagnostic endoscopy

EXCLUDES *Harvesting vein upper extremity (35500)*

Code first (33510-33523)

\+ **33508** **Endoscopy, surgical, including video-assisted harvest of vein(s) for coronary artery bypass procedure (List separately in addition to code for primary procedure)**
0.48 0.48 FUD ZZZ N N1 80
AMA: 1997,Nov,1

33510-33516 Coronary Artery Bypass: Venous Grafts

INCLUDES Obtaining saphenous vein grafts
Venous bypass grafting only

EXCLUDES *Arterial bypass (33533-33536)*
Combined arterial-venous bypass (33517-33523, 33533-33536)
Obtaining vein graft:
Femoropopliteal vein (35572)
Upper extremity vein (35500)
Percutaneous ventricular assist devices ([33995], 33990-33993 [33997])

Code also modifier 80 when assistant at surgery obtains grafts

33510 **Coronary artery bypass, vein only; single coronary venous graft**
56.0 56.0 FUD 090 C 80
AMA: 2018,Jan,8; 2017,Dec,3; 2017,Jan,8; 2016,Jan,13; 2015,Jan,16

33511 **2 coronary venous grafts**
61.4 61.4 FUD 090 C 80
AMA: 2018,Jan,8; 2017,Dec,3; 2017,Jan,8; 2016,Jan,13; 2015,Jan,16

33512 **3 coronary venous grafts**
70.0 70.0 FUD 090 C 80
AMA: 2018,Jan,8; 2017,Dec,3; 2017,Jan,8; 2016,Jan,13; 2015,Jan,16

33513 **4 coronary venous grafts**
71.9 71.9 FUD 090 C 80
AMA: 2018,Jan,8; 2017,Dec,3; 2017,Jan,8; 2016,Jan,13; 2015,Jan,16

33514 **5 coronary venous grafts**
75.6 75.6 FUD 090 C 80
AMA: 2018,Jan,8; 2017,Dec,3; 2017,Jan,8; 2016,Jan,13; 2015,Jan,16

33516 **6 or more coronary venous grafts**
78.1 78.1 FUD 090 C 80
AMA: 2018,Jan,8; 2017,Dec,3; 2017,Jan,8; 2016,Jan,13; 2015,Jan,16

33517-33523 Coronary Artery Bypass: Venous AND Arterial Grafts

INCLUDES Obtaining saphenous vein grafts

EXCLUDES *Obtaining arterial graft:*
Upper extremity (35600)
Obtaining vein graft:
Femoropopliteal vein graft (35572)
Upper extremity (35500)
Percutaneous ventricular assist devices ([33995], 33990-33993 [33997])

Code also modifier 80 when assistant at surgery obtains grafts
Code first (33533-33536)

\+ **33517** **Coronary artery bypass, using venous graft(s) and arterial graft(s); single vein graft (List separately in addition to code for primary procedure)**
5.44 5.44 FUD ZZZ C 80
AMA: 2018,Jan,8; 2017,Jan,8; 2016,Jan,13; 2015,Jan,16

\+ **33518** **2 venous grafts (List separately in addition to code for primary procedure)**
11.9 11.9 FUD ZZZ C 80
AMA: 2018,Jan,8; 2017,Jan,8; 2016,Jan,13; 2015,Jan,16

\+ **33519** **3 venous grafts (List separately in addition to code for primary procedure)**
15.8 15.8 FUD ZZZ C 80
AMA: 2018,Jan,8; 2017,Jan,8; 2016,Jan,13; 2015,Jan,16

\+ **33521** **4 venous grafts (List separately in addition to code for primary procedure)**
18.9 18.9 FUD ZZZ C 80
AMA: 2018,Jan,8; 2017,Jan,8; 2016,Jan,13; 2015,Jan,16

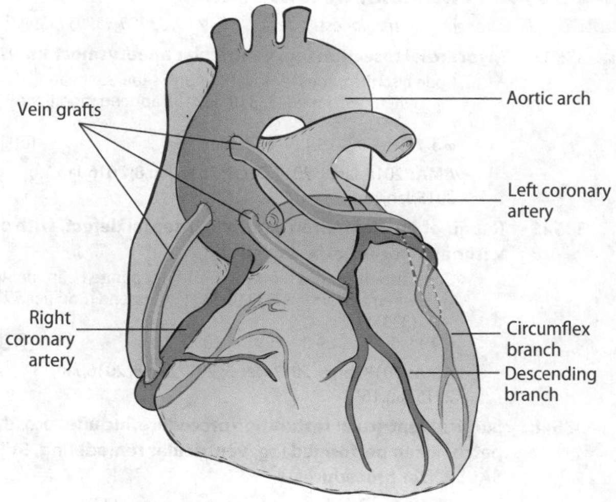

\+ **33522** **5 venous grafts (List separately in addition to code for primary procedure)**
21.2 21.2 FUD ZZZ C 80
AMA: 2018,Jan,8; 2017,Jan,8; 2016,Jan,13; 2015,Jan,16

\+ **33523** **6 or more venous grafts (List separately in addition to code for primary procedure)**
24.0 24.0 FUD ZZZ C 80
AMA: 2018,Jan,8; 2017,Jan,8; 2016,Jan,13; 2015,Jan,16

33530 Reoperative Coronary Artery Bypass Graft or Valve Procedure

EXCLUDES *Percutaneous ventricular assist devices (33990-33993)*

Code first (33390-33391, 33404-33496, 33510-33536, 33863)

\+ **33530** **Reoperation, coronary artery bypass procedure or valve procedure, more than 1 month after original operation (List separately in addition to code for primary procedure)**
15.2 15.2 FUD ZZZ C 80
AMA: 2018,Jan,8; 2017,Jan,8; 2016,Jan,13; 2015,Jan,16

33533-33536 Coronary Artery Bypass: Arterial Grafts

INCLUDES Obtaining arterial graft (eg, epigastric, internal mammary, gastroepiploic and others)

EXCLUDES *Obtaining arterial graft:*
Upper extremity (35600)
Obtaining venous graft:
Femoropopliteal vein (35572)
Upper extremity (35500)
Percutaneous ventricular assist devices ([33995], 33990-33993 [33997])
Venous bypass (33510-33516)

Code also for combined arterial venous grafts (33517-33523)
Code also modifier 80 when assistant at surgery obtains grafts

33533 **Coronary artery bypass, using arterial graft(s); single arterial graft**
54.1 54.1 FUD 090 C 80
AMA: 2018,Jan,8; 2017,Dec,3; 2017,Jan,8; 2016,Jan,13; 2015,Jan,16

33534 **2 coronary arterial grafts**
63.6 63.6 FUD 090 C 80
AMA: 2018,Jan,8; 2017,Dec,3; 2017,Jan,8; 2016,Jan,13; 2015,Jan,16

33535 **3 coronary arterial grafts**
70.9 70.9 FUD 090 C 80
AMA: 2018,Jan,8; 2017,Dec,3; 2017,Jan,8; 2016,Jan,13; 2015,Jan,16

33536 **4 or more coronary arterial grafts**
76.1 76.1 **FUD** 090 C 80
AMA: 2018,Jan,8; 2017,Dec,3; 2017,Jan,8; 2016,Jan,13; 2015,Jan,16

33542-33548 Ventricular Reconstruction

EXCLUDES *Percutaneous ventricular assist devices ([33995], 33990-33993 [33997])*

33542 **Myocardial resection (eg, ventricular aneurysmectomy)**
Code also thrombus removal through separate heart incision, when performed (33310-33315); append modifier 59 to (33315)
76.1 76.1 **FUD** 090 C 80
AMA: 2018,Jan,8; 2017,Dec,3; 2017,Jan,8; 2016,Jan,13; 2015,Jan,16

33545 **Repair of postinfarction ventricular septal defect, with or without myocardial resection**
Code also thrombus removal through separate heart incision, when performed (33310-33315); append modifier 59 to (33315)
89.0 89.0 **FUD** 090 C 80
AMA: 2018,Jan,8; 2017,Dec,3; 2017,Jan,8; 2016,Jan,13; 2015,Jan,16

33548 **Surgical ventricular restoration procedure, includes prosthetic patch, when performed (eg, ventricular remodeling, SVR, SAVER, Dor procedures)**
EXCLUDES *Batista procedure or pachopexy (33999)*
Cardiotomy, exploratory (33310, 33315)
Temporary pacemaker (33210-33211)
Tube thoracostomy (32551)
85.8 85.8 **FUD** 090 C 80
AMA: 2018,Jan,8; 2017,Dec,3; 2017,Jan,8; 2016,Jan,13; 2015,Jan,16

33572 Endarterectomy with CABG (LAD, RCA, Cx)

Code first (33510-33516, 33533-33536)

\+ **33572** **Coronary endarterectomy, open, any method, of left anterior descending, circumflex, or right coronary artery performed in conjunction with coronary artery bypass graft procedure, each vessel (List separately in addition to primary procedure)**
6.67 6.67 **FUD** ZZZ C 80
AMA: 1997,Nov,1; 1994,Win,1

33600-33622 Repair Aberrant Heart Anatomy

33600 **Closure of atrioventricular valve (mitral or tricuspid) by suture or patch**
49.7 49.7 **FUD** 090 C 80
AMA: 2018,Jan,8; 2017,Dec,3; 2017,Jan,8; 2016,Jan,13; 2015,Jan,16

33602 **Closure of semilunar valve (aortic or pulmonary) by suture or patch**
Code also concurrent systemic-to-pulmonary artery shunt ligation/takedown (33924)
48.2 48.2 **FUD** 090 C 80
AMA: 2017,Dec,3

33606 **Anastomosis of pulmonary artery to aorta (Damus-Kaye-Stansel procedure)**
Code also concurrent systemic-to-pulmonary artery shunt ligation/takedown (33924)
51.4 51.4 **FUD** 090 C 80
AMA: 2017,Dec,3

33608 **Repair of complex cardiac anomaly other than pulmonary atresia with ventricular septal defect by construction or replacement of conduit from right or left ventricle to pulmonary artery**
EXCLUDES *Unifocalization arborization anomalies pulmonary artery (33925, 33926)*
Code also concurrent systemic-to-pulmonary artery shunt ligation/takedown (33924)
52.2 52.2 **FUD** 090 C 80
AMA: 2019,Apr,6; 2017,Dec,3

33610 **Repair of complex cardiac anomalies (eg, single ventricle with subaortic obstruction) by surgical enlargement of ventricular septal defect**
Code also concurrent systemic-to-pulmonary artery shunt ligation/takedown (33924)
51.5 51.5 **FUD** 090 63 C 80
AMA: 2017,Dec,3

33611 **Repair of double outlet right ventricle with intraventricular tunnel repair;**
Code also concurrent systemic-to-pulmonary artery shunt ligation/takedown (33924)
56.5 56.5 **FUD** 090 63 C 80
AMA: 2017,Dec,3

33612 **with repair of right ventricular outflow tract obstruction**
Code also concurrent systemic-to-pulmonary artery shunt ligation/takedown (33924)
58.2 58.2 **FUD** 090 C 80
AMA: 2017,Dec,3

33615 **Repair of complex cardiac anomalies (eg, tricuspid atresia) by closure of atrial septal defect and anastomosis of atria or vena cava to pulmonary artery (simple Fontan procedure)**
Code also concurrent systemic-to-pulmonary artery shunt ligation/takedown (33924)
58.0 58.0 **FUD** 090 C 80
AMA: 2017,Dec,3

33617 **Repair of complex cardiac anomalies (eg, single ventricle) by modified Fontan procedure**
Code also cavopulmonary anastomosis to second superior vena cava (33768)
Code also concurrent systemic-to-pulmonary artery shunt ligation/takedown (33924)
62.6 62.6 **FUD** 090 C 80
AMA: 2017,Dec,3

33619 **Repair of single ventricle with aortic outflow obstruction and aortic arch hypoplasia (hypoplastic left heart syndrome) (eg, Norwood procedure)**
79.2 79.2 **FUD** 090 63 C 80
AMA: 2018,Jan,8; 2017,Dec,3; 2017,Jan,8; 2016,Jul,3; 2016,Jan,13; 2015,Jan,16

33620 **Application of right and left pulmonary artery bands (eg, hybrid approach stage 1)**
EXCLUDES *Banding main pulmonary artery related to septal defect (33690)*
Code also transthoracic insertion catheter for stent placement with catheter removal and closure when performed during same session (33621)
47.7 47.7 **FUD** 090 C 80
AMA: 2018,Jan,8; 2017,Dec,3; 2017,Jan,8; 2016,Jul,3; 2016,Jan,13; 2015,Jan,16

33621 **Transthoracic insertion of catheter for stent placement with catheter removal and closure (eg, hybrid approach stage 1)**
Code also application right and left pulmonary artery bands when performed during same session (33620)
Code also stent placement (37236)
26.9 26.9 **FUD** 090 C 80
AMA: 2018,Jan,8; 2017,Dec,3; 2017,Jan,8; 2016,Jul,3; 2016,Jan,13; 2015,Jan,16

33622 **Reconstruction of complex cardiac anomaly (eg, single ventricle or hypoplastic left heart) with palliation of single ventricle with aortic outflow obstruction and aortic arch hypoplasia, creation of cavopulmonary anastomosis, and removal of right and left pulmonary bands (eg, hybrid approach stage 2, Norwood, bidirectional Glenn, pulmonary artery debanding)**

EXCLUDES *Excision coarctation aorta (33840, 33845, 33851)*
Repair hypoplastic or interrupted aortic arch (33853)
Repair patent ductus arteriosus (33822)
Repair pulmonary artery stenosis by reconstruction with patch or graft (33917)
Repair single ventricle with aortic outflow obstruction and aortic arch hypoplasia (33619)
Shunt; superior vena cava to pulmonary artery for flow to both lungs (33767)

Code also anastomosis, cavopulmonary, second superior vena cava for bilateral bidirectional Glenn procedure (33768)
Code also concurrent systemic-to-pulmonary artery shunt ligation/takedown (33924)
100. 100. FUD 090 C 80
AMA: 2018,Jan,8; 2017,Dec,3; 2017,Jan,8; 2016,Jul,3; 2016,Jan,13; 2015,Jan,16

33641-33645 Closure of Defect: Atrium

Code also thrombus removal through separate heart incision, when performed (33310-33315); append modifier 59 to (33315)

33641 **Repair atrial septal defect, secundum, with cardiopulmonary bypass, with or without patch**
47.3 47.3 FUD 090 C 80
AMA: 2018,Jan,8; 2017,Dec,3; 2017,Jan,8; 2016,Jan,13; 2015,Jan,16

33645 **Direct or patch closure, sinus venosus, with or without anomalous pulmonary venous drainage**

EXCLUDES *Repair isolated partial anomalous pulmonary venous return (33724)*
Repair pulmonary venous stenosis (33726)

50.2 50.2 FUD 090 C 80
AMA: 2017,Dec,3

33647 Closure of Septal Defect: Atrium AND Ventricle

EXCLUDES *Tricuspid atresia repair procedures (33615)*

Code also thrombus removal through separate heart incision, when performed (33310-33315); append modifier 59 to (33315)

33647 **Repair of atrial septal defect and ventricular septal defect, with direct or patch closure**
52.6 52.6 FUD 090 63 C 80
AMA: 2017,Dec,3

33660-33670 Closure of Defect: Atrioventricular Canal

33660 **Repair of incomplete or partial atrioventricular canal (ostium primum atrial septal defect), with or without atrioventricular valve repair**
50.8 50.8 FUD 090 C 80
AMA: 2017,Dec,3

33665 **Repair of intermediate or transitional atrioventricular canal, with or without atrioventricular valve repair**
55.6 55.6 FUD 090 C 80
AMA: 2017,Dec,3

33670 **Repair of complete atrioventricular canal, with or without prosthetic valve**
Code also thrombus removal through separate heart incision, when performed (33310-33315); append modifier 59 to (33315)
57.1 57.1 FUD 090 63 C 80
AMA: 2017,Dec,3

33675-33677 Closure of Multiple Septal Defects: Ventricle

EXCLUDES *Closure single ventricular septal defect (33681, 33684, 33688)*
Insertion or replacement temporary transvenous single chamber cardiac electrode or pacemaker catheter (33210)
Percutaneous closure (93581)
Thoracentesis (32554-32555)
Thoracotomy (32100)
Tube thoracostomy (32551)

33675 **Closure of multiple ventricular septal defects;**
57.1 57.1 FUD 090 C 80
AMA: 2018,Jan,8; 2017,Dec,3; 2017,Jan,8; 2016,Jan,13; 2015,Jan,16

33676 **with pulmonary valvotomy or infundibular resection (acyanotic)**
58.6 58.6 FUD 090 C 80
AMA: 2018,Jan,8; 2017,Dec,3; 2017,Jan,8; 2016,Jan,13; 2015,Jan,16

33677 **with removal of pulmonary artery band, with or without gusset**
60.9 60.9 FUD 090 C 80
AMA: 2018,Jan,8; 2017,Dec,3; 2017,Jan,8; 2016,Jan,13; 2015,Jan,16

33681-33688 Closure of Septal Defect: Ventricle

EXCLUDES *Repair pulmonary vein that requires creating an atrial septal defect (33724)*

33681 **Closure of single ventricular septal defect, with or without patch;**
Code also thrombus removal through separate heart incision, when performed (33310-33315); append modifier 59 to (33315)
53.2 53.2 FUD 090 C 80
AMA: 2018,Jan,8; 2017,Dec,3; 2017,Jan,8; 2016,Jan,13; 2015,Jan,16

33684 **with pulmonary valvotomy or infundibular resection (acyanotic)**
Code also concurrent systemic-to-pulmonary artery shunt ligation/takedown, if performed (33924)
54.7 54.7 FUD 090 C 80
AMA: 2017,Dec,3

33688 **with removal of pulmonary artery band, with or without gusset**
Code also concurrent systemic-to-pulmonary artery shunt ligation/takedown, if performed (33924)
54.8 54.8 FUD 090 C 80
AMA: 2017,Dec,3

33690 Reduce Pulmonary Overcirculation in Septal Defects

EXCLUDES *Left and right pulmonary artery banding in single ventricle (33620)*

33690 **Banding of pulmonary artery**
34.7 34.7 FUD 090 63 C 80
AMA: 2018,Jan,8; 2017,Jan,8; 2016,Jan,13; 2015,Jan,16

33692-33697 Repair of Defects of Tetralogy of Fallot

Code also concurrent systemic-to-pulmonary artery shunt ligation/takedown, when performed (33924)

33692 **Complete repair tetralogy of Fallot without pulmonary atresia;**
56.6 56.6 FUD 090 C 80
AMA: 2017,Dec,3

33694 **with transannular patch**
56.5 56.5 FUD 090 63 C 80
AMA: 2017,Dec,3

33697 **Complete repair tetralogy of Fallot with pulmonary atresia including construction of conduit from right ventricle to pulmonary artery and closure of ventricular septal defect**
59.5 59.5 FUD 090 C 80
AMA: 2018,Jan,8; 2017,Dec,3; 2017,Jan,8; 2016,Jan,13; 2015,Jan,16

33702-33722 Repair Anomalies Sinus of Valsalva

33702 Repair sinus of Valsalva fistula, with cardiopulmonary bypass;
44.2 44.2 FUD 090 C 80
AMA: 2018,Jan,8; 2017,Dec,3; 2017,Jan,8; 2016,Jan,13; 2015,Jan,16

33710 with repair of ventricular septal defect
59.4 59.4 FUD 090 C 80
AMA: 2017,Dec,3

33720 Repair sinus of Valsalva aneurysm, with cardiopulmonary bypass
44.7 44.7 FUD 090 C 80
AMA: 2017,Dec,3

33722 Closure of aortico-left ventricular tunnel
47.1 47.1 FUD 090 C 80
AMA: 2018,Jan,8; 2017,Dec,3; 2017,Jan,8; 2016,Jan,13; 2015,Jan,16

33724-33732 Repair Aberrant Pulmonary Venous Connection

33724 Repair of isolated partial anomalous pulmonary venous return (eg, Scimitar Syndrome)
EXCLUDES *Temporary pacemaker (33210-33211)*
Tube thoracostomy (32551)
44.2 44.2 FUD 090 C 80
AMA: 2018,Jan,8; 2017,Dec,3; 2017,Jan,8; 2016,Jan,13; 2015,Jan,16

33726 Repair of pulmonary venous stenosis
EXCLUDES *Temporary pacemaker (33210-33211)*
Tube thoracostomy (32551)
58.8 58.8 FUD 090 C 80
AMA: 2018,Jan,8; 2017,Dec,3; 2017,Jan,8; 2016,Jan,13; 2015,Jan,16

33730 Complete repair of anomalous pulmonary venous return (supracardiac, intracardiac, or infracardiac types)
EXCLUDES *Partial anomalous pulmonary venous return (33724)*
Repair pulmonary venous stenosis (33726)
58.0 58.0 FUD 090 63 C 80
AMA: 2018,Jan,8; 2017,Dec,3; 2017,Jan,8; 2016,Jan,13; 2015,Jan,16

33732 Repair of cor triatriatum or supravalvular mitral ring by resection of left atrial membrane
47.6 47.6 FUD 090 63 C 80
AMA: 2018,Jan,8; 2017,Dec,3; 2017,Jan,8; 2016,Jan,13; 2015,Jan,16

33735-33737 Creation of Atrial Septal Defect

Code also concurrent systemic-to-pulmonary artery shunt ligation/takedown, when performed (33924)

33735 Atrial septectomy or septostomy; closed heart (Blalock-Hanlon type operation)
37.4 37.4 FUD 090 63 C 80
AMA: 2018,Jan,8; 2017,Jan,8; 2016,Jan,13; 2015,Jan,16

33736 open heart with cardiopulmonary bypass
39.6 39.6 FUD 090 63 C 80
AMA: 2017,Dec,3

33737 open heart, with inflow occlusion
37.6 37.6 FUD 090 C 80
AMA: 2007,Mar,1-3; 1997,Nov,1

33741-33746 Transcatheter Procedures

● **33741 Transcatheter atrial septostomy (TAS) for congenital cardiac anomalies to create effective atrial flow, including all imaging guidance by the proceduralist, when performed, any method (eg, Rashkind, Sang-Park, balloon, cutting balloon, blade)**
INCLUDES Angiography to carry out procedure
Fluoroscopic and ultrasound guidance for access and intervention
Percutaneous access, access sheath placement, advancement transcatheter delivery system, creation effective intracardiac blood flow
EXCLUDES *Left heart catheterization via transseptal puncture (93462)*
Septostomy performed for noncongenital indications (93799)
Code also diagnostic congenital cardiac catheterization procedures when patient's condition (clinical indication) changed since intervention or prior study, no available prior catheter-based diagnostic study in treatment zone, or prior study not adequate, and append modifier 59 (93530-93533)
Code also diagnostic cardiac catheterization, when performed distinctly separate from shunt creation (93451-93453, 93456, 93458, 93460, 93530-93533)
Code also injection, diagnostic angiography, when performed separate from shunt creation and append modifier 59 (93563, 93565-93568)
0.00 0.00 FUD 000 63

● **33745 Transcatheter intracardiac shunt (TIS) creation by stent placement for congenital cardiac anomalies to establish effective intracardiac flow, including all imaging guidance by the proceduralist, when performed, left and right heart diagnostic cardiac catherization for congenital cardiac anomalies, and target zone angioplasty, when performed (eg, atrial septum, Fontan fenestration, right ventricular outflow tract, Mustard/Senning/Warden baffles); initial intracardiac shunt**
INCLUDES Angiography to carry out procedure
Balloon angioplasty(ies) and dilation(s) performed in target lesion
Fluoroscopic and ultrasound guidance for access and intervention
Intracardiac stent(s), including angioplasty before and after placement
Percutaneous access, access sheath placement, advancement transcatheter delivery system, creation effective intracardiac blood flow
EXCLUDES *Right heart catheterization for congenital cardiac anomalies (93530-93533)*
Code also diagnostic cardiac catheterization, when performed distinctly separate from shunt creation (93451-93453, 93456, 93458, 93460, 93530-93533)
Code also injection, diagnostic angiography, when performed separate from shunt creation and append modifier 59 (93563, 93565-93568)

● + **33746 each additional intracardiac shunt location (List separately in addition to code for primary procedure)**
INCLUDES Balloon angioplasty(ies) and dilation(s) performed in target lesion
Intracardiac stent(s), including angioplasty before and after placement
EXCLUDES *Right heart catheterization for congenital cardiac anomalies (93530-93533)*
Code also angioplasty performed in distinctly separate cardiac lesion
Code first (33745)
0.00 0.00 FUD 000

33750-33767 Systemic Vessel to Pulmonary Artery Shunts

Code also concurrent systemic-to-pulmonary artery shunt ligation/takedown, when performed (33924)

33750 Shunt; subclavian to pulmonary artery (Blalock-Taussig type operation)
36.5 36.5 FUD 090 63 C 80
AMA: 2017,Dec,3

33755 ascending aorta to pulmonary artery (Waterston type operation)
🚗 38.0 ⚕ 38.0 **FUD** 090   ⑥③ C 80 ▣
AMA: 2017,Dec,3

33762 descending aorta to pulmonary artery (Potts-Smith type operation)
🚗 37.1 ⚕ 37.1 **FUD** 090   ⑥③ C 80 ▣
AMA: 2017,Dec,3

33764 central, with prosthetic graft
🚗 38.0 ⚕ 38.0 **FUD** 090   C 80 ▣
AMA: 2017,Dec,3

33766 superior vena cava to pulmonary artery for flow to 1 lung (classical Glenn procedure)
🚗 38.6 ⚕ 38.6 **FUD** 090   C 80 ▣
AMA: 2017,Dec,3

33767 superior vena cava to pulmonary artery for flow to both lungs (bidirectional Glenn procedure)
🚗 41.1 ⚕ 41.1 **FUD** 090   C 80 ▣
AMA: 2018,Jan,8; 2017,Dec,3; 2017,Jan,8; 2016,Jul,3

33768 Cavopulmonary Anastomosis to Decrease Volume Load

EXCLUDES Temporary pacemaker (33210-33211)
Tube thoracostomy (32551)
Code first (33478, 33617, 33622, 33767)

+ **33768** Anastomosis, cavopulmonary, second superior vena cava (List separately in addition to primary procedure)
🚗 12.0 ⚕ 12.0 **FUD** ZZZ   C 80 ▣
AMA: 2018,Jan,8; 2017,Jan,8; 2016,Jul,3; 2016,Jan,13; 2015,Jan,16

33770-33783 Repair Aberrant Anatomy: Transposition Great Vessels

Code also concurrent systemic-to-pulmonary artery shunt ligation/takedown, when performed (33924)

33770 Repair of transposition of the great arteries with ventricular septal defect and subpulmonary stenosis; without surgical enlargement of ventricular septal defect
🚗 61.3 ⚕ 61.3 **FUD** 090   C 80 ▣
AMA: 2018,Jan,8; 2017,Dec,3; 2017,Jan,8; 2016,Jan,13; 2015,Jan,16

33771 with surgical enlargement of ventricular septal defect
🚗 63.1 ⚕ 63.1 **FUD** 090   C 80 ▣
AMA: 2017,Dec,3

33774 Repair of transposition of the great arteries, atrial baffle procedure (eg, Mustard or Senning type) with cardiopulmonary bypass;
🚗 52.0 ⚕ 52.0 **FUD** 090   C 80 ▣
AMA: 2017,Dec,3

33775 with removal of pulmonary band
🚗 53.6 ⚕ 53.6 **FUD** 090   C 80 ▣
AMA: 2017,Dec,3

33776 with closure of ventricular septal defect
🚗 56.7 ⚕ 56.7 **FUD** 090   C 80 ▣
AMA: 2017,Dec,3

33777 with repair of subpulmonic obstruction
🚗 54.9 ⚕ 54.9 **FUD** 090   C 80 ▣
AMA: 2017,Dec,3

33778 Repair of transposition of the great arteries, aortic pulmonary artery reconstruction (eg, Jatene type);
🚗 68.0 ⚕ 68.0 **FUD** 090   ⑥③ C 80 ▣
AMA: 2017,Dec,3

33779 with removal of pulmonary band
🚗 67.4 ⚕ 67.4 **FUD** 090   C 80 ▣
AMA: 2017,Dec,3

33780 with closure of ventricular septal defect
🚗 68.6 ⚕ 68.6 **FUD** 090   C 80 ▣
AMA: 2017,Dec,3

33781 with repair of subpulmonic obstruction
🚗 67.0 ⚕ 67.0 **FUD** 090   C 80 ▣
AMA: 2018,Jan,8; 2017,Dec,3; 2017,Jan,8; 2016,Jan,13; 2015,Jan,16

33782 Aortic root translocation with ventricular septal defect and pulmonary stenosis repair (ie, Nikaidoh procedure); without coronary ostium reimplantation
EXCLUDES Closure single ventricular septal defect (33681)
Repair complex cardiac anomaly other than pulmonary atresia (33608)
Repair pulmonary atresia with ventricular septal defect (33920)
Repair transposition great arteries (33770-33771, 33778, 33780)
Replacement, aortic valve (33412-33413)
🚗 93.6 ⚕ 93.6 **FUD** 090   C 80 ▣
AMA: 2017,Dec,3

33783 with reimplantation of 1 or both coronary ostia
🚗 101. ⚕ 101. **FUD** 090   C 80 ▣
AMA: 2017,Dec,3

33786-33788 Repair Aberrant Anatomy: Truncus Arteriosus

33786 Total repair, truncus arteriosus (Rastelli type operation)
Code also concurrent systemic-to-pulmonary artery shunt ligation/takedown, when performed (33924)
🚗 66.0 ⚕ 66.0 **FUD** 090   ⑥③ C 80 ▣
AMA: 2018,Jan,8; 2017,Dec,3; 2017,Jan,8; 2016,Jan,13; 2015,Jan,16

33788 Reimplantation of an anomalous pulmonary artery
EXCLUDES Pulmonary artery banding (33690)
🚗 44.3 ⚕ 44.3 **FUD** 090   C 80 ▣
AMA: 2018,Jan,8; 2017,Dec,3; 2017,Jan,8; 2016,Jan,13; 2015,Jan,16

33800-33853 Repair Aberrant Anatomy: Aorta

33800 Aortic suspension (aortopexy) for tracheal decompression (eg, for tracheomalacia) (separate procedure)
🚗 28.5 ⚕ 28.5 **FUD** 090   C 80 ▣
AMA: 2018,Jan,8; 2017,Jan,8; 2016,Jan,13; 2015,Jan,16

33802 Division of aberrant vessel (vascular ring);
🚗 31.3 ⚕ 31.3 **FUD** 090   C 80 ▣
AMA: 2017,Dec,3

33803 with reanastomosis
🚗 33.4 ⚕ 33.4 **FUD** 090   C 80 ▣
AMA: 2017,Dec,3

33813 Obliteration of aortopulmonary septal defect; without cardiopulmonary bypass
🚗 35.8 ⚕ 35.8 **FUD** 090   C 80 ▣
AMA: 2007,Mar,1-3; 1997,Nov,1

33814 with cardiopulmonary bypass
🚗 44.1 ⚕ 44.1 **FUD** 090   C 80 ▣
AMA: 2017,Dec,3

33820 Repair of patent ductus arteriosus; by ligation
EXCLUDES Percutaneous transcatheter closure patent ductus arteriosus (93582)
🚗 27.9 ⚕ 27.9 **FUD** 090   C 80 ▣
AMA: 2018,Jan,8; 2017,Dec,3; 2017,Jan,8; 2016,Jan,13; 2015,Jan,16

33822 by division, younger than 18 years   Ⓐ
EXCLUDES Percutaneous transcatheter closure patent ductus arteriosus (93582)
🚗 29.6 ⚕ 29.6 **FUD** 090   C 80 ▣
AMA: 2018,Jan,8; 2017,Dec,3; 2017,Jan,8; 2016,Jul,3; 2016,Jan,13; 2015,Jan,16

33824 by division, 18 years and older
EXCLUDES Percutaneous closure patent ductus arteriosus (93582)
🚗 34.2 ⚕ 34.2 **FUD** 090   C 80 ▣
AMA: 2017,Dec,3

● New Code   ▲ Revised Code   ○ Reinstated   ● New Web Release   ▲ Revised Web Release   + Add-on   Unlisted   Not Covered   # Resequenced
⑤⓪ Optum Mod 50 Exempt   Ⓢ AMA Mod 51 Exempt   ⑤① Optum Mod 51 Exempt   ⑥③ Mod 63 Exempt   ✗ Non-FDA Drug   ★ Telemedicine   Ⓜ Maternity   Ⓐ Age Edit

33840 **Excision of coarctation of aorta, with or without associated patent ductus arteriosus; with direct anastomosis**
35.8 35.8 FUD 090 C 80
AMA: 2018,Jan,8; 2017,Dec,3; 2017,Jan,8; 2016,Jul,3

33845 **with graft**
37.9 37.9 FUD 090 C 80
AMA: 2018,Jan,8; 2017,Dec,3; 2017,Jan,8; 2016,Jul,3

33851 **repair using either left subclavian artery or prosthetic material as gusset for enlargement**
36.8 36.8 FUD 090 C 80
AMA: 2018,Jan,8; 2017,Dec,3; 2017,Jan,8; 2016,Jul,3

33852 **Repair of hypoplastic or interrupted aortic arch using autogenous or prosthetic material; without cardiopulmonary bypass**
EXCLUDES *Hypoplastic left heart syndrome repair by excision coarctation of aorta (33619)*
40.5 40.5 FUD 090 C 80
AMA: 2007,Mar,1-3; 1997,Nov,1

33853 **with cardiopulmonary bypass**
EXCLUDES *Hypoplastic left heart syndrome repair by excision coarctation of aorta (33619)*
53.0 53.0 FUD 090 C 80
AMA: 2018,Jan,8; 2017,Dec,3; 2017,Jan,8; 2016,Jul,3; 2016,Jan,13; 2015,Jan,16

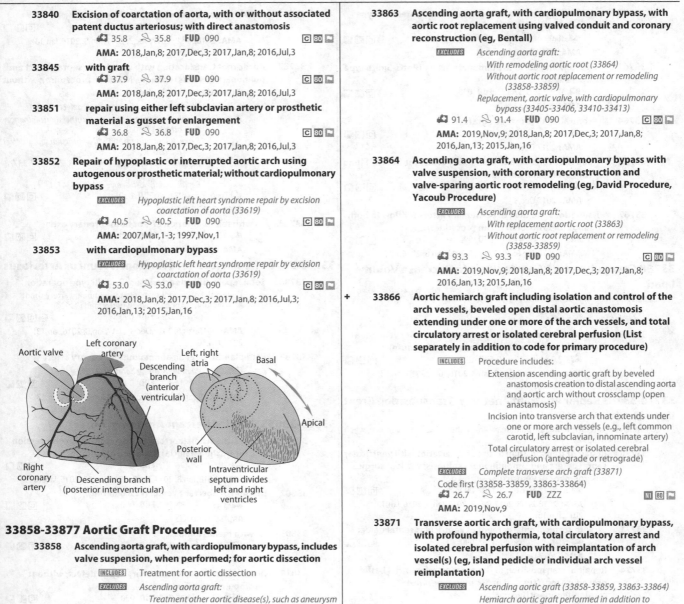

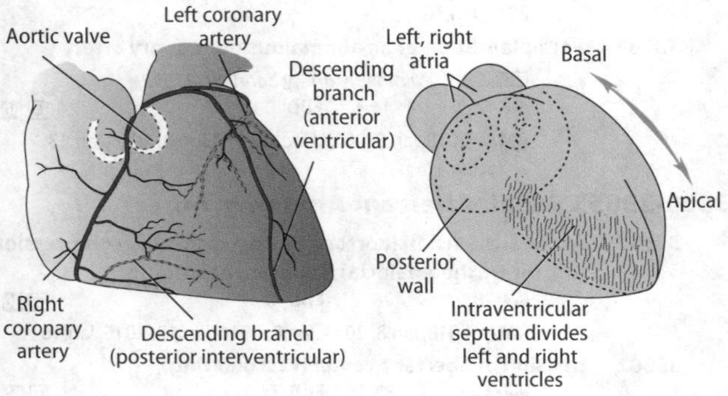

33858-33877 Aortic Graft Procedures

33858 **Ascending aorta graft, with cardiopulmonary bypass, includes valve suspension, when performed; for aortic dissection**
INCLUDES Treatment for aortic dissection
EXCLUDES *Ascending aorta graft:*
Treatment other aortic disease(s), such as aneurysm (33859)
With remodeling aortic root (33864)
With replacement aortic root (33863)
98.5 98.5 FUD 090 80

33859 **for aortic disease other than dissection (eg, aneurysm)**
INCLUDES Treatment of aortic disease(s) other than dissection, such as aneurysm
EXCLUDES *Ascending aorta graft:*
Treatment other aortic dissection (33858)
With remodeling aortic root (33864)
With replacement aortic root (33863)
70.7 70.7 FUD 090 80

33863 **Ascending aorta graft, with cardiopulmonary bypass, with aortic root replacement using valved conduit and coronary reconstruction (eg, Bentall)**
EXCLUDES *Ascending aorta graft:*
With remodeling aortic root (33864)
Without aortic root replacement or remodeling (33858-33859)
Replacement, aortic valve, with cardiopulmonary bypass (33405-33406, 33410-33413)
91.4 91.4 FUD 090 C 80
AMA: 2019,Nov,9; 2018,Jan,8; 2017,Dec,3; 2017,Jan,8; 2016,Jan,13; 2015,Jan,16

33864 **Ascending aorta graft, with cardiopulmonary bypass with valve suspension, with coronary reconstruction and valve-sparing aortic root remodeling (eg, David Procedure, Yacoub Procedure)**
EXCLUDES *Ascending aorta graft:*
With replacement aortic root (33863)
Without aortic root replacement or remodeling (33858-33859)
93.3 93.3 FUD 090 C 80
AMA: 2019,Nov,9; 2018,Jan,8; 2017,Dec,3; 2017,Jan,8; 2016,Jan,13; 2015,Jan,16

\+ **33866** **Aortic hemiarch graft including isolation and control of the arch vessels, beveled open distal aortic anastomosis extending under one or more of the arch vessels, and total circulatory arrest or isolated cerebral perfusion (List separately in addition to code for primary procedure)**
INCLUDES Procedure includes:
Extension ascending aortic graft by beveled anastomosis creation to distal ascending aorta and aortic arch without crossclamp (open anastamosis)
Incision into transverse arch that extends under one or more arch vessels (e.g., left common carotid, left subclavian, innominate artery)
Total circulatory arrest or isolated cerebral perfusion (antegrade or retrograde)
EXCLUDES *Complete transverse arch graft (33871)*
Code first (33858-33859, 33863-33864)
26.7 26.7 FUD ZZZ N1 80
AMA: 2019,Nov,9

33871 **Transverse aortic arch graft, with cardiopulmonary bypass, with profound hypothermia, total circulatory arrest and isolated cerebral perfusion with reimplantation of arch vessel(s) (eg, island pedicle or individual arch vessel reimplantation)**
EXCLUDES *Ascending aortic graft (33858-33859, 33863-33864)*
Hemiarch aortic graft performed in addition to ascending aorta graft (33866)
94.7 94.7 FUD 090 80

33875 **Descending thoracic aorta graft, with or without bypass**
79.5 79.5 FUD 090 C 80
AMA: 2017,Dec,3

26/TC PC/TC Only · A2-Z3 ASC Payment · 50 Bilateral · ♂ Male Only · ♀ Female Only · Facility RVU · Non-Facility RVU · CCI · CLIA
FUD Follow-up Days · CMS: IOM · AMA: CPT Asst · A-Y OPPSI · 80/80 Surg Assist Allowed / w/Doc · Lab Crosswalk · Radiology Crosswalk

33877 Repair of thoracoabdominal aortic aneurysm with graft, with or without cardiopulmonary bypass
105. 105. **FUD** 090 C 80
AMA: 2017,Dec,3

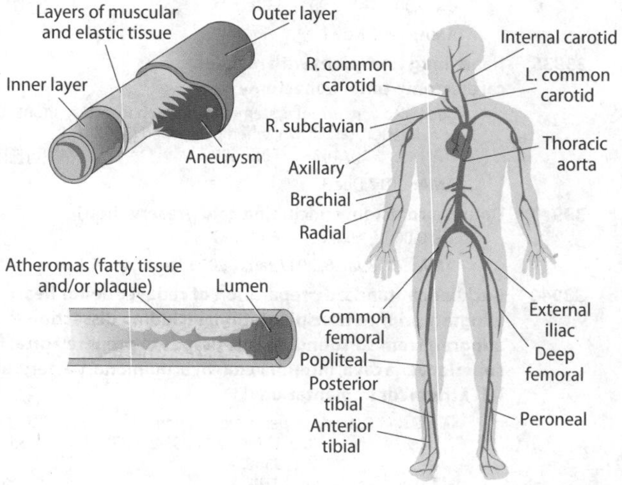

33880-33891 Endovascular Repair Aortic Aneurysm: Thoracic

INCLUDES Balloon angioplasty
Introduction, manipulation, placement, and device deployment
Stent deployment
EXCLUDES *Additional interventional procedures provided during endovascular repair*
Carotid-carotid bypass (33891)
Guidewire and catheter insertion (36140, 36200-36218)
Open exposure artery/subsequent closure ([34812], 34714-34716 [34820, 34833, 34834])
Subclavian to carotid artery transposition (33889)
Substantial artery repair/replacement (35226, 35286)

33880 Endovascular repair of descending thoracic aorta (eg, aneurysm, pseudoaneurysm, dissection, penetrating ulcer, intramural hematoma, or traumatic disruption); involving coverage of left subclavian artery origin, initial endoprosthesis plus descending thoracic aortic extension(s), if required, to level of celiac artery origin
INCLUDES Placement distal extensions in distal thoracic aorta
EXCLUDES *Proximal extensions*
(75956)
52.0 52.0 **FUD** 090 C 80
AMA: 2018,Jan,8; 2017,Dec,3; 2017,Jan,8; 2016,Jan,13; 2015,Jan,16

33881 not involving coverage of left subclavian artery origin, initial endoprosthesis plus descending thoracic aortic extension(s), if required, to level of celiac artery origin
INCLUDES Placement distal extensions in distal thoracic aorta
EXCLUDES *Procedure where extension placement includes coverage left subclavian artery origin (33880)*
Proximal extensions
(75957)
44.6 44.6 **FUD** 090 C 80
AMA: 2018,Jan,8; 2017,Dec,3; 2017,Jan,8; 2016,Jan,13; 2015,Jan,16

33883 Placement of proximal extension prosthesis for endovascular repair of descending thoracic aorta (eg, aneurysm, pseudoaneurysm, dissection, penetrating ulcer, intramural hematoma, or traumatic disruption); initial extension
EXCLUDES *Procedure where extension placement includes coverage left subclavian artery origin (33880)*
(75958)
32.3 32.3 **FUD** 090 C 80
AMA: 2018,Jan,8; 2017,Dec,3; 2017,Jan,8; 2016,Jan,13; 2015,Jan,16

\+ **33884 each additional proximal extension (List separately in addition to code for primary procedure)**
Code first (33883)
(75958)
11.5 11.5 **FUD** ZZZ C 80
AMA: 2018,Jan,8; 2017,Dec,3; 2017,Jan,8; 2016,Jan,13; 2015,Jan,16

33886 Placement of distal extension prosthesis(s) delayed after endovascular repair of descending thoracic aorta
INCLUDES All modules deployed
EXCLUDES *Endovascular repair descending thoracic aorta (33880, 33881)*
(75959)
27.7 27.7 **FUD** 090 C 80
AMA: 2018,Jan,8; 2017,Dec,3; 2017,Jan,8; 2016,Jan,13; 2015,Jan,16

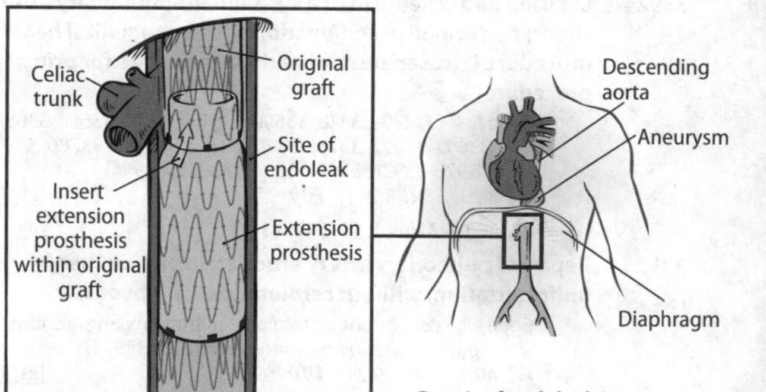

Repair of endoleak in descending thoracic aorta

33889 Open subclavian to carotid artery transposition performed in conjunction with endovascular repair of descending thoracic aorta, by neck incision, unilateral
EXCLUDES *Transposition and/or reimplantation; subclavian to carotid artery (35694)*
22.9 22.9 **FUD** 000 C 80 50
AMA: 2018,Jan,8; 2017,Jan,8; 2016,Jan,13; 2015,Jan,16

33891 Bypass graft, with other than vein, transcervical retropharyngeal carotid-carotid, performed in conjunction with endovascular repair of descending thoracic aorta, by neck incision
EXCLUDES *Bypass graft (35509, 35601)*
28.0 28.0 **FUD** 000 C 80 50
AMA: 2018,Jan,8; 2017,Jan,8; 2016,Jan,13; 2015,Jan,16

33910-33926 Surgical Procedures of Pulmonary Artery

33910 Pulmonary artery embolectomy; with cardiopulmonary bypass
77.1 77.1 **FUD** 090 C 80
AMA: 2018,Jan,8; 2017,Dec,3; 2017,Jan,8; 2016,Jan,13; 2015,Jan,16

33915 without cardiopulmonary bypass
39.8 39.8 **FUD** 090 C 80
AMA: 2018,Jan,8; 2017,Jan,8; 2016,Jan,13; 2015,Jan,16

33916 Pulmonary endarterectomy, with or without embolectomy, with cardiopulmonary bypass
123. 123. **FUD** 090 C 80
AMA: 2018,Jan,8; 2017,Dec,3; 2017,Jan,8; 2016,Jan,13; 2015,Jan,16

33917 Repair of pulmonary artery stenosis by reconstruction with patch or graft
Code also concurrent systemic-to-pulmonary artery shunt ligation/takedown, when performed (33924)
42.1 42.1 **FUD** 090 C 80
AMA: 2018,Jan,8; 2017,Dec,3; 2017,Jan,8; 2016,Jul,3; 2016,Jan,13; 2015,Jan,16

33920 **Repair of pulmonary atresia with ventricular septal defect, by construction or replacement of conduit from right or left ventricle to pulmonary artery**

EXCLUDES *Repair complicated cardiac anomalies by creating/replacing conduit from ventricle to pulmonary artery (33608)*

Code also concurrent systemic-to-pulmonary artery shunt ligation/takedown, when performed (33924)

52.4 52.4 FUD 090 C 80

AMA: 2019,Apr,6; 2018,Jan,8; 2017,Dec,3; 2017,Jan,8; 2016,Jan,13; 2015,Jan,16

33922 **Transection of pulmonary artery with cardiopulmonary bypass**

Code also concurrent systemic-to-pulmonary artery shunt ligation/takedown, when performed (33924)

40.1 40.1 FUD 090 63 C 80

AMA: 2017,Dec,3

+ **33924** **Ligation and takedown of a systemic-to-pulmonary artery shunt, performed in conjunction with a congenital heart procedure (List separately in addition to code for primary procedure)**

Code first (33470-33478, 33600-33617, 33622, 33684-33688, 33692-33697, 33735-33767, 33770-33783, 33786, 33917, 33920-33922, 33925-33926, 33935, 33945)

8.29 8.29 FUD ZZZ C 80

AMA: 1997,Nov,1; 1995,Win,1

33925 **Repair of pulmonary artery arborization anomalies by unifocalization; without cardiopulmonary bypass**

Code also concurrent systemic-to-pulmonary artery shunt ligation/takedown, when performed (33924)

49.7 49.7 FUD 090 C 80

33926 **with cardiopulmonary bypass**

Code also concurrent systemic-to-pulmonary artery shunt ligation/takedown, when performed (33924)

70.3 70.3 FUD 090 C 80

AMA: 2017,Dec,3

33927-33945 Heart and Heart-Lung Transplants

INCLUDES Backbench work to prepare donor heart and/or lungs for transplantation (33933, 33944)
Harvesting donor organs with cold preservation (33930, 33940)
Transplantation heart and/or lungs into recipient (33935, 33945)

33927 **Implantation of a total replacement heart system (artificial heart) with recipient cardiectomy**

EXCLUDES *Implantation ventricular assist device:*
Extracorporeal (33975-33976)
Intracorporeal (33979)
Percutaneous ([33995], 33990-33991)

74.2 74.2 FUD XXX C 80

AMA: 2018,Jun,3

33928 **Removal and replacement of total replacement heart system (artificial heart)**

EXCLUDES *Replacement or revision elements artificial heart (33999)*

0.00 0.00 FUD XXX C 80

AMA: 2018,Jun,3

+ **33929** **Removal of a total replacement heart system (artificial heart) for heart transplantation (List separately in addition to code for primary procedure)**

Code first (33945)

0.00 0.00 FUD ZZZ C 80

AMA: 2018,Jun,3

33930 **Donor cardiectomy-pneumonectomy (including cold preservation)**

0.00 0.00 FUD XXX C

AMA: 1997,Nov,1

33933 **Backbench standard preparation of cadaver donor heart/lung allograft prior to transplantation, including dissection of allograft from surrounding soft tissues to prepare aorta, superior vena cava, inferior vena cava, and trachea for implantation**

0.00 0.00 FUD XXX C 80

AMA: 1997,Nov,1

33935 **Heart-lung transplant with recipient cardiectomy-pneumonectomy**

Code also concurrent systemic-to-pulmonary artery shunt ligation/takedown, when performed (33924)

143. 143. FUD 090 C 80

AMA: 2017,Dec,3

33940 **Donor cardiectomy (including cold preservation)**

0.00 0.00 FUD XXX C

AMA: 2018,Jan,8; 2017,Jan,8; 2016,Jan,13; 2015,Jan,16

33944 **Backbench standard preparation of cadaver donor heart allograft prior to transplantation, including dissection of allograft from surrounding soft tissues to prepare aorta, superior vena cava, inferior vena cava, pulmonary artery, and left atrium for implantation**

EXCLUDES *Procedures performed on donor heart (33300, 33310, 33320, 33390, 33463-33464, 33510, 33641, 35216, 35276, 35685)*

0.00 0.00 FUD XXX C 80

AMA: 1997,Nov,1

33945 **Heart transplant, with or without recipient cardiectomy**

Code also concurrent systemic-to-pulmonary artery shunt ligation/takedown, when performed (33924)

141. 141. FUD 090 C 80

AMA: 2018,Jun,3; 2017,Dec,3

33946-33989 [33962, 33963, 33964, 33965, 33966, 33969, 33984, 33985, 33986, 33987, 33988, 33989] Extracorporeal Circulatory and Respiratory Support

INCLUDES Cannula repositioning and cannula insertion performed during same procedure
Multiple physician and nonphysician team collaboration
Veno-arterial ECMO/ECLS for heart and lung support
Veno-venous ECMO/ECLS for lung support

Code also extensive arterial repair/replacement (35266, 35286, 35371, 35665)

Code also overall daily management services needed to manage patient; report appropriate observation, hospital inpatient, or critical care E/M codes

33946 **Extracorporeal membrane oxygenation (ECMO)/extracorporeal life support (ECLS) provided by physician; initiation, veno-venous**

EXCLUDES *Daily ECMO/ECLS veno-venous management initial service date (33948)*
Repositioning ECMO/ECLS cannula initial service date (33957-33959 [33962, 33963, 33964])

Code also cannula insertion (33951-33956)

8.95 8.95 FUD XXX 63 C

AMA: 2018,Jan,8; 2017,Jan,8; 2016,Mar,5; 2016,Jan,13; 2015,Jul,3

33947 **initiation, veno-arterial**

EXCLUDES *Daily ECMO/ECLS veno-venous management initial service date (33948)*
Repositioning ECMO/ECLS cannula initial service date (33957-33959 [33962, 33963, 33964])

Code also cannula insertion (33951-33956)

9.97 9.97 FUD XXX 63 C

AMA: 2018,Jan,8; 2017,Jan,8; 2016,Mar,5; 2016,Jan,13; 2015,Jul,3

33948 **daily management, each day, veno-venous**

EXCLUDES *ECMO/ECLS initiation, veno-venous (33946)*

6.91 6.91 FUD XXX 63 C

AMA: 2018,Jan,8; 2017,Jan,8; 2016,Mar,5; 2016,Jan,13; 2015,Jul,3

33949 **daily management, each day, veno-arterial**

EXCLUDES *ECMO/ECLS initiation, veno-arterial (33947)*

6.73 6.73 FUD XXX 63 C

AMA: 2018,Jan,8; 2017,Jan,8; 2016,Mar,5; 2016,Jan,13; 2015,Jul,3

33951 **insertion of peripheral (arterial and/or venous) cannula(e), percutaneous, birth through 5 years of age (includes fluoroscopic guidance, when performed)** A

INCLUDES Cannula replacement same vessel
Cannula repositioning during same episode care

Code also cannula removal when new cannula inserted in different vessel with ([33965, 33966, 33969, 33984, 33985, 33986])

Code also ECMO/ECLS initiation or daily management (33946-33947, 33948-33949)

12.3 12.3 **FUD** 000 C 80

AMA: 2018,Jan,8; 2017,Jan,8; 2016,Mar,5; 2016,Jan,13; 2015,Jul,3

33952 **insertion of peripheral (arterial and/or venous) cannula(e), percutaneous, 6 years and older (includes fluoroscopic guidance, when performed)** A

INCLUDES Cannula replacement same vessel
Cannula repositioning during same episode care

Code also cannula removal when new cannula inserted in different vessel with ([33965, 33966, 33969, 33984, 33985, 33986])

Code also ECMO/ECLS initiation or daily management (33946-33947, 33948-33949)

12.4 12.4 **FUD** 000 C 80

AMA: 2018,Jan,8; 2017,Jan,8; 2016,Mar,5; 2016,Jan,13; 2015,Jul,3

33953 **insertion of peripheral (arterial and/or venous) cannula(e), open, birth through 5 years of age** A

INCLUDES Cannula replacement same vessel
Cannula repositioning during same episode care

EXCLUDES *Open artery exposure for delivery/deployment endovascular prosthesis ([34812], 34714-34716 [34820, 34833, 34834], [34820])*

Code also cannula removal when new cannula inserted in different vessel with ([33965, 33966, 33969, 33984, 33985, 33986])

Code also ECMO/ECLS initiation or daily management (33496-33947, 33948-33949)

13.8 13.8 **FUD** 000 C 80

AMA: 2018,Jan,8; 2017,Dec,3; 2017,Jan,8; 2016,Mar,5; 2016,Jan,13; 2015,Jul,3

33954 **insertion of peripheral (arterial and/or venous) cannula(e), open, 6 years and older** A

INCLUDES Cannula replacement same vessel
Cannula repositioning during same episode care

EXCLUDES *Open artery exposure for delivery/deployment endovascular prosthesis ([34812], 34714-34716 [34820, 34833, 34834])*

Code also cannula removal when new cannula inserted in different vessel with ([33965, 33966, 33969, 33984, 33985, 33986])

Code also ECMO/ECLS initiation or daily management (33946-33947, 33948-33949)

13.8 13.8 **FUD** 000 C 80

AMA: 2018,Jan,8; 2017,Dec,3; 2017,Jan,8; 2016,Mar,5; 2016,Jan,13; 2015,Jul,3

33955 **insertion of central cannula(e) by sternotomy or thoracotomy, birth through 5 years of age** A

INCLUDES Cannula replacement same vessel
Cannula repositioning during same episode care

EXCLUDES *Mediastinotomy (39010)*
Thoracotomy (32100)

Code also cannula removal when new cannula inserted in different vessel with ([33965, 33966, 33969, 33984, 33985, 33986])

Code also ECMO/ECLS initiation or daily management (33946-33947, 33948-33949)

24.0 24.0 **FUD** 000 C 80

AMA: 2018,Jan,8; 2017,Jan,8; 2016,Mar,5; 2016,Jan,13; 2015,Jul,3

33956 **insertion of central cannula(e) by sternotomy or thoracotomy, 6 years and older** A

INCLUDES Cannula replacement same vessel
Cannula repositioning during same episode care

EXCLUDES *Mediastinotomy (39010)*
Thoracotomy (32100)

Code also cannula removal when new cannula inserted in different vessel with ([33965, 33966, 33969, 33984, 33985, 33986])

Code also ECMO/ECLS initiation or daily management (33946-33947, 33948-33949)

24.2 24.2 **FUD** 000 C 80

AMA: 2018,Jan,8; 2017,Jan,8; 2016,Mar,5; 2016,Jan,13; 2015,Jul,3

33957 **reposition peripheral (arterial and/or venous) cannula(e), percutaneous, birth through 5 years of age (includes fluoroscopic guidance, when performed)** A

INCLUDES Fluoroscopic guidance

EXCLUDES *ECMO/ECLS initiation, veno-arterial (33947)*
ECMO/ECLS initiation, veno-venous (33946)
ECMO/ECLS insertion cannula (33951-33956)
Percutaneous access and closure femoral artery for endograft delivery (34713)

5.36 5.36 **FUD** 000 C 80

AMA: 2018,Jan,8; 2017,Jan,8; 2016,Mar,5; 2016,Jan,13; 2015,Jul,3

33958 **reposition peripheral (arterial and/or venous) cannula(e), percutaneous, 6 years and older (includes fluoroscopic guidance, when performed)** A

INCLUDES Fluoroscopic guidance

EXCLUDES *ECMO/ECLS initiation, veno-arterial (33947)*
ECMO/ECLS initiation, veno-venous (33946)
ECMO/ECLS insertion of cannula (33951-33956)
Percutaneous access and closure femoral artery for endograft delivery (34713)

5.36 5.36 **FUD** 000 C 80

AMA: 2018,Jan,8; 2017,Jan,8; 2016,Mar,5; 2016,Jan,13; 2015,Jul,3

33959 **reposition peripheral (arterial and/or venous) cannula(e), open, birth through 5 years of age (includes fluoroscopic guidance, when performed)** A

INCLUDES Fluoroscopic guidance

EXCLUDES *ECMO/ECLS initiation, veno-arterial (33947)*
ECMO/ECLS initiation, veno-venous (33946)
ECMO/ECLS insertion of cannula (33951-33956)
Open artery exposure for delivery/deployment endovascular prosthesis ([34812], 34714-34716 [34820, 34833, 34834])

6.84 6.84 **FUD** 000 C 80

AMA: 2018,Jan,8; 2017,Dec,3; 2017,Jan,8; 2016,Mar,5; 2016,Jan,13; 2015,Jul,3

33962 **reposition peripheral (arterial and/or venous) cannula(e), open, 6 years and older (includes fluoroscopic guidance, when performed)** A

INCLUDES Fluoroscopic guidance

EXCLUDES *ECMO/ECLS initiation, veno-arterial (33947)*
ECMO/ECLS initiation, veno-venous (33946)
ECMO/ECLS insertion of cannula (33951-33956)
Open artery exposure for delivery/deployment endovascular prosthesis ([34812], 34714-34716 [34820, 34833, 34834])

6.79 6.79 **FUD** 000 C 80

AMA: 2018,Jan,8; 2017,Dec,3; 2017,Jan,8; 2016,Mar,5; 2016,Jan,13; 2015,Jul,3

33963 **reposition of central cannula(e) by sternotomy or thoracotomy, birth through 5 years of age (includes fluoroscopic guidance, when performed)** A

INCLUDES Fluoroscopic guidance

EXCLUDES *ECMO/ECLS initiation, veno-arterial (33947)*
ECMO/ECLS initiation, veno-venous (33946)
ECMO/ECLS insertion of cannula (33951-33956)
Open artery exposure for delivery/deployment endovascular prosthesis ([34812], 34714-34716 [34820, 34833, 34834])

13.5 13.5 FUD 000 C 80

AMA: 2018,Jan,8; 2017,Jan,8; 2016,Mar,5; 2016,Jan,13; 2015,Jul,3

33964 **reposition central cannula(e) by sternotomy or thoracotomy, 6 years and older (includes fluoroscopic guidance, when performed)** A

INCLUDES Fluoroscopic guidance

EXCLUDES *ECMO/ECLS initiation, veno-arterial (33947)*
ECMO/ECLS initiation, veno-venous (33946)
ECMO/ECLS insertion cannula (33951-33956)
Mediastinotomy (39010)
Thoracotomy (32100)

14.3 14.3 FUD 000 C 80

AMA: 2018,Jan,8; 2017,Jan,8; 2016,Mar,5; 2016,Jan,13; 2015,Jul,3

33965 **removal of peripheral (arterial and/or venous) cannula(e), percutaneous, birth through 5 years of age** A

Code also extensive arterial repair/replacement, when performed (35266, 35286, 35371, 35665)

Code also new cannula insertion into different vessel (33951-33956)

5.36 5.36 FUD 000 C 80

AMA: 2018,Jan,8; 2017,Jan,8; 2016,Mar,5; 2016,Jan,13; 2015,Jul,3

33966 **removal of peripheral (arterial and/or venous) cannula(e), percutaneous, 6 years and older** A

Code also extensive arterial repair/replacement, when performed (35266, 35286, 35371, 35665)

Code also new cannula insertion into different vessel (33951, 33956)

6.87 6.87 FUD 000 C 80

AMA: 2018,Jan,8; 2017,Jan,8; 2016,Mar,5; 2016,Jan,13; 2015,Jul,3

33969 **removal of peripheral (arterial and/or venous) cannula(e), open, birth through 5 years of age** A

EXCLUDES *Open artery exposure for delivery/deployment endovascular prosthesis ([34812], 34714-34716 [34820, 34833, 34834])*
Repair blood vessel (35201, 35206, 35211, 35216, 35226)

Code also extensive arterial repair/replacement, when performed (35266, 35286, 35371, 35665)

Code also new cannula insertion into different vessel (33951-33956)

7.98 7.98 FUD 000 C 80

AMA: 2018,Jan,8; 2017,Dec,3; 2017,Jan,8; 2016,Mar,5; 2016,Jan,13; 2015,Jul,3

33984 **removal of peripheral (arterial and/or venous) cannula(e), open, 6 years and older** A

EXCLUDES *Open artery exposure for delivery/deployment endovascular prosthesis ([34812], 34714-34716 [34820, 34833, 34834])*
Repair blood vessel (35201, 35206, 35211, 35216, 35226)

8.25 8.25 FUD 000 C 80

AMA: 2018,Jan,8; 2017,Dec,3; 2017,Jan,8; 2016,Mar,5; 2016,Jan,13; 2015,Jul,3

33985 **removal of central cannula(e) by sternotomy or thoracotomy, birth through 5 years of age** A

EXCLUDES *Repair blood vessel (35201, 35206, 35211, 35216, 35226)*

Code also extensive arterial repair/replacement, when performed (35266, 35286, 35371, 35665)

Code also new cannula insertion into different vessel (33951-33956)

14.9 14.9 FUD 000 C 80

AMA: 2018,Jan,8; 2017,Jan,8; 2016,Mar,5; 2016,Jan,13; 2015,Jul,3

33986 **removal of central cannula(e) by sternotomy or thoracotomy, 6 years and older** A

EXCLUDES *Repair blood vessel (35201, 35206, 35211, 35216, 35226)*

Code also extensive arterial repair/replacement, when performed (35266, 35286, 35371, 35665)

Code also new cannula insertion into different vessel (33951-33956)

15.1 15.1 FUD 000 C 80

AMA: 2018,Jan,8; 2017,Jan,8; 2016,Mar,5; 2016,Jan,13; 2015,Jul,3

+ # 33987 **Arterial exposure with creation of graft conduit (eg, chimney graft) to facilitate arterial perfusion for ECMO/ECLS (List separately in addition to code for primary procedure)**

EXCLUDES *Open artery exposure for delivery/deployment endovascular prosthesis ([34812], 34714-34716 [34820, 34833, 34834])*

Code first (33953-33956)

6.09 6.09 FUD ZZZ C 80

AMA: 2018,Jan,8; 2017,Dec,3; 2017,Jan,8; 2016,Mar,5; 2016,Jan,13; 2015,Jul,3

33988 **Insertion of left heart vent by thoracic incision (eg, sternotomy, thoracotomy) for ECMO/ECLS**

22.5 22.5 FUD 000 C 80

AMA: 2018,Jan,8; 2017,Jan,8; 2016,Mar,5; 2016,Jan,13; 2015,Jul,3

33989 **Removal of left heart vent by thoracic incision (eg, sternotomy, thoracotomy) for ECMO/ECLS**

14.3 14.3 FUD 000 C 80

AMA: 2018,Jan,8; 2017,Jan,8; 2016,Mar,5; 2016,Jan,13; 2015,Jul,3

33962-33999 [33962, 33963, 33964, 33965, 33966, 33969, 33984, 33985, 33986, 33987, 33988, 33989, 33995, 33997] Mechanical Circulatory Support

33962 **Resequenced code. See code following 33959.**

33963 **Resequenced code. See code following 33959.**

33964 **Resequenced code. See code following 33959.**

33965 **Resequenced code. See code following 33959.**

33966 **Resequenced code. See code following 33959.**

33967 **Insertion of intra-aortic balloon assist device, percutaneous**

7.51 7.51 FUD 000 C 80

AMA: 2018,Jan,8; 2017,Jan,8; 2016,Mar,5; 2016,Jan,13; 2015,Sep,3; 2015,Jul,3; 2015,Jan,16

33968 **Removal of intra-aortic balloon assist device, percutaneous**

EXCLUDES *Removal implantable aortic counterpulsation ventricular assist system (0455T-0458T)*

0.98 0.98 FUD 000 C

AMA: 2018,Jan,8; 2017,Jan,8; 2016,Mar,5; 2016,Jan,13; 2015,Jul,3; 2015,Jan,16

33969 **Resequenced code. See code following 33959.**

33970 **Insertion of intra-aortic balloon assist device through the femoral artery, open approach**

EXCLUDES *Insertion/replacement implantable aortic counterpulsation ventricular assist system (0451T-0454T)*
Percutaneous insertion intra-aortic balloon assist device (33967)

10.2 10.2 FUD 000 C 80

AMA: 2018,Jan,8; 2017,Jan,8; 2016,Mar,5; 2016,Jan,13; 2015,Sep,3; 2015,Jul,3; 2015,Jan,16

33971 **Removal of intra-aortic balloon assist device including repair of femoral artery, with or without graft**

EXCLUDES *Removal implantable aortic counterpulsation ventricular assist system (0455T-0458T)*

20.3 20.3 FUD 090 C

AMA: 2018,Jan,8; 2017,Jan,8; 2016,Mar,5; 2016,Jan,13; 2015,Jul,3; 2015,Jan,16

33973 Insertion of intra-aortic balloon assist device through the ascending aorta

EXCLUDES *Insertion/replacement implantable aortic counterpulsation ventricular assist system (0451T-0454T)*

14.8 | 14.8 | FUD 000 | C 80

AMA: 2018,Jan,8; 2017,Jan,8; 2016,Mar,5; 2016,Jan,13; 2015,Sep,3; 2015,Jul,3; 2015,Jan,16

33974 Removal of intra-aortic balloon assist device from the ascending aorta, including repair of the ascending aorta, with or without graft

EXCLUDES *Removal implantable aortic counterpulsation ventricular assist system (0455T-0458T)*

25.7 | 25.7 | FUD 090 | C

AMA: 2018,Jan,8; 2017,Jan,8; 2016,Mar,5; 2016,Jan,13; 2015,Jul,3; 2015,Jan,16

33975 Insertion of ventricular assist device; extracorporeal, single ventricle

INCLUDES Insertion new pump with de-airing, connection, and initiation
Removal old pump with replacement entire ventricular assist device system, including pump(s) and cannulas
Transthoracic approach

EXCLUDES *Percutaneous approach ([33995], 33990-33991)*

Code also removal thrombus through separate heart incision, when performed (33310-33315); append modifier 59 to (33315)

37.8 | 37.8 | FUD XXX | C 80

AMA: 2018,Jun,3; 2018,Jan,8; 2017,Dec,3; 2017,Jan,8; 2016,Mar,5; 2016,Jan,13; 2015,Jul,3; 2015,Jan,16

33976 extracorporeal, biventricular

INCLUDES Insertion new pump with de-airing, connection, and initiation
Removal with replacement entire ventricular assist device system, including pump(s) and cannulas
Transthoracic approach

EXCLUDES *Percutaneous approach ([33995], 33990-33991)*

Code also removal thrombus through separate heart incision, when performed (33310-33315); append modifier 59 to (33315)

46.0 | 46.0 | FUD XXX | C 80

AMA: 2018,Jun,3; 2018,Jan,8; 2017,Dec,3; 2017,Jan,8; 2016,Mar,5; 2016,Jan,13; 2015,Jul,3; 2015,Jan,16

33977 Removal of ventricular assist device; extracorporeal, single ventricle

INCLUDES Removal entire device and cannulas

EXCLUDES *Removal ventricular assist device when performed same time as new device insertion*

Code also thrombus removal through separate heart incision, when performed (33310-33315); append modifier 59 to (33315)

32.6 | 32.6 | FUD XXX | C 80

AMA: 2018,Jan,8; 2017,Dec,3; 2017,Jan,8; 2016,Mar,5; 2016,Jan,13; 2015,Jul,3; 2015,Jan,16

33978 extracorporeal, biventricular

INCLUDES Removal entire device and cannulas

EXCLUDES *Removal ventricular assist device when performed same time as new device insertion*

Code also thrombus removal through separate heart incision, when performed (33310-33315); append modifier 59 to (33315)

38.5 | 38.5 | FUD XXX | C 80

AMA: 2018,Jan,8; 2017,Dec,3; 2017,Jan,8; 2016,Mar,5; 2016,Jan,13; 2015,Jul,3; 2015,Jan,16

33979 Insertion of ventricular assist device, implantable intracorporeal, single ventricle

INCLUDES New pump insertion with connection, de-airing, and initiation
Removal with replacement entire ventricular assist device system, including pump(s) and cannulas
Transthoracic approach

EXCLUDES *Insertion/replacement implantable aortic counterpulsation ventricular assist system (0451T-0454T)*
Percutaneous approach ([33995], 33990-33991)

Code also thrombus removal through separate heart incision, when performed (33310-33315); append modifier 59 to (33315)

56.5 | 56.5 | FUD XXX | C 80

AMA: 2018,Jun,3; 2018,Jan,8; 2017,Dec,3; 2017,Jan,8; 2016,Mar,5; 2016,Jan,13; 2015,Jul,3; 2015,Jan,16

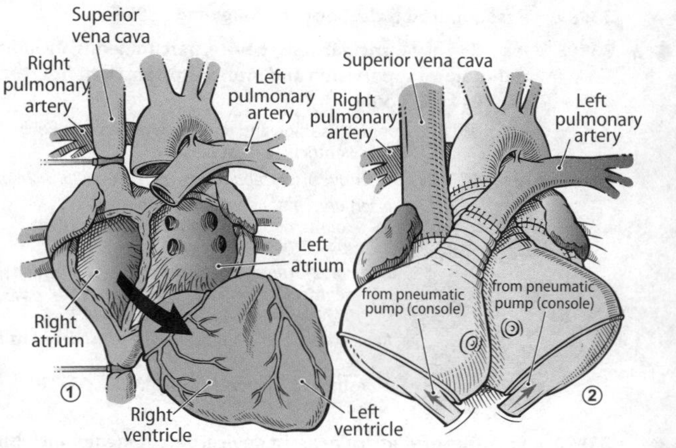

33980 Removal of ventricular assist device, implantable intracorporeal, single ventricle

INCLUDES Removal entire device and cannulas

EXCLUDES *Removal implantable aortic counterpulsation ventricular assist system (0455T-0458T)*
Removal ventricular assist device when performed same time as new device insertion

Code also thrombus removal through separate heart incision, when performed (33310-33315); append modifier 59 to (33315)

51.5 | 51.5 | FUD XXX | C 80

AMA: 2018,Jan,8; 2017,Dec,3; 2017,Jan,8; 2016,Mar,5; 2016,Jan,13; 2015,Jul,3; 2015,Jan,16

33981 Replacement of extracorporeal ventricular assist device, single or biventricular, pump(s), single or each pump

INCLUDES New pump insertion with de-airing, connection, and initiation
Removal old pump

24.3 | 24.3 | FUD XXX | C 80

AMA: 2018,Jan,8; 2017,Jan,8; 2016,Mar,5; 2016,Jan,13; 2015,Jul,3; 2015,Jan,16

33982 Replacement of ventricular assist device pump(s); implantable intracorporeal, single ventricle, without cardiopulmonary bypass

INCLUDES New pump insertion with connection, de-airing, and initiation
Removal old pump

57.1 | 57.1 | FUD XXX | C 80

AMA: 2018,Jan,8; 2017,Jan,8; 2016,Mar,5; 2016,Jan,13; 2015,Jul,3; 2015,Jan,16

33983 **implantable intracorporeal, single ventricle, with cardiopulmonary bypass**

INCLUDES Removal old pump

EXCLUDES *Insertion/replacement implantable aortic counterpulsation ventricular assist system (0451T-0454T)*

Percutaneous transseptal approach (33999)

67.0 67.0 FUD XXX C 80

AMA: 2018,Jan,8; 2017,Dec,3; 2017,Jan,8; 2016,Mar,5; 2016,Jan,13; 2015,Jul,3; 2015,Jan,16

33984 **Resequenced code. See code following 33959.**

33985 **Resequenced code. See code following 33959.**

33986 **Resequenced code. See code following 33959.**

33987 **Resequenced code. See code following 33959.**

33988 **Resequenced code. See code following 33959.**

33989 **Resequenced code. See code following 33959.**

● # **33995** **Insertion of ventricular assist device, percutaneous, including radiological supervision and interpretation; right heart, venous access only**

INCLUDES Initial insertion and replacement percutaneous ventricular assist device

EXCLUDES *Extensive artery repair/replacement (35226, 35286)*

Insertion/replacement implantable aortic counterpulsation ventricular assist system (0451T-0454T)

Open arterial approach to aid insertion percutaneous ventricular assist device, when used ([34812], 34714-34716 [34820, 34833, 34834])

Removal percutaneous ventricular assist device with entire system replacement (33992)

Transthoracic approach (33975-33976, 33979)

0.00 0.00 FUD 000

▲ **33990** **Insertion of ventricular assist device, percutaneous, including radiological supervision and interpretation; left heart, arterial access only**

INCLUDES Initial insertion and replacement percutaneous ventricular assist device

EXCLUDES *Extensive artery repair/replacement (35226, 35286)*

Insertion/replacement implantable aortic counterpulsation ventricular assist system (0451T-0454T)

Open arterial approach to aid insertion percutaneous ventricular assist device, when used ([34812], 34714-34716 [34820, 34833, 34834])

Removal percutaneous ventricular assist device with entire system replacement (33992)

Transthoracic approach (33975-33976, 33979)

12.4 12.4 FUD XXX C 80

AMA: 2018,Jun,3; 2018,Jan,8; 2017,Dec,3; 2017,Jan,8; 2016,Mar,5; 2016,Jan,13; 2015,Sep,3; 2015,Jan,16

▲ **33991** **left heart, both arterial and venous access, with transseptal puncture**

INCLUDES Initial insertion and replacement percutaneous ventricular assist device

EXCLUDES *Extensive artery repair/replacement (35226, 35286)*

Insertion/replacement implantable aortic counterpulsation ventricular assist system (0451T-0454T)

Open arterial approach to aid with insertion percutaneous ventricular assist device, when performed ([34812], 34714-34716 [34820, 34833, 34834])

Removal percutaneous ventricular assist device with entire system replacement (33992)

Transthoracic approach (33975-33976, 33979)

18.1 18.1 FUD XXX C 80

AMA: 2018,Jun,3; 2018,Jan,8; 2017,Dec,3; 2017,Jan,8; 2016,Mar,5; 2016,Jan,13; 2015,Sep,3; 2015,Jan,16

▲ **33992** **Removal of percutaneous left heart ventricular assist device, arterial or arterial and venous cannula(s), at separate and distinct session from insertion**

INCLUDES Removal device and cannulas

EXCLUDES *Removal implantable aortic counterpulsation ventricular assist system (0455T-0458T)*

Code also modifier 59 when percutaneous ventricular assist device removed on same day as insertion, but different session

5.80 5.80 FUD XXX C 80

AMA: 2018,Jan,8; 2017,Jan,8; 2016,Mar,5; 2016,Jan,13; 2015,Sep,3; 2015,Jan,16

● # **33997** **Removal of percutaneous right heart ventricular assist device, venous cannula, at separate and distinct session from insertion**

EXCLUDES *Removal ventricular assist device, open approach, report appropriate vessel repair code(s)*

0.00 0.00 FUD 000

▲ **33993** **Repositioning of percutaneous right or left heart ventricular assist device with imaging guidance at separate and distinct session from insertion**

EXCLUDES *Repositioning percutaneous ventricular assist device without image guidance*

Repositioning device/electrode (0460T-0461T)

Repositioning percutaneous ventricular assist device same session as insertion (33990-33991)

Skin pocket relocation with replacement implantable aortic counterpulsation ventricular assist device and electrodes (0459T)

Code also modifier 59 when percutaneous ventricular assist device repositioned using imaging guidance on same day as insertion, but different session

5.09 5.09 FUD XXX C 80

AMA: 2018,Jan,8; 2017,Jan,8; 2016,Mar,5; 2016,Jan,13; 2015,Sep,3; 2015,Jan,16

33995 **Resequenced code. See code following 33983.**

33997 **Resequenced code. See code following 33992.**

33999 **Unlisted procedure, cardiac surgery**

0.00 0.00 FUD YYY T 80

AMA: 2019,Apr,10; 2019,Jan,14; 2018,Jun,3; 2018,Jan,8; 2017,Jan,8; 2016,May,5; 2016,Jan,13; 2015,Jan,16

34001-34530 Surgical Revascularization: Veins and Arteries

INCLUDES Repair blood vessel

Surgeon's component operative arteriogram

34001 **Embolectomy or thrombectomy, with or without catheter; carotid, subclavian or innominate artery, by neck incision**

27.8 27.8 FUD 090 C 80 50

AMA: 1997,Nov,1

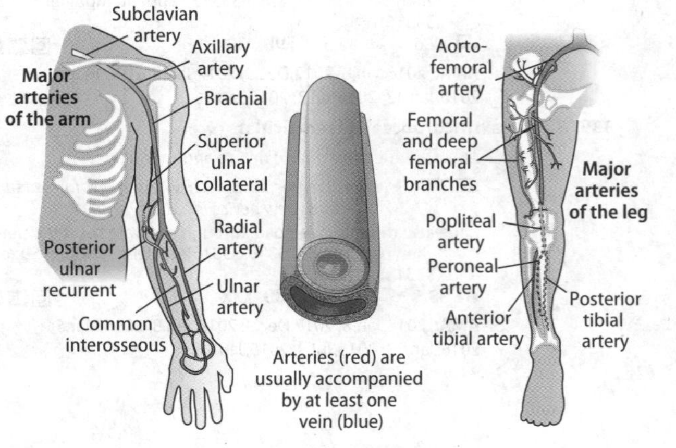

34051 **innominate, subclavian artery, by thoracic incision**

28.6 28.6 FUD 090 C 80 50

AMA: 1997,Nov,1

34101 **axillary, brachial, innominate, subclavian artery, by arm incision**
17.3 17.3 FUD 090 T 80 50
AMA: 1997,Nov,1

34111 **radial or ulnar artery, by arm incision**
17.3 17.3 FUD 090 T 80 50
AMA: 1997,Nov,1

34151 **renal, celiac, mesentery, aortoiliac artery, by abdominal incision**
40.4 40.4 FUD 090 C 80 50
AMA: 1997,Nov,1

34201 **femoropopliteal, aortoiliac artery, by leg incision**
29.8 29.8 FUD 090 T 80 50
AMA: 2018,Jan,8; 2017,Jan,8; 2016,Jan,13; 2015,Jan,16

34203 **popliteal-tibio-peroneal artery, by leg incision**
27.6 27.6 FUD 090 T 80 50
AMA: 1997,Nov,1

34401 **Thrombectomy, direct or with catheter; vena cava, iliac vein, by abdominal incision**
42.4 42.4 FUD 090 C 80 50
AMA: 1997,Nov,1

34421 **vena cava, iliac, femoropopliteal vein, by leg incision**
21.5 21.5 FUD 090 T 80 50
AMA: 2018,Jan,8; 2017,Jan,8; 2016,Jan,13; 2015,Jan,16

34451 **vena cava, iliac, femoropopliteal vein, by abdominal and leg incision**
41.7 41.7 FUD 090 C 80 50
AMA: 1997,Nov,1

34471 **subclavian vein, by neck incision**
31.1 31.1 FUD 090 T 50
AMA: 1997,Nov,1

34490 **axillary and subclavian vein, by arm incision**
18.5 18.5 FUD 090 T 62 50
AMA: 1997,Nov,1

34501 **Valvuloplasty, femoral vein**
25.8 25.8 FUD 090 T 80 50
AMA: 1997,Nov,1

34502 **Reconstruction of vena cava, any method**
44.7 44.7 FUD 090 C 80
AMA: 1997,Nov,1

34510 **Venous valve transposition, any vein donor**
29.6 29.6 FUD 090 T 80 50
AMA: 1997,Nov,1

34520 **Cross-over vein graft to venous system**
28.7 28.7 FUD 090 T 80 50
AMA: 1997,Nov,1

34530 **Saphenopopliteal vein anastomosis**
27.2 27.2 FUD 090 T 80 50
AMA: 1997,Nov,1

34701-34713 [34717, 34718] Abdominal Aorta and Iliac Artery Repairs

INCLUDES Closure artery after endograft delivery using sheath size less than 12 French
Treatment with covered stent for:
- Aneurysm
- Aortic dissection
- Arteriovenous malformation
- Pseudoaneurysm
- Trauma

Treatment zones (vessel(s) in which endograft deployed):
- Iliac artery(ies) (34707-34708, [34717], [34718])
- Infrarenal aorta (34701-34702)
- Infrarenal aorta and both common iliac arteries (34705-34706)
- Infrarenal aorta and ipsilateral common iliac artery (34703-34704)

EXCLUDES *Treatment atherosclerotic occlusive disease with covered stent:*
- *Aorta (37236-37237)*
- *Iliac artery(ies) (37221, 37223)*

Code also open arterial exposure, when appropriate ([34812], 34714 [34820, 34833, 34834], 34715-34716)
Code also percutaneous closure artery when endograft delivered through sheath 12 French or larger (34713)
Code also selective catheterization arteries outside target treatment zone

34701 **Endovascular repair of infrarenal aorta by deployment of an aorto-aortic tube endograft including pre-procedure sizing and device selection, all nonselective catheterization(s), all associated radiological supervision and interpretation, all endograft extension(s) placed in the aorta from the level of the renal arteries to the aortic bifurcation, and all angioplasty/stenting performed from the level of the renal arteries to the aortic bifurcation; for other than rupture (eg, for aneurysm, pseudoaneurysm, dissection, penetrating ulcer)**
INCLUDES Nonselective catheterization
Code also intravascular ultrasound when performed (37252-37253)
36.1 36.1 FUD 090 C 80
AMA: 2019,Nov,6; 2018,Jan,8; 2017,Dec,3

34702 **for rupture including temporary aortic and/or iliac balloon occlusion, when performed (eg, for aneurysm, pseudoaneurysm, dissection, penetrating ulcer, traumatic disruption)**
INCLUDES Nonselective catheterization
Code also decompressive laparotomy for treatment abdominal compartment syndrome (49000)
Code also intravascular ultrasound when performed (37252-37253)
53.9 53.9 FUD 090 C 80
AMA: 2019,Nov,6; 2018,Jan,8; 2017,Dec,3

34703 **Endovascular repair of infrarenal aorta and/or iliac artery(ies) by deployment of an aorto-uni-iliac endograft including pre-procedure sizing and device selection, all nonselective catheterization(s), all associated radiological supervision and interpretation, all endograft extension(s) placed in the aorta from the level of the renal arteries to the iliac bifurcation, and all angioplasty/stenting performed from the level of the renal arteries to the iliac bifurcation; for other than rupture (eg, for aneurysm, pseudoaneurysm, dissection, penetrating ulcer)**
INCLUDES Endograft extensions ending in common iliac arteries
Nonselective catheterization
Code also intravascular ultrasound when performed (37252-37253)
39.8 39.8 FUD 090 C 80
AMA: 2019,Nov,6; 2018,Jan,8; 2017,Dec,3

Cardiovascular, Hemic, and Lymphatic — 34101 — 34703

34704 for rupture including temporary aortic and/or iliac balloon occlusion, when performed (eg, for aneurysm, pseudoaneurysm, dissection, penetrating ulcer, traumatic disruption)

INCLUDES Endograft extensions ending in common iliac arteries
Nonselective catheterization

Code also decompressive laparotomy for treatment abdominal compartment syndrome (49000)

Code also intravascular ultrasound when performed (37252-37253)

66.4 66.4 FUD 090 C 80

AMA: 2019,Nov,6; 2018,Jan,8; 2017,Dec,3

34705 Endovascular repair of infrarenal aorta and/or iliac artery(ies) by deployment of an aorto-bi-iliac endograft including pre-procedure sizing and device selection, all nonselective catheterization(s), all associated radiological supervision and interpretation, all endograft extension(s) placed in the aorta from the level of the renal arteries to the iliac bifurcation, and all angioplasty/stenting performed from the level of the renal arteries to the iliac bifurcation; for other than rupture (eg, for aneurysm, pseudoaneurysm, dissection, penetrating ulcer)

INCLUDES Endograft extensions ending in common iliac arteries
Nonselective catheterization

Code also intravascular ultrasound when performed (37252-37253)

44.5 44.5 FUD 090 C 80

AMA: 2019,Nov,6; 2018,Jan,8; 2017,Dec,3

34706 for rupture including temporary aortic and/or iliac balloon occlusion, when performed (eg, for aneurysm, pseudoaneurysm, dissection, penetrating ulcer, traumatic disruption)

INCLUDES Endograft extensions ending in common iliac arteries
Nonselective catheterization

Code also decompressive laparotomy for treatment abdominal compartment syndrome (49000)

Code also intravascular ultrasound when performed (37252-37253)

67.1 67.1 FUD 090 C 80

AMA: 2019,Nov,6; 2018,Jan,8; 2017,Dec,3

34707 Endovascular repair of iliac artery by deployment of an ilio-iliac tube endograft including pre-procedure sizing and device selection, all nonselective catheterization(s), all associated radiological supervision and interpretation, and all endograft extension(s) proximally to the aortic bifurcation and distally to the iliac bifurcation, and treatment zone angioplasty/stenting, when performed, unilateral; for other than rupture (eg, for aneurysm, pseudoaneurysm, dissection, arteriovenous malformation)

INCLUDES Endograft extensions ending in common iliac arteries
Nonselective catheterization

EXCLUDES *Deployment iliac branched endograft:*
At same time as aorto-iliac graft placement ([34717])
Delayed/separate from aorto-iliac endograft deployment ([34718])

Code also intravascular ultrasound when performed (37252-37253)

33.7 33.7 FUD 090 C 80 50

AMA: 2019,Nov,6; 2018,Jan,8; 2017,Dec,3

34708 for rupture including temporary aortic and/or iliac balloon occlusion, when performed (eg, for aneurysm, pseudoaneurysm, dissection, arteriovenous malformation, traumatic disruption)

INCLUDES Endograft extensions ending in common iliac arteries
Nonselective catheterization

EXCLUDES *Deployment iliac branched endograft:*
At same time as aorto-iliac graft placement ([34717])
Delayed/separate from aorto-iliac endograft deployment ([34718])

Code also decompressive laparotomy for treatment abdominal compartment syndrome (49000)

Code also intravascular ultrasound when performed (37252-37253)

53.8 53.8 FUD 090 C 80 50

AMA: 2019,Nov,6; 2018,Jan,8; 2017,Dec,3

+ # 34717 Endovascular repair of iliac artery at the time of aorto-iliac artery endograft placement by deployment of an iliac branched endograft including pre-procedure sizing and device selection, all ipsilateral selective iliac artery catheterization(s), all associated radiological supervision and interpretation, and all endograft extension(s) proximally to the aortic bifurcation and distally in the internal iliac, external iliac, and common femoral artery(ies), and treatment zone angioplasty/stenting, when performed, for rupture or other than rupture (eg, for aneurysm, pseudoaneurysm, dissection, arteriovenous malformation, penetrating ulcer, traumatic disruption), unilateral (List separately in addition to code for primary procedure)

INCLUDES Endograft extensions into internal and external iliac, and/or common femoral arteries

EXCLUDES *Delayed deployment branched iliac endograft, separate from aorto-iliac endograft placement ([34718])*
Placement prosthesis extensions on same side (34709, 34710-34711)
Reporting with modifier 50. Report once for each side when performed bilaterally

Code first (34703-34706)

12.9 12.9 FUD ZZZ 80

+ 34709 Placement of extension prosthesis(es) distal to the common iliac artery(ies) or proximal to the renal artery(ies) for endovascular repair of infrarenal abdominal aortic or iliac aneurysm, false aneurysm, dissection, penetrating ulcer, including pre-procedure sizing and device selection, all nonselective catheterization(s), all associated radiological supervision and interpretation, and treatment zone angioplasty/stenting, when performed, per vessel treated (List separately in addition to code for primary procedure)

EXCLUDES *Placement covered stent (37236-37237)*
Placement iliac branched endograft ([34717], [34718])
Reporting code more than one time for each vessel treated

Code first (34701-34708, 34845-34848)

9.42 9.42 FUD ZZZ C 80

AMA: 2019,Nov,6; 2018,Jan,8; 2017,Dec,3

\# **34718** **Endovascular repair of iliac artery, not associated with placement of an aorto-iliac artery endograft at the same session, by deployment of an iliac branched endograft, including pre-procedure sizing and device selection, all ipsilateral selective iliac artery catheterization(s), all associated radiological supervision and interpretation, and all endograft extension(s) proximally to the aortic bifurcation and distally in the internal iliac, external iliac, and common femoral artery(ies), and treatment zone angioplasty/stenting, when performed, for other than rupture (eg, for aneurysm, pseudoaneurysm, dissection, arteriovenous malformation, penetrating ulcer), unilateral**

INCLUDES Endograft extensions into internal and external iliac, and/or common femoral arteries

EXCLUDES *Branched iliac endograft deployed same session as aorto-iliac endograft placement (34703-34706, [34717])*

Placement isolated iliac branched endograft, for rupture (37799)

Placement prosthesis extensions on same side (34709, 34710-34711)

36.0 36.0 **FUD** 090 80

34710 **Delayed placement of distal or proximal extension prosthesis for endovascular repair of infrarenal abdominal aortic or iliac aneurysm, false aneurysm, dissection, endoleak, or endograft migration, including pre-procedure sizing and device selection, all nonselective catheterization(s), all associated radiological supervision and interpretation, and treatment zone angioplasty/stenting, when performed; initial vessel treated**

EXCLUDES *Fenestrated endograft repair (34841-34848)*

Initial endovascular repair by endograft (34701-34709)

Reporting code more than one time per procedure

Code also decompressive laparotomy for treatment abdominal compartment syndrome (49000)

23.3 23.3 **FUD** 090 C 80

AMA: 2019,Nov,6; 2018,Jan,8; 2017,Dec,3

\+ **34711** **each additional vessel treated (List separately in addition to code for primary procedure)**

EXCLUDES *Fenestrated endograft repair (34841-34848)*

Initial endovascular repair by endograft (34701-34709)

Reporting code more than one time per procedure

Code first (34710)

8.68 8.68 **FUD** ZZZ C 80

AMA: 2019,Nov,6; 2018,Jan,8; 2017,Dec,3

34712 **Transcatheter delivery of enhanced fixation device(s) to the endograft (eg, anchor, screw, tack) and all associated radiological supervision and interpretation**

EXCLUDES *Reporting code more than one time per procedure*

19.2 19.2 **FUD** 090 C 80

AMA: 2018,Jan,8; 2017,Dec,3

\+ **34713** **Percutaneous access and closure of femoral artery for delivery of endograft through a large sheath (12 French or larger), including ultrasound guidance, when performed, unilateral (List separately in addition to code for primary procedure)**

INCLUDES Ultrasound imaging guidance

Unilateral procedure through large sheath 12 French or larger

EXCLUDES *Reporting with modifier 50. Report once for each side when performed bilaterally*

Code first (33880-33881, 33883-33884, 33886, 34701-34708, [34718], 34710, 34712, 34841-34848)

3.63 3.63 **FUD** ZZZ N N1 80 50

AMA: 2018,Jan,8; 2017,Dec,3

34812-34834 [34717, 34718, 34812, 34820, 34833, 34834] Open Exposure for Endovascular Prosthesis Delivery

INCLUDES Balloon angioplasty/stent deployment within target treatment zone

Introduction, manipulation, placement, and device deployment

Open exposure femoral or iliac artery/subsequent closure

Thromboendarterectomy at site of aneurysm

EXCLUDES *Additional interventional procedures outside target treatment zone*

Guidewire and catheter insertion (36140, 36200, 36245-36248)

Substantial artery repair/replacement (35226, 35286)

\+ # **34812** **Open femoral artery exposure for delivery of endovascular prosthesis, by groin incision, unilateral (List separately in addition to code for primary procedure)**

EXCLUDES *ECMO/ECLS insertion, removal or repositioning (33953-33954, 33959, [33962], [33969], [33984], [33987])*

Extensive repair femoral artery (35226, 35286, 35371)

Reporting with modifier 50. Report once for each side when performed bilaterally

Code first (33880-33881, 33883-33884, 33886, 33990-33991, 34701-34708, [34718], 34710, 34712, 34841-34848)

6.01 6.01 **FUD** ZZZ C 80 50

AMA: 2018,Jan,8; 2017,Dec,3; 2017,Jan,8; 2016,Jan,13; 2015,Jul,3; 2015,Jan,16

\+ **34714** **Open femoral artery exposure with creation of conduit for delivery of endovascular prosthesis or for establishment of cardiopulmonary bypass, by groin incision, unilateral (List separately in addition to code for primary procedure)**

EXCLUDES *Delivery endovascular prosthesis via open femoral artery ([34812])*

ECMO/ECLS insertion, removal or repositioning on same side (33953-33954, 33959, [33962], [33969], [33984])

Reporting with modifier 50. Report once for each side when performed bilaterally

Transcatheter aortic valve replacement via open axillary artery (33362)

Code first (32852, 32854, 33031, 33120, 33251, 33256, 33259, 33261, 33305, 33315, 33322, 33335, 33390-33391, 33404-33406, 33410, [33440], 33411-33417, 33422, 33425-33427, 33430, 33460, 33463-33465, 33468, 33474-33476, 33478, 33496, 33500, 33502, 33504-33507, 33510-33516, 33533-33536, 33542, 33545, 33548, 33600-33688, 33692, 33694, 33697, 33702, 33710, 33720, 33722, 33724, 33726, 33730, 33732, 33736, 33750, 33755, 33762, 33764, 33766-33767, 33770-33783, 33786, 33788, 33802-33803, 33814, 33820, 33822, 33824, 33840, 33845, 33851, 33853, 33858-33859, 33863-33864, 33871, 33875, 33877, 33880-33881, 33883-33884, 33886, 33910, 33916-33917, 33920, 33922, 33926, 33935, 33945, 33975-33980, 33983, 33990-33991, 34701-34708, [34718], 34710, 34712, 34841-34848)

7.87 7.87 **FUD** ZZZ N N1 80 50

AMA: 2018,Jan,8; 2017,Dec,3

\+ # **34820** **Open iliac artery exposure for delivery of endovascular prosthesis or iliac occlusion during endovascular therapy, by abdominal or retroperitoneal incision, unilateral (List separately in addition to code for primary procedure)**

EXCLUDES *ECMO/ECLS insertion, removal or repositioning (33953-33954, 33959, [33962], [33969], [33984])*

Reporting with modifier 50. Report once for each side when performed bilaterally

Code first (33880-33881, 33883-33884, 33886, 33990-33991, 34701-34708, [34718], 34710, 34712, 34841-34848)

10.1 10.1 **FUD** ZZZ C 80 50

AMA: 2018,Jan,8; 2017,Dec,3; 2017,Jan,8; 2016,Jan,13; 2015,Jul,3; 2015,Jan,16

+ # 34833 Open iliac artery exposure with creation of conduit for delivery of endovascular prosthesis or for establishment of cardiopulmonary bypass, by abdominal or retroperitoneal incision, unilateral (List separately in addition to code for primary procedure)

EXCLUDES *Delivery endovascular prosthesis via open iliac artery ([34820])*
ECMO/ECLS insertion, removal or repositioning on same side (33953-33954, 33959, [33962], [33969], [33984])
Reporting with modifier 50. Report once for each side when performed bilaterally
Transcatheter aortic valve replacement via open iliac artery (33364)

Code first (32852, 32854, 33031, 33256, 33259, 33261, 33305, 33315, 33322, 33335, 33390-33391, 33404-33406, 33410, [33440], 33411-33417, 33422, 33425-33427, 33430, 33460, 33463-33465, 33468, 33474-33476, 33478, 33496, 33500, 33502, 33504-33514, 33516, 33533-33536, 33542, 33545, 33548, 33600-33688, 33692, 33694, 33697, 33702, 33710, 33720, 33722, 33724, 33726, 33730, 33732, 33736, 33750, 33755, 33762, 33764, 33766-33767, 33770-33783, 33786, 33788, 33802-33803, 33814, 33820, 33822, 33824, 33840, 33845, 33851, 33853, 33858-33859, 33863-33864, 33871, 33875, 33877, 33880-33881, 33883-33884, 33886, 33910, 33916-33917, 33920, 33922, 33926, 33935, 33945, 33975-33980, 33983, 33990-33991, 34701-34708, [34718], 34710, 34712, 34841-34848)

11.7 11.7 **FUD** ZZZ C 80 50

AMA: 2018,Jan,8; 2017,Dec,3; 2017,Jan,8; 2016,Jan,13; 2015,Jul,3; 2015,Jan,16

+ # 34834 Open brachial artery exposure for delivery of endovascular prosthesis, unilateral (List separately in addition to code for primary procedure)

EXCLUDES *ECMO/ECLS insertion, removal or repositioning (33953-33954, 33959, [33962], [33969], [33984])*
Reporting with modifier 50. Report once for each side when performed bilaterally

Code first (33880-33881, 33883-33884, 33886, 33990-33991, 34701-34708, [34718], 34710, 34712, 34841-34848)

3.75 3.75 **FUD** ZZZ C 80 50

AMA: 2018,Jan,8; 2017,Dec,3; 2017,Jan,8; 2016,Jan,13; 2015,Jul,3; 2015,Jan,16

+ 34715 Open axillary/subclavian artery exposure for delivery of endovascular prosthesis by infraclavicular or supraclavicular incision, unilateral (List separately in addition to code for primary procedure)

EXCLUDES *ECMO/ECLS insertion, removal or repositioning on same side (33953-33954, 33959, [33962], [33969], [33984])*
Implantation or replacement aortic counterpulsation ventricular assist system (0451T-0452T, 0455T-0456T)
Reporting with modifier 50. Report once for each side when performed bilaterally
Transcatheter aortic valve replacement via open axillary artery (33363)

Code first (33880-33881, 33883-33884, 33886, 33990-33991, 34701-34708, [34718], 34710, 34712, 34841-34848)

8.72 8.72 **FUD** ZZZ N N1 80 50

AMA: 2018,Jan,8; 2017,Dec,3

+ 34716 Open axillary/subclavian artery exposure with creation of conduit for delivery of endovascular prosthesis or for establishment of cardiopulmonary bypass, by infraclavicular or supraclavicular incision, unilateral (List separately in addition to code for primary procedure)

EXCLUDES *ECMO/ECLS insertion, removal or repositioning on same side (33953-33954, 33959, [33962], [33969], [33984])*
Implantation or replacement aortic counterpulsation ventricular assist system (0451T-0452T, 0455T-0456T)
Reporting with modifier 50. Report once for each side when performed bilaterally

Code first (32852, 32854, 33031, 33120, 33251, 33256, 33259, 33261, 33305, 33315, 33322, 33335, 33390-33391, 33404-33406, 33410, [33440], 33411-33417, 33422, 33425-33427, 33430, 33460, 33463-33465, 33468, 33474-33476, 33478, 33496, 33500, 33502, 33504-33514, 33516, 33533-33536, 33542, 33545, 33548, 33600-33688, 33692, 33694, 33697, 33702-33722, 33724, 33726, 33730, 33732, 33736, 33750, 33755, 33762, 33764, 33766-33767, 33770-33783, 33786, 33788, 33802-33803, 33814, 33820, 33822, 33824, 33840, 33845, 33851, 33853, 33858-33859, 33863-33864, 33871, 33875, 33877, 33880-33881, 33883-33884, 33886, 33910, 33916-33917, 33920, 33922, 33926, 33935, 33945, 33975-33980, 33983, 33990-33991, 34701-34708, [34718], 34710, 34712, 34841-34848)

10.8 10.8 **FUD** ZZZ N N1 80 50

AMA: 2018,Jan,8; 2017,Dec,3

34717 **Resequenced code. See code following 34708.**

34718 **Resequenced code. See code following 34709.**

+ 34808 Endovascular placement of iliac artery occlusion device (List separately in addition to code for primary procedure)

Code first (34701-34704, 34707-34708, 34709, 34710, 34813, 34841-34844)

5.81 5.81 **FUD** ZZZ C 80

AMA: 2018,Jan,8; 2017,Jan,8; 2016,Jan,13; 2015,Jan,16

34812 **Resequenced code. See code following 34713.**

+ 34813 Placement of femoral-femoral prosthetic graft during endovascular aortic aneurysm repair (List separately in addition to code for primary procedure)

EXCLUDES *Grafting femoral artery (35521, 35533, 35539, 35540, 35556, 35558, 35566, 35621, 35646, 35654-35661, 35666, 35700)*

Code first ([34812])

6.90 6.90 **FUD** ZZZ C 80

AMA: 2018,Jan,8; 2017,Jan,8; 2016,Jan,13; 2015,Jan,16

34820 **Resequenced code. See code following 34714.**

34830 Open repair of infrarenal aortic aneurysm or dissection, plus repair of associated arterial trauma, following unsuccessful endovascular repair; tube prosthesis

51.2 51.2 **FUD** 090 C 80

AMA: 2018,Jan,8; 2017,Jan,8; 2016,Jan,13; 2015,Jan,16

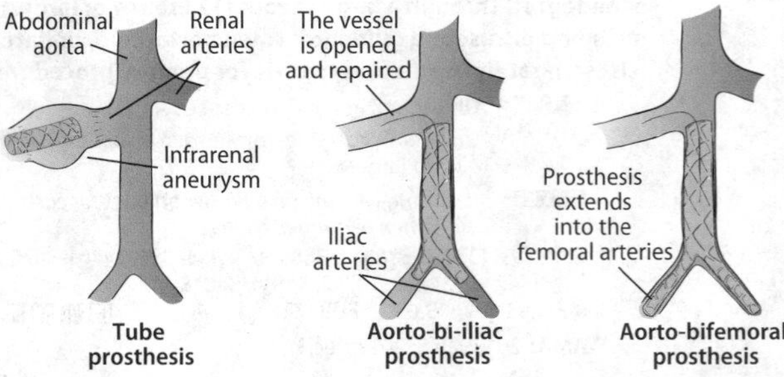

A tube prosthesis is placed and any associated arterial trauma is repaired

34831 aorto-bi-iliac prosthesis

56.0 56.0 **FUD** 090 C 80

AMA: 2018,Jan,8; 2017,Jan,8; 2016,Jan,13; 2015,Jan,16

34832 **aorto-bifemoral prosthesis**
55.0 55.0 **FUD** 090 C 80
AMA: 2018,Jan,8; 2017,Jan,8; 2016,Jan,13; 2015,Jan,16

34833 **Resequenced code. See code following 34714.**

34834 **Resequenced code. See code following 34714.**

34839-34848 Repair Visceral Aorta with Fenestrated Endovascular Grafts

INCLUDES Angiography
Balloon angioplasty before and after graft deployment
Fluoroscopic guidance
Guidewire and catheter insertion vessels in target treatment zone
Radiologic supervision and interpretation
Visceral aorta (34841-34844)
Visceral aorta and associated infrarenal abdominal aorta (34845-34848)

EXCLUDES *Catheterization:*
Arterial families outside treatment zone
Hypogastric arteries
Distal extension prosthesis terminating in common femoral, external iliac, or internal iliac artery (34709-34711 [34718])
Insertion bare metal or covered intravascular stents in visceral branches in target treatment zone (37236-37237)
Interventional procedures outside treatment zone
Open exposure access vessels (34713-34716 [34812, 34820, 34833, 34834])
Placement distal extension prosthesis into internal/external iliac or common femoral artery (34709, [34718], 34710-34711)
Repair abdominal aortic aneurysm without fenestrated graft (34701-34708)
Substantial artery repair (35226, 35286)

Code also associated endovascular repair descending thoracic aorta (33880-33886, 75956-75959)

34839 **Physician planning of a patient-specific fenestrated visceral aortic endograft requiring a minimum of 90 minutes of physician time**

EXCLUDES *3D rendering with interpretation and image reporting (76376-76377)*
Endovascular repair procedure on day of or day after planning (34701-34706, 34841-34848)
Planning on day of or day before endovascular repair procedure
Total planning time less than 90 minutes

0.00 0.00 **FUD** YYY B 80

34841 **Endovascular repair of visceral aorta (eg, aneurysm, pseudoaneurysm, dissection, penetrating ulcer, intramural hematoma, or traumatic disruption) by deployment of a fenestrated visceral aortic endograft and all associated radiological supervision and interpretation, including target zone angioplasty, when performed; including one visceral artery endoprosthesis (superior mesenteric, celiac or renal artery)**

EXCLUDES *Endovascular repair aorta (34701-34706, 34845-34848)*
Physician planning patient-specific fenestrated visceral aortic endograft (34839)

0.00 0.00 **FUD** YYY C 80
AMA: 2018,Jan,8; 2017,Dec,3; 2017,Jul,3; 2017,Jan,8; 2016,Jan,13; 2015,Jan,16

34842 **including two visceral artery endoprostheses (superior mesenteric, celiac and/or renal artery[s])**

INCLUDES Repairs extending from visceral aorta to one or more four visceral artery origins to infrarenal aorta level

EXCLUDES *Endovascular repair aorta (34701-34706, 34845-34848)*
Physician planning patient-specific fenestrated visceral aortic endograft (34839)

0.00 0.00 **FUD** YYY C 80
AMA: 2018,Jan,8; 2017,Dec,3; 2017,Jul,3; 2017,Jan,8; 2016,Jan,13; 2015,Jan,16

34843 **including three visceral artery endoprostheses (superior mesenteric, celiac and/or renal artery[s])**

INCLUDES Repairs extending from visceral aorta to one or more four visceral artery origins to infrarenal aorta level

EXCLUDES *Endovascular repair aorta (34701-34706, 34845-34848)*
Physician planning patient-specific fenestrated visceral aortic endograft (34839)

0.00 0.00 **FUD** YYY C 80
AMA: 2018,Jan,8; 2017,Dec,3; 2017,Jul,3; 2017,Jan,8; 2016,Jan,13; 2015,Jan,16

34844 **including four or more visceral artery endoprostheses (superior mesenteric, celiac and/or renal artery[s])**

INCLUDES Repairs extending from visceral aorta to one or more four visceral artery origins to infrarenal aorta level

EXCLUDES *Endovascular repair aorta (34701-34706, 34845-34848)*
Physician planning patient-specific fenestrated visceral aortic endograft (34839)

0.00 0.00 **FUD** YYY C 80
AMA: 2018,Jan,8; 2017,Dec,3; 2017,Jul,3; 2017,Jan,8; 2016,Jan,13; 2015,Jan,16

34845 **Endovascular repair of visceral aorta and infrarenal abdominal aorta (eg, aneurysm, pseudoaneurysm, dissection, penetrating ulcer, intramural hematoma, or traumatic disruption) with a fenestrated visceral aortic endograft and concomitant unibody or modular infrarenal aortic endograft and all associated radiological supervision and interpretation, including target zone angioplasty, when performed; including one visceral artery endoprosthesis (superior mesenteric, celiac or renal artery)**

INCLUDES Placement device and extensions into common iliac arteries
Repairs extending from visceral aorta to one or more four visceral artery origins to infrarenal aorta level

EXCLUDES *Direct repair aneurysm (35081, 35102)*
Endovascular repair aorta (34701-34706, 34845-34848)
Physician planning patient-specific fenestrated visceral aortic endograft (34839)

Code also iliac artery revascularization when performed outside target treatment zone (37220-37223)

0.00 0.00 **FUD** YYY C 80
AMA: 2018,Jan,8; 2017,Dec,3; 2017,Jul,3; 2017,Jan,8; 2016,Jan,13; 2015,Jan,16

34846 **including two visceral artery endoprostheses (superior mesenteric, celiac and/or renal artery[s])**

INCLUDES Placement device and extensions into common iliac arteries
Repairs extending from visceral aorta to one or more four visceral artery origins to infrarenal aorta level

EXCLUDES *Direct repair aneurysm (35081, 35102)*
Endovascular repair aorta (34701-34706, 34841-34844)
Physician planning patient-specific fenestrated visceral aortic endograft (34839)

Code also iliac artery revascularization when performed outside target treatment zone (37220-37223)

0.00 0.00 **FUD** YYY C 80
AMA: 2018,Jan,8; 2017,Dec,3; 2017,Jul,3; 2017,Jan,8; 2016,Jan,13; 2015,Jan,16

34847 **including three visceral artery endoprostheses (superior mesenteric, celiac and/or renal artery[s])**

INCLUDES Placement device and extensions into common iliac arteries

Repairs extending from visceral aorta to one or more four visceral artery origins to infrarenal aorta level

EXCLUDES *Direct repair aneurysm (35081, 35102)*

Endovascular repair aorta (34701-34706, 34841-34844)

Physician planning patient-specific fenestrated visceral aortic endograft (34839)

Code also iliac artery revascularization when performed outside target treatment zone (37220-37223)

Facility RVU 0.00 Non-Facility RVU 0.00 **FUD** YYY C 80

AMA: 2018,Jan,8; 2017,Dec,3; 2017,Jul,3; 2017,Jan,8; 2016,Jan,13; 2015,Jan,16

34848 **including four or more visceral artery endoprostheses (superior mesenteric, celiac and/or renal artery[s])**

INCLUDES Placement device and extensions into common iliac arteries

Repairs extending from visceral aorta to one or more four visceral artery origins to infrarenal aorta level

EXCLUDES *Direct repair aneurysm (35081, 35102)*

Endovascular repair aorta (34701-34706, 34841-34844)

Physician planning patient-specific fenestrated visceral aortic endograft (34839)

Code also iliac artery revascularization when performed outside target treatment zone (37220-37223)

Facility RVU 0.00 Non-Facility RVU 0.00 **FUD** YYY C 80

AMA: 2018,Jan,8; 2017,Dec,3; 2017,Aug,9; 2017,Jul,3; 2017,Jan,8; 2016,Jul,6; 2016,Jan,13; 2015,Jan,16

35001-35152 Repair Aneurysm, False Aneurysm, Related Arterial Disease

INCLUDES Endarterectomy procedures

EXCLUDES *Endovascular repairs:*

Abdominal aortic aneurysm (34701-34716 [34717, 34718, 34812, 34820, 34833, 34834])

Thoracic aortic aneurysm (33858-33859, 33863-33875)

Intracranial aneurysms (61697-61710)

Repairs related to occlusive disease only (35201-35286)

35001 **Direct repair of aneurysm, pseudoaneurysm, or excision (partial or total) and graft insertion, with or without patch graft; for aneurysm and associated occlusive disease, carotid, subclavian artery, by neck incision**

Facility RVU 32.6 Non-Facility RVU 32.6 **FUD** 090 C 80 50

AMA: 2002,May,7; 2000,Dec,1

35002 **for ruptured aneurysm, carotid, subclavian artery, by neck incision**

Facility RVU 33.0 Non-Facility RVU 33.0 **FUD** 090 C 80 50

AMA: 2002,May,7; 1997,Nov,1

35005 **for aneurysm, pseudoaneurysm, and associated occlusive disease, vertebral artery**

Facility RVU 28.6 Non-Facility RVU 28.6 **FUD** 090 C 80 50

AMA: 2002,May,7; 1997,Nov,1

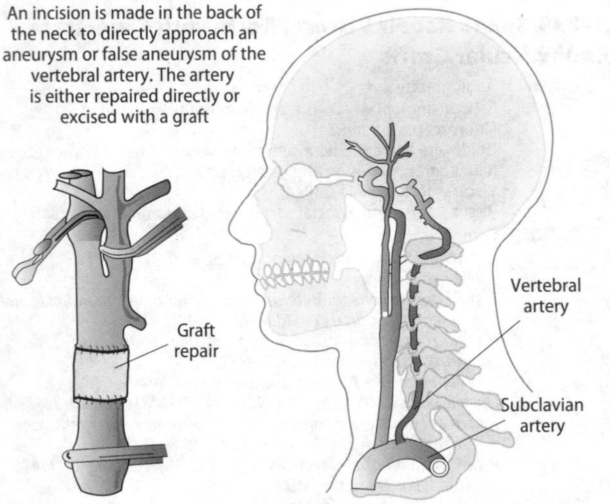

An incision is made in the back of the neck to directly approach an aneurysm or false aneurysm of the vertebral artery. The artery is either repaired directly or excised with a graft
Graft repair
Vertebral artery
Subclavian artery

35011 **for aneurysm and associated occlusive disease, axillary-brachial artery, by arm incision**

Facility RVU 29.0 Non-Facility RVU 29.0 **FUD** 090 T 80 50

AMA: 2002,May,7; 1997,Nov,1

35013 **for ruptured aneurysm, axillary-brachial artery, by arm incision**

Facility RVU 36.6 Non-Facility RVU 36.6 **FUD** 090 C 80 50

AMA: 2002,May,7; 1997,Nov,1

35021 **for aneurysm, pseudoaneurysm, and associated occlusive disease, innominate, subclavian artery, by thoracic incision**

Facility RVU 36.4 Non-Facility RVU 36.4 **FUD** 090 C 80 50

AMA: 2002,May,7; 1997,Nov,1

35022 **for ruptured aneurysm, innominate, subclavian artery, by thoracic incision**

Facility RVU 40.6 Non-Facility RVU 40.6 **FUD** 090 C 80 50

AMA: 2002,May,7; 1997,Nov,1

35045 **for aneurysm, pseudoaneurysm, and associated occlusive disease, radial or ulnar artery**

Facility RVU 28.4 Non-Facility RVU 28.4 **FUD** 090 T 80 50

AMA: 2002,May,7; 1997,Nov,1

35081 **for aneurysm, pseudoaneurysm, and associated occlusive disease, abdominal aorta**

Facility RVU 50.3 Non-Facility RVU 50.3 **FUD** 090 C 80

AMA: 2018,Jan,8; 2017,Jan,8; 2016,Jan,13; 2015,Jan,16

35082 **for ruptured aneurysm, abdominal aorta**

Facility RVU 63.4 Non-Facility RVU 63.4 **FUD** 090 C 80

AMA: 2002,May,7; 1997,Nov,1

35091 **for aneurysm, pseudoaneurysm, and associated occlusive disease, abdominal aorta involving visceral vessels (mesenteric, celiac, renal)**

Facility RVU 52.0 Non-Facility RVU 52.0 **FUD** 090 C 80 50

AMA: 2018,Jan,8; 2017,Jan,8; 2016,Jan,13; 2015,Jan,16

35092 **for ruptured aneurysm, abdominal aorta involving visceral vessels (mesenteric, celiac, renal)**

Facility RVU 75.7 Non-Facility RVU 75.7 **FUD** 090 C 80 50

AMA: 2002,May,7; 1997,Nov,1

35102 **for aneurysm, pseudoaneurysm, and associated occlusive disease, abdominal aorta involving iliac vessels (common, hypogastric, external)**
54.6 54.6 FUD 090 C 80 50
AMA: 2018,Jan,8; 2017,Jan,8; 2016,Jan,13; 2015,Jan,16

35103 **for ruptured aneurysm, abdominal aorta involving iliac vessels (common, hypogastric, external)**
65.0 65.0 FUD 090 C 80 50
AMA: 2002,May,7; 1997,Nov,1

35111 **for aneurysm, pseudoaneurysm, and associated occlusive disease, splenic artery**
38.5 38.5 FUD 090 C 80 50
AMA: 2002,May,7; 1997,Nov,1

35112 **for ruptured aneurysm, splenic artery**
47.4 47.4 FUD 090 C 80 50
AMA: 2002,May,7; 1997,Nov,1

35121 **for aneurysm, pseudoaneurysm, and associated occlusive disease, hepatic, celiac, renal, or mesenteric artery**
45.9 45.9 FUD 090 C 80 50
AMA: 2002,May,7; 1997,Nov,1

35122 **for ruptured aneurysm, hepatic, celiac, renal, or mesenteric artery**
54.9 54.9 FUD 090 C 80 50
AMA: 2002,May,7; 1997,Nov,1

35131 **for aneurysm, pseudoaneurysm, and associated occlusive disease, iliac artery (common, hypogastric, external)**
40.0 40.0 FUD 090 C 80 50
AMA: 2018,Jan,8; 2017,Jan,8; 2016,Jan,13; 2015,Jan,16

35132 **for ruptured aneurysm, iliac artery (common, hypogastric, external)**
47.4 47.4 FUD 090 C 80 50
AMA: 2002,May,7; 1997,Nov,1

35141 **for aneurysm, pseudoaneurysm, and associated occlusive disease, common femoral artery (profunda femoris, superficial femoral)**
32.0 32.0 FUD 090 C 80 50
AMA: 2002,May,7; 1997,Nov,1

35142 **for ruptured aneurysm, common femoral artery (profunda femoris, superficial femoral)**
38.6 38.6 FUD 090 C 80 50
AMA: 2002,May,7; 1997,Nov,1

35151 **for aneurysm, pseudoaneurysm, and associated occlusive disease, popliteal artery**
35.9 35.9 FUD 090 C 80 50
AMA: 2002,May,7; 1997,Nov,1

35152 **for ruptured aneurysm, popliteal artery**
40.5 40.5 FUD 090 C 80 50
AMA: 2002,May,7; 1997,Nov,1

35180-35190 Surgical Repair Arteriovenous Fistula

35180 **Repair, congenital arteriovenous fistula; head and neck**
25.4 25.4 FUD 090 T 80
AMA: 2018,Jan,8; 2017,Jan,8; 2016,Jan,13; 2015,Jan,16

35182 **thorax and abdomen**
51.9 51.9 FUD 090 C 80
AMA: 2018,Jan,8; 2017,Jan,8; 2016,Jan,13; 2015,Jan,16

35184 **extremities**
27.9 27.9 FUD 090 T 80
AMA: 2018,Jan,8; 2017,Jan,8; 2016,Jan,13; 2015,Jan,16

35188 **Repair, acquired or traumatic arteriovenous fistula; head and neck**
36.9 36.9 FUD 090 T A2 80
AMA: 2018,Jan,8; 2017,Jan,8; 2016,Jan,13; 2015,Jan,16

35189 **thorax and abdomen**
43.8 43.8 FUD 090 C 80
AMA: 2018,Jan,8; 2017,Jan,8; 2016,Jan,13; 2015,Jan,16

35190 **extremities**
22.0 22.0 FUD 090 T 80
AMA: 2018,Jan,8; 2017,Jan,8; 2016,Jan,13; 2015,Jan,16

35201-35286 Surgical Repair Artery or Vein

EXCLUDES *Arteriovenous fistula repair (35180-35190)*
Primary open vascular procedures

35201 **Repair blood vessel, direct; neck**
EXCLUDES *Removal ECMO/ECLS cannula ([33969, 33984, 33985, 33986])*
27.3 27.3 FUD 090 T 80 50
AMA: 2019,Dec,5; 2018,Jan,8; 2017,Jan,8; 2016,Jan,13; 2015,Jul,3; 2015,Jan,16

35206 **upper extremity**
EXCLUDES *Removal ECMO/ECLS cannula ([33969, 33984, 33985, 33986])*
22.6 22.6 FUD 090 T 80 50
AMA: 2019,Dec,5; 2018,Jan,8; 2017,Jan,8; 2016,Jan,13; 2015,Jul,3; 2015,Jan,16

35207 **hand, finger**
21.7 21.7 FUD 090 T A2 50
AMA: 2019,Dec,5

35211 **intrathoracic, with bypass**
EXCLUDES *Removal ECMO/ECLS cannula ([33969, 33984, 33985, 33986])*
40.0 40.0 FUD 090 C 80 50
AMA: 2015,Jul,3

35216 **intrathoracic, without bypass**
EXCLUDES *Removal ECMO/ECLS cannula ([33969, 33984, 33985, 33986])*
60.0 60.0 FUD 090 C 80 50
AMA: 2018,Jan,8; 2017,Jan,8; 2016,Jan,13; 2015,Jan,16

35221 **intra-abdominal**
42.4 42.4 FUD 090 C 80 50
AMA: 2012,Apr,3-9; 2003,Feb,1

35226 **lower extremity**
EXCLUDES *Removal ECMO/ECLS cannula ([33969, 33984, 33985, 33986])*
24.1 24.1 FUD 090 T 80 50
AMA: 2019,Jul,10; 2018,Jan,8; 2017,Aug,10; 2017,Jul,3; 2017,Jan,8; 2016,Jul,6; 2016,Jan,13; 2015,Jul,3; 2015,Jan,16

35231 **Repair blood vessel with vein graft; neck**
36.3 36.3 FUD 090 T 80 50
AMA: 2019,Dec,5

35236 **upper extremity**
29.1 29.1 FUD 090 T 80 50
AMA: 2019,Dec,5; 2018,Jan,8; 2017,Jan,8; 2016,Jan,13; 2015,Jan,16

35241 **intrathoracic, with bypass**
41.5 41.5 FUD 090 C 80 50
AMA: 2012,Apr,3-9; 2003,Feb,1

35246 **intrathoracic, without bypass**
45.2 45.2 FUD 090 C 80 50
AMA: 2012,Apr,3-9; 2003,Feb,1

35251 **intra-abdominal**
50.7 50.7 FUD 090 C 80 50
AMA: 2012,Apr,3-9; 2003,Feb,1

35256 **lower extremity**
29.7 29.7 FUD 090 T 80 50
AMA: 2019,Dec,5

35261 **Repair blood vessel with graft other than vein; neck**
28.4 28.4 FUD 090 T 80 50
AMA: 2019,Dec,5

35266 **upper extremity**
25.1 25.1 FUD 090 T 80 50
AMA: 2019,Dec,5; 2018,Jan,8; 2017,Jan,8; 2016,Jan,13; 2015,Jan,16

35271 **intrathoracic, with bypass**
39.9 39.9 FUD 090 C 80 50
AMA: 2012,Apr,3-9; 2003,Feb,1

35276 **intrathoracic, without bypass**
42.1 42.1 FUD 090 C 80 50
AMA: 2012,Apr,3-9; 2003,Feb,1

35281 **intra-abdominal**
47.3 47.3 FUD 090 C 80 50
AMA: 2012,Apr,3-9; 2003,Feb,1

35286 **lower extremity**
27.1 27.1 FUD 090 T 80 50
AMA: 2019,Dec,5; 2019,Jul,10; 2018,Jan,8; 2017,Aug,10; 2017,Jul,3; 2017,Jan,8; 2016,Jul,6; 2016,Jan,13; 2015,Jan,16

35301-35372 Surgical Thromboendarterectomy Peripheral and Visceral Arteries

INCLUDES Obtaining saphenous or arm vein for graft
Thrombectomy/embolectomy

EXCLUDES *Coronary artery bypass procedures (33510-33536, 33572)*
Thromboendarterectomy for vascular occlusion on different vessel during same session

35301 **Thromboendarterectomy, including patch graft, if performed; carotid, vertebral, subclavian, by neck incision**
32.7 32.7 FUD 090 C 80 50
AMA: 2018,Jan,8; 2017,Jan,8; 2016,Jan,13; 2015,Jan,16

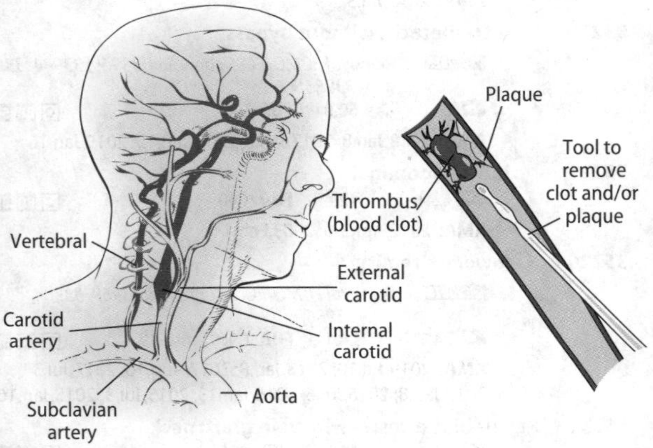

35302 **superficial femoral artery**
EXCLUDES *Revascularization, endovascular, open or percutaneous, femoral, popliteal artery(s) (37225, 37227)*
32.6 32.6 FUD 090 C 80 50
AMA: 2018,Jan,8; 2017,Jan,8; 2016,Jan,13; 2015,Jan,16

35303 **popliteal artery**
EXCLUDES *Revascularization, endovascular, open or percutaneous, femoral, popliteal artery(s) (37225, 37227)*
36.0 36.0 FUD 090 C 80 50
AMA: 2018,Jan,8; 2017,Jan,8; 2016,Jan,13; 2015,Jan,16

35304 **tibioperoneal trunk artery**
EXCLUDES *Revascularization, endovascular, open or percutaneous, tibial/peroneal artery (37229, 37231, 37233, 37235)*
37.0 37.0 FUD 090 C 80 50
AMA: 2018,Jan,8; 2017,Jan,8; 2016,Jan,13; 2015,Jan,16

35305 **tibial or peroneal artery, initial vessel**
EXCLUDES *Revascularization, endovascular, open or percutaneous, tibial/peroneal artery (37229, 37231, 37233, 37235)*
35.6 35.6 FUD 090 C 80 50
AMA: 2018,Jan,8; 2017,Jan,8; 2016,Jan,13; 2015,Jan,16

+ **35306** **each additional tibial or peroneal artery (List separately in addition to code for primary procedure)**
EXCLUDES *Revascularization, endovascular, open or percutaneous, tibial/peroneal artery (37229, 37231, 37233, 37235)*
Code first (35305)
12.9 12.9 FUD ZZZ C 80
AMA: 2018,Jan,8; 2017,Jan,8; 2016,Jan,13; 2015,Jan,16

35311 **subclavian, innominate, by thoracic incision**
45.1 45.1 FUD 090 C 80 50
AMA: 1997,Nov,1

35321 **axillary-brachial**
25.9 25.9 FUD 090 T 80 50
AMA: 1997,Nov,1

35331 **abdominal aorta**
42.3 42.3 FUD 090 C 80 50
AMA: 1997,Nov,1

35341 **mesenteric, celiac, or renal**
39.9 39.9 FUD 090 C 80 50
AMA: 1997,Nov,1

35351 **iliac**
37.3 37.3 FUD 090 C 80 50
AMA: 1997,Nov,1

35355 **iliofemoral**
29.9 29.9 FUD 090 C 80 50
AMA: 1997,Nov,1

35361 **combined aortoiliac**
44.2 44.2 FUD 090 C 80 50
AMA: 1997,Nov,1

35363 **combined aortoiliofemoral**
47.1 47.1 FUD 090 C 80 50
AMA: 1997,Nov,1

35371 **common femoral**
23.7 23.7 FUD 090 C 80 50
AMA: 2018,Jan,8; 2017,Aug,10; 2017,Jul,3; 2017,Jan,8; 2016,Jan,13; 2015,Jan,16

35372 **deep (profunda) femoral**
28.4 28.4 FUD 090 C 80 50
AMA: 2018,Jan,8; 2017,Jan,8; 2016,Jan,13; 2015,Jan,16

35390 Surgical Thromboendarterectomy: Carotid Reoperation

Code first (35301)

+ **35390** **Reoperation, carotid, thromboendarterectomy, more than 1 month after original operation (List separately in addition to code for primary procedure)**
4.65 4.65 FUD ZZZ C 80
AMA: 1997,Nov,1; 1993,Win,1

35400 Endoscopic Visualization of Vessels

Code first therapeutic intervention

+ **35400** **Angioscopy (noncoronary vessels or grafts) during therapeutic intervention (List separately in addition to code for primary procedure)**
4.32 4.32 FUD ZZZ C 80
AMA: 1997,Dec,1; 1997,Nov,1

35500 Obtain Arm Vein for Graft

EXCLUDES *Endoscopic harvest (33508)*
Harvesting multiple vein segments (35682, 35683)

Code first (33510-33536, 35556, 35566, 35570-35571, 35583-35587)

+ **35500** **Harvest of upper extremity vein, 1 segment, for lower extremity or coronary artery bypass procedure (List separately in addition to code for primary procedure)**
9.29 9.29 FUD ZZZ N 80
AMA: 2018,Jan,8; 2017,Jan,8; 2016,Jan,13; 2015,Jan,16

35501-35571 Arterial Bypass Using Vein Grafts

INCLUDES Obtaining saphenous vein grafts

EXCLUDES *Obtaining multiple vein segments (35682, 35683)*
Obtaining vein grafts, upper extremity or femoropopliteal (35500, 35572)
Treatment different sites with different bypass procedures during same operative session

35501 **Bypass graft, with vein; common carotid-ipsilateral internal carotid**
42.4 | 42.4 | FUD 090 | C 80 50
AMA: 2018,Jan,8; 2017,Jan,8; 2016,Jan,13; 2015,Jan,16

35506 **carotid-subclavian or subclavian-carotid**
37.0 | 37.0 | FUD 090 | C 80 50
AMA: 2018,Jan,8; 2017,Jan,8; 2016,Jan,13; 2015,Jan,16

35508 **carotid-vertebral**
INCLUDES Endoscopic procedure
38.5 | 38.5 | FUD 090 | C 80 50
AMA: 1999,Mar,6; 1999,Apr,11

35509 **carotid-contralateral carotid**
40.8 | 40.8 | FUD 090 | C 80 50
AMA: 2018,Jan,8; 2017,Jan,8; 2016,Jan,13; 2015,Jan,16

35510 **carotid-brachial**
35.7 | 35.7 | FUD 090 | C 80 50
AMA: 2018,Jan,8; 2017,Jan,8; 2016,Jan,13; 2015,Jan,16

35511 **subclavian-subclavian**
32.5 | 32.5 | FUD 090 | C 80 50
AMA: 2018,Jan,8; 2017,Jan,8; 2016,Jan,13; 2015,Jan,16

35512 **subclavian-brachial**
35.0 | 35.0 | FUD 090 | C 80 50
AMA: 2018,Jan,8; 2017,Jan,8; 2016,Jan,13; 2015,Jan,16

35515 **subclavian-vertebral**
38.5 | 38.5 | FUD 090 | C 80 50
AMA: 1999,Mar,6; 1999,Apr,11

35516 **subclavian-axillary**
35.4 | 35.4 | FUD 090 | C 80 50
AMA: 1999,Mar,6; 1999,Apr,11

35518 **axillary-axillary**
33.1 | 33.1 | FUD 090 | C 80 50
AMA: 2018,Jan,8; 2017,Jan,8; 2016,Jan,13; 2015,Jan,16

35521 **axillary-femoral**
EXCLUDES *Synthetic graft (35621)*
35.6 | 35.6 | FUD 090 | C 80 50
AMA: 2018,Jan,8; 2017,Jan,8; 2016,Jan,13; 2015,Jan,16

35522 **axillary-brachial**
35.3 | 35.3 | FUD 090 | C 80 50
AMA: 2018,Jan,8; 2017,Jan,8; 2016,Jan,13; 2015,Jan,16

35523 **brachial-ulnar or -radial**
EXCLUDES *Bypass graft using synthetic conduit (37799)*
Bypass graft, with vein; brachial-brachial (35525)
Distal revascularization and interval ligation (DRIL), upper extremity hemodialysis access (steal syndrome) (36838)
Harvest upper extremity vein, 1 segment, for lower extremity or coronary artery bypass procedure (35500)
Repair blood vessel, direct; upper extremity (35206)
37.1 | 37.1 | FUD 090 | C 80 50

35525 **brachial-brachial**
33.0 | 33.0 | FUD 090 | C 80 50
AMA: 2018,Jan,8; 2017,Jan,8; 2016,Jan,13; 2015,Jan,16

35526 **aortosubclavian, aortoinnominate, or aortocarotid**
EXCLUDES *Synthetic graft (35626)*
50.1 | 50.1 | FUD 090 | C 80 50
AMA: 1999,Mar,6; 1999,Apr,11

35531 **aortoceliac or aortomesenteric**
56.6 | 56.6 | FUD 090 | C 80 50
AMA: 1999,Mar,6; 1999,Apr,11

35533 **axillary-femoral-femoral**
EXCLUDES *Synthetic graft (35654)*
43.7 | 43.7 | FUD 090 | C 80 50
AMA: 2012,Apr,3-9; 1999,Mar,6

35535 **hepatorenal**
EXCLUDES *Bypass graft (35536, 35560, 35631, 35636)*
Harvest upper extremity vein, 1 segment, for lower extremity or coronary artery bypass procedure (35500)
Repair blood vessel (35221, 35251, 35281)
55.3 | 55.3 | FUD 090 | C 80 50

35536 **splenorenal**
49.1 | 49.1 | FUD 090 | C 80 50
AMA: 2018,Jan,8; 2017,Jan,8; 2016,Jan,13; 2015,Jan,16

35537 **aortoiliac**
EXCLUDES *Bypass graft, with vein; aortobi-iliac (35538)*
Synthetic graft (35637)
60.6 | 60.6 | FUD 090 | C 80
AMA: 2018,Jan,8; 2017,Jan,8; 2016,Jan,13; 2015,Jan,16

35538 **aortobi-iliac**
EXCLUDES *Bypass graft, with vein; aortoiliac (35537)*
Synthetic graft (35638)
67.9 | 67.9 | FUD 090 | C 80
AMA: 2018,Jan,8; 2017,Jan,8; 2016,Jan,13; 2015,Jan,16

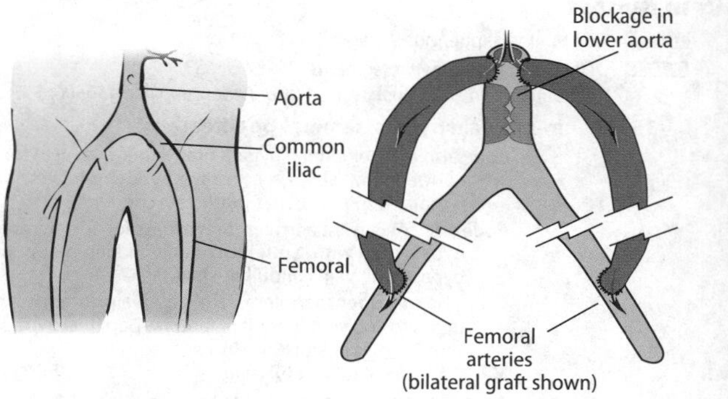

35539 **aortofemoral**
EXCLUDES *Bypass graft, with vein; aortobifemoral (35540)*
Synthetic graft (35647)
63.7 | 63.7 | FUD 090 | C 80 50
AMA: 2018,Jan,8; 2017,Jan,8; 2016,Jan,13; 2015,Jan,16

35540 **aortobifemoral**
EXCLUDES *Bypass graft, with vein; aortofemoral (35539)*
Synthetic graft (35646)
70.6 | 70.6 | FUD 090 | C 50
AMA: 2018,Jan,8; 2017,Jan,8; 2016,Jan,13; 2015,Jan,16

35556 **femoral-popliteal**
40.7 | 40.7 | FUD 090 | C 80 50
AMA: 2018,Jan,8; 2017,Jan,8; 2016,Jan,13; 2015,Jan,16

35558 **femoral-femoral**
35.7 | 35.7 | FUD 090 | C 80 50
AMA: 2012,Apr,3-9; 1999,Mar,6

35560 **aortorenal**
49.2 | 49.2 | FUD 090 | C 80 50
AMA: 2018,Jan,8; 2017,Jan,8; 2016,Jan,13; 2015,Jan,16

35563 **ilioiliac**
38.4 | 38.4 | FUD 090 | C 80 50
AMA: 1999,Mar,6; 1999,Apr,11

35565 **iliofemoral**
38.1 | 38.1 | FUD 090 | C 80 50
AMA: 2012,Apr,3-9; 2004,Oct,6

35566 **femoral-anterior tibial, posterior tibial, peroneal artery or other distal vessels**
48.6 48.6 FUD 090 C 80 50
AMA: 2018,Jan,8; 2017,Jan,8; 2016,Jan,13; 2015,Jan,16

35570 **tibial-tibial, peroneal-tibial, or tibial/peroneal trunk-tibial**
EXCLUDES *Repair blood vessel with graft (35256, 35286)*
42.8 42.8 FUD 090 C 80 50
AMA: 2018,Jan,8; 2017,Jan,8; 2016,Jan,13; 2015,Jan,16

35571 **popliteal-tibial, -peroneal artery or other distal vessels**
38.5 38.5 FUD 090 C 80 50
AMA: 2018,Jan,8; 2017,Jan,8; 2016,Jan,13; 2015,Jan,16

35572 Obtain Femoropopliteal Vein for Graft

EXCLUDES *Reporting with modifier 50. Report once for each side when performed bilaterally*
Code first (33510-33523, 33533-33536, 34502, 34520, 35001-35002, 35011-35022, 35102-35103, 35121-35152, 35231-35256, 35501-35587, 35879-35907)

\+ **35572** **Harvest of femoropopliteal vein, 1 segment, for vascular reconstruction procedure (eg, aortic, vena caval, coronary, peripheral artery) (List separately in addition to code for primary procedure)**
10.0 10.0 FUD ZZZ N N1 80
AMA: 2018,Jan,8; 2017,Jan,8; 2016,Jan,13; 2015,Jan,16

35583-35587 Lower Extremity Revascularization: In-situ Vein Bypass

INCLUDES Obtaining saphenous vein grafts
EXCLUDES *Obtaining multiple vein segments (35682, 35683)*
Obtaining vein graft, upper extremity or femoropopliteal (35500, 35572)

35583 **In-situ vein bypass; femoral-popliteal**
Code also aortobifemoral bypass graft other than vein for aortobifemoral bypass using synthetic conduit and femoral-popliteal bypass with vein conduit in situ (35646)
Code also concurrent aortofemoral bypass for aortofemoral bypass graft with synthetic conduit and femoral-popliteal bypass with vein conduit in-situ (35647)
Code also concurrent aortofemoral bypass (vein) for aortofemoral bypass using vein conduit or femoral-popliteal bypass with vein conduit in-situ (35539)
41.8 41.8 FUD 090 C 80 50
AMA: 2018,Jan,8; 2017,Jan,8; 2016,Jan,13; 2015,Jan,16

35585 **femoral-anterior tibial, posterior tibial, or peroneal artery**
48.6 48.6 FUD 090 C 80 50
AMA: 2018,Jan,8; 2017,Jan,8; 2016,Jan,13; 2015,Jan,16

35587 **popliteal-tibial, peroneal**
39.6 39.6 FUD 090 C 80 50
AMA: 2018,Jan,8; 2017,Jan,8; 2016,Jan,13; 2015,Jan,16

35600 Obtain Arm Artery for Coronary Bypass

EXCLUDES *Transposition and/or reimplantation arteries (35691-35695)*
Code first (33533-33536)

\+ **35600** **Harvest of upper extremity artery, 1 segment, for coronary artery bypass procedure (List separately in addition to code for primary procedure)**
7.43 7.43 FUD ZZZ C 80
AMA: 2018,Jan,8; 2017,Jan,8; 2016,Jan,13; 2015,Jan,16

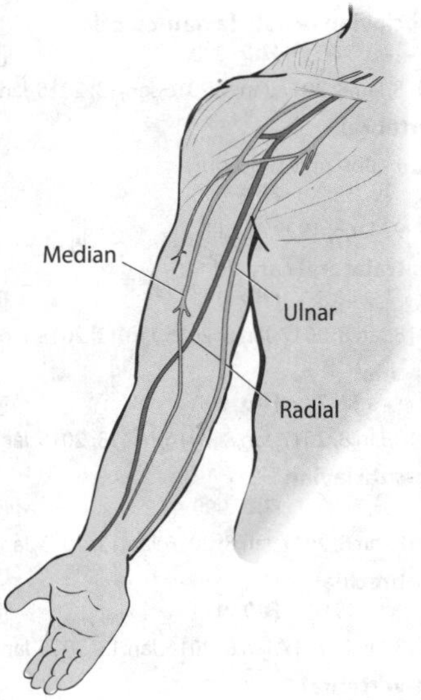
Median
Ulnar
Radial
An upper extremity artery or segment is harvested for a coronary artery bypass procedure

35601-35671 Arterial Bypass: Grafts Other Than Veins

EXCLUDES *Transposition and/or reimplantation arteries (35691-35695)*

35601 **Bypass graft, with other than vein; common carotid-ipsilateral internal carotid**
EXCLUDES *Open transcervical common carotid-common carotid bypass with endovascular repair descending thoracic aorta (33891)*
40.4 40.4 FUD 090 C 80 50
AMA: 2018,Jan,8; 2017,Jan,8; 2016,Jan,13; 2015,Jan,16

35606 **carotid-subclavian**
EXCLUDES *Open subclavian to carotid artery transposition performed with endovascular thoracic aneurysm repair via neck incision (33889)*
34.0 34.0 FUD 090 C 80 50
AMA: 1997,Nov,1

35612 **subclavian-subclavian**
30.3 30.3 FUD 090 C 80 50
AMA: 1997,Nov,1

35616 **subclavian-axillary**
32.0 32.0 FUD 090 C 80 50
AMA: 1997,Nov,1

35621 **axillary-femoral**
31.8 31.8 FUD 090 C 80 50
AMA: 2018,Jan,8; 2017,Jan,8; 2016,Jan,13; 2015,Jan,16

35623 **axillary-popliteal or -tibial**
38.1 38.1 FUD 090 C 80 50
AMA: 2012,Apr,3-9; 1997,Nov,1

35626 **aortosubclavian, aortoinnominate, or aortocarotid**
46.1 46.1 FUD 090 C 80 50
AMA: 1997,Nov,1

26/TC PC/TC Only A2-Z3 ASC Payment 50 Bilateral ♂ Male Only ♀ Female Only Facility RVU Non-Facility RVU CCI CLIA
FUD Follow-up Days CMS: IOM AMA: CPT Asst A-Y OPPSI 80/80 Surg Assist Allowed / w/Doc Lab Crosswalk Radiology Crosswalk

35631 **aortoceliac, aortomesenteric, aortorenal**
53.8 53.8 FUD 090 C 80 50
AMA: 1997,Nov,1

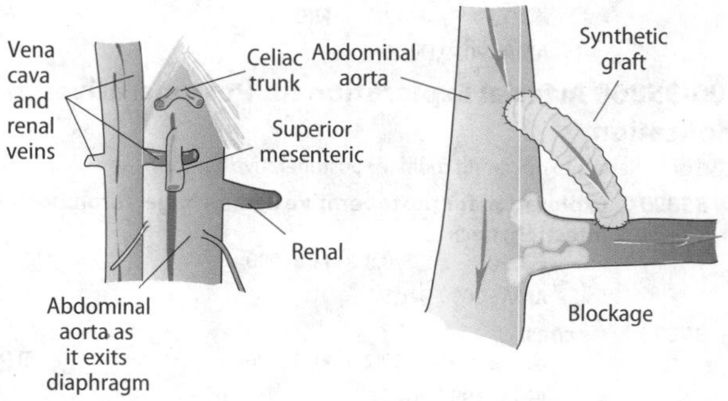

35632 **ilio-celiac**
EXCLUDES *Bypass graft (35531, 35631)*
Repair blood vessel (35221, 35251, 35281)
52.5 52.5 FUD 090 C 80 50

35633 **ilio-mesenteric**
EXCLUDES *Bypass graft (35531, 35631)*
Repair blood vessel (35221, 35251, 35281)
57.6 57.6 FUD 090 C 80 50

35634 **iliorenal**
EXCLUDES *Bypass graft (35536, 35560, 35631)*
Repair blood vessel (35221, 35251, 35281)
51.4 51.4 FUD 090 C 80 50

35636 **splenorenal (splenic to renal arterial anastomosis)**
46.0 46.0 FUD 090 C 80 50
AMA: 1997,Nov,1; 1994,Win,1

35637 **aortoiliac**
EXCLUDES *Bypass graft (35638, 35646)*
47.9 47.9 FUD 090 C 80
AMA: 2018,Jan,8; 2017,Jan,8; 2016,Jan,13; 2015,Jan,16

35638 **aortobi-iliac**
EXCLUDES *Bypass graft (35637, 35646)*
Open placement aorto-bi-iliac prosthesis after failed endovascular repair (34831)
50.7 50.7 FUD 090 C 80
AMA: 2018,Jan,8; 2017,Jan,8; 2016,Jan,13; 2015,Jan,16

35642 **carotid-vertebral**
28.6 28.6 FUD 090 C 80 50
AMA: 1997,Nov,1

35645 **subclavian-vertebral**
27.4 27.4 FUD 090 C 80 50
AMA: 1997,Nov,1

35646 **aortobifemoral**
EXCLUDES *Bypass graft using vein graft (35540)*
Open placement aorto-bi-iliac prosthesis after failed endovascular repair (34831)
49.7 49.7 FUD 090 C 80
AMA: 2018,Jan,8; 2017,Jan,8; 2016,Jan,13; 2015,Jan,16

35647 **aortofemoral**
EXCLUDES *Bypass graft using vein graft (35539)*
44.9 44.9 FUD 090 C 80 50
AMA: 2018,Jan,8; 2017,Jan,8; 2016,Jan,13; 2015,Jan,16

35650 **axillary-axillary**
29.6 29.6 FUD 090 C 80 50
AMA: 1997,Nov,1

35654 **axillary-femoral-femoral**
39.8 39.8 FUD 090 C 80
AMA: 2018,Jan,8; 2017,Jan,8; 2016,Jan,13; 2015,Jan,16

35656 **femoral-popliteal**
31.4 31.4 FUD 090 C 80 50
AMA: 2018,Jan,8; 2017,Jan,8; 2016,Jan,13; 2015,Jan,16

35661 **femoral-femoral**
31.5 31.5 FUD 090 C 80 50
AMA: 2018,Jan,8; 2017,Jan,8; 2016,Jan,13; 2015,Jan,16

35663 **ilioiliac**
35.3 35.3 FUD 090 C 80 50
AMA: 1997,Nov,1

35665 **iliofemoral**
34.1 34.1 FUD 090 C 80 50
AMA: 2018,Jan,8; 2017,Jan,8; 2016,Jan,13; 2015,Jan,16

35666 **femoral-anterior tibial, posterior tibial, or peroneal artery**
37.0 37.0 FUD 090 C 80 50
AMA: 2018,Jan,8; 2017,Jan,8; 2016,Jan,13; 2015,Jan,16

35671 **popliteal-tibial or -peroneal artery**
32.6 32.6 FUD 090 C 80 50
AMA: 2012,Apr,3-9; 1997,Nov,1

35681-35683 Arterial Bypass Using Combination Synthetic and Donor Graft

INCLUDES Acquiring multiple vein segments from sites other than extremity for which arterial bypass performed
Anastomosis vein segments to create bypass graft conduits

+ **35681** **Bypass graft; composite, prosthetic and vein (List separately in addition to code for primary procedure)**
EXCLUDES *Bypass graft (35682, 35683)*
Code first primary procedure
2.36 2.36 FUD ZZZ C 80
AMA: 2018,Jan,8; 2017,Jan,8; 2016,Jan,13; 2015,Jan,16

+ **35682** **autogenous composite, 2 segments of veins from 2 locations (List separately in addition to code for primary procedure)**
EXCLUDES *Bypass graft (35681, 35683)*
Code first (35556, 35566, 35570-35571, 35583-35587)
10.2 10.2 FUD ZZZ C 80
AMA: 2018,Jan,8; 2017,Jan,8; 2016,Jan,13; 2015,Jan,16

+ **35683** **autogenous composite, 3 or more segments of vein from 2 or more locations (List separately in addition to code for primary procedure)**
EXCLUDES *Bypass graft (35681-35682)*
Code first (35556, 35566, 35570-35571, 35583-35587)
11.8 11.8 FUD ZZZ C 80
AMA: 2018,Jan,8; 2017,Jan,8; 2016,Jan,13; 2015,Jan,16

35685-35686 Supplemental Procedures

INCLUDES Additional procedures needed with bypass graft to increase graft patency
EXCLUDES *Composite grafts (35681-35683)*

+ **35685** **Placement of vein patch or cuff at distal anastomosis of bypass graft, synthetic conduit (List separately in addition to code for primary procedure)**
INCLUDES Connection vein segment (cuff or patch) between distal portion synthetic graft and native artery
Code first (35656, 35666, 35671)
5.78 5.78 FUD ZZZ N 80
AMA: 2018,Jan,8; 2017,Jan,8; 2016,Jan,13; 2015,Jan,16

+ **35686** **Creation of distal arteriovenous fistula during lower extremity bypass surgery (non-hemodialysis) (List separately in addition to code for primary procedure)**
INCLUDES Creation fistula between peroneal or tibial artery and vein at or past distal anastomosis site
Code first (35556, 35566, 35570-35571, 35583-35587, 35623, 35656, 35666, 35671)
4.68 4.68 FUD ZZZ N 80
AMA: 2018,Jan,8; 2017,Jan,8; 2016,Jan,13; 2015,Jan,16

35691-35697 Arterial Translocation

CMS: 100-03,160.8 Electroencephalographic Monitoring During Cerebral Vasculature Surgery

35691 **Transposition and/or reimplantation; vertebral to carotid artery**
27.2 27.2 FUD 090 C 80 50
AMA: 1997,Nov,1; 1993,Win,1

35693 **vertebral to subclavian artery**
24.0 24.0 FUD 090 C 80 50
AMA: 1997,Nov,1; 1994,Sum,29

35694 **subclavian to carotid artery**
EXCLUDES *Subclavian to carotid artery transposition procedure (open) with concurrent repair descending thoracic aorta (endovascular) (33889)*
28.5 28.5 FUD 090 C 80 50
AMA: 1997,Nov,1; 1993,Win,1

35695 **carotid to subclavian artery**
29.7 29.7 FUD 090 C 80 50
AMA: 1997,Nov,1; 1993,Win,1

+ **35697** **Reimplantation, visceral artery to infrarenal aortic prosthesis, each artery (List separately in addition to code for primary procedure)**
EXCLUDES *Repair thoracoabdominal aortic aneurysm with graft (33877)*
Code first primary procedure
4.29 4.29 FUD ZZZ C 80
AMA: 1997,Nov,1

35700 Reoperative Bypass Lower Extremities

Code first (35556, 35566, 35570-35571, 35583, 35585, 35587, 35656, 35666, 35671)

+ **35700** **Reoperation, femoral-popliteal or femoral (popliteal)-anterior tibial, posterior tibial, peroneal artery, or other distal vessels, more than 1 month after original operation (List separately in addition to code for primary procedure)**
4.44 4.44 FUD ZZZ C 80
AMA: 2018,Jan,8; 2017,Jan,8; 2016,Jan,13; 2015,Jan,16

35701-35703 Arterial Exploration without Repair

EXCLUDES *Exploration to identify recipient artery for microvascular free graft/flap anastomosis:*
Bone (20955-20962)
Jejunum (43496)
Muscle, skin or fascia (15756-15758)
Omentum (49906)
Osteocutaneous (20969-20973)
Exploration without surgical repair:
Abdominal artery (49000)
Chest artery (32100)
Other arteries not in neck, upper or lower extremities, chest, abdomen, or retroperitoneum (37799)
Retroperitoneal artery (49010)

Code also nonvascular surgical procedures performed in addition to exploration when exploration through separate incision

35701 **Exploration not followed by surgical repair, artery; neck (eg, carotid, subclavian)**
EXCLUDES *Exploration for postoperative hemorrhage, thrombosis or infection (35800)*
Repair blood vessel on same side neck (35201, 35231, 35261)
12.6 12.6 FUD 090 C 80 50
AMA: 2019,Dec,5

35702 **upper extremity (eg, axillary, brachial, radial, ulnar)**
EXCLUDES *Exploration for postoperative hemorrhage, thrombosis or infection in same extremity (35860)*
Repair blood vessel in same extremity (35206-35207, 35236, 35266)
11.9 11.9 FUD 090 80 50
AMA: 2019,Dec,5

35703 **lower extremity (eg, common femoral, deep femoral, superficial femoral, popliteal, tibial, peroneal)**
EXCLUDES *Exploration for postoperative hemorrhage, thrombosis or infection in same extremity (35860)*
Repair blood vessel in same extremity (35256, 35286)
12.0 12.0 FUD 090 80 50
AMA: 2019,Dec,5

35800-35860 Arterial Exploration for Postoperative Complication

INCLUDES Return to operating room for postoperative hemorrhage

35800 **Exploration for postoperative hemorrhage, thrombosis or infection; neck**
20.8 20.8 FUD 090 C 80
AMA: 2019,Dec,5

35820 **chest**
58.2 58.2 FUD 090 C 80
AMA: 1997,Nov,1

35840 **abdomen**
34.8 34.8 FUD 090 C 80
AMA: 1997,May,4; 1997,Nov,1

35860 **extremity**
24.2 24.2 FUD 090 T 80
AMA: 2019,Dec,5; 2018,Jan,8; 2017,Jan,8; 2016,Jan,13; 2015,Jan,16

35870 Repair Secondary Aortoenteric Fistula

35870 **Repair of graft-enteric fistula**
36.1 36.1 FUD 090 C 80
AMA: 1997,Nov,1

35875-35876 Removal of Thrombus from Graft

EXCLUDES *Thrombectomy dialysis fistula or graft (36831, 36833)*
Thrombectomy with blood vessel repair, lower extremity, vein graft (35256)
Thrombectomy with blood vessel repair, lower extremity, with/without patch angioplasty (35226)

35875 **Thrombectomy of arterial or venous graft (other than hemodialysis graft or fistula);**
17.3 17.3 FUD 090 T A2
AMA: 2018,Jan,8; 2017,Jan,8; 2016,Jan,13; 2015,Jan,16

35876 **with revision of arterial or venous graft**
27.5 27.5 FUD 090 T A2 80
AMA: 1999,Mar,6; 1999,Nov,1

35879-35884 Revision Lower Extremity Bypass Graft

EXCLUDES *Removal infected graft (35901-35907)*
Revascularization following removal infected graft(s)
Thrombectomy dialysis fistula or graft (36831, 36833)
Thrombectomy with blood vessel repair, lower extremity, vein graft (35256)
Thrombectomy with blood vessel repair, lower extremity, with/without patch angioplasty (35226)
Thrombectomy with graft revision (35876)

35879 **Revision, lower extremity arterial bypass, without thrombectomy, open; with vein patch angioplasty**
26.8 26.8 FUD 090 T 80 50
AMA: 2018,Jan,8; 2017,Jan,8; 2016,Jan,13; 2015,Jan,16

35881 **with segmental vein interposition**
EXCLUDES *Revision femoral anastomosis synthetic arterial bypass graft (35883-35884)*
29.6 29.6 FUD 090 T 80 50
AMA: 2018,Jan,8; 2017,Jan,8; 2016,Jan,13; 2015,Jan,16

35883 **Revision, femoral anastomosis of synthetic arterial bypass graft in groin, open; with nonautogenous patch graft (eg, Dacron, ePTFE, bovine pericardium)**

EXCLUDES *Reoperation, femoral-popliteal or femoral (popliteal)-anterior tibial, posterior tibial, peroneal artery, or other distal vessels (35700)*
Revision, femoral anastomosis synthetic arterial bypass graft in groin, open; with autogenous vein patch graft (35884)
Thrombectomy arterial or venous graft (35875)

34.8 34.8 FUD 090 T 80 50

AMA: 2018,Jan,8; 2017,Jan,8; 2016,Jan,13; 2015,Jan,16

35884 **with autogenous vein patch graft**

EXCLUDES *Reoperation, femoral-popliteal or femoral (popliteal)-anterior tibial, posterior tibial, peroneal artery, or other distal vessels (35700)*
Revision, femoral anastomosis synthetic arterial bypass graft in groin, open; with autogenous vein patch graft (35883)
Thrombectomy arterial or venous graft (35875-35876)

36.0 36.0 FUD 090 T 80 50

AMA: 2018,Jan,8; 2017,Jan,8; 2016,Jan,13; 2015,Jan,16

35901-35907 Removal of Infected Graft

35901 **Excision of infected graft; neck**

13.6 13.6 FUD 090 C 80

AMA: 1997,Nov,1; 1993,Win,1

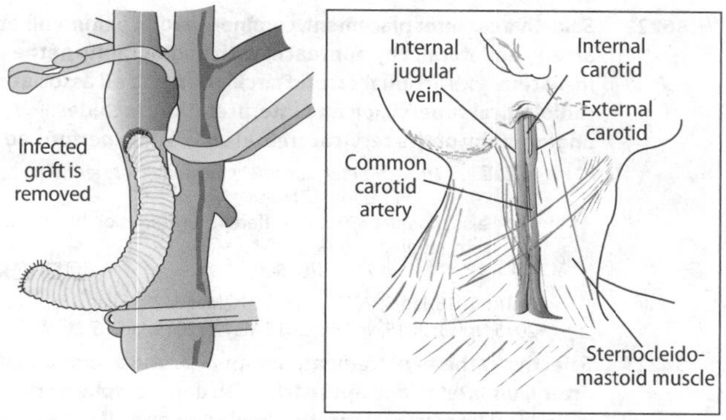

The physician removes an infected graft from the neck and repairs the blood vessel. If a new graft is placed, report the appropriate revascularization code

35903 **extremity**

16.4 16.4 FUD 090 T 80

AMA: 2018,Aug,10

35905 **thorax**

51.4 51.4 FUD 090 C 80

AMA: 1997,Nov,1; 1993,Win,1

35907 **abdomen**

55.3 55.3 FUD 090 C 80

AMA: 1997,Nov,1; 1993,Win,1

36000 Intravenous Access Established

INCLUDES Venous access for phlebotomy, prophylactic intravenous access, infusion therapy, chemotherapy, hydration, transfusion, drug administration, etc., included in primary procedure work value

36000 **Introduction of needle or intracatheter, vein**

0.26 0.79 FUD XXX N N1

AMA: 2019,Aug,8; 2018,Mar,3; 2018,Jan,8; 2017,Jan,8; 2016,Nov,3; 2016,Jan,13; 2015,Jan,16

36002 Injection Treatment of Pseudoaneurysm

INCLUDES Insertion needle or catheter, local anesthesia, contrast injection, power injections, and all pre- and postinjection care provided

EXCLUDES *Arteriotomy site sealant*
Compression repair pseudoaneurysm, ultrasound guided (76936)
Medications, contrast material, catheters

36002 **Injection procedures (eg, thrombin) for percutaneous treatment of extremity pseudoaneurysm**

(76942, 77002, 77012, 77021)

3.04 4.43 FUD 000 T G2 50

AMA: 2018,Mar,3; 2018,Jan,8; 2017,Jan,8; 2016,Nov,3; 2016,Jan,13; 2015,Jan,16

36005-36015 Insertion Needle or Intracatheter: Venous

INCLUDES Insertion needle or catheter, local anesthesia, contrast injection, power injections, and all pre- and postinjection care provided

EXCLUDES *Medications, contrast materials, catheters*

Code also catheterization second order vessels (or higher) supplied by same first order branch, same vascular family (36012)

Code also each vascular family (e.g., bilateral procedures are separate vascular families)

36005 **Injection procedure for extremity venography (including introduction of needle or intracatheter)**

(75820, 75822)

1.38 8.44 FUD 000 N N1 80 50

AMA: 2018,Mar,3; 2018,Jan,8; 2017,Jan,8; 2016,Nov,3; 2016,Jul,6; 2016,Jan,13; 2015,Jan,16

36010 **Introduction of catheter, superior or inferior vena cava**

3.19 15.0 FUD XXX N N1 50

AMA: 2018,Jan,8; 2017,Feb,14; 2017,Jan,8; 2016,Jul,6; 2016,Jan,13; 2015,Jan,16

36011 **Selective catheter placement, venous system; first order branch (eg, renal vein, jugular vein)**

4.54 24.0 FUD XXX N N1 50

AMA: 2018,Jan,8; 2017,Jan,8; 2016,Jul,6; 2016,Jan,13; 2015,Jan,16

36012 **second order, or more selective, branch (eg, left adrenal vein, petrosal sinus)**

5.04 25.0 FUD XXX N N1 50

AMA: 2018,Oct,3; 2018,Jan,8; 2017,Jan,8; 2016,Jul,6; 2016,Jan,13; 2015,Jan,16

36013 **Introduction of catheter, right heart or main pulmonary artery**

3.53 22.7 FUD XXX N N1

AMA: 2019,Jun,3; 2018,Jan,8; 2017,Jan,8; 2016,Jul,6; 2016,Jan,13; 2015,Jan,16

36014 **Selective catheter placement, left or right pulmonary artery**

4.38 23.0 FUD XXX N N1 50

AMA: 2019,Jun,3; 2018,Jan,8; 2017,Jan,8; 2016,Jul,6; 2016,Jan,13; 2015,Jan,16

36015 **Selective catheter placement, segmental or subsegmental pulmonary artery**

EXCLUDES *Placement Swan Ganz/other flow directed catheter for monitoring (93503)*
Selective blood sampling, specific organs (36500)

5.00 25.7 FUD XXX N N1 50

AMA: 2019,Jun,3; 2018,Jan,8; 2017,Jan,8; 2016,Jul,6; 2016,Jan,13; 2015,Jan,16

Cardiovascular, Hemic, and Lymphatic

35883 — 36015

36100-36218 Insertion Needle or Intracatheter: Arterial

INCLUDES Introduction catheter and catheterization all lesser order vessels used for approach
Local anesthesia, placement catheter/needle, contrast injection, power injections, all pre- and postinjection care

EXCLUDES *Angiography (36222-36228, 75600-75774)*
Angioplasty ([37246, 37247])
Chemotherapy injections (96401-96549)
Injection procedures for cardiac catheterizations (93455, 93457, 93459, 93461, 93530-93533, 93564)
Internal mammary artery angiography without left heart catheterization (36216, 36217)
Medications, contrast, catheters
Transcatheter interventions (37200, 37211, 37213-37214, 37241-37244, 61624, 61626)

Code also additional first order or higher catheterization for vascular families when vascular family supplied by first order vessel different from one already coded
Code also catheterization second and third order vessels supplied by same first order branch, same vascular family (36218, 36248)

36100 Introduction of needle or intracatheter, carotid or vertebral artery
4.54 | 14.8 | FUD XXX | N N1 50
AMA: 2000,Oct,4; 1998,Apr,1

36140 Introduction of needle or intracatheter, upper or lower extremity artery
EXCLUDES *Arteriovenous cannula insertion (36810-36821)*
2.60 | 13.6 | FUD XXX | N N1
AMA: 2018,Jan,8; 2017,Jan,8; 2016,Jan,13; 2015,Jan,16

36160 Introduction of needle or intracatheter, aortic, translumbar
3.59 | 14.6 | FUD XXX | N N1
AMA: 2018,Jan,8; 2017,Jan,8; 2016,Jan,13; 2015,Jan,16

36200 Introduction of catheter, aorta
EXCLUDES *Nonselective angiography extracranial carotid and/or cerebral vessels and cervicocerebral arch (36221)*
4.06 | 16.8 | FUD 000 | N N1 50
AMA: 2018,Jan,8; 2017,Mar,3; 2017,Jan,8; 2016,Jul,6; 2016,Jan,13; 2015,Jan,16

36215 Selective catheter placement, arterial system; each first order thoracic or brachiocephalic branch, within a vascular family
INCLUDES Introduction catheter into aorta (36200)
EXCLUDES *Placement catheter for coronary angiography (93454-93461)*
6.13 | 30.7 | FUD 000 | N N1
AMA: 2018,Jan,8; 2017,Mar,3; 2017,Jan,8; 2016,Jul,6; 2016,Jan,13; 2015,Jan,16

36216 initial second order thoracic or brachiocephalic branch, within a vascular family
7.90 | 32.5 | FUD 000 | N N1
AMA: 2018,Jan,8; 2017,Jan,8; 2016,Jul,6; 2016,Jan,13; 2015,Jan,16

36217 initial third order or more selective thoracic or brachiocephalic branch, within a vascular family
9.52 | 53.9 | FUD 000 | N N1
AMA: 2018,Jan,8; 2017,Jan,8; 2016,Jul,6; 2016,Jan,13; 2015,Jan,16

\+ **36218 additional second order, third order, and beyond, thoracic or brachiocephalic branch, within a vascular family (List in addition to code for initial second or third order vessel as appropriate)**
Code also transcatheter therapy procedures (37200, 37211, 37213-37214, 37236-37239, 37241-37244, 61624, 61626)
Code first (36216-36217, 36225-36226)
1.51 | 6.89 | FUD ZZZ | N N1
AMA: 2018,Oct,3; 2018,Jan,8; 2017,Jan,8; 2016,Jul,6; 2016,Jan,13; 2015,Jan,16

36221-36228 Diagnostic Studies: Aortic Arch/Carotid/Vertebral Arteries

INCLUDES Accessing vessel
Arterial contrast injection including arterial, capillary, and venous phase imaging, when performed
Arteriotomy closure (pressure or closure device)
Catheter placement
Radiologic supervision and interpretation
Reporting selective catheter placement based on service intensity in following hierarchy:
36226>36225
36224>36223>36222

EXCLUDES *3D rendering when performed (76376-76377)*
Interventional procedures
Ultrasound guidance (76937)

Code also diagnostic angiography upper extremities/other vascular beds during same session, when performed (75774)

36221 Non-selective catheter placement, thoracic aorta, with angiography of the extracranial carotid, vertebral, and/or intracranial vessels, unilateral or bilateral, and all associated radiological supervision and interpretation, includes angiography of the cervicocerebral arch, when performed
EXCLUDES *Selective catheter placement, common carotid or innominate artery (36222-36226)*
Transcatheter intravascular stent placement common carotid or innominate artery on same side (37217)
5.80 | 29.3 | FUD 000 | 02 N1
AMA: 2018,Jan,8; 2017,Jan,8; 2016,Mar,3; 2016,Jan,13; 2015,Nov,3; 2015,May,7; 2015,Jan,16

36222 Selective catheter placement, common carotid or innominate artery, unilateral, any approach, with angiography of the ipsilateral extracranial carotid circulation and all associated radiological supervision and interpretation, includes angiography of the cervicocerebral arch, when performed
EXCLUDES *Transcatheter placement intravascular stent(s) (37215-37218)*
Code also modifier 59 when different territories on both sides body studied
8.22 | 34.7 | FUD 000 | 02 N1 50
AMA: 2018,Jan,8; 2017,Jan,8; 2016,Mar,3; 2016,Jan,13; 2015,Nov,3; 2015,Nov,10; 2015,May,7; 2015,Jan,16

36223 Selective catheter placement, common carotid or innominate artery, unilateral, any approach, with angiography of the ipsilateral intracranial carotid circulation and all associated radiological supervision and interpretation, includes angiography of the extracranial carotid and cervicocerebral arch, when performed
EXCLUDES *Transcatheter placement intravascular stent(s) (37215-37218)*
Code also modifier 59 when different territories on both sides body studied
9.18 | 43.9 | FUD 000 | 02 N1 50
AMA: 2018,Jan,8; 2017,Jan,8; 2016,Mar,3; 2016,Jan,13; 2015,Nov,3; 2015,Jan,16

36224 Selective catheter placement, internal carotid artery, unilateral, with angiography of the ipsilateral intracranial carotid circulation and all associated radiological supervision and interpretation, includes angiography of the extracranial carotid and cervicocerebral arch, when performed
EXCLUDES *Transcatheter placement intravascular stent(s) (37215-37218)*
Code also modifier 59 when different territories on both sides body studied
10.4 | 56.8 | FUD 000 | 02 N1 50
AMA: 2018,Jan,8; 2017,Jan,8; 2016,Mar,3; 2016,Jan,13; 2015,Nov,3; 2015,Jan,16

36225 **Selective catheter placement, subclavian or innominate artery, unilateral, with angiography of the ipsilateral vertebral circulation and all associated radiological supervision and interpretation, includes angiography of the cervicocerebral arch, when performed**

EXCLUDES *Transcatheter placement intravascular stent(s) (37217)*

9.16 42.3 **FUD** 000 Q2 N1 50

AMA: 2018,Jan,8; 2017,Jan,8; 2016,Mar,3; 2016,Jan,13; 2015,Nov,3; 2015,Jan,16

36226 **Selective catheter placement, vertebral artery, unilateral, with angiography of the ipsilateral vertebral circulation and all associated radiological supervision and interpretation, includes angiography of the cervicocerebral arch, when performed**

EXCLUDES *Transcatheter placement intravascular stent(s) (37217)*

10.3 53.7 **FUD** 000 Q2 N1 50

AMA: 2018,Jan,8; 2017,Jan,8; 2016,Mar,3; 2016,Jan,13; 2015,Nov,3; 2015,Jan,16

\+ **36227** **Selective catheter placement, external carotid artery, unilateral, with angiography of the ipsilateral external carotid circulation and all associated radiological supervision and interpretation (List separately in addition to code for primary procedure)**

EXCLUDES *Reporting with modifier 50. Report once for each side when performed bilaterally*
Transcatheter placement intravascular stent(s) (37217)

Code first (36222-36224)

3.41 7.23 **FUD** ZZZ N N1 50

AMA: 2018,Jan,8; 2017,Jan,8; 2016,Jan,13; 2015,Nov,10; 2015,Jan,16

\+ **36228** **Selective catheter placement, each intracranial branch of the internal carotid or vertebral arteries, unilateral, with angiography of the selected vessel circulation and all associated radiological supervision and interpretation (eg, middle cerebral artery, posterior inferior cerebellar artery) (List separately in addition to code for primary procedure)**

EXCLUDES *Procedure performed more than two times per side*
Reporting with modifier 50. Report once for each side when performed bilaterally

Code first (36223-36226)

7.03 37.6 **FUD** ZZZ N N1 50

AMA: 2018,Jan,8; 2017,Jan,8; 2016,Jan,13; 2015,Nov,3; 2015,Jan,16

36245-36254 Catheter Placement: Arteries of the Lower Body

INCLUDES Introduction catheter and catheterization all lesser order vessels used for approach
Local anesthesia, placement catheter/needle, contrast injection, power injections

EXCLUDES *Angiography (36222-36228, 75600-75774)*
Chemotherapy injections (96401-96549)
Injection procedures for cardiac catheterizations (93455, 93457, 93459, 93461, 93530-93533, 93564)
Internal mammary artery angiography without left heart catheterization (36216-36217)
Medications, contrast, catheters
Transcatheter procedures (37200, 37211, 37213-37214, 37236-37239, 37241-37244, 61624, 61626)

Code also additional first order or higher catheterization for vascular families when vascular family supplied by first order vessel different from vessel already coded

Code also catheterization second and third order vessels supplied by same first order branch, same vascular family (36218, 36248)

(75600-75774)

36245 **Selective catheter placement, arterial system; each first order abdominal, pelvic, or lower extremity artery branch, within a vascular family**

6.89 38.1 **FUD** XXX N N1 50

AMA: 2018,Jan,8; 2017,Jan,8; 2016,Jul,6; 2016,Jan,13; 2015,Jan,16

36246 **initial second order abdominal, pelvic, or lower extremity artery branch, within a vascular family**

7.35 24.5 **FUD** 000 N N1 50

AMA: 2018,Jan,8; 2017,Jan,8; 2016,Jul,6; 2016,Jan,13; 2015,Jan,16

36247 **initial third order or more selective abdominal, pelvic, or lower extremity artery branch, within a vascular family**

8.75 43.2 **FUD** 000 N N1 50

AMA: 2020,Sep,14; 2018,Jan,8; 2017,Jan,8; 2016,Jul,6; 2016,Jan,13; 2015,Jan,16

\+ **36248** **additional second order, third order, and beyond, abdominal, pelvic, or lower extremity artery branch, within a vascular family (List in addition to code for initial second or third order vessel as appropriate)**

Code first (36246, 36247)

1.41 3.92 **FUD** ZZZ N N1

AMA: 2018,Oct,3; 2018,Jan,8; 2017,Jan,8; 2016,Jul,6; 2016,Jan,13; 2015,Jan,16

36251 **Selective catheter placement (first-order), main renal artery and any accessory renal artery(s) for renal angiography, including arterial puncture and catheter placement(s), fluoroscopy, contrast injection(s), image postprocessing, permanent recording of images, and radiological supervision and interpretation, including pressure gradient measurements when performed, and flush aortogram when performed; unilateral**

INCLUDES Closure device placement at vascular access site

EXCLUDES *Transcatheter renal sympathetic denervation, percutaneous approach (0338T-0339T)*

7.55 39.2 **FUD** 000 Q2 N1

AMA: 2018,Jan,8; 2017,Jan,8; 2016,Jan,13; 2015,Jan,16

36252 **bilateral**

INCLUDES Closure device placement at vascular access site

EXCLUDES *Transcatheter renal sympathetic denervation, percutaneous approach (0338T-0339T)*

10.4 42.4 **FUD** 000 Q2 N1

AMA: 2018,Jan,8; 2017,Jan,8; 2016,Jan,13; 2015,Jan,16

36253 **Superselective catheter placement (one or more second order or higher renal artery branches) renal artery and any accessory renal artery(s) for renal angiography, including arterial puncture, catheterization, fluoroscopy, contrast injection(s), image postprocessing, permanent recording of images, and radiological supervision and interpretation, including pressure gradient measurements when performed, and flush aortogram when performed; unilateral**

INCLUDES Closure device placement at vascular access site

EXCLUDES *Procedure performed on same kidney with (36251)*
Transcatheter renal sympathetic denervation, percutaneous approach (0338T-0339T)

10.3 62.6 **FUD** 000 Q2 N1

AMA: 2018,Jan,8; 2017,Jan,8; 2016,Jan,13; 2015,Jan,16

36254 **bilateral**

INCLUDES Closure device placement at vascular access site

EXCLUDES *Selective catheter placement (first-order), main renal artery and any accessory renal artery(s) for renal angiography (36252)*
Transcatheter renal sympathetic denervation, percutaneous approach (0338T-0339T)

12.1 60.8 **FUD** 000 Q2 N1

AMA: 2018,Jan,8; 2017,Jan,8; 2016,Jan,13; 2015,Jan,16

36260-36299 Implanted Infusion Pumps: Intra-arterial

36260 **Insertion of implantable intra-arterial infusion pump (eg, for chemotherapy of liver)**

18.8 18.8 **FUD** 090 T A2

AMA: 2018,Jan,8; 2017,Jan,8; 2016,Jan,13; 2015,Jan,16

36261 **Revision of implanted intra-arterial infusion pump**

11.7 11.7 **FUD** 090 T J8 80

AMA: 2000,Oct,4; 1997,Nov,1

36262 Removal of implanted intra-arterial infusion pump
8.96 | 8.96 | FUD 090 | 02 G2
AMA: 2000,Oct,4; 1997,Nov,1

36299 Unlisted procedure, vascular injection
0.00 | 0.00 | FUD YYY | N 80
AMA: 2000,Oct,4; 1997,Nov,1

36400-36425 Specimen Collection: Phlebotomy

EXCLUDES *Specimen collection from:*
Completely implantable device (36591)
Established catheter (36592)

36400 Venipuncture, younger than age 3 years, necessitating the skill of a physician or other qualified health care professional, not to be used for routine venipuncture; femoral or jugular vein A
0.53 | 0.75 | FUD XXX | N N1
AMA: 2018,Jan,8; 2017,Jan,8; 2016,Jan,13; 2015,Jan,16

36405 scalp vein A
0.44 | 0.66 | FUD XXX | N N1
AMA: 2018,Jan,8; 2017,Jan,8; 2016,Jan,13; 2015,Jan,16

36406 other vein A
0.25 | 0.47 | FUD XXX | N N1
AMA: 2018,Jan,8; 2017,Jan,8; 2016,Jan,13; 2015,Jan,16

36410 Venipuncture, age 3 years or older, necessitating the skill of a physician or other qualified health care professional (separate procedure), for diagnostic or therapeutic purposes (not to be used for routine venipuncture) A
0.27 | 0.49 | FUD XXX | N N1
AMA: 2019,Aug,8; 2018,Mar,3; 2018,Jan,8; 2017,Jan,8; 2016,Nov,3; 2016,Jan,13; 2015,Jan,16

36415 Collection of venous blood by venipuncture
0.00 | 0.00 | FUD XXX | 63 Q
AMA: 2019,Aug,8; 2018,Jan,8; 2017,Jan,8; 2016,Jan,13; 2015,Jan,16

36416 Collection of capillary blood specimen (eg, finger, heel, ear stick)
0.00 | 0.00 | FUD XXX | N N1
AMA: 2008,Apr,-9; 2003,Feb,7

36420 Venipuncture, cutdown; younger than age 1 year A
1.35 | 1.35 | FUD XXX | 63 Q1 N1 80
AMA: 2018,Jan,8; 2017,Jan,8; 2016,Jan,13; 2015,Jan,16

36425 age 1 or over A
EXCLUDES *Endovenous ablation therapy incompetent vein, extremity (36475-36476, 36478-36479)*
1.15 | 1.15 | FUD XXX | Q1 N1
AMA: 2018,Mar,3; 2018,Jan,8; 2017,Jan,8; 2016,Nov,3; 2016,Jan,13; 2015,Jan,16

36430-36460 Transfusions

CMS: 100-01,3,20.5 Blood Deductibles; 100-03,110.16 Transfusion in Kidney Transplants; 100-03,110.7 Blood Transfusions; 100-03,110.8 Blood Platelet Transfusions

36430 Transfusion, blood or blood components
EXCLUDES *Infant partial exchange transfusion (36456)*
0.99 | 0.99 | FUD XXX | S P3
AMA: 2020,Jun,14; 2019,Jun,5; 2018,Jan,8; 2017,Jul,3; 2017,Jan,8; 2016,Jan,13; 2015,Jan,16

36440 Push transfusion, blood, 2 years or younger A
EXCLUDES *Infant partial exchange transfusion (36456)*
1.47 | 1.47 | FUD XXX | S R2 80
AMA: 2018,Jan,8; 2017,Jul,3; 2017,Jan,8; 2016,Jan,13; 2015,Jan,16

36450 Exchange transfusion, blood; newborn A
EXCLUDES *Automated red cell exchange (36512)*
Infant partial exchange transfusion (36456)
4.93 | 4.93 | FUD XXX | 63 S R2 80
AMA: 2018,Jan,8; 2017,Jul,3

36455 other than newborn A
EXCLUDES *Automated red cell exchange (36512)*
3.68 | 3.68 | FUD XXX | S G2
AMA: 2003,Apr,7; 1997,Nov,1

36456 Partial exchange transfusion, blood, plasma or crystalloid necessitating the skill of a physician or other qualified health care professional, newborn A
EXCLUDES *Automated red cell exchange (36512)*
Transfusions other types (36430-36450)
2.93 | 2.93 | FUD XXX | 63 S 80
AMA: 2018,Jan,8; 2017,Jul,3

36460 Transfusion, intrauterine, fetal A ♀
(76941)
10.1 | 10.1 | FUD XXX | 63 S 80
AMA: 2003,Apr,7; 1997,Nov,1

36465-36466 [36465, 36466] Destruction Spider Veins

INCLUDES All supplies, equipment, compression stockings or bandages when performed in physician office

EXCLUDES *Multi-layer compression system applied to leg (29581, 29584)*
Strapping leg: ankle, foot, hip, knee, toes same extremity (29520, 29530, 29540, 29550)
Unna boot (29580)
Reporting code more than one time for each extremity treated
Vascular embolization and occlusion (37241-37244)
Vascular embolization vein in same operative field (37241)

36465 **Resequenced code. See code following 36471.**

36466 **Resequenced code. See code following 36471.**

36468 Injection(s) of sclerosant for spider veins (telangiectasia), limb or trunk
(76942)
0.00 | 0.00 | FUD 000 | Q1 N1 80
AMA: 2018,Mar,3; 2018,Jan,8; 2017,Jan,8; 2016,Nov,3; 2016,Jan,13; 2015,Apr,10; 2015,Jan,16

36470 Injection of sclerosant; single incompetent vein (other than telangiectasia)
EXCLUDES *Injection foam sclerosant with ultrasound guidance for compression maneuvers (36465-36466)*
(76942)
1.10 | 3.10 | FUD 000 | T P3 50
AMA: 2018,Dec,10; 2018,Dec,10; 2018,Mar,3; 2018,Jan,8; 2017,Jan,8; 2016,Nov,3; 2016,Jan,13; 2015,Nov,10; 2015,Apr,10; 2015,Jan,16

36471 multiple incompetent veins (other than telangiectasia), same leg
EXCLUDES *Injection foam sclerosant with ultrasound guidance for compression maneuvers (36465-36466)*
(76942)
2.21 | 5.47 | FUD 000 | T P3 50
AMA: 2018,Dec,10; 2018,Dec,10; 2018,Mar,3; 2018,Jan,8; 2017,Jan,8; 2016,Nov,3; 2016,Jan,13; 2015,Nov,10; 2015,Aug,8; 2015,Apr,10; 2015,Jan,16

36465 Injection of non-compounded foam sclerosant with ultrasound compression maneuvers to guide dispersion of the injectate, inclusive of all imaging guidance and monitoring; single incompetent extremity truncal vein (eg, great saphenous vein, accessory saphenous vein)
EXCLUDES *Ablation vein using chemical adhesive ([36482, 36483])*
Injection foam sclerosant with ultrasound guidance for compression maneuvers (36465-36466)
3.48 | 42.9 | FUD 000 | T P2 50
AMA: 2019,Feb,9; 2018,Dec,10; 2018,Dec,10; 2018,Mar,3

36466 multiple incompetent truncal veins (eg, great saphenous vein, accessory saphenous vein), same leg
EXCLUDES *Ablation vein using chemical adhesive ([36482, 36483])*
Injection foam sclerosant with ultrasound guidance for compression maneuvers (36465-36466)
4.46 | 47.6 | FUD 000 | T P2 50
AMA: 2019,Feb,9; 2018,Dec,10; 2018,Dec,10; 2018,Mar,3

36473-36483 [36482, 36483] Vein Ablation

INCLUDES Multi-layer compression system applied to leg (29581, 29584)
Patient monitoring
Radiological guidance (76000, 76937, 76942, 76998, 77002)
Venous access/injections (36000-36005, 36410, 36425)

EXCLUDES *Duplex scans (93970-93971)*
Strapping leg: ankle, foot, hip, knee, toes same extremity (29520, 29530, 29540, 29550)
Transcatheter embolization (75894)
Unna boot (29580)
Vascular embolization vein in same operative field (37241)

36473 Endovenous ablation therapy of incompetent vein, extremity, inclusive of all imaging guidance and monitoring, percutaneous, mechanochemical; first vein treated

INCLUDES Local anesthesia

EXCLUDES *Laser ablation incompetent vein (36478-36479)*
Radiofrequency ablation incompetent vein (36475-36476)

5.18 | 40.4 | FUD 000 | T P3 50

AMA: 2019,Feb,9; 2018,Mar,3; 2018,Jan,8; 2017,Jan,8; 2016,Nov,3

\+ **36474 subsequent vein(s) treated in a single extremity, each through separate access sites (List separately in addition to code for primary procedure)**

INCLUDES Local anesthesia

EXCLUDES *Laser ablation incompetent vein (36478-36479)*
Radiofrequency ablation incompetent vein (36475-36476)
Reporting code more than one time per extremity

Code first (36473)

2.60 | 8.23 | FUD ZZZ | N N1 50

AMA: 2019,Feb,9; 2018,Mar,3; 2018,Jan,8; 2017,Jan,8; 2016,Nov,3

36475 Endovenous ablation therapy of incompetent vein, extremity, inclusive of all imaging guidance and monitoring, percutaneous, radiofrequency; first vein treated

INCLUDES Tumescent anesthesia

EXCLUDES *Ablation vein using chemical adhesive ([36482, 36483])*
Endovenous ablation therapy incompetent vein (36478-36479)

8.09 | 38.9 | FUD 000 | T A2 50

AMA: 2018,Mar,3; 2018,Jan,8; 2017,Jan,8; 2016,Nov,3; 2016,Aug,3; 2016,Jan,13; 2015,Apr,10; 2015,Jan,16

\+ **36476 subsequent vein(s) treated in a single extremity, each through separate access sites (List separately in addition to code for primary procedure)**

INCLUDES Tumescent anesthesia

EXCLUDES *Ablation vein using chemical adhesive ([36482, 36483])*
Endovenous ablation therapy incompetent vein (36478-36479)
Reporting code more than one time per extremity
Vascular embolization or occlusion (37242-37244)

Code first (36475)

3.92 | 8.81 | FUD ZZZ | N N1 50

AMA: 2018,Mar,3; 2018,Jan,8; 2017,Jan,8; 2016,Nov,3; 2016,Aug,3; 2016,Jan,13; 2015,Apr,10; 2015,Jan,16

36478 Endovenous ablation therapy of incompetent vein, extremity, inclusive of all imaging guidance and monitoring, percutaneous, laser; first vein treated

INCLUDES Tumescent anesthesia

EXCLUDES *Ablation vein using chemical adhesive ([36482, 36483])*
Endovenous ablation therapy incompetent vein (36478-36479)

8.06 | 30.2 | FUD 000 | T A2 50

AMA: 2020,May,13; 2018,Mar,3; 2018,Jan,8; 2017,Jan,8; 2016,Nov,3; 2016,Aug,3; 2016,Jan,13; 2015,Apr,10; 2015,Jan,16

\+ **36479 subsequent vein(s) treated in a single extremity, each through separate access sites (List separately in addition to code for primary procedure)**

INCLUDES Tumescent anesthesia

EXCLUDES *Ablation vein using chemical adhesive ([36482, 36483])*
Endovenous ablation therapy incompetent vein (36478-36479)
Vascular embolization or occlusion (37241)

Code first (36478)

3.96 | 9.28 | FUD ZZZ | N N1 50

AMA: 2020,May,13; 2018,Mar,3; 2018,Jan,8; 2017,Jan,8; 2016,Nov,3; 2016,Aug,3; 2016,Jan,13; 2015,Apr,10; 2015,Jan,16

\# **36482 Endovenous ablation therapy of incompetent vein, extremity, by transcatheter delivery of a chemical adhesive (eg, cyanoacrylate) remote from the access site, inclusive of all imaging guidance and monitoring, percutaneous; first vein treated**

INCLUDES Local anesthesia

EXCLUDES *Laser ablation incompetent vein (36478-36479)*
Radiofrequency ablation incompetent vein (36475-36476)

5.20 | 54.0 | FUD 000 | T P3 50

AMA: 2019,Feb,9; 2018,Mar,3

\+ # **36483 subsequent vein(s) treated in a single extremity, each through separate access sites (List separately in addition to code for primary procedure)**

INCLUDES Local anesthesia

EXCLUDES *Laser ablation incompetent vein (36478-36479)*
Radiofrequency ablation incompetent vein (36475-36476)
Reporting code more than one time per extremity

Code first ([36482])

2.61 | 4.45 | FUD ZZZ | N N1 50

AMA: 2019,Feb,9; 2018,Mar,3

36481-36510 [36482, 36483] Other Venous Catheterization Procedures

EXCLUDES *Specimen collection from:*
Completely implantable device (36591)
Established catheter (36592)

36481 Percutaneous portal vein catheterization by any method

(75885, 75887)

9.56 | 54.6 | FUD 000 | N N1

AMA: 2018,Jan,8; 2017,Jan,8; 2016,Jan,13; 2015,Jan,16

36482 **Resequenced code. See code following 36479.**

36483 **Resequenced code. See code following 36479.**

36500 Venous catheterization for selective organ blood sampling

EXCLUDES *Inferior or superior vena cava catheterization (36010)*

(75893)

5.30 | 5.30 | FUD 000 | N N1

AMA: 2014,Jan,11; 1997,Nov,1

36510 Catheterization of umbilical vein for diagnosis or therapy, newborn A

EXCLUDES *Specimen collection from:*
Capillary blood (36416)
Venipuncture (36415)

1.55 | 2.36 | FUD 000 | 63 N N1 80

AMA: 2018,Jan,8; 2017,Jan,8; 2016,May,3; 2016,Jan,13; 2015,Jan,16

36511-36516 Apheresis

CMS: 100-03,110.14 Apheresis (Therapeutic Pheresis); 100-04,4,231.9 Billing for Pheresis and Apheresis Services

EXCLUDES *Specimen collection for therapeutic treatment from:*
Completely implantable device (36591)
Established catheter (36592)

36511 Therapeutic apheresis; for white blood cells

3.15 | 3.15 | FUD 000 | S G2

AMA: 2018,Jan,8; 2017,Jan,8; 2016,Jan,13; 2015,Jan,16

36512 **for red blood cells**

EXCLUDES *Manual red cell exchange (36450, 36455, 36456)*

3.12 3.12 **FUD** 000 S G2

AMA: 2018,Jan,8; 2017,Jan,8; 2016,Jan,13; 2015,Jan,16

36513 **for platelets**

EXCLUDES *Collection platelets from donors*

3.15 3.15 **FUD** 000 S R2

AMA: 2018,Jan,8; 2017,Jan,8; 2016,Jan,13; 2015,Jan,16

36514 **for plasma pheresis**

2.75 19.1 **FUD** 000 S G2

AMA: 2018,May,10; 2018,Jan,8; 2017,Jan,8; 2016,Jan,13; 2015,Jan,16

36516 **with extracorporeal immunoadsorption, selective adsorption or selective filtration and plasma reinfusion**

Code also modifier 26 for professional evaluation

2.44 55.4 **FUD** 000 S P2

AMA: 2018,Jan,8; 2017,Jan,8; 2016,Jan,13; 2015,Jan,16

36522 Extracorporeal Photopheresis

CMS: 100-03,110.4 Extracorporeal Photopheresis; 100-04,32,190 Billing for Extracorporeal Photopheresis; 100-04,32,190.2 Extracorporeal Photopheresis; 100-04,32,190.3 Medicare Denial Codes; 100-04,4,231.9 Billing for Pheresis and Apheresis Services

36522 **Photopheresis, extracorporeal**

2.79 61.2 **FUD** 000 S G2

AMA: 2018,May,10; 2018,Jan,8; 2017,Jan,8; 2016,Jan,13; 2015,Jan,16

36555-36573 [36572, 36573] Placement of Implantable Venous Access Device

INCLUDES Devices accessed by exposed catheter, or subcutaneous port or pump
Devices inserted via cutdown or percutaneous access:
Centrally (eg, femoral, jugular, subclavian veins, or inferior vena cava)
Peripherally (e.g., basilic, cephalic, saphenous vein)
Devices terminating in brachiocephalic (innominate), iliac, subclavian veins, vena cava, or right atrium

EXCLUDES *Insertion midline catheter (36400, 36406, 36410)*
Maintenance/refilling implantable pump/reservoir (96522)

Code also removal central venous access device (if code available) when new device placed through separate venous access

36555 **Insertion of non-tunneled centrally inserted central venous catheter; younger than 5 years of age** A

EXCLUDES *Peripheral insertion (36568)*

(76937, 77001)

2.44 5.35 **FUD** 000 T A2

AMA: 2019,May,3; 2018,Jan,8; 2017,Jan,8; 2016,Jan,13; 2015,Jan,16

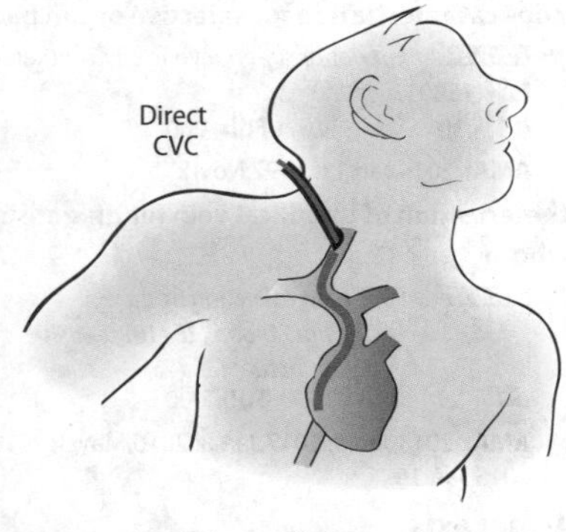

A non-tunneled centrally inserted CVC is inserted

36556 **age 5 years or older** A

EXCLUDES *Peripheral insertion (36569)*

(76937, 77001)

2.46 6.08 **FUD** 000 T A2

AMA: 2019,May,3; 2018,Nov,11; 2018,Jan,8; 2017,Jan,8; 2016,Jan,13; 2015,Jan,16

36557 **Insertion of tunneled centrally inserted central venous catheter, without subcutaneous port or pump; younger than 5 years of age** A

(76937, 77001)

9.25 31.3 **FUD** 010 T A2 80 50

AMA: 2018,Jan,8; 2017,Jan,8; 2016,Jan,13; 2015,Jan,16

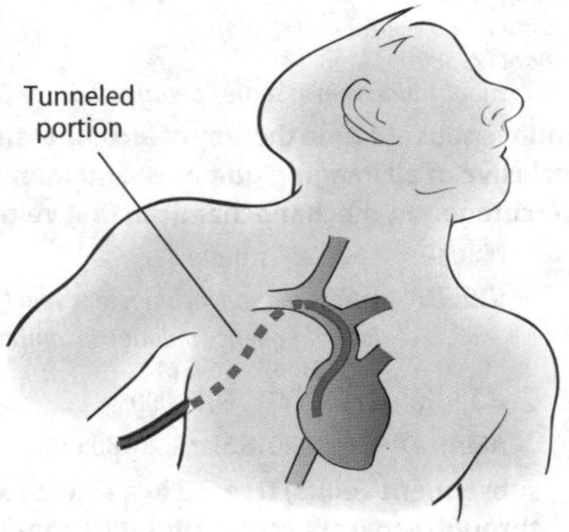

A tunneled centrally inserted CVC is inserted

36558 **age 5 years or older** A

EXCLUDES *Peripheral insertion (36571)*

(76937, 77001)

7.55 23.1 **FUD** 010 T A2 80 50

AMA: 2018,Jan,8; 2017,Jan,8; 2016,Jan,13; 2015,Jan,16; 2015,Jan,13

36560 **Insertion of tunneled centrally inserted central venous access device, with subcutaneous port; younger than 5 years of age** A

EXCLUDES *Peripheral insertion (36570)*

(76937, 77001)

11.0 37.4 **FUD** 010 T G2 80 50

AMA: 2018,Jan,8; 2017,Jan,8; 2016,Jan,13; 2015,Jan,16

36561 **age 5 years or older** A

EXCLUDES *Peripheral insertion (36571)*

(76937, 77001)

9.74 30.6 **FUD** 010 T A2 80 50

AMA: 2018,Jan,8; 2017,Jan,8; 2016,Jan,13; 2015,Jan,16

36563 **Insertion of tunneled centrally inserted central venous access device with subcutaneous pump**

(76937, 77001)

10.6 33.9 **FUD** 010 T A2 80

AMA: 2018,Jan,8; 2017,Jan,8; 2016,Jan,13; 2015,Jan,16

36565 **Insertion of tunneled centrally inserted central venous access device, requiring 2 catheters via 2 separate venous access sites; without subcutaneous port or pump (eg, Tesio type catheter)**

(76937, 77001)

9.71 25.0 **FUD** 010 T A2 80 50

AMA: 2018,Jan,8; 2017,Jan,8; 2016,Jan,13; 2015,Jan,16

36566 **with subcutaneous port(s)**

(76937, 77001)

10.4 132. **FUD** 010 T A2 80 50

AMA: 2018,Jan,8; 2017,Jan,8; 2016,Jan,13; 2015,Jan,16

36568 Insertion of peripherally inserted central venous catheter (PICC), without subcutaneous port or pump, without imaging guidance; younger than 5 years of age **Ⓐ**

> *EXCLUDES* *Centrally inserted placement (36555)*
> *Imaging guidance (76937, 77001)*
> *Peripherally inserted ([36572])*
> *PICC line removal with codes for removal tunneled central venous catheters; report appropriate E/M code*
> 🚑 2.65 ⚕ 2.65 **FUD** 000 Ⓣ A2 🔲
> **AMA:** 2019,May,3; 2018,Jan,8; 2017,Jan,8; 2016,Jan,13; 2015,Jan,16

36569 age 5 years or older **Ⓐ**

> *EXCLUDES* *Centrally inserted placement (36556)*
> *Imaging guidance (76937, 77001)*
> *Peripherally inserted ([36573])*
> *PICC line removal with codes for removal tunneled central venous catheters; report appropriate E/M code*
> 🚑 2.73 ⚕ 2.73 **FUD** 000 Ⓣ A2 🔲
> **AMA:** 2019,May,3; 2018,Jan,8; 2017,Jan,8; 2016,Jan,13; 2015,Jan,16

**36572** Insertion of peripherally inserted central venous catheter (PICC), without subcutaneous port or pump, including all imaging guidance, image documentation, and all associated radiological supervision and interpretation required to perform the insertion; younger than 5 years of age **Ⓐ**

> *INCLUDES* Verification site catheter tip (71045-71048)
> *EXCLUDES* *Centrally inserted placement (36555)*
> *Imaging guidance (76937, 77001)*
> *Peripherally inserted without imaging guidance (36568)*
> 🚑 2.62 ⚕ 12.3 **FUD** 000 G2 🔲
> **AMA:** 2019,May,3; 2019,Mar,10

**36573** age 5 years or older **Ⓐ**

> *INCLUDES* Verification site catheter tip (71045-71048)
> *EXCLUDES* *Centrally inserted placement (36556)*
> *Imaging guidance (76937, 77001)*
> *Peripherally inserted without imaging guidance (36569)*
> 🚑 2.45 ⚕ 11.3 **FUD** 000 G2 🔲
> **AMA:** 2019,May,3; 2019,Mar,10

36570 Insertion of peripherally inserted central venous access device, with subcutaneous port; younger than 5 years of age **Ⓐ**

> *EXCLUDES* *Centrally inserted placement (36560)*
> 🚑 9.61 ⚕ 42.3 **FUD** 010 Ⓣ A2 80 50 🔲
> **AMA:** 2018,Jan,8; 2017,Jan,8; 2016,Jan,13; 2015,Jan,16

36571 age 5 years or older **Ⓐ**

> *EXCLUDES* *Centrally inserted placement (36561)*
> 🚑 9.03 ⚕ 37.0 **FUD** 010 Ⓣ A2 80 50 🔲
> **AMA:** 2018,Jan,8; 2017,Jan,8; 2016,Jan,13; 2015,Jan,16

36572 **Resequenced code. See code following 36569.**

36573 **Resequenced code. See code following 36569.**

36575-36590 Repair, Removal, and Replacement Implantable Venous Access Device

> *EXCLUDES* *Mechanical removal obstructive material, pericatheter/intraluminal (36595, 36596)*
> Code also frequency of two for procedures involving both catheters from multicatheter device

36575 Repair of tunneled or non-tunneled central venous access catheter, without subcutaneous port or pump, central or peripheral insertion site

> *INCLUDES* Repair device without replacing any parts
> 🚑 1.01 ⚕ 4.57 **FUD** 000 Ⓣ A2 80 🔲
> **AMA:** 2018,Jan,8; 2017,Jan,8; 2016,Jan,13; 2015,Jan,16

36576 Repair of central venous access device, with subcutaneous port or pump, central or peripheral insertion site

> *INCLUDES* Repair device without replacing any parts
> 🚑 5.33 ⚕ 9.31 **FUD** 010 Ⓣ A2 80 🔲
> **AMA:** 2018,Jan,8; 2017,Jan,8; 2016,Jan,13; 2015,Jan,16

36578 Replacement, catheter only, of central venous access device, with subcutaneous port or pump, central or peripheral insertion site

> *INCLUDES* Partial replacement (catheter only)
> *EXCLUDES* *Total replacement entire device using same venous access sites (36582-36583)*
> 🚑 5.89 ⚕ 13.4 **FUD** 010 Ⓣ A2 80 🔲
> **AMA:** 2018,Jan,8; 2017,Jan,8; 2016,Jan,13; 2015,Jan,16

36580 Replacement, complete, of a non-tunneled centrally inserted central venous catheter, without subcutaneous port or pump, through same venous access

> *INCLUDES* Complete replacement (replace all components/same access site)
> 🚑 1.91 ⚕ 6.22 **FUD** 000 Ⓣ A2 🔲
> **AMA:** 2018,Jan,8; 2017,Jan,8; 2016,Jan,13; 2015,Jan,16

36581 Replacement, complete, of a tunneled centrally inserted central venous catheter, without subcutaneous port or pump, through same venous access

> *INCLUDES* Complete replacement (replace all components/same access site)
> *EXCLUDES* *Removal old device and insertion new device using separate venous access site*
> 🚑 5.30 ⚕ 22.9 **FUD** 010 Ⓣ A2 80 🔲
> **AMA:** 2018,Jan,8; 2017,Jan,8; 2016,Jan,13; 2015,Jan,16

36582 Replacement, complete, of a tunneled centrally inserted central venous access device, with subcutaneous port, through same venous access

> *INCLUDES* Complete replacement (replace all components/same access site)
> *EXCLUDES* *Removal old device and insertion new device using separate venous access site*
> 🚑 8.40 ⚕ 28.2 **FUD** 010 Ⓣ A2 80 🔲
> **AMA:** 2018,Jan,8; 2017,Jan,8; 2016,Jan,13; 2015,Jan,16

36583 Replacement, complete, of a tunneled centrally inserted central venous access device, with subcutaneous pump, through same venous access

> *INCLUDES* Complete replacement (replace all components/same access site)
> *EXCLUDES* *Removal old device and insertion new device using separate venous access site*
> 🚑 9.44 ⚕ 35.9 **FUD** 010 Ⓣ J8 80 🔲
> **AMA:** 2018,Jan,8; 2017,Jan,8; 2016,Jan,13; 2015,Jan,16

36584 Replacement, complete, of a peripherally inserted central venous catheter (PICC), without subcutaneous port or pump, through same venous access, including all imaging guidance, image documentation, and all associated radiological supervision and interpretation required to perform the replacement

> *INCLUDES* Complete replacement (replace all components/same access site)
> Imaging guidance (76937, 77001)
> Verification site catheter tip (71045-71048)
> *EXCLUDES* *Replacement PICC line without imaging guidance (37799)*
> 🚑 1.73 ⚕ 9.92 **FUD** 000 Ⓣ A2 🔲
> **AMA:** 2019,May,3; 2019,Mar,10; 2018,Jan,8; 2017,Jan,8; 2016,Jan,13; 2015,Jan,16

36585 Replacement, complete, of a peripherally inserted central venous access device, with subcutaneous port, through same venous access

> *INCLUDES* Complete replacement (replace all components/same access site)
> 🚑 7.86 ⚕ 31.4 **FUD** 010 Ⓣ A2 80 🔲
> **AMA:** 2018,Jan,8; 2017,Jan,8; 2016,Jan,13; 2015,Jan,16

● New Code ▲ Revised Code ○ Reinstated ● New Web Release ▲ Revised Web Release + Add-on Unlisted Not Covered # Resequenced
⑤⓪ Optum Mod 50 Exempt Ⓢ AMA Mod 51 Exempt ⑤① Optum Mod 51 Exempt ⑥③ Mod 63 Exempt ✎ Non-FDA Drug ★ Telemedicine Ⓜ Maternity Ⓐ Age Edit

36589 **Removal of tunneled central venous catheter, without subcutaneous port or pump**
INCLUDES Complete removal/all components
EXCLUDES *Non-tunneled central venous catheter removal; report appropriate E/M code*
3.97 4.76 FUD 010 Q2 A2 80
AMA: 2018,Jan,8; 2017,Jan,8; 2016,Jan,13; 2015,Nov,10; 2015,Jan,16

36590 **Removal of tunneled central venous access device, with subcutaneous port or pump, central or peripheral insertion**
INCLUDES Complete removal/all components
EXCLUDES *Non-tunneled central venous catheter removal; report appropriate E/M code*
5.51 6.40 FUD 010 Q2 A2 80
AMA: 2018,Jan,8; 2017,Jan,8; 2016,Jan,13; 2015,Jan,16

36591-36592 Obtain Blood Specimen from Implanted Device or Catheter

EXCLUDES *Use of code with any other service except laboratory services*

36591 **Collection of blood specimen from a completely implantable venous access device**
EXCLUDES *Collection:*
Capillary blood specimen (36416)
Venous blood specimen by venipuncture (36415)
0.70 0.70 FUD XXX Q1 N1 80 TC
AMA: 2019,Aug,8; 2018,Jan,8; 2017,Jan,8; 2016,Jan,13; 2015,Jan,16

36592 **Collection of blood specimen using established central or peripheral catheter, venous, not otherwise specified**
EXCLUDES *Collection blood from established arterial catheter (37799)*
0.77 0.77 FUD XXX Q1 N1 80 TC
AMA: 2018,Jan,8; 2017,Jan,8; 2016,Jan,13; 2015,Jan,16

36593-36596 Restore Patency of Occluded Catheter or Device

EXCLUDES *Venous catheterization (36010-36012)*

36593 **Declotting by thrombolytic agent of implanted vascular access device or catheter**
0.89 0.89 FUD XXX T P3 80 TC
AMA: 2018,Jan,8; 2017,Jan,8; 2016,Jan,13; 2015,Jan,16

36595 **Mechanical removal of pericatheter obstructive material (eg, fibrin sheath) from central venous device via separate venous access**
EXCLUDES *Declotting by thrombolytic agent (36593)*
(75901)
5.30 17.3 FUD 000 T G2
AMA: 2018,Jan,8; 2017,Jan,8; 2016,Jan,13; 2015,Jan,16

36596 **Mechanical removal of intraluminal (intracatheter) obstructive material from central venous device through device lumen**
EXCLUDES *Declotting by thrombolytic agent (36593)*
(75902)
1.26 3.47 FUD 000 T G2
AMA: 2018,Jan,8; 2017,Jan,8; 2016,Jan,13; 2015,Jan,16

36597-36598 Repositioning or Assessment of In Situ Venous Access Device

36597 **Repositioning of previously placed central venous catheter under fluoroscopic guidance**
(76000)
1.75 3.79 FUD 000 T G2
AMA: 2018,Jan,8; 2017,Jan,8; 2016,Jan,13; 2015,Jan,16

36598 **Contrast injection(s) for radiologic evaluation of existing central venous access device, including fluoroscopy, image documentation and report**
EXCLUDES *Complete venography studies (75820, 75825, 75827)*
Fluoroscopy (76000)
Mechanical removal pericatheter obstructive material (36595-36596)
1.07 3.44 FUD 000 T P2 80 50
AMA: 2014,Jan,11

36600-36660 Insertion Needle or Catheter: Artery

36600 **Arterial puncture, withdrawal of blood for diagnosis**
EXCLUDES *Critical care services*
0.45 0.86 FUD XXX Q1 N1
AMA: 2019,Aug,8; 2018,Jan,8; 2017,Jan,8; 2016,Jan,13; 2015,Jan,16

36620 **Arterial catheterization or cannulation for sampling, monitoring or transfusion (separate procedure); percutaneous**
1.28 1.28 FUD 000 N N1
AMA: 2018,Jan,8; 2017,Jan,8; 2016,Jan,13; 2015,Jan,16

36625 **cutdown**
3.06 3.06 FUD 000 N N1
AMA: 2018,Jan,8; 2017,Jan,8; 2016,Jan,13; 2015,Jan,16

36640 **Arterial catheterization for prolonged infusion therapy (chemotherapy), cutdown**
EXCLUDES *Intra-arterial chemotherapy (96420-96425)*
Transcatheter embolization (75894)
3.31 3.31 FUD 000 T A2
AMA: 2018,Jan,8; 2017,Jan,8; 2016,Jan,13; 2015,Jan,16

36660 **Catheterization, umbilical artery, newborn, for diagnosis or therapy** A
1.97 1.97 FUD 000 63 C 80
AMA: 2018,Jan,8; 2017,Jan,8; 2016,Jan,13; 2015,Jan,16

36680 Percutaneous Placement of Catheter/Needle into Bone Marrow Cavity

36680 **Placement of needle for intraosseous infusion**
1.74 1.74 FUD 000 Q1 N1 80
AMA: 2018,Jan,8; 2017,Jan,8; 2016,Jan,13; 2015,Jan,16

36800-36821 Vascular Access for Hemodialysis

36800 **Insertion of cannula for hemodialysis, other purpose (separate procedure); vein to vein**
3.55 3.55 FUD 000 T G2
AMA: 2018,Jan,8; 2017,Jan,8; 2016,Jan,13; 2015,Jan,16

36810 **arteriovenous, external (Scribner type)**
6.11 6.11 FUD 000 T A2
AMA: 2018,Jan,8; 2017,Jan,8; 2016,Jan,13; 2015,Jan,16

36815 **arteriovenous, external revision, or closure**
3.92 3.92 FUD 000 T A2
AMA: 2018,Jan,8; 2017,Jan,8; 2016,Jan,13; 2015,Jan,16

36818 **Arteriovenous anastomosis, open; by upper arm cephalic vein transposition**
INCLUDES Two incisions in upper arm: medial incision over brachial artery and lateral incision for exposure to portion of cephalic vein
EXCLUDES *When performed unilaterally with:*
Arteriovenous anastomosis, open (36819-36820)
Creation arteriovenous fistula by other than direct arteriovenous anastomosis (36830)
Code also modifier 50 or 59, as appropriate, for bilateral procedure
20.1 20.1 FUD 090 T A2 80
AMA: 2018,Jan,8; 2017,Mar,3; 2017,Jan,8; 2016,Mar,10; 2016,Jan,13; 2015,Jan,16

36819 **by upper arm basilic vein transposition**

EXCLUDES *When performed unilaterally with:*
Arteriovenous anastomosis, open (36818, 36820-36821)
Creation arteriovenous fistula by other than direct arteriovenous anastomosis (36830)

Code also modifier 50 or 59, as appropriate, for bilateral procedure

21.2 21.2 **FUD** 090 T A2 80

AMA: 2018,Jan,8; 2017,Mar,3; 2017,Jan,8; 2016,Jan,13; 2015,Jan,16

36820 **by forearm vein transposition**

21.2 21.2 **FUD** 090 T A2 80 50

AMA: 2018,Jan,8; 2017,Mar,3; 2017,Jan,8; 2016,Jan,13; 2015,Jan,16

36821 **direct, any site (eg, Cimino type) (separate procedure)**

19.3 19.3 **FUD** 090 T A2 80

AMA: 2018,Jan,8; 2017,Mar,3; 2017,Jan,8; 2016,Jan,13; 2015,Aug,8; 2015,Jan,16

36823 Vascular Access for Extracorporeal Circulation

INCLUDES Chemotherapy perfusion

EXCLUDES *Chemotherapy administration (96409-96425)*
Maintenance for extracorporeal circulation (33946-33949)

36823 **Insertion of arterial and venous cannula(s) for isolated extracorporeal circulation including regional chemotherapy perfusion to an extremity, with or without hyperthermia, with removal of cannula(s) and repair of arteriotomy and venotomy sites**

40.7 40.7 **FUD** 090 C

AMA: 2018,Jan,8; 2017,Mar,3

36825-36835 Permanent Vascular Access Procedures

36825 **Creation of arteriovenous fistula by other than direct arteriovenous anastomosis (separate procedure); autogenous graft**

EXCLUDES *Direct arteriovenous (AV) anastomosis (36821)*

23.0 23.0 **FUD** 090 T A2 80

AMA: 2018,Jan,8; 2017,Mar,3; 2017,Jan,8; 2016,Jan,13; 2015,Jan,16

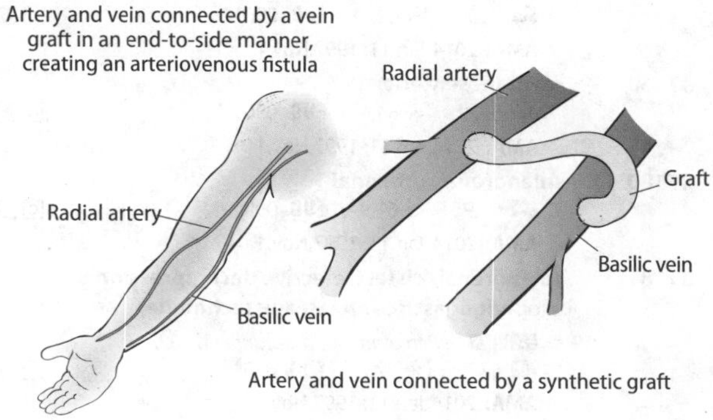
Artery and vein connected by a vein graft in an end-to-side manner, creating an arteriovenous fistula
Radial artery
Graft
Radial artery
Basilic vein
Basilic vein
Artery and vein connected by a synthetic graft

36830 **nonautogenous graft (eg, biological collagen, thermoplastic graft)**

EXCLUDES *Direct arteriovenous (AV) anastomosis (36821)*

19.4 19.4 **FUD** 090 T A2 80

AMA: 2018,Jan,8; 2017,Mar,3; 2017,Jan,8; 2016,Jan,13; 2015,Jan,16; 2015,Jan,13

36831 **Thrombectomy, open, arteriovenous fistula without revision, autogenous or nonautogenous dialysis graft (separate procedure)**

17.9 17.9 **FUD** 090 T A2 80

AMA: 2018,Jan,8; 2017,Mar,3; 2017,Jan,8; 2016,Jan,13; 2015,Jan,16

36832 **Revision, open, arteriovenous fistula; without thrombectomy, autogenous or nonautogenous dialysis graft (separate procedure)**

INCLUDES Revision arteriovenous access fistula or graft

21.9 21.9 **FUD** 090 T A2 80

AMA: 2018,Jan,8; 2017,Mar,3; 2017,Jan,8; 2016,Jan,13; 2015,Jan,16

36833 **with thrombectomy, autogenous or nonautogenous dialysis graft (separate procedure)**

EXCLUDES *Hemodialysis circuit procedures (36901-36906)*

23.5 23.5 **FUD** 090 T A2 80

AMA: 2018,Jan,8; 2017,Mar,3; 2017,Jan,8; 2016,Jan,13; 2015,Jan,16

36835 **Insertion of Thomas shunt (separate procedure)**

13.8 13.8 **FUD** 090 T J8

AMA: 2014,Jan,11; 1997,Nov,1

36838 DRIL Procedure for Ischemic Steal Syndrome

EXCLUDES *Bypass graft, with vein (35512, 35522-35523)*
Ligation (37607, 37618)
Revision, open, arteriovenous fistula (36832)

36838 **Distal revascularization and interval ligation (DRIL), upper extremity hemodialysis access (steal syndrome)**

33.3 33.3 **FUD** 090 T 80 50

AMA: 2014,Jan,11; 1997,Nov,1

36860-36861 Restore Patency of Occluded Cannula or Arteriovenous Fistula

36860 **External cannula declotting (separate procedure); without balloon catheter**

(76000)

3.23 7.05 **FUD** 000 T A2

AMA: 2018,Jan,8; 2017,Jan,8; 2016,Jan,13; 2015,Jan,16

36861 **with balloon catheter**

(76000)

4.05 4.05 **FUD** 000 T A2

AMA: 2018,Jan,8; 2017,Jan,8; 2016,Jan,13; 2015,Jan,16

36901-36909 Hemodialysis Circuit Procedures

EXCLUDES *Arteriography to assess inflow to hemodialysis circuit when performed (76937)*

36901 **Introduction of needle(s) and/or catheter(s), dialysis circuit, with diagnostic angiography of the dialysis circuit, including all direct puncture(s) and catheter placement(s), injection(s) of contrast, all necessary imaging from the arterial anastomosis and adjacent artery through entire venous outflow including the inferior or superior vena cava, fluoroscopic guidance, radiological supervision and interpretation and image documentation and report;**

INCLUDES Access
Catheter advancement (e.g., imaging of accessory veins, assess all circuit sections)
Contrast injection

EXCLUDES *Balloon angioplasty peripheral segment (36902)*
Open revision with thrombectomy arteriovenous fistula (36833)
Percutaneous transluminal procedures peripheral segment (36904-36906)
Stent placement in peripheral segment (36903)
Reporting code more than one time per procedure

4.90 16.9 **FUD** 000 T P3

AMA: 2018,Jan,8; 2017,Mar,3

36902 **with transluminal balloon angioplasty, peripheral dialysis segment, including all imaging and radiological supervision and interpretation necessary to perform the angioplasty**

EXCLUDES *Open revision with thrombectomy arteriovenous fistula (36833)*
Percutaneous transluminal procedures peripheral segment (36904-36906)
Stent placement in peripheral segment (36903)
Reporting code more than one time per procedure

6.94 36.9 FUD 000 J G2

AMA: 2018,Jan,8; 2017,Jul,3; 2017,Mar,3

36903 **with transcatheter placement of intravascular stent(s), peripheral dialysis segment, including all imaging and radiological supervision and interpretation necessary to perform the stenting, and all angioplasty within the peripheral dialysis segment**

INCLUDES Balloon angioplasty peripheral segment (36902)

EXCLUDES *Central hemodialysis circuit procedures (36907-36908)*
Open revision with thrombectomy arteriovenous fistula (36833)
Percutaneous transluminal procedures peripheral segment (36904-36906)
Reporting code more than one time per procedure

9.20 146. FUD 000 J J8

AMA: 2018,Jan,8; 2017,Jul,3; 2017,Mar,3

36904 **Percutaneous transluminal mechanical thrombectomy and/or infusion for thrombolysis, dialysis circuit, any method, including all imaging and radiological supervision and interpretation, diagnostic angiography, fluoroscopic guidance, catheter placement(s), and intraprocedural pharmacological thrombolytic injection(s);**

EXCLUDES *Open thrombectomy arteriovenous fistula with/without revision (36831, 36833)*
Reporting code more than one time per procedure

10.7 54.7 FUD 000 J J8

AMA: 2018,Jan,8; 2017,Jul,3; 2017,Mar,3

36905 **with transluminal balloon angioplasty, peripheral dialysis segment, including all imaging and radiological supervision and interpretation necessary to perform the angioplasty**

INCLUDES Percutaneous mechanical thrombectomy (36904)

EXCLUDES *Reporting code more than one time per procedure*

12.8 68.7 FUD 000 J G2

AMA: 2018,Jan,8; 2017,Jul,3; 2017,Mar,3

36906 **with transcatheter placement of intravascular stent(s), peripheral dialysis segment, including all imaging and radiological supervision and interpretation necessary to perform the stenting, and all angioplasty within the peripheral dialysis circuit**

INCLUDES Percutaneous transluminal balloon angioplasty (36905)
Percutaneous transluminal thrombectomy (36904)

EXCLUDES *Hemodialysis circuit procedures provided by catheter or needle access (36901-36903)*
Reporting code more than one time per procedure

Code also balloon angioplasty central veins, when performed (36907)

Code also stent placement in central veins, when performed (36908)

14.9 193. FUD 000 J J8

AMA: 2018,Jan,8; 2017,Jul,3; 2017,Mar,3

\+ **36907** **Transluminal balloon angioplasty, central dialysis segment, performed through dialysis circuit, including all imaging and radiological supervision and interpretation required to perform the angioplasty (List separately in addition to code for primary procedure)**

INCLUDES All central hemodialysis segment angiography

EXCLUDES *Angiography with stent placement (36908)*

Code first (36818-36833, 36901-36906)

4.25 19.6 FUD ZZZ N N1

AMA: 2018,Jan,8; 2017,Jul,3; 2017,Mar,3

\+ **36908** **Transcatheter placement of intravascular stent(s), central dialysis segment, performed through dialysis circuit, including all imaging and radiological supervision and interpretation required to perform the stenting, and all angioplasty in the central dialysis segment (List separately in addition to code for primary procedure)**

INCLUDES All central hemodialysis segment stent(s) placed
Balloon angioplasty central dialysis segment (36907)

Code first when performed (36818-36833, 36901-36906)

6.02 59.6 FUD ZZZ N N1

AMA: 2018,Jan,8; 2017,Jul,3; 2017,Mar,3

\+ **36909** **Dialysis circuit permanent vascular embolization or occlusion (including main circuit or any accessory veins), endovascular, including all imaging and radiological supervision and interpretation necessary to complete the intervention (List separately in addition to code for primary procedure)**

INCLUDES All embolization/occlusion procedures performed in hemodialysis circuit

EXCLUDES *Banding/ligation arteriovenous fistula (37607)*
Reporting code more than one time per day

Code first (36901-36906)

5.83 56.8 FUD ZZZ N N1

AMA: 2018,Jan,8; 2017,Mar,3

37140-37181 Open Decompression of Portal Circulation

EXCLUDES *Peritoneal-venous shunt (49425)*

37140 **Venous anastomosis, open; portocaval**

67.7 67.7 FUD 090 C

AMA: 2014,Jan,11; 1997,Nov,1

37145 **renoportal**

62.7 62.7 FUD 090 C 80

AMA: 2014,Jan,11; 1997,Nov,1

37160 **caval-mesenteric**

64.4 64.4 FUD 090 C 80

AMA: 2014,Jan,11; 1997,Nov,1

37180 **splenorenal, proximal**

61.9 61.9 FUD 090 C 80

AMA: 2014,Jan,11; 1997,Nov,1

37181 **splenorenal, distal (selective decompression of esophagogastric varices, any technique)**

EXCLUDES *Percutaneous procedure (37182)*

67.7 67.7 FUD 090 C 80

AMA: 2014,Jan,11; 1997,Nov,1

37182-37183 Transvenous Decompression of Portal Circulation

INCLUDES Percutaneous transhepatic portography (75885, 75887)

37182 **Insertion of transvenous intrahepatic portosystemic shunt(s) (TIPS) (includes venous access, hepatic and portal vein catheterization, portography with hemodynamic evaluation, intrahepatic tract formation/dilatation, stent placement and all associated imaging guidance and documentation)**

EXCLUDES *Open procedure (37140)*

23.7 23.7 FUD 000 C 80

AMA: 2018,Jan,8; 2017,Jan,8; 2016,Jan,13; 2015,Jan,16

37183 **Revision of transvenous intrahepatic portosystemic shunt(s) (TIPS) (includes venous access, hepatic and portal vein catheterization, portography with hemodynamic evaluation, intrahepatic tract recanulization/dilatation, stent placement and all associated imaging guidance and documentation)**

EXCLUDES *Arteriovenous (AV) aneurysm repair (36832)*

10.8 176. FUD 000 J 80

AMA: 2018,Jan,8; 2017,Jan,8; 2016,Jan,13; 2015,Jan,16

37184-37188 Removal of Thrombus from Vessel: Percutaneous

INCLUDES Fluoroscopic guidance (76000)
Injection(s) thrombolytics during procedure
Postprocedure evaluation
Pretreatment planning

EXCLUDES *Catheter placement*
Continuous infusion thrombolytics prior to and after procedure (37211-37214)
Diagnostic studies
Intracranial arterial mechanical thrombectomy or infusion (61645)
Mechanical thrombectomy, coronary (92973)
Other interventions performed percutaneously (e.g., balloon angioplasty)
Radiological supervision/interpretation

37184 **Primary percutaneous transluminal mechanical thrombectomy, noncoronary, non-intracranial, arterial or arterial bypass graft, including fluoroscopic guidance and intraprocedural pharmacological thrombolytic injection(s); initial vessel**

EXCLUDES *Intracranial arterial mechanical thrombectomy (61645)*
Mechanical thrombectomy another vascular family/separate access site, append modifier 59 to primary service
Mechanical thrombectomy for embolus/thrombus complicating another percutaneous interventional procedure (37186)
Therapeutic, prophylactic, or diagnostic injection (96374)

12.9 60.2 FUD 000 J J8 50

AMA: 2019,Sep,5; 2018,Jan,8; 2017,Jan,8; 2016,Jul,6; 2016,Mar,3; 2016,Jan,13; 2015,Nov,3; 2015,Apr,10; 2015,Jan,16

\+ **37185** **second and all subsequent vessel(s) within the same vascular family (List separately in addition to code for primary mechanical thrombectomy procedure)**

INCLUDES Treatment second and all succeeding vessel(s) in same vascular family

EXCLUDES *Intravenous drug injections administered subsequent to initial service*
Mechanical thrombectomy another vascular family/separate access site, append modifier 59 to primary service
Therapeutic, prophylactic, or diagnostic injection (96375)

Code first (37184)

4.77 16.9 FUD ZZZ N N1

AMA: 2019,Sep,5; 2018,Jan,8; 2017,Jan,8; 2016,Jul,6; 2016,Jan,13; 2015,Nov,3; 2015,Apr,10; 2015,Jan,16

\+ **37186** **Secondary percutaneous transluminal thrombectomy (eg, nonprimary mechanical, snare basket, suction technique), noncoronary, non-intracranial, arterial or arterial bypass graft, including fluoroscopic guidance and intraprocedural pharmacological thrombolytic injections, provided in conjunction with another percutaneous intervention other than primary mechanical thrombectomy (List separately in addition to code for primary procedure)**

INCLUDES Removal small emboli/thrombi prior to or after another percutaneous procedure

EXCLUDES *Primary percutaneous transluminal mechanical thrombectomy, noncoronary, non-intracranial (37184-37185)*
Therapeutic, prophylactic, or diagnostic injection (96375)

Code first primary procedure

7.10 37.4 FUD ZZZ N N1

AMA: 2019,Sep,5; 2018,Jan,8; 2017,Jan,8; 2016,Jul,6; 2016,Jan,13; 2015,Nov,3; 2015,Jan,16

37187 **Percutaneous transluminal mechanical thrombectomy, vein(s), including intraprocedural pharmacological thrombolytic injections and fluoroscopic guidance**

INCLUDES Secondary or subsequent intravenous injection after another initial service

EXCLUDES *Therapeutic, prophylactic, or diagnostic injection (96375)*

11.4 55.0 FUD 000 J J8 50

AMA: 2018,Jan,8; 2017,Jan,8; 2016,Jul,6; 2016,Mar,3; 2016,Jan,13; 2015,Nov,3; 2015,Jan,16

37188 **Percutaneous transluminal mechanical thrombectomy, vein(s), including intraprocedural pharmacological thrombolytic injections and fluoroscopic guidance, repeat treatment on subsequent day during course of thrombolytic therapy**

EXCLUDES *Therapeutic, prophylactic, or diagnostic injection (96375)*

8.10 46.3 FUD 000 T G2 50

AMA: 2018,Jan,8; 2017,Jan,8; 2016,Jul,6; 2016,Mar,3; 2016,Jan,13; 2015,Nov,3; 2015,Jan,16

37191-37193 Vena Cava Filters

37191 **Insertion of intravascular vena cava filter, endovascular approach including vascular access, vessel selection, and radiological supervision and interpretation, intraprocedural roadmapping, and imaging guidance (ultrasound and fluoroscopy), when performed**

EXCLUDES *Open ligation inferior vena cava via laparotomy or retroperitoneal approach (37619)*

6.49 69.9 FUD 000 T

AMA: 2018,Jan,8; 2017,Feb,14; 2017,Jan,8; 2016,May,11; 2016,Jan,13; 2015,Jan,16

37192 **Repositioning of intravascular vena cava filter, endovascular approach including vascular access, vessel selection, and radiological supervision and interpretation, intraprocedural roadmapping, and imaging guidance (ultrasound and fluoroscopy), when performed**

EXCLUDES *Insertion intravascular vena cava filter (37191)*

9.98 37.4 FUD 000 T

AMA: 2018,Jan,8; 2017,Jan,8; 2016,May,11; 2016,Jan,13; 2015,Jan,16

37193 **Retrieval (removal) of intravascular vena cava filter, endovascular approach including vascular access, vessel selection, and radiological supervision and interpretation, intraprocedural roadmapping, and imaging guidance (ultrasound and fluoroscopy), when performed**

EXCLUDES *Transcatheter retrieval intravascular foreign body, percutaneous (37197)*

10.1 44.0 FUD 000 T

AMA: 2018,Jan,8; 2017,Jan,8; 2016,May,11; 2016,Jan,13; 2015,Jan,16

37195 Intravenous Cerebral Thrombolysis

37195 **Thrombolysis, cerebral, by intravenous infusion**

0.00 0.00 FUD XXX T 80

AMA: 2020,Jan,12

37197-37214 Transcatheter Procedures: Infusions, Biopsy, Foreign Body Removal

37197 **Transcatheter retrieval, percutaneous, of intravascular foreign body (eg, fractured venous or arterial catheter), includes radiological supervision and interpretation, and imaging guidance (ultrasound or fluoroscopy), when performed**

EXCLUDES *Percutaneous vena cava filter retrieval (37193)*
Removal leadless pacemaker system ([33275])

8.78 43.4 FUD 000 T G2

AMA: 2018,Jan,8; 2017,Feb,14; 2017,Jan,8; 2016,May,11; 2016,Jan,13; 2015,Jan,16

37200 Transcatheter biopsy

(75970)
6.30 6.30 FUD 000 T G2

AMA: 2014,Jan,11; 1998,Nov,1

37211 Transcatheter therapy, arterial infusion for thrombolysis other than coronary or intracranial, any method, including radiological supervision and interpretation, initial treatment day

INCLUDES Catheter change or position change
E/M services on day of and related to thrombolysis
First day transcatheter thrombolytic infusion
Fluoroscopic guidance
Follow-up arteriography or venography
Radiologic supervision and interpretation

EXCLUDES *Angiography through existing catheter for follow-up study for transcatheter therapy, embolization, or infusion, other than for thrombolysis (75898)*
Catheter placement
Declotting implanted catheter or vascular access device by thrombolytic agent (36593)
Diagnostic studies
Intracranial arterial mechanical thrombectomy or infusion (61645)
Percutaneous interventions
Procedure performed more than one time per date of service
Ultrasound guidance (76937)

Code also significant, separately identifiable E/M service on day of thrombolysis using modifier 25

11.2 11.2 FUD 000 T G2 50

AMA: 2019,Sep,6; 2018,Jan,8; 2017,Jan,8; 2016,Jul,6; 2016,Mar,3; 2016,Jan,13; 2015,Nov,3; 2015,Jan,16

37212 Transcatheter therapy, venous infusion for thrombolysis, any method, including radiological supervision and interpretation, initial treatment day

INCLUDES Catheter change or position change
E/M services on day of and related to thrombolysis

EXCLUDES *Angiography through existing catheter for follow-up study for transcatheter therapy, embolization, or infusion, other than for thrombolysis (75898)*
Catheter placement
First day transcatheter thrombolytic infusion
Declotting implanted catheter or vascular access device by thrombolytic agent (36593)
Fluoroscopic guidance
Follow-up arteriography or venography
Diagnostic studies
Initiation and completion thrombolysis on same date of service
Percutaneous interventions
Radiologic supervision and interpretation
Procedure performed more than one time per date of service
Ultrasound guidance (76937)

Code also significant, separately identifiable E/M service on day of thrombolysis using modifier 25

9.81 9.81 FUD 000 T G2 50

AMA: 2019,Sep,6; 2018,Jan,8; 2017,Jan,8; 2016,Jul,6; 2016,Mar,3; 2016,Jan,13; 2015,Nov,3; 2015,Jan,16

37213 Transcatheter therapy, arterial or venous infusion for thrombolysis other than coronary, any method, including radiological supervision and interpretation, continued treatment on subsequent day during course of thrombolytic therapy, including follow-up catheter contrast injection, position change, or exchange, when performed;

INCLUDES Continued thrombolytic infusions on subsequent days besides initial and last days of treatment
E/M services on day of and related to thrombolysis
Fluoroscopic guidance
Radiologic supervision and interpretation

EXCLUDES *Angiography through existing catheter for follow-up study for transcatheter therapy, embolization, or infusion, other than for thrombolysis (75898)*
Catheter placement
Declotting implanted catheter or vascular access device by thrombolytic agent (36593)
Diagnostic studies
Percutaneous interventions
Procedure performed more than one time per date of service
Ultrasound guidance (76937)

Code also significant, separately identifiable E/M service on day of thrombolysis using modifier 25

6.76 6.76 FUD 000 T

AMA: 2019,Sep,6; 2018,Jan,8; 2017,Jan,8; 2016,Jul,6; 2016,Mar,3; 2016,Jan,13; 2015,Nov,3; 2015,Jan,16

37214 cessation of thrombolysis including removal of catheter and vessel closure by any method

INCLUDES E/M services on day of and related to thrombolysis
Fluoroscopic guidance
Last day transcatheter thrombolytic infusions
Radiologic supervision and interpretation

EXCLUDES *Angiography through existing catheter for follow-up study for transcatheter therapy, embolization, or infusion, other than for thrombolysis (75898)*
Catheter placement
Declotting implanted catheter or vascular access device by thrombolytic agent (36593)
Diagnostic studies
Percutaneous interventions
Procedure performed more than one time per date of service
Ultrasound guidance (76937)

Code also significant, separately identifiable E/M service on day of thrombolysis using modifier 25

3.57 3.57 FUD 000 T

AMA: 2019,Sep,6; 2018,Jan,8; 2017,Jan,8; 2016,Jul,6; 2016,Mar,3; 2016,Jan,13; 2015,Nov,3; 2015,Jan,16

37215-37216 Stenting of Cervical Carotid Artery with/without Insertion Distal Embolic Protection Device

INCLUDES Carotid stenting, if required
Ipsilateral cerebral and cervical carotid diagnostic imaging/supervision and interpretation
Ipsilateral selective carotid catheterization

EXCLUDES *Carotid catheterization and imaging, if carotid stenting not required*
Selective catheter placement, common carotid or innominate artery (36222-36224)
Transcatheter placement extracranial vertebral artery stents, open or percutaneous (0075T, 0076T)

37215 Transcatheter placement of intravascular stent(s), cervical carotid artery, open or percutaneous, including angioplasty, when performed, and radiological supervision and interpretation; with distal embolic protection

29.2 29.2 **FUD** 090 C 80 50

AMA: 2018,Jan,8; 2017,Jul,3; 2017,Jan,8; 2016,Jan,13; 2015,Jan,16

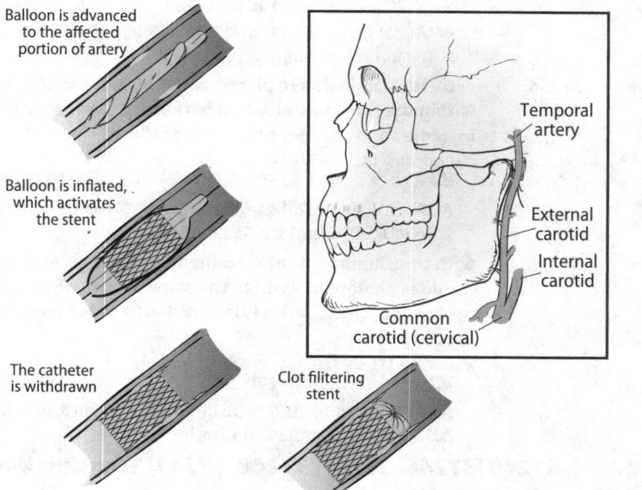
Balloon is advanced to the affected portion of artery
Balloon is inflated, which activates the stent
The catheter is withdrawn
Clot filitering stent
Temporal artery
External carotid
Internal carotid
Common carotid (cervical)

37216 without distal embolic protection

28.2 28.2 **FUD** 090 E

AMA: 2018,Jan,8; 2017,Jul,3; 2017,Jan,8; 2016,Jan,13; 2015,Jan,16

37217-37218 Stenting of Intrathoracic Carotid Artery/Innominate Artery

INCLUDES Access to vessel (open)
Arteriotomy closure by suture
Catheterization vessel (selective) (36222-36227)
Imaging during and after procedure
Radiological supervision and interpretation

EXCLUDES *Carotid artery revascularization procedures when performed during same session*
Transcatheter insertion extracranial vertebral artery stents, open or percutaneous (0075T-0076T)
Transcatheter insertion intracranial stents (61635)
Transcatheter insertion intravascular cervical carotid artery stents, open or percutaneous (37215-37216)

37217 Transcatheter placement of intravascular stent(s), intrathoracic common carotid artery or innominate artery by retrograde treatment, open ipsilateral cervical carotid artery exposure, including angioplasty, when performed, and radiological supervision and interpretation

INCLUDES When performed on same side:
Direct repair blood vessel, neck (35201)
Nonselective catheterization, thoracic aorta (36221)
Transluminal balloon angioplasty (37246-37247 [37246, 37247])

31.3 31.3 **FUD** 090 C 80 50

AMA: 2018,Jan,8; 2017,Jul,3; 2017,Jan,8; 2016,Jan,13; 2015,May,7; 2015,Jan,16

37218 Transcatheter placement of intravascular stent(s), intrathoracic common carotid artery or innominate artery, open or percutaneous antegrade approach, including angioplasty, when performed, and radiological supervision and interpretation

EXCLUDES *Selective catheter placement, common carotid or innominate artery (36222-36224)*

23.7 23.7 **FUD** 090 C 80 50

AMA: 2018,Jan,8; 2017,Jul,3; 2017,Jan,8; 2016,Jan,13; 2015,May,7

37220-37235 Endovascular Revascularization Lower Extremities

INCLUDES Percutaneous and open interventional and associated procedures for lower extremity occlusive disease; unilateral
Accessing vessel
Arteriotomy closure by suturing puncture or pressure with arterial closure device application
Atherectomy (e.g., directional, laser, rotational)
Balloon angioplasty (e.g., cryoplasty, cutting balloon, low-profile)
Catheterization vessel (selective)
Embolic protection
Imaging once procedure complete
Radiological supervision and interpretation
Stenting (e.g., bare metal, balloon-expandable, covered, drug-eluting, self-expanding)
Traversing lesion
Reporting most comprehensive treatment in given vessel according to following hierarchy:
1. Stent and atherectomy
2. Atherectomy
3. Stent
4. PTA
Revascularization procedures for three arterial vascular territories:
Femoral/popliteal vascular territory including common, deep, and superficial femoral arteries, and popliteal artery (one extremity = a single vessel) (37224-37227)
Iliac vascular territory: common iliac, external iliac, internal iliac (37220-37223)
Tibial/peroneal territory: includes anterior tibial, peroneal artery, posterior tibial (37228-37235)

EXCLUDES *Assignment more than one code from this family for each lower extremity vessel treated*
Assignment more than one code when multiple vessels are treated in femoral/popliteal territory (report most complex service for more than one lesion in territory); when contiguous lesion that spans from one territory to another can be opened with single procedure; or when more than one stent deployed in same vessel
Extensive repair or replacement artery (35226, 35286)
Mechanical thrombectomy and/or thrombolysis

Code also add-on codes for different vessels, but not different lesions in same vessel; and for multiple territories in same leg
Code also modifier 59 if same territory(ies) both legs are treated during same surgical session
Code first one primary code for initial service in each leg

37220 Revascularization, endovascular, open or percutaneous, iliac artery, unilateral, initial vessel; with transluminal angioplasty

Code also only when transluminal angioplasty performed outside treatment target zone of (34701-34708, 34709, [34718], 34710-34711, 34845-34848)

11.6 83.7 **FUD** 000 J G2 50

AMA: 2019,Jun,14; 2018,Jan,8; 2017,Jul,3; 2017,Jan,8; 2016,Jul,8; 2016,Jan,13; 2015,Jan,16

37221 with transluminal stent placement(s), includes angioplasty within the same vessel, when performed

Code also only when transluminal angioplasty performed outside treatment target zone of (34701-34708, 34709, [34718], 34710-34711, 34845-34848)

14.3 111. **FUD** 000 J J8 80 50

AMA: 2019,Jun,14; 2018,Jan,8; 2017,Dec,3; 2017,Jul,3; 2017,Jan,8; 2016,Jul,6; 2016,Jul,8; 2016,Jan,13; 2015,Jan,13; 2015,Jan,16

+ **37222** **Revascularization, endovascular, open or percutaneous, iliac artery, each additional ipsilateral iliac vessel; with transluminal angioplasty (List separately in addition to code for primary procedure)**

Code also only when transluminal angioplasty performed outside treatment target zone of (34701-34708, 34709, [34718], 34710-34711, 34845-34848)

Code first (37220-37221)

5.42 21.2 **FUD** ZZZ N N1 80 50

AMA: 2019,Jun,14; 2018,Jan,8; 2017,Jul,3; 2017,Jan,8; 2016,Jul,8; 2016,Jan,13; 2015,Jan,16

+ **37223** **with transluminal stent placement(s), includes angioplasty within the same vessel, when performed (List separately in addition to code for primary procedure)**

Code also only when transluminal angioplasty performed outside treatment target zone of (34701-34708, 34709, [34718], 34710-34711, 34845-34848)

Code first (37221)

6.20 62.6 **FUD** ZZZ N N1 80 50

AMA: 2019,Jun,14; 2018,Jan,8; 2017,Dec,3; 2017,Jul,3; 2017,Jan,8; 2016,Jul,8; 2016,Jul,6; 2016,Jan,13; 2015,Jan,16

37224 **Revascularization, endovascular, open or percutaneous, femoral, popliteal artery(s), unilateral; with transluminal angioplasty**

EXCLUDES *Revascularization with intravascular stent grafts in femoral-popliteal segment (0505T)*

12.9 97.6 **FUD** 000 J J8 80 50

AMA: 2019,Jun,14; 2018,Jan,8; 2017,Jul,3; 2017,Jan,8; 2016,Jul,8; 2016,Jan,13; 2015,Jan,16

37225 **with atherectomy, includes angioplasty within the same vessel, when performed**

EXCLUDES *Revascularization with intravascular stent grafts in femoral-popliteal segment (0505T)*

17.5 320. **FUD** 000 J J8 80 50

AMA: 2019,Jun,14; 2018,Jan,8; 2017,Jul,3; 2017,Jan,8; 2016,Jul,8; 2016,Jan,13; 2015,Jan,16

37226 **with transluminal stent placement(s), includes angioplasty within the same vessel, when performed**

EXCLUDES *Revascularization with intravascular stent grafts in femoral-popliteal segment (0505T)*

15.1 285. **FUD** 000 J J8 80 50

AMA: 2019,Jun,14; 2018,Jan,8; 2017,Jul,3; 2017,Jan,8; 2016,Jul,6; 2016,Jul,8; 2016,Jan,13; 2015,Jan,16

37227 **with transluminal stent placement(s) and atherectomy, includes angioplasty within the same vessel, when performed**

EXCLUDES *Revascularization with intravascular stent grafts in femoral-popliteal segment (0505T)*

21.1 444. **FUD** 000 J J8 80 50

AMA: 2019,Jun,14; 2018,Jan,8; 2017,Jul,3; 2017,Jan,8; 2016,Jul,6; 2016,Jul,8; 2016,Jan,13; 2015,Jan,16

37228 **Revascularization, endovascular, open or percutaneous, tibial, peroneal artery, unilateral, initial vessel; with transluminal angioplasty**

15.7 140. **FUD** 000 J J8 80 50

AMA: 2019,Jun,14; 2018,Jan,8; 2017,Jul,3; 2017,Jan,8; 2016,Jul,8; 2016,Jan,13; 2015,Jan,16

37229 **with atherectomy, includes angioplasty within the same vessel, when performed**

20.4 322. **FUD** 000 J J8 80 50

AMA: 2019,Jun,14; 2018,Jan,8; 2017,Jul,3; 2017,Jan,8; 2016,Jul,8; 2016,Jan,13; 2015,Jan,16

37230 **with transluminal stent placement(s), includes angioplasty within the same vessel, when performed**

20.3 289. **FUD** 000 J J8 80 50

AMA: 2020,Jul,13; 2019,Jun,14; 2018,Jan,8; 2017,Jul,3; 2017,Jan,8; 2016,Jul,6; 2016,Jul,8; 2016,Jan,13; 2015,Jan,16

37231 **with transluminal stent placement(s) and atherectomy, includes angioplasty within the same vessel, when performed**

22.0 401. **FUD** 000 J J8 80 50

AMA: 2019,Jun,14; 2018,Jan,8; 2017,Jul,3; 2017,Jan,8; 2016,Jul,8; 2016,Jul,6; 2016,Jan,13; 2015,Jan,16

+ **37232** **Revascularization, endovascular, open or percutaneous, tibial/peroneal artery, unilateral, each additional vessel; with transluminal angioplasty (List separately in addition to code for primary procedure)**

Code first (37228-37231)

5.83 29.0 **FUD** ZZZ N N1 80 50

AMA: 2019,Jun,14; 2018,Jan,8; 2017,Jul,3; 2017,Jan,8; 2016,Jul,8; 2016,Jan,13; 2015,Jan,16

+ **37233** **with atherectomy, includes angioplasty within the same vessel, when performed (List separately in addition to code for primary procedure)**

Code first (37229, 37231)

9.48 35.7 **FUD** ZZZ N N1 80 50

AMA: 2019,Jun,14; 2018,Jan,8; 2017,Jul,3; 2017,Jan,8; 2016,Jul,8; 2016,Jan,13; 2015,Jan,16

+ **37234** **with transluminal stent placement(s), includes angioplasty within the same vessel, when performed (List separately in addition to code for primary procedure)**

Code first (37229-37231)

8.30 110. **FUD** ZZZ N N1 80 50

AMA: 2019,Jun,14; 2018,Jan,8; 2017,Jul,3; 2017,Jan,8; 2016,Jul,8; 2016,Jul,6; 2016,Jan,13; 2015,Jan,16

+ **37235** **with transluminal stent placement(s) and atherectomy, includes angioplasty within the same vessel, when performed (List separately in addition to code for primary procedure)**

Code first (37231)

11.7 116. **FUD** ZZZ N N1 80 50

AMA: 2019,Jun,14; 2018,Jan,8; 2017,Jul,3; 2017,Jan,8; 2016,Jul,6; 2016,Jul,8; 2016,Jan,13; 2015,Jan,16

37246-37249 [37246, 37247, 37248, 37249] Transluminal Balloon Angioplasty

INCLUDES Open and percutaneous balloon angioplasty
Radiological supervision and interpretation (37220-37235)

EXCLUDES *Angioplasty other vessels:*
Aortic/visceral arteries (with endovascular repair) (34841-34848)
Coronary artery (92920-92944)
Intracranial artery (61630, 61635)
Performed in hemodialysis circuit (36901-36909)
Infusion thrombolytics (37211-37214)
Mechanical thrombectomy (37184-37188)
Pulmonary artery (92997-92998)
Reporting codes more than one time for all services performed in single vessel or treatable with one angioplasty procedure

Code also angioplasty different vessel, when performed ([37247], [37249])
Code also extensive artery repair or replacement, when performed (35226, 35286)
Code also intravascular ultrasound, when performed (37252-37253)

37246 **Transluminal balloon angioplasty (except lower extremity artery(ies) for occlusive disease, intracranial, coronary, pulmonary, or dialysis circuit), open or percutaneous, including all imaging and radiological supervision and interpretation necessary to perform the angioplasty within the same artery; initial artery**

EXCLUDES *Intravascular stent placement except lower extremities (37236-37237)*
Revascularization lower extremities (37220-37235)
Stent placement:
Cervical carotid artery (37215-37216)
Intrathoracic carotid or innominate artery (37217-37218)

Code first (37239)

10.1 58.3 **FUD** 000 J G2 50

AMA: 2018,Jan,8; 2017,Aug,10; 2017,Jul,3

+ # **37247** **each additional artery (List separately in addition to code for primary procedure)**

EXCLUDES *Intravascular stent placement except lower extremities (37236-37237)*
Revascularization lower extremities (37220-37235)
Stent placement:
Cervical carotid artery (37215-37216)
Intrathoracic carotid or innominate artery (37217-37218)

Code first ([37246])

4.97 20.5 FUD ZZZ N N1 50

AMA: 2018,Jan,8; 2017,Aug,10; 2017,Jul,3

37248 **Transluminal balloon angioplasty (except dialysis circuit), open or percutaneous, including all imaging and radiological supervision and interpretation necessary to perform the angioplasty within the same vein; initial vein**

EXCLUDES *Endovascular venous arterialization with intravascular stent graft(s) in tibial-peroneal segment (0620T)*
Placement intravascular (venous) stent in same vein, same session as (37238-37239)
Revascularization with intravascular stent grafts in femoral-popliteal segment (0505T)

8.64 42.9 FUD 000 J G2 50

AMA: 2018,Jan,8; 2017,Aug,10; 2017,Jul,3; 2017,Mar,3

+ # **37249** **each additional vein (List separately in addition to code for primary procedure)**

EXCLUDES *Endovascular venous arterialization with intravascular stent graft(s) in tibial-peroneal segment (0620T)*
Placement intravascular (venous) stent in same vein, same session as (37238-37239)
Revascularization with intravascular stent grafts in femoral-popliteal segment (0505T)

Code first (37239)

4.24 15.6 FUD ZZZ N N1 50

AMA: 2018,Jan,8; 2017,Aug,10; 2017,Jul,3; 2017,Mar,3

37236-37239 Endovascular Revascularization Excluding Lower Extremities

INCLUDES Arteriotomy closure by suturing puncture, pressure, or arterial closure device application
Balloon angioplasty
Post-dilation after stent deployment
Predilation performed as primary or secondary angioplasty
Treatment lesion inside same vessel but outside stented portion
Treatment using different-sized balloons to accomplish procedure
Endovascular revascularization arteries and veins other than carotid, coronary, extracranial, intracranial, lower extremities
Imaging once procedure complete
Radiological supervision and interpretation
Stent placement provided as only treatment

EXCLUDES *Angioplasty in unrelated vessel*
Extensive repair or replacement artery (35226, 35286)
Insertion multiple stents in single vessel using more than one code
Intravascular ultrasound (37252-37253)
Mechanical thrombectomy (37184-37188)
Selective and nonselective catheterization (36005, 36010-36015, 36200, 36215-36218, 36245-36248)
Stent placement in:
Cervical carotid artery (37215-37216)
Extracranial vertebral (0075T-0076T)
Hemodialysis circuit (36903, 36905, 36908)
Intracoronary (92928-92929, 92933-92934, 92937-92938, 92941, 92943-92944)
Intracranial (61635)
Intrathoracic common carotid or innominate artery, retrograde or antegrade approach (37218)
Lower extremity arteries for occlusive disease (37221, 37223, 37226-37227, 37230-37231, 37234-37235)
Visceral arteries with fenestrated aortic repair (34841-34848)
Thrombolytic therapy (37211-37214)
Ultrasound guidance (76937)

Code also add-on codes for different vessels treated during same operative session

37236 **Transcatheter placement of an intravascular stent(s) (except lower extremity artery(s) for occlusive disease, cervical carotid, extracranial vertebral or intrathoracic carotid, intracranial, or coronary), open or percutaneous, including radiological supervision and interpretation and including all angioplasty within the same vessel, when performed; initial artery**

EXCLUDES *Procedures in same target treatment zone with (34841-34848)*

12.9 101. FUD 000 J J8 80 50

AMA: 2018,Jan,8; 2017,Dec,3; 2017,Jul,3; 2017,Jan,8; 2016,Jul,3; 2016,Jul,6; 2016,Mar,5; 2016,Jan,13; 2015,May,7; 2015,Jan,16

+ **37237** **each additional artery (List separately in addition to code for primary procedure)**

EXCLUDES *Procedures in same target treatment zone with (34841-34848)*

Code first (37236)

6.18 53.2 FUD ZZZ N N1 80 50

AMA: 2018,Jan,8; 2017,Dec,3; 2017,Jul,3; 2017,Jan,8; 2016,Jul,6; 2016,Mar,5; 2016,Jan,13; 2015,Jan,16

37238 **Transcatheter placement of an intravascular stent(s), open or percutaneous, including radiological supervision and interpretation and including angioplasty within the same vessel, when performed; initial vein**

EXCLUDES *Endovascular venous arterialization with intravascular stent graft(s) in tibial-peroneal segment (0620T)*
Revascularization with intravascular stent grafts in femoral-popliteal segment (0505T)

8.88 90.3 FUD 000 J J8 80 50

AMA: 2018,Jan,8; 2017,Jul,3; 2017,Mar,3; 2017,Jan,8; 2016,Jul,6; 2016,Jun,8

\+ **37239** **each additional vein (List separately in addition to code for primary procedure)**

EXCLUDES *Endovascular venous arterialization with intravascular stent graft(s) in tibial-peroneal segment (0620T)*
Revascularization with intravascular stent grafts in femoral-popliteal segment (0505T)

Code first (37238)

4.43 41.8 FUD ZZZ N N1 80 50

AMA: 2018,Jan,8; 2017,Jul,3; 2017,Mar,3; 2017,Jan,8; 2016,Jul,6

37241-37249 [37246, 37247, 37248, 37249] Therapeutic Vascular Embolization/Occlusion

INCLUDES Embolization or occlusion arteries, lymphatics, and veins except for head/neck and central nervous system
Imaging once procedure complete
Intraprocedural guidance
Radiological supervision and interpretation
Roadmapping
Stent placement provided as support for embolization

EXCLUDES *Embolization code assigned more than once per operative field*
Head, neck, or central nervous system embolization (61624, 61626, 61710)
Multiple codes for indications that overlap, code only indication needing most immediate attention
Stent deployment as primary aneurysm management, pseudoaneurysm, or vascular extravasation
Vein destruction with sclerosing solution (36468-36471)

Code also additional embolization procedure(s) and appropriate modifiers (e.g., modifier 59) when embolization procedures performed in multiple operative fields

Code also diagnostic angiography and catheter placement using modifier 59 when appropriate

37241 **Vascular embolization or occlusion, inclusive of all radiological supervision and interpretation, intraprocedural roadmapping, and imaging guidance necessary to complete the intervention; venous, other than hemorrhage (eg, congenital or acquired venous malformations, venous and capillary hemangiomas, varices, varicoceles)**

EXCLUDES *Embolization side branch(es) outflow vein from hemodialysis access (36909)*
Procedure in same operative field with:
Endovenous ablation therapy incompetent vein (36475-36479)
Injection sclerosing solution; single vein (36470-36471)
Transcatheter embolization procedures (75894, 75898)
Vein destruction (36468-36479 [36465, 36466])

12.7 140. FUD 000 J P2

AMA: 2019,Sep,6; 2018,Mar,3; 2018,Jan,8; 2017,Mar,3; 2017,Jan,8; 2016,Nov,3; 2016,Jan,13; 2015,Nov,3; 2015,Aug,8; 2015,Apr,10; 2015,Jan,16

37242 **arterial, other than hemorrhage or tumor (eg, congenital or acquired arterial malformations, arteriovenous malformations, arteriovenous fistulas, aneurysms, pseudoaneurysms)**

EXCLUDES *Percutaneous treatment pseudoaneurysm extremity (36002)*

13.8 211. FUD 000 J J8

AMA: 2019,Sep,6; 2018,Jul,14; 2018,Mar,3; 2018,Jan,8; 2017,Jan,8; 2016,Jan,13; 2015,Nov,3; 2015,Jan,16

37243 **for tumors, organ ischemia, or infarction**

INCLUDES Embolization uterine fibroids (37244)

EXCLUDES *Procedure in same operative field:*
Angiography (75898)
Transcatheter embolization in same operative field (75894)

Code also chemotherapy when provided with embolization procedure (96420-96425)

Code also injection radioisotopes when provided with embolization procedure (79445)

16.3 273. FUD 000 J G2

AMA: 2019,Sep,6; 2018,Mar,3; 2018,Jan,8; 2017,Jan,8; 2016,Jan,13; 2015,Nov,3; 2015,Jan,16

37244 **for arterial or venous hemorrhage or lymphatic extravasation**

INCLUDES Embolization uterine arteries for hemorrhage

19.3 200. FUD 000 J

AMA: 2019,Sep,6; 2018,Jul,14; 2018,Mar,3; 2018,Jan,8; 2017,Oct,9; 2017,Jan,8; 2016,Jan,13; 2015,Nov,3; 2015,Jan,16

37246 **Resequenced code. See code following 37235.**

37247 **Resequenced code. See code following 37235.**

37248 **Resequenced code. See code following 37235.**

37249 **Resequenced code. See code following 37235.**

37252-37253 Intravascular Ultrasound: Noncoronary

INCLUDES Manipulation and repositioning transducer prior to and after therapeutic interventional procedures

EXCLUDES *Selective or non-selective catheter placement for access (36005-36248)*
Transcatheter procedures (37200, 37236-37239, 37241-37244, 61624, 61626)
Vena cava filter procedures (37191-37193, 37197)

Code first (33361-33369, 33477, 33880-33886, 34701-34708, 34709, [34718], 34710-34711, 34712, 34841-34848, 36010-36015, 36100-36218, 36221-36228, 36245-36248, 36251-36254, 36481, 36555-36571 [36572, 36573], 36578, 36580-36585, 36595, 36901-36909, 37184-37188, 37200, 37211-37218, 37220-37239 [37246, 37247, 37248, 37249], 37241-37244, 61623, 75600-75635, 75705-75774, 75805, 75807, 75810, 75820-75833, 75860-75872, 75885-75898, 75901-75902, 75956-75959, 75970, 76000, 77001, 0075T-0076T, 0234T-0238T, 0338T)

\+ **37252** **Intravascular ultrasound (noncoronary vessel) during diagnostic evaluation and/or therapeutic intervention, including radiological supervision and interpretation; initial noncoronary vessel (List separately in addition to code for primary procedure)**

Code first primary procedure

2.63 33.2 FUD ZZZ N N1 80

AMA: 2019,Nov,6; 2018,Jan,8; 2017,Dec,3; 2017,Aug,10; 2017,Mar,3; 2017,Jan,8; 2016,Jul,6; 2016,May,11

\+ **37253** **each additional noncoronary vessel (List separately in addition to code for primary procedure)**

Code first (37252)

2.11 5.38 FUD ZZZ N N1 80

AMA: 2019,Nov,6; 2018,Jan,8; 2017,Dec,3; 2017,Aug,10; 2017,Mar,3; 2017,Jan,8; 2016,Jul,6; 2016,May,11

37500-37501 Vascular Endoscopic Procedures

INCLUDES Diagnostic endoscopy

EXCLUDES *Open procedure (37760)*

37500 **Vascular endoscopy, surgical, with ligation of perforator veins, subfascial (SEPS)**

18.3 18.3 FUD 090 T A2 50

AMA: 2018,Jan,8; 2017,Jan,8; 2016,Jan,13; 2015,Jan,16

37501 **Unlisted vascular endoscopy procedure**

0.00 0.00 FUD YYY T 50

AMA: 2014,Jan,11; 1997,Nov,1

37565-37606 Ligation Procedures: Jugular Vein, Carotid Arteries

CMS: 100-03,160.8 Electroencephalographic Monitoring During Cerebral Vasculature Surgery

EXCLUDES *Arterial balloon occlusion, endovascular, temporary (61623)*
Suture arteries and veins (35201-35286)
Transcatheter arterial embolization/occlusion, permanent (61624-61626)
Treatment intracranial aneurysm (61703)

37565 **Ligation, internal jugular vein**

20.7 20.7 FUD 090 T 80 50

AMA: 2014,Jan,11; 1997,Nov,1

37600 **Ligation; external carotid artery**
21.2 21.2 **FUD** 090 T 80
AMA: 2014,Jan,11; 1997,Nov,1

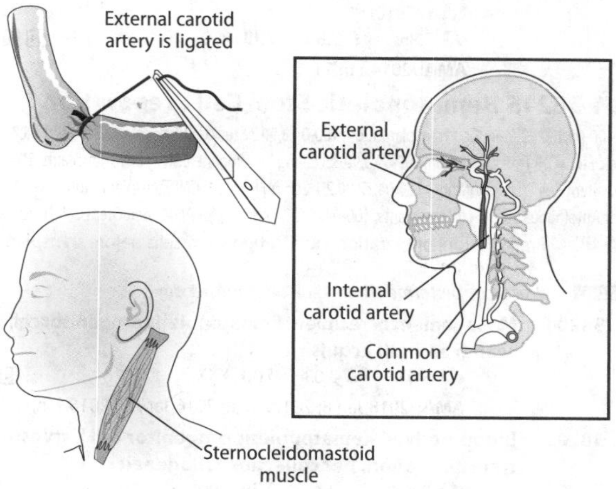

37605 **internal or common carotid artery**
21.4 21.4 **FUD** 090 T 80
AMA: 2014,Jan,11; 1997,Nov,1

37606 **internal or common carotid artery, with gradual occlusion, as with Selverstone or Crutchfield clamp**
20.7 20.7 **FUD** 090 T 80
AMA: 2014,Jan,11; 1997,Nov,1

37607-37609 Ligation Hemodialysis Angioaccess or Temporal Artery

EXCLUDES *Suture arteries and veins (35201-35286)*

37607 **Ligation or banding of angioaccess arteriovenous fistula**
10.8 10.8 **FUD** 090 T A2
AMA: 2014,Jan,11; 1997,Nov,1

37609 **Ligation or biopsy, temporal artery**
5.94 8.94 **FUD** 010 J A2 50
AMA: 2014,Jan,11; 1997,Nov,1

37615-37618 Arterial Ligation, Major Vessel, for Injury/Rupture

EXCLUDES *Suture arteries and veins (35201-35286)*

37615 **Ligation, major artery (eg, post-traumatic, rupture); neck**
INCLUDES Touroff ligation
15.3 15.3 **FUD** 090 T 80
AMA: 2014,Jan,11; 1997,Nov,1

37616 **chest**
INCLUDES Bardenheurer operation
32.0 32.0 **FUD** 090 C 80
AMA: 2014,Jan,11; 1997,Nov,1

37617 **abdomen**
38.6 38.6 **FUD** 090 C 80
AMA: 2018,Jan,8; 2017,Jan,8; 2016,Jan,13; 2015,Jan,16

37618 **extremity**
11.2 11.2 **FUD** 090 C 80
AMA: 2014,Jan,11; 1997,Nov,1

37619 Ligation Inferior Vena Cava

EXCLUDES *Suture arteries and veins (35201-35286)*
Endovascular delivery inferior vena cava filter (37191)

37619 **Ligation of inferior vena cava**
50.1 50.1 **FUD** 090 T 80
AMA: 2018,Jan,8; 2017,Jan,8; 2016,Jan,13; 2015,Jan,16

37650-37660 Venous Ligation, Femoral and Common Iliac

EXCLUDES *Suture arteries and veins (35201-35286)*

37650 **Ligation of femoral vein**
13.2 13.2 **FUD** 090 T A2 50
AMA: 2014,Jan,11; 1997,Nov,1

37660 **Ligation of common iliac vein**
38.3 38.3 **FUD** 090 C 80 50
AMA: 2014,Jan,11; 1997,Nov,1

37700-37785 Treatment of Varicose Veins of Legs

EXCLUDES *Suture arteries and veins (35201-35286)*

37700 **Ligation and division of long saphenous vein at saphenofemoral junction, or distal interruptions**
INCLUDES Babcock operation
EXCLUDES *Ligation, division, and stripping vein (37718, 37722)*
7.08 7.08 **FUD** 090 T A2 50
AMA: 2018,Mar,3; 2018,Jan,8; 2017,Jan,8; 2016,Jan,13; 2015,Jan,16

37718 **Ligation, division, and stripping, short saphenous vein**
EXCLUDES *Ligation, division, and stripping vein (37700, 37735, 37780)*
12.2 12.2 **FUD** 090 T A2 50
AMA: 2018,Mar,3; 2018,Jan,8; 2017,Jan,8

37722 **Ligation, division, and stripping, long (greater) saphenous veins from saphenofemoral junction to knee or below**
EXCLUDES *Ligation, division, and stripping vein (37700, 37718, 37735)*
13.6 13.6 **FUD** 090 T A2 50
AMA: 2018,Mar,3; 2018,Jan,8; 2017,Jan,8

37735 **Ligation and division and complete stripping of long or short saphenous veins with radical excision of ulcer and skin graft and/or interruption of communicating veins of lower leg, with excision of deep fascia**
EXCLUDES *Ligation, division, and stripping vein (37700, 37718, 37722, 37780)*
16.8 16.8 **FUD** 090 T A2 50
AMA: 2018,Mar,3; 2018,Jan,8; 2017,Jan,8; 2016,Jan,13; 2015,Jan,16

37760 **Ligation of perforator veins, subfascial, radical (Linton type), including skin graft, when performed, open, 1 leg**
EXCLUDES *Duplex scan extremity veins (93971)*
Ligation subfascial perforator veins, endoscopic (37500)
Ultrasonic guidance (76937, 76942, 76998)
18.0 18.0 **FUD** 090 T A2 50
AMA: 2018,Mar,3; 2018,Jan,8; 2017,Jan,8; 2016,Jan,13; 2015,Jan,16

37761 **Ligation of perforator vein(s), subfascial, open, including ultrasound guidance, when performed, 1 leg**
INCLUDES Ultrasonic guidance (76937, 76942, 76998)
EXCLUDES *Duplex scan extremity veins (93971)*
Ligation subfascial perforator veins, endoscopic (37500)
15.7 15.7 **FUD** 090 T R2 80 50
AMA: 2018,Mar,3; 2018,Jan,8; 2017,Jan,8; 2016,Jan,13; 2015,Jan,16

37765 **Stab phlebectomy of varicose veins, 1 extremity; 10-20 stab incisions**
EXCLUDES *Fewer than 10 incisions (37799)*
More than 20 incisions (37766)
7.88 12.6 **FUD** 010 T P3 50
AMA: 2018,Mar,3; 2018,Jan,8; 2017,Jan,8; 2016,Nov,3; 2016,Jan,13; 2015,Jan,16

37766 **more than 20 incisions**
EXCLUDES *Fewer than 10 incisions (37799)*
10-20 incisions (37765)
15.8 22.0 **FUD** 090 T P3 50
AMA: 2018,Mar,3; 2018,Jan,8; 2017,Jan,8; 2016,Nov,3; 2016,Jan,13; 2015,Jan,16

37780 **Ligation and division of short saphenous vein at saphenopopliteal junction (separate procedure)**
6.75 6.75 FUD 090 T A2 50
AMA: 2018,Jan,8; 2017,Jan,8; 2016,Jan,13; 2015,Jan,16

37785 **Ligation, division, and/or excision of varicose vein cluster(s), 1 leg**
7.45 10.0 FUD 090 T A2 50
AMA: 2018,Jan,8; 2017,Jan,8; 2016,Jan,13; 2015,Jan,16

37788-37790 Treatment of Vascular Disease of the Penis

37788 **Penile revascularization, artery, with or without vein graft** ♂
36.5 36.5 FUD 090 C 80
AMA: 2014,Jan,11; 1997,Nov,1

37790 **Penile venous occlusive procedure**
14.0 14.0 FUD 090 J A2 80
AMA: 2014,Jan,11; 1997,Nov,1

37799 Unlisted Vascular Surgery Procedures

CMS: 100-04,32,161 Intracranial Percutaneous Transluminal Angioplasty (PTA) With Stenting; 100-04,4,180.3 Unlisted Service or Procedure

37799 **Unlisted procedure, vascular surgery**
0.00 0.00 FUD YYY T 80
AMA: 2019,Dec,5; 2019,Nov,6; 2018,Nov,11; 2018,Jan,8; 2017,Jan,8; 2016,Nov,3; 2016,Jan,13; 2015,Apr,10; 2015,Jan,16

38100-38200 Splenic Procedures

38100 **Splenectomy; total (separate procedure)**
33.5 33.5 FUD 090 C 80
AMA: 2018,Jan,8; 2017,Jan,8; 2016,Jan,13; 2015,Jan,16

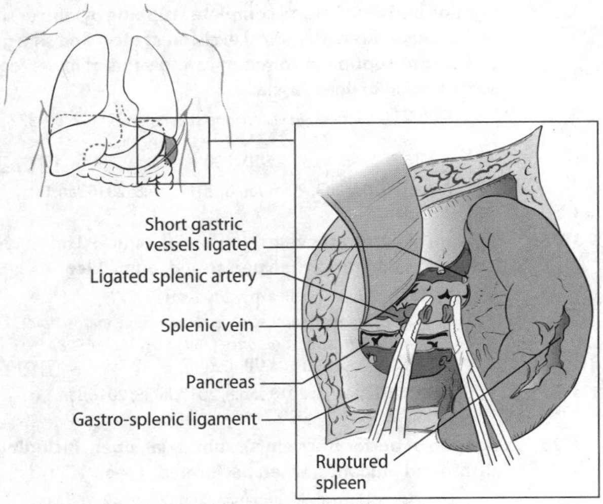

38101 **partial (separate procedure)**
33.5 33.5 FUD 090 C 80
AMA: 2018,Jan,8; 2017,Jan,8; 2016,Jan,13; 2015,Jan,16

\+ **38102** **total, en bloc for extensive disease, in conjunction with other procedure (List in addition to code for primary procedure)**
Code first primary procedure
7.63 7.63 FUD ZZZ C 80
AMA: 2018,Jan,8; 2017,Jan,8; 2016,Jan,13; 2015,Jan,16

38115 **Repair of ruptured spleen (splenorrhaphy) with or without partial splenectomy**
37.1 37.1 FUD 090 C 80
AMA: 2018,Jan,8; 2017,Jan,8; 2016,Jan,13; 2015,Jan,16

38120 **Laparoscopy, surgical, splenectomy**
INCLUDES Diagnostic laparoscopy (49320)
30.6 30.6 FUD 090 J 80
AMA: 2018,Jan,8; 2017,Jan,8; 2016,Jan,13; 2015,Jan,16

38129 **Unlisted laparoscopy procedure, spleen**
0.00 0.00 FUD YYY J 80
AMA: 2018,Jan,8; 2017,Jan,8; 2016,Jan,13; 2015,Jan,16

38200 **Injection procedure for splenoportography**
(75810)
3.85 3.85 FUD 000 N N1 80
AMA: 2014,Jan,11

38204-38215 Hematopoietic Stem Cell Preparation

CMS: 100-03,110.23 Stem Cell Transplantation; 100-04,3,90.3 Stem Cell Transplantation; 100-04,3,90.3.1 Allogeneic Stem Cell Transplantation; 100-04,3,90.3.3 Billing for Allogeneic Stem Cell Transplants; 100-04,32,90 Billing for Stem Cell Transplantation; 100-04,32,90.2.1 Coding for Stem Cell Transplantation; 100-04,4,231.10 Billing for Autologous Stem Cell Transplants; 100-04,4,231.11 Billing for Allogeneic Stem Cell Transplants

INCLUDES Preservation, preparation, purification stem cells before transplant or reinfusion

EXCLUDES *Procedure performed more than one time per day*

38204 **Management of recipient hematopoietic progenitor cell donor search and cell acquisition**
3.03 3.03 FUD XXX N N1
AMA: 2018,Jan,8; 2017,Jan,8; 2016,Jan,13; 2015,Jan,16

38205 **Blood-derived hematopoietic progenitor cell harvesting for transplantation, per collection; allogeneic**
2.44 2.44 FUD 000 B 80
AMA: 2018,May,3; 2018,Jan,8; 2017,Jan,8; 2016,Jan,13; 2015,Jan,16

38206 **autologous**
2.39 2.39 FUD 000 S G2 80
AMA: 2018,May,3; 2018,Jan,8; 2017,Jan,8; 2016,Jan,13; 2015,Jan,16

38207 **Transplant preparation of hematopoietic progenitor cells; cryopreservation and storage**
EXCLUDES *Flow cytometry (88182, 88184-88189)*
(88240)
1.31 1.31 FUD XXX S
AMA: 2018,Jan,8; 2017,Jan,8; 2016,Jan,13; 2015,Jan,16

38208 **thawing of previously frozen harvest, without washing, per donor**
EXCLUDES *Flow cytometry (88182, 88184-88189)*
(88241)
0.83 0.83 FUD XXX S
AMA: 2018,Jan,8; 2017,Jan,8; 2016,Jan,13; 2015,Jan,16

38209 **thawing of previously frozen harvest, with washing, per donor**
EXCLUDES *Flow cytometry (88182, 88184-88189)*
0.35 0.35 FUD XXX S
AMA: 2018,Jan,8; 2017,Jan,8; 2016,Jan,13; 2015,Jan,16

38210 **specific cell depletion within harvest, T-cell depletion**
EXCLUDES *Flow cytometry (88182, 88184-88189)*
2.29 2.29 FUD XXX S
AMA: 2018,Jan,8; 2017,Jan,8; 2016,Jan,13; 2015,Jan,16

38211 **tumor cell depletion**
EXCLUDES *Flow cytometry (88182, 88184-88189)*
2.08 2.08 FUD XXX S
AMA: 2018,Jan,8; 2017,Jan,8; 2016,Jan,13; 2015,Jan,16

38212 **red blood cell removal**
EXCLUDES *Flow cytometry (88182, 88184-88189)*
1.39 1.39 FUD XXX S
AMA: 2018,Jan,8; 2017,Jan,8; 2016,Jan,13; 2015,Jan,16

38213 **platelet depletion**
EXCLUDES *Flow cytometry (88182, 88184-88189)*
0.35 0.35 FUD XXX S
AMA: 2018,Jan,8; 2017,Jan,8; 2016,Jan,13; 2015,Jan,16

38214 **plasma (volume) depletion**
EXCLUDES *Flow cytometry (88182, 88184-88189)*
1.23 1.23 FUD XXX S
AMA: 2018,Jan,8; 2017,Jan,8; 2016,Jan,13; 2015,Jan,16

38215 **cell concentration in plasma, mononuclear, or buffy coat layer**

EXCLUDES *Flow cytometry (88182, 88184-88189)*

1.39 1.39 FUD XXX S

AMA: 2018,Jan,8; 2017,Jan,8; 2016,Jan,13; 2015,Jan,16

38220-38232 Bone Marrow Procedures

CMS: 100-03,110.23 Stem Cell Transplantation; 100-04,3,90.3 Stem Cell Transplantation; 100-04,32,90 Billing for Stem Cell Transplantation; 100-04,4,231.11 Billing for Allogeneic Stem Cell Transplants

38220 **Diagnostic bone marrow; aspiration(s)**

EXCLUDES *Aspiration bone marrow for spinal graft (20939)*
Bone marrow biopsy (38221)
Bone marrow for platelet rich stem cell injection (0232T)

Code also biopsy bone marrow during same session (38222)

1.99 4.71 FUD XXX J P3 80 50

AMA: 2018,May,3; 2018,Jan,8; 2017,Jan,8; 2016,Jan,13; 2015,Mar,9; 2015,Jan,16

38221 **biopsy(ies)**

EXCLUDES *Aspiration and biopsy during same session (38222)*
Aspiration bone marrow (38220)

(88305)

2.00 4.47 FUD XXX J P3 80 50

AMA: 2018,May,3; 2018,Jan,8; 2017,Jan,8; 2016,Jan,13; 2015,Mar,9

38222 **biopsy(ies) and aspiration(s)**

EXCLUDES *Aspiration bone marrow only (38221)*
Biopsy bone marrow only (38220)

(88305)

2.24 4.94 FUD XXX J G2 80 50

AMA: 2018,May,3

38230 **Bone marrow harvesting for transplantation; allogeneic**

EXCLUDES *Aspiration bone marrow for platelet rich stem cell injection (0232T)*
Harvesting blood-derived hematopoietic progenitor cells for transplant (allogeneic) (38205)

5.92 5.92 FUD 000 S G2 80

AMA: 2018,Jan,8; 2017,Jan,8; 2016,Jan,13; 2015,Jan,16

38232 **autologous**

EXCLUDES *Aspiration bone marrow (38220, 38222)*
Aspiration bone marrow for platelet rich stem cell injection (0232T)
Aspiration bone marrow for spinal graft (20939)
Harvesting blood-derived peripheral stem cells for transplant (allogenic/autologous) (38205-38206)

5.75 5.75 FUD 000 S G2 80

AMA: 2018,Jan,8; 2017,Jan,8; 2016,Jan,13; 2015,Jan,16

38240-38243 [38243] Hematopoietic Progenitor Cell Transplantation

CMS: 100-03,110.23 Stem Cell Transplantation; 100-04,3,90.3 Stem Cell Transplantation; 100-04,3,90.3.1 Allogeneic Stem Cell Transplantation; 100-04,3,90.3.2 Autologous Stem Cell Transplantation (AuSCT); 100-04,3,90.3.3 Billing for Allogeneic Stem Cell Transplants; 100-04,32,90 Billing for Stem Cell Transplantation; 100-04,32,90.2 Allogeneic Stem Cell Transplantation; 100-04,32,90.2.1 Coding for Stem Cell Transplantation; 100-04,32,90.3 Autologous Stem Cell Transplantation; 100-04,32,90.4 Edits Stem Cell Transplant; 100-04,32,90.6 Clinical Trials for Stem Cell Transplant for Myelodysplastic Syndrome (; 100-04,4,231.10 Billing for Autologous Stem Cell Transplants; 100-04,4,231.11 Billing for Allogeneic Stem Cell Transplants

INCLUDES Evaluation patient prior to, during, and after infusion
Management uncomplicated adverse reactions such as hives or nausea
Monitoring physiological parameters
Physician presence during infusion
Supervision clinical staff

EXCLUDES *Administration fluids for transplant or incidental hydration separately*
Concurrent administration medications with infusion for transplant
Cryopreservation, freezing, and storage hematopoietic progenitor cells for transplant (38207)
Human leukocyte antigen (HLA) testing (81379-81383, 86812-86821)
Modification, treatment, processing hematopoietic progenitor cell specimens for transplant (38210-38215)
Thawing and expansion hematopoietic progenitor cells for transplant (38208-38209)

Code also administration medications and/or fluids not related to transplant with modifier 59

Code also E/M service for treatment more complicated adverse reactions after infusion, as appropriate

Code also separately identifiable E/M service on same date, appending modifier 25 as appropriate (99211-99215, 99217-99220, [99224, 99225, 99226], 99221-99223, 99231-99239, 99471-99472, 99475-99476)

38240 **Hematopoietic progenitor cell (HPC); allogeneic transplantation per donor**

EXCLUDES *Allogeneic lymphocyte infusions on same date of service with (38242)*
Hematopoietic progenitor cell (HPC); HPC boost on same date of service with ([38243])

6.78 6.78 FUD XXX J 80

AMA: 2018,Jan,8; 2017,Jan,8; 2016,Jan,13; 2015,Jan,16

38241 **autologous transplantation**

5.02 5.02 FUD XXX S G2 80

AMA: 2018,Jan,8; 2017,Jan,8; 2016,Jan,13; 2015,Jan,16

\# **38243** **HPC boost**

EXCLUDES *Allogeneic lymphocyte infusions on same date of service with (38242)*
Hematopoietic progenitor cell (HPC); allogeneic transplantation per donor on same date of service with (38240)

3.47 3.47 FUD 000 S R2 80

AMA: 2018,Jan,8; 2017,Jan,8; 2016,Jan,13; 2015,Feb,10; 2015,Jan,16

38242 **Allogeneic lymphocyte infusions**

EXCLUDES *Aspiration bone marrow (38220, 38222)*
Aspiration bone marrow for platelet rich stem cell injection (0232T)
Aspiration bone marrow for spinal graft (20939)
Hematopoietic progenitor cell (HPC); allogeneic transplantation per donor on same date of service with (38240)
Hematopoietic progenitor cell (HPC); HPC boost on same service date with ([38243])

(81379-81383, 86812-86813, 86816-86817, 86821)

3.63 3.63 FUD 000 S R2 80

AMA: 2018,Jan,8; 2017,Jan,8; 2016,Jan,13; 2015,Jan,16

38243 **Resequenced code. See code following 38241.**

38300-38382 Incision Lymphatic Vessels

38300 **Drainage of lymph node abscess or lymphadenitis; simple**

5.91 9.40 FUD 010 J A2

AMA: 2014,Jan,11

38305 **extensive**

14.1 14.1 FUD 090 J A2

AMA: 2014,Jan,11

38308 **Lymphangiotomy or other operations on lymphatic channels**
13.0 13.0 FUD 090 J A2 80
AMA: 2014,Jan,11

38380 **Suture and/or ligation of thoracic duct; cervical approach**
16.3 16.3 FUD 090 C 80
AMA: 2014,Jan,11

38381 **thoracic approach**
23.2 23.2 FUD 090 C 80
AMA: 2014,Jan,11

38382 **abdominal approach**
19.4 19.4 FUD 090 C 80
AMA: 2014,Jan,11

38500-38555 Biopsy/Excision Lymphatic Vessels

EXCLUDES *Injection for sentinel node identification (38792)*
Percutaneous needle biopsy retroperitoneal mass (49180)

38500 **Biopsy or excision of lymph node(s); open, superficial**
EXCLUDES *Lymphadenectomy (38700-38780)*
7.38 9.68 FUD 010 J A2 50
AMA: 2019,Feb,8; 2018,Jan,8; 2017,Jan,8; 2016,Jan,13; 2015,Jan,16

38505 **by needle, superficial (eg, cervical, inguinal, axillary)**
EXCLUDES *Fine needle aspiration (10004-10012, 10021)*
(88172-88173)
(76942, 77002, 77012, 77021)
2.02 3.55 FUD 000 J A2 50
AMA: 2019,Feb,8; 2018,Jan,8; 2017,Jan,8; 2016,Jan,13; 2015,Jan,16

38510 **open, deep cervical node(s)**
12.0 15.1 FUD 010 J A2 50
AMA: 2019,Feb,8; 2018,Jan,8; 2017,Jan,8; 2016,Jan,13; 2015,Jan,16

38520 **open, deep cervical node(s) with excision scalene fat pad**
13.4 13.4 FUD 090 J A2 50
AMA: 2019,Feb,8; 2018,Jan,8; 2017,Jan,8; 2016,Jan,13; 2015,Jan,16

38525 **open, deep axillary node(s)**
12.6 12.6 FUD 090 J A2 50
AMA: 2019,Feb,8; 2018,Jan,8; 2017,Jan,8; 2016,Jan,13; 2015,Mar,5; 2015,Jan,16

38530 **open, internal mammary node(s)**
EXCLUDES *Fine needle aspiration (10005-10012)*
Lymphadenectomy (38720-38746)
16.3 16.3 FUD 090 J A2 80 50
AMA: 2019,Feb,8; 2018,Jan,8; 2017,Jan,8; 2016,Jan,13; 2015,Jan,16

38531 **open, inguinofemoral node(s)**
12.5 12.5 FUD 090 80 50
AMA: 2019,Feb,8

38542 **Dissection, deep jugular node(s)**
EXCLUDES *Complete cervical lymphadenectomy (38720)*
14.8 14.8 FUD 090 J A2 80 50
AMA: 2019,Feb,8; 2018,Jan,8; 2017,Jan,8; 2016,Jan,13; 2015,Jan,16

38550 **Excision of cystic hygroma, axillary or cervical; without deep neurovascular dissection**
14.9 14.9 FUD 090 J A2 80
AMA: 2014,Jan,11; 1994,Win,1

38555 **with deep neurovascular dissection**
29.5 29.5 FUD 090 J A2 80
AMA: 2014,Jan,11; 1994,Win,1

38562-38564 Limited Lymphadenectomy: Staging

38562 **Limited lymphadenectomy for staging (separate procedure); pelvic and para-aortic**
EXCLUDES *Prostatectomy (55812, 55842)*
Radioactive substance inserted into prostate (55862)
20.4 20.4 FUD 090 C 80
AMA: 2019,Feb,8; 2018,Jan,8; 2017,Jan,8; 2016,Jan,13; 2015,Jan,16

38564 **retroperitoneal (aortic and/or splenic)**
20.4 20.4 FUD 090 C 80
AMA: 2019,Feb,8

38570-38589 Laparoscopic Lymph Node Procedures

INCLUDES Diagnostic laparoscopy (49320)
EXCLUDES *Laparoscopy with draining lymphocele to peritoneal cavity (49323)*
Limited lymphadenectomy:
Pelvic (38562)
Retroperitoneal (38564)

38570 **Laparoscopy, surgical; with retroperitoneal lymph node sampling (biopsy), single or multiple**
14.7 14.7 FUD 010 J A2 80
AMA: 2019,Feb,8; 2018,Jan,8; 2017,Jan,8; 2016,Jan,13; 2015,Jan,16

38571 **with bilateral total pelvic lymphadenectomy**
19.1 19.1 FUD 010 J A2 80
AMA: 2019,Feb,8; 2018,Jan,8; 2017,Jan,8; 2016,Jan,13; 2015,Jan,16

38572 **with bilateral total pelvic lymphadenectomy and peri-aortic lymph node sampling (biopsy), single or multiple**
EXCLUDES *Lymphocele drainage into peritoneal cavity (49323)*
26.3 26.3 FUD 010 J A2 80
AMA: 2019,Feb,8; 2018,Jan,8; 2017,Jan,8; 2016,Jan,13; 2015,Jan,13; 2015,Jan,16

38573 **with bilateral total pelvic lymphadenectomy and peri-aortic lymph node sampling, peritoneal washings, peritoneal biopsy(ies), omentectomy, and diaphragmatic washings, including diaphragmatic and other serosal biopsy(ies), when performed**
EXCLUDES *Laparoscopic hysterectomy procedures (58541-58554)*
Laparoscopic omentopexy (separate procedure) (49326)
Laparoscopy abdomen, diagnostic (separate procedure)(49320)
Laparoscopy unlisted (38589)
Laparoscopy without omentectomy (38570-38572)
Lymphadenectomy for staging (38562-38564)
Omentectomy (separate procedure) (49255)
Pelvic lymphadenectomy external iliac, hypogastric, and obturator nodes (38770)
Retroperitoneal lymphadenectomy aortic, pelvic, and renal nodes (separate procedure) (38780)
33.5 33.5 FUD 010 J G2 80
AMA: 2019,Mar,5; 2018,Apr,10

38589 **Unlisted laparoscopy procedure, lymphatic system**
0.00 0.00 FUD YYY J 80 50
AMA: 2018,Apr,10; 2018,Jan,8; 2017,Jan,8; 2016,Jan,13; 2015,Jan,16

38700-38780 Lymphadenectomy Procedures

INCLUDES Lymph node biopsy/excision (38500)
EXCLUDES *Excision lymphedematous skin and subcutaneous tissue (15004-15005)*
Limited lymphadenectomy
Pelvic (38562)
Retroperitoneal (38564)
Repair lymphedematous skin and tissue (15570-15650)

38700 **Suprahyoid lymphadenectomy**
23.1 23.1 FUD 090 J G2 80 50
AMA: 2019,Feb,8; 2018,Jan,8; 2017,Jan,8; 2016,Jan,13; 2015,Jan,16

38720 Cervical lymphadenectomy (complete)
38.5 38.5 **FUD** 090 J 80 50
AMA: 2020,Apr,10; 2019,Feb,8; 2018,Jan,8; 2017,Jan,8; 2016,Jan,13; 2015,Jan,16

38724 Cervical lymphadenectomy (modified radical neck dissection)
41.5 41.5 **FUD** 090 C 80 50
AMA: 2019,Mar,10; 2019,Feb,8; 2018,Jan,8; 2017,Jan,8; 2016,Jan,13; 2015,Jan,16

38740 Axillary lymphadenectomy; superficial
20.2 20.2 **FUD** 090 J A2 80 50
AMA: 2019,Feb,8; 2018,Jan,8; 2017,Jan,8; 2016,Jan,13; 2015,Jan,16

38745 complete
25.4 25.4 **FUD** 090 J A2 80 50
AMA: 2019,Feb,8

\+ **38746 Thoracic lymphadenectomy by thoracotomy, mediastinal and regional lymphadenectomy (List separately in addition to code for primary procedure)**

INCLUDES Left side
- Aortopulmonary window
- Inferior pulmonary ligament
- Paraesophageal
- Subcarinal

Right side
- Inferior pulmonary ligament
- Paraesophageal
- Paratracheal
- Subcarinal

EXCLUDES *Thoracoscopic mediastinal and regional lymphadenectomy (32674)*

Code first (21601, 31760, 31766, 31786, 32096-32200, 32220-32320, 32440-32491, 32503-32505, 33025, 33030, 33050-33130, 39200-39220, 39560-39561, 43101, 43112, 43117-43118, 43122-43123, 43351, 60270, 60505)
6.22 6.22 **FUD** ZZZ C 80
AMA: 2019,Feb,8; 2018,Jan,8; 2017,Jan,8; 2016,Jan,13; 2015,Jan,16

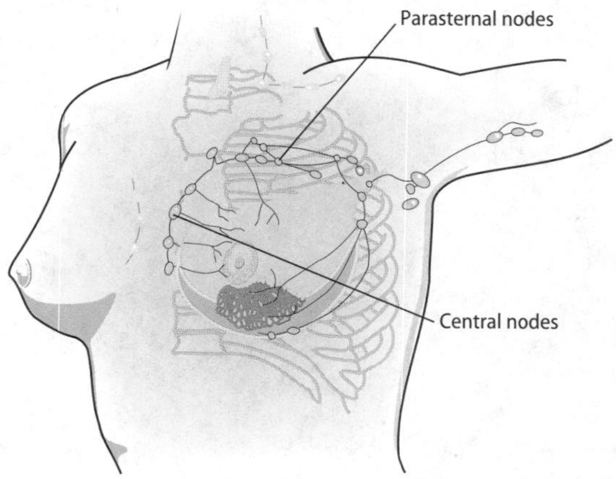

\+ **38747 Abdominal lymphadenectomy, regional, including celiac, gastric, portal, peripancreatic, with or without para-aortic and vena caval nodes (List separately in addition to code for primary procedure)**
Code first primary procedure
7.77 7.77 **FUD** ZZZ C 80
AMA: 2020,Apr,10; 2019,Feb,8

38760 Inguinofemoral lymphadenectomy, superficial, including Cloquet's node (separate procedure)
24.2 24.2 **FUD** 090 J A2 80 50
AMA: 2019,Feb,8; 2018,Jan,8; 2017,Jan,8; 2016,Jan,13; 2015,Jan,16

38765 Inguinofemoral lymphadenectomy, superficial, in continuity with pelvic lymphadenectomy, including external iliac, hypogastric, and obturator nodes (separate procedure)
37.7 37.7 **FUD** 090 C 80 50
AMA: 2019,Feb,8; 2018,Jan,8; 2017,Jan,8; 2016,Jan,13; 2015,Jan,16

38770 Pelvic lymphadenectomy, including external iliac, hypogastric, and obturator nodes (separate procedure)
23.2 23.2 **FUD** 090 C 80 50
AMA: 2019,Feb,8

38780 Retroperitoneal transabdominal lymphadenectomy, extensive, including pelvic, aortic, and renal nodes (separate procedure)
29.9 29.9 **FUD** 090 C 80
AMA: 2019,Feb,8

38790-38999 Cannulation/Injection/Other Procedures

38790 Injection procedure; lymphangiography
(75801-75807)
2.36 2.36 **FUD** 000 N N1 50
AMA: 2014,Jan,11; 1999,Jul,6

38792 radioactive tracer for identification of sentinel node
EXCLUDES *Sentinel node excision (38500-38542)*
Sentinel node(s) identification (mapping) intraoperative with nonradioactive dye injection (38900)
(78195)
0.97 2.37 **FUD** 000 Q1 N1 50
AMA: 2019,Feb,8; 2018,Jan,8; 2017,Jan,8; 2016,Jan,13; 2015,Mar,5; 2015,Jan,16

38794 Cannulation, thoracic duct
8.52 8.52 **FUD** 090 N N1 80
AMA: 2014,Jan,11

\+ **38900 Intraoperative identification (eg, mapping) of sentinel lymph node(s) includes injection of non-radioactive dye, when performed (List separately in addition to code for primary procedure)**
EXCLUDES *Injection tracer for sentinel node identification (38792)*
Code first (19302, 19307, 38500, 38510, 38520, 38525, 38530-38531, 38542, 38562-38564, 38570-38572, 38740, 38745, 38760, 38765, 38770, 38780, 56630-56634, 56637, 56640)
4.03 4.03 **FUD** ZZZ N N1 80 50
AMA: 2019,Feb,8; 2018,Jan,8; 2017,Jan,8; 2016,Jan,13; 2015,Mar,5

38999 Unlisted procedure, hemic or lymphatic system
0.00 0.00 **FUD** YYY S 80
AMA: 2018,Jan,8; 2017,Jan,8; 2016,Jan,13; 2015,Jan,16

39000-39499 Surgical Procedures: Mediastinum

39000 Mediastinotomy with exploration, drainage, removal of foreign body, or biopsy; cervical approach
14.3 14.3 **FUD** 090 C 80
AMA: 2014,Jan,11; 1994,Win,1

39010 transthoracic approach, including either transthoracic or median sternotomy
EXCLUDES *ECMO/ECLS insertion or reposition cannula (33955-33956, [33963, 33964])*
Video-assisted thoracic surgery (VATS) pericardial biopsy (32604)
22.7 22.7 **FUD** 090 C 80
AMA: 2018,Jan,8; 2017,Jan,8; 2016,Jan,13; 2015,Jul,3; 2015,Jan,16

39200 Resection of mediastinal cyst
25.2 25.2 **FUD** 090 C 80
AMA: 2014,Jan,11; 2012,Oct,9-11

39220 Resection of mediastinal tumor

EXCLUDES *Thymectomy (60520)*
Thyroidectomy, substernal (60270)
Video-assisted thoracic surgery (VATS) resection cyst, mass, or tumor of mediastinum (32662)

32.7 32.7 FUD 090 C 80

AMA: 2014,Jan,11; 2012,Oct,9-11

39401 Mediastinoscopy; includes biopsy(ies) of mediastinal mass (eg, lymphoma), when performed

8.93 8.93 FUD 000 J

AMA: 2018,Jan,8; 2017,Jan,8; 2016,Jun,4

39402 with lymph node biopsy(ies) (eg, lung cancer staging)

11.7 11.7 FUD 000 J

AMA: 2018,Jan,8; 2017,Jan,8; 2016,Jun,4

39499 Unlisted procedure, mediastinum

0.00 0.00 FUD YYY C 80

AMA: 2014,Jan,11

39501-39599 Surgical Procedures: Diaphragm

EXCLUDES *Esophagogastric fundoplasty, with fundic patch (43325)*
Repair diaphragmatic (esophageal) hernias:
Laparoscopic with fundoplication (43280-43282)
Laparotomy (43332-43333)
Thoracoabdominal (43336-43337)
Thoracotomy (43334-43335)

39501 Repair, laceration of diaphragm, any approach

24.6 24.6 FUD 090 C 80

AMA: 2018,Jan,8; 2017,Jan,8; 2016,Jan,13; 2015,Jan,16

39503 Repair, neonatal diaphragmatic hernia, with or without chest tube insertion and with or without creation of ventral hernia A

173. 173. FUD 090 63 C 80

AMA: 2018,Jan,8; 2017,Jan,8; 2016,Jan,13; 2015,Jan,16

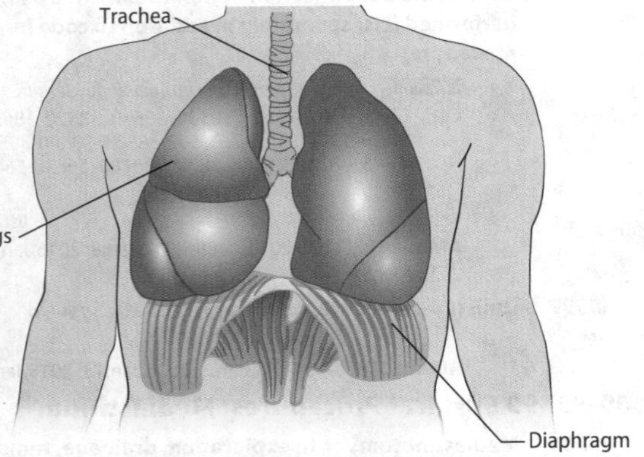

A defect of the diaphragm can allow abdominal contents to herniate into the thoracic cavity

39540 Repair, diaphragmatic hernia (other than neonatal), traumatic; acute

25.3 25.3 FUD 090 C 80

AMA: 2018,Jan,8; 2017,Jan,8; 2016,Jan,13; 2015,Jan,16

39541 chronic

27.3 27.3 FUD 090 C 80

AMA: 2018,Jan,8; 2017,Jan,8; 2016,Jan,13; 2015,Jan,16

39545 Imbrication of diaphragm for eventration, transthoracic or transabdominal, paralytic or nonparalytic

25.8 25.8 FUD 090 C 80

AMA: 2018,Jan,8; 2017,Jan,8; 2016,Jan,13; 2015,Jan,16

39560 Resection, diaphragm; with simple repair (eg, primary suture)

23.1 23.1 FUD 090 C 80

AMA: 2018,Jan,8; 2017,Jan,8; 2016,Jan,13; 2015,Jan,16

39561 with complex repair (eg, prosthetic material, local muscle flap)

35.9 35.9 FUD 090 C 80

AMA: 2018,Jan,8; 2017,Jan,8; 2016,Jan,13; 2015,Jan,16

39599 Unlisted procedure, diaphragm

0.00 0.00 FUD YYY C 80

AMA: 2014,Jan,11

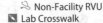

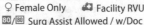

Digestive

Digestive

40490-40799 Resection and Repair Procedures of the Lips

EXCLUDES *Procedures on skin of lips — see integumentary section codes*

40490 Biopsy of lip
2.03 | 3.55 | FUD 000 | T P3
AMA: 2019,Jan,9

40500 Vermilionectomy (lip shave), with mucosal advancement
10.4 | 14.7 | FUD 090 | J A2
AMA: 2014,Jan,11; 2000,Sep,11

40510 Excision of lip; transverse wedge excision with primary closure
EXCLUDES *Excision mucous lesions (40810-40816)*
10.0 | 13.9 | FUD 090 | J A2
AMA: 2014,Jan,11

40520 V-excision with primary direct linear closure
EXCLUDES *Excision mucous lesions (40810-40816)*
10.2 | 14.2 | FUD 090 | J A2
AMA: 2014,Jan,11; 2000,Sep,11

40525 full thickness, reconstruction with local flap (eg, Estlander or fan)
15.8 | 15.8 | FUD 090 | J A2
AMA: 2014,Jan,11

40527 full thickness, reconstruction with cross lip flap (Abbe-Estlander)
INCLUDES Cleft lip repair with cross lip pedicle flap (Abbe-Estlander type), without pedicle sectioning and insertion
EXCLUDES *Cleft lip repair with cross lip pedicle flap (Abbe-Estlander type), with pedicle sectioning and insertion (40761)*
17.7 | 17.7 | FUD 090 | J A2 80
AMA: 2014,Jan,11

40530 Resection of lip, more than one-fourth, without reconstruction
EXCLUDES *Reconstruction (13131-13153)*
11.4 | 15.6 | FUD 090 | J A2
AMA: 2014,Jan,11

40650 Repair lip, full thickness; vermilion only
8.79 | 13.2 | FUD 090 | T A2 80
AMA: 2018,Jan,8; 2017,Jan,8; 2016,Nov,7; 2016,Jan,13; 2015,Jan,16

40652 up to half vertical height
10.2 | 14.5 | FUD 090 | T A2 80
AMA: 2018,Jan,8; 2017,Jan,8; 2016,Nov,7; 2016,Jan,13; 2015,Jan,16

40654 over one-half vertical height, or complex
12.1 | 16.5 | FUD 090 | T A2
AMA: 2018,Jan,8; 2017,Jan,8; 2016,Nov,7

40700 Plastic repair of cleft lip/nasal deformity; primary, partial or complete, unilateral
EXCLUDES *Cleft lip repair with cross lip pedicle flap (Abbe-Estlander type):*
With pedicle sectioning and insertion (40761)
Without pedicle sectioning and insertion (40527)
Rhinoplasty for nasal deformity secondary to congenital cleft lip (30460, 30462)
29.2 | 29.2 | FUD 090 | J A2 80
AMA: 2018,Jan,8; 2017,Jan,8; 2016,Jan,13; 2015,Jan,16

40701 primary bilateral, 1-stage procedure
EXCLUDES *Cleft lip repair with cross lip pedicle flap (Abbe-Estlander type):*
With pedicle sectioning and insertion (40761)
Without pedicle sectioning and insertion (40527)
Rhinoplasty for nasal deformity secondary to congenital cleft lip (30460, 30462)
34.6 | 34.6 | FUD 090 | J A2 80
AMA: 2018,Jan,8; 2017,Jan,8; 2016,Jan,13; 2015,Jan,16

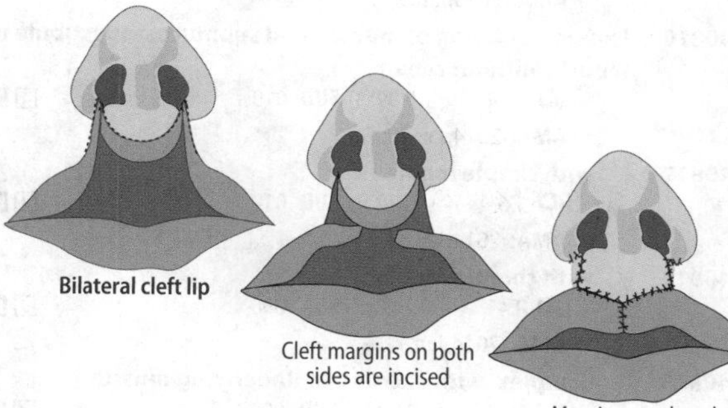
Bilateral cleft lip
Cleft margins on both sides are incised
Margins are closed, correcting cleft

40702 primary bilateral, 1 of 2 stages
EXCLUDES *Cleft lip repair with cross lip pedicle flap (Abbe-Estlander type):*
With pedicle sectioning and insertion (40761)
Without pedicle sectioning and insertion (40527)
Rhinoplasty for nasal deformity secondary to congenital cleft lip (30460, 30462)
29.0 | 29.0 | FUD 090 | J R2 80
AMA: 2018,Jan,8; 2017,Jan,8; 2016,Jan,13; 2015,Jan,16

40720 secondary, by recreation of defect and reclosure
EXCLUDES *Cleft lip repair with cross lip pedicle flap (Abbe-Estlander type):*
With pedicle sectioning and insertion (40761)
Without pedicle sectioning and insertion (40527)
Rhinoplasty for nasal deformity secondary to congenital cleft lip (30460, 30462)
29.8 | 29.8 | FUD 090 | J A2 80 50
AMA: 2018,Jan,8; 2017,Jan,8; 2016,Jan,13; 2015,Jan,16

40761 with cross lip pedicle flap (Abbe-Estlander type), including sectioning and inserting of pedicle
EXCLUDES *Cleft lip repair with cross lip pedicle flap (Abbe-Estlander type) without sectioning and insertion pedicle (40527)*
Cleft palate repair (42200-42225)
Other reconstructive procedures (14060-14061, 15120-15261, 15574, 15576, 15630)
31.3 | 31.3 | FUD 090 | J A2
AMA: 2014,Jan,11

40799 Unlisted procedure, lips
0.00 | 0.00 | FUD YYY | T 80
AMA: 2014,Jan,11

40800-40819 Incision and Resection of Buccal Cavity

INCLUDES Mucosal/submucosal tissue of lips/cheeks
Oral cavity outside dentoalveolar structures

40800 Drainage of abscess, cyst, hematoma, vestibule of mouth; simple
3.56 | 5.96 | FUD 010 | T P3
AMA: 2014,Jan,11

40801 complicated
5.96 | 8.59 | FUD 010 | T A2
AMA: 2014,Jan,11

40804 Removal of embedded foreign body, vestibule of mouth; simple
3.36 | 5.47 | FUD 010 | Q1 N1 80
AMA: 2014,Jan,11

40805 **complicated**
6.43 8.91 FUD 010 T P3 80
AMA: 2014,Jan,11

40806 **Incision of labial frenum (frenotomy)**
0.87 2.84 FUD 000 T P3 80
AMA: 2014,Jan,11

40808 **Biopsy, vestibule of mouth**
2.47 4.54 FUD 010 T P3
AMA: 2019,Jan,9

40810 **Excision of lesion of mucosa and submucosa, vestibule of mouth; without repair**
3.64 5.99 FUD 010 J P3
AMA: 2014,Jan,11

40812 **with simple repair**
5.63 8.30 FUD 010 J P3
AMA: 2014,Jan,11

40814 **with complex repair**
8.41 10.8 FUD 090 J A2
AMA: 2014,Jan,11

40816 **complex, with excision of underlying muscle**
8.81 11.4 FUD 090 J A2
AMA: 2014,Jan,11

40818 **Excision of mucosa of vestibule of mouth as donor graft**
7.78 10.4 FUD 090 T A2 80
AMA: 2014,Jan,11

40819 **Excision of frenum, labial or buccal (frenumectomy, frenulectomy, frenectomy)**
6.07 8.06 FUD 090 T A2 80
AMA: 2020,Aug,14

40820 Destruction of Lesion of Buccal Cavity

CMS: 100-03,140.5 Laser Procedures

INCLUDES Mucosal/submucosal tissue lips/cheeks
Oral cavity outside dentoalveolar structures

40820 **Destruction of lesion or scar of vestibule of mouth by physical methods (eg, laser, thermal, cryo, chemical)**
4.91 7.54 FUD 010 J P3
AMA: 2014,Jan,11; 1997,Nov,1

40830-40899 Repair Procedures of the Buccal Cavity

INCLUDES Mucosal/submucosal tissue lips/cheeks
Oral cavity outside dentoalveolar structures

EXCLUDES *Skin grafts (15002-15630)*

40830 **Closure of laceration, vestibule of mouth; 2.5 cm or less**
4.84 7.98 FUD 010 T G2 80
AMA: 2014,Jan,11

40831 **over 2.5 cm or complex**
6.64 10.1 FUD 010 T A2 80
AMA: 2014,Jan,11

40840 **Vestibuloplasty; anterior**
18.0 23.9 FUD 090 J A2 80
AMA: 2014,Jan,11

40842 **posterior, unilateral**
19.5 26.2 FUD 090 J A2 80
AMA: 2014,Jan,11

40843 **posterior, bilateral**
23.6 30.1 FUD 090 J A2 80
AMA: 2014,Jan,11

40844 **entire arch**
34.2 42.9 FUD 090 J A2 80
AMA: 2014,Jan,11

40845 **complex (including ridge extension, muscle repositioning)**
35.2 42.2 FUD 090 J A2 80
AMA: 2014,Jan,11

40899 **Unlisted procedure, vestibule of mouth**
0.00 0.00 FUD YYY T 80
AMA: 2014,Jan,11

41000-41018 Surgical Incision of Floor of Mouth or Tongue

EXCLUDES *Frenoplasty (41520)*

41000 **Intraoral incision and drainage of abscess, cyst, or hematoma of tongue or floor of mouth; lingual**
3.13 4.54 FUD 010 T P3
AMA: 2014,Jan,11

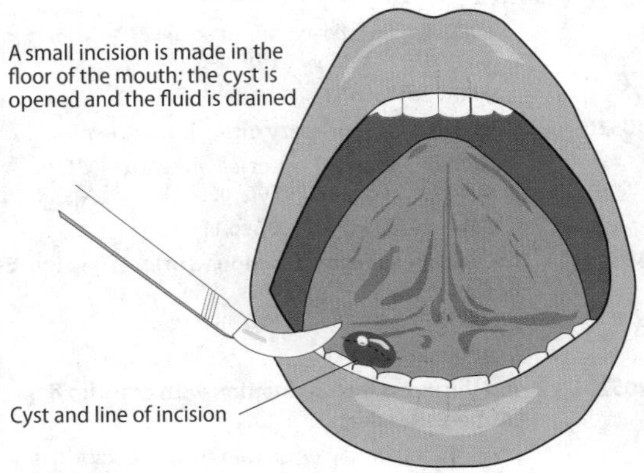
A small incision is made in the floor of the mouth; the cyst is opened and the fluid is drained
Cyst and line of incision

41005 **sublingual, superficial**
3.30 6.20 FUD 010 T A2 80
AMA: 2014,Jan,11

41006 **sublingual, deep, supramylohyoid**
6.85 9.81 FUD 090 T A2 80
AMA: 2014,Jan,11

41007 **submental space**
6.64 9.63 FUD 090 T A2 80
AMA: 2014,Jan,11

41008 **submandibular space**
7.45 10.9 FUD 090 J A2 80
AMA: 2014,Jan,11

41009 **masticator space**
8.19 11.8 FUD 090 T A2 80
AMA: 2014,Jan,11

41010 **Incision of lingual frenum (frenotomy)**
3.09 5.97 FUD 010 T A2 80
AMA: 2020,Aug,14; 2018,Jan,8; 2017,Nov,10; 2017,Sep,14

41015 **Extraoral incision and drainage of abscess, cyst, or hematoma of floor of mouth; sublingual**
8.92 11.6 FUD 090 T A2 80
AMA: 2014,Jan,11

41016 **submental**
9.92 13.0 FUD 090 J A2 80
AMA: 2014,Jan,11

41017 **submandibular**
9.86 12.9 FUD 090 J A2 80
AMA: 2014,Jan,11

41018 **masticator space**
11.4 14.5 FUD 090 T A2 80
AMA: 2014,Jan,11

41019 Placement of Devices for Brachytherapy

EXCLUDES *Application interstitial radioelements (77770-77772, 77778)*
Intracranial brachytherapy radiation sources with stereotactic insertion (61770)

41019 **Placement of needles, catheters, or other device(s) into the head and/or neck region (percutaneous, transoral, or transnasal) for subsequent interstitial radioelement application**
(76942, 77002, 77012, 77021)
13.9 13.9 FUD 000 J G2 80
AMA: 2018,Jan,8; 2017,Jan,8; 2016,Jan,13; 2015,Jan,16

41100-41599 Resection and Repair of the Tongue

41100 **Biopsy of tongue; anterior two-thirds**
3.07 4.94 FUD 010 T P3
AMA: 2019,Jan,9

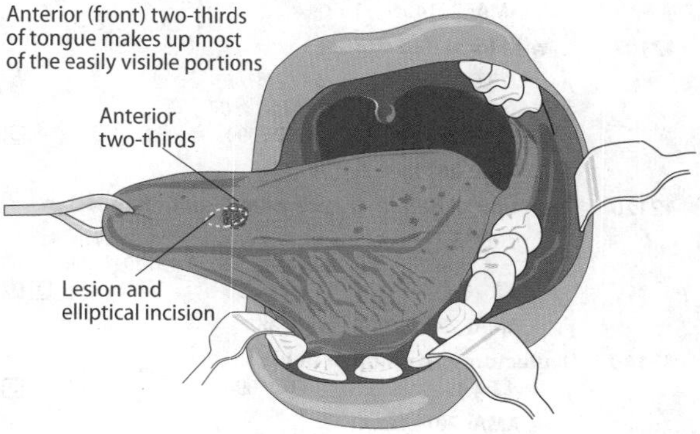
Anterior (front) two-thirds of tongue makes up most of the easily visible portions
Anterior two-thirds
Lesion and elliptical incision

41105 **posterior one-third**
3.11 5.05 FUD 010 J P3
AMA: 2014,Jan,11

41108 **Biopsy of floor of mouth**
2.52 4.43 FUD 010 J P3
AMA: 2019,Jan,9

41110 **Excision of lesion of tongue without closure**
3.73 6.29 FUD 010 J P3
AMA: 2014,Jan,11

41112 **Excision of lesion of tongue with closure; anterior two-thirds**
7.03 9.57 FUD 090 J A2
AMA: 2014,Jan,11

41113 **posterior one-third**
7.98 10.5 FUD 090 J A2
AMA: 2014,Jan,11

41114 **with local tongue flap**
INCLUDES Excision lesion tongue with closure anterior/posterior two-thirds (41112-41113)
17.7 17.7 FUD 090 J A2 80
AMA: 2014,Jan,11

41115 **Excision of lingual frenum (frenectomy)**
4.16 7.25 FUD 010 T P3 80
AMA: 2018,Jan,8; 2017,Nov,10; 2017,Sep,14

41116 **Excision, lesion of floor of mouth**
6.18 9.50 FUD 090 J A2
AMA: 2014,Jan,11

41120 **Glossectomy; less than one-half tongue**
30.3 30.3 FUD 090 J A2 80
AMA: 2018,Jan,8; 2017,Jan,8; 2016,Jan,13; 2015,Jan,16

41130 **hemiglossectomy**
38.0 38.0 FUD 090 C 80
AMA: 2018,Jan,8; 2017,Jan,8; 2016,Jan,13; 2015,Jan,16

41135 **partial, with unilateral radical neck dissection**
62.0 62.0 FUD 090 C 80
AMA: 2018,Jan,8; 2017,Jan,8; 2016,Jan,13; 2015,Jan,16

41140 **complete or total, with or without tracheostomy, without radical neck dissection**
INCLUDES Regnoli's excision
62.3 62.3 FUD 090 C 80
AMA: 2018,Jan,8; 2017,Jan,8; 2016,Jan,13; 2015,Jan,16

41145 **complete or total, with or without tracheostomy, with unilateral radical neck dissection**
78.9 78.9 FUD 090 C 80
AMA: 2018,Jan,8; 2017,Jan,8; 2016,Jan,13; 2015,Jan,16

41150 **composite procedure with resection floor of mouth and mandibular resection, without radical neck dissection**
62.8 62.8 FUD 090 C 80
AMA: 2018,Jan,8; 2017,Jan,8; 2016,Jan,13; 2015,Jan,16

41153 **composite procedure with resection floor of mouth, with suprahyoid neck dissection**
68.8 68.8 FUD 090 C 80
AMA: 2018,Jan,8; 2017,Jan,8; 2016,Jan,13; 2015,Jan,16

41155 **composite procedure with resection floor of mouth, mandibular resection, and radical neck dissection (Commando type)**
86.1 86.1 FUD 090 C 80
AMA: 2018,Jan,8; 2017,Jan,8; 2016,Jan,13; 2015,Jan,16

41250 **Repair of laceration 2.5 cm or less; floor of mouth and/or anterior two-thirds of tongue**
4.43 7.98 FUD 010 Q1 N1 80
AMA: 2014,Jan,11

41251 **posterior one-third of tongue**
5.27 8.83 FUD 010 T A2 80
AMA: 2014,Jan,11

41252 **Repair of laceration of tongue, floor of mouth, over 2.6 cm or complex**
6.01 9.18 FUD 010 T A2 80
AMA: 2014,Jan,11

41510 **Suture of tongue to lip for micrognathia (Douglas type procedure)**
13.0 13.0 FUD 090 J A2 80
AMA: 2018,Jan,8; 2017,Jan,8; 2016,Jan,13; 2015,Jan,16

41512 **Tongue base suspension, permanent suture technique**
EXCLUDES *Suture tongue to lip for micrognathia (41510)*
18.8 18.8 FUD 090 J G2 80
AMA: 2018,Jan,8; 2017,Jan,8; 2016,Jan,13; 2015,Jan,16

41520 **Frenoplasty (surgical revision of frenum, eg, with Z-plasty)**
EXCLUDES *Frenotomy (40806, 41010)*
7.11 10.1 FUD 090 J A2 80
AMA: 2020,Aug,14; 2018,Jan,8; 2017,Nov,10; 2017,Sep,14

41530 **Submucosal ablation of the tongue base, radiofrequency, 1 or more sites, per session**
10.6 27.1 FUD 000 J P3 80
AMA: 2018,Jan,8; 2017,Jan,8; 2016,Jan,13; 2015,Jan,16

41599 **Unlisted procedure, tongue, floor of mouth**
0.00 0.00 FUD YYY T 80
AMA: 2018,Jan,8; 2017,Jan,8; 2016,Jan,13; 2015,Jan,16

41800-41899 Procedures of the Teeth and Supporting Structures

41800 **Drainage of abscess, cyst, hematoma from dentoalveolar structures**
4.35 8.29 FUD 010 Q1 N1
AMA: 2014,Jan,11

41805 **Removal of embedded foreign body from dentoalveolar structures; soft tissues**
5.42 8.45 FUD 010 T P3 80
AMA: 2014,Jan,11

41806 **bone**
7.86 11.4 FUD 010 T P3 80
AMA: 2014,Jan,11

Digestive System

41019 — 41806

● New Code ▲ Revised Code ○ Reinstated ● New Web Release ▲ Revised Web Release + Add-on Unlisted Not Covered # Resequenced
⑩ Optum Mod 50 Exempt ⊘ AMA Mod 51 Exempt ⑪ Optum Mod 51 Exempt ⑬ Mod 63 Exempt Non-FDA Drug ★ Telemedicine M Maternity A Age Edit

41820 Gingivectomy, excision gingiva, each quadrant
0.00 0.00 **FUD** 000 J R2 80
AMA: 2014,Jan,11

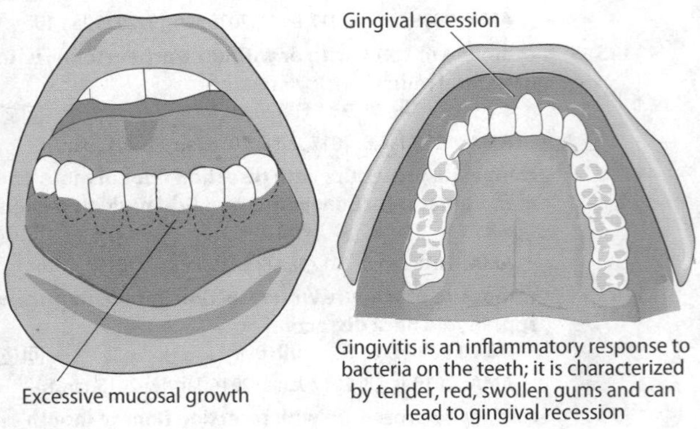

Gingivitis is an inflammatory response to bacteria on the teeth; it is characterized by tender, red, swollen gums and can lead to gingival recession

41821 Operculectomy, excision pericoronal tissues
0.00 0.00 **FUD** 000 T G2 80
AMA: 2014,Jan,11

41822 Excision of fibrous tuberosities, dentoalveolar structures
5.71 9.88 **FUD** 010 T P3 80
AMA: 2014,Jan,11

41823 Excision of osseous tuberosities, dentoalveolar structures
10.2 14.5 **FUD** 090 J P3 80
AMA: 2014,Jan,11

41825 Excision of lesion or tumor (except listed above), dentoalveolar structures; without repair
EXCLUDES *Lesion destruction nonexcisional (41850)*
3.43 6.19 **FUD** 010 J P3
AMA: 2014,Jan,11

41826 with simple repair
EXCLUDES *Lesion destruction nonexcisional (41850)*
5.88 8.96 **FUD** 010 J P3
AMA: 2014,Jan,11

41827 with complex repair
EXCLUDES *Lesion destruction nonexcisional (41850)*
8.59 12.7 **FUD** 090 J A2
AMA: 2014,Jan,11

41828 Excision of hyperplastic alveolar mucosa, each quadrant (specify)
6.43 9.95 **FUD** 010 J P3 80
AMA: 2014,Jan,11; 1994,Win,1

41830 Alveolectomy, including curettage of osteitis or sequestrectomy
8.91 13.0 **FUD** 010 J P3 80
AMA: 2014,Jan,11

41850 Destruction of lesion (except excision), dentoalveolar structures
0.00 0.00 **FUD** 000 T R2 80
AMA: 2014,Jan,11

41870 Periodontal mucosal grafting
0.00 0.00 **FUD** 000 J G2 80
AMA: 2014,Jan,11

41872 Gingivoplasty, each quadrant (specify)
8.54 12.8 **FUD** 090 J P3 80
AMA: 2014,Jan,11; 1994,Win,1

41874 Alveoloplasty, each quadrant (specify)
EXCLUDES *Fracture reduction (21421-21490)*
Laceration closure (40830-40831)
Maxilla osteotomy, segmental (21206)
7.41 11.1 **FUD** 090 J P3 80
AMA: 2014,Jan,11; 1994,Win,1

41899 Unlisted procedure, dentoalveolar structures
0.00 0.00 **FUD** YYY T 80
AMA: 2014,Jan,11

42000-42299 Procedures of the Palate and Uvula

42000 Drainage of abscess of palate, uvula
2.98 4.49 **FUD** 010 T A2 80
AMA: 2014,Jan,11

42100 Biopsy of palate, uvula
3.08 4.22 **FUD** 010 T P3
AMA: 2014,Jan,11

42104 Excision, lesion of palate, uvula; without closure
3.90 6.20 **FUD** 010 J P3
AMA: 2014,Jan,11

42106 with simple primary closure
4.86 7.62 **FUD** 010 J P3
AMA: 2014,Jan,11

42107 with local flap closure
EXCLUDES *Mucosal graft (40818)*
Skin graft (14040-14302)
9.73 13.2 **FUD** 090 J A2
AMA: 2014,Jan,11

42120 Resection of palate or extensive resection of lesion
EXCLUDES *Palate reconstruction using extraoral tissue (14040-14302, 15050, 15120, 15240, 15576)*
28.7 28.7 **FUD** 090 J A2 80
AMA: 2014,Jan,11; 1991,Fall,1

42140 Uvulectomy, excision of uvula
4.46 8.04 **FUD** 090 J A2
AMA: 2014,Jan,11

42145 Palatopharyngoplasty (eg, uvulopalatopharyngoplasty, uvulopharyngoplasty)
EXCLUDES *Excision maxillary torus palatinus (21032)*
Excision torus mandibularis (21031)
19.8 19.8 **FUD** 090 J A2
AMA: 2018,Jan,8; 2017,Jan,8; 2016,Jan,13; 2015,Jan,16

42160 Destruction of lesion, palate or uvula (thermal, cryo or chemical)
4.15 6.71 **FUD** 010 J P3 80
AMA: 2018,Jan,8; 2017,Jan,8; 2016,Jan,13; 2015,Jan,16

42180 Repair, laceration of palate; up to 2 cm
5.28 7.17 **FUD** 010 T A2 80
AMA: 2014,Jan,11

42182 over 2 cm or complex
7.34 9.34 **FUD** 010 J A2 80
AMA: 2014,Jan,11

42200 Palatoplasty for cleft palate, soft and/or hard palate only
27.2 27.2 **FUD** 090 J A2 80
AMA: 2018,Jan,8; 2017,Jan,8; 2016,Jan,13; 2015,Mar,9; 2015,Jan,16

42205 Palatoplasty for cleft palate, with closure of alveolar ridge; soft tissue only
28.4 28.4 **FUD** 090 J A2 80
AMA: 2014,Jan,11

42210 with bone graft to alveolar ridge (includes obtaining graft)
31.7 31.7 **FUD** 090 J A2 80
AMA: 2014,Jan,11

42215 Palatoplasty for cleft palate; major revision
20.7 20.7 **FUD** 090 J A2 80
AMA: 2014,Jan,11

42220 secondary lengthening procedure
17.0 17.0 **FUD** 090 J A2 80
AMA: 2014,Jan,11

42225 attachment pharyngeal flap
28.2 28.2 **FUD** 090 J G2 80
AMA: 2018,Jan,8; 2017,Jan,8; 2016,Jan,13; 2015,Jan,16

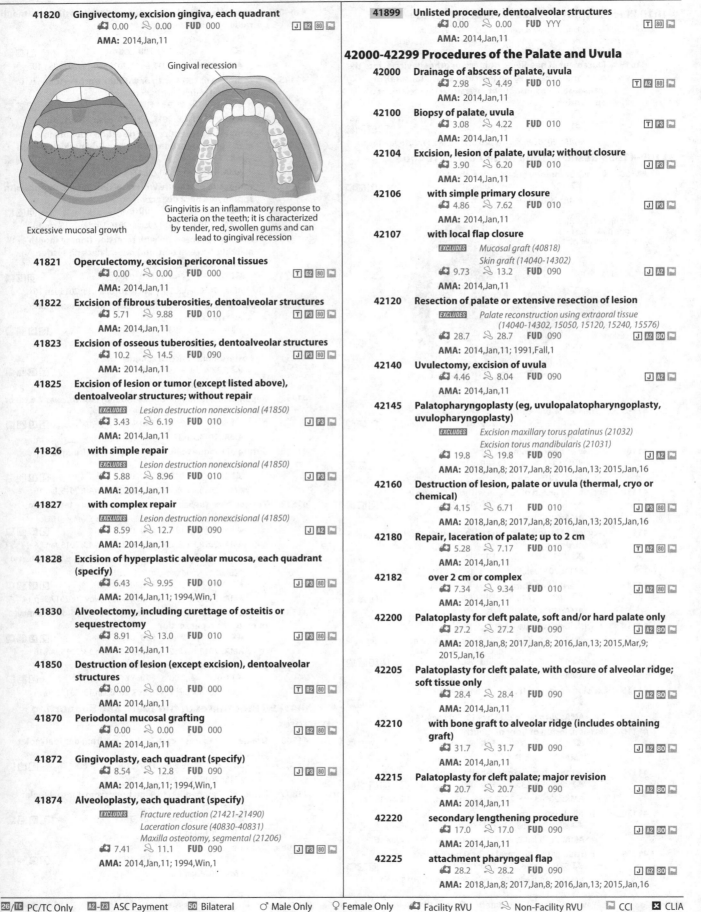

42226 **Lengthening of palate, and pharyngeal flap**
🚑 25.3 ⚕ 25.3 **FUD** 090 `J` `A2` `80` `▣`
AMA: 2014,Jan,11

42227 **Lengthening of palate, with island flap**
🚑 23.6 ⚕ 23.6 **FUD** 090 `J` `G2` `80` `▣`
AMA: 2014,Jan,11

42235 **Repair of anterior palate, including vomer flap**
EXCLUDES *Oronasal fistula repair (30600)*
🚑 20.7 ⚕ 20.7 **FUD** 090 `J` `A2` `80` `▣`
AMA: 2018,Jan,8; 2017,Jan,8; 2016,Jan,13; 2015,Mar,9; 2015,Jan,16

42260 **Repair of nasolabial fistula**
EXCLUDES *Cleft lip repair (40700-40761)*
🚑 18.9 ⚕ 23.8 **FUD** 090 `J` `A2` `80` `▣`
AMA: 2014,Jan,11

42280 **Maxillary impression for palatal prosthesis**
🚑 3.12 ⚕ 5.08 **FUD** 010 `T` `P3` `80` `▣`
AMA: 2014,Jan,11

42281 **Insertion of pin-retained palatal prosthesis**
🚑 4.75 ⚕ 6.56 **FUD** 010 `J` `G2` `80` `▣`
AMA: 2014,Jan,11

42299 **Unlisted procedure, palate, uvula**
🚑 0.00 ⚕ 0.00 **FUD** YYY `T` `80` `▣`
AMA: 2018,Jan,8; 2017,Jan,8; 2016,Jan,13; 2015,Jan,16

42300-42699 Procedures of the Salivary Ducts and Glands

42300 **Drainage of abscess; parotid, simple**
🚑 4.39 ⚕ 6.10 **FUD** 010 `T` `A2` `▣`
AMA: 2014,Jan,11

42305 **parotid, complicated**
🚑 12.2 ⚕ 12.2 **FUD** 090 `J` `A2` `80` `▣`
AMA: 2014,Jan,11

42310 **Drainage of abscess; submaxillary or sublingual, intraoral**
🚑 3.92 ⚕ 5.08 **FUD** 010 `T` `A2` `80` `▣`
AMA: 2014,Jan,11

42320 **submaxillary, external**
🚑 5.03 ⚕ 7.31 **FUD** 010 `T` `A2` `80` `▣`
AMA: 2014,Jan,11

42330 **Sialolithotomy; submandibular (submaxillary), sublingual or parotid, uncomplicated, intraoral**
🚑 4.69 ⚕ 6.63 **FUD** 010 `J` `P3` `▣`
AMA: 2014,Jan,11

42335 **submandibular (submaxillary), complicated, intraoral**
🚑 7.37 ⚕ 11.5 **FUD** 090 `J` `P3` `▣`
AMA: 2014,Jan,11

42340 **parotid, extraoral or complicated intraoral**
🚑 9.65 ⚕ 14.1 **FUD** 090 `J` `A2` `80` `50` `▣`
AMA: 2014,Jan,11

42400 **Biopsy of salivary gland; needle**
EXCLUDES *Fine needle aspiration (10021, [10004, 10005, 10006, 10007, 10008, 10009, 10010, 10011, 10012])*
📷 (76942, 77002, 77012, 77021)
🔬 (88172-88173)
🚑 1.55 ⚕ 2.95 **FUD** 000 `T` `P3` `▣`
AMA: 2019,Apr,4

42405 **incisional**
📷 (76942, 77002, 77012, 77021)
🚑 6.48 ⚕ 8.61 **FUD** 010 `J` `A2`
AMA: 2014,Jan,11

42408 **Excision of sublingual salivary cyst (ranula)**
🚑 10.0 ⚕ 15.0 **FUD** 090 `J` `A2` `80` `▣`
AMA: 2014,Jan,11

42409 **Marsupialization of sublingual salivary cyst (ranula)**
🚑 6.42 ⚕ 10.4 **FUD** 090 `J` `A2` `80` `▣`
AMA: 2014,Jan,11

42410 **Excision of parotid tumor or parotid gland; lateral lobe, without nerve dissection**
EXCLUDES *Facial nerve suture or graft (64864, 64865, 69740, 69745)*
🚑 17.9 ⚕ 17.9 **FUD** 090 `J` `A2` `80` `50` `▣`
AMA: 2014,Jan,11

42415 **lateral lobe, with dissection and preservation of facial nerve**
EXCLUDES *Facial nerve suture or graft (64864, 64865, 69740, 69745)*
🚑 30.2 ⚕ 30.2 **FUD** 090 `J` `A2` `80` `50` `▣`
AMA: 2014,Jan,11

42420 **total, with dissection and preservation of facial nerve**
EXCLUDES *Facial nerve suture or graft (64864, 64865, 69740, 69745)*
🚑 33.9 ⚕ 33.9 **FUD** 090 `J` `A2` `80` `50` `▣`
AMA: 2014,Jan,11; 2010,Aug,3-7

42425 **total, en bloc removal with sacrifice of facial nerve**
EXCLUDES *Facial nerve suture or graft (64864, 64865, 69740, 69745)*
🚑 23.9 ⚕ 23.9 **FUD** 090 `J` `A2` `80` `50` `▣`
AMA: 2014,Jan,11

42426 **total, with unilateral radical neck dissection**
EXCLUDES *Facial nerve suture or graft (64864, 64865, 69740, 69745)*
🚑 38.8 ⚕ 38.8 **FUD** 090 `C` `80` `50` `▣`
AMA: 2018,Jan,8; 2017,Jan,8; 2016,Jan,13; 2015,Jan,16

42440 **Excision of submandibular (submaxillary) gland**
🚑 11.8 ⚕ 11.8 **FUD** 090 `J` `A2` `80` `50` `▣`
AMA: 2014,Jan,11

42450 **Excision of sublingual gland**
🚑 10.3 ⚕ 13.1 **FUD** 090 `J` `A2` `80` `▣`
AMA: 2014,Jan,11

42500 **Plastic repair of salivary duct, sialodochoplasty; primary or simple**
🚑 9.71 ⚕ 12.4 **FUD** 090 `J` `A2` `80` `▣`
AMA: 2014,Jan,11

42505 **secondary or complicated**
🚑 12.9 ⚕ 15.9 **FUD** 090 `J` `A2`
AMA: 2014,Jan,11

42507 **Parotid duct diversion, bilateral (Wilke type procedure);**
🚑 14.4 ⚕ 14.4 **FUD** 090 `J` `A2` `80` `▣`
AMA: 2014,Jan,11

42509 **with excision of both submandibular glands**
🚑 23.6 ⚕ 23.6 **FUD** 090 `J` `A2` `80` `▣`
AMA: 2014,Jan,11

42510 **with ligation of both submandibular (Wharton's) ducts**
🚑 17.5 ⚕ 17.5 **FUD** 090 `J` `A2` `80` `▣`
AMA: 2014,Jan,11

42550 **Injection procedure for sialography**
📷 (70390)
🚑 1.83 ⚕ 4.39 **FUD** 000 `N` `N1` `▣`
AMA: 2014,Jan,11

42600 **Closure salivary fistula**
🚑 9.99 ⚕ 14.5 **FUD** 090 `J` `A2` `80` `▣`
AMA: 2014,Jan,11

42650 **Dilation salivary duct**
🚑 1.65 ⚕ 2.25 **FUD** 000 `T` `P3` `▣`
AMA: 2014,Jan,11

42660 **Dilation and catheterization of salivary duct, with or without injection**
🚑 2.52 ⚕ 3.52 **FUD** 000 `T` `P3` `80` `▣`
AMA: 2014,Jan,11

42665 **Ligation salivary duct, intraoral**
🚑 5.97 ⚕ 9.82 **FUD** 090 `J` `A2` `80` `▣`
AMA: 2014,Jan,11

● New Code   ▲ Revised Code   ○ Reinstated   ● New Web Release   ▲ Revised Web Release   + Add-on   Unlisted   Not Covered   # Resequenced
⑤⓪ Optum Mod 50 Exempt   ⊘ AMA Mod 51 Exempt   ⑤① Optum Mod 51 Exempt   ⑥③ Mod 63 Exempt   ⨍ Non-FDA Drug   ★ Telemedicine   Ⓜ Maternity   Ⓐ Age Edit

42699 **Unlisted procedure, salivary glands or ducts**
0.00 0.00 FUD YYY T 80
AMA: 2014,Jan,11

42700-42999 Procedures of the Adenoids/Throat/Tonsils

42700 **Incision and drainage abscess; peritonsillar**
3.88 5.43 FUD 010 T A2
AMA: 2014,Jan,11

42720 **retropharyngeal or parapharyngeal, intraoral approach**
11.1 12.9 FUD 010 J A2 80
AMA: 2014,Jan,11

42725 **retropharyngeal or parapharyngeal, external approach**
23.0 23.0 FUD 090 J A2 80
AMA: 2014,Jan,11

42800 **Biopsy; oropharynx**
EXCLUDES *Laryngoscopy with biopsy (31510, 31535-31536)*
3.22 4.49 FUD 010 J P3
AMA: 2014,Jan,11

42804 **nasopharynx, visible lesion, simple**
EXCLUDES *Laryngoscopy with biopsy (31510, 31535-31536)*
3.27 5.65 FUD 010 J A2
AMA: 2014,Jan,11

42806 **nasopharynx, survey for unknown primary lesion**
EXCLUDES *Laryngoscopy with biopsy (31510, 31535-31536)*
3.81 6.33 FUD 010 J A2
AMA: 2014,Jan,11

42808 **Excision or destruction of lesion of pharynx, any method**
4.66 6.53 FUD 010 J A2
AMA: 2014,Jan,11

42809 **Removal of foreign body from pharynx**
3.56 5.76 FUD 010 Q1 N1
AMA: 2014,Jan,11

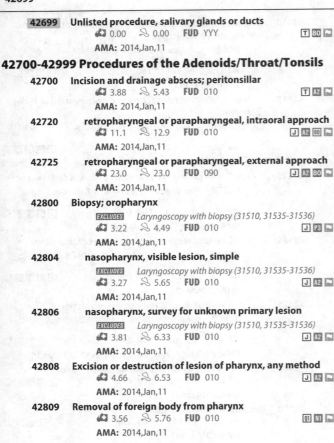

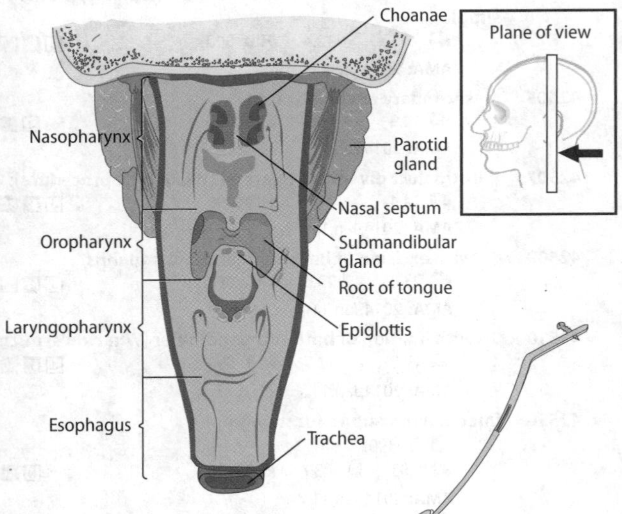

A foreign body is removed from the pharynx

42810 **Excision branchial cleft cyst or vestige, confined to skin and subcutaneous tissues**
8.10 11.0 FUD 090 J A2 80 50
AMA: 2014,Jan,11

42815 **Excision branchial cleft cyst, vestige, or fistula, extending beneath subcutaneous tissues and/or into pharynx**
15.6 15.6 FUD 090 J A2 80 50
AMA: 2014,Jan,11

42820 **Tonsillectomy and adenoidectomy; younger than age 12** A
8.26 8.26 FUD 090 J A2 80
AMA: 2018,Jan,8; 2017,Jan,8; 2016,Jan,13; 2015,Jan,16

42821 **age 12 or over** A
8.62 8.62 FUD 090 J A2 80
AMA: 2018,Jan,8; 2017,Jan,8; 2016,Jan,13; 2015,Jan,16

42825 **Tonsillectomy, primary or secondary; younger than age 12** A
7.52 7.52 FUD 090 J A2 80
AMA: 2018,Jan,8; 2017,Jan,8; 2016,Jan,13; 2015,Jan,16

42826 **age 12 or over** A
7.20 7.20 FUD 090 J A2
AMA: 2018,Jan,8; 2017,Jan,8; 2016,Jan,13; 2015,Jan,16

42830 **Adenoidectomy, primary; younger than age 12** A
5.95 5.95 FUD 090 J A2 80
AMA: 2018,Jan,8; 2017,Jan,8; 2016,Jan,13; 2015,Jan,16

42831 **age 12 or over** A
6.44 6.44 FUD 090 J A2 80
AMA: 2018,Jan,8; 2017,Jan,8; 2016,Jan,13; 2015,Jan,16

42835 **Adenoidectomy, secondary; younger than age 12** A
5.51 5.51 FUD 090 J A2 80
AMA: 2018,Jan,8; 2017,Jan,8; 2016,Jan,13; 2015,Jan,16

42836 **age 12 or over** A
6.89 6.89 FUD 090 J A2 80
AMA: 2018,Jan,8; 2017,Jan,8; 2016,Jan,13; 2015,Jan,16

42842 **Radical resection of tonsil, tonsillar pillars, and/or retromolar trigone; without closure**
28.7 28.7 FUD 090 J 80
AMA: 2018,Jan,8; 2017,Jan,8; 2016,Jan,13; 2015,Jan,16

42844 **closure with local flap (eg, tongue, buccal)**
39.9 39.9 FUD 090 J 80
AMA: 2018,Jan,8; 2017,Jan,8; 2016,Jan,13; 2015,Jan,16

42845 **closure with other flap**
Code also closure with other flap(s)
Code also radical neck dissection when combined (38720)
63.9 63.9 FUD 090 C 80
AMA: 2018,Jan,8; 2017,Jan,8; 2016,Jan,13; 2015,Jan,16

42860 **Excision of tonsil tags**
5.40 5.40 FUD 090 J A2 80
AMA: 2014,Jan,11

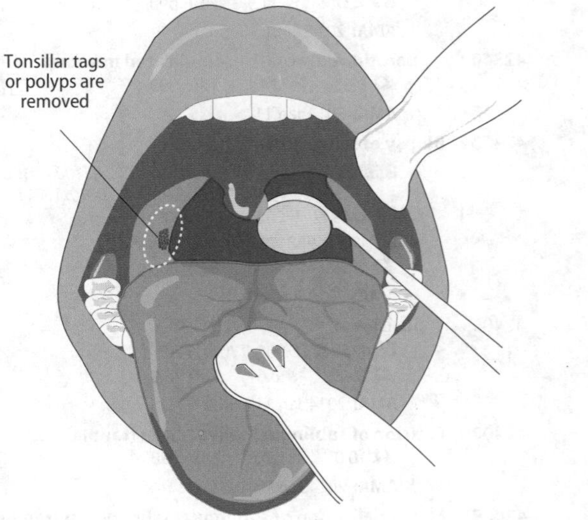

42870 **Excision or destruction lingual tonsil, any method (separate procedure)**

EXCLUDES *Nasopharynx resection (juvenile angiofibroma) by transzygomatic/bicoronal approach (61586, 61600)*

17.0 17.0 FUD 090 J A2 80

AMA: 2014,Jan,11

42890 **Limited pharyngectomy**

Code also radical neck dissection when combined (38720)

40.7 40.7 FUD 090 J A2 80

AMA: 2014,Jan,11; 2010,Aug,3-7

42892 **Resection of lateral pharyngeal wall or pyriform sinus, direct closure by advancement of lateral and posterior pharyngeal walls**

Code also radical neck dissection when combined (38720)

53.6 53.6 FUD 090 J A2 80

AMA: 2018,Jan,8; 2017,Jan,8; 2016,Jan,13; 2015,Jan,16

42894 **Resection of pharyngeal wall requiring closure with myocutaneous or fasciocutaneous flap or free muscle, skin, or fascial flap with microvascular anastomosis**

EXCLUDES *Flap used for reconstruction (15730, 15733-15734, 15756-15758)*

Code also radical neck dissection when combined (38720)

67.7 67.7 FUD 090 C 80

AMA: 2018,Jan,8; 2017,Jan,8; 2016,Jan,13; 2015,Jan,16

42900 **Suture pharynx for wound or injury**

9.56 9.56 FUD 010 T A2 80

AMA: 2014,Jan,11

42950 **Pharyngoplasty (plastic or reconstructive operation on pharynx)**

EXCLUDES *Pharyngeal flap (42225)*

22.8 22.8 FUD 090 J A2 80

AMA: 2019,Oct,10; 2018,Jan,8; 2017,Jan,8; 2016,Apr,8

42953 **Pharyngoesophageal repair**

Code also closure using myocutaneous or other flap

27.3 27.3 FUD 090 C 80

AMA: 2014,Jan,11

42955 **Pharyngostomy (fistulization of pharynx, external for feeding)**

21.7 21.7 FUD 090 T A2 80

AMA: 2014,Jan,11

42960 **Control oropharyngeal hemorrhage, primary or secondary (eg, post-tonsillectomy); simple**

4.83 4.83 FUD 010 T A2 80

AMA: 2014,Jan,11

42961 **complicated, requiring hospitalization**

11.9 11.9 FUD 090 C 80

AMA: 2014,Jan,11

42962 **with secondary surgical intervention**

14.7 14.7 FUD 090 J A2

AMA: 2014,Jan,11

42970 **Control of nasopharyngeal hemorrhage, primary or secondary (eg, postadenoidectomy); simple, with posterior nasal packs, with or without anterior packs and/or cautery**

11.7 11.7 FUD 090 T R2

AMA: 2014,Jan,11; 2002,May,7

42971 **complicated, requiring hospitalization**

12.9 12.9 FUD 090 C 80

AMA: 2014,Jan,11

42972 **with secondary surgical intervention**

14.5 14.5 FUD 090 J A2 80

AMA: 2014,Jan,11

42999 **Unlisted procedure, pharynx, adenoids, or tonsils**

0.00 0.00 FUD YYY T 80

AMA: 2018,Jan,8; 2017,Jan,8; 2016,Jan,13; 2015,Jan,16

43020-43135 Incision/Resection of Esophagus

43020 **Esophagotomy, cervical approach, with removal of foreign body**

EXCLUDES *Laparotomy with esophageal intubation (43510)*

16.2 16.2 FUD 090 T 80

AMA: 2014,Jan,11

43030 **Cricopharyngeal myotomy**

EXCLUDES *Laparotomy with esophageal intubation (43510)*

14.8 14.8 FUD 090 J G2 80

AMA: 2020,Jul,13

43045 **Esophagotomy, thoracic approach, with removal of foreign body**

EXCLUDES *Laparotomy with esophageal intubation (43510)*

37.6 37.6 FUD 090 C 80

AMA: 2014,Jan,11; 1994,Win,1

43100 **Excision of lesion, esophagus, with primary repair; cervical approach**

EXCLUDES *Gastrointestinal reconstruction for previous esophagectomy (43360-43361)*
Wide excision malignant lesion cervical esophagus, with total laryngectomy:
With radical neck dissection (31365, 43107, 43116, 43124)
Without radical neck dissection (31360, 43107, 43116, 43124)

18.0 18.0 FUD 090 C 80

AMA: 2014,Jan,11; 1994,Win,1

43101 **thoracic or abdominal approach**

EXCLUDES *Gastrointestinal reconstruction for previous esophagectomy (43360-43361)*
Wide excision malignant lesion cervical esophagus, with total laryngectomy:
With radical neck dissection (31365, 43107, 43116, 43124)
Without radical neck dissection (31360, 43107, 43116, 43124)

29.1 29.1 FUD 090 C 80

AMA: 2018,Jan,8; 2017,Jan,8; 2016,Jan,13; 2015,Jan,16

43107 **Total or near total esophagectomy, without thoracotomy; with pharyngogastrostomy or cervical esophagogastrostomy, with or without pyloroplasty (transhiatal)**

EXCLUDES *Gastrointestinal reconstruction for previous esophagectomy (43360-43361)*

86.5 86.5 FUD 090 C 80

AMA: 2014,Jan,11; 2010,Aug,3-7

43108 **with colon interposition or small intestine reconstruction, including intestine mobilization, preparation and anastomosis(es)**

EXCLUDES *Gastrointestinal reconstruction for previous esophagectomy (43360-43361)*

129. 129. FUD 090 C 80

AMA: 2014,Jan,11; 2002,May,7

43112 **Total or near total esophagectomy, with thoracotomy; with pharyngogastrostomy or cervical esophagogastrostomy, with or without pyloroplasty (ie, McKeown esophagectomy or tri-incisional esophagectomy)**

EXCLUDES *Gastrointestinal reconstruction for previous esophagectomy (43360-43361)*

101. 101. FUD 090 C 80

AMA: 2018,Jul,7; 2018,Jan,8; 2017,Jan,8; 2016,Jan,13; 2015,Jan,16

43113 **with colon interposition or small intestine reconstruction, including intestine mobilization, preparation, and anastomosis(es)**

EXCLUDES *Gastrointestinal reconstruction for previous esophagectomy (43360-43361)*

126. 126. FUD 090 C 80

AMA: 2014,Jan,11; 2002,May,7

43116 **Partial esophagectomy, cervical, with free intestinal graft, including microvascular anastomosis, obtaining the graft and intestinal reconstruction**

INCLUDES Operating microscope (69990)

EXCLUDES *Free jejunal graft with microvascular anastomosis performed by different physician (43496)*

Gastrointestinal reconstruction for previous esophagectomy (43360-43361)

Code also modifier 52 when intestinal or free jejunal graft with microvascular anastomosis performed by another physician

145. 145. FUD 090 C 80

AMA: 2016,Feb,12

43117 **Partial esophagectomy, distal two-thirds, with thoracotomy and separate abdominal incision, with or without proximal gastrectomy; with thoracic esophagogastrostomy, with or without pyloroplasty (Ivor Lewis)**

EXCLUDES *Esophagogastrectomy (lower third) and vagotomy (43122)*

Gastrointestinal reconstruction for previous esophagectomy (43360-43361)

Total esophagectomy with gastropharyngostomy (43107, 43124)

94.3 94.3 FUD 090 C 80

AMA: 2014,Jan,11; 1994,Win,1

43118 **with colon interposition or small intestine reconstruction, including intestine mobilization, preparation, and anastomosis(es)**

EXCLUDES *Esophagogastrectomy (lower third) and vagotomy (43122)*

Gastrointestinal reconstruction for previous esophagectomy (43360-43361)

Total esophagectomy with gastropharyngostomy (43107, 43124)

105. 105. FUD 090 C 80

AMA: 2014,Jan,11; 2002,May,7

43121 **Partial esophagectomy, distal two-thirds, with thoracotomy only, with or without proximal gastrectomy, with thoracic esophagogastrostomy, with or without pyloroplasty**

Gastrointestinal reconstruction for previous esophagectomy (43360-43361)

82.8 82.8 FUD 090 C 80

AMA: 2014,Jan,11; 1994,Win,1

43122 **Partial esophagectomy, thoracoabdominal or abdominal approach, with or without proximal gastrectomy; with esophagogastrostomy, with or without pyloroplasty**

Gastrointestinal reconstruction for previous esophagectomy (43360-43361)

74.3 74.3 FUD 090 C 80

AMA: 2014,Jan,11; 1994,Win,1

43123 **with colon interposition or small intestine reconstruction, including intestine mobilization, preparation, and anastomosis(es)**

Gastrointestinal reconstruction for previous esophagectomy (43360-43361)

131. 131. FUD 090 C 80

AMA: 2014,Jan,11; 2002,May,7

43124 **Total or partial esophagectomy, without reconstruction (any approach), with cervical esophagostomy**

Gastrointestinal reconstruction for previous esophagectomy (43360-43361)

110. 110. FUD 090 C 80

AMA: 2018,Jan,8; 2017,Jan,8; 2016,Jan,13; 2015,Jan,16

43130 **Diverticulectomy of hypopharynx or esophagus, with or without myotomy; cervical approach**

EXCLUDES *Diverticulectomy hypopharynx or cervical esophagus, endoscopic (43180)*

Gastrointestinal reconstruction for previous esophagectomy (43360-43361)

22.6 22.6 FUD 090 J G2 80

AMA: 2018,Jan,8; 2017,Jan,8; 2016,Jan,13; 2015,Jan,16

43135 **thoracic approach**

EXCLUDES *Diverticulectomy hypopharynx or cervical esophagus, endoscopic (43180)*

Gastrointestinal reconstruction for previous esophagectomy (43360-43361)

42.6 42.6 FUD 090 C 80

AMA: 2018,Jan,8; 2017,Jan,8; 2016,Jan,13; 2015,Jan,16

43180-43233 [43210, 43211, 43212, 43213, 43214, 43233] Endoscopic Procedures: Esophagus

INCLUDES Control bleeding due to endoscopic procedure during same operative session

Diagnostic endoscopy with surgical endoscopy

Examination upper esophageal sphincter (cricopharyngeus muscle) to/including gastroesophageal junction

Retroflexion examination proximal region stomach

43180 **Esophagoscopy, rigid, transoral with diverticulectomy of hypopharynx or cervical esophagus (eg, Zenker's diverticulum), with cricopharyngeal myotomy, includes use of telescope or operating microscope and repair, when performed**

INCLUDES Operating microscope (69990)

EXCLUDES *Esophagogastroduodenoscopy, flexible, transoral; with esophagogastric fundoplasty (43210)*

Open diverticulectomy hypopharynx or esophagus (43130-43135)

15.7 15.7 FUD 090 J G2

AMA: 2018,Jan,8; 2017,Jan,8; 2016,Feb,12; 2016,Jan,13; 2015,Nov,8

43191 **Esophagoscopy, rigid, transoral; diagnostic, including collection of specimen(s) by brushing or washing when performed (separate procedure)**

EXCLUDES *Esophagogastroduodenoscopy, flexible, transoral; with esophagogastric fundoplasty (43210)*

Esophagoscopy:

Flexible, transnasal (43197-43198)

Flexible, transoral (43200)

Rigid, transoral (43192-43196)

4.47 4.47 FUD 000 J G2

AMA: 2018,Jan,8; 2017,Jan,8; 2016,Jan,13; 2015,Nov,8; 2015,Jan,16

43192 **with directed submucosal injection(s), any substance**

EXCLUDES *Esophagoscopy:*

Flexible, transnasal (43197-43198)

Flexible, transoral (43201)

Rigid, transoral (43191)

Injection sclerosis of esophageal varices:

Flexible, transoral (43204)

Rigid, transoral (43499)

4.88 4.88 FUD 000 J G2

AMA: 2018,Jan,8; 2017,Jan,8; 2016,Jan,13; 2015,Jan,16

43193 **with biopsy, single or multiple**

EXCLUDES *Esophagoscopy:*

Flexible, transnasal (43197-43198)

Flexible, transoral (43202)

Rigid, transoral (43191)

4.85 4.85 FUD 000 J G2

AMA: 2018,Jan,8; 2017,Jan,8; 2016,Jan,13; 2015,Jan,16

43194 **with removal of foreign body(s)**

EXCLUDES *Esophagoscopy:*

Flexible, transnasal (43197-43198)

Flexible, transoral (43215)

Rigid, transoral (43191)

(76000)

5.55 5.55 FUD 000 J G2

AMA: 2018,Jan,8; 2017,Jan,8; 2016,Jan,13; 2015,Jan,16

43195 **with balloon dilation (less than 30 mm diameter)**

EXCLUDES *Dilation of esophagus:*
Flexible, with balloon diameter 30 mm or larger (43214, 43233)
Flexible, with balloon diameter less than 30 mm (43220)
Without endoscopic visualization (43450-43453)
Esophagoscopy:
Flexible, transnasal (43197-43198)
Rigid, transoral (43191)

(74360)

5.28 5.28 **FUD** 000 J G2

AMA: 2018,Jan,8; 2017,Jan,8; 2016,Jan,13; 2015,Jan,16

43196 **with insertion of guide wire followed by dilation over guide wire**

EXCLUDES *Esophagoscopy:*
Flexible, transnasal (43197-43198)
Flexible, transoral (43226)
Rigid, transoral (43191)

(74360)

5.63 5.63 **FUD** 000 J G2

AMA: 2018,Jan,8; 2017,Jan,8; 2016,Jan,13; 2015,Jan,16

43197 **Esophagoscopy, flexible, transnasal; diagnostic, including collection of specimen(s) by brushing or washing, when performed (separate procedure)**

EXCLUDES *Esophagogastroduodenoscopy, flexible, transoral (43235-43259 [43233, 43266, 43270])*
Esophagoscopy:
Flexible, transnasal; with biopsy, single or multiple (43198)
Flexible, transoral (43200-43232 [43211, 43212, 43213, 43214])
Rigid, transoral (43191-43196)
Laryngoscopy, flexible fiberoptic; diagnostic (31575)
Nasal endoscopy, diagnostic, unless different type endoscope used (31231)
Nasopharyngoscopy with endoscope (92511)

2.40 5.34 **FUD** 000 T P3

AMA: 2018,Jan,8; 2017,Jul,7; 2017,Jan,8; 2016,Dec,13; 2016,Sep,6; 2016,Jan,13; 2015,Nov,8; 2015,Jan,16

43198 **with biopsy, single or multiple**

EXCLUDES *Esophagogastroduodenoscopy, flexible, transoral (43235-43259 [43233, 43266, 43270])*
Esophagoscopy:
Flexible, transnasal (43197)
Flexible, transoral (43200-43232 [43211, 43212, 43213, 43214])
Rigid, transoral (43191-43196)
Laryngoscopy, flexible fiberoptic; diagnostic (31575)
Nasal endoscopy, diagnostic, unless different type endoscope used (31231)
Nasopharyngoscopy with endoscope (92511)

2.86 6.08 **FUD** 000 T P3

AMA: 2018,Jan,8; 2017,Jul,7; 2017,Jan,8; 2016,Dec,13; 2016,Sep,6; 2016,Jan,13; 2015,Jan,16

43200 **Esophagoscopy, flexible, transoral; diagnostic, including collection of specimen(s) by brushing or washing, when performed (separate procedure)**

EXCLUDES *Esophagogastroduodenoscopy, flexible, transoral (43235)*
Esophagoscopy:
Flexible, transnasal (43197-43198)
Flexible, transoral (43201-43232 [43211, 43212, 43213, 43214])
Rigid, transoral (43191)

2.53 6.50 **FUD** 000 T A2

AMA: 2018,Jan,8; 2017,Jan,8; 2016,Jan,13; 2015,Nov,8; 2015,Jan,16

43201 **with directed submucosal injection(s), any substance**

EXCLUDES *Esophagoscopy:*
Flexible, transnasal (43197-43198)
Flexible, transoral, on same lesion (43200, 43204, 43211, 43227)
Injection sclerosis esophageal varices:
Flexible, transoral (43204)
Rigid, transoral (43192, 43499)

2.98 6.89 **FUD** 000 J A2

AMA: 2018,Jan,8; 2017,Jan,8; 2016,Jan,13; 2015,Jan,16

43202 **with biopsy, single or multiple**

EXCLUDES *Esophagoscopy:*
Flexible, transnasal (43197-43198)
Flexible, transoral; diagnostic (43200)
Flexible, transoral, on same lesion (43211)
Rigid, transoral (43193)

2.97 9.64 **FUD** 000 J A2

AMA: 2018,Jan,8; 2017,Jan,8; 2016,Jan,13; 2015,Jan,16

43204 **with injection sclerosis of esophageal varices**

EXCLUDES *Band ligation non-variceal bleeding (43227)*
Esophagoscopy:
Flexible, transnasal or transoral; diagnostic (43197-43198, 43200)
Flexible, transoral; with control bleeding, any method, on same lesion (43227)
Flexible, transoral; with directed submucosal injection(s), any substance, on same lesion (43201)
Rigid, transoral, with injection esophageal varices (43499)

3.96 3.96 **FUD** 000 J A2

AMA: 2018,Jan,8; 2017,Jan,8; 2016,Jan,13; 2015,Jan,16

43205 **with band ligation of esophageal varices**

EXCLUDES *Band ligation non-variceal bleeding on same lesion (43227)*
Esophagoscopy, flexible, transnasal or transoral; diagnostic (43197-43198, 43200)

4.07 4.07 **FUD** 000 J A2

AMA: 2018,Jan,8; 2017,Jan,8; 2016,Jan,13; 2015,Jan,16

43206 **with optical endomicroscopy**

EXCLUDES *Esophagoscopy, flexible, transnasal or transoral; diagnostic (43197-43198, 43200)*
Optical endomicroscopic image(s), interpretation and report (88375)

Code also contrast agent

3.90 7.85 **FUD** 000 J G2

AMA: 2018,Jan,8; 2017,Nov,10; 2017,Jan,8; 2016,Jan,13; 2015,Jan,16

43210 **Resequenced code. See code following 43259.**

43211 **Resequenced code. See code following 43217.**

43212 **Resequenced code. See code following 43217.**

43213 **Resequenced code. See code following 43220.**

43214 **Resequenced code. See code following 43220.**

43215 **with removal of foreign body(s)**

Esophagoscopy:
Flexible, transnasal or transoral; diagnostic (43197-43198, 43200)
Rigid, transoral (43194)

(76000)

4.14 10.5 **FUD** 000 J A2

AMA: 2018,Jan,8; 2017,Jan,8; 2016,Jan,13; 2015,Jan,16

43216 **with removal of tumor(s), polyp(s), or other lesion(s) by hot biopsy forceps**

EXCLUDES *Esophagoscopy, flexible, transnasal or transoral; diagnostic (43197-43198, 43200)*

3.86 11.1 **FUD** 000 J A2

AMA: 2018,Jan,8; 2017,Jan,8; 2016,Jan,13; 2015,Jan,16

Digestive System

43195 — 43216

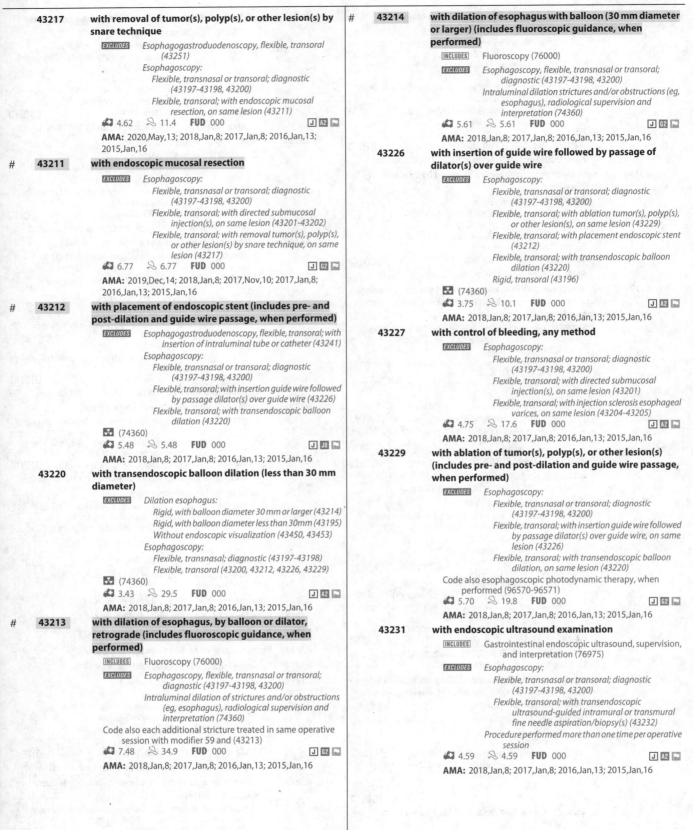

43217 **with removal of tumor(s), polyp(s), or other lesion(s) by snare technique**

EXCLUDES *Esophagogastroduodenoscopy, flexible, transoral (43251)*
Esophagoscopy:
Flexible, transnasal or transoral; diagnostic (43197-43198, 43200)
Flexible, transoral; with endoscopic mucosal resection, on same lesion (43211)

4.62 | 11.4 | FUD 000 | J A2

AMA: 2020,May,13; 2018,Jan,8; 2017,Jan,8; 2016,Jan,13; 2015,Jan,16

\# **43211** **with endoscopic mucosal resection**

EXCLUDES *Esophagoscopy:*
Flexible, transnasal or transoral; diagnostic (43197-43198, 43200)
Flexible, transoral; with directed submucosal injection(s), on same lesion (43201-43202)
Flexible, transoral; with removal tumor(s), polyp(s), or other lesion(s) by snare technique, on same lesion (43217)

6.77 | 6.77 | FUD 000 | J G2

AMA: 2019,Dec,14; 2018,Jan,8; 2017,Nov,10; 2017,Jan,8; 2016,Jan,13; 2015,Jan,16

\# **43212** **with placement of endoscopic stent (includes pre- and post-dilation and guide wire passage, when performed)**

EXCLUDES *Esophagogastroduodenoscopy, flexible, transoral; with insertion of intraluminal tube or catheter (43241)*
Esophagoscopy:
Flexible, transnasal or transoral; diagnostic (43197-43198, 43200)
Flexible, transoral; with insertion guide wire followed by passage dilator(s) over guide wire (43226)
Flexible, transoral; with transendoscopic balloon dilation (43220)

(74360)

5.48 | 5.48 | FUD 000 | J J8

AMA: 2018,Jan,8; 2017,Jan,8; 2016,Jan,13; 2015,Jan,16

43220 **with transendoscopic balloon dilation (less than 30 mm diameter)**

EXCLUDES *Dilation esophagus:*
Rigid, with balloon diameter 30 mm or larger (43214)
Rigid, with balloon diameter less than 30mm (43195)
Without endoscopic visualization (43450, 43453)
Esophagoscopy:
Flexible, transnasal; diagnostic (43197-43198)
Flexible, transoral (43200, 43212, 43226, 43229)

(74360)

3.43 | 29.5 | FUD 000 | J A2

AMA: 2018,Jan,8; 2017,Jan,8; 2016,Jan,13; 2015,Jan,16

\# **43213** **with dilation of esophagus, by balloon or dilator, retrograde (includes fluoroscopic guidance, when performed)**

INCLUDES Fluoroscopy (76000)

EXCLUDES *Esophagoscopy, flexible, transnasal or transoral; diagnostic (43197-43198, 43200)*
Intraluminal dilation of strictures and/or obstructions (eg, esophagus), radiological supervision and interpretation (74360)

Code also each additional stricture treated in same operative session with modifier 59 and (43213)

7.48 | 34.9 | FUD 000 | J G2

AMA: 2018,Jan,8; 2017,Jan,8; 2016,Jan,13; 2015,Jan,16

\# **43214** **with dilation of esophagus with balloon (30 mm diameter or larger) (includes fluoroscopic guidance, when performed)**

INCLUDES Fluoroscopy (76000)

EXCLUDES *Esophagoscopy, flexible, transnasal or transoral; diagnostic (43197-43198, 43200)*
Intraluminal dilation strictures and/or obstructions (eg, esophagus), radiological supervision and interpretation (74360)

5.61 | 5.61 | FUD 000 | J G2

AMA: 2018,Jan,8; 2017,Jan,8; 2016,Jan,13; 2015,Jan,16

43226 **with insertion of guide wire followed by passage of dilator(s) over guide wire**

EXCLUDES *Esophagoscopy:*
Flexible, transnasal or transoral; diagnostic (43197-43198, 43200)
Flexible, transoral; with ablation tumor(s), polyp(s), or other lesion(s), on same lesion (43229)
Flexible, transoral; with placement endoscopic stent (43212)
Flexible, transoral; with transendoscopic balloon dilation (43220)
Rigid, transoral (43196)

(74360)

3.75 | 10.1 | FUD 000 | J A2

AMA: 2018,Jan,8; 2017,Jan,8; 2016,Jan,13; 2015,Jan,16

43227 **with control of bleeding, any method**

EXCLUDES *Esophagoscopy:*
Flexible, transnasal or transoral; diagnostic (43197-43198, 43200)
Flexible, transoral; with directed submucosal injection(s), on same lesion (43201)
Flexible, transoral; with injection sclerosis esophageal varices, on same lesion (43204-43205)

4.75 | 17.6 | FUD 000 | J A2

AMA: 2018,Jan,8; 2017,Jan,8; 2016,Jan,13; 2015,Jan,16

43229 **with ablation of tumor(s), polyp(s), or other lesion(s) (includes pre- and post-dilation and guide wire passage, when performed)**

EXCLUDES *Esophagoscopy:*
Flexible, transnasal or transoral; diagnostic (43197-43198, 43200)
Flexible, transoral; with insertion guide wire followed by passage dilator(s) over guide wire, on same lesion (43226)
Flexible, transoral; with transendoscopic balloon dilation, on same lesion (43220)

Code also esophagoscopic photodynamic therapy, when performed (96570-96571)

5.70 | 19.8 | FUD 000 | J G2

AMA: 2018,Jan,8; 2017,Jan,8; 2016,Jan,13; 2015,Jan,16

43231 **with endoscopic ultrasound examination**

INCLUDES Gastrointestinal endoscopic ultrasound, supervision, and interpretation (76975)

EXCLUDES *Esophagoscopy:*
Flexible, transnasal or transoral; diagnostic (43197-43198, 43200)
Flexible, transoral; with transendoscopic ultrasound-guided intramural or transmural fine needle aspiration/biopsy(s) (43232)
Procedure performed more than one time per operative session

4.59 | 4.59 | FUD 000 | J A2

AMA: 2018,Jan,8; 2017,Jan,8; 2016,Jan,13; 2015,Jan,16

43232 **with transendoscopic ultrasound-guided intramural or transmural fine needle aspiration/biopsy(s)**

INCLUDES Gastrointestinal endoscopic ultrasound, supervision and interpretation (76975)
Ultrasonic guidance (76942)

EXCLUDES *Esophagoscopy:*
Flexible, transnasal or transoral; diagnostic (43197-43198, 43200)
Flexible, transoral; with endoscopic ultrasound examination (43231)
Procedure performed more than one time per operative session

5.75 5.75 FUD 000 J A2

AMA: 2018,Jan,8; 2017,Jan,8; 2016,Jan,13; 2015,Jan,16

43233 **Resequenced code. See code following 43249.**

43235-43210 [43210, 43233, 43266, 43270] Endoscopic Procedures: Esophagogastroduodenoscopy (EGD)

INCLUDES Control bleeding due to endoscopic procedure during same operative session
Diagnostic endoscopy with surgical endoscopy
Exam jejunum distal to anastomosis in surgically altered stomach, including post-gastroenterostomy (Billroth II) and gastric bypass (43235-43259 [43233, 43266, 43270])

EXCLUDES *Exam upper esophageal sphincter (cricopharyngeus muscle) to/including gastroesophageal junction and/or retroflexion exam proximal region stomach (43197-43232 [43211, 43212, 43213, 43214])*

Code also modifier 52 when duodenum not examined either deliberately or due to significant issues and repeat procedure will not be performed

Code also modifier 53 when duodenum not examined either deliberately or due to significant issues and repeat procedure is planned

43235 **Esophagogastroduodenoscopy, flexible, transoral; diagnostic, including collection of specimen(s) by brushing or washing, when performed (separate procedure)**

EXCLUDES *Endoscopy small intestine (44360-44379)*
Esophagogastroduodenoscopy, flexible, transoral; with esophagogastric fundoplasty (43210)
Esophagoscopy, flexible, transnasal; diagnostic (43197-43198)
Procedure performed with surgical endoscopy (43236-43259 [43233, 43266, 43270])

3.54 7.98 FUD 000 T A2

AMA: 2019,Oct,10; 2018,Jul,14; 2018,Jan,8; 2017,Jul,10; 2017,Jan,8; 2016,Jan,13; 2015,Nov,8; 2015,Jan,16

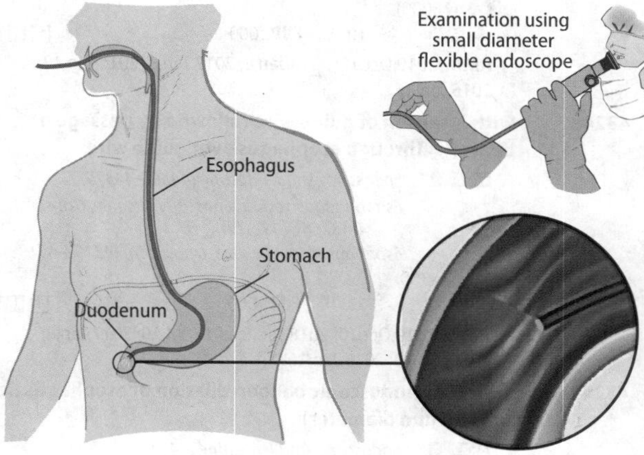

43236 **with directed submucosal injection(s), any substance**

EXCLUDES *Endoscopy small intestine (44360-44379)*
Esophagogastroduodenoscopy, on same lesion:
Flexible, transoral; with control bleeding, any method (43255)
Flexible, transoral; with endoscopic mucosal resection (43254)
Flexible, transoral; with injection sclerosis esophageal/gastric varices (43243)
Esophagoscopy, flexible, transnasal or transoral; diagnostic (43197-43198, 43235)
Injection sclerosis varices, esophageal/gastric (43243)

4.05 10.0 FUD 000 T A2

AMA: 2019,Oct,10; 2018,Jan,8; 2017,Jan,8; 2016,Jan,13; 2015,Jan,16

43237 **with endoscopic ultrasound examination limited to the esophagus, stomach or duodenum, and adjacent structures**

INCLUDES Ultrasonic guidance (76942, 76975)

EXCLUDES *Endoscopy of small intestine (44360-44379)*
Esophagogastroduodenoscopy, flexible, transoral (43238, 43242, 43253, 43259)
Esophagoscopy, flexible, transnasal; diagnostic (43197-43198)
Procedure performed more than one time per operative session

5.73 5.73 FUD 000 J A2

AMA: 2019,Oct,10; 2018,Jan,8; 2017,Jan,8; 2016,Jan,13; 2016,Jan,11; 2015,Jan,16

43238 **with transendoscopic ultrasound-guided intramural or transmural fine needle aspiration/biopsy(s), (includes endoscopic ultrasound examination limited to the esophagus, stomach or duodenum, and adjacent structures)**

INCLUDES Gastrointestinal endoscopic ultrasound, supervision and interpretation (76975)
Ultrasonic guidance (76942)

EXCLUDES *Endoscopy small intestine (44360-44379)*
Esophagogastroduodenoscopy, flexible, transoral (43237, 43242)
Esophagoscopy, flexible, transnasal (43197-43198)
Procedure performed more than one time per operative session

6.70 6.70 FUD 000 J A2

AMA: 2019,Oct,10; 2018,Jan,8; 2017,Jan,8; 2016,Jan,13; 2015,Jan,16

43239 **with biopsy, single or multiple**

EXCLUDES *Endoscopy small intestine (44360-44379)*
Esophagogastroduodenoscopy, flexible, transoral; with endoscopic mucosal resection on same lesion (43254)
Esophagoscopy, flexible, transnasal (43197-43198)

3.99 10.6 FUD 000 T A2

AMA: 2020,Jan,12; 2019,Oct,10; 2018,Jul,14; 2018,Jan,8; 2017,Jan,8; 2016,Jan,13; 2015,Jan,16

43240 **with transmural drainage of pseudocyst (includes placement of transmural drainage catheter[s]/stent[s], when performed, and endoscopic ultrasound, when performed)**

INCLUDES Gastrointestinal endoscopic ultrasound, supervision and interpretation (76975)

EXCLUDES *Endoscopic pancreatic necrosectomy (48999)*
Endoscopy small intestine (44360-44379)
Esophagogastroduodenoscopy:
Flexible, transoral (43242, [43266], 43259)
Flexible, transoral; with transendoscopic ultrasound-guided transmural injection diagnostic or therapeutic substance(s), on same lesion (43253)
Esophagoscopy, flexible, transnasal (43197-43198)
Procedure performed more than one time per operative session

11.5 11.5 **FUD** 000 J J8

AMA: 2019,Oct,10; 2018,Jan,8; 2017,Jan,8; 2016,Jan,13; 2015,Jan,16

43241 **with insertion of intraluminal tube or catheter**

EXCLUDES *Endoscopy small intestine (44360-44379)*
Esophagogastroduodenoscopy, flexible, transoral ([43266])
Esophagoscopy, flexible, transnasal or transoral (43197-43198, 43212)
Insertion long gastrointestinal tube (44500, 74340)
Naso or oro-gastric requiring professional skill and fluoroscopic guidance (43752)

4.17 4.17 **FUD** 000 J A2

AMA: 2019,Oct,10; 2018,Jan,8; 2017,Jan,8; 2016,Jan,13; 2015,Jan,16

43242 **with transendoscopic ultrasound-guided intramural or transmural fine needle aspiration/biopsy(s) (includes endoscopic ultrasound examination of the esophagus, stomach, and either the duodenum or a surgically altered stomach where the jejunum is examined distal to the anastomosis)**

INCLUDES Gastrointestinal endoscopic ultrasound, supervision and interpretation (76975)
Ultrasonic guidance (76942)

EXCLUDES *Endoscopy small intestine (44360-44379)*
Esophagogastroduodenoscopy, flexible, transoral (43237-43238, 43240, 43259)
Esophagoscopy, flexible, transnasal (43197-43198)
Procedure performed more than one time per operative session
Transmural fine needle biopsy/aspiration with ultrasound guidance, transendoscopic, esophagus/stomach/duodenum/neighboring structure (43238)

88172-88173

7.58 7.58 **FUD** 000 J A2

AMA: 2019,Oct,10; 2018,Jan,8; 2017,Jan,8; 2016,Jan,13; 2015,Jan,16

43243 **with injection sclerosis of esophageal/gastric varices**

EXCLUDES *Endoscopy small intestine (44360-44379)*
Esophagogastroduodenoscopy, flexible, transoral on same lesion (43236, 43255)
Esophagoscopy, flexible, transnasal (43197-43198)

6.85 6.85 **FUD** 000 J A2

AMA: 2019,Oct,10; 2018,Jan,8; 2017,Jan,8; 2016,Jan,13; 2015,Jan,16

43244 **with band ligation of esophageal/gastric varices**

EXCLUDES *Band ligation, non-variceal bleeding (43255)*
Endoscopy small intestine (44360-44379)
Esophagoscopy, flexible, transnasal (43197-43198)

7.08 7.08 **FUD** 000 J A2

AMA: 2019,Oct,10; 2018,Jan,8; 2017,Jan,8; 2016,Jan,13; 2015,Jan,16

43245 **with dilation of gastric/duodenal stricture(s) (eg, balloon, bougie)**

EXCLUDES *Endoscopy small intestine (44360-44379)*
Esophagogastroduodenoscopy, flexible, transoral ([43266])
Esophagoscopy, flexible, transnasal (43197-43198)

(74360)

5.13 16.2 **FUD** 000 J A2

AMA: 2019,Oct,10; 2018,Jan,8; 2017,Jan,8; 2016,Jan,13; 2015,Jan,16

43246 **with directed placement of percutaneous gastrostomy tube**

EXCLUDES *Endoscopy small intestine (44360-44372, 44376-44379)*
Esophagoscopy, flexible, transnasal (43197-43198)
Gastrostomy tube replacement without endoscopy or imaging (43762-43763)
Percutaneous insertion gastrostomy tube (49440)

5.86 5.86 **FUD** 000 J A2 80

AMA: 2019,Oct,10; 2019,Feb,5; 2018,Jan,8; 2017,Jan,8; 2016,Jan,13; 2015,Jan,16

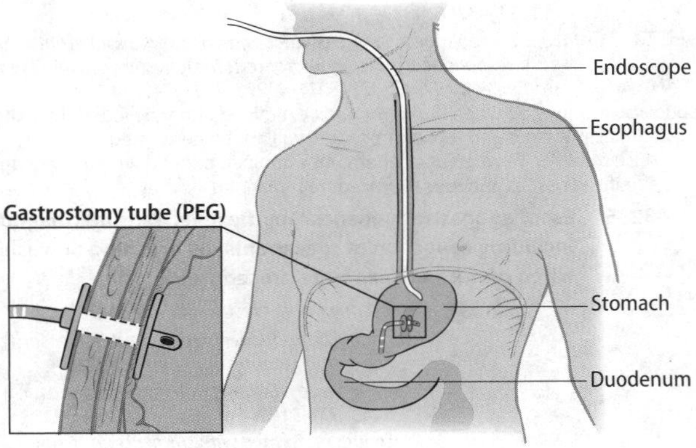

43247 **with removal of foreign body(s)**

EXCLUDES *Endoscopy small intestine (44360-44379)*
Esophagoscopy, flexible, transnasal (43197-43198)

(76000)

5.11 10.5 **FUD** 000 T A2

AMA: 2019,Oct,10; 2018,Jan,8; 2017,Jan,8; 2016,Jan,13; 2015,Jan,16

43248 **with insertion of guide wire followed by passage of dilator(s) through esophagus over guide wire**

EXCLUDES *Endoscopy small intestine (44360-44379)*
Esophagogastroduodenoscopy, flexible, transoral ([43266], [43270])
Esophagoscopy, flexible, transnasal (43197-43198)

(74360)

4.78 11.0 **FUD** 000 T A2

AMA: 2019,Oct,10; 2018,Jan,8; 2017,Jul,10; 2017,Jan,8; 2016,Jan,13; 2015,Jan,16

43249 **with transendoscopic balloon dilation of esophagus (less than 30 mm diameter)**

EXCLUDES *Endoscopy small intestine (44360-44379)*
Esophagogastroduodenoscopy:
Ablation lesion/tumor/polyp, when performed on same lesion ([43270])
With placement endoscopic stent ([43266])
Esophagoscopy, flexible, transnasal (43197-43198)

(74360)

4.42 31.0 **FUD** 000 J A2

AMA: 2019,Oct,10; 2018,Jul,14; 2018,Jan,8; 2017,Jan,8; 2016,Jan,13; 2015,Jan,16

43233   with dilation of esophagus with balloon (30 mm diameter or larger) (includes fluoroscopic guidance, when performed)

INCLUDES   Fluoroscopy (76000)

EXCLUDES   Endoscopy small intestine (44360-44379)

Esophagoscopy, flexible, transnasal (43197-43198)

Intraluminal dilation strictures and/or obstructions (e.g., esophagus), radiological supervision and interpretation (74360)

🚑 6.62   ⚗ 6.62   FUD 000   J G2 ▣

AMA: 2019,Oct,10; 2018,Jan,8; 2017,Jan,8; 2016,Jan,13; 2015,Jan,16

43250   with removal of tumor(s), polyp(s), or other lesion(s) by hot biopsy forceps

EXCLUDES   Endoscopy small intestine (44360-44379)

Esophagoscopy, flexible, transnasal (43197-43198)

🚑 4.97   ⚗ 11.8   FUD 000   J A2 ▣

AMA: 2019,Oct,10; 2018,Jan,8; 2017,Jan,8; 2016,Jan,13; 2015,Jan,16

43251   with removal of tumor(s), polyp(s), or other lesion(s) by snare technique

EXCLUDES   Endoscopic mucosal resection when performed on same lesion (43254)

Endoscopy small intestine (44360-44379)

Esophagoscopy, flexible, transnasal (43197-43198)

🚑 5.66   ⚗ 13.5   FUD 000   J A2 ▣

AMA: 2019,Oct,10; 2018,Jan,8; 2017,Jan,8; 2016,Jan,13; 2015,Jan,16

43252   with optical endomicroscopy

EXCLUDES   Endoscopy small intestine (44360-44379)

Esophagoscopy, flexible, transnasal (43197-43198)

Optical endomicroscopic image(s), interpretation and report (88375)

Code also contrast agent

🚑 4.95   ⚗ 8.96   FUD 000   J G2 ▣

AMA: 2019,Oct,10; 2018,Jan,8; 2017,Jan,8; 2016,Jan,13; 2015,Jan,16

43253   with transendoscopic ultrasound-guided transmural injection of diagnostic or therapeutic substance(s) (eg, anesthetic, neurolytic agent) or fiducial marker(s) (includes endoscopic ultrasound examination of the esophagus, stomach, and either the duodenum or a surgically altered stomach where the jejunum is examined distal to the anastomosis)

INCLUDES   Gastrointestinal endoscopic ultrasound, supervision and interpretation (76975)

Ultrasonic guidance (76942)

EXCLUDES   Endoscopy small intestine (44360-44379)

Esophagogastroduodenoscopy:

Flexible, transoral (43237, 43259)

Flexible, transoral; with transmural drainage pseudocyst on same lesion with (43240)

Esophagoscopy, flexible, transnasal (43197-43198)

Procedure performed more than one time per operative session

Transmural fine needle biopsy/aspiration with ultrasound guidance, transendoscopic, esophagus/stomach/duodenum/neighboring structures (43238, 43242)

🚑 7.70   ⚗ 7.70   FUD 000   J G2 ▣

AMA: 2019,Oct,10; 2018,Apr,10; 2018,Jan,8; 2017,Jan,8; 2016,Jan,13; 2015,Jan,16

43254   with endoscopic mucosal resection

EXCLUDES   Endoscopy small intestine (44360-44379)

Esophagogastroduodenoscopy, flexible, transoral, on same lesion (43236, 43239, 43251)

Esophagoscopy, flexible, transnasal (43197-43198)

🚑 7.80   ⚗ 7.80   FUD 000   J G2 ▣

AMA: 2019,Dec,14; 2019,Oct,10; 2018,Jan,8; 2017,Jan,8; 2016,Jan,13; 2015,Jan,16

43255   with control of bleeding, any method

EXCLUDES   Endoscopy small intestine (44360-44379)

Esophagogastroduodenoscopy, flexible, transoral, on same lesion (43236, 43243-43244)

Esophagoscopy, flexible, transnasal (43197-43198)

🚑 5.79   ⚗ 18.6   FUD 000   J A2 ▣

AMA: 2019,Oct,10; 2018,Jan,8; 2017,Jan,8; 2016,Jan,13; 2015,Jan,16

43266   with placement of endoscopic stent (includes pre- and post-dilation and guide wire passage, when performed)

INCLUDES   When performed:

Balloon dilation esophagus (43249)

Dilation gastric/duodenal stricture (43245)

Insertion guidewire/dilator (43248)

EXCLUDES   Endoscopy small intestine (44360-44379)

Esophagogastroduodenoscopy:

Insertion intraluminal tube or catheter (43241)

Transmural drainage pseudocyst (43240)

Esophagoscopy, flexible, transnasal (43197-43198)

▣ (74360)

🚑 6.39   ⚗ 6.39   FUD 000   J J8 ▣

AMA: 2019,Oct,10; 2018,Jan,8; 2017,Jan,8; 2016,Jan,13; 2015,Jan,16

43257   with delivery of thermal energy to the muscle of lower esophageal sphincter and/or gastric cardia, for treatment of gastroesophageal reflux disease

EXCLUDES   Endoscopy small intestine (44360-44379)

Esophageal lesion ablation (43229, [43270])

Esophagoscopy, flexible, transnasal (43197-43198)

🚑 6.74   ⚗ 6.74   FUD 000   J A2 ▣

AMA: 2019,Oct,10; 2018,Jan,8; 2017,Jan,8; 2016,Jan,13; 2015,Jan,16

43270   with ablation of tumor(s), polyp(s), or other lesion(s) (includes pre- and post-dilation and guide wire passage, when performed)

INCLUDES   Endoscopic dilation performed on same lesion (43248-43249)

EXCLUDES   Endoscopy small intestine (44360-44379)

Esophagoscopy, flexible, transnasal (43197-43198)

Code also photodynamic therapy, when performed (96570-96571)

🚑 6.48   ⚗ 20.3   FUD 000   J G2 ▣

AMA: 2019,Oct,10; 2018,Jan,8; 2017,Jan,8; 2016,Jan,13; 2015,Jan,16

43259   with endoscopic ultrasound examination, including the esophagus, stomach, and either the duodenum or a surgically altered stomach where the jejunum is examined distal to the anastomosis

INCLUDES   Gastrointestinal endoscopic ultrasound, supervision and interpretation (76975)

EXCLUDES   Endoscopy small intestine (44360-44379)

Esophagogastroduodenoscopy, flexible, transoral (43237, 43240, 43242, 43253)

Esophagoscopy, flexible, transnasal (43197-43198)

Procedure performed more than one time per operative session

🚑 6.53   ⚗ 6.53   FUD 000   J A2 ▣

AMA: 2019,Oct,10; 2018,Jan,8; 2017,Jan,8; 2016,Jan,13; 2016,Jan,11; 2015,Jan,16

43210   with esophagogastric fundoplasty, partial or complete, includes duodenoscopy when performed

EXCLUDES   Esophagogastroduodenoscopy:

Flexible, transnasal (43197)

Rigid, transoral (43180, 43191)

Esophagoscopy, flexible, transoral (43200)

🚑 12.5   ⚗ 12.5   FUD 000   J G2 ▣

AMA: 2018,Jan,8; 2017,Jan,8; 2016,Jan,13; 2015,Nov,8

● New Code   ▲ Revised Code   ○ Reinstated   ● New Web Release   ▲ Revised Web Release   + Add-on   Unlisted   Not Covered   # Resequenced

⑤⓪ Optum Mod 50 Exempt   Ⓢ AMA Mod 51 Exempt   ⑤① Optum Mod 51 Exempt   ⑥③ Mod 63 Exempt   ✗ Non-FDA Drug   ★ Telemedicine   M Maternity   A Age Edit

43260-43278 [43266, 43270, 43274, 43275, 43276, 43277, 43278] Endoscopic Procedures: ERCP

INCLUDES Diagnostic endoscopy with surgical endoscopy
Pancreaticobiliary system:
Biliary tree (right and left hepatic ducts, cystic duct/gallbladder, and common bile ducts)
Pancreas (major and minor ducts)

EXCLUDES *ERCP via Roux-en-Y anatomy (for instance post-gastric or bariatric bypass or post total gastrectomy) or via gastrostomy (open or laparoscopic) (47999, 48999)*
Optical endomicroscopy biliary tract and pancreas, report one time per session (0397T)
Percutaneous biliary catheter procedures (47490-47544)

Code also appropriate endoscopy each anatomic site examined
Code also sphincteroplasty or ductal stricture dilation, when necessary to access debris/stones ([43277])
Code also appropriate ERCP procedure when performed on altered postoperative anatomy (i.e., Billroth II gastroenterostomy) (43260, 43262-43265, [43274], [43275], [43276], [43277], [43278], 43273)
(74328-74330)

43260 Endoscopic retrograde cholangiopancreatography (ERCP); diagnostic, including collection of specimen(s) by brushing or washing, when performed (separate procedure)

EXCLUDES *Endoscopic retrograde cholangiopancreatography (ERCP), therapeutic (43261-43265, 43274-43278 [43274, 43275, 43276, 43277, 43278])*

9.31 9.31 **FUD** 000 J A2

AMA: 2018,Jan,8; 2017,Jan,8; 2016,Jan,13; 2015,Dec,3; 2015,Jan,16

43261 with biopsy, single or multiple

INCLUDES Endoscopic retrograde cholangiopancreatography (ERCP); diagnostic (43260)

EXCLUDES *Percutaneous endoluminal biopsy biliary tree (47543)*

9.76 9.76 **FUD** 000 J A2

AMA: 2018,Jan,8; 2017,Jan,8; 2016,Jan,13; 2015,Dec,3; 2015,Jan,16

43262 with sphincterotomy/papillotomy

INCLUDES Endoscopic retrograde cholangiopancreatography (ERCP), diagnostic (43260)

EXCLUDES *Endoscopic retrograde cholangiopancreatography (ERCP):*
With exchange/insertion/removal stent in same location ([43274], [43276])
With trans-endoscopic balloon dilation ampulla/biliary or pancreatic ducts ([43277])
Percutaneous balloon dilation biliary duct or ampulla (47542)

Code also procedure performed with sphincterotomy (43261, 43263-43265, [43275], [43278])

10.3 10.3 **FUD** 000 J A2

AMA: 2018,Jan,8; 2017,Jan,8; 2016,Jan,13; 2015,Dec,3; 2015,Jan,16

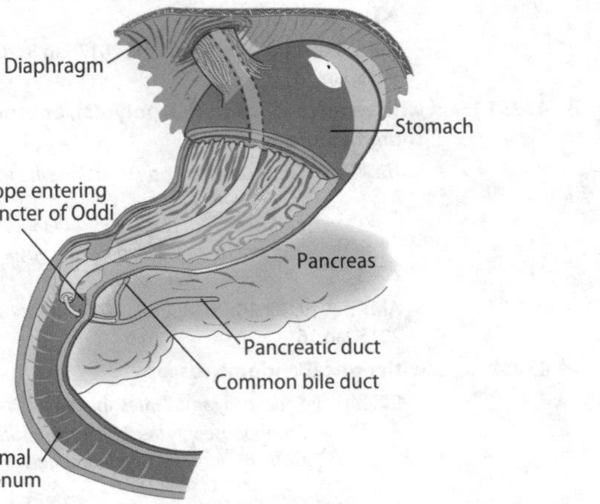

An endoscope is fed through the stomach and into the duodenum
Usually a smaller sub-scope is fed up the sphincter of Oddi and into the ducts that drain the pancreas and the gallbladder (common bile)

43263 with pressure measurement of sphincter of Oddi

INCLUDES Endoscopic retrograde cholangiopancreatography (ERCP); diagnostic (43260)

EXCLUDES *Procedure performed more than one time per session*

10.4 10.4 **FUD** 000 J A2

AMA: 2018,Jan,8; 2017,Jan,8; 2016,Jan,13; 2015,Jan,16

43264 with removal of calculi/debris from biliary/pancreatic duct(s)

INCLUDES Endoscopic retrograde cholangiopancreatography (ERCP); diagnostic (43260)
Incidental dilation due to instrument passage

EXCLUDES *Endoscopic retrograde cholangiopancreatography (ERCP) with calculi destruction (43265)*
Findings without debris or calculi, even when balloon used
Percutaneous calculus/debris removal (47544)

Code also sphincteroplasty when dilation necessary to access debris/stones ([43277])

10.4 10.4 **FUD** 000 J A2

AMA: 2018,Jan,8; 2017,Jan,8; 2016,Jan,13; 2015,Dec,3; 2015,Jan,16

43265 **with destruction of calculi, any method (eg, mechanical, electrohydraulic, lithotripsy)**

> INCLUDES Endoscopic retrograde cholangiopancreatography (ERCP); diagnostic (43260)
> Incidental dilation due to instrument passage
> Stone removal in same ductal system
>
> EXCLUDES *Endoscopic retrograde cholangiopancreatography (ERCP) with removal of calculi/debris from biliary/pancreatic duct(s) (43264)*
> *Findings without debris or calculi, even when balloon used*
> *Percutaneous calculus/debris removal (47544)*
>
> Code also sphincteroplasty when dilation necessary to access debris/stones ([43277])

🚑 12.5   ⚕ 12.5   **FUD** 000   J A2 ▯

AMA: 2018,Jan,8; 2017,Jan,8; 2016,Jan,13; 2015,Dec,3; 2015,Jan,16

43266 Resequenced code. See code following 43255.

43270 Resequenced code. See code following 43257.

43274 **with placement of endoscopic stent into biliary or pancreatic duct, including pre- and post-dilation and guide wire passage, when performed, including sphincterotomy, when performed, each stent**

> INCLUDES Balloon dilation in same duct
> Endoscopic retrograde cholangiopancreatography (ERCP); diagnostic (43260)
> Tube placement for naso-pancreatic or naso-biliary drainage
>
> EXCLUDES *Percutaneous placement biliary stent (47538-47540)*
> *Procedures for stent placement or exchange in same duct (43262, [43275], [43276], [43277])*
>
> Code also for each additional stent placement in different ducts or side by side in same duct same session/day, using modifier 59 with ([43274])

🚑 13.3   ⚕ 13.3   **FUD** 000   J G2 ▯

AMA: 2018,Jan,8; 2017,Jan,8; 2016,Jan,13; 2015,Jan,16

43275 **with removal of foreign body(s) or stent(s) from biliary/pancreatic duct(s)**

> INCLUDES Endoscopic retrograde cholangiopancreatography (ERCP); diagnostic (43260)
>
> EXCLUDES *Endoscopic retrograde cholangiopancreatography (ERCP) with exchange, placement, or removal of stent ([43274], [43276])*
> *Pancreatic or biliary duct stent removal without ERCP (43247)*
> *Percutaneous calculus/debris removal (47544)*
> *Procedure performed more than one time per session*

🚑 11.0   ⚕ 11.0   **FUD** 000   J G2 ▯

AMA: 2018,Jan,8; 2017,Jan,8; 2016,Jan,13; 2015,Jan,16

43276 **with removal and exchange of stent(s), biliary or pancreatic duct, including pre- and post-dilation and guide wire passage, when performed, including sphincterotomy, when performed, each stent exchanged**

> INCLUDES Balloon dilation in same duct
> Endoscopic retrograde cholangiopancreatography (ERCP); diagnostic (43260)
> Stent placement or exchange one stent
>
> EXCLUDES *Endoscopic retrograde cholangiopancreatography (ERCP) with removal foreign body(s) or stent(s) ([43275])*
> *Procedures for stent insertion or exchange stent in same duct (43262, [43274])*
>
> Code also each additional stent exchanged same session/day, using modifier 59 with ([43276])

🚑 13.9   ⚕ 13.9   **FUD** 000   J G2 ▯

AMA: 2018,Jan,8; 2017,Jan,8; 2016,Jan,13; 2015,Jan,16

43277 **with trans-endoscopic balloon dilation of biliary/pancreatic duct(s) or of ampulla (sphincteroplasty), including sphincterotomy, when performed, each duct**

> INCLUDES Endoscopic retrograde cholangiopancreatography (ERCP); diagnostic (43260)
>
> EXCLUDES *Endoscopic retrograde cholangiopancreatography (ERCP):*
> *With ablation tumor(s), polyp(s), or other lesion(s) for same lesion ([43278])*
> *With sphincterotomy/papillotomy (43262)*
> *With stent exchange/removal same biliary/pancreatic duct ([43276])*
> *With stent placement into same biliary/pancreatic duct ([43274])*
> *Percutaneous dilation biliary duct/ampulla (47542)*
> *Removal stone/debris, dilation incidental to instrument passage (43264-43265)*
>
> Code also both right and left hepatic duct (bilateral) balloon dilation, using ([43277]) and append modifier 59 to second procedure
> Code also each additional balloon dilation in different ducts or side by side in same duct same session/day, using modifier 59 with ([43277])
> Code also same session sphincterotomy without sphincteroplasty in different duct, using modifier 59 with (43262)

🚑 10.9   ⚕ 10.9   **FUD** 000   J G2 ▯

AMA: 2018,Jan,8; 2017,Jan,8; 2016,Jan,13; 2015,Dec,3; 2015,Jan,16

43278 **with ablation of tumor(s), polyp(s), or other lesion(s), including pre- and post-dilation and guide wire passage, when performed**

> INCLUDES Endoscopic retrograde cholangiopancreatography (ERCP); diagnostic (43260)
>
> EXCLUDES *Ampullectomy (43254)*
> *Endoscopic retrograde cholangiopancreatography (ERCP); with trans-endoscopic balloon dilation biliary/pancreatic duct(s) or ampulla (sphincteroplasty) in same lesion with ([43277])*

🚑 12.5   ⚕ 12.5   **FUD** 000   J G2 ▯

AMA: 2018,Jan,8; 2017,Jan,8; 2016,Jan,13; 2015,Jan,16

+ **43273** **Endoscopic cannulation of papilla with direct visualization of pancreatic/common bile duct(s) (List separately in addition to code(s) for primary procedure)**

> EXCLUDES *Procedure performed more than one time per session*
> Code first (43260-43265, [43274], [43275], [43276], [43277], [43278])

🚑 3.47   ⚕ 3.47   **FUD** ZZZ   N N1 80 ▯

AMA: 2018,Jan,8; 2017,Jan,8; 2016,Jan,13; 2015,Jan,16

43274 Resequenced code. See code following code 43270.

43275 Resequenced code. See code following code 43270.

43276 Resequenced code. See code following code 43270.

43277 Resequenced code. See code following code 43270.

43278 Resequenced code. See code following code 43270.

43279-43289 Laparoscopic Procedures of Esophagus

> INCLUDES Diagnostic laparoscopy with surgical laparoscopy (49320)

43279 **Laparoscopy, surgical, esophagomyotomy (Heller type), with fundoplasty, when performed**

> EXCLUDES *Esophagomyotomy, open method (43330-43331)*
> *Laparoscopy, surgical, esophagogastric fundoplasty (43280)*

🚑 37.5   ⚕ 37.5   **FUD** 090   C 80 ▯

AMA: 2018,Jan,8; 2017,Aug,6; 2017,Jan,8; 2016,Jan,13; 2015,Jan,16

● New Code   ▲ Revised Code   ○ Reinstated   ● New Web Release   ▲ Revised Web Release   + Add-on   Unlisted   Not Covered   # Resequenced
50 Optum Mod 50 Exempt   Ⓢ AMA Mod 51 Exempt   Ⓢ Optum Mod 51 Exempt   63 Mod 63 Exempt   ✗ Non-FDA Drug   ★ Telemedicine   M Maternity   A Age Edit

43280 Laparoscopy, surgical, esophagogastric fundoplasty (eg, Nissen, Toupet procedures)

EXCLUDES *Esophagogastric fundoplasty, open method (43327-43328)*
Esophagogastroduodenoscopy fundoplasty, transoral (43210)
Laparoscopy, surgical, esophageal sphincter augmentation (43284-43285)
Laparoscopy, surgical, esophagomyotomy (43279)
Laparoscopy, surgical, fundoplasty (43281-43282)

31.4 31.4 **FUD** 090 J 80

AMA: 2018,Jan,8; 2017,Aug,6; 2017,Jan,8; 2016,Jan,13; 2015,Nov,8; 2015,Jan,16

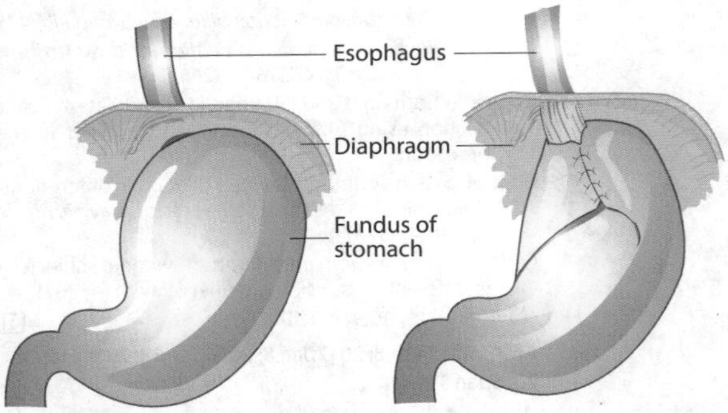

43281 Laparoscopy, surgical, repair of paraesophageal hernia, includes fundoplasty, when performed; without implantation of mesh

EXCLUDES *Dilation esophagus (43450, 43453)*
Implantation mesh or other prosthesis (49568)
Laparoscopy, surgical, esophagogastric fundoplasty (43280)
Transabdominal repair paraesophageal hiatal hernia (43332-43333)
Transthoracic repair diaphragmatic hernia (43334-43335)

44.7 44.7 **FUD** 090 J 80

AMA: 2018,Nov,11; 2018,Sep,14; 2018,Jan,8; 2017,Aug,6; 2017,Jan,8; 2016,Jan,13; 2015,Jan,16

43282 with implantation of mesh

EXCLUDES *Dilation esophagus (43450, 43453)*
Laparoscopy, surgical, esophagogastric fundoplasty (43280)
Transabdominal paraesophageal hernia repair (43332-43333)
Transthoracic paraesophageal hernia repair (43334-43335)

50.6 50.6 **FUD** 090 J 80

AMA: 2018,Jan,8; 2017,Aug,6; 2017,Jan,8; 2016,Aug,9; 2016,Jan,13; 2015,Jan,16

\+ **43283 Laparoscopy, surgical, esophageal lengthening procedure (eg, Collis gastroplasty or wedge gastroplasty) (List separately in addition to code for primary procedure)**

Code first (43280-43282)

4.60 4.60 **FUD** ZZZ C 80

AMA: 2018,Jan,8; 2017,Jan,8; 2016,Jan,13; 2015,Jan,16

43284 Laparoscopy, surgical, esophageal sphincter augmentation procedure, placement of sphincter augmentation device (ie, magnetic band), including cruroplasty when performed

EXCLUDES *Performed during same session (43279-43282)*

18.9 18.9 **FUD** 090 J J8 80

AMA: 2019,Apr,10; 2018,Sep,14; 2018,Jan,8; 2017,Aug,6

43285 Removal of esophageal sphincter augmentation device

19.5 19.5 **FUD** 090 Q2 G2 80

AMA: 2018,Jan,8; 2017,Aug,6

43286 Esophagectomy, total or near total, with laparoscopic mobilization of the abdominal and mediastinal esophagus and proximal gastrectomy, with laparoscopic pyloric drainage procedure if performed, with open cervical pharyngogastrostomy or esophagogastrostomy (ie, laparoscopic transhiatal esophagectomy)

90.9 90.9 **FUD** 090 C 80

AMA: 2018,Jul,7

43287 Esophagectomy, distal two-thirds, with laparoscopic mobilization of the abdominal and lower mediastinal esophagus and proximal gastrectomy, with laparoscopic pyloric drainage procedure if performed, with separate thoracoscopic mobilization of the middle and upper mediastinal esophagus and thoracic esophagogastrostomy (ie, laparoscopic thoracoscopic esophagectomy, Ivor Lewis esophagectomy)

EXCLUDES *Right tube thoracostomy (32551)*

104. 104. **FUD** 090 C 80

AMA: 2018,Jul,7

43288 Esophagectomy, total or near total, with thoracoscopic mobilization of the upper, middle, and lower mediastinal esophagus, with separate laparoscopic proximal gastrectomy, with laparoscopic pyloric drainage procedure if performed, with open cervical pharyngogastrostomy or esophagogastrostomy (ie, thoracoscopic, laparoscopic and cervical incision esophagectomy, McKeown esophagectomy, tri-incisional esophagectomy)

EXCLUDES *Right tube thoracostomy (32551)*

109. 109. **FUD** 090 C 80

AMA: 2018,Jul,7

43289 Unlisted laparoscopy procedure, esophagus

0.00 0.00 **FUD** YYY J 80 50

AMA: 2018,Jul,7; 2018,Jan,8; 2017,Jan,8; 2016,Jan,13; 2015,Jan,16

43300-43425 Open Esophageal Repair Procedures

43300 Esophagoplasty (plastic repair or reconstruction), cervical approach; without repair of tracheoesophageal fistula

17.6 17.6 **FUD** 090 C 80

AMA: 2014,Jan,11; 2013,Jan,11-12

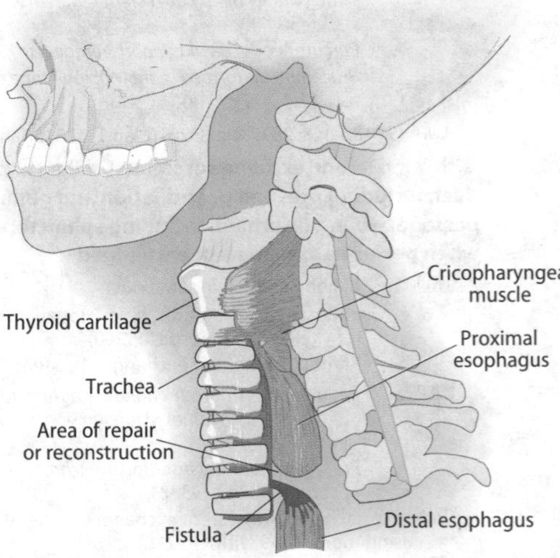

Example of esophageal atresia where the proximal esophagus fails to communicate with the lower portion; note that a fistula has developed from the trachea

43305 with repair of tracheoesophageal fistula

31.3 31.3 **FUD** 090 C 80

AMA: 2014,Jan,11; 2013,Jan,11-12

43310 **Esophagoplasty (plastic repair or reconstruction), thoracic approach; without repair of tracheoesophageal fistula**
42.9 42.9 FUD 090 C 80
AMA: 2014,Jan,11; 2013,Jan,11-12

43312 **with repair of tracheoesophageal fistula**
46.1 46.1 FUD 090 C 80
AMA: 2014,Jan,11; 2013,Jan,11-12

43313 **Esophagoplasty for congenital defect (plastic repair or reconstruction), thoracic approach; without repair of congenital tracheoesophageal fistula**
79.3 79.3 FUD 090 63 C 80
AMA: 2014,Jan,11; 2013,Jan,11-12

43314 **with repair of congenital tracheoesophageal fistula**
85.2 85.2 FUD 090 63 C 80
AMA: 2014,Jan,11; 2013,Jan,11-12

43320 **Esophagogastrostomy (cardioplasty), with or without vagotomy and pyloroplasty, transabdominal or transthoracic approach**
EXCLUDES *Laparoscopic approach (43280)*
40.7 40.7 FUD 090 C 80
AMA: 2014,Jan,11; 2013,Jan,11-12

43325 **Esophagogastric fundoplasty, with fundic patch (Thal-Nissen procedure)**
EXCLUDES *Myotomy, cricopharyngeal (43030)*
39.6 39.6 FUD 090 C 80
AMA: 2014,Jan,11; 2013,Jan,11-12

43327 **Esophagogastric fundoplasty partial or complete; laparotomy**
23.9 23.9 FUD 090 C 80
AMA: 2018,Jan,8; 2017,Jan,8; 2016,Jan,13; 2015,Nov,8; 2015,Jan,16

43328 **thoracotomy**
EXCLUDES *Esophagogastroduodenoscopy fundoplasty, transoral (43210)*
32.6 32.6 FUD 090 C 80
AMA: 2018,Jan,8; 2017,Jan,8; 2016,Jan,13; 2015,Nov,8; 2015,Jan,16

43330 **Esophagomyotomy (Heller type); abdominal approach**
EXCLUDES *Esophagomyotomy, laparoscopic method (43279)*
38.9 38.9 FUD 090 C 80
AMA: 2018,Jan,8; 2017,Jan,8; 2016,Jan,13; 2015,Jan,16

43331 **thoracic approach**
EXCLUDES *Thoracoscopy with esophagomyotomy (32665)*
38.7 38.7 FUD 090 C 80
AMA: 2018,Jan,8; 2017,Jan,8; 2016,Jan,13; 2015,Jan,16

43332 **Repair, paraesophageal hiatal hernia (including fundoplication), via laparotomy, except neonatal; without implantation of mesh or other prosthesis**
EXCLUDES *Neonatal diaphragmatic hernia repair (39503)*
33.7 33.7 FUD 090 C 80
AMA: 2018,Jan,8; 2017,Jan,8; 2016,Jan,13; 2015,Jan,16

43333 **with implantation of mesh or other prosthesis**
EXCLUDES *Neonatal diaphragmatic hernia repair (39503)*
36.8 36.8 FUD 090 C 80
AMA: 2018,Jan,8; 2017,Jan,8; 2016,Jan,13; 2015,Jan,16

43334 **Repair, paraesophageal hiatal hernia (including fundoplication), via thoracotomy, except neonatal; without implantation of mesh or other prosthesis**
EXCLUDES *Neonatal diaphragmatic hernia repair (39503)*
36.2 36.2 FUD 090 C 80
AMA: 2018,Jan,8; 2017,Jan,8; 2016,Jan,13; 2015,Jan,16

43335 **with implantation of mesh or other prosthesis**
EXCLUDES *Neonatal diaphragmatic hernia repair (39503)*
38.7 38.7 FUD 090 C 80
AMA: 2018,Jan,8; 2017,Jan,8; 2016,Jan,13; 2015,Jan,16

43336 **Repair, paraesophageal hiatal hernia, (including fundoplication), via thoracoabdominal incision, except neonatal; without implantation of mesh or other prosthesis**
EXCLUDES *Neonatal diaphragmatic hernia repair (39503)*
42.0 42.0 FUD 090 C 80
AMA: 2018,Jan,8; 2017,Jan,8; 2016,Jan,13; 2015,Jan,16

43337 **with implantation of mesh or other prosthesis**
EXCLUDES *Neonatal diaphragmatic hernia repair (39503)*
44.8 44.8 FUD 090 C 80
AMA: 2018,Jan,8; 2017,Jan,8; 2016,Jan,13; 2015,Jan,16

+ **43338** **Esophageal lengthening procedure (eg, Collis gastroplasty or wedge gastroplasty) (List separately in addition to code for primary procedure)**
Code first (43280, 43327-43337)
3.37 3.37 FUD ZZZ C 80
AMA: 2018,Jan,8; 2017,Jan,8; 2016,Jan,13; 2015,Jan,16

43340 **Esophagojejunostomy (without total gastrectomy); abdominal approach**
40.0 40.0 FUD 090 C 80
AMA: 2014,Jan,11; 2013,Jan,11-12

43341 **thoracic approach**
40.5 40.5 FUD 090 C 80
AMA: 2014,Jan,11; 2013,Jan,11-12

43351 **Esophagostomy, fistulization of esophagus, external; thoracic approach**
38.0 38.0 FUD 090 C 80
AMA: 2014,Jan,11; 2013,Jan,11-12

43352 **cervical approach**
30.8 30.8 FUD 090 C 80
AMA: 2014,Jan,11; 2013,Jan,11-12

43360 **Gastrointestinal reconstruction for previous esophagectomy, for obstructing esophageal lesion or fistula, or for previous esophageal exclusion; with stomach, with or without pyloroplasty**
65.3 65.3 FUD 090 C 80
AMA: 2014,Jan,11; 2013,Jan,11-12

43361 **with colon interposition or small intestine reconstruction, including intestine mobilization, preparation, and anastomosis(es)**
78.6 78.6 FUD 090 C 80
AMA: 2014,Jan,11; 2013,Jan,11-12

43400 **Ligation, direct, esophageal varices**
44.4 44.4 FUD 090 C 80
AMA: 2014,Jan,11; 2013,Jan,11-12

43405 **Ligation or stapling at gastroesophageal junction for pre-existing esophageal perforation**
41.9 41.9 FUD 090 C 80
AMA: 2014,Jan,11; 2013,Jan,11-12

43410 **Suture of esophageal wound or injury; cervical approach**
29.3 29.3 FUD 090 C 80
AMA: 2018,Jan,8; 2017,Jan,8; 2016,Jan,13; 2015,Jan,16

43415 **transthoracic or transabdominal approach**
74.5 74.5 FUD 090 C 80
AMA: 2014,Jan,11; 2013,Jan,11-12

43420 **Closure of esophagostomy or fistula; cervical approach**
EXCLUDES *Paraesophageal hiatal hernia repair:*
Transabdominal (43332-43333)
Transthoracic (43334-43335)
29.1 29.1 FUD 090 J 80
AMA: 2014,Jan,11; 2013,Jan,11-12

43425 **transthoracic or transabdominal approach**
EXCLUDES *Paraesophageal hiatal hernia repair:*
Transabdominal (43332-43333)
Transthoracic (43334-43335)
41.8 41.8 FUD 090 C 80
AMA: 2014,Jan,11; 2013,Jan,11-12

43450-43453 Esophageal Dilation

43450 **Dilation of esophagus, by unguided sound or bougie, single or multiple passes**
(74220, 74360)
2.27 4.87 **FUD** 000 T A2
AMA: 2018,Jan,8; 2017,Jul,10; 2017,Jan,8; 2016,Jan,13; 2015,Jan,16

43453 **Dilation of esophagus, over guide wire**
EXCLUDES *Dilation performed with endoscopic visualization (43195, 43226)*
Endoscopic dilation by dilator or balloon:
Balloon diameter 30 mm or larger (43214, 43233)
Balloon diameter less than 30 mm (43195, 43220, 43249)
(74220, 74360)
2.50 25.4 **FUD** 000 J A2
AMA: 2018,Jan,8; 2017,Jan,8; 2016,Jan,13; 2015,Jan,16

43460-43499 Other/Unlisted Esophageal Procedures

43460 **Esophagogastric tamponade, with balloon (Sengstaken type)**
EXCLUDES *Removal foreign body esophagus with balloon catheter (43499, 74235)*
(74220)
6.13 6.13 **FUD** 000 C
AMA: 2014,Jan,11; 2013,Jan,11-12

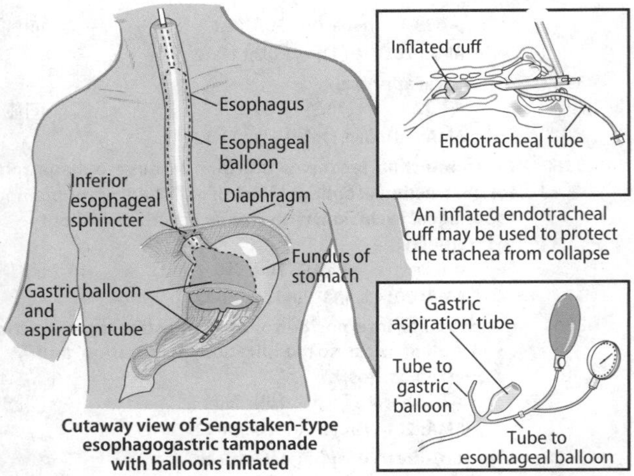

Cutaway view of Sengstaken-type esophagogastric tamponade with balloons inflated

43496 **Free jejunum transfer with microvascular anastomosis**
INCLUDES Operating microscope (69990)
0.00 0.00 **FUD** 090 C 80
AMA: 2019,Dec,5; 2018,Jan,8; 2017,Jan,8; 2016,Feb,12; 2016,Jan,13; 2015,Jan,16

43499 **Unlisted procedure, esophagus**
0.00 0.00 **FUD** YYY T
AMA: 2018,Jul,7; 2018,Jan,8; 2017,Jan,8; 2016,Jan,13; 2015,Nov,10; 2015,Nov,8; 2015,Jan,16

43500-43641 Open Gastric Incisional and Resection Procedures

43500 **Gastrotomy; with exploration or foreign body removal**
22.7 22.7 **FUD** 090 C 80
AMA: 2014,Jan,11; 2013,Jan,11-12

43501 **with suture repair of bleeding ulcer**
39.2 39.2 **FUD** 090 C 80
AMA: 2014,Jan,11; 2013,Jan,11-12

43502 **with suture repair of pre-existing esophagogastric laceration (eg, Mallory-Weiss)**
44.5 44.5 **FUD** 090 C 80
AMA: 2014,Jan,11; 2013,Jan,11-12

43510 **with esophageal dilation and insertion of permanent intraluminal tube (eg, Celestin or Mousseaux-Barbin)**
27.6 27.6 **FUD** 090 T 80
AMA: 2014,Jan,11; 2013,Jan,11-12

43520 **Pyloromyotomy, cutting of pyloric muscle (Fredet-Ramstedt type operation)**
19.9 19.9 **FUD** 090 63 C 80
AMA: 2014,Jan,11; 2013,Jan,11-12

43605 **Biopsy of stomach, by laparotomy**
24.3 24.3 **FUD** 090 C 80
AMA: 2014,Jan,11; 2013,Jan,11-12

43610 **Excision, local; ulcer or benign tumor of stomach**
28.5 28.5 **FUD** 090 C 80
AMA: 2014,Jan,11; 2013,Jan,11-12

43611 **malignant tumor of stomach**
35.6 35.6 **FUD** 090 C 80
AMA: 2014,Jan,11; 2013,Jan,11-12

43620 **Gastrectomy, total; with esophagoenterostomy**
57.8 57.8 **FUD** 090 C 80
AMA: 2014,Jan,11; 2013,Jan,11-12

43621 **with Roux-en-Y reconstruction**
66.2 66.2 **FUD** 090 C 80
AMA: 2014,Jan,11; 2013,Jan,11-12

43622 **with formation of intestinal pouch, any type**
67.5 67.5 **FUD** 090 C 80
AMA: 2014,Jan,11; 2013,Jan,11-12

43631 **Gastrectomy, partial, distal; with gastroduodenostomy**
INCLUDES Billroth operation
42.0 42.0 **FUD** 090 C 80
AMA: 2014,Jan,11; 2013,Jan,11-12

43632 **with gastrojejunostomy**
INCLUDES Polya anastomosis
59.3 59.3 **FUD** 090 C 80
AMA: 2014,Jan,11; 2013,Jan,11-12

43633 **with Roux-en-Y reconstruction**
56.1 56.1 **FUD** 090 C 80
AMA: 2014,Jan,11; 2013,Jan,11-12

43634 **with formation of intestinal pouch**
62.0 62.0 **FUD** 090 C 80
AMA: 2014,Jan,11; 2013,Jan,11-12

+ **43635** **Vagotomy when performed with partial distal gastrectomy (List separately in addition to code[s] for primary procedure)**
Code first as appropriate (43631-43634)
3.29 3.29 **FUD** ZZZ C 80
AMA: 2014,Jan,11; 2013,Jan,11-12

43640 **Vagotomy including pyloroplasty, with or without gastrostomy; truncal or selective**
EXCLUDES *Pyloroplasty (43800)*
Vagotomy (64755, 64760)
34.1 34.1 **FUD** 090 C 80
AMA: 2014,Jan,11; 2013,Jan,11-12

43641 **parietal cell (highly selective)**
EXCLUDES *Upper gastrointestinal endoscopy (43235-43259 [43233, 43266, 43270])*
35.1 35.1 **FUD** 090 C 80
AMA: 2014,Jan,11; 2013,Jan,11-12

43644-43645 Laparoscopic Gastric Bypass with Small Bowel Resection

CMS: 100-03,100.1 Bariatric Surgery for Treatment Co-morbid Conditions Due to Morbid Obesity; 100-04,32,150.1 Bariatric Surgery: Treatment of Co-Morbid Conditions Due to Morbid Obesity; 100-04,32,150.2 HCPCS Procedure Codes for Bariatric Surgery; 100-04,32,150.5 ICD Diagnosis Codes for BMI ≥35; 100-04,32,150.6 Bariatric Surgery Claims Guidance

INCLUDES Diagnostic laparoscopy (49320)

EXCLUDES *Endoscopy, upper gastrointestinal, (esophagus/stomach/duodenum/jejunum) (43235-43259 [43233, 43266, 43270])*

43644 **Laparoscopy, surgical, gastric restrictive procedure; with gastric bypass and Roux-en-Y gastroenterostomy (roux limb 150 cm or less)**

EXCLUDES *Roux limb less than 150 cm (43846)*
Roux limb greater than 150 cm (43645)

50.6 50.6 **FUD** 090 C 80

AMA: 2014,Jan,11; 2013,Jan,11-12

43645 **with gastric bypass and small intestine reconstruction to limit absorption**

EXCLUDES *Roux limb less than 150 cm (43847)*

53.9 53.9 **FUD** 090 C 80

AMA: 2018,Jan,8; 2017,Jan,8; 2016,Jan,13; 2015,Jan,16

43647-43659 Other and Unlisted Laparoscopic Gastric Procedures

INCLUDES Diagnostic laparoscopy (49320)

EXCLUDES *Endoscopy, upper gastrointestinal, (esophagus/stomach/duodenum/jejunum) (43235-43259 [43233, 43266, 43270])*

43647 **Laparoscopy, surgical; implantation or replacement of gastric neurostimulator electrodes, antrum**

EXCLUDES *Electronic analysis/programming gastric neurostimulator (95980-95982)*
Insertion gastric neurostimulator pulse generator, incisional (64590)
Laparoscopy with implantation, removal, or revision gastric neurostimulator electrodes on lesser curvature stomach (43659)
Open method (43881)
Vagus nerve blocking pulse generator and/or neurostimulator electrode array implantation, reprogramming, replacement, revision, or removal at esophagogastric junction performed laparoscopically (0312T-0317T)

0.00 0.00 **FUD** YYY J 80

AMA: 2019,Feb,6; 2018,Jan,8; 2017,Jan,8; 2016,Jan,13; 2015,Jan,16

43648 **revision or removal of gastric neurostimulator electrodes, antrum**

EXCLUDES *Electronic analysis/programming gastric neurostimulator (95980-95982)*
Laparoscopy with implantation, removal, or revision gastric neurostimulator electrodes on lesser curvature stomach (43659)
Open method (43882)
Removal or revision gastric neurostimulator pulse generator (64595)
Vagus nerve blocking pulse generator and/or neurostimulator electrode array implantation, reprogramming, replacement, revision, or removal at esophagogastric junction performed laparoscopically (0312T-0317T)

0.00 0.00 **FUD** YYY J 80

AMA: 2019,Feb,6; 2018,Jan,8; 2017,Jan,8; 2016,Jan,13; 2015,Jan,16

43651 **Laparoscopy, surgical; transection of vagus nerves, truncal**

19.0 19.0 **FUD** 090 J 80

AMA: 2018,Jan,8; 2017,Jan,8; 2016,Jan,13; 2015,Jan,16

43652 **transection of vagus nerves, selective or highly selective**

22.2 22.2 **FUD** 090 J 80

AMA: 2018,Jan,8; 2017,Jan,8; 2016,Jan,13; 2015,Jan,16

43653 **gastrostomy, without construction of gastric tube (eg, Stamm procedure) (separate procedure)**

16.6 16.6 **FUD** 090 J A2 80

AMA: 2018,Jan,8; 2017,Jan,8; 2016,Jan,13; 2015,Jan,16

43659 **Unlisted laparoscopy procedure, stomach**

0.00 0.00 **FUD** YYY J 80 50

AMA: 2018,Jul,7; 2018,Jan,8; 2017,Jan,8; 2016,Jan,13; 2015,Jan,16

43752-43763 Nonsurgical Gastric Tube Procedures

43752 **Naso- or oro-gastric tube placement, requiring physician's skill and fluoroscopic guidance (includes fluoroscopy, image documentation and report)**

EXCLUDES *Critical care services (99291-99292)*
Initial inpatient neonatal/pediatric critical care, per day (99468-99469, 99471-99472)
Insertion long gastrointestinal tube (44500, 74340)
Percutaneous insertion gastrostomy tube (43246, 49440)
Subsequent intensive care, per day, for low birth weight infant (99478-99479)

1.18 1.18 **FUD** 000 Q1 G2

AMA: 2019,Aug,8; 2018,Mar,11; 2018,Jan,8; 2017,Jan,8; 2016,Jan,13; 2015,Jan,16

43753 **Gastric intubation and aspiration(s) therapeutic, necessitating physician's skill (eg, for gastrointestinal hemorrhage), including lavage if performed**

0.63 0.63 **FUD** 000 Q1 N1 80

AMA: 2019,Aug,8; 2018,Jan,8; 2017,Jan,8; 2016,Jan,13; 2015,Jan,16

43754 **Gastric intubation and aspiration, diagnostic; single specimen (eg, acid analysis)**

EXCLUDES *Analysis gastric acid (82930)*
Naso- or oro-gastric tube placement using fluoroscopic guidance (43752)

1.03 5.18 **FUD** 000 Q1 N1 80

AMA: 2018,Jan,8; 2017,Jan,8; 2016,Jan,13; 2015,Jan,16

43755 **collection of multiple fractional specimens with gastric stimulation, single or double lumen tube (gastric secretory study) (eg, histamine, insulin, pentagastrin, calcium, secretin), includes drug administration**

EXCLUDES *Analysis gastric acid (82930)*
Naso- or oro-gastric tube placement using fluoroscopic guidance (43752)

Code also drugs or substances administered

1.74 4.43 **FUD** 000 S G2 80

AMA: 2018,Jan,8; 2017,Jan,8; 2016,Jan,13; 2015,Jan,16

43756 **Duodenal intubation and aspiration, diagnostic, includes image guidance; single specimen (eg, bile study for crystals or afferent loop culture)**

Code also drugs or substances administered

(89049-89240)

1.46 7.11 **FUD** 000 Q1 G2 80

AMA: 2018,Jan,8; 2017,Jan,8; 2016,Jan,13; 2015,Jan,16

43757 **collection of multiple fractional specimens with pancreatic or gallbladder stimulation, single or double lumen tube, includes drug administration**

Code also drugs or substances administered

(89049-89240)

2.20 9.76 **FUD** 000 T G2 80

AMA: 2018,Jan,8; 2017,Jan,8; 2016,Jan,13; 2015,Jan,16

43761 **Repositioning of a naso- or oro-gastric feeding tube, through the duodenum for enteric nutrition**

EXCLUDES *Conversion gastrostomy tube to gastro-jejunostomy tube, percutaneous (49446)*
Gastrostomy tube converted endoscopically to jejunostomy tube (44373)
Insertion long gastrointestinal tube (44500, 74340)

(76000)

2.98 3.43 FUD 000 T A2

AMA: 2018,Jan,8; 2017,Jan,8; 2016,Jan,13; 2015,Jan,16

43762 **Replacement of gastrostomy tube, percutaneous, includes removal, when performed, without imaging or endoscopic guidance; not requiring revision of gastrostomy tract**

1.10 6.45 FUD 000 G2

AMA: 2019,Feb,5

43763 **requiring revision of gastrostomy tract**

EXCLUDES *Gastrostomy tube replacement using fluoroscopy (49450)*
Percutaneous insertion gastrostomy tube (43246)

2.44 9.64 FUD 000 G2

AMA: 2019,Oct,10; 2019,Feb,5

43770-43775 Laparoscopic Bariatric Procedures

CMS: 100-03,100.1 Bariatric Surgery for Treatment Co-morbid Conditions Due to Morbid Obesity; 100-04,32,150.1 Bariatric Surgery: Treatment of Co-Morbid Conditions Due to Morbid Obesity; 100-04,32,150.2 HCPCS Procedure Codes for Bariatric Surgery; 100-04,32,150.5 ICD Diagnosis Codes for BMI ≥35; 100-04,32,150.6 Bariatric Surgery Claims Guidance

INCLUDES Diagnostic laparoscopy (49320)
Stomach/duodenum/jejunum/ileum
Subsequent band adjustments (change gastric band component diameter by injection/aspiration fluid through subcutaneous port component) during postoperative period

43770 **Laparoscopy, surgical, gastric restrictive procedure; placement of adjustable gastric restrictive device (eg, gastric band and subcutaneous port components)**

Code also modifier 52 for placement individual component

32.8 32.8 FUD 090 J 80

AMA: 2018,Jan,8; 2017,Jan,8; 2016,Jan,13; 2015,Jan,16

43771 **revision of adjustable gastric restrictive device component only**

37.2 37.2 FUD 090 C 80

AMA: 2018,Jan,8; 2017,Jan,8; 2016,Jan,13; 2015,Jan,16

43772 **removal of adjustable gastric restrictive device component only**

27.4 27.4 FUD 090 J 80

AMA: 2018,Jan,8; 2017,Jan,8; 2016,Jan,13; 2015,Jan,16

43773 **removal and replacement of adjustable gastric restrictive device component only**

EXCLUDES *Laparoscopy, surgical, gastric restrictive procedure; removal adjustable gastric restrictive device component only (43772)*

37.2 37.2 FUD 090 J 80

AMA: 2018,Jan,8; 2017,Jan,8; 2016,Jan,13; 2015,Jan,16

43774 **removal of adjustable gastric restrictive device and subcutaneous port components**

EXCLUDES *Removal/replacement subcutaneous port components and gastric band (43659)*

27.8 27.8 FUD 090 J 80

AMA: 2018,Jan,8; 2017,Jan,8; 2016,Jan,13; 2015,Jan,16

43775 **longitudinal gastrectomy (ie, sleeve gastrectomy)**

EXCLUDES *Open gastric restrictive procedure for morbid obesity, without gastric bypass, other than vertical-banded gastroplasty (43843)*
Vagus nerve blocking pulse generator and/or neurostimulator electrode array implantation, reprogramming, replacement, revision, or removal at esophagogastric junction performed laparoscopically (0312T-0317T)

32.5 32.5 FUD 090 C 80

AMA: 2019,Oct,10

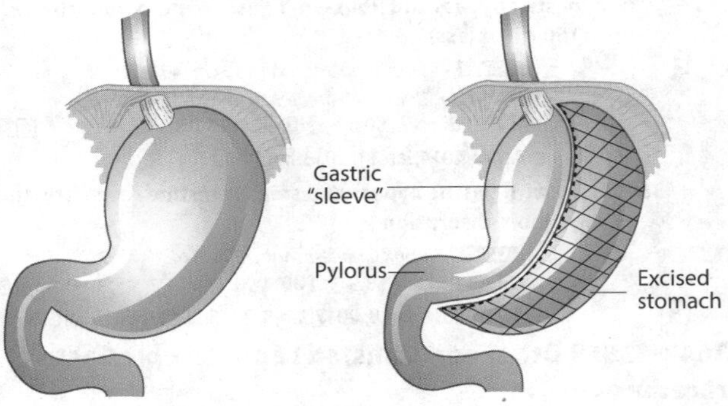

43800-43840 Open Gastric Incisional/Repair/Resection Procedures

43800 **Pyloroplasty**

EXCLUDES *Vagotomy with pyloroplasty (43640)*

27.2 27.2 FUD 090 C 80

AMA: 2014,Jan,11; 2013,Jan,11-12

43810 **Gastroduodenostomy**

29.7 29.7 FUD 090 C 80

AMA: 2014,Jan,11; 2013,Jan,11-12

43820 **Gastrojejunostomy; without vagotomy**

39.1 39.1 FUD 090 C 80

AMA: 2014,Jan,11; 2013,Jan,11-12

43825 **with vagotomy, any type**

37.8 37.8 FUD 090 C 80

AMA: 2014,Jan,11; 2013,Jan,11-12

43830 **Gastrostomy, open; without construction of gastric tube (eg, Stamm procedure) (separate procedure)**

20.4 20.4 FUD 090 J 80

AMA: 2019,Feb,5; 2018,Jan,8; 2017,Jan,8; 2016,Jan,13; 2015,Jan,16

43831 **neonatal, for feeding** A

EXCLUDES *Change gastrostomy tube (43762-43763)*
Gastrostomy tube replacement using fluoroscopy (49450)

17.5 17.5 FUD 090 63 T 80

AMA: 2019,Feb,5; 2018,Jan,8; 2017,Jan,8; 2016,Jan,13; 2015,Jan,16

43832 **with construction of gastric tube (eg, Janeway procedure)**

EXCLUDES *Endoscopic placement percutaneous gastrostomy tube (43246)*

30.3 30.3 FUD 090 C 80

AMA: 2018,Jan,8; 2017,Jan,8; 2016,Jan,13; 2015,Jan,16

43840 **Gastrorrhaphy, suture of perforated duodenal or gastric ulcer, wound, or injury**

39.4 39.4 FUD 090 C 80

AMA: 2014,Jan,11; 2013,Jan,11-12

43842-43848 Open Bariatric Procedures for Morbid Obesity

CMS: 100-03,100.1 Bariatric Surgery for Treatment Co-morbid Conditions Due to Morbid Obesity; 100-04,32,150.1 Bariatric Surgery: Treatment of Co-Morbid Conditions Due to Morbid Obesity; 100-04,32,150.2 HCPCS Procedure Codes for Bariatric Surgery; 100-04,32,150.5 ICD Diagnosis Codes for BMI ≥35; 100-04,32,150.6 Bariatric Surgery Claims Guidance

43842 **Gastric restrictive procedure, without gastric bypass, for morbid obesity; vertical-banded gastroplasty**
33.4 33.4 **FUD** 090 E
AMA: 2018,Jan,8; 2017,Jan,8; 2016,Jan,13; 2015,Jan,16

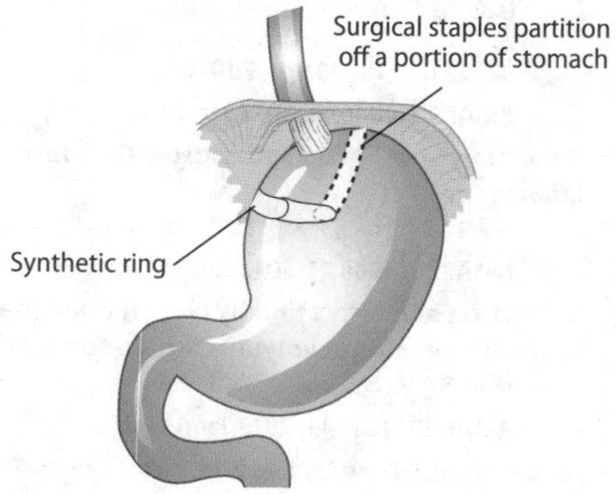

The stomach is surgically restricted to treat morbid obesity; a vertical-banded partitioning technique gives the patient a sensation of fullness, thus decreasing daily caloric intake

43843 **other than vertical-banded gastroplasty**
EXCLUDES *Laparoscopic longitudinal gastrectomy (e.g., sleeve gastrectomy) (43775)*
37.4 37.4 **FUD** 090 C 80
AMA: 2018,Jan,8; 2017,Jan,8; 2016,Jan,13; 2015,Jan,16

43845 **Gastric restrictive procedure with partial gastrectomy, pylorus-preserving duodenoileostomy and ileoileostomy (50 to 100 cm common channel) to limit absorption (biliopancreatic diversion with duodenal switch)**
EXCLUDES *Enteroenterostomy, anastomosis intestine (44130)*
Exploratory laparotomy, exploratory celiotomy (49000)
Gastrectomy, partial, distal; with Roux-en-Y reconstruction (43633)
Gastric restrictive procedure, with gastric bypass for morbid obesity; with small intestine reconstruction (43847)
56.8 56.8 **FUD** 090 C 80
AMA: 2018,Jan,8; 2017,Jan,8; 2016,Jan,13; 2015,Jan,16

43846 **Gastric restrictive procedure, with gastric bypass for morbid obesity; with short limb (150 cm or less) Roux-en-Y gastroenterostomy**
EXCLUDES *Performed laparoscopically (43644)*
Roux limb more than 150 cm (43847)
47.3 47.3 **FUD** 090 C 80
AMA: 2018,Jan,8; 2017,Jan,8; 2016,Jan,13; 2015,Jan,16

43847 **with small intestine reconstruction to limit absorption**
EXCLUDES *Performed laparoscopically (43645)*
52.4 52.4 **FUD** 090 C 80
AMA: 2018,Jan,8; 2017,Jan,8; 2016,Jan,13; 2015,Jan,16

43848 **Revision, open, of gastric restrictive procedure for morbid obesity, other than adjustable gastric restrictive device (separate procedure)**
EXCLUDES *Gastric restrictive port procedures (43886-43888)*
Procedures for adjustable gastric restrictive devices (43770-43774)
56.4 56.4 **FUD** 090 C 80
AMA: 2018,Jan,8; 2017,Jan,8; 2016,Jan,13; 2015,Jan,16

43850-43882 Open Gastric Procedures: Closure/Implantation/Replacement/Revision

43850 **Revision of gastroduodenal anastomosis (gastroduodenostomy) with reconstruction; without vagotomy**
47.5 47.5 **FUD** 090 C 80
AMA: 2014,Jan,11; 2013,Jan,11-12

43855 **with vagotomy**
49.1 49.1 **FUD** 090 C 80
AMA: 2014,Jan,11; 2013,Jan,11-12

43860 **Revision of gastrojejunal anastomosis (gastrojejunostomy) with reconstruction, with or without partial gastrectomy or intestine resection; without vagotomy**
47.7 47.7 **FUD** 090 C 80
AMA: 2014,Jan,11; 2013,Jan,11-12

43865 **with vagotomy**
49.9 49.9 **FUD** 090 C 80
AMA: 2014,Jan,11; 2013,Jan,11-12

43870 **Closure of gastrostomy, surgical**
20.6 20.6 **FUD** 090 J A2 80
AMA: 2018,Jul,14

43880 **Closure of gastrocolic fistula**
46.1 46.1 **FUD** 090 C 80
AMA: 2014,Jan,11; 2013,Jan,11-12

43881 **Implantation or replacement of gastric neurostimulator electrodes, antrum, open**
EXCLUDES *Electronic analysis and programming (95980-95982)*
Implantation/removal/revision gastric neurostimulator electrodes, lesser curvature or vagal trunk (EGJ):
Laparoscopically (43659)
Open, lesser curvature (43999)
Implantation/replacement performed laparoscopically (43647)
Insertion gastric neurostimulator pulse generator (64590)
Vagus nerve blocking pulse generator and/or neurostimulator electrode array implantation, reprogramming, replacement, revision, or removal at esophagogastric junction performed laparoscopically (0312T-0317T)
0.00 0.00 **FUD** YYY C 80
AMA: 2019,Feb,6; 2018,Jan,8; 2017,Jan,8; 2016,Jan,13; 2015,Jan,16

43882 **Revision or removal of gastric neurostimulator electrodes, antrum, open**
EXCLUDES *Electronic analysis and programming (95980-95982)*
Implantation/removal/revision gastric neurostimulator electrodes, lesser curvature or vagal trunk (EGJ):
Laparoscopic (43659)
Open, lesser curvature (43999)
Revision/removal gastric neurostimulator electrodes, antrum, performed laparoscopically (43648)
Revision/removal gastric neurostimulator pulse generator (64595)
Vagus nerve blocking pulse generator and/or neurostimulator electrode array implantation, reprogramming, replacement, revision, or removal at esophagogastric junction performed laparoscopically (0312T-0317T)
0.00 0.00 **FUD** YYY C 80
AMA: 2019,Feb,6; 2018,Jan,8; 2017,Jan,8; 2016,Jan,13; 2015,Jan,16

43886-43999 Bariatric Procedures: Removal/Replacement/Revision Port Components

CMS: 100-04,32,150.1 Bariatric Surgery: Treatment of Co-Morbid Conditions Due to Morbid Obesity; 100-04,32,150.2 HCPCS Procedure Codes for Bariatric Surgery; 100-04,32,150.5 ICD Diagnosis Codes for BMI ≥35; 100-04,32,150.6 Bariatric Surgery Claims Guidance

43886 **Gastric restrictive procedure, open; revision of subcutaneous port component only**
10.5 10.5 FUD 090 T G2 80
AMA: 2018,Jan,8; 2017,Jan,8; 2016,Jan,13; 2015,Jan,16

43887 **removal of subcutaneous port component only**
EXCLUDES *Gastric band and subcutaneous port components:*
Removal and replacement performed laparoscopically (43659)
Removal performed laparoscopically (43774)
9.52 9.52 FUD 090 Q2 G2 80
AMA: 2018,Jan,8; 2017,Jan,8; 2016,Jan,13; 2015,Jan,16

43888 **removal and replacement of subcutaneous port component only**
EXCLUDES *Gastric band and subcutaneous port components:*
Removal and replacement performed laparoscopically (43659)
Removal performed laparoscopically (43774)
Gastric restrictive procedure, open; removal subcutaneous port component only (43887)
13.4 13.4 FUD 090 T G2 80
AMA: 2018,Jan,8; 2017,Jan,8; 2016,Jan,13; 2015,Jan,16

43999 **Unlisted procedure, stomach**
0.00 0.00 FUD YYY T 80
AMA: 2018,Dec,10; 2018,Dec,10; 2018,Jul,14; 2018,Jan,8; 2017,Jan,8; 2016,Jan,13; 2015,Jan,16

44005-44130 Incisional and Resection Procedures of Bowel

44005 **Enterolysis (freeing of intestinal adhesion) (separate procedure)**
EXCLUDES *Enterolysis performed laparoscopically (44180)*
Excision ileoanal reservoir with ileostomy (45136)
31.7 31.7 FUD 090 C 80
AMA: 2018,Feb,11; 2018,Jan,8; 2017,Jan,8; 2016,Jan,13; 2015,Jan,16

44010 **Duodenotomy, for exploration, biopsy(s), or foreign body removal**
24.8 24.8 FUD 090 C 80
AMA: 2014,Jan,11; 2013,Jan,11-12

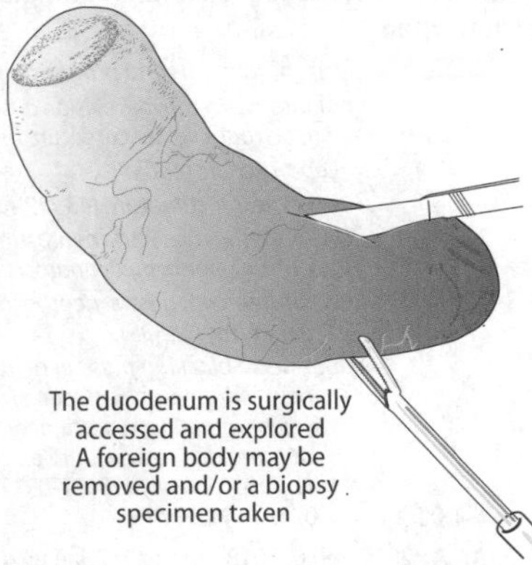
The duodenum is surgically accessed and explored
A foreign body may be removed and/or a biopsy specimen taken

\+ **44015** **Tube or needle catheter jejunostomy for enteral alimentation, intraoperative, any method (List separately in addition to primary procedure)**
Code first primary procedure
4.15 4.15 FUD ZZZ C 80
AMA: 2018,Jan,8; 2017,Jan,8; 2016,Jan,13; 2015,Jan,16

44020 **Enterotomy, small intestine, other than duodenum; for exploration, biopsy(s), or foreign body removal**
28.2 28.2 FUD 090 C 80
AMA: 2014,Jan,11; 2013,Jan,11-12

44021 **for decompression (eg, Baker tube)**
28.3 28.3 FUD 090 C 80
AMA: 2014,Jan,11; 2013,Jan,11-12

44025 **Colotomy, for exploration, biopsy(s), or foreign body removal**
INCLUDES Amussat's operation
EXCLUDES *Intestine exteriorization (Mikulicz resection with crushing of spur) (44602-44605)*
28.6 28.6 FUD 090 C 80
AMA: 2014,Jan,11; 2013,Jan,11-12

44050 **Reduction of volvulus, intussusception, internal hernia, by laparotomy**
27.2 27.2 FUD 090 C 80
AMA: 2014,Jan,11; 2013,Jan,11-12

44055 **Correction of malrotation by lysis of duodenal bands and/or reduction of midgut volvulus (eg, Ladd procedure)**
43.4 43.4 FUD 090 63 C 80
AMA: 2014,Jan,11; 2013,Jan,11-12

44100 **Biopsy of intestine by capsule, tube, peroral (1 or more specimens)**
3.11 3.11 FUD 000 T A2
AMA: 2014,Jan,11; 2013,Jan,11-12

44110 **Excision of 1 or more lesions of small or large intestine not requiring anastomosis, exteriorization, or fistulization; single enterotomy**
24.6 24.6 FUD 090 C 80
AMA: 2014,Jan,11; 2013,Jan,11-12

44111 **multiple enterotomies**
28.5 28.5 FUD 090 C 80
AMA: 2014,Jan,11; 2013,Jan,11-12

44120 **Enterectomy, resection of small intestine; single resection and anastomosis**
35.6 35.6 FUD 090 C 80
AMA: 2018,Nov,11; 2018,Jan,8; 2017,Jan,8; 2016,Jan,13; 2015,Jan,16

\+ **44121** **each additional resection and anastomosis (List separately in addition to code for primary procedure)**
Code first (44120)
7.04 7.04 FUD ZZZ C 80
AMA: 2014,Jan,11; 2013,Jan,11-12

44125 **with enterostomy**
34.3 34.3 FUD 090 C 80
AMA: 2014,Jan,11; 2013,Jan,11-12

44126 **Enterectomy, resection of small intestine for congenital atresia, single resection and anastomosis of proximal segment of intestine; without tapering**
71.3 71.3 FUD 090 63 C 80
AMA: 2014,Jan,11; 2013,Jan,11-12

44127 **with tapering**
83.3 83.3 FUD 090 63 C 80
AMA: 2014,Jan,11; 2013,Jan,11-12

\+ **44128** **each additional resection and anastomosis (List separately in addition to code for primary procedure)**
Code first single resection small intestine (44126, 44127)
7.10 7.10 FUD ZZZ 63 C 80
AMA: 2014,Jan,11; 2013,Jan,11-12

44130 **Enteroenterostomy, anastomosis of intestine, with or without cutaneous enterostomy (separate procedure)**
38.2 38.2 FUD 090 C 80
AMA: 2014,Jan,11; 2013,Jan,11-12

44132-44137 Intestine Transplant Procedures

CMS: 100-03,260.5 Intestinal and Multi-Visceral Transplantation; 100-04,3,90.6 Intestinal and Multi-Visceral Transplants

44132 **Donor enterectomy (including cold preservation), open; from cadaver donor**

INCLUDES Graft:
Cold preservation
Harvest

EXCLUDES Preparation/reconstruction backbench intestinal graft (44715, 44720-44721)

🔹 0.00 ⚕ 0.00 **FUD** XXX   C 80 ▣

AMA: 2014,Jan,11; 2013,Jan,11-12

44133 **partial, from living donor**

INCLUDES Donor care
Graft:
Cold preservation
Harvest

EXCLUDES Preparation/reconstruction backbench intestinal graft (44715, 44720-44721)

🔹 0.00 ⚕ 0.00 **FUD** XXX   C 80 ▣

AMA: 2014,Jan,11; 2013,Jan,11-12

44135 **Intestinal allotransplantation; from cadaver donor**

INCLUDES Allograft transplantation
Recipient care

🔹 0.00 ⚕ 0.00 **FUD** XXX   C 80 ▣

AMA: 2014,Jan,11; 2013,Jan,11-12

44136 **from living donor**

INCLUDES Allograft transplantation
Recipient care

🔹 0.00 ⚕ 0.00 **FUD** XXX   C 80 ▣

AMA: 2014,Jan,11; 2013,Jan,11-12

44137 **Removal of transplanted intestinal allograft, complete**

EXCLUDES Partial removal transplant allograft (44120-44121, 44140)

🔹 0.00 ⚕ 0.00 **FUD** XXX   C 80 ▣

AMA: 2014,Jan,11; 2013,Jan,11-12

44139-44160 Colon Resection Procedures

+ **44139** **Mobilization (take-down) of splenic flexure performed in conjunction with partial colectomy (List separately in addition to primary procedure)**

Code first partial colectomy (44140-44147)

🔹 3.52 ⚕ 3.52 **FUD** ZZZ   C 80 ▣

AMA: 2014,Jan,11; 2013,Jan,11-12

44140 **Colectomy, partial; with anastomosis**

EXCLUDES Laparoscopic method (44204)

🔹 39.0 ⚕ 39.0 **FUD** 090   C 80 ▣

AMA: 2020,Apr,10; 2018,Jan,8; 2017,Jan,8; 2016,Jan,13; 2015,Jan,16

44141 **with skin level cecostomy or colostomy**

🔹 53.0 ⚕ 53.0 **FUD** 090   C 80 ▣

AMA: 2018,Jan,8; 2017,Jan,8; 2016,Jan,13; 2015,Jan,16

44143 **with end colostomy and closure of distal segment (Hartmann type procedure)**

EXCLUDES Laparoscopic method (44206)

🔹 48.4 ⚕ 48.4 **FUD** 090   C 80 ▣

AMA: 2018,Jan,8; 2017,Jan,8; 2016,Jan,13; 2015,Jan,16

44144 **with resection, with colostomy or ileostomy and creation of mucofistula**

🔹 51.3 ⚕ 51.3 **FUD** 090   C 80 ▣

AMA: 2018,Jan,8; 2017,Jan,8; 2016,Jan,13; 2015,Jan,16

44145 **with coloproctostomy (low pelvic anastomosis)**

EXCLUDES Laparoscopic method (44207)

🔹 48.0 ⚕ 48.0 **FUD** 090   C 80 ▣

AMA: 2014,Jan,11; 2013,Jan,11-12

44146 **with coloproctostomy (low pelvic anastomosis), with colostomy**

EXCLUDES Laparoscopic method (44208)

🔹 61.2 ⚕ 61.2 **FUD** 090   C 80 ▣

AMA: 2018,Jun,11; 2018,Jan,8; 2017,Jan,8; 2016,Jan,13; 2015,Jan,16

44147 **abdominal and transanal approach**

🔹 56.3 ⚕ 56.3 **FUD** 090   C 80 ▣

AMA: 2018,Jan,8; 2017,Jan,8; 2016,Jan,13; 2015,Jan,16

44150 **Colectomy, total, abdominal, without proctectomy; with ileostomy or ileoproctostomy**

INCLUDES Lane's operation

EXCLUDES Laparoscopic method (44210)

🔹 54.0 ⚕ 54.0 **FUD** 090   C 80 ▣

AMA: 2014,Jan,11; 2013,Jan,11-12

44151 **with continent ileostomy**

🔹 62.9 ⚕ 62.9 **FUD** 090   C 80 ▣

AMA: 2014,Jan,11; 2013,Jan,11-12

44155 **Colectomy, total, abdominal, with proctectomy; with ileostomy**

INCLUDES Miles' colectomy

EXCLUDES Laparoscopic method (44212)

🔹 60.0 ⚕ 60.0 **FUD** 090   C 80 ▣

AMA: 2014,Jan,11; 2013,Jan,11-12

44156 **with continent ileostomy**

🔹 67.4 ⚕ 67.4 **FUD** 090   C 80 ▣

AMA: 2014,Jan,11; 2013,Jan,11-12

44157 **with ileoanal anastomosis, includes loop ileostomy, and rectal mucosectomy, when performed**

🔹 63.9 ⚕ 63.9 **FUD** 090   C 80 ▣

AMA: 2014,Jan,11; 2013,Jan,11-12

44158 **with ileoanal anastomosis, creation of ileal reservoir (S or J), includes loop ileostomy, and rectal mucosectomy, when performed**

EXCLUDES Laparoscopic method (44211)

🔹 65.5 ⚕ 65.5 **FUD** 090   C 80 ▣

AMA: 2014,Jan,11; 2013,Jan,11-12

44160 **Colectomy, partial, with removal of terminal ileum with ileocolostomy**

EXCLUDES Laparoscopic method (44205)

🔹 36.0 ⚕ 36.0 **FUD** 090   C 80 ▣

AMA: 2018,Jan,8; 2017,Jan,8; 2016,Jan,13; 2015,Jan,16

44180 Laparoscopic Enterolysis

INCLUDES Diagnostic laparoscopy (49320)
EXCLUDES Laparoscopic salpingolysis/ovariolysis (58660)

44180 **Laparoscopy, surgical, enterolysis (freeing of intestinal adhesion) (separate procedure)**

🔹 26.6 ⚕ 26.6 **FUD** 090   J 80 ▣

AMA: 2018,Feb,11; 2018,Jan,8; 2017,Jan,8; 2016,Jan,13; 2015,Jan,16

44186-44238 Laparoscopic Enterostomy Procedures

INCLUDES Diagnostic laparoscopy (49320)

44186 **Laparoscopy, surgical; jejunostomy (eg, for decompression or feeding)**

🔹 18.9 ⚕ 18.9 **FUD** 090   J 80 ▣

AMA: 2018,Jan,8; 2017,Jan,8; 2016,Jan,13; 2015,Jan,16

44187 **ileostomy or jejunostomy, non-tube**

EXCLUDES Open method (44310)

🔹 31.8 ⚕ 31.8 **FUD** 090   C 80 ▣

AMA: 2019,Sep,10; 2018,Jan,8; 2017,Jan,8; 2016,Jan,13; 2015,Jan,16

● New Code   ▲ Revised Code   ○ Reinstated   ● New Web Release   ▲ Revised Web Release   + Add-on   Unlisted   Not Covered   # Resequenced
50 Optum Mod 50 Exempt   ⊘ AMA Mod 51 Exempt   51 Optum Mod 51 Exempt   63 Mod 63 Exempt   ∥ Non-FDA Drug   ★ Telemedicine   M Maternity   A Age Edit

44188 Laparoscopy, surgical, colostomy or skin level cecostomy

EXCLUDES *Laparoscopy, surgical, appendectomy (44970)*
Open method (44320)

35.4 35.4 FUD 090 C 80

AMA: 2018,Jan,8; 2017,Jan,8; 2016,Jan,13; 2015,Jan,16

44202 Laparoscopy, surgical; enterectomy, resection of small intestine, single resection and anastomosis

EXCLUDES *Open method (44120)*

40.1 40.1 FUD 090 C 80

AMA: 2020,Jul,13; 2018,Jan,8; 2017,Jan,8; 2016,Jan,13; 2015,Jan,16

+ **44203 each additional small intestine resection and anastomosis (List separately in addition to code for primary procedure)**

EXCLUDES *Open method (44121)*

Code first single resection small intestine (44202)

7.00 7.00 FUD ZZZ C 80

AMA: 2018,Jan,8; 2017,Jan,8; 2016,Jan,13; 2015,Jan,16

44204 colectomy, partial, with anastomosis

EXCLUDES *Open method (44140)*

44.7 44.7 FUD 090 C 80

AMA: 2018,Jan,8; 2017,Dec,14; 2017,Jan,8; 2016,Jan,13; 2015,Jan,16

44205 colectomy, partial, with removal of terminal ileum with ileocolostomy

EXCLUDES *Open method (44160)*

38.8 38.8 FUD 090 C 80

AMA: 2018,Jan,8; 2017,Jan,8; 2016,Jan,13; 2015,Jan,16

44206 colectomy, partial, with end colostomy and closure of distal segment (Hartmann type procedure)

EXCLUDES *Open method (44143)*

50.7 50.7 FUD 090 C 80

AMA: 2018,Jan,8; 2017,Jan,8; 2016,Jan,13; 2015,Jan,16

44207 colectomy, partial, with anastomosis, with coloproctostomy (low pelvic anastomosis)

EXCLUDES *Open method (44145)*

52.6 52.6 FUD 090 C 80

AMA: 2018,Jan,8; 2017,Jan,8; 2016,Jan,13; 2015,Jan,16

44208 colectomy, partial, with anastomosis, with coloproctostomy (low pelvic anastomosis) with colostomy

EXCLUDES *Open method (44146)*

57.4 57.4 FUD 090 C 80

AMA: 2018,Jan,8; 2017,Jan,8; 2016,Jan,13; 2015,Jan,16

44210 colectomy, total, abdominal, without proctectomy, with ileostomy or ileoproctostomy

EXCLUDES *Open method (44150)*

51.3 51.3 FUD 090 C 80

AMA: 2018,Jan,8; 2017,Jan,8; 2016,Jan,13; 2015,Jan,16

44211 colectomy, total, abdominal, with proctectomy, with ileoanal anastomosis, creation of ileal reservoir (S or J), with loop ileostomy, includes rectal mucosectomy, when performed

EXCLUDES *Open method (44157-44158)*

61.2 61.2 FUD 090 C 80

AMA: 2018,Jan,8; 2017,Jan,8; 2016,Jan,13; 2015,Jan,16

44212 colectomy, total, abdominal, with proctectomy, with ileostomy

EXCLUDES *Open method (44155)*

59.0 59.0 FUD 090 C 80

AMA: 2018,Jan,8; 2017,Jan,8; 2016,Jan,13; 2015,Jan,16

+ **44213 Laparoscopy, surgical, mobilization (take-down) of splenic flexure performed in conjunction with partial colectomy (List separately in addition to primary procedure)**

EXCLUDES *Open method (44139)*

Code first partial colectomy (44204-44208)

5.43 5.43 FUD ZZZ C 80

AMA: 2018,Jan,8; 2017,Jan,8; 2016,Jan,13; 2015,Jan,16

44227 Laparoscopy, surgical, closure of enterostomy, large or small intestine, with resection and anastomosis

EXCLUDES *Open method (44625-44626)*

48.4 48.4 FUD 090 C 80

AMA: 2018,Jan,8; 2017,Jan,8; 2016,Jan,13; 2015,Jan,16

44238 Unlisted laparoscopy procedure, intestine (except rectum)

0.00 0.00 FUD YYY J 80 50

AMA: 2020,Jul,13; 2019,Oct,10; 2018,Jan,8; 2017,Jul,10; 2017,Jan,8; 2016,Jan,13; 2015,Jan,16

44300-44346 Open Enterostomy Procedures

44300 Placement, enterostomy or cecostomy, tube open (eg, for feeding or decompression) (separate procedure)

EXCLUDES *Intraoperative lavage, colon (44701)*
Other gastrointestinal tube(s) placed percutaneously with fluoroscopic imaging guidance (49441-49442)

24.5 24.5 FUD 090 C 80

AMA: 2018,Jan,8; 2017,Jan,8; 2016,Jan,13; 2015,Jan,16

44310 Ileostomy or jejunostomy, non-tube

EXCLUDES *Colectomy, partial; with resection, with colostomy or ileostomy and creation mucofistula (44144)*
Colectomy, total, abdominal (44150-44151, 44155-44156)
Excision ileoanal reservoir with ileostomy (45136)
Laparoscopic method (44187)
Proctectomy (45113, 45119)

30.2 30.2 FUD 090 C 80

AMA: 2018,Jan,8; 2017,Jan,8; 2016,Jan,13; 2015,Jan,16

44312 Revision of ileostomy; simple (release of superficial scar) (separate procedure)

17.1 17.1 FUD 090 T A2 80

AMA: 2014,Jan,11; 2013,Jan,11-12

44314 complicated (reconstruction in-depth) (separate procedure)

29.1 29.1 FUD 090 C 80

AMA: 2014,Jan,11; 2013,Jan,11-12

44316 Continent ileostomy (Kock procedure) (separate procedure)

EXCLUDES *Fiberoptic evaluation (44385)*

41.2 41.2 FUD 090 C 80

AMA: 2014,Jan,11; 2013,Jan,11-12

44320 Colostomy or skin level cecostomy;

EXCLUDES *Closure fistula (45805, 45825, 57307)*
Colectomy, partial (44141, 44144, 44146)
Exploration, repair, and presacral drainage (45563)
Laparoscopic method (44188)
Pelvic exenteration (45126, 51597, 58240)
Proctectomy (45110, 45119)
Suture large intestine (44605)
Ureterosigmoidostomy (50810)

34.9 34.9 FUD 090 C 80

AMA: 2018,Jan,8; 2017,Jan,8; 2016,Jan,13; 2015,Jan,16

44322 with multiple biopsies (eg, for congenital megacolon) (separate procedure)

29.2 29.2 FUD 090 C 80

AMA: 2014,Jan,11; 2013,Jan,11-12

44340 Revision of colostomy; simple (release of superficial scar) (separate procedure)

18.0 18.0 FUD 090 T A2

AMA: 2014,Jan,11; 2013,Jan,11-12

44345 **complicated (reconstruction in-depth) (separate procedure)**

30.4 30.4 FUD 090 C 80

AMA: 2014,Jan,11; 2013,Jan,11-12

44346 **with repair of paracolostomy hernia (separate procedure)**

34.3 34.3 FUD 090 C 80

AMA: 2018,Jan,8; 2017,Jan,8; 2016,Jan,13; 2015,Jan,16

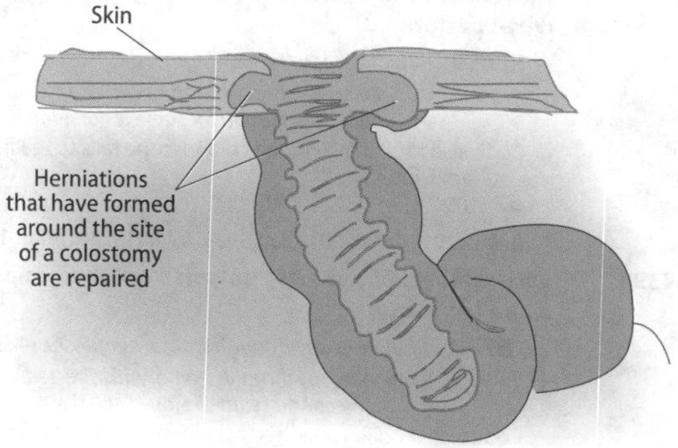
Skin
Herniations that have formed around the site of a colostomy are repaired

The colon is mobilized, trimmed if necessary, and a new stoma is often created

44360-44379 Endoscopy of Small Intestine

INCLUDES Control bleeding due to endoscopic procedure during same operative session

44360 **Small intestinal endoscopy, enteroscopy beyond second portion of duodenum, not including ileum; diagnostic, including collection of specimen(s) by brushing or washing, when performed (separate procedure)**

EXCLUDES *Esophagogastroduodenoscopy, flexible, transoral (43235-43259 [43233, 43266, 43270])*

4.14 4.14 FUD 000 J A2

AMA: 2019,Oct,10; 2018,Jan,8; 2017,Jan,8; 2016,Jan,13; 2015,Jan,16

44361 **with biopsy, single or multiple**

EXCLUDES *Esophagogastroduodenoscopy, flexible, transoral (43235-43259 [43233, 43266, 43270])*

4.65 4.65 FUD 000 J A2

AMA: 2019,Oct,10

44363 **with removal of foreign body(s)**

EXCLUDES *Esophagogastroduodenoscopy, flexible, transoral (43235-43259 [43233, 43266, 43270])*

5.54 5.54 FUD 000 J A2 80

AMA: 2019,Oct,10

44364 **with removal of tumor(s), polyp(s), or other lesion(s) by snare technique**

EXCLUDES *Esophagogastroduodenoscopy, flexible, transoral (43235-43259 [43233, 43266, 43270])*

5.90 5.90 FUD 000 J A2 80

AMA: 2019,Oct,10

44365 **with removal of tumor(s), polyp(s), or other lesion(s) by hot biopsy forceps or bipolar cautery**

EXCLUDES *Esophagogastroduodenoscopy, flexible, transoral (43235-43259 [43233, 43266, 43270])*

5.24 5.24 FUD 000 J A2 80

AMA: 2019,Oct,10

44366 **with control of bleeding (eg, injection, bipolar cautery, unipolar cautery, laser, heater probe, stapler, plasma coagulator)**

EXCLUDES *Esophagogastroduodenoscopy, flexible, transoral (43235-43259 [43233, 43266, 43270])*

6.93 6.93 FUD 000 J A2

AMA: 2019,Oct,10; 2018,Jan,8; 2017,Jan,8; 2016,Jan,13; 2015,Jan,16

44369 **with ablation of tumor(s), polyp(s), or other lesion(s) not amenable to removal by hot biopsy forceps, bipolar cautery or snare technique**

EXCLUDES *Esophagogastroduodenoscopy, flexible, transoral (43235-43259 [43233, 43266, 43270])*

7.10 7.10 FUD 000 J A2 80

AMA: 2019,Oct,10

44370 **with transendoscopic stent placement (includes predilation)**

EXCLUDES *Esophagogastroduodenoscopy, flexible, transoral (43235-43259 [43233, 43266, 43270])*

7.69 7.69 FUD 000 J J8 80

AMA: 2019,Oct,10; 2018,Jan,8; 2017,Jan,8; 2016,Jan,13; 2015,Jan,16

44372 **with placement of percutaneous jejunostomy tube**

EXCLUDES *Esophagogastroduodenoscopy, flexible, transoral (43235-43259 [43233, 43266, 43270])*

7.02 7.02 FUD 000 J A2

AMA: 2019,Oct,10; 2018,Jan,8; 2017,Jan,8; 2016,Jan,13; 2015,Jan,16

44373 **with conversion of percutaneous gastrostomy tube to percutaneous jejunostomy tube**

EXCLUDES *Esophagogastroduodenoscopy, flexible, transoral (43235-43259 [43233, 43266, 43270])*

5.62 5.62 FUD 000 J A2

AMA: 2019,Oct,10; 2018,Jan,8; 2017,Jan,8; 2016,Jan,13; 2015,Jan,16

44376 **Small intestinal endoscopy, enteroscopy beyond second portion of duodenum, including ileum; diagnostic, with or without collection of specimen(s) by brushing or washing (separate procedure)**

EXCLUDES *Small intestinal endoscopy, enteroscopy (44360-44373)*

8.33 8.33 FUD 000 J A2 80

AMA: 2018,Jan,8; 2017,Jan,8; 2016,Jan,13; 2015,Jan,16

44377 **with biopsy, single or multiple**

EXCLUDES *Small intestinal endoscopy, enteroscopy (44360-44373)*

8.63 8.63 FUD 000 J A2 80

AMA: 2018,Jan,8; 2017,Jan,8; 2016,Jan,13; 2015,Jan,16

44378 **with control of bleeding (eg, injection, bipolar cautery, unipolar cautery, laser, heater probe, stapler, plasma coagulator)**

EXCLUDES *Small intestinal endoscopy, enteroscopy (44360-44373)*

11.2 11.2 FUD 000 J A2 80

AMA: 2018,Jan,8; 2017,Jan,8; 2016,Jan,13; 2015,Jan,16

44379 **with transendoscopic stent placement (includes predilation)**

EXCLUDES *Small intestinal endoscopy, enteroscopy (44360-44373)*

11.8 11.8 FUD 000 J A2 80

AMA: 2018,Jan,8; 2017,Jan,8; 2016,Jan,13; 2015,Jan,16

44380-44384 [44381] Ileoscopy Via Stoma

INCLUDES Control bleeding due to endoscopic procedure during same operative session

EXCLUDES *Computed tomographic colonography (74261-74263)*

Code also exam nonfunctional distal colon/rectum, when performed, with:
- Anoscopy (46600, 46604-46606, 46608-46615)
- Proctosigmoidoscopy (45300-45327)
- Sigmoidoscopy (45330-45347 [45346])

44380 **Ileoscopy, through stoma; diagnostic, including collection of specimen(s) by brushing or washing, when performed (separate procedure)**

EXCLUDES *Ileoscopy, through stoma (44382-44384 [44381])*

1.61 5.20 FUD 000 T A2

AMA: 2018,Jan,8; 2017,Jan,8; 2016,Jan,13; 2015,Jan,16

44381 **Resequenced code. See code following 44382.**

44382 **with biopsy, single or multiple**

EXCLUDES *Ileoscopy, through stoma; diagnostic (44380)*

2.10 8.14 FUD 000 T A2

AMA: 2018,Jan,8; 2017,Jan,8; 2016,Jan,13; 2015,Jan,16

44381 **with transendoscopic balloon dilation**

EXCLUDES *Ileoscopy, through stoma (44380, 44384)*

Code also each additional stricture dilated in same session, using modifier 59 with (44381)

(74360)

2.44 | 27.0 | FUD 000 | J G2

AMA: 2018,Jan,8; 2017,Jan,8; 2016,Jan,13; 2015,Jan,16

44384 **with placement of endoscopic stent (includes pre- and post-dilation and guide wire passage, when performed)**

EXCLUDES *Ileoscopy, through stoma (44380-44381)*

(74360)

4.44 | 4.44 | FUD 000 | J G2

AMA: 2018,Jan,8; 2017,Jan,8; 2016,Jan,13; 2015,Jan,16

44385-44386 Endoscopy of Small Intestinal Pouch

INCLUDES Control bleeding due to endoscopic procedure during same operative session

EXCLUDES *Computed tomographic colonography (74261-74263)*

44385 **Endoscopic evaluation of small intestinal pouch (eg, Kock pouch, ileal reservoir [S or J]); diagnostic, including collection of specimen(s) by brushing or washing, when performed (separate procedure)**

EXCLUDES *Endoscopic evaluation small intestinal pouch (44386)*

2.09 | 5.60 | FUD 000 | T A2

AMA: 2018,Jan,8; 2017,Jan,8; 2016,Jan,13; 2015,Jan,16

44386 **with biopsy, single or multiple**

EXCLUDES *Endoscopic evaluation small intestinal pouch (44385)*

2.57 | 8.54 | FUD 000 | T A2

AMA: 2018,Jan,8; 2017,Jan,8; 2016,Jan,13; 2015,Jan,16

44388-44408 [44401] Colonoscopy Via Stoma

INCLUDES Control bleeding due to endoscopic procedure during same operative session

EXCLUDES *Colonoscopy via rectum (45378, 45392-45393 [45390, 45398])*
Computed tomographic colonography (74261-74263)

Code also exam nonfunctional distal colon/rectum, when performed, with:
Anoscopy (46600, 46604-46606, 46608-46615)
Proctosigmoidoscopy (45300-45327)
Sigmoidoscopy (45330-45347 [45346])

44388 **Colonoscopy through stoma; diagnostic, including collection of specimen(s) by brushing or washing, when performed (separate procedure)**

EXCLUDES *Colonoscopy through stoma (44389-44408 [44401])*

Code also modifier 53 when planned total colonoscopy cannot be completed

4.52 | 8.69 | FUD 000 | T A2

AMA: 2018,Jan,8; 2017,Jan,8; 2016,Jan,13; 2015,Jan,16

44389 **with biopsy, single or multiple**

EXCLUDES *Colonoscopy through stoma; diagnostic (44388)*
Colonoscopy through stoma; with endoscopic mucosal resection on same lesion (44403)

Code also modifier 52 when colonoscope fails to reach junction small intestine

4.97 | 11.4 | FUD 000 | T A2

AMA: 2018,Jan,8; 2017,Jan,8; 2016,Jan,13; 2015,Jan,16

44390 **with removal of foreign body(s)**

EXCLUDES *Colonoscopy through stoma; diagnostic (44388)*

Code also modifier 52 when colonoscope fails to reach junction small intestine

(76000)

6.07 | 11.2 | FUD 000 | T A2

AMA: 2018,Jan,8; 2017,Jan,8; 2016,Jan,13; 2015,Jan,16

44391 **with control of bleeding, any method**

EXCLUDES *Colonoscopy through stoma; diagnostic (44388)*
Colonoscopy through stoma; with directed submucosal injection(s) in same lesion (44404)

Code also modifier 52 when colonoscope fails to reach junction small intestine

6.65 | 19.2 | FUD 000 | T A2

AMA: 2018,Jan,8; 2017,Jan,8; 2016,Jan,13; 2015,Jan,16

44392 **with removal of tumor(s), polyp(s), or other lesion(s) by hot biopsy forceps**

EXCLUDES *Colonoscopy through stoma; diagnostic (44388)*

Code also modifier 52 when colonoscope fails to reach junction small intestine

5.82 | 10.2 | FUD 000 | T A2

AMA: 2018,Jan,8; 2017,Jan,8; 2016,Jan,13; 2015,Jan,16

44401 **with ablation of tumor(s), polyp(s), or other lesion(s) (includes pre-and post-dilation and guide wire passage, when performed)**

EXCLUDES *Colonoscopy through stoma; diagnostic (44388)*
Colonoscopy through stoma; with transendoscopic balloon dilation for same lesion (44405)

Code also modifier 52 when colonoscope fails to reach junction small intestine

7.00 | 80.2 | FUD 000 | T G2

AMA: 2018,Jan,8; 2017,Jan,8; 2016,Jan,13; 2015,Jan,16

44394 **with removal of tumor(s), polyp(s), or other lesion(s) by snare technique**

EXCLUDES *Colonoscopy through stoma; diagnostic (44388)*
Colonoscopy through stoma; with directed submucosal injection(s) same lesion (44403)

Code also modifier 52 when colonoscope fails to reach junction small intestine

6.60 | 11.7 | FUD 000 | T A2

AMA: 2018,Jan,8; 2017,Jan,8; 2016,Jan,13; 2015,Jan,16

44401 **Resequenced code. See code following 44392.**

44402 **with endoscopic stent placement (including pre- and post-dilation and guide wire passage, when performed)**

EXCLUDES *Colonoscopy through stoma (44388, 44405)*

Code also modifier 52 when colonoscope fails to reach junction small intestine

(74360)

7.56 | 7.56 | FUD 000 | J J8

AMA: 2018,Jan,8; 2017,Jan,8; 2016,Jan,13; 2015,Jan,16

44403 **with endoscopic mucosal resection**

EXCLUDES *Colonoscopy through stoma; diagnostic (44388)*
Colonoscopy through stoma for same lesion (44389, 44394, 44404)

Code also modifier 52 when colonoscope fails to reach junction small intestine

8.77 | 8.77 | FUD 000 | T G2

AMA: 2019,Dec,14; 2018,Jan,8; 2017,Jan,8; 2016,Jan,13; 2015,Jan,16

44404 **with directed submucosal injection(s), any substance**

EXCLUDES *Colonoscopy through stoma; diagnostic (44388)*
Colonoscopy through stoma for same lesion (44391, 44403)

Code also modifier 52 when colonoscope fails to reach small intestine junction

4.97 | 11.3 | FUD 000 | T G2

AMA: 2018,Jan,8; 2017,Jan,8; 2016,Jan,13; 2015,Jan,16

44405 **with transendoscopic balloon dilation**

EXCLUDES *Colonoscopy through stoma (44388, [44401], 44402)*

Code also each additional stricture dilated same session, using modifier 59 with (44405)

Code also modifier 52 when colonoscope fails to reach small intestine junction

(74360)

5.28 | 15.9 | FUD 000 | T G2

AMA: 2018,Jan,8; 2017,Jan,8; 2016,Jan,13; 2015,Jan,16

44406 **with endoscopic ultrasound examination, limited to the sigmoid, descending, transverse, or ascending colon and cecum and adjacent structures**

INCLUDES Gastrointestinal endoscopic ultrasound, supervision and interpretation (76975)

EXCLUDES *Colonoscopy through stoma (44388, 44407)*
Procedure performed more than one time per operative session

Code also modifier 52 when colonoscope fails to reach small intestine junction

6.62 6.62 FUD 000 T G2

AMA: 2018,Jan,8; 2017,Jan,8; 2016,Jan,13; 2015,Jan,16

44407 **with transendoscopic ultrasound guided intramural or transmural fine needle aspiration/biopsy(s), includes endoscopic ultrasound examination limited to the sigmoid, descending, transverse, or ascending colon and cecum and adjacent structures**

INCLUDES Gastrointestinal endoscopic ultrasound, supervision and interpretation (76975)
Ultrasonic guidance (76942)

EXCLUDES *Colonoscopy through stoma (44388, 44406)*
Procedure performed more than one time per operative session

Code also modifier 52 when colonoscope fails to reach small intestine junction

8.08 8.08 FUD 000 T G2

AMA: 2018,Jan,8; 2017,Jan,8; 2016,Jan,13; 2015,Jan,16

44408 **with decompression (for pathologic distention) (eg, volvulus, megacolon), including placement of decompression tube, when performed**

EXCLUDES *Colonoscopy through stoma; diagnostic (44388)*
Procedure performed more than one time per operative session

6.68 6.68 FUD 000 T G2

AMA: 2018,Jan,8; 2017,Jan,8; 2016,Jan,13; 2015,Jan,16

44500 Gastrointestinal Intubation

44500 **Introduction of long gastrointestinal tube (eg, Miller-Abbott) (separate procedure)**

EXCLUDES *Placement oro- or naso-gastric tube (43752)*

(74340)

0.56 0.56 FUD 000 ⊘ T G2 80

AMA: 2020,Aug,9; 2018,Jan,8; 2017,Jan,8; 2016,Sep,9; 2016,Jan,13; 2015,Jan,16

44602-44680 Open Repair Procedures of Intestines

44602 **Suture of small intestine (enterorrhaphy) for perforated ulcer, diverticulum, wound, injury or rupture; single perforation**

41.0 41.0 FUD 090 C 80

AMA: 2020,Feb,13

44603 **multiple perforations**

47.1 47.1 FUD 090 C 80

AMA: 2014,Jan,11; 2013,Dec,3

44604 **Suture of large intestine (colorrhaphy) for perforated ulcer, diverticulum, wound, injury or rupture (single or multiple perforations); without colostomy**

30.7 30.7 FUD 090 C 80

AMA: 2014,Jan,11; 2013,Dec,3

44605 **with colostomy**

37.9 37.9 FUD 090 C 80

AMA: 2014,Jan,11; 2013,Dec,3

44615 **Intestinal strictureplasty (enterotomy and enterorrhaphy) with or without dilation, for intestinal obstruction**

31.1 31.1 FUD 090 C 80

AMA: 2014,Jan,11; 2013,Dec,3

44620 **Closure of enterostomy, large or small intestine;**

EXCLUDES *Laparoscopic method (44227)*

25.1 25.1 FUD 090 C 80

AMA: 2014,Jan,11; 2013,Dec,3

44625 **with resection and anastomosis other than colorectal**

EXCLUDES *Laparoscopic method (44227)*

29.3 29.3 FUD 090 C 80

AMA: 2014,Jan,11; 2013,Dec,3

44626 **with resection and colorectal anastomosis (eg, closure of Hartmann type procedure)**

EXCLUDES *Laparoscopic method (44227)*

46.5 46.5 FUD 090 C 80

AMA: 2014,Jan,11; 2013,Dec,3

44640 **Closure of intestinal cutaneous fistula**

40.6 40.6 FUD 090 C 80

AMA: 2014,Jan,11; 2013,Dec,3

44650 **Closure of enteroenteric or enterocolic fistula**

42.0 42.0 FUD 090 C 80

AMA: 2014,Jan,11; 2013,Dec,3

44660 **Closure of enterovesical fistula; without intestinal or bladder resection**

EXCLUDES *Closure fistula:*
Gastrocolic (43880)
Rectovesical (45800, 45805)
Renocolic (50525-50526)

38.7 38.7 FUD 090 C 80

AMA: 2014,Jan,11; 2013,Dec,3

44661 **with intestine and/or bladder resection**

EXCLUDES *Closure fistula:*
Gastrocolic (43880)
Rectovesical (45800, 45805)
Renocolic (50525-50526)

45.0 45.0 FUD 090 C 80

AMA: 2014,Jan,11; 2013,Dec,3

44680 **Intestinal plication (separate procedure)**

INCLUDES Noble intestinal plication

30.8 30.8 FUD 090 C 80

AMA: 2014,Jan,11; 2013,Dec,3

44700-44705 Other Intestinal Procedures

44700 **Exclusion of small intestine from pelvis by mesh or other prosthesis, or native tissue (eg, bladder or omentum)**

EXCLUDES *Therapeutic radiation clinical treatment (77261-77799 [77295, 77385, 77386, 77387, 77424, 77425])*

29.1 29.1 FUD 090 C 80

AMA: 2014,Jan,11; 2013,Dec,3

+ **44701** **Intraoperative colonic lavage (List separately in addition to code for primary procedure)**

EXCLUDES *Appendectomy (44950-44960)*

Code first as appropriate (44140, 44145, 44150, 44604)

4.94 4.94 FUD ZZZ N N1 80

AMA: 2014,Jan,11; 2013,Dec,3

44705 **Preparation of fecal microbiota for instillation, including assessment of donor specimen**

EXCLUDES *Fecal instillation by enema or oro-nasogastric tube (44799)*
Therapeutic enema (74283)

2.16 3.25 FUD XXX B

AMA: 2018,Jan,8; 2017,Jan,8; 2016,Jan,13; 2015,Jan,16

44715-44799 Backbench Transplant Procedures

CMS: 100-04,3,90.6 Intestinal and Multi-Visceral Transplants

44715 **Backbench standard preparation of cadaver or living donor intestine allograft prior to transplantation, including mobilization and fashioning of the superior mesenteric artery and vein**

INCLUDES Mobilization/fashioning of superior mesenteric vein/artery

0.00 0.00 FUD XXX C 80

AMA: 2014,Jan,11; 2013,Dec,3

44720 **Backbench reconstruction of cadaver or living donor intestine allograft prior to transplantation; venous anastomosis, each**
8.02 8.02 FUD XXX C 80
AMA: 2014,Jan,11; 2013,Dec,3

44721 **arterial anastomosis, each**
11.2 11.2 FUD XXX C 80
AMA: 2018,Jan,8; 2017,Jan,8; 2016,Jan,13; 2015,Jan,16

44799 **Unlisted procedure, small intestine**
EXCLUDES *Unlisted colon procedure (45399)*
Unlisted intestinal procedure performed laparoscopically (44238)
Unlisted rectal procedure (45499, 45999)
0.00 0.00 FUD YYY T
AMA: 2018,Jan,8; 2017,Jan,8; 2016,Jan,13; 2015,Jan,16

44800-44899 Meckel's Diverticulum and Mesentery Procedures

44800 **Excision of Meckel's diverticulum (diverticulectomy) or omphalomesenteric duct**
22.3 22.3 FUD 090 C 80
AMA: 2014,Jan,11; 2013,Dec,3

44820 **Excision of lesion of mesentery (separate procedure)**
EXCLUDES *Resection intestine (44120-44128, 44140-44160)*
24.3 24.3 FUD 090 C 80
AMA: 2014,Jan,11; 2013,Dec,3

44850 **Suture of mesentery (separate procedure)**
EXCLUDES *Internal hernia repair/reduction (44050)*
21.7 21.7 FUD 090 C 80
AMA: 2014,Jan,11; 2013,Dec,3

44899 **Unlisted procedure, Meckel's diverticulum and the mesentery**
0.00 0.00 FUD YYY C 80
AMA: 2020,Jul,13

44900-44979 Open and Endoscopic Appendix Procedures

44900 **Incision and drainage of appendiceal abscess, open**
EXCLUDES *Image guided percutaneous catheter drainage (49406)*
22.4 22.4 FUD 090 C 80
AMA: 2014,Jan,11; 2013,Nov,9

44950 **Appendectomy;**
INCLUDES Battle's operation
EXCLUDES *Procedure performed with other intra-abdominal procedure(s) when appendectomy incidental*
18.7 18.7 FUD 090 J 80
AMA: 2018,Jan,8; 2017,Jan,8; 2016,Jan,13; 2015,Jan,16

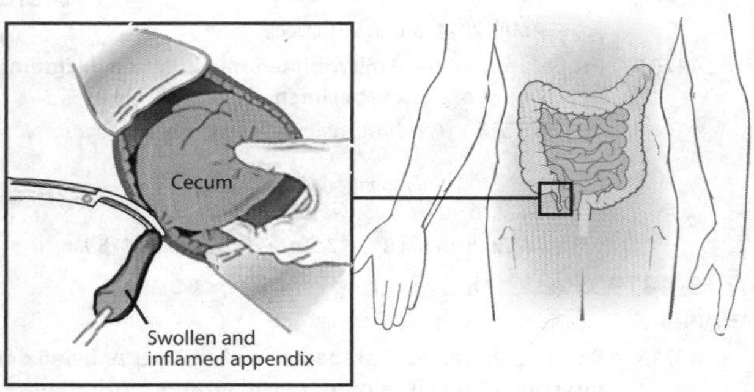

\+ **44955** **when done for indicated purpose at time of other major procedure (not as separate procedure) (List separately in addition to code for primary procedure)**
Code first primary procedure
2.45 2.45 FUD ZZZ N 80
AMA: 2018,Jan,8; 2017,Jan,8; 2016,Jan,13; 2015,Jan,16

44960 **for ruptured appendix with abscess or generalized peritonitis**
INCLUDES Battle's operation
25.5 25.5 FUD 090 C 80
AMA: 2019,Dec,12; 2018,Jan,8; 2017,Jan,8; 2016,Jan,13; 2015,Jan,16

44970 **Laparoscopy, surgical, appendectomy**
INCLUDES Diagnostic laparoscopy
17.4 17.4 FUD 090 J 80
AMA: 2019,Dec,12; 2018,Jan,8; 2017,Jan,8; 2016,Jan,13; 2015,Mar,3; 2015,Jan,16

44979 **Unlisted laparoscopy procedure, appendix**
0.00 0.00 FUD YYY J 80 50
AMA: 2018,Jan,8; 2017,Jan,8; 2016,Jan,13; 2015,Jan,16

45000-45190 Open and Transrectal Procedures of Rectum

45000 **Transrectal drainage of pelvic abscess**
EXCLUDES *Image guided transrectal catheter drainage (49407)*
12.2 12.2 FUD 090 T A2
AMA: 2014,Jan,11; 2013,Nov,9

45005 **Incision and drainage of submucosal abscess, rectum**
4.69 8.38 FUD 010 T A2
AMA: 2014,Jan,11; 2013,Dec,3

45020 **Incision and drainage of deep supralevator, pelvirectal, or retrorectal abscess**
EXCLUDES *Incision and drainage perianal, ischiorectal, intramural abscess (46050, 46060)*
16.5 16.5 FUD 090 J A2
AMA: 2014,Jan,11; 2013,Dec,3

45100 **Biopsy of anorectal wall, anal approach (eg, congenital megacolon)**
EXCLUDES *Biopsy performed endoscopically (45305)*
8.65 8.65 FUD 090 J A2
AMA: 2014,Jan,11; 2013,Dec,3

45108 **Anorectal myomectomy**
10.7 10.7 FUD 090 J A2
AMA: 2014,Jan,11; 2013,Dec,3

45110 **Proctectomy; complete, combined abdominoperineal, with colostomy**
EXCLUDES *Laparoscopic method (45395)*
53.1 53.1 FUD 090 C 80
AMA: 2014,Jan,11; 2013,Dec,3

45111 **partial resection of rectum, transabdominal approach**
INCLUDES Luschka proctectomy
31.4 31.4 FUD 090 C 80
AMA: 2014,Jan,11; 2013,Dec,3

45112 **Proctectomy, combined abdominoperineal, pull-through procedure (eg, colo-anal anastomosis)**
EXCLUDES *Proctectomy for colo-anal anastomosis with colonic pouch or reservoir creation (45119)*
53.9 53.9 FUD 090 C 80
AMA: 2014,Jan,11; 2013,Dec,3

45113 **Proctectomy, partial, with rectal mucosectomy, ileoanal anastomosis, creation of ileal reservoir (S or J), with or without loop ileostomy**
54.7 54.7 FUD 090 C 80
AMA: 2014,Jan,11; 2013,Dec,3

45114 **Proctectomy, partial, with anastomosis; abdominal and transsacral approach**
53.0 53.0 FUD 090 C 80
AMA: 2014,Jan,11; 2013,Dec,3

45116 **transsacral approach only (Kraske type)**
45.1 45.1 FUD 090 C 80
AMA: 2014,Jan,11; 2013,Dec,3

210 CPT © 2020 American Medical Association. All Rights Reserved. © 2020 Optum360, LLC

45119 **Proctectomy, combined abdominoperineal pull-through procedure (eg, colo-anal anastomosis), with creation of colonic reservoir (eg, J-pouch), with diverting enterostomy when performed**

EXCLUDES *Laparoscopic method (45397)*

55.9 55.9 FUD 090 C 80

AMA: 2018,Jan,8; 2017,Jan,8; 2016,Jan,13; 2015,Jan,16

45120 **Proctectomy, complete (for congenital megacolon), abdominal and perineal approach; with pull-through procedure and anastomosis (eg, Swenson, Duhamel, or Soave type operation)**

46.5 46.5 FUD 090 C 80

AMA: 2014,Jan,11; 2013,Dec,3

45121 **with subtotal or total colectomy, with multiple biopsies**

50.5 50.5 FUD 090 C 80

AMA: 2014,Jan,11; 2013,Dec,3

45123 **Proctectomy, partial, without anastomosis, perineal approach**

32.4 32.4 FUD 090 C 80

AMA: 2014,Jan,11; 2013,Dec,3

45126 **Pelvic exenteration for colorectal malignancy, with proctectomy (with or without colostomy), with removal of bladder and ureteral transplantations, and/or hysterectomy, or cervicectomy, with or without removal of tube(s), with or without removal of ovary(s), or any combination thereof**

80.1 80.1 FUD 090 C 80

AMA: 2014,Jan,11; 2013,Dec,3

45130 **Excision of rectal procidentia, with anastomosis; perineal approach**

INCLUDES Altemeier procedure

31.3 31.3 FUD 090 C 80

AMA: 2014,Jan,11; 2013,Dec,3

45135 **abdominal and perineal approach**

INCLUDES Altemeier procedure

37.6 37.6 FUD 090 C 80

AMA: 2014,Jan,11; 2013,Dec,3

45136 **Excision of ileoanal reservoir with ileostomy**

EXCLUDES *Enterolysis (44005)*

Ileostomy or jejunostomy, non-tube (44310)

51.8 51.8 FUD 090 C 80

AMA: 2014,Jan,11; 2013,Dec,3

45150 **Division of stricture of rectum**

12.1 12.1 FUD 090 T A2 80

AMA: 2014,Jan,11; 2013,Dec,3

45160 **Excision of rectal tumor by proctotomy, transsacral or transcoccygeal approach**

29.7 29.7 FUD 090 J A2 80

AMA: 2014,Jan,11; 2013,Dec,3

45171 **Excision of rectal tumor, transanal approach; not including muscularis propria (ie, partial thickness)**

EXCLUDES *Transanal destruction rectal tumor (45190)*

Transanal endoscopic microsurgical tumor excision (TEMS) (0184T)

17.5 17.5 FUD 090 J G2 80

AMA: 2018,Jan,8; 2017,Jan,8; 2016,Jan,13; 2015,Jan,16

45172 **including muscularis propria (ie, full thickness)**

EXCLUDES *Transanal destruction rectal tumor (45190)*

Transanal endoscopic microsurgical tumor excision (TEMS) (0184T)

23.5 23.5 FUD 090 J G2 80

AMA: 2018,Feb,11; 2018,Jan,8; 2017,Jan,8; 2016,Jan,13; 2015,Jan,16

45190 **Destruction of rectal tumor (eg, electrodesiccation, electrosurgery, laser ablation, laser resection, cryosurgery) transanal approach**

EXCLUDES *Transanal endoscopic microsurgical tumor excision (TEMS) (0184T)*

Transanal excision rectal tumor (45171-45172)

20.2 20.2 FUD 090 J A2

AMA: 2018,Jan,8; 2017,Jan,8; 2016,Jan,13; 2015,Jan,16

45300-45327 Rigid Proctosigmoidoscopy Procedures

INCLUDES Control bleeding due to endoscopic procedure during same operative session

Exam:

Entire rectum

Portion sigmoid colon

EXCLUDES *Computed tomographic colonography (74261-74263)*

Code also examination colon through stoma:

Colonoscopy via stoma (44388-44408 [44401])

Ileoscopy via stoma (44380-44384 [44381])

45300 **Proctosigmoidoscopy, rigid; diagnostic, with or without collection of specimen(s) by brushing or washing (separate procedure)**

(74360)

1.38 3.52 FUD 000 T P3

AMA: 2018,Jan,8; 2017,Jan,8; 2016,Jan,13; 2015,Jan,16

45303 **with dilation (eg, balloon, guide wire, bougie)**

(74360)

2.45 27.2 FUD 000 T P2

AMA: 2018,Jan,8; 2017,Jan,8; 2016,Jan,13; 2015,Jan,16

45305 **with biopsy, single or multiple**

2.10 4.63 FUD 000 T A2

AMA: 2018,Jan,8; 2017,Jan,8; 2016,Jan,13; 2015,Jan,16

45307 **with removal of foreign body**

2.81 5.33 FUD 000 J A2 80

AMA: 2018,Jan,8; 2017,Jan,8; 2016,Jan,13; 2015,Jan,16

45308 **with removal of single tumor, polyp, or other lesion by hot biopsy forceps or bipolar cautery**

2.44 5.25 FUD 000 J A2

AMA: 2018,Jan,8; 2017,Jan,8; 2016,Jan,13; 2015,Jan,16

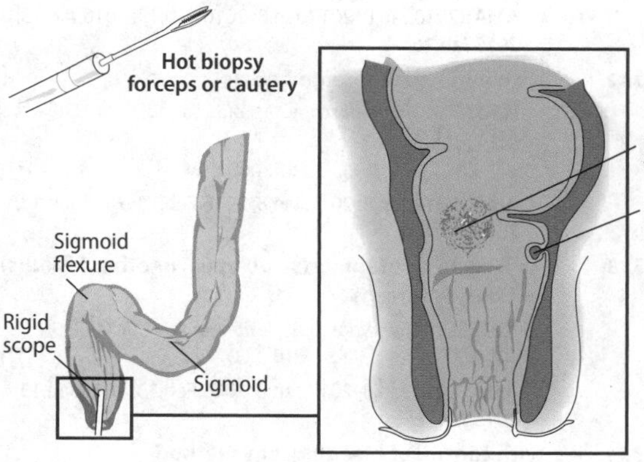

A rigid proctosigmoid procedure of the rectum and sigmoid is performed

45309 **with removal of single tumor, polyp, or other lesion by snare technique**

2.60 5.43 FUD 000 T A2

AMA: 2018,Jan,8; 2017,Jan,8; 2016,Jan,13; 2015,Jan,16

45315 **with removal of multiple tumors, polyps, or other lesions by hot biopsy forceps, bipolar cautery or snare technique**

3.08 5.93 FUD 000 T A2

AMA: 2018,Jan,8; 2017,Jan,8; 2016,Jan,13; 2015,Jan,16

45317 **with control of bleeding (eg, injection, bipolar cautery, unipolar cautery, laser, heater probe, stapler, plasma coagulator)**
3.24 5.52 FUD 000 T A2
AMA: 2018,Jan,8; 2017,Jan,8; 2016,Jan,13; 2015,Jan,16

45320 **with ablation of tumor(s), polyp(s), or other lesion(s) not amenable to removal by hot biopsy forceps, bipolar cautery or snare technique (eg, laser)**
3.05 5.78 FUD 000 J A2
AMA: 2018,Jan,8; 2017,Jan,8; 2016,Jan,13; 2015,Jan,16

45321 **with decompression of volvulus**
3.01 3.01 FUD 000 J A2
AMA: 2018,Jan,8; 2017,Jan,8; 2016,Jan,13; 2015,Jan,16

45327 **with transendoscopic stent placement (includes predilation)**
3.41 3.41 FUD 000 J J8
AMA: 2018,Jan,8; 2017,Jan,8; 2016,Jan,13; 2015,Jan,16

45330-45350 [45346] Flexible Sigmoidoscopy Procedures

INCLUDES Control bleeding due to endoscopic procedure during same operative session
Exam:
Entire rectum
Entire sigmoid colon
Portion descending colon (when performed)

EXCLUDES *Computed tomographic colonography (74261-74263)*

Code also examination colon through stoma when appropriate:
Colonoscopy (44388-44408 [44401])
Ileoscopy (44380-44384 [44381])

45330 **Sigmoidoscopy, flexible; diagnostic, including collection of specimen(s) by brushing or washing, when performed (separate procedure)**
EXCLUDES *Sigmoidoscopy, flexible (45331-45350 [45346])*
1.61 4.98 FUD 000 T P3
AMA: 2018,Jan,8; 2017,Jan,8; 2016,Feb,13; 2016,Jan,13; 2015,Sep,12; 2015,Jan,16

45331 **with biopsy, single or multiple**
EXCLUDES *Sigmoidoscopy, flexible; with endoscopic mucosal resection same lesion (45349)*
2.08 7.60 FUD 000 T A2
AMA: 2018,Jan,8; 2017,Jan,8; 2016,Feb,13; 2016,Jan,13; 2015,Jan,16

45332 **with removal of foreign body(s)**
EXCLUDES *Sigmoidoscopy, flexible; diagnostic (45330)*
(76000)
3.06 7.36 FUD 000 T A2
AMA: 2018,Jan,8; 2017,Jan,8; 2016,Feb,13; 2016,Jan,13; 2015,Jan,16

45333 **with removal of tumor(s), polyp(s), or other lesion(s) by hot biopsy forceps**
EXCLUDES *Sigmoidoscopy, flexible; diagnostic (45330)*
2.71 8.92 FUD 000 T A2
AMA: 2018,Jan,8; 2017,Jan,8; 2016,Feb,13; 2016,Jan,13; 2015,Jan,16

45334 **with control of bleeding, any method**
EXCLUDES *Sigmoidoscopy, flexible; diagnostic (45330)*
Sigmoidoscopy, flexible; with band ligation same lesion (45350)
Sigmoidoscopy, flexible; with directed submucosal injection same lesion (45335)
3.44 15.3 FUD 000 T A2
AMA: 2018,Jan,8; 2017,Jan,8; 2016,Feb,13; 2016,Jan,13; 2015,Jan,16

45335 **with directed submucosal injection(s), any substance**
EXCLUDES *Sigmoidoscopy, flexible; diagnostic (45330)*
Sigmoidoscopy, flexible; with control bleeding same lesion (45334)
Sigmoidoscopy, flexible; with endoscopic mucosal resection same lesion (45349)
1.91 7.58 FUD 000 T A2
AMA: 2018,Jan,8; 2017,Jan,8; 2016,Feb,13; 2016,Jan,13; 2015,Jan,16

45337 **with decompression (for pathologic distention) (eg, volvulus, megacolon), including placement of decompression tube, when performed**
EXCLUDES *Procedure performed more than one time per operative session*
Sigmoidoscopy, flexible; diagnostic (45330)
3.37 3.37 FUD 000 T A2
AMA: 2018,Jan,8; 2017,Jan,8; 2016,Feb,13; 2016,Jan,13; 2015,Jan,16

45338 **with removal of tumor(s), polyp(s), or other lesion(s) by snare technique**
EXCLUDES *Sigmoidoscopy, flexible; diagnostic (45330)*
Sigmoidoscopy, flexible; with endoscopic mucosal resection same lesion (45349)
3.47 8.07 FUD 000 T A2
AMA: 2018,Jan,8; 2017,Jan,8; 2016,Feb,13; 2016,Jan,13; 2015,Jan,16

45346 **with ablation of tumor(s), polyp(s), or other lesion(s) (includes pre- and post-dilation and guide wire passage, when performed)**
EXCLUDES *Sigmoidoscopy, flexible; diagnostic (45330)*
Sigmoidoscopy, flexible; with transendoscopic balloon dilation same lesion (45340)
4.70 82.3 FUD 000 T G2
AMA: 2018,Jan,8; 2017,Jan,8; 2016,Feb,13; 2016,Jan,13; 2015,Jan,16

45340 **with transendoscopic balloon dilation**
EXCLUDES *Sigmoidoscopy, flexible (45330, [45346], 45347)*
Code also each additional stricture dilated same session, using modifier 59 with (45340)
(74360)
2.24 12.9 FUD 000 T A2
AMA: 2018,Jan,8; 2017,Jan,8; 2016,Feb,13; 2016,Jan,13; 2015,Jan,16

45341 **with endoscopic ultrasound examination**
INCLUDES Gastrointestinal endoscopic ultrasound, supervision, and interpretation (76975)
Ultrasound, transrectal (76872)
EXCLUDES *Procedure performed more than one time per operative session*
Sigmoidoscopy, flexible (45330, 45342)
3.57 3.57 FUD 000 T A2
AMA: 2018,Jan,8; 2017,Jan,8; 2016,Feb,13; 2016,Jan,13; 2015,Jan,16

45342 **with transendoscopic ultrasound guided intramural or transmural fine needle aspiration/biopsy(s)**
INCLUDES Gastrointestinal endoscopic ultrasound, supervision and interpretation (76975)
Ultrasonic guidance (76942)
Ultrasound, transrectal (76872)
EXCLUDES *Sigmoidoscopy, flexible (45330, 45341)*
Procedure performed more than one time per operative session
4.89 4.89 FUD 000 T A2
AMA: 2018,Jan,8; 2017,Jan,8; 2016,Feb,13; 2016,Jan,13; 2015,Jan,16

45346 **Resequenced code. See code following 45338.**

45347 **with placement of endoscopic stent (includes pre- and post-dilation and guide wire passage, when performed)**

EXCLUDES *Sigmoidoscopy, flexible (45330, 45340)*

(74360)

4.44 4.44 FUD 000 J J8

AMA: 2018,Jan,8; 2017,Jan,8; 2016,Feb,13; 2016,Jan,13; 2015,Jan,16

45349 **with endoscopic mucosal resection**

EXCLUDES *Procedure performed same lesion with (45331, 45335, 45338, 45350)*

Sigmoidoscopy, flexible; diagnostic (45330)

5.73 5.73 FUD 000 T G2

AMA: 2020,May,13; 2019,Dec,14; 2018,Jan,8; 2017,Jan,8; 2016,Jan,13; 2015,Jan,16

45350 **with band ligation(s) (eg, hemorrhoids)**

EXCLUDES *Hemorrhoidectomy, internal, by rubber band ligation (46221)*

Procedure performed more than one time per operative session

Sigmoidoscopy, flexible; diagnostic (45330)

Sigmoidoscopy, flexible; with control bleeding same lesion (45334)

Sigmoidoscopy, flexible; with endoscopic mucosal resection (45349)

2.92 17.8 FUD 000 T G2

AMA: 2020,Feb,11; 2018,Jan,8; 2017,Jan,8; 2016,Jan,13; 2015,Jan,16

45378-45398 [45388, 45390, 45398] Flexible and Rigid Colonoscopy Procedures

INCLUDES Control bleeding due to endoscopic procedure during same operative session

Exam:

Entire colon (rectum to cecum)

Terminal ileum (when performed)

EXCLUDES *Computed tomographic colonography (74261-74263)*

Code also modifier 53 (physician), or 73, 74 (facility) for incomplete colonoscopy

45378 **Colonoscopy, flexible; diagnostic, including collection of specimen(s) by brushing or washing, when performed (separate procedure)**

EXCLUDES *Colonoscopy, flexible (45379-45393 [45388, 45390, 45398])*

Decompression for pathological distention (45393)

5.35 9.42 FUD 000 T A2

AMA: 2018,Jan,7; 2018,Jan,8; 2017,Sep,14; 2017,Jan,8; 2016,Jan,13; 2015,Sep,12; 2015,Jan,16

45379 **with removal of foreign body(s)**

EXCLUDES *Colonoscopy, flexible; diagnostic (45378)*

Code also modifier 52 when colonoscope fails to reach small intestine junction

(76000)

6.91 12.1 FUD 000 T A2

AMA: 2018,Jan,8; 2017,Jan,8; 2016,Jan,13; 2015,Jan,16

45380 **with biopsy, single or multiple**

EXCLUDES *Colonoscopy, flexible; diagnostic (45378)*

Colonoscopy, flexible; with endoscopic mucosal resection same lesion (45390)

Code also modifier 52 when colonoscope fails to reach small intestine junction

5.87 11.7 FUD 000 T A2

AMA: 2018,Jan,8; 2017,Jan,8; 2016,Jan,13; 2015,Jan,16

45381 **with directed submucosal injection(s), any substance**

EXCLUDES *Colonoscopy, flexible; diagnostic (45378)*

Colonoscopy, flexible; with control bleeding same lesion (45382)

Colonoscopy, flexible; with endoscopic mucosal resection same lesion (45390)

Code also modifier 52 when colonoscope fails to reach small intestine junction

5.87 11.5 FUD 000 T A2

AMA: 2018,Jan,8; 2017,Jan,8; 2017,Jan,6; 2016,Jan,13; 2015,Jan,16

45382 **with control of bleeding, any method**

EXCLUDES *Colonoscopy, flexible; diagnostic (45378)*

Colonoscopy, flexible; with band ligation same lesion ([45398])

Colonoscopy, flexible; with directed submucosal injection same lesion (45381)

Code also modifier 52 when colonoscope fails to reach small intestine junction

7.48 20.0 FUD 000 T A2

AMA: 2018,Jan,8; 2017,Jan,8; 2016,Jan,13; 2015,Jan,16

45388 **with ablation of tumor(s), polyp(s), or other lesion(s) (includes pre- and post-dilation and guide wire passage, when performed)**

EXCLUDES *Colonoscopy, flexible (45378, 45386)*

7.83 82.9 FUD 000 T G2

AMA: 2018,Jan,8; 2017,Jan,8; 2016,Jan,13; 2015,Jan,16

45384 **with removal of tumor(s), polyp(s), or other lesion(s) by hot biopsy forceps**

EXCLUDES *Colonoscopy, flexible; diagnostic (45378)*

Code also modifier 52 when colonoscope fails to reach small intestine junction

6.68 13.1 FUD 000 T A2

AMA: 2018,Jan,8; 2017,Jan,8; 2016,Jan,13; 2015,Jun,10; 2015,Jan,16

45385 **with removal of tumor(s), polyp(s), or other lesion(s) by snare technique**

EXCLUDES *Colonoscopy, flexible; diagnostic (45378)*

Colonoscopy, flexible; with endoscopic mucosal resection same lesion (45390)

7.35 12.6 FUD 000 T A2

AMA: 2018,Jan,8; 2017,Jan,8; 2017,Jan,6; 2016,Jan,13; 2015,Jan,16

45386 **with transendoscopic balloon dilation**

EXCLUDES *Colonoscopy, flexible (45378, [45388], 45389)*

Code also each additional stricture dilated same operative session, using modifier 59 with (45386)

(74360)

6.20 17.0 FUD 000 T A2

AMA: 2018,Jan,8; 2017,Jan,8; 2016,Jan,13; 2015,Jan,16

45388 **Resequenced code. See code following 45382.**

45389 **with endoscopic stent placement (includes pre- and post-dilation and guide wire passage, when performed)**

EXCLUDES *Colonoscopy, flexible (45378, 45386)*

(74360)

8.37 8.37 FUD 000 J J8

AMA: 2018,Jan,8; 2017,Jan,8; 2016,Jan,13; 2015,Jan,16

45390 **Resequenced code. See code following 45392.**

45391 **with endoscopic ultrasound examination limited to the rectum, sigmoid, descending, transverse, or ascending colon and cecum, and adjacent structures**

INCLUDES Gastrointestinal endoscopic ultrasound, supervision and interpretation (76975)

Ultrasound, transrectal (76872)

EXCLUDES *Colonoscopy, flexible (45378, 45392)*

Procedure performed more than one time per operative session

7.43 7.43 FUD 000 T A2

AMA: 2018,Jan,8; 2017,Jan,8; 2016,Jan,13; 2015,Jan,16

Digestive System

45347 — 45391

● New Code ▲ Revised Code ○ Reinstated ● New Web Release ▲ Revised Web Release + Add-on Unlisted Not Covered # Resequenced

(50) Optum Mod 50 Exempt ⊘ AMA Mod 51 Exempt (51) Optum Mod 51 Exempt (63) Mod 63 Exempt Non-FDA Drug ★ Telemedicine M Maternity A Age Edit

45392 **with transendoscopic ultrasound guided intramural or transmural fine needle aspiration/biopsy(s), includes endoscopic ultrasound examination limited to the rectum, sigmoid, descending, transverse, or ascending colon and cecum, and adjacent structures**

INCLUDES Gastrointestinal endoscopic ultrasound, supervision and interpretation (76975)
Ultrasonic guidance (76942)
Ultrasound, transrectal (76872)

EXCLUDES *Colonoscopy, flexible (45378, 45391)*
Procedure performed more than one time per operative session

8.78 8.78 FUD 000 T A2

AMA: 2018,Jan,8; 2017,Jan,8; 2016,Jan,13; 2015,Jan,16

45390 **with endoscopic mucosal resection**

EXCLUDES *Colonoscopy, flexible; diagnostic (45378)*
Colonoscopy, flexible; with band ligation same lesion ([45398])
Colonoscopy, flexible; with biopsy same lesion (45380-45381)
Colonoscopy, flexible; with removal tumor(s), polyp(s), or other lesion(s) by snare technique same lesion (45385)

9.74 9.74 FUD 000 T G2

AMA: 2020,May,13; 2019,Dec,14; 2018,Jan,8; 2017,Jan,6; 2017,Jan,8; 2016,Jan,13; 2015,Jan,16

45393 **with decompression (for pathologic distention) (eg, volvulus, megacolon), including placement of decompression tube, when performed**

EXCLUDES *Colonoscopy, flexible; diagnostic (45378)*
Procedure performed more than one time per operative session

7.31 7.31 FUD 000 T G2

AMA: 2018,Jan,8; 2017,Jan,8; 2016,Jan,13; 2015,Jan,16

45398 **with band ligation(s) (eg, hemorrhoids)**

EXCLUDES *Bleeding control by band ligation (45382)*
Colonoscopy, flexible (45378, 45390)
Hemorrhoidectomy, internal, by rubber band ligation (46221)
Procedure performed more than one time per operative session

Code also modifier 52 when colonoscope fails to reach small intestine junction

6.83 22.3 FUD 000 T G2

AMA: 2020,Feb,11; 2018,Jan,8; 2018,Jan,7; 2017,Sep,14; 2017,Jan,8; 2016,Jan,13; 2015,Jan,16

45395-45499 [45398, 45399] Laparoscopic Procedures of Rectum

INCLUDES Diagnostic laparoscopy

45395 **Laparoscopy, surgical; proctectomy, complete, combined abdominoperineal, with colostomy**

EXCLUDES *Open method (45110)*

56.8 56.8 FUD 090 C 80

AMA: 2018,Jan,8; 2017,Jan,8; 2016,Jan,13; 2015,Jan,16

45397 **proctectomy, combined abdominoperineal pull-through procedure (eg, colo-anal anastomosis), with creation of colonic reservoir (eg, J-pouch), with diverting enterostomy, when performed**

EXCLUDES *Open method (45119)*

61.8 61.8 FUD 090 C 80

AMA: 2018,Jan,8; 2017,Jan,8; 2016,Jan,13; 2015,Jan,16

45398 **Resequenced code. See code following 45393.**

45399 **Resequenced code. See code before 45990.**

45400 **Laparoscopy, surgical; proctopexy (for prolapse)**

EXCLUDES *Open method (45540-45541)*

32.8 32.8 FUD 090 C 80

AMA: 2018,Jan,8; 2017,Jan,8; 2016,Jan,13; 2015,Jan,16

45402 **proctopexy (for prolapse), with sigmoid resection**

EXCLUDES *Open method (45550)*

43.8 43.8 FUD 090 C 80

AMA: 2018,Jan,8; 2017,Jan,8; 2016,Jan,13; 2015,Jan,16

45499 **Unlisted laparoscopy procedure, rectum**

EXCLUDES *Unlisted rectal procedure performed via open technique (45999)*

0.00 0.00 FUD YYY J 80

AMA: 2014,Jan,11; 2013,Jan,11-12

45500-45825 Open Repairs of Rectum

45500 **Proctoplasty; for stenosis**

16.3 16.3 FUD 090 J A2 80

AMA: 2014,Jan,11; 2013,Jan,11-12

45505 **for prolapse of mucous membrane**

17.2 17.2 FUD 090 J A2

AMA: 2018,Jan,8; 2017,Jan,8; 2016,Jan,13; 2015,Mar,9; 2015,Jan,16

45520 **Perirectal injection of sclerosing solution for prolapse**

1.16 4.41 FUD 000 Q1 N1

AMA: 2018,Jan,8; 2017,Jan,8; 2016,Jan,13; 2015,Jan,16

45540 **Proctopexy (eg, for prolapse); abdominal approach**

EXCLUDES *Laparoscopic method (45400)*

30.6 30.6 FUD 090 C 80

AMA: 2014,Jan,11; 2013,Jan,11-12

45541 **perineal approach**

27.3 27.3 FUD 090 J G2 80

AMA: 2014,Jan,11; 2013,Jan,11-12

45550 **with sigmoid resection, abdominal approach**

INCLUDES Frickman proctopexy

EXCLUDES *Laparoscopic method (45402)*

42.3 42.3 FUD 090 C 80

AMA: 2014,Jan,11; 2013,Jan,11-12

45560 **Repair of rectocele (separate procedure)**

EXCLUDES *Posterior colporrhaphy with rectocele repair (57250)*

19.8 19.8 FUD 090 J A2 80

AMA: 2014,Jan,11; 2013,Jan,11-12

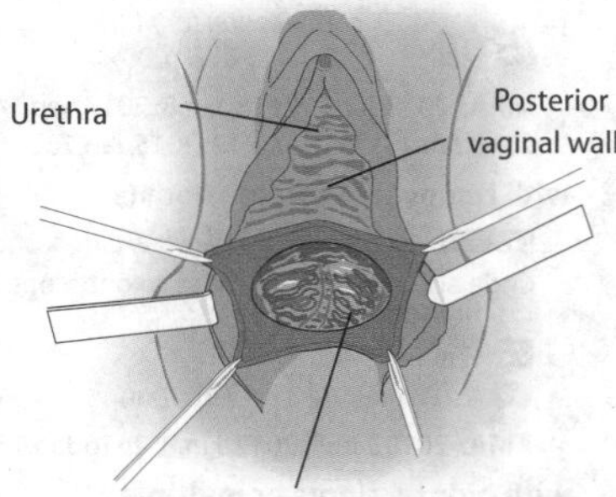

The posterior wall of the vagina is opened directly over the rectocele; the walls of both structures are repaired; a rectocele is a herniated protrusion of part of the rectum into the vagina

45562 **Exploration, repair, and presacral drainage for rectal injury;**

32.7 32.7 FUD 090 C 80

AMA: 2014,Jan,11; 2013,Jan,11-12

45563 **with colostomy**

INCLUDES Maydl colostomy

48.3 48.3 FUD 090 C 80

AMA: 2014,Jan,11; 2013,Jan,11-12

45800 **Closure of rectovesical fistula;**

36.4 36.4 FUD 090 C 80

AMA: 2014,Jan,11; 2013,Jan,11-12

45805 **with colostomy**

42.8 42.8 FUD 090 C 80

AMA: 2014,Jan,11; 2013,Jan,11-12

45820 **Closure of rectourethral fistula;**

EXCLUDES *Closure fistula, rectovaginal (57300-57308)*

37.0 37.0 FUD 090 C 80

AMA: 2014,Jan,11; 2013,Jan,11-12

45825 **with colostomy**

EXCLUDES *Closure fistula, rectovaginal (57300-57308)*

44.4 44.4 FUD 090 C 80

AMA: 2014,Jan,11; 2013,Jan,11-12

45900-45999 [45399] Closed Procedures of Rectum With Anesthesia

45900 **Reduction of procidentia (separate procedure) under anesthesia**

6.14 6.14 FUD 010 T A2 80

AMA: 2014,Jan,11; 2013,Jan,11-12

45905 **Dilation of anal sphincter (separate procedure) under anesthesia other than local**

4.86 4.86 FUD 010 T A2

AMA: 2014,Jan,11; 2013,Jan,11-12

45910 **Dilation of rectal stricture (separate procedure) under anesthesia other than local**

5.54 5.54 FUD 010 T A2

AMA: 2014,Jan,11; 2013,Jan,11-12

45915 **Removal of fecal impaction or foreign body (separate procedure) under anesthesia**

6.65 9.90 FUD 010 T A2

AMA: 2018,Jan,8; 2017,Jan,8; 2016,Jan,13; 2015,Jan,16

\# **45399** **Unlisted procedure, colon**

0.00 0.00 FUD YYY T

AMA: 2018,Jan,8; 2017,Jan,8; 2016,Jan,13; 2015,Jan,16

45990 **Anorectal exam, surgical, requiring anesthesia (general, spinal, or epidural), diagnostic**

INCLUDES Diagnostic:
- Anoscopy
- Proctoscopy, rigid

Exam:
- Pelvic (when performed)
- Perineal, external
- Rectal, digital

EXCLUDES *Anogenital examination (99170)*
Anoscopy; diagnostic (46600)
Pelvic examination under anesthesia (57410)
Proctosigmoidoscopy, rigid (45300-45327)

3.09 3.09 FUD 000 J A2 80

AMA: 2018,Jan,8; 2017,Jan,8; 2016,Jan,13; 2015,Jan,16

45999 **Unlisted procedure, rectum**

EXCLUDES *Unlisted rectal procedure performed laparoscopically (45499)*

0.00 0.00 FUD YYY T 80

AMA: 2018,Jan,8; 2017,Jan,8; 2016,Jan,13; 2015,Jan,16

46020-46083 Surgical Incision of Anus

EXCLUDES *Cryosurgical destruction hemorrhoid(s) (46999)*
Fistulotomy, subcutaneous (46270)
Hemorrhoidopexy ([46947])
Injection hemorrhoid(s) (46500)
Thermal energy destruction internal hemorrhoid(s) (46930)

46020 **Placement of seton**

EXCLUDES *Anoscopy; diagnostic (46600)*
Incision and drainage ischiorectal or intramural abscess (46060)
Surgical anal fistula treatment (46280)

6.82 8.10 FUD 010 J A2

AMA: 2014,Jan,11; 2013,Jan,11-12

46030 **Removal of anal seton, other marker**

2.59 4.13 FUD 010 T A2 80

AMA: 2014,Jan,11; 2013,Jan,11-12

46040 **Incision and drainage of ischiorectal and/or perirectal abscess (separate procedure)**

12.1 15.7 FUD 090 T A2

AMA: 2014,Jan,11; 2013,Jan,11-12

46045 **Incision and drainage of intramural, intramuscular, or submucosal abscess, transanal, under anesthesia**

12.6 12.6 FUD 090 J A2

AMA: 2014,Jan,11; 2013,Jan,11-12

46050 **Incision and drainage, perianal abscess, superficial**

EXCLUDES *Incision and drainage abscess:*
Ischiorectal/intramural (46060)
Supralevator/pelvirectal/retrorectal (45020)

2.85 6.27 FUD 010 T A2

AMA: 2014,Jan,11; 2013,Jan,11-12

46060 **Incision and drainage of ischiorectal or intramural abscess, with fistulectomy or fistulotomy, submuscular, with or without placement of seton**

EXCLUDES *Incision and drainage abscess:*
Supralevator/pelvirectal/retrorectal (45020)
Placement seton (46020)

13.8 13.8 FUD 090 J A2

AMA: 2014,Jan,11; 2013,Jan,11-12

46070 **Incision, anal septum (infant)** A

EXCLUDES *Anoplasty (46700-46705)*

7.52 7.52 FUD 090 63 J G2 80

AMA: 2014,Jan,11; 2013,Jan,11-12

46080 **Sphincterotomy, anal, division of sphincter (separate procedure)**

4.60 7.74 FUD 010 J A2

AMA: 2014,Jan,11; 2013,Jan,11-12

46083 **Incision of thrombosed hemorrhoid, external**

3.08 5.24 FUD 010 T P2

AMA: 2018,Jan,8; 2017,Jan,8; 2016,Jan,13; 2015,Jan,16

46200-46262 [46220, 46320, 46945, 46946, 46948] Anal Resection and Hemorrhoidectomies

EXCLUDES *Cryosurgical destruction hemorrhoid(s) (46999)*
Hemorrhoidopexy ([46947])
Injection hemorrhoid(s) (46500)
Thermal energy destruction internal hemorrhoid(s) (46930)

46200 **Fissurectomy, including sphincterotomy, when performed**

9.45 13.0 FUD 090 J A2

AMA: 2014,Jan,11; 2013,Jan,11-12

46220 **Resequenced code. See code before 46230.**

46221 **Hemorrhoidectomy, internal, by rubber band ligation(s)**

EXCLUDES *Colonoscopy or sigmoidoscopy, flexible; with band ligation (45350, [45398])*
Transanal hemorrhoidal dearterialization, two or more columns/groups ([46948])

5.51 7.77 FUD 010 T P3

AMA: 2020,Feb,11; 2018,Jan,8; 2018,Jan,7; 2017,Sep,14; 2017,Jan,8; 2016,Jan,13; 2015,Apr,10; 2015,Jan,16

\# **46945** **Hemorrhoidectomy, internal, by ligation other than rubber band; single hemorrhoid column/group, without imaging guidance**

EXCLUDES *Transanal hemorrhoidal dearterialization, two or more columns/groups ([46948])*
Ultrasonic guidance (76942)
Ultrasonic guidance, intraoperative (76998)
Ultrasound, transrectal (76872)

6.54 9.08 FUD 090 J R2

AMA: 2020,Feb,11; 2018,Jan,8; 2017,Jan,8; 2016,Jan,13; 2015,Apr,10

Digestive System

45820 — 46945

● New Code ▲ Revised Code ○ Reinstated ● New Web Release ▲ Revised Web Release + Add-on Unlisted Not Covered # Resequenced
50 Optum Mod 50 Exempt ⊘ AMA Mod 51 Exempt 51 Optum Mod 51 Exempt 63 Mod 63 Exempt Non-FDA Drug ★ Telemedicine M Maternity A Age Edit

46946 2 or more hemorrhoid columns/groups, without imaging guidance

EXCLUDES *Transanal hemorrhoidal dearterialization, two or more columns/groups ([46948])*
Ultrasonic guidance (76942)
Ultrasonic guidance, intraoperative (76998)
Ultrasound, transrectal (76872)

6.50 9.17 **FUD** 090 J A2

AMA: 2020,Feb,11; 2018,Jan,8; 2017,Jan,8; 2016,Jan,13; 2015,Apr,10

46948 **Hemorrhoidectomy, internal, by transanal hemorrhoidal dearterialization, 2 or more hemorrhoid columns/groups, including ultrasound guidance, with mucopexy, when performed**

INCLUDES Ultrasonic guidance (76872, 76942, 76998)
EXCLUDES *Transanal hemorrhoidal dearterialization, single column/group (46999)*

12.7 12.7 **FUD** 090 G2

AMA: 2020,Feb,11

46220 **Excision of single external papilla or tag, anus**

3.43 6.54 **FUD** 010 T A2

AMA: 2014,Jan,11; 2013,Jan,11-12

46230 **Excision of multiple external papillae or tags, anus**

5.00 8.43 **FUD** 010 J A2

AMA: 2014,Jan,11; 2013,Jan,11-12

46320 **Excision of thrombosed hemorrhoid, external**

3.22 5.65 **FUD** 010 T P3

AMA: 2014,Jan,11; 2013,Jan,11-12

46250 **Hemorrhoidectomy, external, 2 or more columns/groups**

EXCLUDES *Hemorrhoidectomy, external, single column/group (46999)*
Transanal hemorrhoidal dearterialization, two or more columns/groups ([46948])

9.19 13.6 **FUD** 090 J A2

AMA: 2014,Jan,11; 2013,Jan,11-12

46255 **Hemorrhoidectomy, internal and external, single column/group;**

EXCLUDES *Transanal hemorrhoidal dearterialization, two or more columns/groups ([46948])*

10.3 14.8 **FUD** 090 J A2

AMA: 2018,Jan,8; 2017,Jan,8; 2016,Jan,13; 2015,Jan,16

46257 **with fissurectomy**

EXCLUDES *Transanal hemorrhoidal dearterialization, two or more columns/groups ([46948])*

12.3 12.3 **FUD** 090 J A2

AMA: 2014,Jan,11; 2013,Jan,11-12

46258 **with fistulectomy, including fissurectomy, when performed**

EXCLUDES *Transanal hemorrhoidal dearterialization, two or more columns/groups ([46948])*

13.7 13.7 **FUD** 090 J A2 80

AMA: 2014,Jan,11; 2013,Jan,11-12

46260 **Hemorrhoidectomy, internal and external, 2 or more columns/groups;**

INCLUDES Whitehead hemorrhoidectomy
EXCLUDES *Transanal hemorrhoidal dearterialization, two or more columns/groups ([46948])*

13.8 13.8 **FUD** 090 J A2

AMA: 2014,Jan,11; 2013,Jan,11-12

46261 **with fissurectomy**

EXCLUDES *Transanal hemorrhoidal dearterialization, two or more columns/groups ([46948])*

15.1 15.1 **FUD** 090 J A2

AMA: 2014,Jan,11; 2013,Jan,11-12

46262 **with fistulectomy, including fissurectomy, when performed**

EXCLUDES *Transanal hemorrhoidal dearterialization, two or more columns/groups ([46948])*

16.0 16.0 **FUD** 090 J A2

AMA: 2018,Jan,8; 2017,Jan,8; 2016,Jan,13; 2015,Jan,16

46270-46320 [46320] Resection of Anal Fistula

46270 **Surgical treatment of anal fistula (fistulectomy/fistulotomy); subcutaneous**

11.3 14.8 **FUD** 090 J A2

AMA: 2014,Jan,11; 2013,Jan,11-12

46275 **intersphincteric**

11.9 15.6 **FUD** 090 J A2

AMA: 2014,Jan,11; 2013,Jan,11-12

46280 **transsphincteric, suprasphincteric, extrasphincteric or multiple, including placement of seton, when performed**

EXCLUDES *Placement seton (46020)*

13.7 13.7 **FUD** 090 J A2

AMA: 2014,Jan,11; 2013,Jan,11-12

46285 **second stage**

12.0 15.7 **FUD** 090 J A2

AMA: 2014,Jan,11; 2013,Jan,11-12

46288 **Closure of anal fistula with rectal advancement flap**

15.8 15.8 **FUD** 090 J A2

AMA: 2014,Jan,11; 2013,Jan,11-12

46320 **Resequenced code. See code following 46230.**

46500 Other Hemorrhoid Procedures

EXCLUDES *Anoscopic injection bulking agent, submucosal, for fecal incontinence (46999)*

46500 **Injection of sclerosing solution, hemorrhoids**

5.20 8.54 **FUD** 010 T P3

AMA: 2018,Jan,8; 2017,Jan,8; 2016,Jan,13; 2015,Jan,16

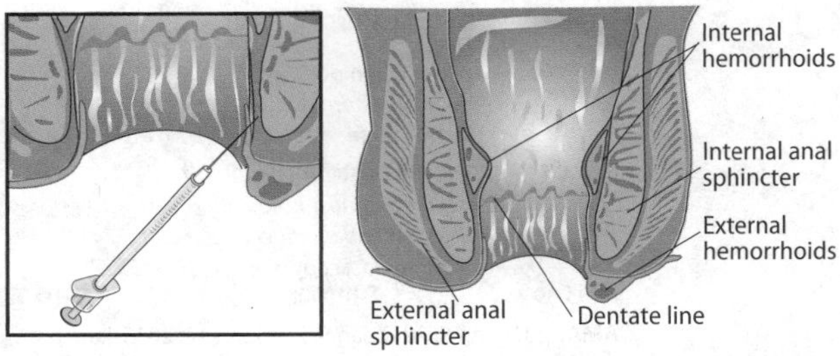

A sclerosing agent is injected into the tissues underlying hemorrhoids

46505 Chemodenervation Anal Sphincter

EXCLUDES *Chemodenervation:*
Extremity muscles (64642-64645)
Muscles/facial nerve (64612)
Neck muscles (64616)
Other peripheral nerve/branch (64640)
Pudendal nerve (64630)
Trunk muscles (64646-64647)

Code also drug(s)/substance(s) given

46505 **Chemodenervation of internal anal sphincter**

7.00 8.55 **FUD** 010 T G2 50

AMA: 2019,Apr,9; 2018,Jan,8; 2017,Jan,8; 2016,Jan,13; 2015,Jan,16

46600-46615 Anoscopic Procedures

EXCLUDES *Delivery thermal energy via anoscope to anal canal muscle (46999)*
Injection bulking agent, submucosal, for fecal incontinence (46999)

46600 **Anoscopy; diagnostic, including collection of specimen(s) by brushing or washing, when performed (separate procedure)**

EXCLUDES *Excision rectal tumor, transanal endoscopic microsurgical approach (i.e., TEMS) (0184T)*
High-resolution anoscopy (HRA), diagnostic (46601)
Surgical incision anus (46020-46761 [46220, 46320, 46320, 46945, 46946, 46947, 46948])

1.17 2.94 FUD 000 Q1 N1

AMA: 2018,Jan,7; 2018,Jan,8; 2017,Jan,8; 2016,Jan,13; 2015,Jan,16

46601 **diagnostic, with high-resolution magnification (HRA) (eg, colposcope, operating microscope) and chemical agent enhancement, including collection of specimen(s) by brushing or washing, when performed**

INCLUDES Operating microscope (69990)

2.70 3.97 FUD 000 Q1 N1

AMA: 2018,Oct,11; 2016,Feb,12

46604 **with dilation (eg, balloon, guide wire, bougie)**

1.90 18.3 FUD 000 T P2

AMA: 2018,Jan,8; 2017,Jan,8; 2016,Jan,13; 2015,Jan,16

46606 **with biopsy, single or multiple**

EXCLUDES *High resolution anoscopy (HRA) with biopsy (46607)*

2.17 7.31 FUD 000 T P3

AMA: 2019,Sep,10; 2018,Jan,8; 2017,Jan,8; 2016,Jan,13; 2015,Jan,16

46607 **with high-resolution magnification (HRA) (eg, colposcope, operating microscope) and chemical agent enhancement, with biopsy, single or multiple**

INCLUDES Operating microscope (69990)

3.65 5.75 FUD 000 T G2

AMA: 2019,Dec,12; 2018,Oct,11; 2016,Feb,12

46608 **with removal of foreign body**

2.44 7.68 FUD 000 T A2

AMA: 2018,Jan,8; 2017,Jan,8; 2016,Jan,13; 2015,Jan,16

46610 **with removal of single tumor, polyp, or other lesion by hot biopsy forceps or bipolar cautery**

2.34 7.30 FUD 000 J A2

AMA: 2018,Jan,8; 2017,Jan,8; 2016,Jan,13; 2015,Jan,16

46611 **with removal of single tumor, polyp, or other lesion by snare technique**

2.31 5.78 FUD 000 T A2

AMA: 2018,Jan,8; 2017,Jan,8; 2016,Jan,13; 2015,Jan,16

46612 **with removal of multiple tumors, polyps, or other lesions by hot biopsy forceps, bipolar cautery or snare technique**

2.76 8.90 FUD 000 J A2

AMA: 2018,Jan,8; 2017,Jan,8; 2016,Jan,13; 2015,Jan,16

46614 **with control of bleeding (eg, injection, bipolar cautery, unipolar cautery, laser, heater probe, stapler, plasma coagulator)**

1.85 4.21 FUD 000 T P3

AMA: 2018,Jan,8; 2017,Jan,8; 2016,Jan,13; 2015,Jan,16

46615 **with ablation of tumor(s), polyp(s), or other lesion(s) not amenable to removal by hot biopsy forceps, bipolar cautery or snare technique**

2.64 4.34 FUD 000 J A2

AMA: 2018,Jan,8; 2017,Jan,8; 2016,Jan,13; 2015,Jan,16

46700-46947 [46947] Anal Repairs and Stapled Hemorrhoidopexy

46700 **Anoplasty, plastic operation for stricture; adult**

18.9 18.9 FUD 090 J A2

AMA: 2014,Jan,11; 2013,Jan,11-12

46705 **infant** A

EXCLUDES *Anal septum incision (46070)*

16.1 16.1 FUD 090 63 C 80

AMA: 2014,Jan,11; 2013,Jan,11-12

46706 **Repair of anal fistula with fibrin glue**

5.14 5.14 FUD 010 J A2

AMA: 2014,Jan,11; 2013,Jan,11-12

46707 **Repair of anorectal fistula with plug (eg, porcine small intestine submucosa [SIS])**

14.4 14.4 FUD 090 J G2 80

AMA: 2018,Jan,8; 2017,Jan,8; 2016,Jan,13; 2015,Jan,16

46710 **Repair of ileoanal pouch fistula/sinus (eg, perineal or vaginal), pouch advancement; transperineal approach**

32.3 32.3 FUD 090 C 80

AMA: 2018,Jan,8; 2017,Jan,8; 2016,Jan,13; 2015,Jan,16

46712 **combined transperineal and transabdominal approach**

65.0 65.0 FUD 090 C 80

AMA: 2018,Jan,8; 2017,Jan,8; 2016,Jan,13; 2015,Jan,16

46715 **Repair of low imperforate anus; with anoperineal fistula (cut-back procedure)**

15.9 15.9 FUD 090 63 C 80

AMA: 2014,Jan,11; 2013,Jan,11-12

46716 **with transposition of anoperineal or anovestibular fistula**

35.4 35.4 FUD 090 63 C 80

AMA: 2014,Jan,11; 2013,Jan,11-12

46730 **Repair of high imperforate anus without fistula; perineal or sacroperineal approach**

57.4 57.4 FUD 090 63 C 80

AMA: 2014,Jan,11; 2013,Jan,11-12

46735 **combined transabdominal and sacroperineal approaches**

66.2 66.2 FUD 090 63 C 80

AMA: 2014,Jan,11; 2013,Jan,11-12

46740 **Repair of high imperforate anus with rectourethral or rectovaginal fistula; perineal or sacroperineal approach**

62.7 62.7 FUD 090 63 C 80

AMA: 2014,Jan,11; 2013,Jan,11-12

46742 **combined transabdominal and sacroperineal approaches**

72.7 72.7 FUD 090 63 C 80

AMA: 2014,Jan,11; 2013,Jan,11-12

46744 **Repair of cloacal anomaly by anorectovaginoplasty and urethroplasty, sacroperineal approach** ♀

103. 103. FUD 090 63 C 80

AMA: 2014,Jan,11; 2013,Jan,11-12

46746 **Repair of cloacal anomaly by anorectovaginoplasty and urethroplasty, combined abdominal and sacroperineal approach;** ♀

113. 113. FUD 090 C 80

AMA: 2014,Jan,11; 2013,Jan,11-12

46748 **with vaginal lengthening by intestinal graft or pedicle flaps** ♀

123. 123. FUD 090 C 80

AMA: 2014,Jan,11; 2013,Jan,11-12

46750 **Sphincteroplasty, anal, for incontinence or prolapse; adult**

21.7 21.7 FUD 090 J A2 80

AMA: 2014,Jan,11; 2013,Jan,11-12

46751 **child** A

19.2 19.2 FUD 090 C 80

AMA: 2014,Jan,11; 2013,Jan,11-12

46753 **Graft (Thiersch operation) for rectal incontinence and/or prolapse**

17.7 17.7 FUD 090 J A2

AMA: 2014,Jan,11; 2013,Jan,11-12

46754 **Removal of Thiersch wire or suture, anal canal**
6.76 9.30 FUD 010 J A2 80
AMA: 2014,Jan,11; 2013,Jan,11-12

46760 **Sphincteroplasty, anal, for incontinence, adult; muscle transplant**
31.6 31.6 FUD 090 J A2 80
AMA: 2014,Jan,11; 2013,Jan,11-12

46761 **levator muscle imbrication (Park posterior anal repair)**
26.6 26.6 FUD 090 J A2 80
AMA: 2014,Jan,11; 2013,Jan,11-12

46947 **Hemorrhoidopexy (eg, for prolapsing internal hemorrhoids) by stapling**
11.1 11.1 FUD 090 J A2
AMA: 2018,Jan,8; 2017,Jan,8; 2016,Jan,13; 2015,Jan,16

46900-46999 [46945, 46946, 46947, 46948] Destruction Procedures: Anus

46900 **Destruction of lesion(s), anus (eg, condyloma, papilloma, molluscum contagiosum, herpetic vesicle), simple; chemical**
3.92 6.76 FUD 010 T P2
AMA: 2014,Jan,11; 2013,Jan,11-12

46910 **electrodesiccation**
3.84 7.39 FUD 010 T P3
AMA: 2019,Dec,12

46916 **cryosurgery**
4.06 7.00 FUD 010 T P2
AMA: 2014,Jan,11; 2013,Jan,11-12

46917 **laser surgery**
3.68 11.9 FUD 010 J A2
AMA: 2014,Jan,11; 2013,Jan,11-12

46922 **surgical excision**
3.92 8.00 FUD 010 J A2
AMA: 2014,Jan,11; 2013,Jan,11-12

46924 **Destruction of lesion(s), anus (eg, condyloma, papilloma, molluscum contagiosum, herpetic vesicle), extensive (eg, laser surgery, electrosurgery, cryosurgery, chemosurgery)**
5.21 15.1 FUD 010 J A2
AMA: 2014,Jan,11; 2013,Jan,11-12

46930 **Destruction of internal hemorrhoid(s) by thermal energy (eg, infrared coagulation, cautery, radiofrequency)**
EXCLUDES *Other hemorrhoid procedures:*
Cryosurgery destruction (46999)
Excision ([46320], 46250-46262)
Hemorrhoidopexy ([46947])
Incision (46083)
Injection sclerosing solution (46500)
Ligation (46221, [46945, 46946])
4.33 6.12 FUD 090 T P3 80
AMA: 2018,Jan,8; 2017,Jan,8; 2016,Jul,8; 2016,Jan,13; 2015,Apr,10

46940 **Curettage or cautery of anal fissure, including dilation of anal sphincter (separate procedure); initial**
4.20 6.79 FUD 010 J P3
AMA: 2014,Jan,11; 2013,Jan,11-12

46942 **subsequent**
3.74 6.72 FUD 010 T P3 80
AMA: 2014,Jan,11; 2013,Jan,11-12

46945 **Resequenced code. See code following 46221.**

46946 **Resequenced code. See code following resequenced code 46945.**

46947 **Resequenced code. See code following 46761.**

46948 **Resequenced code. See code before resequenced code 46220.**

46999 **Unlisted procedure, anus**
0.00 0.00 FUD YYY T 80
AMA: 2020,Feb,11; 2018,Oct,11; 2018,Jan,8; 2017,Jan,8; 2016,Jan,13; 2015,Apr,10; 2015,Jan,16

47000-47001 Needle Biopsy of Liver

EXCLUDES *Fine needle aspiration (10021, [10004, 10005, 10006, 10007, 10008, 10009, 10010, 10011, 10012])*

47000 **Biopsy of liver, needle; percutaneous**
(76942, 77002, 77012, 77021)
(88172-88173)
2.56 8.85 FUD 000 J A2
AMA: 2019,Apr,4; 2018,Jan,8; 2017,Jan,8; 2016,Jan,13; 2015,Jan,16

+ **47001** **when done for indicated purpose at time of other major procedure (List separately in addition to code for primary procedure)**
Code first primary procedure
(76942, 77002)
(88172-88173)
3.04 3.04 FUD ZZZ N N1
AMA: 2018,Jan,8; 2017,Jan,8; 2016,Jan,13; 2015,Jan,16

47010-47130 Open Incisional and Resection Procedures of Liver

47010 **Hepatotomy, for open drainage of abscess or cyst, 1 or 2 stages**
EXCLUDES *Image guided percutaneous catheter drainage (49505)*
35.2 35.2 FUD 090 C 80
AMA: 2014,Jan,11; 2013,Nov,9

47015 **Laparotomy, with aspiration and/or injection of hepatic parasitic (eg, amoebic or echinococcal) cyst(s) or abscess(es)**
33.9 33.9 FUD 090 C 80
AMA: 2014,Jan,11; 2013,Jan,11-12

47100 **Biopsy of liver, wedge**
24.6 24.6 FUD 090 C 80
AMA: 2014,Jan,11; 2013,Jan,11-12

47120 **Hepatectomy, resection of liver; partial lobectomy**
68.0 68.0 FUD 090 C 80
AMA: 2018,Jan,8; 2017,Jan,8; 2016,Oct,11; 2016,Jan,13; 2015,Jan,16

47122 **trisegmentectomy**
100. 100. FUD 090 C 80
AMA: 2014,Jan,11; 2013,Jan,11-12

47125 **total left lobectomy**
89.8 89.8 FUD 090 C 80
AMA: 2014,Jan,11; 2013,Jan,11-12

47130 **total right lobectomy**
96.4 96.4 FUD 090 C 80
AMA: 2014,Jan,11; 2013,Jan,11-12

47133-47147 Liver Transplant Procedures

CMS: 100-03,260.1 Adult Liver Transplantation; 100-03,260.2 Pediatric Liver Transplantation; 100-04,3,90.4 Liver Transplants; 100-04,3,90.4.1 Standard Liver Acquisition Charge; 100-04,3,90.4.2 Billing for Liver Transplant and Acquisition Services; 100-04,3,90.6 Intestinal and Multi-Visceral Transplants

47133 **Donor hepatectomy (including cold preservation), from cadaver donor**
INCLUDES Graft:
Cold preservation
Harvest
0.00 0.00 FUD XXX C
AMA: 2014,Jan,11; 2013,Jan,11-12

47135 **Liver allotransplantation, orthotopic, partial or whole, from cadaver or living donor, any age**

INCLUDES Partial/whole recipient hepatectomy
Partial/whole transplant allograft
Recipient care

157. 157. FUD 090 C 80

AMA: 2018,Jan,8; 2017,Jan,8; 2016,Jan,13; 2015,Jan,16

47140 **Donor hepatectomy (including cold preservation), from living donor; left lateral segment only (segments II and III)**

INCLUDES Donor care
Graft:
Cold preservation
Harvest

103. 103. FUD 090 C 80

AMA: 2018,Jan,8; 2017,Jan,8; 2016,Jan,13; 2015,Jan,16

47141 **total left lobectomy (segments II, III and IV)**

INCLUDES Donor care
Graft:
Cold preservation
Harvest

124. 124. FUD 090 C 80

AMA: 2014,Jan,11; 2013,Jan,11-12

47142 **total right lobectomy (segments V, VI, VII and VIII)**

INCLUDES Donor care
Graft:
Cold preservation
Harvest

136. 136. FUD 090 C 80

AMA: 2014,Jan,11; 2013,Jan,11-12

47143 **Backbench standard preparation of cadaver donor whole liver graft prior to allotransplantation, including cholecystectomy, if necessary, and dissection and removal of surrounding soft tissues to prepare the vena cava, portal vein, hepatic artery, and common bile duct for implantation; without trisegment or lobe split**

EXCLUDES *Cholecystectomy (47600, 47610)*
Hepatectomy (47120-47125)

0.00 0.00 FUD XXX C 80

AMA: 2018,Jan,8; 2017,Jan,8; 2016,Jan,13; 2015,Jan,16

47144 **with trisegment split of whole liver graft into 2 partial liver grafts (ie, left lateral segment [segments II and III] and right trisegment [segments I and IV through VIII])**

EXCLUDES *Cholecystectomy (47600, 47610)*
Hepatectomy (47120-47125)

0.00 0.00 FUD 090 C 80

AMA: 2014,Jan,11; 2013,Jan,11-12

47145 **with lobe split of whole liver graft into 2 partial liver grafts (ie, left lobe [segments II, III, and IV] and right lobe [segments I and V through VIII])**

EXCLUDES *Cholecystectomy (47600, 47610)*
Hepatectomy (47120-47125)

0.00 0.00 FUD XXX C 80

AMA: 2014,Jan,11; 2013,Jan,11-12

47146 **Backbench reconstruction of cadaver or living donor liver graft prior to allotransplantation; venous anastomosis, each**

EXCLUDES *Cholecystectomy (47600, 47610)*
Hepatectomy (47120-47125)

9.43 9.43 FUD XXX C 80

AMA: 2014,Jan,11; 2013,Jan,11-12

47147 **arterial anastomosis, each**

EXCLUDES *Cholecystectomy (47600, 47610)*
Hepatectomy (47120-47125)

11.1 11.1 FUD XXX C 80

AMA: 2014,Jan,11; 2013,Jan,11-12

47300-47362 Open Repair of Liver

47300 **Marsupialization of cyst or abscess of liver**

32.9 32.9 FUD 090 C 80

AMA: 2014,Jan,11; 2013,Jan,11-12

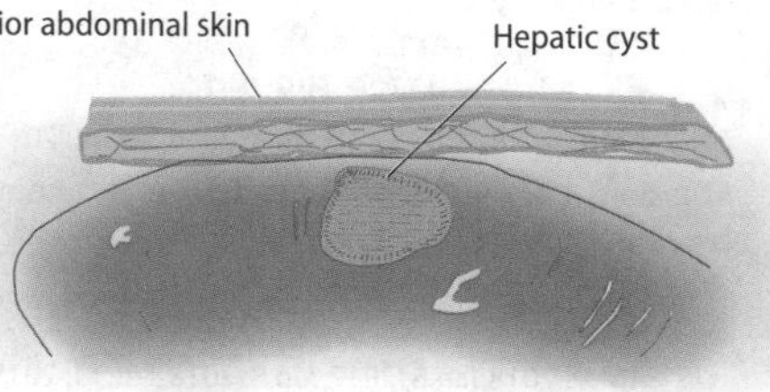

Cutaway view of liver

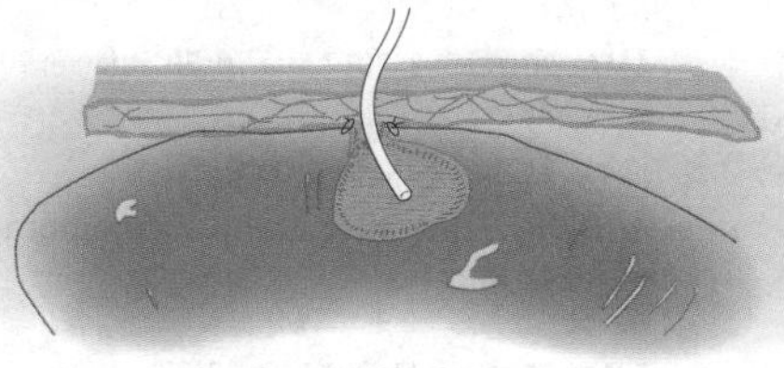

Marsupialization of cyst

A liver cyst or abscess is marsupialized; this method involves surgical access to the cyst and making an incision into it; the edges of the cyst are sutured to the abdominal wall and drainage, open or closed, is placed into the cyst

47350 **Management of liver hemorrhage; simple suture of liver wound or injury**

39.7 39.7 FUD 090 C 80

AMA: 2014,Jan,11; 2013,Jan,11-12

47360 **complex suture of liver wound or injury, with or without hepatic artery ligation**

54.8 54.8 FUD 090 C 80

AMA: 2014,Jan,11; 2013,Jan,11-12

47361 **exploration of hepatic wound, extensive debridement, coagulation and/or suture, with or without packing of liver**

88.0 88.0 FUD 090 C 80

AMA: 2014,Jan,11; 2013,Jan,11-12

47362 **re-exploration of hepatic wound for removal of packing**

42.1 42.1 FUD 090 C 80

AMA: 2020,Jan,6

47370-47379 Laparoscopic Ablation Liver Tumors

INCLUDES Diagnostic laparoscopy (49320)

47370 **Laparoscopy, surgical, ablation of 1 or more liver tumor(s); radiofrequency**

(76940)

36.4 36.4 FUD 090 J 80

AMA: 2018,Jan,8; 2017,Jan,8; 2016,Jan,13; 2015,Jan,16

47371 **cryosurgical**

(76940)

36.5 36.5 FUD 090 J 80

AMA: 2014,Jan,11; 2013,Jan,11-12

47379 **Unlisted laparoscopic procedure, liver**

0.00 0.00 FUD YYY J 80

AMA: 2018,Aug,10; 2018,Jan,8; 2017,Jan,8; 2016,Jan,13; 2015,Jan,16

47380-47399 Open/Percutaneous Ablation Liver Tumors

47380 **Ablation, open, of 1 or more liver tumor(s); radiofrequency**

(76940)

42.1 42.1 FUD 090 C 80

AMA: 2018,Jan,8; 2017,Jan,8; 2016,Jan,13; 2015,Jan,16

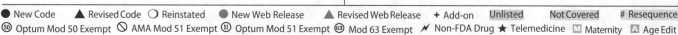

47381 **cryosurgical**
(76940)
43.2 43.2 FUD 090 C 80
AMA: 2014,Jan,11; 2013,Jan,11-12

47382 **Ablation, 1 or more liver tumor(s), percutaneous, radiofrequency**
(76940, 77013, 77022)
21.4 125. FUD 010 J G2
AMA: 2018,Jan,8; 2017,Jan,8; 2016,Jan,13; 2015,Jan,16

47383 **Ablation, 1 or more liver tumor(s), percutaneous, cryoablation**
(76940, 77013, 77022)
13.1 195. FUD 010 J J8
AMA: 2018,Jan,8; 2017,Jan,8; 2016,Jan,13; 2015,Jan,16

47399 **Unlisted procedure, liver**
0.00 0.00 FUD YYY T
AMA: 2018,Jan,8; 2017,Mar,10; 2017,Jan,8; 2016,Jan,13; 2015,Jan,16

47400-47490 Biliary Tract Procedures

47400 **Hepaticotomy or hepaticostomy with exploration, drainage, or removal of calculus**
62.9 62.9 FUD 090 C 80
AMA: 2014,Jan,11; 2013,Jan,11-12

47420 **Choledochotomy or choledochostomy with exploration, drainage, or removal of calculus, with or without cholecystotomy; without transduodenal sphincterotomy or sphincteroplasty**
39.1 39.1 FUD 090 C 80
AMA: 2014,Jan,11; 2013,Jan,11-12

47425 **with transduodenal sphincterotomy or sphincteroplasty**
39.9 39.9 FUD 090 C 80
AMA: 2014,Jan,11; 2013,Jan,11-12

47460 **Transduodenal sphincterotomy or sphincteroplasty, with or without transduodenal extraction of calculus (separate procedure)**
37.0 37.0 FUD 090 C 80
AMA: 2014,Jan,11; 2013,Jan,11-12

47480 **Cholecystotomy or cholecystostomy, open, with exploration, drainage, or removal of calculus (separate procedure)**
EXCLUDES *Percutaneous cholecystostomy (47490)*
25.4 25.4 FUD 090 C 80
AMA: 2018,Jan,8; 2017,Jan,8; 2016,Jan,13; 2015,Jan,16

47490 **Cholecystostomy, percutaneous, complete procedure, including imaging guidance, catheter placement, cholecystogram when performed, and radiological supervision and interpretation**
INCLUDES Radiological guidance (75989, 76942, 77002, 77012, 77021)
EXCLUDES *Injection procedure for cholangiography (47531-47532)*
Open cholecystostomy (47480)
9.56 9.56 FUD 010 J
AMA: 2018,Jan,8; 2017,Jan,8; 2016,Jan,13; 2015,Dec,3; 2015,Jan,16

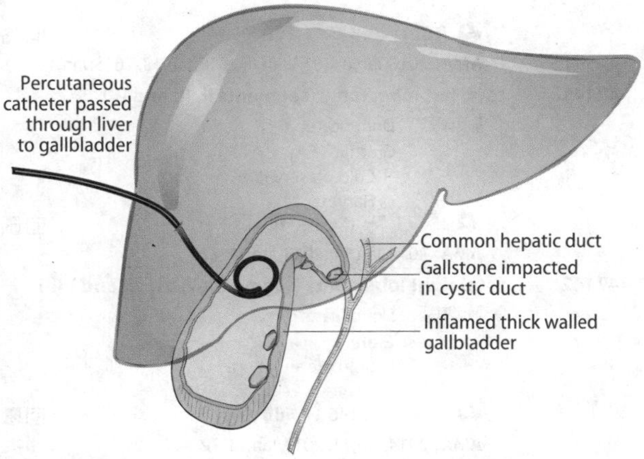

47531-47532 Injection/Insertion Procedures of Biliary Tract

INCLUDES Contrast material injection
Radiologic supervision and interpretation
EXCLUDES *Intraoperative cholangiography (74300-74301)*
Procedures performed via same access (47490, 47533-47541)

47531 **Injection procedure for cholangiography, percutaneous, complete diagnostic procedure including imaging guidance (eg, ultrasound and/or fluoroscopy) and all associated radiological supervision and interpretation; existing access**
2.07 9.00 FUD 000 Q2 N1
AMA: 2018,Jan,8; 2017,Jan,8; 2015,Dec,3

47532 **new access (eg, percutaneous transhepatic cholangiogram)**
6.18 22.6 FUD 000 Q2 N1
AMA: 2018,Jan,8; 2017,Jan,8; 2015,Dec,3

47533-47544 Percutaneous Procedures of the Biliary Tract

47533 **Placement of biliary drainage catheter, percutaneous, including diagnostic cholangiography when performed, imaging guidance (eg, ultrasound and/or fluoroscopy), and all associated radiological supervision and interpretation; external**
EXCLUDES *Conversion to internal-external drainage catheter (47535)*
Percutaneous placement stent bile duct (47538)
Placement stent bile duct, new access (47540)
Replacement existing internal drainage catheter (47536)
7.77 35.0 FUD 000 J G2
AMA: 2018,Jan,8; 2017,Jan,8; 2015,Dec,3

47534 **internal-external**
EXCLUDES *Conversion to external only drainage catheter (47536)*
Percutaneous placement stent bile duct (47538)
Placement stent bile duct, new access (47540)
10.8 41.0 FUD 000 J G2
AMA: 2018,Jan,8; 2017,Jan,8; 2015,Dec,3

47535 **Conversion of external biliary drainage catheter to internal-external biliary drainage catheter, percutaneous, including diagnostic cholangiography when performed, imaging guidance (eg, fluoroscopy), and all associated radiological supervision and interpretation**

5.76 28.8 **FUD** 000 J G2

AMA: 2018,Jan,8; 2017,Jan,8; 2015,Dec,3

47536 **Exchange of biliary drainage catheter (eg, external, internal-external, or conversion of internal-external to external only), percutaneous, including diagnostic cholangiography when performed, imaging guidance (eg, fluoroscopy), and all associated radiological supervision and interpretation**

INCLUDES Exchange one drainage catheter

EXCLUDES *Placement stent(s) into bile duct, percutaneous (47538)*

Code also exchange additional catheters same session with modifier 59 (47536)

3.86 19.5 **FUD** 000 J G2

AMA: 2018,Jan,8; 2017,Jan,8; 2015,Dec,3

47537 **Removal of biliary drainage catheter, percutaneous, requiring fluoroscopic guidance (eg, with concurrent indwelling biliary stents), including diagnostic cholangiography when performed, imaging guidance (eg, fluoroscopy), and all associated radiological supervision and interpretation**

EXCLUDES *Placement stent(s) into bile duct via same access (47538)*

Removal without fluoroscopic guidance; report with appropriate E/M service code

2.80 10.4 **FUD** 000 Q2 G2

AMA: 2018,Jan,8; 2017,Jan,8; 2015,Dec,3

47538 **Placement of stent(s) into a bile duct, percutaneous, including diagnostic cholangiography, imaging guidance (eg, fluoroscopy and/or ultrasound), balloon dilation, catheter exchange(s) and catheter removal(s) when performed, and all associated radiological supervision and interpretation; existing access**

EXCLUDES *Drainage catheter inserted following stent placement (47536)*

Procedures performed via same access (47536-47537)

Treatment same lesion same operative session ([43277], 47542, 47555-47556)

Code also multiple stents placed during same session when: (47538-47540)

Serial stents placed within same bile duct

Stent placement via two or more percutaneous access sites or space between two other stents

Two or more stents inserted through same percutaneous access

6.88 121. **FUD** 000 J J8

AMA: 2018,Jan,8; 2017,Jan,8; 2016,Mar,10; 2015,Dec,3

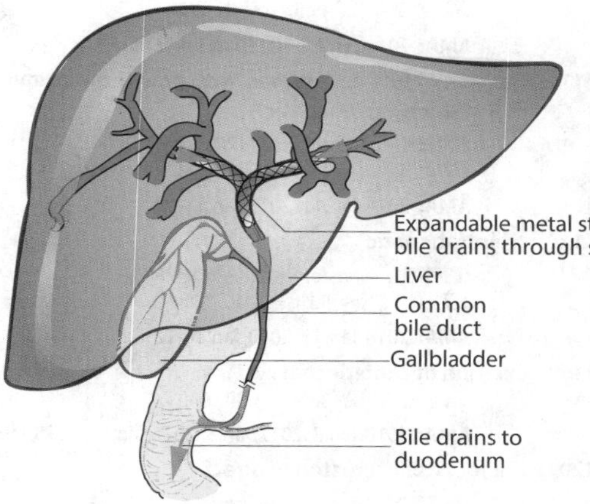

47539 **new access, without placement of separate biliary drainage catheter**

EXCLUDES *Treatment same lesion same operative session ([43277], 47542, 47555-47556)*

Code also multiple stents placed during same session when: (47538-47540)

Serial stents placed within same bile duct

Stent placement via two or more percutaneous access sites or space between two other stents

Two or more stents inserted through same percutaneous access

12.4 135. **FUD** 000 J G2

AMA: 2018,Jan,8; 2017,Jan,8; 2016,Mar,10; 2015,Dec,3

47540 **new access, with placement of separate biliary drainage catheter (eg, external or internal-external)**

EXCLUDES *Procedures performed via same access (47533-47534)*

Treatment same lesion same operative session ([43277], 47542, 47555-47556)

Code also multiple stents placed during same session when: (47538-47540)

Serial stents placed within same bile duct

Stent placement via two or more percutaneous access sites or space between two other stents

Two or more stents inserted through same percutaneous access

12.8 139. **FUD** 000 J J8

AMA: 2018,Jan,8; 2017,Jan,8; 2016,Mar,10; 2015,Dec,3

47541 **Placement of access through the biliary tree and into small bowel to assist with an endoscopic biliary procedure (eg, rendezvous procedure), percutaneous, including diagnostic cholangiography when performed, imaging guidance (eg, ultrasound and/or fluoroscopy), and all associated radiological supervision and interpretation, new access**

EXCLUDES *Access through biliary tree into small bowel for endoscopic biliary procedure (47535-47537)*

Conversion, exchange, or removal external biliary drainage catheter (47535-47537)

Injection procedure for cholangiography (47531-47532)

Placement biliary drainage catheter (47533-47534)

Placement stent(s) into bile duct (47538-47540)

Procedure performed when previous catheter access exists

9.69 33.3 **FUD** 000 J G2

AMA: 2018,Jan,8; 2017,Jan,8; 2015,Dec,3

\+ **47542** **Balloon dilation of biliary duct(s) or of ampulla (sphincteroplasty), percutaneous, including imaging guidance (eg, fluoroscopy), and all associated radiological supervision and interpretation, each duct (List separately in addition to code for primary procedure)**

EXCLUDES *Biliary endoscopy, with dilation of biliary duct stricture (47555-47556)*

Endoscopic balloon dilation ([43277], 47555-47556)

Endoscopic retrograde cholangiopancreatography (ERCP) (43262, [43277])

Placement stent(s) into a bile duct (47538-47540)

Procedure performed with balloon to remove calculi, debris, sludge without dilation (47544)

Code also one additional dilation code when more than one dilation performed same session, using modifier 59 with (47542)

Code first (47531-47537, 47541)

3.95 13.1 **FUD** ZZZ N N1

AMA: 2018,Jan,8; 2017,Jan,8; 2015,Dec,3

+ 47543 Endoluminal biopsy(ies) of biliary tree, percutaneous, any method(s) (eg, brush, forceps, and/or needle), including imaging guidance (eg, fluoroscopy), and all associated radiological supervision and interpretation, single or multiple (List separately in addition to code for primary procedure)

EXCLUDES *Endoscopic biopsy (46261, 47553)*
Endoscopic brushings (43260, 47552)
Procedure performed more than one time per session

Code first (47531-47540)

4.20 | 13.3 | FUD ZZZ | N N1

AMA: 2018,Jan,8; 2017,Jan,8; 2015,Dec,3

+ 47544 Removal of calculi/debris from biliary duct(s) and/or gallbladder, percutaneous, including destruction of calculi by any method (eg, mechanical, electrohydraulic, lithotripsy) when performed, imaging guidance (eg, fluoroscopy), and all associated radiological supervision and interpretation (List separately in addition to code for primary procedure)

EXCLUDES *Device deployment without finding calculi/debris*
Endoscopic calculi removal/destruction (43264-43265, 47554)
Endoscopic retrograde cholangiopancreatography (ERCP); with removal calculi/debris from biliary/pancreatic duct(s) (43264)
Procedures with removal incidental debris (47531-47543)

Code first when debris removal not incidental, as appropriate (47531-47540)

4.61 | 29.2 | FUD ZZZ | N N1

AMA: 2018,Jan,8; 2017,Jan,8; 2015,Dec,3

47550-47556 Endoscopic Procedures of the Biliary Tract

INCLUDES Diagnostic endoscopy (49320)

EXCLUDES *Endoscopic retrograde cholangiopancreatography (ERCP) (43260-43265, [43274], [43275], [43276], [43277], [43278], 74328-74330, 74363)*

+ 47550 Biliary endoscopy, intraoperative (choledochoscopy) (List separately in addition to code for primary procedure)

Code first primary procedure

4.80 | 4.80 | FUD ZZZ | C 80

AMA: 2014,Jan,11; 2013,Jan,11-12

47552 Biliary endoscopy, percutaneous via T-tube or other tract; diagnostic, with collection of specimen(s) by brushing and/or washing, when performed (separate procedure)

9.01 | 9.01 | FUD 000 | J A2

AMA: 2018,Jan,8; 2017,Jan,8; 2016,Jan,13; 2015,Dec,3; 2015,Jan,16

47553 with biopsy, single or multiple

8.91 | 8.91 | FUD 000 | J A2

AMA: 2018,Jan,8; 2017,Jan,8; 2016,Jan,13; 2015,Dec,3; 2015,Jan,16

47554 with removal of calculus/calculi

14.9 | 14.9 | FUD 000 | J A2

AMA: 2018,Jan,8; 2017,Jan,8; 2016,Jan,13; 2015,Dec,3; 2015,Jan,16

47555 with dilation of biliary duct stricture(s) without stent

(74363)

9.46 | 9.46 | FUD 000 | J A2

AMA: 2018,Jan,8; 2017,Jan,8; 2016,Jan,13; 2015,Dec,3; 2015,Jan,16

47556 with dilation of biliary duct stricture(s) with stent

(74363)

10.7 | 10.7 | FUD 000 | J J8

AMA: 2018,Jan,8; 2017,Jan,8; 2016,Jan,13; 2015,Dec,3; 2015,Jan,16

47562-47579 Laparoscopic Gallbladder Procedures

INCLUDES Diagnostic laparoscopy (49320)

47562 Laparoscopy, surgical; cholecystectomy

19.0 | 19.0 | FUD 090 | J G2 80

AMA: 2020,Aug,14; 2018,Jan,8; 2017,Jan,8; 2016,Jan,13; 2015,Jan,16

47563 cholecystectomy with cholangiography

EXCLUDES *Percutaneous cholangiography (47531-47532)*

Code also intraoperative radiology supervision and interpretation (74300-74301)

20.7 | 20.7 | FUD 090 | J G2 80

AMA: 2019,Mar,10; 2018,Jan,8; 2017,Jan,8; 2016,Jan,13; 2015,Jan,16

47564 cholecystectomy with exploration of common duct

32.2 | 32.2 | FUD 090 | J G2 80

AMA: 2018,Jan,8; 2017,Jan,8; 2016,Jan,13; 2015,Jan,16

47570 cholecystoenterostomy

22.5 | 22.5 | FUD 090 | C 80

AMA: 2018,Jan,8; 2017,Jan,8; 2016,Jan,13; 2015,Jan,16

47579 Unlisted laparoscopy procedure, biliary tract

0.00 | 0.00 | FUD YYY | J 80 50

AMA: 2018,Jan,8; 2017,Jan,8; 2016,Jan,13; 2015,Jan,16

47600-47620 Open Gallbladder Procedures

47600 Cholecystectomy;

EXCLUDES *Laparoscopic method (47562-47564)*

30.9 | 30.9 | FUD 090 | C 80

AMA: 2018,Jan,8; 2017,Jan,8; 2016,Jan,13; 2015,Jan,16

47605 with cholangiography

EXCLUDES *Laparoscopic method (47563-47564)*

32.6 | 32.6 | FUD 090 | C 80

AMA: 2018,Jan,8; 2017,Jan,8; 2016,Jan,13; 2015,Jan,16

47610 Cholecystectomy with exploration of common duct;

EXCLUDES *Laparoscopic method (47564)*

Code also biliary endoscopy when performed in conjunction with cholecystectomy with exploration common duct (47550)

36.3 | 36.3 | FUD 090 | C 80

AMA: 2018,Jan,8; 2017,Jan,8; 2016,Jan,13; 2015,Jan,16

47612 with choledochoenterostomy

36.6 | 36.6 | FUD 090 | C 80

AMA: 2014,Jan,11; 2013,Jan,11-12

47620 with transduodenal sphincterotomy or sphincteroplasty, with or without cholangiography

40.0 | 40.0 | FUD 090 | C 80

AMA: 2014,Jan,11; 2013,Jan,11-12

47700-47999 Open Resection and Repair of Biliary Tract

47700 Exploration for congenital atresia of bile ducts, without repair, with or without liver biopsy, with or without cholangiography

30.6 | 30.6 | FUD 090 | 63 C 80

AMA: 2014,Jan,11; 2013,Jan,11-12

47701 Portoenterostomy (eg, Kasai procedure)

49.5 | 49.5 | FUD 090 | 63 C 80

AMA: 2014,Jan,11; 2013,Jan,11-12

47711 Excision of bile duct tumor, with or without primary repair of bile duct; extrahepatic

EXCLUDES *Anastomosis (47760-47800)*

45.1 | 45.1 | FUD 090 | C 80

AMA: 2014,Jan,11; 2013,Jan,11-12

47712 intrahepatic

EXCLUDES *Anastomosis (47760-47800)*

58.1 | 58.1 | FUD 090 | C 80

AMA: 2014,Jan,11; 2013,Jan,11-12

47715 Excision of choledochal cyst

38.8 | 38.8 | FUD 090 | C 80

AMA: 2018,Jan,8; 2017,Jan,8; 2016,Jan,13; 2015,Jan,16

47720 Cholecystoenterostomy; direct

EXCLUDES *Laparoscopic method (47570)*

33.4 | 33.4 | FUD 090 | C 80

AMA: 2018,Jan,8; 2017,Jan,8; 2016,Jan,13; 2015,Jan,16

47721 **with gastroenterostomy**
39.3 39.3 **FUD** 090 C 80
AMA: 2014,Jan,11; 2013,Jan,11-12

47740 **Roux-en-Y**
37.7 37.7 **FUD** 090 C 80
AMA: 2014,Jan,11; 2013,Jan,11-12

47741 **Roux-en-Y with gastroenterostomy**
42.8 42.8 **FUD** 090 C 80
AMA: 2014,Jan,11; 2013,Jan,11-12

47760 **Anastomosis, of extrahepatic biliary ducts and gastrointestinal tract**
65.4 65.4 **FUD** 090 C 80
AMA: 2014,Jan,11; 2013,Jan,11-12

47765 **Anastomosis, of intrahepatic ducts and gastrointestinal tract**
INCLUDES Longmire anastomosis
87.9 87.9 **FUD** 090 C 80
AMA: 2014,Jan,11; 2013,Jan,11-12

47780 **Anastomosis, Roux-en-Y, of extrahepatic biliary ducts and gastrointestinal tract**
71.8 71.8 **FUD** 090 C 80
AMA: 2014,Jan,11; 2013,Jan,11-12

47785 **Anastomosis, Roux-en-Y, of intrahepatic biliary ducts and gastrointestinal tract**
94.4 94.4 **FUD** 090 C 80
AMA: 2014,Jan,11; 2013,Jan,11-12

47800 **Reconstruction, plastic, of extrahepatic biliary ducts with end-to-end anastomosis**
45.5 45.5 **FUD** 090 C 80
AMA: 2014,Jan,11; 2013,Jan,11-12

47801 **Placement of choledochal stent**
32.3 32.3 **FUD** 090 C 80
AMA: 2018,Jan,8; 2017,Jan,8; 2016,Jan,13; 2015,Jan,16

47802 **U-tube hepaticoenterostomy**
44.3 44.3 **FUD** 090 C 80
AMA: 2014,Jan,11; 2013,Jan,11-12

47900 **Suture of extrahepatic biliary duct for pre-existing injury (separate procedure)**
39.7 39.7 **FUD** 090 C 80
AMA: 2014,Jan,11; 2013,Jan,11-12

47999 **Unlisted procedure, biliary tract**
0.00 0.00 **FUD** YYY T
AMA: 2018,Jan,8; 2017,Jan,8; 2016,Jan,13; 2015,Jan,16

48000-48548 Open Procedures of the Pancreas

EXCLUDES *Peroral pancreatic procedures performed endoscopically (43260-43265, [43274], [43275], [43276], [43277], [43278])*

48000 **Placement of drains, peripancreatic, for acute pancreatitis;**
54.6 54.6 **FUD** 090 C 80
AMA: 2014,Jan,11; 2013,Jan,11-12

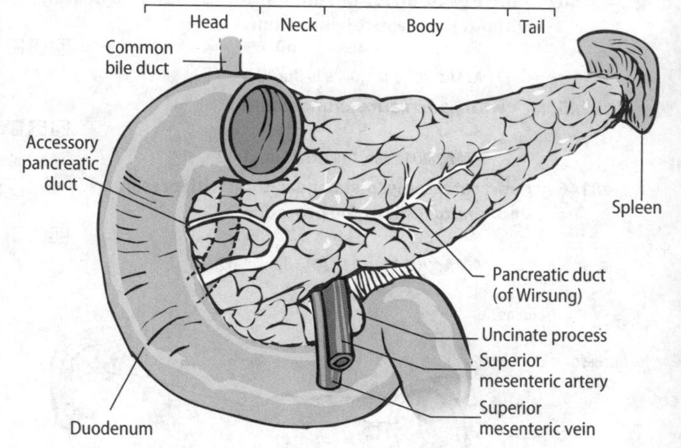

48001 **with cholecystostomy, gastrostomy, and jejunostomy**
67.1 67.1 **FUD** 090 C 80
AMA: 2014,Jan,11; 2013,Jan,11-12

48020 **Removal of pancreatic calculus**
34.1 34.1 **FUD** 090 C 80
AMA: 2014,Jan,11; 2013,Jan,11-12

48100 **Biopsy of pancreas, open (eg, fine needle aspiration, needle core biopsy, wedge biopsy)**
25.8 25.8 **FUD** 090 C 80
AMA: 2014,Jan,11; 2013,Jan,11-12

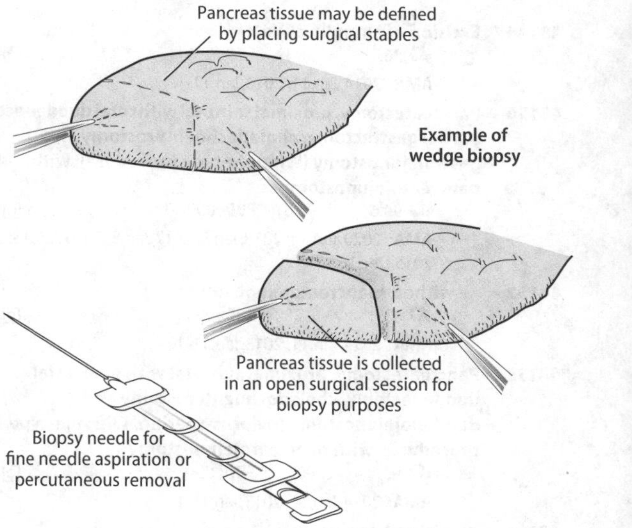

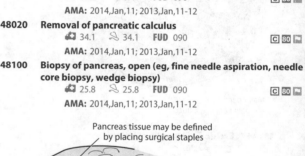

48102 **Biopsy of pancreas, percutaneous needle**
EXCLUDES *Fine needle aspiration ([10005, 10006, 10007, 10008, 10009, 10010, 10011, 10012])*
(76942, 77002, 77012, 77021)
(88172-88173)
6.95 15.2 **FUD** 010 J A2
AMA: 2019,Apr,4

48105 **Resection or debridement of pancreas and peripancreatic tissue for acute necrotizing pancreatitis**
82.4 82.4 FUD 090 C 80
AMA: 2014,Jan,11; 2013,Jan,11-12

48120 **Excision of lesion of pancreas (eg, cyst, adenoma)**
32.0 32.0 FUD 090 C 80
AMA: 2014,Jan,11; 2013,Jan,11-12

48140 **Pancreatectomy, distal subtotal, with or without splenectomy; without pancreaticojejunostomy**
45.4 45.4 FUD 090 C 80
AMA: 2018,Jan,8; 2017,Jul,10

48145 **with pancreaticojejunostomy**
47.3 47.3 FUD 090 C 80
AMA: 2014,Jan,11; 2013,Jan,11-12

48146 **Pancreatectomy, distal, near-total with preservation of duodenum (Child-type procedure)**
54.5 54.5 FUD 090 C 80
AMA: 2014,Jan,11; 2013,Jan,11-12

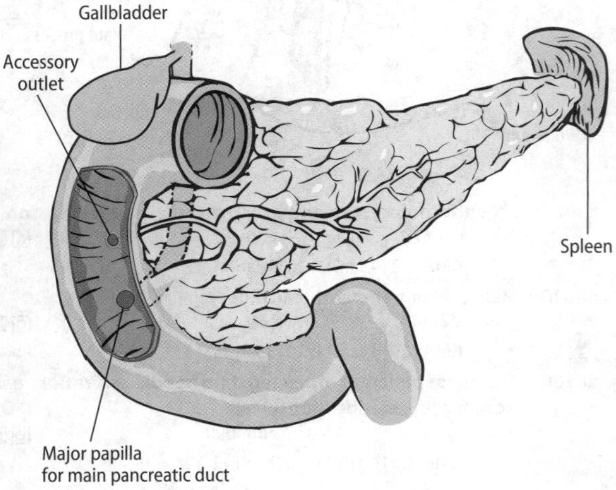

48148 **Excision of ampulla of Vater**
36.1 36.1 FUD 090 C 80
AMA: 2014,Jan,11; 2013,Jan,11-12

48150 **Pancreatectomy, proximal subtotal with total duodenectomy, partial gastrectomy, choledochoenterostomy and gastrojejunostomy (Whipple-type procedure); with pancreatojejunostomy**
90.6 90.6 FUD 090 C 80
AMA: 2020,Jun,14; 2018,Jan,8; 2017,Jan,8; 2016,Jan,13; 2015,Dec,16

48152 **without pancreatojejunostomy**
83.8 83.8 FUD 090 C 80
AMA: 2014,Jan,11; 2013,Jan,11-12

48153 **Pancreatectomy, proximal subtotal with near-total duodenectomy, choledochoenterostomy and duodenojejunostomy (pylorus-sparing, Whipple-type procedure); with pancreatojejunostomy**
90.1 90.1 FUD 090 C 80
AMA: 2014,Jan,11; 2013,Jan,11-12

48154 **without pancreatojejunostomy**
84.3 84.3 FUD 090 C 80
AMA: 2014,Jan,11; 2013,Jan,11-12

48155 **Pancreatectomy, total**
52.6 52.6 FUD 090 C 80
AMA: 2014,Jan,11; 2013,Jan,11-12

48160 **Pancreatectomy, total or subtotal, with autologous transplantation of pancreas or pancreatic islet cells**
EXCLUDES *Laparoscopic pancreatic islet cell transplantation (0585T)*
Open pancreatic islet cell transplantation (0586T)
Percutaneous pancreatic islet cell transplantation (0584T)
0.00 0.00 FUD XXX E
AMA: 2014,Jan,11; 2013,Jan,11-12

\+ **48400** **Injection procedure for intraoperative pancreatography (List separately in addition to code for primary procedure)**
Code first primary procedure
(74300-74301)
3.12 3.12 FUD ZZZ C 80
AMA: 2018,Jan,8; 2017,Jan,8; 2016,Jan,13; 2015,Jan,16

48500 **Marsupialization of pancreatic cyst**
33.4 33.4 FUD 090 C 80
AMA: 2014,Jan,11; 2013,Jan,11-12

48510 **External drainage, pseudocyst of pancreas, open**
EXCLUDES *Image guided percutaneous catheter drainage (49405)*
31.8 31.8 FUD 090 C 80
AMA: 2014,Jan,11; 2013,Nov,9

48520 **Internal anastomosis of pancreatic cyst to gastrointestinal tract; direct**
31.5 31.5 FUD 090 C 80
AMA: 2014,Jan,11; 2013,Jan,11-12

48540 **Roux-en-Y**
37.8 37.8 FUD 090 C 80
AMA: 2014,Jan,11; 2013,Jan,11-12

48545 **Pancreatorrhaphy for injury**
39.0 39.0 FUD 090 C 80
AMA: 2014,Jan,11; 2013,Jan,11-12

48547 **Duodenal exclusion with gastrojejunostomy for pancreatic injury**
51.9 51.9 FUD 090 C 80
AMA: 2014,Jan,11; 2013,Jan,11-12

48548 **Pancreaticojejunostomy, side-to-side anastomosis (Puestow-type operation)**
48.5 48.5 FUD 090 C 80
AMA: 2014,Jan,11; 2013,Jan,11-12

48550-48999 Pancreas Transplant Procedures

CMS: 100-03,260.3 Pancreas Transplants; 100-04,3,90.5 Pancreas Transplants with Kidney Transplants; 100-04,3,90.5.1 Pancreas Transplants Alone

48550 **Donor pancreatectomy (including cold preservation), with or without duodenal segment for transplantation**
INCLUDES Graft:
Cold preservation
Harvest (with or without duodenal segment)
0.00 0.00 FUD XXX E
AMA: 2018,Jan,8; 2017,Jan,8; 2016,Jan,13; 2015,Jan,16

48551 Backbench standard preparation of cadaver donor pancreas allograft prior to transplantation, including dissection of allograft from surrounding soft tissues, splenectomy, duodenotomy, ligation of bile duct, ligation of mesenteric vessels, and Y-graft arterial anastomoses from iliac artery to superior mesenteric artery and to splenic artery

EXCLUDES
- Biopsy pancreas (48100-48102)
- Bypass graft, with vein (35531, 35563)
- Duodenotomy (44010)
- Endoscopic procedures biliary tract (47550-47556)
- Excision lesion mesentery (44820)
- Excision lesion pancreas (48120)
- Pancreatorrhaphy for injury (48545)
- Placement vein patch or cuff at distal anastomosis bypass graft (35685)
- Resection or debridement pancreas (48105)
- Splenectomy (38100-38102)
- Suture mesentery (44850)
- Transduodenal sphincterotomy, sphincteroplasty (47460)

0.00   0.00   **FUD** XXX   C 80

AMA: 2014,Jan,11; 2013,Jan,11-12

48552 Backbench reconstruction of cadaver donor pancreas allograft prior to transplantation, venous anastomosis, each

EXCLUDES
- Biopsy pancreas (48100-48102)
- Bypass graft, with vein (35531, 35563)
- Duodenotomy (44010)
- Endoscopic procedures biliary tract (47550-47556)
- Excision lesion mesentery (44820)
- Excision lesion pancreas (48120)
- Pancreatorrhaphy for injury (48545)
- Placement vein patch or cuff at distal anastomosis bypass graft (35685)
- Resection or debridement pancreas (48105)
- Splenectomy (38100-38102)
- Suture mesentery (44850)
- Transduodenal sphincterotomy, sphincteroplasty (47460)

6.87   6.87   **FUD** XXX   C 80

AMA: 2014,Jan,11; 2013,Jan,11-12

48554 Transplantation of pancreatic allograft

INCLUDES
- Allograft transplant
- Recipient care

74.4   74.4   **FUD** 090   C 80

AMA: 2014,Jan,11; 2013,Jan,11-12

48556 Removal of transplanted pancreatic allograft

37.1   37.1   **FUD** 090   C 80

AMA: 2014,Jan,11; 2013,Jan,11-12

48999 Unlisted procedure, pancreas

0.00   0.00   **FUD** YYY   T 80

AMA: 2018,Jan,8; 2017,Jan,8; 2016,Jan,13; 2015,Jan,16

49000-49084 Exploratory and Drainage Procedures: Abdomen/Peritoneum

49000 Exploratory laparotomy, exploratory celiotomy with or without biopsy(s) (separate procedure)

EXCLUDES
- Exploration penetrating wound without laparotomy (20102)

22.3   22.3   **FUD** 090   C 80

AMA: 2020,Jan,6; 2019,Dec,5; 2018,Jan,8; 2017,Dec,3; 2017,Jan,8; 2016,Jan,13; 2015,Jan,16

49002 Reopening of recent laparotomy

EXCLUDES
- Hepatic wound re-exploration for packing removal (47362)
- Pelvic wound re-exploration for packing removal/repacking (49014)

30.4   30.4   **FUD** 090   C 80

AMA: 2020,Jan,6; 2018,Jan,8; 2017,Jan,8; 2016,Jan,13; 2015,Jan,16

49010 Exploration, retroperitoneal area with or without biopsy(s) (separate procedure)

EXCLUDES
- Exploration penetrating wound without laparotomy (20102)

26.8   26.8   **FUD** 090   C 80

AMA: 2020,Jan,6; 2019,Dec,5

49013 Preperitoneal pelvic packing for hemorrhage associated with pelvic trauma, including local exploration

12.7   12.7   **FUD** 000

AMA: 2020,Jan,6

49014 Re-exploration of pelvic wound with removal of preperitoneal pelvic packing, including repacking, when performed

10.5   10.5   **FUD** 000

AMA: 2020,Jan,6

49020 Drainage of peritoneal abscess or localized peritonitis, exclusive of appendiceal abscess, open

EXCLUDES
- Appendiceal abscess (44900)
- Image-guided percutaneous catheter drainage abscess/peritonitis via catheter (49406)
- Image-guided transrectal/transvaginal drainage peritoneal abscess via catheter (49407)

46.3   46.3   **FUD** 090   C 80

AMA: 2014,Jan,11; 2013,Nov,9

49040 Drainage of subdiaphragmatic or subphrenic abscess, open

EXCLUDES
- Image-guided percutaneous drainage subdiaphragmatic/subphrenic abscess via catheter (49406)

29.1   29.1   **FUD** 090   C 80

AMA: 2014,Jan,11; 2013,Nov,9

49060 Drainage of retroperitoneal abscess, open

EXCLUDES
- Image-guided percutaneous drainage retroperitoneal abscess via catheter (49406)
- Transrectal/transvaginal image-guided drainage retroperitoneal abscess via catheter (49407)

32.0   32.0   **FUD** 090   C

AMA: 2018,Jan,8; 2017,Jan,8; 2016,Jan,13; 2015,Jan,16

49062 Drainage of extraperitoneal lymphocele to peritoneal cavity, open

EXCLUDES
- Drainage lymphocele to peritoneal cavity, laparoscopic (49323)
- Image-guided percutaneous drainage retroperitoneal lymphocele via catheter (49406)

21.3   21.3   **FUD** 090   C 80

AMA: 2018,Jan,8; 2017,Jan,8; 2016,Jan,13; 2015,Jan,16

49082 Abdominal paracentesis (diagnostic or therapeutic); without imaging guidance

2.12   5.67   **FUD** 000   T 62

AMA: 2018,Jan,8; 2017,Jan,8; 2016,Jan,13; 2015,Jan,16

49083 with imaging guidance

INCLUDES
- Radiological guidance (76942, 77002, 77012, 77021)

EXCLUDES
- Image-guided percutaneous drainage retroperitoneal abscess via catheter (49406)

3.11   8.44   **FUD** 000   T 62

AMA: 2018,Jan,8; 2017,Jan,8; 2016,Jan,13; 2015,Jan,16

49084 Peritoneal lavage, including imaging guidance, when performed

INCLUDES
- Radiological guidance (76942, 77002, 77012, 77021)

EXCLUDES
- Image-guided percutaneous drainage retroperitoneal abscess via catheter (49406)

3.13   3.13   **FUD** 000   T 62

AMA: 2018,Jan,8; 2017,Jan,8; 2016,Jan,13; 2015,Jan,16

● New Code   ▲ Revised Code   ○ Reinstated   ● New Web Release   ▲ Revised Web Release   + Add-on   Unlisted   Not Covered   # Resequenced
⑤⓪ Optum Mod 50 Exempt   ⊘ AMA Mod 51 Exempt   ⑤① Optum Mod 51 Exempt   ㊿ Mod 63 Exempt   ✗ Non-FDA Drug   ★ Telemedicine   Ⓜ Maternity   Ⓐ Age Edit

49180 Biopsy of Mass: Abdomen/Retroperitoneum

EXCLUDES *Fine needle aspiration (10021, [10004, 10005, 10006, 10007, 10008, 10009, 10010, 10011, 10012])*
Lysis intestinal adhesions (44005)

49180 Biopsy, abdominal or retroperitoneal mass, percutaneous needle
(76942, 77002, 77012, 77021)
(88172-88173)
2.43 4.86 FUD 000 J A2
AMA: 2019,Feb,8; 2019,Apr,4; 2018,Jan,8; 2017,Jan,8; 2016,Jan,13; 2015,Jan,16

49185 Sclerotherapy of a Fluid Collection

49185 Sclerotherapy of a fluid collection (eg, lymphocele, cyst, or seroma), percutaneous, including contrast injection(s), sclerosant injection(s), diagnostic study, imaging guidance (eg, ultrasound, fluoroscopy) and radiological supervision and interpretation when performed
INCLUDES Multiple lesions treated via same access
EXCLUDES *Contrast injection for assessment abscess or cyst (49424)*
Pleurodesis (32560)
Radiologic examination, abscess, fistula or sinus tract stud (76080)
Sclerosis veins/endovenous ablation incompetent veins extremity (36468, 36470-36471, 36475-36476, 36478-36479)
Sclerotherapy lymphatic/vascular malformation (37241)
Code also access or drainage via needle or catheter (10030, 10160, 49405-49407, 50390)
Code also existing catheter exchange pre- or post-sclerosant injection (49423, 75984)
Code also modifier 59 for treatment multiple lesions same session via separate access
3.47 33.4 FUD 000 T
AMA: 2018,Jan,8; 2017,Jan,8; 2016,Mar,10

49203-49205 Open Destruction or Excision: Abdominal Tumors

EXCLUDES *Ablation, open, one or more renal mass lesion(s), cryosurgical*
Biopsy kidney or ovary (50205, 58900)
Cryoablation renal tumor (50250, 50593)
Excision perinephric cyst (50290)
Excision presacral or sacrococcygeal tumor (49215)
Exploration, renal or retroperitoneal area (49010, 50010)
Exploratory laparotomy (49000)
Laparotomy, for staging or restaging ovarian, tubal, or primary peritoneal malignancy (58960)
Nephrectomy (50225, 50236)
Oophorectomy (58940-58958)
Ovarian cystectomy (58925)
Pelvic or retroperitoneal lymphadenectomy (38770, 38780)
Primary, recurrent ovarian, uterine, or tubal resection (58957-58958)
Wedge resection or bisection ovary (58920)
Code also colectomy (44140)
Code also nephrectomy (50220, 50240)
Code also small bowel resection (44120)
Code also vena caval resection with reconstruction (37799)

49203 Excision or destruction, open, intra-abdominal tumors, cysts or endometriomas, 1 or more peritoneal, mesenteric, or retroperitoneal primary or secondary tumors; largest tumor 5 cm diameter or less
34.7 34.7 FUD 090 C 80
AMA: 2018,Jan,8; 2017,Jan,8; 2016,Jan,13; 2015,Jan,16

49204 largest tumor 5.1-10.0 cm diameter
44.2 44.2 FUD 090 C 80
AMA: 2018,Jan,8; 2017,Jan,8; 2016,Jan,13; 2015,Jan,16

49205 largest tumor greater than 10.0 cm diameter
50.6 50.6 FUD 090 C 80
AMA: 2018,Jan,8; 2017,Jan,8; 2016,Jan,13; 2015,Jan,16

49215 Resection Presacral/Sacrococcygeal Tumor

49215 Excision of presacral or sacrococcygeal tumor
64.2 64.2 FUD 090 63 C 80
AMA: 2014,Jan,11; 2013,Jan,11-12

49220-49255 Other Open Abdominal Procedures

EXCLUDES *Lysis intestinal adhesions (44005)*

49220 ~~Staging laparotomy for Hodgkins disease or lymphoma (includes splenectomy, needle or open biopsies of both liver lobes, possibly also removal of abdominal nodes, abdominal node and/or bone marrow biopsies, ovarian repositioning)~~

49250 Umbilectomy, omphalectomy, excision of umbilicus (separate procedure)
16.9 16.9 FUD 090 J A2
AMA: 2014,Jan,11; 2013,Jan,11-12

49255 Omentectomy, epiploectomy, resection of omentum (separate procedure)
22.8 22.8 FUD 090 C 80
AMA: 2018,Mar,11; 2018,Jan,8; 2017,Jan,8; 2016,Jan,13; 2015,Jan,16

49320-49329 Laparoscopic Procedures of the Abdomen/Peritoneum/Omentum

INCLUDES Diagnostic laparoscopy (49320)
EXCLUDES *Fulguration/excision lesions ovary/pelvic viscera/peritoneal surface, performed laparoscopically (58662)*

49320 Laparoscopy, abdomen, peritoneum, and omentum, diagnostic, with or without collection of specimen(s) by brushing or washing (separate procedure)
9.54 9.54 FUD 010 J A2 80
AMA: 2018,Jan,8; 2017,Apr,7; 2017,Jan,8; 2016,Jan,13; 2015,Dec,16; 2015,Jan,16

49321 Laparoscopy, surgical; with biopsy (single or multiple)
10.0 10.0 FUD 010 J A2 80
AMA: 2018,Aug,10; 2018,Jan,8; 2017,Jan,8; 2016,Jan,13; 2015,Jan,16

49322 with aspiration of cavity or cyst (eg, ovarian cyst) (single or multiple)
10.8 10.8 FUD 010 J A2 80
AMA: 2018,Jan,8; 2017,Jan,8; 2016,Jan,13; 2015,Jan,16

49323 with drainage of lymphocele to peritoneal cavity
EXCLUDES *Open drainage lymphocele to peritoneal cavity (49062)*
18.3 18.3 FUD 090 J 80
AMA: 2018,Jan,8; 2017,Jan,8; 2016,Jan,13; 2015,Jan,16

49324 with insertion of tunneled intraperitoneal catheter
EXCLUDES *Open approach (49421)*
Code also insertion subcutaneous extension to intraperitoneal cannula with remote chest exit site, when appropriate (49435)
11.3 11.3 FUD 010 J G2 80
AMA: 2014,Jan,11; 2013,Jan,11-12

49325 with revision of previously placed intraperitoneal cannula or catheter, with removal of intraluminal obstructive material if performed
12.1 12.1 FUD 010 J G2 80
AMA: 2014,Jan,11; 2013,Jan,11-12

\+ **49326 with omentopexy (omental tacking procedure) (List separately in addition to code for primary procedure)**
Code first laparoscopy with permanent intraperitoneal cannula or catheter insertion or revision previously placed catheter/cannula (49324, 49325)
5.52 5.52 FUD ZZZ N N1 80
AMA: 2014,Jan,11; 2013,Jan,11-12

+ **49327** **with placement of interstitial device(s) for radiation therapy guidance (eg, fiducial markers, dosimeter), intra-abdominal, intrapelvic, and/or retroperitoneum, including imaging guidance, if performed, single or multiple (List separately in addition to code for primary procedure)**

EXCLUDES *Open approach (49412)*
Percutaneous approach (49411)

Code first laparoscopic abdominal, pelvic or retroperitoneal procedures

3.81 3.81 FUD ZZZ N N1 80

AMA: 2014,Jan,11; 2013,Jan,11-12

49329 **Unlisted laparoscopy procedure, abdomen, peritoneum and omentum**

0.00 0.00 FUD YYY J 80 50

AMA: 2020,Feb,13; 2019,Mar,10; 2018,Jan,8; 2017,Jan,8; 2016,Jan,13; 2015,Jan,16

49400-49436 Peritoneal and Visceral Procedures: Drainage/Insertion/Modifications/Removal

49400 **Injection of air or contrast into peritoneal cavity (separate procedure)**

(74190)

2.68 3.93 FUD 000 N N1

AMA: 2018,Jan,8; 2017,Jan,8; 2016,Jan,13; 2015,Jan,16

49402 **Removal of peritoneal foreign body from peritoneal cavity**

EXCLUDES *Enterolysis (44005)*
Percutaneous or open drainage or lavage (49020, 49040, 49082-49084, 49406)
Percutaneous tunneled intraperitoneal catheter insertion without subcutaneous port (49418)

24.9 24.9 FUD 090 J A2

AMA: 2014,Jan,11; 2013,Jan,11-12

49405 **Image-guided fluid collection drainage by catheter (eg, abscess, hematoma, seroma, lymphocele, cyst); visceral (eg, kidney, liver, spleen, lung/mediastinum), percutaneous**

INCLUDES Radiological guidance (75989, 76942, 77002-77003, 77012, 77021)

EXCLUDES *Open drainage (47010, 48510, 50020)*
Percutaneous cholecystostomy (47490)
Percutaneous pleural drainage (32556-32557)
Pneumonostomy (32200)
Thoracentesis (32554-32555)

Code also each individual collection drained per separate catheter

5.71 25.1 FUD 000 J

AMA: 2020,Feb,13; 2018,Jan,8; 2017,Jan,8; 2016,Jan,13; 2015,Jan,16

49406 **peritoneal or retroperitoneal, percutaneous**

INCLUDES Radiological guidance (75989, 76942, 77002-77003, 77012, 77021)

EXCLUDES *Diagnostic or therapeutic percutaneous abdominal paracentesis (49082-49083)*
Open peritoneal/retroperitoneal drainage (44900, 49020-49062, 49084, 50020, 58805, 58822)
Open transrectal drainage pelvic abscess (45000)
Percutaneous tunneled intraperitoneal catheter insertion without subcutaneous port (49418)
Transrectal/transvaginal image-guided peritoneal/retroperitoneal drainage via catheter (49407)

Code also each individual collection drained per separate catheter

5.70 25.1 FUD 000 J G2

AMA: 2020,Feb,13; 2018,Jan,8; 2017,Jan,8; 2016,Jan,13; 2015,Jan,16

49407 **peritoneal or retroperitoneal, transvaginal or transrectal**

INCLUDES Radiological guidance (75989, 76942, 77002-77003, 77012, 77021)

EXCLUDES *Image-guided percutaneous catheter drainage soft tissue (eg, abdominal wall, neck, extremity) (10030)*
Open transrectal/transvaginal drainage (45000, 58800, 58820)
Percutaneous pleural drainage (32556-32557)
Peritoneal drainage or lavage, open or percutaneous (49020, 49040, 49060)
Thoracentesis (32554-32555)

Code also each individual collection drained per separate catheter

6.05 20.6 FUD 000 J G2

AMA: 2018,Jan,8; 2017,Jan,8; 2016,Jan,13; 2015,Jan,16

49411 **Placement of interstitial device(s) for radiation therapy guidance (eg, fiducial markers, dosimeter), percutaneous, intra-abdominal, intra-pelvic (except prostate), and/or retroperitoneum, single or multiple**

EXCLUDES *Placement (percutaneous) interstitial device(s) for intrathoracic radiation therapy guidance (32553)*

Code also supply device

(76942, 77002, 77012, 77021)

5.33 13.9 FUD 000 S P3 80

AMA: 2018,Jan,8; 2017,Jan,8; 2016,Jun,3; 2016,Jan,13; 2015,Jan,16

+ **49412** **Placement of interstitial device(s) for radiation therapy guidance (eg, fiducial markers, dosimeter), open, intra-abdominal, intrapelvic, and/or retroperitoneum, including image guidance, if performed, single or multiple (List separately in addition to code for primary procedure)**

EXCLUDES *Laparoscopic approach (49327)*
Percutaneous approach (49411)

Code first open abdominal, pelvic or retroperitoneal procedure(s)

2.41 2.41 FUD ZZZ C 80

AMA: 2014,Jan,11; 2013,Jan,11-12

49418 **Insertion of tunneled intraperitoneal catheter (eg, dialysis, intraperitoneal chemotherapy instillation, management of ascites), complete procedure, including imaging guidance, catheter placement, contrast injection when performed, and radiological supervision and interpretation, percutaneous**

5.88 34.1 FUD 000 J G2 80

AMA: 2014,Jan,11; 2013,Nov,9

49419 **Insertion of tunneled intraperitoneal catheter, with subcutaneous port (ie, totally implantable)**

EXCLUDES *Removal catheter/cannula (49422)*

12.5 12.5 FUD 090 T A2

AMA: 2014,Jan,11; 2013,Jan,11-12

49421 **Insertion of tunneled intraperitoneal catheter for dialysis, open**

EXCLUDES *Laparoscopic approach (49324)*

Code also insertion subcutaneous extension to intraperitoneal cannula with remote chest exit site, when appropriate (49435)

6.65 6.65 FUD 000 J G2

AMA: 2018,Jan,8; 2017,Jan,8; 2016,Jan,13; 2015,Jan,16

49422 **Removal of tunneled intraperitoneal catheter**

EXCLUDES *Removal temporary catheter or cannula (Report appropriate E/M code)*

6.46 6.46 FUD 000 Q2 A2

AMA: 2014,Jan,11; 2013,Jan,11-12

49423 **Exchange of previously placed abscess or cyst drainage catheter under radiological guidance (separate procedure)**

(75984)

2.05 16.9 FUD 000 J G2 80

AMA: 2018,Jan,8; 2017,Jan,8; 2016,Jan,13; 2015,Jan,16

49424 **Contrast injection for assessment of abscess or cyst via previously placed drainage catheter or tube (separate procedure)**
(76080)
1.10 4.35 FUD 000 N N1 80
AMA: 2018,Jan,8; 2017,Jan,8; 2016,Jan,13; 2015,Jan,16

49425 **Insertion of peritoneal-venous shunt**
20.7 20.7 FUD 090 C 80
AMA: 2014,Jan,11; 2013,Jan,11-12

49426 **Revision of peritoneal-venous shunt**
EXCLUDES *Shunt patency test (78291)*
19.4 19.4 FUD 090 J A2
AMA: 2014,Jan,11; 2013,Jan,11-12

49427 **Injection procedure (eg, contrast media) for evaluation of previously placed peritoneal-venous shunt**
(75809, 78291)
1.13 1.13 FUD 000 N N1 80
AMA: 2014,Jan,11; 2013,Jan,11-12

49428 **Ligation of peritoneal-venous shunt**
12.5 12.5 FUD 010 C
AMA: 2014,Jan,11; 2013,Jan,11-12

49429 **Removal of peritoneal-venous shunt**
13.3 13.3 FUD 010 Q2 G2
AMA: 2014,Jan,11; 2013,Jan,11-12

+ **49435** **Insertion of subcutaneous extension to intraperitoneal cannula or catheter with remote chest exit site (List separately in addition to code for primary procedure)**
Code first permanent insertion intraperitoneal catheter/cannula (49324, 49421)
3.50 3.50 FUD ZZZ N N1 80
AMA: 2014,Jan,11; 2013,Jan,11-12

49436 **Delayed creation of exit site from embedded subcutaneous segment of intraperitoneal cannula or catheter**
5.42 5.42 FUD 010 J G2 80
AMA: 2014,Jan,11; 2013,Jan,11-12

49440-49442 Insertion of Percutaneous Gastrointestinal Tube

EXCLUDES *Naso- or oro-gastric tube placement (43752)*

49440 **Insertion of gastrostomy tube, percutaneous, under fluoroscopic guidance including contrast injection(s), image documentation and report**
INCLUDES Needle placement with fluoroscopic guidance (77002)
Code also gastrostomy to gastro-jejunostomy tube conversion with initial gastrostomy tube insertion, when performed (49446)
5.93 26.6 FUD 010 J G2 80
AMA: 2018,Jan,8; 2017,Jan,8; 2016,Jan,13; 2015,Jan,16

49441 **Insertion of duodenostomy or jejunostomy tube, percutaneous, under fluoroscopic guidance including contrast injection(s), image documentation and report**
EXCLUDES *Gastrostomy tube to gastrojejunostomy tube conversion (49446)*
7.00 30.6 FUD 010 J G2 80
AMA: 2018,Jan,8; 2017,Jan,8; 2016,Jan,13; 2015,Jan,16

49442 **Insertion of cecostomy or other colonic tube, percutaneous, under fluoroscopic guidance including contrast injection(s), image documentation and report**
6.00 25.2 FUD 010 T G2 80
AMA: 2018,Jan,8; 2017,Jan,8; 2016,Jan,13; 2015,Jan,16

49446 Percutaneous Conversion: Gastrostomy to Gastro-jejunostomy Tube

EXCLUDES *Code also initial gastrostomy tube insertion (49440) when conversion performed same time*

49446 **Conversion of gastrostomy tube to gastro-jejunostomy tube, percutaneous, under fluoroscopic guidance including contrast injection(s), image documentation and report**
4.30 25.6 FUD 000 J G2 80
AMA: 2018,Jan,8; 2017,Jan,8; 2016,Jan,13; 2015,Jan,16

49450-49452 Replacement Gastrointestinal Tube

EXCLUDES *Placement new tube whether gastrostomy, jejunostomy, duodenostomy, gastro-jejunostomy, or cecostomy different percutaneous site (49440-49442)*

49450 **Replacement of gastrostomy or cecostomy (or other colonic) tube, percutaneous, under fluoroscopic guidance including contrast injection(s), image documentation and report**
EXCLUDES *Change gastrostomy tube, percutaneous, without imaging or endoscopic guidance (43762-43763)*
1.91 18.7 FUD 000 T G2 80
AMA: 2019,Feb,5; 2018,Jan,8; 2017,Jan,8; 2016,Jan,13; 2015,Jan,16

49451 **Replacement of duodenostomy or jejunostomy tube, percutaneous, under fluoroscopic guidance including contrast injection(s), image documentation and report**
2.61 20.3 FUD 000 T G2 80
AMA: 2018,Jan,8; 2017,Jan,8; 2016,Jan,13; 2015,Jan,16

49452 **Replacement of gastro-jejunostomy tube, percutaneous, under fluoroscopic guidance including contrast injection(s), image documentation and report**
4.01 25.1 FUD 000 T G2 80
AMA: 2018,Jan,8; 2017,Jan,8; 2016,Jan,13; 2015,Jan,16

49460-49465 Removal of Obstruction/Injection for Contrast Through Gastrointestinal Tube

49460 **Mechanical removal of obstructive material from gastrostomy, duodenostomy, jejunostomy, gastro-jejunostomy, or cecostomy (or other colonic) tube, any method, under fluoroscopic guidance including contrast injection(s), if performed, image documentation and report**
INCLUDES Contrast injection (49465)
EXCLUDES *Replacement gastrointestinal tube (49450-49452)*
1.39 20.4 FUD 000 T G2 80
AMA: 2018,Jan,8; 2017,Jan,8; 2016,Jan,13; 2015,Jan,16

49465 **Contrast injection(s) for radiological evaluation of existing gastrostomy, duodenostomy, jejunostomy, gastro-jejunostomy, or cecostomy (or other colonic) tube, from a percutaneous approach including image documentation and report**
EXCLUDES *Mechanical removal obstructive material from gastrointestinal tube (49460)*
Replacement gastrointestinal tube (49450-49452)
0.89 4.48 FUD 000 Q1 G2 80
AMA: 2018,Jan,8; 2017,Jan,8; 2016,Jan,13; 2015,Jan,16

49491-49492 Inguinal Hernia Repair on Premature Infant

INCLUDES Hernia repairs done on preterm infants younger than or equal to 50 weeks postconception age and younger than 6 months
Initial repair: no previous repair required
Mesh or other prosthesis
EXCLUDES *Abdominal wall debridement (11042, 11043)*
Intra-abdominal hernia repair/reduction (44050)
Code also repair or excision testicle(s), intestine, ovaries, when performed (44120, 54520, 58940)

49491 **Repair, initial inguinal hernia, preterm infant (younger than 37 weeks gestation at birth), performed from birth up to 50 weeks postconception age, with or without hydrocelectomy; reducible** A
23.2 23.2 FUD 090 63 J 80 50
AMA: 2018,Jan,8; 2017,Jan,8; 2016,Jan,13; 2015,Jan,16

49492 **incarcerated or strangulated** A
27.9 27.9 **FUD** 090 63 J 80 50
AMA: 2018,Jan,8; 2017,Jan,8; 2016,Jan,13; 2015,Jan,16

49495-49557 Hernia Repair: Femoral/Inguinal /Lumbar

INCLUDES Initial repair: no previous repair required
Mesh or other prosthesis
Recurrent repair: required previous repair(s)
EXCLUDES *Abdominal wall debridement (11042, 11043)*
Intra-abdominal hernia repair/reduction (44050)
Code also repair or excision testicle(s), intestine, ovaries, when performed (44120, 54520, 58940)

49495 **Repair, initial inguinal hernia, full term infant younger than age 6 months, or preterm infant older than 50 weeks postconception age and younger than age 6 months at the time of surgery, with or without hydrocelectomy; reducible** A
INCLUDES Hernia repairs done on preterm infants older than 50 weeks postconception age and younger than 6 months
11.8 11.8 **FUD** 090 63 J A2 80 50
AMA: 2018,Jan,8; 2017,Jan,8; 2016,Jan,13; 2015,Jan,16

49496 **incarcerated or strangulated** A
INCLUDES Hernia repairs done on preterm infants older than 50 weeks postconception age and younger than 6 months
17.7 17.7 **FUD** 090 63 J A2 80 50
AMA: 2018,Jan,8; 2017,Jan,8; 2016,Jan,13; 2015,Jan,16

49500 **Repair initial inguinal hernia, age 6 months to younger than 5 years, with or without hydrocelectomy; reducible** A
INCLUDES Repairs performed on patients 6 months to younger than 5 years old
11.9 11.9 **FUD** 090 J A2 80 50
AMA: 2018,Jan,8; 2017,Jan,8; 2016,Jan,13; 2015,Jan,16

49501 **incarcerated or strangulated** A
INCLUDES Repairs performed on patients 6 months to younger than 5 years old
17.6 17.6 **FUD** 090 J A2 80 50
AMA: 2018,Jan,8; 2017,Jan,8; 2016,Jan,13; 2015,Jan,16

49505 **Repair initial inguinal hernia, age 5 years or older; reducible** A
INCLUDES MacEwen hernia repair
Code also when performed:
Excision hydrocele (55040)
Excision spermatocele (54840)
Simple orchiectomy (54520)
15.0 15.0 **FUD** 090 J A2 80 50
AMA: 2018,Jan,8; 2017,Jan,8; 2016,Jan,13; 2015,Jan,16

49507 **incarcerated or strangulated** A
Code also when performed:
Excision hydrocele (55040)
Excision spermatocele (54840)
Simple orchiectomy (54520)
17.0 17.0 **FUD** 090 J A2 80 50
AMA: 2018,Jan,8; 2017,Jan,8; 2016,Jan,13; 2015,Jan,16

49520 **Repair recurrent inguinal hernia, any age; reducible**
18.3 18.3 **FUD** 090 J A2 80 50
AMA: 2018,Jan,8; 2017,Jan,8; 2016,Jan,13; 2015,Jan,16

49521 **incarcerated or strangulated**
20.8 20.8 **FUD** 090 J A2 80 50
AMA: 2018,Jan,8; 2017,Jan,8; 2016,Jan,13; 2015,Jan,16

49525 **Repair inguinal hernia, sliding, any age**
EXCLUDES *Inguinal hernia repair, incarcerated/strangulated (49496, 49501, 49507, 49521)*
16.7 16.7 **FUD** 090 J A2 80 50
AMA: 2018,Jan,8; 2017,Jan,8; 2016,Jan,13; 2015,Jan,16

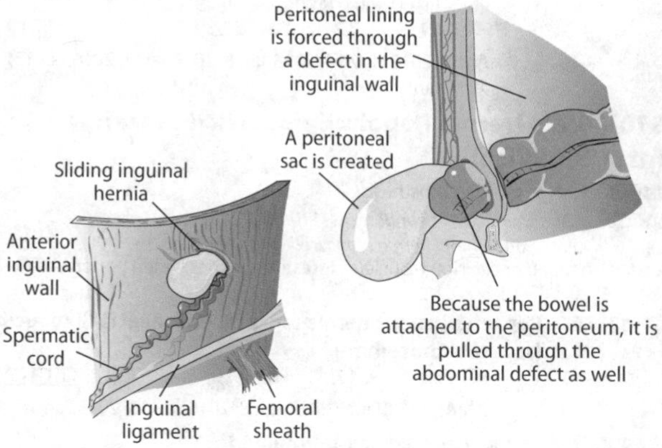
Peritoneal lining is forced through a defect in the inguinal wall
A peritoneal sac is created
Sliding inguinal hernia
Anterior inguinal wall
Spermatic cord
Inguinal ligament
Femoral sheath
Because the bowel is attached to the peritoneum, it is pulled through the abdominal defect as well

49540 **Repair lumbar hernia**
19.5 19.5 **FUD** 090 J A2 80 50
AMA: 2018,Jan,8; 2017,Jan,8; 2016,Jan,13; 2015,Jan,16

49550 **Repair initial femoral hernia, any age; reducible**
16.7 16.7 **FUD** 090 J A2 80 50
AMA: 2018,Jan,8; 2017,Jan,8; 2016,Jan,13; 2015,Jan,16

49553 **incarcerated or strangulated**
18.3 18.3 **FUD** 090 J A2 80 50
AMA: 2018,Jan,8; 2017,Jan,8; 2016,Jan,13; 2015,Jan,16

49555 **Repair recurrent femoral hernia; reducible**
17.5 17.5 **FUD** 090 J A2 80 50
AMA: 2018,Jan,8; 2017,Jan,8; 2016,Jan,13; 2015,Jan,16

49557 **incarcerated or strangulated**
21.0 21.0 **FUD** 090 J A2 80 50
AMA: 2018,Jan,8; 2017,Jan,8; 2016,Jan,13; 2015,Jan,16

49560-49568 Hernia Repair: Incisional/Ventral

INCLUDES Initial repair: no previous repair required
Recurrent repair: required previous repair(s)
EXCLUDES *Abdominal wall debridement (11042, 11043)*
Intra-abdominal hernia repair/reduction (44050)
Code also repair or excision testicle(s), intestine, ovaries, when performed (44120, 54520, 58940)

49560 **Repair initial incisional or ventral hernia; reducible**
Code also implantation mesh or other prosthesis, when performed (49568)
21.5 21.5 **FUD** 090 J A2 80 50
AMA: 2019,Nov,14; 2018,Jan,8; 2017,Jan,8; 2016,Jan,13; 2015,Jan,16

49561 **incarcerated or strangulated**
Code also implantation mesh or other prosthesis, when performed (49568)
27.0 27.0 **FUD** 090 J A2 80 50
AMA: 2019,Nov,14; 2018,Jul,14; 2018,Mar,11; 2018,Jan,8; 2017,Jan,8; 2016,Jan,13; 2015,Jan,16

49565 **Repair recurrent incisional or ventral hernia; reducible**
Code also implantation mesh or other prosthesis, when performed (49568)
22.3 22.3 **FUD** 090 J A2 80 50
AMA: 2019,Nov,14; 2018,Jan,8; 2017,Jan,8; 2016,Jan,13; 2015,Jan,16

49566 **incarcerated or strangulated**
Code also implantation mesh or other prosthesis, when performed (49568)
27.3 27.3 **FUD** 090 J A2 80 50
AMA: 2019,Nov,14; 2018,Jan,8; 2017,Jan,8; 2016,Jan,13; 2015,Jan,16

+ **49568** **Implantation of mesh or other prosthesis for open incisional or ventral hernia repair or mesh for closure of debridement for necrotizing soft tissue infection (List separately in addition to code for the incisional or ventral hernia repair)**
EXCLUDES *Reporting with modifier 50. Report once for each side when performed bilaterally*
Code first (11004-11006, 49560-49566)
7.77 7.77 FUD ZZZ N N1 80
AMA: 2019,Nov,14; 2018,Jan,8; 2017,Jan,8; 2016,Jan,13; 2015,Jan,16

49570-49590 Hernia Repair: Epigastric/Lateral Ventral/Umbilical

INCLUDES Mesh or other prosthesis
EXCLUDES *Abdominal wall debridement (11042, 11043)*
Intra-abdominal hernia repair/reduction (44050)
Code also repair or excision testicle(s), intestine, ovaries, when performed (44120, 54520, 58940)

49570 **Repair epigastric hernia (eg, preperitoneal fat); reducible (separate procedure)**
12.1 12.1 FUD 090 J A2 80 50
AMA: 2018,Jan,8; 2017,Jan,8; 2016,Jan,13; 2015,Jan,16

49572 **incarcerated or strangulated**
14.9 14.9 FUD 090 J A2 80 50
AMA: 2018,Jan,8; 2017,Jan,8; 2016,Jan,13; 2015,Jan,16

49580 **Repair umbilical hernia, younger than age 5 years; reducible** A
9.69 9.69 FUD 090 J A2 80
AMA: 2018,Jan,8; 2017,Jan,8; 2016,Jan,13; 2015,Jan,16

49582 **incarcerated or strangulated** A
14.0 14.0 FUD 090 J A2 80
AMA: 2018,Jan,8; 2017,Jan,8; 2016,Jan,13; 2015,Jan,16

49585 **Repair umbilical hernia, age 5 years or older; reducible** A
INCLUDES Mayo hernia repair
12.9 12.9 FUD 090 J A2 80
AMA: 2018,Jan,8; 2017,Jan,8; 2016,Jan,13; 2015,Jan,16

49587 **incarcerated or strangulated** A
13.7 13.7 FUD 090 J A2 80
AMA: 2018,Jan,8; 2017,Jan,8; 2016,Jan,13; 2015,Jan,16

49590 **Repair spigelian hernia**
16.5 16.5 FUD 090 J A2 80 50
AMA: 2018,Jan,8; 2017,Jan,8; 2016,Jan,13; 2015,Jan,16

49600-49611 Repair Birth Defect Abdominal Wall: Omphalocele/Gastroschisis

INCLUDES Mesh or other prosthesis
EXCLUDES *Abdominal wall debridement (11042, 11043)*
Intra-abdominal hernia repair/reduction (44050)
Repair:
Diaphragmatic or hiatal hernia (39503, 43332-43337)
Omentum (49999)

49600 **Repair of small omphalocele, with primary closure**
21.2 21.2 FUD 090 63 J A2 80
AMA: 2018,Jan,8; 2017,Jan,8; 2016,Jan,13; 2015,Jan,16

49605 **Repair of large omphalocele or gastroschisis; with or without prosthesis**
144. 144. FUD 090 63 C 80
AMA: 2018,Jan,8; 2017,Jan,8; 2016,Jan,13; 2015,Jan,16

49606 **with removal of prosthesis, final reduction and closure, in operating room**
32.9 32.9 FUD 090 63 C 80
AMA: 2018,Jan,8; 2017,Jan,8; 2016,Jan,13; 2015,Jan,16

49610 **Repair of omphalocele (Gross type operation); first stage**
20.1 20.1 FUD 090 63 C 80
AMA: 2018,Jan,8; 2017,Jan,8; 2016,Jan,13; 2015,Jan,16

49611 **second stage**
17.7 17.7 FUD 090 63 C 80
AMA: 2018,Jan,8; 2017,Jan,8; 2016,Jan,13; 2015,Jan,16

49650-49659 Laparoscopic Hernia Repair

INCLUDES Diagnostic laparoscopy (49320)
Mesh or other prosthesis (49568)

49650 **Laparoscopy, surgical; repair initial inguinal hernia**
12.5 12.5 FUD 090 J A2 80 50
AMA: 2018,Jan,8; 2017,Jan,8; 2016,Jan,13; 2015,Jan,16

49651 **repair recurrent inguinal hernia**
16.2 16.2 FUD 090 J A2 80 50
AMA: 2018,Jan,8; 2017,Jan,8; 2016,Jan,13; 2015,Jan,16

49652 **Laparoscopy, surgical, repair, ventral, umbilical, spigelian or epigastric hernia (includes mesh insertion, when performed); reducible**
INCLUDES Laparoscopy, surgical, enterolysis (44180)
21.5 21.5 FUD 090 J G2 80 50
AMA: 2014,Jan,11; 2013,Jan,11-12

49653 **incarcerated or strangulated**
INCLUDES Laparoscopy, surgical, enterolysis (44180)
27.0 27.0 FUD 090 J G2 80 50
AMA: 2014,Jan,11; 2013,Jan,11-12

49654 **Laparoscopy, surgical, repair, incisional hernia (includes mesh insertion, when performed); reducible**
INCLUDES Laparoscopy, surgical, enterolysis (44180)
24.6 24.6 FUD 090 J G2 80 50
AMA: 2018,Jan,7

49655 **incarcerated or strangulated**
INCLUDES Laparoscopy, surgical, enterolysis (44180)
29.9 29.9 FUD 090 J G2 80 50
AMA: 2018,Jan,7

49656 **Laparoscopy, surgical, repair, recurrent incisional hernia (includes mesh insertion, when performed); reducible**
INCLUDES Laparoscopy, surgical, enterolysis (44180)
26.7 26.7 FUD 090 J G2 80 50
AMA: 2014,Jan,11; 2013,Jan,11-12

49657 **incarcerated or strangulated**
INCLUDES Laparoscopy, surgical, enterolysis (44180)
38.2 38.2 FUD 090 J G2 80 50
AMA: 2014,Jan,11; 2013,Jan,11-12

49659 **Unlisted laparoscopy procedure, hernioplasty, herniorrhaphy, herniotomy**
0.00 0.00 FUD YYY J 80 50
AMA: 2018,Jan,8; 2017,Jul,10; 2017,Jan,8; 2016,Jan,13; 2015,Jan,16

49900 Surgical Repair Abdominal Wall

EXCLUDES *Abdominal wall debridement (11042, 11043)*
Suture ruptured diaphragm (39540-39541)

49900 **Suture, secondary, of abdominal wall for evisceration or dehiscence**
23.7 23.7 FUD 090 C 80
AMA: 2018,Jan,8; 2017,Jan,8; 2016,Jan,13; 2015,Jan,16

49904-49999 Harvesting of Omental Flap

49904 **Omental flap, extra-abdominal (eg, for reconstruction of sternal and chest wall defects)**
INCLUDES Harvest and transfer
EXCLUDES *Omental flap harvest by second surgeon: both surgeons report code with modifier 62*
40.5 40.5 FUD 090 C
AMA: 2014,Jan,11; 2013,Jan,11-12

+ **49905** **Omental flap, intra-abdominal (List separately in addition to code for primary procedure)**
EXCLUDES *Exclusion small intestine from pelvis by mesh, other prosthesis, or native tissue (44700)*
Code first primary procedure
10.3 10.3 FUD ZZZ C 80
AMA: 2020,Feb,13; 2018,Jan,8; 2017,Jan,8; 2016,Jan,13; 2015,Jan,16

49906 **Free omental flap with microvascular anastomosis**

INCLUDES Operating microscope (69990)

0.00 0.00 **FUD** 090 C

AMA: 2019,Dec,5; 2018,Jan,8; 2017,Jan,8; 2016,Feb,12; 2016,Jan,13; 2015,Jan,16

49999 **Unlisted procedure, abdomen, peritoneum and omentum**

0.00 0.00 **FUD** YYY T

AMA: 2020,Jun,14; 2019,Nov,14; 2018,Jan,8; 2017,Jan,8; 2016,Jan,13; 2015,Jan,16

50010-50045 Kidney Procedures for Exploration or Drainage

EXCLUDES *Donor nephrectomy performed laparoscopically (50547)*
Retroperitoneal
Abscess drainage (49060)
Exploration (49010)
Tumor/cyst excision (49203-49205)

50010   Renal exploration, not necessitating other specific procedures

EXCLUDES *Laparoscopic ablation mass lesions of kidney (50542)*
⚕ 21.2   ⚕ 21.2   **FUD** 090   C 80 50 ▣
AMA: 2014,Jan,11; 2008,Aug,7-9

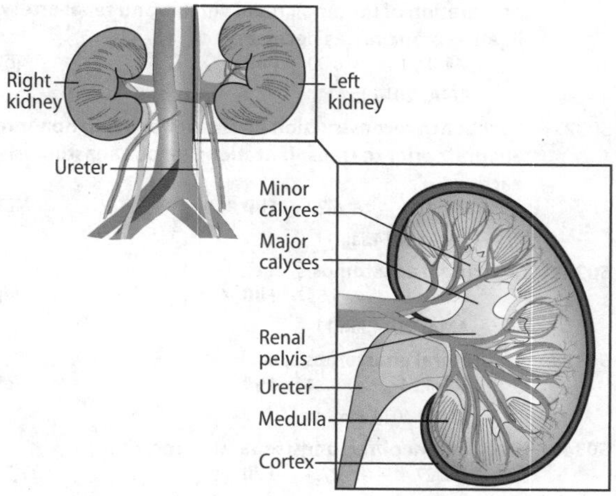

Right kidney
Left kidney
Ureter
Minor calyces
Major calyces
Renal pelvis
Ureter
Medulla
Cortex

50020   Drainage of perirenal or renal abscess, open

EXCLUDES *Image-guided percutaneous drainage perirenal or renal abscess (49405)*
⚕ 29.2   ⚕ 29.2   **FUD** 090   J ▣
AMA: 2018,Jan,8; 2017,Jan,8; 2016,Jan,13; 2015,Jan,16

50040   Nephrostomy, nephrotomy with drainage
⚕ 26.6   ⚕ 26.6   **FUD** 090   C 50 ▣
AMA: 2018,Jan,8; 2017,Jan,8; 2016,Jan,13; 2015,Jan,16

50045   Nephrotomy, with exploration

EXCLUDES *Renal endoscopy through nephrotomy (50570-50580)*
⚕ 26.9   ⚕ 26.9   **FUD** 090   C 80 50 ▣
AMA: 2018,Jan,8; 2017,Jan,8; 2016,Jan,13; 2015,Jan,16

50060-50081 Treatment of Kidney Stones

CMS: 100-03,230.1 NCD for Treatment of Kidney Stones

EXCLUDES *Retroperitoneal:*
Abscess drainage (49060)
Exploration (49010)
Tumor/cyst excision (49203-49205)

50060   Nephrolithotomy; removal of calculus
⚕ 32.9   ⚕ 32.9   **FUD** 090   C 80 50 ▣
AMA: 2018,Jan,8; 2017,Jan,8; 2016,Jan,13; 2015,Jan,16

50065   secondary surgical operation for calculus
⚕ 34.9   ⚕ 34.9   **FUD** 090   C 80 50 ▣
AMA: 2018,Jan,8; 2017,Jan,8; 2016,Jan,13; 2015,Jan,16

50070   complicated by congenital kidney abnormality
⚕ 34.2   ⚕ 34.2   **FUD** 090   C 80 50 ▣
AMA: 2018,Jan,8; 2017,Jan,8; 2016,Jan,13; 2015,Jan,16

50075   removal of large staghorn calculus filling renal pelvis and calyces (including anatrophic pyelolithotomy)
⚕ 42.1   ⚕ 42.1   **FUD** 090   C 80 50 ▣
AMA: 2018,Jan,8; 2017,Jan,8; 2016,Jan,13; 2015,Jan,16

50080   Percutaneous nephrostolithotomy or pyelostolithotomy, with or without dilation, endoscopy, lithotripsy, stenting, or basket extraction; up to 2 cm

EXCLUDES *Dilation existing tract by same provider ([50436, 50437])*
Nephrostomy without nephrostolithotomy (50040, [50432, 50433], 52334)
⚕ (76000)
⚕ 25.0   ⚕ 25.0   **FUD** 090   J 62 50 ▣
AMA: 2018,Jan,8; 2017,Jan,8; 2016,Jan,13; 2015,Jan,16

50081   over 2 cm

EXCLUDES *Dilation existing tract by same provider ([50436, 50437])*
Nephrostomy without nephrostolithotomy (50040, [50432, 50433], 52334)
⚕ (76000)
⚕ 36.9   ⚕ 36.9   **FUD** 090   J 62 80 50 ▣
AMA: 2018,Jan,8; 2017,Jan,8; 2016,Jan,13; 2015,Jan,16

50100 Repair of Anomalous Vessels of the Kidney

EXCLUDES *Retroperitoneal:*
Abscess drainage (49060)
Exploration (49010)
Tumor/cyst excision (49203-49205)

50100   Transection or repositioning of aberrant renal vessels (separate procedure)
⚕ 31.4   ⚕ 31.4   **FUD** 090   C 80 50 ▣
AMA: 2018,Jan,8; 2017,Jan,8; 2016,Jan,13; 2015,Jan,16

50120-50135 Procedures of Renal Pelvis

EXCLUDES *Retroperitoneal:*
Abscess drainage (49060)
Exploration (49010)
Tumor/cyst excision (49203-49205)

50120   Pyelotomy; with exploration

INCLUDES Gol-Vernet pyelotomy

EXCLUDES *Renal endoscopy through pyelotomy (50570-50580)*
⚕ 27.4   ⚕ 27.4   **FUD** 090   C 80 50 ▣
AMA: 2018,Jan,8; 2017,Jan,8; 2016,Jan,13; 2015,Jan,16

50125   with drainage, pyelostomy
⚕ 28.3   ⚕ 28.3   **FUD** 090   C 80 50 ▣
AMA: 2018,Jan,8; 2017,Jan,8; 2016,Jan,13; 2015,Jan,16

50130   with removal of calculus (pyelolithotomy, pelviolithotomy, including coagulum pyelolithotomy)
⚕ 29.8   ⚕ 29.8   **FUD** 090   C 80 50 ▣
AMA: 2018,Jan,8; 2017,Jan,8; 2016,Jan,13; 2015,Jan,16

50135   complicated (eg, secondary operation, congenital kidney abnormality)
⚕ 32.4   ⚕ 32.4   **FUD** 090   C 80 50 ▣
AMA: 2018,Jan,8; 2017,Jan,8; 2016,Jan,13; 2015,Jan,16

50200-50205 Biopsy of Kidney

EXCLUDES *Laparoscopic renal mass lesion ablation (50542)*
Retroperitoneal tumor/cyst excision (49203-49205)

50200   Renal biopsy; percutaneous, by trocar or needle

EXCLUDES *Fine needle aspiration ([10005, 10006, 10007, 10008, 10009, 10010, 10011, 10012])*
⚕ (76942, 77002, 77012, 77021)
⚕ (88172-88173)
⚕ 3.70   ⚕ 15.4   **FUD** 000   J A2 50 ▣
AMA: 2019,Apr,4; 2018,Jan,8; 2017,Jan,8; 2016,Jan,13; 2015,Jan,16

50205   by surgical exposure of kidney
⚕ 21.9   ⚕ 21.9   **FUD** 090   C 80 50 ▣
AMA: 2018,Jan,8; 2017,Jan,8; 2016,Jan,13; 2015,Jan,16

50220-50240 Nephrectomy Procedures

EXCLUDES *Laparoscopic renal mass lesion ablation (50542)*
Retroperitoneal tumor/cyst excision (49203-49205)

50220   Nephrectomy, including partial ureterectomy, any open approach including rib resection;
⚕ 30.3   ⚕ 30.3   **FUD** 090   C 80 50 ▣
AMA: 2018,Jan,8; 2017,Jan,8; 2016,Jan,13; 2015,Jan,16

● New Code   ▲ Revised Code   ○ Reinstated   ● New Web Release   ▲ Revised Web Release   + Add-on   Unlisted   Not Covered   # Resequenced
50 Optum Mod 50 Exempt   ⊘ AMA Mod 51 Exempt   51 Optum Mod 51 Exempt   63 Mod 63 Exempt   ⩘ Non-FDA Drug   ★ Telemedicine   M Maternity   A Age Edit

50225 **complicated because of previous surgery on same kidney**
34.7 34.7 FUD 090 C 80 50
AMA: 2018,Jan,8; 2017,Jan,8; 2016,Jan,13; 2015,Jan,16

50230 **radical, with regional lymphadenectomy and/or vena caval thrombectomy**
EXCLUDES *Vena caval resection with reconstruction (37799)*
37.0 37.0 FUD 090 C 80 50
AMA: 2018,Jan,8; 2017,Jan,8; 2016,Jan,13; 2015,Jan,16

50234 **Nephrectomy with total ureterectomy and bladder cuff; through same incision**
37.6 37.6 FUD 090 C 80 50
AMA: 2018,Jan,8; 2017,Jan,8; 2016,Jan,13; 2015,Jan,16

50236 **through separate incision**
42.3 42.3 FUD 090 C 80 50
AMA: 2018,Jan,8; 2017,Jan,8; 2016,Jan,13; 2015,Jan,16

50240 **Nephrectomy, partial**
EXCLUDES *Laparoscopic partial nephrectomy (50543)*
38.2 38.2 FUD 090 C 80 50
AMA: 2018,Jan,8; 2017,Jan,8; 2016,Jan,13; 2015,Jan,16

50250-50290 Open Removal Kidney Lesions

EXCLUDES *Open destruction or excision intra-abdominal tumors (49203-49205)*

50250 **Ablation, open, 1 or more renal mass lesion(s), cryosurgical, including intraoperative ultrasound guidance and monitoring, if performed**
EXCLUDES *Laparoscopic renal mass lesion ablation (50542)*
Percutaneous renal tumor ablation (50592-50593)
35.1 35.1 FUD 090 C 80
AMA: 2018,Jan,8; 2017,Jan,8; 2016,Jan,13; 2015,Jan,16

50280 **Excision or unroofing of cyst(s) of kidney**
EXCLUDES *Renal cyst laparoscopic ablation (50541)*
27.6 27.6 FUD 090 C 80 50
AMA: 2018,Jan,8; 2017,Jan,8; 2016,Jan,13; 2015,Jan,16

50290 **Excision of perinephric cyst**
25.9 25.9 FUD 090 C 80
AMA: 2018,Jan,8; 2017,Jan,8; 2016,Jan,13; 2015,Jan,16

50300-50380 Kidney Transplant Procedures

CMS: 100-04,3,90.1 Kidney Transplant - General; 100-04,3,90.1.1 Standard Kidney Acquisition Charge; 100-04,3,90.1.2 Billing for Kidney Transplant and Acquisition Services; 100-04,3,90.5 Pancreas Transplants with Kidney Transplants

EXCLUDES *Dialysis procedures (90935-90999)*
Lymphocele drainage to peritoneal cavity performed laparoscopically (49323)

50300 **Donor nephrectomy (including cold preservation); from cadaver donor, unilateral or bilateral**
INCLUDES Graft:
Cold preservation
Harvesting
EXCLUDES *Donor nephrectomy performed laparoscopically (50547)*
0.00 0.00 FUD XXX C
AMA: 2018,Jan,8; 2017,Jan,8; 2016,Jan,13; 2015,Jan,16

50320 **open, from living donor**
INCLUDES Donor care
Graft:
Cold preservation
Harvesting
EXCLUDES *Donor nephrectomy performed laparoscopically (50547)*
43.7 43.7 FUD 090 C 80 50
AMA: 2018,Jan,8; 2017,Jan,8; 2016,Jan,13; 2015,Jan,16

50323 **Backbench standard preparation of cadaver donor renal allograft prior to transplantation, including dissection and removal of perinephric fat, diaphragmatic and retroperitoneal attachments, excision of adrenal gland, and preparation of ureter(s), renal vein(s), and renal artery(s), ligating branches, as necessary**
EXCLUDES *Adrenalectomy (60540, 60545)*
0.00 0.00 FUD XXX C 80
AMA: 2018,Jan,8; 2017,Jan,8; 2016,Jan,13; 2015,Jan,16

50325 **Backbench standard preparation of living donor renal allograft (open or laparoscopic) prior to transplantation, including dissection and removal of perinephric fat and preparation of ureter(s), renal vein(s), and renal artery(s), ligating branches, as necessary**
0.00 0.00 FUD XXX C 80
AMA: 2014,Jan,11

50327 **Backbench reconstruction of cadaver or living donor renal allograft prior to transplantation; venous anastomosis, each**
6.29 6.29 FUD XXX C 80
AMA: 2014,Jan,11

50328 **arterial anastomosis, each**
5.53 5.53 FUD XXX C 80
AMA: 2014,Jan,11

50329 **ureteral anastomosis, each**
5.24 5.24 FUD XXX C 80
AMA: 2014,Jan,11

50340 **Recipient nephrectomy (separate procedure)**
27.4 27.4 FUD 090 C 80 50
AMA: 2014,Jan,11

50360 **Renal allotransplantation, implantation of graft; without recipient nephrectomy**
INCLUDES Allograft transplantation
Recipient care
Code also backbench work (50323, 50325, 50327-50329)
Code also donor nephrectomy (cadaver or living donor) (50300, 50320, 50547)
70.0 70.0 FUD 090 C 80
AMA: 2014,Jan,11; 1994,Win,1

50365 **with recipient nephrectomy**
INCLUDES Allograft transplantation
Recipient care
83.5 83.5 FUD 090 C 80 50
AMA: 2018,Jan,8; 2017,Jan,8; 2016,Jan,13; 2015,Jan,16

50370 **Removal of transplanted renal allograft**
35.0 35.0 FUD 090 C 80
AMA: 2014,Jan,11; 2002,Oct,5

50380 **Renal autotransplantation, reimplantation of kidney**
INCLUDES Reimplantation autograft
EXCLUDES *Secondary procedures:*
Nephrolithotomy (50060-50075)
Partial nephrectomy (50240, 50543)
58.4 58.4 FUD 090 C 80
AMA: 2019,Sep,10; 2018,Jan,8; 2017,Jan,8; 2016,Jan,13; 2015,Jan,16

50382-50386 Removal With/Without Replacement Internal Ureteral Stent

INCLUDES Radiological supervision and interpretation

50382 **Removal (via snare/capture) and replacement of internally dwelling ureteral stent via percutaneous approach, including radiological supervision and interpretation**

EXCLUDES *Dilation existing tract, percutaneous for endourologic procedure ([50436, 50437])*
Removal and replacement internally dwelling ureteral stent using transurethral approach (50385)

7.46 31.3 FUD 000 J G2 50

AMA: 2018,Jan,8; 2017,Jan,8; 2016,Jan,13; 2016,Jan,3; 2015,Jan,16

50384 **Removal (via snare/capture) of internally dwelling ureteral stent via percutaneous approach, including radiological supervision and interpretation**

EXCLUDES *Dilation existing tract, percutaneous for endourologic procedure ([50436, 50437])*
Removal internally dwelling ureteral stent using transurethral approach (50386)

6.71 24.8 FUD 000 Q2 G2 50

AMA: 2018,Jan,8; 2017,Jan,8; 2016,Jan,13; 2016,Jan,3; 2015,Jan,16

50385 **Removal (via snare/capture) and replacement of internally dwelling ureteral stent via transurethral approach, without use of cystoscopy, including radiological supervision and interpretation**

6.34 30.7 FUD 000 J G2 80 50

AMA: 2018,Jan,8; 2017,Jan,8; 2016,Jan,13; 2016,Jan,3; 2015,Jan,16

50386 **Removal (via snare/capture) of internally dwelling ureteral stent via transurethral approach, without use of cystoscopy, including radiological supervision and interpretation**

4.70 20.3 FUD 000 Q2 P3 80 50

AMA: 2018,Jan,8; 2017,Jan,8; 2016,Jan,3; 2016,Jan,13; 2015,Jan,16

50387 Remove/Replace Accessible Ureteral Stent

EXCLUDES *Removal and replacement ureteral stent through ureterostomy tube or ileal conduit (50688)*
Removal without replacement externally accessible ureteral stent without fluoroscopic guidance, report with appropriate E/M code

50387 **Removal and replacement of externally accessible nephroureteral catheter (eg, external/internal stent) requiring fluoroscopic guidance, including radiological supervision and interpretation**

2.43 14.6 FUD 000 J G2 80 50

AMA: 2018,Jan,8; 2017,Jan,8; 2016,Mar,10; 2016,Jan,13; 2016,Jan,3; 2015,Oct,5; 2015,Jan,16

50389-50435 [50430, 50431, 50432, 50433, 50434, 50435, 50436, 50437] Percutaneous and Injection Procedures With/Without Indwelling Tube/Catheter Access

50389 **Removal of nephrostomy tube, requiring fluoroscopic guidance (eg, with concurrent indwelling ureteral stent)**

EXCLUDES *Nephrostomy tube removal without fluoroscopic guidance, report with appropriate E/M code*

1.56 9.49 FUD 000 Q2 G2 50

AMA: 2018,Jan,8; 2017,Jan,8; 2016,Jan,13; 2016,Jan,3; 2015,Oct,5; 2015,Jan,16

50390 **Aspiration and/or injection of renal cyst or pelvis by needle, percutaneous**

EXCLUDES *Antegrade nephrostogram/pyelogram ([50430, 50431])*
(74425, 74470, 76942, 77002, 77012, 77021)

2.78 2.78 FUD 000 T A2 50

AMA: 2018,Jan,8; 2017,Jan,8; 2016,Jan,13; 2015,Oct,5; 2015,Jan,16

50391 **Instillation(s) of therapeutic agent into renal pelvis and/or ureter through established nephrostomy, pyelostomy or ureterostomy tube (eg, anticarcinogenic or antifungal agent)**

Code also therapeutic agent

2.84 3.52 FUD 000 T P3 50

AMA: 2018,Jan,8; 2017,Jan,8; 2016,Jan,13; 2015,Oct,5; 2015,Jan,16

50436 **Dilation of existing tract, percutaneous, for an endourologic procedure including imaging guidance (eg, ultrasound and/or fluoroscopy) and all associated radiological supervision and interpretation, with postprocedure tube placement, when performed**

EXCLUDES *Percutaneous nephrostolithotomy (50080-50081)*
Procedure performed for same renal collecting system/ureter ([50430, 50431, 50432, 50433], 52334, 74485)
Removal, replacement internally dwelling ureteral stent (50382, 50384)

4.35 4.35 FUD 000 G2 50

50437 **including new access into the renal collecting system**

EXCLUDES *Percutaneous nephrostolithotomy (50080-50081)*
Procedure performed for same renal collecting system/ureter ([50430, 50431, 50432, 50433], 52334, 74485)
Removal, replacement internally dwelling ureteral stent (50382, 50384)

7.29 7.29 FUD 000 G2 50

50396 **Manometric studies through nephrostomy or pyelostomy tube, or indwelling ureteral catheter**

(74425)

3.38 3.38 FUD 000 J A2 80 50

AMA: 2018,Jan,8; 2017,Jan,8; 2016,Jan,13; 2015,Jan,16

50430 **Injection procedure for antegrade nephrostogram and/or ureterogram, complete diagnostic procedure including imaging guidance (eg, ultrasound and fluoroscopy) and all associated radiological supervision and interpretation; new access**

INCLUDES Renal pelvis and associated ureter as single element

EXCLUDES *Procedure performed for same renal collecting system/ureter ([50432, 50433, 50434, 50435], 50693-50695, 74425)*

4.47 13.0 FUD 000 Q2 N1 80 50

AMA: 2018,Jan,8; 2017,Jan,8; 2016,Jan,3; 2016,Jan,13; 2015,Oct,5

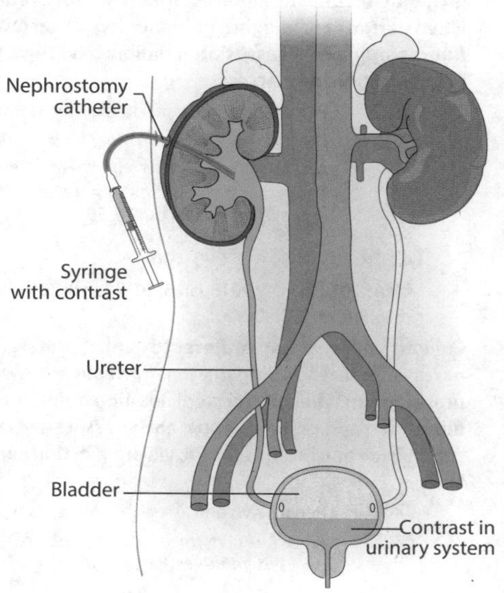

Urinary System

50382 — 50430

\# **50431** **existing access**

INCLUDES Renal pelvis and associated ureter as single element

EXCLUDES *Procedure performed for same renal collecting system/ureter ([50432, 50433, 50434, 50435], 50693-50695, 74425)*

1.90 6.03 **FUD** 000 02 N1 50

AMA: 2018,Jan,8; 2017,Jan,8; 2016,Jan,3; 2016,Jan,13; 2015,Oct,5

\# **50432** **Placement of nephrostomy catheter, percutaneous, including diagnostic nephrostogram and/or ureterogram when performed, imaging guidance (eg, ultrasound and/or fluoroscopy) and all associated radiological supervision and interpretation**

INCLUDES Renal pelvis and associated ureter as single element

EXCLUDES *Dilation nephroureteral catheter tract ([50436, 50437])*

Procedure performed for same renal collecting system/ureter ([50430, 50431], [50433], 50694-50695, 74425)

5.99 21.9 **FUD** 000 J G2 50

AMA: 2018,Mar,11; 2018,Jan,8; 2017,Jan,8; 2016,Jan,3; 2016,Jan,13; 2015,Oct,5

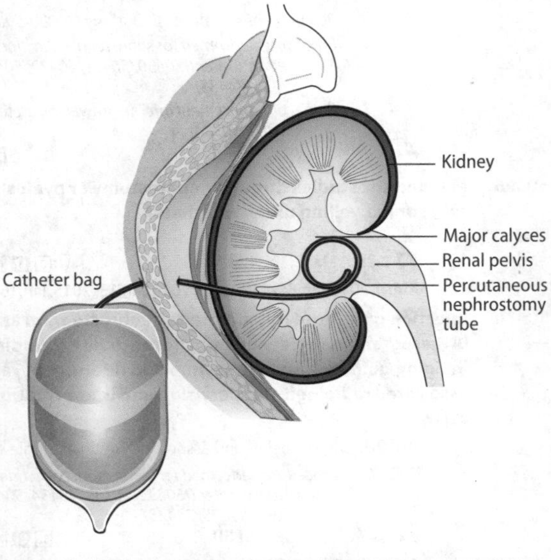

\# **50433** **Placement of nephroureteral catheter, percutaneous, including diagnostic nephrostogram and/or ureterogram when performed, imaging guidance (eg, ultrasound and/or fluoroscopy) and all associated radiological supervision and interpretation, new access**

INCLUDES Renal pelvis and associated ureter as single element

EXCLUDES *Dilation nephroureteral catheter tract ([50436, 50437])*

Nephroureteral catheter removal/replacement (50387)

Procedures performed for same renal collecting system/ureter ([50430, 50431, 50432], 50693-50695, 74425)

7.48 30.0 **FUD** 000 J G2 50

AMA: 2018,Mar,11; 2018,Jan,8; 2017,Jan,8; 2016,Jan,3; 2016,Jan,13; 2015,Oct,5

\# **50434** **Convert nephrostomy catheter to nephroureteral catheter, percutaneous, including diagnostic nephrostogram and/or ureterogram when performed, imaging guidance (eg, ultrasound and/or fluoroscopy) and all associated radiological supervision and interpretation, via pre-existing nephrostomy tract**

INCLUDES Renal pelvis and associated ureter as single element

EXCLUDES *Procedure performed for same renal collecting system/ureter ([50430, 50431], [50435], 50684, 50693, 74425)*

5.63 23.5 **FUD** 000 J J8 50

AMA: 2018,Jan,8; 2017,Jan,8; 2016,Jan,3; 2016,Jan,13; 2015,Oct,5

\# **50435** **Exchange nephrostomy catheter, percutaneous, including diagnostic nephrostogram and/or ureterogram when performed, imaging guidance (eg, ultrasound and/or fluoroscopy) and all associated radiological supervision and interpretation**

INCLUDES Renal pelvis and associated ureter as single element

EXCLUDES *Procedure performed for same renal collecting system/ureter ([50430, 50431], [50434], 50693, 74425)*

Removal nephrostomy catheter requiring fluoroscopic guidance (50389)

2.91 13.4 **FUD** 000 J G2 50

AMA: 2018,Mar,11; 2018,Jan,8; 2017,Jan,8; 2016,Jan,3; 2016,Jan,13; 2015,Oct,5

50400-50540 [50430, 50431, 50432, 50433, 50434, 50435, 50436, 50437] Open Surgical Procedures of Kidney

50400 **Pyeloplasty (Foley Y-pyeloplasty), plastic operation on renal pelvis, with or without plastic operation on ureter, nephropexy, nephrostomy, pyelostomy, or ureteral splinting; simple**

EXCLUDES *Laparoscopic pyeloplasty (50544)*

33.5 33.5 **FUD** 090 C 80 50

AMA: 2018,Jan,8; 2017,Jan,8; 2016,Jan,13; 2015,Jan,16

50405 **complicated (congenital kidney abnormality, secondary pyeloplasty, solitary kidney, calycoplasty)**

EXCLUDES *Laparoscopic pyeloplasty (50544)*

40.3 40.3 **FUD** 090 C 80 50

AMA: 2018,Jan,8; 2017,Jan,8; 2016,Jan,13; 2015,Jan,16

50430 **Resequenced code. See code following 50396.**

50431 **Resequenced code. See code following 50396.**

50432 **Resequenced code. See code following 50396.**

50433 **Resequenced code. See code following 50396.**

50434 **Resequenced code. See code following 50396.**

50435 **Resequenced code. See code following 50396.**

50436 **Resequenced code. See code following 50391.**

50437 **Resequenced code. See code following 50391.**

50500 **Nephrorrhaphy, suture of kidney wound or injury**

37.3 37.3 **FUD** 090 C 80

AMA: 2014,Jan,11

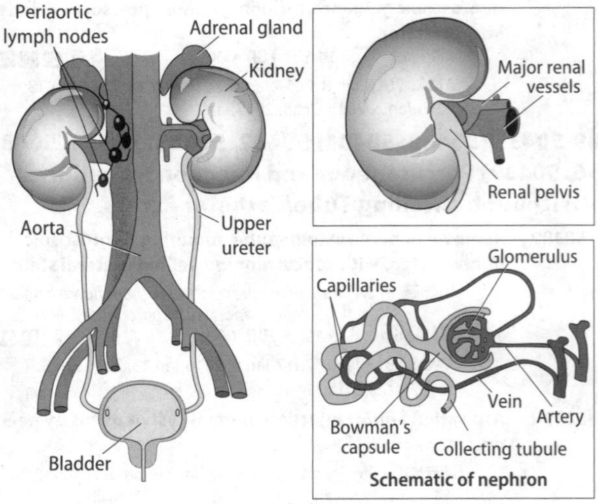

50520 **Closure of nephrocutaneous or pyelocutaneous fistula**

33.6 33.6 **FUD** 090 C 80

AMA: 2014,Jan,11; 2000,Oct,8

50525 **Closure of nephrovisceral fistula (eg, renocolic), including visceral repair; abdominal approach**
42.6 42.6 FUD 090 C 80
AMA: 2014,Jan,11

50526 **thoracic approach**
45.7 45.7 FUD 090 C 80
AMA: 2014,Jan,11

50540 **Symphysiotomy for horseshoe kidney with or without pyeloplasty and/or other plastic procedure, unilateral or bilateral (1 operation)**
33.2 33.2 FUD 090 C 80
AMA: 2014,Jan,11; 2000,Oct,8

50541-50549 Laparoscopic Surgical Procedures of the Kidney

INCLUDES Diagnostic laparoscopy (49320)

EXCLUDES *Laparoscopic drainage lymphocele to peritoneal cavity (49323)*

50541 **Laparoscopy, surgical; ablation of renal cysts**
26.5 26.5 FUD 090 J 80 50
AMA: 2018,Jan,8; 2017,Jan,8; 2016,Jan,13; 2015,Jan,16

50542 **ablation of renal mass lesion(s), including intraoperative ultrasound guidance and monitoring, when performed**
EXCLUDES *Open ablation renal mass lesions (50250)*
Percutaneous ablation renal tumors (50592-50593)
33.7 33.7 FUD 090 J 80 50
AMA: 2018,Jan,8; 2017,Jan,8; 2016,Jan,13; 2015,Jan,16

50543 **partial nephrectomy**
EXCLUDES *Partial nephrectomy, open approach (50240)*
43.0 43.0 FUD 090 J 80 50
AMA: 2018,Jan,8; 2017,Jan,8; 2016,Jan,13; 2015,Jan,16

50544 **pyeloplasty**
36.0 36.0 FUD 090 J 80 50
AMA: 2018,Jan,8; 2017,Jan,8; 2016,Jan,13; 2015,Jan,16

50545 **radical nephrectomy (includes removal of Gerota's fascia and surrounding fatty tissue, removal of regional lymph nodes, and adrenalectomy)**
EXCLUDES *Radical nephrectomy, open approach (50230)*
38.7 38.7 FUD 090 C 80 50
AMA: 2018,Jan,8; 2017,Jan,8; 2016,Jan,13; 2015,Jan,16

50546 **nephrectomy, including partial ureterectomy**
34.8 34.8 FUD 090 C 80 50
AMA: 2018,Jan,8; 2017,Jan,8; 2016,Jan,13; 2015,Jan,16

50547 **donor nephrectomy (including cold preservation), from living donor**
INCLUDES Donor care
Graft:
Cold preservation
Harvesting
EXCLUDES *Backbench reconstruction renal allograft prior to transplantation (50327-50329)*
Backbench standard preparation living donor renal allograft prior to transplantation (50325)
Donor nephrectomy, open approach (50320)
46.4 46.4 FUD 090 C 80 50
AMA: 2018,Jan,8; 2017,Jan,8; 2016,Jan,13; 2015,Jan,16

50548 **nephrectomy with total ureterectomy**
EXCLUDES *Nephrectomy, open approach (50234, 50236)*
38.9 38.9 FUD 090 C 80 50
AMA: 2018,Jan,8; 2017,Jan,8; 2016,Jan,13; 2015,Jan,16

50549 **Unlisted laparoscopy procedure, renal**
0.00 0.00 FUD YYY J 80 50
AMA: 2018,Jan,8; 2017,Jan,8; 2016,Jan,13; 2015,Jan,16

50551-50562 Endoscopic Procedures of Kidney via Established Nephrostomy/Pyelostomy Access

50551 **Renal endoscopy through established nephrostomy or pyelostomy, with or without irrigation, instillation, or ureteropyelography, exclusive of radiologic service;**
8.54 10.4 FUD 000 J A2 80 50
AMA: 2018,Jan,8; 2017,Jan,8; 2016,Jan,13; 2015,Jan,16

50553 **with ureteral catheterization, with or without dilation of ureter**
EXCLUDES *Image-guided ureter dilation without endoscopic guidance (50706)*
9.09 11.1 FUD 000 J A2 50
AMA: 2018,Jan,8; 2017,Jan,8; 2016,Jan,3; 2016,Jan,13; 2015,Jan,16

50555 **with biopsy**
EXCLUDES *Image-guided biopsy ureter/renal pelvis without endoscopic guidance (50606)*
9.88 11.9 FUD 000 J A2 80 50
AMA: 2018,Jan,8; 2017,Jan,8; 2016,Jan,3; 2016,Jan,13; 2015,Jan,16

50557 **with fulguration and/or incision, with or without biopsy**
10.0 12.1 FUD 000 J A2 80 50
AMA: 2018,Jan,8; 2017,Jan,8; 2016,Jan,13; 2015,Jan,16

50561 **with removal of foreign body or calculus**
11.4 13.7 FUD 000 J A2 80 50
AMA: 2018,Jan,8; 2017,Jan,8; 2016,Jan,13; 2015,Jan,16

50562 **with resection of tumor**
16.8 16.8 FUD 090 J G2 80
AMA: 2018,Jan,8; 2017,Jan,8; 2016,Jan,13; 2015,Jan,16

50570-50580 Endoscopic Procedures of Kidney via Nephrotomy/Pyelotomy Access

Code also when provided service significant and identifiable (50045, 50120)

50570 **Renal endoscopy through nephrotomy or pyelotomy, with or without irrigation, instillation, or ureteropyelography, exclusive of radiologic service;**
14.2 14.2 FUD 000 J G2 80 50
AMA: 2018,Jan,8; 2017,Jan,8; 2016,Jan,13; 2015,Jan,16

50572 **with ureteral catheterization, with or without dilation of ureter**
EXCLUDES *Image-guided ureter dilation without endoscopic guidance (50706)*
15.3 15.3 FUD 000 T G2 80 50
AMA: 2018,Jan,8; 2017,Jan,8; 2016,Jan,3; 2016,Jan,13; 2015,Jan,16

50574 **with biopsy**
EXCLUDES *Image-guide ureter/renal pelvis biopsy without endoscopic guidance (50606)*
16.3 16.3 FUD 000 J G2 80 50
AMA: 2018,Jan,8; 2017,Jan,8; 2016,Jan,3; 2016,Jan,13; 2015,Jan,16

50575 **with endopyelotomy (includes cystoscopy, ureteroscopy, dilation of ureter and ureteral pelvic junction, incision of ureteral pelvic junction and insertion of endopyelotomy stent)**
20.6 20.6 FUD 000 J G2 50
AMA: 2018,Jan,8; 2017,Jan,8; 2016,Jan,13; 2015,Jan,16

50576 **with fulguration and/or incision, with or without biopsy**
16.3 16.3 FUD 000 J G2 80 50
AMA: 2018,Jan,8; 2017,Jan,8; 2016,Jan,13; 2015,Jan,16

50580 **with removal of foreign body or calculus**
17.5 17.5 FUD 000 J G2 80 50
AMA: 2018,Jan,8; 2017,Jan,8; 2016,Jan,13; 2015,Jan,16

50590-50593 Noninvasive and Minimally Invasive Procedures of the Kidney

50590 Lithotripsy, extracorporeal shock wave
16.4 | 21.1 | FUD 090 | J G2 50
AMA: 2018,Jan,8; 2017,Jan,8; 2016,Jan,13; 2015,Jan,16

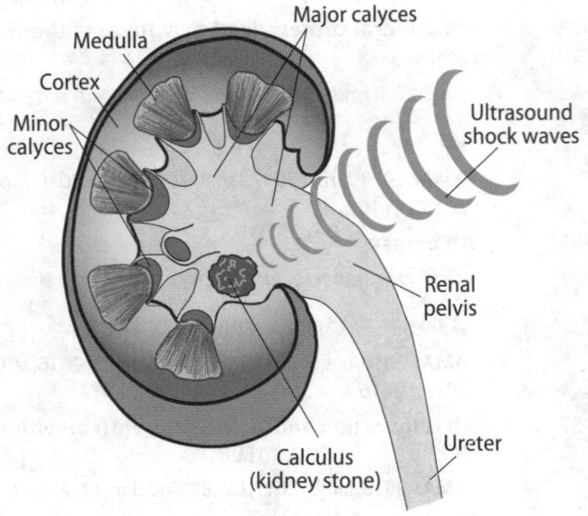

50592 Ablation, 1 or more renal tumor(s), percutaneous, unilateral, radiofrequency
(76940, 77013, 77022)
9.93 | 92.3 | FUD 010 | J G2 50
AMA: 2014,Jan,11

50593 Ablation, renal tumor(s), unilateral, percutaneous, cryotherapy
(76940, 77013, 77022)
13.3 | 125. | FUD 010 | J J8 80 50
AMA: 2018,Jan,8

50600-50940 Open and Injection Procedures of Ureter

50600 Ureterotomy with exploration or drainage (separate procedure)
Code also ureteral endoscopy through ureterotomy when procedures constitute significant identifiable service (50970-50980)
27.1 | 27.1 | FUD 090 | C 80 50
AMA: 2014,Jan,11; 2000,Oct,8

50605 Ureterotomy for insertion of indwelling stent, all types
28.6 | 28.6 | FUD 090 | C 80 50
AMA: 2018,Jan,8; 2017,Jan,8; 2016,Jan,13; 2015,Jan,16

+ **50606 Endoluminal biopsy of ureter and/or renal pelvis, non-endoscopic, including imaging guidance (eg, ultrasound and/or fluoroscopy) and all associated radiological supervision and interpretation (List separately in addition to code for primary procedure)**
INCLUDES Renal pelvis and associated ureter as single element
EXCLUDES *Procedure performed for same renal collecting system/associated ureter with (50555, 50574, 50955, 50974, 52007, 74425)*
Code first (50382-50389, [50430, 50431, 50432, 50433, 50434, 50435], 50684, 50688, 50690, 50693-50695, 51610)
4.46 | 19.9 | FUD ZZZ | N N1 50
AMA: 2018,Jan,8; 2017,Jan,8; 2016,Jan,3

50610 Ureterolithotomy; upper one-third of ureter
EXCLUDES *Cystotomy with calculus basket extraction ureteral calculus (51065)*
Transvesical ureterolithotomy (51060)
Ureteral calculus manipulation/extraction performed endoscopically (50080-50081, 50561, 50961, 50980, 52320-52330, 52352-52353, [52356])
Ureterolithotomy performed laparoscopically (50945)
27.3 | 27.3 | FUD 090 | C 80 50
AMA: 2018,Jan,8; 2017,Jan,8; 2016,Jan,13; 2015,Jan,16

50620 middle one-third of ureter
EXCLUDES *Cystotomy with calculus basket extraction ureteral calculus (51065)*
Transvesical ureterolithotomy (51060)
Ureteral calculus manipulation/extraction performed endoscopically (50080-50081, 50561, 50961, 50980, 52320-52330, 52352-52353, [52356])
Ureterolithotomy performed laparoscopically (50945)
26.1 | 26.1 | FUD 090 | C 80 50
AMA: 2018,Jan,8; 2017,Jan,8; 2016,Jan,13; 2015,Jan,16

50630 lower one-third of ureter
EXCLUDES *Cystotomy with calculus basket extraction ureteral calculus (51065)*
Transvesical ureterolithotomy (51060)
Ureteral calculus manipulation/extraction performed endoscopically (50080-50081, 50561, 50961, 50980, 52320-52330, 52352-52353, [52356])
Ureterolithotomy performed laparoscopically (50945)
25.8 | 25.8 | FUD 090 | C 80 50
AMA: 2018,Jan,8; 2017,Jan,8; 2016,Jan,13; 2015,Jan,16

50650 Ureterectomy, with bladder cuff (separate procedure)
EXCLUDES *Ureterocele (51535, 52300)*
30.0 | 30.0 | FUD 090 | C 80 50
AMA: 2014,Jan,11

50660 Ureterectomy, total, ectopic ureter, combination abdominal, vaginal and/or perineal approach
EXCLUDES *Ureterocele (51535, 52300)*
33.0 | 33.0 | FUD 090 | C 80
AMA: 2014,Jan,11

50684 Injection procedure for ureterography or ureteropyelography through ureterostomy or indwelling ureteral catheter
EXCLUDES *Placement nephroureteral catheter ([50433, 50434])*
Placement ureteral stent (50693-50695)
(74425)
1.45 | 3.10 | FUD 000 | N N1 50
AMA: 2018,Jan,8; 2017,Jan,8; 2016,Jan,3; 2015,Oct,5

50686 Manometric studies through ureterostomy or indwelling ureteral catheter
2.55 | 3.99 | FUD 000 | S P2 80
AMA: 2014,Jan,11

50688 Change of ureterostomy tube or externally accessible ureteral stent via ileal conduit
(75984)
2.25 | 2.25 | FUD 010 | J A2
AMA: 2018,Jan,8; 2017,Jan,8; 2016,Jan,3

50690 Injection procedure for visualization of ileal conduit and/or ureteropyelography, exclusive of radiologic service
Code also radiological supervision and interpretation:
antegrade (74425)
retrograde (74420)
(74420, 74425)
2.02 | 2.87 | FUD 000 | N N1
AMA: 2018,Jan,8; 2017,Jan,8; 2016,Jan,3

50693 **Placement of ureteral stent, percutaneous, including diagnostic nephrostogram and/or ureterogram when performed, imaging guidance (eg, ultrasound and/or fluoroscopy), and all associated radiological supervision and interpretation; pre-existing nephrostomy tract**

INCLUDES Renal pelvis and associated ureter as single element

EXCLUDES *Procedure performed for same renal collecting system/ureter ([50430, 50431, 50432, 50433, 50434, 50435], 50684, 74425)*

5.94 28.0 **FUD** 000 J G2 50

AMA: 2018,Jan,8; 2017,Jan,8; 2016,Jan,3; 2016,Jan,13; 2015,Oct,5

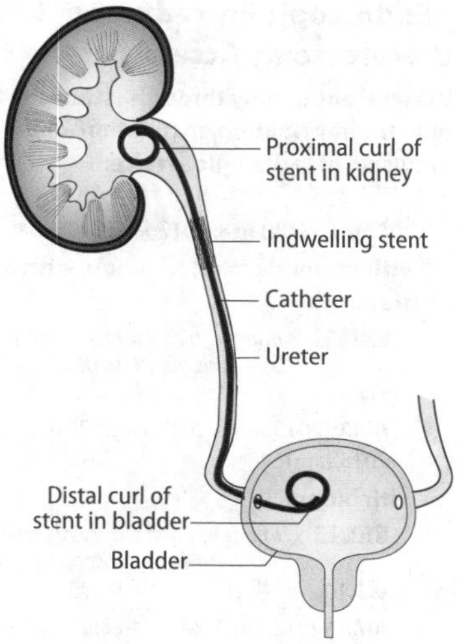

50694 **new access, without separate nephrostomy catheter**

INCLUDES Renal pelvis and associated ureter as single element

EXCLUDES *Procedure performed for same renal collecting system/ureter ([50430, 50431, 50432, 50433, 50434, 50435], 50684, 74425)*

7.78 30.8 **FUD** 000 J G2 50

AMA: 2018,Jan,8; 2017,Jan,8; 2016,Jan,3; 2016,Jan,13; 2015,Oct,5

50695 **new access, with separate nephrostomy catheter**

INCLUDES Placement separate ureteral stent and nephrostomy catheter into ureter/associated renal pelvis through new access

Renal pelvis and associated ureter as single element

EXCLUDES *Procedure performed for same renal collecting system/ureter ([50430, 50431, 50432, 50433, 50434, 50435], 50684, 74425)*

9.96 37.8 **FUD** 000 J G2 50

AMA: 2018,Jan,8; 2017,Jan,8; 2016,Jan,3; 2016,Jan,13; 2015,Oct,5

50700 **Ureteroplasty, plastic operation on ureter (eg, stricture)**

26.7 26.7 **FUD** 090 C 80 50

AMA: 2014,Jan,11

\+ **50705** **Ureteral embolization or occlusion, including imaging guidance (eg, ultrasound and/or fluoroscopy) and all associated radiological supervision and interpretation (List separately in addition to code for primary procedure)**

INCLUDES Renal pelvis and associated ureter as single element

Code also when performed:

Additional catheter insertions

Diagnostic pyelography/ureterography

Other interventions

Code first (50382-50389, [50430, 50431, 50432, 50433, 50434, 50435], 50684, 50688, 50690, 50693-50695, 51610)

5.70 54.9 **FUD** ZZZ N N1 50

AMA: 2018,Jan,8; 2017,Jan,8; 2016,Jan,3

\+ **50706** **Balloon dilation, ureteral stricture, including imaging guidance (eg, ultrasound and/or fluoroscopy) and all associated radiological supervision and interpretation (List separately in addition to code for primary procedure)**

INCLUDES Dilation nephrostomy, ureters, or urethra (74485)

Renal pelvis and associated ureter as single element

EXCLUDES *Cystourethroscopy (52341, 52344-52345)*

Renal endoscopy (50553, 50572)

Ureteral endoscopy (50953, 50972)

Code also when performed:

Additional catheter insertions

Diagnostic pyelography/ureterography

Other interventions

Code first (50382-50389, [50430, 50431, 50432, 50433, 50434, 50435], 50684, 50688, 50690, 50693-50695, 51610)

5.33 28.0 **FUD** ZZZ N N1 50

AMA: 2018,Jan,8; 2017,Jan,8; 2016,Jan,3

50715 **Ureterolysis, with or without repositioning of ureter for retroperitoneal fibrosis**

35.2 35.2 **FUD** 090 C 80 50

AMA: 2014,Jan,11

50722 **Ureterolysis for ovarian vein syndrome** ♀

29.0 29.0 **FUD** 090 C 80

AMA: 2014,Jan,11

50725 **Ureterolysis for retrocaval ureter, with reanastomosis of upper urinary tract or vena cava**

31.9 31.9 **FUD** 090 C 80

AMA: 2014,Jan,11

50727 **Revision of urinary-cutaneous anastomosis (any type urostomy);**

14.7 14.7 **FUD** 090 J G2 80

AMA: 2014,Jan,11; 1992,Win,1

50728 **with repair of fascial defect and hernia**

21.2 21.2 **FUD** 090 C 80

AMA: 2014,Jan,11; 1992,Win,1

50740 **Ureteropyelostomy, anastomosis of ureter and renal pelvis**

35.4 35.4 **FUD** 090 C 80 50

AMA: 2018,Jan,8; 2017,Jan,8; 2016,Jan,13; 2015,Jan,16

50750 **Ureterocalycostomy, anastomosis of ureter to renal calyx**

33.3 33.3 **FUD** 090 C 80 50

AMA: 2018,Jan,8; 2017,Jan,8; 2016,Jan,13; 2015,Jan,16

50760 **Ureteroureterostomy**

32.6 32.6 **FUD** 090 C 80 50

AMA: 2018,Jan,8; 2017,Jan,8; 2016,Jan,13; 2015,Jan,16

50770 **Transureteroureterostomy, anastomosis of ureter to contralateral ureter**

33.3 33.3 **FUD** 090 C 80

AMA: 2014,Jan,11

50780 **Ureteroneocystostomy; anastomosis of single ureter to bladder**

INCLUDES Minor procedures to prevent vesicoureteral reflux

EXCLUDES *Cystourethroplasty with ureteroneocystostomy (51820)*

31.9 31.9 **FUD** 090 C 80 50

AMA: 2018,Feb,11; 2018,Jan,8; 2017,Jan,8; 2016,Jan,13; 2015,Jan,16

50782 **anastomosis of duplicated ureter to bladder**

INCLUDES Minor procedures to prevent vesicoureteral reflux

31.1 31.1 **FUD** 090 C 80 50

AMA: 2018,Jan,8; 2017,Jan,8; 2016,Jan,13; 2015,Jan,16

50783 **with extensive ureteral tailoring**

INCLUDES Minor procedures to prevent vesicoureteral reflux

32.6 32.6 **FUD** 090 C 80 50

AMA: 2018,Jan,8; 2017,Jan,8; 2016,Jan,13; 2015,Jan,16

50785 **with vesico-psoas hitch or bladder flap**

INCLUDES Minor procedures to prevent vesicoureteral reflux

35.1 35.1 **FUD** 090 C 80 50

AMA: 2018,Jan,8; 2017,Jan,8; 2016,Jan,13; 2015,Jan,16

50800 **Ureteroenterostomy, direct anastomosis of ureter to intestine**

EXCLUDES *Cystectomy with ureterosigmoidostomy/ureteroileal conduit (51580-51595)*

26.7 26.7 FUD 090 C 80 50

AMA: 2018,Jan,8; 2017,Jan,8; 2016,Jan,13; 2015,Jan,16

50810 **Ureterosigmoidostomy, with creation of sigmoid bladder and establishment of abdominal or perineal colostomy, including intestine anastomosis**

EXCLUDES *Cystectomy with ureterosigmoidostomy/ureteroileal conduit (51580-51595)*

40.5 40.5 FUD 090 C 80

AMA: 2018,Jan,8; 2017,Jan,8; 2016,Jan,13; 2015,Jan,16

50815 **Ureterocolon conduit, including intestine anastomosis**

EXCLUDES *Cystectomy with ureterosigmoidostomy/ureteroileal conduit (51580-51595)*

35.3 35.3 FUD 090 C 80 50

AMA: 2018,Jan,8; 2017,Jan,8; 2016,Jan,13; 2015,Jan,16

50820 **Ureteroileal conduit (ileal bladder), including intestine anastomosis (Bricker operation)**

EXCLUDES *Cystectomy with ureterosigmoidostomy/ureteroileal conduit (51580-51595)*

38.0 38.0 FUD 090 C 80 50

AMA: 2018,Jan,8; 2017,Jan,8; 2016,Jan,13; 2015,Jan,16

50825 **Continent diversion, including intestine anastomosis using any segment of small and/or large intestine (Kock pouch or Camey enterocystoplasty)**

48.0 48.0 FUD 090 C 80

AMA: 2018,Jan,8; 2017,Jan,8; 2016,Jan,13; 2015,Jan,16

50830 **Urinary undiversion (eg, taking down of ureteroileal conduit, ureterosigmoidostomy or ureteroenterostomy with ureteroureterostomy or ureteroneocystostomy)**

52.0 52.0 FUD 090 C 80

AMA: 2018,Jan,8; 2017,Jan,8; 2016,Jan,13; 2015,Jan,16

50840 **Replacement of all or part of ureter by intestine segment, including intestine anastomosis**

35.5 35.5 FUD 090 C 80 50

AMA: 2018,Jan,8; 2017,Jan,8; 2016,Jan,13; 2015,Jan,16

50845 **Cutaneous appendico-vesicostomy**

INCLUDES Mitrofanoff operation

36.1 36.1 FUD 090 C 80

AMA: 2014,Jan,11; 1993,Win,1

50860 **Ureterostomy, transplantation of ureter to skin**

27.3 27.3 FUD 090 C 80 50

AMA: 2014,Jan,11; 2001,Oct,8

50900 **Ureterorrhaphy, suture of ureter (separate procedure)**

24.3 24.3 FUD 090 C 80 50

AMA: 2014,Jan,11; 2001,Oct,8

50920 **Closure of ureterocutaneous fistula**

25.3 25.3 FUD 090 C 80

AMA: 2014,Jan,11; 2001,Oct,8

50930 **Closure of ureterovisceral fistula (including visceral repair)**

31.8 31.8 FUD 090 C 80

AMA: 2014,Jan,11; 2001,Oct,8

50940 **Deligation of ureter**

EXCLUDES *Ureteroplasty/ureterolysis (50700-50860)*

25.6 25.6 FUD 090 C 80 50

AMA: 2014,Jan,11; 2001,Oct,8

50945-50949 Laparoscopic Procedures of Ureter

INCLUDES Diagnostic laparoscopy (49320)

EXCLUDES *Ureteroneocystostomy, open approach (50780-50785)*

50945 **Laparoscopy, surgical; ureterolithotomy**

28.1 28.1 FUD 090 J 80 50

AMA: 2018,Jan,8; 2017,Jan,8; 2016,Jan,13; 2015,Jan,16

50947 **ureteroneocystostomy with cystoscopy and ureteral stent placement**

40.1 40.1 FUD 090 J A2 80 50

AMA: 2018,Jan,8; 2017,Jan,8; 2016,Jan,13; 2015,Jan,16

50948 **ureteroneocystostomy without cystoscopy and ureteral stent placement**

36.9 36.9 FUD 090 J A2 80 50

AMA: 2018,Jan,8; 2017,Jan,8; 2016,Jan,13; 2015,Jan,16

50949 **Unlisted laparoscopy procedure, ureter**

0.00 0.00 FUD YYY J 80 50

AMA: 2018,Jan,8; 2017,Jan,8; 2016,Jan,13; 2015,Jan,16

50951-50961 Endoscopic Procedures of Ureter via Established Ureterostomy Access

50951 **Ureteral endoscopy through established ureterostomy, with or without irrigation, instillation, or ureteropyelography, exclusive of radiologic service;**

8.89 10.9 FUD 000 J A2 80 50

AMA: 2018,Jan,8; 2017,Jan,8; 2016,Jan,13; 2015,Jan,16

50953 **with ureteral catheterization, with or without dilation of ureter**

EXCLUDES *Image-guided ureter dilation without endoscopic guidance (50706)*

9.46 11.5 FUD 000 J A2 80 50

AMA: 2018,Jan,8; 2017,Jan,8; 2016,Jan,13; 2016,Jan,3; 2015,Jan,16

50955 **with biopsy**

EXCLUDES *Image-guided biopsy of ureter and/or renal pelvis without endoscopic guidance (50606)*

10.2 12.3 FUD 000 J A2 80 50

AMA: 2018,Jan,8; 2017,Jan,8; 2016,Jan,13; 2016,Jan,3; 2015,Jan,16

50957 **with fulguration and/or incision, with or without biopsy**

10.2 12.4 FUD 000 J A2 80 50

AMA: 2018,Jan,8; 2017,Jan,8; 2016,Jan,13; 2015,Jan,16

50961 **with removal of foreign body or calculus**

9.17 11.1 FUD 000 J A2 80 50

AMA: 2018,Jan,8; 2017,Jan,8; 2016,Jan,13; 2015,Jan,16

50970-50980 Endoscopic Procedures of Ureter via Ureterotomy

EXCLUDES *Ureterotomy (50600)*

50970 **Ureteral endoscopy through ureterotomy, with or without irrigation, instillation, or ureteropyelography, exclusive of radiologic service;**

10.7 10.7 FUD 000 J A2 80 50

AMA: 2018,Jan,8; 2017,Jan,8; 2016,Jan,13; 2015,Jan,16

50972 **with ureteral catheterization, with or without dilation of ureter**

EXCLUDES *Image-guided ureter dilation without endoscopic guidance (50706)*

10.3 10.3 FUD 000 J A2 80 50

AMA: 2018,Jan,8; 2017,Jan,8; 2016,Jan,3; 2016,Jan,13; 2015,Jan,16

50974 **with biopsy**

EXCLUDES *Image-guided biopsy of ureter and/or renal pelvis without endoscopic guidance (50606)*

13.6 13.6 FUD 000 J A2 80 50

AMA: 2018,Jan,8; 2017,Jan,8; 2016,Jan,3; 2016,Jan,13; 2015,Jan,16

50976 **with fulguration and/or incision, with or without biopsy**

13.5 13.5 FUD 000 J A2 80 50

AMA: 2018,Jan,8; 2017,Jan,8; 2016,Jan,13; 2015,Jan,16

50980 **with removal of foreign body or calculus**

10.3 10.3 FUD 000 J A2 80 50

AMA: 2018,Jan,8; 2017,Jan,8; 2016,Jan,13; 2015,Jan,16

51020-51080 Open Incisional Procedures of Bladder

51020 **Cystotomy or cystostomy; with fulguration and/or insertion of radioactive material**
13.5 13.5 FUD 090 J A2 80
AMA: 2014,Jan,11

51030 **with cryosurgical destruction of intravesical lesion**
13.6 13.6 FUD 090 J A2 80
AMA: 2014,Jan,11

51040 **Cystostomy, cystotomy with drainage**
8.36 8.36 FUD 090 J A2 80
AMA: 2014,Jan,11

51045 **Cystotomy, with insertion of ureteral catheter or stent (separate procedure)**
14.2 14.2 FUD 090 J A2 80
AMA: 2014,Jan,11

51050 **Cystolithotomy, cystotomy with removal of calculus, without vesical neck resection**
13.6 13.6 FUD 090 J A2 80
AMA: 2014,Jan,11

51060 **Transvesical ureterolithotomy**
16.8 16.8 FUD 090 J 80
AMA: 2014,Jan,11

51065 **Cystotomy, with calculus basket extraction and/or ultrasonic or electrohydraulic fragmentation of ureteral calculus**
16.7 16.7 FUD 090 J A2 80
AMA: 2014,Jan,11; 2002,May,7

51080 **Drainage of perivesical or prevesical space abscess**
EXCLUDES *Image-guided percutaneous catheter drainage (49406)*
11.8 11.8 FUD 090 J A2 80
AMA: 2014,Jan,11

51100-51102 Bladder Aspiration Procedures

51100 **Aspiration of bladder; by needle**
(76942, 77002, 77012)
1.12 1.95 FUD 000 T P3
AMA: 2018,Jan,8; 2017,Jan,8; 2016,Jan,13; 2015,Jan,16

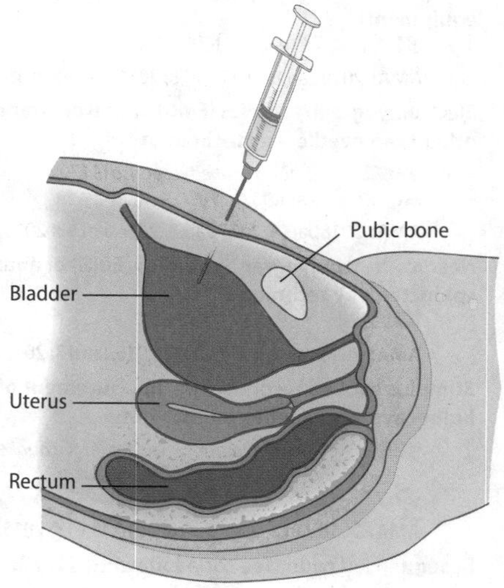

51101 **by trocar or intracatheter**
(76942, 77002, 77012)
1.50 3.79 FUD 000 S P3
AMA: 2018,Jan,8; 2017,Jan,8; 2016,Jan,13; 2015,Jan,16

51102 **with insertion of suprapubic catheter**
(76942, 77002, 77012)
4.18 6.60 FUD 000 J A2
AMA: 2018,Jan,8; 2017,Jan,8; 2016,Jan,13; 2015,Jan,16

51500-51597 Open Excisional Procedures of Bladder

51500 **Excision of urachal cyst or sinus, with or without umbilical hernia repair**
18.4 18.4 FUD 090 J A2 80
AMA: 2014,Jan,11

51520 **Cystotomy; for simple excision of vesical neck (separate procedure)**
17.2 17.2 FUD 090 J A2 80
AMA: 2014,Jan,11

51525 **for excision of bladder diverticulum, single or multiple (separate procedure)**
EXCLUDES *Transurethral resection (52305)*
24.8 24.8 FUD 090 C 80
AMA: 2014,Jan,11

51530 **for excision of bladder tumor**
EXCLUDES *Transurethral resection (52234-52240, 52305)*
22.2 22.2 FUD 090 C 80
AMA: 2014,Jan,11

51535 **Cystotomy for excision, incision, or repair of ureterocele**
EXCLUDES *Transurethral excision (52300)*
22.5 22.5 FUD 090 J 62 80 50
AMA: 2014,Jan,11; 1993,Sum,25

51550 **Cystectomy, partial; simple**
27.9 27.9 FUD 090 C 80
AMA: 2014,Jan,11

51555 **complicated (eg, postradiation, previous surgery, difficult location)**
36.6 36.6 FUD 090 C 80
AMA: 2014,Jan,11

51565 **Cystectomy, partial, with reimplantation of ureter(s) into bladder (ureteroneocystostomy)**
37.5 37.5 FUD 090 C 80
AMA: 2014,Jan,11

51570 **Cystectomy, complete; (separate procedure)**
42.6 42.6 FUD 090 C 80
AMA: 2014,Jan,11; 1993,Spr,34

51575 **with bilateral pelvic lymphadenectomy, including external iliac, hypogastric, and obturator nodes**
52.7 52.7 FUD 090 C 80
AMA: 2014,Jan,11; 1993,Spr,34

51580 **Cystectomy, complete, with ureterosigmoidostomy or ureterocutaneous transplantations;**
54.8 54.8 FUD 090 C 80
AMA: 2014,Jan,11; 1993,Spr,34

51585 **with bilateral pelvic lymphadenectomy, including external iliac, hypogastric, and obturator nodes**
61.0 61.0 FUD 090 C 80
AMA: 2014,Jan,11; 1993,Spr,34

51590 **Cystectomy, complete, with ureteroileal conduit or sigmoid bladder, including intestine anastomosis;**
55.9 55.9 FUD 090 C 80
AMA: 2014,Jan,11; 2002,May,7

51595 **with bilateral pelvic lymphadenectomy, including external iliac, hypogastric, and obturator nodes**
63.3 63.3 FUD 090 C 80
AMA: 2014,Jan,11; 2002,May,7

51596 **Cystectomy, complete, with continent diversion, any open technique, using any segment of small and/or large intestine to construct neobladder**
68.1 68.1 FUD 090 C 80
AMA: 2014,Jan,11; 2002,May,7

51597 **Pelvic exenteration, complete, for vesical, prostatic or urethral malignancy, with removal of bladder and ureteral transplantations, with or without hysterectomy and/or abdominoperineal resection of rectum and colon and colostomy, or any combination thereof**

EXCLUDES *Pelvic exenteration for gynecologic malignancy (58240)*

66.3 66.3 **FUD** 090 C 80

AMA: 2014,Jan,11

51600-51720 Injection/Insertion/Instillation Procedures of Bladder

51600 **Injection procedure for cystography or voiding urethrocystography**

(74430, 74455)

1.29 5.57 **FUD** 000 N N1

AMA: 2019,Oct,10

51605 **Injection procedure and placement of chain for contrast and/or chain urethrocystography**

(74430)

1.12 1.12 **FUD** 000 N N1

AMA: 2014,Jan,11

51610 **Injection procedure for retrograde urethrocystography**

(74450)

1.85 3.21 **FUD** 000 N N1

AMA: 2019,Oct,10; 2018,Jan,8; 2017,Jan,8; 2016,Jan,3

51700 **Bladder irrigation, simple, lavage and/or instillation**

0.87 2.12 **FUD** 000 T P3

AMA: 2014,Jan,11

51701 **Insertion of non-indwelling bladder catheter (eg, straight catheterization for residual urine)**

EXCLUDES *Catheterization for specimen collection (P9612)*
Insertion catheter as another procedure component

0.73 1.27 **FUD** 000 Q1 N1

AMA: 2018,Jan,8; 2017,Jan,8; 2016,Jan,13; 2015,Jan,16

51702 **Insertion of temporary indwelling bladder catheter; simple (eg, Foley)**

EXCLUDES *Focused ultrasound ablation uterine leiomyomata (0071T-0072T)*
Insertion catheter as another procedure component

0.73 1.76 **FUD** 000 Q1 N1

AMA: 2018,Jan,8; 2017,Jan,8; 2016,Jan,13; 2015,Jan,16

51703 **complicated (eg, altered anatomy, fractured catheter/balloon)**

2.23 3.78 **FUD** 000 S P2

AMA: 2018,Jan,8; 2017,Jan,8; 2016,Jan,13; 2015,Jan,16

51705 **Change of cystostomy tube; simple**

1.50 2.67 **FUD** 000 T P3

AMA: 2018,Jan,8; 2017,Jan,8; 2016,Jan,13; 2015,Jan,16

51710 **complicated**

(75984)

2.30 3.69 **FUD** 000 T A2

AMA: 2018,Jan,8; 2017,Jan,8; 2016,Jan,13; 2015,Jan,16

51715 **Endoscopic injection of implant material into the submucosal tissues of the urethra and/or bladder neck**

EXCLUDES *Injection bulking agent (submucosal) for fecal incontinence, via anoscope (46999)*

5.76 9.07 **FUD** 000 J J8 80

AMA: 2014,Jan,11; 1993,Win,1

51720 **Bladder instillation of anticarcinogenic agent (including retention time)**

Code also bacillus Calmette-Guerin vaccine (BCG) (90586)

1.27 2.40 **FUD** 000 T P3

AMA: 2020,Jan,11; 2018,Jan,8; 2017,Jan,8; 2016,Jan,13; 2015,Jan,16

51725-51798 [51797] Uroflowmetric Evaluations

INCLUDES Equipment
Fees for technician services
Medications
Supplies

Code also modifier 26 when physician/other qualified health care professional provides only interpretation results and/or operates equipment

51725 **Simple cystometrogram (CMG) (eg, spinal manometer)**

5.69 5.69 **FUD** 000 T P2 80

AMA: 2018,Jan,8; 2017,Jan,8; 2016,Jan,13; 2015,Jan,16

51726 **Complex cystometrogram (ie, calibrated electronic equipment);**

8.23 8.23 **FUD** 000 T A2

AMA: 2018,Jan,8; 2017,Jan,8; 2016,Jan,13; 2015,Jan,16

51727 **with urethral pressure profile studies (ie, urethral closure pressure profile), any technique**

9.88 9.88 **FUD** 000 T P3 80

AMA: 2018,Jan,8; 2017,Jan,8; 2016,Jan,13; 2015,Jan,16

51728 **with voiding pressure studies (ie, bladder voiding pressure), any technique**

9.55 9.55 **FUD** 000 T P3 80

AMA: 2018,Jan,8; 2017,Jan,8; 2016,Jan,13; 2015,Jan,16

51729 **with voiding pressure studies (ie, bladder voiding pressure) and urethral pressure profile studies (ie, urethral closure pressure profile), any technique**

10.6 10.6 **FUD** 000 T P3 80

AMA: 2018,Jan,8; 2017,Jan,8; 2016,Jan,13; 2015,Jan,16

\+ # **51797** **Voiding pressure studies, intra-abdominal (ie, rectal, gastric, intraperitoneal) (List separately in addition to code for primary procedure)**

Code first (51728-51729)

4.61 4.61 **FUD** ZZZ N N1 80

AMA: 2018,Jan,8; 2017,Jan,8; 2016,Jan,13; 2015,Jan,16

51736 **Simple uroflowmetry (UFR) (eg, stop-watch flow rate, mechanical uroflowmeter)**

0.40 0.40 **FUD** XXX Q1 N1 80

AMA: 2018,Jan,8; 2017,Jan,8; 2016,Jan,13; 2015,Jan,16

51741 **Complex uroflowmetry (eg, calibrated electronic equipment)**

0.41 0.41 **FUD** XXX Q1 N1

AMA: 2018,Jan,8; 2017,Jan,8; 2016,Jan,13; 2015,Jan,16

51784 **Electromyography studies (EMG) of anal or urethral sphincter, other than needle, any technique**

EXCLUDES *Stimulus evoked response (51792)*

1.93 1.93 **FUD** XXX S P3

AMA: 2018,Jan,8; 2017,Jan,8; 2016,Jan,13; 2015,Jan,16

51785 **Needle electromyography studies (EMG) of anal or urethral sphincter, any technique**

9.17 9.17 **FUD** XXX T A2 80

AMA: 2018,Jan,8; 2017,Jan,8; 2016,Jan,13; 2015,Jan,16

51792 **Stimulus evoked response (eg, measurement of bulbocavernosus reflex latency time)**

EXCLUDES *Electromyography studies (EMG) anal or urethral sphincter (51784)*

7.04 7.04 **FUD** 000 Q1 N1 80

AMA: 2018,Jan,8; 2017,Jan,8; 2016,Jan,13; 2015,Jan,16

51797 **Resequenced code. See code following 51729.**

51798 **Measurement of post-voiding residual urine and/or bladder capacity by ultrasound, non-imaging**

0.36 0.36 **FUD** XXX Q1 N1 80 TC

AMA: 2018,Jun,11; 2018,Jan,8; 2017,Jan,8; 2016,Jan,13; 2015,Jan,16

CPT © 2020 American Medical Association. All Rights Reserved. © 2020 Optum360, LLC

51800-51980 Open Repairs Urinary System

51800 Cystoplasty or cystourethroplasty, plastic operation on bladder and/or vesical neck (anterior Y-plasty, vesical fundus resection), any procedure, with or without wedge resection of posterior vesical neck
30.3 30.3 FUD 090 C 80
AMA: 2014,Jan,11

51820 Cystourethroplasty with unilateral or bilateral ureteroneocystostomy
31.3 31.3 FUD 090 C 80
AMA: 2014,Jan,11

51840 Anterior vesicourethropexy, or urethropexy (eg, Marshall-Marchetti-Krantz, Burch); simple
EXCLUDES *Pereyra type urethropexy (57289)*
19.3 19.3 FUD 090 C 80
AMA: 2018,Jan,8; 2017,Jan,8; 2016,Jan,13; 2015,Jan,16

51841 complicated (eg, secondary repair)
EXCLUDES *Pereyra type urethropexy (57289)*
22.4 22.4 FUD 090 C 80
AMA: 2018,Jan,8; 2017,Jan,8; 2016,Jan,13; 2015,Jan,16

51845 Abdomino-vaginal vesical neck suspension, with or without endoscopic control (eg, Stamey, Raz, modified Pereyra) ♀
16.8 16.8 FUD 090 J 80
AMA: 2018,Jan,8; 2017,Jan,8; 2016,Jan,13; 2015,Jan,16

51860 Cystorrhaphy, suture of bladder wound, injury or rupture; simple
21.5 21.5 FUD 090 J 80
AMA: 2014,Jan,11

51865 complicated
25.9 25.9 FUD 090 C 80
AMA: 2014,Jan,11

51880 Closure of cystostomy (separate procedure)
13.5 13.5 FUD 090 J A2 80
AMA: 2014,Jan,11

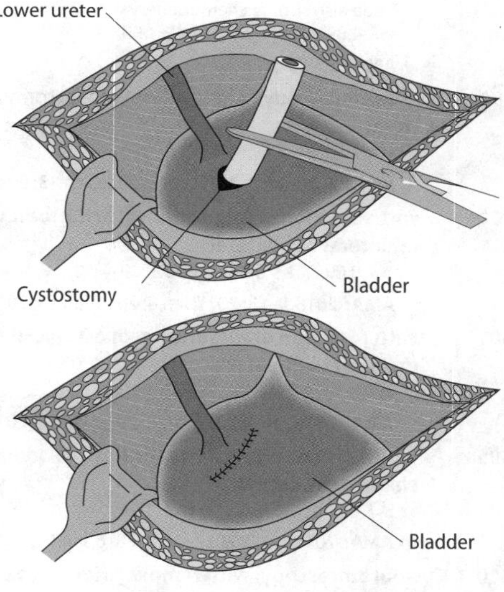

Physician removes a cystostomy tube

51900 Closure of vesicovaginal fistula, abdominal approach ♀
EXCLUDES *Vesicovaginal fistula closure, vaginal approach (57320-57330)*
23.9 23.9 FUD 090 C 80
AMA: 2014,Jan,11

51920 Closure of vesicouterine fistula; ♀
EXCLUDES *Enterovesical fistula closure (44660-44661)*
Rectovesical fistula closure (45800-45805)
22.0 22.0 FUD 090 C 80
AMA: 2014,Jan,11

51925 with hysterectomy ♀
EXCLUDES *Enterovesical fistula closure (44660-44661)*
Rectovesical fistula closure (45800-45805)
29.5 29.5 FUD 090 C 80
AMA: 2014,Jan,11

51940 Closure, exstrophy of bladder
EXCLUDES *Epispadias reconstruction with exstrophy bladder (54390)*
47.5 47.5 FUD 090 C 80
AMA: 2014,Jan,11; 2002,May,7

51960 Enterocystoplasty, including intestinal anastomosis
40.1 40.1 FUD 090 C 80
AMA: 2014,Jan,11; 2002,May,7

51980 Cutaneous vesicostomy
20.6 20.6 FUD 090 C 80
AMA: 2014,Jan,11

51990-51999 Laparoscopic Procedures of Urinary System

CMS: 100-03,230.10 Incontinence Control Devices
INCLUDES Diagnostic laparoscopy (49320)

51990 Laparoscopy, surgical; urethral suspension for stress incontinence
21.6 21.6 FUD 090 J 80
AMA: 2019,Feb,10; 2018,Jan,8; 2017,Jan,8; 2016,Jan,13; 2015,Jan,16

51992 sling operation for stress incontinence (eg, fascia or synthetic)
EXCLUDES *Removal/revision sling for stress incontinence (57287)*
Sling operation for stress incontinence, open approach (57288)
24.0 24.0 FUD 090 J J8 80
AMA: 2019,Feb,10; 2018,Jan,8; 2017,Jan,8; 2016,Jan,13; 2015,Jan,16

51999 Unlisted laparoscopy procedure, bladder
0.00 0.00 FUD YYY J 80
AMA: 2018,Jan,8; 2017,Dec,14

52000-52318 Endoscopic Procedures via Urethra: Bladder and Urethra

INCLUDES Diagnostic and therapeutic endoscopy bowel segments utilized as replacements for native bladder

52000 Cystourethroscopy (separate procedure)
EXCLUDES *Cystourethroscopy (52001, 52320, 52325, 52327, 52330, 52332, 52334, 52341-52343, [52356], 57240, 57260, 57265)*
2.34 5.39 FUD 000 T A2
AMA: 2019,Feb,10; 2018,Nov,10; 2018,Jan,8; 2017,Oct,9; 2017,Jan,8; 2016,Jan,13; 2015,Jan,16

52001 Cystourethroscopy with irrigation and evacuation of multiple obstructing clots
INCLUDES Cystourethroscopy (separate procedure) (52000)
8.31 11.3 FUD 000 J A2
AMA: 2014,Jan,11; 2001,May,5

52005 Cystourethroscopy, with ureteral catheterization, with or without irrigation, instillation, or ureteropyelography, exclusive of radiologic service;
INCLUDES Howard test
3.81 8.37 FUD 000 J A2
AMA: 2019,Mar,10; 2018,Jan,8; 2017,Jan,8; 2016,Jan,13; 2015,Jan,16

52007 **with brush biopsy of ureter and/or renal pelvis**
EXCLUDES *Image-guided ureter/renal pelvis biopsy without endoscopic guidance (50606)*
4.80 13.1 FUD 000 J A2 50
AMA: 2018,Jan,8; 2017,Jan,8; 2016,Jan,13; 2016,Jan,3; 2015,Jan,16

52010 **Cystourethroscopy, with ejaculatory duct catheterization, with or without irrigation, instillation, or duct radiography, exclusive of radiologic service** ♂
(74440)
4.79 10.9 FUD 000 T A2
AMA: 2018,Jan,8; 2017,Jan,8; 2016,Jan,13; 2015,Jan,16

52204 **Cystourethroscopy, with biopsy(s)**
4.08 10.8 FUD 000 J A2
AMA: 2018,Jan,8; 2017,Jan,8; 2016,May,12; 2016,Jan,13; 2015,Jan,16

52214 **Cystourethroscopy, with fulguration (including cryosurgery or laser surgery) of trigone, bladder neck, prostatic fossa, urethra, or periurethral glands**
Code also modifier 78 when performed by same physician:
- During postoperative period (52601, 52630)
- During postoperative period related surgical procedure
- For postoperative bleeding

5.10 20.0 FUD 000 J A2
AMA: 2018,Jan,8; 2017,Jan,8; 2016,May,12; 2016,Jan,13; 2015,Jan,16

52224 **Cystourethroscopy, with fulguration (including cryosurgery or laser surgery) or treatment of MINOR (less than 0.5 cm) lesion(s) with or without biopsy**
5.89 20.9 FUD 000 J A2
AMA: 2018,Jan,8; 2017,Jan,8; 2016,May,12; 2016,Jan,13; 2015,Jan,16

52234 **Cystourethroscopy, with fulguration (including cryosurgery or laser surgery) and/or resection of; SMALL bladder tumor(s) (0.5 up to 2.0 cm)**
EXCLUDES *Bladder tumor excision through cystotomy (51530)*
7.12 7.12 FUD 000 J A2
AMA: 2018,Jan,8; 2017,Jan,8; 2016,May,12; 2016,Jan,13; 2015,Jan,16

52235 **MEDIUM bladder tumor(s) (2.0 to 5.0 cm)**
EXCLUDES *Bladder tumor excision through cystotomy (51530)*
8.34 8.34 FUD 000 J A2
AMA: 2018,Jan,8; 2017,Jan,8; 2016,May,12; 2016,Jan,13; 2015,Jan,16

52240 **LARGE bladder tumor(s)**
EXCLUDES *Bladder tumor excision through cystotomy (51530)*
11.3 11.3 FUD 000 J A2
AMA: 2018,Jan,8; 2017,Jan,8; 2016,May,12; 2016,Jan,13; 2015,Jan,16

52250 **Cystourethroscopy with insertion of radioactive substance, with or without biopsy or fulguration**
6.92 6.92 FUD 000 J A2
AMA: 2018,Jan,8; 2017,Jan,8; 2016,Jan,13; 2015,Jan,16

52260 **Cystourethroscopy, with dilation of bladder for interstitial cystitis; general or conduction (spinal) anesthesia**
6.07 6.07 FUD 000 J A2
AMA: 2018,Jan,8; 2017,Jan,8; 2016,Jan,13; 2015,Jan,16

52265 **local anesthesia**
4.67 10.6 FUD 000 J P3
AMA: 2018,Jan,8; 2017,Jan,8; 2016,Jan,13; 2015,Jan,16

52270 **Cystourethroscopy, with internal urethrotomy; female** ♀
5.27 10.9 FUD 000 J A2
AMA: 2018,Jan,8; 2017,Jan,8; 2016,Jan,13; 2015,Jan,16

52275 **male** ♂
7.19 14.4 FUD 000 J A2
AMA: 2018,Jan,8; 2017,Jan,8; 2016,Jan,13; 2015,Jan,16

52276 **Cystourethroscopy with direct vision internal urethrotomy**
7.65 7.65 FUD 000 J A2
AMA: 2019,Feb,10; 2018,Jan,8; 2017,Jan,8; 2016,Jan,13; 2015,Jan,16

52277 **Cystourethroscopy, with resection of external sphincter (sphincterotomy)**
9.35 9.35 FUD 000 J A2 80
AMA: 2018,Jan,8; 2017,Jan,8; 2016,Jan,13; 2015,Jan,16

52281 **Cystourethroscopy, with calibration and/or dilation of urethral stricture or stenosis, with or without meatotomy, with or without injection procedure for cystography, male or female**
EXCLUDES *Urethral delivery therapeutic drug (0499T)*
4.40 8.53 FUD 000 J A2
AMA: 2018,Jan,8; 2017,Oct,9; 2017,Jan,8; 2016,Jan,13; 2015,Jan,16

52282 **Cystourethroscopy, with insertion of permanent urethral stent**
EXCLUDES *Placement temporary prostatic urethral stent (53855)*
9.76 9.76 FUD 000 J A2
AMA: 2018,Jan,8; 2017,Jan,8; 2016,Jan,13; 2015,Jun,5; 2015,Jan,16

52283 **Cystourethroscopy, with steroid injection into stricture**
5.83 8.68 FUD 000 J A2
AMA: 2019,Feb,10; 2018,Jan,8; 2017,Jan,8; 2016,Jan,13; 2015,Mar,9; 2015,Jan,16

52285 **Cystourethroscopy for treatment of the female urethral syndrome with any or all of the following: urethral meatotomy, urethral dilation, internal urethrotomy, lysis of urethrovaginal septal fibrosis, lateral incisions of the bladder neck, and fulguration of polyp(s) of urethra, bladder neck, and/or trigone** ♀
5.66 8.66 FUD 000 J A2
AMA: 2018,Jan,8; 2017,Jan,8; 2016,Jan,13; 2015,Jan,16

52287 **Cystourethroscopy, with injection(s) for chemodenervation of the bladder**
Code also supply chemodenervation agent
4.89 9.65 FUD 000 J G2
AMA: 2019,Apr,9

52290 **Cystourethroscopy; with ureteral meatotomy, unilateral or bilateral**
7.10 7.10 FUD 000 J A2
AMA: 2018,Jan,8; 2017,Jan,8; 2016,Jan,13; 2015,Jan,16

52300 **with resection or fulguration of orthotopic ureterocele(s), unilateral or bilateral**
8.09 8.09 FUD 000 J A2 80
AMA: 2018,Jan,8; 2017,Jan,8; 2016,Jan,13; 2015,Jan,16

52301 **with resection or fulguration of ectopic ureterocele(s), unilateral or bilateral**
8.38 8.38 FUD 000 J A2 80
AMA: 2018,Jan,8; 2017,Jan,8; 2016,Jan,13; 2015,Jan,16

52305 **with incision or resection of orifice of bladder diverticulum, single or multiple**
8.06 8.06 FUD 000 J A2
AMA: 2018,Jan,8; 2017,Jan,8; 2016,Jan,13; 2015,Jan,16

52310 **Cystourethroscopy, with removal of foreign body, calculus, or ureteral stent from urethra or bladder (separate procedure); simple**
Code also modifier 58 for removal self-retaining, indwelling ureteral stent
4.39 7.03 FUD 000 J A2
AMA: 2018,Jan,8; 2017,Jan,8; 2016,Jan,13; 2015,Jun,5; 2015,Jan,16

52315 **complicated**
Code also modifier 58 for removal self-retaining, indwelling ureteral stent
7.94 12.6 FUD 000 J A2
AMA: 2018,Jan,8; 2017,Jan,8; 2016,Jan,13; 2015,Jan,16

52317 **Lithopaxy: crushing or fragmentation of calculus by any means in bladder and removal of fragments; simple or small (less than 2.5 cm)**

10.0 24.1 FUD 000 J A2

AMA: 2018,Jan,8; 2017,Jan,8; 2016,Jan,13; 2015,Jan,16

52318 **complicated or large (over 2.5 cm)**

13.7 13.7 FUD 000 J A2

AMA: 2018,Jan,8; 2017,Jan,8; 2016,Jan,13; 2015,Jan,16

52320-52356 [52356] Endoscopic Procedures via Urethra: Renal Pelvis and Ureter

INCLUDES Diagnostic cystourethroscopy when performed with therapeutic cystourethroscopy

Insertion/removal temporary ureteral catheter (52005)

EXCLUDES *Self-retaining/indwelling ureteral stent removal by cystourethroscope, with modifier 58 when appropriate (52310, 52315)*

Code also insertion indwelling stent performed in addition to other procedures within this section (52332)

52320 **Cystourethroscopy (including ureteral catheterization); with removal of ureteral calculus**

INCLUDES Cystourethroscopy (separate procedure) (52000)

7.13 7.13 FUD 000 J A2 50

AMA: 2018,Jan,8; 2017,Jan,8; 2016,Jan,13; 2015,Jan,16

52325 **with fragmentation of ureteral calculus (eg, ultrasonic or electro-hydraulic technique)**

INCLUDES Cystourethroscopy (separate procedure) (52000)

9.27 9.27 FUD 000 J A2 50

AMA: 2018,Jan,8; 2017,Jan,8; 2016,Jan,13; 2015,Jan,16

52327 **with subureteric injection of implant material**

INCLUDES Cystourethroscopy (separate procedure) (52000)

7.59 7.59 FUD 000 J J8 50

AMA: 2018,Jan,8; 2017,Jan,8; 2016,Jan,13; 2015,Jan,16

52330 **with manipulation, without removal of ureteral calculus**

INCLUDES Cystourethroscopy (separate procedure) (52000)

7.63 15.4 FUD 000 J A2 50

AMA: 2018,Jan,8; 2017,Jan,8; 2016,Jan,13; 2015,Jan,16

52332 **Cystourethroscopy, with insertion of indwelling ureteral stent (eg, Gibbons or double-J type)**

INCLUDES Cystourethroscopy (separate procedure) (52000)

EXCLUDES *Cystourethroscopy, with ureteroscopy and/or pyeloscopy; with lithotripsy when performed on same side with (52353, [52356])*

4.50 13.5 FUD 000 J A2 50

AMA: 2019,Dec,12; 2018,Jan,8; 2017,Jan,8; 2016,Jan,13; 2015,Jan,16

52334 **Cystourethroscopy with insertion of ureteral guide wire through kidney to establish a percutaneous nephrostomy, retrograde**

INCLUDES Cystourethroscopy (separate procedure) (52000)

EXCLUDES *Cystourethroscopy with incision/fulguration/resection congenital posterior urethral valves/obstructive hypertrophic mucosal folds (52400)*

Cystourethroscopy with pyeloscopy and/or ureteroscopy (52351-52353 [52356])

Dilation nephroureteral catheter tract ([50436], [50437])

Nephrostomy tract establishment only ([50432, 50433])

Percutaneous nephrostolithotomy (50080, 50081)

5.30 5.30 FUD 000 J A2

AMA: 2018,Jan,8; 2017,Jan,8; 2016,Jan,13; 2015,Jan,16

52341 **Cystourethroscopy; with treatment of ureteral stricture (eg, balloon dilation, laser, electrocautery, and incision)**

INCLUDES Diagnostic cystourethroscopy (52351)

EXCLUDES *Balloon dilation with imaging guidance (50706)*

Cystourethroscopy, separate procedure (52000)

(74485)

8.21 8.21 FUD 000 J A2 50

AMA: 2018,Jan,8; 2017,Jan,8; 2016,Jan,13; 2016,Jan,3; 2015,Jan,16

52342 **with treatment of ureteropelvic junction stricture (eg, balloon dilation, laser, electrocautery, and incision)**

INCLUDES Diagnostic cystourethroscopy (52351)

EXCLUDES *Balloon dilation with imaging guidance (50706)*

Cystourethroscopy (separate procedure) (52000)

(74485)

8.93 8.93 FUD 000 J A2 50

AMA: 2018,Jan,8; 2017,Jan,8; 2016,Jan,13; 2015,Jan,16

52343 **with treatment of intra-renal stricture (eg, balloon dilation, laser, electrocautery, and incision)**

INCLUDES Diagnostic cystourethroscopy (52351)

EXCLUDES *Balloon dilation with imaging guidance (50706)*

Cystourethroscopy (separate procedure) (52000)

(74485)

9.96 9.96 FUD 000 J A2 50

AMA: 2018,Jan,8; 2017,Jan,8; 2016,Jan,13; 2015,Jan,16

52344 **Cystourethroscopy with ureteroscopy; with treatment of ureteral stricture (eg, balloon dilation, laser, electrocautery, and incision)**

INCLUDES Diagnostic cystourethroscopy (52351)

EXCLUDES *Balloon dilation, ureteral stricture (50706)*

Cystourethroscopy with transurethral resection or incision ejaculatory ducts (52402)

(74485)

10.6 10.6 FUD 000 J A2 50

AMA: 2018,Jan,8; 2017,Jan,8; 2016,Jan,13; 2016,Jan,3; 2015,Jan,16

52345 **with treatment of ureteropelvic junction stricture (eg, balloon dilation, laser, electrocautery, and incision)**

INCLUDES Diagnostic cystourethroscopy (52351)

EXCLUDES *Balloon dilation, ureteral stricture (50706)*

Cystourethroscopy with transurethral resection or incision ejaculatory ducts (52402)

(74485)

11.4 11.4 FUD 000 J A2 80 50

AMA: 2018,Jan,8; 2017,Jan,8; 2016,Jan,13; 2016,Jan,3; 2015,Jan,16

52346 **with treatment of intra-renal stricture (eg, balloon dilation, laser, electrocautery, and incision)**

INCLUDES Diagnostic cystourethroscopy (52351)

EXCLUDES *Balloon dilation with imaging guidance (50706)*

Cystourethroscopy with transurethral resection or incision ejaculatory ducts (52402)

(74485)

12.9 12.9 FUD 000 J A2 80 50

AMA: 2018,Jan,8; 2017,Jan,8; 2016,Jan,13; 2015,Jan,16

52351 **Cystourethroscopy, with ureteroscopy and/or pyeloscopy; diagnostic**

EXCLUDES *Cystourethroscopy (52341-52346, 52352-52353 [52356])*

8.75 8.75 FUD 000 J A2

AMA: 2018,Jan,8; 2017,Jan,8; 2016,Jan,13; 2015,Jan,16

52352 **with removal or manipulation of calculus (ureteral catheterization is included)**
INCLUDES Diagnostic cystourethroscopy (52351)
10.2 10.2 FUD 000 J A2 50
AMA: 2018,Jan,8; 2017,Jan,8; 2016,Jan,13; 2015,Jan,16

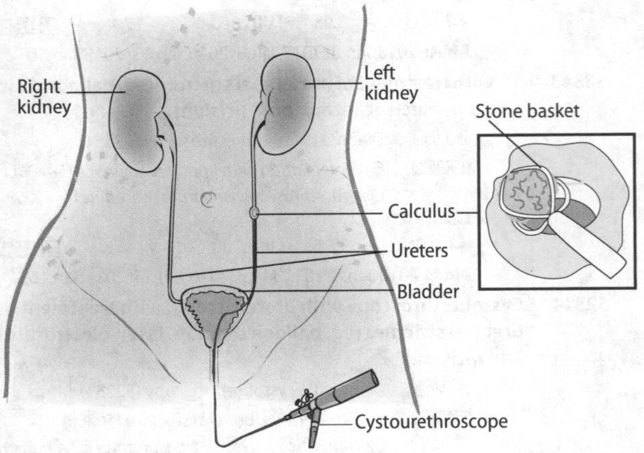

52353 **with lithotripsy (ureteral catheterization is included)**
INCLUDES Diagnostic cystourethroscopy (52351)
EXCLUDES *Cystourethroscopy when performed on same side (52332, [52356])*
11.3 11.3 FUD 000 J A2 50
AMA: 2019,Dec,12; 2018,Jan,8; 2017,Jan,8; 2016,Jan,13; 2015,Jan,16

52356 **with lithotripsy including insertion of indwelling ureteral stent (eg, Gibbons or double-J type)**
INCLUDES Diagnostic cystourethroscopy (52351)
EXCLUDES *Cystourethroscopy (separate procedure) (52000)*
When performed on same side:
Cystourethroscopy, with insertion indwelling ureteral stent (e.g., Gibbons or double-J type) (52332)
Cystourethroscopy, with ureteroscopy and/or pyeloscopy; with lithotripsy (ureteral catheterization is included) (52353)
12.0 12.0 FUD 000 J G2 50
AMA: 2019,Dec,12; 2018,Jan,8; 2017,Jan,8; 2016,Jan,13; 2015,Jan,16

52354 **with biopsy and/or fulguration of ureteral or renal pelvic lesion**
INCLUDES Diagnostic cystourethroscopy (52351)
EXCLUDES *Image guided biopsy without endoscopic guidance (50606)*
12.0 12.0 FUD 000 J A2 50
AMA: 2018,Jan,8; 2017,Jan,8; 2016,Jan,13; 2015,Jan,16

52355 **with resection of ureteral or renal pelvic tumor**
INCLUDES Diagnostic cystourethroscopy (52351)
13.5 13.5 FUD 000 J A2 50
AMA: 2018,Jan,8; 2017,Jan,8; 2016,Jan,13; 2015,Jan,16

52356 **Resequenced code. See code following 52353.**

52400-52700 Endoscopic Procedures via Urethra: Prostate and Vesical Neck

52400 **Cystourethroscopy with incision, fulguration, or resection of congenital posterior urethral valves, or congenital obstructive hypertrophic mucosal folds**
13.8 13.8 FUD 090 J A2
AMA: 2018,Jan,8; 2017,Jan,8; 2016,Jan,13; 2015,Jan,16

52402 **Cystourethroscopy with transurethral resection or incision of ejaculatory ducts** ♂
7.73 7.73 FUD 000 J A2
AMA: 2014,Jan,11; 2001,Apr,4

52441 **Cystourethroscopy, with insertion of permanent adjustable transprostatic implant; single implant**
6.55 36.1 FUD 000 B
AMA: 2018,Jan,8; 2017,Jan,8; 2016,Jan,13; 2015,Jun,5

\+ **52442** **each additional permanent adjustable transprostatic implant (List separately in addition to code for primary procedure)**
EXCLUDES *Permanent urethral stent insertion (52282)*
Removal stent, calculus, or foreign body (implant) (52310)
Temporary prostatic urethral stent insertion (53855)
Code first (52441)
1.75 27.1 FUD ZZZ B
AMA: 2018,Jan,8; 2017,Jan,8; 2016,Jan,13; 2015,Jun,5

52450 **Transurethral incision of prostate** ♂
13.5 13.5 FUD 090 J A2
AMA: 2018,Jan,8; 2017,Jan,8; 2016,Jan,13; 2015,Jun,5; 2015,Jan,16

52500 **Transurethral resection of bladder neck (separate procedure)**
14.1 14.1 FUD 090 J A2
AMA: 2018,Jan,8; 2017,Jan,8; 2016,Jan,13; 2015,Jan,16

52601 **Transurethral electrosurgical resection of prostate, including control of postoperative bleeding, complete (vasectomy, meatotomy, cystourethroscopy, urethral calibration and/or dilation, and internal urethrotomy are included)** ♂
INCLUDES Stage 1 partial transurethral resection prostate
EXCLUDES *Ablation by waterjet (0421T)*
Excision prostate (55801-55845)
Transurethral fulguration prostate (52214)
Code also modifier 58 for stage 2 partial transurethral resection prostate
21.0 21.0 FUD 090 J A2
AMA: 2018,Jan,8; 2017,Jan,8; 2016,Jan,13; 2015,Jun,5; 2015,Jan,16

52630 **Transurethral resection; residual or regrowth of obstructive prostate tissue including control of postoperative bleeding, complete (vasectomy, meatotomy, cystourethroscopy, urethral calibration and/or dilation, and internal urethrotomy are included)** ♂
EXCLUDES *Ablation by waterjet (0421T)*
Excision prostate (55801-55845)
Code also modifier 78 when performed by same physician within postoperative period related procedure
11.5 11.5 FUD 090 J A2
AMA: 2018,Jan,8; 2017,Jan,8; 2016,Jan,13; 2015,Jan,16

52640 **of postoperative bladder neck contracture**
EXCLUDES *Excision prostate (55801-55845)*
9.14 9.14 FUD 090 J A2
AMA: 2018,Jan,8; 2017,Jan,8; 2016,Jan,13; 2015,Jan,16

52647 **Laser coagulation of prostate, including control of postoperative bleeding, complete (vasectomy, meatotomy, cystourethroscopy, urethral calibration and/or dilation, and internal urethrotomy are included if performed)** ♂
18.7 46.2 FUD 090 J A2
AMA: 2018,Jan,8; 2017,Jan,8; 2016,Jan,13; 2015,Jan,16

52648 **Laser vaporization of prostate, including control of postoperative bleeding, complete (vasectomy, meatotomy, cystourethroscopy, urethral calibration and/or dilation, internal urethrotomy and transurethral resection of prostate are included if performed)** ♂
19.9 47.7 FUD 090 J A2
AMA: 2018,Jan,8; 2017,Jan,8; 2016,Jan,13; 2015,Jun,5; 2015,Jan,16

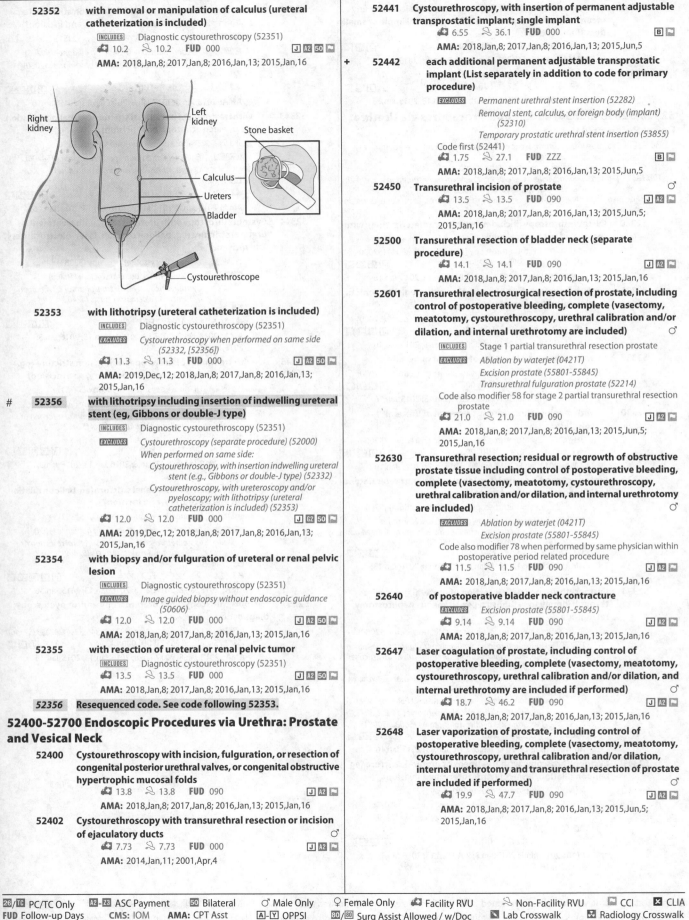

52649 Laser enucleation of the prostate with morcellation, including control of postoperative bleeding, complete (vasectomy, meatotomy, cystourethroscopy, urethral calibration and/or dilation, internal urethrotomy and transurethral resection of prostate are included if performed) ♂

INCLUDES Cystourethroscopy (52000, 52276, 52281)
Laser coagulation prostate (52647-52648)
Meatotomy (53020)
Transurethral resection of prostate (52601)
Vasectomy (55250)

🔪 23.8 ⚕ 23.8 **FUD** 090 [J] [G2] [80] ▣

AMA: 2018,Jan,8; 2017,Jan,8; 2016,Jan,13; 2015,Jun,5

52700 Transurethral drainage of prostatic abscess ♂

EXCLUDES Litholapaxy (52317, 52318)
🔪 12.7 ⚕ 12.7 **FUD** 090 [J] [A2] [80] ▣

AMA: 2018,Jan,8; 2017,Jan,8; 2016,Jan,13; 2015,Jan,16

Bladder — Prostate — Urethra

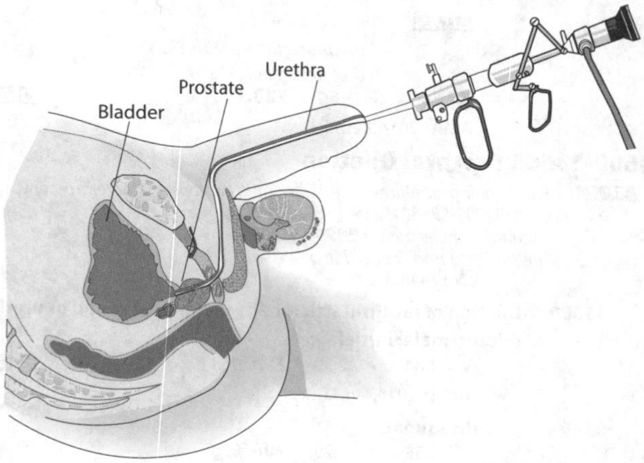

53000-53520 Open Surgical Procedures of Urethra

EXCLUDES Endoscopic procedures; cystoscopy, urethroscopy, cystourethroscopy
(52000-52700 [52356])
Urethrocystography injection procedure (51600-51610)

53000 Urethrotomy or urethrostomy, external (separate procedure); pendulous urethra
🔪 4.28 ⚕ 4.28 **FUD** 010 [J] [A2] ▣
AMA: 2014,Jan,11

53010 perineal urethra, external
🔪 8.51 ⚕ 8.51 **FUD** 090 [J] [A2] ▣
AMA: 2014,Jan,11

53020 Meatotomy, cutting of meatus (separate procedure); except infant
🔪 2.80 ⚕ 2.80 **FUD** 000 [J] [A2] ▣
AMA: 2014,Jan,11

53025 infant [A]
🔪 1.97 ⚕ 1.97 **FUD** 000 [63] [J] [R2] [80] ▣
AMA: 2014,Jan,11

53040 Drainage of deep periurethral abscess
EXCLUDES Incision and drainage subcutaneous abscess
(10060-10061)
🔪 11.3 ⚕ 11.3 **FUD** 090 [J] [A2] [80] ▣
AMA: 2014,Jan,11

53060 Drainage of Skene's gland abscess or cyst
🔪 4.70 ⚕ 5.25 **FUD** 010 [J] [P3] ▣
AMA: 2014,Jan,11

53080 Drainage of perineal urinary extravasation; uncomplicated (separate procedure)
🔪 12.1 ⚕ 12.1 **FUD** 090 [J] [A2] ▣
AMA: 2014,Jan,11

53085 complicated
🔪 18.7 ⚕ 18.7 **FUD** 090 [J] [G2] [80] ▣
AMA: 2014,Jan,11

53200 Biopsy of urethra
🔪 4.12 ⚕ 4.55 **FUD** 000 [J] [A2] ▣
AMA: 2014,Jan,11

53210 Urethrectomy, total, including cystostomy; female ♀
🔪 22.2 ⚕ 22.2 **FUD** 090 [J] [A2] [80] ▣
AMA: 2014,Jan,11

53215 male ♂
🔪 26.8 ⚕ 26.8 **FUD** 090 [J] [A2] [80] ▣
AMA: 2014,Jan,11

53220 Excision or fulguration of carcinoma of urethra
🔪 13.0 ⚕ 13.0 **FUD** 090 [J] [A2] [80] ▣
AMA: 2014,Jan,11

53230 Excision of urethral diverticulum (separate procedure); female ♀
🔪 17.5 ⚕ 17.5 **FUD** 090 [J] [A2] [80] ▣
AMA: 2014,Jan,11

53235 male ♂
🔪 18.3 ⚕ 18.3 **FUD** 090 [J] [A2] [80] ▣
AMA: 2014,Jan,11

53240 Marsupialization of urethral diverticulum, male or female
🔪 12.2 ⚕ 12.2 **FUD** 090 [J] [A2] ▣
AMA: 2014,Jan,11

53250 Excision of bulbourethral gland (Cowper's gland)
🔪 11.4 ⚕ 11.4 **FUD** 090 [J] [A2] ▣
AMA: 2014,Jan,11

53260 Excision or fulguration; urethral polyp(s), distal urethra
EXCLUDES Endoscopic method (52214, 52224)
🔪 5.20 ⚕ 5.83 **FUD** 010 [J] [A2] ▣
AMA: 2014,Jan,11

53265 urethral caruncle
EXCLUDES Endoscopic method (52214, 52224)
🔪 5.38 ⚕ 6.36 **FUD** 010 [J] [A2] ▣
AMA: 2014,Jan,11

53270 Skene's glands
EXCLUDES Endoscopic method (52214, 52224)
🔪 5.32 ⚕ 5.98 **FUD** 010 [J] [A2] ▣
AMA: 2014,Jan,11

53275 urethral prolapse
EXCLUDES Endoscopic method (52214, 52224)
🔪 7.58 ⚕ 7.58 **FUD** 010 [J] [A2] ▣
AMA: 2014,Jan,11

53400 Urethroplasty; first stage, for fistula, diverticulum, or stricture (eg, Johannsen type)
EXCLUDES Hypospadias repair (54300-54352)
🔪 23.1 ⚕ 23.1 **FUD** 090 [J] [A2] [80] ▣
AMA: 2014,Jan,11

53405 second stage (formation of urethra), including urinary diversion
EXCLUDES Hypospadias repair (54300-54352)
🔪 25.2 ⚕ 25.2 **FUD** 090 [J] [A2] [80] ▣
AMA: 2014,Jan,11

53410 Urethroplasty, 1-stage reconstruction of male anterior urethra ♂
EXCLUDES Hypospadias repair (54300-54352)
🔪 28.3 ⚕ 28.3 **FUD** 090 [J] [A2] [80] ▣
AMA: 2014,Jan,11

53415 Urethroplasty, transpubic or perineal, 1-stage, for reconstruction or repair of prostatic or membranous urethra ♂
🔪 32.8 ⚕ 32.8 **FUD** 090 [C] [80] ▣
AMA: 2014,Jan,11

● New Code ▲ Revised Code ○ Reinstated ● New Web Release ▲ Revised Web Release ＋ Add-on Unlisted Not Covered # Resequenced
⑤⓪ Optum Mod 50 Exempt ⊘ AMA Mod 51 Exempt ⑤ Optum Mod 51 Exempt ⑥³ Mod 63 Exempt ✗ Non-FDA Drug ★ Telemedicine M Maternity [A] Age Edit

53420 **Urethroplasty, 2-stage reconstruction or repair of prostatic or membranous urethra; first stage** ♂
24.3 | 24.3 | FUD 090 | J A2
AMA: 2014,Jan,11

53425 **second stage** ♂
27.1 | 27.1 | FUD 090 | J A2 80
AMA: 2014,Jan,11

53430 **Urethroplasty, reconstruction of female urethra** ♀
27.9 | 27.9 | FUD 090 | J A2 80
AMA: 2014,Jan,11

53431 **Urethroplasty with tubularization of posterior urethra and/or lower bladder for incontinence (eg, Tenago, Leadbetter procedure)**
33.3 | 33.3 | FUD 090 | J A2 80
AMA: 2014,Jan,11

53440 **Sling operation for correction of male urinary incontinence (eg, fascia or synthetic)** ♂
21.7 | 21.7 | FUD 090 | J J8 80
AMA: 2020,Aug,6

53442 **Removal or revision of sling for male urinary incontinence (eg, fascia or synthetic)** ♂
22.6 | 22.6 | FUD 090 | J A2 80
AMA: 2020,Aug,6

53444 **Insertion of tandem cuff (dual cuff)**
22.9 | 22.9 | FUD 090 | J J8 80
AMA: 2014,Jan,11

53445 **Insertion of inflatable urethral/bladder neck sphincter, including placement of pump, reservoir, and cuff**
21.7 | 21.7 | FUD 090 | J J8 80
AMA: 2020,Aug,6

53446 **Removal of inflatable urethral/bladder neck sphincter, including pump, reservoir, and cuff**
18.5 | 18.5 | FUD 090 | Q2 A2 80
AMA: 2020,Aug,6

53447 **Removal and replacement of inflatable urethral/bladder neck sphincter including pump, reservoir, and cuff at the same operative session**
23.3 | 23.3 | FUD 090 | J J8 80
AMA: 2020,Aug,6

53448 **Removal and replacement of inflatable urethral/bladder neck sphincter including pump, reservoir, and cuff through an infected field at the same operative session including irrigation and debridement of infected tissue**
INCLUDES Debridement (11042, 11043)
36.9 | 36.9 | FUD 090 | C 80
AMA: 2020,Aug,6

53449 **Repair of inflatable urethral/bladder neck sphincter, including pump, reservoir, and cuff**
17.6 | 17.6 | FUD 090 | J A2 80
AMA: 2020,Aug,6

53450 **Urethromeatoplasty, with mucosal advancement**
EXCLUDES *Meatotomy (53020, 53025)*
11.8 | 11.8 | FUD 090 | J A2
AMA: 2018,Jan,8; 2017,Jan,8; 2016,Jan,13; 2015,Jan,16

53460 **Urethromeatoplasty, with partial excision of distal urethral segment (Richardson type procedure)**
13.2 | 13.2 | FUD 090 | J A2 80
AMA: 2014,Jan,11

53500 **Urethrolysis, transvaginal, secondary, open, including cystourethroscopy (eg, postsurgical obstruction, scarring)**
INCLUDES Cystourethroscopy (separate procedure) (52000)
EXCLUDES *Retropubic approach (53899)*
21.5 | 21.5 | FUD 090 | J 80
AMA: 2018,Jan,8; 2017,Jan,8; 2016,Jan,13; 2015,Jan,16

53502 **Urethrorrhaphy, suture of urethral wound or injury, female** ♀
14.0 | 14.0 | FUD 090 | J A2
AMA: 2014,Jan,11

53505 **Urethrorrhaphy, suture of urethral wound or injury; penile** ♂
14.0 | 14.0 | FUD 090 | J A2 80
AMA: 2014,Jan,11

53510 **perineal** ♂
18.2 | 18.2 | FUD 090 | J A2 80
AMA: 2014,Jan,11

53515 **prostatomembranous** ♂
23.0 | 23.0 | FUD 090 | J A2 80
AMA: 2014,Jan,11

53520 **Closure of urethrostomy or urethrocutaneous fistula, male (separate procedure)** ♂
EXCLUDES *Closure fistula:*
Urethrorectal (45820, 45825)
Urethrovaginal (57310)
16.1 | 16.1 | FUD 090 | J A2
AMA: 2014,Jan,11

53600-53665 Urethral Dilation

EXCLUDES *Endoscopic procedures; cystoscopy, urethroscopy, cystourethroscopy (52000-52700 [52356])*
Urethral catheterization (51701-51703)
Urethrocystography injection procedure (51600-51610)
(74485)

53600 **Dilation of urethral stricture by passage of sound or urethral dilator, male; initial** ♂
1.84 | 2.39 | FUD 000 | T P3
AMA: 2014,Jan,11

53601 **subsequent** ♂
1.55 | 2.29 | FUD 000 | Q1 N1
AMA: 2014,Jan,11

53605 **Dilation of urethral stricture or vesical neck by passage of sound or urethral dilator, male, general or conduction (spinal) anesthesia** ♂
EXCLUDES *Procedure performed under local anesthesia (53600-53601, 53620-53621)*
1.87 | 1.87 | FUD 000 | J A2
AMA: 2014,Jan,11

53620 **Dilation of urethral stricture by passage of filiform and follower, male; initial** ♂
2.52 | 3.79 | FUD 000 | T P3
AMA: 2014,Jan,11; 1996,Nov,1

53621 **subsequent** ♂
2.09 | 3.56 | FUD 000 | T P3
AMA: 2014,Jan,11

53660 **Dilation of female urethra including suppository and/or instillation; initial** ♀
1.20 | 2.02 | FUD 000 | S P3
AMA: 2014,Jan,11

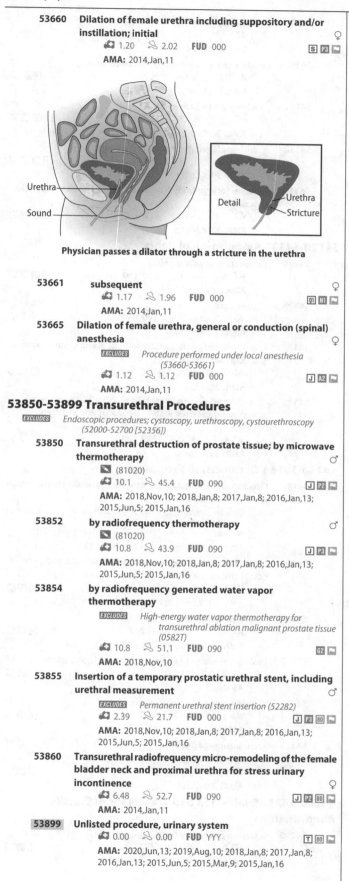

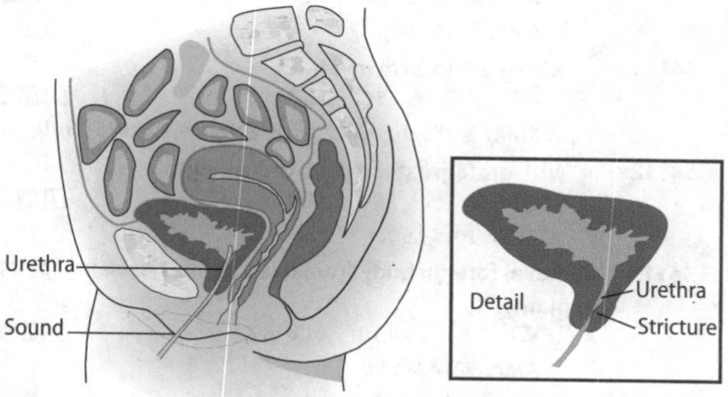

Physician passes a dilator through a stricture in the urethra

53661 **subsequent** ♀
1.17 | 1.96 | FUD 000 | Q1 N1
AMA: 2014,Jan,11

53665 **Dilation of female urethra, general or conduction (spinal) anesthesia** ♀
EXCLUDES *Procedure performed under local anesthesia (53660-53661)*
1.12 | 1.12 | FUD 000 | J A2
AMA: 2014,Jan,11

53850-53899 Transurethral Procedures

EXCLUDES *Endoscopic procedures; cystoscopy, urethroscopy, cystourethroscopy (52000-52700 [52356])*

53850 **Transurethral destruction of prostate tissue; by microwave thermotherapy** ♂
(81020)
10.1 | 45.4 | FUD 090 | J P2
AMA: 2018,Nov,10; 2018,Jan,8; 2017,Jan,8; 2016,Jan,13; 2015,Jun,5; 2015,Jan,16

53852 **by radiofrequency thermotherapy** ♂
(81020)
10.8 | 43.9 | FUD 090 | J P3
AMA: 2018,Nov,10; 2018,Jan,8; 2017,Jan,8; 2016,Jan,13; 2015,Jun,5; 2015,Jan,16

53854 **by radiofrequency generated water vapor thermotherapy**
EXCLUDES *High-energy water vapor thermotherapy for transurethral ablation malignant prostate tissue (0582T)*
10.8 | 51.1 | FUD 090 | G2
AMA: 2018,Nov,10

53855 **Insertion of a temporary prostatic urethral stent, including urethral measurement** ♂
EXCLUDES *Permanent urethral stent insertion (52282)*
2.39 | 21.7 | FUD 000 | J P3 80
AMA: 2018,Nov,10; 2018,Jan,8; 2017,Jan,8; 2016,Jan,13; 2015,Jun,5; 2015,Jan,16

53860 **Transurethral radiofrequency micro-remodeling of the female bladder neck and proximal urethra for stress urinary incontinence** ♀
6.48 | 52.7 | FUD 090 | J P2 80
AMA: 2014,Jan,11

53899 **Unlisted procedure, urinary system**
0.00 | 0.00 | FUD YYY | T 80
AMA: 2020,Jun,13; 2019,Aug,10; 2018,Jan,8; 2017,Jan,8; 2016,Jan,13; 2015,Jun,5; 2015,Mar,9; 2015,Jan,16

54000-54015 Procedures of Penis: Incisional

EXCLUDES *Debridement abdominal perineal gangrene (11004-11006)*

54000 **Slitting of prepuce, dorsal or lateral (separate procedure); newborn** A ♂
Facility RVU 3.14 Non-Facility RVU 4.40 FUD 010 63 J A2 80
AMA: 2014,Jan,11

54001 **except newborn** ♂
Facility RVU 4.02 Non-Facility RVU 5.44 FUD 010 J A2
AMA: 2014,Jan,11

54015 **Incision and drainage of penis, deep** ♂
EXCLUDES *Abscess, skin/subcutaneous (10060-10160)*
Facility RVU 8.92 Non-Facility RVU 8.92 FUD 010 J A2 80
AMA: 2014,Jan,11

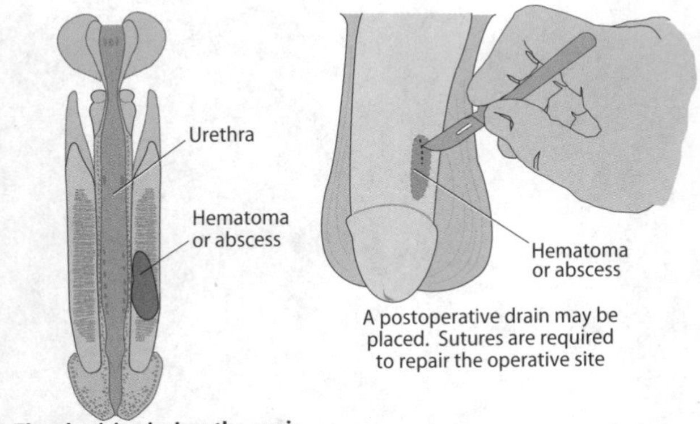
Urethra
Hematoma
or abscess
Hematoma
or abscess
A postoperative drain may be
placed. Sutures are required
to repair the operative site

The physician incises the penis to drain an abscess or hematoma

54050-54065 Destruction of Penis Lesions: Multiple Methods

EXCLUDES *Excision/destruction other lesions (11420-11426, 11620-11626, 17000-17250, 17270-17276)*

54050 **Destruction of lesion(s), penis (eg, condyloma, papilloma, molluscum contagiosum, herpetic vesicle), simple; chemical** ♂
Facility RVU 3.05 Non-Facility RVU 3.80 FUD 010 Q1 N1
AMA: 2014,Jan,11; 1997,Nov,1

54055 **electrodesiccation** ♂
Facility RVU 2.69 Non-Facility RVU 3.49 FUD 010 T P3
AMA: 2014,Jan,11; 1997,Nov,1

54056 **cryosurgery** ♂
Facility RVU 3.18 Non-Facility RVU 4.03 FUD 010 Q1 N1
AMA: 2014,Jan,11; 1997,Nov,1

54057 **laser surgery** ♂
Facility RVU 2.76 Non-Facility RVU 3.97 FUD 010 T A2
AMA: 2014,Jan,11; 1997,Nov,1

54060 **surgical excision** ♂
Facility RVU 3.76 Non-Facility RVU 5.29 FUD 010 T A2
AMA: 2014,Jan,11

54065 **Destruction of lesion(s), penis (eg, condyloma, papilloma, molluscum contagiosum, herpetic vesicle), extensive (eg, laser surgery, electrosurgery, cryosurgery, chemosurgery)** ♂
Facility RVU 4.90 Non-Facility RVU 6.27 FUD 010 T A2
AMA: 2014,Jan,11; 1997,Nov,1

54100-54115 Procedures of Penis: Excisional

54100 **Biopsy of penis; (separate procedure)** ♂
Facility RVU 3.50 Non-Facility RVU 5.67 FUD 000 J A2
AMA: 2019,Jan,9; 2018,Jan,8; 2017,Jan,8; 2016,Jan,13; 2015,Jan,16

54105 **deep structures** ♂
Facility RVU 6.16 Non-Facility RVU 7.68 FUD 010 J A2
AMA: 2014,Jan,11

54110 **Excision of penile plaque (Peyronie disease);** ♂
Facility RVU 18.0 Non-Facility RVU 18.0 FUD 090 J A2 80
AMA: 2014,Jan,11

54111 **with graft to 5 cm in length** ♂
Facility RVU 23.1 Non-Facility RVU 23.1 FUD 090 J A2 80
AMA: 2018,Jan,8; 2017,Jan,8; 2016,Jan,13; 2015,Jan,16

54112 **with graft greater than 5 cm in length** ♂
Facility RVU 27.0 Non-Facility RVU 27.0 FUD 090 J A2 80
AMA: 2014,Jan,11

54115 **Removal foreign body from deep penile tissue (eg, plastic implant)** ♂
Facility RVU 12.2 Non-Facility RVU 13.0 FUD 090 J A2 80
AMA: 2014,Jan,11

54120-54135 Amputation of Penis

54120 **Amputation of penis; partial** ♂
Facility RVU 18.2 Non-Facility RVU 18.2 FUD 090 J A2 80
AMA: 2014,Jan,11

54125 **complete** ♂
Facility RVU 23.5 Non-Facility RVU 23.5 FUD 090 C 80
AMA: 2014,Jan,11

54130 **Amputation of penis, radical; with bilateral inguinofemoral lymphadenectomy** ♂
Facility RVU 34.5 Non-Facility RVU 34.5 FUD 090 C 80
AMA: 2014,Jan,11

54135 **in continuity with bilateral pelvic lymphadenectomy, including external iliac, hypogastric and obturator nodes** ♂
Facility RVU 43.6 Non-Facility RVU 43.6 FUD 090 C 80
AMA: 2014,Jan,11

54150-54164 Circumcision Procedures

54150 **Circumcision, using clamp or other device with regional dorsal penile or ring block** ♂
Code also modifier 52 when performed without dorsal penile or ring block
Facility RVU 2.84 Non-Facility RVU 4.40 FUD 000 63 J A2 80
AMA: 2018,Jan,8; 2017,Jan,8; 2016,Jan,13; 2015,Jan,16

54160 **Circumcision, surgical excision other than clamp, device, or dorsal slit; neonate (28 days of age or less)** A ♂
Facility RVU 4.17 Non-Facility RVU 6.29 FUD 010 63 J A2
AMA: 2018,Jan,8; 2017,Jan,8; 2016,Jan,13; 2015,Jan,16

54161 **older than 28 days of age** A ♂
Facility RVU 5.70 Non-Facility RVU 5.70 FUD 010 J A2
AMA: 2018,Jan,8; 2017,Jan,8; 2016,Jan,13; 2015,Jan,16

54162 **Lysis or excision of penile post-circumcision adhesions** ♂
Facility RVU 5.77 Non-Facility RVU 7.42 FUD 010 J A2
AMA: 2014,Jan,11

54163 **Repair incomplete circumcision** ♂
Facility RVU 6.31 Non-Facility RVU 6.31 FUD 010 J A2
AMA: 2014,Jan,11

54164 **Frenulotomy of penis** ♂
EXCLUDES *Circumcision (54150-54163)*
Facility RVU 5.54 Non-Facility RVU 5.54 FUD 010 J A2
AMA: 2014,Jan,11

54200-54250 Evaluation and Treatment of Erectile Abnormalities

54200 **Injection procedure for Peyronie disease;** ♂
Facility RVU 2.41 Non-Facility RVU 3.17 FUD 010 T P3
AMA: 2014,Jan,11

54205 **with surgical exposure of plaque** ♂
15.4 15.4 **FUD** 090 J A2 80
AMA: 2014,Jan,11

54220 **Irrigation of corpora cavernosa for priapism** ♂
3.86 6.07 **FUD** 000 T A2
AMA: 2014,Jan,11

54230 **Injection procedure for corpora cavernosography** ♂
(74445)
2.28 2.87 **FUD** 000 N N1
AMA: 2014,Jan,11

54231 **Dynamic cavernosometry, including intracavernosal injection of vasoactive drugs (eg, papaverine, phentolamine)** ♂
3.34 4.07 **FUD** 000 J P3
AMA: 2014,Jan,11; 1994,Sum,29

54235 **Injection of corpora cavernosa with pharmacologic agent(s) (eg, papaverine, phentolamine)** ♂
2.10 2.53 **FUD** 000 T P3
AMA: 2018,Jan,8; 2017,Jan,8; 2016,Jan,13; 2015,Jan,16

54240 **Penile plethysmography** ♂
2.97 2.97 **FUD** 000 S P3 80
AMA: 2014,Jan,11

54250 **Nocturnal penile tumescence and/or rigidity test** ♂
3.50 3.50 **FUD** 000 T P3 80
AMA: 2014,Jan,11

54300-54390 Hypospadias Repair and Related Procedures

EXCLUDES *Other urethroplasties (53400-53430)*
Revascularization penis (37788)

54300 **Plastic operation of penis for straightening of chordee (eg, hypospadias), with or without mobilization of urethra** ♂
18.6 18.6 **FUD** 090 J A2 80
AMA: 2018,Jan,8; 2017,Jan,8; 2016,Jan,13; 2015,Jan,16

54304 **Plastic operation on penis for correction of chordee or for first stage hypospadias repair with or without transplantation of prepuce and/or skin flaps** ♂
21.6 21.6 **FUD** 090 J A2 80
AMA: 2014,Jan,11

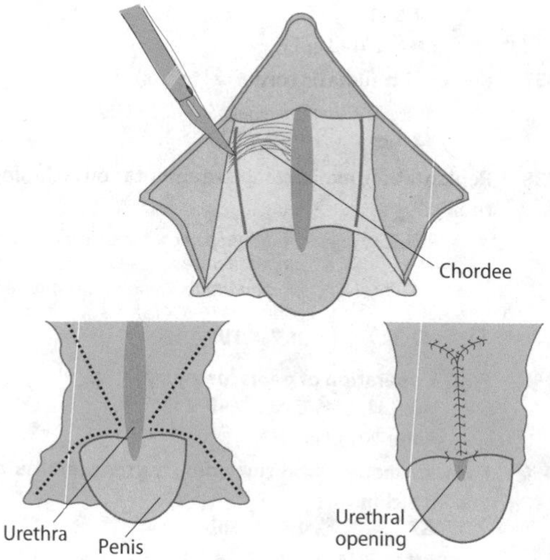

The foreskin is used in either a free graft or a flap graft to cover the ventral skin defects created to correct the chordee

54308 **Urethroplasty for second stage hypospadias repair (including urinary diversion); less than 3 cm** ♂
20.6 20.6 **FUD** 090 J A2 80
AMA: 2014,Jan,11

54312 **greater than 3 cm** ♂
23.6 23.6 **FUD** 090 J A2 80
AMA: 2014,Jan,11

54316 **Urethroplasty for second stage hypospadias repair (including urinary diversion) with free skin graft obtained from site other than genitalia** ♂
28.8 28.8 **FUD** 090 J A2 80
AMA: 2014,Jan,11

54318 **Urethroplasty for third stage hypospadias repair to release penis from scrotum (eg, third stage Cecil repair)** ♂
20.5 20.5 **FUD** 090 J A2 80
AMA: 2014,Jan,11

54322 **1-stage distal hypospadias repair (with or without chordee or circumcision); with simple meatal advancement (eg, Magpi, V-flap)** ♂
22.5 22.5 **FUD** 090 J A2 80
AMA: 2014,Jan,11

54324 **with urethroplasty by local skin flaps (eg, flip-flap, prepucial flap)** ♂
INCLUDES Browne's operation
27.9 27.9 **FUD** 090 J A2 80
AMA: 2014,Jan,11

54326 **with urethroplasty by local skin flaps and mobilization of urethra** ♂
27.2 27.2 **FUD** 090 J A2 80
AMA: 2014,Jan,11

54328 **with extensive dissection to correct chordee and urethroplasty with local skin flaps, skin graft patch, and/or island flap** ♂
EXCLUDES *Urethroplasty/straightening chordee (54308)*
27.1 27.1 **FUD** 090 J A2 80
AMA: 2018,Jan,8; 2017,Jan,8; 2016,Jan,13; 2015,Jan,16

54332 **1-stage proximal penile or penoscrotal hypospadias repair requiring extensive dissection to correct chordee and urethroplasty by use of skin graft tube and/or island flap** ♂
29.3 29.3 **FUD** 090 J 80
AMA: 2018,Jan,8; 2017,Jan,8; 2016,Jan,13; 2015,Jan,16

54336 **1-stage perineal hypospadias repair requiring extensive dissection to correct chordee and urethroplasty by use of skin graft tube and/or island flap** ♂
34.4 34.4 **FUD** 090 J 80
AMA: 2018,Jan,8; 2017,Jan,8; 2016,Jan,13; 2015,Jan,16

54340 **Repair of hypospadias complications (ie, fistula, stricture, diverticula); by closure, incision, or excision, simple** ♂
16.4 16.4 **FUD** 090 J A2 80
AMA: 2014,Jan,11

54344 **requiring mobilization of skin flaps and urethroplasty with flap or patch graft** ♂
27.3 27.3 **FUD** 090 J A2 80
AMA: 2014,Jan,11

54348 **requiring extensive dissection and urethroplasty with flap, patch or tubed graft (includes urinary diversion)** ♂
29.2 29.2 **FUD** 090 J A2 80
AMA: 2014,Jan,11

54352 **Repair of hypospadias cripple requiring extensive dissection and excision of previously constructed structures including re-release of chordee and reconstruction of urethra and penis by use of local skin as grafts and island flaps and skin brought in as flaps or grafts** ♂
40.9 40.9 **FUD** 090 J A2 80
AMA: 2014,Jan,11

54360 **Plastic operation on penis to correct angulation** ♂
20.8 20.8 **FUD** 090 J A2 80
AMA: 2014,Jan,11

54380 **Plastic operation on penis for epispadias distal to external sphincter;** ♂
INCLUDES Lowsley's operation
23.1 23.1 FUD 090 J A2 80
AMA: 2014,Jan,11

54385 **with incontinence** ♂
26.8 26.8 FUD 090 J A2 80
AMA: 2014,Jan,11

54390 **with exstrophy of bladder** ♂
35.8 35.8 FUD 090 C 80
AMA: 2014,Jan,11

54400-54417 Procedures to Treat Impotence

CMS: 100-03,230.4 Diagnosis and Treatment of Impotence
EXCLUDES *Other urethroplasties (53400-53430)*
Revascularization penis (37788)

54400 **Insertion of penile prosthesis; non-inflatable (semi-rigid)** ♂
EXCLUDES *Replacement/removal penile prosthesis (54415, 54416)*
15.3 15.3 FUD 090 J J8
AMA: 2014,Jan,11

54401 **inflatable (self-contained)** ♂
EXCLUDES *Replacement/removal penile prosthesis (54415, 54416)*
18.9 18.9 FUD 090 J J8
AMA: 2014,Jan,11

54405 **Insertion of multi-component, inflatable penile prosthesis, including placement of pump, cylinders, and reservoir** ♂
Code also modifier 52 for reduced services
23.4 23.4 FUD 090 J J8 80
AMA: 2014,Jan,11

54406 **Removal of all components of a multi-component, inflatable penile prosthesis without replacement of prosthesis** ♂
Code also modifier 52 for reduced services
21.1 21.1 FUD 090 02 A2 80
AMA: 2014,Jan,11

54408 **Repair of component(s) of a multi-component, inflatable penile prosthesis** ♂
22.8 22.8 FUD 090 J A2 80
AMA: 2014,Jan,11

54410 **Removal and replacement of all component(s) of a multi-component, inflatable penile prosthesis at the same operative session** ♂
24.8 24.8 FUD 090 J J8 80
AMA: 2014,Jan,11

54411 **Removal and replacement of all components of a multi-component inflatable penile prosthesis through an infected field at the same operative session, including irrigation and debridement of infected tissue** ♂
INCLUDES Debridement (11042, 11043)
Code also modifier 52 for reduced services
29.7 29.7 FUD 090 J 80
AMA: 2014,Jan,11

54415 **Removal of non-inflatable (semi-rigid) or inflatable (self-contained) penile prosthesis, without replacement of prosthesis** ♂
15.3 15.3 FUD 090 02 A2 80
AMA: 2014,Jan,11

54416 **Removal and replacement of non-inflatable (semi-rigid) or inflatable (self-contained) penile prosthesis at the same operative session** ♂
20.5 20.5 FUD 090 J J8 80
AMA: 2014,Jan,11

54417 **Removal and replacement of non-inflatable (semi-rigid) or inflatable (self-contained) penile prosthesis through an infected field at the same operative session, including irrigation and debridement of infected tissue** ♂
INCLUDES Debridement (11042, 11043)
25.9 25.9 FUD 090 J 80
AMA: 2014,Jan,11

54420-54450 Other Procedures of the Penis

EXCLUDES *Other urethroplasties (53400-53430)*
Revascularization penis (37788)

54420 **Corpora cavernosa-saphenous vein shunt (priapism operation), unilateral or bilateral** ♂
20.3 20.3 FUD 090 J A2 80
AMA: 2014,Jan,11

54430 **Corpora cavernosa-corpus spongiosum shunt (priapism operation), unilateral or bilateral** ♂
18.5 18.5 FUD 090 C 80
AMA: 2014,Jan,11

Cross section of penis

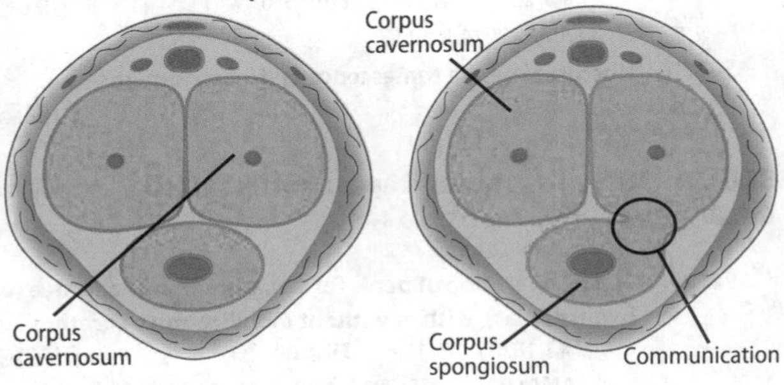

The physician creates a communication between the corpus cavernosum and the corpus spongiosum

54435 **Corpora cavernosa-glans penis fistulization (eg, biopsy needle, Winter procedure, rongeur, or punch) for priapism** ♂
12.0 12.0 FUD 090 J A2
AMA: 2014,Jan,11

54437 **Repair of traumatic corporeal tear(s)** ♂
EXCLUDES *Urethral repair (53410, 53415)*
19.4 19.4 FUD 090 J G2 80

54438 **Replantation, penis, complete amputation including urethral repair** ♂
EXCLUDES *Replantation/repair corporeal tear in incomplete amputation penis (54437)*
Replantation/urethral repair in incomplete amputation penis (53410-53415)
38.7 38.7 FUD 090 C 80

54440 **Plastic operation of penis for injury** ♂
0.00 0.00 FUD 090 J A2 80
AMA: 2014,Jan,11

54450 **Foreskin manipulation including lysis of preputial adhesions and stretching** ♂
1.66 1.98 FUD 000 T A2
AMA: 2014,Jan,11

54500-54560 Testicular Procedures: Incisional

EXCLUDES *Debridement abdominal perineal gangrene (11004-11006)*

54500 **Biopsy of testis, needle (separate procedure)** ♂
EXCLUDES *Fine needle aspiration (10021, [10004, 10005, 10006, 10007, 10008, 10009, 10010, 10011, 10012])*
(88172-88173)
2.15 2.15 FUD 000 J A2 80 50
AMA: 2019,Apr,4

54505 Biopsy of testis, incisional (separate procedure) ♂

Code also when combined with epididymogram, seminal vesiculogram or vasogram (55300)

6.07 6.07 **FUD** 010 J A2 80 50

AMA: 2018,Jan,8; 2017,Jan,8; 2016,Jan,13; 2015,Jan,16

54512 Excision of extraparenchymal lesion of testis ♂

15.6 15.6 **FUD** 090 J A2 50

AMA: 2018,Jan,8; 2017,Jan,8; 2016,Jan,13; 2015,Jan,16

54520 Orchiectomy, simple (including subcapsular), with or without testicular prosthesis, scrotal or inguinal approach ♂

INCLUDES Huggins' orchiectomy

EXCLUDES *Lymphadenectomy, radical retroperitoneal (38780)*

Code also hernia repair, when performed (49505, 49507)

9.45 9.45 **FUD** 090 J A2 50

AMA: 2018,Jan,8; 2017,Jan,8; 2016,Jan,13; 2015,Jan,16

54522 Orchiectomy, partial ♂

EXCLUDES *Lymphadenectomy, radical retroperitoneal (38780)*

17.0 17.0 **FUD** 090 J A2 80 50

AMA: 2018,Jan,8; 2017,Jan,8; 2016,Jan,13; 2015,Jan,16

54530 Orchiectomy, radical, for tumor; inguinal approach ♂

EXCLUDES *Lymphadenectomy, radical retroperitoneal (38780)*

14.6 14.6 **FUD** 090 J A2 80 50

AMA: 2018,Jan,8; 2017,Jan,8; 2016,Jan,13; 2015,Jan,16

54535 with abdominal exploration ♂

EXCLUDES *Lymphadenectomy, radical retroperitoneal (38780)*

21.4 21.4 **FUD** 090 J 80 50

AMA: 2018,Jan,8; 2017,Jan,8; 2016,Jan,13; 2015,Jan,16

54550 Exploration for undescended testis (inguinal or scrotal area) ♂

14.2 14.2 **FUD** 090 J A2 80 50

AMA: 2018,Jan,8; 2017,Mar,10; 2017,Jan,8; 2016,Jan,13; 2015,Jan,16

54560 Exploration for undescended testis with abdominal exploration ♂

19.8 19.8 **FUD** 090 J G2 80 50

AMA: 2018,Jan,8; 2017,Jan,8; 2016,Jan,13; 2015,Jan,16

54600-54699 Open and Laparoscopic Testicular Procedures

54600 Reduction of torsion of testis, surgical, with or without fixation of contralateral testis ♂

13.1 13.1 **FUD** 090 J A2 50

AMA: 2018,Jan,8; 2017,Jan,8; 2016,Jan,13; 2015,Jan,16

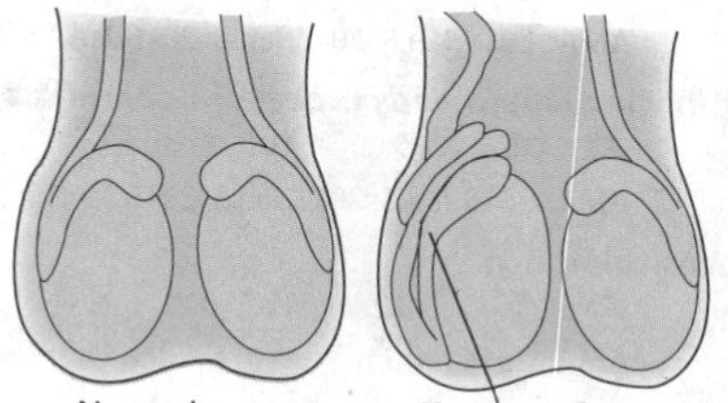

Normal testes Torsion of testis

54620 Fixation of contralateral testis (separate procedure) ♂

8.64 8.64 **FUD** 010 J A2 50

AMA: 2014,Jan,11

54640 Orchiopexy, inguinal or scrotal approach ♂

INCLUDES Bevan's operation
Koop inguinal orchiopexy
Prentice orchiopexy

EXCLUDES *Repair inguinal hernia with inguinal orchiopexy (49495-49525)*

13.8 13.8 **FUD** 090 J A2 80 50

AMA: 2018,Jan,8; 2017,Mar,10; 2017,Jan,8; 2016,Jan,13; 2015,Jan,16

54650 Orchiopexy, abdominal approach, for intra-abdominal testis (eg, Fowler-Stephens) ♂

EXCLUDES *Laparoscopic orchiopexy (54692)*

20.5 20.5 **FUD** 090 J 80 50

AMA: 2018,Jan,8; 2017,Jan,8; 2016,Jan,13; 2015,Jan,16

54660 Insertion of testicular prosthesis (separate procedure) ♂

10.3 10.3 **FUD** 090 J J8 80 50

AMA: 2018,Jan,8; 2017,Jan,8; 2016,Jan,13; 2015,Jan,16

54670 Suture or repair of testicular injury ♂

11.7 11.7 **FUD** 090 J A2 80 50

AMA: 2018,Jan,8; 2017,Jan,8; 2016,Jan,13; 2015,Jan,16

54680 Transplantation of testis(es) to thigh (because of scrotal destruction) ♂

22.7 22.7 **FUD** 090 J A2 80 50

AMA: 2018,Jan,8; 2017,Jan,8; 2016,Jan,13; 2015,Jan,16

54690 Laparoscopy, surgical; orchiectomy ♂

INCLUDES Diagnostic laparoscopy (49320)

18.9 18.9 **FUD** 090 J A2 80 50

AMA: 2019,Feb,10; 2018,Jan,8; 2017,Jan,8; 2016,Jan,13; 2015,Jan,16

54692 orchiopexy for intra-abdominal testis ♂

INCLUDES Diagnostic laparoscopy (49320)

21.9 21.9 **FUD** 090 J G2 50

AMA: 2018,Jan,8; 2017,Jan,8; 2016,Jan,13; 2015,Jan,16

54699 Unlisted laparoscopy procedure, testis ♂

0.00 0.00 **FUD** YYY J 80 50

AMA: 2018,Jan,8; 2017,Jan,8; 2016,Jan,13; 2015,Jan,16

54700-54901 Open Procedures of the Epididymis

54700 Incision and drainage of epididymis, testis and/or scrotal space (eg, abscess or hematoma) ♂

EXCLUDES *Debridement genitalia for necrotizing soft tissue infection (11004-11006)*

6.16 6.16 **FUD** 010 J A2 50

AMA: 2018,Jan,8; 2017,Jan,8; 2016,Jan,13; 2015,Jan,16

54800 Biopsy of epididymis, needle ♂

EXCLUDES *Fine needle aspiration (10021, [10004, 10005, 10006, 10007, 10008, 10009, 10010, 10011, 10012])*

88172-88173

3.64 3.64 **FUD** 000 J A2 80 50

AMA: 2019,Apr,4; 2018,Jan,8; 2017,Jan,8; 2016,Jan,13; 2015,Jan,16

54830 Excision of local lesion of epididymis ♂

10.7 10.7 **FUD** 090 J A2 80 50

AMA: 2018,Jan,8; 2017,Jan,8; 2016,Jan,13; 2015,Jan,16

54840 Excision of spermatocele, with or without epididymectomy ♂

9.29 9.29 **FUD** 090 J A2 50

AMA: 2018,Jan,8; 2017,Jan,8; 2016,Jan,13; 2015,Jan,16

54860 Epididymectomy; unilateral ♂

12.1 12.1 **FUD** 090 J A2

AMA: 2014,Jan,11

54861 bilateral ♂

16.3 16.3 **FUD** 090 J A2 80

AMA: 2014,Jan,11

54865 Exploration of epididymis, with or without biopsy ♂

10.3 10.3 **FUD** 090 J A2 80

AMA: 2014,Jan,11; 2007,Jul,5

54900 Epididymovasostomy, anastomosis of epididymis to vas deferens; unilateral ♂

EXCLUDES *Operating microscope (69990)*

23.1 23.1 **FUD** 090 J A2 80

AMA: 2018,Jan,8; 2017,Jan,8; 2016,Jan,13; 2015,Jan,16

54901 **bilateral** ♂

EXCLUDES *Operating microscope (69990)*

30.5 30.5 **FUD** 090 J A2 80

AMA: 2018,Jan,8; 2017,Jan,8; 2016,Jan,13; 2015,Jan,16

55000-55180 Procedures of the Tunica Vaginalis and Scrotum

55000 **Puncture aspiration of hydrocele, tunica vaginalis, with or without injection of medication** ♂

2.44 3.39 **FUD** 000 T P3 50

AMA: 2014,Jan,11

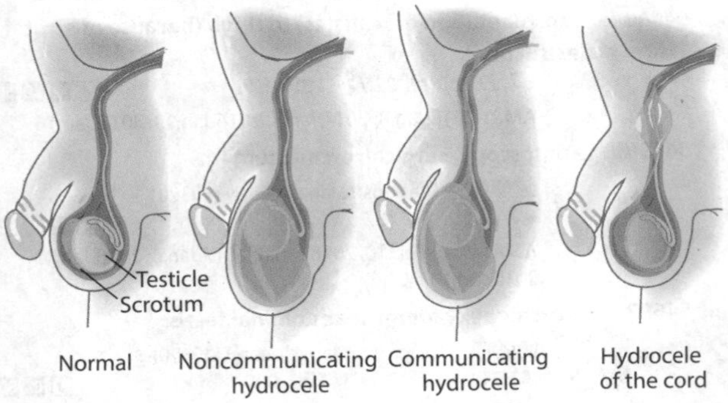

55040 **Excision of hydrocele; unilateral** ♂

EXCLUDES *Repair hernia with hydrocelectomy (49495-49501)*

9.77 9.77 **FUD** 090 J A2

AMA: 2018,Jan,8; 2017,Nov,10; 2017,Jan,8; 2016,Jan,13; 2015,Jan,16

55041 **bilateral** ♂

EXCLUDES *Repair hernia with hydrocelectomy (49495-49501)*

14.7 14.7 **FUD** 090 J A2

AMA: 2014,Jan,11

55060 **Repair of tunica vaginalis hydrocele (Bottle type)** ♂

11.0 11.0 **FUD** 090 J A2 80 50

AMA: 2018,Jan,8; 2017,Jan,8; 2016,Jan,13; 2015,Jan,16

55100 **Drainage of scrotal wall abscess** ♂

EXCLUDES *Debridement genitalia for necrotizing soft tissue infection (11004-11006)*

Incision and drainage scrotal space (54700)

4.80 6.28 **FUD** 010 J A2

AMA: 2014,Jan,11

55110 **Scrotal exploration** ♂

11.1 11.1 **FUD** 090 J A2

AMA: 2014,Jan,11

55120 **Removal of foreign body in scrotum** ♂

10.1 10.1 **FUD** 090 J A2 80

AMA: 2014,Jan,11

55150 **Resection of scrotum** ♂

EXCLUDES *Lesion excision skin, scrotum (11420-11426, 11620-11626)*

14.2 14.2 **FUD** 090 J A2 80

AMA: 2014,Jan,11

55175 **Scrotoplasty; simple** ♂

10.5 10.5 **FUD** 090 J A2 80

AMA: 2018,Jan,8; 2017,Jan,8; 2016,Jan,13; 2015,Jan,16

55180 **complicated** ♂

20.0 20.0 **FUD** 090 J A2 80

AMA: 2014,Jan,11

55200-55680 Procedures of Other Male Genital Ducts and Glands

55200 **Vasotomy, cannulization with or without incision of vas, unilateral or bilateral (separate procedure)** ♂

8.00 11.7 **FUD** 090 J A2 80

AMA: 2014,Jan,11

55250 **Vasectomy, unilateral or bilateral (separate procedure), including postoperative semen examination(s)** ♂

6.58 10.6 **FUD** 090 J A2

AMA: 2018,Jan,8; 2017,Jan,8; 2016,Jan,13; 2015,Jan,16

55300 **Vasotomy for vasograms, seminal vesiculograms, or epididymograms, unilateral or bilateral** ♂

Code also biopsy testis and modifier 51 when combined (54505)

(74440)

5.39 5.39 **FUD** 000 N N1 80

AMA: 2014,Jan,11

55400 **Vasovasostomy, vasovasorrhaphy** ♂

EXCLUDES *Operating microscope (69990)*

14.4 14.4 **FUD** 090 J A2 80 50

AMA: 2018,Jan,8; 2017,Jan,8; 2016,Jan,13; 2015,Jan,16

55500 **Excision of hydrocele of spermatic cord, unilateral (separate procedure)** ♂

11.3 11.3 **FUD** 090 J A2 80 50

AMA: 2018,Jan,8; 2017,Jan,8; 2016,Jan,13; 2015,Jan,16

55520 **Excision of lesion of spermatic cord (separate procedure)** ♂

13.2 13.2 **FUD** 090 J A2 80 50

AMA: 2018,Jan,8; 2017,Jan,8; 2016,Jan,13; 2015,Jan,16

55530 **Excision of varicocele or ligation of spermatic veins for varicocele; (separate procedure)** ♂

10.1 10.1 **FUD** 090 J A2 50

AMA: 2018,Jan,8; 2017,Jan,8; 2016,Jan,13; 2015,Jan,16

55535 **abdominal approach** ♂

12.4 12.4 **FUD** 090 J A2 80 50

AMA: 2018,Jan,8; 2017,Jan,8; 2016,Jan,13; 2015,Jan,16

55540 **with hernia repair** ♂

16.0 16.0 **FUD** 090 J A2 50

AMA: 2018,Jan,8; 2017,Jan,8; 2016,Jan,13; 2015,Jan,16

55550 **Laparoscopy, surgical, with ligation of spermatic veins for varicocele** ♂

INCLUDES Diagnostic laparoscopy (49320)

12.3 12.3 **FUD** 090 J A2 80 50

AMA: 2018,Jan,8; 2017,Jan,8; 2016,Jan,13; 2015,Jan,16

55559 **Unlisted laparoscopy procedure, spermatic cord** ♂

0.00 0.00 **FUD** YYY J 80 50

AMA: 2018,Jan,8; 2017,Jan,8; 2016,Jan,13; 2015,Jan,16

55600 **Vesiculotomy;** ♂

12.1 12.1 **FUD** 090 J R2 80 50

AMA: 2014,Jan,11

55605 **complicated** ♂

15.0 15.0 **FUD** 090 C 80 50

AMA: 2014,Jan,11

55650 **Vesiculectomy, any approach** ♂

20.7 20.7 **FUD** 090 C 80 50

AMA: 2014,Jan,11

55680 **Excision of Mullerian duct cyst** ♂

EXCLUDES *Injection procedure (52010, 55300)*

9.99 9.99 **FUD** 090 J A2 80 50

AMA: 2014,Jan,11

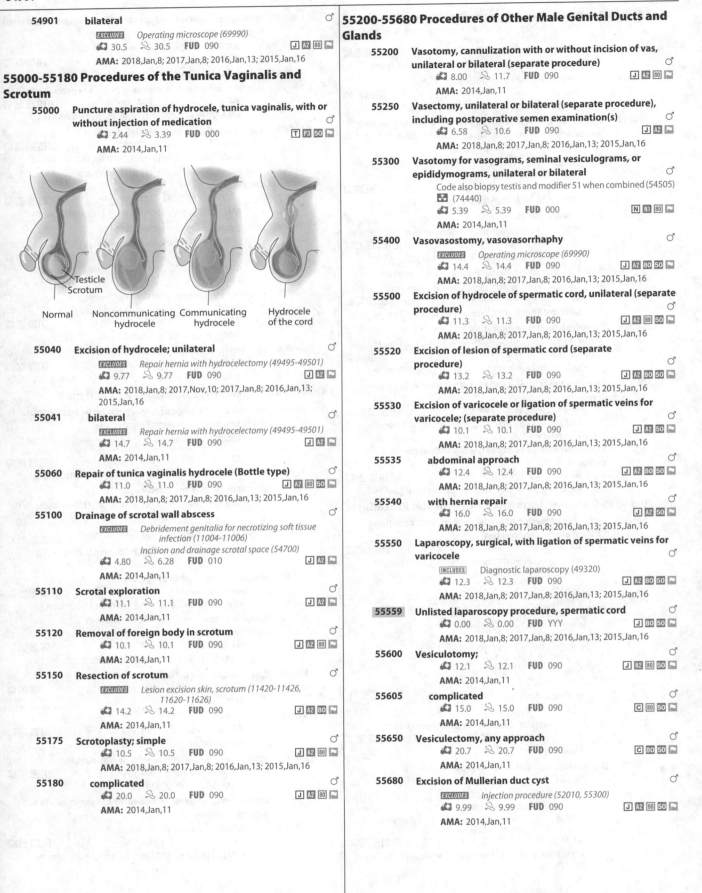

55700-55725 Procedures of Prostate: Incisional

55700 **Biopsy, prostate; needle or punch, single or multiple, any approach** ♂

EXCLUDES *Fine needle aspiration (10021, [10004, 10005, 10006, 10007, 10008, 10009, 10010, 10011, 10012])*
Needle biopsy prostate, saturation sampling for prostate mapping (55706)

(76942, 77002, 77012, 77021)
(88172-88173)
3.77 | 7.12 | **FUD** 000 | J A2
AMA: 2018,Jul,11; 2018,Jan,8; 2017,Jan,8; 2016,Jan,13; 2015,Jan,16

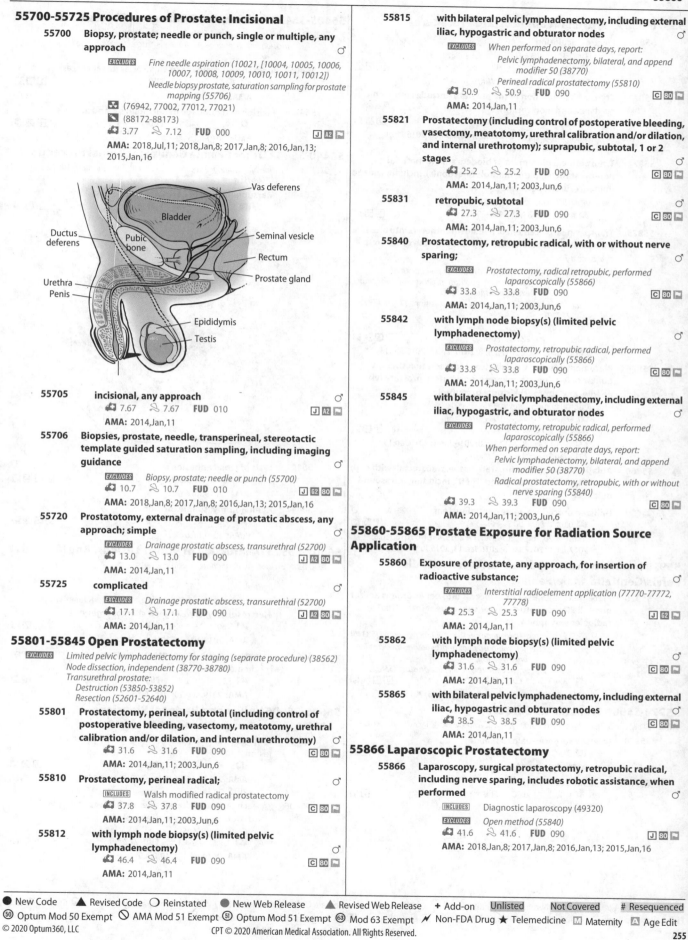

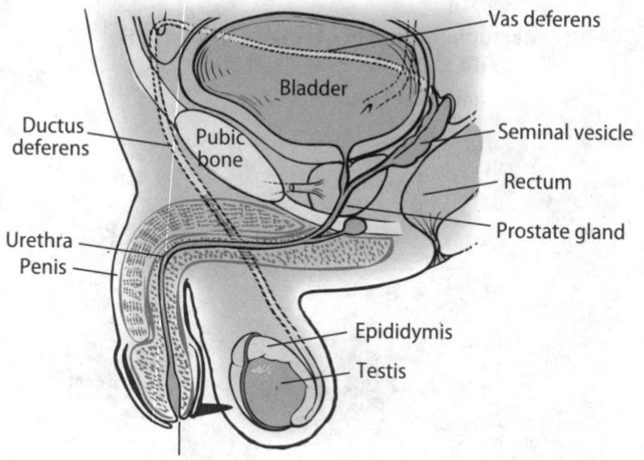

55705 **incisional, any approach** ♂
7.67 | 7.67 | **FUD** 010 | J A2
AMA: 2014,Jan,11

55706 **Biopsies, prostate, needle, transperineal, stereotactic template guided saturation sampling, including imaging guidance** ♂

EXCLUDES *Biopsy, prostate; needle or punch (55700)*

10.7 | 10.7 | **FUD** 010 | J G2 80
AMA: 2018,Jan,8; 2017,Jan,8; 2016,Jan,13; 2015,Jan,16

55720 **Prostatotomy, external drainage of prostatic abscess, any approach; simple** ♂

EXCLUDES *Drainage prostatic abscess, transurethral (52700)*

13.0 | 13.0 | **FUD** 090 | J A2 80
AMA: 2014,Jan,11

55725 **complicated** ♂

EXCLUDES *Drainage prostatic abscess, transurethral (52700)*

17.1 | 17.1 | **FUD** 090 | J A2 80
AMA: 2014,Jan,11

55801-55845 Open Prostatectomy

EXCLUDES *Limited pelvic lymphadenectomy for staging (separate procedure) (38562)*
Node dissection, independent (38770-38780)
Transurethral prostate:
Destruction (53850-53852)
Resection (52601-52640)

55801 **Prostatectomy, perineal, subtotal (including control of postoperative bleeding, vasectomy, meatotomy, urethral calibration and/or dilation, and internal urethrotomy)** ♂
31.6 | 31.6 | **FUD** 090 | C 80
AMA: 2014,Jan,11; 2003,Jun,6

55810 **Prostatectomy, perineal radical;** ♂

INCLUDES Walsh modified radical prostatectomy

37.8 | 37.8 | **FUD** 090 | C 80
AMA: 2014,Jan,11; 2003,Jun,6

55812 **with lymph node biopsy(s) (limited pelvic lymphadenectomy)** ♂
46.4 | 46.4 | **FUD** 090 | C 80
AMA: 2014,Jan,11

55815 **with bilateral pelvic lymphadenectomy, including external iliac, hypogastric and obturator nodes** ♂

EXCLUDES *When performed on separate days, report:*
Pelvic lymphadenectomy, bilateral, and append modifier 50 (38770)
Perineal radical prostatectomy (55810)

50.9 | 50.9 | **FUD** 090 | C 80
AMA: 2014,Jan,11

55821 **Prostatectomy (including control of postoperative bleeding, vasectomy, meatotomy, urethral calibration and/or dilation, and internal urethrotomy); suprapubic, subtotal, 1 or 2 stages** ♂
25.2 | 25.2 | **FUD** 090 | C 80
AMA: 2014,Jan,11; 2003,Jun,6

55831 **retropubic, subtotal** ♂
27.3 | 27.3 | **FUD** 090 | C 80
AMA: 2014,Jan,11; 2003,Jun,6

55840 **Prostatectomy, retropubic radical, with or without nerve sparing;** ♂

EXCLUDES *Prostatectomy, radical retropubic, performed laparoscopically (55866)*

33.8 | 33.8 | **FUD** 090 | C 80
AMA: 2014,Jan,11; 2003,Jun,6

55842 **with lymph node biopsy(s) (limited pelvic lymphadenectomy)** ♂

EXCLUDES *Prostatectomy, retropubic radical, performed laparoscopically (55866)*

33.8 | 33.8 | **FUD** 090 | C 80
AMA: 2014,Jan,11; 2003,Jun,6

55845 **with bilateral pelvic lymphadenectomy, including external iliac, hypogastric, and obturator nodes** ♂

EXCLUDES *Prostatectomy, retropubic radical, performed laparoscopically (55866)*
When performed on separate days, report:
Pelvic lymphadenectomy, bilateral, and append modifier 50 (38770)
Radical prostatectomy, retropubic, with or without nerve sparing (55840)

39.3 | 39.3 | **FUD** 090 | C 80
AMA: 2014,Jan,11; 2003,Jun,6

55860-55865 Prostate Exposure for Radiation Source Application

55860 **Exposure of prostate, any approach, for insertion of radioactive substance;** ♂

EXCLUDES *Interstitial radioelement application (77770-77772, 77778)*

25.3 | 25.3 | **FUD** 090 | J G2
AMA: 2014,Jan,11

55862 **with lymph node biopsy(s) (limited pelvic lymphadenectomy)** ♂
31.6 | 31.6 | **FUD** 090 | C 80
AMA: 2014,Jan,11

55865 **with bilateral pelvic lymphadenectomy, including external iliac, hypogastric and obturator nodes** ♂
38.5 | 38.5 | **FUD** 090 | C 80
AMA: 2014,Jan,11

55866 Laparoscopic Prostatectomy

55866 **Laparoscopy, surgical prostatectomy, retropubic radical, including nerve sparing, includes robotic assistance, when performed** ♂

INCLUDES Diagnostic laparoscopy (49320)
EXCLUDES *Open method (55840)*

41.6 | 41.6 | **FUD** 090 | J 80
AMA: 2018,Jan,8; 2017,Jan,8; 2016,Jan,13; 2015,Jan,16

55870-55899 Miscellaneous Prostate Procedures

55870 Electroejaculation ♂

EXCLUDES *Artificial insemination (58321-58322)*

4.10 5.04 **FUD** 000 T P3

AMA: 2014,Jan,11; 1991,Win,1

55873 Cryosurgical ablation of the prostate (includes ultrasonic guidance and monitoring) ♂

22.0 175. **FUD** 090 J J8

AMA: 2019,Sep,10; 2018,Jan,8; 2017,Jan,8; 2016,Jan,13; 2015,Sep,12; 2015,Jan,16

55874 Transperineal placement of biodegradable material, peri-prostatic, single or multiple injection(s), including image guidance, when performed ♂

INCLUDES Ultrasound guidance (76942)

4.77 87.0 **FUD** 000 T G2

55875 Transperineal placement of needles or catheters into prostate for interstitial radioelement application, with or without cystoscopy ♂

EXCLUDES *Placement needles/catheters for interstitial radioelement application, pelvic organs/genitalia, except prostate (55920)*

Code also interstitial radioelement application (77770-77772, 77778)

(76965)

22.2 22.2 **FUD** 090 J A2 80

AMA: 2018,Jan,8; 2017,Jan,8; 2016,Jan,13; 2015,Jan,16

55876 Placement of interstitial device(s) for radiation therapy guidance (eg, fiducial markers, dosimeter), prostate (via needle, any approach), single or multiple ♂

Code also supply device

(76942, 77002, 77012, 77021)

2.91 4.16 **FUD** 000 S P3

AMA: 2018,Jan,8; 2017,Jan,8; 2016,Jun,3; 2016,Jan,13; 2015,Jan,16

● **55880 Ablation of malignant prostate tissue, transrectal, with high intensity-focused ultrasound (HIFU), including ultrasound guidance**

55899 Unlisted procedure, male genital system ♂

0.00 0.00 **FUD** YYY T 80

AMA: 2020,Aug,6; 2019,Dec,12; 2019,Jun,14; 2018,Jan,8; 2017,Jan,8; 2017,Jan,6; 2016,Jan,13; 2015,Jun,5; 2015,Jan,16

55920 Insertion Brachytherapy Catheters/Needles Pelvis/Genitalia, Male/Female

55920 Placement of needles or catheters into pelvic organs and/or genitalia (except prostate) for subsequent interstitial radioelement application

EXCLUDES *Insertion Heyman capsules for brachytherapy (58346)*
Insertion vaginal ovoids and/or uterine tandems for brachytherapy (57155)
Placement catheters or needles, prostate (55875)

13.0 13.0 **FUD** 000 J G2 80

AMA: 2018,Jan,8; 2017,Jan,8; 2016,Jan,13; 2015,Jan,16

55970-55980 Transsexual Surgery

CMS: 100-02,16,10 Exclusions from Coverage; 100-02,16,180 Services Related to Noncovered Procedures

55970 Intersex surgery; male to female ♂

0.00 0.00 **FUD** YYY J

AMA: 2014,Jan,11

55980 female to male ♀

0.00 0.00 **FUD** YYY J

AMA: 2014,Jan,11

56405-56420 Incision and Drainage of Abscess

EXCLUDES *Incision and drainage Skene's gland cyst/abscess (53060)*
Incision and drainage subcutaneous abscess/cyst/furuncle (10040, 10060, 10061)

56405 Incision and drainage of vulva or perineal abscess ♀

3.43 3.69 **FUD** 010 T P3

AMA: 2019,Jul,6

56420 Incision and drainage of Bartholin's gland abscess ♀

2.97 4.47 **FUD** 010 T P2

AMA: 2019,Jul,6

56440-56442 Other Female Genital Incisional Procedures

EXCLUDES *Incision and drainage subcutaneous abscess/cyst/furuncle (10040, 10060, 10061)*

56440 Marsupialization of Bartholin's gland cyst ♀

5.25 5.25 **FUD** 010 J A2

AMA: 2019,Jul,6

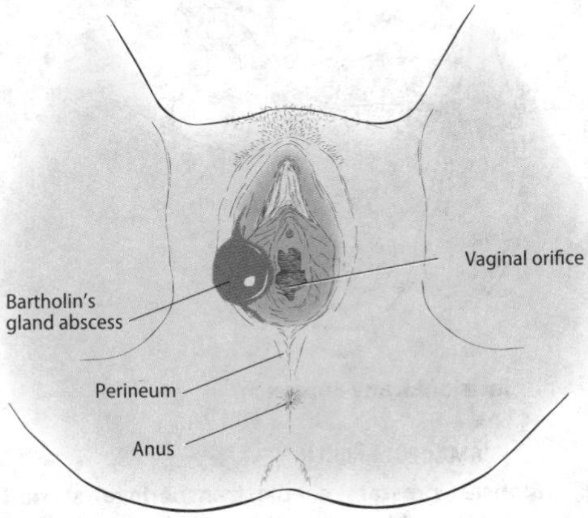

56441 Lysis of labial adhesions ♀

4.09 4.33 **FUD** 010 J A2 80

AMA: 2019,Jul,6

56442 Hymenotomy, simple incision ♀

1.36 1.36 **FUD** 000 J A2 80

AMA: 2019,Jul,6

56501-56515 Destruction of Vulvar Lesions, Any Method

EXCLUDES *Excision/fulguration/destruction:*
Skene's glands (53270)
Urethral caruncle (53265)

56501 Destruction of lesion(s), vulva; simple (eg, laser surgery, electrosurgery, cryosurgery, chemosurgery) ♀

3.60 4.69 **FUD** 010 T P3

AMA: 2019,Aug,10; 2019,Jul,6

56515 extensive (eg, laser surgery, electrosurgery, cryosurgery, chemosurgery) ♀

5.97 7.25 **FUD** 010 T A2

AMA: 2019,Aug,10; 2019,Jul,6

56605-56606 Vulvar and Perineal Biopsies

EXCLUDES *Excision local lesion (11420-11426, 11620-11626)*

56605 Biopsy of vulva or perineum (separate procedure); 1 lesion ♀

1.71 2.43 **FUD** 000 T P3

AMA: 2019,Jul,6; 2019,Jan,9; 2018,Jan,8; 2017,Jan,8; 2016,Jan,13; 2015,Jan,16

+ **56606 each separate additional lesion (List separately in addition to code for primary procedure)** ♀

Code first (56605)

0.86 1.11 **FUD** ZZZ N N1

AMA: 2019,Jul,6; 2019,Jan,9

56620-56640 Vulvectomy Procedures

INCLUDES Removal:
Greater than 80% vulvar area - complete procedure
Less than 80% vulvar area - partial procedure
Skin and deep subcutaneous tissue - radical procedure
Skin and superficial subcutaneous tissues - simple procedure

EXCLUDES *Skin graft (15004-15005, 15120-15121, 15240-15241)*

56620 **Vulvectomy simple; partial** ♀
15.9 15.9 FUD 090 J A2 80
AMA: 2019,Jul,6; 2019,Jan,14; 2018,Jan,8; 2017,Jan,8; 2016,Jan,13; 2015,Jan,16

56625 **complete** ♀
18.6 18.6 FUD 090 J A2 80
AMA: 2019,Jul,6

56630 **Vulvectomy, radical, partial;** ♀
Code also lymph node biopsy/excision when partial radical vulvectomy with inguinofemoral lymph node biopsy without inguinofemoral lymphadenectomy performed (38531)
27.0 27.0 FUD 090 C 80
AMA: 2019,Jul,6; 2019,Feb,8

56631 **with unilateral inguinofemoral lymphadenectomy** ♀
INCLUDES Bassett's operation
34.4 34.4 FUD 090 C 80
AMA: 2019,Jul,6; 2019,Feb,8

56632 **with bilateral inguinofemoral lymphadenectomy** ♀
INCLUDES Bassett's operation
40.2 40.2 FUD 090 C 80
AMA: 2019,Jul,6; 2019,Feb,8

56633 **Vulvectomy, radical, complete;** ♀
INCLUDES Bassett's operation
34.9 34.9 FUD 090 C 80
AMA: 2019,Jul,6; 2019,Feb,8

56634 **with unilateral inguinofemoral lymphadenectomy** ♀
INCLUDES Bassett's operation
36.8 36.8 FUD 090 C 80
AMA: 2019,Jul,6; 2019,Feb,8

56637 **with bilateral inguinofemoral lymphadenectomy** ♀
INCLUDES Bassett's operation
Code also lymph node biopsy/excision when complete radical vulvectomy with inguinofemoral lymph node biopsy without inguinofemoral lymphadenectomy performed (38531)
43.9 43.9 FUD 090 C 80
AMA: 2019,Jul,6; 2019,Feb,8

56640 **Vulvectomy, radical, complete, with inguinofemoral, iliac, and pelvic lymphadenectomy** ♀
INCLUDES Bassett's operation
EXCLUDES *Lymphadenectomy (38760-38780)*
43.3 43.3 FUD 090 C 80 50
AMA: 2019,Jul,6; 2019,Feb,8

56700-56740 Other Excisional Procedures: External Female Genitalia

56700 **Partial hymenectomy or revision of hymenal ring** ♀
5.38 5.38 FUD 010 J A2 80
AMA: 2019,Jul,6

56740 **Excision of Bartholin's gland or cyst** ♀
EXCLUDES *Excision/fulguration/marsupialization:*
Skene's glands (53270)
Urethral carcinoma (53220)
Urethral caruncle (53265)
Urethral diverticulum (53230, 53240)
8.92 8.92 FUD 010 J A2 50
AMA: 2019,Jul,6

56800-56810 Repair/Reconstruction External Female Genitalia

EXCLUDES *Repair urethra for mucosal prolapse (53275)*

56800 **Plastic repair of introitus** ♀
INCLUDES Emmet's operation
7.17 7.17 FUD 010 J A2 80
AMA: 2019,Jul,6

56805 **Clitoroplasty for intersex state** ♀
33.6 33.6 FUD 090 J G2 80
AMA: 2019,Jul,6

56810 **Perineoplasty, repair of perineum, nonobstetrical (separate procedure)** ♀
INCLUDES Emmet's operation
EXCLUDES *Genitalia wound repair (12001-12007, 12041-12047, 13131-13133)*
Introitus plastic repair (56800)
Sphincteroplasty, anal (46750-46751)
Vaginal/perineum recent injury repair, nonobstetrical (57210)
7.72 7.72 FUD 010 J A2 80
AMA: 2019,Jul,6

56820-56821 Vulvar Colposcopy with/without Biopsy

EXCLUDES *Colposcopic procedures and/or examinations:*
Cervix (57452-57461)
Vagina (57420-57421)

56820 **Colposcopy of the vulva;** ♀
2.46 3.28 FUD 000 T P3
AMA: 2019,Jul,6; 2018,Jan,8; 2017,Jan,8; 2016,Jan,13; 2015,Jan,16

56821 **with biopsy(s)** ♀
3.28 4.36 FUD 000 T P3
AMA: 2019,Jul,6; 2018,Jan,8; 2017,Jan,8; 2016,Jan,13; 2015,Jan,16

57000-57023 Incisional Procedures: Vagina

57000 **Colpotomy; with exploration** ♀
5.44 5.44 FUD 010 J A2 80
AMA: 2019,Jul,6; 2018,Jan,8; 2017,Jan,8; 2016,Jan,13; 2015,Jan,16

57010 **with drainage of pelvic abscess** ♀
INCLUDES Laroyenne operation
12.9 12.9 FUD 090 J A2 80
AMA: 2019,Jul,6

57020 **Colpocentesis (separate procedure)** ♀
2.35 3.17 FUD 000 J A2 80
AMA: 2019,Jul,6

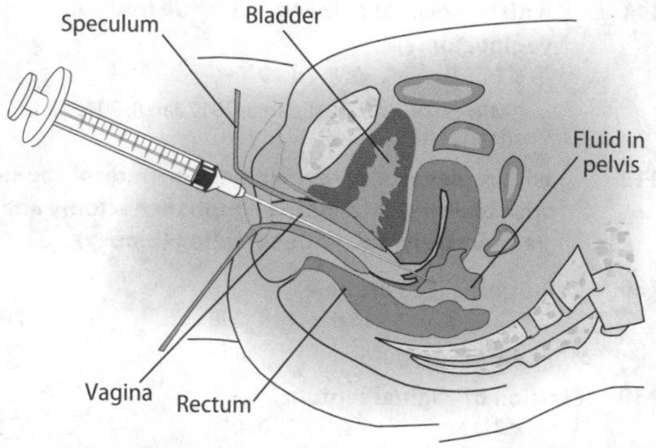

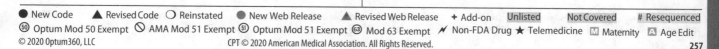

The physician aspirates matter from the pelvis through a needle inserted through the vaginal wall

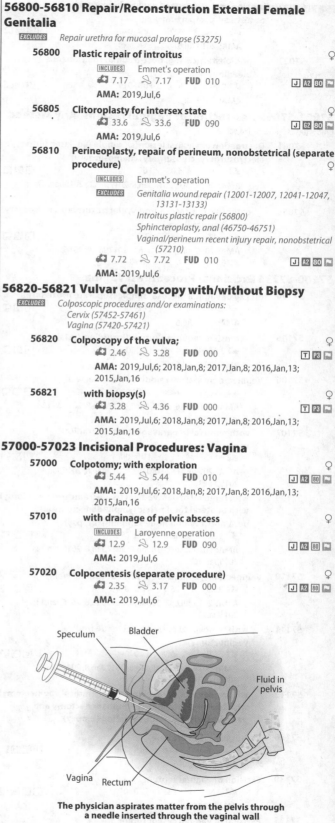

57022 **Incision and drainage of vaginal hematoma; obstetrical/postpartum** ♀
4.86 4.86 FUD 010 J R2 80
AMA: 2019,Jul,6

57023 **non-obstetrical (eg, post-trauma, spontaneous bleeding)** ♀
9.16 9.16 FUD 010 J A2 80
AMA: 2019,Jul,6

57061-57065 Destruction of Vaginal Lesions, Any Method

CMS: 100-03,140.5 Laser Procedures

57061 **Destruction of vaginal lesion(s); simple (eg, laser surgery, electrosurgery, cryosurgery, chemosurgery)** ♀
3.09 4.05 FUD 010 J P3
AMA: 2019,Jul,6; 2018,Jan,8; 2017,Jan,8; 2016,Jan,13; 2015,Jan,16

57065 **extensive (eg, laser surgery, electrosurgery, cryosurgery, chemosurgery)** ♀
5.08 5.88 FUD 010 J A2
AMA: 2019,Jul,6; 2018,Jan,8; 2017,Jan,8; 2016,Jan,13; 2015,Jan,16

57100-57135 Excisional Procedures: Vagina

57100 **Biopsy of vaginal mucosa; simple (separate procedure)** ♀
1.90 2.76 FUD 000 T P3
AMA: 2019,Jul,6

57105 **extensive, requiring suture (including cysts)** ♀
3.75 4.19 FUD 010 J A2
AMA: 2019,Jul,6

57106 **Vaginectomy, partial removal of vaginal wall;** ♀
14.5 14.5 FUD 090 J 80
AMA: 2019,Jul,6; 2018,Jan,8; 2017,Jan,8; 2016,Jan,13; 2015,Jan,16

57107 **with removal of paravaginal tissue (radical vaginectomy)** ♀
41.5 41.5 FUD 090 J 80
AMA: 2019,Jul,6; 2018,Jan,8; 2017,Jan,8; 2016,Jan,13; 2015,Jan,16

57109 **with removal of paravaginal tissue (radical vaginectomy) with bilateral total pelvic lymphadenectomy and para-aortic lymph node sampling (biopsy)** ♀
50.8 50.8 FUD 090 J 80
AMA: 2019,Jul,6; 2018,Jan,8; 2017,Jan,8; 2016,Jan,13; 2015,Jan,16

57110 **Vaginectomy, complete removal of vaginal wall;** ♀
25.3 25.3 FUD 090 C 80
AMA: 2019,Jul,6; 2018,Jan,8; 2017,Jan,8; 2016,Jan,13; 2015,Jan,16

57111 **with removal of paravaginal tissue (radical vaginectomy)** ♀
50.9 50.9 FUD 090 C 80
AMA: 2019,Jul,6; 2018,Jan,8; 2017,Jan,8; 2016,Jan,13; 2015,Jan,16

57112 ~~**with removal of paravaginal tissue (radical vaginectomy) with bilateral total pelvic lymphadenectomy and para-aortic lymph node sampling (biopsy)**~~

57120 **Colpocleisis (Le Fort type)** ♀
14.6 14.6 FUD 090 J G2 80
AMA: 2019,Jul,6

57130 **Excision of vaginal septum** ♀
4.60 5.32 FUD 010 J A2 80
AMA: 2019,Jul,6

57135 **Excision of vaginal cyst or tumor** ♀
5.05 5.80 FUD 010 J A2
AMA: 2019,Jul,6

57150-57180 Irrigation/Insertion/Introduction Vaginal Medication or Supply

57150 **Irrigation of vagina and/or application of medicament for treatment of bacterial, parasitic, or fungoid disease** ♀
0.78 1.54 FUD 000 01 N1
AMA: 2019,Jul,6

57155 **Insertion of uterine tandem and/or vaginal ovoids for clinical brachytherapy** ♀
EXCLUDES *Insertion radioelement sources or ribbons (77761-77763, 77770-77772)*
Placement needles or catheters into pelvic organs and/or genitalia (except prostate) for interstitial radioelement application (55920)
8.09 10.6 FUD 000 J A2
AMA: 2019,Jul,6; 2018,Jan,8; 2017,Jan,8; 2016,Jan,13; 2015,Jan,16

57156 **Insertion of a vaginal radiation afterloading apparatus for clinical brachytherapy** ♀
4.27 5.92 FUD 000 T G2 80
AMA: 2019,Jul,6

57160 **Fitting and insertion of pessary or other intravaginal support device** ♀
1.33 1.79 FUD 000 T P3
AMA: 2019,Jul,6; 2018,Jan,8; 2017,Jan,8; 2016,Jan,13; 2015,Jan,16

57170 **Diaphragm or cervical cap fitting with instructions** ♀
1.37 1.85 FUD 000 T P3 80
AMA: 2019,Jul,6

57180 **Introduction of any hemostatic agent or pack for spontaneous or traumatic nonobstetrical vaginal hemorrhage (separate procedure)** ♀
3.11 4.37 FUD 010 T A2
AMA: 2019,Jul,6; 2018,Jan,8; 2017,Jan,8; 2016,Jan,13; 2015,Jan,16

57200-57335 Vaginal Repair and Reconstruction

EXCLUDES *Marshall-Marchetti-Kranz type urethral suspension, abdominal approach (51840-51841)*
Urethral suspension performed laparoscopically (51990)

57200 **Colporrhaphy, suture of injury of vagina (nonobstetrical)** ♀
8.87 8.87 FUD 090 J A2 80
AMA: 2019,Jul,6

57210 **Colpoperineorrhaphy, suture of injury of vagina and/or perineum (nonobstetrical)** ♀
10.6 10.6 FUD 090 J A2 80
AMA: 2019,Jul,6

57220 **Plastic operation on urethral sphincter, vaginal approach (eg, Kelly urethral plication)** ♀
9.24 9.24 FUD 090 J A2 80
AMA: 2019,Jul,6

57230 **Plastic repair of urethrocele** ♀
11.3 11.3 FUD 090 J A2 80
AMA: 2019,Jul,6

57240 **Anterior colporrhaphy, repair of cystocele with or without repair of urethrocele, including cystourethroscopy, when performed** ♀
INCLUDES Cystourethroscopy (52000)
17.0 17.0 FUD 090 J A2 80
AMA: 2019,Jul,6; 2018,Jan,8; 2017,Jan,8; 2016,Jan,13; 2015,Jan,16

57250 Posterior colporrhaphy, repair of rectocele with or without perineorrhaphy ♀

INCLUDES Rectocele repair (separate procedure) without posterior colporrhaphy (45560)

17.0 17.0 FUD 090 J A2 80

AMA: 2019,Jul,6; 2018,Jan,8; 2017,Jan,8; 2016,Jan,13; 2015,Jan,16

57260 Combined anteroposterior colporrhaphy, including cystourethroscopy, when performed; ♀

INCLUDES Cystourethroscopy (52000)

21.7 21.7 FUD 090 J A2 80

AMA: 2019,Jul,6; 2018,Jan,8; 2017,Jan,8; 2016,Jan,13; 2015,Jan,16

57265 with enterocele repair ♀

INCLUDES Cystourethroscopy (52000)

24.4 24.4 FUD 090 J A2 80

AMA: 2019,Jul,6; 2018,Jan,8; 2017,Jan,8; 2016,Jan,13; 2015,Jan,16

+ **57267 Insertion of mesh or other prosthesis for repair of pelvic floor defect, each site (anterior, posterior compartment), vaginal approach (List separately in addition to code for primary procedure)** ♀

Code first (45560, 57240-57265, 57285)

7.25 7.25 FUD ZZZ N N1 80

AMA: 2019,Jul,6; 2018,Jan,8; 2017,Jan,8; 2016,Jan,13; 2015,Jan,16

57268 Repair of enterocele, vaginal approach (separate procedure) ♀

13.9 13.9 FUD 090 J A2 80

AMA: 2019,Jul,6; 2018,Jan,8; 2017,Jan,8; 2016,Jan,13; 2015,Jan,16

57270 Repair of enterocele, abdominal approach (separate procedure) ♀

23.0 23.0 FUD 090 C 80

AMA: 2019,Jul,6; 2018,Jan,8; 2017,Jan,8; 2016,Jan,13; 2015,Jan,16

57280 Colpopexy, abdominal approach ♀

27.2 27.2 FUD 090 C 80

AMA: 2019,Jul,6; 2018,Jan,8; 2017,Jan,8; 2016,Jan,13; 2015,Jan,16

57282 Colpopexy, vaginal; extra-peritoneal approach (sacrospinous, iliococcygeus) ♀

15.1 15.1 FUD 090 J 80

AMA: 2019,Jul,6; 2018,Jan,8; 2017,Jan,8; 2016,Jan,13; 2015,Jan,16

57283 intra-peritoneal approach (uterosacral, levator myorrhaphy) ♀

EXCLUDES *Excision cervical stump (57556)*
Vaginal hysterectomy (58263, 58270, 58280, 58292, 58294)

19.6 19.6 FUD 090 J 80

AMA: 2019,Jul,6; 2018,Jan,8; 2017,Jan,8; 2016,Jan,13; 2015,Jan,16

57284 Paravaginal defect repair (including repair of cystocele, if performed); open abdominal approach ♀

EXCLUDES *Anterior colporrhaphy (57240)*
Anterior vesicourethropexy (51840-51841)
Combined anteroposterior colporrhaphy (57260-57265)
Hysterectomy (58152, 58267)
Laparoscopy, surgical; urethral suspension for stress incontinence (51990)

23.8 23.8 FUD 090 J 80

AMA: 2019,Jul,6; 2018,Jan,8; 2017,Jan,8; 2016,Jan,13; 2015,Jan,16

57285 vaginal approach ♀

EXCLUDES *Anterior colporrhaphy (57240)*
Combined anteroposterior colporrhaphy (57260-57265)
Laparoscopy, surgical; urethral suspension for stress incontinence (51990)
Vaginal hysterectomy (58267)

19.2 19.2 FUD 090 J 80

AMA: 2019,Jul,6; 2018,Jan,8; 2017,Jan,8; 2016,Jan,13; 2015,Jan,16

57287 Removal or revision of sling for stress incontinence (eg, fascia or synthetic) ♀

20.6 20.6 FUD 090 02 G2 80

AMA: 2019,Jul,6; 2018,Jan,8; 2017,Jan,8; 2016,Jan,13; 2015,Jan,16

57288 Sling operation for stress incontinence (eg, fascia or synthetic) ♀

INCLUDES Millin-Read operation

EXCLUDES *Sling operation for stress incontinence performed laparoscopically (51992)*

21.1 21.1 FUD 090 J J8 80

AMA: 2019,Jul,6; 2019,Feb,10; 2018,Jan,8; 2017,Jan,8; 2016,Jan,13; 2015,Jan,16

57289 Pereyra procedure, including anterior colporrhaphy ♀

21.7 21.7 FUD 090 J A2 80

AMA: 2019,Jul,6; 2018,Jan,8; 2017,Jan,8; 2016,Jan,13; 2015,Jan,16

57291 Construction of artificial vagina; without graft ♀

INCLUDES McIndoe vaginal construction

15.6 15.6 FUD 090 J A2 80

AMA: 2019,Jul,6

57292 with graft ♀

23.9 23.9 FUD 090 J 80

AMA: 2019,Jul,6

57295 Revision (including removal) of prosthetic vaginal graft; vaginal approach ♀

EXCLUDES *Laparoscopic approach (57426)*

14.2 14.2 FUD 090 J G2 80

AMA: 2019,Jul,6

57296 open abdominal approach ♀

EXCLUDES *Laparoscopic approach (57426)*

27.4 27.4 FUD 090 C 80

AMA: 2019,Jul,6

57300 Closure of rectovaginal fistula; vaginal or transanal approach ♀

17.0 17.0 FUD 090 J A2 80

AMA: 2019,Jul,6

57305 abdominal approach ♀

27.9 27.9 FUD 090 C 80

AMA: 2019,Jul,6

57307 abdominal approach, with concomitant colostomy ♀

30.3 30.3 FUD 090 C 80

AMA: 2019,Jul,6

57308 transperineal approach, with perineal body reconstruction, with or without levator plication ♀

19.0 19.0 FUD 090 C 80

AMA: 2019,Jul,6

57310 Closure of urethrovaginal fistula; ♀

13.8 13.8 FUD 090 J G2 80

AMA: 2019,Jul,6

57311 with bulbocavernosus transplant ♀

15.6 15.6 FUD 090 C 80

AMA: 2019,Jul,6

Genital System

57320 — 57460

57320 Closure of vesicovaginal fistula; vaginal approach ♀

EXCLUDES *Cystostomy, concomitant (51020-51040, 51101-51102)*

15.8 15.8 FUD 090 J G2 80

AMA: 2019,Jul,6

57330 transvesical and vaginal approach ♀

EXCLUDES *Vesicovaginal fistula closure, abdominal approach (51900)*

21.8 21.8 FUD 090 J 80

AMA: 2019,Jul,6

57335 Vaginoplasty for intersex state ♀

33.9 33.9 FUD 090 J 80

AMA: 2019,Jul,6

57400-57415 Treatment of Vaginal Disorders Under Anesthesia

57400 Dilation of vagina under anesthesia (other than local) ♀

3.81 3.81 FUD 000 J A2 80

AMA: 2019,Jul,6

57410 Pelvic examination under anesthesia (other than local) ♀

3.05 3.05 FUD 000 J A2

AMA: 2019,Jul,6; 2018,Jan,8; 2017,Jan,8; 2016,Jan,13; 2015,Jan,16

57415 Removal of impacted vaginal foreign body (separate procedure) under anesthesia (other than local) ♀

EXCLUDES *Removal impacted vaginal foreign body without anesthesia, report with appropriate E/M code*

4.89 4.89 FUD 010 J A2 80

AMA: 2019,Jul,6

57420-57426 Endoscopic Vaginal Procedures

57420 Colposcopy of the entire vagina, with cervix if present; ♀

EXCLUDES *Colposcopic procedures and/or examinations:*
Cervix (57452-57461)
Vulva (56820-56821)

Code also computer-aided cervical mapping during colposcopy (57465)

Code also endometrial sampling (biopsy) performed same time as colposcopy (58110)

Code also modifier 51 for colposcopic procedures different sites, as appropriate

2.62 3.61 FUD 000 T P3

AMA: 2019,Jul,6; 2018,Jan,8; 2017,Jan,8; 2016,Jan,13; 2015,Jan,16

57421 with biopsy(s) of vagina/cervix ♀

EXCLUDES *Colposcopic procedures and/or examinations:*
Cervix (57452-57461)
Vulva (56820-56821)

Code also computer-aided cervical mapping during colposcopy (57465)

Code also endometrial sampling (biopsy) performed same time as colposcopy (58110)

Code also modifier 51 for colposcopic procedures multiple sites, as appropriate

3.55 4.86 FUD 000 T P3

AMA: 2019,Jul,6; 2018,Jan,8; 2017,Jan,8; 2016,Jan,13; 2015,Jan,16

57423 Paravaginal defect repair (including repair of cystocele, if performed), laparoscopic approach ♀

EXCLUDES *Anterior colporrhaphy (57240)*
Anterior vesicourethropexy (51840-51841)
Combined anteroposterior colporrhaphy (57260)
Diagnostic laparoscopy (49320)
Hysterectomy (58152, 58267)
Laparoscopy, surgical; urethral suspension for stress incontinence (51990)

26.8 26.8 FUD 090 J 80

AMA: 2019,Jul,6; 2018,Jan,8; 2017,Jan,8; 2016,Jan,13; 2015,Jan,16

57425 Laparoscopy, surgical, colpopexy (suspension of vaginal apex) ♀

27.6 27.6 FUD 090 J 80

AMA: 2019,Jul,6

57426 Revision (including removal) of prosthetic vaginal graft, laparoscopic approach ♀

EXCLUDES *Open abdominal approach (57296)*
Vaginal approach (57295)

24.8 24.8 FUD 090 J G2 80

AMA: 2019,Jul,6

57452-57465 Endoscopic Cervical Procedures

EXCLUDES *Colposcopic procedures and/or examinations:*
Vagina (57420-57421)
Vulva (56820-56821)

Code also endometrial sampling (biopsy) performed same time as colposcopy (58110)

57452 Colposcopy of the cervix including upper/adjacent vagina; ♀

Code also computer-aided cervical mapping during colposcopy (57465)

2.64 3.45 FUD 000 T P3

AMA: 2019,Jul,6; 2018,Jan,8; 2017,Jan,8; 2016,Jan,13; 2015,Jan,16

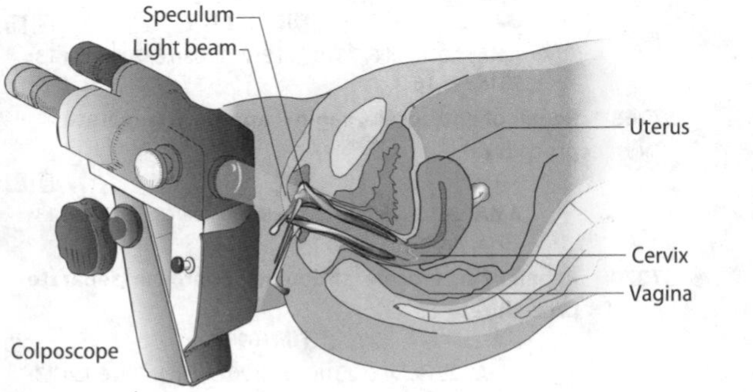

57454 with biopsy(s) of the cervix and endocervical curettage ♀

INCLUDES Colposcopy cervix (57452)

Code also computer-aided cervical mapping during colposcopy (57465)

3.89 4.71 FUD 000 T P3

AMA: 2019,Jul,6; 2018,Jan,8; 2017,Jan,8; 2016,Jan,13; 2015,Jan,16

57455 with biopsy(s) of the cervix ♀

INCLUDES Colposcopy cervix (57452)

Code also computer-aided cervical mapping during colposcopy (57465)

3.19 4.44 FUD 000 T P3

AMA: 2019,Jul,6; 2018,Jan,8; 2017,Jan,8; 2016,Jan,13; 2015,Jan,16

57456 with endocervical curettage ♀

INCLUDES Colposcopy cervix (57452)

EXCLUDES *Colposcopy cervix including upper/adjacent vagina; with loop electrode conization cervix (57461)*

Code also computer-aided cervical mapping during colposcopy (57465)

2.90 3.95 FUD 000 T P3

AMA: 2019,Jul,6; 2018,Jan,8; 2017,Jan,8; 2016,Jan,13; 2015,Jan,16

57460 with loop electrode biopsy(s) of the cervix ♀

INCLUDES Colposcopy cervix (57452)

Code also computer-aided cervical mapping during colposcopy (57465)

4.66 8.78 FUD 000 J P3

AMA: 2019,Jul,6; 2018,Jan,8; 2017,Jan,8; 2016,Jan,13; 2015,Jan,16

57461 **with loop electrode conization of the cervix** ♀

INCLUDES Colposcopy cervix (57452)

EXCLUDES *Colposcopy cervix including upper/adjacent vagina; with endocervical curettage (57456)*

Code also computer-aided cervical mapping during colposcopy (57465)

5.39 | 9.85 | FUD 000 | J P3

AMA: 2019,Jul,6; 2018,Jan,8; 2017,Jan,8; 2016,Jan,13; 2015,Jan,16

● + **57465** **Computer-aided mapping of cervix uteri during colposcopy, including optical dynamic spectral imaging and algorithmic quantification of the acetowhitening effect (List separately in addition to code for primary procedure)**

Code first (57420-57421, 57452-57461)

0.00 | 0.00 | FUD 000

57500-57556 Cervical Procedures: Multiple Techniques

EXCLUDES *Radical surgical procedures (58200-58240)*

57500 **Biopsy of cervix, single or multiple, or local excision of lesion, with or without fulguration (separate procedure)** ♀

2.17 | 4.11 | FUD 000 | T P3

AMA: 2019,Jul,6

57505 **Endocervical curettage (not done as part of a dilation and curettage)** ♀

2.90 | 3.69 | FUD 010 | T P3

AMA: 2019,Jul,6; 2018,Jan,8; 2017,Jan,8; 2016,Jan,13; 2015,Jan,16

57510 **Cautery of cervix; electro or thermal** ♀

3.29 | 4.33 | FUD 010 | J P3

AMA: 2019,Jul,6

57511 **cryocautery, initial or repeat** ♀

3.86 | 4.43 | FUD 010 | T P3

AMA: 2019,Jul,6

57513 **laser ablation** ♀

4.05 | 5.08 | FUD 010 | J A2

AMA: 2019,Jul,6

57520 **Conization of cervix, with or without fulguration, with or without dilation and curettage, with or without repair; cold knife or laser** ♀

EXCLUDES *Dilation and curettage, diagnostic/therapeutic, nonobstetrical (58120)*

8.23 | 9.59 | FUD 090 | J A2

AMA: 2019,Jul,6; 2018,Jan,8; 2017,Jan,8; 2016,Jan,13; 2015,Jan,16

57522 **loop electrode excision** ♀

7.21 | 8.25 | FUD 090 | J A2

AMA: 2019,Jul,6; 2018,Jan,8; 2017,Jan,8; 2016,Jan,13; 2015,Jan,16

57530 **Trachelectomy (cervicectomy), amputation of cervix (separate procedure)** ♀

10.0 | 10.0 | FUD 090 | J A2 80

AMA: 2019,Jul,6

57531 **Radical trachelectomy, with bilateral total pelvic lymphadenectomy and para-aortic lymph node sampling biopsy, with or without removal of tube(s), with or without removal of ovary(s)** ♀

EXCLUDES *Radical hysterectomy (58210)*

52.9 | 52.9 | FUD 090 | C 80

AMA: 2019,Jul,6

57540 **Excision of cervical stump, abdominal approach;** ♀

22.8 | 22.8 | FUD 090 | C 80

AMA: 2019,Jul,6

57545 **with pelvic floor repair** ♀

24.0 | 24.0 | FUD 090 | C 80

AMA: 2019,Jul,6

57550 **Excision of cervical stump, vaginal approach;** ♀

12.1 | 12.1 | FUD 090 | J A2 80

AMA: 2019,Jul,6

57555 **with anterior and/or posterior repair** ♀

17.7 | 17.7 | FUD 090 | J 80

AMA: 2019,Jul,6

57556 **with repair of enterocele** ♀

EXCLUDES *Insertion hemostatic agent/pack for spontaneous/traumatic nonobstetrical vaginal hemorrhage (57180)*

Intrauterine device insertion (58300)

16.8 | 16.8 | FUD 090 | J A2 80

AMA: 2019,Jul,6

57558-57800 Cervical Procedures: Dilation, Suturing, or Instrumentation

57558 **Dilation and curettage of cervical stump** ♀

EXCLUDES *Radical surgical procedures (58200-58240)*

3.33 | 3.80 | FUD 010 | J A2

AMA: 2019,Jul,6

57700 **Cerclage of uterine cervix, nonobstetrical** ♀

INCLUDES McDonald cerclage

Shirodker operation

9.13 | 9.13 | FUD 090 | J A2 80

AMA: 2019,Jul,6

57720 **Trachelorrhaphy, plastic repair of uterine cervix, vaginal approach** ♀

INCLUDES Emmet operation

9.33 | 9.33 | FUD 090 | J A2 80

AMA: 2019,Jul,6

57800 **Dilation of cervical canal, instrumental (separate procedure)** ♀

1.39 | 2.01 | FUD 000 | J P3

AMA: 2019,Jul,6

58100-58120 Procedures Involving the Endometrium

58100 **Endometrial sampling (biopsy) with or without endocervical sampling (biopsy), without cervical dilation, any method (separate procedure)** ♀

EXCLUDES *Endocervical curettage only (57505)*

Endometrial sampling (biopsy) performed in conjunction with colposcopy (58110)

1.86 | 2.80 | FUD 000 | T P3

AMA: 2019,Jul,6

\+ **58110** **Endometrial sampling (biopsy) performed in conjunction with colposcopy (List separately in addition to code for primary procedure)** ♀

Code first colposcopy (57420-57421, 57452-57461)

1.19 | 1.46 | FUD ZZZ | N N1 80

AMA: 2019,Jul,6; 2018,Jan,8; 2017,Jan,8; 2016,Jan,13; 2015,Jan,16

57461 — 58110

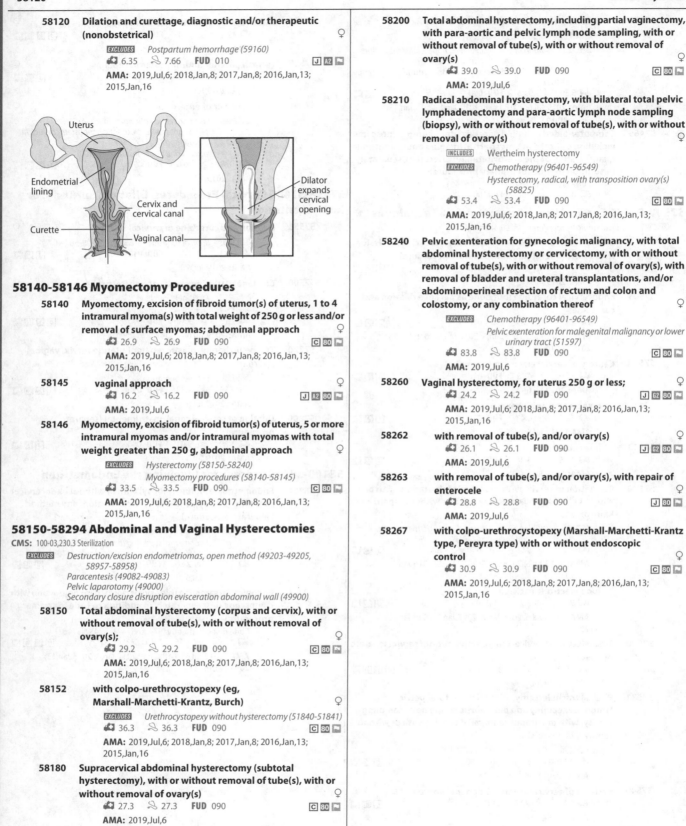

58120 **Dilation and curettage, diagnostic and/or therapeutic (nonobstetrical)** ♀

EXCLUDES *Postpartum hemorrhage (59160)*

Facility RVU 6.35 Non-Facility RVU 7.66 FUD 010 J A2 CCI

AMA: 2019,Jul,6; 2018,Jan,8; 2017,Jan,8; 2016,Jan,13; 2015,Jan,16

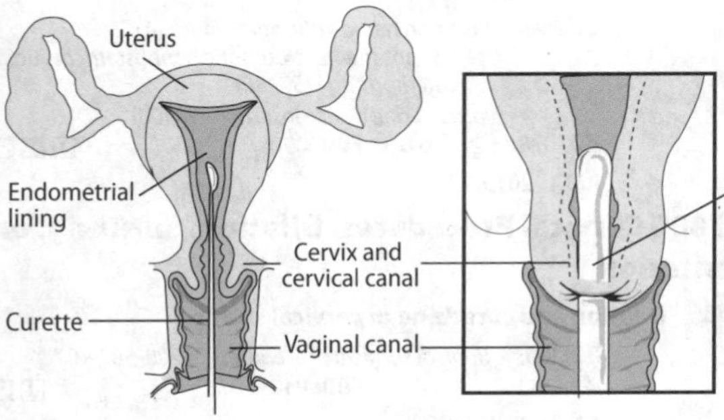

58140-58146 Myomectomy Procedures

58140 **Myomectomy, excision of fibroid tumor(s) of uterus, 1 to 4 intramural myoma(s) with total weight of 250 g or less and/or removal of surface myomas; abdominal approach** ♀

Facility RVU 26.9 Non-Facility RVU 26.9 FUD 090 C 80 CCI

AMA: 2019,Jul,6; 2018,Jan,8; 2017,Jan,8; 2016,Jan,13; 2015,Jan,16

58145 **vaginal approach** ♀

Facility RVU 16.2 Non-Facility RVU 16.2 FUD 090 J A2 80 CCI

AMA: 2019,Jul,6

58146 **Myomectomy, excision of fibroid tumor(s) of uterus, 5 or more intramural myomas and/or intramural myomas with total weight greater than 250 g, abdominal approach** ♀

EXCLUDES *Hysterectomy (58150-58240)*
Myomectomy procedures (58140-58145)

Facility RVU 33.5 Non-Facility RVU 33.5 FUD 090 C 80 CCI

AMA: 2019,Jul,6; 2018,Jan,8; 2017,Jan,8; 2016,Jan,13; 2015,Jan,16

58150-58294 Abdominal and Vaginal Hysterectomies

CMS: 100-03,230.3 Sterilization

EXCLUDES *Destruction/excision endometriomas, open method (49203-49205, 58957-58958)*
Paracentesis (49082-49083)
Pelvic laparotomy (49000)
Secondary closure disruption evisceration abdominal wall (49900)

58150 **Total abdominal hysterectomy (corpus and cervix), with or without removal of tube(s), with or without removal of ovary(s);** ♀

Facility RVU 29.2 Non-Facility RVU 29.2 FUD 090 C 80 CCI

AMA: 2019,Jul,6; 2018,Jan,8; 2017,Jan,8; 2016,Jan,13; 2015,Jan,16

58152 **with colpo-urethrocystopexy (eg, Marshall-Marchetti-Krantz, Burch)** ♀

EXCLUDES *Urethrocystopexy without hysterectomy (51840-51841)*

Facility RVU 36.3 Non-Facility RVU 36.3 FUD 090 C 80 CCI

AMA: 2019,Jul,6; 2018,Jan,8; 2017,Jan,8; 2016,Jan,13; 2015,Jan,16

58180 **Supracervical abdominal hysterectomy (subtotal hysterectomy), with or without removal of tube(s), with or without removal of ovary(s)** ♀

Facility RVU 27.3 Non-Facility RVU 27.3 FUD 090 C 80 CCI

AMA: 2019,Jul,6

58200 **Total abdominal hysterectomy, including partial vaginectomy, with para-aortic and pelvic lymph node sampling, with or without removal of tube(s), with or without removal of ovary(s)** ♀

Facility RVU 39.0 Non-Facility RVU 39.0 FUD 090 C 80 CCI

AMA: 2019,Jul,6

58210 **Radical abdominal hysterectomy, with bilateral total pelvic lymphadenectomy and para-aortic lymph node sampling (biopsy), with or without removal of tube(s), with or without removal of ovary(s)** ♀

INCLUDES Wertheim hysterectomy

EXCLUDES *Chemotherapy (96401-96549)*
Hysterectomy, radical, with transposition ovary(s) (58825)

Facility RVU 53.4 Non-Facility RVU 53.4 FUD 090 C 80 CCI

AMA: 2019,Jul,6; 2018,Jan,8; 2017,Jan,8; 2016,Jan,13; 2015,Jan,16

58240 **Pelvic exenteration for gynecologic malignancy, with total abdominal hysterectomy or cervicectomy, with or without removal of tube(s), with or without removal of ovary(s), with removal of bladder and ureteral transplantations, and/or abdominoperineal resection of rectum and colon and colostomy, or any combination thereof** ♀

EXCLUDES *Chemotherapy (96401-96549)*
Pelvic exenteration for male genital malignancy or lower urinary tract (51597)

Facility RVU 83.8 Non-Facility RVU 83.8 FUD 090 C 80 CCI

AMA: 2019,Jul,6

58260 **Vaginal hysterectomy, for uterus 250 g or less;** ♀

Facility RVU 24.2 Non-Facility RVU 24.2 FUD 090 J G2 80 CCI

AMA: 2019,Jul,6; 2018,Jan,8; 2017,Jan,8; 2016,Jan,13; 2015,Jan,16

58262 **with removal of tube(s), and/or ovary(s)** ♀

Facility RVU 26.1 Non-Facility RVU 26.1 FUD 090 J G2 80 CCI

AMA: 2019,Jul,6

58263 **with removal of tube(s), and/or ovary(s), with repair of enterocele** ♀

Facility RVU 28.8 Non-Facility RVU 28.8 FUD 090 J 80 CCI

AMA: 2019,Jul,6

58267 **with colpo-urethrocystopexy (Marshall-Marchetti-Krantz type, Pereyra type) with or without endoscopic control** ♀

Facility RVU 30.9 Non-Facility RVU 30.9 FUD 090 C 80 CCI

AMA: 2019,Jul,6; 2018,Jan,8; 2017,Jan,8; 2016,Jan,13; 2015,Jan,16

58270   **with repair of enterocele**   ♀

> *EXCLUDES* *Vaginal hysterectomy with repair enterocele and removal tubes and/or ovaries (58263)*

🚑 25.8   ⚕ 25.8   **FUD** 090   J 80 ▣

AMA: 2019,Jul,6

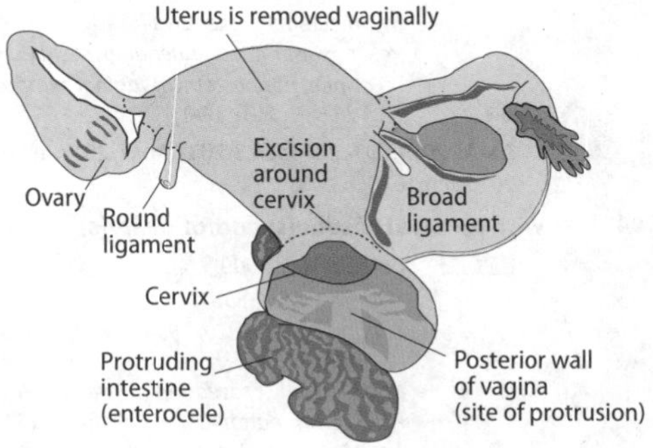

Uterus is removed vaginally

Excision around cervix

Ovary

Round ligament

Broad ligament

Cervix

Protruding intestine (enterocele)

Posterior wall of vagina (site of protrusion)

Repair of enterocele

Posterior vaginal wall

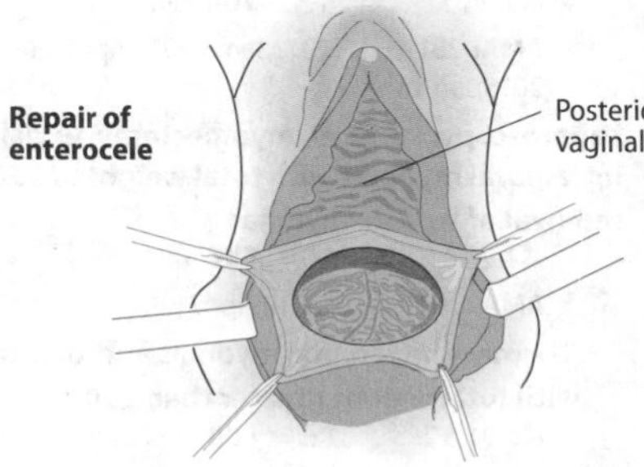

58275   **Vaginal hysterectomy, with total or partial vaginectomy;**   ♀

🚑 28.6   ⚕ 28.6   **FUD** 090   C 80 ▣

AMA: 2019,Jul,6

58280   **with repair of enterocele**   ♀

🚑 29.7   ⚕ 29.7   **FUD** 090   C 80 ▣

AMA: 2019,Jul,6

58285   **Vaginal hysterectomy, radical (Schauta type operation)**   ♀

🚑 41.8   ⚕ 41.8   **FUD** 090   C 80 ▣

AMA: 2019,Jul,6; 2018,Jan,8; 2017,Jan,8; 2016,Jan,13; 2015,Jan,16

58290   **Vaginal hysterectomy, for uterus greater than 250 g;**   ♀

🚑 33.4   ⚕ 33.4   **FUD** 090   J 80 ▣

AMA: 2019,Jul,6

58291   **with removal of tube(s) and/or ovary(s)**   ♀

🚑 36.2   ⚕ 36.2   **FUD** 090   J 80 ▣

AMA: 2019,Jul,6

58292   **with removal of tube(s) and/or ovary(s), with repair of enterocele**   ♀

🚑 38.2   ⚕ 38.2   **FUD** 090   J 80 ▣

AMA: 2019,Jul,6

58293   ~~with colpo-urethrocystopexy (Marshall-Marchetti-Krantz type, Pereyra type) with or without endoscopic control~~

58294   **with repair of enterocele**   ♀

🚑 34.2   ⚕ 34.2   **FUD** 090   J 80 ▣

AMA: 2019,Jul,6

58300-58323 Contraception and Reproduction Procedures

58300   **Insertion of intrauterine device (IUD)**   ♀

> *EXCLUDES* *Insertion and/or removal implantable contraceptive capsules (11976, 11981-11983)*

🚑 1.49   ⚕ 2.60   **FUD** XXX   E ▣

AMA: 2019,Jul,6; 2018,Jan,8; 2017,Jan,8; 2016,Jan,13; 2015,Jan,16

58301   **Removal of intrauterine device (IUD)**   ♀

> *EXCLUDES* *Insertion and/or removal implantable contraceptive capsules (11976, 11981-11983)*

🚑 1.95   ⚕ 2.91   **FUD** 000   02 P3 80 ▣

AMA: 2019,Jul,6; 2018,Jan,8; 2017,Jan,8; 2016,Jan,13; 2015,Jan,16

58321   **Artificial insemination; intra-cervical**   ♀

🚑 1.40   ⚕ 2.26   **FUD** 000   T P3 80 ▣

AMA: 2019,Jul,6

58322   **intra-uterine**   ♀

🚑 1.70   ⚕ 2.56   **FUD** 000   T P3 80 ▣

AMA: 2019,Jul,6

58323   **Sperm washing for artificial insemination**   ♀

🚑 0.37   ⚕ 0.45   **FUD** 000   T P3 80 ▣

AMA: 2019,Jul,6

58340-58350 Fallopian Tube Patency and Brachytherapy Procedures

58340   **Catheterization and introduction of saline or contrast material for saline infusion sonohysterography (SIS) or hysterosalpingography**   ♀

🔗 (74740, 76831)

🚑 1.65   ⚕ 5.53   **FUD** 000   N M1 ▣

AMA: 2019,Jul,6; 2018,Jan,8; 2017,Jan,8; 2016,Jan,13; 2015,Jan,16

58345   **Transcervical introduction of fallopian tube catheter for diagnosis and/or re-establishing patency (any method), with or without hysterosalpingography**   ♀

🔗 (74742)

🚑 8.27   ⚕ 8.27   **FUD** 010   J R2 80 50 ▣

AMA: 2019,Jul,6; 2018,Jan,8; 2017,Jan,8; 2016,Jan,13; 2015,Jan,16

58346   **Insertion of Heyman capsules for clinical brachytherapy**   ♀

> *EXCLUDES* *Insertion radioelement sources or ribbons (77761-77763, 77770-77772)*
>
> *Placement needles or catheters into pelvic organs and/or genitalia (except prostate) for interstitial radioelement application (55920)*

🚑 13.2   ⚕ 13.2   **FUD** 090   J A2 ▣

AMA: 2019,Jul,6; 2018,Jan,8; 2017,Jan,8; 2016,Jan,13; 2015,Jan,16

58350   **Chromotubation of oviduct, including materials**   ♀

🚑 2.51   ⚕ 3.62   **FUD** 010   J A2 50 ▣

AMA: 2019,Jul,6; 2018,Jan,8; 2017,Jan,8; 2016,Jan,13; 2015,Jan,16

58353-58356 Ablation of Endometrium

> *EXCLUDES* *Destruction/excision endometriomas, open method (49203-49205)*

58353   **Endometrial ablation, thermal, without hysteroscopic guidance**   ♀

> *EXCLUDES* *Endometrial ablation performed hysteroscopically (58563)*

🚑 6.54   ⚕ 28.5   **FUD** 010   J A2 ▣

AMA: 2019,Jul,6; 2018,Jan,8; 2017,Jan,8; 2016,Jan,13; 2015,Jan,16

58356   **Endometrial cryoablation with ultrasonic guidance, including endometrial curettage, when performed**   ♀

> *EXCLUDES* *Dilation and curettage (58120)*
> *Endometrial biopsy (58100)*
> *Hysterosalpingography (58340)*
> *Ultrasound (76700, 76856)*

🚑 10.2   ⚕ 52.0   **FUD** 010   J P3 80 ▣

AMA: 2019,Jul,6

● New Code   ▲ Revised Code   ○ Reinstated   ● New Web Release   ▲ Revised Web Release   + Add-on   Unlisted   Not Covered   # Resequenced
50 Optum Mod 50 Exempt   Ⓝ AMA Mod 51 Exempt   51 Optum Mod 51 Exempt   63 Mod 63 Exempt   ✗ Non-FDA Drug   ★ Telemedicine   M Maternity   A Age Edit

58400-58540 Uterine Repairs: Vaginal and Abdominal

58400 Uterine suspension, with or without shortening of round ligaments, with or without shortening of sacrouterine ligaments; (separate procedure) ♀

INCLUDES Alexander's operation
Baldy-Webster operation
Manchester colporrhaphy

EXCLUDES *Anastomosis tubes to uterus (58752)*

13.1 13.1 FUD 090 C 80

AMA: 2019,Jul,6

58410 with presacral sympathectomy ♀

INCLUDES Alexander's operation

EXCLUDES *Anastomosis tubes to uterus (58752)*

23.5 23.5 FUD 090 C 80

AMA: 2019,Jul,6; 2018,Jan,8; 2017,Jan,8; 2016,Jan,13; 2015,Jan,16

58520 Hysterorrhaphy, repair of ruptured uterus (nonobstetrical) ♀

23.0 23.0 FUD 090 C 80

AMA: 2019,Jul,6

58540 Hysteroplasty, repair of uterine anomaly (Strassman type) ♀

INCLUDES Strassman type

EXCLUDES *Vesicouterine fistula closure (51920)*

26.5 26.5 FUD 090 C 80

AMA: 2019,Jul,6

58674-58554 [58674] Laparoscopic Procedures of the Uterus

INCLUDES Diagnostic laparoscopy

EXCLUDES *Hysteroscopy (58555-58565)*

\# **58674 Laparoscopy, surgical, ablation of uterine fibroid(s) including intraoperative ultrasound guidance and monitoring, radiofrequency** ♀

INCLUDES Intraoperative ultrasound (76998)

EXCLUDES *Laparoscopy (49320, 58541-58554, 58570-58573)*

23.6 23.6 FUD 090 J G2 80

AMA: 2019,Jul,6; 2018,Jan,8; 2017,Apr,7; 2017,Feb,14

58541 Laparoscopy, surgical, supracervical hysterectomy, for uterus 250 g or less; ♀

EXCLUDES *Colpotomy (57000)*
Hysteroscopy (58561)
Laparoscopy (49320, 58545-58546, 58661, 58670-58671)
Myomectomy procedures (58140-58146)
Pelvic examination under anesthesia (57410)
Treatment nonobstetrical vaginal hemorrhage (57180)

21.0 21.0 FUD 090 J G2 80

AMA: 2019,Jul,6; 2018,Jan,8; 2017,Apr,7; 2017,Jan,8; 2016,Jan,13; 2015,Jan,16

58542 with removal of tube(s) and/or ovary(s) ♀

EXCLUDES *Colpotomy (57000)*
Hysteroscopy (58561)
Laparoscopy (49320, 58545-58546, 58661, 58670-58671)
Myomectomy procedures (58140-58146)
Pelvic examination under anesthesia (57410)
Treatment nonobstetrical vaginal hemorrhage (57180)

23.9 23.9 FUD 090 J G2 80

AMA: 2019,Jul,6; 2018,Jan,8; 2017,Apr,7; 2017,Jan,8; 2016,Jan,13; 2015,Jan,16

58543 Laparoscopy, surgical, supracervical hysterectomy, for uterus greater than 250 g; ♀

EXCLUDES *Colpotomy (57000)*
Hysteroscopy (58561)
Laparoscopy (49320, 58545-58546, 58661, 58670-58671)
Myomectomy procedures (58140-58146)
Pelvic examination under anesthesia (57410)
Treatment nonobstetrical vaginal hemorrhage (57180)

24.3 24.3 FUD 090 J G2 80

AMA: 2019,Jul,6; 2018,Jan,8; 2017,Apr,7; 2017,Jan,8; 2016,Jan,13; 2015,Jan,16

58544 with removal of tube(s) and/or ovary(s) ♀

EXCLUDES *Colpotomy (57000)*
Hysteroscopy (58561)
Laparoscopy (49320, 58545-58546, 58661, 58670-58671)
Myomectomy procedures (58140-58146)
Pelvic examination under anesthesia (57410)
Treatment nonobstetrical vaginal hemorrhage (57180)

26.2 26.2 FUD 090 J G2 80

AMA: 2019,Jul,6; 2018,Jan,8; 2017,Apr,7; 2017,Jan,8; 2016,Jan,13; 2015,Jan,16

58545 Laparoscopy, surgical, myomectomy, excision; 1 to 4 intramural myomas with total weight of 250 g or less and/or removal of surface myomas ♀

26.0 26.0 FUD 090 J A2 80

AMA: 2019,Jul,6; 2017,Apr,7

58546 5 or more intramural myomas and/or intramural myomas with total weight greater than 250 g ♀

31.6 31.6 FUD 090 J A2 80

AMA: 2019,Jul,6; 2018,Jan,8; 2017,Apr,7; 2017,Jan,8; 2016,Jan,13; 2015,Jan,16

58548 Laparoscopy, surgical, with radical hysterectomy, with bilateral total pelvic lymphadenectomy and para-aortic lymph node sampling (biopsy), with removal of tube(s) and ovary(s), if performed ♀

EXCLUDES *Laparoscopy (38570-38572, 58550-58554)*
Radical hysterectomy (58210, 58285)

53.9 53.9 FUD 090 C 80

AMA: 2019,Jul,6; 2019,Mar,5; 2018,Jan,8; 2017,Apr,7; 2017,Jan,8; 2016,Jan,13; 2015,Sep,12; 2015,Jan,16

58550 Laparoscopy, surgical, with vaginal hysterectomy, for uterus 250 g or less; ♀

EXCLUDES *Colpotomy (57000)*
Hysteroscopy (58561)
Laparoscopy (49320, 58545-58546, 58661, 58670-58671)
Myomectomy procedures (58140-58146)
Pelvic examination under anesthesia (57410)
Treatment nonobstetrical vaginal hemorrhage (57180)

25.5 25.5 FUD 090 J A2 80

AMA: 2019,Jul,6; 2018,Jan,8; 2017,Apr,7; 2017,Jan,8; 2016,Jan,13; 2015,Jan,16

58552 with removal of tube(s) and/or ovary(s) ♀

EXCLUDES *Colpotomy (57000)*
Hysteroscopy (58561)
Laparoscopy (49320, 58545-58546, 58661, 58670-58671)
Myomectomy procedures (58140-58146)
Pelvic examination under anesthesia (57410)
Treatment nonobstetrical vaginal hemorrhage (57180)

28.0 28.0 FUD 090 J G2 80

AMA: 2019,Jul,6; 2018,Jan,8; 2017,Apr,7; 2017,Jan,8; 2016,Jan,13; 2015,Jan,16

58553 **Laparoscopy, surgical, with vaginal hysterectomy, for uterus greater than 250 g;** ♀

EXCLUDES *Colpotomy (57000)*
Hysteroscopy (58561)
Laparoscopy (49320, 58545-58546, 58661, 58670-58671)
Myomectomy procedures (58140-58146)
Pelvic examination under anesthesia (57410)
Treatment nonobstetrical vaginal hemorrhage (57180)

31.8 31.8 **FUD** 090 J G2 80

AMA: 2019,Jul,6; 2018,Jan,8; 2017,Apr,7

58554 **with removal of tube(s) and/or ovary(s)** ♀

EXCLUDES *Colpotomy (57000)*
Hysteroscopy (58561)
Laparoscopy (49320, 58545-58546, 58661, 58670-58671)
Myomectomy procedures (58140-58146)
Pelvic examination under anesthesia (57410)
Treatment nonobstetrical vaginal hemorrhage (57180)

38.1 38.1 **FUD** 090 J G2 80

AMA: 2019,Jul,6; 2018,Jan,8; 2017,Apr,7

58555-58565 Hysteroscopy

INCLUDES Diagnostic hysteroscopy (58555)
EXCLUDES *Laparoscopy (58541-58554, 58570-58578)*

58555 **Hysteroscopy, diagnostic (separate procedure)** ♀

4.35 8.40 **FUD** 000 J A2 80

AMA: 2019,Jul,6; 2018,Jan,8; 2017,Jan,8; 2016,Jan,13; 2015,Jan,16

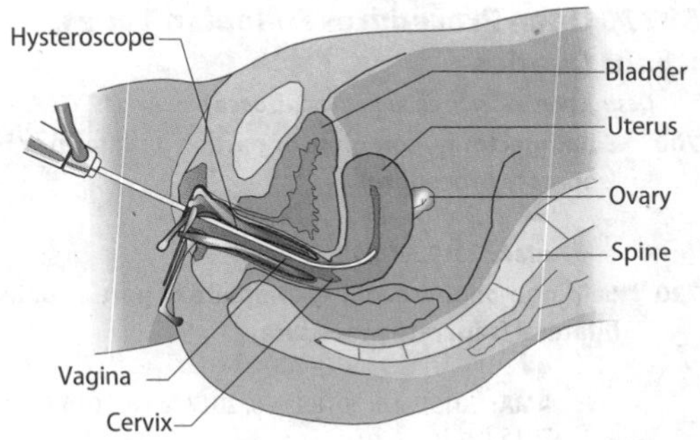

58558 **Hysteroscopy, surgical; with sampling (biopsy) of endometrium and/or polypectomy, with or without D & C** ♀

6.74 39.6 **FUD** 000 J A2

AMA: 2019,Jul,6; 2018,Jan,8; 2017,Jan,8; 2016,Jan,13; 2015,Jan,16

58559 **with lysis of intrauterine adhesions (any method)** ♀

8.33 8.33 **FUD** 000 J A2

AMA: 2019,Jul,6; 2018,Jan,8; 2017,Jan,8; 2016,Jan,13; 2015,Jan,16

58560 **with division or resection of intrauterine septum (any method)** ♀

9.16 9.16 **FUD** 000 J A2 80

AMA: 2019,Jul,6; 2018,Jan,8; 2017,Jan,8; 2016,Jan,13; 2015,Jan,16

58561 **with removal of leiomyomata** ♀

10.4 10.4 **FUD** 000 J A2 80

AMA: 2019,Jul,6; 2018,Jan,8; 2017,Jan,8; 2016,Jan,13; 2015,Jan,16

58562 **with removal of impacted foreign body** ♀

6.34 10.3 **FUD** 000 J A2

AMA: 2019,Jul,6; 2018,Jan,8; 2017,Jan,8; 2016,Jan,13; 2015,Jan,16

58563 **with endometrial ablation (eg, endometrial resection, electrosurgical ablation, thermoablation)** ♀

7.18 55.6 **FUD** 000 J A2 80

AMA: 2019,Jul,6; 2018,Jan,8; 2017,Jan,8; 2016,Jan,13; 2015,Jan,16; 2015,Jan,13

58565 **with bilateral fallopian tube cannulation to induce occlusion by placement of permanent implants** ♀

EXCLUDES *Diagnostic hysteroscopy (58555)*
Dilation cervical canal (57800)

Code also modifier 52 when unilateral procedure performed

12.9 51.6 **FUD** 090 J A2

AMA: 2019,Jul,6; 2018,Jan,8; 2017,Jan,8; 2016,Jan,13; 2015,Jan,16

58570-58579 Other Uterine Endoscopy

INCLUDES Diagnostic laparoscopy
EXCLUDES *Hysteroscopy (58555-58565)*

58570 **Laparoscopy, surgical, with total hysterectomy, for uterus 250 g or less;** ♀

EXCLUDES *Colpotomy (57000)*
Hysteroscopy (58561)
Laparoscopy (49320, 58545-58546, 58661, 58670-58671)
Myomectomy procedures (58140-58146)
Pelvic examination under anesthesia (57410)
Total abdominal hysterectomy (58150)
Treatment nonobstetrical vaginal hemorrhage (57180)

22.9 22.9 **FUD** 090 J G2 80

AMA: 2019,Jul,6; 2018,Jan,8; 2017,Apr,7

58571 **with removal of tube(s) and/or ovary(s)** ♀

EXCLUDES *Colpotomy (57000)*
Hysteroscopy (58561)
Laparoscopy (49320, 58545-58546, 58661, 58670-58671)
Myomectomy procedures (58140-58146)
Pelvic examination under anesthesia (57410)
Total abdominal hysterectomy (58150)
Treatment nonobstetrical vaginal hemorrhage (57180)

25.9 25.9 **FUD** 090 J G2 80

AMA: 2019,Jul,6; 2018,Feb,11; 2018,Jan,8; 2017,Apr,7; 2017,Jan,8; 2016,Jan,13; 2015,Jan,16

58572 **Laparoscopy, surgical, with total hysterectomy, for uterus greater than 250 g;** ♀

EXCLUDES *Colpotomy (57000)*
Hysteroscopy (58561)
Laparoscopy (49320, 58545-58546, 58661, 58670-58671)
Myomectomy procedures (58140-58146)
Pelvic examination under anesthesia (57410)
Total abdominal hysterectomy (58150)
Treatment nonobstetrical vaginal hemorrhage (57180)

29.3 29.3 **FUD** 090 J G2 80

AMA: 2019,Jul,6; 2018,Jan,8; 2017,Apr,7

58573 **with removal of tube(s) and/or ovary(s)** ♀

EXCLUDES *Colpotomy (57000)*
Hysteroscopy (58561)
Laparoscopy (49320, 58545-58546, 58661, 58670-58671)
Myomectomy procedures (58140-58146)
Pelvic examination under anesthesia (57410)
Total abdominal hysterectomy (58150)
Treatment nonobstetrical vaginal hemorrhage (57180)

35.0 35.0 **FUD** 090 J G2 80

AMA: 2019,Jul,6; 2019,Mar,5; 2018,Apr,10; 2018,Feb,11; 2018,Jan,8; 2017,Apr,7; 2017,Jan,8; 2016,Jan,13; 2015,Jan,16

58575 **Laparoscopy, surgical, total hysterectomy for resection of malignancy (tumor debulking), with omentectomy including salpingo-oophorectomy, unilateral or bilateral, when performed** ♀

EXCLUDES *Laparoscopy (49320-49321, 58570-58573, 58661)*
Omentectomy (49255)

54.9 54.9 FUD 090 C 80

AMA: 2019,Jul,6; 2019,Mar,5

58578 **Unlisted laparoscopy procedure, uterus** ♀

0.00 0.00 FUD YYY J 80 50

AMA: 2019,Jul,6; 2018,Jan,8; 2017,Jan,8; 2016,Jan,13; 2015,Jan,16

58579 **Unlisted hysteroscopy procedure, uterus** ♀

0.00 0.00 FUD YYY T 80 50

AMA: 2019,Jul,6; 2018,Jan,8; 2017,Jan,8; 2016,Jan,13; 2015,Jan,16

58600-58615 Sterilization by Tubal Interruption

CMS: 100-03,230.3 Sterilization

EXCLUDES *Destruction/excision endometriomas, open method (49203-49205)*

58600 **Ligation or transection of fallopian tube(s), abdominal or vaginal approach, unilateral or bilateral** ♀

INCLUDES Madlener operation

10.6 10.6 FUD 090 J G2 80

AMA: 2019,Jul,6; 2018,Jan,8; 2017,Jan,8; 2016,Jan,13; 2015,Jan,16

58605 **Ligation or transection of fallopian tube(s), abdominal or vaginal approach, postpartum, unilateral or bilateral, during same hospitalization (separate procedure)** ♀

EXCLUDES *Laparoscopic methods (58670-58671)*

9.65 9.65 FUD 090 C 80

AMA: 2019,Jul,6; 2018,Jan,8; 2017,Jan,8; 2016,Jan,13; 2015,Jan,16

\+ **58611** **Ligation or transection of fallopian tube(s) when done at the time of cesarean delivery or intra-abdominal surgery (not a separate procedure) (List separately in addition to code for primary procedure)** ♀

Code first primary procedure

2.24 2.24 FUD ZZZ C 80

AMA: 2019,Jul,6

58615 **Occlusion of fallopian tube(s) by device (eg, band, clip, Falope ring) vaginal or suprapubic approach** ♀

EXCLUDES *Laparoscopic method (58671)*
Lysis adnexal adhesions (58740)

7.24 7.24 FUD 010 J G2 80

AMA: 2019,Jul,6; 2018,Jan,8; 2017,Jan,8; 2016,Jan,13; 2015,Jan,16

58660-58679 [58674] Endoscopic Procedures Fallopian Tubes and/or Ovaries

CMS: 100-03,230.3 Sterilization

INCLUDES Diagnostic laparoscopy (49320)

EXCLUDES *Laparoscopy with biopsy fallopian tube or ovary (49321)*
Laparoscopy with ovarian cyst aspiration (49322)

58660 **Laparoscopy, surgical; with lysis of adhesions (salpingolysis, ovariolysis) (separate procedure)** ♀

19.6 19.6 FUD 090 J A2 80

AMA: 2019,Jul,6; 2018,Jan,8; 2017,Jan,8; 2016,Jan,13; 2015,Jan,16

58661 **with removal of adnexal structures (partial or total oophorectomy and/or salpingectomy)** ♀

18.8 18.8 FUD 010 J A2 80 50

AMA: 2020,Jan,12; 2019,Jul,6; 2018,Jan,8; 2017,Jan,8; 2016,Jan,13; 2015,Jan,16

58662 **with fulguration or excision of lesions of the ovary, pelvic viscera, or peritoneal surface by any method** ♀

20.6 20.6 FUD 090 J A2 80

AMA: 2019,Jul,6; 2018,Jan,8; 2017,Dec,14; 2017,Jan,8; 2016,Jan,13; 2015,Jan,16

58670 **with fulguration of oviducts (with or without transection)** ♀

10.3 10.3 FUD 090 J A2

AMA: 2019,Jul,6; 2018,Jan,8; 2017,Jan,8; 2016,Jan,13; 2015,Jan,16

58671 **with occlusion of oviducts by device (eg, band, clip, or Falope ring)** ♀

10.6 10.6 FUD 090 J A2

AMA: 2019,Jul,6; 2018,Jan,8; 2017,Jan,8; 2016,Jan,13; 2015,Jan,16

58672 **with fimbrioplasty** ♀

21.3 21.3 FUD 090 J A2 80 50

AMA: 2019,Jul,6; 2018,Jan,8; 2017,Jan,8; 2016,Jan,13; 2015,Jan,16

58673 **with salpingostomy (salpingoneostomy)** ♀

23.1 23.1 FUD 090 J A2 80 50

AMA: 2019,Jul,6; 2018,Jan,8; 2017,Jan,8; 2016,Jan,13; 2015,Jan,16

58674 **Resequenced code. See code before 58541.**

58679 **Unlisted laparoscopy procedure, oviduct, ovary** ♀

0.00 0.00 FUD YYY J 80 50

AMA: 2019,Jul,6; 2018,Jan,8; 2017,Jan,8; 2016,Jan,13; 2015,Jan,16

58700-58770 Open Procedures Fallopian Tubes, with/without Ovaries

EXCLUDES *Destruction/excision endometriomas, open method (49203-49205)*

58700 **Salpingectomy, complete or partial, unilateral or bilateral (separate procedure)** ♀

22.3 22.3 FUD 090 C 80

AMA: 2019,Jul,6; 2018,Sep,14

58720 **Salpingo-oophorectomy, complete or partial, unilateral or bilateral (separate procedure)** ♀

21.5 21.5 FUD 090 C 80

AMA: 2019,Jul,6; 2018,Jan,8; 2017,Jan,8; 2016,Jan,13; 2015,Jan,16

58740 **Lysis of adhesions (salpingolysis, ovariolysis)** ♀

EXCLUDES *Excision/fulguration lesions performed laparoscopically (58662)*
Laparoscopic method (58660)

25.9 25.9 FUD 090 C 80

AMA: 2019,Jul,6; 2018,Jan,8; 2017,Jan,8; 2016,Jan,13; 2015,Jan,16

58750 Tubotubal anastomosis ♀

26.3 26.3 FUD 090 C 80 50

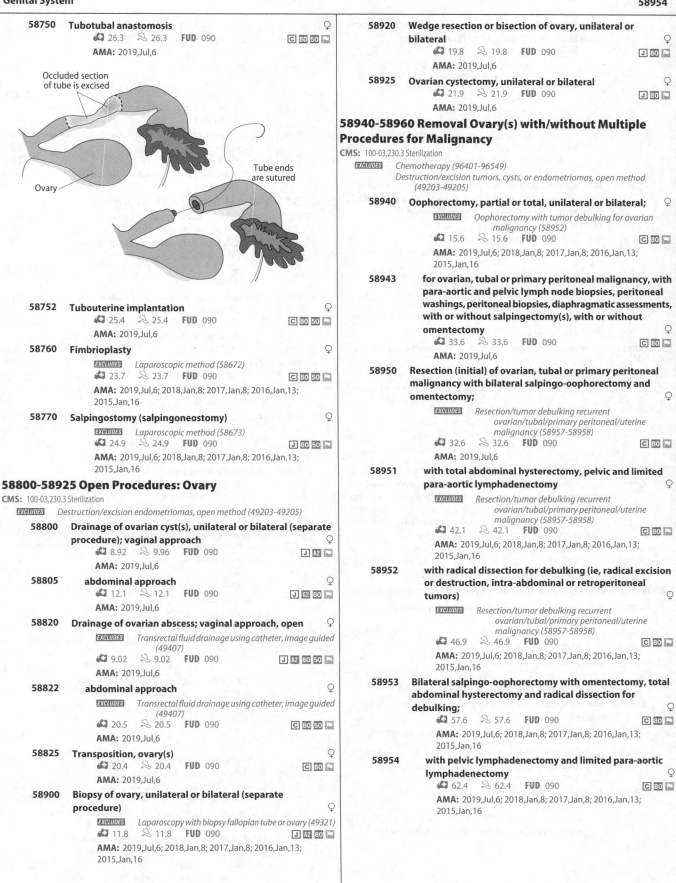

AMA: 2019,Jul,6

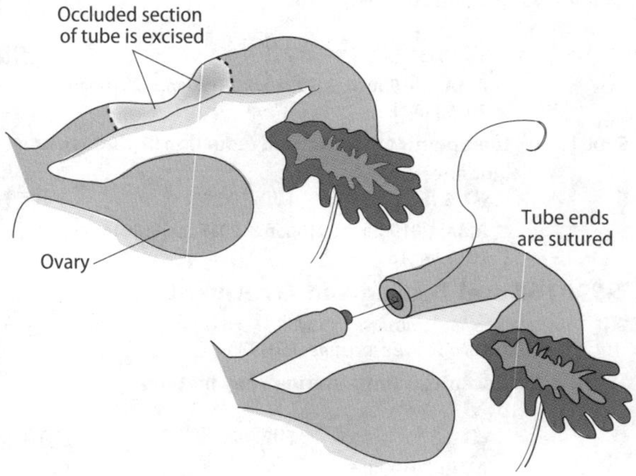

58752 Tubouterine implantation ♀

25.4 25.4 FUD 090 C 80 50

AMA: 2019,Jul,6

58760 Fimbrioplasty ♀

EXCLUDES *Laparoscopic method (58672)*

23.7 23.7 FUD 090 C 80 50

AMA: 2019,Jul,6; 2018,Jan,8; 2017,Jan,8; 2016,Jan,13; 2015,Jan,16

58770 Salpingostomy (salpingoneostomy) ♀

EXCLUDES *Laparoscopic method (58673)*

24.9 24.9 FUD 090 J 80 50

AMA: 2019,Jul,6; 2018,Jan,8; 2017,Jan,8; 2016,Jan,13; 2015,Jan,16

58800-58925 Open Procedures: Ovary

CMS: 100-03,230.3 Sterilization

EXCLUDES *Destruction/excision endometriomas, open method (49203-49205)*

58800 Drainage of ovarian cyst(s), unilateral or bilateral (separate procedure); vaginal approach ♀

8.92 9.96 FUD 090 J A2

AMA: 2019,Jul,6

58805 abdominal approach ♀

12.1 12.1 FUD 090 J G2 80

AMA: 2019,Jul,6

58820 Drainage of ovarian abscess; vaginal approach, open ♀

EXCLUDES *Transrectal fluid drainage using catheter, image guided (49407)*

9.02 9.02 FUD 090 J A2 80 50

AMA: 2019,Jul,6

58822 abdominal approach ♀

EXCLUDES *Transrectal fluid drainage using catheter, image guided (49407)*

20.5 20.5 FUD 090 C 80 50

AMA: 2019,Jul,6

58825 Transposition, ovary(s) ♀

20.4 20.4 FUD 090 C 80

AMA: 2019,Jul,6

58900 Biopsy of ovary, unilateral or bilateral (separate procedure) ♀

EXCLUDES *Laparoscopy with biopsy fallopian tube or ovary (49321)*

11.8 11.8 FUD 090 J A2 80

AMA: 2019,Jul,6; 2018,Jan,8; 2017,Jan,8; 2016,Jan,13; 2015,Jan,16

58920 Wedge resection or bisection of ovary, unilateral or bilateral ♀

19.8 19.8 FUD 090 J 80

AMA: 2019,Jul,6

58925 Ovarian cystectomy, unilateral or bilateral ♀

21.9 21.9 FUD 090 J 80

AMA: 2019,Jul,6

58940-58960 Removal Ovary(s) with/without Multiple Procedures for Malignancy

CMS: 100-03,230.3 Sterilization

EXCLUDES *Chemotherapy (96401-96549)*

Destruction/excision tumors, cysts, or endometriomas, open method (49203-49205)

58940 Oophorectomy, partial or total, unilateral or bilateral; ♀

EXCLUDES *Oophorectomy with tumor debulking for ovarian malignancy (58952)*

15.6 15.6 FUD 090 C 80

AMA: 2019,Jul,6; 2018,Jan,8; 2017,Jan,8; 2016,Jan,13; 2015,Jan,16

58943 for ovarian, tubal or primary peritoneal malignancy, with para-aortic and pelvic lymph node biopsies, peritoneal washings, peritoneal biopsies, diaphragmatic assessments, with or without salpingectomy(s), with or without omentectomy ♀

33.6 33.6 FUD 090 C 80

AMA: 2019,Jul,6

58950 Resection (initial) of ovarian, tubal or primary peritoneal malignancy with bilateral salpingo-oophorectomy and omentectomy; ♀

EXCLUDES *Resection/tumor debulking recurrent ovarian/tubal/primary peritoneal/uterine malignancy (58957-58958)*

32.6 32.6 FUD 090 C 80

AMA: 2019,Jul,6

58951 with total abdominal hysterectomy, pelvic and limited para-aortic lymphadenectomy ♀

EXCLUDES *Resection/tumor debulking recurrent ovarian/tubal/primary peritoneal/uterine malignancy (58957-58958)*

42.1 42.1 FUD 090 C 80

AMA: 2019,Jul,6; 2018,Jan,8; 2017,Jan,8; 2016,Jan,13; 2015,Jan,16

58952 with radical dissection for debulking (ie, radical excision or destruction, intra-abdominal or retroperitoneal tumors) ♀

EXCLUDES *Resection/tumor debulking recurrent ovarian/tubal/primary peritoneal/uterine malignancy (58957-58958)*

46.9 46.9 FUD 090 C 80

AMA: 2019,Jul,6; 2018,Jan,8; 2017,Jan,8; 2016,Jan,13; 2015,Jan,16

58953 Bilateral salpingo-oophorectomy with omentectomy, total abdominal hysterectomy and radical dissection for debulking; ♀

57.6 57.6 FUD 090 C 80

AMA: 2019,Jul,6; 2018,Jan,8; 2017,Jan,8; 2016,Jan,13; 2015,Jan,16

58954 with pelvic lymphadenectomy and limited para-aortic lymphadenectomy ♀

62.4 62.4 FUD 090 C 80

AMA: 2019,Jul,6; 2018,Jan,8; 2017,Jan,8; 2016,Jan,13; 2015,Jan,16

58956 **Bilateral salpingo-oophorectomy with total omentectomy, total abdominal hysterectomy for malignancy** ♀

EXCLUDES *Biopsy ovary (58900)*
Hysterectomy (58150, 58180, 58262-58263)
Laparoscopy (58550, 58661)
Omentectomy (49255)
Oophorectomy (58940)
Ovarian cystectomy (58925)
Resection malignancy (58957-58958)
Salpingectomy salpingo-oophorectomy, (58700, 58720)

39.1 39.1 FUD 090 C 80

AMA: 2019,Jul,6; 2018,Jan,8; 2017,Jan,8; 2016,Jan,13; 2015,Jan,16

58957 **Resection (tumor debulking) of recurrent ovarian, tubal, primary peritoneal, uterine malignancy (intra-abdominal, retroperitoneal tumors), with omentectomy, if performed;** ♀

EXCLUDES *Biopsy ovary (58900)*
Destruction, excision cysts, endometriomas, or tumors (49203-49215)
Enterolysis (44005)
Exploratory laparotomy (49000)
Lymphadenectomy (38770, 38780)
Omentectomy (49255)

45.4 45.4 FUD 090 C 80

AMA: 2019,Jul,6

58958 **with pelvic lymphadenectomy and limited para-aortic lymphadenectomy** ♀

EXCLUDES *Biopsy ovary (58900)*
Destruction, excision cysts, endometriomas, or tumors (49203-49215)
Enterolysis (44005)
Exploratory laparotomy (49000)
Lymphadenectomy (38770, 38780)
Omentectomy (49255)

51.2 51.2 FUD 090 C 80

AMA: 2019,Jul,6

58960 **Laparotomy, for staging or restaging of ovarian, tubal, or primary peritoneal malignancy (second look), with or without omentectomy, peritoneal washing, biopsy of abdominal and pelvic peritoneum, diaphragmatic assessment with pelvic and limited para-aortic lymphadenectomy** ♀

EXCLUDES *Resection malignancy (58957-58958)*

27.9 27.9 FUD 090 C 80

AMA: 2019,Jul,6

58970-58999 Procedural Components: In Vitro Fertilization

58970 **Follicle puncture for oocyte retrieval, any method** M ♀

(76948)

5.62 6.43 FUD 000 T A2 80

AMA: 2019,Jul,6

58974 **Embryo transfer, intrauterine** M ♀

0.00 0.00 FUD 000 T A2 80

AMA: 2019,Jul,6

58976 **Gamete, zygote, or embryo intrafallopian transfer, any method** M ♀

EXCLUDES *Adnexal procedures performed laparoscopically (58660-58673)*

6.06 7.05 FUD 000 T A2 80

AMA: 2019,Jul,6; 2018,Jan,8; 2017,Jan,8; 2016,Jan,13; 2015,Jan,16

58999 **Unlisted procedure, female genital system (nonobstetrical)** ♀

0.00 0.00 FUD YYY T

AMA: 2019,Jul,6; 2018,Jan,8; 2017,Jan,8; 2016,Jan,13; 2015,Jan,16

59000-59001 Aspiration of Amniotic Fluid

EXCLUDES *Intrauterine fetal transfusion (36460)*
Unlisted fetal invasive procedure (59897)

59000 **Amniocentesis; diagnostic** M ♀

(76946)

2.33 3.47 FUD 000 T P3

AMA: 2019,Jul,6; 2018,Jan,8; 2017,Jan,8; 2016,Jan,13; 2015,Jan,16

59001 **therapeutic amniotic fluid reduction (includes ultrasound guidance)** M ♀

5.18 5.18 FUD 000 T R2

AMA: 2019,Jul,6; 2018,Jan,8; 2017,Jan,8; 2016,Jan,13; 2015,Jan,16

59012-59076 Fetal Testing and Treatment

EXCLUDES *Intrauterine fetal transfusion (36460)*
Unlisted fetal invasive procedures (59897)

59012 **Cordocentesis (intrauterine), any method** M ♀

(76941)

5.87 5.87 FUD 000 T G2 80

AMA: 2019,Jul,6

59015 **Chorionic villus sampling, any method** M ♀

(76945)

3.82 4.51 FUD 000 T P3 80

AMA: 2019,Jul,6; 2018,Jan,8; 2017,Jan,8; 2016,Jan,13; 2015,Jan,16

59020 **Fetal contraction stress test** M ♀

1.99 1.99 FUD 000 T P3 80

AMA: 2019,Jul,6; 2018,Jan,8; 2017,Jan,8; 2016,Jan,13; 2015,Jan,16

59025 **Fetal non-stress test** M ♀

1.37 1.37 FUD 000 T P3 80

AMA: 2019,Jul,6; 2018,Jan,8; 2017,Jan,8; 2016,Jan,13; 2015,Jan,16

59030 **Fetal scalp blood sampling** M ♀

Code also modifier 76 or 77, as appropriate, for repeat fetal scalp blood sampling

3.28 3.28 FUD 000 T 80

AMA: 2019,Jul,6

59050 **Fetal monitoring during labor by consulting physician (ie, non-attending physician) with written report; supervision and interpretation** M ♀

1.49 1.49 FUD XXX M 80

AMA: 2019,Jul,6

59051 **interpretation only** M ♀

1.23 1.23 FUD XXX B 80

AMA: 2019,Jul,6

59070 **Transabdominal amnioinfusion, including ultrasound guidance** M ♀

8.99 11.6 FUD 000 T G2 80

AMA: 2019,Jul,6; 2018,Jan,8; 2017,Jan,8; 2016,Jan,13; 2015,Jan,16

59072 **Fetal umbilical cord occlusion, including ultrasound guidance** M ♀

15.0 15.0 FUD 000 T J8

AMA: 2019,Jul,6; 2018,Jan,8; 2017,Jan,8; 2016,Jan,13; 2015,Jan,16

59074 **Fetal fluid drainage (eg, vesicocentesis, thoracocentesis, paracentesis), including ultrasound guidance** M ♀

8.92 11.1 FUD 000 T G2 80

AMA: 2019,Jul,6; 2018,Jan,8; 2017,Jan,8; 2016,Jan,13; 2015,Jan,16

59076 **Fetal shunt placement, including ultrasound guidance** M ♀

15.2 15.2 FUD 000 T G2 80

AMA: 2019,Jul,6; 2018,Jan,8; 2017,Jan,8; 2016,Jan,13; 2015,Jan,16

59100-59151 Tubal Pregnancy/Hysterotomy Procedures

CMS: 100-03,230.3 Sterilization

59100 **Hysterotomy, abdominal (eg, for hydatidiform mole, abortion)** M ♀
Code also ligation fallopian tubes when performed same time as hysterotomy (58611)
24.1 24.1 **FUD** 090 J R2 80
AMA: 2019,Jul,6

59120 **Surgical treatment of ectopic pregnancy; tubal or ovarian, requiring salpingectomy and/or oophorectomy, abdominal or vaginal approach** M ♀
23.4 23.4 **FUD** 090 C 80
AMA: 2019,Jul,6

59121 **tubal or ovarian, without salpingectomy and/or oophorectomy** M ♀
23.0 23.0 **FUD** 090 C 80
AMA: 2019,Jul,6

59130 **abdominal pregnancy** M ♀
26.8 26.8 **FUD** 090 C 80
AMA: 2019,Jul,6

59135 **interstitial, uterine pregnancy requiring total hysterectomy** M ♀
27.0 27.0 **FUD** 090 C 80
AMA: 2019,Jul,6

59136 **interstitial, uterine pregnancy with partial resection of uterus** M ♀
25.9 25.9 **FUD** 090 C 80
AMA: 2019,Jul,6

59140 **cervical, with evacuation** M ♀
11.9 11.9 **FUD** 090 C 80
AMA: 2019,Jul,6

59150 **Laparoscopic treatment of ectopic pregnancy; without salpingectomy and/or oophorectomy** M ♀
22.7 22.7 **FUD** 090 J G2 80
AMA: 2019,Jul,6; 2018,Jan,8; 2017,Jan,8; 2016,Jan,13; 2015,Jan,16

59151 **with salpingectomy and/or oophorectomy** M ♀
21.7 21.7 **FUD** 090 J G2 80
AMA: 2019,Jul,6

59160-59200 Procedures of Uterus Prior To/After Delivery

59160 **Curettage, postpartum** M ♀
5.11 6.21 **FUD** 010 J A2 80
AMA: 2019,Jul,6; 2018,Jan,8; 2017,Jan,8; 2016,Jan,13; 2015,Jan,16

59200 **Insertion of cervical dilator (eg, laminaria, prostaglandin) (separate procedure)** M ♀
EXCLUDES *Fetal transfusion, intrauterine (36460)*
Hypertonic solution/prostaglandin introduction for labor initiation (59850-59857)
1.30 2.56 **FUD** 000 T P3
AMA: 2019,Jul,6; 2018,Jan,8; 2017,Dec,14; 2017,Jan,8; 2016,Jan,13; 2015,Jan,16

59300-59350 Postpartum Vaginal/Cervical/Uterine Repairs

EXCLUDES *Nonpregnancy-related cerclage (57700)*

59300 **Episiotomy or vaginal repair, by other than attending** M ♀
4.26 6.15 **FUD** 000 J P3 80
AMA: 2019,Jul,6

59320 **Cerclage of cervix, during pregnancy; vaginal** M ♀
4.37 4.37 **FUD** 000 J A2 80
AMA: 2019,Jul,6; 2018,Jan,8; 2017,Jan,8; 2016,Jan,13; 2015,Jan,16

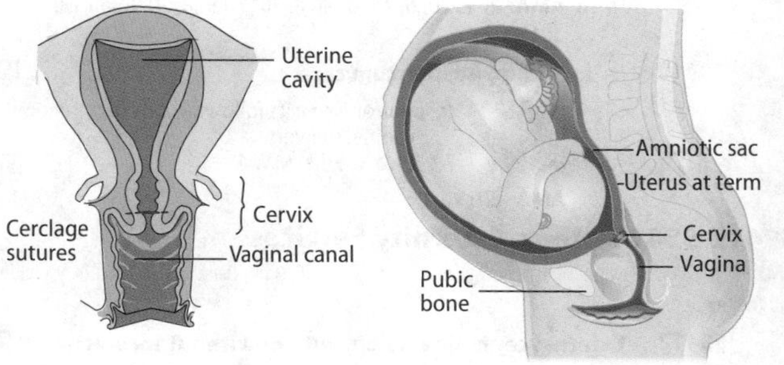

59325 **abdominal** M ♀
6.96 6.96 **FUD** 000 C 80
AMA: 2019,Jul,6; 2018,Jan,8; 2017,Jan,8; 2016,Jan,13; 2015,Jan,16

59350 **Hysterorrhaphy of ruptured uterus** M ♀
8.08 8.08 **FUD** 000 C 80
AMA: 2019,Jul,6

59400-59410 Vaginal Delivery: Comprehensive and Component Services

CMS: 100-02,15,180 Nurse-Midwife (CNM) Services; 100-02,15,20.1 Physician Expense for Surgery, Childbirth, and Treatment for Infertility

INCLUDES Care provided for uncomplicated pregnancy including delivery, antepartum, and postpartum care:
- Admission history
- Admission to hospital
- Artificial rupture membranes
- Management uncomplicated labor
- Physical exam
- Vaginal delivery with or without episiotomy or forceps

EXCLUDES *Medical complications pregnancy, labor, and delivery:*
- *Cardiac problems*
- *Diabetes*
- *Hyperemesis*
- *Hypertension*
- *Neurological problems*
- *Premature rupture membranes*
- *Pre-term labor*
- *Toxemia*
- *Trauma*

Newborn circumcision (54150, 54160)
Services incidental to or unrelated to pregnancy

59400 **Routine obstetric care including antepartum care, vaginal delivery (with or without episiotomy, and/or forceps) and postpartum care** M ♀
INCLUDES Fetal heart tones
Hospital/office visits following cesarean section or vaginal delivery
Initial/subsequent history
Physical exams
Recording weight/blood pressures
Routine chemical urinalysis
Routine prenatal visits:
- Each month up to 28 weeks gestation
- Every other week from 29 to 36 weeks gestation
- Weekly from 36 weeks until delivery

60.4 60.4 **FUD** MMM B
AMA: 2019,Jul,6; 2018,Jan,8; 2017,Jan,8; 2016,Jan,13; 2015,Jan,16

59409 Vaginal delivery only (with or without episiotomy and/or forceps); M ♀

Code also inpatient management after delivery/discharge services (99217-99239 [99224, 99225, 99226])

23.3 23.3 FUD MMM J 80

AMA: 2019,Jul,6; 2018,Jan,8; 2017,Jan,8; 2016,Jan,13; 2015,Jan,16

59410 including postpartum care M ♀

INCLUDES Hospital/office visits following cesarean section or vaginal delivery

29.9 29.9 FUD MMM B

AMA: 2019,Jul,6

59412-59414 Other Maternity Services

CMS: 100-02,15,180 Nurse-Midwife (CNM) Services; 100-02,15,20.1 Physician Expense for Surgery, Childbirth, and Treatment for Infertility

59412 External cephalic version, with or without tocolysis M ♀

Code also delivery code(s)

2.95 2.95 FUD MMM J G2 80

AMA: 2019,Jul,6

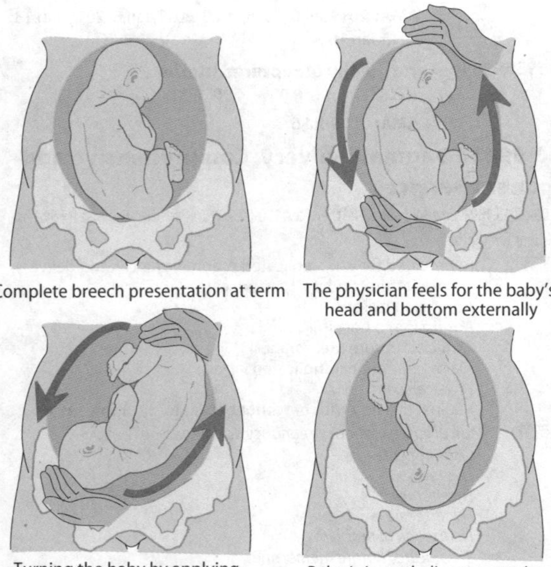

Complete breech presentation at term

The physician feels for the baby's head and bottom externally

Turning the baby by applying external pressure

Baby is in cephalic presentation, engaged for normal delivery

59414 Delivery of placenta (separate procedure) M ♀

2.66 2.66 FUD MMM J G2 80

AMA: 2019,Jul,6; 2018,Jan,8; 2017,Jan,8; 2016,Jan,13; 2015,Jan,16

59425-59430 Prenatal and Postpartum Visits

CMS: 100-02,15,180 Nurse-Midwife (CNM) Services; 100-02,15,20.1 Physician Expense for Surgery, Childbirth, and Treatment for Infertility

INCLUDES Physician/other qualified health care professional providing all or portion antepartum/postpartum care, but no delivery due to:
- Referral to another physician for delivery
- Termination pregnancy by abortion

EXCLUDES *Antepartum care, one to three visits, report with appropriate E/M service code*
Medical complications pregnancy, labor, and delivery:
- *Cardiac problems*
- *Diabetes*
- *Hyperemesis*
- *Hypertension*
- *Neurological problems*
- *Premature rupture membranes*
- *Pre-term labor*
- *Toxemia*
- *Trauma*

Newborn circumcision (54150, 54160)
Services incidental to or unrelated to pregnancy

59425 Antepartum care only; 4-6 visits M ♀

INCLUDES Fetal heart tones
Initial/subsequent history
Physical exams
Recording weight/blood pressures
Routine chemical urinalysis
Routine prenatal visits:
- Each month up to 28 weeks gestation
- Every other week from 29 to 36 weeks gestation
- Weekly from 36 weeks until delivery

10.3 13.5 FUD MMM B 80

AMA: 2019,Jul,6; 2018,Jan,8; 2017,Jan,8; 2016,Jan,13; 2015,Jan,16

59426 7 or more visits M ♀

INCLUDES Biweekly visits to 36 weeks gestation
Fetal heart tones
Initial/subsequent history
Monthly visits up to 28 weeks gestation
Physical exams
Recording weight/blood pressures
Routine chemical urinalysis
Weekly visits until delivery

17.9 23.5 FUD MMM B 80

AMA: 2019,Jul,6; 2018,Jan,8; 2017,Jan,8; 2016,Jan,13; 2015,Jan,16

59430 Postpartum care only (separate procedure) M ♀

INCLUDES Office/other outpatient visits following cesarean section or vaginal delivery

4.05 5.96 FUD MMM B

AMA: 2019,Jul,6; 2018,Jan,8; 2017,Jan,8; 2016,Jan,13; 2015,Jan,16

59510-59525 Cesarean Section Delivery: Comprehensive and Components of Care

CMS: 100-02,15,20.1 Physician Expense for Surgery, Childbirth, and Treatment for Infertility

INCLUDES Classic cesarean section
Low cervical cesarean section

EXCLUDES *Infant standby attendance (99360)*
Medical complications pregnancy, labor, and delivery:
Cardiac problems
Diabetes
Hyperemesis
Hypertension
Neurological problems
Premature rupture membranes
Pre-term labor
Toxemia
Trauma
Newborn circumcision (54150, 54160)
Services incidental to or unrelated to pregnancy
Vaginal delivery after prior cesarean section (59610-59614)

59510 **Routine obstetric care including antepartum care, cesarean delivery, and postpartum care** M ♀

INCLUDES Admission history
Admission to hospital
Cesarean delivery
Fetal heart tones
Hospital/office visits following cesarean section
Initial/subsequent history
Management uncomplicated labor
Physical exam
Recording weight/blood pressures
Routine chemical urinalysis
Routine prenatal visits:
Each month up to 28 weeks gestation
Every other week 29 to 36 weeks gestation
Weekly from 36 weeks until delivery

67.0 67.0 **FUD** MMM B

AMA: 2019,Jul,6; 2018,Jan,8; 2017,Jan,8; 2016,Jan,13; 2015,Jan,16

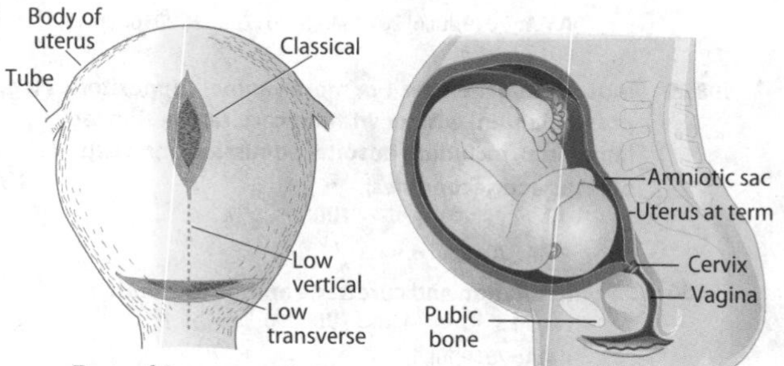

Types of Cesarean section are classified by uterine incision

59514 **Cesarean delivery only;** M ♀

INCLUDES Admission history
Admission to hospital
Cesarean delivery
Management uncomplicated labor
Physical exam

Code also inpatient management after delivery/discharge services (99217-99239 [99224, 99225, 99226])

26.5 26.5 **FUD** MMM C 80

AMA: 2019,Jul,6; 2018,Jan,8; 2017,Jan,8; 2016,Jan,13; 2015,Jan,16

59515 **including postpartum care** M ♀

INCLUDES Admission history
Admission to hospital
Cesarean delivery
Hospital/office visits following cesarean section or vaginal delivery
Management uncomplicated labor
Physical exam

36.8 36.8 **FUD** MMM B

AMA: 2019,Jul,6; 2018,Jan,8; 2017,Jan,8; 2016,Jan,13; 2015,Jan,16

\+ **59525** **Subtotal or total hysterectomy after cesarean delivery (List separately in addition to code for primary procedure)** M ♀

Code first cesarean delivery (59510, 59514, 59515, 59618, 59620, 59622)

14.1 14.1 **FUD** ZZZ C 80

AMA: 2019,Jul,6

59610-59614 Vaginal Delivery After Prior Cesarean Section: Comprehensive and Components of Care

CMS: 100-02,15,180 Nurse-Midwife (CNM) Services; 100-02,15,20.1 Physician Expense for Surgery, Childbirth, and Treatment for Infertility

INCLUDES Admission history
Admission to hospital
Management uncomplicated labor
Patients with previous cesarean delivery who present with vaginal delivery expectation
Physical exam
Successful vaginal delivery after previous cesarean delivery (VBAC)
Vaginal delivery with or without episiotomy or forceps

EXCLUDES *Elective cesarean delivery (59510, 59514, 59515)*
Medical complications pregnancy, labor, and delivery:
Cardiac problems
Diabetes
Hyperemesis
Hypertension
Neurological problems
Premature rupture membranes
Pre-term labor
Toxemia
Trauma
Newborn circumcision (54150, 54160)
Services incidental to or unrelated to pregnancy

59610 **Routine obstetric care including antepartum care, vaginal delivery (with or without episiotomy, and/or forceps) and postpartum care, after previous cesarean delivery** M ♀

INCLUDES Fetal heart tones
Hospital/office visits following cesarean section or vaginal delivery
Initial/subsequent history
Physical exams
Recording weight/blood pressures
Routine chemical urinalysis
Routine prenatal visits:
Each month up to 28 weeks gestation
Every other week 29 to 36 weeks gestation
Weekly from 36 weeks until delivery

63.4 63.4 **FUD** MMM B 80

AMA: 2019,Jul,6; 2018,Jan,8; 2017,Jan,8; 2016,Jan,13; 2015,Jan,16

59612 **Vaginal delivery only, after previous cesarean delivery (with or without episiotomy and/or forceps);** M ♀

Code also inpatient management after delivery/discharge services (99217-99239 [99224, 99225, 99226])

26.3 26.3 **FUD** MMM J 80

AMA: 2019,Jul,6; 2018,Jan,8; 2017,Jan,8; 2016,Jan,13; 2015,Jan,16

59614 **including postpartum care** M ♀

INCLUDES Hospital/office visits following cesarean section or vaginal delivery

32.6 32.6 **FUD** MMM B 80

AMA: 2019,Jul,6; 2018,Jan,8; 2017,Jan,8; 2016,Jan,13; 2015,Jan,16

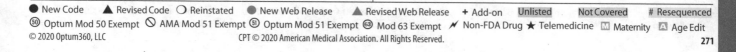

59618-59622 Cesarean Section After Attempted Vaginal Birth/Prior C-Section

CMS: 100-02,15,20.1 Physician Expense for Surgery, Childbirth, and Treatment for Infertility

INCLUDES Admission history
Admission to hospital
Cesarean delivery
Cesarean delivery following unsuccessful vaginal delivery attempt after previous cesarean delivery
Management uncomplicated labor
Patients with previous cesarean delivery who present with vaginal delivery expectation
Physical exam

EXCLUDES *Elective cesarean delivery (59510, 59514, 59515)*
Medical complications of pregnancy, labor, and delivery:
Cardiac problems
Diabetes
Hyperemesis
Hypertension
Neurological problems
Premature rupture of membranes
Pre-term labor
Toxemia
Trauma
Newborn circumcision (54150, 54160)
Services incidental to or unrelated to the pregnancy

59618 **Routine obstetric care including antepartum care, cesarean delivery, and postpartum care, following attempted vaginal delivery after previous cesarean delivery** M ♀
INCLUDES Fetal heart tones
Hospital/office visits following cesarean section or vaginal delivery
Initial/subsequent history
Physical exams
Recording weight/blood pressures
Routine chemical urinalysis
Routine prenatal visits:
Each month up to 28 weeks gestation
Every two weeks 29 to 36 weeks gestation
Weekly from 36 weeks until delivery
69.1 69.1 **FUD** MMM B 80
AMA: 2019,Jul,6; 2018,Jan,8; 2017,Jan,8; 2016,Jan,13; 2015,Jan,16

59620 **Cesarean delivery only, following attempted vaginal delivery after previous cesarean delivery;** M ♀
Code also inpatient management after delivery/discharge services (99217-99239 [99224, 99225, 99226])
27.0 27.0 **FUD** MMM C 80
AMA: 2019,Jul,6; 2018,Jan,8; 2017,Jan,8; 2016,Jan,13; 2015,Jan,16

59622 **including postpartum care** M ♀
INCLUDES Hospital/office visits following cesarean section or vaginal delivery
37.4 37.4 **FUD** MMM B 80
AMA: 2019,Jul,6; 2018,Jan,8; 2017,Jan,8; 2016,Jan,13; 2015,Jan,16

59812-59830 Treatment of Miscarriage

CMS: 100-02,15,20.1 Physician Expense for Surgery, Childbirth, and Treatment for Infertility

EXCLUDES *Medical treatment spontaneous complete abortion, any trimester (99202-99233 [99224, 99225, 99226])*

59812 **Treatment of incomplete abortion, any trimester, completed surgically** M ♀
INCLUDES Surgical treatment spontaneous abortion
8.79 9.89 **FUD** 090 J A2
AMA: 2019,Jul,6; 2018,Jan,8; 2017,Jan,8; 2016,Jan,13; 2015,Jan,16

59820 **Treatment of missed abortion, completed surgically; first trimester** M ♀
10.4 11.2 **FUD** 090 J A2
AMA: 2019,Jul,6; 2018,Jan,8; 2017,Jan,8; 2016,Jan,13; 2015,Jan,16

59821 **second trimester** M ♀
10.6 11.8 **FUD** 090 J A2 80
AMA: 2019,Jul,6; 2018,Jan,8; 2017,Jan,8; 2016,Jan,13; 2015,Jan,16

59830 **Treatment of septic abortion, completed surgically** M ♀
12.7 12.7 **FUD** 090 C 80
AMA: 2019,Jul,6; 2018,Jan,8; 2017,Jan,8; 2016,Jan,13; 2015,Jan,16

59840-59866 Elective Abortions

CMS: 100-02,1,90 Termination of Pregnancy; 100-02,15,20.1 Physician Expense for Surgery, Childbirth, and Treatment for Infertility; 100-03,140.1 Abortion; 100-04,3,100.1 Billing for Abortion Services

59840 **Induced abortion, by dilation and curettage** M ♀
6.08 6.50 **FUD** 010 J A2 80
AMA: 2019,Jul,6; 2018,Jan,8; 2017,Jan,8; 2016,Jan,13; 2015,Jan,16

59841 **Induced abortion, by dilation and evacuation** M ♀
10.6 11.7 **FUD** 010 J A2 80
AMA: 2019,Jul,6; 2018,Jan,8; 2017,Jan,8; 2016,Jan,13; 2015,Jan,16

59850 **Induced abortion, by 1 or more intra-amniotic injections (amniocentesis-injections), including hospital admission and visits, delivery of fetus and secundines;** M ♀
EXCLUDES *Cervical dilator insertion (59200)*
10.1 10.1 **FUD** 090 C 80
AMA: 2019,Jul,6; 2018,Jan,8; 2017,Jan,8; 2016,Jan,13; 2015,Jan,16

59851 **with dilation and curettage and/or evacuation** M ♀
EXCLUDES *Cervical dilator insertion (59200)*
10.9 10.9 **FUD** 090 C 80
AMA: 2019,Jul,6; 2018,Jan,8; 2017,Jan,8; 2016,Jan,13; 2015,Jan,16

59852 **with hysterotomy (failed intra-amniotic injection)** M ♀
EXCLUDES *Cervical dilator insertion (59200)*
15.0 15.0 **FUD** 090 C 80
AMA: 2019,Jul,6; 2018,Jan,8; 2017,Jan,8; 2016,Jan,13; 2015,Jan,16

59855 **Induced abortion, by 1 or more vaginal suppositories (eg, prostaglandin) with or without cervical dilation (eg, laminaria), including hospital admission and visits, delivery of fetus and secundines;** M ♀
12.2 12.2 **FUD** 090 C 80
AMA: 2019,Jul,6

59856 **with dilation and curettage and/or evacuation** M ♀
14.3 14.3 **FUD** 090 C 80
AMA: 2019,Jul,6

59857 **with hysterotomy (failed medical evacuation)** M ♀
15.0 15.0 **FUD** 090 C 80
AMA: 2019,Jul,6

59866 **Multifetal pregnancy reduction(s) (MPR)** M ♀
6.22 6.22 **FUD** 000 T G2 80
AMA: 2019,Jul,6

59870-59899 Miscellaneous Obstetrical Procedures

CMS: 100-02,15,20.1 Physician Expense for Surgery, Childbirth, and Treatment for Infertility

59870 **Uterine evacuation and curettage for hydatidiform mole** M ♀
14.7 14.7 **FUD** 090 J A2 80
AMA: 2019,Jul,6; 2018,Jan,8; 2017,Jan,8; 2016,Jan,13; 2015,Jan,16

59871 **Removal of cerclage suture under anesthesia (other than local)** M ♀
3.82 3.82 **FUD** 000 Q2 A2 80
AMA: 2019,Jul,6; 2018,Jan,8; 2017,Jan,8; 2016,Jan,13; 2015,Jan,16

59897 **Unlisted fetal invasive procedure, including ultrasound guidance, when performed**

0.00 0.00 **FUD** YYY

AMA: 2019,Jul,6

59898 **Unlisted laparoscopy procedure, maternity care and delivery**

0.00 0.00 **FUD** YYY

AMA: 2019,Jul,6; 2018,Jan,8; 2017,Jan,8; 2016,Jan,13; 2015,Jan,16

59899 **Unlisted procedure, maternity care and delivery**

0.00 0.00 **FUD** YYY

AMA: 2019,Jul,6; 2018,Jan,8; 2017,Jan,8; 2016,Jan,13; 2015,Jan,16

60000 I&D of Infected Thyroglossal Cyst

60000 Incision and drainage of thyroglossal duct cyst, infected
4.37 4.99 FUD 010 T A2 80
AMA: 2014,Jan,11; 2002,May,7

60100 Core Needle Biopsy: Thyroid

EXCLUDES *Fine needle aspiration (10021, [10004, 10005, 10006, 10007, 10008, 10009, 10010, 10011, 10012])*

60100 Biopsy thyroid, percutaneous core needle
(76942, 77002, 77012, 77021)
(88172-88173)
2.25 3.18 FUD 000 T P3
AMA: 2019,Apr,4; 2018,Jan,8; 2017,Jan,8; 2016,Jan,13; 2015,Jan,16

60200 Surgical Removal Thyroid Cyst or Mass; Division of Isthmus

60200 Excision of cyst or adenoma of thyroid, or transection of isthmus
19.0 19.0 FUD 090 J A2 80
AMA: 2018,Jan,8; 2017,Jan,8; 2016,Jan,13; 2015,Jan,16

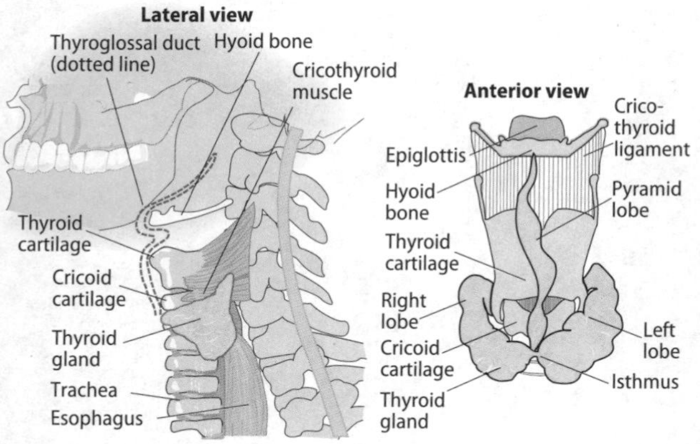

60210-60225 Subtotal Thyroidectomy

60210 Partial thyroid lobectomy, unilateral; with or without isthmusectomy
20.3 20.3 FUD 090 J G2 80
AMA: 2018,Jan,8; 2017,Jan,8; 2016,Jan,13; 2015,Jan,16

60212 with contralateral subtotal lobectomy, including isthmusectomy
29.0 29.0 FUD 090 J G2 80
AMA: 2018,Jan,8; 2017,Jan,8; 2016,Jan,13; 2015,Jan,16

60220 Total thyroid lobectomy, unilateral; with or without isthmusectomy
20.3 20.3 FUD 090 J G2 80
AMA: 2020,Aug,14; 2018,Jan,8; 2017,Jan,8; 2016,Jan,13; 2015,Jan,16

60225 with contralateral subtotal lobectomy, including isthmusectomy
26.8 26.8 FUD 090 J G2 80
AMA: 2018,Jan,8; 2017,Jan,8; 2016,Jan,13; 2015,Jan,16

60240-60271 Complete Thyroidectomy Procedures

60240 Thyroidectomy, total or complete
EXCLUDES *Subtotal or partial thyroidectomy (60271)*
26.5 26.5 FUD 090 J G2 80
AMA: 2018,Jan,8; 2017,Jan,8; 2016,Jan,13; 2015,Jan,16

60252 Thyroidectomy, total or subtotal for malignancy; with limited neck dissection
38.0 38.0 FUD 090 J 80
AMA: 2018,Jan,8; 2017,Jan,8; 2016,Jan,13; 2015,Jan,16

60254 with radical neck dissection
48.1 48.1 FUD 090 C 80
AMA: 2018,Jan,8; 2017,Jan,8; 2016,Jan,13; 2015,Jan,16

60260 Thyroidectomy, removal of all remaining thyroid tissue following previous removal of a portion of thyroid
31.4 31.4 FUD 090 J 80 50
AMA: 2018,Jan,8; 2017,Jan,8; 2016,Jan,13; 2015,Jan,16

60270 Thyroidectomy, including substernal thyroid; sternal split or transthoracic approach
39.4 39.4 FUD 090 C 80
AMA: 2018,Jan,8; 2017,Jan,8; 2016,Jan,13; 2015,Jan,16

60271 cervical approach
30.4 30.4 FUD 090 J 80
AMA: 2020,Aug,14; 2018,Jan,8; 2017,Jan,8; 2016,Jan,13; 2015,Jan,16

60280-60300 Treatment of Cyst/Sinus of Thyroid

60280 Excision of thyroglossal duct cyst or sinus;
EXCLUDES *Thyroid ultrasound (76536)*
12.6 12.6 FUD 090 J A2 80
AMA: 2014,Jan,11

60281 recurrent
EXCLUDES *Thyroid ultrasound (76536)*
16.8 16.8 FUD 090 J A2 80
AMA: 2014,Jan,11; 1994,Win,1

60300 Aspiration and/or injection, thyroid cyst
EXCLUDES *Fine needle aspiration (10021, [10004, 10005, 10006, 10007, 10008, 10009, 10010, 10011, 10012])*
(76942, 77012)
1.42 3.24 FUD 000 T P3
AMA: 2014,Jan,11

60500-60512 Parathyroid Procedures

60500 Parathyroidectomy or exploration of parathyroid(s);
27.9 27.9 FUD 090 J G2 80
AMA: 2018,Jan,8; 2017,Jan,8; 2016,Jan,13; 2015,Jan,16

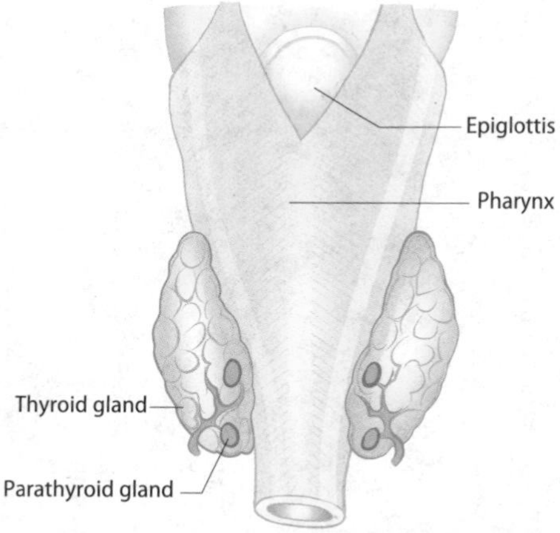

Posterior view of pharynx, thyroid glands, and parathyroid glands

60502 re-exploration
37.2 37.2 FUD 090 J 80
AMA: 2018,Jan,8; 2017,Jan,8; 2016,Jan,13; 2015,Jan,16

60505 with mediastinal exploration, sternal split or transthoracic approach
40.1 40.1 FUD 090 C 80
AMA: 2018,Jan,8; 2017,Jan,8; 2016,Jan,13; 2015,Jan,16

\+ **60512 Parathyroid autotransplantation (List separately in addition to code for primary procedure)**

Code first (60212, 60225, 60240, 60252, 60254, 60260, 60270-60271, 60500, 60502, 60505)

7.03 7.03 **FUD** ZZZ N 80

AMA: 2018,Jan,8; 2017,Jan,8; 2017,Jan,6; 2016,Jan,13; 2015,Jan,16

60520-60522 Thymus Procedures

EXCLUDES *Surgical thoracoscopy (video-assisted thoracic surgery (VATS) thymectomy (32673)*

60520 Thymectomy, partial or total; transcervical approach (separate procedure)

30.2 30.2 **FUD** 090 J 80

AMA: 2019,Mar,10

60521 sternal split or transthoracic approach, without radical mediastinal dissection (separate procedure)

32.4 32.4 **FUD** 090 C 80

AMA: 2018,Jan,8; 2017,Jan,8; 2016,Jan,13; 2015,Jan,16

60522 sternal split or transthoracic approach, with radical mediastinal dissection (separate procedure)

39.5 39.5 **FUD** 090 C 80

AMA: 2014,Jan,11; 2012,Oct,9-11

60540-60545 Adrenal Gland Procedures

EXCLUDES *Laparoscopic approach (60650)*
Removal remote or disseminated pheochromocytoma (49203-49205)
Standard backbench preparation cadaver donor (50323)

60540 Adrenalectomy, partial or complete, or exploration of adrenal gland with or without biopsy, transabdominal, lumbar or dorsal (separate procedure);

30.8 30.8 **FUD** 090 C 80 50

AMA: 2014,Jan,11; 1998,Nov,1

60545 with excision of adjacent retroperitoneal tumor

35.3 35.3 **FUD** 090 C 80 50

AMA: 2014,Jan,11; 1998,Nov,1

60600-60605 Carotid Body Procedures

60600 Excision of carotid body tumor; without excision of carotid artery

39.6 39.6 **FUD** 090 C 80

AMA: 2014,Jan,11

60605 with excision of carotid artery

48.2 48.2 **FUD** 090 C 80

AMA: 2018,Sep,9; 2017,Sep,13; 2016,Nov,8; 2016,Oct,10; 2016,Sep,8; 2016,Jul,10

60650-60699 Laparoscopic and Unlisted Procedures

INCLUDES Diagnostic laparoscopy (49320)

60650 Laparoscopy, surgical, with adrenalectomy, partial or complete, or exploration of adrenal gland with or without biopsy, transabdominal, lumbar or dorsal

EXCLUDES *Peritoneoscopy performed as separate procedure (49320)*

34.5 34.5 **FUD** 090 C 80 50

AMA: 2018,Jan,8; 2017,Jan,8; 2016,Jan,13; 2015,Jan,16

60659 Unlisted laparoscopy procedure, endocrine system

0.00 0.00 **FUD** YYY J 80 50

AMA: 2018,Jan,8; 2017,Jan,8; 2016,Jan,13; 2015,Jan,16

60699 Unlisted procedure, endocrine system

0.00 0.00 **FUD** YYY J 80

AMA: 2018,Jan,8; 2017,Jan,8; 2016,Jan,13; 2015,Jan,16

Endocrine System

60512 — 60699

61000-61253 Transcranial Access via Puncture, Burr Hole, Twist Hole, or Trephine

EXCLUDES *Injection for cerebral angiography (36100-36218)*

61000 **Subdural tap through fontanelle, or suture, infant, unilateral or bilateral; initial** A

EXCLUDES *Injection for:*
Pneumoencephalography (61055)
Ventriculography (61026, 61120)

3.33 3.33 **FUD** 000 T R2

AMA: 2014,Jan,11

Overhead view of newborn skull

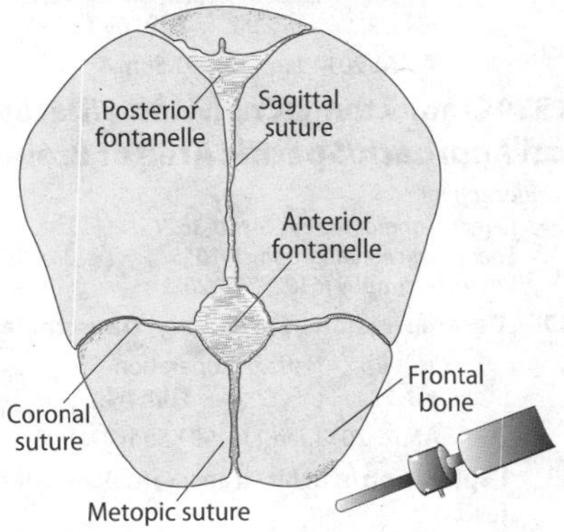

An initial tap through to the subdural level is performed on an infant via a fontanelle or suture, either unilateral or bilateral

61001 **subsequent taps** A
3.16 3.16 **FUD** 000 T R2
AMA: 2014,Jan,11

61020 **Ventricular puncture through previous burr hole, fontanelle, suture, or implanted ventricular catheter/reservoir; without injection**
2.87 2.87 **FUD** 000 T A2
AMA: 2014,Jan,11

61026 **with injection of medication or other substance for diagnosis or treatment**
INCLUDES Injection for ventriculography
3.05 3.05 **FUD** 000 T A2
AMA: 2014,Jan,11; 2002,May,7

61050 **Cisternal or lateral cervical (C1-C2) puncture; without injection (separate procedure)**
2.44 2.44 **FUD** 000 T A2 80
AMA: 2014,Jan,11; 1991,Win,1

61055 **with injection of medication or other substance for diagnosis or treatment**
INCLUDES Injection for pneumoencephalography
EXCLUDES *Myelography via lumbar injection (62302-62305)*
Radiology procedures except when furnished by different provider
3.62 3.62 **FUD** 000 T A2
AMA: 2014,Sep,3; 2014,Jan,11

61070 **Puncture of shunt tubing or reservoir for aspiration or injection procedure**
(75809)
1.63 1.63 **FUD** 000 T A2
AMA: 2018,Jan,8; 2017,Jan,8; 2016,Jan,13; 2015,Jan,16

61105 **Twist drill hole for subdural or ventricular puncture**
13.5 13.5 **FUD** 090 C 80
AMA: 2014,Jan,11

61107 **Twist drill hole(s) for subdural, intracerebral, or ventricular puncture; for implanting ventricular catheter, pressure recording device, or other intracerebral monitoring device**
Code also intracranial neuroendoscopic ventricular catheter insertion or reinsertion, when performed (62160)
9.20 9.20 **FUD** 000 ⊘ C
AMA: 2014,Jan,11; 2007,Jun,10-11

61108 **for evacuation and/or drainage of subdural hematoma**
25.8 25.8 **FUD** 090 C
AMA: 2014,Jan,11

61120 **Burr hole(s) for ventricular puncture (including injection of gas, contrast media, dye, or radioactive material)**
INCLUDES Injection for ventriculography
21.8 21.8 **FUD** 090 C 80
AMA: 2014,Jan,11

61140 **Burr hole(s) or trephine; with biopsy of brain or intracranial lesion**
36.9 36.9 **FUD** 090 C 80
AMA: 2014,Jan,11

61150 **with drainage of brain abscess or cyst**
39.8 39.8 **FUD** 090 C
AMA: 2014,Jan,11

61151 **with subsequent tapping (aspiration) of intracranial abscess or cyst**
29.1 29.1 **FUD** 090 C
AMA: 2014,Jan,11

61154 **Burr hole(s) with evacuation and/or drainage of hematoma, extradural or subdural**
36.6 36.6 **FUD** 090 C 80 50
AMA: 2014,Jan,11

61156 **Burr hole(s); with aspiration of hematoma or cyst, intracerebral**
36.5 36.5 **FUD** 090 C 80
AMA: 2014,Jan,11

61210 **for implanting ventricular catheter, reservoir, EEG electrode(s), pressure recording device, or other cerebral monitoring device (separate procedure)**
Code also intracranial neuroendoscopic ventricular catheter insertion or reinsertion, when performed (62160)
10.8 10.8 **FUD** 000 C
AMA: 2018,Jan,8; 2017,Jan,8; 2016,Jan,13; 2015,Jan,16

61215 **Insertion of subcutaneous reservoir, pump or continuous infusion system for connection to ventricular catheter**
EXCLUDES *Chemotherapy (96450)*
Refilling and maintenance implantable infusion pump (95990)
14.8 14.8 **FUD** 090 J A2
AMA: 2018,Jan,8; 2017,Jan,8; 2016,Jan,13; 2015,Jan,16

61250 **Burr hole(s) or trephine, supratentorial, exploratory, not followed by other surgery**
EXCLUDES *Burr hole or trephine followed by craniotomy same operative session (61304-61321)*
25.2 25.2 **FUD** 090 C 80 50
AMA: 2014,Jan,11

61253 **Burr hole(s) or trephine, infratentorial, unilateral or bilateral**
EXCLUDES *Burr hole or trephine followed by craniotomy same operative session (61304-61321)*
28.8 28.8 **FUD** 090 C 80
AMA: 2018,Jan,8; 2017,Jan,8; 2016,Jan,13; 2015,Jan,16

61304-61323 Craniectomy/Craniotomy: By Indication/Specific Area of Brain

EXCLUDES *Injection for:*
Cerebral angiography (36100-36218)
Pneumoencephalography (61055)
Ventriculography (61026, 61120)

61304 Craniectomy or craniotomy, exploratory; supratentorial
EXCLUDES *Other craniectomy/craniotomy procedures when performed same anatomical site and during same surgical encounter*
48.1 48.1 FUD 090 C 80
AMA: 2014,Jan,11; 2002,Sep,10

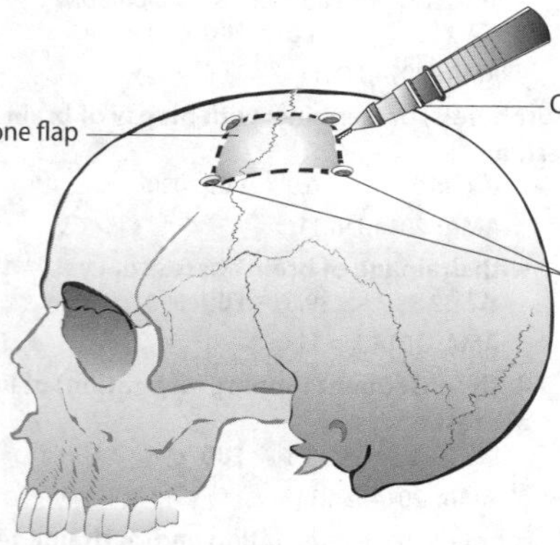

61305 infratentorial (posterior fossa)
EXCLUDES *Other craniectomy/craniotomy procedures when performed same anatomical site and during same surgical encounter*
58.6 58.6 FUD 090 C 80
AMA: 2014,Jan,11; 2002,Sep,10

61312 Craniectomy or craniotomy for evacuation of hematoma, supratentorial; extradural or subdural
60.8 60.8 FUD 090 C 80
AMA: 2018,Jan,8; 2017,Jan,8; 2016,Jan,13; 2015,Jan,16

61313 intracerebral
58.0 58.0 FUD 090 C 80
AMA: 2014,Jan,11; 2002,Sep,10

61314 Craniectomy or craniotomy for evacuation of hematoma, infratentorial; extradural or subdural
53.2 53.2 FUD 090 C 80
AMA: 2014,Jan,11; 2002,Sep,10

61315 intracerebellar
60.4 60.4 FUD 090 C 80
AMA: 2014,Jan,11; 2002,Sep,10

+ **61316 Incision and subcutaneous placement of cranial bone graft (List separately in addition to code for primary procedure)**
Code first (61304, 61312-61313, 61322-61323, 61340, 61570-61571, 61680-61705)
2.60 2.60 FUD ZZZ C
AMA: 2014,Jan,11; 2002,Sep,10

61320 Craniectomy or craniotomy, drainage of intracranial abscess; supratentorial
55.5 55.5 FUD 090 C 80
AMA: 2014,Jan,11; 2002,Sep,10

61321 infratentorial
61.7 61.7 FUD 090 C 80
AMA: 2014,Jan,11; 2002,Sep,10

61322 Craniectomy or craniotomy, decompressive, with or without duraplasty, for treatment of intracranial hypertension, without evacuation of associated intraparenchymal hematoma; without lobectomy
EXCLUDES *Craniectomy or craniotomy for evacuation hematoma (61313)*
Subtemporal decompression (61340)
69.7 69.7 FUD 090 C 80
AMA: 2020,May,13; 2018,Aug,10

61323 with lobectomy
EXCLUDES *Craniectomy or craniotomy for evacuation hematoma (61313)*
Subtemporal decompression (61340)
69.2 69.2 FUD 090 C 80
AMA: 2014,Jan,11; 1991,Sum,4

61330-61530 Craniectomy/Craniotomy/Decompression Brain By Surgical Approach/Specific Area of Brain

EXCLUDES *Injection for:*
Cerebral angiography (36100-36218)
Pneumoencephalography (61055)
Ventriculography (61026, 61120)

61330 Decompression of orbit only, transcranial approach
INCLUDES Naffziger operation
52.8 52.8 FUD 090 J G2 80 50
AMA: 2014,Jan,11; 1991,Sum,4

61333 Exploration of orbit (transcranial approach); with removal of lesion
59.6 59.6 FUD 090 C 80 50
AMA: 2014,Jan,11; 1991,Sum,4

61340 Subtemporal cranial decompression (pseudotumor cerebri, slit ventricle syndrome)
EXCLUDES *Decompression craniotomy or craniectomy for intracranial hypertension, without hematoma removal (61322-61323)*
42.4 42.4 FUD 090 C 80 50
AMA: 2020,May,13

61343 Craniectomy, suboccipital with cervical laminectomy for decompression of medulla and spinal cord, with or without dural graft (eg, Arnold-Chiari malformation)
63.4 63.4 FUD 090 C 80
AMA: 2014,Jan,11; 1991,Sum,4

61345 Other cranial decompression, posterior fossa
EXCLUDES *Kroenlein procedure*
Orbital decompression using lateral wall approach (67445)
60.1 60.1 FUD 090 C 80
AMA: 2014,Jan,11; 1991,Sum,4

61450 Craniectomy, subtemporal, for section, compression, or decompression of sensory root of gasserian ganglion
INCLUDES Frazier-Spiller procedure
Hartley-Krause
Krause decompression
Taarnhoj procedure
56.0 56.0 FUD 090 C 80
AMA: 2014,Jan,11; 1991,Sum,4

61458 Craniectomy, suboccipital; for exploration or decompression of cranial nerves
INCLUDES Jannetta decompression
58.8 58.8 FUD 090 C 80
AMA: 2014,Jan,11; 1991,Sum,4

61460 **for section of 1 or more cranial nerves**
61.7 61.7 **FUD** 090
AMA: 2014,Jan,11; 1991,Sum,4

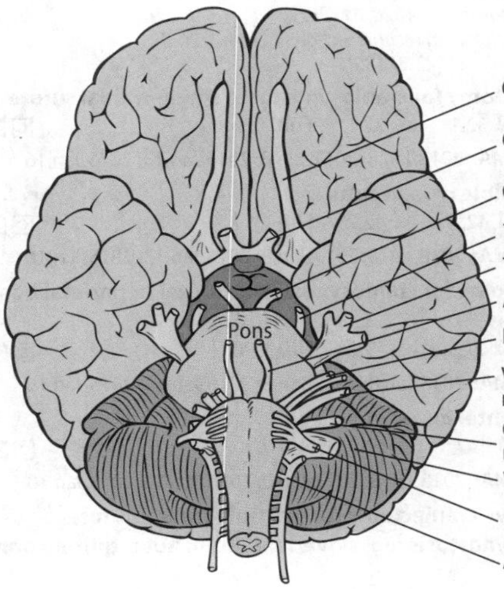

61500 **Craniectomy; with excision of tumor or other bone lesion of skull**
38.2 38.2 **FUD** 090
AMA: 2018,Jan,8; 2017,Jan,8; 2016,Jan,13; 2015,Jan,16

61501 **for osteomyelitis**
32.8 32.8 **FUD** 090
AMA: 2018,Jan,8; 2017,Jan,8; 2016,Jan,13; 2015,Jan,16

61510 **Craniectomy, trephination, bone flap craniotomy; for excision of brain tumor, supratentorial, except meningioma**
64.0 64.0 **FUD** 090
AMA: 2014,Jan,11; 1991,Sum,4

61512 **for excision of meningioma, supratentorial**
74.8 74.8 **FUD** 090
AMA: 2014,Jan,11; 1991,Sum,4

61514 **for excision of brain abscess, supratentorial**
55.9 55.9 **FUD** 090
AMA: 2014,Jan,11; 1991,Sum,4

61516 **for excision or fenestration of cyst, supratentorial**
EXCLUDES *Craniopharyngioma (61545)*
Pituitary tumor removal (61546, 61548)
54.4 54.4 **FUD** 090
AMA: 2014,Jan,11; 1991,Sum,4

\+ **61517** **Implantation of brain intracavitary chemotherapy agent (List separately in addition to code for primary procedure)**
EXCLUDES *Intracavity radioelement source or ribbon implantation (77770-77772)*
Code first (61510, 61518)
2.59 2.59 **FUD** ZZZ
AMA: 2014,Jan,11; 1991,Sum,4

61518 **Craniectomy for excision of brain tumor, infratentorial or posterior fossa; except meningioma, cerebellopontine angle tumor, or midline tumor at base of skull**
79.9 79.9 **FUD** 090
AMA: 2014,Jan,11; 1991,Sum,4

61519 **meningioma**
86.7 86.7 **FUD** 090
AMA: 2014,Jan,11; 1991,Sum,4

61520 **cerebellopontine angle tumor**
110. 110. **FUD** 090
AMA: 2014,Jan,11; 1991,Sum,4

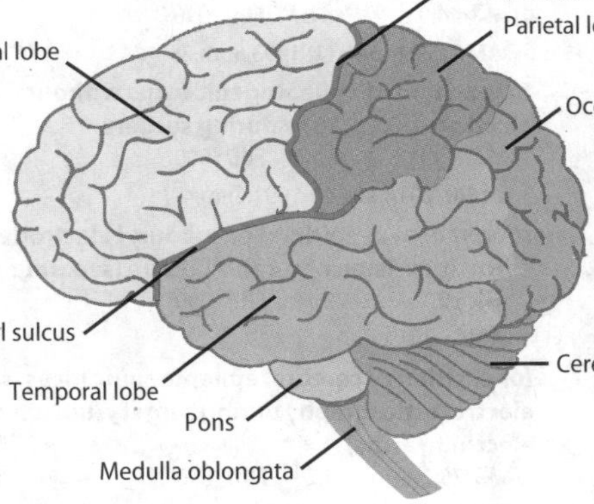

61521 **midline tumor at base of skull**
93.7 93.7 **FUD** 090
AMA: 2018,Jan,8; 2017,Jan,8; 2016,Jan,13; 2015,Jan,16

61522 **Craniectomy, infratentorial or posterior fossa; for excision of brain abscess**
62.9 62.9 **FUD** 090
AMA: 2014,Jan,11; 1991,Sum,4

61524 **for excision or fenestration of cyst**
60.1 60.1 **FUD** 090
AMA: 2014,Jan,11; 1991,Sum,4

61526 **Craniectomy, bone flap craniotomy, transtemporal (mastoid) for excision of cerebellopontine angle tumor;**
97.9 97.9 **FUD** 090
AMA: 2018,Mar,11; 2018,Jan,8; 2017,Jan,8; 2016,Jan,13; 2015,Jan,16

61530 **combined with middle/posterior fossa craniotomy/craniectomy**
91.0 91.0 **FUD** 090
AMA: 2014,Jan,11; 1991,Sum,4

61531-61545 Procedures for Seizures/Implanted Electrodes/Choroid Plexus/Craniopharyngioma

EXCLUDES *Craniotomy for:*
Multiple subpial transections during procedure (61567)
Selective amygdalohippocampectomy (61566)
Injection for:
Cerebral angiography (36100-36218)
Pneumoencephalography (61055)
Ventriculography (61026, 61120)

61531 **Subdural implantation of strip electrodes through 1 or more burr or trephine hole(s) for long-term seizure monitoring**
EXCLUDES *Continuous EEG observation ([95700, 95705, 95706, 95707, 95708, 95709, 95710, 95711, 95712, 95713, 95714, 95715, 95716, 95717, 95718, 95719, 95720, 95721, 95722, 95723, 95724, 95725, 95726])*
Craniotomy for intracranial arteriovenous malformation removal (61680-61692)
Stereotactic insertion electrodes (61760)
35.2 35.2 **FUD** 090
AMA: 2019,Jul,10

Nervous System

61460 — 61531

61533 **Craniotomy with elevation of bone flap; for subdural implantation of an electrode array, for long-term seizure monitoring**

EXCLUDES *Continuous EEG monitoring ([95700, 95705, 95706, 95707, 95708, 95709, 95710, 95711, 95712, 95713, 95714, 95715, 95716, 95717, 95718, 95719, 95720, 95721, 95722, 95723, 95724, 95725, 95726])*

44.0 44.0 **FUD** 090 C 80

AMA: 2014,Jan,11; 1993,Sum,25

61534 **for excision of epileptogenic focus without electrocorticography during surgery**

47.4 47.4 **FUD** 090 C 80

AMA: 2014,Jan,11; 1991,Sum,4

61535 **for removal of epidural or subdural electrode array, without excision of cerebral tissue (separate procedure)**

29.1 29.1 **FUD** 090 C 80

AMA: 2019,Jul,10

61536 **for excision of cerebral epileptogenic focus, with electrocorticography during surgery (includes removal of electrode array)**

75.2 75.2 **FUD** 090 C 80

AMA: 2014,Jan,11; 1991,Sum,4

61537 **for lobectomy, temporal lobe, without electrocorticography during surgery**

72.4 72.4 **FUD** 090 C 80

AMA: 2014,Jan,11; 1991,Sum,4

61538 **for lobectomy, temporal lobe, with electrocorticography during surgery**

77.1 77.1 **FUD** 090 C 80

AMA: 2019,Mar,6

61539 **for lobectomy, other than temporal lobe, partial or total, with electrocorticography during surgery**

68.2 68.2 **FUD** 090 C 80

AMA: 2019,Mar,6

61540 **for lobectomy, other than temporal lobe, partial or total, without electrocorticography during surgery**

62.9 62.9 **FUD** 090 C 80

AMA: 2014,Jan,11; 1991,Sum,4

61541 **for transection of corpus callosum**

63.3 63.3 **FUD** 090 C 80

AMA: 2014,Jan,11; 1991,Sum,4

61543 **for partial or subtotal (functional) hemispherectomy**

64.0 64.0 **FUD** 090 C 80

AMA: 2014,Jan,11; 1991,Sum,4

61544 **for excision or coagulation of choroid plexus**

54.8 54.8 **FUD** 090 C 80

AMA: 2014,Jan,11; 1991,Sum,4

61545 **for excision of craniopharyngioma**

92.3 92.3 **FUD** 090 C 80

AMA: 2014,Jan,11; 1991,Sum,4

61546-61548 Removal Pituitary Gland/Tumor

EXCLUDES *Injection for:*
Cerebral angiography (36100-36218)
Pneumoencephalography (61055)
Ventriculography (61026, 61120)

61546 **Craniotomy for hypophysectomy or excision of pituitary tumor, intracranial approach**

67.4 67.4 **FUD** 090 C 80

AMA: 2014,Jan,11; 1991,Sum,4

61548 **Hypophysectomy or excision of pituitary tumor, transnasal or transseptal approach, nonstereotactic**

INCLUDES Operating microscope (69990)

45.8 45.8 **FUD** 090 C 80

AMA: 2019,Dec,12; 2016,Feb,12

61550-61559 Craniosynostosis Procedures

EXCLUDES *Injection for:*
Cerebral angiography (36100-36218)
Pneumoencephalography (61055)
Ventriculography (61026, 61120)
Orbital hypertelorism reconstruction (21260-21263)
Reconstruction (21172-21180)

61550 **Craniectomy for craniosynostosis; single cranial suture**

32.1 32.1 **FUD** 090 C 80

AMA: 2018,Jan,8; 2017,Jan,8; 2016,Jan,13; 2015,Jan,16

61552 **multiple cranial sutures**

42.7 42.7 **FUD** 090 C 80

AMA: 2018,Jan,8; 2017,Jan,8; 2016,Jan,13; 2015,Jan,16

61556 **Craniotomy for craniosynostosis; frontal or parietal bone flap**

49.2 49.2 **FUD** 090 C 80

AMA: 2018,Jan,8; 2017,Jan,8; 2016,Jan,13; 2015,Jan,16

61557 **bifrontal bone flap**

49.4 49.4 **FUD** 090 C 80

AMA: 2018,Jan,8; 2017,Jan,8; 2016,Jan,13; 2015,Jan,16

61558 **Extensive craniectomy for multiple cranial suture craniosynostosis (eg, cloverleaf skull); not requiring bone grafts**

55.2 55.2 **FUD** 090 C 80

AMA: 2018,Jan,8; 2017,Jan,8; 2016,Jan,13; 2015,Jan,16

61559 **recontouring with multiple osteotomies and bone autografts (eg, barrel-stave procedure) (includes obtaining grafts)**

70.5 70.5 **FUD** 090 C 80

AMA: 2018,Jan,8; 2017,Jan,8; 2016,Jan,13; 2015,Jan,16

61563-61564 Removal Cranial Bone Tumor With/Without Optic Nerve Decompression

EXCLUDES *Injection for:*
Cerebral angiography (36100-36218)
Pneumoencephalography (61055)
Ventriculography (61026, 61120)
Reconstruction (21181-21183)

61563 **Excision, intra and extracranial, benign tumor of cranial bone (eg, fibrous dysplasia); without optic nerve decompression**

57.5 57.5 **FUD** 090 C 80

AMA: 2014,Jan,11; 1991,Sum,4

61564 **with optic nerve decompression**

69.5 69.5 **FUD** 090 C 80 50

AMA: 2014,Jan,11; 1991,Sum,4

61566-61567 Craniotomy for Seizures

EXCLUDES *Injection for:*
Cerebral angiography (36100-36218)
Pneumoencephalography (61055)
Ventriculography (61026, 61120)

61566 **Craniotomy with elevation of bone flap; for selective amygdalohippocampectomy**

64.8 64.8 **FUD** 090 C 80

AMA: 2018,Nov,7

61567 **for multiple subpial transections, with electrocorticography during surgery**

72.9 72.9 **FUD** 090 C 80

AMA: 2014,Jan,11; 1991,Sum,4

61570-61571 Removal of Foreign Body from Brain

EXCLUDES *Injection for:*
Cerebral angiography (36100-36218)
Pneumoencephalography (61055)
Ventriculography (61026, 61120)
Sequestrectomy for osteomyelitis (61501)

61570 **Craniectomy or craniotomy; with excision of foreign body from brain**

53.9 53.9 **FUD** 090 C 80

AMA: 2014,Jan,11; 1991,Sum,4

61571   with treatment of penetrating wound of brain
🚗 57.4   ⚕ 57.4   **FUD** 090   C 80 ▣
AMA: 2014,Jan,11; 1991,Sum,4

61575-61576 Transoral Approach Posterior Cranial Fossa/Upper Cervical Cord

EXCLUDES   Arthrodesis (22548)
Injection for:
Cerebral angiography (36100-36218)
Pneumoencephalography (61055)
Ventriculography (61026, 61120)

61575   Transoral approach to skull base, brain stem or upper spinal cord for biopsy, decompression or excision of lesion;
🚗 72.4   ⚕ 72.4   **FUD** 090   C 80 ▣
AMA: 2014,Jan,11; 1991,Sum,4

61576   requiring splitting of tongue and/or mandible (including tracheostomy)
🚗 121.   ⚕ 121.   **FUD** 090   C 80 ▣
AMA: 2014,Jan,11; 1991,Sum,4

61580-61598 Surgical Approach: Cranial Fossae

EXCLUDES   Definitive surgery (61600-61616)
Dural repair and/or reconstruction (61618-61619)
Injection for:
Cerebral angiography (36100-36218)
Pneumoencephalography (61055)
Ventriculography (61026, 61120)
Primary closure (15730, 15733, 15756-15758)

61580   Craniofacial approach to anterior cranial fossa; extradural, including lateral rhinotomy, ethmoidectomy, sphenoidectomy, without maxillectomy or orbital exenteration
🚗 70.3   ⚕ 70.3   **FUD** 090   C 50 ▣
AMA: 2018,Jan,8; 2017,Jan,8; 2016,Jan,13; 2015,Jan,16

61581   extradural, including lateral rhinotomy, orbital exenteration, ethmoidectomy, sphenoidectomy and/or maxillectomy
🚗 76.6   ⚕ 76.6   **FUD** 090   C 50 ▣
AMA: 2018,Jan,8; 2017,Jan,8; 2016,Jan,13; 2015,Jan,16

61582   extradural, including unilateral or bifrontal craniotomy, elevation of frontal lobe(s), osteotomy of base of anterior cranial fossa
🚗 88.5   ⚕ 88.5   **FUD** 090   C 80 ▣
AMA: 2018,Jan,8; 2017,Jan,8; 2016,Jan,13; 2015,Jan,16

61583   intradural, including unilateral or bifrontal craniotomy, elevation or resection of frontal lobe, osteotomy of base of anterior cranial fossa
🚗 84.2   ⚕ 84.2   **FUD** 090   C 80 ▣
AMA: 2018,Jan,8; 2017,Dec,13; 2017,Jan,8; 2016,Jan,13; 2015,Jan,16

61584   Orbitocranial approach to anterior cranial fossa, extradural, including supraorbital ridge osteotomy and elevation of frontal and/or temporal lobe(s); without orbital exenteration
🚗 83.7   ⚕ 83.7   **FUD** 090   C 80 50 ▣
AMA: 2018,Jan,8; 2017,Jan,8; 2016,Jan,13; 2015,Jan,16

61585   with orbital exenteration
🚗 95.1   ⚕ 95.1   **FUD** 090   C 80 50 ▣
AMA: 2018,Jan,8; 2017,Jan,8; 2016,Jan,13; 2015,Jan,16

61586   Bicoronal, transzygomatic and/or LeFort I osteotomy approach to anterior cranial fossa with or without internal fixation, without bone graft
🚗 70.5   ⚕ 70.5   **FUD** 090   C 80 ▣
AMA: 2014,Jan,11; 1997,Nov,1

61590   Infratemporal pre-auricular approach to middle cranial fossa (parapharyngeal space, infratemporal and midline skull base, nasopharynx), with or without disarticulation of the mandible, including parotidectomy, craniotomy, decompression and/or mobilization of the facial nerve and/or petrous carotid artery
🚗 88.1   ⚕ 88.1   **FUD** 090   C 80 50 ▣
AMA: 2020,Apr,10; 2018,Jan,8; 2017,Jan,8; 2016,Jan,13; 2015,Jan,16

61591   Infratemporal post-auricular approach to middle cranial fossa (internal auditory meatus, petrous apex, tentorium, cavernous sinus, parasellar area, infratemporal fossa) including mastoidectomy, resection of sigmoid sinus, with or without decompression and/or mobilization of contents of auditory canal or petrous carotid artery
🚗 89.1   ⚕ 89.1   **FUD** 090   C 80 50 ▣
AMA: 2018,Jan,8; 2017,Jan,8; 2016,Jan,13; 2015,Jan,16

61592   Orbitocranial zygomatic approach to middle cranial fossa (cavernous sinus and carotid artery, clivus, basilar artery or petrous apex) including osteotomy of zygoma, craniotomy, extra- or intradural elevation of temporal lobe
🚗 92.5   ⚕ 92.5   **FUD** 090   C 80 50 ▣
AMA: 2018,Jan,8; 2017,Jan,8; 2016,Jan,13; 2015,Jan,16

61595   Transtemporal approach to posterior cranial fossa, jugular foramen or midline skull base, including mastoidectomy, decompression of sigmoid sinus and/or facial nerve, with or without mobilization
🚗 68.1   ⚕ 68.1   **FUD** 090   C 50 ▣
AMA: 2018,Mar,11; 2018,Jan,8; 2017,Jan,8; 2016,Jan,13; 2015,Jan,16

61596   Transcochlear approach to posterior cranial fossa, jugular foramen or midline skull base, including labyrinthectomy, decompression, with or without mobilization of facial nerve and/or petrous carotid artery
🚗 70.1   ⚕ 70.1   **FUD** 090   C 80 50 ▣
AMA: 2018,Jan,8; 2017,Jan,8; 2016,Jan,13; 2015,Jan,16

61597   Transcondylar (far lateral) approach to posterior cranial fossa, jugular foramen or midline skull base, including occipital condylectomy, mastoidectomy, resection of C1-C3 vertebral body(s), decompression of vertebral artery, with or without mobilization
🚗 85.5   ⚕ 85.5   **FUD** 090   C 80 50 ▣
AMA: 2018,Jan,8; 2017,Jan,8; 2016,Jan,13; 2015,Jan,16

61598   Transpetrosal approach to posterior cranial fossa, clivus or foramen magnum, including ligation of superior petrosal sinus and/or sigmoid sinus
🚗 82.9   ⚕ 82.9   **FUD** 090   C 80 ▣
AMA: 2018,Jan,8; 2017,Jan,8; 2016,Jan,13; 2015,Jan,16

61600-61616 Definitive Procedures: Cranial Fossae

EXCLUDES   Dural repair and/or reconstruction (61618-61619)
Injection for:
Cerebral angiography (36100-36218)
Pneumoencephalography (61055)
Ventriculography (61026, 61120)
Primary closure (15730, 15733, 15756-15758)
Surgical approach (61580-61598)

61600   Resection or excision of neoplastic, vascular or infectious lesion of base of anterior cranial fossa; extradural
🚗 61.5   ⚕ 61.5   **FUD** 090   C 80 ▣
AMA: 2018,Jan,8; 2017,Jan,8; 2016,Jan,13; 2015,Jan,16

61601   intradural, including dural repair, with or without graft
🚗 70.1   ⚕ 70.1   **FUD** 090   C 80 ▣
AMA: 2018,Jan,8; 2017,Jan,8; 2016,Jan,13; 2015,Jan,16

61605   Resection or excision of neoplastic, vascular or infectious lesion of infratemporal fossa, parapharyngeal space, petrous apex; extradural
🚗 62.1   ⚕ 62.1   **FUD** 090   C 80 ▣
AMA: 2020,Apr,10; 2018,Jan,8; 2017,Jan,8; 2016,Jan,13; 2015,Jan,16

● New Code   ▲ Revised Code   ○ Reinstated   ● New Web Release   ▲ Revised Web Release   + Add-on   Unlisted   Not Covered   # Resequenced
50 Optum Mod 50 Exempt   ⊘ AMA Mod 51 Exempt   51 Optum Mod 51 Exempt   63 Mod 63 Exempt   ✗ Non-FDA Drug   ★ Telemedicine   M Maternity   A Age Edit

61606 **intradural, including dural repair, with or without graft**
85.7 85.7 **FUD** 090 C 80
AMA: 2018,Jan,8; 2017,Jan,8; 2016,Jan,13; 2015,Jan,16

61607 **Resection or excision of neoplastic, vascular or infectious lesion of parasellar area, cavernous sinus, clivus or midline skull base; extradural**
77.8 77.8 **FUD** 090 C 80
AMA: 2018,Jan,8; 2017,Jan,8; 2016,Jan,13; 2015,Jan,16

61608 **intradural, including dural repair, with or without graft**
95.7 95.7 **FUD** 090 C 80
AMA: 2018,Jan,8; 2017,Jan,8; 2016,Jan,13; 2015,Jan,16

\+ **61611** **Transection or ligation, carotid artery in petrous canal; without repair (List separately in addition to code for primary procedure)**
Code first (61605-61608)
13.8 13.8 **FUD** ZZZ C 80
AMA: 2018,Jan,8; 2017,Jan,8; 2016,Jan,13; 2015,Jan,16

61613 **Obliteration of carotid aneurysm, arteriovenous malformation, or carotid-cavernous fistula by dissection within cavernous sinus**
96.9 96.9 **FUD** 090 C 80 50
AMA: 2018,Jan,8; 2017,Jan,8; 2016,Jan,13; 2015,Jan,16

61615 **Resection or excision of neoplastic, vascular or infectious lesion of base of posterior cranial fossa, jugular foramen, foramen magnum, or C1-C3 vertebral bodies; extradural**
81.9 81.9 **FUD** 090 C 80
AMA: 2018,Jan,8; 2017,Jan,8; 2016,Jan,13; 2015,Jan,16

61616 **intradural, including dural repair, with or without graft**
96.0 96.0 **FUD** 090 C 80
AMA: 2018,Mar,11; 2018,Jan,8; 2017,Jan,8; 2016,Jan,13; 2015,Jan,16

61618-61619 Reconstruction Post-Surgical Cranial Fossae Defects

EXCLUDES *Definitive surgery (61600-61616)*
Injection for:
Cerebral angiography (36100-36218)
Pneumoencephalography (61055)
Ventriculography (61026, 61120)
Primary closure (15730, 15733, 15756-15758)
Surgical approach (61580-61598)

61618 **Secondary repair of dura for cerebrospinal fluid leak, anterior, middle or posterior cranial fossa following surgery of the skull base; by free tissue graft (eg, pericranium, fascia, tensor fascia lata, adipose tissue, homologous or synthetic grafts)**
37.5 37.5 **FUD** 090 C 80
AMA: 2018,Jan,8; 2017,Jan,8; 2016,Jan,13; 2015,Jan,16

61619 **by local or regionalized vascularized pedicle flap or myocutaneous flap (including galea, temporalis, frontalis or occipitalis muscle)**
41.3 41.3 **FUD** 090 C 80
AMA: 2018,Jan,8; 2017,Jan,8; 2016,Jan,13; 2015,Jan,16

61623-61651 Neurovascular Interventional Procedures

61623 **Endovascular temporary balloon arterial occlusion, head or neck (extracranial/intracranial) including selective catheterization of vessel to be occluded, positioning and inflation of occlusion balloon, concomitant neurological monitoring, and radiologic supervision and interpretation of all angiography required for balloon occlusion and to exclude vascular injury post occlusion**

EXCLUDES *Diagnostic angiography target artery just before temporary occlusion; report only radiological supervision and interpretation*
Selective catheterization and angiography artery besides the target artery; report catheterization and radiological supervision and interpretation codes as appropriate

16.6 16.6 **FUD** 000 J
AMA: 2018,Jan,8; 2017,Jan,8; 2016,Jan,13; 2015,Jan,16

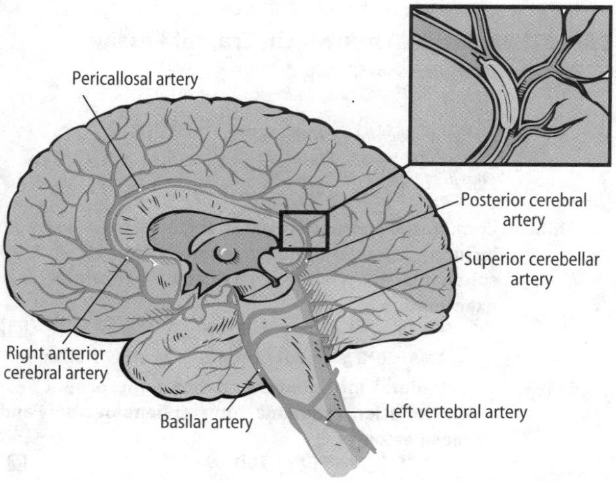

61624 **Transcatheter permanent occlusion or embolization (eg, for tumor destruction, to achieve hemostasis, to occlude a vascular malformation), percutaneous, any method; central nervous system (intracranial, spinal cord)**

EXCLUDES *Non-central nervous system transcatheter occlusion or embolization other than head or neck (37241-37244)*

(75894)
33.3 33.3 **FUD** 000 C
AMA: 2019,Sep,6; 2018,Jan,8; 2017,Jan,8; 2016,Jan,13; 2015,Jan,16

61626 **non-central nervous system, head or neck (extracranial, brachiocephalic branch)**

EXCLUDES *Non-central nervous system transcatheter occlusion or embolization other than head or neck (37241-37244)*

(75894)
25.5 25.5 **FUD** 000 J
AMA: 2019,Sep,6; 2018,Jan,8; 2017,Jan,8; 2016,Jan,13; 2015,Jan,16

61630 Balloon angioplasty, intracranial (eg, atherosclerotic stenosis), percutaneous

INCLUDES Diagnostic arteriogram when stent or angioplasty necessary
Radiology services for arteriography target vascular territory
Selective catheterization target vascular territory

EXCLUDES *Diagnostic arteriogram when stent or angioplasty not necessary (report applicable code for selective catheterization and radiology services)*
Percutaneous arterial transluminal mechanical thrombectomy and/or infusion for thrombolysis performed same vascular territory (61645)

40.6 40.6 FUD XXX C 80

AMA: 2018,Jan,8; 2017,Jul,3; 2017,Apr,9; 2017,Jan,8; 2016,Mar,3; 2016,Jan,13; 2015,Nov,3; 2015,Jan,16

61635 Transcatheter placement of intravascular stent(s), intracranial (eg, atherosclerotic stenosis), including balloon angioplasty, if performed

INCLUDES Diagnostic arteriogram when stent or angioplasty necessary
Radiology services for arteriography target vascular territory
Selective catheterization target vascular territory

EXCLUDES *Diagnostic arteriogram when stent or angioplasty not necessary (report applicable code for selective catheterization and radiology services)*
Percutaneous arterial transluminal mechanical thrombectomy and/or infusion for thrombolysis performed same vascular territory (61645)

42.6 42.6 FUD XXX C 80

AMA: 2018,Jan,8; 2017,Jul,3; 2017,Jan,8; 2016,Mar,3; 2016,Jan,13; 2015,Nov,3; 2015,Jan,16

61640 Balloon dilatation of intracranial vasospasm, percutaneous; initial vessel

INCLUDES Angiography after dilation vessel
Fluoroscopic guidance
Injection contrast material
Roadmapping
Selective catheterization target vessel
Vessel analysis

EXCLUDES *Endovascular intracranial prolonged administration pharmacologic agent performed same vascular territory (61650-61651)*

Code first (61640)

14.0 14.0 FUD 000 E

AMA: 2018,Jan,8; 2017,Jan,8; 2016,Mar,3; 2016,Jan,13; 2015,Nov,3; 2015,Jan,16

+ **61641 each additional vessel in same vascular territory (List separately in addition to code for primary procedure)**

INCLUDES Angiography after dilation vessel
Fluoroscopic guidance
Injection contrast material
Roadmapping
Selective catheterization target vessel
Vessel analysis

EXCLUDES *Endovascular intracranial prolonged administration pharmacologic agent performed same vascular territory (61640)*

Code first (61640)

4.92 4.92 FUD ZZZ E

AMA: 2018,Jan,8; 2017,Jan,8; 2016,Mar,3; 2016,Jan,13; 2015,Nov,3; 2015,Jan,16

+ **61642 each additional vessel in different vascular territory (List separately in addition to code for primary procedure))**

INCLUDES Angiography after dilation vessel
Fluoroscopic guidance
Injection contrast material
Roadmapping
Selective catheterization target vessel
Vessel analysis

EXCLUDES *Endovascular intracranial prolonged administration pharmacologic agent performed same vascular territory (61650-61651)*

Code first (61640)

9.84 9.84 FUD ZZZ E

AMA: 2018,Jan,8; 2017,Jan,8; 2016,Mar,3; 2016,Jan,13; 2015,Nov,3; 2015,Jan,16

61645 Percutaneous arterial transluminal mechanical thrombectomy and/or infusion for thrombolysis, intracranial, any method, including diagnostic angiography, fluoroscopic guidance, catheter placement, and intraprocedural pharmacological thrombolytic injection(s)

INCLUDES Interventions performed in intracranial artery including:
Angiography with radiologic supervision and interpretation (diagnostic and subsequent)
Closure arteriotomy by any method
Fluoroscopy
Patient monitoring
Procedures performed in vascular territories:
Left carotid
Right carotid
Vertebro-basilar

EXCLUDES *Procedure performed same vascular target area:*
Balloon angioplasty, intracranial (61630)
Diagnostic studies: aortic arch, carotid, and vertebral arteries (36221-36226)
Endovascular intracranial prolonged administration pharmacologic agent (61650-61651)
Transcatheter placement intravascular stent (61635)
Transluminal thrombectomy (37184, 37186)
Reporting code more than one time for treatment each intracranial vascular territory
Venous thrombectomy or thrombolysis (37187-37188, 37212, 37214)

24.0 24.0 FUD 000 C 80 50

AMA: 2019,Sep,6; 2019,Sep,5; 2018,Jan,8; 2017,Jan,8; 2016,Mar,3; 2016,Jan,13; 2015,Dec,18; 2015,Nov,3

61650 **Endovascular intracranial prolonged administration of pharmacologic agent(s) other than for thrombolysis, arterial, including catheter placement, diagnostic angiography, and imaging guidance; initial vascular territory**

INCLUDES Interventions performed in intracranial artery, including:
- Angiography with radiologic supervision and interpretation (diagnostic and subsequent)
- Closure arteriotomy by any method
- Fluoroscopy
- Patient monitoring
- Procedures performed in vascular territories:
  - Left carotid
  - Right carotid
  - Vertebro-basilar

Prolonged (at least 10 minutes) arterial administration nonthrombolytic agents

EXCLUDES *Procedure performed same vascular target area:*
- *Balloon dilatation intracranial vasospasm (61640-61642)*
- *Chemotherapy administration (96420-96425)*
- *Diagnostic studies: aortic arch, carotid, and vertebral arteries (36221-36228)*
- *Transluminal thrombectomy (37184, 37186, 61645)*

Reporting code more than one time for treatment each intracranial vascular territory
Treatment iatrogenic condition
Venous thrombectomy or thrombolysis

15.6 15.6 **FUD** 000 C

AMA: 2019,Sep,6; 2018,Jan,8; 2017,Jan,8; 2016,Mar,3; 2016,Jan,13; 2015,Nov,3

\+ **61651** **each additional vascular territory (List separately in addition to code for primary procedure)**

INCLUDES Interventions performed in intracranial artery, including:
- Angiography with radiologic supervision and interpretation (diagnostic and subsequent)
- Closure arteriotomy by any method
- Fluoroscopy
- Patient monitoring
- Procedures performed in vascular territories:
  - Left carotid
  - Right carotid
  - Vertebro-basilar

Prolonged (at least 10 minutes) arterial administration nonthrombolytic agents

EXCLUDES *Procedure performed same vascular target area:*
- *Balloon dilatation intracranial vasospasm (61640-61642)*
- *Chemotherapy administration (96420-96425)*
- *Diagnostic studies: aortic arch, carotid, and vertebral arteries (36221-36228)*
- *Transluminal thrombectomy (37184, 37186, 61645)*

Reporting code more than one time for treatment each intracranial vascular territory
Treatment iatrogenic condition
Venous thrombectomy or thrombolysis

Code first (61650)

6.65 6.65 **FUD** ZZZ C

AMA: 2019,Sep,6; 2018,Jan,8; 2017,Jan,8; 2016,Mar,3; 2016,Jan,13; 2015,Nov,3

61680-61692 Surgical Treatment of Arteriovenous Malformation of the Brain

INCLUDES Craniotomy

61680 **Surgery of intracranial arteriovenous malformation; supratentorial, simple**

65.1 65.1 **FUD** 090 C 80

AMA: 2014,Jan,11

61682 **supratentorial, complex**

123. 123. **FUD** 090 C 80

AMA: 2018,Jan,8; 2017,Jan,8; 2016,Jan,13; 2015,Jan,16

61684 **infratentorial, simple**

84.0 84.0 **FUD** 090 C 80

AMA: 2014,Jan,11

61686 **infratentorial, complex**

134. 134. **FUD** 090 C 80

AMA: 2018,Jan,8; 2017,Jan,8; 2016,Jan,13; 2015,Jan,16

61690 **dural, simple**

63.0 63.0 **FUD** 090 C 80

AMA: 2014,Jan,11

61692 **dural, complex**

106. 106. **FUD** 090 C 80

AMA: 2018,Jan,8; 2017,Jan,8; 2016,Jan,13; 2015,Jan,16

61697-61703 Surgical Treatment Brain Aneurysm

INCLUDES Craniotomy

61697 **Surgery of complex intracranial aneurysm, intracranial approach; carotid circulation**

INCLUDES
- Aneurysms bigger than 15 mm
- Calcification aneurysm neck
- Inclusion normal vessels in aneurysm neck
- Surgery needing temporary vessel occlusion, trapping, or cardiopulmonary bypass to treat aneurysm

125. 125. **FUD** 090 C 80

AMA: 2018,Jan,8; 2017,Dec,13

61698 **vertebrobasilar circulation**

INCLUDES
- Aneurysm bigger than 15 mm
- Calcification aneurysm neck
- Inclusion normal vessels in aneurysm neck
- Surgery needing temporary vessel occlusion, trapping, or cardiopulmonary bypass to treat aneurysm

141. 141. **FUD** 090 C 80

AMA: 2014,Jan,11

61700 **Surgery of simple intracranial aneurysm, intracranial approach; carotid circulation**

100. 100. **FUD** 090 C 80

AMA: 2018,Jan,8; 2017,Dec,13; 2017,Jan,8; 2016,Jan,13; 2015,Jan,16

61702 **vertebrobasilar circulation**

117. 117. **FUD** 090 C 80

AMA: 2014,Jan,11

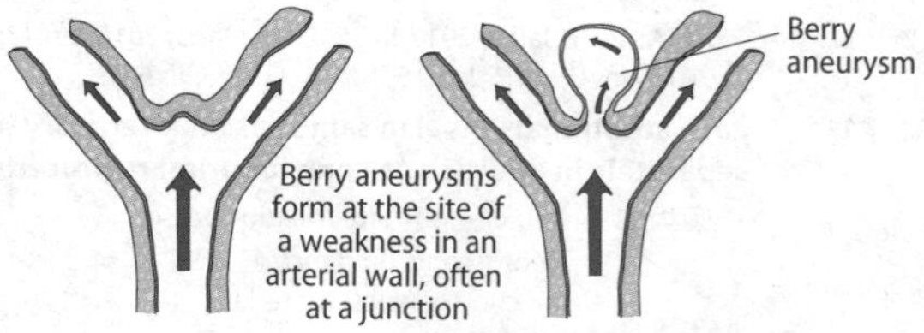

Common sites of berry aneurysms in the circle of Willis arteries

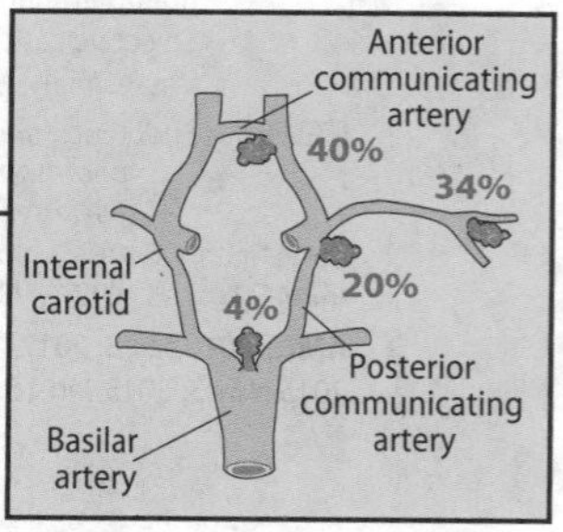

61703 **Surgery of intracranial aneurysm, cervical approach by application of occluding clamp to cervical carotid artery (Selverstone-Crutchfield type)**

EXCLUDES *Cervical approach for direct ligation carotid artery (37600-37606)*

39.0 39.0 **FUD** 090 C 80

AMA: 2014,Jan,11

61705-61710 Other Procedures for Aneurysm, Arteriovenous Malformation, and Carotid-Cavernous Fistula

INCLUDES Craniotomy

61705 **Surgery of aneurysm, vascular malformation or carotid-cavernous fistula; by intracranial and cervical occlusion of carotid artery**
73.6 73.6 **FUD** 090 C 80
AMA: 2014,Jan,11

61708 **by intracranial electrothrombosis**
EXCLUDES *Ligation or gradual occlusion internal or common carotid artery (37605-37606)*
75.1 75.1 **FUD** 090 C 80
AMA: 2014,Jan,11; 2000,Sep,11

61710 **by intra-arterial embolization, injection procedure, or balloon catheter**
63.3 63.3 **FUD** 090 C 80
AMA: 2018,Jan,8; 2017,Jan,8; 2016,Jan,13; 2015,Jan,16

61711 Extracranial-Intracranial Bypass

CMS: 100-02,16,10 Exclusions from Coverage; 100-03,20.2 Extracranial-intracranial (EC-IC) Arterial Bypass Surgery

INCLUDES Craniotomy
EXCLUDES *Carotid or vertebral thromboendarterectomy (35301)*
Code also operating microscope when appropriate (69990)

61711 **Anastomosis, arterial, extracranial-intracranial (eg, middle cerebral/cortical) arteries**
75.8 75.8 **FUD** 090 C 80
AMA: 2014,Jan,11

61720-61791 Stereotactic Procedures of the Brain

61720 **Creation of lesion by stereotactic method, including burr hole(s) and localizing and recording techniques, single or multiple stages; globus pallidus or thalamus**
37.3 37.3 **FUD** 090 J
AMA: 2018,Jan,8; 2017,Jan,8; 2016,Jan,13; 2015,Jan,16

61735 **subcortical structure(s) other than globus pallidus or thalamus**
46.8 46.8 **FUD** 090 C
AMA: 2014,Jul,8; 2014,Jan,11

61750 **Stereotactic biopsy, aspiration, or excision, including burr hole(s), for intracranial lesion;**
40.6 40.6 **FUD** 090 C
AMA: 2018,Jan,8; 2017,Jan,8; 2016,Jan,13; 2015,Jan,16

61751 **with computed tomography and/or magnetic resonance guidance**
(70450, 70460, 70470, 70551-70553)
39.7 39.7 **FUD** 090 C
AMA: 2018,Jan,8; 2017,Jan,8; 2016,Jan,13; 2015,Jan,16

61760 **Stereotactic implantation of depth electrodes into the cerebrum for long-term seizure monitoring**
46.0 46.0 **FUD** 090 C
AMA: 2014,Jul,8; 2014,Jan,11

61770 **Stereotactic localization, including burr hole(s), with insertion of catheter(s) or probe(s) for placement of radiation source**
46.8 46.8 **FUD** 090 J 62
AMA: 2018,Jan,8; 2017,Jan,8; 2016,Jan,13; 2015,Jan,16

\+ **61781** **Stereotactic computer-assisted (navigational) procedure; cranial, intradural (List separately in addition to code for primary procedure)**
EXCLUDES *Creation lesion by stereotactic method (61720-61791)*
Extradural stereotactic computer-assisted procedure for same surgical session by same individual (61782)
Radiation treatment delivery, stereotactic radiosurgery (SRS) (77371-77373)
Stereotactic implantation neurostimulator electrode array (61863-61868)
Stereotactic radiation treatment management (77432)
Stereotactic radiosurgery (61796-61799)
Ventriculocisternostomy (62201)
Code first primary procedure
6.94 6.94 **FUD** ZZZ N N1 80
AMA: 2018,Jan,8; 2017,Jan,8; 2016,Jan,13; 2015,Jan,16

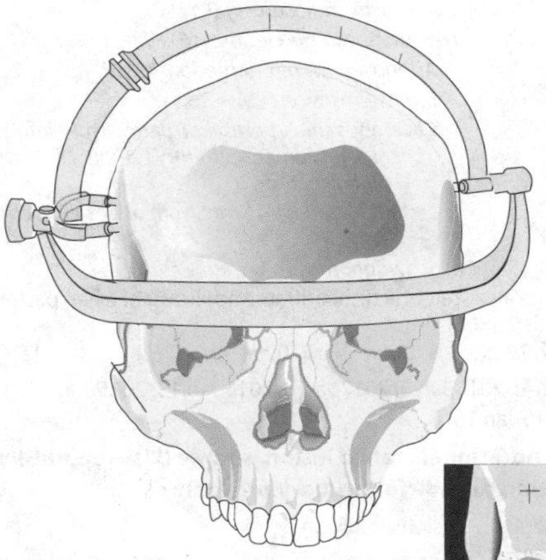
Stereotactic guide in place

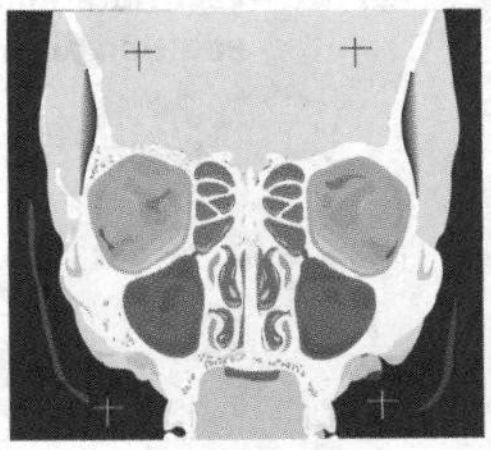
Computer assitance determines precise coordinates for a stereotactic intracranial procedure

CT or MRI scan

\+ **61782** **cranial, extradural (List separately in addition to code for primary procedure)**
EXCLUDES *Intradural stereotactic computer-assisted procedure for same surgical session by same individual (61781)*
Stereotactic radiosurgery (61796-61799)
Code first primary procedure
5.02 5.02 **FUD** ZZZ N N1 80
AMA: 2018,Apr,3; 2018,Jan,8; 2017,Jan,8; 2016,Jan,13; 2015,Jan,16

\+ **61783** **spinal (List separately in addition to code for primary procedure)**
EXCLUDES *Stereotactic radiosurgery (61796-61799, 63620-63621)*
Code first primary procedure
6.80 6.80 **FUD** ZZZ N N1 80
AMA: 2018,Jan,8; 2017,Jan,8; 2016,Jan,13; 2015,Jan,16

61790 **Creation of lesion by stereotactic method, percutaneous, by neurolytic agent (eg, alcohol, thermal, electrical, radiofrequency); gasserian ganglion**
25.7 25.7 **FUD** 090 J A2 50
AMA: 2014,Jul,8; 2014,Jan,11

61791 **trigeminal medullary tract**
32.4 32.4 **FUD** 090 J A2 80 50
AMA: 2018,Jan,8; 2017,Jan,8; 2016,Jan,13; 2015,Jan,16

61796-61800 Stereotactic Radiosurgery (SRS): Brain

INCLUDES Planning, dosimetry, targeting, positioning, or blocking performed by neurosurgeon

EXCLUDES *Application cranial tongs, caliper, or stereotactic frame (20660)*
Intensity modulated beam delivery plan and treatment (77301, 77385-77386)
Radiation treatment management and radiosurgery by same provider (77427-77435)
Stereotactic body radiation therapy (77373, 77435)
Stereotactic radiosurgery more than once per lesion per treatment course
Treatment planning, physics and dosimetry, and treatment delivery performed by radiation oncologist

61796 **Stereotactic radiosurgery (particle beam, gamma ray, or linear accelerator); 1 simple cranial lesion**

INCLUDES Lesions < 3.5 cm

EXCLUDES *Reporting code more than one time per treatment course*
Stereotactic computer-assisted procedures (61781-61783)
Stereotactic radiosurgery (61798)
Treatment complex lesions: (61798-61799)
Arteriovenous malformations (AVM)
Brainstem lesions
Cavernous sinus/parasellar/petroclival tumors, glomus tumors, pituitary tumors, and tumors pineal region
Lesions located <= 5 mm from optic nerve, chasm, or tract
Schwannomas

Code also stereotactic headframe application, when performed (61800)

Facility RVU 29.2 Non-Facility RVU 29.2 FUD 090 B 80

AMA: 2018,Jan,8; 2017,Jan,8; 2016,Jan,13; 2015,Jun,6; 2015,Jan,16

+ **61797** **each additional cranial lesion, simple (List separately in addition to code for primary procedure)**

INCLUDES Lesions < 3.5 cm

EXCLUDES *Reporting code for additional stereotactic radiosurgery more than four times in total per treatment course when used alone or in combination with (61799)*
Stereotactic computer-assisted procedures (61781-61783)
Treatment complex lesions: (61798-61799)
Arteriovenous malformations (AVM)
Brainstem lesion
Cavernous sinus/parasellar/petroclival tumors, glomus tumors, pituitary tumors, and tumors pineal region
Lesions located <= 5 mm from optic nerve, chasm, or tract
Schwannomas

Code first (61796, 61798)

Facility RVU 6.35 Non-Facility RVU 6.35 FUD ZZZ B 80

AMA: 2018,Jan,8; 2017,Jan,8; 2016,Jan,13; 2015,Jun,6; 2015,Jan,16

61798 **1 complex cranial lesion**

INCLUDES All therapeutic lesion creation procedures
Treatment complex lesions:
Arteriovenous malformations (AVM)
Brainstem lesions
Cavernous sinus, parasellar, petroclival, glomus, pineal region, and pituitary tumors
Lesions located <= 5 mm from optic nerve, chasm, or tract
Lesions >= 3.5 cm
Schwannomas
Treatment multiple lesions when at least one considered complex

EXCLUDES *Reporting code more than one time per treatment course*
Stereotactic computer-assisted procedures (61781-61783)
Stereotactic radiosurgery (61796)

Code also stereotactic headframe application, when performed (61800)

Facility RVU 40.5 Non-Facility RVU 40.5 FUD 090 B 80

AMA: 2018,Jan,8; 2017,Jan,8; 2016,Jan,13; 2015,Jun,6; 2015,Jan,16

+ **61799** **each additional cranial lesion, complex (List separately in addition to code for primary procedure)**

INCLUDES All therapeutic lesion creation procedures
Treatment complex lesions:
Arteriovenous malformations (AVM)
Brainstem lesions
Cavernous sinus, parasellar, petroclival, glomus, pineal region, and pituitary tumors
Lesions located <= 5 mm from optic nerve, chasm, or tract
Lesions >= 3.5 cm
Schwannomas

EXCLUDES *Reporting code for additional stereotactic radiosurgery more than four times in total per treatment course when used alone or in combination with (61797)*
Stereotactic computer-assisted procedures (61781-61783)

Code first (61798)

Facility RVU 8.98 Non-Facility RVU 8.98 FUD ZZZ B 80

AMA: 2018,Jan,8; 2017,Jan,8; 2016,Jan,13; 2015,Jun,6; 2015,Jan,16

+ **61800** **Application of stereotactic headframe for stereotactic radiosurgery (List separately in addition to code for primary procedure)**

Code first (61796, 61798)

Facility RVU 4.40 Non-Facility RVU 4.40 FUD ZZZ B 80

AMA: 2018,Jan,8; 2017,Jan,8; 2016,Jan,13; 2015,Jun,6; 2015,Jan,16

61850-61888 Intracranial Neurostimulation

INCLUDES Analysis system at implantation (95970)
Microelectrode recording by operating surgeon

EXCLUDES *Electronic analysis and reprogramming neurostimulator pulse generator (95970, 95976-95977, [95983, 95984])*
Neurophysiological mapping by another physician/qualified health care professional (95961-95962)

61850 **Twist drill or burr hole(s) for implantation of neurostimulator electrodes, cortical**

Facility RVU 28.1 Non-Facility RVU 28.1 FUD 090 C 80

AMA: 2019,Feb,6; 2018,Jan,8; 2017,Jan,8; 2016,Jan,13; 2015,Jan,16

61860 **Craniectomy or craniotomy for implantation of neurostimulator electrodes, cerebral, cortical**

Facility RVU 45.7 Non-Facility RVU 45.7 FUD 090 C 80

AMA: 2019,Feb,6; 2018,Jan,8; 2017,Jan,8; 2016,Jan,13; 2015,Jan,16

61863 **Twist drill, burr hole, craniotomy, or craniectomy with stereotactic implantation of neurostimulator electrode array in subcortical site (eg, thalamus, globus pallidus, subthalamic nucleus, periventricular, periaqueductal gray), without use of intraoperative microelectrode recording; first array**
43.3 43.3 FUD 090 C 80 50
AMA: 2019,Feb,6; 2018,Jan,8; 2017,Jan,8; 2016,Jan,13; 2015,Jan,16

+ 61864 **each additional array (List separately in addition to primary procedure)**
Code first (61863)
8.36 8.36 FUD ZZZ C 80
AMA: 2019,Feb,6

61867 **Twist drill, burr hole, craniotomy, or craniectomy with stereotactic implantation of neurostimulator electrode array in subcortical site (eg, thalamus, globus pallidus, subthalamic nucleus, periventricular, periaqueductal gray), with use of intraoperative microelectrode recording; first array**
65.9 65.9 FUD 090 C 80 50
AMA: 2019,Feb,6

+ 61868 **each additional array (List separately in addition to primary procedure)**
Code first (61867)
14.7 14.7 FUD ZZZ C 80
AMA: 2019,Feb,6; 2018,Jan,8; 2017,Jan,8; 2016,Jan,13; 2015,Jan,16

~~61870~~ ~~**Craniectomy for implantation of neurostimulator electrodes, cerebellar, cortical**~~

61880 **Revision or removal of intracranial neurostimulator electrodes**
16.6 16.6 FUD 090 02 G2 80 50
AMA: 2019,Feb,6

61885 **Insertion or replacement of cranial neurostimulator pulse generator or receiver, direct or inductive coupling; with connection to a single electrode array**
EXCLUDES *Percutaneous procedure to place cranial nerve neurostimulator electrode(s) (64553)*
Revision or replacement cranial nerve neurostimulator electrode array (64569)
14.9 14.9 FUD 090 J J8 80 50
AMA: 2019,Feb,6; 2018,Jan,8; 2017,Jan,8; 2016,Jan,13; 2015,Jan,16

61886 **with connection to 2 or more electrode arrays**
EXCLUDES *Percutaneous procedure to place cranial nerve neurostimulator electrode(s) (64553)*
Revision or replacement cranial nerve neurostimulator electrode array (64569)
24.7 24.7 FUD 090 J J8 80
AMA: 2019,Feb,6; 2018,Jan,8; 2017,Jan,8; 2016,Jan,13; 2015,Jan,16

61888 **Revision or removal of cranial neurostimulator pulse generator or receiver**
EXCLUDES *Insertion or replacement cranial neurostimulator pulse generator or receiver (61885-61886)*
11.5 11.5 FUD 010 J J8 50
AMA: 2019,Feb,6; 2018,Jan,8; 2017,Jan,8; 2016,Jan,13; 2015,Jan,16

62000-62148 Repair of Skull and/or Cerebrospinal Fluid Leaks

62000 **Elevation of depressed skull fracture; simple, extradural**
29.7 29.7 FUD 090 J
AMA: 2014,Jan,11

62005 **compound or comminuted, extradural**
36.6 36.6 FUD 090 C 80
AMA: 2014,Jan,11

62010 **with repair of dura and/or debridement of brain**
44.2 44.2 FUD 090 C 80
AMA: 2014,Jan,11

62100 **Craniotomy for repair of dural/cerebrospinal fluid leak, including surgery for rhinorrhea/otorrhea**
EXCLUDES *Repair spinal fluid leak (63707, 63709)*
46.4 46.4 FUD 090 C 80
AMA: 2014,Jan,11; 2002,May,7

62115 **Reduction of craniomegalic skull (eg, treated hydrocephalus); not requiring bone grafts or cranioplasty**
48.4 48.4 FUD 090 C 80
AMA: 2014,Jan,11

62117 **requiring craniotomy and reconstruction with or without bone graft (includes obtaining grafts)**
57.8 57.8 FUD 090 C 80
AMA: 2014,Jan,11

62120 **Repair of encephalocele, skull vault, including cranioplasty**
61.9 61.9 FUD 090 C 80
AMA: 2014,Jan,11

62121 **Craniotomy for repair of encephalocele, skull base**
45.7 45.7 FUD 090 C 80
AMA: 2014,Jan,11

62140 **Cranioplasty for skull defect; up to 5 cm diameter**
29.9 29.9 FUD 090 C 80
AMA: 2018,Jan,8; 2017,Jan,8; 2016,Jan,13; 2015,Jan,16

62141 **larger than 5 cm diameter**
33.1 33.1 FUD 090 C 80
AMA: 2018,Jan,8; 2017,Jan,8; 2016,Jan,13; 2015,Jan,16

62142 **Removal of bone flap or prosthetic plate of skull**
25.8 25.8 FUD 090 C 80
AMA: 2018,Jan,8; 2017,Jan,8; 2016,Jan,13; 2015,Jan,16

62143 **Replacement of bone flap or prosthetic plate of skull**
30.0 30.0 FUD 090 C 80
AMA: 2018,Jan,8; 2017,Jan,8; 2016,Jan,13; 2015,Jan,16

62145 **Cranioplasty for skull defect with reparative brain surgery**
41.0 41.0 FUD 090 C 80
AMA: 2018,Jan,8; 2017,Jan,8; 2016,Jan,13; 2015,Jan,16

62146 **Cranioplasty with autograft (includes obtaining bone grafts); up to 5 cm diameter**
34.2 34.2 FUD 090 C 80
AMA: 2018,Jan,8; 2017,Jan,8; 2016,Jan,13; 2015,Jan,16

62147 **larger than 5 cm diameter**
41.9 41.9 FUD 090 C 80
AMA: 2018,Jan,8; 2017,Jan,8; 2016,Jan,13; 2015,Jan,16

+ 62148 **Incision and retrieval of subcutaneous cranial bone graft for cranioplasty (List separately in addition to code for primary procedure)**
Code first (62140-62147)
3.73 3.73 FUD ZZZ C
AMA: 2014,Jan,11

62160-62165 Neuroendoscopic Brain Procedures

INCLUDES Diagnostic endoscopy

+ 62160 **Neuroendoscopy, intracranial, for placement or replacement of ventricular catheter and attachment to shunt system or external drainage (List separately in addition to code for primary procedure)**
Code first (61107, 61210, 62220-62230, 62258)
5.61 5.61 FUD ZZZ N N1
AMA: 2018,Jan,8; 2017,Jan,8; 2016,Jan,13; 2015,Jan,16

62161 **Neuroendoscopy, intracranial; with dissection of adhesions, fenestration of septum pellucidum or intraventricular cysts (including placement, replacement, or removal of ventricular catheter)**
44.1 44.1 FUD 090 C 80
AMA: 2014,Jan,11

62162 **with fenestration or excision of colloid cyst, including placement of external ventricular catheter for drainage**
55.3 55.3 FUD 090 C 80
AMA: 2014,Jan,11

Nervous System

61863 — 62162

~~62163 with retrieval of foreign body~~

62164 **with excision of brain tumor, including placement of external ventricular catheter for drainage**
61.0 61.0 FUD 090 C 80
AMA: 2014,Jan,11

62165 **with excision of pituitary tumor, transnasal or trans-sphenoidal approach**
44.6 44.6 FUD 090 C 80
AMA: 2019,Dec,12; 2018,Jan,8; 2017,Dec,14

62180-62258 Cerebrospinal Fluid Diversion Procedures

62180 **Ventriculocisternostomy (Torkildsen type operation)**
47.0 47.0 FUD 090 C 80
AMA: 2014,Jan,11

62190 **Creation of shunt; subarachnoid/subdural-atrial, -jugular, -auricular**
27.1 27.1 FUD 090 C
AMA: 2014,Jan,11; 2000,Dec,12

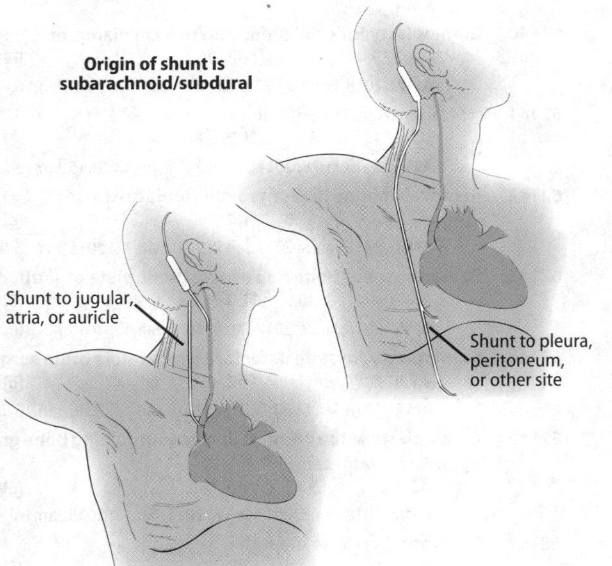

62192 **subarachnoid/subdural-peritoneal, -pleural, other terminus**
28.5 28.5 FUD 090 C 80
AMA: 2014,Jan,11

62194 **Replacement or irrigation, subarachnoid/subdural catheter**
14.1 14.1 FUD 010 J A2 80
AMA: 2018,Jan,8; 2017,Jan,8; 2016,Jan,13; 2015,Jan,16

62200 **Ventriculocisternostomy, third ventricle;**
INCLUDES Dandy ventriculocisternostomy
40.2 40.2 FUD 090 C 80
AMA: 2014,Jan,11

62201 **stereotactic, neuroendoscopic method**
EXCLUDES *Intracranial neuroendoscopic surgery (62161-62165)*
34.8 34.8 FUD 090 C
AMA: 2018,Jan,8; 2017,Jan,8; 2016,Jan,13; 2015,Jan,16

62220 **Creation of shunt; ventriculo-atrial, -jugular, -auricular**
Code also intracranial neuroendoscopic ventricular catheter insertion, when performed (62160)
29.2 29.2 FUD 090 C 80
AMA: 2014,Jan,11; 2007,Jun,10-11

62223 **ventriculo-peritoneal, -pleural, other terminus**
Code also intracranial neuroendoscopic ventricular catheter insertion, when performed (62160)
30.0 30.0 FUD 090 C 80
AMA: 2014,Jan,11; 2007,Jun,10-11

62225 **Replacement or irrigation, ventricular catheter**
Code also intracranial neuroendoscopic ventricular catheter insertion, when performed (62160)
15.3 15.3 FUD 090 J A2
AMA: 2018,Jan,8; 2017,Jan,8; 2016,Jan,13; 2015,Jan,16

62230 **Replacement or revision of cerebrospinal fluid shunt, obstructed valve, or distal catheter in shunt system**
Code also intracranial neuroendoscopic ventricular catheter insertion, when performed (62160)
Code also when proximal catheter and valve replaced (62225)
24.5 24.5 FUD 090 J A2 80
AMA: 2018,Jan,8; 2017,Jan,8; 2016,Jan,13; 2015,Jan,16

62252 **Reprogramming of programmable cerebrospinal shunt**
2.34 2.34 FUD XXX S P3 80
AMA: 2014,Jan,11; 2002,May,7

62256 **Removal of complete cerebrospinal fluid shunt system; without replacement**
EXCLUDES *Reprogramming cerebrospinal fluid (CSF) shunt (62252)*
17.3 17.3 FUD 090 C 80
AMA: 2014,Jan,11; 2002,May,7

62258 **with replacement by similar or other shunt at same operation**
EXCLUDES *Aspiration or irrigation shunt reservoir (61070)*
Reprogramming cerebrospinal fluid (CSF) shunt (62252)
Code also intracranial neuroendoscopic ventricular catheter insertion, when performed (62160)
32.5 32.5 FUD 090 C 80
AMA: 2018,Jan,8; 2017,Jan,8; 2016,Jan,13; 2015,Jan,16

62263-62264 Lysis of Epidural Lesions with Injection of Solution/Mechanical Methods

INCLUDES Epidurography (72275)
Fluoroscopic guidance (77003)
Percutaneous mechanical lysis

62263 **Percutaneous lysis of epidural adhesions using solution injection (eg, hypertonic saline, enzyme) or mechanical means (eg, catheter) including radiologic localization (includes contrast when administered), multiple adhesiolysis sessions; 2 or more days**
INCLUDES All adhesiolysis treatments, injections, and infusions during treatment course
Percutaneous epidural catheter insertion and removal for neurolytic agent injections during treatment sessions series
EXCLUDES *Procedure performed more than one time for complete series spanning two or more treatment days*
8.92 17.1 FUD 010 T A2
AMA: 2018,Jan,8; 2017,Jan,8; 2016,Jan,13; 2015,Jan,16

62264 **1 day**
INCLUDES Multiple treatment sessions performed same day
EXCLUDES *Percutaneous lysis epidural adhesions using solution injection,two or more treatment days (62263)*
6.89 12.2 FUD 010 T A2
AMA: 2018,Jan,8; 2017,Jan,8; 2016,Jan,13; 2015,Jan,16

62267-62269 Percutaneous Procedures of Spinal Cord

62267 **Percutaneous aspiration within the nucleus pulposus, intervertebral disc, or paravertebral tissue for diagnostic purposes**

EXCLUDES *Bone biopsy (20225)*
Decompression intervertebral disc (62287)
Fine needle aspiration ([10005, 10006, 10007, 10008, 10009, 10010, 10011, 10012]
Injection for discography (62290-62291)

Code also fluoroscopic guidance (77003)
4.54 7.60 FUD 000 T G2 80

AMA: 2019,Apr,4; 2018,Jan,8; 2017,Feb,12; 2017,Jan,8; 2016,Jan,13; 2015,Jan,16

62268 **Percutaneous aspiration, spinal cord cyst or syrinx**

(76942, 77002, 77012)
7.40 7.40 FUD 000 T A2

AMA: 2018,Jan,8; 2017,Dec,13

62269 **Biopsy of spinal cord, percutaneous needle**

EXCLUDES *Fine needle aspiration [(10005, 1006, 1007, 1008, 1009, 10010, 10011, 10012)]*

(76942, 77002, 77012)
(88172-88173)
7.66 7.66 FUD 000 J A2 80

AMA: 2019,Apr,4

62270-62329 [62328, 62329] Spinal Puncture, Subarachnoid Space, Diagnostic/Therapeutic

62270 **Spinal puncture, lumbar, diagnostic;**

EXCLUDES *Radiological guidance (77003, 77012)*

Code also ultrasound or MRI guidance (76942, 77021)
2.23 4.22 FUD 000 T A2

AMA: 2020,Jun,10; 2018,Jan,8; 2017,Jan,8; 2016,Jan,13; 2015,Jan,16

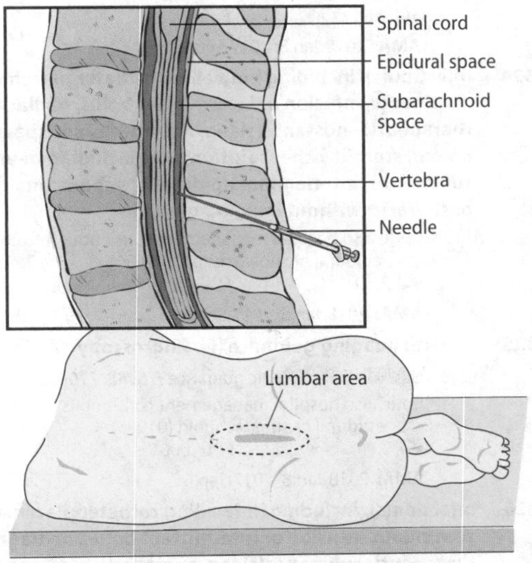

Common position to access vertebral interspace

\# **62328** **with fluoroscopic or CT guidance**

INCLUDES Radiological guidance (77003, 77012)

Code also ultrasound or MRI guidance (76942, 77021)
2.59 7.40 FUD 000 G2

AMA: 2020,Jun,10

62272 **Spinal puncture, therapeutic, for drainage of cerebrospinal fluid (by needle or catheter);**

EXCLUDES *Radiological guidance (77003, 77012)*

Code also ultrasound or MRI guidance (76942, 77021)
2.41 5.57 FUD 000 T A2

AMA: 2020,Jun,10; 2018,Jan,8; 2017,Jan,8; 2016,Jan,13; 2015,Jan,16

\# **62329** **with fluoroscopic or CT guidance**

INCLUDES Radiological guidance (77003, 77012)

Code also ultrasound or MRI guidance (76942, 77021)
3.26 9.19 FUD 000 G2

AMA: 2020,Jul,15; 2020,Jun,10

62273 Epidural Blood Patch

CMS: 100-03,10.5 NCD for Autogenous Epidural Blood Graft (10.5)

EXCLUDES *Injection diagnostic or therapeutic material (62320-62327)*

Code also fluoroscopic guidance (77003)

62273 **Injection, epidural, of blood or clot patch**

3.26 4.93 FUD 000 T A2

AMA: 2018,Jan,8; 2017,Jan,8; 2016,Jan,13; 2015,Jan,16

62280-62282 Neurolysis

INCLUDES Contrast injection during fluoroscopic guidance/localization

EXCLUDES *Injection diagnostic or therapeutic material only (62320-62327)*

Code also fluoroscopic guidance and localization unless formal contrast study performed (77003)

62280 **Injection/infusion of neurolytic substance (eg, alcohol, phenol, iced saline solutions), with or without other therapeutic substance; subarachnoid**

4.76 9.45 FUD 010 T A2

AMA: 2018,Jan,8; 2017,Jan,8; 2016,Jan,13; 2015,Jan,16

62281 **epidural, cervical or thoracic**

4.58 6.94 FUD 010 T A2

AMA: 2018,Jan,8; 2017,Jan,8; 2016,Jan,13; 2015,Jan,16

62282 **epidural, lumbar, sacral (caudal)**

4.16 8.63 FUD 010 T A2

AMA: 2018,Jan,8; 2017,Jan,8; 2016,Jan,13; 2015,Jan,16

62284-62294 Injection/Aspiration of Spine, Diagnostic/Therapeutic

62284 **Injection procedure for myelography and/or computed tomography, lumbar**

EXCLUDES *Injection C1-C2 (61055)*
Myelography (62302-62305, 72240, 72255, 72265, 72270)

Code also fluoroscopic guidance (77003)
2.54 5.61 FUD 000 N N1

AMA: 2018,Jan,8; 2017,Jan,8; 2016,Jan,13; 2015,Jan,16

62287 **Decompression procedure, percutaneous, of nucleus pulposus of intervertebral disc, any method utilizing needle based technique to remove disc material under fluoroscopic imaging or other form of indirect visualization, with discography and/or epidural injection(s) at the treated level(s), when performed, single or multiple levels, lumbar**

INCLUDES Endoscopic approach

EXCLUDES *Injection for discography (62290)*
Injection diagnostic or therapeutic substance(s) (62322)
Lumbar discography (72295)
Percutaneous aspiration, diagnostic (62267)
Percutaneous decompression nucleus pulposus intervertebral disc, non-needle based technique (0274T-0275T)
Radiological guidance (77003, 77012)

16.7 16.7 FUD 090 J A2

AMA: 2019,Dec,12; 2018,Jan,8; 2017,Feb,12; 2017,Jan,8; 2016,Jan,13; 2015,Mar,9; 2015,Jan,16

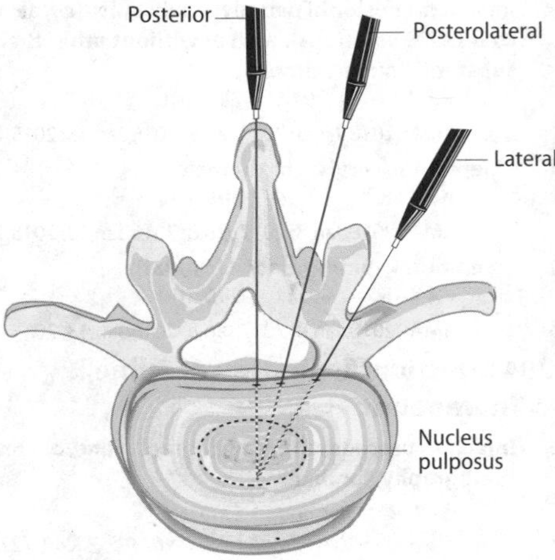

62290 **Injection procedure for discography, each level; lumbar**

(72295)

4.81 9.62 FUD 000 N N1

AMA: 2018,Jan,8; 2017,Feb,12; 2017,Jan,8; 2016,Jan,13; 2015,Jan,16

62291 **cervical or thoracic**

(72285)

4.65 9.28 FUD 000 N N1

AMA: 2018,Jan,8; 2017,Jan,8; 2016,Jan,13; 2015,Jan,16

62292 **Injection procedure for chemonucleolysis, including discography, intervertebral disc, single or multiple levels, lumbar**

16.4 16.4 FUD 090 J R2 80

AMA: 2018,Jan,8; 2017,Jan,8; 2016,Jan,13; 2015,Jan,16

62294 **Injection procedure, arterial, for occlusion of arteriovenous malformation, spinal**

27.8 27.8 FUD 090 T A2

AMA: 2014,Jan,11; 2000,Jan,1

62302-62305 Myelography

EXCLUDES *Injection C1-C2 (61055)*
Lumbar myelogram furnished by other providers (62284, 72240, 72255, 72265, 72270)

62302 **Myelography via lumbar injection, including radiological supervision and interpretation; cervical**

EXCLUDES *Myelography (62303-62305)*

3.51 7.13 FUD 000 Q2 N1

62303 **thoracic**

EXCLUDES *Myelography (62302, 62304-62305)*

3.51 7.29 FUD 000 Q2 N1

62304 **lumbosacral**

EXCLUDES *Myelography (62302-62303, 62305)*

3.45 7.04 FUD 000 Q2 N1

62305 **2 or more regions (eg, lumbar/thoracic, cervical/thoracic, lumbar/cervical, lumbar/thoracic/cervical)**

EXCLUDES *Myelography (62302-62305)*

3.60 7.65 FUD 000 Q2 N1

62320-62329 [62328, 62329] Injection/Infusion Diagnostic/Therapeutic Material

EXCLUDES *Epidurography (72275)*
Reporting code more than one time even when catheter tip or injected drug travels into different spinal area
Transforaminal epidural injection (64479-64484)

62320 **Injection(s), of diagnostic or therapeutic substance(s) (eg, anesthetic, antispasmodic, opioid, steroid, other solution), not including neurolytic substances, including needle or catheter placement, interlaminar epidural or subarachnoid, cervical or thoracic; without imaging guidance**

2.87 4.73 FUD 000 T G2

AMA: 2018,Jan,8; 2017,Sep,6

62321 **with imaging guidance (ie, fluoroscopy or CT)**

INCLUDES Radiologic guidance (76942, 77003, 77012)

3.08 7.05 FUD 000 T G2

AMA: 2018,Jan,8; 2017,Sep,6

62322 **Injection(s), of diagnostic or therapeutic substance(s) (eg, anesthetic, antispasmodic, opioid, steroid, other solution), not including neurolytic substances, including needle or catheter placement, interlaminar epidural or subarachnoid, lumbar or sacral (caudal); without imaging guidance**

2.49 4.44 FUD 000 T G2

AMA: 2018,Jan,8; 2017,Sep,6; 2017,Feb,12

62323 **with imaging guidance (ie, fluoroscopy or CT)**

INCLUDES Radiologic guidance (76942, 77003, 77012)

2.84 7.11 FUD 000 T G2

AMA: 2018,Jan,8; 2017,Sep,6

62324 **Injection(s), including indwelling catheter placement, continuous infusion or intermittent bolus, of diagnostic or therapeutic substance(s) (eg, anesthetic, antispasmodic, opioid, steroid, other solution), not including neurolytic substances, interlaminar epidural or subarachnoid, cervical or thoracic; without imaging guidance**

Code also hospital management continuous infusion drug, epidural or subarachnoid (01996)

2.60 4.14 FUD 000 T G2

AMA: 2018,Jan,8; 2017,Sep,6

62325 **with imaging guidance (ie, fluoroscopy or CT)**

INCLUDES Radiologic guidance (76942, 77003, 77012)

Code also hospital management continuous infusion drug, epidural or subarachnoid (01996)

3.00 6.27 FUD 000 T G2

AMA: 2018,Jan,8; 2017,Sep,6

62326 **Injection(s), including indwelling catheter placement, continuous infusion or intermittent bolus, of diagnostic or therapeutic substance(s) (eg, anesthetic, antispasmodic, opioid, steroid, other solution), not including neurolytic substances, interlaminar epidural or subarachnoid, lumbar or sacral (caudal); without imaging guidance**

Code also hospital management continuous infusion drug, epidural or subarachnoid (01996)

2.58 4.36 FUD 000 T G2

AMA: 2018,Jan,8; 2017,Sep,6

62327 **with imaging guidance (ie, fluoroscopy or CT)**

INCLUDES Radiologic guidance (76942, 77003, 77012)

Code also hospital management continuous infusion drug, epidural or subarachnoid (01996)

2.78 6.69 FUD 000 T G2

AMA: 2018,Jan,8; 2017,Sep,6

62328 **Resequenced code. See code following 62270.**

62329 **Resequenced code. See code following 62272.**

62350-62370 Procedures Related to Epidural and Intrathecal Catheters

EXCLUDES *Epidural blood patch (62273)*
Injection epidural/subarachnoid diagnostic/therapeutic drugs ([62328], [62329], 62320-62327)
Injection for lumbar computed tomography/myelography (62284)
Injection/infusion neurolytic substances (62280-62282)
Spinal puncture (62270-62272)

62350 Implantation, revision or repositioning of tunneled intrathecal or epidural catheter, for long-term medication administration via an external pump or implantable reservoir/infusion pump; without laminectomy

EXCLUDES *Maintenance and refilling infusion pumps for CNS drug therapy (95990-95991)*

11.5 11.5 FUD 010 J J8

AMA: 2018,Jan,8; 2017,Jan,8; 2016,Jan,13; 2015,Jan,16

62351 with laminectomy

EXCLUDES *Maintenance and refilling infusion pumps for CNS drug therapy (95990-95991)*

24.8 24.8 FUD 090 J 80

AMA: 2018,Jan,8; 2017,Jan,8; 2016,Jan,13; 2015,Jan,16

62355 Removal of previously implanted intrathecal or epidural catheter

7.73 7.73 FUD 010 Q2 A2 80

AMA: 2014,Jan,11; 1995,Win,1

62360 Implantation or replacement of device for intrathecal or epidural drug infusion; subcutaneous reservoir

9.13 9.13 FUD 010 J J8 80

AMA: 2014,Jan,11; 1995,Win,1

62361 nonprogrammable pump

12.4 12.4 FUD 010 J J8 80

AMA: 2014,Jan,11; 1995,Win,1

62362 programmable pump, including preparation of pump, with or without programming

11.0 11.0 FUD 010 J J8 80

AMA: 2018,Jan,8; 2017,Jan,8; 2016,Jan,13; 2015,Jan,16

62365 Removal of subcutaneous reservoir or pump, previously implanted for intrathecal or epidural infusion

8.52 8.52 FUD 010 Q2 A2 80

AMA: 2014,Jan,11; 1995,Win,1

62367 Electronic analysis of programmable, implanted pump for intrathecal or epidural drug infusion (includes evaluation of reservoir status, alarm status, drug prescription status); without reprogramming or refill

EXCLUDES *Maintenance and refilling infusion pumps for CNS drug therapy (95990-95991)*

0.72 1.14 FUD XXX S P3

AMA: 2018,Jan,8; 2017,Jan,8; 2016,Jan,13; 2015,Jan,16

62368 with reprogramming

EXCLUDES *Maintenance and refilling infusion pumps for CNS drug therapy (95990-95991)*

1.01 1.57 FUD XXX S P3

AMA: 2018,Jan,8; 2017,Jan,8; 2016,Jan,13; 2015,Jan,16

62369 with reprogramming and refill

EXCLUDES *Maintenance and refilling infusion pumps for CNS drug therapy (95990-95991)*

1.01 3.34 FUD XXX S P3

AMA: 2018,Jan,8; 2017,Jan,8; 2016,Jan,13; 2015,Jan,16

62370 with reprogramming and refill (requiring skill of a physician or other qualified health care professional)

EXCLUDES *Maintenance and refilling infusion pumps for CNS drug therapy (95990-95991)*

1.33 3.47 FUD XXX S P3

AMA: 2018,Jan,8; 2017,Jan,8; 2016,Jan,13; 2015,Jan,16

62380 Endoscopic Decompression/Laminectomy/Laminotomy

EXCLUDES *Open decompression (63030, 63056)*
Percutaneous decompression (62267, 0274T-0275T)

62380 Endoscopic decompression of spinal cord, nerve root(s), including laminotomy, partial facetectomy, foraminotomy, discectomy and/or excision of herniated intervertebral disc, 1 interspace, lumbar

0.00 0.00 FUD 090 J G2 80 50

AMA: 2018,Jan,8; 2017,Feb,12

63001-63048 Posterior Midline Approach: Laminectomy/Laminotomy/Decompression

INCLUDES Endoscopic assistance through open and direct visualization
EXCLUDES *Arthrodesis (22590-22614)*
Percutaneous decompression (62287, 0274T, 0275T)

63001 Laminectomy with exploration and/or decompression of spinal cord and/or cauda equina, without facetectomy, foraminotomy or discectomy (eg, spinal stenosis), 1 or 2 vertebral segments; cervical

36.0 36.0 FUD 090 J G2 80

AMA: 2018,Jan,8; 2017,Mar,7; 2017,Jan,8; 2016,Jan,13; 2015,Jan,16

63003 thoracic

36.0 36.0 FUD 090 J G2 80

AMA: 2018,Jan,8; 2017,Mar,7; 2017,Jan,8; 2016,Jan,13; 2015,Jan,16

63005 lumbar, except for spondylolisthesis

34.4 34.4 FUD 090 J G2 80

AMA: 2018,Jan,8; 2017,Mar,7; 2017,Feb,9; 2017,Jan,8; 2016,Jan,13; 2015,Jan,16

63011 sacral

31.6 31.6 FUD 090 J 80

AMA: 2018,Jan,8; 2017,Mar,7; 2017,Jan,8; 2016,Jan,13; 2015,Jan,16

63012 Laminectomy with removal of abnormal facets and/or pars inter-articularis with decompression of cauda equina and nerve roots for spondylolisthesis, lumbar (Gill type procedure)

34.6 34.6 FUD 090 J 80

AMA: 2019,Dec,12; 2018,Jan,8; 2017,Mar,7; 2017,Feb,9; 2017,Jan,8; 2016,Jan,13; 2015,Jan,16

63015 Laminectomy with exploration and/or decompression of spinal cord and/or cauda equina, without facetectomy, foraminotomy or discectomy (eg, spinal stenosis), more than 2 vertebral segments; cervical

43.2 43.2 FUD 090 J 80

AMA: 2018,Jan,8; 2017,Mar,7; 2017,Jan,8; 2016,Jan,13; 2015,Jan,16

63016 thoracic

44.0 44.0 FUD 090 J 80

AMA: 2018,Jan,8; 2017,Mar,7; 2017,Jan,8; 2016,Jan,13; 2015,Jan,16

63017 **lumbar**
36.7 36.7 **FUD** 090 J 80
AMA: 2018,Jan,8; 2017,Mar,7; 2017,Feb,9; 2017,Jan,8; 2016,Jan,13; 2015,Jan,16

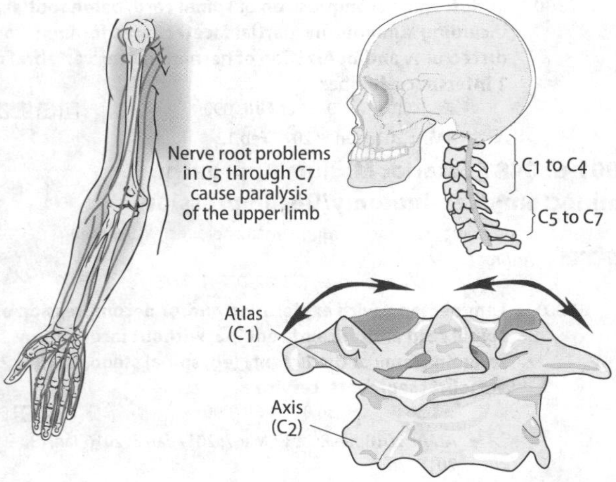

Nerve root problems in C5 through C7 cause paralysis of the upper limb
C1 to C4
C5 to C7
Atlas (C1)
Axis (C2)

The specialized atlas allows for rotary motion, which turns the head

63020 **Laminotomy (hemilaminectomy), with decompression of nerve root(s), including partial facetectomy, foraminotomy and/or excision of herniated intervertebral disc; 1 interspace, cervical**
33.6 33.6 **FUD** 090 J G2 80 50
AMA: 2018,Jan,8; 2017,Mar,7; 2017,Jan,8; 2016,Jan,13; 2015,Jan,16

63030 **1 interspace, lumbar**
28.2 28.2 **FUD** 090 J G2 80 50
AMA: 2020,May,13; 2019,Nov,14; 2018,Jan,8; 2017,Mar,7; 2017,Feb,12; 2017,Feb,9; 2017,Jan,8; 2016,May,13; 2016,Jan,13; 2015,Jan,16

\+ 63035 **each additional interspace, cervical or lumbar (List separately in addition to code for primary procedure)**
EXCLUDES *Reporting with modifier 50. Report once for each side when performed bilaterally*
Code first (63020-63030)
5.58 5.58 **FUD** ZZZ N 80 50
AMA: 2018,Jan,8; 2017,Feb,9; 2017,Jan,8; 2016,Jan,13; 2015,Jan,16

63040 **Laminotomy (hemilaminectomy), with decompression of nerve root(s), including partial facetectomy, foraminotomy and/or excision of herniated intervertebral disc, reexploration, single interspace; cervical**
40.4 40.4 **FUD** 090 J 80 50
AMA: 2020,May,13; 2018,Jan,8; 2017,Mar,7; 2017,Jan,8; 2016,Jan,13; 2015,Jan,16

63042 **lumbar**
37.5 37.5 **FUD** 090 J G2 80 50
AMA: 2020,May,13; 2018,Jan,8; 2017,Mar,7; 2017,Feb,9; 2017,Jan,8; 2016,Jan,13; 2015,Jan,16

\+ 63043 **each additional cervical interspace (List separately in addition to code for primary procedure)**
EXCLUDES *Reporting with modifier 50. Report once for each side when performed bilaterally*
Code first (63040)
0.00 0.00 **FUD** ZZZ N 80 50
AMA: 2020,May,13; 2018,Jan,8; 2017,Jan,8; 2016,Jan,13; 2015,Jan,16

\+ 63044 **each additional lumbar interspace (List separately in addition to code for primary procedure)**
EXCLUDES *Reporting with modifier 50. Report once for each side when performed bilaterally*
Code first (63042)
0.00 0.00 **FUD** ZZZ N N1 80 50
AMA: 2020,May,13; 2018,Jan,8; 2017,Feb,9; 2017,Jan,8; 2016,Jan,13; 2015,Jan,16

63045 **Laminectomy, facetectomy and foraminotomy (unilateral or bilateral with decompression of spinal cord, cauda equina and/or nerve root[s], [eg, spinal or lateral recess stenosis]), single vertebral segment; cervical**
37.1 37.1 **FUD** 090 J G2 80
AMA: 2018,Jan,8; 2017,Mar,7; 2017,Jan,8; 2016,Jan,13; 2015,Jan,16

63046 **thoracic**
35.4 35.4 **FUD** 090 J G2 80
AMA: 2018,Jan,8; 2017,Mar,7; 2017,Jan,8; 2016,Jan,13; 2015,Jan,16

63047 **lumbar**
31.9 31.9 **FUD** 090 J G2 80
AMA: 2020,May,13; 2019,Dec,12; 2018,May,10; 2018,May,9; 2018,Jan,8; 2017,Mar,7; 2017,Feb,9; 2017,Feb,12; 2017,Jan,8; 2016,Oct,11; 2016,Jan,13; 2015,Jan,16

\+ 63048 **each additional segment, cervical, thoracic, or lumbar (List separately in addition to code for primary procedure)**
Code first (63045-63047)
6.13 6.13 **FUD** ZZZ N 80
AMA: 2018,Jan,8; 2017,Feb,9; 2017,Jan,8; 2016,Jan,13; 2015,Jan,16

63050-63051 Cervical Laminoplasty: Posterior Midline Approach

EXCLUDES *Procedure performed on same vertebral segment(s) (22600, 22614, 22840-22842, 63001, 63015, 63045, 63048, 63295)*

63050 **Laminoplasty, cervical, with decompression of the spinal cord, 2 or more vertebral segments;**
43.5 43.5 **FUD** 090 C 80
AMA: 2018,Jan,8; 2017,Mar,7; 2017,Jan,8; 2016,Jan,13; 2015,Jan,16

63051 **with reconstruction of the posterior bony elements (including the application of bridging bone graft and non-segmental fixation devices [eg, wire, suture, mini-plates], when performed)**
49.3 49.3 **FUD** 090 C 80
AMA: 2018,Jan,8; 2017,Mar,7; 2017,Jan,8; 2016,Jan,13; 2015,Jan,16

63055-63066 Spinal Cord/Nerve Root Decompression: Costovertebral or Transpedicular Approach

63055 **Transpedicular approach with decompression of spinal cord, equina and/or nerve root(s) (eg, herniated intervertebral disc), single segment; thoracic**
47.0 47.0 **FUD** 090 J G2 80
AMA: 2018,Jan,8; 2017,Mar,7; 2017,Jan,8; 2016,Jan,13; 2015,Jan,16

63056 **lumbar (including transfacet, or lateral extraforaminal approach) (eg, far lateral herniated intervertebral disc)**
43.2 43.2 **FUD** 090 J G2 80
AMA: 2019,Nov,14; 2018,Jan,8; 2017,Mar,7; 2017,Feb,12; 2017,Jan,8; 2016,Jan,13; 2015,Jan,16

\+ 63057 **each additional segment, thoracic or lumbar (List separately in addition to code for primary procedure)**
Code first (63055-63056)
9.28 9.28 **FUD** ZZZ N 80
AMA: 2018,Jan,8; 2017,Jan,8; 2016,Jan,13; 2015,Jan,16

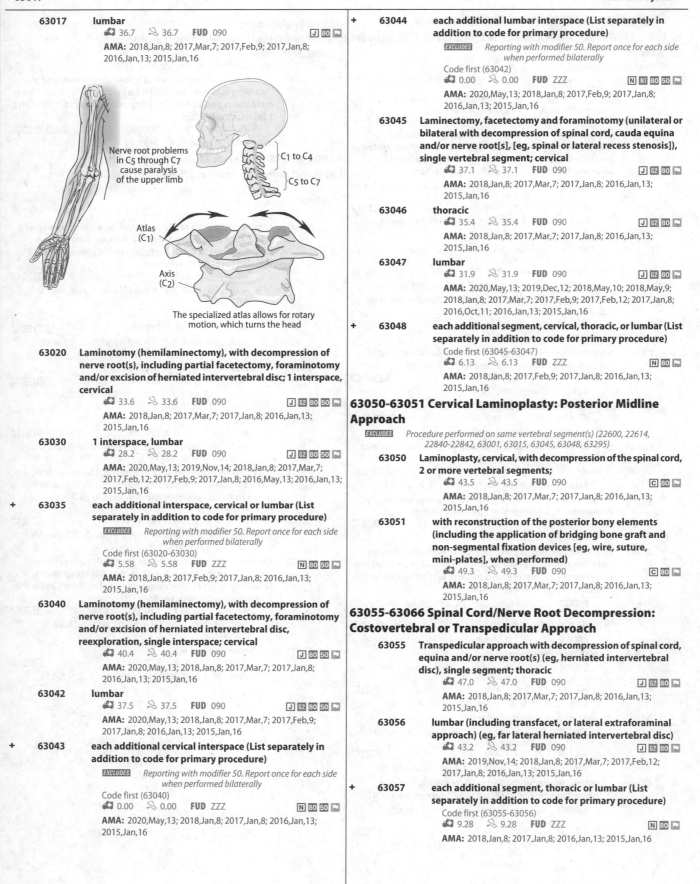

63064 Costovertebral approach with decompression of spinal cord or nerve root(s) (eg, herniated intervertebral disc), thoracic; single segment

> EXCLUDES Laminectomy with intraspinal thoracic lesion removal (63266, 63271, 63276, 63281, 63286)

51.5   51.5   **FUD** 090   J 80 ▢

AMA: 2018,Jan,8; 2017,Mar,7; 2017,Jan,8; 2016,Jan,13; 2015,Jan,16

+ 63066 each additional segment (List separately in addition to code for primary procedure)

> EXCLUDES Laminectomy with intraspinal thoracic lesion removal (63266, 63271, 63276, 63281, 63286)

Code first (63064)

5.97   5.97   **FUD** ZZZ   N 80 ▢

AMA: 2014,Jan,11; 1996,Feb,6

63075-63078 Discectomy: Anterior or Anterolateral Approach

> INCLUDES Operating microscope (69990)

63075 Discectomy, anterior, with decompression of spinal cord and/or nerve root(s), including osteophytectomy; cervical, single interspace

> EXCLUDES Anterior cervical discectomy and anterior interbody fusion at same level during same operative session (22551)
> Anterior interbody arthrodesis (even by another provider) (22554)

39.1   39.1   **FUD** 090   J 80 ▢

AMA: 2018,Jan,8; 2017,Mar,7; 2017,Jan,8; 2016,Feb,12; 2016,Jan,13; 2015,Apr,7; 2015,Jan,16

+ 63076 cervical, each additional interspace (List separately in addition to code for primary procedure)

> EXCLUDES Anterior cervical discectomy and anterior interbody fusion at same level during same operative session (22552)
> Anterior interbody arthrodesis (even by another provider) (22554)

Code first (63075)

7.20   7.20   **FUD** ZZZ   N 80 ▢

AMA: 2018,Jan,8; 2017,Jan,8; 2016,Feb,12; 2016,Jan,13; 2015,Jan,16

63077 thoracic, single interspace

43.6   43.6   **FUD** 090   C 80 ▢

AMA: 2018,Jan,8; 2017,Mar,7; 2017,Jan,8; 2016,Feb,12; 2016,Jan,13; 2015,Jan,16

+ 63078 thoracic, each additional interspace (List separately in addition to code for primary procedure)

Code first (63077)

6.01   6.01   **FUD** ZZZ   C 80 ▢

AMA: 2018,Jan,8; 2017,Jan,8; 2016,Feb,12; 2016,Jan,13; 2015,Jan,16

63081-63091 Vertebral Corpectomy, All Levels, Anterior Approach

> INCLUDES Disc removal level below and/or above vertebral segment
> Partial removal:
>   Cervical: Removal ≥ 1/2 vertebral body
>   Lumbar: Removal ≥ 1/3 vertebral body
>   Thoracic: Removal ≥ 1/3 vertebral body
> EXCLUDES Arthrodesis (22548-22812)

Code also reconstruction (20930-20938, 22548-22812, 22840-22855 [22859])

63081 Vertebral corpectomy (vertebral body resection), partial or complete, anterior approach with decompression of spinal cord and/or nerve root(s); cervical, single segment

> EXCLUDES Transoral approach (61575-61576)

50.9   50.9   **FUD** 090   C 80 ▢

AMA: 2018,Jan,8; 2017,Mar,7; 2017,Jan,8; 2016,Apr,8; 2016,Jan,13; 2015,Jun,10; 2015,Jan,16

+ 63082 cervical, each additional segment (List separately in addition to code for primary procedure)

> EXCLUDES Transoral approach (61575-61576)

Code first (63081)

7.72   7.72   **FUD** ZZZ   C 80 ▢

AMA: 2018,Jan,8; 2017,Jan,8; 2016,Apr,8; 2016,Jan,13; 2015,Jan,16

63085 Vertebral corpectomy (vertebral body resection), partial or complete, transthoracic approach with decompression of spinal cord and/or nerve root(s); thoracic, single segment

55.7   55.7   **FUD** 090   C 80 ▢

AMA: 2018,Jan,8; 2017,Mar,7; 2017,Jan,8; 2016,Apr,8; 2016,Jan,13; 2015,Jan,16

+ 63086 thoracic, each additional segment (List separately in addition to code for primary procedure)

Code first (63085)

5.53   5.53   **FUD** ZZZ   C 80 ▢

AMA: 2018,Jan,8; 2017,Jan,8; 2016,Apr,8; 2016,Jan,13; 2015,Jan,16

63087 Vertebral corpectomy (vertebral body resection), partial or complete, combined thoracolumbar approach with decompression of spinal cord, cauda equina or nerve root(s), lower thoracic or lumbar; single segment

69.8   69.8   **FUD** 090   C 80 ▢

AMA: 2018,Jan,8; 2017,Mar,7; 2017,Jan,8; 2016,Apr,8; 2016,Jan,13; 2015,Jan,16

+ 63088 each additional segment (List separately in addition to code for primary procedure)

Code first (63087)

7.43   7.43   **FUD** ZZZ   C 80 ▢

AMA: 2018,Jan,8; 2017,Jan,8; 2016,Apr,8; 2016,Jan,13; 2015,Jan,16

63090 Vertebral corpectomy (vertebral body resection), partial or complete, transperitoneal or retroperitoneal approach with decompression of spinal cord, cauda equina or nerve root(s), lower thoracic, lumbar, or sacral; single segment

56.8   56.8   **FUD** 090   C 80 ▢

AMA: 2018,Jan,8; 2017,Mar,7; 2017,Jan,8; 2016,Apr,8; 2016,Jan,13; 2015,Jan,16

+ 63091 each additional segment (List separately in addition to code for primary procedure)

Code first (63090)

5.18   5.18   **FUD** ZZZ   C 80 ▢

AMA: 2018,Jan,8; 2017,Jan,8; 2016,Apr,8; 2016,Jan,13; 2015,Jan,16

63101-63103 Corpectomy: Lateral Extracavitary Approach

> INCLUDES Partial removal:
>   Cervical: Removal ≥ 1/2 vertebral body
>   Lumbar: Removal ≥ 1/3 vertebral body
>   Thoracic: Removal ≥ 1/3 vertebral body

63101 Vertebral corpectomy (vertebral body resection), partial or complete, lateral extracavitary approach with decompression of spinal cord and/or nerve root(s) (eg, for tumor or retropulsed bone fragments); thoracic, single segment

67.2   67.2   **FUD** 090   C 80 ▢

AMA: 2018,Jan,8; 2017,Mar,7; 2017,Jan,8; 2016,Jan,13; 2015,Jan,16

63102 lumbar, single segment

65.5   65.5   **FUD** 090   C 80 ▢

AMA: 2018,Jan,8; 2017,Mar,7; 2017,Jan,8; 2016,Jan,13; 2015,Jan,16

+ 63103 thoracic or lumbar, each additional segment (List separately in addition to code for primary procedure)

Code first (63101-63102)

8.53   8.53   **FUD** ZZZ   C 80 ▢

AMA: 2014,Jan,11

● New Code   ▲ Revised Code   ○ Reinstated   ● New Web Release   ▲ Revised Web Release   + Add-on   Unlisted   Not Covered   # Resequenced

50 Optum Mod 50 Exempt   ⊘ AMA Mod 51 Exempt   51 Optum Mod 51 Exempt   63 Mod 63 Exempt   ⚕ Non-FDA Drug   ★ Telemedicine   M Maternity   A Age Edit

63170-63295 Laminectomies

63170 **Laminectomy with myelotomy (eg, Bischof or DREZ type), cervical, thoracic, or thoracolumbar**
45.9 45.9 FUD 090 C 80
AMA: 2018,Jan,8; 2017,Mar,7; 2017,Jan,8; 2016,Jan,13; 2015,Jan,16

63172 **Laminectomy with drainage of intramedullary cyst/syrinx; to subarachnoid space**
40.0 40.0 FUD 090 C 80
AMA: 2018,Jan,8; 2017,Mar,7; 2017,Jan,8; 2016,Jan,13; 2015,Jan,16

63173 **to peritoneal or pleural space**
49.7 49.7 FUD 090 C 80
AMA: 2018,Jan,8; 2017,Mar,7; 2017,Jan,8; 2016,Jan,13; 2015,Jan,16

63180 **~~Laminectomy and section of dentate ligaments, with or without dural graft, cervical; 1 or 2 segments~~**

63182 **~~more than 2 segments~~**

63185 **Laminectomy with rhizotomy; 1 or 2 segments**
INCLUDES Dana rhizotomy
Stoffel rhizotomy
33.1 33.1 FUD 090 C 80
AMA: 2018,Jan,8; 2017,Mar,7; 2017,Jan,8; 2016,Jan,13; 2015,Jan,16

63190 **more than 2 segments**
36.0 36.0 FUD 090 C 80
AMA: 2018,Jan,8; 2017,Mar,7; 2017,Jan,8; 2016,Jan,13; 2015,Jan,16

63191 **Laminectomy with section of spinal accessory nerve**
EXCLUDES *Division sternocleidomastoid muscle for torticollis (21720)*
39.7 39.7 FUD 090 C 80 50
AMA: 2018,Jan,8; 2017,Mar,7; 2017,Jan,8; 2016,Jan,13; 2015,Jan,16

63194 **Laminectomy with cordotomy, with section of 1 spinothalamic tract, 1 stage; cervical**
46.0 46.0 FUD 090 C 80
AMA: 2018,Jan,8; 2017,Mar,7; 2017,Jan,8; 2016,Jan,13; 2015,Jan,16

63195 **thoracic**
44.2 44.2 FUD 090 C 80
AMA: 2018,Jan,8; 2017,Mar,7; 2017,Jan,8; 2016,Jan,13; 2015,Jan,16

63196 **Laminectomy with cordotomy, with section of both spinothalamic tracts, 1 stage; cervical**
51.3 51.3 FUD 090 C 80
AMA: 2018,Jan,8; 2017,Mar,7; 2017,Jan,8; 2016,Jan,13; 2015,Jan,16

63197 **thoracic**
49.3 49.3 FUD 090 C 80
AMA: 2018,Jan,8; 2017,Mar,7; 2017,Jan,8; 2016,Jan,13; 2015,Jan,16

63198 **Laminectomy with cordotomy with section of both spinothalamic tracts, 2 stages within 14 days; cervical**
INCLUDES Keen laminectomy
60.3 60.3 FUD 090 C 80
AMA: 2018,Jan,8; 2017,Mar,7; 2017,Jan,8; 2016,Jan,13; 2015,Jan,16

63199 **thoracic**
63.2 63.2 FUD 090 C 80
AMA: 2018,Jan,8; 2017,Mar,7; 2017,Jan,8; 2016,Jan,13; 2015,Jan,16

63200 **Laminectomy, with release of tethered spinal cord, lumbar**
44.1 44.1 FUD 090 C 80
AMA: 2018,Jan,8; 2017,Mar,7; 2017,Jan,8; 2016,Jan,13; 2015,Jan,16

63250 **Laminectomy for excision or occlusion of arteriovenous malformation of spinal cord; cervical**
87.8 87.8 FUD 090 C 80
AMA: 2018,Jan,8; 2017,Mar,7; 2017,Jan,8; 2016,Jan,13; 2015,Jan,16

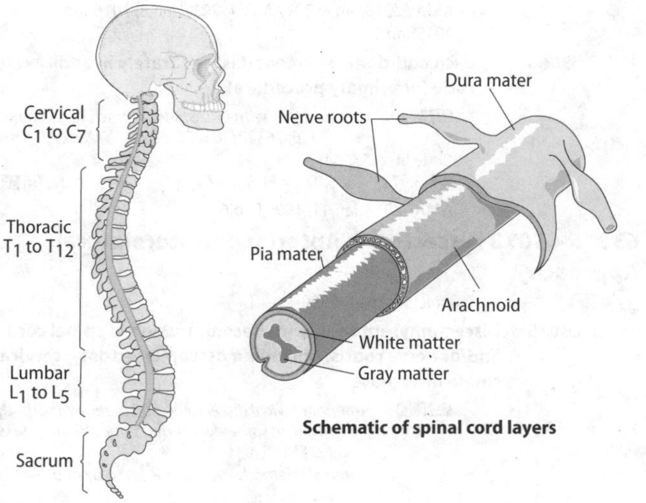

Schematic of spinal cord layers

63251 **thoracic**
87.8 87.8 FUD 090 C 80
AMA: 2018,Jan,8; 2017,Mar,7; 2017,Jan,8; 2016,Jan,13; 2015,Jan,16

63252 **thoracolumbar**
87.8 87.8 FUD 090 C 80
AMA: 2018,Jan,8; 2017,Mar,7; 2017,Jan,8; 2016,Jan,13; 2015,Jan,16

63265 **Laminectomy for excision or evacuation of intraspinal lesion other than neoplasm, extradural; cervical**
48.2 48.2 FUD 090 C 80
AMA: 2018,Jan,8; 2017,Mar,7; 2017,Jan,8; 2016,Jan,13; 2015,Jan,16

63266 **thoracic**
49.7 49.7 FUD 090 C 80
AMA: 2017,Mar,7

63267 **lumbar**
39.6 39.6 FUD 090 C 80
AMA: 2018,Jan,8; 2017,Mar,7; 2017,Jan,8; 2016,Jan,13; 2015,Jan,16

63268 **sacral**
40.9 40.9 FUD 090 C 80
AMA: 2018,Jan,8; 2017,Mar,7; 2017,Jan,8; 2016,Jan,13; 2015,Jan,16

63270 **Laminectomy for excision of intraspinal lesion other than neoplasm, intradural; cervical**
61.1 61.1 FUD 090 C 80
AMA: 2018,Jan,8; 2017,Mar,7; 2017,Jan,8; 2016,Jan,13; 2015,Jan,16

63271 **thoracic**
59.8 59.8 FUD 090 C 80
AMA: 2018,Jan,8; 2017,Mar,7; 2017,Jan,8; 2016,Jan,13; 2015,Jan,16

63272 **lumbar**
54.5 54.5 FUD 090 C 80
AMA: 2018,Jan,8; 2017,Mar,7; 2017,Jan,8; 2016,Jan,13; 2015,Jan,16

63273 **sacral**
53.8 53.8 FUD 090 C 80
AMA: 2018,Jan,8; 2017,Mar,7; 2017,Jan,8; 2016,Jan,13; 2015,Jan,16

63275 **Laminectomy for biopsy/excision of intraspinal neoplasm; extradural, cervical**
52.1 52.1 FUD 090 C 80
AMA: 2018,Jan,8; 2017,Mar,7; 2017,Jan,8; 2016,Jan,13; 2015,Jan,16

63276 **extradural, thoracic**
51.7 51.7 FUD 090 C 80
AMA: 2018,Jan,8; 2017,Mar,7; 2017,Jan,8; 2016,Jan,13; 2015,Jan,16

63277 **extradural, lumbar**
45.3 45.3 FUD 090 C 80
AMA: 2018,Jan,8; 2017,Mar,7; 2017,Jan,8; 2016,Jan,13; 2015,Jan,16

63278 **extradural, sacral**
45.9 45.9 FUD 090 C 80
AMA: 2018,Jan,8; 2017,Mar,7; 2017,Jan,8; 2016,Jan,13; 2015,Jan,16

63280 **intradural, extramedullary, cervical**
61.2 61.2 FUD 090 C 80
AMA: 2018,Jan,8; 2017,Mar,7; 2017,Jan,8; 2016,Jan,13; 2015,Jan,16

63281 **intradural, extramedullary, thoracic**
60.5 60.5 FUD 090 C 80
AMA: 2018,Jan,8; 2017,Mar,7; 2017,Jan,8; 2016,Jan,13; 2015,Jan,16

63282 **intradural, extramedullary, lumbar**
57.7 57.7 FUD 090 C 80
AMA: 2018,Jan,8; 2017,Mar,7; 2017,Jan,8; 2016,Jan,13; 2015,Jan,16

63283 **intradural, sacral**
54.8 54.8 FUD 090 C 80
AMA: 2018,Jan,8; 2017,Mar,7; 2017,Jan,8; 2016,Jan,13; 2015,Jan,16

63285 **intradural, intramedullary, cervical**
77.2 77.2 FUD 090 C 80
AMA: 2018,Jan,8; 2017,Mar,7; 2017,Jan,8; 2016,Jan,13; 2015,Jan,16

63286 **intradural, intramedullary, thoracic**
74.7 74.7 FUD 090 C 80
AMA: 2018,Jan,8; 2017,Mar,7; 2017,Jan,8; 2016,Jan,13; 2015,Jan,16

63287 **intradural, intramedullary, thoracolumbar**
81.0 81.0 FUD 090 C 80
AMA: 2018,Jan,8; 2017,Mar,7; 2017,Jan,8; 2016,Jan,13; 2015,Jan,16

63290 **combined extradural-intradural lesion, any level**
EXCLUDES *Drainage intramedullary cyst or syrinx (63172-63173)*
80.7 80.7 FUD 090 C 80
AMA: 2018,Jan,8; 2017,Mar,7; 2017,Jan,8; 2016,Jan,13; 2015,Jan,16

+ **63295** **Osteoplastic reconstruction of dorsal spinal elements, following primary intraspinal procedure (List separately in addition to code for primary procedure)**
EXCLUDES *Procedure performed same vertebral segment(s) (22590-22614, 22840-22844, 63050-63051)*
Code first (63172-63173, 63185, 63190, 63200-63290)
9.55 9.55 FUD ZZZ C 80
AMA: 2014,Jan,11

63300-63308 Vertebral Corpectomy for Intraspinal Lesion: Anterior/Anterolateral Approach

INCLUDES Partial removal:
Cervical: Removal ≥ 1/2 vertebral body
Lumbar: Removal ≥ 1/3 vertebral body
Thoracic: Removal ≥ 1/3 vertebral body

EXCLUDES *Arthrodesis (22548-22585)*
Spinal reconstruction (20930-20938)

63300 **Vertebral corpectomy (vertebral body resection), partial or complete, for excision of intraspinal lesion, single segment; extradural, cervical**
53.1 53.1 FUD 090 C 80
AMA: 2018,Jan,8; 2017,Mar,7; 2017,Jan,8; 2016,Jan,13; 2015,Jan,16

63301 **extradural, thoracic by transthoracic approach**
63.7 63.7 FUD 090 C 80
AMA: 2018,Jan,8; 2017,Mar,7; 2017,Jan,8; 2016,Jan,13; 2015,Jan,16

63302 **extradural, thoracic by thoracolumbar approach**
62.9 62.9 FUD 090 C 80
AMA: 2018,Jan,8; 2017,Mar,7; 2017,Jan,8; 2016,Jan,13; 2015,Jan,16

63303 **extradural, lumbar or sacral by transperitoneal or retroperitoneal approach**
63.1 63.1 FUD 090 C 80
AMA: 2018,Jan,8; 2017,Mar,7; 2017,Jan,8; 2016,Jan,13; 2015,Jan,16

63304 **intradural, cervical**
67.8 67.8 FUD 090 C 80
AMA: 2018,Jan,8; 2017,Mar,7; 2017,Jan,8; 2016,Jan,13; 2015,Jan,16

63305 **intradural, thoracic by transthoracic approach**
73.7 73.7 FUD 090 C 80
AMA: 2018,Jan,8; 2017,Mar,7; 2017,Jan,8; 2016,Jan,13; 2015,Jan,16

63306 **intradural, thoracic by thoracolumbar approach**
71.0 71.0 FUD 090 C 80
AMA: 2018,Jan,8; 2017,Mar,7; 2017,Jan,8; 2016,Jan,13; 2015,Jan,16

63307 **intradural, lumbar or sacral by transperitoneal or retroperitoneal approach**
69.5 69.5 FUD 090 C 80
AMA: 2018,Jan,8; 2017,Mar,7; 2017,Jan,8; 2016,Jan,13; 2015,Jan,16

+ **63308** **each additional segment (List separately in addition to codes for single segment)**
Code first (63300-63307)
9.37 9.37 FUD ZZZ C 80
AMA: 2014,Jan,11; 2002,Feb,4

63600-63610 Stereotactic Procedures of the Spinal Cord

63600 **Creation of lesion of spinal cord by stereotactic method, percutaneous, any modality (including stimulation and/or recording)**
32.0 32.0 FUD 090 J A2 80
AMA: 2014,Jan,11; 2000,Dec,12

63610 **Stereotactic stimulation of spinal cord, percutaneous, separate procedure not followed by other surgery**
17.1 17.1 FUD 000 J J8 80
AMA: 2014,Jan,11

Nervous System

63275 — 63610

● New Code ▲ Revised Code ○ Reinstated ● New Web Release ▲ Revised Web Release + Add-on Unlisted Not Covered # Resequenced
⑤⓪ Optum Mod 50 Exempt ⊘ AMA Mod 51 Exempt ⑤① Optum Mod 51 Exempt ⑥③ Mod 63 Exempt ✓ Non-FDA Drug ★ Telemedicine M Maternity A Age Edit

63620-63621 Stereotactic Radiosurgery (SRS): Spine

INCLUDES Computer assisted planning
Planning dosimetry, targeting, positioning, or blocking by neurosurgeon

EXCLUDES *Arteriovenous malformations (see Radiation Oncology Section)*
Intensity modulated beam delivery plan and treatment (77301, 77385-77386)
Radiation treatment management by same provider (77427-77432)
Stereotactic body radiation therapy (77373, 77435)
Stereotactic computer-assisted procedures (61781-61783)
Treatment planning, physics, dosimetry, treatment delivery and management provided by radiation oncologist (77261-77790 [77295, 77385, 77386, 77387, 77424, 77425])

63620 Stereotactic radiosurgery (particle beam, gamma ray, or linear accelerator); 1 spinal lesion

EXCLUDES *Reporting code more than one time per entire treatment course*

32.2 32.2 FUD 090 B 80

AMA: 2018,Jan,8; 2017,Jan,8; 2016,Jan,13; 2015,Jun,6; 2015,Jan,16

\+ **63621 each additional spinal lesion (List separately in addition to code for primary procedure)**

EXCLUDES *Reporting code more than one time per lesion*
Reporting code more than two times per entire treatment course

Code first (63620)

7.30 7.30 FUD ZZZ B 80

AMA: 2018,Jan,8; 2017,Jan,8; 2016,Jan,13; 2015,Jun,6; 2015,Jan,16

63650-63688 Spinal Neurostimulation

INCLUDES Analysis system at implantation (95970)
Complex and simple neurostimulators

EXCLUDES *Analysis and programming neurostimulator pulse generator (95970-95972)*

63650 Percutaneous implantation of neurostimulator electrode array, epidural

INCLUDES Neurostimulator system components:
Multiple contacts which four or more provide electrical stimulation in epidural space
Contacts on catheter-type lead (array)
Extension
External controller
Implanted neurostimulator

11.9 54.1 FUD 010 J J8

AMA: 2019,Feb,6; 2018,Oct,11; 2018,Jan,8; 2017,Dec,13; 2017,Jan,8; 2016,Jan,13; 2016,Jan,11; 2015,Dec,18; 2015,Jan,16

63655 Laminectomy for implantation of neurostimulator electrodes, plate/paddle, epidural

INCLUDES Neurostimulator system components:
Multiple contacts which four or more provide electrical stimulation in epidural space
Contacts on catheter-type lead (array)
Extension
External controller
Implanted neurostimulator

24.0 24.0 FUD 090 J J8 80

AMA: 2019,Feb,6; 2018,Jan,8; 2017,Jan,8; 2016,Jan,13; 2015,Jan,16

63661 Removal of spinal neurostimulator electrode percutaneous array(s), including fluoroscopy, when performed

INCLUDES Neurostimulator system components:
Multiple contacts which four or more provide electrical stimulation in epidural space
Contacts on catheter-type lead (array)
Extension
External controller
Implanted neurostimulator

EXCLUDES *Reporting code when removing or replacing temporary array placed percutaneously for external generator*

9.33 18.3 FUD 010 Q2 G2 80

AMA: 2019,Feb,6; 2018,Jan,8; 2017,Jan,8; 2016,Jan,13; 2015,Jan,16

63662 Removal of spinal neurostimulator electrode plate/paddle(s) placed via laminotomy or laminectomy, including fluoroscopy, when performed

INCLUDES Neurostimulator system components:
Multiple contacts which four or more provide electrical stimulation in epidural space
Contacts on catheter-type lead (array)
Extension
External controller
Implanted neurostimulator

24.3 24.3 FUD 090 Q2 G2 80

AMA: 2019,Feb,6; 2018,Jan,8; 2017,Jan,8; 2016,Jan,13; 2015,Jan,16

63663 Revision including replacement, when performed, of spinal neurostimulator electrode percutaneous array(s), including fluoroscopy, when performed

INCLUDES Neurostimulator system components:
Multiple contacts which four or more provide electrical stimulation in epidural space
Contacts on catheter-type lead (array)
Extension
External controller
Implanted neurostimulator

EXCLUDES *Removal of spinal neurostimulator electrode percutaneous array(s), plate/paddle(s) at same level (63661-63662)*
Reporting code when removing or replacing temporary array placed percutaneously for external generator

12.9 23.4 FUD 010 J J8 80

AMA: 2019,Feb,6; 2018,Jan,8; 2017,Jan,8; 2016,Jan,13; 2015,Jan,16

63664 Revision including replacement, when performed, of spinal neurostimulator electrode plate/paddle(s) placed via laminotomy or laminectomy, including fluoroscopy, when performed

INCLUDES Neurostimulator system components:
Multiple contacts which four or more provide electrical stimulation in epidural space
Contacts on catheter-type lead (array)
Extension
External controller
Implanted neurostimulator

EXCLUDES *Removal spinal neurostimulator electrode percutaneous array(s), plate/paddle(s) at same level (63661-63662)*

25.2 25.2 FUD 090 J J8 80

AMA: 2019,Feb,6; 2018,Jan,8; 2017,Jan,8; 2016,Jan,13; 2015,Jan,16

63685 Insertion or replacement of spinal neurostimulator pulse generator or receiver, direct or inductive coupling

EXCLUDES *Reporting code for insertion/replacement with code for revision/removal (63688)*

10.3 10.3 FUD 010 J J8 80

AMA: 2019,Feb,6; 2018,Jan,8; 2017,Dec,13; 2017,Jan,8; 2016,Jan,13; 2015,Jan,16

63688 Revision or removal of implanted spinal neurostimulator pulse generator or receiver

EXCLUDES *Reporting code for revision/removal with code for insertion/replacement (63685)*

10.7 10.7 FUD 010 Q2 A2

AMA: 2019,Feb,6; 2018,Jan,8; 2017,Jan,8; 2016,Jan,13; 2015,Jan,16

63700-63706 Repair Congenital Neural Tube Defects

EXCLUDES *Complex skin repair (see appropriate integumentary closure code)*

63700 **Repair of meningocele; less than 5 cm diameter**
37.6 37.6 FUD 090 63 C 80
AMA: 2014,Jan,11

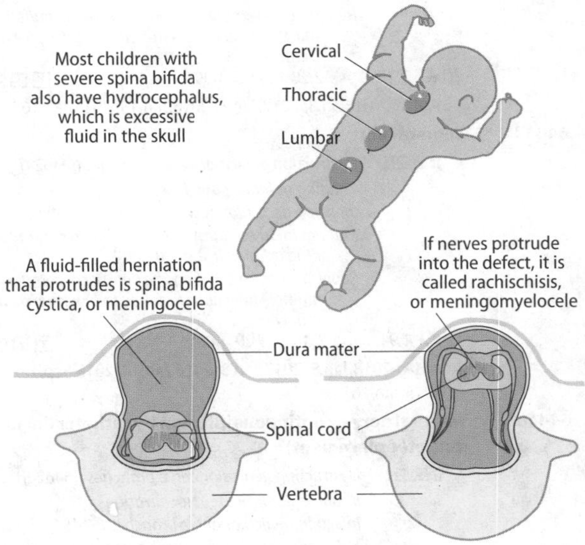
Most children with severe spina bifida also have hydrocephalus, which is excessive fluid in the skull
Cervical
Thoracic
Lumbar
A fluid-filled herniation that protrudes is spina bifida cystica, or meningocele
If nerves protrude into the defect, it is called rachischisis, or meningomyelocele
Dura mater
Spinal cord
Vertebra

63702 **larger than 5 cm diameter**
41.8 41.8 FUD 090 63 C 80
AMA: 2014,Jan,11

63704 **Repair of myelomeningocele; less than 5 cm diameter**
47.7 47.7 FUD 090 63 C 80
AMA: 2014,Jan,11

63706 **larger than 5 cm diameter**
53.1 53.1 FUD 090 63 C 80
AMA: 2014,Jan,11

63707-63710 Repair Dural Cerebrospinal Fluid Leak

63707 **Repair of dural/cerebrospinal fluid leak, not requiring laminectomy**
26.8 26.8 FUD 090 C 80
AMA: 2014,Jan,11; 2002,May,7

63709 **Repair of dural/cerebrospinal fluid leak or pseudomeningocele, with laminectomy**
32.0 32.0 FUD 090 C 80
AMA: 2014,Jan,11; 2002,May,7

63710 **Dural graft, spinal**
31.6 31.6 FUD 090 C 80
AMA: 2014,Jan,11

63740-63746 Cerebrospinal Fluid (CSF) Shunt: Lumbar

EXCLUDES *Placement subarachnoid catheter with reservoir and/or pump:*
Not requiring laminectomy (62350, 62360-62362)
With laminectomy (62351, 62360-62362)

63740 **Creation of shunt, lumbar, subarachnoid-peritoneal, -pleural, or other; including laminectomy**
28.1 28.1 FUD 090 C 80
AMA: 2014,Jan,11; 2000,Dec,12

63741 **percutaneous, not requiring laminectomy**
19.7 19.7 FUD 090 J 80
AMA: 2014,Jan,11; 1990,Win,4

63744 **Replacement, irrigation or revision of lumbosubarachnoid shunt**
19.1 19.1 FUD 090 J A2 80
AMA: 2014,Jan,11

63746 **Removal of entire lumbosubarachnoid shunt system without replacement**
17.6 17.6 FUD 090 02 A2 80
AMA: 2014,Jan,11

64400-64463 [64461, 64462, 64463] Nerve Blocks

EXCLUDES *Epidural or subarachnoid injection (62320-62327)*
Nerve destruction (62280-62282, 64600-64681 [64624, 64625, 64633, 64634, 64635, 64636])

64400 **Injection(s), anesthetic agent(s) and/or steroid; trigeminal nerve, each branch (ie, ophthalmic, maxillary, mandibular)**
EXCLUDES *Destruction genicular nerve branches ([64624])*
Imaging guidance and localization
Injection genicular nerve branches (64454)
Reporting code more than one time per encounter when multiple injections required to block nerve and branches
1.44 3.05 FUD 000 T P3 50
AMA: 2018,Jan,8; 2017,Jan,8; 2016,Jan,13; 2015,Jan,16

64405 **greater occipital nerve**
EXCLUDES *Destruction genicular nerve branches ([64624])*
Imaging guidance and localization
Injection genicular nerve branches (64454)
Reporting code more than one time per encounter when multiple injections required to block nerve and branches
1.55 2.07 FUD 000 T P3 50
AMA: 2018,Jan,8; 2017,Jan,8; 2016,Oct,11; 2016,Jan,13; 2015,Jan,16

64408 **vagus nerve**
EXCLUDES *Destruction genicular nerve branches ([64624])*
Imaging guidance and localization
Injection genicular nerve branches (64454)
Reporting code more than one time per encounter when multiple injections required to block nerve and branches
2.44 3.35 FUD 000 T P3 80 50
AMA: 2018,Jan,8; 2017,Jan,8; 2016,Jan,13; 2015,Jan,16

64415 **brachial plexus**
EXCLUDES *Destruction genicular nerve branches ([64624])*
Imaging guidance and localization
Injection genicular nerve branches (64454)
Reporting code more than one time per encounter when multiple injections required to block nerve and branches
1.83 3.22 FUD 000 T A2 50
AMA: 2018,Jan,8; 2017,Jan,8; 2016,Jan,13; 2015,Jan,16

64416 **brachial plexus, continuous infusion by catheter (including catheter placement)**
EXCLUDES *Destruction genicular nerve branches ([64624])*
Imaging guidance and localization
Injection genicular nerve branches (64454)
Management epidural or subarachnoid continuous drug administration (01996)
Reporting code more than one time per encounter when multiple injections required to block nerve and branches
1.85 1.85 FUD 000 T G2 50
AMA: 2018,Jan,8; 2017,Jan,8; 2016,Jan,13; 2015,Jan,16

64417 **axillary nerve**
EXCLUDES *Destruction genicular nerve branches ([64624])*
Imaging guidance and localization
Injection genicular nerve branches (64454)
Reporting code more than one time per encounter when multiple injections required to block nerve and branches
2.02 3.76 FUD 000 T A2 50
AMA: 2018,Jan,8; 2017,Jan,8; 2016,Jan,13; 2015,Jan,16

64418 **suprascapular nerve**

EXCLUDES *Destruction genicular nerve branches ([64624])*
Imaging guidance and localization
Injection genicular nerve branches (64454)
Reporting code more than one time per encounter when multiple injections required to block nerve and branches

1.64 2.42 **FUD** 000 T P3 50

AMA: 2018,Jan,8; 2017,Jan,8; 2016,Jan,13; 2015,Jan,16

64420 **intercostal nerve, single level**

EXCLUDES *Destruction genicular nerve branches ([64624])*
Imaging guidance and localization
Injection genicular nerve branches (64454)
Reporting code more than one time per encounter when multiple injections required to block nerve and branches

1.72 2.85 **FUD** 000 T A2 50

AMA: 2018,Jan,8; 2017,Jan,8; 2016,Jan,9; 2016,Jan,13; 2015,Jun,3; 2015,Jan,16

\+ **64421** **intercostal nerve, each additional level (List separately in addition to code for primary procedure)**

EXCLUDES *Destruction genicular nerve branches ([64624])*
Imaging guidance and localization
Injection genicular nerve branches (64454)
Reporting code more than one time per encounter when multiple injections required to block nerve and branches
Reporting with modifier 50. Report once for each side when performed bilaterally

Code first (64420)

0.73 0.97 **FUD** ZZZ T A2 50

AMA: 2018,Jan,8; 2017,Jan,8; 2016,Jan,9; 2016,Jan,13; 2015,Jun,3; 2015,Jan,16

64425 **ilioinguinal, iliohypogastric nerves**

EXCLUDES *Destruction genicular nerve branches ([64624])*
Imaging guidance and localization
Injection genicular nerve branches (64454)
Reporting code more than one time per encounter when multiple injections required to block nerve and branches

1.60 3.19 **FUD** 000 T P3 50

AMA: 2018,Jan,8; 2017,Jan,8; 2016,Jan,13; 2015,Jun,3; 2015,Jan,16

64430 **pudendal nerve**

EXCLUDES *Destruction genicular nerve branches ([64624])*
Imaging guidance and localization
Injection genicular nerve branches (64454)
Reporting code more than one time per encounter when multiple injections required to block nerve and branches

2.30 4.14 **FUD** 000 T A2 50

AMA: 2018,Jan,8; 2017,Jan,8; 2016,Jan,13; 2015,Jan,16

64435 **paracervical (uterine) nerve** ♀

EXCLUDES *Destruction genicular nerve branches ([64624])*
Imaging guidance and localization
Injection genicular nerve branches (64454)
Reporting code more than one time per encounter when multiple injections required to block nerve and branches

2.35 4.00 **FUD** 000 T P3 50

AMA: 2018,Jan,8; 2017,Jan,8; 2016,Jan,13; 2015,Jan,16

64445 **sciatic nerve**

EXCLUDES *Destruction genicular nerve branches ([64624])*
Imaging guidance and localization
Injection genicular nerve branches (64454)
Reporting code more than one time per encounter when multiple injections required to block nerve and branches

2.09 3.89 **FUD** 000 T P3 50

AMA: 2018,Jan,8; 2017,Jan,8; 2016,Jan,13; 2015,Jan,16

64446 **sciatic nerve, continuous infusion by catheter (including catheter placement)**

EXCLUDES *Destruction genicular nerve branches ([64624])*
Imaging guidance and localization
Injection genicular nerve branches (64454)
Management epidural or subarachnoid continuous drug administration (01996)
Reporting code more than one time per encounter when multiple injections required to block nerve and branches

2.28 2.28 **FUD** 000 T G2 50

AMA: 2018,Jan,8; 2017,Jan,8; 2016,Jan,13; 2015,Jan,16

64447 **femoral nerve**

EXCLUDES *Destruction genicular nerve branches ([64624])*
Imaging guidance and localization
Injection genicular nerve branches (64454)
Management epidural or subarachnoid continuous drug administration (01996)
Reporting code more than one time per encounter when multiple injections required to block nerve and branches

1.91 3.46 **FUD** 000 T P3 50

AMA: 2018,Jan,8; 2017,Jan,8; 2016,Jan,13; 2015,Sep,12; 2015,Jan,16

64448 **femoral nerve, continuous infusion by catheter (including catheter placement)**

EXCLUDES *Destruction genicular nerve branches ([64624])*
Imaging guidance and localization
Injection genicular nerve branches (64454)
Management epidural or subarachnoid continuous drug administration (01996)
Reporting code more than one time per encounter when multiple injections required to block nerve and branches

2.05 2.05 **FUD** 000 T G2 50

AMA: 2018,Jan,8; 2017,Jan,8; 2016,Jan,13; 2015,Sep,12; 2015,Jan,16

64449 **lumbar plexus, posterior approach, continuous infusion by catheter (including catheter placement)**

EXCLUDES *Destruction genicular nerve branches ([64624])*
Imaging guidance and localization
Injection genicular nerve branches (64454)
Management epidural or subarachnoid continuous drug administration (01996)
Reporting code more than one time per encounter when multiple injections required to block nerve and branches

2.44 2.44 **FUD** 000 T G2 50

AMA: 2018,Jan,8; 2017,Jan,8; 2016,Jan,13; 2015,Jan,16

64450 **other peripheral nerve or branch**

EXCLUDES *Destruction genicular nerve branches ([64624])*
Imaging guidance and localization
Injection genicular nerve branches (64454)
Injection nerves innervating the sacroiliac joint (64451)
Reporting code more than one time per encounter when multiple injections required to block nerve and branches

1.28 2.19 **FUD** 000 T P3 50

AMA: 2019,Nov,14; 2018,Nov,10; 2018,Jan,8; 2017,Jan,8; 2016,Oct,11; 2016,Jan,13; 2015,Nov,10; 2015,Sep,12; 2015,Jun,3; 2015,Jan,16

64451 **nerves innervating the sacroiliac joint, with image guidance (ie, fluoroscopy or computed tomography)**

INCLUDES Imaging guidance and any contrast injection

EXCLUDES *Destruction genicular nerve branches ([64624])*
Injection genicular nerve branches (64454)
Injection nerves innervating paravertebral facet joint (64493-64495)
Injection with ultrasound (76999)
Reporting code more than one time per encounter when multiple injections required to block nerve and branches

2.29 5.99 **FUD** 000 G2 50

AMA: 2020,Jul,13

64454 **genicular nerve branches, including imaging guidance, when performed**

INCLUDES Imaging guidance and any contrast injection

EXCLUDES *Destruction genicular nerve branches ([64624])*
Injection genicular nerve branches (64454)
Reporting code more than one time per encounter when multiple injections required to block nerve and branches

Code also modifier 52 for injection fewer than following all genicular nerve branches: superolateral, superomedial, and inferomedial

2.36 6.05 **FUD** 000 P3 50

AMA: 2019,Dec,8

▲ **64455** **plantar common digital nerve(s) (eg, Morton's neuroma)**

INCLUDES Single or multiple injections on the same site

EXCLUDES *Destruction by neurolytic agent; plantar common digital nerve (64632)*
Destruction genicular nerve branches ([64624])
Imaging guidance and localization
Injection genicular nerve branches (64454)
Reporting code more than one time per encounter when multiple injections required to block nerve and branches

1.00 1.36 **FUD** 000 T P3 80 50

AMA: 2018,Jan,8; 2017,Jan,8; 2016,Jan,13; 2015,Jan,16

64461 **Resequenced code. See code following 64484.**

64462 **Resequenced code. See code following 64484.**

64463 **Resequenced code. See code following 64484.**

64479-64484 Transforaminal Injection

INCLUDES Imaging guidance (fluoroscopy or CT) and contrast injection

EXCLUDES *Epidural or subarachnoid injection (62320-62327)*
Nerve destruction (62280-62282, 64600-64681 [64624, 64625, 64633, 64634, 64635, 64636])

▲ **64479** **transforaminal epidural, with imaging guidance (fluoroscopy or CT), cervical or thoracic, single level**

INCLUDES Imaging guidance and any contrast injection
Single or multiple injections same site
Transforaminal epidural injection T12-L1 level

3.76 6.95 **FUD** 000 T A2 50

AMA: 2018,Jan,8; 2017,Jan,8; 2016,Jan,13; 2016,Jan,9; 2015,Jan,16

Thoracic vertebra (superior view)

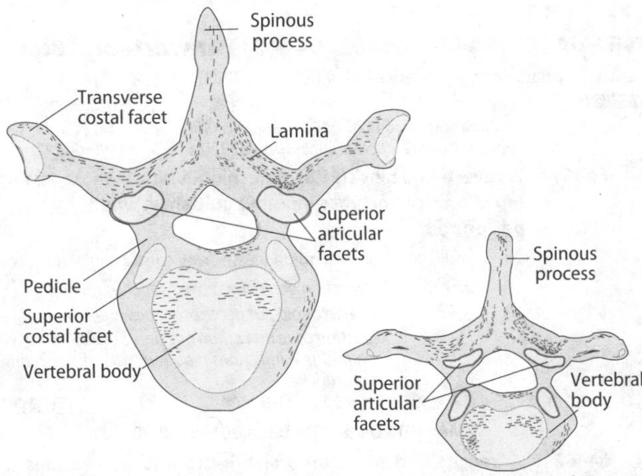

Superior view of C7

▲ + **64480** **transforaminal epidural, with imaging guidance (fluoroscopy or CT), cervical or thoracic, each additional level (List separately in addition to code for primary procedure)**

INCLUDES Imaging guidance and any contrast injection
Single or multiple injections same site

EXCLUDES *Destruction genicular nerve branches ([64624])*
Injection genicular nerve branches (64454)
Reporting with modifier 50. Report once for each side when performed bilaterally
Transforaminal epidural injection T12-L1 level
Reporting code more than one time per encounter when multiple injections required to block nerve and branches

Code first (64479)

1.80 3.42 **FUD** ZZZ N N1 50

AMA: 2018,Jan,8; 2017,Jan,8; 2016,Jan,9; 2016,Jan,13; 2015,Jan,16

▲ **64483** **transforaminal epidural, with imaging guidance (fluoroscopy or CT), lumbar or sacral, single level**

INCLUDES Imaging guidance and any contrast injection
Single or multiple injections same site

EXCLUDES *Destruction genicular nerve branches ([64624])*
Injection genicular nerve branches (64454)
Reporting code more than one time per encounter when multiple injections required to block nerve and branches

3.19 6.44 **FUD** 000 T A2 50

AMA: 2018,Jan,8; 2017,Jan,8; 2016,Oct,11; 2016,Jan,13; 2016,Jan,9; 2015,Jan,16

▲ + 64484 **transforaminal epidural, with imaging guidance (fluoroscopy or CT), lumbar or sacral, each additional level (List separately in addition to code for primary procedure)**

INCLUDES Imaging guidance and any contrast injection
Single or multiple injections same site

EXCLUDES *Destruction genicular nerve branches ([64624])*
Injection genicular nerve branches (64454)
Reporting code more than one time per encounter when multiple injections required to block nerve and branches
Reporting with modifier 50. Report once for each side when performed bilaterally

Code first (64483)

1.49 2.79 FUD ZZZ N N1 50

AMA: 2018,Jan,8; 2017,Jan,8; 2016,Jan,9; 2016,Jan,13; 2015,Jan,16

64461-64463 [64461, 64462, 64463] Paravertebral Blocks

INCLUDES Radiological guidance (76942, 77002-77003)

EXCLUDES *Injection:*
Anesthetic agent (64420-64421, 64479-64480)
Diagnostic or therapeutic substance (62320, 62324, 64490-64492)

64461 **Paravertebral block (PVB) (paraspinous block), thoracic; single injection site (includes imaging guidance, when performed)**

INCLUDES Imaging guidance and any contrast injection

EXCLUDES *Destruction genicular nerve branches ([64624])*
Injection genicular nerve branches (64454)
Reporting code more than one time per encounter when multiple injections required to block nerve and branches

2.50 4.22 FUD 000 T G2 50

AMA: 2018,Dec,8; 2018,Dec,8; 2018,Jan,8; 2017,Jan,8; 2016,Jan,9

+ # 64462 **second and any additional injection site(s) (includes imaging guidance, when performed) (List separately in addition to code for primary procedure)**

INCLUDES Imaging guidance and any contrast injection

EXCLUDES *Destruction genicular nerve branches ([64624])*
Injection genicular nerve branches (64454)
Procedure performed more than one time per day
Reporting with modifier 50. Report once for each side when performed bilaterally

Code first (64461)

1.54 2.32 FUD ZZZ N N1 50

AMA: 2018,Dec,8; 2018,Dec,8; 2018,Jan,8; 2017,Jan,8; 2016,Jan,9

64463 **continuous infusion by catheter (includes imaging guidance, when performed)**

INCLUDES Imaging guidance and any contrast injection

EXCLUDES *Destruction genicular nerve branches ([64624])*
Injection genicular nerve branches (64454)
Reporting code more than one time per encounter when multiple injections required to block nerve and branches

2.47 4.51 FUD 000 T G2 50

AMA: 2018,Dec,8; 2018,Dec,8; 2018,Jan,8; 2017,Jan,8; 2016,Jan,9

64486-64489 Transversus Abdominis Plane (TAP) Block

64486 **Transversus abdominis plane (TAP) block (abdominal plane block, rectus sheath block) unilateral; by injection(s) (includes imaging guidance, when performed)**

INCLUDES Imaging guidance and any contrast injection

EXCLUDES *Destruction genicular nerve branches ([64624])*
Injection genicular nerve branches (64454)
Reporting code more than one time per encounter when multiple injections required to block nerve and branches

1.61 3.12 FUD 000 N N1 50

AMA: 2018,Jan,8; 2017,Jan,8; 2016,Jan,13; 2015,Jun,3

64487 **by continuous infusion(s) (includes imaging guidance, when performed)**

INCLUDES Imaging guidance and any contrast injection

EXCLUDES *Destruction genicular nerve branches ([64624])*
Injection genicular nerve branches (64454)
Reporting code more than one time per encounter when multiple injections required to block nerve and branches

1.87 4.49 FUD 000 N N1 50

AMA: 2018,Jan,8; 2017,Jan,8; 2016,Jan,13; 2015,Jun,3

64488 **Transversus abdominis plane (TAP) block (abdominal plane block, rectus sheath block) bilateral; by injections (includes imaging guidance, when performed)**

INCLUDES Imaging guidance and any contrast injection

EXCLUDES *Destruction genicular nerve branches ([64624])*
Injection genicular nerve branches (64454)
Reporting code more than one time per encounter when multiple injections required to block nerve and branches

2.02 3.83 FUD 000 N N1

AMA: 2018,Jan,8; 2017,Jan,8; 2016,Jan,13; 2015,Jun,3

64489 **by continuous infusions (includes imaging guidance, when performed)**

INCLUDES Imaging guidance and any contrast injection

EXCLUDES *Destruction genicular nerve branches ([64624])*
Injection genicular nerve branches (64454)
Reporting code more than one time per encounter when multiple injections required to block nerve and branches

2.27 6.65 FUD 000 N N1

AMA: 2018,Jan,8; 2017,Jan,8; 2016,Jan,13; 2015,Jun,3

64490-64495 Paraspinal Nerve Injections

INCLUDES Image guidance (CT or fluoroscopy) and any contrast injection

EXCLUDES *Injection without imaging (20552-20553)*
Ultrasonic guidance (0213T-0218T)

64490 **Injection(s), diagnostic or therapeutic agent, paravertebral facet (zygapophyseal) joint (or nerves innervating that joint) with image guidance (fluoroscopy or CT), cervical or thoracic; single level**

INCLUDES Injection T12-L1 joint and nerves that innervate joint

3.03 5.39 FUD 000 T G2 80 50

AMA: 2018,Jan,8; 2017,Jan,8; 2016,Jan,9; 2016,Jan,13; 2015,Jan,16

+ 64491 **second level (List separately in addition to code for primary procedure)**

EXCLUDES *Reporting with modifier 50. Report once for each side when performed bilaterally*

Code first (64490)

1.72 2.68 FUD ZZZ N N1 80 50

AMA: 2018,Jan,8; 2017,Jan,8; 2016,Jan,9; 2016,Jan,13; 2015,Jan,16

+ 64492 **third and any additional level(s) (List separately in addition to code for primary procedure)**

EXCLUDES *Procedure performed more than one time per day*
Reporting with modifier 50. Report once for each side when performed bilaterally

Code also when appropriate (64491)

Code first (64490)

1.74 2.70 FUD ZZZ N N1 80 50

AMA: 2018,Jan,8; 2017,Jan,8; 2016,Jan,9; 2016,Jan,13; 2015,Jan,16

64493 **Injection(s), diagnostic or therapeutic agent, paravertebral facet (zygapophyseal) joint (or nerves innervating that joint) with image guidance (fluoroscopy or CT), lumbar or sacral; single level**

EXCLUDES *Injection nerves innervating sacroiliac joint (64451)*

2.58 4.91 FUD 000 T G2 80 50

AMA: 2020,Jul,13; 2018,May,10; 2018,Jan,8; 2017,Jan,8; 2016,Jan,13; 2015,Jan,16

\+ **64494** **second level (List separately in addition to code for primary procedure)**

EXCLUDES *Reporting with modifier 50. Report once for each side when performed bilaterally*

Code first (64493)

1.49 2.49 **FUD** ZZZ N N1 80 50

AMA: 2020,Jul,13; 2018,May,10; 2018,Jan,8; 2017,Jan,8; 2016,Jan,13; 2015,Jan,16

\+ **64495** **third and any additional level(s) (List separately in addition to code for primary procedure)**

EXCLUDES *Procedure performed more than one time per day*

Reporting with modifier 50. Report once for each side when performed bilaterally

Code also when appropriate (64494)

Code first (64493)

1.51 2.49 **FUD** ZZZ N N1 80 50

AMA: 2018,May,10; 2018,Jan,8; 2017,Jan,8; 2016,Jan,13; 2015,Jan,16

64505-64530 Sympathetic Nerve Blocks

64505 **Injection, anesthetic agent; sphenopalatine ganglion**

2.69 3.36 **FUD** 000 T P3 50

AMA: 2018,Jan,8; 2017,Jan,8; 2016,Jan,13; 2015,Jan,16

64510 **stellate ganglion (cervical sympathetic)**

2.13 3.78 **FUD** 000 T A2 50

AMA: 2018,Jan,8; 2017,Jan,8; 2016,Jan,13; 2015,Jan,16

64517 **superior hypogastric plexus**

3.60 5.47 **FUD** 000 T A2

AMA: 2018,Jan,8; 2017,Jan,8; 2016,Jan,13; 2015,Jan,16

64520 **lumbar or thoracic (paravertebral sympathetic)**

2.34 5.75 **FUD** 000 T A2 50

AMA: 2018,Jan,8; 2017,Jan,8; 2016,Jan,13; 2015,Jan,16

64530 **celiac plexus, with or without radiologic monitoring**

EXCLUDES *Transmural anesthetic injection with transendoscopic ultrasound-guidance (43253)*

2.63 5.73 **FUD** 000 T A2

AMA: 2018,Jan,8; 2017,Jan,8; 2016,Jan,13; 2015,Jan,16

64553-64570 Electrical Nerve Stimulation: Insertion/Replacement/Removal/Revision

INCLUDES Analysis system at implantation (95970)

Simple and complex neurostimulators

EXCLUDES *Analysis and programming neurostimulator pulse generator (95970-95972)*

TENS therapy (97014, 97032)

64553 **Percutaneous implantation of neurostimulator electrode array; cranial nerve**

INCLUDES Temporary and permanent percutaneous array placement

EXCLUDES *Open procedure (61885-61886)*

Percutaneous electrical stimulation peripheral nerve with needle or needle electrodes (64999)

10.1 48.8 **FUD** 010 J J8 80

AMA: 2019,Feb,6; 2018,Oct,8; 2018,Jan,8; 2017,Jan,8; 2016,Jan,13; 2015,Jan,16

64555 **peripheral nerve (excludes sacral nerve)**

INCLUDES Temporary and permanent percutaneous array placement

EXCLUDES *Percutaneous electrical stimulation cranial nerve with needle or needle electrodes (64999)*

Posterior tibial neurostimulation (64566)

9.85 44.3 **FUD** 010 J J8

AMA: 2019,Feb,6; 2018,Oct,8; 2018,Aug,10; 2018,Jan,8; 2017,Dec,13; 2017,Jan,8; 2016,Feb,13; 2016,Jan,13; 2015,Jan,16; 2015,Jan,13

64561 **sacral nerve (transforaminal placement) including image guidance, if performed**

INCLUDES Temporary and permanent percutaneous array placement

EXCLUDES *Percutaneous electrical stimulation or neuromodulation with needle or needle electrodes (64999)*

8.75 20.9 **FUD** 010 J J8 50

AMA: 2019,Feb,6; 2018,Oct,8; 2018,Jan,8; 2017,Jan,8; 2016,Jan,13; 2015,Jan,16

64566 **Posterior tibial neurostimulation, percutaneous needle electrode, single treatment, includes programming**

EXCLUDES *Electronic analysis implanted neurostimulator pulse generator system (95970-95972)*

Percutaneous implantation neurostimulator electrode array; peripheral nerve (64555)

0.87 3.62 **FUD** 000 T P3 80

AMA: 2019,Feb,6; 2018,Oct,8; 2018,Jan,8; 2017,Jan,8; 2016,Jan,13; 2015,Jan,16

64568 **Incision for implantation of cranial nerve (eg, vagus nerve) neurostimulator electrode array and pulse generator**

EXCLUDES *Insertion chest wall respiratory sensor electrode or array with pulse generator connection (0466T)*

Insertion, replacement cranial neurostimulator pulse generator or receiver (61885-61886)

Removal neurostimulator electrode array and pulse generator (64570)

18.4 18.4 **FUD** 090 J J8 80 50

AMA: 2019,Feb,6; 2018,Mar,9; 2018,Jan,8; 2017,Jan,8; 2016,Nov,6; 2016,Jan,13; 2015,Jan,16

64569 **Revision or replacement of cranial nerve (eg, vagus nerve) neurostimulator electrode array, including connection to existing pulse generator**

EXCLUDES *Removal neurostimulator electrode array and pulse generator (64570)*

Replacement pulse generator (61885)

Revision or replacement chest wall respiratory sensor electrode with pulse generator connection (0467T)

Revision, removal pulse generator (61888)

22.1 22.1 **FUD** 090 J J8 80 50

AMA: 2019,Feb,6; 2018,Mar,9; 2018,Jan,8; 2017,Jan,8; 2016,Nov,6; 2016,Jan,13; 2015,Jan,16

64570 **Removal of cranial nerve (eg, vagus nerve) neurostimulator electrode array and pulse generator**

EXCLUDES *Laparoscopic revision, replacement, removal, or implantation vagus nerve blocking neurostimulator pulse generator and/or electrode array at esophagogastric junction (0312T-0317T)*

Removal chest wall respiratory sensor electrode or array (0468T)

Revision, removal pulse generator (61888)

21.2 21.2 **FUD** 090 Q2 G2 80 50

AMA: 2019,Feb,6; 2018,Mar,9; 2018,Jan,8; 2017,Jan,8; 2016,Nov,6; 2016,Jan,13; 2015,Jan,16

64575-64595 Implantation/Revision/Removal Neurostimulators: Incisional

INCLUDES Simple and complex neurostimulators

EXCLUDES *Analysis and programming neurostimulator pulse generator (95970-95972)*

64575 **Incision for implantation of neurostimulator electrode array; peripheral nerve (excludes sacral nerve)**

9.60 9.60 **FUD** 090 J J8

AMA: 2019,Feb,6

64580 **neuromuscular**

8.97 8.97 **FUD** 090 J J8 80

AMA: 2019,Feb,6

64581 **sacral nerve (transforaminal placement)**

19.0 19.0 **FUD** 090 J J8

AMA: 2019,Feb,6; 2018,Jan,8; 2017,Jan,8; 2016,Jan,13; 2015,Jan,16

64585 **Revision or removal of peripheral neurostimulator electrode array**
4.14 | 7.03 | **FUD** 010 | Q2 A2
AMA: 2019,Feb,6

64590 **Insertion or replacement of peripheral or gastric neurostimulator pulse generator or receiver, direct or inductive coupling**
EXCLUDES *Revision, removal neurostimulator pulse generator (64595)*
4.64 | 7.60 | **FUD** 010 | J J8
AMA: 2019,Feb,6; 2018,Aug,10; 2018,Jan,8; 2017,Dec,13; 2017,Jan,8; 2016,Jan,13; 2015,Jan,13; 2015,Jan,16

64595 **Revision or removal of peripheral or gastric neurostimulator pulse generator or receiver**
EXCLUDES *Insertion, replacement neurostimulator pulse generator (64590)*
3.63 | 6.89 | **FUD** 010 | Q2 A2
AMA: 2019,Feb,6; 2018,Jan,8; 2017,Jan,8; 2016,Jan,13; 2015,Jan,16

64600-64610 Chemical Denervation Trigeminal Nerve

INCLUDES Injection therapeutic medication
EXCLUDES *Electromyography or muscle electric stimulation guidance (95873-95874)*
Nerve destruction:
Anal sphincter (46505)
Bladder (52287)
Strabismus involving extraocular muscles (67345)
Treatments that do not destroy target nerve (64999)
Code also chemodenervation agent

64600 **Destruction by neurolytic agent, trigeminal nerve; supraorbital, infraorbital, mental, or inferior alveolar branch**
6.66 | 12.3 | **FUD** 010 | T A2
AMA: 2019,Apr,9; 2018,Jan,8; 2017,Jan,8; 2016,Jan,13; 2015,Jan,16

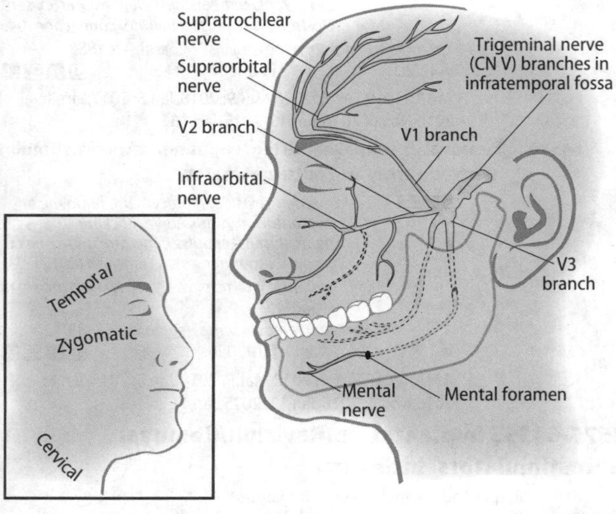

64605 **second and third division branches at foramen ovale**
10.1 | 17.8 | **FUD** 010 | J A2 80 50
AMA: 2019,Apr,9; 2018,Jan,8; 2017,Jan,8; 2016,Jan,13; 2015,Jan,16

64610 **second and third division branches at foramen ovale under radiologic monitoring**
14.2 | 22.0 | **FUD** 010 | J A2 50
AMA: 2019,Apr,9; 2018,Jan,8; 2017,Apr,9; 2017,Jan,8; 2016,Jan,13; 2015,Jan,16

64624 [64624] Chemical Denervation Genicular Nerve Branches

\# **64624** **Destruction by neurolytic agent, genicular nerve branches including imaging guidance, when performed**
EXCLUDES *Injection genicular nerve branches (64454)*
Code also modifier 52 for destruction fewer than all genicular nerve branches: superolateral, superomedial, and inferomedial
4.23 | 11.5 | **FUD** 010 | P3 80 50
AMA: 2019,Dec,8

64625 [64625] Radiofrequency Ablation Sacroiliac Joint Nerves

\# **64625** **Radiofrequency ablation, nerves innervating the sacroiliac joint, with image guidance (ie, fluoroscopy or computed tomography)**
INCLUDES CT needle guidance (77012)
Electrical stimulation or needle electromyelograph for guidance (95873-95874)
Fluoroscopic needle guidance or localization (77002-77003)
EXCLUDES *Destruction by neurolytic agent, paravertebral facet joint nerve ([64635])*
Radiofrequency ablation with ultrasound (76999)
5.59 | 14.1 | **FUD** 010 | G2 50
AMA: 2020,Jun,14; 2019,Dec,8

64611-64617 Chemical Denervation Procedures Head and Neck

INCLUDES Injection therapeutic medication
EXCLUDES *Electromyography or muscle electric stimulation guidance (95873-95874)*
Nerve destruction:
Anal sphincter (46505)
Bladder (52287)
Extraocular muscles to treat strabismus (67345)
Treatments that do not destroy target nerve (64999)

64611 **Chemodenervation of parotid and submandibular salivary glands, bilateral**
Code also modifier 52 for injection of fewer than four salivary glands
3.03 | 3.45 | **FUD** 010 | T P3 80
AMA: 2019,Apr,9; 2018,Jan,8; 2017,Jan,8; 2016,Jan,13; 2015,Jan,16

64612 **Chemodenervation of muscle(s); muscle(s) innervated by facial nerve, unilateral (eg, for blepharospasm, hemifacial spasm)**
3.39 | 3.83 | **FUD** 010 | T P3 50
AMA: 2019,Apr,9; 2018,Jan,8; 2017,Jan,8; 2016,Jan,13; 2015,Jan,16

64615 **muscle(s) innervated by facial, trigeminal, cervical spinal and accessory nerves, bilateral (eg, for chronic migraine)**
EXCLUDES *Chemodenervation (64612, 64616-64617, 64642-64647)*
Procedure performed more than one time per session
Code also any guidance by muscle electrical stimulation or needle electromyography but report only once (95873-95874)
3.58 | 4.27 | **FUD** 010 | T P3
AMA: 2019,Apr,9; 2018,Jan,8; 2017,Jan,8; 2016,Jan,13; 2015,Jan,16

64616 **neck muscle(s), excluding muscles of the larynx, unilateral (eg, for cervical dystonia, spasmodic torticollis)**
Code also guidance by muscle electrical stimulation or needle electromyography, but report only once (95873-95874)
3.18 | 3.80 | **FUD** 010 | T P3 50
AMA: 2019,Apr,9; 2018,Jan,8; 2017,Jan,8; 2016,Jan,13; 2015,Jan,16

64617 **larynx, unilateral, percutaneous (eg, for spasmodic dysphonia), includes guidance by needle electromyography, when performed**

EXCLUDES *Chemodenervation larynx via direct laryngoscopy (31570-31571)*
Diagnostic needle electromyography larynx (95865)
Electrical stimulation guidance for chemodenervation (95873-95874)

3.14 4.62 FUD 010 T P3 50

AMA: 2019,Apr,9; 2018,Jan,8; 2017,Jan,8; 2016,Jan,13; 2015,Jan,16

64620-64640 [64624, 64625, 64633, 64634, 64635, 64636] Chemical Denervation Intercostal, Facet Joint, Plantar, and Pudendal Nerve(s)

INCLUDES Injection therapeutic medication

64620 **Destruction by neurolytic agent, intercostal nerve**

5.00 5.91 FUD 010 T A2

AMA: 2019,Nov,14; 2019,Apr,9; 2018,Jan,8; 2017,Jan,8; 2016,Jan,13; 2015,Jan,16

64624 **Resequenced code. See code following 64610.**

64625 **Resequenced code. See code before 64611.**

\# **64633** **Destruction by neurolytic agent, paravertebral facet joint nerve(s), with imaging guidance (fluoroscopy or CT); cervical or thoracic, single facet joint**

INCLUDES Paravertebral facet destruction T12-L1 joint or nerve(s) that innervate joint
Radiological guidance (77003, 77012)

EXCLUDES *Denervation performed using chemical, low grade thermal, or pulsed radiofrequency methods (64999)*
Destruction paravertebral facet joint nerve(s) without imaging guidance (64999)

6.43 11.8 FUD 010 J G2 50

AMA: 2019,Apr,9; 2018,Jan,8; 2017,Jan,8; 2016,Jan,13; 2015,Feb,9; 2015,Jan,16

\+ # **64634** **cervical or thoracic, each additional facet joint (List separately in addition to code for primary procedure)**

INCLUDES Radiological guidance (77003, 77012)

EXCLUDES *Denervation performed using chemical, low grade thermal, or pulsed radiofrequency methods (64999)*
Destruction paravertebral facet joint nerve(s) without imaging guidance (64999)
Reporting with modifier 50. Report once for each side when performed bilaterally

Code first ([64633])

1.95 5.34 FUD ZZZ N N1 50

AMA: 2019,Apr,9; 2018,Jan,8; 2017,Jan,8; 2016,Jan,13; 2015,Feb,9; 2015,Jan,16

\# **64635** **lumbar or sacral, single facet joint**

INCLUDES Radiological guidance (77003, 77012)

EXCLUDES *Denervation performed using chemical, low grade thermal, or pulsed radiofrequency methods (64999)*
Destruction individual nerves, sacroiliac joint, by neurolytic agent (64640)
Destruction paravertebral facet joint nerve(s) without imaging guidance (64999)

6.34 11.7 FUD 010 J G2 50

AMA: 2020,May,13; 2019,Dec,8; 2019,Apr,9; 2018,Jan,8; 2017,Jan,8; 2016,Jan,13; 2015,Feb,9; 2015,Jan,16

\+ # **64636** **lumbar or sacral, each additional facet joint (List separately in addition to code for primary procedure)**

INCLUDES Radiological guidance (77003, 77012)

EXCLUDES *Denervation performed using chemical, low grade thermal, or pulsed radiofrequency methods (64999)*
Destruction individual nerves, sacroiliac joint, by neurolytic agent (64640)
Destruction paravertebral facet joint nerve(s) without imaging guidance (64999)
Radiofrequency ablation nerves innervating sacroiliac joint with imaging ([64625])
Reporting with modifier 50. Report once for each side when performed bilaterally

Code first ([64635])

1.71 4.85 FUD ZZZ N N1 50

AMA: 2020,May,13; 2019,Apr,9; 2018,Jan,8; 2017,Jan,8; 2016,Jan,13; 2015,Feb,9; 2015,Jan,16

64630 **Destruction by neurolytic agent; pudendal nerve**

5.44 6.94 FUD 010 T A2 80

AMA: 2019,Apr,9; 2018,Jan,8; 2017,Oct,9; 2017,Jan,8; 2016,Jan,13; 2015,Jan,16

64632 **plantar common digital nerve**

EXCLUDES *Injection(s), anesthetic agent and/or steroid (64455)*

1.96 2.45 FUD 010 T P3 80 50

AMA: 2019,Apr,9; 2018,Jan,8; 2017,Oct,9; 2017,Jan,8; 2016,Jan,13; 2015,Jul,10; 2015,Jan,16

64633 **Resequenced code. See code following 64620.**

64634 **Resequenced code. See code following 64620.**

64635 **Resequenced code. See code following 64620.**

64636 **Resequenced code. See code before 64630.**

64640 **other peripheral nerve or branch**

INCLUDES Neurolytic destruction of nerves of sacroiliac joint

2.69 3.86 FUD 010 T P3 50

AMA: 2019,Apr,9; 2018,Jan,8; 2018,Jan,7; 2017,Oct,9; 2017,Jan,8; 2016,Jan,13; 2015,Jan,16

64642-64645 Chemical Denervation Extremity Muscles

INCLUDES Trunk muscles include erector spine, obliques, paraspinal, and rectus abdominus. Remaining muscles considered neck, head or extremity muscles

EXCLUDES *Chemodenervation with needle-guided electromyography or with guidance provided by muscle electrical stimulation (95873-95874)*
Procedure performed more than once per extremity

Code also other extremities when appropriate, up to total four units per patient (when all extremities injected) (64642-64645)

64642 **Chemodenervation of one extremity; 1-4 muscle(s)**

EXCLUDES *Reporting more than one base code per session (64642)*

3.12 4.15 FUD 000 T P3

AMA: 2019,Aug,10; 2019,Apr,9; 2018,Jan,8; 2017,Jan,8; 2016,Jan,13; 2015,Jan,16

\+ **64643** **each additional extremity, 1-4 muscle(s) (List separately in addition to code for primary procedure)**

Code first (64642, 64644)

2.08 2.65 FUD ZZZ N N1

AMA: 2019,Aug,10; 2019,Apr,9; 2018,Jan,8; 2017,Jan,8; 2016,Jan,13; 2015,Jan,16

64644 **Chemodenervation of one extremity; 5 or more muscles**

EXCLUDES *Reporting more than one base code per session (64644)*

3.42 4.82 FUD 000 T P3

AMA: 2019,Aug,10; 2019,Apr,9; 2018,Jan,8; 2017,Jan,8; 2016,Jan,13; 2015,Jan,16

\+ **64645** **each additional extremity, 5 or more muscles (List separately in addition to code for primary procedure)**

Code first (64644)

2.40 3.33 FUD ZZZ N N1

AMA: 2019,Aug,10; 2019,Apr,9; 2018,Jan,8; 2017,Jan,8; 2016,Jan,13; 2015,Jan,16

64646-64647 Chemical Denervation Trunk Muscles

EXCLUDES *Procedure performed more than once per session*

64646 Chemodenervation of trunk muscle(s); 1-5 muscle(s)
3.34 | 4.35 | FUD 000 | T P3
AMA: 2019,Apr,9; 2018,Jan,8; 2017,Jan,8; 2016,Jan,13; 2015,Jan,16

64647 6 or more muscles
3.96 | 5.12 | FUD 000 | T P3
AMA: 2019,Apr,9; 2018,Jan,8; 2017,Jan,8; 2016,Jan,13; 2015,Jan,16

64650-64653 Chemical Denervation Eccrine Glands

INCLUDES Injection therapeutic medication

EXCLUDES *Bladder chemodenervation (52287)*
Chemodenervation extremities (64999)

Code also drugs or other substances used

64650 Chemodenervation of eccrine glands; both axillae
1.21 | 2.25 | FUD 000 | T P3 80
AMA: 2019,Apr,9; 2018,Jan,8; 2017,Jan,8; 2016,Jan,13; 2015,Jan,16

64653 other area(s) (eg, scalp, face, neck), per day
1.53 | 2.79 | FUD 000 | T P3 80
AMA: 2019,Apr,9; 2018,Jan,8; 2017,Jan,8; 2016,Jan,13; 2015,Jan,16

64680-64681 Neurolysis: Celiac Plexus, Superior Hypogastric Plexus

INCLUDES Injection therapeutic medication

64680 Destruction by neurolytic agent, with or without radiologic monitoring; celiac plexus
EXCLUDES *Transmural neurolytic agent injection with transendoscopic ultrasound guidance (43253)*
4.66 | 9.55 | FUD 010 | T A2
AMA: 2019,Apr,9; 2018,Jan,8; 2017,Jan,8; 2016,Jan,13; 2015,Jan,16

64681 superior hypogastric plexus
7.87 | 16.4 | FUD 010 | T A2
AMA: 2019,Apr,9; 2018,Jan,8; 2017,Jan,8; 2016,Jan,13; 2015,Jan,16

64702-64727 Decompression and/or Transposition of Nerve

INCLUDES External neurolysis and/or transposition to repair or restore nerve
Neuroplasty with nerve wrapping
Surgical decompression/freeing nerve from scar tissue

EXCLUDES *Facial nerve decompression (69720)*
Percutaneous neurolysis (62263-62264, 62280-62282)
Reporting with tissue expander insertion (11960)

64702 Neuroplasty; digital, 1 or both, same digit
14.4 | 14.4 | FUD 090 | J A2
AMA: 2018,Jan,8; 2017,Jan,8; 2016,Jan,13; 2015,Jan,16

64704 nerve of hand or foot
9.23 | 9.23 | FUD 090 | J A2 80
AMA: 2018,Jan,8; 2017,Jan,8; 2016,Jan,13; 2015,Jan,16

64708 Neuroplasty, major peripheral nerve, arm or leg, open; other than specified
14.4 | 14.4 | FUD 090 | J G2 80
AMA: 2018,Jan,8; 2017,Nov,10; 2017,Jan,8; 2016,Jan,13; 2015,Jan,16

64712 sciatic nerve
16.9 | 16.9 | FUD 090 | J G2 80 50
AMA: 2018,Jan,8; 2017,Jan,8; 2016,Jan,13; 2015,Jan,16

64713 brachial plexus
22.5 | 22.5 | FUD 090 | J G2 80 50
AMA: 2018,Jan,8; 2017,Jan,8; 2016,Jan,13; 2015,Jan,16

64714 lumbar plexus
21.1 | 21.1 | FUD 090 | J G2 80 50
AMA: 2018,Jan,8; 2017,Jan,8; 2016,Jan,13; 2015,Jan,16

64716 Neuroplasty and/or transposition; cranial nerve (specify)
15.0 | 15.0 | FUD 090 | J A2 80
AMA: 2018,Jan,8; 2017,Jan,8; 2016,Jan,13; 2015,Jan,16

64718 ulnar nerve at elbow
17.0 | 17.0 | FUD 090 | J A2 80 50
AMA: 2020,Jun,14; 2018,Jan,8; 2017,Jan,8; 2016,Jan,13; 2015,Jan,16

64719 ulnar nerve at wrist
11.5 | 11.5 | FUD 090 | J A2 50
AMA: 2018,Jan,8; 2017,Jan,8; 2016,Jan,13; 2015,Jan,16

64721 median nerve at carpal tunnel
EXCLUDES *Endoscopic procedure (29848)*
12.3 | 12.4 | FUD 090 | J A2 50
AMA: 2018,Jan,8; 2017,Jan,8; 2016,Jan,13; 2015,Jul,10; 2015,Jan,16

64722 Decompression; unspecified nerve(s) (specify)
10.3 | 10.3 | FUD 090 | J A2 80
AMA: 2018,Jan,8; 2017,Jan,8; 2016,Jan,13; 2015,Jan,16

64726 plantar digital nerve
7.80 | 7.80 | FUD 090 | J A2
AMA: 2018,Jan,8; 2017,Jan,8; 2016,Jan,13; 2015,Jan,16

+ **64727 Internal neurolysis, requiring use of operating microscope (List separately in addition to code for neuroplasty) (Neuroplasty includes external neurolysis)**
INCLUDES Operating microscope (69990)
Code first neuroplasty (64702-64721)
5.31 | 5.31 | FUD ZZZ | N N1
AMA: 2018,Jan,8; 2017,Jan,8; 2016,Feb,12; 2016,Jan,13; 2015,Jan,16

64732-64772 Surgical Avulsion/Transection of Nerve

EXCLUDES *Stereotactic lesion gasserian ganglion (61790)*

64732 Transection or avulsion of; supraorbital nerve
12.7 | 12.7 | FUD 090 | J A2 80 50
AMA: 2018,Jan,8; 2017,Jan,8; 2016,Jan,13; 2015,Jan,16

64734 infraorbital nerve
14.5 | 14.5 | FUD 090 | J A2 80 50
AMA: 2014,Jan,11

64736 mental nerve
10.7 | 10.7 | FUD 090 | J A2 80 50
AMA: 2014,Jan,11

64738 inferior alveolar nerve by osteotomy
13.0 | 13.0 | FUD 090 | J A2 80 50
AMA: 2014,Jan,11

64740 lingual nerve
14.0 | 14.0 | FUD 090 | J A2 80 50
AMA: 2014,Jan,11

64742 facial nerve, differential or complete
14.0 | 14.0 | FUD 090 | J A2 80 50
AMA: 2014,Jan,11

64744 greater occipital nerve
14.2 | 14.2 | FUD 090 | J A2 80 50
AMA: 2014,Jan,11

64746 phrenic nerve
12.4 | 12.4 | FUD 090 | J A2 80 50
AMA: 2014,Jan,11

64755 vagus nerves limited to proximal stomach (selective proximal vagotomy, proximal gastric vagotomy, parietal cell vagotomy, supra- or highly selective vagotomy)
EXCLUDES *Laparoscopic procedure (43652)*
26.8 | 26.8 | FUD 090 | C 80
AMA: 2018,Jan,8; 2017,Jan,8; 2016,Jan,13; 2015,Jan,16

64760 vagus nerve (vagotomy), abdominal
EXCLUDES *Laparoscopic procedure (43651)*
14.7 | 14.7 | FUD 090 | C 80
AMA: 2018,Jan,8; 2017,Jan,8; 2016,Jan,13; 2015,Jan,16

64763 **Transection or avulsion of obturator nerve, extrapelvic, with or without adductor tenotomy**
14.8 14.8 FUD 090 J G2 80 50
AMA: 2014,Jan,11

64766 **Transection or avulsion of obturator nerve, intrapelvic, with or without adductor tenotomy**
18.2 18.2 FUD 090 J G2 80 50
AMA: 2014,Jan,11

64771 **Transection or avulsion of other cranial nerve, extradural**
17.5 17.5 FUD 090 J A2 80
AMA: 2014,Jan,11

64772 **Transection or avulsion of other spinal nerve, extradural**
EXCLUDES *Removal tender scar and soft tissue including neuroma when necessary (11400-11446, 13100-13153)*
16.2 16.2 FUD 090 J A2 80
AMA: 2018,Jan,8; 2017,Jan,8; 2016,Jan,13; 2015,Apr,10

64774-64823 Excisional Nerve Procedures

EXCLUDES *Morton neuroma excision (28080)*

64774 **Excision of neuroma; cutaneous nerve, surgically identifiable**
11.7 11.7 FUD 090 J A2
AMA: 2014,Jan,11

64776 **digital nerve, 1 or both, same digit**
11.1 11.1 FUD 090 J A2 80
AMA: 2014,Jan,11

\+ **64778** **digital nerve, each additional digit (List separately in addition to code for primary procedure)**
Code first (64776)
5.30 5.30 FUD ZZZ N N1
AMA: 2014,Jan,11

64782 **hand or foot, except digital nerve**
13.2 13.2 FUD 090 J A2
AMA: 2014,Jan,11

\+ **64783** **hand or foot, each additional nerve, except same digit (List separately in addition to code for primary procedure)**
Code first (64782)
6.33 6.33 FUD ZZZ N N1
AMA: 2014,Jan,11

64784 **major peripheral nerve, except sciatic**
20.9 20.9 FUD 090 J A2 80
AMA: 2014,Jan,11

64786 **sciatic nerve**
29.2 29.2 FUD 090 J A2 80 50
AMA: 2014,Jan,11

\+ **64787** **Implantation of nerve end into bone or muscle (List separately in addition to neuroma excision)**
Code also, when appropriate (64774-64786)
6.96 6.96 FUD ZZZ N N1 80
AMA: 2014,Jan,11

64788 **Excision of neurofibroma or neurolemmoma; cutaneous nerve**
11.5 11.5 FUD 090 J A2
AMA: 2018,Jan,8; 2017,Jan,8; 2016,Apr,3

64790 **major peripheral nerve**
24.1 24.1 FUD 090 J A2 80
AMA: 2018,Jan,8; 2017,Jan,8; 2016,Apr,3

64792 **extensive (including malignant type)**
EXCLUDES *Destruction neurofibroma skin (0419T-0420T)*
31.4 31.4 FUD 090 J A2 80
AMA: 2018,Jan,8; 2017,Jan,8; 2016,Apr,3

64795 **Biopsy of nerve**
5.64 5.64 FUD 000 J A2
AMA: 2014,Jan,11

64802 **Sympathectomy, cervical**
24.3 24.3 FUD 090 J A2 80 50
AMA: 2014,Jan,11

64804 **Sympathectomy, cervicothoracic**
34.1 34.1 FUD 090 J 80 50
AMA: 2014,Jan,11

64809 **Sympathectomy, thoracolumbar**
INCLUDES Leriche sympathectomy
31.8 31.8 FUD 090 C 80 50
AMA: 2014,Jan,11

64818 **Sympathectomy, lumbar**
22.5 22.5 FUD 090 C 80 50
AMA: 2014,Jan,11

64820 **Sympathectomy; digital arteries, each digit**
INCLUDES Operating microscope (69990)
21.0 21.0 FUD 090 J G2
AMA: 2018,Jan,8; 2017,Jan,8; 2016,Feb,12; 2016,Jan,13; 2015,Jan,16

64821 **radial artery**
INCLUDES Operating microscope (69990)
20.0 20.0 FUD 090 J A2 50
AMA: 2016,Feb,12

64822 **ulnar artery**
INCLUDES Operating microscope (69990)
20.0 20.0 FUD 090 J G2 50
AMA: 2016,Feb,12

64823 **superficial palmar arch**
INCLUDES Operating microscope (69990)
22.7 22.7 FUD 090 J G2 50
AMA: 2016,Feb,12

64831-64907 Nerve Repair: Suture and Nerve Grafts

64831 **Suture of digital nerve, hand or foot; 1 nerve**
19.7 19.7 FUD 090 J A2 50
AMA: 2018,Jan,8; 2017,Jan,8; 2016,Jan,13; 2015,Jan,16

\+ **64832** **each additional digital nerve (List separately in addition to code for primary procedure)**
Code first (64831)
9.73 9.73 FUD ZZZ N N1 80
AMA: 2018,Jan,8; 2017,Jan,8; 2016,Jan,13; 2015,Jan,16

64834 **Suture of 1 nerve; hand or foot, common sensory nerve**
21.3 21.3 FUD 090 J A2 80 50
AMA: 2014,Jan,11

64835 **median motor thenar**
23.4 23.4 FUD 090 J A2 80 50
AMA: 2014,Jan,11

64836 **ulnar motor**
23.5 23.5 FUD 090 J A2 80 50
AMA: 2014,Jan,11

\+ **64837** **Suture of each additional nerve, hand or foot (List separately in addition to code for primary procedure)**
Code first (64834-64836)
10.6 10.6 FUD ZZZ N N1 80
AMA: 2014,Jan,11

64840 **Suture of posterior tibial nerve**
27.8 27.8 FUD 090 J A2 80 50
AMA: 2014,Jan,11

64856 **Suture of major peripheral nerve, arm or leg, except sciatic; including transposition**
29.2 29.2 FUD 090 J A2
AMA: 2014,Jan,11

64857 **without transposition**
30.4 30.4 FUD 090 J A2 80
AMA: 2014,Jan,11

64858 **Suture of sciatic nerve**
34.0 34.0 FUD 090 J A2 80 50
AMA: 2014,Jan,11

+ **64859** **Suture of each additional major peripheral nerve (List separately in addition to code for primary procedure)**
Code first (64856-64857)
7.19 7.19 FUD ZZZ N N1 80
AMA: 2014,Jan,11

64861 **Suture of; brachial plexus**
43.7 43.7 FUD 090 J A2 80 50
AMA: 2014,Jan,11

64862 **lumbar plexus**
39.3 39.3 FUD 090 J A2 80 50
AMA: 2014,Jan,11

64864 **Suture of facial nerve; extracranial**
24.9 24.9 FUD 090 J A2 80
AMA: 2014,Jan,11

64865 **infratemporal, with or without grafting**
31.4 31.4 FUD 090 J A2 80
AMA: 2014,Jan,11

64866 **Anastomosis; facial-spinal accessory**
36.7 36.7 FUD 090 C 80
AMA: 2014,Jan,11

64868 **facial-hypoglossal**
INCLUDES Korte-Ballance anastomosis
28.8 28.8 FUD 090 C 80
AMA: 2014,Jan,11

+ **64872** **Suture of nerve; requiring secondary or delayed suture (List separately in addition to code for primary neurorrhaphy)**
Code first (64831-64865)
3.39 3.39 FUD ZZZ N N1 80
AMA: 2014,Jan,11

+ **64874** **requiring extensive mobilization, or transposition of nerve (List separately in addition to code for nerve suture)**
Code first (64831-64865)
5.05 5.05 FUD ZZZ N N1 80
AMA: 2014,Jan,11

+ **64876** **requiring shortening of bone of extremity (List separately in addition to code for nerve suture)**
Code first (64831-64865)
5.71 5.71 FUD ZZZ N N1 80
AMA: 2014,Jan,11; 2003,Jan,1

64885 **Nerve graft (includes obtaining graft), head or neck; up to 4 cm in length**
32.1 32.1 FUD 090 J A2 80
AMA: 2018,Jan,8; 2017,Dec,12; 2017,Jan,8; 2016,Jan,13; 2015,Jan,16

64886 **more than 4 cm length**
37.2 37.2 FUD 090 J A2 80
AMA: 2018,Jan,8; 2017,Dec,12; 2017,Jan,8; 2016,Jan,13; 2015,Jan,16

64890 **Nerve graft (includes obtaining graft), single strand, hand or foot; up to 4 cm length**
31.2 31.2 FUD 090 J A2 80
AMA: 2018,Jan,8; 2017,Dec,12; 2017,Jan,8; 2016,Jan,13; 2015,Aug,8; 2015,Apr,10

64891 **more than 4 cm length**
33.2 33.2 FUD 090 J J8 80
AMA: 2018,Jan,8; 2017,Dec,12

64892 **Nerve graft (includes obtaining graft), single strand, arm or leg; up to 4 cm length**
30.1 30.1 FUD 090 J A2 80
AMA: 2018,Jan,8; 2017,Dec,12

64893 **more than 4 cm length**
32.4 32.4 FUD 090 J G2 80
AMA: 2018,Jan,8; 2017,Dec,12

64895 **Nerve graft (includes obtaining graft), multiple strands (cable), hand or foot; up to 4 cm length**
38.2 38.2 FUD 090 J A2 80
AMA: 2018,Jan,8; 2017,Dec,12; 2017,Jan,8; 2016,Jan,13; 2015,Jan,16

64896 **more than 4 cm length**
41.4 41.4 FUD 090 J A2 80
AMA: 2018,Jan,8; 2017,Dec,12; 2017,Jan,8; 2016,Jan,13; 2015,Jan,16

64897 **Nerve graft (includes obtaining graft), multiple strands (cable), arm or leg; up to 4 cm length**
36.4 36.4 FUD 090 J G2 80
AMA: 2018,Jan,8; 2017,Dec,12; 2017,Jan,8; 2016,Jan,13; 2015,Jan,16

64898 **more than 4 cm length**
39.6 39.6 FUD 090 J A2 80
AMA: 2018,Jan,8; 2017,Dec,12; 2017,Jan,8; 2016,Jan,13; 2015,Jan,16

+ **64901** **Nerve graft, each additional nerve; single strand (List separately in addition to code for primary procedure)**
Code first (64885-64893)
17.4 17.4 FUD ZZZ N N1 80
AMA: 2018,Jan,8; 2017,Dec,12; 2017,Jan,8; 2016,Jan,13; 2015,Jan,16

+ **64902** **multiple strands (cable) (List separately in addition to code for primary procedure)**
Code first (64885-64886, 64895-64898)
20.1 20.1 FUD ZZZ N N1 80
AMA: 2018,Jan,8; 2017,Dec,12; 2017,Jan,8; 2016,Jan,13; 2015,Jan,16

64905 **Nerve pedicle transfer; first stage**
29.4 29.4 FUD 090 J A2 80
AMA: 2018,Jan,8; 2017,Dec,12

64907 **second stage**
37.7 37.7 FUD 090 J A2 80
AMA: 2018,Jan,8; 2017,Dec,12

64910-64999 Nerve Repair: Synthetic and Vein Grafts

64910 Nerve repair; with synthetic conduit or vein allograft (eg, nerve tube), each nerve

INCLUDES Operating microscope (69990)

22.7 22.7 FUD 090 J J8 80

AMA: 2018,Jan,8; 2017,Dec,12; 2017,Jan,8; 2016,Jan,13; 2015,Aug,8; 2015,Apr,10; 2015,Jan,16

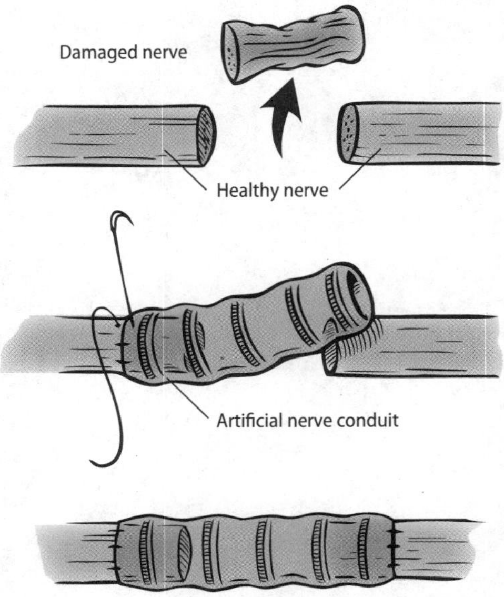

A synthetic "bridge" is affixed to each end of a severed nerve with sutures
The procedure is performed using an operating microscope

64911 with autogenous vein graft (includes harvest of vein graft), each nerve

INCLUDES Operating microscope (69990)

29.5 29.5 FUD 090 J 80

AMA: 2018,Jan,8; 2017,Dec,12; 2017,Jan,8; 2016,Jan,13; 2015,Jan,16

64912 with nerve allograft, each nerve, first strand (cable)

INCLUDES Operating microscope (69990)

26.3 26.3 FUD 090 J J8 80

AMA: 2018,Jan,8; 2017,Dec,12

\+ **64913 with nerve allograft, each additional strand (List separately in addition to code for primary procedure)**

INCLUDES Operating microscope (69990)

Code first (64912)

5.16 5.16 FUD ZZZ N N1 80

AMA: 2018,Jan,8; 2017,Dec,12

64999 Unlisted procedure, nervous system

0.00 0.00 FUD YYY T 80

AMA: 2020,Jun,14; 2020,Feb,13; 2019,Dec,12; 2019,Jul,10; 2019,May,10; 2019,Apr,9; 2018,Dec,8; 2018,Dec,8; 2018,Oct,11; 2018,Oct,8; 2018,Aug,10; 2018,Mar,9; 2018,Jan,8; 2018,Jan,7; 2017,Dec,12; 2017,Dec,13; 2017,Dec,14; 2017,Jan,8; 2016,Nov,6; 2016,Oct,11; 2016,Feb,13; 2016,Jan,13; 2015,Oct,9; 2015,Aug,8; 2015,Jul,10; 2015,Apr,10; 2015,Feb,9; 2015,Jan,16

65091-65093 Surgical Removal of Eyeball Contents

INCLUDES Operating microscope (69990)

65091 **Evisceration of ocular contents; without implant**
18.4 18.4 FUD 090 J A2 80 50
AMA: 2016,Feb,12

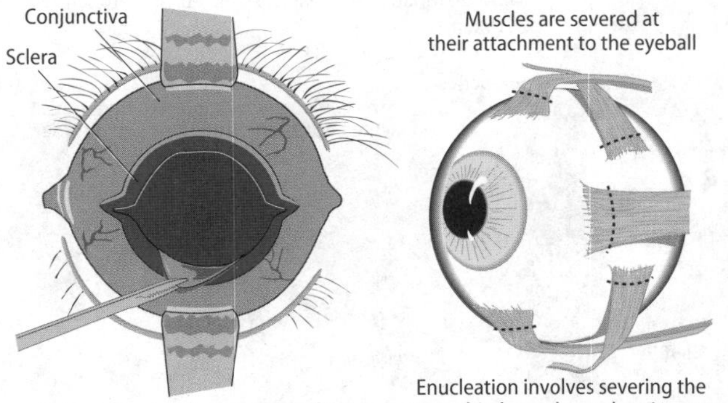

Evisceration involves removal of the contents of the eyeball: the vitreous; retina; choroid; lens; iris; and ciliary muscle. Only the scleral shell remains. A temporary or permanent implant is usually inserted

Enucleation involves severing the extraorbital muscles and optic nerve with removal of the eyeball. An implant is usually inserted and, if permanent, may involve attachment to the severed extraorbital muscles

65093 **with implant**
18.2 18.2 FUD 090 J A2 50
AMA: 2016,Feb,12

65101-65105 Surgical Removal of Eyeball

INCLUDES Operating microscope (69990)

EXCLUDES *Conjunctivoplasty following enucleation (68320-68328)*

65101 **Enucleation of eye; without implant**
21.3 21.3 FUD 090 J A2 50
AMA: 2016,Feb,12

65103 **with implant, muscles not attached to implant**
22.2 22.2 FUD 090 J A2 50
AMA: 2016,Feb,12

65105 **with implant, muscles attached to implant**
24.4 24.4 FUD 090 J A2 80 50
AMA: 2016,Feb,12

65110-65114 Surgical Removal of Orbital Contents

INCLUDES Operating microscope (69990)

EXCLUDES *Free full thickness graft (15260-15261)*
Repair more extensive than skin (67930-67975)
Skin graft (15120-15121)

65110 **Exenteration of orbit (does not include skin graft), removal of orbital contents; only**
36.0 36.0 FUD 090 J A2 80 50
AMA: 2016,Feb,12

65112 **with therapeutic removal of bone**
40.5 40.5 FUD 090 J A2 80 50
AMA: 2016,Feb,12

65114 **with muscle or myocutaneous flap**
43.4 43.4 FUD 090 J A2 80 50
AMA: 2016,Feb,12

65125-65175 Implant Procedures: Insertion, Removal, and Revision

INCLUDES Ocular implant procedures (inside muscle cone)
Operating microscope (69990)

EXCLUDES *Orbital implant insertion (outside muscle cone) (67550)*
Orbital implant removal or revision (outside muscle cone) (67560)

65125 **Modification of ocular implant with placement or replacement of pegs (eg, drilling receptacle for prosthesis appendage) (separate procedure)**
8.26 12.9 FUD 090 J G2 50
AMA: 2016,Feb,12

65130 **Insertion of ocular implant secondary; after evisceration, in scleral shell**
21.1 21.1 FUD 090 J A2 50
AMA: 2016,Feb,12

65135 **after enucleation, muscles not attached to implant**
22.6 22.6 FUD 090 J A2 50
AMA: 2016,Feb,12

65140 **after enucleation, muscles attached to implant**
23.3 23.3 FUD 090 J A2 50
AMA: 2016,Feb,12

65150 **Reinsertion of ocular implant; with or without conjunctival graft**
18.0 18.0 FUD 090 J A2 80 50
AMA: 2016,Feb,12

65155 **with use of foreign material for reinforcement and/or attachment of muscles to implant**
24.4 24.4 FUD 090 J A2 50
AMA: 2016,Feb,12

65175 **Removal of ocular implant**
19.0 19.0 FUD 090 J A2 50
AMA: 2016,Feb,12

65205-65265 Foreign Body Removal By Area of Eye

INCLUDES Operating microscope (69990)

EXCLUDES *Removal foreign body:*
Eyelid (67938)
Lacrimal system (68530)
Orbit:
Frontal approach (67413)
Lateral approach (67430)
Removal implant:
Anterior segment (65920)
Ocular (65175)
Orbital (67560)
Posterior segment (67120)

65205 **Removal of foreign body, external eye; conjunctival superficial**
(70030, 76529)
1.02 1.31 FUD 000 Q1 N1 50
AMA: 2018,Jan,8; 2017,Jan,8; 2016,Feb,12; 2016,Jan,13; 2015,Jan,16

65210 **conjunctival embedded (includes concretions), subconjunctival, or scleral nonperforating**
(70030, 76529)
1.04 1.30 FUD 000 Q1 N1 50
AMA: 2016,Feb,12

65220 **corneal, without slit lamp**
EXCLUDES *Repair corneal wound with foreign body (65275)*
(70030, 76529)
1.19 1.68 FUD 000 Q1 N1 50
AMA: 2018,Jan,8; 2017,Jan,8; 2016,Feb,12; 2016,Jan,13; 2015,Jan,16

65222 **corneal, with slit lamp**
EXCLUDES *Repair corneal wound with foreign body (65275)*
(70030, 76529)
1.48 1.93 FUD 000 Q1 N1 50
AMA: 2018,Jan,8; 2017,Jan,8; 2016,Feb,12; 2016,Jan,13; 2015,Jan,16

65235 **Removal of foreign body, intraocular; from anterior chamber of eye or lens**
EXCLUDES *Removal implanted material from anterior segment (65920)*
(70030, 76529)
20.2 20.2 FUD 090 J A2 80 50
AMA: 2018,Jan,8; 2017,Jan,8; 2016,Feb,12; 2016,Jan,13; 2015,Jan,16

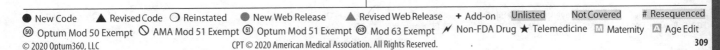

65260 **from posterior segment, magnetic extraction, anterior or posterior route**

EXCLUDES *Removal implanted material from posterior segment (67120)*

(70030, 76529)

27.4 27.4 FUD 090 J A2 80 50

AMA: 2016,Feb,12

65265 **from posterior segment, nonmagnetic extraction**

EXCLUDES *Removal implanted material from posterior segment (67120)*

(70030, 76529)

30.9 30.9 FUD 090 J A2 80 50

AMA: 2016,Feb,12

65270-65290 Laceration Repair External Eye

INCLUDES Conjunctival flap
Operating microscope (69990)
Restoration anterior chamber with air or saline injection

EXCLUDES *Repair:*
Ciliary body or iris (66680)
Eyelid laceration (12011-12018, 12051-12057, 13151-13160, 67930, 67935)
Lacrimal system injury (68700)
Surgical wound (66250)
Treatment orbit fracture (21385-21408)

65270 **Repair of laceration; conjunctiva, with or without nonperforating laceration sclera, direct closure**

4.01 7.79 FUD 010 J A2 80 50

AMA: 2018,Jan,8; 2017,Jan,8; 2016,Feb,12; 2016,Jan,13; 2015,Jan,16

65272 **conjunctiva, by mobilization and rearrangement, without hospitalization**

10.0 14.5 FUD 090 J A2 50

AMA: 2016,Feb,12

65273 **conjunctiva, by mobilization and rearrangement, with hospitalization**

10.8 10.8 FUD 090 C 50

AMA: 2016,Feb,12

65275 **cornea, nonperforating, with or without removal foreign body**

13.1 16.5 FUD 090 J A2 80 50

AMA: 2016,Feb,12

65280 **cornea and/or sclera, perforating, not involving uveal tissue**

EXCLUDES *Procedure performed for surgical wound repair*

19.1 19.1 FUD 090 J A2 80 50

AMA: 2018,Jan,8; 2017,Jan,8; 2016,Feb,12; 2016,Jan,13; 2015,Jan,16

65285 **cornea and/or sclera, perforating, with reposition or resection of uveal tissue**

EXCLUDES *Procedure performed for surgical wound repair*

31.4 31.4 FUD 090 J A2 50

AMA: 2018,Jan,8; 2017,Jan,8; 2016,Feb,12; 2016,Jan,13; 2015,Jan,16

65286 **application of tissue glue, wounds of cornea and/or sclera**

14.1 20.0 FUD 090 J P3 50

AMA: 2018,Jan,8; 2017,Jan,8; 2016,Feb,12; 2016,Jan,13; 2015,Jan,16

65290 **Repair of wound, extraocular muscle, tendon and/or Tenon's capsule**

13.9 13.9 FUD 090 J A2 50

AMA: 2016,Feb,12

65400-65600 Removal Corneal Lesions

INCLUDES Operating microscope (69990)

65400 **Excision of lesion, cornea (keratectomy, lamellar, partial), except pterygium**

17.1 19.4 FUD 090 T A2 50

AMA: 2018,Jan,8; 2017,Jan,8; 2016,Feb,12; 2016,Jan,13; 2015,Jan,16

65410 **Biopsy of cornea**

2.96 4.11 FUD 000 J A2 80 50

AMA: 2018,Jan,8; 2017,Jan,8; 2016,Feb,12; 2016,Jan,13; 2015,Jan,16

65420 **Excision or transposition of pterygium; without graft**

10.7 14.9 FUD 090 J A2 50

AMA: 2018,Jan,8; 2017,Jan,8; 2016,Feb,12; 2016,Jan,13; 2015,Jan,16

The conjunctiva is subject to numerous acute and chronic irritations and disorders

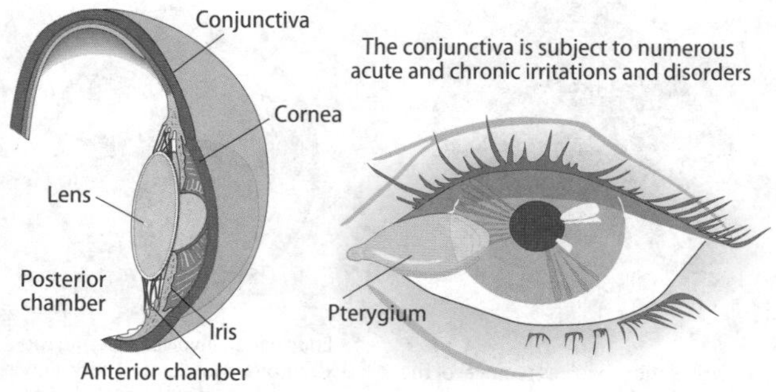

65426 **with graft**

13.6 18.7 FUD 090 J A2 50

AMA: 2018,May,10; 2018,Jan,8; 2017,Jan,8; 2016,Feb,12; 2016,Jan,13; 2015,Jan,16

65430 **Scraping of cornea, diagnostic, for smear and/or culture**

2.90 3.28 FUD 000 Q1 N1 50

AMA: 2016,Feb,12

65435 **Removal of corneal epithelium; with or without chemocauterization (abrasion, curettage)**

EXCLUDES *Collagen cross-linking, cornea (0402T)*

1.98 2.32 FUD 000 T P3 50

AMA: 2018,Jan,8; 2017,Jan,8; 2016,Feb,12; 2016,Jan,13; 2015,Jan,16

65436 **with application of chelating agent (eg, EDTA)**

10.4 10.9 FUD 090 J P3 50

AMA: 2016,Feb,12

65450 **Destruction of lesion of cornea by cryotherapy, photocoagulation or thermocauterization**

9.15 9.30 FUD 090 T G2 50

AMA: 2016,Feb,12

65600 **Multiple punctures of anterior cornea (eg, for corneal erosion, tattoo)**

9.74 11.3 FUD 090 J P3 50

AMA: 2016,Feb,12

65710-65757 Corneal Transplants

CMS: 100-03,80.7 Refractive Keratoplasty

INCLUDES Operating microscope (69990)

EXCLUDES *Computerized corneal topography (92025)*
Processing, preserving, and transporting corneal tissue (V2785)

65710 **Keratoplasty (corneal transplant); anterior lamellar**

INCLUDES Use and preparation fresh or preserved graft

EXCLUDES *Refractive keratoplasty surgery (65760-65767)*

31.7 31.7 FUD 090 J A2 80 50

AMA: 2018,Jan,8; 2017,Jan,8; 2016,Feb,12; 2016,Jan,13; 2015,Jan,16

65730 **penetrating (except in aphakia or pseudophakia)**

INCLUDES Use and preparation fresh or preserved graft

EXCLUDES *Refractive keratoplasty surgery (65760-65767)*

35.1 35.1 FUD 090 J A2 80 50

AMA: 2018,Jan,8; 2017,Jan,8; 2016,Feb,12; 2016,Jan,13; 2015,Jan,16

310 CPT © 2020 American Medical Association. All Rights Reserved. © 2020 Optum360, LLC

65750 **penetrating (in aphakia)**

INCLUDES Use and preparation fresh or preserved graft

EXCLUDES *Refractive keratoplasty surgery (65760-65767)*

35.4 35.4 FUD 090 J A2 80 50

AMA: 2018,Jan,8; 2017,Jan,8; 2016,Feb,12; 2016,Jan,13; 2015,Jan,16

65755 **penetrating (in pseudophakia)**

INCLUDES Use and preparation fresh or preserved graft

EXCLUDES *Refractive keratoplasty surgery (65760-65767)*

35.1 35.1 FUD 090 J A2 80 50

AMA: 2018,Jan,8; 2017,Jan,8; 2016,Feb,12; 2016,Jan,13; 2015,Jan,16

65756 **endothelial**

EXCLUDES *Refractive keratoplasty surgery (65760-65767)*

Code also donor material

Code also when appropriate (65757)

33.6 33.6 FUD 090 J G2 80 50

AMA: 2018,Jan,8; 2017,Jan,8; 2016,Feb,12; 2016,Jan,13; 2015,Jan,16

\+ **65757** **Backbench preparation of corneal endothelial allograft prior to transplantation (List separately in addition to code for primary procedure)**

Code first (65756)

0.00 0.00 FUD ZZZ N N1 80

AMA: 2018,Jan,8; 2017,Jan,8; 2016,Feb,12; 2016,Jan,13; 2015,Jan,16

65760-65785 Corneal Refractive Procedures

CMS: 100-03,80.7 Refractive Keratoplasty

INCLUDES Operating microscope (69990)

EXCLUDES *Unlisted corneal procedures (66999)*

65760 **Keratomileusis**

EXCLUDES *Computerized corneal topography (92025)*

0.00 0.00 FUD XXX E

AMA: 2016,Feb,12

65765 **Keratophakia**

EXCLUDES *Computerized corneal topography (92025)*

0.00 0.00 FUD XXX E

AMA: 2016,Feb,12

65767 **Epikeratoplasty**

EXCLUDES *Computerized corneal topography (92025)*

0.00 0.00 FUD XXX E

AMA: 2016,Feb,12

65770 **Keratoprosthesis**

EXCLUDES *Computerized corneal topography (92025)*

39.6 39.6 FUD 090 J J8 80 50

AMA: 2016,Feb,12

65771 **Radial keratotomy**

EXCLUDES *Computerized corneal topography (92025)*

0.00 0.00 FUD XXX E

AMA: 2016,Feb,12

65772 **Corneal relaxing incision for correction of surgically induced astigmatism**

11.5 12.8 FUD 090 T A2 50

AMA: 2016,Feb,12

65775 **Corneal wedge resection for correction of surgically induced astigmatism**

EXCLUDES *Fitting contact lens to treat disease (92071-92072)*

15.8 15.8 FUD 090 J A2 50

AMA: 2018,Jan,8; 2017,Jan,8; 2016,Feb,12; 2016,Jan,13; 2015,Jan,16

65778 **Placement of amniotic membrane on the ocular surface; without sutures**

EXCLUDES *Ocular surface reconstruction (65780)*
Removal corneal epithelium (65435)
Scraping cornea, diagnostic (65430)
Using tissue glue to place amniotic membrane (66999)

1.58 40.0 FUD 000 Q2 N1 80 50

AMA: 2018,Feb,11; 2018,Jan,8; 2017,Jan,8; 2016,Feb,12; 2016,Jan,13; 2015,Jan,16

65779 **single layer, sutured**

EXCLUDES *Ocular surface reconstruction (65780)*
Removal corneal epithelium (65435)
Scraping cornea, diagnostic (65430)
Using tissue glue to place amniotic membrane (66999)

4.32 34.5 FUD 000 Q2 N1 80 50

AMA: 2018,Feb,11; 2018,Jan,8; 2017,Jan,8; 2016,Feb,12; 2016,Jan,13; 2015,Jan,16

65780 **Ocular surface reconstruction; amniotic membrane transplantation, multiple layers**

EXCLUDES *Placement amniotic membrane without reconstruction without sutures or single layer sutures (65778-65779)*

18.9 18.9 FUD 090 J A2 50

AMA: 2018,Feb,11; 2018,Jan,8; 2017,Jan,8; 2016,Feb,12; 2016,Jan,13; 2015,Jan,16

65781 **limbal stem cell allograft (eg, cadaveric or living donor)**

37.9 37.9 FUD 090 J A2 80 50

AMA: 2018,Jan,8; 2017,Jan,8; 2016,Feb,12; 2016,Jan,13; 2015,Jan,16

65782 **limbal conjunctival autograft (includes obtaining graft)**

EXCLUDES *Conjunctival allograft harvest from living donor (68371)*

32.6 32.6 FUD 090 J A2 50

AMA: 2018,Jan,8; 2017,Jan,8; 2016,Feb,12; 2016,Jan,13; 2015,Jan,16

65785 **Implantation of intrastromal corneal ring segments**

12.6 71.4 FUD 090 J P2 50

AMA: 2016,Feb,12

65800-66030 Anterior Segment Procedures

INCLUDES Operating microscope (69990)

EXCLUDES *Unlisted procedures anterior segment (66999)*

65800 **Paracentesis of anterior chamber of eye (separate procedure); with removal of aqueous**

EXCLUDES *Insertion ocular telescope prosthesis (0308T)*

2.58 3.39 FUD 000 J A2 50

AMA: 2018,Jan,8; 2017,Jan,8; 2016,Feb,12; 2016,Jan,13; 2015,Jan,16

65810 **with removal of vitreous and/or discission of anterior hyaloid membrane, with or without air injection**

EXCLUDES *Insertion ocular telescope prosthesis (0308T)*

13.2 13.2 FUD 090 J A2 50

AMA: 2018,Jan,8; 2017,Jan,8; 2016,Feb,12; 2016,Jan,13; 2015,Jan,16

65815 **with removal of blood, with or without irrigation and/or air injection**

EXCLUDES *Injection only (66020-66030)*
Insertion ocular telescope prosthesis (0308T)
Removal blood clot only (65930)

13.5 18.2 FUD 090 J A2 50

AMA: 2018,Jan,8; 2017,Jan,8; 2016,Feb,12; 2016,Jan,13; 2015,Jan,16

65820 **Goniotomy**

INCLUDES Barkan's operation

Code also ophthalmic endoscope if used (66990)

21.5 21.5 FUD 090 63 J A2 80 50

AMA: 2019,Sep,10; 2018,Dec,8; 2018,Dec,8; 2018,Jul,3; 2018,Jan,8; 2017,Jan,8; 2016,Feb,12; 2016,Jan,13; 2015,Jan,16

65850 Trabeculotomy ab externo
23.8 23.8 FUD 090 J A2 50
AMA: 2016,Feb,12

65855 Trabeculoplasty by laser surgery
EXCLUDES *Severing adhesions anterior segment (65860-65880)*
Trabeculectomy ab externo (66170)
5.87 6.99 FUD 010 T P3 50
AMA: 2018,Jan,8; 2017,Jan,8; 2016,Feb,12; 2016,Jan,13; 2015,Jan,16

65860 Severing adhesions of anterior segment, laser technique (separate procedure)
7.18 8.81 FUD 090 T P3 80 50
AMA: 2016,Feb,12

65865 Severing adhesions of anterior segment of eye, incisional technique (with or without injection of air or liquid) (separate procedure); goniosynechiae
EXCLUDES *Laser trabeculectomy (65855)*
13.4 13.4 FUD 090 J A2 50
AMA: 2016,Feb,12

65870 anterior synechiae, except goniosynechiae
16.7 16.7 FUD 090 J A2 50
AMA: 2016,Feb,12

65875 posterior synechiae
Code also ophthalmic endoscope when used (66990)
17.9 17.9 FUD 090 J A2 50
AMA: 2018,Jan,8; 2017,Jan,8; 2016,Feb,12; 2016,Jan,13; 2015,Jan,16

65880 corneovitreal adhesions
EXCLUDES *Laser procedure (66821)*
18.8 18.8 FUD 090 J A2 50
AMA: 2016,Feb,12

65900 Removal of epithelial downgrowth, anterior chamber of eye
27.6 27.6 FUD 090 J A2 80 50
AMA: 2016,Feb,12

65920 Removal of implanted material, anterior segment of eye
Code also ophthalmic endoscope when used (66990)
22.3 22.3 FUD 090 J A2 50
AMA: 2018,Jan,8; 2017,Jan,8; 2016,Feb,12; 2016,Jan,13; 2015,Jan,16

65930 Removal of blood clot, anterior segment of eye
18.1 18.1 FUD 090 J A2 50
AMA: 2016,Feb,12

66020 Injection, anterior chamber of eye (separate procedure); air or liquid
EXCLUDES *Insertion ocular telescope prosthesis (0308T)*
3.74 5.43 FUD 010 J A2 50
AMA: 2018,Jan,8; 2017,Jan,8; 2016,Feb,12; 2016,Jan,13; 2015,Jan,16

66030 medication
EXCLUDES *Insertion ocular telescope prosthesis (0308T)*
3.16 4.87 FUD 010 J A2 50
AMA: 2016,Feb,12

66130 Excision Scleral Lesion

INCLUDES Operating microscope (69990)
EXCLUDES *Removal intraocular foreign body (65235)*
Surgery on posterior sclera (67250, 67255)

66130 Excision of lesion, sclera
16.1 19.9 FUD 090 J A2 80 50
AMA: 2016,Feb,12

66150-66185 Procedures for Glaucoma

INCLUDES Operating microscope (69990)
EXCLUDES *Removal intraocular foreign body (65235)*
Surgery on posterior sclera (67250, 67255)

66150 Fistulization of sclera for glaucoma; trephination with iridectomy
24.9 24.9 FUD 090 J A2 50
AMA: 2018,Jul,3; 2016,Feb,12

66155 thermocauterization with iridectomy
24.8 24.8 FUD 090 J A2 50
AMA: 2018,Jul,3; 2016,Feb,12

66160 sclerectomy with punch or scissors, with iridectomy
INCLUDES Knapp's operation
28.1 28.1 FUD 090 J A2 50
AMA: 2018,Jul,3; 2016,Feb,12

66170 trabeculectomy ab externo in absence of previous surgery
EXCLUDES *Repair surgical wound (66250)*
Trabeculectomy ab externo (65850)
30.9 30.9 FUD 090 J A2 80 50
AMA: 2018,Dec,8; 2018,Dec,10; 2018,Dec,8; 2018,Dec,10; 2018,Jul,3; 2018,Jan,8; 2017,Jan,8; 2016,Feb,12; 2016,Jan,13; 2015,Jan,16

66172 trabeculectomy ab externo with scarring from previous ocular surgery or trauma (includes injection of antifibrotic agents)
33.9 33.9 FUD 090 J A2 80 50
AMA: 2019,Apr,7; 2018,Dec,10; 2018,Dec,10; 2018,Jul,3; 2018,Jan,8; 2017,Jan,8; 2016,Feb,12; 2016,Jan,13; 2015,Jan,16

66174 Transluminal dilation of aqueous outflow canal; without retention of device or stent
26.9 26.9 FUD 090 J A2 80 50
AMA: 2019,Sep,10; 2018,Dec,8; 2018,Dec,8; 2016,Feb,12

66175 with retention of device or stent
28.2 28.2 FUD 090 J A2 80 50
AMA: 2016,Feb,12

66179 Aqueous shunt to extraocular equatorial plate reservoir, external approach; without graft
30.6 30.6 FUD 090 J G2 80 50
AMA: 2018,Jul,3; 2018,Jan,8; 2017,Jan,8; 2016,Feb,12; 2016,Jan,13; 2015,Jan,10

66180 with graft
EXCLUDES *Scleral reinforcement (67255)*
32.3 32.3 FUD 090 J J8 80 50
AMA: 2018,Jul,3; 2018,Jan,8; 2017,Jan,8; 2016,Feb,12; 2016,Jan,13; 2015,Jan,16; 2015,Jan,10

66183 Insertion of anterior segment aqueous drainage device, without extraocular reservoir, external approach
29.2 29.2 FUD 090 J J8 80 50
AMA: 2020,Jun,14; 2018,Jul,3; 2018,Jan,8; 2017,Jan,8; 2016,Feb,12; 2016,Jan,13; 2015,Jan,16

66184 Revision of aqueous shunt to extraocular equatorial plate reservoir; without graft
22.3 22.3 FUD 090 J G2 80 50
AMA: 2018,Jan,8; 2017,Jan,8; 2016,Feb,12; 2016,Jan,13; 2015,Jan,10

66185 with graft
EXCLUDES *Removal implanted shunt (67120)*
Scleral reinforcement (67255)
23.9 23.9 FUD 090 J A2 80 50
AMA: 2018,Jan,8; 2017,Jan,8; 2016,Feb,12; 2016,Jan,13; 2015,Jan,10

66225 Staphyloma Repair

INCLUDES Operating microscope (69990)

EXCLUDES *Scleral procedures with retinal procedures (67101-67228)*
Scleral reinforcement (67250, 67255)

66225 **Repair of scleral staphyloma; with graft**
26.5 26.5 FUD 090 J A2 50
AMA: 2016,Feb,12

66250 Anterior Segment Operative Wound Revision or Repair

INCLUDES Operating microscope (69990)

EXCLUDES *Unlisted procedures anterior sclera (66999)*

66250 **Revision or repair of operative wound of anterior segment, any type, early or late, major or minor procedure**
15.8 21.4 FUD 090 J A2 50
AMA: 2018,Dec,8; 2018,Dec,8; 2018,Jan,8; 2017,Jan,8; 2016,Feb,12; 2016,Jan,13; 2015,Jan,16

66500-66505 Iridotomy With/Without Transfixion

INCLUDES Operating microscope (69990)

EXCLUDES *Photocoagulation iridotomy (66761)*

66500 **Iridotomy by stab incision (separate procedure); except transfixion**
10.5 10.5 FUD 090 J A2 50
AMA: 2016,Feb,12

66505 **with transfixion as for iris bombe**
11.5 11.5 FUD 090 J A2 50
AMA: 2016,Feb,12

66600-66635 Iridectomy Procedures

INCLUDES Operating microscope (69990)

EXCLUDES *Insertion ocular telescope prosthesis (0308T)*
Photocoagulation coreoplasty (66762)

66600 **Iridectomy, with corneoscleral or corneal section; for removal of lesion**
23.9 23.9 FUD 090 J A2 50
AMA: 2016,Feb,12

66605 **with cyclectomy**
30.3 30.3 FUD 090 J A2 50
AMA: 2016,Feb,12

66625 **peripheral for glaucoma (separate procedure)**
12.2 12.2 FUD 090 J A2 50
AMA: 2016,Feb,12

66630 **sector for glaucoma (separate procedure)**
16.1 16.1 FUD 090 J A2 50
AMA: 2016,Feb,12

66635 **optical (separate procedure)**
16.2 16.2 FUD 090 J A2 50
AMA: 2016,Feb,12

66680-66770 Other Procedures of the Uveal Tract

INCLUDES Operating microscope (69990)

EXCLUDES *Unlisted procedures ciliary body or iris (66999)*

66680 **Repair of iris, ciliary body (as for iridodialysis)**
EXCLUDES *Resection/repositioning uveal tissue for perforating laceration, cornea and/or sclera (65285)*
14.7 14.7 FUD 090 J A2 50
AMA: 2016,Feb,12

66682 **Suture of iris, ciliary body (separate procedure) with retrieval of suture through small incision (eg, McCannel suture)**
19.0 19.0 FUD 090 J A2 50
AMA: 2016,Feb,12

66700 **Ciliary body destruction; diathermy**
INCLUDES Heine's operation
11.1 12.8 FUD 090 J A2 80 50
AMA: 2016,Feb,12

66710 **cyclophotocoagulation, transscleral**
11.0 12.5 FUD 090 J A2 50
AMA: 2018,Jan,8; 2017,Jan,8; 2016,Feb,12; 2016,Jan,13; 2015,Jan,16

66711 **cyclophotocoagulation, endoscopic, without concomitant removal of crystalline lens**
EXCLUDES *Endoscopic cyclophotocoagulation performed in conjunction with extracapsular cataract removal with insertion lens ([66987], [66988])*
18.2 18.2 FUD 090 J A2 50
AMA: 2019,Dec,6; 2018,Jan,8; 2017,Jan,8; 2016,Feb,12; 2016,Jan,13; 2015,Jan,16

66720 **cryotherapy**
11.6 13.1 FUD 090 J A2 50
AMA: 2016,Feb,12

66740 **cyclodialysis**
11.1 12.5 FUD 090 J A2 50
AMA: 2016,Feb,12

66761 **Iridotomy/iridectomy by laser surgery (eg, for glaucoma) (per session)**
EXCLUDES *Insertion ocular telescope prosthesis (0308T)*
6.71 8.50 FUD 010 T P3 50
AMA: 2018,Jan,8; 2017,Jan,8; 2016,Feb,12; 2016,Jan,13; 2015,Jan,16

66762 **Iridoplasty by photocoagulation (1 or more sessions) (eg, for improvement of vision, for widening of anterior chamber angle)**
12.0 13.5 FUD 090 T P2 50
AMA: 2018,Jan,8; 2017,Jan,8; 2016,Feb,12; 2016,Jan,13; 2015,Jan,16

66770 **Destruction of cyst or lesion iris or ciliary body (nonexcisional procedure)**
EXCLUDES *Excision:*
Epithelial downgrowth (65900)
Iris, ciliary body lesion (66600-66605)
13.6 15.0 FUD 090 T P2 50
AMA: 2016,Feb,12

66820-66825 Post-Cataract Surgery Procedures

INCLUDES Operating microscope (69990)

66820 **Discission of secondary membranous cataract (opacified posterior lens capsule and/or anterior hyaloid); stab incision technique (Ziegler or Wheeler knife)**
12.1 12.1 FUD 090 J G2 50
AMA: 2016,Feb,12

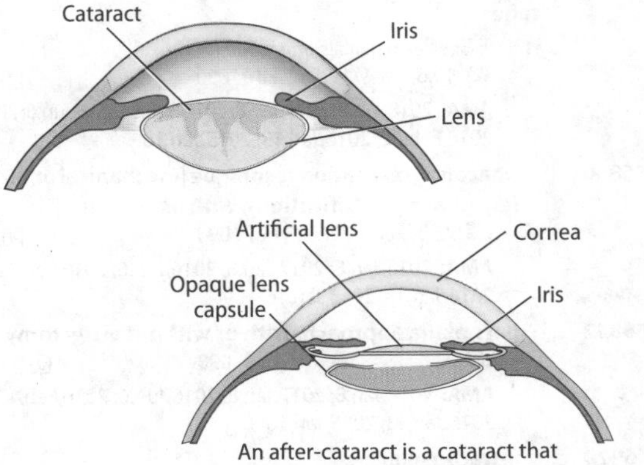

An after-cataract is a cataract that develops in a lens tissue that remains after most of the lens has already been removed

66821 **laser surgery (eg, YAG laser) (1 or more stages)**
8.81 9.40 FUD 090 T A2 50
AMA: 2016,Feb,12

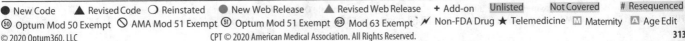

66825 **Repositioning of intraocular lens prosthesis, requiring an incision (separate procedure)**

EXCLUDES *Insertion ocular telescope prosthesis (0308T)*

21.8 21.8 **FUD** 090 J A2 80 50

AMA: 2016,Feb,12

66830-66940 Cataract Extraction; Without Insertion Intraocular Lens

CMS: 100-03,80.10 Phacoemulsification Procedure--Cataract Extraction

INCLUDES Anterior and/or posterior capsulotomy
Enzymatic zonulysis
Iridectomy/iridotomy
Lateral canthotomy
Medications
Operating microscope (69990)
Subconjunctival injection
Subtenon injection
Using viscoelastic material

EXCLUDES *Removal intralenticular foreign body without lens excision (65235)*
Repair surgical laceration (66250)

66830 **Removal of secondary membranous cataract (opacified posterior lens capsule and/or anterior hyaloid) with corneo-scleral section, with or without iridectomy (iridocapsulotomy, iridocapsulectomy)**

INCLUDES Graefe's operation

20.1 20.1 **FUD** 090 J A2 50

AMA: 2016,Feb,12

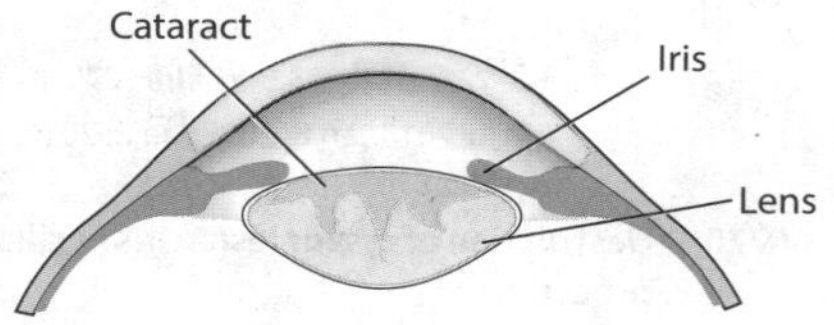

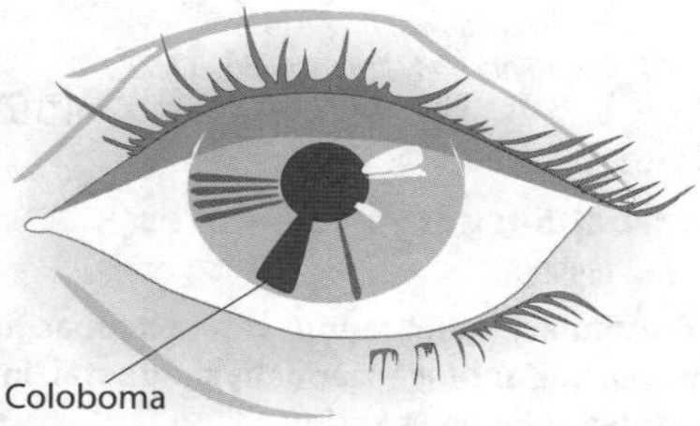

A congenital keyhole pupil is also called a coloboma of the iris

66840 **Removal of lens material; aspiration technique, 1 or more stages**

INCLUDES Fukala's operation

19.6 19.6 **FUD** 090 J A2 50

AMA: 2018,Jan,8; 2017,Jan,8; 2016,Sep,9; 2016,Jun,6; 2016,Apr,8; 2016,Feb,12; 2016,Jan,13; 2015,Jan,16

66850 **phacofragmentation technique (mechanical or ultrasonic) (eg, phacoemulsification), with aspiration**

22.3 22.3 **FUD** 090 J A2 50

AMA: 2018,Jan,8; 2017,Jan,8; 2016,Jun,6; 2016,Feb,12; 2016,Jan,13; 2015,Jan,16

66852 **pars plana approach, with or without vitrectomy**

23.8 23.8 **FUD** 090 J A2 80 50

AMA: 2018,Jan,8; 2017,Jan,8; 2016,Jun,6; 2016,Feb,12; 2016,Jan,13; 2015,Jan,16

66920 **intracapsular**

21.4 21.4 **FUD** 090 J A2 80 50

AMA: 2018,Jan,8; 2017,Jan,8; 2016,Feb,12; 2016,Jan,13; 2015,Jan,16

66930 **intracapsular, for dislocated lens**

24.3 24.3 **FUD** 090 J A2 80 50

AMA: 2018,Jan,8; 2017,Jan,8; 2016,Feb,12; 2016,Jan,13; 2015,Jan,16

66940 **extracapsular (other than 66840, 66850, 66852)**

22.1 22.1 **FUD** 090 J A2 80 50

AMA: 2018,Jan,8; 2017,Jan,8; 2016,Jun,6; 2016,Feb,12; 2016,Jan,13; 2015,Jan,16

66982-66988 [66987, 66988] Cataract Extraction: With Insertion Intraocular Lens

INCLUDES Anterior or posterior capsulotomy
Enzymatic zonulysis
Iridectomy/iridotomy
Lateral canthotomy
Medications
Operating microscope (69990)
Subconjunctival injection
Subtenon injection
Using viscoelastic material

EXCLUDES *Implanted material removal from anterior segment (65920)*
Insertion ocular telescope prosthesis (0308T)
Secondary fixation (66682)
Supply intraocular lens

66982 **Extracapsular cataract removal with insertion of intraocular lens prosthesis (1-stage procedure), manual or mechanical technique (eg, irrigation and aspiration or phacoemulsification), complex, requiring devices or techniques not generally used in routine cataract surgery (eg, iris expansion device, suture support for intraocular lens, or primary posterior capsulorrhexis) or performed on patients in the amblyogenic developmental stage; without endoscopic cyclophotocoagulation**

EXCLUDES *Complex extracapsular cataract removal in conjunction with endoscopic cyclophotocoagulation ([66987])*

(76519)

21.2 21.2 **FUD** 090 J A2 50

AMA: 2019,Dec,6; 2018,Dec,6; 2018,Dec,6; 2018,Jan,8; 2017,Dec,14; 2017,Jan,8; 2016,Mar,10; 2016,Feb,12; 2016,Jan,13; 2015,Jan,16

\# **66987** **with endoscopic cyclophotocoagulation**

EXCLUDES *Complex extracapsular cataract removal without endoscopic cyclophotocoagulation (66982)*

0.00 0.00 **FUD** 090 J8 80 50

AMA: 2019,Dec,6

66983 **Intracapsular cataract extraction with insertion of intraocular lens prosthesis (1 stage procedure)**

(76519)

21.0 21.0 **FUD** 090 J A2 50

AMA: 2019,Dec,6; 2018,Jan,8; 2017,Jan,8; 2016,Feb,12; 2016,Jan,13; 2015,Jan,16

66984 **Extracapsular cataract removal with insertion of intraocular lens prosthesis (1 stage procedure), manual or mechanical technique (eg, irrigation and aspiration or phacoemulsification); without endoscopic cyclophotocoagulation**

EXCLUDES *Complex extracapsular cataract removal (66982)*
Extracapsular cataract removal in conjunction with endoscopic cyclophotocoagulation ([66988])

(76519)

18.1 18.1 **FUD** 090 J A2 50

AMA: 2019,Dec,6; 2018,Dec,6; 2018,Dec,6; 2018,Jan,8; 2017,Jan,8; 2016,Feb,12; 2016,Jan,13; 2015,Jan,16

\# **66988** **with endoscopic cyclophotocoagulation**

EXCLUDES *Complex extracapsular cataract removal in conjunction with endoscopic cyclophotocoagulation (66987 [66987])*
Extracapsular cataract removal without endoscopic cyclophotocoagulation (66984)

0.00 0.00 **FUD** 090 J8 80 50

AMA: 2019,Dec,6

66985-66988 [66987, 66988] Secondary Insertion or Replacement of Intraocular Lens

INCLUDES Operating microscope (69990)

EXCLUDES *Implanted material removal from anterior segment (65920)*
Insertion ocular telescope prosthesis (0308T)
Secondary fixation (66682)
Supply intraocular lens

Code also ophthalmic endoscope if used (66990)

66985 Insertion of intraocular lens prosthesis (secondary implant), not associated with concurrent cataract removal

EXCLUDES *Implanted material removal from anterior segment (65920)*
Insertion lens at time of cataract procedure (66982-66984)
Insertion ocular telescope prosthesis (0308T)
Secondary fixation (66682)
Supply intraocular lens

(76519)

21.8 21.8 **FUD** 090 J A2 50

AMA: 2018,Jan,8; 2017,Jan,8; 2016,Feb,12; 2016,Jan,13; 2015,Jan,16

66986 Exchange of intraocular lens

(76519)

25.6 25.6 **FUD** 090 J A2 50

AMA: 2018,Jan,8; 2017,Jan,8; 2016,Feb,12; 2016,Jan,13; 2015,Jan,16

66987 **Resequenced code. See code following 66982.**

66988 **Resequenced code. See code following 66984.**

66990-66999 Ophthalmic Endoscopy

INCLUDES Operating microscope (69990)

\+ **66990 Use of ophthalmic endoscope (List separately in addition to code for primary procedure)**

Code first (65820, 65875, 65920, 66985-66986, 67036, 67039-67043, 67113)

2.55 2.55 **FUD** ZZZ N N1

AMA: 2018,Jul,3; 2018,Jan,8; 2017,Jan,8; 2016,Sep,5; 2016,Feb,12; 2016,Jan,13; 2015,Jan,16

66999 Unlisted procedure, anterior segment of eye

0.00 0.00 **FUD** YYY J 80 50

AMA: 2018,Jan,8; 2017,Jan,8; 2016,Apr,8; 2016,Feb,12; 2016,Jan,13; 2015,Jan,16

67005-67015 Vitrectomy: Partial and Subtotal

INCLUDES Operating microscope (69990)

67005 Removal of vitreous, anterior approach (open sky technique or limbal incision); partial removal

EXCLUDES *Anterior chamber vitrectomy by paracentesis (65810)*
Severing corneovitreal adhesions (65880)

13.4 13.4 **FUD** 090 J A2 50

AMA: 2018,Jan,8; 2017,Jan,8; 2016,Feb,12; 2016,Jan,13; 2015,Jan,16

67010 subtotal removal with mechanical vitrectomy

EXCLUDES *Anterior chamber vitrectomy by paracentesis (65810)*
Severing corneovitreal adhesions (65880)

15.3 15.3 **FUD** 090 J A2 50

AMA: 2018,Jan,8; 2017,Jan,8; 2016,Feb,12; 2016,Jan,13; 2015,Jan,16

67015 Aspiration or release of vitreous, subretinal or choroidal fluid, pars plana approach (posterior sclerotomy)

16.7 16.7 **FUD** 090 J A2 50

AMA: 2018,Jan,8; 2017,Jan,8; 2016,Sep,5; 2016,Jun,6; 2016,Feb,12

67025-67028 Intravitreal Injection/Implantation

INCLUDES Operating microscope (69990)

67025 Injection of vitreous substitute, pars plana or limbal approach (fluid-gas exchange), with or without aspiration (separate procedure)

17.8 20.9 **FUD** 090 J A2 50

AMA: 2019,Aug,10; 2018,Feb,3; 2016,Feb,12

67027 Implantation of intravitreal drug delivery system (eg, ganciclovir implant), includes concomitant removal of vitreous

EXCLUDES *Removal drug delivery system (67121)*

24.0 24.0 **FUD** 090 J A2 80 50

AMA: 2018,Feb,3; 2018,Jan,8; 2017,Jan,8; 2016,Feb,12; 2016,Jan,13; 2015,Jan,16

67028 Intravitreal injection of a pharmacologic agent (separate procedure)

2.79 2.86 **FUD** 000 S P3 50

AMA: 2018,Feb,3; 2018,Jan,8; 2017,Jan,8; 2016,Feb,12; 2016,Jan,13; 2015,Jan,16

67030-67031 Incision of Vitreous Strands/Membranes

INCLUDES Operating microscope (69990)

67030 Discission of vitreous strands (without removal), pars plana approach

15.2 15.2 **FUD** 090 J A2 50

AMA: 2016,Feb,12

67031 Severing of vitreous strands, vitreous face adhesions, sheets, membranes or opacities, laser surgery (1 or more stages)

10.1 11.1 **FUD** 090 T A2 50

AMA: 2016,Feb,12

67036-67043 Pars Plana Mechanical Vitrectomy

INCLUDES Operating microscope (69990)

EXCLUDES *Lens removal (66850)*
Removal foreign body (65260, 65265)
Unlisted vitreal procedures (67299)
Vitrectomy in retinal detachment (67108, 67113)

Code also ophthalmic endoscope if used (66990)

67036 Vitrectomy, mechanical, pars plana approach;

25.4 25.4 **FUD** 090 J A2 80 50

AMA: 2018,Jan,8; 2017,Jan,8; 2016,Sep,5; 2016,Feb,12; 2016,Jan,13; 2015,Jan,16

67039 with focal endolaser photocoagulation

27.2 27.2 **FUD** 090 J A2 80 50

AMA: 2018,Jan,8; 2017,Jan,8; 2016,Sep,5; 2016,Feb,12; 2016,Jan,13; 2015,Jan,16

67040 with endolaser panretinal photocoagulation

29.4 29.4 **FUD** 090 J A2 80 50

AMA: 2018,Jan,8; 2017,Jan,8; 2016,Sep,5; 2016,Feb,12; 2016,Jan,13; 2015,Jan,16

67041 with removal of preretinal cellular membrane (eg, macular pucker)

32.7 32.7 **FUD** 090 J G2 80 50

AMA: 2018,Jan,8; 2017,Jan,8; 2016,Sep,5; 2016,Feb,12; 2016,Jan,13; 2015,Jan,16

67042 with removal of internal limiting membrane of retina (eg, for repair of macular hole, diabetic macular edema), includes, if performed, intraocular tamponade (ie, air, gas or silicone oil)

32.7 32.7 **FUD** 090 J G2 80 50

AMA: 2018,Jan,8; 2017,Jan,8; 2016,Sep,5; 2016,Feb,12; 2016,Jan,13; 2015,Jan,16

67043 with removal of subretinal membrane (eg, choroidal neovascularization), includes, if performed, intraocular tamponade (ie, air, gas or silicone oil) and laser photocoagulation

34.5 34.5 **FUD** 090 J G2 80 50

AMA: 2018,Jan,8; 2017,Jan,8; 2016,Sep,5; 2016,Feb,12; 2016,Jan,13; 2015,Jan,16

67101-67115 Detached Retina Repair

INCLUDES Operating microscope (69990)
Primary technique when cryotherapy and/or diathermy and/or photocoagulation are used in combination

67101 **Repair of retinal detachment, including drainage of subretinal fluid when performed; cryotherapy**
8.10 | 9.40 | **FUD** 010 | J P3 50
AMA: 2018,Jan,8; 2017,Feb,14; 2017,Jan,8; 2016,Sep,5; 2016,Jun,6; 2016,Feb,12; 2016,Jan,13; 2015,Jan,16

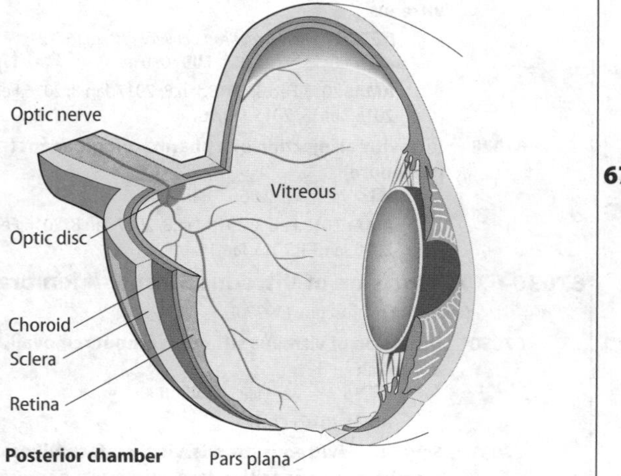

67105 **photocoagulation**
7.82 | 8.45 | **FUD** 010 | T P3 50
AMA: 2018,Jan,8; 2017,Feb,14; 2017,Jan,8; 2016,Sep,5; 2016,Jun,6; 2016,Feb,12; 2016,Jan,13; 2015,Jan,16

67107 **Repair of retinal detachment; scleral buckling (such as lamellar scleral dissection, imbrication or encircling procedure), including, when performed, implant, cryotherapy, photocoagulation, and drainage of subretinal fluid**
INCLUDES Gonin's operation
32.1 | 32.1 | **FUD** 090 | J G2 80 50
AMA: 2019,Aug,10; 2018,Jan,8; 2017,Jan,8; 2016,Sep,5; 2016,Jun,6; 2016,Feb,12

67108 **with vitrectomy, any method, including, when performed, air or gas tamponade, focal endolaser photocoagulation, cryotherapy, drainage of subretinal fluid, scleral buckling, and/or removal of lens by same technique**
34.1 | 34.1 | **FUD** 090 | J G2 80 50
AMA: 2018,Jan,8; 2017,Jan,8; 2016,Sep,5; 2016,Jun,6; 2016,Feb,12; 2016,Jan,13; 2015,Jan,16

67110 **by injection of air or other gas (eg, pneumatic retinopexy)**
23.1 | 25.0 | **FUD** 090 | J P3 50
AMA: 2018,Jan,8; 2017,Jan,8; 2016,Sep,5; 2016,Jun,6; 2016,Feb,12

67113 **Repair of complex retinal detachment (eg, proliferative vitreoretinopathy, stage C-1 or greater, diabetic traction retinal detachment, retinopathy of prematurity, retinal tear of greater than 90 degrees), with vitrectomy and membrane peeling, including, when performed, air, gas, or silicone oil tamponade, cryotherapy, endolaser photocoagulation, drainage of subretinal fluid, scleral buckling, and/or removal of lens**
EXCLUDES *Vitrectomy for other than retinal detachment, pars plana approach (67036-67043)*
Code also ophthalmic endoscope if used (66990)
38.0 | 38.0 | **FUD** 090 | J G2 80 50
AMA: 2018,Jan,8; 2017,Jan,8; 2016,Sep,5; 2016,Jun,6; 2016,Feb,12; 2016,Jan,13; 2015,Jan,16

67115 **Release of encircling material (posterior segment)**
14.1 | 14.1 | **FUD** 090 | J A2 50
AMA: 2016,Feb,12

67120-67121 Removal of Previously Implanted Prosthetic Device

INCLUDES Operating microscope (69990)
EXCLUDES *Foreign body removal (65260, 65265)*
Removal implanted material anterior segment (65920)

67120 **Removal of implanted material, posterior segment; extraocular**
15.8 | 18.8 | **FUD** 090 | J A2 50
AMA: 2016,Feb,12

67121 **intraocular**
25.6 | 25.6 | **FUD** 090 | J A2 80 50
AMA: 2016,Feb,12

67141-67145 Retinal Detachment: Preventative Procedures

INCLUDES Operating microscope (69990)
Treatment at one or more sessions that may occur at different encounters
EXCLUDES *Procedure performed more than one time during defined period of treatment*

67141 **Prophylaxis of retinal detachment (eg, retinal break, lattice degeneration) without drainage, 1 or more sessions; cryotherapy, diathermy**
13.8 | 14.9 | **FUD** 090 | T A2 50
AMA: 2018,Jan,8; 2017,Jan,8; 2016,Sep,5; 2016,Feb,12; 2016,Jan,13; 2015,Jan,16

67145 **photocoagulation (laser or xenon arc)**
14.0 | 14.9 | **FUD** 090 | T P2 50
AMA: 2018,Jan,8; 2017,Jan,8; 2016,Sep,5; 2016,Feb,12; 2016,Jan,13; 2015,Jan,16

67208-67218 Destruction of Retinal Lesions

INCLUDES Operating microscope (69990)
Treatment at one or more sessions that may occur at different encounters
EXCLUDES *Procedure performed more than one time during defined period of treatment*
Unlisted retinal procedures (67299)

67208 **Destruction of localized lesion of retina (eg, macular edema, tumors), 1 or more sessions; cryotherapy, diathermy**
16.4 | 17.0 | **FUD** 090 | T P2 50
AMA: 2018,Jan,8; 2017,Jan,8; 2016,Feb,12; 2016,Jan,13; 2015,Jan,16

67210 **photocoagulation**
14.1 | 14.6 | **FUD** 090 | T P2 50
AMA: 2018,Jan,8; 2017,Jan,8; 2016,Feb,12; 2016,Jan,13; 2015,Jan,16

67218 **radiation by implantation of source (includes removal of source)**
39.3 | 39.3 | **FUD** 090 | J A2 50
AMA: 2018,Jan,8; 2017,Jan,8; 2016,Feb,12; 2016,Jan,13; 2015,Jan,16

67220-67225 Destruction of Choroidal Lesions

INCLUDES Operating microscope (69990)

67220 **Destruction of localized lesion of choroid (eg, choroidal neovascularization); photocoagulation (eg, laser), 1 or more sessions**
INCLUDES Treatment at one or more sessions that may occur at different encounters
EXCLUDES *Procedure performed more than one time during defined period of treatment*
14.1 | 15.0 | **FUD** 090 | T P2 50
AMA: 2018,Jan,8; 2017,Jan,8; 2016,Feb,12; 2016,Jan,13; 2015,Jan,16

67221 **photodynamic therapy (includes intravenous infusion)**
6.05 | 8.07 | **FUD** 000 | T P3
AMA: 2018,Feb,10; 2018,Jan,8; 2017,Jan,8; 2016,Feb,12; 2016,Jan,13; 2015,Jan,16

\+ **67225** **photodynamic therapy, second eye, at single session (List separately in addition to code for primary eye treatment)**
Code first (67221)
0.81 0.85 **FUD** ZZZ N N1
AMA: 2018,Jan,8; 2017,Jan,8; 2016,Feb,12; 2016,Jan,13; 2015,Jan,16

67227-67229 Destruction Retinopathy

INCLUDES Operating microscope (69990)
EXCLUDES *Unlisted retinal procedures (67299)*

67227 **Destruction of extensive or progressive retinopathy (eg, diabetic retinopathy), cryotherapy, diathermy**
7.24 8.33 **FUD** 010 J P3 50
AMA: 2018,Jan,8; 2017,Jan,8; 2016,Feb,12; 2016,Jan,13; 2015,Jan,16

67228 **Treatment of extensive or progressive retinopathy (eg, diabetic retinopathy), photocoagulation**
8.72 9.73 **FUD** 010 T P3 50
AMA: 2018,Jan,8; 2017,Jan,8; 2016,Feb,12; 2016,Jan,13; 2015,Jan,16

67229 **Treatment of extensive or progressive retinopathy, 1 or more sessions, preterm infant (less than 37 weeks gestation at birth), performed from birth up to 1 year of age (eg, retinopathy of prematurity), photocoagulation or cryotherapy**
INCLUDES Treatment at one or more sessions that may occur at different encounters
EXCLUDES *Procedure performed more than one time during defined period of treatment*
33.1 33.1 **FUD** 090 T R2 50
AMA: 2018,Jan,8; 2017,Jan,8; 2016,Feb,12; 2016,Jan,13; 2015,Jan,16

67250-67255 Reinforcement of Posterior Sclera

INCLUDES Operating microscope (69990)
EXCLUDES *Removal scleral lesion (66130)*
Repair scleral staphyloma (66225)

67250 **Scleral reinforcement (separate procedure); without graft**
22.6 22.6 **FUD** 090 J A2 50
AMA: 2016,Feb,12

67255 **with graft**
EXCLUDES *Aqueous shunt to extraocular equatorial plate reservoir (66180)*
Revision aqueous shunt to extraocular equatorial plate reservoir; with graft (66185)
19.3 19.3 **FUD** 090 J A2 80 50
AMA: 2018,Jan,8; 2017,Jan,8; 2016,Feb,12; 2016,Jan,13; 2015,Jan,16; 2015,Jan,10

67299 Unlisted Posterior Segment Procedure

CMS: 100-04,4,180.3 Unlisted Service or Procedure
INCLUDES Operating microscope (69990)

67299 **Unlisted procedure, posterior segment**
0.00 0.00 **FUD** YYY J 80 50
AMA: 2018,Jan,8; 2017,Jan,8; 2016,Feb,12; 2016,Jan,13; 2015,Jan,16

67311-67334 Strabismus Procedures on Extraocular Muscles

INCLUDES Operating microscope (69990)
Code also adjustable sutures (67335)

67311 **Strabismus surgery, recession or resection procedure; 1 horizontal muscle**
16.9 16.9 **FUD** 090 J A2 50
AMA: 2018,Jan,8; 2017,Jan,8; 2017,Jan,6; 2016,Feb,12; 2016,Jan,13; 2015,Jan,16

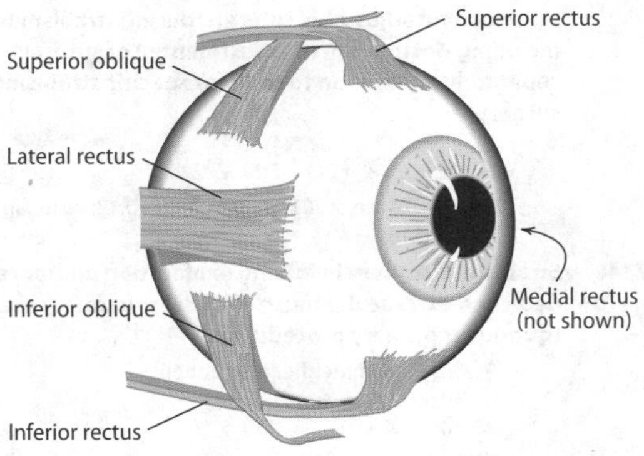

Muscles of the eyeball (right eye shown)

67312 **2 horizontal muscles**
20.3 20.3 **FUD** 090 J A2 50
AMA: 2018,Jan,8; 2017,Jan,8; 2016,Feb,12; 2016,Jan,13; 2015,Jan,16

67314 **1 vertical muscle (excluding superior oblique)**
19.1 19.1 **FUD** 090 J A2 50
AMA: 2018,Jan,8; 2017,Jan,8; 2016,Feb,12; 2016,Jan,13; 2015,Jan,16

67316 **2 or more vertical muscles (excluding superior oblique)**
22.7 22.7 **FUD** 090 J A2 80 50
AMA: 2018,Jan,8; 2017,Jan,8; 2016,Feb,12; 2016,Jan,13; 2015,Jan,16

67318 **Strabismus surgery, any procedure, superior oblique muscle**
19.9 19.9 **FUD** 090 J A2 50
AMA: 2018,Jan,8; 2017,Jan,8; 2016,Feb,12; 2016,Jan,13; 2015,Jan,16

\+ **67320** **Transposition procedure (eg, for paretic extraocular muscle), any extraocular muscle (specify) (List separately in addition to code for primary procedure)**
Code first (67311-67318)
9.10 9.10 **FUD** ZZZ N N1
AMA: 2018,Jan,8; 2017,Jan,8; 2016,Feb,12; 2016,Jan,13; 2015,Jan,16

\+ **67331** **Strabismus surgery on patient with previous eye surgery or injury that did not involve the extraocular muscles (List separately in addition to code for primary procedure)**
Code first (67311-67318)
8.70 8.70 **FUD** ZZZ N N1 50
AMA: 2018,Jan,8; 2017,Jan,8; 2016,Feb,12; 2016,Jan,13; 2015,Jan,16

\+ **67332** **Strabismus surgery on patient with scarring of extraocular muscles (eg, prior ocular injury, strabismus or retinal detachment surgery) or restrictive myopathy (eg, dysthyroid ophthalmopathy) (List separately in addition to code for primary procedure)**
Code first (67311-67318)
9.37 9.37 **FUD** ZZZ N N1 50
AMA: 2018,Jan,8; 2017,Jan,8; 2016,Feb,12; 2016,Jan,13; 2015,Jan,16

+ **67334 Strabismus surgery by posterior fixation suture technique, with or without muscle recession (List separately in addition to code for primary procedure)**
Code first (67311-67318)
8.52 8.52 FUD ZZZ N N1 50
AMA: 2018,Jan,8; 2017,Jan,8; 2016,Feb,12; 2016,Jan,13; 2015,Jan,16

67335-67399 Other Procedures of Extraocular Muscles

INCLUDES Operating microscope (69990)

+ **67335 Placement of adjustable suture(s) during strabismus surgery, including postoperative adjustment(s) of suture(s) (List separately in addition to code for specific strabismus surgery)**
Code first (67311-67334)
4.21 4.21 FUD ZZZ N N1 50
AMA: 2018,Jan,8; 2017,Jan,8; 2016,Feb,12; 2016,Jan,13; 2015,Jan,16

+ **67340 Strabismus surgery involving exploration and/or repair of detached extraocular muscle(s) (List separately in addition to code for primary procedure)**
INCLUDES Hummelsheim operation
Code first (67311-67334)
10.1 10.1 FUD ZZZ N N1 80
AMA: 2018,Jan,8; 2017,Jan,8; 2016,Feb,12; 2016,Jan,13; 2015,Jan,16

67343 Release of extensive scar tissue without detaching extraocular muscle (separate procedure)
Code also when performed on other than affected muscle (67311-67340)
18.5 18.5 FUD 090 J A2 50
AMA: 2018,Jan,8; 2017,Jan,8; 2016,Feb,12; 2016,Jan,13; 2015,Jan,16

67345 Chemodenervation of extraocular muscle
EXCLUDES *Nerve destruction for blepharospasm and other neurological disorders (64612, 64616)*
6.22 6.96 FUD 010 T P3 50
AMA: 2019,Apr,9; 2018,Jan,8; 2017,Jan,8; 2016,Feb,12; 2016,Jan,13; 2015,Jan,16

67346 Biopsy of extraocular muscle
EXCLUDES *Repair laceration extraocular muscle, tendon, or Tenon's capsule (65290)*
5.50 5.50 FUD 000 J A2 80 50
AMA: 2016,Feb,12

67399 Unlisted procedure, extraocular muscle
0.00 0.00 FUD YYY T 80 50
AMA: 2018,Jan,8; 2017,Jul,10; 2016,Feb,12

67400-67415 Frontal Orbitotomy

INCLUDES Operating microscope (69990)

67400 Orbitotomy without bone flap (frontal or transconjunctival approach); for exploration, with or without biopsy
27.8 27.8 FUD 090 J A2 50
AMA: 2016,Feb,12

67405 with drainage only
22.8 22.8 FUD 090 J A2 50
AMA: 2018,Jan,8; 2017,Jan,8; 2016,Feb,12; 2016,Jan,13; 2015,Jan,16

67412 with removal of lesion
24.6 24.6 FUD 090 J A2 50
AMA: 2016,Feb,12

67413 with removal of foreign body
25.8 25.8 FUD 090 J A2 80 50
AMA: 2016,Feb,12

67414 with removal of bone for decompression
38.1 38.1 FUD 090 J G2 80 50
AMA: 2018,Jan,8; 2017,Jan,8; 2016,Feb,12; 2016,Jan,13; 2015,Jan,16

67415 Fine needle aspiration of orbital contents
EXCLUDES *Decompression optic nerve (67570)*
Exenteration, enucleation, and repair (65101-65175)
2.96 2.96 FUD 000 J A2 80 50
AMA: 2016,Feb,12

67420-67450 Lateral Orbitotomy

INCLUDES Operating microscope (69990)
EXCLUDES *Orbital implant (67550, 67560)*
Surgical removal all or some orbital contents or repair after removal (65091-65175)
Transcranial approach orbitotomy (61330, 61333)

67420 Orbitotomy with bone flap or window, lateral approach (eg, Kroenlein); with removal of lesion
46.2 46.2 FUD 090 J A2 80 50
AMA: 2016,Feb,12

67430 with removal of foreign body
37.3 37.3 FUD 090 J A2 80 50
AMA: 2016,Feb,12

67440 with drainage
36.1 36.1 FUD 090 J A2 80 50
AMA: 2016,Feb,12

67445 with removal of bone for decompression
EXCLUDES *Decompression optic nerve sheath (67570)*
41.6 41.6 FUD 090 J A2 80 50
AMA: 2019,Dec,14; 2016,Feb,12

67450 for exploration, with or without biopsy
37.5 37.5 FUD 090 J A2 80 50
AMA: 2016,Feb,12

67500-67515 Eye Injections

INCLUDES Operating microscope (69990)

67500 Retrobulbar injection; medication (separate procedure, does not include supply of medication)
1.73 2.02 FUD 000 T G2 50
AMA: 2018,Jan,8; 2017,Jan,8; 2016,Feb,12; 2016,Jan,13; 2015,Jan,16

67505 alcohol
2.03 2.38 FUD 000 T P3 50
AMA: 2016,Feb,12

67515 Injection of medication or other substance into Tenon's capsule
EXCLUDES *Subconjunctival injection (68200)*
2.06 2.24 FUD 000 T P3 50
AMA: 2018,Jan,8; 2017,Jan,8; 2016,Feb,12; 2016,Jan,13; 2015,Jan,16

67550-67560 Orbital Implant

INCLUDES Operating microscope (69990)
EXCLUDES *Fracture repair malar area, orbit (21355-21408)*
Ocular implant inside muscle cone (65093-65105, 65130-65175)

67550 Orbital implant (implant outside muscle cone); insertion
27.8 27.8 FUD 090 J A2 50
AMA: 2016,Feb,12

67560 removal or revision
28.5 28.5 FUD 090 J A2 80 50
AMA: 2016,Feb,12

67570-67599 Other and Unlisted Orbital Procedures

INCLUDES Operating microscope (69990)

67570 Optic nerve decompression (eg, incision or fenestration of optic nerve sheath)
33.9 33.9 FUD 090 J A2 80 50
AMA: 2016,Feb,12

67599 Unlisted procedure, orbit
0.00 0.00 FUD YYY T 80 50
AMA: 2016,Feb,12

67700-67810 [67810] Incisional Procedures of Eyelids

INCLUDES Operating microscope (69990)

67700 **Blepharotomy, drainage of abscess, eyelid**
3.31 7.82 FUD 010 T P2 50
AMA: 2018,Jan,8; 2017,Jan,8; 2016,Feb,12; 2016,Jan,13; 2015,Jan,16

67710 **Severing of tarsorrhaphy**
2.77 6.56 FUD 010 T P3 50
AMA: 2018,Jan,8; 2017,Jan,8; 2016,Feb,12; 2016,Jan,13; 2015,Jan,16

67715 **Canthotomy (separate procedure)**
EXCLUDES *Canthoplasty (67950)*
Symblepharon division (68340)
3.08 7.07 FUD 010 J A2 50
AMA: 2018,Jan,8; 2017,Jan,8; 2016,Feb,12; 2016,Jan,13; 2015,Jan,16

67810 **Incisional biopsy of eyelid skin including lid margin**
EXCLUDES *Biopsy eyelid skin (11102-11107)*
2.03 4.99 FUD 000 T P2 50
AMA: 2019,Jan,9; 2018,Jan,8; 2017,Jan,8; 2016,Feb,12; 2016,Jan,13; 2015,Jan,16

67800-67808 Excision of Chalazion (Meibomian Cyst)

INCLUDES Lesion removal requiring more than skin:
- Lid margin
- Palpebral conjunctiva
- Tarsus

Operating microscope (69990)

EXCLUDES *Blepharoplasty, graft, or reconstructive procedures (67930-67975)*
Excision/destruction skin lesion eyelid (11310-11313, 11440-11446, 11640-11646, 17000-17004)

67800 **Excision of chalazion; single**
2.93 3.64 FUD 010 T P3
AMA: 2018,Jan,8; 2017,Jan,8; 2016,Feb,12; 2016,Jan,13; 2015,Jan,16

67801 **multiple, same lid**
3.79 4.64 FUD 010 T P3
AMA: 2016,Feb,12

67805 **multiple, different lids**
4.67 5.76 FUD 010 T P3
AMA: 2018,Jan,8; 2017,Jan,8; 2016,Feb,12; 2016,Jan,13; 2015,Jan,16

67808 **under general anesthesia and/or requiring hospitalization, single or multiple**
10.4 10.4 FUD 090 J A2
AMA: 2016,Feb,12

67810-67850 [67810] Other Eyelid Procedures

INCLUDES Operating microscope (69990)

67810 **Resequenced code. See code following 67715.**

67820 **Correction of trichiasis; epilation, by forceps only**
0.99 0.93 FUD 000 Q1 N1 50
AMA: 2018,Jan,8; 2017,Jan,8; 2016,Feb,12; 2016,Jan,13; 2015,Jan,16

67825 **epilation by other than forceps (eg, by electrosurgery, cryotherapy, laser surgery)**
3.43 3.77 FUD 010 T P3 50
AMA: 2018,Jan,8; 2017,Jan,8; 2016,Feb,12; 2016,Jan,13; 2015,Jan,16

67830 **incision of lid margin**
3.92 7.64 FUD 010 T A2 50
AMA: 2016,Feb,12

67835 **incision of lid margin, with free mucous membrane graft**
12.4 12.4 FUD 090 J A2 80 50
AMA: 2016,Feb,12

67840 **Excision of lesion of eyelid (except chalazion) without closure or with simple direct closure**
EXCLUDES *Eyelid resection and reconstruction (67961, 67966)*
4.49 7.91 FUD 010 T P3 50
AMA: 2019,Jan,14; 2016,Feb,12

67850 **Destruction of lesion of lid margin (up to 1 cm)**
EXCLUDES *Mohs micro procedures (17311-17315)*
Topical chemotherapy (99202-99215)
3.84 6.13 FUD 010 T P3 50
AMA: 2016,Feb,12

67875-67882 Suturing of the Eyelids

INCLUDES Operating microscope (69990)

EXCLUDES *Canthoplasty (67950)*
Canthotomy (67715)
Severing of tarsorrhaphy (67710)

67875 **Temporary closure of eyelids by suture (eg, Frost suture)**
2.72 5.01 FUD 000 T G2 50
AMA: 2016,Feb,12

67880 **Construction of intermarginal adhesions, median tarsorrhaphy, or canthorrhaphy;**
10.3 13.1 FUD 090 J A2 50
AMA: 2016,Feb,12

67882 **with transposition of tarsal plate**
13.4 16.1 FUD 090 J A2 50
AMA: 2016,Feb,12

67900-67912 Repair of Ptosis/Retraction Eyelids, Eyebrows

INCLUDES Operating microscope (69990)

67900 **Repair of brow ptosis (supraciliary, mid-forehead or coronal approach)**
EXCLUDES *Forehead rhytidectomy (15824)*
14.4 18.2 FUD 090 J A2 50
AMA: 2018,Jan,8; 2017,Jan,8; 2016,Feb,12; 2016,Jan,13; 2015,Jan,16

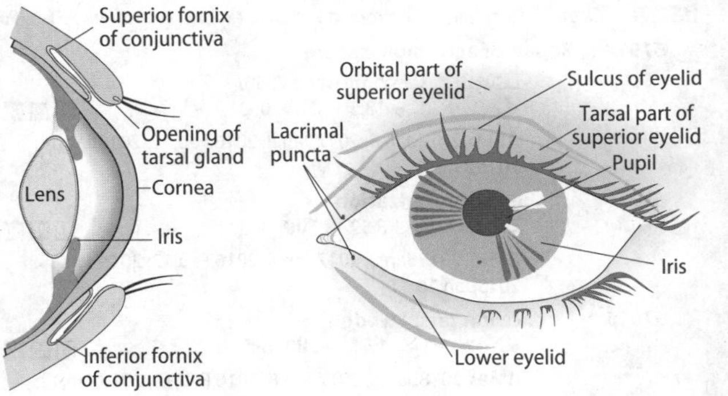

67901 **Repair of blepharoptosis; frontalis muscle technique with suture or other material (eg, banked fascia)**
16.5 21.9 FUD 090 J A2 50
AMA: 2018,Jan,8; 2017,Jul,10; 2017,Jan,8; 2016,Feb,12; 2016,Jan,13; 2015,Jan,16

67902 **frontalis muscle technique with autologous fascial sling (includes obtaining fascia)**
20.5 20.5 FUD 090 J A2 50
AMA: 2018,Jan,8; 2017,Jan,8; 2016,Feb,12; 2016,Jan,13; 2015,Jan,16

67903 **(tarso) levator resection or advancement, internal approach**
13.7 16.9 FUD 090 J A2 50
AMA: 2018,Jan,8; 2017,Jan,8; 2016,Feb,12; 2016,Jan,13; 2015,Jan,16

67904 **(tarso) levator resection or advancement, external approach**

INCLUDES Everbusch's operation

16.9 20.9 FUD 090 J A2 50

AMA: 2018,Jan,8; 2017,Jan,8; 2016,Feb,12; 2016,Jan,13; 2015,Jan,16

67906 **superior rectus technique with fascial sling (includes obtaining fascia)**

14.4 14.4 FUD 090 J A2 50

AMA: 2018,Jan,8; 2017,Jan,8; 2016,Feb,12; 2016,Jan,13; 2015,Jan,16

67908 **conjunctivo-tarso-Muller's muscle-levator resection (eg, Fasanella-Servat type)**

12.1 14.1 FUD 090 J A2 50

AMA: 2018,Jan,8; 2017,Jan,8; 2016,Feb,12; 2016,Jan,13; 2015,Jan,16

67909 **Reduction of overcorrection of ptosis**

12.4 15.3 FUD 090 J A2 50

AMA: 2018,Jan,8; 2017,Jan,8; 2016,Feb,12; 2016,Jan,13; 2015,Jan,16

67911 **Correction of lid retraction**

EXCLUDES *Autologous graft harvest ([15769], 20920, 20922)*
Lid defect correction using fat obtained via liposuction (15773-15774)
Mucous membrane graft repair trichiasis (67835)

15.8 15.8 FUD 090 J A2 50

AMA: 2018,Jan,8; 2017,Jan,8; 2016,Feb,12; 2016,Jan,13; 2015,Jan,16

67912 **Correction of lagophthalmos, with implantation of upper eyelid lid load (eg, gold weight)**

13.8 25.4 FUD 090 J A2 50

AMA: 2018,Jan,8; 2017,Jan,8; 2016,Feb,12; 2016,Jan,13; 2015,Jan,16

67914-67924 Repair Ectropion/Entropion

INCLUDES Operating microscope (69990)

EXCLUDES *Cicatricial ectropion or entropion with scar excision or graft (67961-67966)*

67914 **Repair of ectropion; suture**

INCLUDES Canthoplasty (67950)

9.29 13.5 FUD 090 J A2 50

AMA: 2018,Jan,8; 2017,Jan,8; 2016,Feb,12; 2016,Jan,13; 2015,Jan,16

67915 **thermocauterization**

5.62 8.52 FUD 090 J P3 50

AMA: 2018,Jan,8; 2017,Jan,8; 2016,Feb,12; 2016,Jan,13; 2015,Jan,16

67916 **excision tarsal wedge**

12.1 17.1 FUD 090 J A2 50

AMA: 2018,Jan,8; 2017,Jan,8; 2016,Feb,12; 2016,Jan,13; 2015,Jan,16

67917 **extensive (eg, tarsal strip operations)**

EXCLUDES *Repair everted punctum (68705)*

13.0 17.3 FUD 090 J A2 50

AMA: 2020,Feb,13; 2018,Jan,8; 2017,Jan,8; 2016,Feb,12; 2016,Jan,13; 2015,Jan,16

67921 **Repair of entropion; suture**

8.82 13.2 FUD 090 J A2 50

AMA: 2018,Jan,8; 2017,Jan,8; 2016,Feb,12; 2016,Jan,13; 2015,Jan,16

67922 **thermocauterization**

5.52 8.42 FUD 090 J P3 50

AMA: 2018,Jan,8; 2017,Jan,8; 2016,Feb,12; 2016,Jan,13; 2015,Jan,16

67923 **excision tarsal wedge**

12.1 17.1 FUD 090 J A2 50

AMA: 2018,Jan,8; 2017,Jan,8; 2016,Feb,12; 2016,Jan,13; 2015,Jan,16

67924 **extensive (eg, tarsal strip or capsulopalpebral fascia repairs operation)**

INCLUDES Canthoplasty (67950)

12.9 18.2 FUD 090 J A2 50

AMA: 2018,Jan,8; 2017,Jan,8; 2016,Feb,12; 2016,Jan,13; 2015,Jan,16

67930-67935 Repair Eyelid Wound

INCLUDES Operating microscope (69990)
Repairs involving more than skin:
- Lid margin
- Palpebral conjunctiva
- Tarsus

EXCLUDES *Blepharoplasty for entropion or ectropion (67916-67917, 67923-67924)*
Correction lid retraction and blepharoptosis (67901-67911)
Free graft (15120-15121, 15260-15261)
Graft preparation (15004)
Plastic repair lacrimal canaliculi (68700)
Removal eyelid lesion (67800 [67810], 67840-67850)
Repair blepharochalasis (15820-15823)
Repair involving eyelid skin (12011-12018, 12051-12057, 13151-13153)
Skin adjacent tissue transfer (14060-14061)
Tarsorrhaphy, canthorrhaphy (67880, 67882)

67930 **Suture of recent wound, eyelid, involving lid margin, tarsus, and/or palpebral conjunctiva direct closure; partial thickness**

6.78 10.4 FUD 010 J P3 50

AMA: 2016,Feb,12

67935 **full thickness**

12.5 16.9 FUD 090 J A2 50

AMA: 2016,Feb,12

67938-67999 Eyelid Reconstruction/Repair/Removal Deep Foreign Body

INCLUDES Operating microscope (69990)

EXCLUDES *Blepharoplasty for entropion or ectropion (67916-67917, 67923-67924)*
Correction lid retraction and blepharoptosis (67901-67911)
Free graft (15120-15121, 15260-15261)
Graft preparation (15004)
Plastic repair lacrimal canaliculi (68700)
Removal eyelid lesion (67800-67808, 67840-67850)
Repair blepharochalasis (15820-15823)
Repair involving eyelid skin (12011-12018, 12051-12057, 13151-13153)
Skin adjacent tissue transfer (14060-14061)
Tarsorrhaphy, canthorrhaphy (67880, 67882)

67938 **Removal of embedded foreign body, eyelid**

3.28 7.36 FUD 010 T P2 50

AMA: 2018,Jan,8; 2017,Jan,8; 2016,Feb,12; 2016,Jan,13; 2015,Jan,16

67950 **Canthoplasty (reconstruction of canthus)**

13.1 16.4 FUD 090 J A2 50

AMA: 2016,Feb,12

67961 **Excision and repair of eyelid, involving lid margin, tarsus, conjunctiva, canthus, or full thickness, may include preparation for skin graft or pedicle flap with adjacent tissue transfer or rearrangement; up to one-fourth of lid margin**

INCLUDES Canthoplasty (67950)

EXCLUDES *Delay flap (15630)*
Flap attachment (15650)
Free skin grafts (15120-15121, 15260-15261)
Tubed pedicle flap preparation (15576)

12.8 16.4 FUD 090 J A2 80 50

AMA: 2018,Jan,8; 2017,Jan,8; 2016,Feb,12; 2016,Jan,13; 2015,Jan,16

67966 **over one-fourth of lid margin**

INCLUDES Canthoplasty (67950)

EXCLUDES *Delay flap (15630)*
Flap attachment (15650)
Free skin grafts (15120-15121, 15260-15261)
Tubed pedicle flap preparation (15576)

18.7 21.9 FUD 090 J A2 50

AMA: 2018,Jan,8; 2017,Jan,8; 2016,Feb,12; 2016,Jan,13; 2015,Jan,16

67971 Reconstruction of eyelid, full thickness by transfer of tarsoconjunctival flap from opposing eyelid; up to two-thirds of eyelid, 1 stage or first stage

INCLUDES Dupuy-Dutemp reconstruction
Landboldt's operation

20.4 20.4 FUD 090 J A2 50

AMA: 2016,Feb,12

67973 total eyelid, lower, 1 stage or first stage

INCLUDES Landboldt's operation

26.3 26.3 FUD 090 J A2 80 50

AMA: 2016,Feb,12

67974 total eyelid, upper, 1 stage or first stage

INCLUDES Landboldt's operation

26.2 26.2 FUD 090 J A2 80 50

AMA: 2016,Feb,12

67975 second stage

INCLUDES Landboldt's operation

19.4 19.4 FUD 090 J A2 50

AMA: 2016,Feb,12

67999 Unlisted procedure, eyelids

0.00 0.00 FUD YYY T 80 50

AMA: 2018,Jan,8; 2017,Jul,10; 2017,Jan,8; 2016,Feb,12; 2016,Jan,13; 2015,Jan,16

68020-68200 Conjunctival Biopsy/Injection/Treatment of Lesions

INCLUDES Operating microscope (69990)

EXCLUDES *Foreign body removal (65205-65265)*

68020 Incision of conjunctiva, drainage of cyst

3.11 3.41 FUD 010 T P3 50

AMA: 2016,Feb,12

68040 Expression of conjunctival follicles (eg, for trachoma)

EXCLUDES *Automated evacuation meibomian glands with heat/pressure (0207T)*
Manual evacuation meibomian glands ([0563T])

1.40 1.78 FUD 000 T P3 50

AMA: 2018,Jan,8; 2017,Jan,8; 2016,Feb,12; 2016,Jan,13; 2015,Jan,16

68100 Biopsy of conjunctiva

2.75 4.97 FUD 000 J P3 50

AMA: 2019,Jan,9; 2016,Feb,12

68110 Excision of lesion, conjunctiva; up to 1 cm

4.18 6.63 FUD 010 J P3 50

AMA: 2018,Feb,11; 2018,Jan,8; 2017,Jan,6; 2016,Feb,12

68115 over 1 cm

5.18 9.19 FUD 010 J A2 50

AMA: 2018,Feb,11; 2016,Feb,12

68130 with adjacent sclera

11.6 15.5 FUD 090 J A2 50

AMA: 2016,Feb,12

68135 Destruction of lesion, conjunctiva

4.24 4.46 FUD 010 J P3 50

AMA: 2016,Feb,12

68200 Subconjunctival injection

EXCLUDES *Retrobulbar or Tenon's capsule injection (67500-67515)*

0.99 1.19 FUD 000 Q1 N1 50

AMA: 2018,Jan,8; 2017,Jan,8; 2016,Feb,12; 2016,Jan,13; 2015,Jan,16

68320-68340 Conjunctivoplasty Procedures

INCLUDES Operating microscope (69990)

EXCLUDES *Conjunctival foreign body removal (65205, 65210)*
Laceration repair (65270-65273)

68320 Conjunctivoplasty; with conjunctival graft or extensive rearrangement

15.3 20.8 FUD 090 J A2 50

AMA: 2018,Jan,8; 2017,Jan,8; 2016,Feb,12; 2016,Jan,13; 2015,Jan,16

68325 with buccal mucous membrane graft (includes obtaining graft)

18.5 18.5 FUD 090 J A2 50

AMA: 2016,Feb,12

68326 Conjunctivoplasty, reconstruction cul-de-sac; with conjunctival graft or extensive rearrangement

18.3 18.3 FUD 090 J A2 50

AMA: 2016,Feb,12

68328 with buccal mucous membrane graft (includes obtaining graft)

20.1 20.1 FUD 090 J A2 80 50

AMA: 2016,Feb,12

68330 Repair of symblepharon; conjunctivoplasty, without graft

13.0 17.4 FUD 090 J A2 80 50

AMA: 2016,Feb,12

68335 with free graft conjunctiva or buccal mucous membrane (includes obtaining graft)

18.4 18.4 FUD 090 J A2 50

AMA: 2016,Feb,12

68340 division of symblepharon, with or without insertion of conformer or contact lens

11.2 16.4 FUD 090 J A2 80 50

AMA: 2016,Feb,12

68360-68399 Conjunctival Flaps and Unlisted Procedures

INCLUDES Operating microscope (69990)

68360 Conjunctival flap; bridge or partial (separate procedure)

EXCLUDES *Conjunctival flap for injury (65280, 65285)*
Conjunctival foreign body removal (65205, 65210)
Surgical wound repair (66250)

11.7 15.3 FUD 090 J A2 50

AMA: 2016,Feb,12

68362 total (such as Gunderson thin flap or purse string flap)

EXCLUDES *Conjunctival flap for injury (65280, 65285)*
Conjunctival foreign body removal (65205, 65210)
Surgical wound repair (66250)

18.5 18.5 FUD 090 J A2 50

AMA: 2018,Jan,8; 2017,Jan,8; 2016,Feb,12; 2016,Jan,13; 2015,Jan,16

68371 Harvesting conjunctival allograft, living donor

11.7 11.7 FUD 010 J A2 50

AMA: 2018,Jan,8; 2017,Jan,8; 2016,Feb,12; 2016,Jan,13; 2015,Jan,16

68399 Unlisted procedure, conjunctiva

0.00 0.00 FUD YYY T 80 50

AMA: 2018,Jan,8; 2017,Jan,8; 2016,Feb,12; 2016,Jan,13; 2015,Jan,16

68400-68899 Nasolacrimal System Procedures

INCLUDES Operating microscope (69990)

68400 Incision, drainage of lacrimal gland
3.76 8.24 FUD 010 T P3 50
AMA: 2016,Feb,12

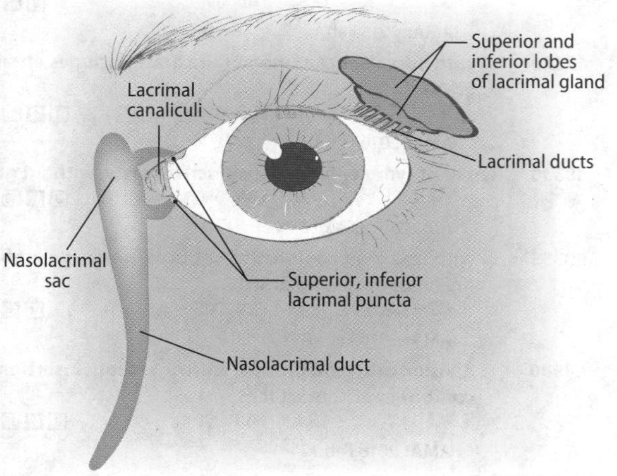

68420 Incision, drainage of lacrimal sac (dacryocystotomy or dacryocystostomy)
4.75 9.35 FUD 010 J P3 50
AMA: 2016,Feb,12

68440 Snip incision of lacrimal punctum
2.80 2.92 FUD 010 T P3 50
AMA: 2016,Feb,12

68500 Excision of lacrimal gland (dacryoadenectomy), except for tumor; total
28.6 28.6 FUD 090 J A2 50
AMA: 2016,Feb,12

68505 partial
28.5 28.5 FUD 090 J A2 50
AMA: 2016,Feb,12

68510 Biopsy of lacrimal gland
8.26 12.9 FUD 000 J A2 80 50
AMA: 2016,Feb,12

68520 Excision of lacrimal sac (dacryocystectomy)
20.0 20.0 FUD 090 J A2 80 50
AMA: 2016,Feb,12

68525 Biopsy of lacrimal sac
7.52 7.52 FUD 000 J A2 50
AMA: 2016,Feb,12

68530 Removal of foreign body or dacryolith, lacrimal passages
INCLUDES Meller's excision
7.23 12.2 FUD 010 T P2 50
AMA: 2016,Feb,12

68540 Excision of lacrimal gland tumor; frontal approach
27.0 27.0 FUD 090 J A2 50
AMA: 2016,Feb,12

68550 involving osteotomy
33.3 33.3 FUD 090 J A2 50
AMA: 2016,Feb,12

68700 Plastic repair of canaliculi
17.0 17.0 FUD 090 J A2 50
AMA: 2016,Feb,12

68705 Correction of everted punctum, cautery
4.68 7.19 FUD 010 T P2 50
AMA: 2020,Feb,13; 2018,Jan,8; 2017,Jan,8; 2016,Feb,12; 2016,Jan,13; 2015,Jan,16

68720 Dacryocystorhinostomy (fistulization of lacrimal sac to nasal cavity)
22.1 22.1 FUD 090 J A2 80 50
AMA: 2018,Jan,8; 2017,Jan,8; 2016,Feb,12; 2016,Jan,13; 2015,Jan,16

68745 Conjunctivorhinostomy (fistulization of conjunctiva to nasal cavity); without tube
22.2 22.2 FUD 090 J A2 80 50
AMA: 2016,Feb,12

68750 with insertion of tube or stent
22.4 22.4 FUD 090 J A2 80 50
AMA: 2018,Jan,8; 2017,Jan,8; 2016,Feb,12; 2016,Jan,13; 2015,Jan,16

68760 Closure of the lacrimal punctum; by thermocauterization, ligation, or laser surgery
4.11 6.07 FUD 010 T P2 50
AMA: 2016,Feb,12

68761 by plug, each
EXCLUDES *Drug-eluting lacrimal implant (0356T)*
Drug-eluting ocular insert (0444T-0445T)
3.32 4.20 FUD 010 T P3 80 50
AMA: 2018,Jan,8; 2017,Jan,8; 2016,Feb,12; 2016,Jan,13; 2015,Jan,16

68770 Closure of lacrimal fistula (separate procedure)
17.7 17.7 FUD 090 J A2 80 50
AMA: 2016,Feb,12

68801 Dilation of lacrimal punctum, with or without irrigation
2.18 2.60 FUD 010 Q1 N1 50
AMA: 2016,Feb,12

68810 Probing of nasolacrimal duct, with or without irrigation;
EXCLUDES *Ophthalmological exam under anesthesia (92018)*
3.64 4.47 FUD 010 T A2 50
AMA: 2018,Jan,8; 2017,Jan,8; 2016,Feb,12; 2016,Jan,13; 2015,Jan,16

68811 requiring general anesthesia
EXCLUDES *Ophthalmological exam under anesthesia (92018)*
3.82 3.82 FUD 010 J A2 50
AMA: 2018,Jan,8; 2017,Jan,8; 2016,Feb,12; 2016,Jan,13; 2015,Jan,16

68815 with insertion of tube or stent
EXCLUDES *Drug-eluting lacrimal implant (0356T)*
Drug-eluting ocular insert (0444T-0445T)
Ophthalmological exam under anesthesia (92018)
6.27 11.0 FUD 010 J A2 50
AMA: 2018,Jan,8; 2017,Jan,8; 2016,Feb,12; 2016,Jan,13; 2015,Jan,16

68816 with transluminal balloon catheter dilation
EXCLUDES *Probing nasolacrimal duct (68810-68811, 68815)*
4.45 22.2 FUD 010 J G2 50
AMA: 2018,Jan,8; 2017,Jan,8; 2016,Feb,12; 2016,Jan,13; 2015,Jan,16

68840 Probing of lacrimal canaliculi, with or without irrigation
3.27 3.70 FUD 010 T P3 50
AMA: 2016,Feb,12

68850 Injection of contrast medium for dacryocystography
(70170, 78660)
1.59 1.80 FUD 000 N N1 50
AMA: 2018,Jan,8; 2017,Jan,8; 2016,Feb,12; 2016,Jan,13; 2015,Jan,16

68899 Unlisted procedure, lacrimal system
0.00 0.00 FUD YYY T 80 50
AMA: 2014,Jan,11; 1991,Sum,17

69000-69020 Treatment External Abscess/Hematoma

69000 **Drainage external ear, abscess or hematoma; simple**
3.47 5.34 **FUD** 010 T P3 50
AMA: 2018,Jan,8; 2017,Jan,8; 2016,Jan,13; 2015,Jan,16

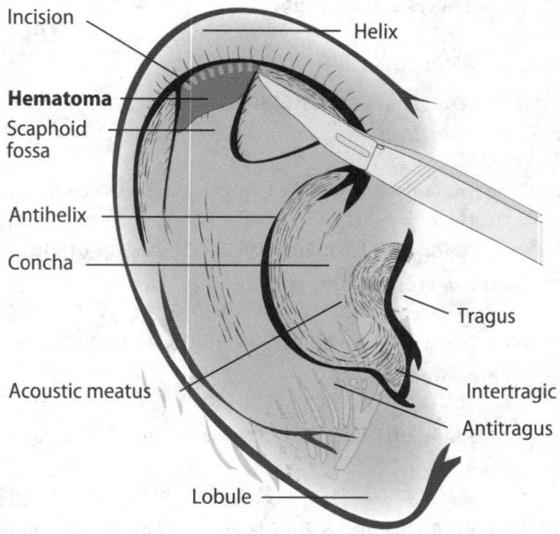

An incision is made to drain the contents of an abscess or hematoma

69005 **complicated**
4.50 6.13 **FUD** 010 J P3 50
AMA: 2014,Jan,11; 1999,Oct,10

69020 **Drainage external auditory canal, abscess**
4.03 6.57 **FUD** 010 T P3 50
AMA: 2018,Jan,8; 2017,Jan,8; 2016,Jan,13; 2015,Jan,16

69090 Cosmetic Ear Piercing

CMS: 100-02,16,10 Exclusions from Coverage; 100-02,16,120 Cosmetic Procedures

69090 **Ear piercing**
0.00 0.00 **FUD** XXX E
AMA: 2014,Jan,11; 1999,Oct,10

69100-69222 External Ear/Auditory Canal Procedures

EXCLUDES *Reconstruction ear (see integumentary section codes)*

69100 **Biopsy external ear**
1.37 2.79 **FUD** 000 T P3
AMA: 2019,Jan,9

69105 **Biopsy external auditory canal**
1.78 4.00 **FUD** 000 T P3 50
AMA: 2014,Jan,11; 1999,Oct,10

69110 **Excision external ear; partial, simple repair**
9.21 13.0 **FUD** 090 J A2 50
AMA: 2014,Jan,11; 1999,Oct,10

69120 **complete amputation**
11.1 11.1 **FUD** 090 J A2
AMA: 2014,Jan,11; 1999,Oct,10

69140 **Excision exostosis(es), external auditory canal**
24.8 24.8 **FUD** 090 J A2 80 50
AMA: 2014,Jan,11; 1999,Oct,10

69145 **Excision soft tissue lesion, external auditory canal**
7.04 11.1 **FUD** 090 J A2 50
AMA: 2019,Dec,14

69150 **Radical excision external auditory canal lesion; without neck dissection**
EXCLUDES *Skin graft (15004-15261)*
Temporal bone resection (69535)
29.5 29.5 **FUD** 090 J A2
AMA: 2014,Jan,11; 2003,Jan,1

69155 **with neck dissection**
EXCLUDES *Skin graft (15004-15261)*
Temporal bone resection (69535)
47.0 47.0 **FUD** 090 C 80
AMA: 2014,Jan,11; 1999,Oct,10

69200 **Removal foreign body from external auditory canal; without general anesthesia**
1.35 2.31 **FUD** 000 Q1 N1 50
AMA: 2014,Jan,11; 1999,Oct,10

69205 **with general anesthesia**
2.77 2.77 **FUD** 010 J A2 50
AMA: 2018,Jan,8; 2017,Jan,8; 2016,Jan,13; 2015,Jan,16

69209 **Removal impacted cerumen using irrigation/lavage, unilateral**
EXCLUDES *Removal impacted cerumen using instrumentation (69210)*
Removal nonimpacted cerumen (see appropriate E/M code(s)) (99202-99233 [99224, 99225, 99226], 99241-99255, 99281-99285, 99304-99318, 99324-99337, 99341-99350)
0.40 0.40 **FUD** 000 Q1 N1 50
AMA: 2018,Jan,8; 2017,Jan,8; 2016,Mar,10; 2016,Feb,13; 2016,Jan,7

69210 **Removal impacted cerumen requiring instrumentation, unilateral**
EXCLUDES *Removal impacted cerumen using irrigation or lavage (69209)*
Removal nonimpacted cerumen (see appropriate E/M code(s)) (99202-99233 [99224, 99225, 99226], 99241-99255, 99281-99285, 99304-99318, 99324-99337, 99341-99350)
0.96 1.36 **FUD** 000 Q1 N1
AMA: 2018,Jan,8; 2017,Jan,8; 2016,Mar,10; 2016,Feb,13; 2016,Jan,13; 2016,Jan,7; 2015,Jan,16

69220 **Debridement, mastoidectomy cavity, simple (eg, routine cleaning)**
1.46 2.25 **FUD** 000 Q1 N1 50
AMA: 2014,Jan,11; 1999,Oct,10

69222 **Debridement, mastoidectomy cavity, complex (eg, with anesthesia or more than routine cleaning)**
3.81 6.02 **FUD** 010 T P3 50
AMA: 2014,Jan,11; 1999,Oct,10

69300 Plastic Surgery for Prominent Ears

CMS: 100-02,16,120 Cosmetic Procedures; 100-02,16,180 Services Related to Noncovered Procedures

EXCLUDES *Suture laceration external ear (12011-14302)*

69300 **Otoplasty, protruding ear, with or without size reduction**
13.8 18.1 **FUD** YYY J A2 80 50
AMA: 2014,Jan,11; 1999,Oct,10

69310-69399 Reconstruction Auditory Canal: Postaural Approach

EXCLUDES *Suture laceration external ear (12011-14302)*

69310 **Reconstruction of external auditory canal (meatoplasty) (eg, for stenosis due to injury, infection) (separate procedure)**
30.9 30.9 **FUD** 090 J A2 50
AMA: 2018,Jan,8; 2017,Jan,8; 2016,Jan,13; 2015,Jan,16

69320 **Reconstruction external auditory canal for congenital atresia, single stage**
EXCLUDES *Other reconstruction surgery with graft (13151-15760, 21230-21235)*
Tympanoplasty (69631, 69641)
43.4 43.4 **FUD** 090 J A2 80 50
AMA: 2014,Jan,11; 1999,Oct,10

69399 **Unlisted procedure, external ear**
EXCLUDES *Otoscopy under general anesthesia (92502)*
0.00 0.00 **FUD** YYY T 80
AMA: 2014,Jan,11; 1999,Oct,10

69420-69450 Ear Drum Procedures

69420 Myringotomy including aspiration and/or eustachian tube inflation

3.39 5.31 **FUD** 010 T P2 50

AMA: 2018,Jan,8; 2017,Jan,8; 2016,Jan,13; 2015,Jan,16

69421 Myringotomy including aspiration and/or eustachian tube inflation requiring general anesthesia

4.21 4.21 **FUD** 010 J A2 50

AMA: 2018,Jan,8; 2017,Jan,8; 2016,Jan,13; 2015,Jan,16

69424 Ventilating tube removal requiring general anesthesia

EXCLUDES
Cochlear device implantation (69930)
Eardrum repair (69610-69646)
Foreign body removal (69205)
Implantation, replacement electromagnetic bone conduction hearing device in temporal bone (69710-69745)
Labyrinth procedures (69801-69915)
Mastoid obliteration (69670)
Myringotomy (69420-69421)
Polyp, glomus tumor removal (69535-69554)
Removal impacted cerumen requiring instrumentation (69210)
Repair window (69666-69667)
Revised mastoidectomy (69601-69604)
Stapes procedures (69650-69662)
Transmastoid excision (69501-69530)
Tympanic neurectomy (69676)
Tympanostomy, tympanolysis (69433-69450)

1.73 3.62 **FUD** 000 Q2 P3 50

AMA: 2018,Jan,8; 2017,Jan,8; 2016,Jan,13; 2015,Jan,16

69433 Tympanostomy (requiring insertion of ventilating tube), local or topical anesthesia

EXCLUDES *Tympanostomy with tube insertion using iontophoresis and automated tube delivery system (0583T)*

3.72 5.62 **FUD** 010 T P3 50

AMA: 2018,Feb,11; 2018,Jan,8; 2017,Jan,8; 2016,Jan,13; 2015,Jan,16

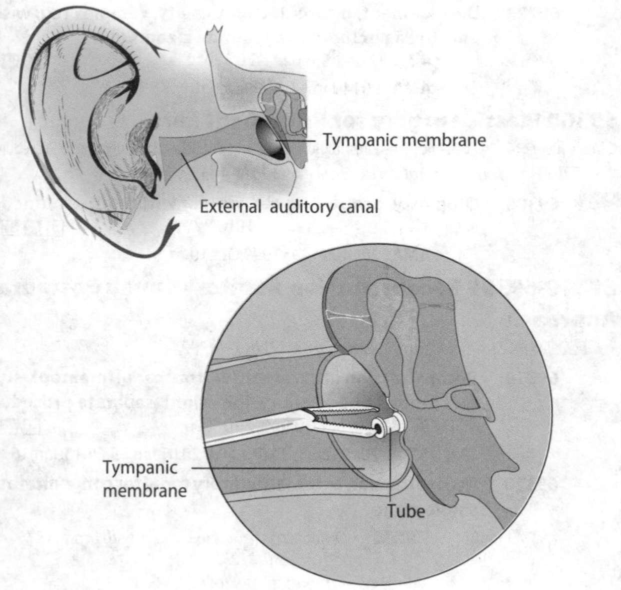

69436 Tympanostomy (requiring insertion of ventilating tube), general anesthesia

4.51 4.51 **FUD** 010 T A2 50

AMA: 2018,Feb,11; 2018,Jan,8; 2017,Jan,8; 2016,Jan,13; 2015,Jan,16

69440 Middle ear exploration through postauricular or ear canal incision

EXCLUDES *Atticotomy (69601-69604)*

19.5 19.5 **FUD** 090 J A2 50

AMA: 2014,Jan,11; 2008,Sep,10-11

69450 Tympanolysis, transcanal

15.4 15.4 **FUD** 090 J A2 80 50

AMA: 2014,Jan,11; 2008,Sep,10-11

69501-69530 Transmastoid Excision

EXCLUDES
Mastoidectomy cavity debridement (69220, 69222)
Skin graft (15004-15770)

69501 Transmastoid antrotomy (simple mastoidectomy)

20.3 20.3 **FUD** 090 J A2 50

AMA: 2018,Jan,8; 2017,Jan,8; 2016,Jan,13; 2015,Jan,16

69502 Mastoidectomy; complete

27.3 27.3 **FUD** 090 J A2 80 50

AMA: 2018,Jan,8; 2017,Jan,8; 2016,Jan,13; 2015,Jan,16

69505 modified radical

34.2 34.2 **FUD** 090 J A2 80 50

AMA: 2018,Jan,8; 2017,Jan,8; 2016,Jan,13; 2015,Jan,16

69511 radical

35.0 35.0 **FUD** 090 J A2 80 50

AMA: 2018,Jan,8; 2017,Jan,8; 2016,Jan,13; 2015,Jan,16

69530 Petrous apicectomy including radical mastoidectomy

47.1 47.1 **FUD** 090 J A2 80 50

AMA: 2014,Jan,11; 1999,Oct,10

69535-69554 Polyp and Glomus Tumor Removal

69535 Resection temporal bone, external approach

EXCLUDES *Middle fossa approach (69950-69970)*

75.4 75.4 **FUD** 090 C 50

AMA: 2014,Jan,11; 1999,Oct,10

69540 Excision aural polyp

3.58 5.83 **FUD** 010 T P3 50

AMA: 2014,Jan,11; 1999,Oct,10

69550 Excision aural glomus tumor; transcanal

29.5 29.5 **FUD** 090 J A2 80 50

AMA: 2014,Jan,11; 1999,Oct,10

69552 transmastoid

44.6 44.6 **FUD** 090 J A2 80 50

AMA: 2014,Jan,11; 1999,Oct,10

69554 extended (extratemporal)

71.5 71.5 **FUD** 090 C 80 50

AMA: 2014,Jan,11; 1999,Oct,10

69601-69605 Revised Mastoidectomy

EXCLUDES *Skin graft (15120-15121, 15260-15261)*

69601 Revision mastoidectomy; resulting in complete mastoidectomy

29.5 29.5 **FUD** 090 J A2 80 50

AMA: 2018,Jan,8; 2017,Jan,8; 2016,Jan,13; 2015,Jan,16

69602 resulting in modified radical mastoidectomy

30.8 30.8 **FUD** 090 J A2 80 50

AMA: 2018,Jan,8; 2017,Jan,8; 2016,Jan,13; 2015,Jan,16

69603 resulting in radical mastoidectomy

35.9 35.9 **FUD** 090 J A2 80 50

AMA: 2018,Jan,8; 2017,Jan,8; 2016,Jan,13; 2015,Jan,16

69604 resulting in tympanoplasty

EXCLUDES *Secondary tympanoplasty following mastoidectomy (69631-69632)*

31.5 31.5 **FUD** 090 J A2 50

AMA: 2018,Jan,8; 2017,Jan,8; 2016,Jan,13; 2015,Jan,16

69605 ~~with apicectomy~~

69610-69646 Eardrum Repair with/without Other Procedures

69610 **Tympanic membrane repair, with or without site preparation of perforation for closure, with or without patch**
8.27 10.8 FUD 010 J P3 50
AMA: 2018,Jan,8; 2017,Jan,8; 2016,Jan,13; 2015,May,10; 2015,Apr,10; 2015,Jan,16

69620 **Myringoplasty (surgery confined to drumhead and donor area)**
13.9 20.0 FUD 090 J A2 50
AMA: 2018,Jan,8; 2017,Jan,8; 2016,Jan,13; 2015,May,10; 2015,Apr,10; 2015,Jan,16

69631 **Tympanoplasty without mastoidectomy (including canalplasty, atticotomy and/or middle ear surgery), initial or revision; without ossicular chain reconstruction**
25.0 25.0 FUD 090 J A2 50
AMA: 2018,Jan,8; 2017,Jan,8; 2016,Jan,13; 2015,Jan,16

69632 **with ossicular chain reconstruction (eg, postfenestration)**
30.5 30.5 FUD 090 J A2 50
AMA: 2018,Jan,8; 2017,Jan,8; 2016,Jan,13; 2015,Jan,16

69633 **with ossicular chain reconstruction and synthetic prosthesis (eg, partial ossicular replacement prosthesis [PORP], total ossicular replacement prosthesis [TORP])**
29.6 29.6 FUD 090 J A2 50
AMA: 2018,Jan,8; 2017,Jan,8; 2016,Jan,13; 2015,Jan,16

69635 **Tympanoplasty with antrotomy or mastoidotomy (including canalplasty, atticotomy, middle ear surgery, and/or tympanic membrane repair); without ossicular chain reconstruction**
35.3 35.3 FUD 090 J A2 50
AMA: 2018,Jan,8; 2017,Jan,8; 2016,Jan,13; 2015,Jan,16

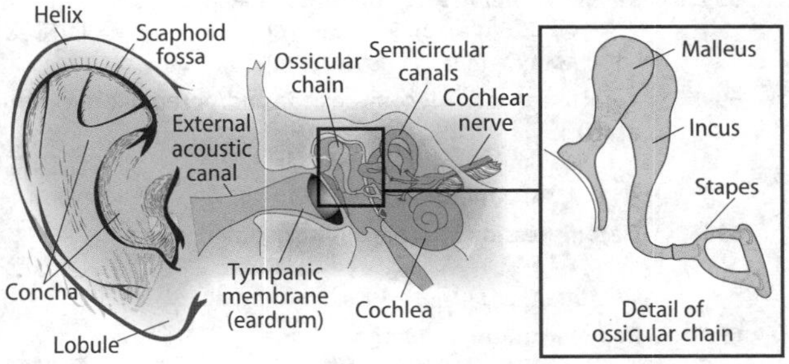

69636 **with ossicular chain reconstruction**
39.3 39.3 FUD 090 J A2 80 50
AMA: 2018,Jan,8; 2017,Jan,8; 2016,Jan,13; 2015,Jan,16

69637 **with ossicular chain reconstruction and synthetic prosthesis (eg, partial ossicular replacement prosthesis [PORP], total ossicular replacement prosthesis [TORP])**
39.9 39.9 FUD 090 J A2 80 50
AMA: 2018,Jan,8; 2017,Jan,8; 2016,Jan,13; 2015,Jan,16

69641 **Tympanoplasty with mastoidectomy (including canalplasty, middle ear surgery, tympanic membrane repair); without ossicular chain reconstruction**
29.6 29.6 FUD 090 J A2 50
AMA: 2018,Jan,8; 2017,Jan,8; 2016,Jan,13; 2015,Jan,16

69642 **with ossicular chain reconstruction**
38.0 38.0 FUD 090 J A2 50
AMA: 2018,Jan,8; 2017,Jan,8; 2016,Jan,13; 2015,Jan,16

69643 **with intact or reconstructed wall, without ossicular chain reconstruction**
34.7 34.7 FUD 090 J A2 50
AMA: 2018,Jan,8; 2017,Jan,8; 2016,Jan,13; 2015,Jan,16

69644 **with intact or reconstructed canal wall, with ossicular chain reconstruction**
42.1 42.1 FUD 090 J A2 50
AMA: 2018,Jan,8; 2017,Jan,8; 2016,Jan,13; 2015,Jan,16

69645 **radical or complete, without ossicular chain reconstruction**
41.4 41.4 FUD 090 J A2 50
AMA: 2018,Jan,8; 2017,Jan,8; 2016,Jan,13; 2015,Jan,16

69646 **radical or complete, with ossicular chain reconstruction**
44.1 44.1 FUD 090 J A2 80 50
AMA: 2018,Jan,8; 2017,Jan,8; 2016,Jan,13; 2015,Jan,16

69650-69662 Stapes Procedures

69650 **Stapes mobilization**
22.8 22.8 FUD 090 J A2 50
AMA: 2014,Jan,11; 1999,Oct,10

69660 **Stapedectomy or stapedotomy with reestablishment of ossicular continuity, with or without use of foreign material;**
26.3 26.3 FUD 090 J A2 50
AMA: 2014,Jan,11; 1999,Oct,10

69661 **with footplate drill out**
34.3 34.3 FUD 090 J A2 80 50
AMA: 2014,Jan,11; 1999,Oct,10

69662 **Revision of stapedectomy or stapedotomy**
32.9 32.9 FUD 090 J A2 50
AMA: 2014,Jan,11; 1999,Oct,10

69666-69706 Other Inner Ear Procedures

69666 **Repair oval window fistula**
22.9 22.9 FUD 090 J A2 80 50
AMA: 2014,Jan,11; 1999,Oct,10

69667 **Repair round window fistula**
23.0 23.0 FUD 090 J A2 80 50
AMA: 2014,Jan,11; 1999,Oct,10

69670 **Mastoid obliteration (separate procedure)**
26.8 26.8 FUD 090 J A2 80 50
AMA: 2014,Jan,11; 1999,Oct,10

69676 **Tympanic neurectomy**
23.6 23.6 FUD 090 J A2 50
AMA: 2014,Jan,11; 1999,Oct,10

69700 **Closure postauricular fistula, mastoid (separate procedure)**
19.3 19.3 FUD 090 T A2 50
AMA: 2014,Jan,11; 1999,Oct,10

● **69705** **Nasopharyngoscopy, surgical, with dilation of eustachian tube (ie, balloon dilation); unilateral**
EXCLUDES *Nasal endoscopy, diagnostic (31231)*
Nasopharyngoscopy with endoscope (92511)

● **69706** **bilateral**
EXCLUDES *Nasal endoscopy, diagnostic (31231)*
Nasopharyngoscopy with endoscope (92511)

69710-69718 Procedures Related to Hearing Aids/Auditory Implants

CMS: 100-02,16,100 Hearing Devices

69710 **Implantation or replacement of electromagnetic bone conduction hearing device in temporal bone**
INCLUDES Removal existing device when performing replacement procedure
0.00 0.00 FUD XXX E
AMA: 2014,Jan,11; 1999,Oct,10

69711 **Removal or repair of electromagnetic bone conduction hearing device in temporal bone**
24.2 24.2 FUD 090 J A2 80 50
AMA: 2014,Jan,11; 1999,Oct,10

69714 **Implantation, osseointegrated implant, temporal bone, with percutaneous attachment to external speech processor/cochlear stimulator; without mastoidectomy**
30.4 30.4 FUD 090 J J8 50
AMA: 2018,Jan,8; 2017,Jan,8; 2016,Jan,13; 2015,Jan,16

69715 **with mastoidectomy**
37.6 37.6 FUD 090 J J8 50
AMA: 2014,Jan,11; 1999,Oct,10

69717 **Replacement (including removal of existing device), osseointegrated implant, temporal bone, with percutaneous attachment to external speech processor/cochlear stimulator; without mastoidectomy**
31.9 31.9 FUD 090 J J8 50
AMA: 2014,Jan,11; 1999,Oct,10

69718 **with mastoidectomy**
38.0 38.0 FUD 090 J G2 50
AMA: 2014,Jan,11; 1999,Oct,10

69720-69799 Procedures of the Facial Nerve

EXCLUDES *Extracranial suture facial nerve (64864)*

69720 **Decompression facial nerve, intratemporal; lateral to geniculate ganglion**
34.1 34.1 FUD 090 J A2 80 50
AMA: 2014,Jan,11; 1999,Oct,10

69725 **including medial to geniculate ganglion**
53.5 53.5 FUD 090 J 80 50
AMA: 2014,Jan,11; 1999,Oct,10

69740 **Suture facial nerve, intratemporal, with or without graft or decompression; lateral to geniculate ganglion**
33.2 33.2 FUD 090 J A2 80 50
AMA: 2014,Jan,11; 1999,Oct,10

69745 **including medial to geniculate ganglion**
35.2 35.2 FUD 090 J A2 80 50
AMA: 2014,Jan,11; 1999,Oct,10

69799 **Unlisted procedure, middle ear**
0.00 0.00 FUD YYY T 80 50
AMA: 2019,Jan,14; 2018,Jan,8; 2017,Jan,8; 2016,Jan,13; 2015,Jan,16

69801-69915 Procedures of the Labyrinth

69801 **Labyrinthotomy, with perfusion of vestibuloactive drug(s), transcanal**
EXCLUDES *Myringotomy, tympanostomy on same ear (69420-69421, 69433, 69436)*
Procedure performed more than one time per day
3.55 6.05 FUD 000 T P3 80 50
AMA: 2018,Jan,8; 2017,Jan,8; 2016,Jan,13; 2015,Jan,16

69805 **Endolymphatic sac operation; without shunt**
29.8 29.8 FUD 090 J A2 80 50
AMA: 2014,Jan,11; 1999,Oct,10

69806 **with shunt**
26.6 26.6 FUD 090 J A2 50
AMA: 2014,Jan,11; 1999,Oct,10

69905 **Labyrinthectomy; transcanal**
26.0 26.0 FUD 090 J A2 50
AMA: 2014,Jan,11; 1999,Oct,10

69910 **with mastoidectomy**
28.7 28.7 FUD 090 J A2 80 50
AMA: 2014,Jan,11; 1999,Oct,10

69915 **Vestibular nerve section, translabyrinthine approach**
EXCLUDES *Transcranial approach (69950)*
43.6 43.6 FUD 090 J A2 80 50
AMA: 2014,Jan,11; 1999,Oct,10

69930-69949 Cochlear Implantation

CMS: 100-02,16,100 Hearing Devices

69930 **Cochlear device implantation, with or without mastoidectomy**
34.8 34.8 FUD 090 J J8 80 50
AMA: 2014,Jan,11; 1999,Oct,10

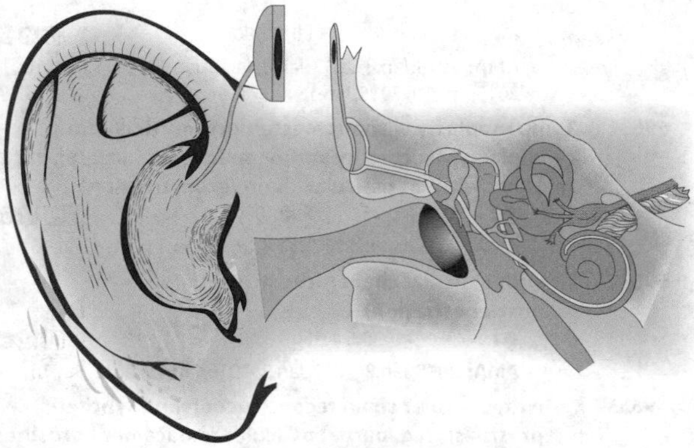

The internal coil is secured to the temporal bone and an electrode is fed through the round window into the cochlea

69949 **Unlisted procedure, inner ear**
0.00 0.00 FUD YYY T 80 50
AMA: 2014,Jan,11; 1999,Oct,10

69950-69979 Inner Ear Procedures via Craniotomy

EXCLUDES *External approach (69535)*

69950 **Vestibular nerve section, transcranial approach**
50.6 50.6 FUD 090 C 80 50
AMA: 2014,Jan,11; 1999,Oct,10

69955 **Total facial nerve decompression and/or repair (may include graft)**
56.1 56.1 FUD 090 J 80 50
AMA: 2014,Jan,11; 1999,Oct,10

69960 **Decompression internal auditory canal**
54.2 54.2 FUD 090 J 80 50
AMA: 2014,Jan,11; 1999,Oct,10

69970 **Removal of tumor, temporal bone**
60.8 60.8 FUD 090 J 80 50
AMA: 2014,Jan,11; 1999,Oct,10

69979 **Unlisted procedure, temporal bone, middle fossa approach**
0.00 0.00 FUD YYY T 80 50
AMA: 2018,Jan,8; 2017,Jan,8; 2016,Jan,13; 2015,Jan,16

69990 Operating Microscope

EXCLUDES *Magnifying loupes*
Reporting code with (15756-15758, 15842, 19364, 19368, 20955-20962, 20969-20973, 22551-22552, 22856-22857 [22858], 22861, 26551-26554, 26556, 31526, 31531, 31536, 31541-31546, 31561, 31571, 43116, 43180, 43496, 46601, 46607, 49906, 61548, 63075-63078, 64727, 64820-64823, 64912-64913, 65091-68850 [66987, 66988, 67810], 0184T, 0308T, 0402T, 0583T)

+ **69990** **Microsurgical techniques, requiring use of operating microscope (List separately in addition to code for primary procedure)**
Code first primary procedure
6.30 6.30 FUD ZZZ N N1 80
AMA: 2018,Feb,11; 2018,Jan,8; 2017,Dec,12; 2017,Dec,13; 2017,Dec,14; 2017,Jan,8; 2016,Feb,12; 2016,Jan,13; 2015,Jan,16

Radiology

Radiology

70010-70015 Radiography: Neurodiagnostic

70010 **Myelography, posterior fossa, radiological supervision and interpretation**
1.73 1.73 FUD XXX Q2 N1 80
AMA: 2018,Jan,8; 2017,Jan,8; 2016,Jan,13; 2015,Jan,16

70015 **Cisternography, positive contrast, radiological supervision and interpretation**
4.35 4.35 FUD XXX Q2 N1 80
AMA: 2014,Jan,11; 2012,Feb,9-10

70030-70390 Radiography: Head, Neck, Orofacial Structures

INCLUDES Minimum number views or more views when needed to adequately complete study
Radiographs repeated during encounter due to substandard quality; only one unit reported

EXCLUDES *Obtaining more films after initial film review, based on radiologist discretion, order for test, and change in patient's condition*

70030 **Radiologic examination, eye, for detection of foreign body**
0.87 0.87 FUD XXX Q1 N1 80
AMA: 2014,Jan,11; 2012,Feb,9-10

70100 **Radiologic examination, mandible; partial, less than 4 views**
1.03 1.03 FUD XXX Q1 N1 80
AMA: 2014,Jan,11; 2012,Feb,9-10

70110 **complete, minimum of 4 views**
1.13 1.13 FUD XXX Q1 N1 80
AMA: 2014,Jan,11; 2012,Feb,9-10

70120 **Radiologic examination, mastoids; less than 3 views per side**
1.03 1.03 FUD XXX Q1 N1 80
AMA: 2014,Jan,11; 2012,Feb,9-10

70130 **complete, minimum of 3 views per side**
1.68 1.68 FUD XXX Q1 N1 80
AMA: 2014,Jan,11; 2012,Feb,9-10

70134 **Radiologic examination, internal auditory meati, complete**
1.59 1.59 FUD XXX Q1 N1 80
AMA: 2014,Jan,11; 2012,Feb,9-10

70140 **Radiologic examination, facial bones; less than 3 views**
0.88 0.88 FUD XXX Q1 N1 80
AMA: 2014,Jan,11; 2012,Feb,9-10

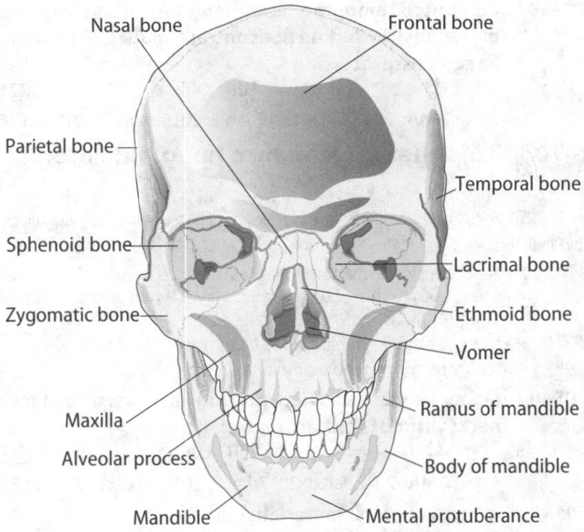

70150 **complete, minimum of 3 views**
1.23 1.23 FUD XXX Q1 N1 80
AMA: 2014,Jan,11; 2012,Feb,9-10

70160 **Radiologic examination, nasal bones, complete, minimum of 3 views**
1.02 1.02 FUD XXX Q1 N1 80
AMA: 2014,Jan,11; 2012,Feb,9-10

70170 **Dacryocystography, nasolacrimal duct, radiological supervision and interpretation**
EXCLUDES *Injection contrast (68850)*
0.00 0.00 FUD XXX Q2 N1 80
AMA: 2014,Jan,11; 2012,Feb,9-10

70190 **Radiologic examination; optic foramina**
1.08 1.08 FUD XXX Q1 N1 80
AMA: 2014,Jan,11; 2012,Feb,9-10

70200 **orbits, complete, minimum of 4 views**
1.31 1.31 FUD XXX Q1 N1 80
AMA: 2014,Jan,11; 2012,Feb,9-10

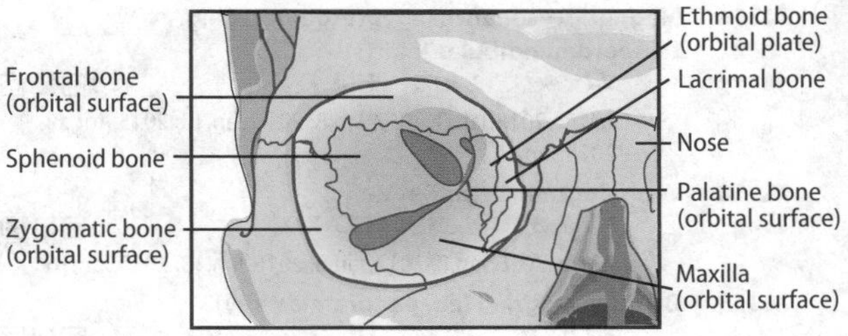

70210 **Radiologic examination, sinuses, paranasal, less than 3 views**
0.89 0.89 FUD XXX Q1 N1 80
AMA: 2014,Jan,11; 2012,Feb,9-10

70220 **Radiologic examination, sinuses, paranasal, complete, minimum of 3 views**
1.10 1.10 FUD XXX Q1 N1 80
AMA: 2014,Jan,11; 2012,Feb,9-10

70240 **Radiologic examination, sella turcica**
0.94 0.94 FUD XXX Q1 N1 80
AMA: 2014,Jan,11; 2012,Feb,9-10

70250 **X-ray of skull, fewer than 4 views**
1.07 1.07 FUD XXX Q1 N1 80
AMA: 2014,Jan,11; 2012,Feb,9-10

70260 **complete, minimum of 4 views**
1.24 1.24 FUD XXX Q1 N1 80
AMA: 2014,Jan,11; 2012,Feb,9-10

70300 **Radiologic examination, teeth; single view**
0.39 0.39 FUD XXX Q1 N1 80
AMA: 2014,Jan,11; 2012,Feb,9-10

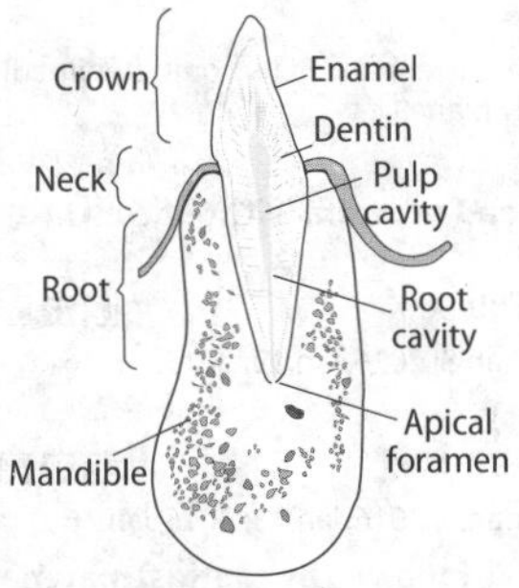

Section of incisor

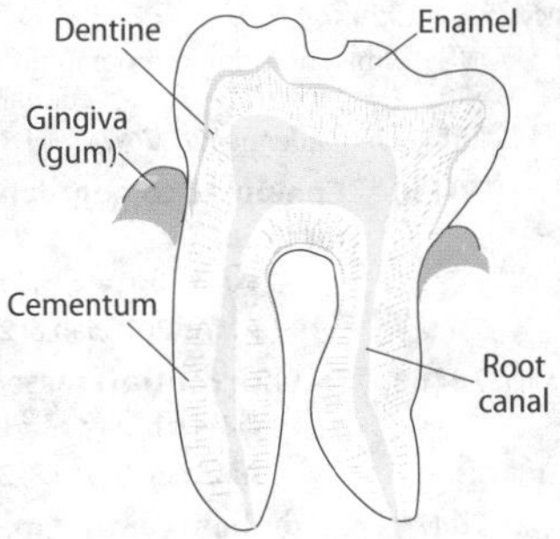

Section of molar

70310 **partial examination, less than full mouth**
1.10 1.10 FUD XXX Q1 N1 80
AMA: 2014,Jan,11; 2012,Feb,9-10

70320 **complete, full mouth**
1.56 1.56 FUD XXX Q1 N1 80
AMA: 2014,Jan,11; 2012,Feb,9-10

70328 **Radiologic examination, temporomandibular joint, open and closed mouth; unilateral**
0.94 0.94 FUD XXX Q1 N1 80
AMA: 2014,Jan,11; 2012,Feb,9-10

70330 **bilateral**
1.45 1.45 FUD XXX Q1 N1 80
AMA: 2018,Jan,8; 2017,Jan,8; 2016,Jan,13; 2015,Jan,16

70332 **Temporomandibular joint arthrography, radiological supervision and interpretation**
INCLUDES Fluoroscopic guidance (77002)
2.15 2.15 FUD XXX Q2 N1 80
AMA: 2018,Jan,8; 2017,Jan,8; 2016,Jan,13; 2015,Jan,16

70336 **Magnetic resonance (eg, proton) imaging, temporomandibular joint(s)**
8.86 8.86 FUD XXX Q3 Z2 80
AMA: 2018,Jan,8; 2017,Jan,8; 2016,Jan,13; 2015,Aug,6; 2015,Jan,16

70350 **Cephalogram, orthodontic**
0.53 0.53 FUD XXX Q1 N1 80
AMA: 2018,Jan,8; 2017,Jan,8; 2016,Jan,13; 2015,Jan,16

70355 **Orthopantogram (eg, panoramic x-ray)**
0.54 0.54 FUD XXX Q1 N1 80
AMA: 2014,Jan,11; 2012,Feb,9-10

70360 **Radiologic examination; neck, soft tissue**
0.86 0.86 FUD XXX Q1 N1 80
AMA: 2014,Jan,11; 2012,Feb,9-10

70370 **pharynx or larynx, including fluoroscopy and/or magnification technique**
2.49 2.49 FUD XXX Q1 N1 80
AMA: 2014,Jan,11; 2012,Feb,9-10

70371 **Complex dynamic pharyngeal and speech evaluation by cine or video recording**
EXCLUDES *Laryngeal computed tomography (70490-70492)*
3.03 3.03 FUD XXX Q1 N1 80
AMA: 2018,Jan,8; 2017,Jan,8; 2016,Jan,13; 2015,Jan,16

70380 **Radiologic examination, salivary gland for calculus**
0.95 0.95 FUD XXX Q1 N1 80
AMA: 2014,Jan,11; 2012,Feb,9-10

70390 **Sialography, radiological supervision and interpretation**
3.16 3.16 FUD XXX Q2 N1 80
AMA: 2014,Jan,11; 2012,Feb,9-10

70450-70492 Computerized Tomography: Head, Neck, Face

CMS: 100-04,4,250.16 Multiple Procedure Payment Reduction: Certain Diagnostic Imaging Procedures Rendered by Physicians

INCLUDES Imaging using tomographic technique enhanced by computer imaging to create cross-sectional body plane view
EXCLUDES *3D rendering (76376-76377)*

70450 **Computed tomography, head or brain; without contrast material**
3.26 3.26 FUD XXX Q3 Z2 80
AMA: 2018,Jan,8; 2017,Jan,8; 2016,Jan,13; 2015,Jan,16

70460 **with contrast material(s)**
4.61 4.61 FUD XXX Q3 Z2 80
AMA: 2018,Jan,8; 2017,Jan,8; 2016,Jan,13; 2015,Jan,16

70470 **without contrast material, followed by contrast material(s) and further sections**
5.38 5.38 FUD XXX Q3 Z2 80
AMA: 2018,Jan,8; 2017,Jan,8; 2016,Jan,13; 2015,Jan,16

70480 **Computed tomography, orbit, sella, or posterior fossa or outer, middle, or inner ear; without contrast material**
5.64 5.64 FUD XXX Q3 Z2 80
AMA: 2018,Jan,8; 2017,Jan,8; 2016,Jan,13; 2015,Jan,16

70481 **with contrast material(s)**
7.76 7.76 FUD XXX Q3 Z2 80
AMA: 2018,Jan,8; 2017,Jan,8; 2016,Jan,13; 2015,Jan,16

70482 **without contrast material, followed by contrast material(s) and further sections**
6.97 6.97 FUD XXX Q3 Z2 80
AMA: 2014,Jan,11; 2012,Feb,9-10

70486 **Computed tomography, maxillofacial area; without contrast material**
3.92 3.92 FUD XXX Q3 Z2 80
AMA: 2018,Jan,8; 2017,Jan,8; 2016,Jan,13; 2015,Jan,16

70487 **with contrast material(s)**
4.70 4.70 FUD XXX Q3 Z2 80
AMA: 2014,Jan,11; 2012,Feb,9-10

70488 **without contrast material, followed by contrast material(s) and further sections**
5.73 5.73 FUD XXX Q3 Z2 80
AMA: 2014,Jan,11; 2012,Feb,9-10

70490 **Computed tomography, soft tissue neck; without contrast material**
EXCLUDES *CT cervical spine (72125)*
4.63 4.63 FUD XXX Q3 Z2 80
AMA: 2014,Jan,11; 2012,Feb,9-10

70491 **with contrast material(s)**
EXCLUDES *CT cervical spine (72125)*
5.71 5.71 FUD XXX Q3 Z2 80
AMA: 2014,Jan,11; 2012,Feb,9-10

70492 **without contrast material followed by contrast material(s) and further sections**
EXCLUDES *CT cervical spine (72125)*
6.89 6.89 FUD XXX Q3 Z2 80
AMA: 2014,Jan,11; 2012,Feb,9-10

70496-70498 Computerized Tomographic Angiography: Head and Neck

CMS: 100-04,4,250.16 Multiple Procedure Payment Reduction: Certain Diagnostic Imaging Procedures Rendered by Physicians

INCLUDES Computed tomography to visualize arterial and venous vessels

70496 **Computed tomographic angiography, head, with contrast material(s), including noncontrast images, if performed, and image postprocessing**
8.31 8.31 FUD XXX Q3 Z2 80
AMA: 2018,Jan,8; 2017,Jan,8; 2016,Jan,13; 2015,Jan,16

70498 **Computed tomographic angiography, neck, with contrast material(s), including noncontrast images, if performed, and image postprocessing**
8.29 8.29 FUD XXX Q3 Z2 80
AMA: 2018,Jan,8; 2017,Jan,8; 2016,Jan,13; 2015,Jan,16

70540-70543 Magnetic Resonance Imaging: Face, Neck, Orbits

CMS: 100-04,4,250.16 Multiple Procedure Payment Reduction: Certain Diagnostic Imaging Procedures Rendered by Physicians

INCLUDES Three-dimensional imaging that measures response oatomic nuclei in soft tissues to high-frequency radio waves when strong magnetic field applied
EXCLUDES *Magnetic resonance angiography head/neck (70544-70549)*
Procedure performed more than one time per session

70540 **Magnetic resonance (eg, proton) imaging, orbit, face, and/or neck; without contrast material(s)**
7.34 7.34 FUD XXX Q3 Z2 80
AMA: 2018,Jan,8; 2017,Jan,8; 2016,Jan,13; 2015,Jan,16

70542 **with contrast material(s)**
8.72 8.72 FUD XXX Q3 Z2 80
AMA: 2018,Jan,8; 2017,Jan,8; 2016,Jan,13; 2015,Jan,16

70543 **without contrast material(s), followed by contrast material(s) and further sequences**
11.1 11.1 FUD XXX Q3 Z2 80
AMA: 2018,Jan,8; 2017,Jan,8; 2016,Jan,13; 2015,Jan,16

70544-70549 Magnetic Resonance Angiography: Head and Neck

CMS: 100-04,13,40.1.1 Magnetic Resonance Angiography; 100-04,13,40.1.2 HCPCS Coding Requirements; 100-04,4,250.16 Multiple Procedure Payment Reduction: Certain Diagnostic Imaging Procedures Rendered by Physicians

INCLUDES Magnetic fields and radio waves to produce detailed cross-sectional internal body structure images

EXCLUDES *Reporting code with following unless separate diagnostic MRI performed (70551-70553)*

70544 **Magnetic resonance angiography, head; without contrast material(s)**
7.84 7.84 **FUD** XXX Q3 Z2 80
AMA: 2018,Jan,8; 2017,Jan,8; 2016,Jan,13; 2015,Jan,16

70545 **with contrast material(s)**
7.21 7.21 **FUD** XXX Q3 Z2 80
AMA: 2018,Jan,8; 2017,Jan,8; 2016,Jan,13; 2015,Jan,16

70546 **without contrast material(s), followed by contrast material(s) and further sequences**
10.4 10.4 **FUD** XXX Q3 Z2 80
AMA: 2018,Jan,8; 2017,Jan,8; 2016,Jan,13; 2015,Jan,16

70547 **Magnetic resonance angiography, neck; without contrast material(s)**
6.93 6.93 **FUD** XXX Q3 Z2 80
AMA: 2018,Jan,8; 2017,Jan,8; 2016,Jan,13; 2015,Jan,16

70548 **with contrast material(s)**
7.74 7.74 **FUD** XXX Q3 Z2 80
AMA: 2018,Jan,8; 2017,Jan,8; 2016,Jan,13; 2015,Jan,16

70549 **without contrast material(s), followed by contrast material(s) and further sequences**
10.9 10.9 **FUD** XXX Q3 Z2 80
AMA: 2018,Jan,8; 2017,Jan,8; 2016,Jan,13; 2015,Jan,16

70551-70553 Magnetic Resonance Imaging: Brain and Brain Stem

CMS: 100-04,4,200.3.2 Multi-Source Photon Stereotactic RadiosurgeryPlanning and Delivery; 100-04,4,250.16 Multiple Procedure Payment Reduction: Certain Diagnostic Imaging Procedures Rendered by Physicians

INCLUDES Three-dimensional imaging that measures response oatomic nuclei in soft tissues to high-frequency radio waves when strong magnetic field applied

EXCLUDES *Magnetic spectroscopy (76390)*

70551 **Magnetic resonance (eg, proton) imaging, brain (including brain stem); without contrast material**
6.28 6.28 **FUD** XXX Q3 Z2 80
AMA: 2018,Jan,8; 2017,Jan,8; 2016,Jan,13; 2015,Jan,16

70552 **with contrast material(s)**
8.69 8.69 **FUD** XXX Q3 Z2 80
AMA: 2018,Jan,8; 2017,Jan,8; 2016,Jan,13; 2015,Jan,16

70553 **without contrast material, followed by contrast material(s) and further sequences**
10.4 10.4 **FUD** XXX Q3 Z2 80
AMA: 2018,Jan,8; 2017,Jan,8; 2016,Jan,13; 2015,Jan,16

70554-70555 Magnetic Resonance Imaging: Brain Mapping

INCLUDES Neuroimaging technique using MRI to identify and map signals related to brain activity

EXCLUDES *Reporting code with following unless separate diagnostic MRI performed (70551-70553)*

70554 **Magnetic resonance imaging, brain, functional MRI; including test selection and administration of repetitive body part movement and/or visual stimulation, not requiring physician or psychologist administration**
EXCLUDES *Functional brain mapping (96020)*
Testing performed by physician or psychologist (70555)
12.4 12.4 **FUD** XXX Q3 Z2 80
AMA: 2018,Jan,8; 2017,Jan,8; 2016,Jan,13; 2015,Jan,16

70555 **requiring physician or psychologist administration of entire neurofunctional testing**
EXCLUDES *Testing performed by technologist, nonphysician, or nonpsychologist (70554)*
Code also (96020)
0.00 0.00 **FUD** XXX S Z2 80
AMA: 2018,Jan,8; 2017,Jan,8; 2016,Jan,13; 2015,Jan,16

70557-70559 Magnetic Resonance Imaging: Intraoperative

EXCLUDES *Intracranial lesion stereotaxic biopsy with magnetic resonance guidance (61751, 77021-77022)*
Procedures performed more than one time per surgical encounter
Reporting codes unless separate report generated

Code also stereotactic biopsy, aspiration, or excision, when performed with MRI (61751)

70557 **Magnetic resonance (eg, proton) imaging, brain (including brain stem and skull base), during open intracranial procedure (eg, to assess for residual tumor or residual vascular malformation); without contrast material**
0.00 0.00 **FUD** XXX S Z2 80
AMA: 2014,Jan,11; 2012,Feb,9-10

70558 **with contrast material(s)**
0.00 0.00 **FUD** XXX S Z2 80
AMA: 2014,Jan,11; 2012,Feb,9-10

70559 **without contrast material(s), followed by contrast material(s) and further sequences**
0.00 0.00 **FUD** XXX S Z2 80
AMA: 2014,Jan,11; 2012,Feb,9-10

71045-71130 Radiography: Thorax

71045 **Radiologic examination, chest; single view**
EXCLUDES *Acute abdomen series, complete (2 or more views) including chest view (74022)*
Remotely performed CAD (0175T)
Code also concurrent computer-aided detection (CAD) (0174T)
0.70 0.70 **FUD** XXX Q3 Z3 80
AMA: 2019,Aug,8; 2019,May,10; 2019,Mar,10; 2018,Apr,7

71046 **2 views**
EXCLUDES *Acute abdomen series, complete (2 or more views) including chest view (74022)*
Remotely performed CAD (0175T)
Code also concurrent computer-aided detection (CAD) (0174T)
0.89 0.89 **FUD** XXX Q3 Z3 80
AMA: 2019,Aug,8; 2019,Mar,10; 2018,Apr,7

71047 **3 views**
EXCLUDES *Acute abdomen series, complete (2 or more views) including chest view (74022)*
Remotely performed CAD (0175T)
Code also concurrent computer-aided detection (CAD) (0174T)
1.12 1.12 **FUD** XXX Q1 N1 80
AMA: 2019,Mar,10; 2018,Apr,7

71048 **4 or more views**
EXCLUDES *Acute abdomen series, complete (2 or more views) including chest view (74022)*
Remotely performed CAD (0175T)
Code also concurrent computer-aided detection (CAD) (0174T)
1.21 1.21 **FUD** XXX Q1 N1 80
AMA: 2019,Mar,10; 2018,Apr,7

71100 Radiologic examination, ribs, unilateral; 2 views
1.00 1.00 FUD XXX Q1 N1 80
AMA: 2014,Jan,11; 2012,Feb,9-10

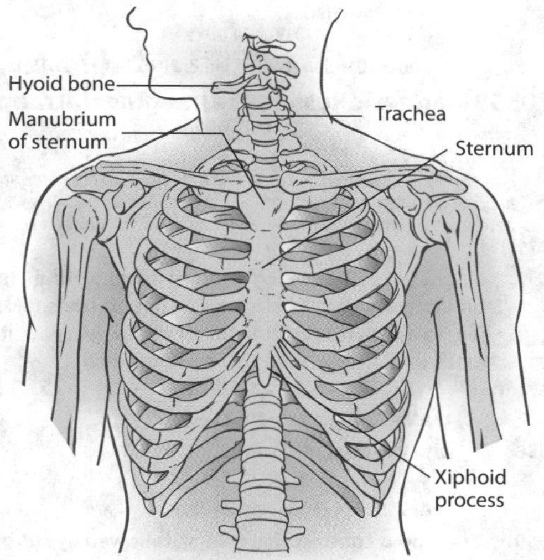

71101 including posteroanterior chest, minimum of 3 views
1.11 1.11 FUD XXX Q1 N1 80
AMA: 2014,Jan,11; 2012,Feb,9-10

71110 Radiologic examination, ribs, bilateral; 3 views
1.21 1.21 FUD XXX Q1 N1 80
AMA: 2014,Jan,11; 2012,Feb,9-10

71111 including posteroanterior chest, minimum of 4 views
1.38 1.38 FUD XXX Q1 N1 80
AMA: 2014,Jan,11; 2012,Feb,9-10

71120 Radiologic examination; sternum, minimum of 2 views
0.88 0.88 FUD XXX Q1 N1 80
AMA: 2014,Jan,11; 2012,Feb,9-10

71130 sternoclavicular joint or joints, minimum of 3 views
1.12 1.12 FUD XXX Q1 N1 80
AMA: 2014,Jan,11; 2012,Feb,9-10

71250-71271 Computerized Tomography: Thorax

INCLUDES Imaging using tomographic technique enhanced by computer imaging to create cross-sectional body plane view

EXCLUDES *3D rendering (76376-76377)*
CT breast (0633T-0638T)
CT heart (75571-75574)

▲ **71250 Computed tomography, thorax, diagnostic; without contrast material**
EXCLUDES *CT thorax with contrast (71260-71270)*
CT thorax for lung cancer screening (71271)
4.47 4.47 FUD XXX Q3 Z2 80
AMA: 2020,Sep,11; 2018,Jan,8; 2017,Jan,8; 2016,Jan,13; 2015,Jan,16

▲ **71260 with contrast material(s)**
EXCLUDES *CT thorax for lung cancer screening (71271)*
CT thorax without contrast (71250, 71270)
5.52 5.52 FUD XXX Q3 Z2 80
AMA: 2020,Sep,11; 2018,Jan,8; 2017,Jan,8; 2016,Jan,13; 2015,Jan,16

▲ **71270 without contrast material, followed by contrast material(s) and further sections**
EXCLUDES *CT thorax for lung cancer screening (71271)*
CT thorax with or without contrast only (71250, 71260)
6.53 6.53 FUD XXX Q3 Z2 80
AMA: 2020,Sep,11; 2018,Jan,8; 2017,Jan,8; 2016,Jan,13; 2015,Jan,16

● **71271 Computed tomography, thorax, low dose for lung cancer screening, without contrast material(s)**
EXCLUDES *CT thorax not for lung cancer screening (71250, 71260, 71270)*

71275 Computerized Tomographic Angiography: Thorax

CMS: 100-04,4,250.16 Multiple Procedure Payment Reduction: Certain Diagnostic Imaging Procedures Rendered by Physicians

INCLUDES Multiple rapid thin section CT scans to create cross-sectional bone, organ, and tissue images

EXCLUDES *CT angiography coronary arteries including calcification score and/or cardiac morphology (75574)*

71275 Computed tomographic angiography, chest (noncoronary), with contrast material(s), including noncontrast images, if performed, and image postprocessing
8.53 8.53 FUD XXX Q3 Z2 80
AMA: 2020,Sep,11; 2018,Jan,8; 2017,Jan,8; 2016,Jan,13; 2015,Jan,16

71550-71552 Magnetic Resonance Imaging: Thorax

CMS: 100-04,4,250.16 Multiple Procedure Payment Reduction: Certain Diagnostic Imaging Procedures Rendered by Physicians

INCLUDES Three-dimensional imaging that measures response atomic nuclei in soft tissues to high-frequency radio waves when strong magnetic field applied

EXCLUDES *MRI of the breast (77046-77049)*

71550 Magnetic resonance (eg, proton) imaging, chest (eg, for evaluation of hilar and mediastinal lymphadenopathy); without contrast material(s)
11.1 11.1 FUD XXX Q3 Z2 80
AMA: 2018,Jan,8; 2017,Jan,8; 2016,Jan,13; 2015,Jan,16

71551 with contrast material(s)
12.3 12.3 FUD XXX Q3 Z2 80
AMA: 2018,Jan,8; 2017,Jan,8; 2016,Jan,13; 2015,Jan,16

71552 without contrast material(s), followed by contrast material(s) and further sequences
15.5 15.5 FUD XXX Q3 Z2 80
AMA: 2018,Jan,8; 2017,Jan,8; 2016,Jan,13; 2015,Jan,16

71555 Magnetic Resonance Angiography: Thorax

CMS: 100-04,13,40.1.1 Magnetic Resonance Angiography; 100-04,13,40.1.2 HCPCS Coding Requirements; 100-04,4,250.16 Multiple Procedure Payment Reduction: Certain Diagnostic Imaging Procedures Rendered by Physicians

71555 Magnetic resonance angiography, chest (excluding myocardium), with or without contrast material(s)
10.8 10.8 FUD XXX B 80
AMA: 2018,Jan,8; 2017,Jan,8; 2016,Jan,13; 2015,Jan,16

72020-72120 Radiography: Spine

INCLUDES Minimum number views or more views when needed to adequately complete study
Radiographs repeated during encounter due to substandard quality; only one unit reported

EXCLUDES *Obtaining more films after initial film review, based on the radiologist discretion, an order for the test, and change in patient's condition*

72020 Radiologic examination, spine, single view, specify level
EXCLUDES *Single view entire thoracic and lumbar spine (72081)*
0.65 0.65 FUD XXX Q1 N1 80
AMA: 2018,Jan,8; 2017,Jan,8; 2016,Sep,4; 2016,Jan,13; 2015,Oct,9; 2015,Jan,16

72040 **Radiologic examination, spine, cervical; 2 or 3 views**
1.03 1.03 FUD XXX Q1 N1 80
AMA: 2018,Aug,10; 2018,Jan,8; 2017,Jan,8; 2016,Jan,13; 2015,Jan,16

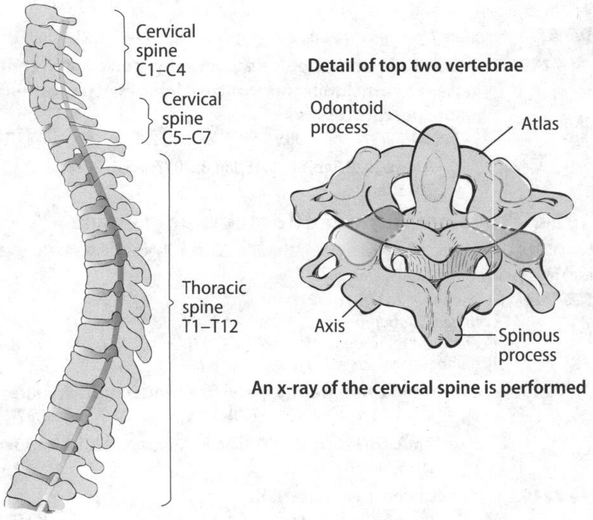

An x-ray of the cervical spine is performed

72050 **4 or 5 views**
1.42 1.42 FUD XXX Q1 N1 80
AMA: 2014,Jan,11; 2012,Feb,9-10

72052 **6 or more views**
1.69 1.69 FUD XXX Q1 N1 80
AMA: 2014,Jan,11; 2012,Feb,9-10

72070 **Radiologic examination, spine; thoracic, 2 views**
0.89 0.89 FUD XXX Q1 N1 80
AMA: 2018,Jan,8; 2017,Jan,8; 2016,Jan,13; 2015,Jan,16

72072 **thoracic, 3 views**
1.08 1.08 FUD XXX Q1 N1 80
AMA: 2018,Jan,8; 2017,Jan,8; 2016,Jan,13; 2015,Jan,16

72074 **thoracic, minimum of 4 views**
1.21 1.21 FUD XXX Q1 N1 80
AMA: 2018,Jan,8; 2017,Jan,8; 2016,Jan,13; 2015,Jan,16

72080 **thoracolumbar junction, minimum of 2 views**
EXCLUDES *Single view thoracolumbar junction (72020)*
0.95 0.95 FUD XXX Q1 N1 80
AMA: 2018,Jan,8; 2017,Jan,8; 2016,Sep,4; 2016,Jan,13; 2015,Oct,9; 2015,Jan,16

72081 **Radiologic examination, spine, entire thoracic and lumbar, including skull, cervical and sacral spine if performed (eg, scoliosis evaluation); one view**
1.17 1.17 FUD XXX Q1 N1 80
AMA: 2018,Jan,8; 2017,Jan,8; 2016,Sep,4

72082 **2 or 3 views**
1.90 1.90 FUD XXX Q1 N1 80
AMA: 2018,Jan,8; 2017,Jan,8; 2016,Sep,4

72083 **4 or 5 views**
2.21 2.21 FUD XXX S Z2 80
AMA: 2018,Jan,8; 2017,Jan,8; 2016,Sep,4

72084 **minimum of 6 views**
2.62 2.62 FUD XXX S Z2 80
AMA: 2018,Jan,8; 2017,Jan,8; 2016,Sep,4

72100 **Radiologic examination, spine, lumbosacral; 2 or 3 views**
1.07 1.07 FUD XXX Q1 N1 80
AMA: 2018,Jan,8; 2017,Jan,8; 2016,Jan,13; 2015,Jan,16

72110 **minimum of 4 views**
1.36 1.36 FUD XXX Q1 N1 80
AMA: 2018,Jan,8; 2017,Jan,8; 2016,Jan,13; 2015,Jan,16

72114 **complete, including bending views, minimum of 6 views**
1.64 1.64 FUD XXX Q1 N1 80
AMA: 2014,Jan,11; 2012,Feb,9-10

72120 **bending views only, 2 or 3 views**
1.11 1.11 FUD XXX Q1 N1 80
AMA: 2018,Jan,8; 2017,Jan,8; 2016,Aug,7

72125-72133 Computerized Tomography: Spine

CMS: 100-04,12,20.4.7 Services Not Meeting National Electrical Manufacturers Association (NEMA) Standard; 100-04,4,20.6.12 Use of HCPCS Modifier – CT; 100-04,4,250.16 Multiple Procedure Payment Reduction: Certain Diagnostic Imaging Procedures Rendered by Physicians

INCLUDES Imaging using tomographic technique enhanced by computer imaging to create cross-sectional body plane view
EXCLUDES *3D rendering (76376-76377)*
Code also intrathecal injection procedure when performed (61055, 62284)

72125 **Computed tomography, cervical spine; without contrast material**
5.18 5.18 FUD XXX Q3 Z2 80
AMA: 2020,Sep,11

72126 **with contrast material**
6.40 6.40 FUD XXX Q3 Z3 80
AMA: 2020,Sep,11; 2018,Jan,8; 2017,Jan,8; 2016,Jan,13; 2015,Jan,16

72127 **without contrast material, followed by contrast material(s) and further sections**
6.48 6.48 FUD XXX Q3 Z2 80
AMA: 2020,Sep,11

72128 **Computed tomography, thoracic spine; without contrast material**
5.08 5.08 FUD XXX Q3 Z2 80
AMA: 2020,Sep,11

72129 **with contrast material**
5.54 5.54 FUD XXX Q3 Z2 80
AMA: 2020,Sep,11; 2019,Jan,14; 2018,Jan,8; 2017,Jan,8; 2016,Jan,13; 2015,Jan,16

72130 **without contrast material, followed by contrast material(s) and further sections**
7.59 7.59 FUD XXX Q3 Z2 80
AMA: 2020,Sep,11

72131 **Computed tomography, lumbar spine; without contrast material**
4.36 4.36 FUD XXX Q3 Z2 80
AMA: 2020,Sep,11

72132 **with contrast material**
5.51 5.51 FUD XXX Q3 Z3 80
AMA: 2020,Sep,11; 2019,Jan,14; 2018,Jan,8; 2017,Jan,8; 2016,Jan,13; 2015,Jan,16

72133 **without contrast material, followed by contrast material(s) and further sections**
6.45 6.45 FUD XXX Q3 Z2 80
AMA: 2020,Sep,11

72141-72158 Magnetic Resonance Imaging: Spine

CMS: 100-04,4,250.16 Multiple Procedure Payment Reduction: Certain Diagnostic Imaging Procedures Rendered by Physicians

INCLUDES Three-dimensional imaging that measures response atomic nuclei in soft tissues to high-frequency radio waves when strong magnetic field applied
EXCLUDES *MR spectroscopy (0609T-0610T)*
Code also intrathecal injection procedure when performed (61055, 62284)

72141 **Magnetic resonance (eg, proton) imaging, spinal canal and contents, cervical; without contrast material**
6.11 6.11 FUD XXX Q3 Z2 80
AMA: 2018,Jan,8; 2017,Jan,8; 2016,Jan,13; 2015,Jan,16

72142 **with contrast material(s)**
EXCLUDES *MRI cervical spinal canal performed without contrast followed by repeating study with contrast (72156)*
8.88 8.88 FUD XXX Q3 Z2 80
AMA: 2018,Jan,8; 2017,Jan,8; 2016,Jan,13; 2015,Jan,16

72146 **Magnetic resonance (eg, proton) imaging, spinal canal and contents, thoracic; without contrast material**
6.23 6.23 FUD XXX Q3 Z2 80
AMA: 2018,Jan,8; 2017,Jan,8; 2016,Jan,13; 2015,Jan,16

72147 **with contrast material(s)**
EXCLUDES *MRI thoracic spinal canal performed without contrast followed by repeating study with contrast (72157)*
8.82 8.82 FUD XXX Q3 Z2 80
AMA: 2018,Jan,8; 2017,Jan,8; 2016,Jan,13; 2015,Jan,16

72148 **Magnetic resonance (eg, proton) imaging, spinal canal and contents, lumbar; without contrast material**
6.23 6.23 FUD XXX Q3 Z2 80
AMA: 2018,Jan,8; 2017,Jan,8; 2016,Jan,13; 2015,Jan,16

72149 **with contrast material(s)**
EXCLUDES *MRI lumbar spinal canal performed without contrast followed by repeating study with contrast (72158)*
8.92 8.92 FUD XXX Q3 Z2 80
AMA: 2014,Jan,11; 2012,Feb,9-10

72156 **Magnetic resonance (eg, proton) imaging, spinal canal and contents, without contrast material, followed by contrast material(s) and further sequences; cervical**
10.3 10.3 FUD XXX Q3 Z2 80
AMA: 2014,Jan,11; 2012,Feb,9-10

72157 **thoracic**
10.5 10.5 FUD XXX Q3 Z2 80
AMA: 2014,Jan,11; 2012,Feb,9-10

72158 **lumbar**
10.3 10.3 FUD XXX Q3 Z2 80
AMA: 2014,Jan,11; 2012,Feb,9-10

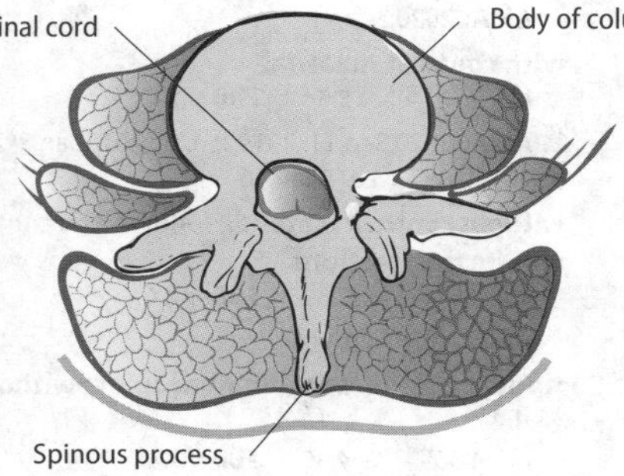

Superior view of thoracic spine and surrounding paraspinal muscles

72159 Magnetic Resonance Angiography: Spine

CMS: 100-04,13,40.1.1 Magnetic Resonance Angiography; 100-04,13,40.1.2 HCPCS Coding Requirements; 100-04,4,250.16 Multiple Procedure Payment Reduction: Certain Diagnostic Imaging Procedures Rendered by Physicians

72159 **Magnetic resonance angiography, spinal canal and contents, with or without contrast material(s)**
11.2 11.2 FUD XXX B 80
AMA: 2018,Jan,8; 2017,Jan,8; 2016,Jan,13; 2015,Jan,16

72170-72190 Radiography: Pelvis

INCLUDES Minimum number views or more views when needed to adequately complete study
Radiographs repeated during encounter due to substandard quality; only one unit reported

EXCLUDES *Combined CT or CT angiography abdomen and pelvis (74174, 74176-74178)*
Obtaining more films after initial film review, based on radiologist discretion, order for test, and change in patient's condition
Pelvimetry (74710)
Second interpretation by requesting physician (included in E/M service)

72170 **Radiologic examination, pelvis; 1 or 2 views**
0.80 0.80 FUD XXX Q1 N1 80
AMA: 2018,Jan,8; 2017,Jan,8; 2016,Aug,7; 2016,Jun,5; 2016,Jan,13; 2015,Jan,16

72190 **complete, minimum of 3 views**
1.12 1.12 FUD XXX Q1 N1 80
AMA: 2016,Jun,5

72191 Computerized Tomographic Angiography: Pelvis

CMS: 100-04,4,250.16 Multiple Procedure Payment Reduction: Certain Diagnostic Imaging Procedures Rendered by Physicians

EXCLUDES *Computed tomographic angiography (73706, 74174-74175, 75635)*

72191 **Computed tomographic angiography, pelvis, with contrast material(s), including noncontrast images, if performed, and image postprocessing**
9.08 9.08 FUD XXX Q3 Z2 80
AMA: 2020,Sep,11; 2018,Jan,8; 2017,Jan,8; 2016,Jan,13; 2015,Jan,16

72192-72194 Computerized Tomography: Pelvis

CMS: 100-04,4,250.16 Multiple Procedure Payment Reduction: Certain Diagnostic Imaging Procedures Rendered by Physicians

EXCLUDES *3D rendering (76376-76377)*
Combined CT abdomen and pelvis (74176-74178)
CT colonography, diagnostic (74261-74262)
CT colonography, screening (74263)

72192 **Computed tomography, pelvis; without contrast material**
4.10 4.10 FUD XXX Q3 Z2 80
AMA: 2020,Sep,11; 2018,Jan,8; 2017,Jan,8; 2016,Jan,13; 2015,Jan,16

72193 **with contrast material(s)**
6.59 6.59 FUD XXX Q3 Z2 80
AMA: 2020,Sep,11; 2018,Jan,8; 2017,Jan,8; 2016,Jan,13; 2015,Jan,16

72194 **without contrast material, followed by contrast material(s) and further sections**
7.48 7.48 FUD XXX Q3 Z2 80
AMA: 2020,Sep,11; 2018,Jan,8; 2017,Jan,8; 2016,Jan,13; 2015,Jan,16

72195-72197 Magnetic Resonance Imaging: Pelvis

CMS: 100-04,4,250.16 Multiple Procedure Payment Reduction: Certain Diagnostic Imaging Procedures Rendered by Physicians

INCLUDES Three-dimensional imaging that measures response atomic nuclei in soft tissues to high-frequency radio waves when strong magnetic field applied

EXCLUDES *MRI fetus(es) (74712-74713)*

72195 **Magnetic resonance (eg, proton) imaging, pelvis; without contrast material(s)**
7.62 7.62 FUD XXX Q3 Z2 80
AMA: 2018,Jul,11; 2018,Jan,8; 2017,Jan,8; 2016,Jun,5; 2016,Jan,13; 2015,Jan,16

72196 **with contrast material(s)**
8.74 8.74 FUD XXX Q3 Z2 80
AMA: 2018,Jul,11; 2018,Jan,8; 2017,Jan,8; 2016,Jun,5; 2016,Jan,13; 2015,Jan,16

72197 **without contrast material(s), followed by contrast material(s) and further sequences**
10.9 10.9 FUD XXX Q3 Z2 80
AMA: 2018,Jul,11; 2018,Jan,8; 2017,Jan,8; 2016,Jun,5; 2016,Jan,13; 2015,Jan,16

72198 Magnetic Resonance Angiography: Pelvis

CMS: 100-04,13,40.1.1 Magnetic Resonance Angiography; 100-04,13,40.1.2 HCPCS Coding Requirements; 100-04,4,250.16 Multiple Procedure Payment Reduction: Certain Diagnostic Imaging Procedures Rendered by Physicians

INCLUDES Magnetic fields and radio waves to produce detailed cross-sectional images arteries and veins

72198 **Magnetic resonance angiography, pelvis, with or without contrast material(s)**
11.0 11.0 FUD XXX B 80
AMA: 2018,Jan,8; 2017,Jan,8; 2016,Jan,13; 2015,Jan,16

72200-72220 Radiography: Pelvisacral

INCLUDES Minimum number views or more views when needed to adequately complete study
Radiographs repeated during encounter due to substandard quality; only one unit reported

EXCLUDES *Obtaining more films after initial film review, based on radiologist discretion, order for, and change in patient's condition*
Second interpretation by requesting physician (included in E/M service)

72200 Radiologic examination, sacroiliac joints; less than 3 views
0.90 0.90 **FUD** XXX Q1 N1 80
AMA: 2014,Jan,11; 2012,Feb,9-10

72202 3 or more views
0.98 0.98 **FUD** XXX Q1 N1 80
AMA: 2014,Jan,11; 2012,Feb,9-10

72220 Radiologic examination, sacrum and coccyx, minimum of 2 views
0.88 0.88 **FUD** XXX Q1 N1 80
AMA: 2014,Jan,11; 2012,Feb,9-10

72240-72270 Myelography with Contrast: Spinal Cord

CMS: 100-04,13,30.1.3.1 Payment for Low Osmolar Contrast Material

EXCLUDES *Injection procedure for myelography (62284)*
Myelography (62302-62305)

Code also injection at C1-C2 for complete myelography (61055)

72240 Myelography, cervical, radiological supervision and interpretation
3.14 3.14 **FUD** XXX Q2 N1 80
AMA: 2018,Jan,8; 2017,Jan,8; 2016,Jan,13; 2015,Jan,16

72255 Myelography, thoracic, radiological supervision and interpretation
3.19 3.19 **FUD** XXX Q2 N1 80
AMA: 2018,Jan,8; 2017,Jan,8; 2016,Jan,13; 2015,Jan,16

72265 Myelography, lumbosacral, radiological supervision and interpretation
2.90 2.90 **FUD** XXX Q2 N1 80
AMA: 2018,Jan,8; 2017,Jan,8; 2016,Jan,13; 2015,Jan,16

72270 Myelography, 2 or more regions (eg, lumbar/thoracic, cervical/thoracic, lumbar/cervical, lumbar/thoracic/cervical), radiological supervision and interpretation
4.00 4.00 **FUD** XXX Q2 N1 80
AMA: 2018,Jan,8; 2017,Jan,8; 2016,Jan,13; 2015,Jan,16

72275 Radiography: Epidural Space

INCLUDES Epidurogram, image documentation, and formal written report
Fluoroscopic guidance (77003)

EXCLUDES *Arthrodesis (22586)*
Second interpretation by requesting physician (included in E/M service)

Code also injection procedure as appropriate (62280-62282, 62320-62327, 64479-64480, 64483-64484)

72275 Epidurography, radiological supervision and interpretation
3.48 3.48 **FUD** XXX N N1 80
AMA: 2018,Jan,8; 2017,Jan,8; 2016,Jan,13; 2015,Jan,16

72285 Radiography: Intervertebral Disc (Cervical/Thoracic)

CMS: 100-04,13,30.1.3.1 Payment for Low Osmolar Contrast Material

Code also discography injection procedure (62291)

72285 Discography, cervical or thoracic, radiological supervision and interpretation
3.32 3.32 **FUD** XXX Q2 N1 80
AMA: 2018,Jan,8; 2017,Jan,8; 2016,Jan,13; 2015,Jan,16

72295 Radiography: Intervertebral Disc (Lumbar)

CMS: 100-04,13,30.1.3.1 Payment for Low Osmolar Contrast Material

Code also discography injection procedure (62290)

72295 Discography, lumbar, radiological supervision and interpretation
2.90 2.90 **FUD** XXX Q2 N1 80
AMA: 2018,Jan,8; 2017,Feb,12; 2017,Jan,8; 2016,Jan,13; 2015,Jan,16

73000-73085 Radiography: Shoulder and Upper Arm

INCLUDES Minimum number views or more views when needed to adequately complete study
Radiographs repeated during encounter due to substandard quality; only one unit reported

EXCLUDES *Obtaining more films after initial film review, based on radiologist discretion, order for test, and change in patient's condition*
Second interpretation by requesting physician (included in E/M service)
Stress views upper body joint(s), when performed (77071)

73000 Radiologic examination; clavicle, complete
0.88 0.88 **FUD** XXX Q1 N1 80
AMA: 2014,Jan,11; 2012,Feb,9-10

Radiograph

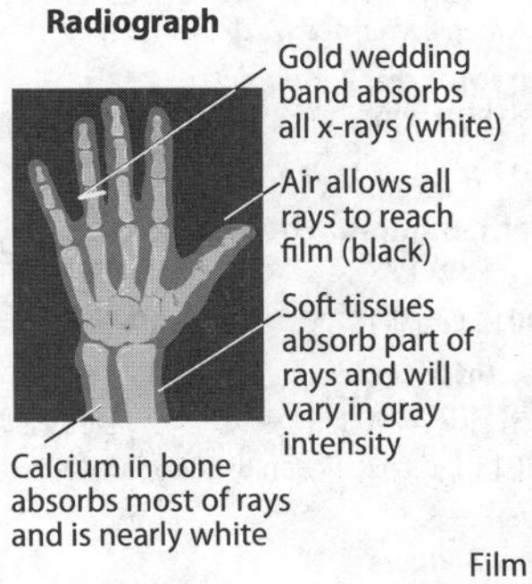
Gold wedding band absorbs all x-rays (white)
Air allows all rays to reach film (black)
Soft tissues absorb part of rays and will vary in gray intensity
Calcium in bone absorbs most of rays and is nearly white

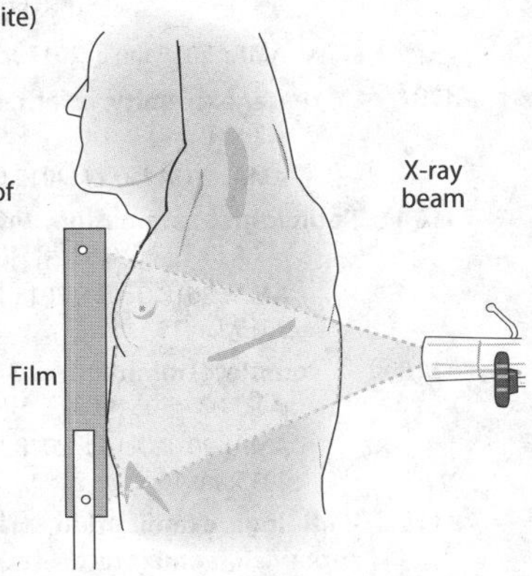
X-ray beam
Film

Posterioranterior (PA) chest study; lateral views also common

73010 scapula, complete
0.90 0.90 **FUD** XXX Q1 N1 80
AMA: 2014,Jan,11; 2012,Feb,9-10

73020 Radiologic examination, shoulder; 1 view
0.67 0.67 **FUD** XXX Q1 N1 80
AMA: 2014,Jan,11; 2012,Feb,9-10

73030 complete, minimum of 2 views
0.85 0.85 **FUD** XXX Q1 N1 80
AMA: 2014,Jan,11; 2012,Feb,9-10

73040 Radiologic examination, shoulder, arthrography, radiological supervision and interpretation
INCLUDES Fluoroscopic guidance (77002)
Code also arthrography injection procedure (23350)
3.12 3.12 **FUD** XXX Q2 N1 80
AMA: 2018,Jan,8; 2017,Jan,8; 2016,Jan,13; 2015,Jan,16

73050 Radiologic examination; acromioclavicular joints, bilateral, with or without weighted distraction
1.05 1.05 **FUD** XXX Q1 N1 80
AMA: 2014,Jan,11; 2012,Feb,9-10

73060 humerus, minimum of 2 views
0.88 0.88 **FUD** XXX Q1 N1 80
AMA: 2014,Jan,11; 2012,Feb,9-10

73070 Radiologic examination, elbow; 2 views
0.76 0.76 **FUD** XXX Q1 N1 80
AMA: 2018,Jan,8; 2017,Jan,8; 2016,Jan,13; 2015,Jan,16

73080 complete, minimum of 3 views
0.84 0.84 **FUD** XXX Q1 N1 80
AMA: 2014,Jan,11; 2012,Feb,9-10

73085 **Radiologic examination, elbow, arthrography, radiological supervision and interpretation**

INCLUDES Fluoroscopic guidance (77002)

Code also arthrography injection procedure (24220)

3.18 3.18 FUD XXX Q2 N1 80

AMA: 2018,Jan,8; 2017,Jan,8; 2016,Jan,13; 2015,Jan,16

73090-73140 Radiography: Forearm and Hand

INCLUDES Minimum number views or more views when needed to adequately complete study

Radiographs repeated during encounter due to substandard quality; only one unit reported

EXCLUDES *Obtaining more films after initial film review, based on radiologist discretion, order for test, and change in patient's condition*

Second interpretation by requesting physician (included in E/M service)

Stress views upper body joint(s), when performed (77071)

73090 **Radiologic examination; forearm, 2 views**

0.79 0.79 FUD XXX Q1 N1 80

AMA: 2018,Jan,8; 2017,Jan,8; 2016,Jan,13; 2015,Jan,16

73092 **upper extremity, infant, minimum of 2 views** A

0.81 0.81 FUD XXX Q1 N1 80

AMA: 2014,Jan,11; 2012,Feb,9-10

73100 **Radiologic examination, wrist; 2 views**

0.92 0.92 FUD XXX Q1 N1 80

AMA: 2018,Oct,11; 2018,Jan,8; 2017,Jan,8; 2016,Jan,13; 2015,Jan,16

73110 **complete, minimum of 3 views**

1.03 1.03 FUD XXX Q1 N1 80

AMA: 2018,Oct,11; 2018,Jan,8; 2017,Jan,8; 2016,Jan,13; 2015,Jan,16

73115 **Radiologic examination, wrist, arthrography, radiological supervision and interpretation**

INCLUDES Fluoroscopic guidance (77002)

Code also arthrography injection procedure (25246)

3.33 3.33 FUD XXX Q2 N1 80

AMA: 2018,Jan,8; 2017,Jan,8; 2016,Jan,13; 2015,Jan,16

73120 **Radiologic examination, hand; 2 views**

0.85 0.85 FUD XXX Q1 N1 80

AMA: 2018,Oct,11

73130 **minimum of 3 views**

0.98 0.98 FUD XXX Q1 N1 80

AMA: 2014,Jan,11; 2012,Feb,9-10

73140 **Radiologic examination, finger(s), minimum of 2 views**

1.00 1.00 FUD XXX Q1 N1 80

AMA: 2018,Jan,8; 2017,Jan,8; 2016,Jan,13; 2015,Jan,16

73200-73202 Computerized Tomography: Shoulder, Arm, Hand

CMS: 100-04,4,250.16 Multiple Procedure Payment Reduction: Certain Diagnostic Imaging Procedures Rendered by Physicians

INCLUDES Imaging using tomographic technique enhanced by computer imaging to create cross-sectional body plane view

Intravascular, intrathecal, or intra-articular contrast materials when noted in code descriptor

EXCLUDES *3D rendering (76376-76377)*

73200 **Computed tomography, upper extremity; without contrast material**

5.03 5.03 FUD XXX Q3 Z2 80

AMA: 2018,Jan,8; 2017,Jan,8; 2016,Jan,13; 2015,Jan,16

73201 **with contrast material(s)**

6.26 6.26 FUD XXX Q3 Z3 80

AMA: 2018,Jan,8; 2017,Jan,8; 2016,Jan,13; 2015,Aug,6; 2015,Jan,16

73202 **without contrast material, followed by contrast material(s) and further sections**

7.82 7.82 FUD XXX Q3 Z2 80

AMA: 2014,Jan,11; 2012,Feb,9-10

73206 Computerized Tomographic Angiography: Shoulder, Arm, and Hand

CMS: 100-04,4,250.16 Multiple Procedure Payment Reduction: Certain Diagnostic Imaging Procedures Rendered by Physicians

INCLUDES Intravascular, intrathecal, or intra-articular contrast materials when noted in code descriptor

Multiple rapid thin section CT scans to create cross-sectional images arteries and veins

73206 **Computed tomographic angiography, upper extremity, with contrast material(s), including noncontrast images, if performed, and image postprocessing**

9.24 9.24 FUD XXX Q3 Z2 80

AMA: 2018,Jan,8; 2017,Jan,8; 2016,Jan,13; 2015,Jan,16

73218-73223 Magnetic Resonance Imaging: Shoulder, Arm, Hand

CMS: 100-04,4,250.16 Multiple Procedure Payment Reduction: Certain Diagnostic Imaging Procedures Rendered by Physicians

INCLUDES Three-dimensional imaging that measures response atomic nuclei in soft tissues to high-frequency radio waves when strong magnetic field applied

Intravascular, intrathecal, or intra-articular contrast materials when noted in code descriptor

73218 **Magnetic resonance (eg, proton) imaging, upper extremity, other than joint; without contrast material(s)**

9.93 9.93 FUD XXX Q3 Z2 80

AMA: 2018,Jan,8; 2017,Jan,8; 2016,Jan,13; 2015,Jan,16

73219 **with contrast material(s)**

10.9 10.9 FUD XXX Q3 Z2 80

AMA: 2018,Jan,8; 2017,Jan,8; 2016,Jan,13; 2015,Jan,16

73220 **without contrast material(s), followed by contrast material(s) and further sequences**

13.7 13.7 FUD XXX Q3 Z2 80

AMA: 2018,Jan,8; 2017,Jan,8; 2016,Jan,13; 2015,Jan,16

73221 **Magnetic resonance (eg, proton) imaging, any joint of upper extremity; without contrast material(s)**

6.57 6.57 FUD XXX Q3 Z2 80

AMA: 2018,Jan,8; 2017,Jan,8; 2016,Jan,13; 2015,Jan,16

73222 **with contrast material(s)**

10.2 10.2 FUD XXX Q3 Z3 80

AMA: 2018,Jan,8; 2017,Jan,8; 2016,Jan,13; 2015,Aug,6; 2015,Jan,16

73223 **without contrast material(s), followed by contrast material(s) and further sequences**

12.7 12.7 FUD XXX Q3 Z2 80

AMA: 2018,Jan,8; 2017,Jan,8; 2016,Jan,13; 2015,Jan,16

73225 Magnetic Resonance Angiography: Shoulder, Arm, Hand

CMS: 100-04,13,40.1.1 Magnetic Resonance Angiography; 100-04,4,250.16 Multiple Procedure Payment Reduction: Certain Diagnostic Imaging Procedures Rendered by Physicians

INCLUDES Intravascular, intrathecal, or intra-articular contrast materials when noted in code descriptor

Magnetic fields and radio waves to produce detailed cross-sectional images arteries and veins

73225 **Magnetic resonance angiography, upper extremity, with or without contrast material(s)**

11.1 11.1 FUD XXX B 80

AMA: 2018,Jan,8; 2017,Jan,8; 2016,Jan,13; 2015,Jan,16

73501-73552 Radiography: Pelvic Region and Thigh

EXCLUDES *Stress views lower body joint(s), when performed (77071)*

73501 **Radiologic examination, hip, unilateral, with pelvis when performed; 1 view**

0.89 0.89 FUD XXX Q1 N1 80

AMA: 2018,Jan,8; 2017,Jan,8; 2016,Aug,7; 2016,Jun,8; 2016,Jan,13; 2015,Oct,9

73502 **2-3 views**
1.27 1.27 FUD XXX Q1 N1 80
AMA: 2018,Jan,8; 2017,Jan,8; 2016,Aug,7; 2016,Jun,8; 2016,Jan,13; 2015,Oct,9

73503 **minimum of 4 views**
1.57 1.57 FUD XXX Q1 N1 80
AMA: 2018,Jan,8; 2017,Jan,8; 2016,Aug,7; 2016,Jun,8; 2016,Jan,13; 2015,Oct,9

73521 **Radiologic examination, hips, bilateral, with pelvis when performed; 2 views**
1.12 1.12 FUD XXX Q1 N1 80
AMA: 2018,Jan,8; 2017,Jan,8; 2016,Aug,7; 2016,Jun,8; 2016,Jan,13; 2015,Oct,9

73522 **3-4 views**
1.46 1.46 FUD XXX Q1 N1 80
AMA: 2018,Jan,8; 2017,Jan,8; 2016,Aug,7; 2016,Jun,8; 2016,Jan,13; 2015,Oct,9

73523 **minimum of 5 views**
1.66 1.66 FUD XXX S N1 80
AMA: 2018,Jan,8; 2017,Jan,8; 2016,Aug,7; 2016,Jun,8; 2016,Jan,13; 2015,Oct,9

73525 **Radiologic examination, hip, arthrography, radiological supervision and interpretation**
INCLUDES Fluoroscopic guidance (77002)
3.47 3.47 FUD XXX Q2 N1 80
AMA: 2018,Jan,8; 2017,Jan,8; 2016,Nov,10; 2016,Aug,7; 2016,Jan,13; 2015,Jan,16

73551 **Radiologic examination, femur; 1 view**
0.82 0.82 FUD XXX Q1 N1 80
AMA: 2018,Jan,8; 2017,Jan,8; 2016,Aug,7

73552 **minimum 2 views**
0.97 0.97 FUD XXX Q1 N1 80
AMA: 2018,Jan,8; 2017,Nov,10; 2017,Jan,8; 2016,Aug,7

73560-73660 Radiography: Lower Leg, Ankle, and Foot

EXCLUDES *Stress views lower body joint(s), when performed (77071)*

73560 **Radiologic examination, knee; 1 or 2 views**
0.94 0.94 FUD XXX Q1 N1 80
AMA: 2018,Jan,8; 2017,Jan,8; 2016,Jan,13; 2015,May,10; 2015,Feb,10

73562 **3 views**
1.05 1.05 FUD XXX Q1 N1 80
AMA: 2014,Jan,11; 2012,Feb,9-10

73564 **complete, 4 or more views**
1.17 1.17 FUD XXX Q1 N1 80
AMA: 2018,Jan,8; 2017,Jan,8; 2016,Jan,13; 2015,May,10; 2015,Feb,10; 2015,Jan,16

73565 **both knees, standing, anteroposterior**
1.05 1.05 FUD XXX Q1 N1 80
AMA: 2018,Jan,8; 2017,Jan,8; 2016,Jan,13; 2015,May,10; 2015,Feb,10

73580 **Radiologic examination, knee, arthrography, radiological supervision and interpretation**
INCLUDES Fluoroscopic guidance (77002)
3.59 3.59 FUD XXX Q2 N1 80
AMA: 2019,Aug,7; 2018,Jan,8; 2017,Jan,8; 2016,Jan,13; 2015,Aug,6; 2015,Jan,16

73590 **Radiologic examination; tibia and fibula, 2 views**
0.86 0.86 FUD XXX Q1 N1 80
AMA: 2018,Jan,8; 2017,Nov,10; 2017,Jan,8; 2016,Jan,13; 2015,Jan,16

73592 **lower extremity, infant, minimum of 2 views** A
0.81 0.81 FUD XXX Q1 N1 80
AMA: 2018,Jan,8; 2017,Nov,10

73600 **Radiologic examination, ankle; 2 views**
0.87 0.87 FUD XXX Q1 N1 80
AMA: 2018,Jan,8; 2017,Jan,8; 2016,Jan,13; 2015,Jan,16

73610 **complete, minimum of 3 views**
0.98 0.98 FUD XXX Q1 N1 80
AMA: 2018,Jan,8; 2017,Jan,8; 2016,Jan,13; 2015,Jan,16

73615 **Radiologic examination, ankle, arthrography, radiological supervision and interpretation**
INCLUDES Fluoroscopic guidance (77002)
3.34 3.34 FUD XXX Q2 N1 80
AMA: 2018,Jan,8; 2017,Jan,8; 2016,Jan,13; 2015,Jan,16

73620 **Radiologic examination, foot; 2 views**
0.78 0.78 FUD XXX Q1 N1 80
AMA: 2018,Jan,8; 2017,Jan,8; 2016,Jan,13; 2015,Jan,16

73630 **complete, minimum of 3 views**
0.88 0.88 FUD XXX Q1 N1 80
AMA: 2014,Jan,11; 2012,Feb,9-10

73650 **Radiologic examination; calcaneus, minimum of 2 views**
0.76 0.76 FUD XXX Q1 N1 80
AMA: 2014,Jan,11; 2012,Feb,9-10

73660 **toe(s), minimum of 2 views**
0.79 0.79 FUD XXX Q1 N1 80
AMA: 2014,Jan,11; 2012,Feb,9-10

73700-73702 Computerized Tomography: Leg, Ankle, and Foot

CMS: 100-04,4,250.16 Multiple Procedure Payment Reduction: Certain Diagnostic Imaging Procedures Rendered by Physicians

EXCLUDES *3D rendering (76376-76377)*

73700 **Computed tomography, lower extremity; without contrast material**
4.36 4.36 FUD XXX Q3 Z2 80
AMA: 2018,Jan,8; 2017,Jan,8; 2016,Jan,13; 2015,Jan,16

73701 **with contrast material(s)**
6.36 6.36 FUD XXX Q3 Z2 80
AMA: 2019,Aug,7; 2018,Jan,8; 2017,Jan,8; 2016,Jan,13; 2015,Jan,16

73702 **without contrast material, followed by contrast material(s) and further sections**
6.56 6.56 FUD XXX Q3 Z2 80
AMA: 2019,Aug,7; 2018,Jan,8; 2017,Jan,8; 2016,Jan,13; 2015,Jan,16

73706 Computerized Tomographic Angiography: Leg, Ankle, and Foot

CMS: 100-04,4,250.16 Multiple Procedure Payment Reduction: Certain Diagnostic Imaging Procedures Rendered by Physicians

EXCLUDES *CT angiography for aorto-iliofemoral runoff (75635)*

73706 **Computed tomographic angiography, lower extremity, with contrast material(s), including noncontrast images, if performed, and image postprocessing**
10.0 10.0 FUD XXX Q3 Z2 80
AMA: 2018,Jan,8; 2017,Jan,8; 2016,Jan,13; 2015,Jan,16

73718-73723 Magnetic Resonance Imaging: Leg, Ankle, and Foot

CMS: 100-04,4,250.16 Multiple Procedure Payment Reduction: Certain Diagnostic Imaging Procedures Rendered by Physicians

73718 **Magnetic resonance (eg, proton) imaging, lower extremity other than joint; without contrast material(s)**
7.39 7.39 FUD XXX Q3 Z2 80
AMA: 2018,Jan,8; 2017,Jan,8; 2016,Jan,13; 2015,Jan,16

73719 **with contrast material(s)**
8.58 8.58 FUD XXX Q3 Z2 80
AMA: 2019,Aug,7; 2018,Jan,8; 2017,Jan,8; 2016,Jan,13; 2015,Jan,16

73720 **without contrast material(s), followed by contrast material(s) and further sequences**
11.2 11.2 FUD XXX Q3 Z2 80
AMA: 2019,Aug,7; 2018,Jan,8; 2017,Jan,8; 2016,Jan,13; 2015,Jan,16

73721 **Magnetic resonance (eg, proton) imaging, any joint of lower extremity; without contrast material**
6.44 | 6.44 | **FUD** XXX | Q3 Z2 80
AMA: 2018,Jan,8; 2017,Jan,8; 2016,Jan,13; 2015,Jan,16

73722 **with contrast material(s)**
10.5 | 10.5 | **FUD** XXX | Q3 Z3 80
AMA: 2019,Aug,7; 2018,Jan,8; 2017,Jan,8; 2016,Jan,13; 2015,Aug,6; 2015,Jan,16

73723 **without contrast material(s), followed by contrast material(s) and further sequences**
12.7 | 12.7 | **FUD** XXX | Q3 Z2 80
AMA: 2019,Aug,7; 2018,Jan,8; 2017,Jan,8; 2016,Jan,13; 2015,Jan,16

73725 Magnetic Resonance Angiography: Leg, Ankle, and Foot

CMS: 100-04,13,40.1.2 HCPCS Coding Requirements; 100-04,4,250.16 Multiple Procedure Payment Reduction: Certain Diagnostic Imaging Procedures Rendered by Physicians

73725 **Magnetic resonance angiography, lower extremity, with or without contrast material(s)**
11.1 | 11.1 | **FUD** XXX | B 80
AMA: 2018,Jan,8; 2017,Jan,8; 2016,Jan,13; 2015,Jan,16

74018-74022 Radiography: Abdomen--General

74018 **Radiologic examination, abdomen; 1 view**
0.80 | 0.80 | **FUD** XXX | Q1 N1 80
AMA: 2020,Apr,10; 2019,May,10; 2018,Apr,7

74019 **2 views**
0.98 | 0.98 | **FUD** XXX | Q1 N1 80
AMA: 2018,Apr,7

74021 **3 or more views**
1.17 | 1.17 | **FUD** XXX | Q1 N1 80
AMA: 2018,Apr,7

74022 **Radiologic examination, complete acute abdomen series, including 2 or more views of the abdomen (eg, supine, erect, decubitus), and a single view chest**
1.36 | 1.36 | **FUD** XXX | Q1 N1 80
AMA: 2019,May,10; 2018,Apr,7; 2016,Jun,5

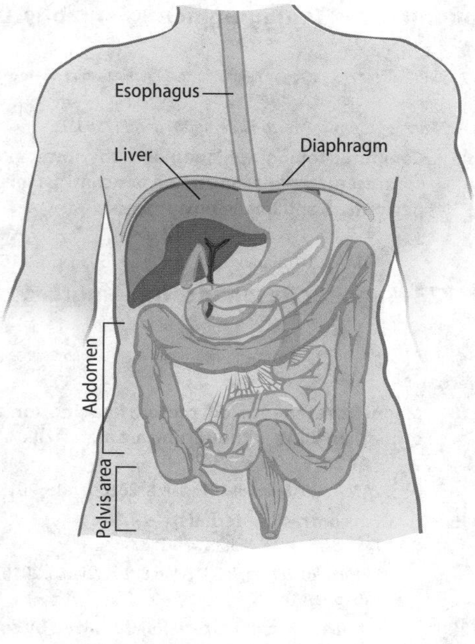

74150-74170 Computerized Tomography: Abdomen–General

CMS: 100-04,4,250.16 Multiple Procedure Payment Reduction: Certain Diagnostic Imaging Procedures Rendered by Physicians

EXCLUDES *3D rendering (76376-76377)*
Combined CT abdomen and pelvis (74176-74178)
CT colonography, diagnostic (74261-74262)
CT colonography, screening (74263)

74150 **Computed tomography, abdomen; without contrast material**
4.20 | 4.20 | **FUD** XXX | Q3 Z2 80
AMA: 2020,Sep,11; 2018,Jan,8; 2017,Jan,8; 2016,Jun,5; 2016,Jan,13; 2015,Jan,16

74160 **with contrast material(s)**
6.72 | 6.72 | **FUD** XXX | Q3 Z2 80
AMA: 2020,Sep,11; 2018,Jan,8; 2017,Jan,8; 2016,Jun,5; 2016,Jan,13; 2015,Jan,16

74170 **without contrast material, followed by contrast material(s) and further sections**
7.62 | 7.62 | **FUD** XXX | Q3 Z2 80
AMA: 2020,Sep,11; 2018,Jan,8; 2017,Jan,8; 2016,Jun,5; 2016,Jan,13; 2015,Jan,16

74174-74175 Computerized Tomographic Angiography: Abdomen and Pelvis

CMS: 100-04,4,250.16 Multiple Procedure Payment Reduction: Certain Diagnostic Imaging Procedures Rendered by Physicians

EXCLUDES *CT angiography for aorto-iliofemoral runoff (75635)*
CT angiography, lower extremity (73706)
CT angiography, pelvis (72191)

74174 **Computed tomographic angiography, abdomen and pelvis, with contrast material(s), including noncontrast images, if performed, and image postprocessing**
EXCLUDES *3D rendering (76376-76377)*
CT angiography abdomen (74175)
11.1 | 11.1 | **FUD** XXX | S Z2 80
AMA: 2020,Sep,11

74175 **Computed tomographic angiography, abdomen, with contrast material(s), including noncontrast images, if performed, and image postprocessing**
9.10 | 9.10 | **FUD** XXX | Q3 Z2 80
AMA: 2020,Sep,11; 2018,Jan,8; 2017,Jan,8; 2016,Jan,13; 2015,Jan,16

74176-74178 Computerized Tomography: Abdomen and Pelvis

CMS: 100-04,4,250.16 Multiple Procedure Payment Reduction: Certain Diagnostic Imaging Procedures Rendered by Physicians

EXCLUDES *CT abdomen or pelvis alone (72192-72194, 74150-74170)*
Procedure performed more than one time for each combined abdomen and pelvis examination

74176 **Computed tomography, abdomen and pelvis; without contrast material**
5.63 | 5.63 | **FUD** XXX | Q3 Z3
AMA: 2020,Sep,11; 2018,Jan,8; 2017,Jan,8; 2016,Jan,13; 2015,Jan,16

74177 **with contrast material(s)**
8.99 | 8.99 | **FUD** XXX | Q3 Z2
AMA: 2020,Sep,11; 2018,Jan,8; 2017,Jan,8; 2016,Jan,13; 2015,Jan,16

74178 **without contrast material in one or both body regions, followed by contrast material(s) and further sections in one or both body regions**
10.3 | 10.3 | **FUD** XXX | Q3 Z2
AMA: 2020,Sep,11; 2018,Jan,8; 2017,Jan,8; 2016,Jan,13; 2015,Jan,16

74181-74183 Magnetic Resonance Imaging: Abdomen–General

CMS: 100-04,4,250.16 Multiple Procedure Payment Reduction: Certain Diagnostic Imaging Procedures Rendered by Physicians

74181 **Magnetic resonance (eg, proton) imaging, abdomen; without contrast material(s)**
6.34 6.34 **FUD** XXX Q3 Z2 80
AMA: 2018,Mar,11; 2018,Jan,8; 2017,Jan,8; 2016,Jan,13; 2015,Jan,16

74182 **with contrast material(s)**
9.90 9.90 **FUD** XXX Q3 Z2 80
AMA: 2018,Mar,11; 2018,Jan,8; 2017,Jan,8; 2016,Jan,13; 2015,Jan,16

74183 **without contrast material(s), followed by with contrast material(s) and further sequences**
11.0 11.0 **FUD** XXX Q3 Z2 80
AMA: 2018,Mar,11; 2018,Jan,8; 2017,Jan,8; 2016,Jan,13; 2015,Jan,16

74185 Magnetic Resonance Angiography: Abdomen–General

CMS: 100-04,13,40.1.1 Magnetic Resonance Angiography; 100-04,13,40.1.2 HCPCS Coding Requirements; 100-04,4,250.16 Multiple Procedure Payment Reduction: Certain Diagnostic Imaging Procedures Rendered by Physicians

74185 **Magnetic resonance angiography, abdomen, with or without contrast material(s)**
11.1 11.1 **FUD** XXX B 80
AMA: 2018,Jan,8; 2017,Jan,8; 2016,Jan,13; 2015,Jan,16

74190 Peritoneography

74190 **Peritoneogram (eg, after injection of air or contrast), radiological supervision and interpretation**
EXCLUDES *CT pelvis or abdomen (72192, 74150)*
Code also injection procedure (49400)
0.00 0.00 **FUD** XXX Q2 N1 80
AMA: 2018,Jan,8; 2017,Jan,8; 2016,Jan,13; 2015,Jan,16

74210-74235 Radiography: Throat and Esophagus

EXCLUDES *Percutaneous placement gastrostomy tube, endoscopic (43246)*
Percutaneous placement gastrostomy tube, fluoroscopic guidance (49440)

74210 **Radiologic examination, pharynx and/or cervical esophagus, including scout neck radiograph(s) and delayed image(s), when performed, contrast (eg, barium) study**
2.49 2.49 **FUD** XXX Q1 N1 80
AMA: 2020,Aug,9

74220 **Radiologic examination, esophagus, including scout chest radiograph(s) and delayed image(s), when performed; single-contrast (eg, barium) study**
EXCLUDES *Double-contrast study (74221)*
Small bowel follow-through (74248)
Upper GI tract studies (74240-74246)
2.71 2.71 **FUD** XXX Q1 N1 80
AMA: 2020,Aug,9

74221 **double-contrast (eg, high-density barium and effervescent agent) study**
EXCLUDES *Single-contrast study (74220)*
Small bowel follow-through (74248)
Upper GI tract studies (74240-74246)
3.06 3.06 **FUD** XXX 80
AMA: 2020,Aug,9

74230 **Radiologic examination, swallowing function, with cineradiography/videoradiography, including scout neck radiograph(s) and delayed image(s), when performed, contrast (eg, barium) study**
EXCLUDES *Swallowing function motion fluoroscopic examination (92611)*
3.64 3.64 **FUD** XXX Q1 Z2 80
AMA: 2020,Aug,9; 2018,Jan,8; 2017,Jan,8; 2016,Jan,13; 2015,Jan,16

74235 **Removal of foreign body(s), esophageal, with use of balloon catheter, radiological supervision and interpretation**
Code also procedure (43499)
0.00 0.00 **FUD** XXX N N1 80
AMA: 2014,Jan,11; 2012,Feb,9-10

74240-74283 Radiography: Intestines

EXCLUDES *Percutaneous placement gastrostomy tube, endoscopic (43246)*
Percutaneous placement gastrostomy tube, fluoroscopic guidance (49440)

74240 **Radiologic examination, upper gastrointestinal tract, including scout abdominal radiograph(s) and delayed image(s), when performed; single-contrast (eg, barium) study**
INCLUDES Upper GI with KUB
EXCLUDES *Double-contrast study (74246)*
Esophagus studies (74220-74221)
Code also small bowel follow-through when performed (74248)
3.45 3.45 **FUD** XXX Q1 Z3 80
AMA: 2020,Aug,9; 2018,Jan,8; 2017,Jan,8; 2016,Sep,7

74246 **double-contrast (eg, high-density barium and effervescent agent) study, including glucagon, when administered**
INCLUDES Upper GI with KUB
EXCLUDES *Esophagus studies (74220-74221)*
Single-contrast study (74240)
3.84 3.84 **FUD** XXX Q1 Z2 80
AMA: 2020,Aug,9; 2018,Jan,8; 2017,Jan,8; 2016,Sep,7

\+ **74248** **Radiologic small intestine follow-through study, including multiple serial images (List separately in addition to code for primary procedure for upper GI radiologic examination)**
EXCLUDES *Single- or double-contrast small intestine studies (74250-74251)*
Code first (74240, 74246)
2.32 2.32 **FUD** ZZZ 80
AMA: 2020,Aug,9

74250 **Radiologic examination, small intestine, including multiple serial images and scout abdominal radiograph(s), when performed; single-contrast (eg, barium) study**
EXCLUDES *Double-contrast study (74251)*
Small bowel follow-through (74248)
3.41 3.41 **FUD** XXX Q1 Z3 80
AMA: 2020,Aug,9; 2018,Jan,8; 2017,Jan,8; 2016,Sep,7

74251 **double-contrast (eg, high-density barium and air via enteroclysis tube) study, including glucagon, when administered**
EXCLUDES *Single-contrast study (74250)*
Small bowel follow-through (74248)
Code also insertion long gastrointestinal tube (44500, 74340)
11.3 11.3 **FUD** XXX S Z2 80
AMA: 2020,Aug,9; 2018,Jan,8; 2017,Jan,8; 2016,Sep,7

74261 **Computed tomographic (CT) colonography, diagnostic, including image postprocessing; without contrast material**
EXCLUDES *3D rendering (76376-76377)*
CT abdomen or pelvis alone (72192-72194, 74150-74170)
Screening CT colonography (74263)
13.4 13.4 **FUD** XXX Q3 Z2 80
AMA: 2020,Sep,11; 2020,Feb,13; 2018,Jan,8; 2017,Jan,8; 2016,Jan,13; 2015,Jan,16

74262 **with contrast material(s) including non-contrast images, if performed**
EXCLUDES *3D rendering (76376-76377)*
CT abdomen or pelvis alone (72192-72194, 74150-74170)
Screening CT colonography (74263)
15.1 15.1 **FUD** XXX Q3 Z2 80
AMA: 2020,Sep,11; 2020,Feb,13; 2018,Jan,8; 2017,Jan,8; 2016,Jan,13; 2015,Jan,16

74263 **Computed tomographic (CT) colonography, screening, including image postprocessing**

EXCLUDES *3D rendering (76376-76377)*
CT abdomen or pelvis alone (72192-72194, 74150-74170)
CT colonography (74261-74262)

21.1 21.1 FUD XXX E

AMA: 2020,Sep,11; 2020,Feb,13; 2018,Jan,8; 2017,Jan,8; 2016,Jan,13; 2015,Jan,16

74270 **Radiologic examination, colon, including scout abdominal radiograph(s) and delayed image(s), when performed; single-contrast (eg, barium) study**

EXCLUDES *Double-contrast study (74280)*

4.34 4.34 FUD XXX Q1 N1 80

AMA: 2020,Aug,9; 2018,Jan,8; 2017,Jan,8; 2016,Jan,13; 2015,Jan,16

74280 **double-contrast (eg, high density barium and air) study, including glucagon, when administered**

EXCLUDES *Single-contrast study (74270)*

6.41 6.41 FUD XXX S N1 80

AMA: 2020,Aug,9

74283 **Therapeutic enema, contrast or air, for reduction of intussusception or other intraluminal obstruction (eg, meconium ileus)**

7.00 7.00 FUD XXX S Z2 80

AMA: 2014,Jan,11; 2012,Feb,9-10

74290-74330 Radiography: Biliary Tract

74290 **Cholecystography, oral contrast**

2.15 2.15 FUD XXX Q1 N1 80

AMA: 2014,Jan,11; 2012,Feb,9-10

74300 **Cholangiography and/or pancreatography; intraoperative, radiological supervision and interpretation**

0.00 0.00 FUD XXX N N1 80

AMA: 2018,Jan,8; 2017,Jan,8; 2016,Jan,13; 2015,Dec,3; 2015,Jan,16

\+ **74301** **additional set intraoperative, radiological supervision and interpretation (List separately in addition to code for primary procedure)**

Code first (74300)

0.00 0.00 FUD ZZZ N N1 80

AMA: 2015,Dec,3

74328 **Endoscopic catheterization of the biliary ductal system, radiological supervision and interpretation**

Code also ERCP (43261-43265, 43274-43278 [43274, 43275, 43276, 43277, 43278])

0.00 0.00 FUD XXX N N1 80

AMA: 2018,Jan,8; 2017,Jan,8; 2016,Jan,13; 2015,Jan,16

74329 **Endoscopic catheterization of the pancreatic ductal system, radiological supervision and interpretation**

Code also ERCP (43261-43265, 43274-43278 [43274, 43275, 43276, 43277, 43278])

0.00 0.00 FUD XXX N N1 80

AMA: 2014,Jan,11; 2012,Feb,9-10

74330 **Combined endoscopic catheterization of the biliary and pancreatic ductal systems, radiological supervision and interpretation**

Code also ERCP (43261-43265, 43274-43278 [43274, 43275, 43276, 43277, 43278])

0.00 0.00 FUD XXX N N1 80

AMA: 2014,Jan,11; 2012,Feb,9-10

74340-74363 Radiography: Bilidigestive Intubation

EXCLUDES *Percutaneous placement gastrostomy tube, endoscopic (43246)*
Percutaneous placement gastrotomy tube, fluoroscopic guidance (49440)

74340 **Introduction of long gastrointestinal tube (eg, Miller-Abbott), including multiple fluoroscopies and images, radiological supervision and interpretation**

Code also placement tube (44500)

0.00 0.00 FUD XXX N N1 80

AMA: 2020,Aug,9; 2018,Jan,8; 2017,Jan,8; 2016,Sep,9

74355 **Percutaneous placement of enteroclysis tube, radiological supervision and interpretation**

INCLUDES Fluoroscopic guidance (77002)

0.00 0.00 FUD XXX N N1 80

AMA: 2018,Jan,8; 2017,Jan,8; 2016,Jan,13; 2015,Jan,16

74360 **Intraluminal dilation of strictures and/or obstructions (eg, esophagus), radiological supervision and interpretation**

EXCLUDES *Esophagogastroduodenoscopy, flexible, transoral; with dilation esophagus (43233)*
Esophagoscopy, flexible, transoral; with dilation esophagus (43213-43214)

0.00 0.00 FUD XXX N N1 80

AMA: 2018,Jan,8; 2017,Jan,8; 2016,Jan,13; 2015,Jan,16

74363 **Percutaneous transhepatic dilation of biliary duct stricture with or without placement of stent, radiological supervision and interpretation**

EXCLUDES *Surgical procedure (47555-47556)*

0.00 0.00 FUD XXX N N1 80

AMA: 2014,Jan,11; 2012,Feb,9-10

74400-74775 Radiography: Urogenital

74400 **Urography (pyelography), intravenous, with or without KUB, with or without tomography**

3.36 3.36 FUD XXX S Z2 80

AMA: 2014,Jan,11; 2012,Feb,9-10

74410 **Urography, infusion, drip technique and/or bolus technique;**

3.66 3.66 FUD XXX S Z2 80

AMA: 2014,Jan,11; 2012,Feb,9-10

74415 **with nephrotomography**

4.28 4.28 FUD XXX S Z2 80

AMA: 2014,Jan,11; 2012,Feb,9-10

74420 **Urography, retrograde, with or without KUB**

2.08 2.08 FUD XXX S Z2 80

AMA: 2018,Jan,8; 2017,Jan,8; 2016,Jan,13; 2015,Jan,16

▲ **74425 Urography, antegrade, radiological supervision and interpretation**

EXCLUDES *Injection for antegrade nephrostogram and/or ureterogram ([50430, 50431, 50432, 50433, 50434, 50435])*

Ureteral stent placement (50693-50695)

Code also aspiration/injection renal cyst or pelvis, percutaneous (50390)

Code also injection procedure:

ureterography or ureteropyelography (50684)

visualization ileal conduit/ureteropyelography (50690)

Code also manometric study through nephrostomy or pyelostomy tube (50396)

3.66 3.66 FUD XXX Q2 N1 80

AMA: 2018,Jan,8; 2017,Jan,8; 2016,Jan,13; 2016,Jan,3; 2015,Oct,5; 2015,Jan,16

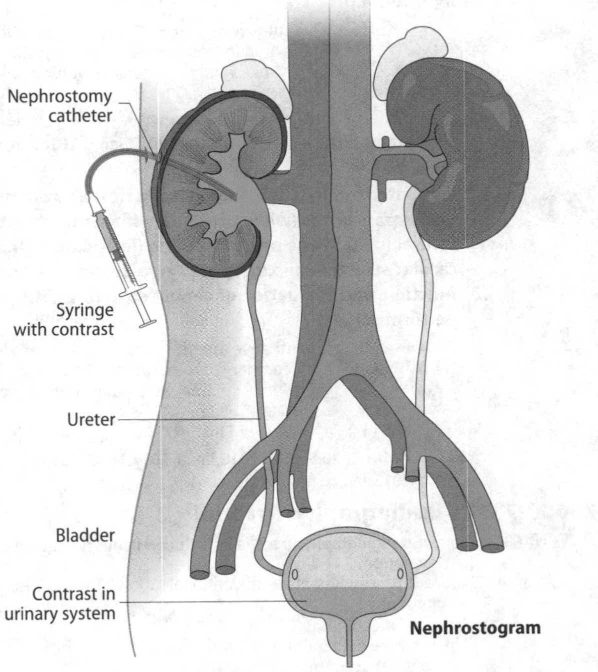

Nephrostogram

74430 Cystography, minimum of 3 views, radiological supervision and interpretation

1.13 1.13 FUD XXX Q2 N1 80

AMA: 2014,Jan,11; 2012,Feb,9-10

74440 Vasography, vesiculography, or epididymography, radiological supervision and interpretation ♂

2.44 2.44 FUD XXX Q2 N1 80

AMA: 2014,Jan,11; 2012,Feb,9-10

74445 Corpora cavernosography, radiological supervision and interpretation ♂

INCLUDES Needle placement with fluoroscopic guidance (77002)

0.00 0.00 FUD XXX Q2 N1 80

AMA: 2018,Jan,8; 2017,Jan,8; 2016,Jan,13; 2015,Jan,16

74450 Urethrocystography, retrograde, radiological supervision and interpretation

0.00 0.00 FUD XXX Q2 N1 80

AMA: 2019,Oct,10

74455 Urethrocystography, voiding, radiological supervision and interpretation

2.55 2.55 FUD XXX Q2 N1 80

AMA: 2019,Oct,10

74470 Radiologic examination, renal cyst study, translumbar, contrast visualization, radiological supervision and interpretation

INCLUDES Needle placement with fluoroscopic guidance (77002)

0.00 0.00 FUD XXX Q2 N1 80

AMA: 2018,Jan,8; 2017,Jan,8; 2016,Jan,13; 2015,Jan,16

74485 Dilation of ureter(s) or urethra, radiological supervision and interpretation

EXCLUDES *Change pyelostomy/nephrostomy tube ([50435])*

Nephrostomy tract dilation for procedure ([50436, 50437])

Ureter dilation without radiologic guidance (52341, 52344)

3.19 3.19 FUD XXX Q2 N1 80

AMA: 2018,Jan,8; 2017,Jan,8; 2016,Jan,13; 2016,Jan,3; 2015,Oct,5; 2015,Jan,16

74710 Pelvimetry, with or without placental localization ♀

EXCLUDES *Imaging procedures on abdomen and pelvis (72170-72190, 74018-74019, 74021-74022, 74150-74170)*

1.08 1.08 FUD XXX Q1 N1 80

AMA: 2014,Jan,11; 2012,Feb,9-10

74712 Magnetic resonance (eg, proton) imaging, fetal, including placental and maternal pelvic imaging when performed; single or first gestation ♀

EXCLUDES *Imaging maternal pelvis or placenta without fetal imaging (72195-72197)*

13.3 13.3 FUD XXX S Z2 80

AMA: 2018,Jan,8; 2017,Jan,8; 2016,Jun,5

\+ **74713 each additional gestation (List separately in addition to code for primary procedure)** ♀

EXCLUDES *Imaging maternal pelvis or placenta without fetal imaging (72195-72197)*

Code first (74712)

6.46 6.46 FUD ZZZ N N1 80

AMA: 2018,Jan,8; 2017,Jan,8; 2016,Jun,5

74740 Hysterosalpingography, radiological supervision and interpretation ♀

EXCLUDES *Imaging procedures abdomen and pelvis (72170-72190, 74018-74019, 74021-74022, 74150-74170)*

Code also injection saline/contrast (58340)

2.32 2.32 FUD XXX Q2 N1 80

AMA: 2018,Jan,8; 2017,Jan,8; 2016,Jan,13; 2015,Jan,16

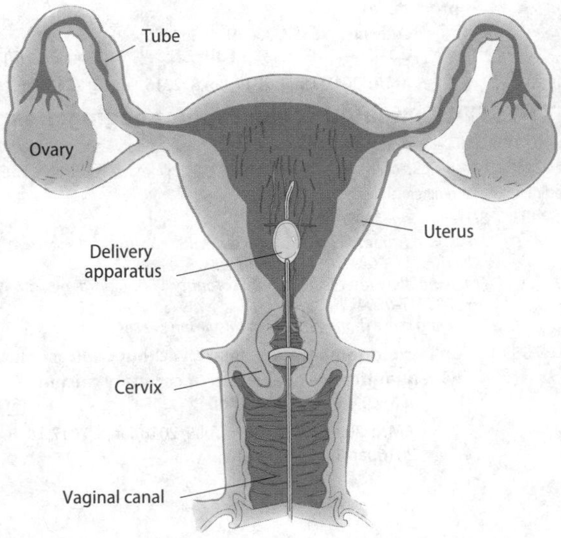

Hysterosalpingography (imaging of the uterus and tubes) is performed. Report for radiological supervision and interpretation

74742 Transcervical catheterization of fallopian tube, radiological supervision and interpretation ♀

EXCLUDES *Imaging procedures abdomen and pelvis (72170-72190, 74018-74019, 74021-74022, 74150-74170)*

Code also transcervical fallopian tube catheter (58345)

Facility RVU 0.00 Non-Facility RVU 0.00 **FUD** XXX N N1 80

AMA: 2018,Jan,8; 2017,Jan,8; 2016,Jan,13; 2015,Jan,16

74775 Perineogram (eg, vaginogram, for sex determination or extent of anomalies) M ♀

EXCLUDES *Imaging procedures abdomen and pelvis (72170-72190, 74018-74019, 74021-74022, 74150-74170)*

Facility RVU 0.00 Non-Facility RVU 0.00 **FUD** XXX S Z2 80

AMA: 2014,Jan,11; 2012,Feb,9-10

75557-75565 Magnetic Resonance Imaging: Heart Structure and Physiology

INCLUDES Physiologic evaluation cardiac function

EXCLUDES *3D rendering (76376-76377)*
Cardiac catheterization procedures (93451-93572)
Reporting more than one code in this group per session

Code also separate vascular injection (36000-36299)

75557 Cardiac magnetic resonance imaging for morphology and function without contrast material;

Facility RVU 9.01 Non-Facility RVU 9.01 **FUD** XXX Q3 Z2 80

AMA: 2018,Jan,8; 2017,Jan,8; 2016,Jan,13; 2015,Jan,16

75559 with stress imaging

INCLUDES Pharmacologic wall motion stress evaluation without contrast

Code also stress testing when performed (93015-93018)

Facility RVU 12.7 Non-Facility RVU 12.7 **FUD** XXX Q3 Z2 80

AMA: 2018,Jan,8; 2017,Jan,8; 2016,Jan,13; 2015,Jan,16

75561 Cardiac magnetic resonance imaging for morphology and function without contrast material(s), followed by contrast material(s) and further sequences;

Facility RVU 12.0 Non-Facility RVU 12.0 **FUD** XXX Q3 Z2 80

AMA: 2018,Jan,8; 2017,Jan,8; 2016,Jan,13; 2015,Jan,16

75563 with stress imaging

INCLUDES Pharmacologic perfusion stress evaluation with contrast

Code also stress testing when performed (93015-93018)

Facility RVU 14.2 Non-Facility RVU 14.2 **FUD** XXX Q3 Z2 80

AMA: 2018,Jan,8; 2017,Jan,8; 2016,Jan,13; 2015,Jan,16

+ **75565 Cardiac magnetic resonance imaging for velocity flow mapping (List separately in addition to code for primary procedure)**

Code first (75557, 75559, 75561, 75563)

Facility RVU 1.48 Non-Facility RVU 1.48 **FUD** ZZZ N N1 80

AMA: 2018,Jan,8; 2017,Jan,8; 2016,Jan,13; 2015,Jan,16

75571-75574 Computed Tomographic Imaging: Heart

CMS: 100-04,12,20.4.7 Services Not Meeting National Electrical Manufacturers Association (NEMA) Standard; 100-04,4,20.6.12 Use of HCPCS Modifier – CT; 100-04,4,250.16 Multiple Procedure Payment Reduction: Certain Diagnostic Imaging Procedures Rendered by Physicians

EXCLUDES *3D rendering (76376-76377)*
Automated quantification/characterization coronary atherosclerotic plaque ([0623T, 0624T, 0625T, 0626T])
Fractional flow reserve (FFR) from coronary CT angiography data (0501T-0504T)
Reporting more than one code in this group per session

75571 Computed tomography, heart, without contrast material, with quantitative evaluation of coronary calcium

Facility RVU 2.92 Non-Facility RVU 2.92 **FUD** XXX Q1 N1 80

AMA: 2020,Sep,11; 2020,Jul,5; 2018,Jan,8; 2017,Jan,8; 2016,Jan,13; 2015,Jan,16

75572 Computed tomography, heart, with contrast material, for evaluation of cardiac structure and morphology (including 3D image postprocessing, assessment of cardiac function, and evaluation of venous structures, if performed)

INCLUDES Quantitative assessment(s) such as quantification coronary percentage stenosis, ejection fraction, stroke volume, ventricular volume, when performed

Facility RVU 7.01 Non-Facility RVU 7.01 **FUD** XXX S Z2 80

AMA: 2020,Sep,11; 2018,Jan,8; 2017,Jan,8; 2016,Jan,13; 2015,Jan,16

75573 Computed tomography, heart, with contrast material, for evaluation of cardiac structure and morphology in the setting of congenital heart disease (including 3D image postprocessing, assessment of LV cardiac function, RV structure and function and evaluation of venous structures, if performed)

INCLUDES Quantitative assessment(s) such as quantification coronary percentage stenosis, ejection fraction, stroke volume, ventricular volume, when performed

Facility RVU 9.43 Non-Facility RVU 9.43 **FUD** XXX S Z2 80

AMA: 2020,Sep,11; 2018,Jan,8; 2017,Jan,8; 2016,Jan,13; 2015,Jan,16

75574 Computed tomographic angiography, heart, coronary arteries and bypass grafts (when present), with contrast material, including 3D image postprocessing (including evaluation of cardiac structure and morphology, assessment of cardiac function, and evaluation of venous structures, if performed)

INCLUDES Quantitative assessment(s) such as quantification coronary percentage stenosis, ejection fraction, stroke volume, ventricular volume, when performed

Facility RVU 11.0 Non-Facility RVU 11.0 **FUD** XXX S Z2 80

AMA: 2020,Sep,11; 2018,Jan,8; 2017,Jan,8; 2016,Jan,13; 2015,Jan,16

75600-75774 Radiography: Arterial

INCLUDES Diagnostic angiography specifically included in interventional code description
Diagnostic procedures with interventional supervision and interpretation:
- Angiography
- Contrast injection
- Fluoroscopic guidance for intervention
- Post-angioplasty/atherectomy/stent angiography
- Roadmapping
- Vessel measurement

EXCLUDES *Catheterization codes for diagnostic angiography lower extremity when access site other than site used for therapy required*
Diagnostic angiogram during separate encounter from interventional procedure
Diagnostic angiography with interventional procedure if:
1. No previous catheter-based angiogram accessible and complete diagnostic procedure performed, and decision to proceed with interventional procedure based on diagnostic service, OR
2. Previous diagnostic angiogram accessible but documentation in medical record specifies that:
A. patient's condition has changed
B. insufficient imaging patient's anatomy and/or disease, OR
C. clinical change during procedure that necessitates new examination away from intervention site
3. Modifier 59 appended to code(s) for diagnostic radiological supervision and interpretation service to indicate guidelines were met
Intra-arterial procedures (36100-36248)
Intravenous procedures (36000, 36005-36015)

75600 Aortography, thoracic, without serialography, radiological supervision and interpretation

EXCLUDES *Supravalvular aortography (93567)*

Facility RVU 5.63 Non-Facility RVU 5.63 **FUD** XXX Q2 N1 80

AMA: 2014,Jan,11; 2012,Feb,9-10

75605 Aortography, thoracic, by serialography, radiological supervision and interpretation

EXCLUDES *Supravalvular aortography (93567)*

Facility RVU 3.67 Non-Facility RVU 3.67 **FUD** XXX Q2 N1 80

AMA: 2018,Jan,8; 2017,Jan,8; 2016,Jan,13; 2015,Jan,16

75625 Aortography, abdominal, by serialography, radiological supervision and interpretation

EXCLUDES *Supravalvular aortography (93567)*

3.73 3.73 FUD XXX Q2 N1 80

AMA: 2020,Sep,14; 2018,Jan,8; 2017,Jan,8; 2016,Jan,13; 2015,Jan,16

75630 Aortography, abdominal plus bilateral iliofemoral lower extremity, catheter, by serialography, radiological supervision and interpretation

EXCLUDES *Supravalvular aortography (93567)*

4.81 4.81 FUD XXX Q2 N1 80

AMA: 2020,Sep,14; 2018,Jan,8; 2017,Jan,8; 2016,Jan,13; 2015,Jan,16

75635 Computed tomographic angiography, abdominal aorta and bilateral iliofemoral lower extremity runoff, with contrast material(s), including noncontrast images, if performed, and image postprocessing

EXCLUDES *3D rendering (76376-76377)*

CT angiography, abdomen, lower extremity, pelvis (72191, 73706, 74174-74175)

12.4 12.4 FUD XXX Q2 N1 80

AMA: 2020,Sep,11; 2018,Jan,8; 2017,Jan,8; 2016,Jan,13; 2015,Jan,16

75705 Angiography, spinal, selective, radiological supervision and interpretation

7.09 7.09 FUD XXX Q2 N1 80

AMA: 2014,Jan,11; 2012,Feb,9-10

75710 Angiography, extremity, unilateral, radiological supervision and interpretation

4.63 4.63 FUD XXX Q2 N1 80

AMA: 2018,Jan,8; 2017,Mar,3; 2017,Jan,8; 2016,Jan,13; 2015,Jan,16

75716 Angiography, extremity, bilateral, radiological supervision and interpretation

5.04 5.04 FUD XXX Q2 N1 80

AMA: 2020,Sep,14; 2018,Jan,8; 2017,Jan,8; 2016,Jan,13; 2015,Jan,16

75726 Angiography, visceral, selective or supraselective (with or without flush aortogram), radiological supervision and interpretation

EXCLUDES *Selective angiography, each additional visceral vessel examined after basic examination (75774)*

5.20 5.20 FUD XXX Q2 N1 80

AMA: 2014,Jan,11; 2012,Feb,9-10

75731 Angiography, adrenal, unilateral, selective, radiological supervision and interpretation

4.73 4.73 FUD XXX Q2 Z3 80

AMA: 2014,Jan,11; 2012,Feb,9-10

75733 Angiography, adrenal, bilateral, selective, radiological supervision and interpretation

5.09 5.09 FUD XXX Q2 N1 80

AMA: 2014,Jan,11; 2012,Feb,9-10

75736 Angiography, pelvic, selective or supraselective, radiological supervision and interpretation

4.38 4.38 FUD XXX Q2 N1 80

AMA: 2014,Jan,11; 2012,Feb,9-10

75741 Angiography, pulmonary, unilateral, selective, radiological supervision and interpretation

4.03 4.03 FUD XXX Q2 N1 80

AMA: 2019,Jun,3; 2018,Jan,8; 2017,Jan,8; 2016,Jan,13; 2015,Jan,16

75743 Angiography, pulmonary, bilateral, selective, radiological supervision and interpretation

4.55 4.55 FUD XXX Q2 N1 80

AMA: 2019,Jun,3; 2018,Jan,8; 2017,Jan,8; 2016,Jan,13; 2015,Jan,16

75746 Angiography, pulmonary, by nonselective catheter or venous injection, radiological supervision and interpretation

EXCLUDES *Nonselective injection procedure or catheter introduction with cardiac cath (93568)*

4.07 4.07 FUD XXX Q2 Z3 80

AMA: 2019,Jun,3

75756 Angiography, internal mammary, radiological supervision and interpretation

EXCLUDES *Internal mammary angiography with cardiac cath (93455, 93457, 93459, 93461, 93564)*

4.62 4.62 FUD XXX Q2 N1 80

AMA: 2018,Jan,8; 2017,Jan,8; 2016,Jan,13; 2015,Jan,16

\+ **75774 Angiography, selective, each additional vessel studied after basic examination, radiological supervision and interpretation (List separately in addition to code for primary procedure)**

EXCLUDES *Angiography (75600-75756)*

Cardiac cath procedures (93452-93462, 93531-93533, 93563-93568)

Catheterizations (36215-36248)

Dialysis circuit angiography (current access), report modifier 52 with (36901)

Nonselective catheter placement, thoracic aorta (36221-36228)

Code also diagnostic angiography upper extremities and other vascular beds (except cervicocerebral vessels), when appropriate

Code first initial vessel

3.04 3.04 FUD ZZZ N N1 80

AMA: 2020,Sep,14; 2018,Jan,8; 2017,Jan,8; 2016,Jan,13; 2015,Jan,16

75801-75893 Radiography: Lymphatic and Venous

INCLUDES Diagnostic venography specifically included in interventional code description

Diagnostic procedures with interventional supervision and interpretation:

- Contrast injection
- Fluoroscopic guidance for intervention
- Post-angioplasty/venography
- Roadmapping
- Venography
- Vessel measurement

EXCLUDES *Diagnostic venogram during separate encounter from interventional procedure*

Diagnostic venography with interventional procedure if:

1. No previous catheter-based venogram accessible and complete diagnostic procedure performed and decision to proceed with interventional procedure based on diagnostic service, OR

2. Previous diagnostic venogram accessible but documentation in medical record specifies that:

A. patient's condition has changed

B. insufficient imaging patient's anatomy and/or disease, OR

C. clinical change during procedure that necessitates new examination away from intervention site

Intravenous procedures (36000-36015, 36400-36510 [36465, 36466, 36482, 36483])

Lymphatic injection procedures (38790)

75801 Lymphangiography, extremity only, unilateral, radiological supervision and interpretation

0.00 0.00 FUD XXX Q2 N1 80

AMA: 2014,Jan,11; 2012,Feb,9-10

75803 Lymphangiography, extremity only, bilateral, radiological supervision and interpretation

0.00 0.00 FUD XXX Q2 Z2 80

AMA: 2014,Jan,11; 2012,Feb,9-10

75805 Lymphangiography, pelvic/abdominal, unilateral, radiological supervision and interpretation

0.00 0.00 FUD XXX Q2 Z2 80

AMA: 2014,Jan,11; 2012,Feb,9-10

75807 Lymphangiography, pelvic/abdominal, bilateral, radiological supervision and interpretation

0.00 0.00 FUD XXX Q2 N1 80

AMA: 2014,Jan,11; 2012,Feb,9-10

75809 **Shuntogram for investigation of previously placed indwelling nonvascular shunt (eg, LeVeen shunt, ventriculoperitoneal shunt, indwelling infusion pump), radiological supervision and interpretation**
Code also surgical procedure (49427, 61070)
2.69 2.69 FUD XXX Q2 N1 80
AMA: 2018,Jan,8; 2017,Jan,8; 2016,Jan,13; 2015,Jan,16

75810 **Splenoportography, radiological supervision and interpretation**
0.00 0.00 FUD XXX Q2 Z2 80
AMA: 2018,Jan,8; 2017,Jan,8; 2016,Jan,13; 2015,Jan,16

75820 **Venography, extremity, unilateral, radiological supervision and interpretation**
3.15 3.15 FUD XXX Q2 N1 80
AMA: 2019,Mar,6; 2018,Jan,8; 2017,Jan,8; 2016,May,5; 2016,Jan,13; 2015,May,3; 2015,Jan,16

75822 **Venography, extremity, bilateral, radiological supervision and interpretation**
3.56 3.56 FUD XXX Q2 Z3 80
AMA: 2014,Jan,11; 2012,Feb,9-10

75825 **Venography, caval, inferior, with serialography, radiological supervision and interpretation**
3.55 3.55 FUD XXX Q2 N1 80
AMA: 2018,Jan,8; 2017,Feb,14; 2017,Jan,8; 2016,Jan,13; 2015,Jan,16

75827 **Venography, caval, superior, with serialography, radiological supervision and interpretation**
3.82 3.82 FUD XXX Q2 N1 80
AMA: 2018,Jan,8; 2017,Jan,8; 2016,Jan,13; 2015,Jan,16

75831 **Venography, renal, unilateral, selective, radiological supervision and interpretation**
3.70 3.70 FUD XXX Q2 N1 80
AMA: 2014,Jan,11; 2012,Feb,9-10

75833 **Venography, renal, bilateral, selective, radiological supervision and interpretation**
4.55 4.55 FUD XXX Q2 N1 80
AMA: 2014,Jan,11; 2012,Feb,9-10

75840 **Venography, adrenal, unilateral, selective, radiological supervision and interpretation**
4.08 4.08 FUD XXX Q2 N1 80
AMA: 2014,Jan,11; 2012,Feb,9-10

75842 **Venography, adrenal, bilateral, selective, radiological supervision and interpretation**
4.95 4.95 FUD XXX Q2 N1 80
AMA: 2014,Jan,11; 2012,Feb,9-10

75860 **Venography, venous sinus (eg, petrosal and inferior sagittal) or jugular, catheter, radiological supervision and interpretation**
3.99 3.99 FUD XXX Q2 N1 80
AMA: 2014,Jan,11; 2012,Feb,9-10

75870 **Venography, superior sagittal sinus, radiological supervision and interpretation**
5.30 5.30 FUD XXX Q2 Z3 80
AMA: 2014,Jan,11; 2012,Feb,9-10

75872 **Venography, epidural, radiological supervision and interpretation**
4.08 4.08 FUD XXX Q2 N1 80
AMA: 2014,Jan,11; 2012,Feb,9-10

75880 **Venography, orbital, radiological supervision and interpretation**
3.44 3.44 FUD XXX Q2 N1 80
AMA: 2014,Jan,11; 2012,Feb,9-10

75885 **Percutaneous transhepatic portography with hemodynamic evaluation, radiological supervision and interpretation**
4.21 4.21 FUD XXX Q2 N1 80
AMA: 2018,Jan,8; 2017,Jan,8; 2016,Jan,13; 2015,Jan,16

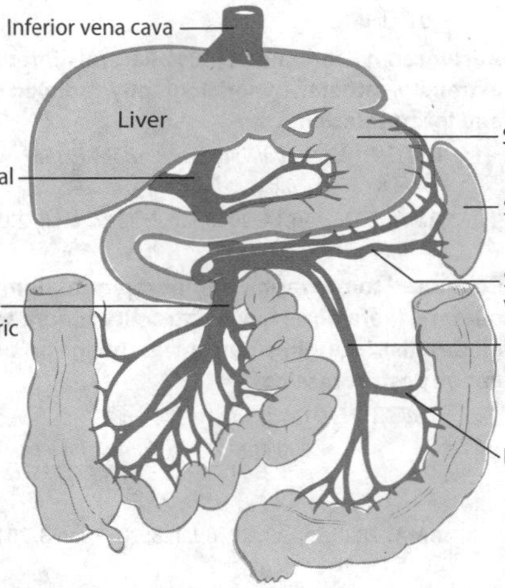

Schematic showing the portal vein

75887 **Percutaneous transhepatic portography without hemodynamic evaluation, radiological supervision and interpretation**
4.24 4.24 FUD XXX Q2 Z3 80
AMA: 2018,Jan,8; 2017,Jan,8; 2016,Jan,13; 2015,Jan,16

75889 **Hepatic venography, wedged or free, with hemodynamic evaluation, radiological supervision and interpretation**
3.81 3.81 FUD XXX Q2 N1 80
AMA: 2014,Jan,11; 2012,Feb,9-10

75891 **Hepatic venography, wedged or free, without hemodynamic evaluation, radiological supervision and interpretation**
3.87 3.87 FUD XXX Q2 N1 80
AMA: 2014,Jan,11; 2012,Feb,9-10

75893 **Venous sampling through catheter, with or without angiography (eg, for parathyroid hormone, renin), radiological supervision and interpretation**
Code also surgical procedure (36500)
3.32 3.32 FUD XXX Q2 N1 80
AMA: 2014,Jan,11; 2012,Feb,9-10

75894-75902 Transcatheter Procedures

INCLUDES Diagnostic procedures with interventional supervision and interpretation:
- Angiography/venography
- Completion angiography/venography except for those services allowed by (75898)
- Contrast injection
- Fluoroscopic guidance for intervention
- Roadmapping
- Vessel measurement

EXCLUDES *Diagnostic angiography/venography performed same session as transcatheter therapy unless specifically included in code descriptor or excluded in venography/angiography notes (75600-75893)*

75894 **Transcatheter therapy, embolization, any method, radiological supervision and interpretation**
EXCLUDES *Endovenous ablation therapy incompetent vein (36478-36479)*
Transluminal balloon angioplasty (36475-36476)
Vascular embolization or occlusion (37241-37244)
0.00 0.00 FUD XXX N N1 80
AMA: 2018,Mar,3; 2018,Jan,8; 2017,Jan,8; 2016,Nov,3; 2016,Jan,13; 2015,Jan,16

75898 **Angiography through existing catheter for follow-up study for transcatheter therapy, embolization or infusion, other than for thrombolysis**

EXCLUDES *Percutaneous arterial transluminal mechanical thrombectomy (61645)*
Prolonged endovascular intracranial administration pharmacologic agent(s) (61650-61651)
Transcatheter therapy, arterial infusion for thrombolysis (37211-37214)
Vascular embolization or occlusion (37241-37244)

0.00 0.00 **FUD** XXX Q2 Z2 80

AMA: 2019,Sep,6; 2018,Jan,8; 2017,Jan,8; 2016,Jan,13; 2015,Nov,3; 2015,Jan,16

75901 **Mechanical removal of pericatheter obstructive material (eg, fibrin sheath) from central venous device via separate venous access, radiologic supervision and interpretation**

EXCLUDES *Venous catheterization (36010-36012)*

Code also surgical procedure (36595)

6.15 6.15 **FUD** XXX N N1 80

AMA: 2018,Jan,8; 2017,Jan,8; 2016,Jan,13; 2015,Jan,16

75902 **Mechanical removal of intraluminal (intracatheter) obstructive material from central venous device through device lumen, radiologic supervision and interpretation**

EXCLUDES *Venous catheterization (36010-36012)*

Code also surgical procedure (36596)

2.40 2.40 **FUD** XXX N N1 80

AMA: 2018,Jan,8; 2017,Jan,8; 2016,Jan,13; 2015,Jan,16

75956-75959 Endovascular Aneurysm Repair

INCLUDES Diagnostic procedures with interventional supervision and interpretation:
- Angiography/venography
- Completion angiography/venography except for those services allowed by (75898)
- Contrast injection
- Fluoroscopic guidance for intervention
- Injection procedure only for transcatheter therapy or biopsy (36100-36299)
- Percutaneous needle biopsy;
  - Pancreas (48102)
  - Retroperitoneal lymph node/mass (49180)
- Roadmapping
- Vessel measurement

EXCLUDES *Diagnostic angiography/venography performed same session as transcatheter therapy unless specifically included in code descriptor (75600-75893)*
Radiological supervision and interpretation for transluminal angioplasty in:
Femoral/popliteal arteries (37224-37227)
Iliac artery (37220-37223)
Tibial/peroneal artery (37228-37235)

75956 **Endovascular repair of descending thoracic aorta (eg, aneurysm, pseudoaneurysm, dissection, penetrating ulcer, intramural hematoma, or traumatic disruption); involving coverage of left subclavian artery origin, initial endoprosthesis plus descending thoracic aortic extension(s), if required, to level of celiac artery origin, radiological supervision and interpretation**

Code also endovascular graft implantation (33880)

0.00 0.00 **FUD** XXX C 80

AMA: 2018,Jan,8; 2017,Jan,8; 2016,Jan,13; 2015,Jan,16

75957 **not involving coverage of left subclavian artery origin, initial endoprosthesis plus descending thoracic aortic extension(s), if required, to level of celiac artery origin, radiological supervision and interpretation**

Code also endovascular graft implantation (33881)

0.00 0.00 **FUD** XXX C 80

AMA: 2018,Jan,8; 2017,Jan,8; 2016,Jan,13; 2015,Jan,16

75958 **Placement of proximal extension prosthesis for endovascular repair of descending thoracic aorta (eg, aneurysm, pseudoaneurysm, dissection, penetrating ulcer, intramural hematoma, or traumatic disruption), radiological supervision and interpretation**

Code also placement each additional proximal extension(s) (75958)

Code also proximal endovascular extension implantation (33883-33884)

0.00 0.00 **FUD** XXX C 80

AMA: 2018,Jan,8; 2017,Jan,8; 2016,Jan,13; 2015,Jan,16

75959 **Placement of distal extension prosthesis(s) (delayed) after endovascular repair of descending thoracic aorta, as needed, to level of celiac origin, radiological supervision and interpretation**

INCLUDES Corresponding services for placement distal thoracic endovascular extension(s) placed during procedure following principal procedure

EXCLUDES *Endovascular repair descending thoracic aorta (75956-75957)*
Reporting code more than one time no matter how many modules are deployed

Code also placement distal endovascular extension (33886)

0.00 0.00 **FUD** XXX C 80

AMA: 2018,Jan,8; 2017,Jan,8; 2016,Jan,13; 2015,Jan,16

75970 Percutaneous Transluminal Angioplasty

INCLUDES Diagnostic procedures with interventional supervision and interpretation:
- Angiography/venography
- Completion angiography/venography except for those services allowed by (75898)
- Contrast injection
- Fluoroscopic guidance for intervention
- Roadmapping
- Vessel measurement

EXCLUDES *Diagnostic angiography/venography performed same session as transcatheter therapy unless specifically included in code descriptor (75600-75893)*
Injection procedure only for transcatheter therapy or biopsy (36100-36299)
Percutaneous needle biopsy (48102)
Pancreas (48102)
Retroperitoneal lymph node/mass (49180)
Radiological supervision and interpretation for transluminal balloon angioplasty in:
Femoral/popliteal arteries (37224-37227)
Iliac artery (37220-37223)
Tibial/peroneal artery (37228-37235)
Transcatheter renal/ureteral biopsy (52007)

75970 **Transcatheter biopsy, radiological supervision and interpretation**

0.00 0.00 **FUD** XXX N N1 80

AMA: 2018,Jan,8

75984-75989 Percutaneous Drainage

75984 **Change of percutaneous tube or drainage catheter with contrast monitoring (eg, genitourinary system, abscess), radiological supervision and interpretation**

EXCLUDES *Change only nephrostomy/pyelostomy tube ([50435])*
Cholecystostomy, percutaneous (47490)
Introduction procedure only for percutaneous biliary drainage (47531-47544)
Nephrostolithotomy/pyelostolithotomy, percutaneous (50080-50081)
Percutaneous replacement gastrointestinal tube using fluoroscopic guidance (49450-49452)
Removal and/or replacement internal ureteral stent using transurethral approach (50385-50386)

2.89 2.89 **FUD** XXX N N1 80

AMA: 2014,Jan,11; 2012,Feb,9-10

75989 Radiological guidance (ie, fluoroscopy, ultrasound, or computed tomography), for percutaneous drainage (eg, abscess, specimen collection), with placement of catheter, radiological supervision and interpretation

INCLUDES Imaging guidance

EXCLUDES *Cholecystostomy (47490)*
Image-guided fluid collection drainage by catheter (10030, 49405-49407)
Pericardial drainage (33017-33019)
Thoracentesis (32554-32557)

3.42 3.42 FUD XXX N N1 80

AMA: 2020,Jan,7; 2018,Jan,8; 2017,Jan,8; 2016,Jan,13; 2015,Dec,3; 2015,Jan,16

76000-76145 Miscellaneous Techniques

EXCLUDES *Arthrography:*
Ankle (73615)
Elbow (73085)
Hip (73525)
Knee (73580)
Shoulder (73040)
Wrist (73115)
CT cerebral perfusion test (0042T)

76000 Fluoroscopy (separate procedure), up to 1 hour physician or other qualified health care professional time

EXCLUDES *Extracorporeal membrane oxygenation (ECMO)/extracorporeal life support (ECLS) (33957-33959, [33962, 33963, 33964])*
Insertion/removal/replacement wireless cardiac stimulator (0515T-0520T)
Insertion/replacement/removal leadless pacemaker ([33274, 33275])

1.18 1.18 FUD XXX S Z3 80

AMA: 2019,Sep,10; 2019,Sep,5; 2019,Jun,3; 2019,Mar,6; 2018,Apr,7; 2018,Mar,3; 2018,Jan,8; 2017,Jan,8; 2016,Nov,3; 2016,Aug,5; 2016,May,5; 2016,May,13; 2016,Mar,5; 2016,Jan,11; 2016,Jan,13; 2015,Nov,3; 2015,Sep,3; 2015,May,3; 2015,Jan,16

76010 Radiologic examination from nose to rectum for foreign body, single view, child A

0.77 0.77 FUD XXX Q1 N1 80

AMA: 2018,Jan,8; 2017,Jan,8; 2016,Jan,13; 2015,Jan,16

76080 Radiologic examination, abscess, fistula or sinus tract study, radiological supervision and interpretation

EXCLUDES *Contrast injections, radiology evaluation, and guidance via fluoroscopy for gastrostomy, duodenostomy, jejunostomy, gastro-jejunostomy, or cecostomy tube (49465)*

1.67 1.67 FUD XXX Q2 N1 80

AMA: 2018,Jan,8; 2017,Jan,8; 2016,Jan,13; 2015,Jan,16

76098 Radiological examination, surgical specimen

EXCLUDES *Breast biopsy with placement breast localization device(s) (19081-19086)*

0.47 0.47 FUD XXX Q2 N1 80

AMA: 2012,Feb,9-10; 1997,Nov,1

76100 Radiologic examination, single plane body section (eg, tomography), other than with urography

2.75 2.75 FUD XXX Q1 N1 80

AMA: 2012,Feb,9-10; 1997,Nov,1

76101 Radiologic examination, complex motion (ie, hypercycloidal) body section (eg, mastoid polytomography), other than with urography; unilateral

EXCLUDES *Nephrotomography (74415)*
Panoramic x-ray (70355)
Procedure performed more than one time per day

2.77 2.77 FUD XXX Q1 Z2 80

AMA: 2012,Feb,9-10; 1997,Nov,1

76102 bilateral

EXCLUDES *Nephrotomography (74415)*
Panoramic x-ray (70355)
Procedure performed more than one time per day

4.88 4.88 FUD XXX S Z2 80

AMA: 2012,Feb,9-10; 1997,Nov,1

76120 Cineradiography/videoradiography, except where specifically included

2.87 2.87 FUD XXX Q1 N1 80

AMA: 2018,Jan,8; 2017,Jan,8; 2016,Jan,13; 2015,Jan,16

+ **76125 Cineradiography/videoradiography to complement routine examination (List separately in addition to code for primary procedure)**

Code first primary procedure

0.00 0.00 FUD ZZZ N N1 80

AMA: 2018,Jan,8; 2017,Jan,8; 2016,Jan,13; 2015,Jan,16

76140 Consultation on X-ray examination made elsewhere, written report

0.00 0.00 FUD XXX E

AMA: 2018,Jan,8; 2017,Jan,8; 2016,Jan,13; 2015,Jan,16

● **76145 Medical physics dose evaluation for radiation exposure that exceeds institutional review threshold, including report**

76376-76377 Three-dimensional Manipulation

INCLUDES 3D manipulation volumetric data set
Concurrent physician supervision image postprocessing
Rendering image

EXCLUDES *Anatomic guide 3D-printed and designed from image data set (0561T-0562T)*
Anatomic model 3D-printed from image data set (0559T-0560T)
Arthrography:
Ankle (73615)
Elbow (73085)
Hip (73525)
Knee (73580)
Shoulder (73040)
Wrist (73115)
Automated quantification/characterization coronary atherosclerotic plaque ([0623T, 0624T, 0625T, 0626T])
Cardiac MRI (75557, 75559, 75561, 75563, 75565)
Computer-aided detection MRI data for lesion, breast MRI (77046-77049)
CT angiography (70496, 70498, 71275, 72191, 73206, 73706, 74174-74175, 74261-74263, 75571-75574, 75635)
CT breast (0633T-0638T)
CT cerebral perfusion test (0042T)
Digital breast tomosynthesis (77061-77063)
Echocardiography, transesophageal (TEE) for guidance (93355)
Magnetic resonance angiography (70544-70549, 71555, 72198, 73225, 73725, 74185)
Nuclear radiology procedures (78012-78999 [78429, 78430, 78431, 78432, 78433, 78434, 78804, 78830, 78831, 78832, 78835])
Physician planning patient-specific fenestrated visceral aortic endograft (34839)

Code also base imaging procedure(s)

76376 3D rendering with interpretation and reporting of computed tomography, magnetic resonance imaging, ultrasound, or other tomographic modality with image postprocessing under concurrent supervision; not requiring image postprocessing on an independent workstation

EXCLUDES *3D rendering (76377)*
Bronchoscopy, with computer-assisted, image-guided navigation (31627)

0.65 0.65 FUD XXX N N1 80

AMA: 2019,Oct,10; 2019,Sep,10; 2019,Aug,5; 2018,Jul,11; 2018,Jan,8; 2017,Jan,8; 2016,Apr,8; 2016,Jan,13; 2015,Jan,16

76377 requiring image postprocessing on an independent workstation

EXCLUDES *3D rendering (76376)*

2.01 2.01 FUD XXX N N1 80

AMA: 2019,Oct,10; 2019,Sep,10; 2019,Aug,5; 2018,Jul,11; 2018,Jan,8; 2017,Jan,8; 2016,Apr,8; 2016,Jan,13; 2015,Jan,16

76380 Computerized Tomography: Delimited

EXCLUDES *Arthrography:*
Ankle (73615)
Elbow (73085)
Hip (73525)
Knee (73580)
Shoulder (73040)
Wrist (73115)
CT cerebral perfusion test (0042T)

76380 Computed tomography, limited or localized follow-up study
4.07 4.07 FUD XXX Q1 N1 80
AMA: 2019,Mar,10; 2018,Jan,8; 2017,Jan,8; 2016,Jan,13; 2015,Jan,16

76390-76391 Magnetic Resonance Spectroscopy

EXCLUDES *Arthrography:*
Ankle (73615)
Elbow (73085)
Hip (73525)
Knee (73580)
Shoulder (73040)
Wrist (73115)
CT cerebral perfusion test (0042T)

76390 Magnetic resonance spectroscopy
EXCLUDES *MRI*
MR spectroscopy for discogenic pain (0609T-0610T)
11.9 11.9 FUD XXX E
AMA: 2012,Feb,9-10; 1997,Nov,1

76391 Magnetic resonance (eg, vibration) elastography
6.54 6.54 FUD XXX Z2 80
AMA: 2019,Aug,3

76496-76499 Unlisted Radiology Procedures

76496 Unlisted fluoroscopic procedure (eg, diagnostic, interventional)
0.00 0.00 FUD XXX Q1 N1 80
AMA: 2012,Feb,9-10; 1997,Nov,1

76497 Unlisted computed tomography procedure (eg, diagnostic, interventional)
0.00 0.00 FUD XXX Q1 N1 80
AMA: 2018,Sep,10; 2018,Jan,8; 2017,Jan,8; 2016,Jan,13; 2015,Jan,16

76498 Unlisted magnetic resonance procedure (eg, diagnostic, interventional)
0.00 0.00 FUD XXX S Z2 80
AMA: 2019,Aug,5; 2018,Jul,11; 2018,Jan,8; 2017,Jan,8; 2016,Jan,13; 2015,Jan,16

76499 Unlisted diagnostic radiographic procedure
0.00 0.00 FUD XXX Q1 N1 80
AMA: 2018,Jan,8; 2017,Jan,8; 2016,Dec,15; 2016,Jul,8; 2016,Jan,13; 2015,Jan,16

76506 Ultrasound: Brain

INCLUDES Required permanent documentation ultrasound images except when diagnostic purpose is biometric measurement
Written documentation

EXCLUDES *Noninvasive vascular studies, diagnostic (93880-93990)*
Ultrasound not including thorough assessment organ or site, recorded image, and written report

76506 Echoencephalography, real time with image documentation (gray scale) (for determination of ventricular size, delineation of cerebral contents, and detection of fluid masses or other intracranial abnormalities), including A-mode encephalography as secondary component where indicated
3.25 3.25 FUD XXX Q1 N1 80
AMA: 2018,Jan,8; 2017,Jan,8; 2016,Jan,13; 2015,Jan,16

76510-76529 Ultrasound: Eyes

INCLUDES Required permanent documentation ultrasound images except when diagnostic purpose is biometric measurement
Written documentation

76510 Ophthalmic ultrasound, diagnostic; B-scan and quantitative A-scan performed during the same patient encounter
2.56 2.56 FUD XXX Q1 N1 80
AMA: 2018,Jan,8; 2017,Jan,8; 2016,Jan,13; 2015,Jan,16

76511 quantitative A-scan only
1.75 1.75 FUD XXX Q1 N1 80
AMA: 2019,Jan,12; 2018,Jan,8; 2017,Jan,8; 2016,Jan,13; 2015,Jan,16

76512 B-scan (with or without superimposed non-quantitative A-scan)
1.73 1.73 FUD XXX Q1 N1 80
AMA: 2019,Jan,12; 2018,Jan,8; 2017,Jan,8; 2016,Jan,13; 2015,Jan,16

▲ **76513 anterior segment ultrasound, immersion (water bath) B-scan or high resolution biomicroscopy, unilateral or bilateral**
EXCLUDES *Computerized ophthalmic testing other than by ultrasound (92132-92134)*
2.78 2.78 FUD XXX Q1 N1 80
AMA: 2019,Jan,12; 2018,Jan,8; 2017,Jan,8; 2016,Jan,13; 2015,Jan,16

76514 corneal pachymetry, unilateral or bilateral (determination of corneal thickness)
INCLUDES Biometric measurement for which permanent image documentation not required
EXCLUDES *Collagen cross-linking cornea (0402T)*
0.34 0.34 FUD XXX Q1 N1 80
AMA: 2019,Jan,12; 2018,Jan,8; 2017,Jan,8; 2016,Feb,12; 2016,Jan,13; 2015,Jan,16

76516 Ophthalmic biometry by ultrasound echography, A-scan;
INCLUDES Biometric measurement for which permanent image documentation not required
1.36 1.36 FUD XXX Q1 N1 80
AMA: 2019,Jan,12; 2018,Jan,8; 2017,Jan,8; 2016,Jan,13; 2015,Jan,16

76519 with intraocular lens power calculation
INCLUDES Biometric measurement for which permanent image documentation not required
Written prescription that satisfies requirement for written report
EXCLUDES *Partial coherence interferometry (92136)*
1.88 1.88 FUD XXX Q1 N1 80
AMA: 2019,Jan,12; 2018,Jan,8; 2017,Jan,8; 2016,Jan,13; 2015,Jan,16

76529 Ophthalmic ultrasonic foreign body localization
2.33 2.33 FUD XXX Q1 N1 80
AMA: 2019,Jan,12; 2018,Jan,8; 2017,Jan,8; 2016,Jan,13; 2015,Jan,16

76536-76800 Ultrasound: Neck, Thorax, Abdomen, and Spine

INCLUDES Required permanent documentation ultrasound images except when diagnostic purpose is biometric measurement
Written documentation

EXCLUDES *Focused ultrasound ablation uterine leiomyomata (0071T-0072T)*
Ultrasound exam not including thorough assessment organ or site, recorded image, and written report

76536 Ultrasound, soft tissues of head and neck (eg, thyroid, parathyroid, parotid), real time with image documentation
3.27 3.27 FUD XXX Q1 N1 80
AMA: 2018,Jan,8; 2017,Oct,9; 2017,Jan,8; 2016,Jan,13; 2015,Jan,16

76604 Ultrasound, chest (includes mediastinum), real time with image documentation
2.23 2.23 FUD XXX Q1 N1 80
AMA: 2018,Jan,8; 2017,Oct,9; 2017,Jan,8; 2016,Jan,13; 2015,Jan,16

76641 **Ultrasound, breast, unilateral, real time with image documentation, including axilla when performed; complete**

INCLUDES Complete examination all four quadrants, retroareolar region, and axilla when performed

EXCLUDES *Procedure performed more than one time per breast per session*

3.02 3.02 FUD XXX Q1 N1 80 50

AMA: 2018,Jan,8; 2017,Oct,9; 2017,Jan,8; 2016,Jan,13; 2015,Aug,8

76642 **limited**

INCLUDES Examination not including all complete examination elements

EXCLUDES *Procedure performed more than one time per breast per session*

2.47 2.47 FUD XXX Q1 N1 80 50

AMA: 2018,Jan,8; 2017,Oct,9

76700 **Ultrasound, abdominal, real time with image documentation; complete**

INCLUDES Real time scans:
- Common bile duct
- Gallbladder
- Inferior vena cava
- Kidneys
- Liver
- Pancreas
- Spleen
- Upper abdominal aorta

3.47 3.47 FUD XXX Q3 Z2 80

AMA: 2018,Jan,8; 2017,Oct,9; 2017,Jan,8; 2016,Jan,13; 2015,Jan,16

76705 **limited (eg, single organ, quadrant, follow-up)**

2.56 2.56 FUD XXX Q3 Z2 80

AMA: 2018,Jan,8; 2017,Oct,9; 2017,Jan,8; 2016,Jan,13; 2015,Jan,16

76706 **Ultrasound, abdominal aorta, real time with image documentation, screening study for abdominal aortic aneurysm (AAA)**

EXCLUDES *Diagnostic ultrasound aorta (76770-76775)*
Duplex scan aorta (93978-93979)

3.21 3.21 FUD XXX S 80

AMA: 2018,Jan,8; 2017,Sep,11

76770 **Ultrasound, retroperitoneal (eg, renal, aorta, nodes), real time with image documentation; complete**

INCLUDES Complete assessment kidneys and bladder when history indicates urinary pathology
Real time scans:
- Abdominal aorta
- Common iliac artery origins
- Inferior vena cava
- Kidneys

3.18 3.18 FUD XXX Q3 Z2 80

AMA: 2018,Jan,8; 2017,Oct,9; 2017,Jan,8; 2016,Jan,13; 2015,Jan,16

76775 **limited**

1.66 1.66 FUD XXX Q1 N1 80

AMA: 2018,Jan,8; 2017,Oct,9; 2017,Jan,8; 2016,Jan,13; 2015,Jan,16

76776 **Ultrasound, transplanted kidney, real time and duplex Doppler with image documentation**

EXCLUDES *Abdominal/pelvic/scrotal contents/retroperitoneal duplex scan (93975-93976)*
Transplanted kidney ultrasound without duplex doppler (76775)

4.41 4.41 FUD XXX Q3 Z2 80

AMA: 2018,Jan,8; 2017,Jan,8; 2016,Jan,13; 2015,Jan,16

76800 **Ultrasound, spinal canal and contents**

4.04 4.04 FUD XXX Q1 N1 80

AMA: 2018,Jan,8; 2017,Jan,8; 2016,Jan,13; 2015,Jan,16

76801-76802 Ultrasound: Pregnancy Less Than 14 Weeks

INCLUDES Determination number gestational sacs and fetuses
Gestational sac/fetal measurement appropriate for gestational age (younger than 14 weeks 0 days)
Inspection maternal uterus and adnexa
Quality analysis amniotic fluid volume/gestational sac shape
Visualization fetal and placental anatomic formation
Written documentation each exam component

EXCLUDES *Focused ultrasound ablation uterine leiomyomata (0071T-0072T)*
Ultrasound exam not including thorough assessment organ or site, recorded image, and written report

76801 **Ultrasound, pregnant uterus, real time with image documentation, fetal and maternal evaluation, first trimester (< 14 weeks 0 days), transabdominal approach; single or first gestation** M ♀

EXCLUDES *Fetal nuchal translucency measurement, first trimester (76813)*

3.45 3.45 FUD XXX S Z2 80

AMA: 2018,Jan,8; 2017,Jan,8; 2016,Jan,13; 2015,Jan,16

+ **76802** **each additional gestation (List separately in addition to code for primary procedure)** M ♀

EXCLUDES *Fetal nuchal translucency measurement, first trimester (76814)*

Code first (76801)

1.78 1.78 FUD ZZZ N N1 80

AMA: 2018,Jan,8; 2017,Jan,8; 2016,Jan,13; 2015,Jan,16

76805-76810 Ultrasound: Pregnancy of 14 Weeks or More

INCLUDES Determination number gestational/chorionic sacs and fetuses
Evaluation:
- Amniotic fluid
- Four chambered heart
- Intracranial, spinal, abdominal anatomy
- Placenta location
- Umbilical cord insertion site

Examination maternal adnexa if visible
Gestational sac/fetal measurement appropriate for gestational age (older than or equal to 14 weeks 0 days)
Written documentation each exam component

EXCLUDES *Focused ultrasound ablation uterine leiomyomata (0071T-0072T)*
Ultrasound exam not including thorough assessment organ or site, recorded image, and written report

76805 **Ultrasound, pregnant uterus, real time with image documentation, fetal and maternal evaluation, after first trimester (> or = 14 weeks 0 days), transabdominal approach; single or first gestation** M ♀

3.97 3.97 FUD XXX S Z2 80

AMA: 2018,Jan,8; 2017,Jan,8; 2016,Jan,13; 2015,Jan,16

+ **76810** **each additional gestation (List separately in addition to code for primary procedure)** M ♀

Code first (76805)

2.59 2.59 FUD ZZZ N N1 80

AMA: 2018,Jan,8; 2017,Jan,8; 2016,Jan,13; 2015,Jan,16

76811-76812 Ultrasound: Pregnancy, with Additional Studies of Fetus

INCLUDES Determination number gestational/chorionic sacs and fetuses
Evaluation:
Amniotic fluid
Examination maternal adnexa if visible
Focused ultrasound ablation uterine leiomyomata (0071T-0072T)
Four-chambered heart
Gestational sac/fetal measurement appropriate for gestational age (older than or equal to 14 weeks 0 days)
Intracranial, spinal, abdominal anatomy
Placenta location
Ultrasound exam not including thorough assessment organ or site, recorded image, and written report
Umbilical cord insertion site
Written documentation each exam component
Examination of maternal adnexa if visible
Gestational sac/fetal measurement appropriate for gestational age (older than or equal to 14 weeks 0 days)
Written documentation of each component of exam, including reason for nonvisualization, when applicable

EXCLUDES *Focused ultrasound ablation of uterine leiomyomata (0071T-0072T)*
Ultrasound exam that does not include thorough assessment organ or site, recorded image, and written report

76811 Ultrasound, pregnant uterus, real time with image documentation, fetal and maternal evaluation plus detailed fetal anatomic examination, transabdominal approach; single or first gestation M ♀
5.12 5.12 FUD XXX S Z3 80
AMA: 2018,Jan,8; 2017,Jan,8; 2016,Jan,13; 2015,Jan,16

\+ **76812 each additional gestation (List separately in addition to code for primary procedure)** M ♀
Code first (76811)
5.72 5.72 FUD ZZZ N N1 80
AMA: 2018,Jan,8; 2017,Jan,8; 2016,Jan,13; 2015,Jan,16

76813-76828 Ultrasound: Other Fetal Evaluations

INCLUDES Required permanent documentation ultrasound images except when diagnostic purpose is biometric measurement
Written documentation

EXCLUDES *Focused ultrasound ablation uterine leiomyomata (0071T-0072T)*
Ultrasound exam not including thorough assessment organ or site, recorded image, and written report

76813 Ultrasound, pregnant uterus, real time with image documentation, first trimester fetal nuchal translucency measurement, transabdominal or transvaginal approach; single or first gestation M ♀
3.45 3.45 FUD XXX Q1 N1 80
AMA: 2018,Jan,8; 2017,Jan,8; 2016,Jan,13; 2015,Jan,16

\+ **76814 each additional gestation (List separately in addition to code for primary procedure)** M ♀
Code first (76813)
2.27 2.27 FUD XXX N N1 80
AMA: 2018,Jan,8; 2017,Jan,8; 2016,Jan,13; 2015,Jan,16

76815 Ultrasound, pregnant uterus, real time with image documentation, limited (eg, fetal heart beat, placental location, fetal position and/or qualitative amniotic fluid volume), 1 or more fetuses M ♀
INCLUDES Exam concentrating on one or more elements
Reporting only one time per exam, not per element
EXCLUDES *Fetal nuchal translucency measurement, first trimester (76813-76814)*
2.37 2.37 FUD XXX Q1 N1 80
AMA: 2018,Jan,8; 2017,Jan,8; 2016,Jan,13; 2015,Jan,16

76816 Ultrasound, pregnant uterus, real time with image documentation, follow-up (eg, re-evaluation of fetal size by measuring standard growth parameters and amniotic fluid volume, re-evaluation of organ system(s) suspected or confirmed to be abnormal on a previous scan), transabdominal approach, per fetus M ♀
INCLUDES Re-evaluation fetal size, interval growth, or aberrancies noted on prior ultrasound
Code also modifier 59 for examination each additional fetus
3.19 3.19 FUD XXX Q1 N1 80
AMA: 2018,Jan,8; 2017,Jan,8; 2016,Jan,13; 2015,Jan,16

76817 Ultrasound, pregnant uterus, real time with image documentation, transvaginal M ♀
EXCLUDES *Transvaginal ultrasound, non-obstetrical (76830)*
Code also transabdominal obstetrical ultrasound, when performed
2.73 2.73 FUD XXX Q1 N1 80
AMA: 2018,Jan,8; 2017,Jan,8; 2016,Jan,13; 2015,Jan,16

76818 Fetal biophysical profile; with non-stress testing M ♀
Code also modifier 59 for each additional fetus
3.44 3.44 FUD XXX S Z2 80
AMA: 2018,Jan,8; 2017,Jan,8; 2016,Jan,13; 2015,Jan,16

76819 without non-stress testing M ♀
EXCLUDES *Amniotic fluid index without non-stress test (76815)*
Code also modifier 59 for each additional fetus
2.45 2.45 FUD XXX S Z3 80
AMA: 2018,Jan,8; 2017,Jan,8; 2016,Jan,13; 2015,Jan,16

76820 Doppler velocimetry, fetal; umbilical artery M
1.35 1.35 FUD XXX Q1 N1 80
AMA: 2018,Jan,8; 2017,Jan,8; 2016,Jul,8; 2016,Jan,13; 2015,Jan,16

76821 middle cerebral artery M
2.55 2.55 FUD XXX Q1 N1 80
AMA: 2018,Jan,8; 2017,Jan,8; 2016,Jan,13; 2015,Jan,16

76825 Echocardiography, fetal, cardiovascular system, real time with image documentation (2D), with or without M-mode recording; M ♀
7.79 7.79 FUD XXX S Z3 80
AMA: 2018,Jan,8; 2017,Sep,14; 2017,Jan,8; 2016,Jan,13; 2015,Jan,16

76826 follow-up or repeat study M ♀
4.58 4.58 FUD XXX S Z2 80
AMA: 2018,Jan,8; 2017,Sep,14

76827 Doppler echocardiography, fetal, pulsed wave and/or continuous wave with spectral display; complete M ♀
2.07 2.07 FUD XXX Q1 N1 80
AMA: 2018,Jan,8; 2017,Jan,8; 2016,Jan,13; 2015,Jan,16

76828 follow-up or repeat study M ♀
EXCLUDES *Color mapping (93325)*
1.47 1.47 FUD XXX Q1 N1 80
AMA: 2018,Jan,8; 2017,Jan,8; 2016,Jan,13; 2015,Jan,16

76830-76873 Ultrasound: Male and Female Genitalia

INCLUDES Required permanent documentation ultrasound images except when diagnostic purpose is biometric measurement
Written documentation

EXCLUDES *Focused ultrasound ablation uterine leiomyomata (0071T-0072T)*
Ultrasound exam not including thorough assessment organ or site, recorded image, and written report

76830 Ultrasound, transvaginal ♀

EXCLUDES *Transvaginal ultrasound, obstetric (76817)*

Code also transabdominal nonobstetrical ultrasound, when performed

3.47 3.47 **FUD** XXX S Z2 80

AMA: 2018,Jan,8; 2017,Oct,9; 2017,Jan,8; 2016,Jan,13; 2015,Jan,16

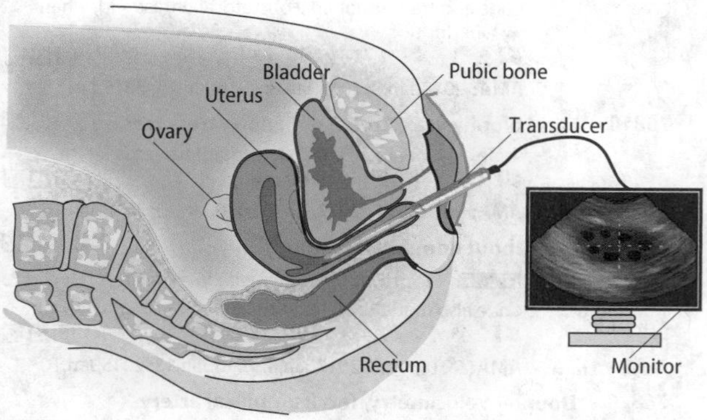

Ultrasound is performed in real time with image documentation by a transvaginal approach

76831 Saline infusion sonohysterography (SIS), including color flow Doppler, when performed ♀

Code also saline introduction for saline infusion sonohysterography (58340)

3.36 3.36 **FUD** XXX Q3 Z3 80

AMA: 2018,Jan,8; 2017,Jan,8; 2016,Jan,13; 2015,Jan,16

76856 Ultrasound, pelvic (nonobstetric), real time with image documentation; complete

INCLUDES Total examination female pelvic anatomy including:
- Bladder measurement
- Description and measurement uterus and adnexa
- Description any pelvic pathology
- Measurement, endometrium

Total examination male pelvis including:
- Bladder measurement
- Description any pelvic pathology
- Evaluation prostate and seminal vesicles

3.09 3.09 **FUD** XXX Q3 Z2 80

AMA: 2018,Jan,8; 2017,Oct,9; 2017,Jan,8; 2016,Aug,9; 2016,Jan,13; 2015,Jan,16

76857 limited or follow-up (eg, for follicles)

INCLUDES Focused evaluation limited to:
- Evaluation one or more elements listed in 76856 and/or
- Re-evaluation one or more pelvic aberrancies noted on prior ultrasound

Urinary bladder alone

EXCLUDES *Bladder volume or post-voided residual measurement without bladder imaging (51798)*
Urinary bladder and kidneys (76770)

1.38 1.38 **FUD** XXX Q3 Z3 80

AMA: 2018,Jan,8; 2017,Oct,9; 2017,Jan,8; 2016,Jan,13; 2015,Jan,16

76870 Ultrasound, scrotum and contents ♂

2.97 2.97 **FUD** XXX Q1 N1 80

AMA: 2018,Jan,8; 2017,Oct,9

76872 Ultrasound, transrectal;

EXCLUDES *Colonoscopy (45391-45392)*
Cystourethroscopy with transurethral anterior prostate commissurotomy/drug delivery (0619T)
Hemorrhoidectomy by transanal hemorrhoidal dearterialization ([46948])
Sigmoidoscopy (45341-45342)
Transurethral prostate ablation (0421T)

4.43 4.43 **FUD** XXX S Z2 80

AMA: 2020,Feb,11; 2018,Nov,10; 2018,Jul,11; 2018,Jan,8; 2017,Oct,9; 2017,Jan,8; 2016,Jan,13; 2015,Jan,16

76873 prostate volume study for brachytherapy treatment planning (separate procedure) ♂

4.91 4.91 **FUD** XXX S Z2 80

AMA: 2018,Jan,8; 2017,Jan,8; 2016,Jan,13; 2015,Jan,16

76881-76886 Ultrasound: Extremities

EXCLUDES *Doppler studies extremities (93925-93926, 93930-93931, 93970-93971)*

76881 Ultrasound, complete joint (ie, joint space and peri-articular soft tissue structures) real-time with image documentation

INCLUDES Real-time scans specific joint including assessment:
- Joint space
- Muscles
- Other soft tissue
- Tendons

Required permanent image documentation
Stress manipulations and dynamic imaging when performed
Written documentation including explanation any joint components not visualized

2.51 2.51 **FUD** XXX S Z3 80

AMA: 2018,Jan,8; 2017,Oct,9; 2017,Jan,8; 2016,Sep,9

76882 Ultrasound, limited, joint or other nonvascular extremity structure(s) (eg, joint space, peri-articular tendon[s], muscle[s], nerve[s], other soft tissue structure[s], or soft tissue mass[es]), real-time with image documentation

INCLUDES Limited joint examination or evaluation due to mass or other abnormality not requiring all complete joint evaluation components (76881)

Real-time scans specific joint including assessment:
- Joint space
- Muscles
- Other soft tissue
- Tendons

Required permanent image documentation
Written documentation including explanation any joint components not visualized

1.61 1.61 **FUD** XXX Q1 N1 80

AMA: 2018,Jan,8; 2017,Oct,9; 2017,Jan,8; 2016,Sep,9

76885 Ultrasound, infant hips, real time with imaging documentation; dynamic (requiring physician or other qualified health care professional manipulation) A

4.05 4.05 **FUD** XXX Q1 N1 80

AMA: 2012,Feb,9-10; 2002,May,7

76886 limited, static (not requiring physician or other qualified health care professional manipulation) A

2.97 2.97 **FUD** XXX Q1 N1 80

AMA: 2012,Feb,9-10; 2002,May,7

76932-76970 Imaging Guidance: Ultrasound

INCLUDES Required permanent documentation ultrasound images except when diagnostic purpose is biometric measurement
Written documentation

EXCLUDES *Focused ultrasound ablation uterine leiomyomata (0071T-0072T)*
Ultrasound exam not including thorough assessment organ or site, recorded image, and written report

76932 Ultrasonic guidance for endomyocardial biopsy, imaging supervision and interpretation

0.00 0.00 **FUD** YYY N N1 80

AMA: 2012,Feb,9-10; 2001,Sep,4

76936 Ultrasound guided compression repair of arterial pseudoaneurysm or arteriovenous fistulae (includes diagnostic ultrasound evaluation, compression of lesion and imaging)

7.60 7.60 FUD XXX S Z2 80

AMA: 2012,Feb,9-10; 2002,May,7

+ **76937 Ultrasound guidance for vascular access requiring ultrasound evaluation of potential access sites, documentation of selected vessel patency, concurrent realtime ultrasound visualization of vascular needle entry, with permanent recording and reporting (List separately in addition to code for primary procedure)**

INCLUDES Ultrasound guidance, needle placement (76942)

EXCLUDES *Endovascular venous arterialization, tibial or peroneal vein ([0620T])*
Endovenous femoral-popliteal arterial revascularization (0505T)
Extremity venous noninvasive vascular diagnostic study performed separately from venous access guidance (93970-93971)
Insertion or replacement peripherally inserted central venous catheter (36568-36569, [36572, 36573], 36584)
Insertion, removal, or replacement permanent leadless pacemaker ([33274, 33275])
Insertion, removal, or repositioning vena cava filter (37191-37193)
Ligation perforator veins (37760-37761)

Code first primary procedure

0.96 0.96 FUD ZZZ N N1 80

AMA: 2019,May,3; 2019,Mar,6; 2018,Mar,3; 2018,Jan,8; 2017,Dec,3; 2017,Aug,10; 2017,Jul,3; 2017,Mar,3; 2017,Jan,8; 2016,Nov,3; 2016,Jul,6; 2016,Jan,13; 2015,Jul,10; 2015,Jan,16

76940 Ultrasound guidance for, and monitoring of, parenchymal tissue ablation

EXCLUDES *Ablation (20982-20983, [32994], 32998, 47370-47383, 50250, 50542, 50592-50593, 0582T, 0600T-0601T)*
Ultrasound guidance:
Intraoperative (76998)
Needle placement (76942)

0.00 0.00 FUD YYY N N1 80

AMA: 2018,Jan,8; 2017,Nov,8; 2017,Jan,8; 2016,Jan,13; 2015,Jul,8; 2015,Jan,16

76941 Ultrasonic guidance for intrauterine fetal transfusion or cordocentesis, imaging supervision and interpretation M ♀

Code also surgical procedure (36460, 59012)

0.00 0.00 FUD XXX N N1 80

AMA: 2012,Feb,9-10; 2001,Sep,4

76942 Ultrasonic guidance for needle placement (eg, biopsy, aspiration, injection, localization device), imaging supervision and interpretation

EXCLUDES *Arthrocentesis (20604, 20606, 20611)*
Autologous WBC injection (0481T)
Breast biopsy with placement localization device(s) (19083)
Core needle biopsy, lung or mediastinum (32408)
Esophagogastroduodenoscopy (43237, 43242)
Esophagoscopy (43232)
Fine needle aspiration biopsy ([10004, 10005, 10006], 10021)
Gastrointestinal endoscopic ultrasound (76975)
Hemorrhoidectomy by transanal hemorrhoidal dearterialization ([46948])
Image-guided fluid collection drainage by catheter (10030)
Injection procedures (27096, 64479-64484, 0232T)
Ligation (37760-37761)
Paravertebral facet joint injections (64490-64491, 64493-64495, 0213T-0218T)
Placement breast localization device(s) (19285)
Sigmoidoscopy (45341-45342)
Thoracentesis (32554-32557)
Transperineal placement, periprostatic biodegradable material (55874)
Transurethral ablation, malignant prostate tissue (0582T)

1.61 1.61 FUD XXX N N1 80

AMA: 2020,Jun,10; 2020,Feb,11; 2020,Feb,9; 2020,Jan,7; 2019,Aug,10; 2019,Apr,4; 2019,Feb,8; 2018,Jul,11; 2018,Mar,3; 2018,Jan,8; 2017,Dec,13; 2017,Sep,6; 2017,Jun,10; 2017,Jan,8; 2016,Nov,3; 2016,Jun,3; 2016,Jan,13; 2016,Jan,9; 2015,Dec,3; 2015,Nov,10; 2015,Aug,8; 2015,Feb,6; 2015,Jan,16

76945 Ultrasonic guidance for chorionic villus sampling, imaging supervision and interpretation M ♀

Code also surgical procedure (59015)

0.00 0.00 FUD XXX N N1 80

AMA: 2012,Feb,9-10; 2001,Sep,4

76946 Ultrasonic guidance for amniocentesis, imaging supervision and interpretation M ♀

0.91 0.91 FUD XXX N N1 80

AMA: 2012,Feb,9-10; 2001,Sep,4

76948 Ultrasonic guidance for aspiration of ova, imaging supervision and interpretation M ♀

2.15 2.15 FUD XXX N N1 80

AMA: 2012,Feb,9-10; 2001,Sep,4

76965 Ultrasonic guidance for interstitial radioelement application

2.62 2.62 FUD XXX N N1 80

AMA: 2012,Feb,9-10; 1997,Nov,1

~~**76970 Ultrasound study follow-up (specify)**~~

76975 Endoscopic Ultrasound

INCLUDES Required permanent documentation ultrasound images except when diagnostic purpose is biometric measurement
Written documentation

EXCLUDES *Focused ultrasound ablation uterine leiomyomata (0071T-0072T)*
Ultrasound exam not including thorough assessment organ or site, recorded image, and written report

76975 Gastrointestinal endoscopic ultrasound, supervision and interpretation

INCLUDES Ultrasonic guidance (76942)

EXCLUDES *Colonoscopy (44406-44407, 45391-45392)*
Esophagogastroduodenoscopy (43237-43238, 43240, 43242, 43259)
Esophagoscopy (43231-43232)
Sigmoidoscopy (45341-45342)

0.00 0.00 FUD XXX 02 N1 80

AMA: 2018,Jan,8; 2017,Jan,8; 2016,Jan,13; 2015,Jan,16

Radiology

76936 — 76975

76977 Bone Density Measurements: Ultrasound

CMS: 100-02,15,80.5.5 Frequency Standards

INCLUDES Required permanent documentation ultrasound images except when diagnostic purpose is biometric measurement
Written documentation

EXCLUDES *Ultrasound exam not including thorough assessment organ or site, recorded image, and written report*

76977 Ultrasound bone density measurement and interpretation, peripheral site(s), any method
0.21 0.21 **FUD** XXX S Z3 80
AMA: 2012,Feb,9-10; 1998,Nov,1

76978-76979 Targeted Dynamic Microbubble Sonographic Contrast Characterization: Ultrasound

INCLUDES Intravenous injection (96374)

76978 Ultrasound, targeted dynamic microbubble sonographic contrast characterization (non-cardiac); initial lesion
9.21 9.21 **FUD** XXX Z2 80
AMA: 2019,Jun,9

+ **76979 each additional lesion with separate injection (List separately in addition to code for primary procedure)**
Code first (76978)
6.23 6.23 **FUD** ZZZ N1 80
AMA: 2019,Jun,9

76981-76983 Elastography: Ultrasound

EXCLUDES *Shear wave liver elastography (91200)*

76981 Ultrasound, elastography; parenchyma (eg, organ)
EXCLUDES *Reporting code more than one time each session for same parenchymal organ and/or parenchymal organ and lesion*
3.04 3.04 **FUD** XXX Z2 80
AMA: 2019,Aug,3

76982 first target lesion
2.71 2.71 **FUD** XXX Z2 80
AMA: 2019,Aug,3

+ **76983 each additional target lesion (List separately in addition to code for primary procedure)**
EXCLUDES *Reporting code more than one time each session for same parenchymal organ and/or parenchymal organ and lesion*
Code first (76982)
1.67 1.67 **FUD** ZZZ N1 80
AMA: 2019,Aug,3

76998-76999 Imaging Guidance During Surgery: Ultrasound

INCLUDES Required permanent documentation ultrasound images except when diagnostic purpose is biometric measurement
Written documentation

EXCLUDES *Focused ultrasound ablation uterine leiomyomata (0071T-0072T)*
Ultrasound exam not including thorough assessment organ or site, recorded image, and written report

76998 Ultrasonic guidance, intraoperative
EXCLUDES *Ablation (47370-47371, 47380-47382)*
Endovenous ablation therapy incompetent vein (36475, 36479)
Hemorrhoidectomy by transanal hemorrhoidal dearterialization ([46948])
Ligation (37760-37761)
Wireless cardiac stimulator (0515T-0520T)
0.00 0.00 **FUD** XXX N N1 80
AMA: 2020,Feb,11; 2018,Mar,3; 2018,Jan,8; 2017,Apr,7; 2017,Jan,8; 2016,Nov,3; 2016,Jan,13; 2015,Aug,8; 2015,Jan,16

76999 Unlisted ultrasound procedure (eg, diagnostic, interventional)
0.00 0.00 **FUD** XXX Q1 N1 80
AMA: 2019,Dec,8; 2018,Jul,11; 2018,Jan,8; 2017,Jan,8; 2016,Jan,13; 2015,Jan,16

77001-77022 Imaging Guidance Techniques

EXCLUDES *Imaging guidance, breast localization device(s) (19081, 19281, 19283)*

+ **77001 Fluoroscopic guidance for central venous access device placement, replacement (catheter only or complete), or removal (includes fluoroscopic guidance for vascular access and catheter manipulation, any necessary contrast injections through access site or catheter with related venography radiologic supervision and interpretation, and radiographic documentation of final catheter position) (List separately in addition to code for primary procedure)**
INCLUDES Fluoroscopic guidance for needle placement (77002)
EXCLUDES *Any procedure codes that include fluoroscopic guidance in code descriptor*
Extracorporeal membrane oxygenation (ECMO)/extracorporeal life support (ECLS) (33957-33959, [33962, 33963, 33964])
Formal extremity venography performed separately from venous access and interpreted separately (36005, 75820, 75822, 75825, 75827)
Insertion peripherally inserted central venous catheter (PICC) (36568-36569, [36572, 36573])
Replacement peripherally inserted central venous catheter (PICC) (36584)
Code first primary procedure
2.71 2.71 **FUD** ZZZ N N1 80
AMA: 2019,May,3; 2018,Jan,8; 2017,Jan,8; 2016,Jan,13; 2015,Jan,16

+ **77002 Fluoroscopic guidance for needle placement (eg, biopsy, aspiration, injection, localization device) (List separately in addition to code for primary procedure)**
EXCLUDES *Ablation therapy (20982-20983)*
Any procedure codes that include fluoroscopic guidance in code descriptor:
Radiological guidance for percutaneous drainage by catheter (75989)
Transhepatic portography (75885, 75887)
Arthrography procedure(s) (70332, 73040, 73085, 73115, 73525, 73580, 73615)
Biopsy, breast, with placement breast localization device(s) (19081-19086)
Image-guided fluid collection drainage by catheter (10030)
Placement breast localization device(s) (19281-19288)
Platelet rich plasma injection(s) (0232T)
Thoracentesis (32554-32557)
Code first surgical procedure (10160, 20206, 20220, 20225, 20520, 20525-20526, 20550, 20551, 20552, 20553, 20555, 20600, 20605, 20610, 20612, 20615, 21116, 21550, 23350, 24220, 25246, 27093-27095, 27369, 27648, 32400, 32553, 36002, 38220-38222, 38505, 38794, 41019, 42400-42405, 47000-47001, 48102, 49180, 49411, 50200, 50390, 51100-51102, 55700, 55876, 60100, 62268-62269, 64400-64448, 64450, 64455, 64505, 64600-64605)
2.86 2.86 **FUD** ZZZ N N1 80
AMA: 2020,Feb,9; 2020,Jan,7; 2019,Dec,8; 2019,Dec,12; 2019,Aug,7; 2019,Mar,6; 2019,Apr,4; 2019,Feb,8; 2018,Dec,10; 2018,Dec,10; 2018,Jan,8; 2017,Jun,10; 2017,Jan,8; 2016,Sep,9; 2016,Aug,7; 2016,Jun,3; 2016,Jan,9; 2016,Jan,13; 2015,Dec,3; 2015,Aug,6; 2015,Jul,8; 2015,Feb,6; 2015,Feb,10; 2015,Jan,16

+ **77003 Fluoroscopic guidance and localization of needle or catheter tip for spine or paraspinous diagnostic or therapeutic injection procedures (epidural or subarachnoid) (List separately in addition to code for primary procedure)**

EXCLUDES *Any procedure codes that include fluoroscopic guidance in code descriptor*
Arthrodesis (22586)
Image-guided fluid collection drainage by catheter (10030)
Injection allogenic cellular and/or tissue-based product, intervertebral disc (0627T-0628T)
Injection medication (subarachnoid/interlaminar epidural) (62320-62327)
Spinal puncture (62270, [62328], 62272, [62329])

Code first (61050-61055, 62267, 62273, 62280-62284, 64449, 64510, 64517, 64520, 64610, 96450)

2.85 2.85 **FUD** ZZZ N N1 80

AMA: 2020,Jun,10; 2019,Dec,8; 2018,Jan,8; 2017,Dec,13; 2017,Sep,6; 2017,Feb,9; 2017,Feb,12; 2017,Jan,8; 2016,Jan,11; 2016,Jan,9; 2016,Jan,13; 2015,Jan,16

77011 Computed tomography guidance for stereotactic localization

EXCLUDES *Arthrodesis (22586)*

6.47 6.47 **FUD** XXX N N1

AMA: 2018,Jan,8; 2017,Jan,8; 2016,Jan,13; 2015,Jan,16

77012 Computed tomography guidance for needle placement (eg, biopsy, aspiration, injection, localization device), radiological supervision and interpretation

EXCLUDES *Arthrodesis (22586)*
Autologous white blood cell concentrate (0481T)
Core needle biopsy, lung or mediastinum (32408)
Destruction paravertebral facet joint nerve by neurolysis ([64633, 64634, 64635, 64636])
Fine needle aspiration biopsy using CT guidance ([10009, 10010])
Image-guided fluid collection drainage by catheter (10030)
Injection allogenic cellular and/or tissue-based product, intervertebral disc (0629T-0630T)
Injection, paravertebral facet joint (64490-64495)
Platelet rich plasma injection(s) (0232T)
Sacroiliac joint arthrography (27096)
Spinal puncture (62270, [62328], 62272, [62329])
Thoracentesis (32554-32557)
Transforaminal epidural needle placement/injection (64479-64480, 64483-64484)

4.27 4.27 **FUD** XXX N N1

AMA: 2020,Jun,10; 2020,Jan,7; 2019,Dec,8; 2019,Apr,4; 2019,Feb,8; 2018,Jan,8; 2017,Sep,6; 2017,Feb,12; 2017,Jan,8; 2016,Jun,3; 2016,Jan,13; 2015,Dec,3; 2015,Feb,6; 2015,Jan,16

77013 Computed tomography guidance for, and monitoring of, parenchymal tissue ablation

EXCLUDES *Ablation therapy (20982-20983, [32994], 32998, 47382-47383, 50592-50593)*
Ablation, irreversible electroporation (0600T)

0.00 0.00 **FUD** XXX N N1 80

AMA: 2018,Jan,8; 2017,Nov,8; 2017,Jan,8; 2016,Jan,13; 2015,Jul,8; 2015,Jan,16

77014 Computed tomography guidance for placement of radiation therapy fields

Code also placement interstitial device(s) for radiation therapy guidance (31627, 32553, 49411, 55876)

3.45 3.45 **FUD** XXX N N1

AMA: 2018,Jan,8; 2017,Jan,8; 2016,Feb,3; 2016,Jan,13; 2015,Apr,10; 2015,Jan,16

77021 Magnetic resonance imaging guidance for needle placement (eg, for biopsy, needle aspiration, injection, or placement of localization device) radiological supervision and interpretation

EXCLUDES *Autologous white blood cell concentrate (0481T)*
Biopsy, breast, with placement breast localization device(s) (19085)
Core needle biopsy, lung or mediastinum (32408)
Fine needle aspiration biopsy using MR guidance ([10011, 10012])
Image-guided fluid collection drainage by catheter (10030)
Placement breast localization device(s) (19287)
Platelet rich plasma injection(s) (0232T)
Surgical procedure
Thoracentesis (32554-32557)

13.1 13.1 **FUD** XXX N N1

AMA: 2020,Jun,10; 2020,Feb,9; 2020,Jan,7; 2019,Apr,4; 2019,Feb,8; 2018,Jul,11; 2018,Jan,8; 2017,Jun,10; 2017,Jan,8; 2016,Jun,3; 2016,Jan,13; 2015,Dec,3; 2015,Feb,6; 2015,Jan,16

77022 Magnetic resonance imaging guidance for, and monitoring of, parenchymal tissue ablation

EXCLUDES *Ablation:*
Irreversible electroporation (0600T)
Percutaneous radiofrequency ([32994], 32998, 47382-47383, 50592-50593)
Reduction or eradication one or more bone tumors (20982-20983)
Uterine leiomyomata by focused ablation (0071T-0072T)

0.00 0.00 **FUD** XXX N N1 80

AMA: 2019,Sep,10; 2018,Mar,3; 2018,Jan,8; 2017,Nov,8; 2017,Jan,8; 2016,Nov,3; 2016,Jan,13; 2015,Jul,8; 2015,Jan,16

77046-77067 Radiography: Breast

77046 Magnetic resonance imaging, breast, without contrast material; unilateral

7.02 7.02 **FUD** XXX Z2 80

AMA: 2019,Aug,5

77047 bilateral

7.08 7.08 **FUD** XXX Z2 80

AMA: 2019,Aug,5

77048 Magnetic resonance imaging, breast, without and with contrast material(s), including computer-aided detection (CAD real-time lesion detection, characterization and pharmacokinetic analysis), when performed; unilateral

11.1 11.1 **FUD** XXX 80

AMA: 2019,Dec,14; 2019,Aug,5

77049 bilateral

11.1 11.1 **FUD** XXX 80

AMA: 2019,Dec,14; 2019,Aug,5

77053 Mammary ductogram or galactogram, single duct, radiological supervision and interpretation

Code also injection procedure (19030)

1.60 1.60 **FUD** XXX Q2 N1

AMA: 2018,Jan,8; 2017,Jan,8; 2016,Jan,13; 2015,Jan,16

77054 Mammary ductogram or galactogram, multiple ducts, radiological supervision and interpretation

2.07 2.07 **FUD** XXX Q2 N1

AMA: 2018,Jan,8; 2017,Jan,8; 2016,Jan,13; 2015,Jan,16

77061 Diagnostic digital breast tomosynthesis; unilateral

EXCLUDES *3D rendering (76376-76377)*
Screening mammography (77067)

0.00 0.00 **FUD** XXX E

AMA: 2020,Sep,14; 2018,Jan,8

77062 bilateral

EXCLUDES *3D rendering (76376-76377)*
Screening mammography (77067)

0.00 0.00 **FUD** XXX E

AMA: 2020,Sep,14; 2018,Jan,8; 2017,Jan,8; 2016,Dec,15

+ **77063 Screening digital breast tomosynthesis, bilateral (List separately in addition to code for primary procedure)**
 EXCLUDES *3D rendering (76376-76377)*
 Diagnostic mammography (77065-77066)
 Code first (77067)
 1.55 1.55 FUD ZZZ A
 AMA: 2020,Sep,14; 2018,Jan,8; 2017,Jan,8; 2016,Dec,15

77065 Diagnostic mammography, including computer-aided detection (CAD) when performed; unilateral
 3.78 3.78 FUD XXX A 80
 AMA: 2020,Sep,14; 2019,Aug,5; 2018,Jan,8; 2017,Jan,8; 2016,Dec,15

77066 bilateral
 4.76 4.76 FUD XXX A 80
 AMA: 2020,Sep,14; 2019,Aug,5; 2018,Jan,8; 2017,Jan,8; 2016,Dec,15

77067 Screening mammography, bilateral (2-view study of each breast), including computer-aided detection (CAD) when performed
 EXCLUDES *Breast scan, electrical impedance (76499)*
 3.86 3.86 FUD XXX A 80
 AMA: 2020,Sep,14; 2019,Aug,5; 2018,Jan,8; 2017,Jan,8; 2016,Dec,15

77071-77086 [77085, 77086] Additional Evaluations of Bones and Joints

77071 Manual application of stress performed by physician or other qualified health care professional for joint radiography, including contralateral joint if indicated
 Code also interpretation stressed images according to anatomical site and number of views
 1.43 1.43 FUD XXX Q1 N1 80 26
 AMA: 2018,Jan,8; 2017,Jan,8; 2016,Jan,13; 2015,Jan,16

77072 Bone age studies
 0.71 0.71 FUD XXX Q1 N1 80
 AMA: 2018,Jan,8; 2017,Jan,8; 2016,Jan,13; 2015,Jan,16

77073 Bone length studies (orthoroentgenogram, scanogram)
 1.06 1.06 FUD XXX Q1 N1 80
 AMA: 2018,Jan,8; 2017,Jan,8; 2016,Jan,13; 2015,Jan,16

77074 Radiologic examination, osseous survey; limited (eg, for metastases)
 1.78 1.78 FUD XXX Q1 N1 80
 AMA: 2018,Jan,8; 2017,Jan,8; 2016,Jan,13; 2015,Jan,16

77075 complete (axial and appendicular skeleton)
 2.60 2.60 FUD XXX Q1 N1 80
 AMA: 2018,Jan,8; 2017,Jan,8; 2016,Jan,13; 2015,Jan,16

77076 Radiologic examination, osseous survey, infant
 2.85 2.85 FUD XXX Q1 N1 80
 AMA: 2018,Jan,8; 2017,Jan,8; 2016,Jan,13; 2015,Jan,16

77077 Joint survey, single view, 2 or more joints (specify)
 1.29 1.29 FUD XXX Q1 N1 80
 AMA: 2018,Jan,8; 2017,Jan,8; 2016,Jan,13; 2015,Jan,16

77078 Computed tomography, bone mineral density study, 1 or more sites, axial skeleton (eg, hips, pelvis, spine)
 3.24 3.24 FUD XXX S Z2 80
 AMA: 2018,Jan,8; 2017,Jan,8; 2016,Jan,13; 2015,Jan,16

77080 Dual-energy X-ray absorptiometry (DXA), bone density study, 1 or more sites; axial skeleton (eg, hips, pelvis, spine)
 EXCLUDES *Dual-energy x-ray absorptiometry (DXA), bone density study ([77085])*
 Vertebral fracture assessment via dual-energy x-ray absorptiometry (DXA) ([77086])
 1.13 1.13 FUD XXX S Z3 80
 AMA: 2018,Jan,8; 2017,Jan,8; 2016,Jan,13; 2015,Jan,16

77081 appendicular skeleton (peripheral) (eg, radius, wrist, heel)
 0.91 0.91 FUD XXX S Z3 80
 AMA: 2018,Jan,8; 2017,Jan,8; 2016,Jan,13; 2015,Jan,16

77085 axial skeleton (eg, hips, pelvis, spine), including vertebral fracture assessment
 EXCLUDES *Dual-energy x-ray absorptiometry (DXA), bone density study (77080)*
 Vertebral fracture assessment via dual-energy x-ray absorptiometry (DXA) ([77086])
 1.54 1.54 FUD XXX Q1 N1 80

77086 Vertebral fracture assessment via dual-energy X-ray absorptiometry (DXA)
 EXCLUDES *Dual-energy x-ray absorptiometry (DXA), bone density study (77080)*
 Therapy performed more than one time for treatment to specific area
 Vertebral fracture assessment via dual-energy X-ray absorptiometry (DXA) ([77085])
 0.99 0.99 FUD XXX Q1 N1 80

77084 Magnetic resonance (eg, proton) imaging, bone marrow blood supply
 10.7 10.7 FUD XXX S Z2 80
 AMA: 2018,Jan,8; 2017,Jan,8; 2016,Jan,13; 2015,Jan,16

77085 **Resequenced code. See code following 77081.**

77086 **Resequenced code. See code before 77084.**

77261-77263 Therapeutic Radiology: Treatment Planning

INCLUDES Determination:
 Appropriate treatment devices
 Number and size treatment ports
 Treatment method
 Treatment time/dosage
 Treatment volume
 Interpretation special testing
 Tumor localization
EXCLUDES *Brachytherapy (0394T-0395T)*
 Radiation treatment delivery, superficial (77401)

77261 Therapeutic radiology treatment planning; simple
 INCLUDES Planning for single treatment area included in single port or simple parallel opposed ports with simple or no blocking
 2.03 2.03 FUD XXX B 80 26
 AMA: 2018,Jan,8; 2017,Jan,8; 2016,Feb,3; 2016,Jan,13; 2015,Jan,16

77262 intermediate
 INCLUDES Planning for three or more converging ports, two separate treatment sites, multiple blocks, or special time dose constraints
 3.06 3.06 FUD XXX B 80 26
 AMA: 2018,Jan,8; 2017,Jan,8; 2016,Feb,3; 2016,Jan,13; 2015,Jan,16

77263 complex
 INCLUDES Planning for very complex blocking, custom shielding blocks, tangential ports, special wedges or compensators, three or more separate treatment areas, rotational or special beam considerations, treatment modality combinations
 4.78 4.78 FUD XXX B 80 26
 AMA: 2018,Jan,8; 2017,Jan,8; 2016,Feb,3; 2016,Jan,13; 2015,Jan,16

77280-77299 [77295] Radiation Therapy Simulation

77280 Therapeutic radiology simulation-aided field setting; simple
 INCLUDES Simulation single treatment site
 7.85 7.85 FUD XXX S Z2 80
 AMA: 2018,Jan,8; 2017,Jan,8; 2016,Jan,13; 2015,Apr,10; 2015,Jan,16

77285 intermediate
 INCLUDES Two different treatment sites
 12.9 12.9 FUD XXX S Z2 80
 AMA: 2018,Jan,8; 2017,Jan,8; 2016,Jan,13; 2015,Apr,10; 2015,Jan,16

77290 **complex**

INCLUDES Brachytherapy
Complex blocking
Contrast material
Custom shielding blocks
Hyperthermia probe verification
Rotation, arc or particle therapy
Simulation to ≥ 3 treatment sites

🚑 14.4   ⚖ 14.4   **FUD** XXX   S Z2 80 ▣

AMA: 2018,Jan,8; 2017,Jan,8; 2016,Sep,9; 2016,Jan,13; 2015,Apr,10; 2015,Jan,16

+ 77293 **Respiratory motion management simulation (List separately in addition to code for primary procedure)**

Code first (77295, 77301)

🚑 12.7   ⚖ 12.7   **FUD** ZZZ   N N1 80 ▣

AMA: 2018,Jan,8; 2017,Jan,8; 2016,Jan,13; 2015,Dec,16

77295 Resequenced code. See code before 77300.

77299 **Unlisted procedure, therapeutic radiology clinical treatment planning**

🚑 0.00   ⚖ 0.00   **FUD** XXX   S Z2 80 ▣

AMA: 2018,Jan,8; 2017,Jan,8; 2016,Jan,13; 2015,Jan,16

77295-77370 [77295] Radiation Physics Services

 # 77295 **3-dimensional radiotherapy plan, including dose-volume histograms**

🚑 13.9   ⚖ 13.9   **FUD** XXX   S Z3 80 ▣

AMA: 2018,Jan,8; 2017,Jan,8; 2016,Jan,13; 2015,Dec,16; 2015,Jun,6; 2015,Jan,16

77300 **Basic radiation dosimetry calculation, central axis depth dose calculation, TDF, NSD, gap calculation, off axis factor, tissue inhomogeneity factors, calculation of non-ionizing radiation surface and depth dose, as required during course of treatment, only when prescribed by the treating physician**

EXCLUDES Brachytherapy (77316-77318, 77767-77772, 0394T-0395T)
Teletherapy plan (77306-77307, 77321)

🚑 1.88   ⚖ 1.88   **FUD** XXX   S Z3 80 ▣

AMA: 2018,Jan,8; 2017,Jan,8; 2016,Jan,13; 2015,Jan,16

77301 **Intensity modulated radiotherapy plan, including dose-volume histograms for target and critical structure partial tolerance specifications**

🚑 55.0   ⚖ 55.0   **FUD** XXX   S Z2 80 ▣

AMA: 2018,Jan,8; 2017,Jan,8; 2016,Jan,13; 2015,Jan,16

77306 **Teletherapy isodose plan; simple (1 or 2 unmodified ports directed to a single area of interest), includes basic dosimetry calculation(s)**

EXCLUDES Brachytherapy (0394T-0395T)
Radiation dosimetry calculation (77300)
Radiation treatment delivery (77401)
Therapy performed more than one time for treatment to specific area

🚑 4.25   ⚖ 4.25   **FUD** XXX   S Z3 80 ▣

AMA: 2018,Jan,8; 2017,Jan,8; 2016,Feb,3

77307 **complex (multiple treatment areas, tangential ports, the use of wedges, blocking, rotational beam, or special beam considerations), includes basic dosimetry calculation(s)**

EXCLUDES Brachytherapy (0394T-0395T)
Radiation dosimetry calculation (77300)
Radiation treatment delivery (77401)
Therapy performed more than one time for treatment to specific area

🚑 8.20   ⚖ 8.20   **FUD** XXX   S Z3 80 ▣

AMA: 2018,Jan,8; 2017,Jan,8; 2016,Feb,3

77316 **Brachytherapy isodose plan; simple (calculation[s] made from 1 to 4 sources, or remote afterloading brachytherapy, 1 channel), includes basic dosimetry calculation(s)**

EXCLUDES Brachytherapy (0394T-0395T)
Radiation dosimetry calculation (77300)
Radiation treatment delivery (77401)

🚑 6.17   ⚖ 6.17   **FUD** XXX   S Z3 80 ▣

AMA: 2018,Jan,8; 2017,Jan,8; 2016,Feb,3

77317 **intermediate (calculation[s] made from 5 to 10 sources, or remote afterloading brachytherapy, 2-12 channels), includes basic dosimetry calculation(s)**

EXCLUDES Brachytherapy (0394T-0395T)
Radiation dosimetry calculation (77300)
Radiation treatment delivery (77401)

🚑 8.09   ⚖ 8.09   **FUD** XXX   S Z2 80 ▣

AMA: 2018,Jan,8; 2017,Jan,8

77318 **complex (calculation[s] made from over 10 sources, or remote afterloading brachytherapy, over 12 channels), includes basic dosimetry calculation(s)**

EXCLUDES Brachytherapy (0394T-0395T)
Radiation dosimetry calculation (77300)
Radiation treatment delivery (77401)

🚑 11.5   ⚖ 11.5   **FUD** XXX   S Z2 80 ▣

AMA: 2018,Jan,8; 2017,Jan,8; 2016,Feb,3

77321 **Special teletherapy port plan, particles, hemibody, total body**

🚑 2.68   ⚖ 2.68   **FUD** XXX   S Z3 80 ▣

AMA: 2018,Jan,8; 2017,Jan,8; 2016,Jan,13; 2015,Jan,16

77331 **Special dosimetry (eg, TLD, microdosimetry) (specify), only when prescribed by the treating physician**

🚑 1.84   ⚖ 1.84   **FUD** XXX   S Z3 80 ▣

AMA: 2018,Jan,8; 2017,Jan,8; 2016,Jan,13; 2015,Jun,6; 2015,Jan,16

77332 **Treatment devices, design and construction; simple (simple block, simple bolus)**

EXCLUDES Brachytherapy (0394T-0395T)
Radiation treatment delivery (77401)

🚑 1.49   ⚖ 1.49   **FUD** XXX   S Z3 80 ▣

AMA: 2018,Jan,8; 2017,Jan,8; 2016,Feb,3; 2016,Jan,13; 2015,Jan,16

77333 **intermediate (multiple blocks, stents, bite blocks, special bolus)**

EXCLUDES Brachytherapy (0394T-0395T)
Radiation treatment delivery (77401)

🚑 3.10   ⚖ 3.10   **FUD** XXX   S Z2 80 ▣

AMA: 2018,Jan,8; 2017,Jan,8; 2016,Feb,3; 2016,Jan,13; 2015,Jan,16

77334 **complex (irregular blocks, special shields, compensators, wedges, molds or casts)**

EXCLUDES Brachytherapy (0394T-0395T)
Radiation treatment delivery (77401)

🚑 3.61   ⚖ 3.61   **FUD** XXX   S Z3 80 ▣

AMA: 2018,Jan,8; 2017,Jan,8; 2016,Sep,9; 2016,Feb,3; 2016,Jan,13; 2015,Dec,16; 2015,Jan,16

77336 **Continuing medical physics consultation, including assessment of treatment parameters, quality assurance of dose delivery, and review of patient treatment documentation in support of the radiation oncologist, reported per week of therapy**

EXCLUDES Brachytherapy (0394T-0395T)
Radiation treatment delivery (77401)

🚑 2.26   ⚖ 2.26   **FUD** XXX   S Z2 80 TC ▣

AMA: 2018,Jan,8; 2017,Jan,8; 2016,Feb,3; 2016,Jan,13; 2015,Jan,16

● New Code   ▲ Revised Code   ○ Reinstated   ● New Web Release   ▲ Revised Web Release   + Add-on   Unlisted   Not Covered   # Resequenced
50 Optum Mod 50 Exempt   ⊘ AMA Mod 51 Exempt   51 Optum Mod 51 Exempt   63 Mod 63 Exempt   ✓ Non-FDA Drug   ★ Telemedicine   M Maternity   A Age Edit

77338 **Multi-leaf collimator (MLC) device(s) for intensity modulated radiation therapy (IMRT), design and construction per IMRT plan**

EXCLUDES *Immobilization in IMRT treatment (77332-77334)*
Intensity modulated radiation treatment delivery (IMRT) (77385)
Reporting code more than one time per IMRT plan

13.7 13.7 FUD XXX S Z2 80

AMA: 2018,Jan,8; 2017,Jan,8; 2016,Jan,13; 2015,Jan,16

77370 **Special medical radiation physics consultation**

3.52 3.52 FUD XXX S Z2 80 TC

AMA: 2018,Jan,8; 2017,Jan,8; 2016,Feb,3; 2016,Jan,13; 2015,Jun,6; 2015,Jan,16

77371-77399 [77385, 77386, 77387] Stereotactic Radiosurgery (SRS) Planning and Delivery

77371 **Radiation treatment delivery, stereotactic radiosurgery (SRS), complete course of treatment of cranial lesion(s) consisting of 1 session; multi-source Cobalt 60 based**

EXCLUDES *Guidance with computed tomography for radiation therapy field placement (77014)*

0.00 0.00 FUD XXX J 80 TC

AMA: 2018,Jan,8; 2017,Jan,8; 2016,Jan,13; 2015,Jan,16

77372 **linear accelerator based**

EXCLUDES *Guidance with computed tomography for radiation therapy field placement (77014)*
Radiation treatment supervision (77432)

30.2 30.2 FUD XXX J 80 TC

AMA: 2018,Jan,8; 2017,Jan,8; 2016,Jan,13; 2015,Jan,16

77373 **Stereotactic body radiation therapy, treatment delivery, per fraction to 1 or more lesions, including image guidance, entire course not to exceed 5 fractions**

EXCLUDES *Guidance with computed tomography for radiation therapy field placement (77014)*
Intensity modulated radiation treatment delivery (IMRT) (77385-77386)
Radiation treatment delivery (77401-77402, 77407, 77412)
Single fraction cranial lesion(s) (77371-77372)

36.6 36.6 FUD XXX S 80 TC

AMA: 2018,Jan,8; 2017,Jan,8; 2016,Jan,13; 2015,Jun,6; 2015,Jan,16

77385 **Resequenced code. See code following 77417.**

77386 **Resequenced code. See code following 77417.**

77387 **Resequenced code. See code following 77417.**

77399 **Unlisted procedure, medical radiation physics, dosimetry and treatment devices, and special services**

0.00 0.00 FUD XXX S Z2 80

AMA: 2018,Jan,8; 2017,Jan,8; 2016,Jan,13; 2015,Jan,16

77401-77425 [77385, 77386, 77387, 77424, 77425] Radiation Treatment

INCLUDES Technical component and assorted energy levels

77401 **Radiation treatment delivery, superficial and/or ortho voltage, per day**

EXCLUDES *Continuing medical physics consultation (77336)*
Isodose plan:
Brachytherapy (77316-77318)
Teletherapy (77306-77307)
Management:
Intraoperative radiation treatment (77469-77470)
Radiation therapy (77431-77432)
Radiation treatment (77427)
Stereotactic body radiation therapy (77435)
Stereotactic body radiation therapy, treatment delivery (77373)
Unlisted procedure, therapeutic radiology treatment management (77499)
Therapeutic radiology treatment planning (77261-77263)
Treatment devices, design and construction (77332-77334)

Code also E/M services when performed alone, as appropriate

0.70 0.70 FUD XXX S Z3 80 TC

AMA: 2018,Jan,8; 2017,Jan,8; 2016,Feb,3; 2016,Jan,13; 2015,Dec,14; 2015,Jan,16

77402 **Radiation treatment delivery, ≥1 MeV; simple**

EXCLUDES *Stereotactic body radiation therapy, treatment delivery (77373)*

0.00 0.00 FUD XXX S Z2 80 TC

AMA: 2018,Jan,8; 2017,Jan,8; 2016,Jun,9; 2016,Mar,7; 2016,Feb,3; 2016,Jan,13; 2015,Dec,14; 2015,Jan,16

77407 **intermediate**

EXCLUDES *Stereotactic body radiation therapy, treatment delivery (77373)*

0.00 0.00 FUD XXX S Z2 80 TC

AMA: 2018,Jan,8; 2017,Jan,8; 2016,Jun,9; 2016,Mar,7; 2016,Feb,3; 2016,Jan,13; 2015,Dec,14; 2015,Jan,16

77412 **complex**

0.00 0.00 FUD XXX S Z2 80 TC

AMA: 2018,Jan,8; 2017,Jan,8; 2016,Jun,9; 2016,Mar,7; 2016,Feb,3; 2016,Jan,13; 2015,Dec,14; 2015,Jan,16

77417 **Therapeutic radiology port image(s)**

0.32 0.32 FUD XXX N N1 80 TC

AMA: 2018,Jan,8; 2017,Dec,14; 2017,Jan,8; 2016,Jan,13; 2015,Dec,14; 2015,Jan,16

77385 **Intensity modulated radiation treatment delivery (IMRT), includes guidance and tracking, when performed; simple**

0.00 0.00 FUD XXX S Z2 80 TC

AMA: 2018,Jan,8; 2017,Jan,8; 2016,Feb,3

77386 **complex**

0.00 0.00 FUD XXX S Z2 80 TC

AMA: 2018,Jan,8; 2017,Jan,8; 2016,Feb,3

77387 **Guidance for localization of target volume for delivery of radiation treatment, includes intrafraction tracking, when performed**

0.00 0.00 FUD XXX N N1 80

AMA: 2018,Jan,8; 2017,Jan,8; 2016,Feb,3; 2016,Jan,13; 2015,Dec,16; 2015,Dec,14

77424 **Intraoperative radiation treatment delivery, x-ray, single treatment session**

0.00 0.00 FUD XXX J Z2

AMA: 2018,Jan,8; 2017,Jan,8; 2016,Jan,13; 2015,Dec,14

77425 **Intraoperative radiation treatment delivery, electrons, single treatment session**

0.00 0.00 FUD XXX J Z2

AMA: 2018,Jan,8; 2017,Jan,8; 2016,Jan,13; 2015,Dec,14; 2015,Jan,16

77423-77425 [77424, 77425] Neutron Therapy

77423 **High energy neutron radiation treatment delivery, 1 or more isocenter(s) with coplanar or non-coplanar geometry with blocking and/or wedge, and/or compensator(s)**
 0.00   0.00   **FUD** XXX   S Z3 80 TC ☐
AMA: 2018,Jan,8; 2017,Jan,8; 2016,Jan,13; 2015,Dec,14; 2015,Jan,16

77424 Resequenced code. See code following 77417.

77425 Resequenced code. See code following 77417.

77427-77499 Radiation Therapy Management

INCLUDES Assessment patient for medical evaluation and management (at least one per treatment management service) including:
  Coordination care/treatment
  Evaluation patient's response to treatment
  Review:
    Dose delivery
    Dosimetry
    Lab tests
    Patient treatment set-up
    Port film
    Treatment parameters
    X-rays
  Five fractions or treatment sessions regardless of time. Two or more fractions performed same day can be reported separately provided a distinct break in service exists between sessions and fractions are usually furnished on different days
EXCLUDES High dose rate electronic brachytherapy (0394T-0395T)
Radiation treatment delivery (77401)

77427 **Radiation treatment management, 5 treatments**
 5.37   5.37   **FUD** XXX   B 26 ☐
AMA: 2018,Jan,8; 2017,Jan,8; 2016,Feb,3; 2016,Jan,13; 2015,Jun,6; 2015,Jan,16

77431 **Radiation therapy management with complete course of therapy consisting of 1 or 2 fractions only**
 2.96   2.96   **FUD** XXX   B 80 26 ☐
AMA: 2018,Jan,8; 2017,Jan,8; 2016,Feb,3; 2016,Jan,13; 2015,Jun,6; 2015,Jan,16

77432 **Stereotactic radiation treatment management of cranial lesion(s) (complete course of treatment consisting of 1 session)**
 12.0   12.0   **FUD** XXX   B 80 26 ☐
AMA: 2018,Jan,8; 2017,Jan,8; 2016,Feb,3; 2016,Jan,13; 2015,Dec,14; 2015,Dec,16; 2015,Jun,6; 2015,Jan,16

77435 **Stereotactic body radiation therapy, treatment management, per treatment course, to 1 or more lesions, including image guidance, entire course not to exceed 5 fractions**
 18.1   18.1   **FUD** XXX   N N1 80 26 ☐
AMA: 2018,Jan,8; 2017,Jan,8; 2016,Feb,3; 2016,Jan,13; 2015,Dec,14; 2015,Jun,6; 2015,Jan,16

77469 **Intraoperative radiation treatment management**
 9.00   9.00   **FUD** XXX   B 80 ☐
AMA: 2018,Jan,8; 2017,Jan,8; 2016,Feb,3; 2015,Jun,6

77470 **Special treatment procedure (eg, total body irradiation, hemibody radiation, per oral or endocavitary irradiation)**
 3.75   3.75   **FUD** XXX   S Z3 80 ☐
AMA: 2018,Jan,8; 2017,Jan,8; 2016,Feb,3; 2016,Jan,13; 2015,Jun,6; 2015,Jan,16

77499 **Unlisted procedure, therapeutic radiology treatment management**
 0.00   0.00   **FUD** XXX   B 80 ☐
AMA: 2018,Jan,8; 2017,Jan,8; 2016,Feb,3; 2016,Jan,13; 2015,Jun,6; 2015,Jan,16

77520-77525 Proton Therapy

EXCLUDES High dose rate electronic brachytherapy, per fraction (0394T-0395T)

77520 **Proton treatment delivery; simple, without compensation**
 0.00   0.00   **FUD** XXX   S Z2 80 TC ☐
AMA: 2018,Jan,8; 2017,Jan,8; 2016,Jan,13; 2015,Jan,16

77522 **simple, with compensation**
 0.00   0.00   **FUD** XXX   S Z2 80 TC ☐
AMA: 2012,Feb,9-10; 2010,Oct,3-4

77523 **intermediate**
 0.00   0.00   **FUD** XXX   S Z2 80 TC ☐
AMA: 2018,Jan,8; 2017,Jan,8; 2016,Jan,13; 2015,Jan,16

77525 **complex**
 0.00   0.00   **FUD** XXX   S Z2 80 TC ☐
AMA: 2012,Feb,9-10; 2010,Oct,3-4

77600-77620 Hyperthermia Treatment

CMS: 100-03,110.1 Hyperthermia for Treatment of Cancer
INCLUDES Heat generating devices
Interstitial insertion temperature sensors
Management during course therapy
Normal follow-up care for three months after completion
Physics planning
EXCLUDES Initial E/M service
Radiation therapy treatment (77371-77373, 77401-77412, 77423)

77600 **Hyperthermia, externally generated; superficial (ie, heating to a depth of 4 cm or less)**
 13.1   13.1   **FUD** XXX   S Z2 80 ☐
AMA: 2018,Jan,8; 2017,Jan,8; 2016,Jan,13; 2015,Jan,16

77605 **deep (ie, heating to depths greater than 4 cm)**
 24.0   24.0   **FUD** XXX   S Z2 80 ☐
AMA: 2018,Jan,8; 2017,Jan,8; 2016,Jan,13; 2015,Jan,16

77610 **Hyperthermia generated by interstitial probe(s); 5 or fewer interstitial applicators**
 19.2   19.2   **FUD** XXX   S Z2 80 ☐
AMA: 2018,Jan,8; 2017,Jan,8; 2016,Jan,13; 2015,Jan,16

77615 **more than 5 interstitial applicators**
 30.0   30.0   **FUD** XXX   S Z2 80 ☐
AMA: 2018,Jan,8; 2017,Jan,8; 2016,Jan,13; 2015,Jan,16

77620 **Hyperthermia generated by intracavitary probe(s)**
 14.6   14.6   **FUD** XXX   S Z2 80 ☐
AMA: 2018,Jan,8; 2017,Jan,8; 2016,Jan,13; 2015,Jan,16

77750-77799 Brachytherapy

CMS: 100-04,13,70.4 Clinical Brachytherapy; 100-04,13,70.5 Radiation Physics Services; 100-04,4,61.4.4 Billing for Brachytherapy Source Supervision, Handling and Loading Costs
INCLUDES Hospital admission and daily visits
EXCLUDES Placement:
  Heyman capsules (58346)
  Ovoids and tandems (57155)

77750 **Infusion or instillation of radioelement solution (includes 3-month follow-up care)**
 10.7   10.7   **FUD** 090   S Z2 80 ☐
AMA: 2018,Jan,8; 2017,Jan,8; 2016,Jan,13; 2015,Jan,16

77761 **Intracavitary radiation source application; simple**
 11.4   11.4   **FUD** 090   S Z3 80 ☐
AMA: 2018,Jan,8; 2017,Jan,8; 2016,Jan,13; 2015,Jan,16

77762 **intermediate**
 15.0   15.0   **FUD** 090   S Z3 80 ☐
AMA: 2018,Jan,8; 2017,Jan,8; 2016,Jan,13; 2015,Jan,16

77763 **complex**
 21.4   21.4   **FUD** 090   S Z3 80 ☐
AMA: 2018,Jan,8; 2017,Jan,8; 2016,Jan,13; 2015,Jan,16

77767 **Remote afterloading high dose rate radionuclide skin surface brachytherapy, includes basic dosimetry, when performed; lesion diameter up to 2.0 cm or 1 channel**
 6.78   6.78   **FUD** XXX   S Z2 80 ☐

77768 **lesion diameter over 2.0 cm and 2 or more channels, or multiple lesions**
 10.1   10.1   **FUD** XXX   S Z2 80 ☐

77770 **Remote afterloading high dose rate radionuclide interstitial or intracavitary brachytherapy, includes basic dosimetry, when performed; 1 channel**
 9.51   9.51   **FUD** XXX   S Z3 80 ☐

● New Code   ▲ Revised Code   ○ Reinstated   ● New Web Release   ▲ Revised Web Release   + Add-on   Unlisted   Not Covered   # Resequenced
50 Optum Mod 50 Exempt   ⊘ AMA Mod 51 Exempt   51 Optum Mod 51 Exempt   63 Mod 63 Exempt   ✗ Non-FDA Drug   ★ Telemedicine   M Maternity   A Age Edit

77771 **2-12 channels**
16.9 | 16.9 | FUD XXX | S Z2 80

77772 **over 12 channels**
25.5 | 25.5 | FUD XXX | S Z2 80

77778 **Interstitial radiation source application, complex, includes supervision, handling, loading of radiation source, when performed**
24.0 | 24.0 | FUD 000 | S Z2 80
AMA: 2018,Jan,8; 2017,Jan,8; 2016,Jan,13; 2015,Jan,16

77789 **Surface application of low dose rate radionuclide source**
3.49 | 3.49 | FUD 000 | S Z2 80
AMA: 2018,Jan,8; 2017,Jan,8; 2016,Jan,13; 2015,Jan,16

77790 **Supervision, handling, loading of radiation source**
0.43 | 0.43 | FUD XXX | N N1 80 TC
AMA: 2018,Jan,8; 2017,Jan,8; 2016,Jan,13; 2015,Jan,16

77799 **Unlisted procedure, clinical brachytherapy**
0.00 | 0.00 | FUD XXX | S Z2 80
AMA: 2018,Jan,8; 2017,Jan,8; 2016,Jan,13; 2015,Jan,16

78012-78099 Nuclear Radiology: Thyroid, Parathyroid, Adrenal

EXCLUDES *Diagnostic services (see appropriate sections)*
Follow-up care (see appropriate section)
Code also radiopharmaceutical(s) and/or drug(s) supplied

78012 **Thyroid uptake, single or multiple quantitative measurement(s) (including stimulation, suppression, or discharge, when performed)**
2.34 | 2.34 | FUD XXX | S Z2 80
AMA: 2018,Jan,8; 2017,Jan,8; 2016,Jan,13; 2015,Jan,16

78013 **Thyroid imaging (including vascular flow, when performed);**
5.54 | 5.54 | FUD XXX | S Z2 80
AMA: 2018,Jan,8; 2017,Jan,8; 2016,Jan,13; 2015,Jan,16

78014 **with single or multiple uptake(s) quantitative measurement(s) (including stimulation, suppression, or discharge, when performed)**
6.95 | 6.95 | FUD XXX | S Z2 80
AMA: 2018,Jan,8; 2017,Jan,8; 2016,Jan,13; 2015,Jan,16

78015 **Thyroid carcinoma metastases imaging; limited area (eg, neck and chest only)**
6.47 | 6.47 | FUD XXX | S Z2 80
AMA: 2018,Jan,8; 2017,Jan,8; 2016,Jan,13; 2015,Jan,16

78016 **with additional studies (eg, urinary recovery)**
8.08 | 8.08 | FUD XXX | S Z2 80
AMA: 2018,Jan,8; 2017,Jan,8; 2016,Jan,13; 2015,Jan,16

78018 **whole body**
8.96 | 8.96 | FUD XXX | S Z2 80
AMA: 2018,Jan,8; 2017,Jan,8; 2016,Jan,13; 2015,Jan,16

+ **78020** **Thyroid carcinoma metastases uptake (List separately in addition to code for primary procedure)**
2.41 | 2.41 | FUD ZZZ | N N1 80
AMA: 2018,Jan,8; 2017,Jan,8; 2016,Jan,13; 2015,Jan,16

78070 **Parathyroid planar imaging (including subtraction, when performed);**
EXCLUDES *Distribution radiopharmaceutical agents or tumor localization (78800-78802, [78804], 78803)*
Radiopharmaceutical quantification measurements ([78835])
SPECT with concurrently acquired CT transmission scan ([78830, 78831, 78832])
8.48 | 8.48 | FUD XXX | S Z2 80
AMA: 2018,Jan,8; 2017,Jan,8; 2016,Dec,9; 2016,Dec,16; 2016,Jan,13; 2015,Jan,16

78071 **with tomographic (SPECT)**
EXCLUDES *Distribution radiopharmaceutical agents or tumor localization (78800-78802, [78804], 78803)*
Radiopharmaceutical quantification measurements ([78835])
SPECT with concurrently acquired CT transmission scan ([78830, 78831, 78832])
10.1 | 10.1 | FUD XXX | S Z2 80
AMA: 2018,Jan,8; 2017,Jan,8; 2016,Dec,16; 2016,Dec,9

78072 **with tomographic (SPECT), and concurrently acquired computed tomography (CT) for anatomical localization**
EXCLUDES *Distribution radiopharmaceutical agents or tumor localization (78800-78802, [78804], 78803)*
Radiopharmaceutical quantification measurements ([78835])
SPECT with concurrently acquired CT transmission scan ([78830, 78831, 78832])
11.2 | 11.2 | FUD XXX | S Z2 80
AMA: 2018,Jan,8; 2017,Jan,8; 2016,Dec,16; 2016,Dec,9

78075 **Adrenal imaging, cortex and/or medulla**
13.0 | 13.0 | FUD XXX | S Z2 80
AMA: 2018,Jan,8; 2017,Jan,8; 2016,Jan,13; 2015,Jan,16

78099 **Unlisted endocrine procedure, diagnostic nuclear medicine**
0.00 | 0.00 | FUD XXX | S Z2 80
AMA: 2018,Jan,8; 2017,Jan,8; 2016,Dec,9; 2016,Jan,13; 2015,Jan,16

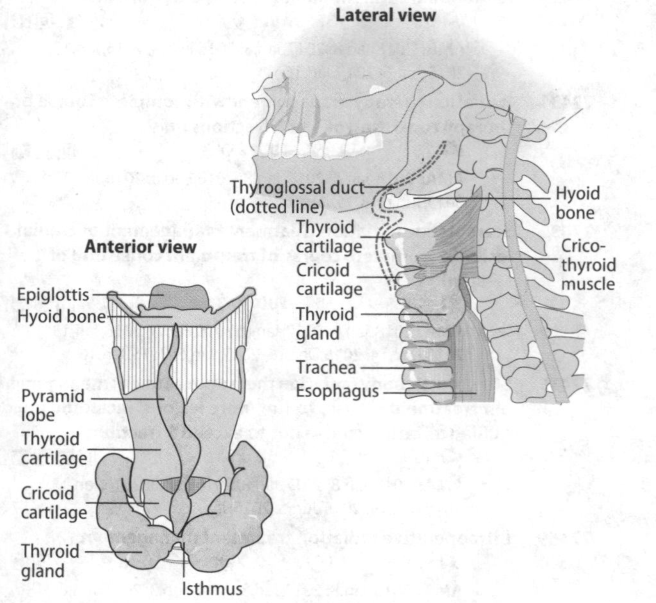

78102-78199 Nuclear Radiology: Blood Forming Organs

EXCLUDES *Diagnostic services (see appropriate sections)*
Follow-up care (see appropriate section)
Radioimmunoassays (82009-84999 [82042, 82652])
Code also radiopharmaceutical(s) and/or drug(s) supplied

78102 **Bone marrow imaging; limited area**
4.89 | 4.89 | FUD XXX | S Z2 80
AMA: 2018,Jan,8; 2017,Jan,8; 2016,Jan,13; 2015,Jan,16

78103 **multiple areas**
6.20 | 6.20 | FUD XXX | S Z2 80
AMA: 2012,Feb,9-10; 2007,Jan,28-31

78104 **whole body**
7.14 | 7.14 | FUD XXX | S Z2 80
AMA: 2012,Feb,9-10; 2007,Jan,28-31

78110 **Plasma volume, radiopharmaceutical volume-dilution technique (separate procedure); single sampling**
1.99 1.99 **FUD** XXX S Z2 80
AMA: 2012,Feb,9-10; 2007,Jan,28-31

78111 **multiple samplings**
2.11 2.11 **FUD** XXX S Z2 80
AMA: 2012,Feb,9-10; 2007,Jan,28-31

78120 **Red cell volume determination (separate procedure); single sampling**
2.04 2.04 **FUD** XXX S Z2 80
AMA: 2012,Feb,9-10; 2007,Jan,28-31

78121 **multiple samplings**
2.23 2.23 **FUD** XXX S Z2 80
AMA: 2012,Feb,9-10; 2007,Jan,28-31

78122 **Whole blood volume determination, including separate measurement of plasma volume and red cell volume (radiopharmaceutical volume-dilution technique)**
2.75 2.75 **FUD** XXX S Z2 80
AMA: 2012,Feb,9-10; 2007,Jan,28-31

▲ **78130** **Red cell survival study**
3.59 3.59 **FUD** XXX S Z2 80
AMA: 2012,Feb,9-10; 2007,Jan,28-31

~~**78135** **differential organ/tissue kinetics (eg, splenic and/or hepatic sequestration)**~~

78140 **Labeled red cell sequestration, differential organ/tissue (eg, splenic and/or hepatic)**
3.19 3.19 **FUD** XXX S Z2 80
AMA: 2012,Feb,9-10; 2007,Jan,28-31

78185 **Spleen imaging only, with or without vascular flow**
EXCLUDES *Liver imaging (78215-78216)*
4.87 4.87 **FUD** XXX S Z2 80
AMA: 2012,Feb,9-10; 2007,Jan,28-31

78191 **Platelet survival study**
3.56 3.56 **FUD** XXX S Z2 80
AMA: 2012,Feb,9-10; 2007,Jan,28-31

78195 **Lymphatics and lymph nodes imaging**
EXCLUDES *Sentinel node identification without scintigraphy (38792)*
Sentinel node removal (38500-38542)
10.2 10.2 **FUD** XXX S Z2 80
AMA: 2018,Jan,8; 2017,Jan,8; 2016,Jan,13; 2015,Jan,16

78199 **Unlisted hematopoietic, reticuloendothelial and lymphatic procedure, diagnostic nuclear medicine**
0.00 0.00 **FUD** XXX S Z2 80
AMA: 2018,Jan,8; 2017,Jan,8; 2016,Jan,13; 2015,Jan,16

78201-78299 Nuclear Radiology: Digestive System

EXCLUDES *Diagnostic services (see appropriate sections)*
Follow-up care (see appropriate section)
Code also radiopharmaceutical(s) and/or drug(s) supplied

78201 **Liver imaging; static only**
EXCLUDES *Spleen imaging only (78185)*
5.49 5.49 **FUD** XXX S Z2 80
AMA: 2018,Jan,8; 2017,Jan,8; 2016,Jan,13; 2015,Jan,16

78202 **with vascular flow**
EXCLUDES *Spleen imaging only (78185)*
5.82 5.82 **FUD** XXX S Z2 80
AMA: 2012,Feb,9-10; 2007,Jan,28-31

78215 **Liver and spleen imaging; static only**
5.59 5.59 **FUD** XXX S Z2 80
AMA: 2012,Feb,9-10; 2007,Jan,28-31

78216 **with vascular flow**
3.68 3.68 **FUD** XXX S Z2 80
AMA: 2012,Feb,9-10; 2007,Jan,28-31

78226 **Hepatobiliary system imaging, including gallbladder when present;**
9.38 9.38 **FUD** XXX S Z2 80
AMA: 2012,Feb,9-10

78227 **with pharmacologic intervention, including quantitative measurement(s) when performed**
12.8 12.8 **FUD** XXX S Z2 80
AMA: 2012,Feb,9-10

78230 **Salivary gland imaging;**
4.99 4.99 **FUD** XXX S Z2 80
AMA: 2012,Feb,9-10; 2007,Jan,28-31

78231 **with serial images**
2.98 2.98 **FUD** XXX S Z2 80
AMA: 2012,Feb,9-10; 2007,Jan,28-31

78232 **Salivary gland function study**
2.96 2.96 **FUD** XXX S Z2 80
AMA: 2012,Feb,9-10; 2007,Jan,28-31

78258 **Esophageal motility**
6.19 6.19 **FUD** XXX S Z2 80
AMA: 2012,Feb,9-10; 2007,Jan,28-31

78261 **Gastric mucosa imaging**
5.83 5.83 **FUD** XXX S Z2 80
AMA: 2012,Feb,9-10; 2007,Jan,28-31

78262 **Gastroesophageal reflux study**
6.86 6.86 **FUD** XXX S Z2 80
AMA: 2018,Jan,8; 2017,Jan,8; 2016,Jan,13; 2015,Dec,11

78264 **Gastric emptying imaging study (eg, solid, liquid, or both);**
EXCLUDES *Procedure performed more than one time per study*
9.65 9.65 **FUD** XXX S Z2 80
AMA: 2018,Jan,8; 2017,Jan,8; 2016,Jan,13; 2015,Dec,11

78265 **with small bowel transit**
EXCLUDES *Procedure performed more than one time per study*
11.2 11.2 **FUD** XXX S Z2 80
AMA: 2018,Jan,8; 2017,Jan,8; 2015,Dec,11

78266 **with small bowel and colon transit, multiple days**
EXCLUDES *Procedure performed more than one time per study*
12.3 12.3 **FUD** XXX S Z2 80
AMA: 2018,Jan,8; 2017,Jan,8; 2015,Dec,11

78267 **Urea breath test, C-14 (isotopic); acquisition for analysis**
EXCLUDES *Breath hydrogen/methane test (91065)*
0.00 0.00 **FUD** XXX A
AMA: 2020,OctSE,1; 2018,Jan,8; 2017,Jan,8; 2016,Jan,13; 2015,Jan,16

78268 **analysis**
EXCLUDES *Breath hydrogen/methane test (91065)*
0.00 0.00 **FUD** XXX A
AMA: 2020,OctSE,1; 2018,Jan,8; 2017,Jan,8; 2016,Jan,13; 2015,Jan,16

78278 **Acute gastrointestinal blood loss imaging**
9.97 9.97 **FUD** XXX S Z2 80
AMA: 2012,Feb,9-10; 2007,Jan,28-31

78282 **Gastrointestinal protein loss**
0.00 0.00 **FUD** XXX S Z2 80
AMA: 2018,Jul,14

78290 **Intestine imaging (eg, ectopic gastric mucosa, Meckel's localization, volvulus)**
9.44 9.44 **FUD** XXX S Z2 80
AMA: 2012,Feb,9-10; 2007,Jan,28-31

78291 **Peritoneal-venous shunt patency test (eg, for LeVeen, Denver shunt)**
Code also (49427)
7.39 7.39 **FUD** XXX S Z2 80
AMA: 2012,Feb,9-10; 2007,Jan,28-31

78299 **Unlisted gastrointestinal procedure, diagnostic nuclear medicine**
0.00 0.00 FUD XXX S Z2 80
AMA: 2018,Jan,8; 2017,Jan,8; 2016,Jan,13; 2015,Jan,16

78300-78399 Nuclear Radiology: Bones and Joints

EXCLUDES *Diagnostic services (see appropriate sections)*
Follow-up care (see appropriate section)
Code also radiopharmaceutical(s) and/or drug(s) supplied

78300 **Bone and/or joint imaging; limited area**
6.56 6.56 FUD XXX S Z2 80
AMA: 2018,Jan,8; 2017,Jan,8; 2016,Jan,13; 2015,Jan,16

78305 **multiple areas**
7.95 7.95 FUD XXX S Z2 80
AMA: 2018,Jan,8; 2017,Jan,8; 2016,Jan,13; 2015,Jan,16

78306 **whole body**
8.62 8.62 FUD XXX S Z2 80
AMA: 2018,Jan,8; 2017,Jan,8; 2016,Jan,13; 2015,Jan,16

78315 **3 phase study**
9.98 9.98 FUD XXX S Z2 80
AMA: 2018,Jan,8; 2017,Jan,8; 2016,Jan,13; 2015,Jan,16

78350 **Bone density (bone mineral content) study, 1 or more sites; single photon absorptiometry**
0.91 0.91 FUD XXX E
AMA: 2012,Feb,9-10; 2007,Jan,28-31

78351 **dual photon absorptiometry, 1 or more sites**
0.44 0.44 FUD XXX E
AMA: 2012,Feb,9-10; 2007,Jan,28-31

78399 **Unlisted musculoskeletal procedure, diagnostic nuclear medicine**
0.00 0.00 FUD XXX S Z2 80
AMA: 2018,Jan,8; 2017,Jan,8; 2016,Jan,13; 2015,Jan,16

78414-78499 [78429, 78430, 78431, 78432, 78433, 78434] Nuclear Radiology: Heart and Vascular

EXCLUDES *Diagnostic services (see appropriate sections)*
Follow-up care (see appropriate section)
Code also radiopharmaceutical(s) and/or drug(s) supplied

78414 **Determination of central c-v hemodynamics (non-imaging) (eg, ejection fraction with probe technique) with or without pharmacologic intervention or exercise, single or multiple determinations**
0.00 0.00 FUD XXX S Z2 80
AMA: 2018,Jan,8; 2017,Jan,8; 2016,Jan,13; 2015,Jan,16

78428 **Cardiac shunt detection**
5.29 5.29 FUD XXX S Z2 80
AMA: 2018,Jan,8; 2017,Jan,8; 2016,Jan,13; 2015,Jan,16

78429 **Resequenced code. See code following 78459.**

78430 **Resequenced code. See code following 78491.**

78431 **Resequenced code. See code following 78492.**

78432 **Resequenced code. See code following 78492.**

78433 **Resequenced code. See code following 78492.**

78434 **Resequenced code. See code following 78492.**

78445 **Non-cardiac vascular flow imaging (ie, angiography, venography)**
5.38 5.38 FUD XXX S Z2 80
AMA: 2018,Jan,8; 2017,Jan,8; 2016,Jan,13; 2015,Jan,16

78451 **Myocardial perfusion imaging, tomographic (SPECT) (including attenuation correction, qualitative or quantitative wall motion, ejection fraction by first pass or gated technique, additional quantification, when performed); single study, at rest or stress (exercise or pharmacologic)**
EXCLUDES *Distribution radiopharmaceutical agents or tumor localization (78800-78802, [78804], 78803)*
Radiopharmaceutical quantification measurements ([78835])
SPECT with concurrently acquired CT transmission scan ([78830, 78831, 78832])
Code also stress testing when performed (93015-93018)
9.63 9.63 FUD XXX S Z2 80
AMA: 2020,Jul,5; 2018,Jan,8; 2017,Jan,8; 2016,Jan,13; 2015,Jan,16

78452 **multiple studies, at rest and/or stress (exercise or pharmacologic) and/or redistribution and/or rest reinjection**
EXCLUDES *Distribution radiopharmaceutical agents or tumor localization (78800-78802, [78804], 78803)*
Radiopharmaceutical quantification measurements ([78835])
SPECT with concurrently acquired CT transmission scan ([78830, 78831, 78832])
Code also stress testing when performed (93015-93018)
13.4 13.4 FUD XXX S Z2 80
AMA: 2020,Jul,5; 2018,Jan,8; 2017,Jan,8; 2016,Jan,13; 2015,Jan,16

78453 **Myocardial perfusion imaging, planar (including qualitative or quantitative wall motion, ejection fraction by first pass or gated technique, additional quantification, when performed); single study, at rest or stress (exercise or pharmacologic)**
Code also stress testing when performed (93015-93018)
8.66 8.66 FUD XXX S Z2 80
AMA: 2020,Jul,5; 2018,Jan,8; 2017,Jan,8; 2016,Jan,13; 2015,Jan,16

78454 **multiple studies, at rest and/or stress (exercise or pharmacologic) and/or redistribution and/or rest reinjection**
Code also stress testing when performed (93015-93018)
12.5 12.5 FUD XXX S Z2 80
AMA: 2020,Jul,5; 2018,Jan,8; 2017,Jan,8; 2016,Jan,13; 2015,Jan,16

78456 **Acute venous thrombosis imaging, peptide**
8.93 8.93 FUD XXX S Z2
AMA: 2018,Jan,8; 2017,Jan,8; 2016,Jan,13; 2015,Jan,16

78457 **Venous thrombosis imaging, venogram; unilateral**
5.52 5.52 FUD XXX S Z2 80
AMA: 2018,Jan,8; 2017,Jan,8; 2016,Jan,13; 2015,Jan,16

78458 **bilateral**
5.88 5.88 FUD XXX S Z2 80
AMA: 2018,Jan,8; 2017,Jan,8; 2016,Jan,13; 2015,Jan,16

78459 **Myocardial imaging, positron emission tomography (PET), metabolic evaluation study (including ventricular wall motion[s] and/or ejection fraction[s], when performed), single study;**
INCLUDES Examination CT transmission images for field of view anatomy review
EXCLUDES *CT coronary calcium scoring (75571)*
CT for other than attenuation correction/anatomical localization; report site-specific CT code with modifier 59
Myocardial perfusion studies (78491-78492)
0.00 0.00 FUD XXX S Z2 80
AMA: 2020,Jul,5; 2018,Jan,8; 2017,Jan,8; 2016,Jan,13; 2015,Jan,16

78429 with concurrently acquired computed tomography transmission scan

INCLUDES Examination CT transmission images for field of view anatomy review

EXCLUDES *CT coronary calcium scoring (75571)*

CT for other than attenuation correction/anatomical localization; report site-specific CT code with modifier 59

0.00 0.00 FUD XXX Z2 80

AMA: 2020,Jul,5

78466 Myocardial imaging, infarct avid, planar; qualitative or quantitative

5.72 5.72 FUD XXX S Z2 80

AMA: 2012,Feb,9-10; 2010,May,5-6

78468 with ejection fraction by first pass technique

5.88 5.88 FUD XXX S Z2 80

AMA: 2018,Jan,8; 2017,Jan,8; 2016,Jan,13; 2015,Jan,16

78469 tomographic SPECT with or without quantification

EXCLUDES *Distribution radiopharmaceutical agents or tumor localization (78800-78802, [78804], 78803)*

Myocardial sympathetic innervation imaging (0331T-0332T)

Radiopharmaceutical quantification measurements ([78835])

SPECT with concurrently acquired CT transmission scan ([78830, 78831, 78832])

6.39 6.39 FUD XXX S Z2 80

AMA: 2018,Nov,11; 2018,Jan,8; 2017,Jan,8; 2016,Jan,13; 2015,Jan,16

78472 Cardiac blood pool imaging, gated equilibrium; planar, single study at rest or stress (exercise and/or pharmacologic), wall motion study plus ejection fraction, with or without additional quantitative processing

EXCLUDES *Cardiac blood pool imaging (78481, 78483, 78494)*

Myocardial perfusion imaging (78451-78454)

Right ventricular ejection fraction by first pass technique (78496)

Code also stress testing when performed (93015-93018)

6.59 6.59 FUD XXX S Z2 80

AMA: 2018,Jan,8; 2017,Jan,8; 2016,Jan,13; 2015,Jan,16

78473 multiple studies, wall motion study plus ejection fraction, at rest and stress (exercise and/or pharmacologic), with or without additional quantification

EXCLUDES *Cardiac blood pool imaging (78481, 78483, 78494)*

Myocardial perfusion imaging (78451-78454)

Code also stress testing when performed (93015-93018)

8.32 8.32 FUD XXX S Z2 80

AMA: 2018,Jan,8; 2017,Jan,8; 2016,Jan,13; 2015,Jan,16

78481 Cardiac blood pool imaging (planar), first pass technique; single study, at rest or with stress (exercise and/or pharmacologic), wall motion study plus ejection fraction, with or without quantification

EXCLUDES *Myocardial perfusion imaging (78451-78454)*

Code also stress testing when performed (93015-93018)

5.03 5.03 FUD XXX S Z2 80

AMA: 2018,Jan,8; 2017,Jan,8; 2016,Jan,13; 2015,Jan,16

78483 multiple studies, at rest and with stress (exercise and/or pharmacologic), wall motion study plus ejection fraction, with or without quantification

EXCLUDES *Blood flow studies brain (78610)*

Myocardial perfusion imaging (78451-78454)

Code also stress testing when performed (93015-93018)

6.89 6.89 FUD XXX S Z2 80

AMA: 2018,Jan,8; 2017,Jan,8; 2016,Jan,13; 2015,Jan,16

78491 Myocardial imaging, positron emission tomography (PET), perfusion study (including ventricular wall motion[s] and/or ejection fraction[s], when performed); single study, at rest or stress (exercise or pharmacologic)

Code also stress testing when performed (93015-93018)

0.00 0.00 FUD XXX S Z2 80

AMA: 2020,Jul,5; 2018,Jan,8; 2017,Jan,8; 2016,Jan,13; 2015,Jan,16

 # 78430 single study, at rest or stress (exercise or pharmacologic), with concurrently acquired computed tomography transmission scan

INCLUDES Examination CT transmission images for field of view anatomy review

Code also stress testing when performed (93015-93018)

0.00 0.00 FUD XXX Z2 80

AMA: 2020,Jul,5

78492 multiple studies at rest and stress (exercise or pharmacologic)

Code also stress testing when performed (93015-93018)

0.00 0.00 FUD XXX S Z2 80

AMA: 2020,Jul,5; 2018,Jan,8; 2017,Jan,8; 2016,Jan,13; 2015,Jan,16

 # 78431 multiple studies at rest and stress (exercise or pharmacologic), with concurrently acquired computed tomography transmission scan

INCLUDES Examination CT transmission images for field of view anatomy review

Code also stress testing when performed (93015-93018)

2.62 2.62 FUD XXX Z2 80

AMA: 2020,Jul,5

 # 78432 Myocardial imaging, positron emission tomography (PET), combined perfusion with metabolic evaluation study (including ventricular wall motion[s] and/or ejection fraction[s], when performed), dual radiotracer (eg, myocardial viability);

Code also stress testing when performed (93015-93018)

0.00 0.00 FUD XXX Z2 80

AMA: 2020,Jul,5

 # 78433 with concurrently acquired computed tomography transmission scan

INCLUDES Examination CT transmission images for field of view anatomy review

EXCLUDES *CT for other than attenuation correction/anatomical localization; use site-specific CT code with modifier 59*

Code also stress testing when performed (93015-93018)

0.00 0.00 FUD XXX Z2 80

AMA: 2020,Jul,5

+ # 78434 Absolute quantitation of myocardial blood flow (AQMBF), positron emission tomography (PET), rest and pharmacologic stress (List separately in addition to code for primary procedure)

EXCLUDES *CT coronary calcium scoring (75571)*

Myocardial imaging by planar or SPECT (78451-78454)

Code first ([78431], 78492)

0.00 0.00 FUD ZZZ N1 80

AMA: 2020,Jul,5

78494 Cardiac blood pool imaging, gated equilibrium, SPECT, at rest, wall motion study plus ejection fraction, with or without quantitative processing

EXCLUDES *Distribution radiopharmaceutical agents or tumor localization (78800-78802, [78804], 78803)*

Radiopharmaceutical quantification measurements ([78835])

SPECT with concurrently acquired CT transmission scan ([78830, 78831, 78832])

6.51 6.51 FUD XXX S Z2 80

AMA: 2018,Jan,8; 2017,Jan,8; 2016,Jan,13; 2015,Jan,16

Radiology

78429 — 78494

+ **78496 Cardiac blood pool imaging, gated equilibrium, single study, at rest, with right ventricular ejection fraction by first pass technique (List separately in addition to code for primary procedure)**

Code first (78472)

1.25 1.25 FUD ZZZ N N1 80

AMA: 2018,Jan,8; 2017,Jan,8; 2016,Jan,13; 2015,Jan,16

78499 Unlisted cardiovascular procedure, diagnostic nuclear medicine

0.00 0.00 FUD XXX S Z2 80

AMA: 2018,Jan,8; 2017,Jan,8; 2016,Jan,13; 2015,Jan,16

78579-78599 Nuclear Radiology: Lungs

EXCLUDES *Diagnostic services (see appropriate sections)*
Follow-up care (see appropriate sections)

Code also radiopharmaceutical(s) and/or drug(s) supplied

78579 Pulmonary ventilation imaging (eg, aerosol or gas)

EXCLUDES *Procedure performed more than one time per imaging session*

5.36 5.36 FUD XXX S Z2 80

AMA: 2012,Feb,9-10

78580 Pulmonary perfusion imaging (eg, particulate)

EXCLUDES *Myocardial perfusion imaging (78451-78454)*
Procedure performed more than one time per imaging session

6.87 6.87 FUD XXX S Z2 80

AMA: 2018,Jan,8; 2017,Jan,8; 2016,Jan,13; 2015,Jan,16

78582 Pulmonary ventilation (eg, aerosol or gas) and perfusion imaging

EXCLUDES *Myocardial perfusion imaging (78451-78454)*
Procedure performed more than one time per imaging session

9.54 9.54 FUD XXX S Z2 80

AMA: 2012,Feb,9-10

78597 Quantitative differential pulmonary perfusion, including imaging when performed

EXCLUDES *Myocardial perfusion imaging (78451-78454)*
Procedure performed more than one time per imaging session

5.74 5.74 FUD XXX S Z2 80

AMA: 2012,Feb,9-10

78598 Quantitative differential pulmonary perfusion and ventilation (eg, aerosol or gas), including imaging when performed

EXCLUDES *Myocardial perfusion imaging (78451-78454)*
Procedure performed more than one time per imaging session

8.80 8.80 FUD XXX S Z2 80

AMA: 2012,Feb,9-10

78599 Unlisted respiratory procedure, diagnostic nuclear medicine

0.00 0.00 FUD XXX S Z2 80

AMA: 2018,Jan,8; 2017,Jan,8; 2016,Jan,13; 2015,Jan,16

78600-78650 Nuclear Radiology: Brain/Cerebrospinal Fluid

EXCLUDES *Diagnostic services (see appropriate sections)*
Follow-up care (see appropriate section)

Code also radiopharmaceutical(s) and/or drug(s) supplied

78600 Brain imaging, less than 4 static views;

5.32 5.32 FUD XXX S Z2 80

AMA: 2018,Jan,8; 2017,Jan,8; 2016,Jan,13; 2015,Jan,16

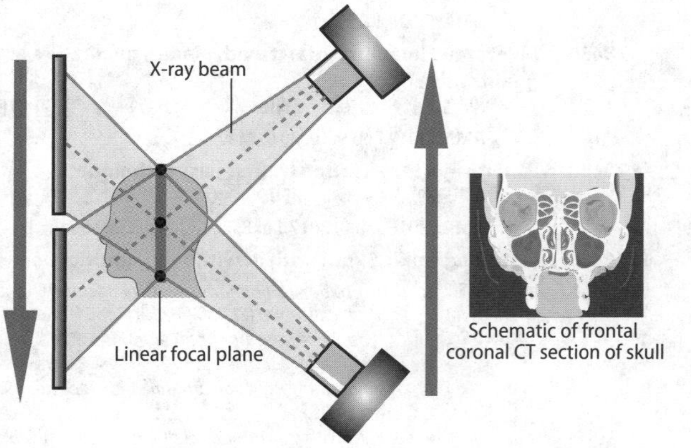

78601 with vascular flow

6.25 6.25 FUD XXX S Z2 80

AMA: 2012,Feb,9-10; 2007,Jan,28-31

78605 Brain imaging, minimum 4 static views;

5.71 5.71 FUD XXX S Z2 80

AMA: 2012,Feb,9-10; 2007,Jan,28-31

78606 with vascular flow

9.45 9.45 FUD XXX S Z2 80

AMA: 2012,Feb,9-10; 2007,Jan,28-31

78608 Brain imaging, positron emission tomography (PET); metabolic evaluation

0.00 0.00 FUD XXX S Z2 80

AMA: 2012,Feb,9-10; 2007,Jan,28-31

78609 perfusion evaluation

2.16 2.16 FUD XXX E

AMA: 2012,Feb,9-10; 2007,Jan,28-31

78610 Brain imaging, vascular flow only

5.04 5.04 FUD XXX S Z2 80

AMA: 2012,Feb,9-10; 2007,Jan,28-31

78630 Cerebrospinal fluid flow, imaging (not including introduction of material); cisternography

Code also injection procedure (61000-61070, 62270-62327)

9.74 9.74 FUD XXX S Z2 80

AMA: 2018,Jan,8

78635 ventriculography

Code also injection procedure (61000-61070, 62270-62294)

9.77 9.77 FUD XXX S Z2 80

AMA: 2012,Feb,9-10; 2007,Jan,28-31

78645 shunt evaluation

Code also injection procedure (61000-61070, 62270-62294)

9.28 9.28 FUD XXX S Z2 80

AMA: 2012,Feb,9-10; 2007,Jan,28-31

78650 Cerebrospinal fluid leakage detection and localization

Code also injection procedure (61000-61070, 62270-62294)

7.89 7.89 FUD XXX S Z2 80

AMA: 2012,Feb,9-10; 2007,Jan,28-31

78660-78699 Nuclear Radiology: Lacrimal Duct System

Code also radiopharmaceutical(s) and/or drug(s) supplied

78660 Radiopharmaceutical dacryocystography

5.26 5.26 FUD XXX S Z2 80

AMA: 2012,Feb,9-10; 2007,Jan,28-31

78699 Unlisted nervous system procedure, diagnostic nuclear medicine

    0.00   0.00   **FUD** XXX   [S] [Z2] [80] [▭]

    AMA: 2018,Jan,8; 2017,Jan,8; 2016,Jan,13; 2015,Jan,16

78700-78725 Nuclear Radiology: Renal Anatomy and Function

> *EXCLUDES*   Diagnostic services (see appropriate sections)
> Follow-up care (see appropriate section)
> Renal endoscopy with insertion radioactive substances (77778)
> Code also radiopharmaceutical(s) and/or drug(s) supplied

78700 Kidney imaging morphology;

    4.92   4.92   **FUD** XXX   [S] [Z2] [80] [▭]

    AMA: 2018,Jan,8; 2017,Jan,8; 2016,Jan,13; 2015,Jan,16

78701 with vascular flow

    6.25   6.25   **FUD** XXX   [S] [Z2] [80] [▭]

    AMA: 2012,Feb,9-10; 2007,Mar,7-8

78707 with vascular flow and function, single study without pharmacological intervention

    6.66   6.66   **FUD** XXX   [S] [Z2] [80] [▭]

    AMA: 2018,Jan,8; 2017,Jan,8; 2016,Jan,13; 2015,Jan,16

78708 with vascular flow and function, single study, with pharmacological intervention (eg, angiotensin converting enzyme inhibitor and/or diuretic)

    5.09   5.09   **FUD** XXX   [S] [Z2] [80] [▭]

    AMA: 2018,Jan,8; 2017,Jan,8; 2016,Jan,13; 2015,Jan,16

78709 with vascular flow and function, multiple studies, with and without pharmacological intervention (eg, angiotensin converting enzyme inhibitor and/or diuretic)

    10.5   10.5   **FUD** XXX   [S] [Z2] [80] [▭]

    AMA: 2018,Jan,8; 2017,Jan,8; 2016,Jan,13; 2015,Jan,16

78725 Kidney function study, non-imaging radioisotopic study

    3.10   3.10   **FUD** XXX   [S] [Z2] [80] [▭]

    AMA: 2012,Feb,9-10; 2007,Jan,28-31

78730-78799 Nuclear Radiology: Urogenital

> *EXCLUDES*   Diagnostic services (see appropriate sections)
> Follow-up care (see appropriate section)
> Code also radiopharmaceutical(s) and/or drug(s) supplied

+   **78730** Urinary bladder residual study (List separately in addition to code for primary procedure)

> *EXCLUDES*   Measurement postvoid residual urine and /or bladder capacity using ultrasound (51798)
> Ultrasound imaging bladder only with measurement postvoid residual urine (76857)

    Code first (78740)

    2.22   2.22   **FUD** ZZZ   [N] [N1] [80] [▭]

    AMA: 2018,Jan,8; 2017,Jan,8; 2016,Jan,13; 2015,Jan,16

78740 Ureteral reflux study (radiopharmaceutical voiding cystogram)

> *EXCLUDES*   Catheterization (51701-51703)

    Code also urinary bladder residual study (78730)

    6.29   6.29   **FUD** XXX   [S] [Z2] [80] [▭]

    AMA: 2012,Feb,9-10; 2007,Jan,28-31

78761 Testicular imaging with vascular flow   ♂

    6.08   6.08   **FUD** XXX   [S] [Z2] [80] [▭]

    AMA: 2018,Jan,8; 2017,Jan,8; 2016,Jan,13; 2015,Jan,16

78799 Unlisted genitourinary procedure, diagnostic nuclear medicine

    0.00   0.00   **FUD** XXX   [S] [Z2] [80] [▭]

    AMA: 2018,Jan,8; 2017,Jan,8; 2016,Jan,13; 2015,Jan,16

78800-78835 [78804, 78830, 78831, 78832, 78835] Nuclear Radiology: Tumor Localization

> *EXCLUDES*   CSF studies requiring injection procedure (61055, 61070, 62320-62323)
> Code also radiopharmaceutical(s) and/or drug(s) supplied

78800 Radiopharmaceutical localization of tumor, inflammatory process or distribution of radiopharmaceutical agent(s) (includes vascular flow and blood pool imaging, when performed); planar, single area (eg, head, neck, chest, pelvis), single day imaging

> *INCLUDES*   Ocular radiophosphorus tumor identification
> *EXCLUDES*   Specific organ (see appropriate site)

    5.61   5.61   **FUD** XXX   [S] [Z2] [80] [▭]

    AMA: 2018,Nov,11; 2018,Jan,8; 2017,Jan,8; 2016,Jan,13; 2015,Jan,16

78801 planar, 2 or more areas (eg, abdomen and pelvis, head and chest), 1 or more days imaging or single area imaging over 2 or more days

    7.42   7.42   **FUD** XXX   [S] [Z2] [80] [▭]

    AMA: 2018,Jan,8; 2017,Jan,8; 2016,Jan,13; 2015,Jan,16

78802 planar, whole body, single day imaging

    9.29   9.29   **FUD** XXX   [S] [Z2] [80] [▭]

    AMA: 2012,Feb,9-10; 2007,Jan,28-31

**78804** planar, whole body, requiring 2 or more days imaging

    16.3   16.3   **FUD** XXX   [S] [Z2] [80] [▭]

    AMA: 2012,Feb,9-10; 2007,Jan,28-31

78803 tomographic (SPECT), single area (eg, head, neck, chest, pelvis), single day imaging

    11.1   11.1   **FUD** XXX   [S] [Z2] [80] [▭]

    AMA: 2018,Nov,11; 2018,Jan,8; 2017,Jan,8; 2016,Dec,9; 2016,Dec,16; 2016,Jan,13; 2015,Oct,9

78804 Resequenced code. See code following 78802.

**78830** tomographic (SPECT) with concurrently acquired computed tomography (CT) transmission scan for anatomical review, localization and determination/detection of pathology, single area (eg, head, neck, chest, pelvis), single day imaging

    14.0   14.0   **FUD** XXX   [Z2] [80] [▭]

**78831** tomographic (SPECT), minimum 2 areas (eg, pelvis and knees, abdomen and pelvis), single day imaging, or single area imaging over 2 or more days

    20.3   20.3   **FUD** XXX   [Z2] [80] [▭]

**78832** tomographic (SPECT) with concurrently acquired computed tomography (CT) transmission scan for anatomical review, localization and determination/detection of pathology, minimum 2 areas (eg, pelvis and knees, abdomen and pelvis), single day imaging, or single area imaging over 2 or more days

    26.4   26.4   **FUD** XXX   [Z2] [80] [▭]

+ #   **78835** Radiopharmaceutical quantification measurement(s) single area (List separately in addition to code for primary procedure)

    2.95   2.95   **FUD** ZZZ   [80]

78808 Intravenous Injection for Radiopharmaceutical Localization

> Code also radiopharmaceutical(s) and/or drug(s) supplied

78808 Injection procedure for radiopharmaceutical localization by non-imaging probe study, intravenous (eg, parathyroid adenoma)

    1.12   1.12   **FUD** XXX   [Q1] [N1] [80] [▭]

    AMA: 2018,Jan,8; 2017,Jan,8; 2016,Dec,9

● New Code   ▲ Revised Code   ○ Reinstated   ● New Web Release   ▲ Revised Web Release   + Add-on   Unlisted   Not Covered   # Resequenced

⑤⓪ Optum Mod 50 Exempt   ⊘ AMA Mod 51 Exempt   ⑤① Optum Mod 51 Exempt   ⑥③ Mod 63 Exempt   ✗ Non-FDA Drug   ★ Telemedicine   Ⓜ Maternity   Ⓐ Age Edit

78811-78999 [78830, 78831, 78832, 78835] Nuclear Radiology: Diagnosis, Staging, Restaging or Monitoring Cancer

CMS: 100-03,220.6.17 Positron Emission Tomography (FDG) for Oncologic Conditions; 100-03,220.6.19 NaF-18 PET to Identify Bone Metastasis of Cancer; 100-03,220.6.9 FDG PET for Refractory Seizures; 100-04,13,60 Positron Emission Tomography (PET) Scans - General Information; 100-04,13,60.13 Billing for PET Scans for Specific Indications of Cervical Cancer; 100-04,13,60.15 Billing for CMS-Approved Clinical Trials for PET Scans; 100-04,13,60.16 Billing and Coverage for PET Scans; 100-04,13,60.17 Billing and Coverage Changes for PET Scans for Cervical Cancer; 100-04,13,60.18 Billing and Coverage for PET (NaF-18) Scans to Identify Bone Metastasis; 100-04,13,60.2 Use of Gamma Cameras, Full and Partial Ring PET Scanners; 100-04,13,60.3 PET Scan Qualifying Conditions; 100-04,13,60.3.1 Appropriate Codes for PET Scans; 100-04,13,60.3.2 Tracer Codes Required for Positron Emission Tomography (PET) Scans

EXCLUDES *CT scan performed for other than attenuation correction and anatomical localization (report with appropriate site-specific CT code and modifier 59)*
Ocular radiophosphorus tumor identification (78800)
PET brain scan (78608-78609)
PET myocardial imaging (78459, 78491-78492)
Procedure performed more than one time per imaging session

Code also radiopharmaceutical(s) and/or drug(s) supplied

78811 Positron emission tomography (PET) imaging; limited area (eg, chest, head/neck)
0.00 0.00 **FUD** XXX S Z2 80
AMA: 2018,Jan,8; 2017,Jan,8; 2016,Jan,13; 2015,Jan,16

78812 skull base to mid-thigh
0.00 0.00 **FUD** XXX S Z2 80
AMA: 2018,Jan,8; 2017,Jan,8; 2016,Jan,13; 2015,Jan,16

78813 whole body
0.00 0.00 **FUD** XXX S Z2 80
AMA: 2018,Jan,8; 2017,Jan,8; 2016,Jan,13; 2015,Jan,16

78814 Positron emission tomography (PET) with concurrently acquired computed tomography (CT) for attenuation correction and anatomical localization imaging; limited area (eg, chest, head/neck)
0.00 0.00 **FUD** XXX S Z2 80
AMA: 2018,Jan,8; 2017,Jan,8; 2016,Jan,13; 2015,Jan,16

78815 skull base to mid-thigh
0.00 0.00 **FUD** XXX S Z2 80
AMA: 2018,Jan,8; 2017,Jan,8; 2016,Jan,13; 2015,Jan,16

78816 whole body
0.00 0.00 **FUD** XXX S Z2 80
AMA: 2020,Sep,11; 2018,Jan,8; 2017,Jan,8; 2016,Jan,13; 2015,Jan,16

***78830* Resequenced code. See code following code 78803.**

***78831* Resequenced code. See code following code 78803.**

***78832* Resequenced code. See code following code 78803.**

***78835* Resequenced code. See code following code 78803.**

78999 Unlisted miscellaneous procedure, diagnostic nuclear medicine
0.00 0.00 **FUD** XXX S Z2 80
AMA: 2018,Jan,8; 2017,Jan,8; 2016,Dec,9; 2016,Dec,16; 2016,Jan,13; 2015,Oct,9; 2015,Jan,16

79005-79999 Systemic Radiopharmaceutical Therapy

EXCLUDES *Imaging guidance*
Injection into artery, body cavity, or joint (see appropriate injection codes)
Radiological supervision and interpretation

79005 Radiopharmaceutical therapy, by oral administration
EXCLUDES *Monoclonal antibody treatment (79403)*
3.92 3.92 **FUD** XXX S Z3 80
AMA: 2018,Jan,8; 2017,Jan,8; 2016,Jan,13; 2015,Jan,16

79101 Radiopharmaceutical therapy, by intravenous administration
EXCLUDES *Administration nonantibody radioelement solution including follow-up care (77750)*
Hydration infusion (96360)
Intravenous injection, IV push (96374-96375, 96409)
Radiolabeled monoclonal antibody IV infusion (79403)
Venipuncture (36400, 36410)
4.18 4.18 **FUD** XXX S Z3 80
AMA: 2018,Jan,8; 2017,Jan,8; 2016,Jan,13; 2015,Jan,16

79200 Radiopharmaceutical therapy, by intracavitary administration
3.86 3.86 **FUD** XXX S Z3 80
AMA: 2018,Jan,8; 2017,Jan,8; 2016,Jan,13; 2015,Jan,16

79300 Radiopharmaceutical therapy, by interstitial radioactive colloid administration
0.00 0.00 **FUD** XXX S Z2 80
AMA: 2018,Jan,8; 2017,Jan,8; 2016,Jan,13; 2015,Jan,16

79403 Radiopharmaceutical therapy, radiolabeled monoclonal antibody by intravenous infusion
EXCLUDES *Intravenous radiopharmaceutical therapy (79101)*
5.39 5.39 **FUD** XXX S Z3 80
AMA: 2018,Jan,8; 2017,Jan,8; 2016,Jan,13; 2015,Jan,16

79440 Radiopharmaceutical therapy, by intra-articular administration
3.48 3.48 **FUD** XXX S Z3 80
AMA: 2018,Jan,8; 2017,Jan,8; 2016,Jan,13; 2015,Jan,16

79445 Radiopharmaceutical therapy, by intra-arterial particulate administration
EXCLUDES *Intra-arterial injections (96373, 96420)*
Procedural and radiological supervision and interpretation for angiographic and interventional procedures before intra-arterial radiopharmaceutical therapy
0.00 0.00 **FUD** XXX S Z2 80
AMA: 2018,Jan,8; 2017,Jan,8; 2016,Jan,13; 2015,Jan,16

79999 Radiopharmaceutical therapy, unlisted procedure
0.00 0.00 **FUD** XXX S Z2 80
AMA: 2018,Jan,8; 2017,Jan,8; 2016,Jan,13; 2015,Jan,16

80047-80081 [80081] Multi-test Laboratory Panels

INCLUDES Specified test grous that may be reported in a panel

EXCLUDES *Reporting two or more panel codes including same tests; report panel with most tests in common to meet panel code definition*

Code also individual tests not part included in panel, when appropriate

80047 Basic metabolic panel (Calcium, ionized)

INCLUDES Calcium, ionized (82330)
Carbon dioxide (bicarbonate) (82374)
Chloride (82435)
Creatinine (82565)
Glucose (82947)
Potassium (84132)
Sodium (84295)
Urea nitrogen (BUN) (84520)

🚑 0.00   ⚕ 0.00   **FUD** XXX   ☒ ◙ ▭

AMA: 2020,Jun,3; 2018,Jan,8; 2017,Jan,8; 2016,Jan,13; 2015,Jan,16

80048 Basic metabolic panel (Calcium, total)

INCLUDES Calcium, total (82310)
Carbon dioxide (bicarbonate) (82374)
Chloride (82435)
Creatinine (82565)
Glucose (82947)
Potassium (84132)
Sodium (84295)
Urea nitrogen (BUN) (84520)

🚑 0.00   ⚕ 0.00   **FUD** XXX   ☒ ◙ ▭

AMA: 2018,Jan,8; 2017,Jan,8; 2016,Jan,13; 2015,Jan,16

80050 General health panel

INCLUDES Complete blood count (CBC), automated, with:
Manual differential WBC count
Blood smear with manual differential AND complete (CBC), automated (85007, 85027)
Manual differential WBC count, buffy coat AND complete (CBC), automated (85009, 85027)
OR
Automated differential WBC count
Automated differential WBC count AND complete (CBC), automated/automated differential WBC count (85004, 85025)
Automated differential WBC count AND complete (CBC), automated (85004, 85027)
Comprehensive metabolic profile (80053)
Thyroid stimulating hormone (84443)

🚑 0.00   ⚕ 0.00   **FUD** XXX   E ▭

AMA: 2018,Jan,8; 2017,Jan,8; 2016,Jan,13; 2015,Jan,16

80051 Electrolyte panel

INCLUDES Carbon dioxide (bicarbonate) (82374)
Chloride (82435)
Potassium (84132)
Sodium (84295)

🚑 0.00   ⚕ 0.00   **FUD** XXX   ☒ ◙ ▭

AMA: 2018,Jan,8; 2017,Jan,8; 2016,Jan,13; 2015,Jan,16

80053 Comprehensive metabolic panel

INCLUDES Albumin (82040)
Bilirubin, total (82247)
Calcium, total (82310)
Carbon dioxide (bicarbonate) (82374)
Chloride (82435)
Creatinine (82565)
Glucose (82947)
Phosphatase, alkaline (84075)
Potassium (84132)
Protein, total (84155)
Sodium (84295)
Transferase, alanine amino (ALT) (SGPT) (84460)
Transferase, aspartate amino (AST) (SGOT) (84450)
Urea nitrogen (BUN) (84520)

🚑 0.00   ⚕ 0.00   **FUD** XXX   ☒ ◙ ▭

AMA: 2018,Jan,8; 2017,Jan,8; 2016,Jan,13; 2015,Jan,16

80055 Obstetric panel Ⓜ ♀

INCLUDES Complete blood count (CBC), automated, with:
Manual differential WBC count
Blood smear with manual differential AND complete (CBC), automated (85007, 85027)
Manual differential WBC count, buffy coat AND complete (CBC), automated (85009, 85027)
OR
Automated differential WBC count
Automated differential WBC count AND complete (CBC), automated/automated differential WBC count (85004, 85025)
Automated differential WBC count AND complete (CBC), automated (85004, 85027)
Blood typing, ABO and Rh (86900-86901)
Hepatitis B surface antigen (HBsAg) (87340)
RBC antibody screen, each serum technique (86850)
Rubella antibody (86762)
Syphilis test, non-treponemal antibody qualitative (86592)

EXCLUDES *Reporting code when syphilis screening provided using treponemal antibody approach. Instead, assign individual codes for tests performed in OB panel (86780)*

🚑 0.00   ⚕ 0.00   **FUD** XXX   ◙ ▭

AMA: 2018,Jan,8; 2017,Jan,8; 2016,Jan,13; 2015,Jan,16

80081 Obstetric panel (includes HIV testing) Ⓜ ♀

INCLUDES Complete blood count (CBC), automated, with:
Manual differential WBC count
Blood smear with manual differential AND complete (CBC), automated (85007, 85027)
Manual differential WBC count, buffy count AND complete (CBC), automated (85009, 85027)
OR
Automated differential WBC count
Automated differential WBC count AND complete (CBC), automated/automated differential WBC count (85004, 85025)
Automated differential WBC count AND complete (CBC), automated (85004, 85027)
Blood typing, ABO and Rh (86900-86901)
Hepatitis B surface antigen (HBsAg) (87340)
HIV-1 antigens, with HIV-1 and HIV-2 antibodies, single result (87389)
RBC antibody screen, each serum technique (86850)
Rubella antibody (86762)
Syphilis test, non-treponemal antibody qualitative (86592)

EXCLUDES *Reporting code when syphilis screening provided using treponemal antibody approach. Instead, assign individual codes for tests performed in OB panel (86780)*

🚑 0.00   ⚕ 0.00   **FUD** XXX   ◙ ▭

AMA: 2018,Jan,8; 2017,Jan,8; 2016,Jan,13

80061 Lipid panel

INCLUDES Cholesterol, serum, total (82465)
Lipoprotein, direct measurement, high density cholesterol (HDL cholesterol) (83718)
Triglycerides (84478)

🚑 0.00   ⚕ 0.00   **FUD** XXX   ☒ A ▭

AMA: 2018,Jan,8; 2017,Sep,11; 2017,Jan,8; 2016,Jan,13; 2015,Jan,16

80069 Renal function panel

INCLUDES Albumin (82040)
Calcium, total (82310)
Carbon dioxide (bicarbonate) (82374)
Chloride (82435)
Creatinine (82565)
Glucose (82947)
Phosphorus inorganic (phosphate) (84100)
Potassium (84132)
Sodium (84295)
Urea nitrogen (BUN) (84520)

🚑 0.00   ⚕ 0.00   **FUD** XXX   ☒ ◙ ▭

AMA: 2018,Jan,8; 2017,Jan,8; 2016,Jan,13; 2015,Jan,16

80074 **Acute hepatitis panel**

INCLUDES Hepatitis A antibody (HAAb) IgM (86709)
Hepatitis B core antibody (HBcAb), IgM (86705)
Hepatitis B surface antigen (HBsAg) (87340)
Hepatitis C antibody (86803)

0.00 0.00 **FUD** XXX

AMA: 2018,Jan,8; 2017,Jan,8; 2016,Jan,13; 2015,Jan,16

80076 **Hepatic function panel**

INCLUDES Albumin (82040)
Bilirubin, direct (82248)
Bilirubin, total (82247)
Phosphatase, alkaline (84075)
Protein, total (84155)
Transferase, alanine amino (ALT) (SGPT) (84460)
Transferase, aspartate amino (AST) (SGOT) (84450)

0.00 0.00 **FUD** XXX

AMA: 2018,Jan,8; 2017,Jan,8; 2016,Jan,13; 2015,Jan,16

80081 **Resequenced code. See code following 80055.**

80305-80307 [80305, 80306, 80307] Nonspecific Drug Screening

INCLUDES All class testing procedures performed per modality
Validation testing

EXCLUDES *Confirmatory drug testing ([80320, 80321, 80322, 80323, 80324, 80325, 80326, 80327, 80328, 80329, 80330, 80331, 80332, 80333, 80334, 80335, 80336, 80337, 80338, 80339, 80340, 80341, 80342, 80343, 80344, 80345, 80346, 80347, 80348, 80349, 80350, 80351, 80352, 80353, 80354, 80355, 80356, 80357, 80358, 80359, 80360, 80361, 80362, 80363, 80364, 80365, 80366, 80367, 80368, 80369, 80370, 80371, 80372, 80373, 80374, 80375, 80376, 80377, 83992], [83992])*

\# **80305** **Drug test(s), presumptive, any number of drug classes, any number of devices or procedures; capable of being read by direct optical observation only (eg, utilizing immunoassay [eg, dipsticks, cups, cards, or cartridges]), includes sample validation when performed, per date of service**

0.00 0.00 **FUD** XXX

AMA: 2018,Jul,14; 2018,Jan,8; 2017,Mar,6

\# **80306** **read by instrument assisted direct optical observation (eg, utilizing immunoassay [eg, dipsticks, cups, cards, or cartridges]), includes sample validation when performed, per date of service**

0.00 0.00 **FUD** XXX

AMA: 2018,Jan,8; 2017,Mar,6

\# **80307** **by instrument chemistry analyzers (eg, utilizing immunoassay [eg, EIA, ELISA, EMIT, FPIA, IA, KIMS, RIA]), chromatography (eg, GC, HPLC), and mass spectrometry either with or without chromatography, (eg, DART, DESI, GC-MS, GC-MS/MS, LC-MS, LC-MS/MS, LDTD, MALDI, TOF) includes sample validation when performed, per date of service**

0.00 0.00 **FUD** XXX

AMA: 2018,Jan,8; 2017,Mar,6

80320-80377 [80320, 80321, 80322, 80323, 80324, 80325, 80326, 80327, 80328, 80329, 80330, 80331, 80332, 80333, 80334, 80335, 80336, 80337, 80338, 80339, 80340, 80341, 80342, 80343, 80344, 80345, 80346, 80347, 80348, 80349, 80350, 80351, 80352, 80353, 80354, 80355, 80356, 80357, 80358, 80359, 80360, 80361, 80362, 80363, 80364, 80365, 80366, 80367, 80368, 80369, 80370, 80371, 80372, 80373, 80374, 80375, 80376, 80377, 83992] Confirmatory Drug Testing

INCLUDES Antihistamine drug tests ([80375, 80376, 80377])
Detection specific drugs using methods other than immunoassay or enzymatic technique

EXCLUDES *Definitive drug testing for any drug class not specified; report with NOS codes ([80375, 80376, 80377])*
Metabolites separate from code for drug except when distinct code available

\# **80320** **Alcohols**

EXCLUDES *Alcohol (ethanol) therapeutic drug assay (82077)*

0.00 0.00 **FUD** XXX

AMA: 2018,Jan,8; 2017,Jan,8; 2016,Jan,13; 2015,Apr,3

\# **80321** **Alcohol biomarkers; 1 or 2**

0.00 0.00 **FUD** XXX

AMA: 2015,Apr,3

\# **80322** **3 or more**

0.00 0.00 **FUD** XXX

AMA: 2015,Apr,3

\# **80323** **Alkaloids, not otherwise specified**

0.00 0.00 **FUD** XXX

AMA: 2015,Apr,3

\# **80324** **Amphetamines; 1 or 2**

0.00 0.00 **FUD** XXX

AMA: 2015,Apr,3

\# **80325** **3 or 4**

0.00 0.00 **FUD** XXX

AMA: 2015,Apr,3

\# **80326** **5 or more**

0.00 0.00 **FUD** XXX

AMA: 2015,Apr,3

\# **80327** **Anabolic steroids; 1 or 2**

0.00 0.00 **FUD** XXX

AMA: 2015,Apr,3

\# **80328** **3 or more**

EXCLUDES *Analysis dihydrotestosterone for monitoring, endogenous levels of hormone (82642)*

0.00 0.00 **FUD** XXX

AMA: 2015,Apr,3

\# **80329** **Analgesics, non-opioid; 1 or 2**

EXCLUDES *Acetaminophen therapeutic drug assay (80143)*
Salicylate therapeutic drug assay ([80179])

0.00 0.00 **FUD** XXX

AMA: 2015,Apr,3

\# **80330** **3-5**

EXCLUDES *Acetaminophen therapeutic drug assay (80143)*
Salicylate therapeutic drug assay ([80179])

0.00 0.00 **FUD** XXX

AMA: 2015,Apr,3

\# **80331** **6 or more**

EXCLUDES *Acetaminophen therapeutic drug assay (80143)*
Salicylate therapeutic drug assay ([80179])

0.00 0.00 **FUD** XXX

AMA: 2015,Apr,3

\# **80332** **Antidepressants, serotonergic class; 1 or 2**

0.00 0.00 **FUD** XXX

AMA: 2015,Apr,3

\# **80333** **3-5**
0.00 0.00 FUD XXX B
AMA: 2015,Apr,3

\# **80334** **6 or more**
0.00 0.00 FUD XXX B
AMA: 2015,Apr,3

\# **80335** **Antidepressants, tricyclic and other cyclicals; 1 or 2**
0.00 0.00 FUD XXX B
AMA: 2015,Apr,3

\# **80336** **3-5**
0.00 0.00 FUD XXX B
AMA: 2015,Apr,3

\# **80337** **6 or more**
0.00 0.00 FUD XXX B
AMA: 2015,Apr,3

\# **80338** **Antidepressants, not otherwise specified**
0.00 0.00 FUD XXX B
AMA: 2015,Apr,3

\# **80339** **Antiepileptics, not otherwise specified; 1-3**
0.00 0.00 FUD XXX B
AMA: 2015,Apr,3

\# **80340** **4-6**
0.00 0.00 FUD XXX B
AMA: 2015,Apr,3

\# **80341** **7 or more**
EXCLUDES *Carbamazepine therapeutic drug assay (80156, 80157, [80161])*
Definitive drug testing for antihistamines ([80375, 80376, 80377])
0.00 0.00 FUD XXX B
AMA: 2015,Apr,3

\# **80342** **Antipsychotics, not otherwise specified; 1-3**
0.00 0.00 FUD XXX B
AMA: 2015,Apr,3

\# **80343** **4-6**
0.00 0.00 FUD XXX B
AMA: 2015,Apr,3

\# **80344** **7 or more**
0.00 0.00 FUD XXX B
AMA: 2015,Apr,3

\# **80345** **Barbiturates**
0.00 0.00 FUD XXX B
AMA: 2015,Apr,3

\# **80346** **Benzodiazepines; 1-12**
0.00 0.00 FUD XXX B
AMA: 2015,Apr,3

\# **80347** **13 or more**
0.00 0.00 FUD XXX B
AMA: 2015,Apr,3

\# **80348** **Buprenorphine**
0.00 0.00 FUD XXX B
AMA: 2015,Apr,3

\# **80349** **Cannabinoids, natural**
0.00 0.00 FUD XXX B
AMA: 2015,Apr,3

\# **80350** **Cannabinoids, synthetic; 1-3**
0.00 0.00 FUD XXX B
AMA: 2015,Apr,3

\# **80351** **4-6**
0.00 0.00 FUD XXX B
AMA: 2015,Apr,3

\# **80352** **7 or more**
0.00 0.00 FUD XXX B
AMA: 2015,Apr,3

\# **80353** **Cocaine**
0.00 0.00 FUD XXX B
AMA: 2015,Apr,3

\# **80354** **Fentanyl**
0.00 0.00 FUD XXX B
AMA: 2015,Apr,3

\# **80355** **Gabapentin, non-blood**
EXCLUDES *Therapeutic drug assay ([80171])*
0.00 0.00 FUD XXX B
AMA: 2018,Jan,8; 2017,Jan,8; 2016,Jan,13; 2015,Apr,3

\# **80356** **Heroin metabolite**
0.00 0.00 FUD XXX B
AMA: 2015,Apr,3

\# **80357** **Ketamine and norketamine**
0.00 0.00 FUD XXX B
AMA: 2015,Apr,3

\# **80358** **Methadone**
0.00 0.00 FUD XXX B
AMA: 2015,Apr,3

\# **80359** **Methylenedioxyamphetamines (MDA, MDEA, MDMA)**
0.00 0.00 FUD XXX B
AMA: 2015,Apr,3

\# **80360** **Methylphenidate**
0.00 0.00 FUD XXX B
AMA: 2015,Apr,3

\# **80361** **Opiates, 1 or more**
0.00 0.00 FUD XXX B
AMA: 2015,Apr,3

\# **80362** **Opioids and opiate analogs; 1 or 2**
0.00 0.00 FUD XXX B
AMA: 2015,Apr,3

\# **80363** **3 or 4**
0.00 0.00 FUD XXX B
AMA: 2015,Apr,3

\# **80364** **5 or more**
0.00 0.00 FUD XXX B
AMA: 2015,Apr,3

\# **80365** **Oxycodone**
0.00 0.00 FUD XXX B
AMA: 2015,Apr,3

\# **83992** **Phencyclidine (PCP)**
0.00 0.00 FUD XXX E
AMA: 2018,Jan,8; 2017,Jan,8; 2016,Jan,13; 2015,Jun,10; 2015,Apr,3

\# **80366** **Pregabalin**
0.00 0.00 FUD XXX B
AMA: 2015,Apr,3

\# **80367** **Propoxyphene**
0.00 0.00 FUD XXX B
AMA: 2015,Apr,3

\# **80368** **Sedative hypnotics (non-benzodiazepines)**
0.00 0.00 FUD XXX B
AMA: 2015,Apr,3

\# **80369** **Skeletal muscle relaxants; 1 or 2**
0.00 0.00 FUD XXX B
AMA: 2015,Apr,3

\# **80370** **3 or more**
0.00 0.00 FUD XXX B
AMA: 2015,Apr,3

80371 Stimulants, synthetic
0.00 0.00 FUD XXX
AMA: 2015,Apr,3

80372 Tapentadol
0.00 0.00 FUD XXX
AMA: 2015,Apr,3

80373 Tramadol
0.00 0.00 FUD XXX
AMA: 2015,Apr,3

80374 Stereoisomer (enantiomer) analysis, single drug class
Code also index drug analysis when appropriate
0.00 0.00 FUD XXX
AMA: 2015,Apr,3

80375 Drug(s) or substance(s), definitive, qualitative or quantitative, not otherwise specified; 1-3
0.00 0.00 FUD XXX
AMA: 2018,Jan,8; 2017,Jan,8; 2016,Jan,13; 2015,Apr,3

80376 4-6
0.00 0.00 FUD XXX
AMA: 2018,Jan,8; 2017,Jan,8; 2016,Jan,13; 2015,Apr,3

80377 7 or more
EXCLUDES *Definitive drug testing for antihistamines ([80375, 80376, 80377])*
0.00 0.00 FUD XXX
AMA: 2018,Jan,8; 2017,Jan,8; 2016,Jan,13; 2015,Apr,3

80143-80377 [80161, 80164, 80165, 80167, 80171, 80176, 80179, 80181, 80189, 80193, 80204, 80210, 80230, 80235, 80280, 80285, 80305, 80306, 80307, 80320, 80321, 80322, 80323, 80324, 80325, 80326, 80327, 80328, 80329, 80330, 80331, 80332, 80333, 80334, 80335, 80336, 80337, 80338, 80339, 80340, 80341, 80342, 80343, 80344, 80345, 80346, 80347, 80348, 80349, 80350, 80351, 80352, 80353, 80354, 80355, 80356, 80357, 80358, 80359, 80360, 80361, 80362, 80363, 80364, 80365, 80366, 80367, 80368, 80369, 80370, 80371, 80372, 80373, 80374, 80375, 80376, 80377]

Therapeutic Drug Levels

INCLUDES Monitoring known, prescribed or over-the-counter medication levels
Testing drug and metabolite(s) in primary code
Tests on specimens from blood, blood components, and spinal fluid

● 80143 Acetaminophen
EXCLUDES *Acetaminophen confirmatory drug testing ([80329, 80330, 80331])*

80145 Adalimumab
0.00 0.00 FUD XXX

80150 Amikacin
0.00 0.00 FUD XXX
AMA: 2018,Jan,8; 2017,Jan,8; 2016,Jan,13; 2015,Apr,3; 2015,Jan,16

● 80151 Amiodarone

80155 Caffeine
0.00 0.00 FUD XXX
AMA: 2015,Apr,3

80156 Carbamazepine; total
0.00 0.00 FUD XXX
AMA: 2018,Jan,8; 2017,Jan,8; 2016,Jan,13; 2015,Apr,3; 2015,Jan,16

80157 free
0.00 0.00 FUD XXX
AMA: 2018,Jan,8; 2017,Jan,8; 2016,Jan,13; 2015,Apr,3; 2015,Jan,16

● # 80161 Carbamazepine; -10,11-epoxide
0.00 0.00 FUD 000

80158 Cyclosporine
0.00 0.00 FUD XXX
AMA: 2018,Jan,8; 2017,Jan,8; 2016,Jan,13; 2015,Apr,3; 2015,Jan,16

80159 Clozapine
0.00 0.00 FUD XXX
AMA: 2015,Apr,3

80161 Resequenced code. See code following 80157.

80162 Digoxin; total
0.00 0.00 FUD XXX
AMA: 2018,Jan,8; 2017,Jan,8; 2016,Jan,13; 2015,Apr,3; 2015,Jan,16

80163 free
0.00 0.00 FUD XXX
AMA: 2018,Jan,8; 2017,Jan,8; 2016,Jan,13; 2015,Apr,3

80164 Resequenced code. See code following 80201.

80165 Resequenced code. See code following 80201.

80167 Resequenced code. See code following 80169.

80168 Ethosuximide
0.00 0.00 FUD XXX
AMA: 2018,Jan,8; 2017,Jan,8; 2016,Jan,13; 2015,Apr,3; 2015,Jan,16

80169 Everolimus
0.00 0.00 FUD XXX
AMA: 2015,Apr,3

● # 80167 Felbamate
0.00 0.00 FUD 000

● # 80181 Flecainide
0.00 0.00 FUD 000

80171 Gabapentin, whole blood, serum, or plasma
0.00 0.00 FUD XXX
AMA: 2018,Jan,8; 2017,Jan,8; 2016,Jan,13; 2015,Apr,3

80170 Gentamicin
0.00 0.00 FUD XXX
AMA: 2018,Jan,8; 2017,Jan,8; 2016,Jan,13; 2015,Apr,3; 2015,Jan,16

80171 Resequenced code. See code before 80170.

80173 Haloperidol
0.00 0.00 FUD XXX
AMA: 2018,Jan,8; 2017,Jan,8; 2016,Jan,13; 2015,Apr,3; 2015,Jan,16

80230 Infliximab
0.00 0.00 FUD XXX

● # 80189 Itraconazole
0.00 0.00 FUD 000

80235 Lacosamide
0.00 0.00 FUD XXX

80175 Lamotrigine
0.00 0.00 FUD XXX
AMA: 2015,Apr,3

80176 Resequenced code. See code following 80177.

● # 80193 Leflunomide
0.00 0.00 FUD 000

80177 Levetiracetam
0.00 0.00 FUD XXX
AMA: 2015,Apr,3

80176 Lidocaine
0.00 0.00 FUD XXX
AMA: 2018,Jan,8; 2017,Jan,8; 2016,Jan,13; 2015,Apr,3; 2015,Jan,16

80178 Lithium
🚑 0.00   ⚕ 0.00   **FUD** XXX   ☒ 🔲 🔲
AMA: 2018,Jan,8; 2017,Jan,8; 2016,Jan,13; 2015,Apr,3; 2015,Jan,16

● # **80204 Methotrexate**
🚑 0.00   ⚕ 0.00   **FUD** 000

80179 Resequenced code. See code before 80195.

80180 Mycophenolate (mycophenolic acid)
🚑 0.00   ⚕ 0.00   **FUD** XXX   🔲 🔲
AMA: 2015,Apr,3

80181 Resequenced code. See code following resequenced code 80167.

80183 Oxcarbazepine
🚑 0.00   ⚕ 0.00   **FUD** XXX   🔲 🔲
AMA: 2015,Apr,3

80184 Phenobarbital
🚑 0.00   ⚕ 0.00   **FUD** XXX   🔲 🔲
AMA: 2018,Jan,8; 2017,Jan,8; 2016,Jan,13; 2015,Apr,3; 2015,Jan,16

80185 Phenytoin; total
🚑 0.00   ⚕ 0.00   **FUD** XXX   🔲 🔲
AMA: 2018,Jan,8; 2017,Jan,8; 2016,Jan,13; 2015,Apr,3; 2015,Jan,16

80186   free
🚑 0.00   ⚕ 0.00   **FUD** XXX   🔲 🔲
AMA: 2018,Jan,8; 2017,Jan,8; 2016,Jan,13; 2015,Apr,3; 2015,Jan,16

80187 Posaconazole
🚑 0.00   ⚕ 0.00   **FUD** XXX

80188 Primidone
🚑 0.00   ⚕ 0.00   **FUD** XXX   🔲 🔲
AMA: 2018,Jan,8; 2017,Jan,8; 2016,Jan,13; 2015,Apr,3; 2015,Jan,16

80189 Resequenced code. See code following resequenced code 80230.

80190 Procainamide;
🚑 0.00   ⚕ 0.00   **FUD** XXX   🔲 🔲
AMA: 2018,Jan,8; 2017,Jan,8; 2016,Jan,13; 2015,Apr,3; 2015,Jan,16

80192   with metabolites (eg, n-acetyl procainamide)
🚑 0.00   ⚕ 0.00   **FUD** XXX   🔲 🔲
AMA: 2018,Jan,8; 2017,Jan,8; 2016,Jan,13; 2015,Apr,3; 2015,Jan,16

80193 Resequenced code. See code before 80177.

80194 Quinidine
🚑 0.00   ⚕ 0.00   **FUD** XXX   🔲 🔲
AMA: 2018,Jan,8; 2017,Jan,8; 2016,Jan,13; 2015,Apr,3; 2015,Jan,16

● # **80210 Rufinamide**
🚑 0.00   ⚕ 0.00   **FUD** 000

● # **80179 Salicylate**
EXCLUDES   *Salicylate confirmatory drug testing ([80329, 80330, 80331])*
🚑 0.00   ⚕ 0.00   **FUD** 000

80195 Sirolimus
🚑 0.00   ⚕ 0.00   **FUD** XXX   🔲 🔲
AMA: 2018,Jan,8; 2017,Jan,8; 2016,Jan,13; 2015,Apr,3; 2015,Jan,16

80197 Tacrolimus
🚑 0.00   ⚕ 0.00   **FUD** XXX   🔲 🔲
AMA: 2018,Jan,8; 2017,Jan,8; 2016,Jan,13; 2015,Apr,3; 2015,Jan,16

80198 Theophylline
🚑 0.00   ⚕ 0.00   **FUD** XXX   🔲 🔲
AMA: 2018,Jan,8; 2017,Jan,8; 2016,Jan,13; 2015,Apr,3; 2015,Jan,16

80199 Tiagabine
🚑 0.00   ⚕ 0.00   **FUD** XXX   🔲 🔲
AMA: 2015,Apr,3

80200 Tobramycin
🚑 0.00   ⚕ 0.00   **FUD** XXX   🔲 🔲
AMA: 2018,Jan,8; 2017,Jan,8; 2016,Jan,13; 2015,Apr,3; 2015,Jan,16

80201 Topiramate
🚑 0.00   ⚕ 0.00   **FUD** XXX   🔲 🔲
AMA: 2018,Jan,8; 2017,Jan,8; 2016,Jan,13; 2015,Apr,3; 2015,Jan,16

80164 Valproic acid (dipropylacetic acid); total
🚑 0.00   ⚕ 0.00   **FUD** XXX   🔲 🔲
AMA: 2018,Jan,8; 2017,Jan,8; 2016,Jan,13; 2015,Apr,3; 2015,Jan,16

80165   free
🚑 0.00   ⚕ 0.00   **FUD** XXX   🔲 🔲
AMA: 2018,Jan,8; 2017,Jan,8; 2016,Jan,13; 2015,Apr,3

80202 Vancomycin
🚑 0.00   ⚕ 0.00   **FUD** XXX   🔲 🔲
AMA: 2018,Jan,8; 2017,Jan,8; 2016,Jan,13; 2015,Apr,3; 2015,Jan,16

80280 Vedolizumab
🚑 0.00   ⚕ 0.00   **FUD** XXX

80285 Voriconazole
🚑 0.00   ⚕ 0.00   **FUD** XXX

80203 Zonisamide
🚑 0.00   ⚕ 0.00   **FUD** XXX   🔲 🔲
AMA: 2015,Apr,3

80204 Resequenced code. See code following 80178.
80210 Resequenced code. See code following 80194.
80230 Resequenced code. See code following 80173.
80235 Resequenced code. See code before 80175.
80280 Resequenced code. See code following 80202.
80285 Resequenced code. See code before 80203.

80299 Quantitation of therapeutic drug, not elsewhere specified
🚑 0.00   ⚕ 0.00   **FUD** XXX   🔲 🔲
AMA: 2018,Jan,8; 2017,Jan,8; 2016,Jan,13; 2015,Apr,3; 2015,Jan,16

80305 Resequenced code. See code before 80143.
80306 Resequenced code. See code before 80143.
80307 Resequenced code. See code before 80143.
80320 Resequenced code. See code before 80143.
80321 Resequenced code. See code before 80143.
80322 Resequenced code. See code before 80143.
80323 Resequenced code. See code before 80143.
80324 Resequenced code. See code before 80143.
80325 Resequenced code. See code before 80143.
80326 Resequenced code. See code before 80143.
80327 Resequenced code. See code before 80143.
80328 Resequenced code. See code before 80143.
80329 Resequenced code. See code before 80143.
80330 Resequenced code. See code before 80143.
80331 Resequenced code. See code before 80143.
80332 Resequenced code. See code before 80143.
80333 Resequenced code. See code before 80143.

● New Code   ▲ Revised Code   ○ Reinstated   ● New Web Release   ▲ Revised Web Release   + Add-on   Unlisted   Not Covered   # Resequenced
⑤⓪ Optum Mod 50 Exempt   ⊘ AMA Mod 51 Exempt   ⑤① Optum Mod 51 Exempt   ⑥③ Mod 63 Exempt   ✗ Non-FDA Drug   ★ Telemedicine   Ⓜ Maternity   Ⓐ Age Edit

80334 **Resequenced code. See code before 80143.**

80335 **Resequenced code. See code before 80143.**

80336 **Resequenced code. See code before 80143.**

80337 **Resequenced code. See code before 80143.**

80338 **Resequenced code. See code before 80143.**

80339 **Resequenced code. See code before 80143.**

80340 **Resequenced code. See code before 80143.**

80341 **Resequenced code. See code before 80143.**

80342 **Resequenced code. See code before 80143.**

80343 **Resequenced code. See code before 80143.**

80344 **Resequenced code. See code before 80143.**

80345 **Resequenced code. See code before 80143.**

80346 **Resequenced code. See code before 80143.**

80347 **Resequenced code. See code before 80143.**

80348 **Resequenced code. See code before 80143.**

80349 **Resequenced code. See code before 80143.**

80350 **Resequenced code. See code before 80143.**

80351 **Resequenced code. See code before 80143.**

80352 **Resequenced code. See code before 80143.**

80353 **Resequenced code. See code before 80143.**

80354 **Resequenced code. See code before 80143.**

80355 **Resequenced code. See code before 80143.**

80356 **Resequenced code. See code before 80143.**

80357 **Resequenced code. See code before 80143.**

80358 **Resequenced code. See code before 80143.**

80359 **Resequenced code. See code before 80143.**

80360 **Resequenced code. See code before 80143.**

80361 **Resequenced code. See code before 80143.**

80362 **Resequenced code. See code before 80143.**

80363 **Resequenced code. See code before 80143.**

80364 **Resequenced code. See code before 80143.**

80365 **Resequenced code. See code before 80143.**

80366 **Resequenced code. See code before 80143.**

80367 **Resequenced code. See code before 80143.**

80368 **Resequenced code. See code before 80143.**

80369 **Resequenced code. See code before 80143.**

80370 **Resequenced code. See code before 80143.**

80371 **Resequenced code. See code before 80143.**

80372 **Resequenced code. See code before 80143.**

80373 **Resequenced code. See code before 80143.**

80374 **Resequenced code. See code before 80143.**

80375 **Resequenced code. See code before 80143.**

80376 **Resequenced code. See code before 80143.**

80377 **Resequenced code. See code before 80143.**

80400-80439 Stimulation and Suppression Test Panels

EXCLUDES *Administration evocative or suppressive material (96365-96368, 96372, 96374-96376, C8957)*
Evocative or suppression test substances, when applicable
Physician monitoring and attendance during test (see E/M services)

80400 ACTH stimulation panel; for adrenal insufficiency

INCLUDES Cortisol x 2 (82533)

0.00 0.00 **FUD** XXX

AMA: 2018,Jan,8; 2017,Jan,8; 2016,Jan,13; 2015,Jan,16

80402 for 21 hydroxylase deficiency

INCLUDES 17 hydroxyprogesterone X 2 (83498)
Cortisol x 2 (82533)

0.00 0.00 **FUD** XXX

AMA: 2014,Jan,11; 2005,Jul,11-12

80406 for 3 beta-hydroxydehydrogenase deficiency

INCLUDES 17 hydroxypregnenolone x 2 (84143)
Cortisol x 2 (82533)

0.00 0.00 **FUD** XXX

AMA: 2014,Jan,11; 2005,Jul,11-12

80408 Aldosterone suppression evaluation panel (eg, saline infusion)

INCLUDES Aldosterone x 2 (82088)
Renin x 2 (84244)

0.00 0.00 **FUD** XXX

AMA: 2014,Jan,11; 2005,Jul,11-12

80410 Calcitonin stimulation panel (eg, calcium, pentagastrin)

INCLUDES Calcitonin x 3 (82308)

0.00 0.00 **FUD** XXX

AMA: 2014,Jan,11; 2005,Jul,11-12

80412 Corticotropic releasing hormone (CRH) stimulation panel

INCLUDES Adrenocorticotropic hormone (ACTH) x 6 (82024)
Cortisol x 6 (82533)

0.00 0.00 **FUD** XXX

AMA: 2014,Jan,11; 2005,Jul,11-12

80414 Chorionic gonadotropin stimulation panel; testosterone response

INCLUDES Testosterone x 2 on three pooled blood samples (84403)

0.00 0.00 **FUD** XXX

AMA: 2014,Jan,11; 2005,Jul,11-12

▲ **80415 estradiol response**

INCLUDES Estradiol x 2 on three pooled blood samples (82670)

0.00 0.00 **FUD** XXX

AMA: 2014,Jan,11; 2005,Jul,11-12

80416 Renal vein renin stimulation panel (eg, captopril)

INCLUDES Renin x 6 (84244)

0.00 0.00 **FUD** XXX

AMA: 2014,Jan,11; 2005,Jul,11-12

80417 Peripheral vein renin stimulation panel (eg, captopril)

INCLUDES Renin x 2 (84244)

0.00 0.00 **FUD** XXX

AMA: 2014,Jan,11; 2005,Jul,11-12

80418 Combined rapid anterior pituitary evaluation panel

INCLUDES Adrenocorticotropic hormone (ACTH) x 4 (82024)
Cortisol x 4 (82533)
Follicle stimulating hormone (FSH) x 4 (83001)
Human growth hormone x 4 (83003)
Luteinizing hormone (LH) x 4 (83002)
Prolactin x 4 (84146)
Thyroid stimulating hormone (TSH) x 4 (84443)

0.00 0.00 **FUD** XXX

AMA: 2014,Jan,11; 2005,Jul,11-12

80420 Dexamethasone suppression panel, 48 hour

INCLUDES Cortisol x 2 (82533)
Free cortisol, urine x 2 (82530)
Volume measurement for timed collection x 2 (81050)

EXCLUDES *Single dose dexamethasone (82533)*

0.00 0.00 **FUD** XXX

AMA: 2014,Jan,11; 2005,Jul,11-12

80422 Glucagon tolerance panel; for insulinoma

INCLUDES Glucose x 3 (82947)
Insulin x 3 (83525)

0.00 0.00 **FUD** XXX

AMA: 2014,Jan,11; 2005,Jul,11-12

80424 **for pheochromocytoma**
INCLUDES Catecholamines, fractionated x 2 (82384)
0.00 0.00 FUD XXX
AMA: 2014,Jan,11; 2005,Jul,11-12

80426 **Gonadotropin releasing hormone stimulation panel**
INCLUDES Follicle stimulating hormone (FSH) x 4 (83001)
Luteinizing hormone (LH) x 4 (83002)
0.00 0.00 FUD XXX
AMA: 2014,Jan,11; 2005,Jul,11-12

80428 **Growth hormone stimulation panel (eg, arginine infusion, l-dopa administration)**
INCLUDES Human growth hormone (HGH) x 4 (83003)
0.00 0.00 FUD XXX
AMA: 2014,Jan,11; 2005,Jul,11-12

80430 **Growth hormone suppression panel (glucose administration)**
INCLUDES Glucose x 3 (82947)
Human growth hormone (HGH) x 4 (83003)
0.00 0.00 FUD XXX
AMA: 2014,Jan,11; 2005,Jul,11-12

80432 **Insulin-induced C-peptide suppression panel**
INCLUDES C-peptide x 5 (84681)
Glucose x 5 (82947)
Insulin (83525)
0.00 0.00 FUD XXX
AMA: 2014,Jan,11; 2005,Jul,11-12

80434 **Insulin tolerance panel; for ACTH insufficiency**
INCLUDES Cortisol x 5 (82533)
Glucose x 5 (82947)
0.00 0.00 FUD XXX
AMA: 2014,Jan,11; 2005,Jul,11-12

80435 **for growth hormone deficiency**
INCLUDES Glucose x 5 (82947)
Human growth hormone (HGH) x 5 (83003)
0.00 0.00 FUD XXX
AMA: 2014,Jan,11; 2005,Aug,9-10

80436 **Metyrapone panel**
INCLUDES 11 deoxycortisol x 2 (82634)
Cortisol x 2 (82533)
0.00 0.00 FUD XXX
AMA: 2014,Jan,11; 2005,Jul,11-12

80438 **Thyrotropin releasing hormone (TRH) stimulation panel; 1 hour**
INCLUDES Thyroid stimulating hormone (TSH) x 3 (84443)
0.00 0.00 FUD XXX
AMA: 2014,Jan,11; 2005,Jul,11-12

80439 **2 hour**
INCLUDES Thyroid stimulating hormone (TSH) x 4 (84443)
0.00 0.00 FUD XXX
AMA: 2014,Jan,11; 2005,Jul,11-12

80500-80502 Consultation By Clinical Pathologist

INCLUDES Pharmacokinetic consultations
Written report by pathologist for tests requiring additional medical judgment and requested by physician or other qualified health care professional
EXCLUDES *Consultations including patient examination*
Reporting code when medical interpretive assessment not provided

80500 **Clinical pathology consultation; limited, without review of patient's history and medical records**
0.56 0.65 FUD XXX
AMA: 2018,Jan,8; 2017,Jan,8; 2016,Jan,13; 2015,Jan,16

80502 **comprehensive, for a complex diagnostic problem, with review of patient's history and medical records**
2.02 2.11 FUD XXX
AMA: 2018,Jan,8; 2017,Jan,8; 2016,Jan,13; 2015,Jan,16

81000-81099 Urine Tests

81000 **Urinalysis, by dip stick or tablet reagent for bilirubin, glucose, hemoglobin, ketones, leukocytes, nitrite, pH, protein, specific gravity, urobilinogen, any number of these constituents; non-automated, with microscopy**
0.00 0.00 FUD XXX
AMA: 2018,Jul,14; 2018,Jan,8; 2017,Jan,8; 2016,Jan,13; 2015,Jan,16

81001 **automated, with microscopy**
0.00 0.00 FUD XXX
AMA: 2014,Jan,11; 2005,Jul,11-12

81002 **non-automated, without microscopy**
INCLUDES Mosenthal test
0.00 0.00 FUD XXX
AMA: 2018,Jan,8; 2017,Jan,8; 2016,Jan,13; 2015,Jan,16

81003 **automated, without microscopy**
0.00 0.00 FUD XXX
AMA: 2018,Jan,8; 2017,Jan,8; 2016,Jan,13; 2015,Jan,16

81005 **Urinalysis; qualitative or semiquantitative, except immunoassays**
INCLUDES Benedict test for dextrose
EXCLUDES *Immunoassay, qualitative or semiquantitative (83518)*
Microalbumin (82043-82044)
Nonimmunoassay reagent strip analysis (81000, 81002)
0.00 0.00 FUD XXX
AMA: 2018,Jan,8; 2017,Jan,8; 2016,Jan,13; 2015,Jan,16

81007 **bacteriuria screen, except by culture or dipstick**
EXCLUDES *Culture (87086-87088)*
Dipstick (81000, 81002)
0.00 0.00 FUD XXX
AMA: 2014,Jan,11; 2005,Jul,11-12

81015 **microscopic only**
EXCLUDES *Sperm evaluation for retrograde ejaculation (89331)*
0.00 0.00 FUD XXX
AMA: 2018,Jan,8; 2017,Nov,10

81020 **2 or 3 glass test**
INCLUDES Valentine's test
0.00 0.00 FUD XXX
AMA: 2014,Jan,11; 2005,Jul,11-12

81025 **Urine pregnancy test, by visual color comparison methods**
M ♀
0.00 0.00 FUD XXX
AMA: 2018,Jan,8; 2017,Jan,8; 2016,Jan,13; 2015,Jan,16

81050 **Volume measurement for timed collection, each**
0.00 0.00 FUD XXX
AMA: 2014,Jan,11; 2005,Jul,11-12

81099 **Unlisted urinalysis procedure**
0.00 0.00 FUD XXX
AMA: 2018,Jan,8; 2017,Jan,8; 2016,Jan,13; 2015,Jan,16

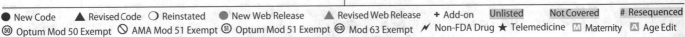

81105-81364 [81105, 81106, 81107, 81108, 81109, 81110, 81111, 81112, 81120, 81121, 81161, 81162, 81163, 81164, 81165, 81166, 81167, 81168, 81173, 81174, 81184, 81185, 81186, 81187, 81188, 81189, 81190, 81191, 81192, 81193, 81194, 81200, 81201, 81202, 81203, 81204, 81205, 81206, 81207, 81208, 81209, 81210, 81219, 81227, 81230, 81231, 81233, 81234, 81238, 81239, 81245, 81246, 81250, 81257, 81258, 81259, 81261, 81262, 81263, 81264, 81265, 81266, 81267, 81268, 81269, 81271, 81274, 81277, 81278, 81279, 81283, 81284, 81285, 81286, 81287, 81288, 81289, 81291, 81292, 81293, 81294, 81295, 81301, 81302, 81303, 81304, 81306, 81307, 81308, 81309, 81312, 81320, 81324, 81325, 81326, 81332, 81334, 81336, 81337, 81338, 81339, 81343, 81344, 81345, 81347, 81348, 81351, 81352, 81353, 81357, 81361, 81362, 81363, 81364] Gene Analysis: Tier 1 Procedures

INCLUDES All analytical procedures in evaluation:
- Amplification
- Cell lysis
- Detection
- Digestion
- Extraction
- Nucleic acid stabilization

Code selection based on specific gene being reviewed
Evaluation constitutional or somatic gene variations
Evaluation gene variant presence using common gene variant name
Gene specific and genomic testing
Generally, all listed gene variants in code description (lists not all inclusive)
Genes described using Human Genome Organization (HUGO) approved names
Protein or disease examples in code description not all inclusive
Qualitative results unless otherwise stated
Tier 1 molecular pathology codes (81105-81254 [81161, 81162, 81163, 81164, 81165, 81166, 81167, 81173, 81174, 81184, 81185, 81186, 81187, 81188, 81189, 81190, 81200, 81201, 81202, 81203, 81204, 81205, 81206, 81207, 81208, 81209, 81210, 81219, 81227, 81230, 81231, 81233, 81234, 81238, 81239, 81245, 81246, 81250, 81257, 81258, 81259, 81265, 81266, 81267, 81268, 81269, 81284, 81285, 81286, 81289, 81361, 81362, 81363, 81364])

EXCLUDES *Full gene sequencing using separate gene variant assessment codes unless specifically stated in code description*
In situ hybridization analyses (88271-88275, 88365-88368 [88364, 88373, 88374])
Microbial identification (87149-87153, 87471-87801 [87623, 87624, 87625], 87900-87904 [87906, 87910, 87912])
Other related gene variants not listed in code description
Tier 1 molecular pathology codes (81370-81383)
Tier 2 codes (81400-81408)
Unlisted molecular pathology procedures ([81479])

Code also modifier 26 when only interpretation and report performed
Code also services required before cell lysis

81105 **Resequenced code. See code before 81260.**

81106 **Resequenced code. See code before 81260.**

81107 **Resequenced code. See code before 81260.**

81108 **Resequenced code. See code before 81260.**

81109 **Resequenced code. See code before 81260.**

81110 **Resequenced code. See code before 81260.**

81111 **Resequenced code. See code before 81260.**

81112 **Resequenced code. See code before 81260.**

81120 **Resequenced code. See code before 81260.**

81121 **Resequenced code. See code before 81260.**

81161 **Resequenced code. See code following 81231.**

81162 **Resequenced code. See code following resequenced code 81210.**

81163 **Resequenced code. See code following resequenced code 81210.**

81164 **Resequenced code. See code before 81212.**

81165 **Resequenced code. See code following 81212.**

81166 **Resequenced code. See code following 81212.**

81167 **Resequenced code. See code following 81216.**

81168 **Resequenced code. See code before 81218.**

81170 ***ABL1 (ABL proto-oncogene 1, non-receptor tyrosine kinase)*** **(eg, acquired imatinib tyrosine kinase inhibitor resistance), gene analysis, variants in the kinase domain**
Facility RVU 0.00 Non-Facility RVU 0.00 FUD XXX A CCI
AMA: 2018,Jan,8; 2017,Jan,8; 2016,Aug,9

81171 ***AFF2 (AF4/FMR2 family, member 2 [FMR2])*** **(eg, fragile X mental retardation 2 [FRAXE]) gene analysis; evaluation to detect abnormal (eg, expanded) alleles**
Facility RVU 0.00 Non-Facility RVU 0.00 FUD XXX CCI

81172 **characterization of alleles (eg, expanded size and methylation status)**
Facility RVU 0.00 Non-Facility RVU 0.00 FUD XXX CCI

81173 **Resequenced code. See code following resequenced code 81204.**

81174 **Resequenced code. See code following resequenced code 81204.**

\# 81201 ***APC (adenomatous polyposis coli)*** **(eg, familial adenomatosis polyposis [FAP], attenuated FAP) gene analysis; full gene sequence**
Facility RVU 0.00 Non-Facility RVU 0.00 FUD XXX A CCI
AMA: 2020,OctSE,1; 2018,Nov,9; 2018,Jan,8; 2017,Jan,8; 2016,Aug,9; 2016,Jan,13; 2015,Jan,16

\# 81202 **known familial variants**
Facility RVU 0.00 Non-Facility RVU 0.00 FUD XXX A CCI
AMA: 2020,OctSE,1; 2018,Nov,9; 2018,Jan,8; 2017,Jan,8; 2016,Aug,9; 2016,Jan,13; 2015,Jan,16

\# 81203 **duplication/deletion variants**
Facility RVU 0.00 Non-Facility RVU 0.00 FUD XXX A CCI
AMA: 2020,OctSE,1; 2018,Nov,9; 2018,Jan,8; 2017,Jan,8; 2016,Aug,9; 2016,Jan,13; 2015,Jan,16

\# 81204 ***AR (androgen receptor)*** **(eg, spinal and bulbar muscular atrophy, Kennedy disease, X chromosome inactivation) gene analysis; characterization of alleles (eg, expanded size or methylation status)**
Facility RVU 0.00 Non-Facility RVU 0.00 FUD XXX CCI
AMA: 2020,OctSE,1; 2018,Nov,9

\# 81173 **full gene sequence**
Facility RVU 0.00 Non-Facility RVU 0.00 FUD XXX CCI

\# 81174 **known familial variant**
Facility RVU 0.00 Non-Facility RVU 0.00 FUD XXX CCI

\# 81200 ***ASPA (aspartoacylase)*** **(eg, Canavan disease) gene analysis, common variants (eg, E285A, Y231X)**
Facility RVU 0.00 Non-Facility RVU 0.00 FUD XXX A CCI
AMA: 2020,OctSE,1; 2018,Nov,9; 2018,Jan,8; 2017,Jan,8; 2016,Aug,9; 2016,Jan,13; 2015,Jan,16

81175 ***ASXL1 (additional sex combs like 1, transcriptional regulator)*** **(eg, myelodysplastic syndrome, myeloproliferative neoplasms, chronic myelomonocytic leukemia), gene analysis; full gene sequence**
Facility RVU 0.00 Non-Facility RVU 0.00 FUD XXX A CCI

81176 **targeted sequence analysis (eg, exon 12)**
Facility RVU 0.00 Non-Facility RVU 0.00 FUD XXX A CCI

81177 ***ATN1 (atrophin 1)*** **(eg, dentatorubral-pallidoluysian atrophy) gene analysis, evaluation to detect abnormal (eg, expanded) alleles**
Facility RVU 0.00 Non-Facility RVU 0.00 FUD XXX CCI

81178 ***ATXN1 (ataxin 1)*** **(eg, spinocerebellar ataxia) gene analysis, evaluation to detect abnormal (eg, expanded) alleles**
Facility RVU 0.00 Non-Facility RVU 0.00 FUD XXX CCI
AMA: 2019,Sep,7

81179 ***ATXN2 (ataxin 2)*** **(eg, spinocerebellar ataxia) gene analysis, evaluation to detect abnormal (eg, expanded) alleles**
0.00 0.00 FUD XXX
AMA: 2019,Sep,7

81180 ***ATXN3 (ataxin 3)*** **(eg, spinocerebellar ataxia, Machado-Joseph disease) gene analysis, evaluation to detect abnormal (eg, expanded) alleles**
0.00 0.00 FUD XXX
AMA: 2019,Sep,7

81181 ***ATXN7 (ataxin 7)*** **(eg, spinocerebellar ataxia) gene analysis, evaluation to detect abnormal (eg, expanded) alleles**
0.00 0.00 FUD XXX
AMA: 2019,Sep,7

81182 ***ATXN8OS (ATXN8 opposite strand [non-protein coding])*** **(eg, spinocerebellar ataxia) gene analysis, evaluation to detect abnormal (eg, expanded) alleles**
0.00 0.00 FUD XXX
AMA: 2019,Sep,7

81183 ***ATXN10 (ataxin 10)*** **(eg, spinocerebellar ataxia) gene analysis, evaluation to detect abnormal (eg, expanded) alleles**
0.00 0.00 FUD XXX
AMA: 2019,Sep,7

81184 **Resequenced code. See code following resequenced code 81233.**

81185 **Resequenced code. See code following resequenced code 81233.**

81186 **Resequenced code. See code following resequenced code 81233.**

81187 **Resequenced code. See code following resequenced code 81268.**

81188 **Resequenced code. See code following resequenced code 81266.**

81189 **Resequenced code. See code following resequenced code 81266.**

81190 **Resequenced code. See code following resequenced code 81266.**

81191 **Resequenced code. See code following numeric code 81312.**

81192 **Resequenced code. See code following numeric code 81312.**

81193 **Resequenced code. See code following numeric code 81312.**

81194 **Resequenced code. See code following numeric code 81312.**

81200 **Resequenced code. See code before 81175.**

81201 **Resequenced code. See code following code 81174.**

81202 **Resequenced code. See code following code 81174.**

81203 **Resequenced code. See code following code 81174.**

81204 **Resequenced code. See code following code 81174.**

81205 **Resequenced code. See code following code 81210.**

81206 **Resequenced code. See code following code 81210.**

81207 **Resequenced code. See code following code 81210.**

81208 **Resequenced code. See code following code 81210.**

81209 **Resequenced code. See code following code 81210.**

81210 **Resequenced code. See code following resequenced code 81209.**

\# **81205** ***BCKDHB (branched-chain keto acid dehydrogenase E1, beta polypeptide)*** **(eg, maple syrup urine disease) gene analysis, common variants (eg, R183P, G278S, E422X)**
0.00 0.00 FUD XXX A
AMA: 2020,OctSE,1; 2018,Nov,9; 2018,Jan,8; 2017,Jan,8; 2016,Aug,9; 2016,Jan,13; 2015,Jan,16

\# **81206** ***BCR/ABL1 (t(9;22))*** **(eg, chronic myelogenous leukemia) translocation analysis; major breakpoint, qualitative or quantitative**
0.00 0.00 FUD XXX A
AMA: 2020,OctSE,1; 2018,Nov,9; 2018,Jan,8; 2017,Jan,8; 2016,Aug,9; 2016,Jan,13; 2015,Jan,16

\# **81207** **minor breakpoint, qualitative or quantitative**
0.00 0.00 FUD XXX A
AMA: 2020,OctSE,1; 2018,Nov,9; 2018,Jan,8; 2017,Jan,8; 2016,Aug,9; 2016,Jan,13; 2015,Jan,16

\# **81208** **other breakpoint, qualitative or quantitative**
0.00 0.00 FUD XXX A
AMA: 2020,OctSE,1; 2018,Nov,9; 2018,Jan,8; 2017,Jan,8; 2016,Aug,9; 2016,Jan,13; 2015,Jan,16

\# **81209** ***BLM (Bloom syndrome, RecQ helicase-like)*** **(eg, Bloom syndrome) gene analysis, 2281del6ins7 variant**
0.00 0.00 FUD XXX A
AMA: 2020,OctSE,1; 2018,Nov,9; 2018,Jan,8; 2017,Jan,8; 2016,Aug,9; 2016,Jan,13; 2015,Jan,16

\# **81210** ***BRAF (B-Raf proto-oncogene, serine/threonine kinase)*** **(eg, colon cancer, melanoma), gene analysis, V600 variant(s)**
0.00 0.00 FUD XXX A
AMA: 2020,OctSE,1; 2018,Nov,9; 2018,Jan,8; 2017,Jan,8; 2016,Aug,9; 2016,Jan,13; 2015,Jan,16

\# **81162** ***BRCA1 (BRCA1, DNA repair associated), BRCA2 (BRCA2, DNA repair associated)*** **(eg, hereditary breast and ovarian cancer) gene analysis; full sequence analysis and full duplication/deletion analysis (ie, detection of large gene rearrangements)**

EXCLUDES *BRCA1 common duplication/deletion variant ([81479])*
BRCA1, BRCA2 full duplication/deletion analysis only (81164, 81166-81167, 81216)
BRCA1, BRCA2 full sequence analysis only (81163, 81165)
BRCA1, BRCA2 known familial variant only (81215, 81217)
Hereditary breast cancer genomic sequence analysis panel (81432)

0.00 0.00 FUD XXX A
AMA: 2019,May,5; 2018,Jan,8; 2017,Jan,8; 2016,Aug,9

\# **81163** **full sequence analysis**

EXCLUDES *BRCA1 common duplication/deletion variant ([81479])*
BRCA1, BRCA2 full duplication/deletion analysis only (81164, 81216)
BRCA1, BRCA2 full sequence analysis and full duplication/deletion analysis (81162)
BRCA1, BRCA2 full sequence analysis only (81165)
Hereditary breast cancer genomic sequence analysis panel (81432)

0.00 0.00 FUD XXX
AMA: 2019,May,5

\# **81164** **full duplication/deletion analysis (ie, detection of large gene rearrangements)**

EXCLUDES *BRCA1 common duplication/deletion variant ([81479])*
BRCA1, BRCA2 full sequence analysis and full duplication/deletion analysis (81162)
BRCA1, BRCA2 full sequence analysis only (81163)
BRCA1, BRCA2 full duplication/deletion analysis only (81166-81167)
BRCA1, BRCA2 known familial variant only (81217)

0.00 0.00 FUD XXX
AMA: 2019,May,5

81212 **185delAG, 5385insC, 6174delT variants**
0.00 0.00 FUD XXX A
AMA: 2020,OctSE,1; 2019,May,5; 2018,Nov,9; 2018,Jan,8; 2017,Jan,8; 2016,Aug,9; 2016,Jan,13; 2015,Jan,16

81165 **_BRCA1 (BRCA1, DNA repair associated)_ (eg, hereditary breast and ovarian cancer) gene analysis; full sequence analysis**

EXCLUDES *BRCA1 common duplication/deletion variant ([81479])*
BRCA1, BRCA2 full sequence analysis and full duplication/deletion analysis (81162)
BRCA1, BRCA2 full sequence analysis only (81163)
Hereditary breast cancer genomic sequence analysis panel (81432)

0.00 0.00 FUD XXX

AMA: 2019,May,5

81166 **full duplication/deletion analysis (ie, detection of large gene rearrangements)**

EXCLUDES *BRCA1 common duplication/deletion variant ([81479])*
BRCA1, BRCA2 full duplication/deletion analysis only (81164)
BRCA1, BRCA2 full sequence analysis and full duplication/deletion analysis (81162)

0.00 0.00 FUD XXX

AMA: 2019,May,5

81215 **known familial variant**

EXCLUDES *BRCA1 common duplication/deletion variant ([81479])*

0.00 0.00 FUD XXX

AMA: 2020,OctSE,1; 2019,May,5; 2018,Nov,9; 2018,Jan,8; 2017,Jan,8; 2016,Aug,9; 2016,Jan,13; 2015,Jan,16

81216 **_BRCA2 (BRCA2, DNA repair associated)_ (eg, hereditary breast and ovarian cancer) gene analysis; full sequence analysis**

EXCLUDES *BRCA1, BRCA2 full sequence analysis only (81163)*
BRCA1, BRCA2 full sequence analysis and full duplication/deletion analysis (81162)
Hereditary breast cancer genomic sequence analysis panel (81432)

0.00 0.00 FUD XXX

AMA: 2020,OctSE,1; 2019,May,5; 2018,Nov,9; 2018,Jan,8; 2017,Jan,8; 2016,Aug,9; 2016,Jan,13; 2015,Jan,16

81167 **full duplication/deletion analysis (ie, detection of large gene rearrangements)**

EXCLUDES *BRCA1, BRCA2 full duplication/deletion analysis only (81164, 81167)*
BRCA1, BRCA2 full sequence analysis and full duplication/deletion analysis (81162)

0.00 0.00 FUD XXX

AMA: 2019,May,5

81217 **known familial variant**

EXCLUDES *BRCA1, BRCA2 full duplication/deletion analysis only (81164, 81167)*
BRCA1, BRCA2 full sequence analysis and full duplication/deletion analysis (81162)

0.00 0.00 FUD XXX

AMA: 2020,OctSE,1; 2019,May,5; 2018,Nov,9; 2018,Jan,8; 2017,Jan,8; 2016,Aug,9; 2016,Jan,13; 2015,Jan,16

81233 **_BTK (Bruton's tyrosine kinase)_ (eg, chronic lymphocytic leukemia) gene analysis, common variants (eg, C481S, C481R, C481F)**

0.00 0.00 FUD XXX

AMA: 2020,OctSE,1; 2018,Nov,9

81184 **_CACNA1A (calcium voltage-gated channel subunit alpha1 A)_ (eg, spinocerebellar ataxia) gene analysis; evaluation to detect abnormal (eg, expanded) alleles**

0.00 0.00 FUD XXX

81185 **full gene sequence**

0.00 0.00 FUD XXX

81186 **known familial variant**

0.00 0.00 FUD XXX

81219 **_CALR (calreticulin)_ (eg, myeloproliferative disorders), gene analysis, common variants in exon 9**

0.00 0.00 FUD XXX

AMA: 2020,OctSE,1; 2018,Nov,9; 2018,Jan,8; 2017,Jan,8; 2016,Aug,9

● # 81168 **_CCND1/IGH (t(11;14))_ (eg, mantle cell lymphoma) translocation analysis, major breakpoint, qualitative and quantitative, if performed**

0.00 0.00 FUD 000

81218 **_CEBPA (CCAAT/enhancer binding protein [C/EBP], alpha)_ (eg, acute myeloid leukemia), gene analysis, full gene sequence**

0.00 0.00 FUD XXX

AMA: 2020,OctSE,1; 2018,Nov,9; 2018,Jan,8; 2017,Jan,8; 2016,Aug,9

81219 **Resequenced code. See code before 81218.**

81220 **_CFTR (cystic fibrosis transmembrane conductance regulator)_ (eg, cystic fibrosis) gene analysis; common variants (eg, ACMG/ACOG guidelines)**

EXCLUDES *Excludes Intron 8 poly-T analysis performed in conjunction with 81220 in R117H positive patient*

0.00 0.00 FUD XXX

AMA: 2020,OctSE,1; 2018,Nov,9; 2018,Jan,8; 2017,Jan,8; 2016,Aug,9; 2016,Jan,13; 2015,Jan,16

81221 **known familial variants**

0.00 0.00 FUD XXX

AMA: 2020,OctSE,1; 2018,Nov,9; 2018,Jan,8; 2017,Jan,8; 2016,Aug,9; 2016,Jan,13; 2015,Jan,16

81222 **duplication/deletion variants**

0.00 0.00 FUD XXX

AMA: 2020,OctSE,1; 2018,Nov,9; 2018,Jan,8; 2017,Jan,8; 2016,Aug,9; 2016,Jan,13; 2015,Jan,16

81223 **full gene sequence**

0.00 0.00 FUD XXX

AMA: 2020,OctSE,1; 2018,Nov,9; 2018,Jan,8; 2017,Jan,8; 2016,Aug,9; 2016,Jan,13; 2015,Jan,16

81224 **intron 8 poly-T analysis (eg, male infertility)**

0.00 0.00 FUD XXX

AMA: 2020,OctSE,1; 2018,Nov,9; 2018,Jan,8; 2017,Jan,8; 2016,Aug,9; 2016,Jan,13; 2015,Jan,16

81267 **Chimerism (engraftment) analysis, post transplantation specimen (eg, hematopoietic stem cell), includes comparison to previously performed baseline analyses; without cell selection**

0.00 0.00 FUD XXX

AMA: 2020,OctSE,1; 2018,Nov,9; 2018,Jan,8; 2017,Jan,8; 2016,Aug,9; 2016,Jan,13; 2015,Jan,16

81268 **with cell selection (eg, CD3, CD33), each cell type**

0.00 0.00 FUD XXX

AMA: 2020,OctSE,1; 2018,Nov,9; 2018,Jan,8; 2017,Jan,8; 2016,Aug,9; 2016,Jan,13; 2015,Jan,16

81187 **_CNBP (CCHC-type zinc finger nucleic acid binding protein)_ (eg, myotonic dystrophy type 2) gene analysis, evaluation to detect abnormal (eg, expanded) alleles**

0.00 0.00 FUD XXX

81265 **Comparative analysis using Short Tandem Repeat (STR) markers; patient and comparative specimen (eg, pre-transplant recipient and donor germline testing, post-transplant non-hematopoietic recipient germline [eg, buccal swab or other germline tissue sample] and donor testing, twin zygosity testing, or maternal cell contamination of fetal cells)**

0.00 0.00 FUD XXX

AMA: 2020,OctSE,1; 2018,Nov,9; 2018,Jan,8; 2017,Jan,8; 2016,Aug,9; 2016,Jan,13; 2015,Jan,16

+ # 81266 **each additional specimen (eg, additional cord blood donor, additional fetal samples from different cultures, or additional zygosity in multiple birth pregnancies) (List separately in addition to code for primary procedure)**

0.00 0.00 FUD XXX

AMA: 2020,OctSE,1; 2018,Nov,9; 2018,Jan,8; 2017,Jan,8; 2016,Aug,9; 2016,Jan,13; 2015,Jan,16

\# 81188 *CSTB (cystatin B)* (eg, Unverricht-Lundborg disease) gene analysis; evaluation to detect abnormal (eg, expanded) alleles
🚑 0.00 ⚕ 0.00 **FUD** XXX ▣

\# 81189 full gene sequence
🚑 0.00 ⚕ 0.00 **FUD** XXX ▣

\# 81190 known familial variant(s)
🚑 0.00 ⚕ 0.00 **FUD** XXX ▣

\# 81227 *CYP2C9 (cytochrome P450, family 2, subfamily C, polypeptide 9)* (eg, drug metabolism), gene analysis, common variants (eg, *2, *3, *5, *6)
🚑 0.00 ⚕ 0.00 **FUD** XXX A ▣
AMA: 2020,OctSE,1; 2018,Nov,9; 2018,Jan,8; 2017,Jan,8; 2016,Aug,9; 2016,Jan,13; 2015,Jan,16

81225 *CYP2C19 (cytochrome P450, family 2, subfamily C, polypeptide 19)* (eg, drug metabolism), gene analysis, common variants (eg, *2, *3, *4, *8, *17)
🚑 0.00 ⚕ 0.00 **FUD** XXX A ▣
AMA: 2020,OctSE,1; 2018,Nov,9; 2018,Jan,8; 2017,Jan,8; 2016,Aug,9; 2016,Jan,13; 2015,Jan,16

81226 *CYP2D6 (cytochrome P450, family 2, subfamily D, polypeptide 6)* (eg, drug metabolism), gene analysis, common variants (eg, *2, *3, *4, *5, *6, *9, *10, *17, *19, *29, *35, *41, *1XN, *2XN, *4XN)
🚑 0.00 ⚕ 0.00 **FUD** XXX A ▣
AMA: 2020,OctSE,1; 2018,Nov,9; 2018,Jan,8; 2017,Jan,8; 2016,Aug,9; 2016,Jan,13; 2015,Jan,16

81227 **Resequenced code. See code following resequenced code 81190.**

\# 81230 *CYP3A4 (cytochrome P450 family 3 subfamily A member 4)* (eg, drug metabolism), gene analysis, common variant(s) (eg, *2, *22)
🚑 0.00 ⚕ 0.00 **FUD** XXX A ▣
AMA: 2020,OctSE,1; 2018,Nov,9

\# 81231 *CYP3A5 (cytochrome P450 family 3 subfamily A member 5)* (eg, drug metabolism), gene analysis, common variants (eg, *2, *3, *4, *5, *6, *7)
🚑 0.00 ⚕ 0.00 **FUD** XXX A ▣
AMA: 2020,OctSE,1; 2018,Nov,9

81228 Cytogenomic constitutional (genome-wide) microarray analysis; interrogation of genomic regions for copy number variants (eg, bacterial artificial chromosome [BAC] or oligo-based comparative genomic hybridization [CGH] microarray analysis)
EXCLUDES *Analyte-specific molecular pathology procedures included in microarray analysis*
When performed in conjunction with single nucleotide polymorphism interrogation (81229)
🚑 0.00 ⚕ 0.00 **FUD** XXX A ▣
AMA: 2020,OctSE,1; 2018,Nov,9; 2018,Jan,8; 2017,Apr,3; 2017,Jan,8; 2016,Aug,9; 2016,Jan,13; 2015,Jan,16

81229 interrogation of genomic regions for copy number and single nucleotide polymorphism (SNP) variants for chromosomal abnormalities
EXCLUDES *Analyte-specific molecular pathology procedures included in microarray analysis*
Copy number variant detection using oligonucleotide interrogation only (81228)
Fetal genomic sequencing or other molecular multianalyte assays using circulating cell-free DNA in maternal blood ([81479], 81420, 81422)
Molecular cytogenetics; DNA probe (88271)
Specific code for targeted cytogenomic constitutional microarray analysis
Unlisted molecular pathology procedures ([81479])
🚑 0.00 ⚕ 0.00 **FUD** XXX A ▣
AMA: 2020,OctSE,1; 2018,Nov,9; 2018,Jan,8; 2017,Apr,3; 2017,Jan,8; 2016,Aug,9; 2016,Jan,13; 2015,Jan,16

\# 81277 Cytogenomic neoplasia (genome-wide) microarray analysis, interrogation of genomic regions for copy number and loss-of-heterozygosity variants for chromosomal abnormalities
EXCLUDES *Analyte-specific molecular pathology procedures included in microarray analysis for neoplasia*
Molecular cytogenetics; DNA probe (88271)
🚑 0.00 ⚕ 0.00 **FUD** XXX ▣
AMA: 2020,OctSE,1; 2020,Feb,10

81230 **Resequenced code. See code following code 81227.**

81231 **Resequenced code. See code following code 81227.**

\# 81161 *DMD (dystrophin)* (eg, Duchenne/Becker muscular dystrophy) deletion analysis, and duplication analysis, if performed
🚑 0.00 ⚕ 0.00 **FUD** XXX A ▣
AMA: 2020,OctSE,1; 2018,Nov,9; 2018,Jan,8; 2017,Jan,8; 2016,Aug,9

\# 81234 *DMPK (DM1 protein kinase)* (eg, myotonic dystrophy type 1) gene analysis; evaluation to detect abnormal (expanded) alleles
🚑 0.00 ⚕ 0.00 **FUD** XXX ▣
AMA: 2020,OctSE,1; 2018,Nov,9

\# 81239 characterization of alleles (eg, expanded size)
🚑 0.00 ⚕ 0.00 **FUD** XXX ▣
AMA: 2020,OctSE,1; 2018,Nov,9

81232 *DPYD (dihydropyrimidine dehydrogenase)* (eg, 5-fluorouracil/5-FU and capecitabine drug metabolism), gene analysis, common variant(s) (eg, *2A, *4, *5, *6)
🚑 0.00 ⚕ 0.00 **FUD** XXX A ▣
AMA: 2020,OctSE,1; 2018,Nov,9

81233 **Resequenced code. See code following 81217.**

81234 **Resequenced code. See code following code 81231.**

81235 *EGFR (epidermal growth factor receptor)* (eg, non-small cell lung cancer) gene analysis, common variants (eg, exon 19 LREA deletion, L858R, T790M, G719A, G719S, L861Q)
🚑 0.00 ⚕ 0.00 **FUD** XXX A ▣
AMA: 2020,OctSE,1; 2018,Nov,9; 2018,Jan,8; 2017,Jan,8; 2016,Aug,9; 2016,Jan,13; 2015,Jan,16

81236 *EZH2 (enhancer of zeste 2 polycomb repressive complex 2 subunit)* (eg, myelodysplastic syndrome, myeloproliferative neoplasms) gene analysis, full gene sequence
🚑 0.00 ⚕ 0.00 **FUD** XXX ▣
AMA: 2020,OctSE,1; 2019,Jul,3; 2018,Nov,9

81237 *EZH2 (enhancer of zeste 2 polycomb repressive complex 2 subunit)* (eg, diffuse large B-cell lymphoma) gene analysis, common variant(s) (eg, codon 646)
🚑 0.00 ⚕ 0.00 **FUD** XXX ▣
AMA: 2020,OctSE,1; 2019,Jul,3; 2018,Nov,9

81238 **Resequenced code. See code following 81241.**

81239 **Resequenced code. See code before 81232.**

81240 *F2 (prothrombin, coagulation factor II)* (eg, hereditary hypercoagulability) gene analysis, 20210G>A variant
🚑 0.00 ⚕ 0.00 **FUD** XXX A ▣
AMA: 2020,OctSE,1; 2018,Nov,9; 2018,Jan,8; 2017,Jan,8; 2016,Aug,9; 2016,Jan,13; 2015,Jan,16

81241 *F5 (coagulation factor V)* (eg, hereditary hypercoagulability) gene analysis, Leiden variant
🚑 0.00 ⚕ 0.00 **FUD** XXX A ▣
AMA: 2020,OctSE,1; 2018,Nov,9; 2018,Jan,8; 2017,Jan,8; 2016,Aug,9; 2016,Jan,13; 2015,Jan,16

\# 81238 *F9 (coagulation factor IX)* (eg, hemophilia B), full gene sequence
🚑 0.00 ⚕ 0.00 **FUD** XXX A ▣
AMA: 2020,OctSE,1; 2018,Nov,9

● New Code ▲ Revised Code ○ Reinstated ● New Web Release ▲ Revised Web Release + Add-on Unlisted Not Covered # Resequenced
50 Optum Mod 50 Exempt ⊘ AMA Mod 51 Exempt 51 Optum Mod 51 Exempt 63 Mod 63 Exempt ✗ Non-FDA Drug ★ Telemedicine M Maternity A Age Edit

81242 ***FANCC (Fanconi anemia, complementation group C)*** **(eg, Fanconi anemia, type C) gene analysis, common variant (eg, IVS4+4A>T)**
0.00 0.00 FUD XXX
AMA: 2020,OctSE,1; 2018,Nov,9; 2018,Jan,8; 2017,Jan,8; 2016,Aug,9; 2016,Jan,13; 2015,Jan,16

\# **81245** ***FLT3 (fms-related tyrosine kinase 3)*** **(eg, acute myeloid leukemia), gene analysis; internal tandem duplication (ITD) variants (ie, exons 14, 15)**
0.00 0.00 FUD XXX
AMA: 2020,OctSE,1; 2018,Nov,9; 2018,Jan,8; 2017,Jan,8; 2016,Aug,9; 2016,Jan,13; 2015,Jan,16; 2015,Jan,3

\# **81246** **tyrosine kinase domain (TKD) variants (eg, D835, I836)**
0.00 0.00 FUD XXX
AMA: 2020,OctSE,1; 2018,Nov,9; 2018,Jan,8; 2017,Jan,8; 2016,Aug,9; 2016,Jan,13; 2015,Jan,3

81243 ***FMR1 (fragile X mental retardation 1)*** **(eg, fragile X mental retardation) gene analysis; evaluation to detect abnormal (eg, expanded) alleles**
INCLUDES Evaluation to detect and characterize abnormal alleles using single assay [i.e., PCR]
EXCLUDES *Evaluation to detect and characterize abnormal alleles (81244)*
0.00 0.00 FUD XXX
AMA: 2020,OctSE,1; 2019,Jul,3; 2018,Nov,9; 2018,Jan,8; 2017,Jan,8; 2016,Aug,9; 2016,Jan,13; 2015,Jan,16

81244 **characterization of alleles (eg, expanded size and promoter methylation status)**
EXCLUDES *Evaluation to detect and characterize abnormal alleles using single assay [i.e., PCR] (81243)*
0.00 0.00 FUD XXX
AMA: 2020,OctSE,1; 2019,Jul,3; 2018,Nov,9; 2018,Jan,8; 2017,Jan,8; 2016,Aug,9; 2016,Jan,13; 2015,Jan,16

81245 **Resequenced code. See code following 81242.**

81246 **Resequenced code. See code following 81242.**

\# **81284** ***FXN (frataxin)*** **(eg, Friedreich ataxia) gene analysis; evaluation to detect abnormal (expanded) alleles**
0.00 0.00 FUD XXX
AMA: 2020,OctSE,1; 2018,Nov,9

\# **81285** **characterization of alleles (eg, expanded size)**
0.00 0.00 FUD XXX
AMA: 2020,OctSE,1; 2018,Nov,9

\# **81286** **full gene sequence**
0.00 0.00 FUD XXX
AMA: 2020,OctSE,1; 2018,Nov,9

\# **81289** **known familial variant(s)**
0.00 0.00 FUD XXX
AMA: 2020,OctSE,1; 2018,Nov,9

\# **81250** ***G6PC (glucose-6-phosphatase, catalytic subunit)*** **(eg, Glycogen storage disease, type 1a, von Gierke disease) gene analysis, common variants (eg, R83C, Q347X)**
0.00 0.00 FUD XXX
AMA: 2020,OctSE,1; 2018,Nov,9; 2018,Jan,8; 2017,Jan,8; 2016,Aug,9; 2016,Jan,13; 2015,Jan,16

81247 ***G6PD (glucose-6-phosphate dehydrogenase)*** **(eg, hemolytic anemia, jaundice), gene analysis; common variant(s) (eg, A, A-)**
0.00 0.00 FUD XXX
AMA: 2020,OctSE,1; 2018,Nov,9

81248 **known familial variant(s)**
0.00 0.00 FUD XXX
AMA: 2020,OctSE,1; 2018,Nov,9

81249 **full gene sequence**
0.00 0.00 FUD XXX
AMA: 2020,OctSE,1; 2018,Nov,9

81250 **Resequenced code. See code before 81247.**

81251 ***GBA (glucosidase, beta, acid)*** **(eg, Gaucher disease) gene analysis, common variants (eg, N370S, 84GG, L444P, IVS2+1G>A)**
0.00 0.00 FUD XXX
AMA: 2020,OctSE,1; 2018,Nov,9; 2018,Jan,8; 2017,Jan,8; 2016,Aug,9; 2016,Jan,13; 2015,Jan,16

81252 ***GJB2 (gap junction protein, beta 2, 26kDa, connexin 26)*** **(eg, nonsyndromic hearing loss) gene analysis; full gene sequence**
0.00 0.00 FUD XXX
AMA: 2020,OctSE,1; 2018,Nov,9; 2018,Jan,8; 2017,Jan,8; 2016,Aug,9; 2016,Jan,13; 2015,Jan,16

81253 **known familial variants**
0.00 0.00 FUD XXX
AMA: 2020,OctSE,1; 2018,Nov,9; 2018,Jan,8; 2017,Jan,8; 2016,Aug,9; 2016,Jan,13; 2015,Jan,16

81254 ***GJB6 (gap junction protein, beta 6, 30kDa, connexin 30)*** **(eg, nonsyndromic hearing loss) gene analysis, common variants (eg, 309kb [del(GJB6-D13S1830)] and 232kb [del(GJB6-D13S1854)])**
0.00 0.00 FUD XXX
AMA: 2020,OctSE,1; 2018,Nov,9; 2018,Jan,8; 2017,Jan,8; 2016,Aug,9; 2016,Jan,13; 2015,Jan,16

\# **81257** ***HBA1/HBA2 (alpha globin 1 and alpha globin 2)*** **(eg, alpha thalassemia, Hb Bart hydrops fetalis syndrome, HbH disease), gene analysis; common deletions or variant (eg, Southeast Asian, Thai, Filipino, Mediterranean, alpha3.7, alpha4.2, alpha20.5, Constant Spring)**
0.00 0.00 FUD XXX
AMA: 2020,OctSE,1; 2018,Nov,9; 2018,Jan,8; 2017,Jan,8; 2016,Aug,9; 2016,Jan,13; 2015,Jan,16

\# **81258** **known familial variant**
0.00 0.00 FUD XXX
AMA: 2020,OctSE,1; 2018,Nov,9

\# **81259** **full gene sequence**
0.00 0.00 FUD XXX
AMA: 2020,OctSE,1; 2018,Nov,9

\# **81269** **duplication/deletion variants**
0.00 0.00 FUD XXX
AMA: 2020,OctSE,1; 2018,Nov,9

\# **81361** ***HBB (hemoglobin, subunit beta)*** **(eg, sickle cell anemia, beta thalassemia, hemoglobinopathy); common variant(s) (eg, HbS, HbC, HbE)**
0.00 0.00 FUD XXX
AMA: 2020,OctSE,1; 2018,Nov,9

\# **81362** **known familial variant(s)**
0.00 0.00 FUD XXX
AMA: 2020,OctSE,1; 2018,Nov,9

\# **81363** **duplication/deletion variant(s)**
0.00 0.00 FUD XXX
AMA: 2020,OctSE,1; 2018,Nov,9; 2018,Sep,14

\# **81364** **full gene sequence**
0.00 0.00 FUD XXX
AMA: 2020,OctSE,1; 2018,Nov,9; 2018,Sep,14

81255 ***HEXA (hexosaminidase A [alpha polypeptide])*** **(eg, Tay-Sachs disease) gene analysis, common variants (eg, 1278insTATC, 1421+1G>C, G269S)**
0.00 0.00 FUD XXX
AMA: 2020,OctSE,1; 2018,Nov,9; 2018,Jan,8; 2017,Jan,8; 2016,Aug,9; 2016,Jan,13; 2015,Jan,16

81256 ***HFE (hemochromatosis)*** **(eg, hereditary hemochromatosis) gene analysis, common variants (eg, C282Y, H63D)**
0.00 0.00 FUD XXX
AMA: 2020,OctSE,1; 2018,Nov,9; 2018,Jan,8; 2017,Jan,8; 2016,Aug,9; 2016,Jan,13; 2015,Jan,16

81257 **Resequenced code. See code following 81254.**

81258 **Resequenced code. See code following 81254.**

81259 **Resequenced code. See code following 81254.**

\# **81271** *HTT (huntingtin)* (eg, Huntington disease) gene analysis; evaluation to detect abnormal (eg, expanded) alleles
0.00 0.00 FUD XXX
AMA: 2020,OctSE,1; 2018,Nov,9

\# **81274** characterization of alleles (eg, expanded size)
0.00 0.00 FUD XXX
AMA: 2020,OctSE,1; 2018,Nov,9

\# **81105** *Human Platelet Antigen 1 genotyping (HPA-1), ITGB3 (integrin, beta 3 [platelet glycoprotein IIIa], antigen CD61 [GPIIIa])* (eg, neonatal alloimmune thrombocytopenia [NAIT], post-transfusion purpura), gene analysis, common variant, HPA-1a/b (L33P)
0.00 0.00 FUD XXX

\# **81106** *Human Platelet Antigen 2 genotyping (HPA-2), GP1BA (glycoprotein Ib [platelet], alpha polypeptide [GPIba])* (eg, neonatal alloimmune thrombocytopenia [NAIT], post-transfusion purpura), gene analysis, common variant, HPA-2a/b (T145M)
0.00 0.00 FUD XXX

\# **81107** *Human Platelet Antigen 3 genotyping (HPA-3), ITGA2B (integrin, alpha 2b [platelet glycoprotein IIb of IIb/IIIa complex], antigen CD41 [GPIIb])* (eg, neonatal alloimmune thrombocytopenia [NAIT], post-transfusion purpura), gene analysis, common variant, HPA-3a/b (I843S)
0.00 0.00 FUD XXX

\# **81108** *Human Platelet Antigen 4 genotyping (HPA-4), ITGB3 (integrin, beta 3 [platelet glycoprotein IIIa], antigen CD61 [GPIIIa])* (eg, neonatal alloimmune thrombocytopenia [NAIT], post-transfusion purpura), gene analysis, common variant, HPA-4a/b (R143Q)
0.00 0.00 FUD XXX

\# **81109** *Human Platelet Antigen 5 genotyping (HPA-5), ITGA2 (integrin, alpha 2 [CD49B, alpha 2 subunit of VLA-2 receptor] [GPIa])* (eg, neonatal alloimmune thrombocytopenia [NAIT], post-transfusion purpura), gene analysis, common variant (eg, HPA-5a/b (K505E))
0.00 0.00 FUD XXX

\# **81110** *Human Platelet Antigen 6 genotyping (HPA-6w), ITGB3 (integrin, beta 3 [platelet glycoprotein IIIa, antigen CD61] [GPIIIa])* (eg, neonatal alloimmune thrombocytopenia [NAIT], post-transfusion purpura), gene analysis, common variant, HPA-6a/b (R489Q)
0.00 0.00 FUD XXX

\# **81111** *Human Platelet Antigen 9 genotyping (HPA-9w), ITGA2B (integrin, alpha 2b [platelet glycoprotein IIb of IIb/IIIa complex, antigen CD41] [GPIIb])* (eg, neonatal alloimmune thrombocytopenia [NAIT], post-transfusion purpura), gene analysis, common variant, HPA-9a/b (V837M)
0.00 0.00 FUD XXX

\# **81112** *Human Platelet Antigen 15 genotyping (HPA-15), CD109 (CD109 molecule)* (eg, neonatal alloimmune thrombocytopenia [NAIT], post-transfusion purpura), gene analysis, common variant, HPA-15a/b (S682Y)
0.00 0.00 FUD XXX

\# **81120** *IDH1 (isocitrate dehydrogenase 1 [NADP+], soluble)* (eg, glioma), common variants (eg, R132H, R132C)
0.00 0.00 FUD XXX

\# **81121** *IDH2 (isocitrate dehydrogenase 2 [NADP+], mitochondrial)* (eg, glioma), common variants (eg, R140W, R172M)
0.00 0.00 FUD XXX

\# **81283** *IFNL3 (interferon, lambda 3)* (eg, drug response), gene analysis, rs12979860 variant
0.00 0.00 FUD XXX
AMA: 2020,OctSE,1; 2018,Nov,9

\# **81261** *IGH@ (Immunoglobulin heavy chain locus)* (eg, leukemias and lymphomas, B-cell), gene rearrangement analysis to detect abnormal clonal population(s); amplified methodology (eg, polymerase chain reaction)
0.00 0.00 FUD XXX
AMA: 2020,OctSE,1; 2018,Nov,9; 2018,Jan,8; 2017,Jan,8; 2016,Aug,9; 2016,Jan,13; 2015,Jan,16

\# **81262** direct probe methodology (eg, Southern blot)
0.00 0.00 FUD XXX
AMA: 2020,OctSE,1; 2018,Nov,9; 2018,Jan,8; 2017,Jan,8; 2016,Aug,9; 2016,Jan,13; 2015,Jan,16

\# **81263** *IGH@ (Immunoglobulin heavy chain locus)* (eg, leukemia and lymphoma, B-cell), variable region somatic mutation analysis
0.00 0.00 FUD XXX
AMA: 2020,OctSE,1; 2018,Nov,9; 2018,Jan,8; 2017,Jan,8; 2016,Aug,9; 2016,Jan,13; 2015,Jan,16

● # **81278** *IGH@/BCL2 (t(14;18))* (eg, follicular lymphoma) translocation analysis, major breakpoint region (MBR) and minor cluster region (mcr) breakpoints, qualitative or quantitative
0.00 0.00 FUD 000

\# **81264** *IGK@ (Immunoglobulin kappa light chain locus)* (eg, leukemia and lymphoma, B-cell), gene rearrangement analysis, evaluation to detect abnormal clonal population(s)
0.00 0.00 FUD XXX
AMA: 2020,OctSE,1; 2018,Nov,9; 2018,Jan,8; 2017,Jan,8; 2016,Aug,9; 2016,Jan,13; 2015,Jan,16

81260 *IKBKAP (inhibitor of kappa light polypeptide gene enhancer in B-cells, kinase complex-associated protein)* (eg, familial dysautonomia) gene analysis, common variants (eg, 2507+6T>C, R696P)
0.00 0.00 FUD XXX
AMA: 2020,OctSE,1; 2018,Nov,9; 2018,Jan,8; 2017,Jan,8; 2016,Aug,9; 2016,Jan,13; 2015,Jan,16

81261 **Resequenced code. See code before 81260.**

81262 **Resequenced code. See code before 81260.**

81263 **Resequenced code. See code following resequenced code 81262.**

81264 **Resequenced code. See code before 81260.**

81265 **Resequenced code. See code following resequenced code 81187.**

81266 **Resequenced code. See code following resequenced code 81265.**

81267 **Resequenced code. See code following 81224.**

81268 **Resequenced code. See code following 81224.**

81269 **Resequenced code. See code following resequenced code 81259.**

81270 *JAK2 (Janus kinase 2)* (eg, myeloproliferative disorder) gene analysis, p.Val617Phe (V617F) variant
0.00 0.00 FUD XXX
AMA: 2020,OctSE,1; 2018,Nov,9; 2018,Jan,8; 2017,Jan,8; 2016,Aug,9; 2016,Jan,13; 2015,Jan,16

● # **81279** *JAK2 (Janus kinase 2)* (eg, myeloproliferative disorder) targeted sequence analysis (eg, exons 12 and 13)
0.00 0.00 FUD 000

81271 **Resequenced code. See code following code 81259.**

81272 *KIT (v-kit Hardy-Zuckerman 4 feline sarcoma viral oncogene homolog)* (eg, gastrointestinal stromal tumor [GIST], acute myeloid leukemia, melanoma), gene analysis, targeted sequence analysis (eg, exons 8, 11, 13, 17, 18)
0.00 0.00 FUD XXX
AMA: 2020,OctSE,1; 2018,Nov,9; 2018,Jan,8; 2017,Jan,8; 2016,Aug,9

81273 ***KIT (v-kit Hardy-Zuckerman 4 feline sarcoma viral oncogene homolog)*** **(eg, mastocytosis), gene analysis, D816 variant**
0.00 0.00 FUD XXX
AMA: 2020,OctSE,1; 2018,Nov,9; 2018,Jan,8; 2017,Jan,8; 2016,Aug,9

81274 **Resequenced code. See code following resequenced code 81271.**

81275 ***KRAS (Kirsten rat sarcoma viral oncogene homolog)*** **(eg, carcinoma) gene analysis; variants in exon 2 (eg, codons 12 and 13)**
0.00 0.00 FUD XXX
AMA: 2020,OctSE,1; 2018,Nov,9; 2018,Jan,8; 2017,Jan,8; 2016,Aug,9; 2016,Jan,13; 2015,Jan,16

81276 **additional variant(s) (eg, codon 61, codon 146)**
0.00 0.00 FUD XXX
AMA: 2020,OctSE,1; 2018,Nov,9; 2018,Jan,8; 2017,Jan,8; 2016,Aug,9

81277 **Resequenced code. See code following 81229.**

81278 **Resequenced code. See code following resequenced code 81263.**

81279 **Resequenced code. See code following 81270.**

81283 **Resequenced code. See code following resequenced code 81121.**

81284 **Resequenced code. See code following code 81246.**

81285 **Resequenced code. See code following code 81246.**

81286 **Resequenced code. See code following code 81246.**

81287 **Resequenced code. See code following resequenced code 81304.**

81288 **Resequenced code. See code following resequenced code 81292.**

81289 **Resequenced code. See code following code 81246.**

81290 ***MCOLN1 (mucolipin 1)*** **(eg, Mucolipidosis, type IV) gene analysis, common variants (eg, IVS3-2A>G, del6.4kb)**
0.00 0.00 FUD XXX
AMA: 2020,OctSE,1; 2018,Nov,9; 2018,Jan,8; 2017,Jan,8; 2016,Aug,9; 2016,Jan,13; 2015,Jan,16

\# **81302** ***MECP2 (methyl CpG binding protein 2)*** **(eg, Rett syndrome) gene analysis; full sequence analysis**
0.00 0.00 FUD XXX
AMA: 2020,OctSE,1; 2018,Nov,9; 2018,Jan,8; 2017,Jan,8; 2016,Aug,9; 2016,Jan,13; 2015,Jan,16

\# **81303** **known familial variant**
0.00 0.00 FUD XXX
AMA: 2020,OctSE,1; 2018,Nov,9; 2018,Jan,8; 2017,Jan,8; 2016,Aug,9; 2016,Jan,13; 2015,Jan,16

\# **81304** **duplication/deletion variants**
0.00 0.00 FUD XXX
AMA: 2020,OctSE,1; 2018,Nov,9; 2018,Jan,8; 2017,Jan,8; 2016,Aug,9; 2016,Jan,13; 2015,Jan,16

\# **81287** ***MGMT (O-6-methylguanine-DNA methyltransferase)*** **(eg, glioblastoma multiforme), promoter methylation analysis**
0.00 0.00 FUD XXX
AMA: 2020,OctSE,1; 2019,Jul,3; 2018,Dec,10; 2018,Dec,10; 2018,Nov,9; 2018,Jan,8; 2017,Jan,8; 2016,Aug,9

\# **81301** **Microsatellite instability analysis (eg, hereditary non-polyposis colorectal cancer, Lynch syndrome) of markers for mismatch repair deficiency (eg, BAT25, BAT26), includes comparison of neoplastic and normal tissue, if performed**
0.00 0.00 FUD XXX
AMA: 2020,OctSE,1; 2018,Nov,9; 2018,Jan,8; 2017,Jan,8; 2016,Aug,9; 2016,Jan,13; 2015,Jan,16

\# **81292** ***MLH1 (mutL homolog 1, colon cancer, nonpolyposis type 2)*** **(eg, hereditary non-polyposis colorectal cancer, Lynch syndrome) gene analysis; full sequence analysis**
0.00 0.00 FUD XXX
AMA: 2020,OctSE,1; 2018,Nov,9; 2018,Jan,8; 2017,Jan,8; 2016,Aug,9; 2016,Jan,13; 2015,Jan,16; 2015,Jan,3

\# **81288** **promoter methylation analysis**
0.00 0.00 FUD XXX
AMA: 2020,OctSE,1; 2018,Nov,9; 2018,Jan,8; 2017,Jan,8; 2016,Aug,9; 2016,Jan,13; 2015,Jan,3

\# **81293** **known familial variants**
0.00 0.00 FUD XXX
AMA: 2020,OctSE,1; 2018,Nov,9; 2018,Jan,8; 2017,Jan,8; 2016,Aug,9; 2016,Jan,13; 2015,Jan,16

\# **81294** **duplication/deletion variants**
0.00 0.00 FUD XXX
AMA: 2020,OctSE,1; 2018,Nov,9; 2018,Jan,8; 2017,Jan,8; 2016,Aug,9; 2016,Jan,13; 2015,Jan,16

● # **81338** ***MPL (MPL proto-oncogene, thrombopoietin receptor)*** **(eg, myeloproliferative disorder) gene analysis; common variants (eg, W515A, W515K, W515L, W515R)**
0.00 0.00 FUD 000

● # **81339** **sequence analysis, exon 10**
0.00 0.00 FUD 000

\# **81295** ***MSH2 (mutS homolog 2, colon cancer, nonpolyposis type 1)*** **(eg, hereditary non-polyposis colorectal cancer, Lynch syndrome) gene analysis; full sequence analysis**
0.00 0.00 FUD XXX
AMA: 2020,OctSE,1; 2018,Nov,9; 2018,Jan,8; 2017,Jan,8; 2016,Aug,9; 2016,Jan,13; 2015,Jan,16

81291 **Resequenced code. See code before 81305.**

81292 **Resequenced code. See code before code 81291.**

81293 **Resequenced code. See code before code 81291.**

81294 **Resequenced code. See code before code 81291.**

81295 **Resequenced code. See code before code 81291.**

81296 **known familial variants**
0.00 0.00 FUD XXX
AMA: 2020,OctSE,1; 2018,Nov,9; 2018,Jan,8; 2017,Jan,8; 2016,Aug,9; 2016,Jan,13; 2015,Jan,16

81297 **duplication/deletion variants**
0.00 0.00 FUD XXX
AMA: 2020,OctSE,1; 2018,Nov,9; 2018,Jan,8; 2017,Jan,8; 2016,Aug,9; 2016,Jan,13; 2015,Jan,16

81298 ***MSH6 (mutS homolog 6 [E. coli])*** **(eg, hereditary non-polyposis colorectal cancer, Lynch syndrome) gene analysis; full sequence analysis**
0.00 0.00 FUD XXX
AMA: 2020,OctSE,1; 2018,Nov,9; 2018,Jan,8; 2017,Jan,8; 2016,Aug,9; 2016,Jan,13; 2015,Jan,16

81299 **known familial variants**
0.00 0.00 FUD XXX
AMA: 2020,OctSE,1; 2018,Nov,9; 2018,Jan,8; 2017,Jan,8; 2016,Aug,9; 2016,Jan,13; 2015,Jan,16

81300 **duplication/deletion variants**
0.00 0.00 FUD XXX
AMA: 2020,OctSE,1; 2018,Nov,9; 2018,Jan,8; 2017,Jan,8; 2016,Aug,9; 2016,Jan,13; 2015,Jan,16

81301 **Resequenced code. See code following resequenced code 81287.**

81302 **Resequenced code. See code following 81290.**

81303 **Resequenced code. See code following 81290.**

81304 **Resequenced code. See code following 81290.**

\# **81291** ***MTHFR (5,10-methylenetetrahydrofolate reductase)*** **(eg, hereditary hypercoagulability) gene analysis, common variants (eg, 677T, 1298C)**
0.00 0.00 FUD XXX
AMA: 2020,OctSE,1; 2018,Nov,9; 2018,Jan,8; 2017,Jan,8; 2016,Aug,9; 2016,Jan,13; 2015,Jan,16

81305 ***MYD88 (myeloid differentiation primary response 88)*** **(eg, Waldenstrom's macroglobulinemia, lymphoplasmacytic leukemia) gene analysis, p.Leu265Pro (L265P) variant**
0.00 0.00 FUD XXX
AMA: 2020,OctSE,1; 2019,Jul,3; 2018,Nov,9

81306 **Resequenced code. See code following code 81312.**

81307 **Resequenced code. See code before 81313.**

81308 **Resequenced code. See code before 81313.**

81309 **Resequenced code. See code following 81314.**

81310 ***NPM1 (nucleophosmin)*** **(eg, acute myeloid leukemia) gene analysis, exon 12 variants**
0.00 0.00 FUD XXX
AMA: 2020,OctSE,1; 2018,Nov,9; 2018,Jan,8; 2017,Jan,8; 2016,Aug,9; 2016,Jan,13; 2015,Jan,16

81311 ***NRAS (neuroblastoma RAS viral [v-ras] oncogene homolog)*** **(eg, colorectal carcinoma), gene analysis, variants in exon 2 (eg, codons 12 and 13) and exon 3 (eg, codon 61)**
0.00 0.00 FUD XXX
AMA: 2020,OctSE,1; 2018,Nov,9; 2018,Jan,8; 2017,Jan,8; 2016,Aug,9

81312 **Resequenced code. See code before resequenced code 81307.**

● # **81191** ***NTRK1 (neurotrophic receptor tyrosine kinase 1)*** **(eg, solid tumors) translocation analysis**
0.00 0.00 FUD 000

● # **81192** ***NTRK2 (neurotrophic receptor tyrosine kinase 2)*** **(eg, solid tumors) translocation analysis**
0.00 0.00 FUD 000

● # **81193** ***NTRK3 (neurotrophic receptor tyrosine kinase 3)*** **(eg, solid tumors) translocation analysis**
0.00 0.00 FUD 000

● # **81194** ***NTRK (neurotrophic-tropomyosin receptor tyrosine kinase 1, 2, and 3)*** **(eg, solid tumors) translocation analysis**
INCLUDES Analysis NTRK1, NTRK2, and NTRK3 by single assay
0.00 0.00 FUD 000

\# **81306** ***NUDT15 (nudix hydrolase 15)*** **(eg, drug metabolism) gene analysis, common variant(s) (eg, *2, *3, *4, *5, *6)**
0.00 0.00 FUD XXX
AMA: 2020,OctSE,1; 2019,Jul,3; 2018,Nov,9

\# **81312** ***PABPN1 (poly[A] binding protein nuclear 1)*** **(eg, oculopharyngeal muscular dystrophy) gene analysis, evaluation to detect abnormal (eg, expanded) alleles**
0.00 0.00 FUD XXX
AMA: 2020,OctSE,1; 2018,Nov,9

\# **81307** ***PALB2 (partner and localizer of BRCA2)*** **(eg, breast and pancreatic cancer) gene analysis; full gene sequence**
0.00 0.00 FUD XXX
AMA: 2020,OctSE,1

\# **81308** **known familial variant**
0.00 0.00 FUD XXX
AMA: 2020,OctSE,1

81313 ***PCA3/KLK3 (prostate cancer antigen 3 [non-protein coding]/kallikrein-related peptidase 3 [prostate specific antigen])*** **ratio (eg, prostate cancer)**
0.00 0.00 FUD XXX
AMA: 2020,OctSE,1; 2018,Nov,9; 2018,Jan,8; 2017,Jan,8; 2016,Aug,9; 2016,Jan,13; 2015,Jan,3

81314 ***PDGFRA (platelet-derived growth factor receptor, alpha polypeptide)*** **(eg, gastrointestinal stromal tumor [GIST]), gene analysis, targeted sequence analysis (eg, exons 12, 18)**
0.00 0.00 FUD XXX
AMA: 2020,OctSE,1; 2018,Nov,9; 2018,Jan,8; 2017,Jan,8; 2016,Aug,9

\# **81309** ***PIK3CA (phosphatidylinositol-4, 5-biphosphate 3-kinase, catalytic subunit alpha)*** **(eg, colorectal and breast cancer) gene analysis, targeted sequence analysis (eg, exons 7, 9, 20)**
0.00 0.00 FUD XXX
AMA: 2020,OctSE,1; 2020,Apr,10

\# **81320** ***PLCG2 (phospholipase C gamma 2)*** **(eg, chronic lymphocytic leukemia) gene analysis, common variants (eg, R665W, S707F, L845F)**
0.00 0.00 FUD XXX
AMA: 2020,OctSE,1; 2019,Jul,3; 2018,Nov,9

81315 ***PML/RARalpha, (t(15;17)), (promyelocytic leukemia/retinoic acid receptor alpha)*** **(eg, promyelocytic leukemia) translocation analysis; common breakpoints (eg, intron 3 and intron 6), qualitative or quantitative**
0.00 0.00 FUD XXX
AMA: 2020,OctSE,1; 2018,Nov,9; 2018,Jan,8; 2017,Jan,8; 2016,Aug,9; 2016,Jan,13; 2015,Jan,16

81316 **single breakpoint (eg, intron 3, intron 6 or exon 6), qualitative or quantitative**
0.00 0.00 FUD XXX
AMA: 2020,OctSE,1; 2018,Nov,9; 2018,Jan,8; 2017,Jan,8; 2016,Aug,9; 2016,Jan,13; 2015,Jan,16

\# **81324** ***PMP22 (peripheral myelin protein 22)*** **(eg, Charcot-Marie-Tooth, hereditary neuropathy with liability to pressure palsies) gene analysis; duplication/deletion analysis**
0.00 0.00 FUD XXX
AMA: 2020,OctSE,1; 2018,Nov,9; 2018,Jan,8; 2017,Jan,8; 2016,Aug,9; 2016,Jan,13; 2015,Jan,16

\# **81325** **full sequence analysis**
0.00 0.00 FUD XXX
AMA: 2020,OctSE,1; 2018,Nov,9; 2018,May,6; 2018,Jan,8; 2017,Jan,8; 2016,Aug,9; 2016,Jan,13; 2015,Jan,16

\# **81326** **known familial variant**
0.00 0.00 FUD XXX
AMA: 2020,OctSE,1; 2018,Nov,9; 2018,Jan,8; 2017,Jan,8; 2016,Aug,9; 2016,Jan,13; 2015,Jan,16

81317 ***PMS2 (postmeiotic segregation increased 2 [S. cerevisiae])*** **(eg, hereditary non-polyposis colorectal cancer, Lynch syndrome) gene analysis; full sequence analysis**
0.00 0.00 FUD XXX
AMA: 2020,OctSE,1; 2018,Nov,9; 2018,Jan,8; 2017,Jan,8; 2016,Aug,9; 2016,Jan,13; 2015,Jan,16

81318 **known familial variants**
0.00 0.00 FUD XXX
AMA: 2020,OctSE,1; 2018,Nov,9; 2018,Jan,8; 2017,Jan,8; 2016,Aug,9; 2016,Jan,13; 2015,Jan,16

81319 **duplication/deletion variants**
0.00 0.00 FUD XXX
AMA: 2020,OctSE,1; 2018,Nov,9; 2018,Jan,8; 2017,Jan,8; 2016,Aug,9; 2016,Jan,13; 2015,Jan,16

81320 **Resequenced code. See code before 81315.**

\# **81343** ***PPP2R2B (protein phosphatase 2 regulatory subunit Bbeta)*** **(eg, spinocerebellar ataxia) gene analysis, evaluation to detect abnormal (eg, expanded) alleles**
0.00 0.00 FUD XXX
AMA: 2020,OctSE,1; 2018,Nov,9

81321 ***PTEN (phosphatase and tensin homolog)*** **(eg, Cowden syndrome, PTEN hamartoma tumor syndrome) gene analysis; full sequence analysis**
0.00 0.00 FUD XXX [A]
AMA: 2020,OctSE,1; 2018,Nov,9; 2018,Jan,8; 2017,Jan,8; 2016,Aug,9; 2016,Jan,13; 2015,Jan,16

81322 **known familial variant**
0.00 0.00 FUD XXX [A]
AMA: 2020,OctSE,1; 2018,Nov,9; 2018,Jan,8; 2017,Jan,8; 2016,Aug,9; 2016,Jan,13; 2015,Jan,16

81323 **duplication/deletion variant**
0.00 0.00 FUD XXX [A]
AMA: 2020,OctSE,1; 2018,Nov,9; 2018,Jan,8; 2017,Jan,8; 2016,Aug,9; 2016,Jan,13; 2015,Jan,16

81324 **Resequenced code. See code following 81316.**

81325 **Resequenced code. See code following 81316.**

81326 **Resequenced code. See code following 81316.**

\# **81334** ***RUNX1 (runt related transcription factor 1)*** **(eg, acute myeloid leukemia, familial platelet disorder with associated myeloid malignancy), gene analysis, targeted sequence analysis (eg, exons 3-8)**
0.00 0.00 FUD XXX [A]
AMA: 2020,OctSE,1; 2018,Nov,9

81327 ***SEPT9 (Septin9)*** **(eg, colorectal cancer) promoter methylation analysis**
0.00 0.00 FUD XXX [A]
AMA: 2020,OctSE,1; 2019,Jul,3; 2018,Nov,9

\# **81332** ***SERPINA1 (serpin peptidase inhibitor, clade A, alpha-1 antiproteinase, antitrypsin, member 1)*** **(eg, alpha-1-antitrypsin deficiency), gene analysis, common variants (eg, *S and *Z)**
0.00 0.00 FUD XXX [A]
AMA: 2020,OctSE,1; 2018,Nov,9; 2018,Jan,8; 2017,Jan,8; 2016,Aug,9; 2016,Jan,13; 2015,Jan,16

● # **81347** ***SF3B1 (splicing factor [3b] subunit B1)*** **(eg, myelodysplastic syndrome/acute myeloid leukemia) gene analysis, common variants (eg, A672T, E622D, L833F, R625C, R625L)**
0.00 0.00 FUD 000

81328 ***SLCO1B1 (solute carrier organic anion transporter family, member 1B1)*** **(eg, adverse drug reaction), gene analysis, common variant(s) (eg, *5)**
0.00 0.00 FUD XXX [A]
AMA: 2020,OctSE,1; 2018,Nov,9

81329 ***SMN1 (survival of motor neuron 1, telomeric)*** **(eg, spinal muscular atrophy) gene analysis; dosage/deletion analysis (eg, carrier testing), includes SMN2 (survival of motor neuron 2, centromeric) analysis, if performed**
0.00 0.00 FUD XXX
AMA: 2020,OctSE,1; 2019,Jul,3; 2018,Nov,9

\# **81336** **full gene sequence**
0.00 0.00 FUD XXX
AMA: 2020,OctSE,1; 2019,Jul,3; 2018,Nov,9

\# **81337** **known familial sequence variant(s)**
0.00 0.00 FUD XXX
AMA: 2020,OctSE,1; 2019,Jul,3; 2018,Nov,9

81330 ***SMPD1(sphingomyelin phosphodiesterase 1, acid lysosomal)*** **(eg, Niemann-Pick disease, Type A) gene analysis, common variants (eg, R496L, L302P, fsP330)**
0.00 0.00 FUD XXX [A]
AMA: 2020,OctSE,1; 2018,Nov,9; 2018,Jan,8; 2017,Jan,8; 2016,Aug,9; 2016,Jan,13; 2015,Jan,16

81331 ***SNRPN/UBE3A (small nuclear ribonucleoprotein polypeptide N and ubiquitin protein ligase E3A)*** **(eg, Prader-Willi syndrome and/or Angelman syndrome), methylation analysis**
0.00 0.00 FUD XXX [A]
AMA: 2020,OctSE,1; 2018,Nov,9; 2018,Jan,8; 2017,Jan,8; 2016,Aug,9; 2016,Jan,13; 2015,Jan,16

81332 **Resequenced code. See code following 81327.**

● # **81348** ***SRSF2 (serine and arginine-rich splicing factor 2)*** **(eg, myelodysplastic syndrome, acute myeloid leukemia) gene analysis, common variants (eg, P95H, P95L)**
0.00 0.00 FUD 000

\# **81344** ***TBP (TATA box binding protein)*** **(eg, spinocerebellar ataxia) gene analysis, evaluation to detect abnormal (eg, expanded) alleles**
0.00 0.00 FUD XXX
AMA: 2020,OctSE,1; 2018,Nov,9

\# **81345** ***TERT (telomerase reverse transcriptase)*** **(eg, thyroid carcinoma, glioblastoma multiforme) gene analysis, targeted sequence analysis (eg, promoter region)**
0.00 0.00 FUD XXX
AMA: 2020,OctSE,1; 2019,Jul,3; 2018,Nov,9

81333 ***TGFBI (transforming growth factor beta-induced)*** **(eg, corneal dystrophy) gene analysis, common variants (eg, R124H, R124C, R124L, R555W, R555Q)**
0.00 0.00 FUD XXX
AMA: 2020,OctSE,1; 2019,Jul,3; 2018,Nov,9

81334 **Resequenced code. See code following code 81326.**

● # **81351** ***TP53 (tumor protein 53)*** **(eg, Li-Fraumeni syndrome) gene analysis; full gene sequence**
0.00 0.00 FUD 000

● # **81352** **targeted sequence analysis (eg, 4 oncology)**
0.00 0.00 FUD 000

● # **81353** **known familial variant**
0.00 0.00 FUD 000

81335 ***TPMT (thiopurine S-methyltransferase)*** **(eg, drug metabolism), gene analysis, common variants (eg, *2, *3)**
0.00 0.00 FUD XXX [A]
AMA: 2020,OctSE,1; 2018,Nov,9

81336 **Resequenced code. See code following 81329.**

81337 **Resequenced code. See code following 81329.**

81338 **Resequenced code. See code following resequenced code 81294.**

81339 **Resequenced code. See code fbefore resequenced code 81295.**

81340 ***TRB@ (T cell antigen receptor, beta)*** **(eg, leukemia and lymphoma), gene rearrangement analysis to detect abnormal clonal population(s); using amplification methodology (eg, polymerase chain reaction)**
0.00 0.00 FUD XXX [A]
AMA: 2020,OctSE,1; 2018,Nov,9; 2018,Jan,8; 2017,Jan,8; 2016,Aug,9; 2016,Jan,13; 2015,Jan,16

81341 **using direct probe methodology (eg, Southern blot)**
0.00 0.00 FUD XXX [A]
AMA: 2020,OctSE,1; 2018,Nov,9; 2018,Jan,8; 2017,Jan,8; 2016,Aug,9; 2016,Jan,13; 2015,Jan,16

81342 ***TRG@ (T cell antigen receptor, gamma)*** **(eg, leukemia and lymphoma), gene rearrangement analysis, evaluation to detect abnormal clonal population(s)**
0.00 0.00 FUD XXX [A]
AMA: 2020,OctSE,1; 2018,Nov,9; 2018,Jan,8; 2017,Jan,8; 2016,Aug,9; 2016,Jan,13; 2015,Jan,16

81343 **Resequenced code. See code following code 81320.**

81344 **Resequenced code. See code following code 81320.**

81345 **Resequenced code. See code following code 81320.**

81346 ***TYMS (thymidylate synthetase)*** **(eg, 5-fluorouracil/5-FU drug metabolism), gene analysis, common variant(s) (eg, tandem repeat variant)**
0.00 0.00 FUD XXX [A]
AMA: 2020,OctSE,1; 2018,Nov,9

81347 **Resequenced code. See code before 81328.**

81348 **Resequenced code. See code following 81331.**

● # 81357 ***U2AF1 (U2 small nuclear RNA auxiliary factor 1)*** **(eg, myelodysplastic syndrome, acute myeloid leukemia) gene analysis, common variants (eg, S34F, S34Y, Q157R, Q157P)**
0.00 0.00 FUD 000

81350 ***UGT1A1 (UDP glucuronosyltransferase 1 family, polypeptide A1)*** **(eg, drug metabolism, hereditary unconjugated hyperbilirubinemia [Gilbert syndrome]) gene analysis, common variants (eg, *28, *36, *37)**
0.00 0.00 FUD XXX A
AMA: 2020,OctSE,1; 2020,Apr,9; 2018,Nov,9; 2018,Jan,8; 2017,Jan,8; 2016,Aug,9; 2016,Jan,13; 2015,Jan,16

81351 **Resequenced code. See code following 81333.**

81352 **Resequenced code. See code following 81333.**

81353 **Resequenced code. See code following 81333.**

81355 ***VKORC1 (vitamin K epoxide reductase complex, subunit 1)*** **(eg, warfarin metabolism), gene analysis, common variant(s) (eg, -1639G>A, c.173+1000C>T)**
0.00 0.00 FUD XXX A
AMA: 2020,OctSE,1; 2018,Nov,9; 2018,Jan,8; 2017,Jan,8; 2016,Aug,9; 2016,Jan,13; 2015,Jan,16

81357 **Resequenced code. See code following 81346.**

● 81360 ***ZRSR2 (zinc finger CCCH-type, RNA binding motif and serine/arginine-rich 2)*** **(eg, myelodysplastic syndrome, acute myeloid leukemia) gene analysis, common variant(s) (eg, E65fs, E122fs, R448fs)**

81361 **Resequenced code. See code following resequenced code 81269.**

81362 **Resequenced code. See code following resequenced code 81269.**

81363 **Resequenced code. See code following resequenced code 81269.**

81364 **Resequenced code. See code following resequenced code 81269.**

81370-81383 Human Leukocyte Antigen (HLA) Testing

INCLUDES Additional testing performed to resolve ambiguous allele combinations for high-resolution typing
All analytical procedures in evaluation:
- Amplification
- Cell lysis
- Detection
- Digestion
- Extraction
- Nucleic acid stabilization

Analysis to identify human leukocyte antigen (HLA) alleles and allele groups connected to specific diseases and individual response to drug therapy in addition to other clinical uses
Code selection based on specific gene being reviewed
Evaluation gene variant presence using common gene variant name
Generally, all listed gene variants in code description tested (lists not all inclusive)
Genes described using Human Genome Organization (HUGO) approved names
High-resolution typing resolves common well-defined (CWD) alleles usually identified by at least four-digits. Some instances when high-resolution typing may include ambiguities for rare alleles may be reported as string of alleles or National Marrow Donor Program (NMDP) code
Histocompatibility antigen testing
Intermediate resolution HLA testing identified by string of alleles or NMDP code
Low and intermediate resolution considered low resolution for code assignment
Low-resolution HLA type reporting identified by two-digit HLA name
Multiple variant alleles or allele groups identified by typing
One or more HLA genes in specific clinical circumstances
Protein or disease examples in code description not all inclusive
Qualitative results unless otherwise stated
Typing performed to determine recipient compatibility and potential donors undergoing solid organ or hematopoietic stem cell pretransplantation testing

EXCLUDES *Full gene sequencing using separate gene variant assessment codes unless specifically stated in code description*
HLA antigen typing by nonmolecular pathology methods (86812-86821)
In situ hybridization analyses (88271-88275, 88368-88375 [88377])
Microbial identification (87149-87153, 87471-87801 [87623, 87624, 87625], 87900-87904 [87906, 87910, 87912])
Other related gene variants not listed in code description
Tier 1 molecular pathology codes (81105-81254 [81161, 81162, 81163, 81164, 81165, 81166, 81167, 81173, 81174, 81184, 81185, 81186, 81187, 81188, 81189, 81190, 81200, 81201, 81202, 81203, 81204, 81205, 81206, 81207, 81208, 81209, 81210, 81219, 81227, 81230, 81231, 81233, 81234, 81238, 81239, 81245, 81246, 81250, 81257, 81258, 81259, 81265, 81266, 81267, 81268, 81269, 81284, 81285, 81286, 81289, 81361, 81362, 81363, 81364])
Tier 2 and unlisted molecular pathology procedures (81400-81408, [81479])

Code also modifier 26 when only interpretation and report performed
Code also services required before cell lysis

81370 **HLA Class I and II typing, low resolution (eg, antigen equivalents);** ***HLA-A, -B, -C, -DRB1/3/4/5, and -DQB1***
0.00 0.00 FUD XXX A
AMA: 2020,OctSE,1; 2018,Nov,9; 2018,Jan,8; 2017,Jan,8; 2016,Aug,9; 2016,Jan,13; 2015,Jan,16

81371 ***HLA-A, -B, and -DRB1*** **(eg, verification typing)**
0.00 0.00 FUD XXX A
AMA: 2020,OctSE,1; 2018,Nov,9; 2018,Jan,8; 2017,Jan,8; 2016,Aug,9; 2016,Jan,13; 2015,Jan,16

81372 **HLA Class I typing, low resolution (eg, antigen equivalents); complete** ***(ie, HLA-A, -B, and -C)***
EXCLUDES *Class I and II low-resolution HLA typing for HLA-A, -B, -C, -DRB1/3/4/5, and -DQB1 (81370)*
0.00 0.00 FUD XXX A
AMA: 2020,OctSE,1; 2018,Nov,9; 2018,Jan,8; 2017,Jan,8; 2016,Aug,9; 2016,Jan,13; 2015,Jan,16

81373 **one locus** ***(eg, HLA-A, -B, or -C)*****, each**
EXCLUDES *Complete Class 1 (HLA-A, -B, and -C) low-resolution typing (81372)*
Reporting presence or absence single antigen equivalent using low-resolution methodology (81374)
0.00 0.00 FUD XXX A
AMA: 2020,OctSE,1; 2018,Nov,9; 2018,Jan,8; 2017,Jan,8; 2016,Aug,9; 2016,Jan,13; 2015,Jan,16

81374 **one antigen equivalent *(eg, B*27)*, each**

EXCLUDES *Testing for presence or absence more than two antigen equivalents at locus, report for each locus test (81373)*

0.00 0.00 FUD XXX A

AMA: 2020,OctSE,1; 2018,Nov,9; 2018,Jan,8; 2017,Jan,8; 2016,Aug,9; 2016,Jan,13; 2015,Jan,16

81375 **HLA Class II typing, low resolution (eg, antigen equivalents); *HLA-DRB1/3/4/5 and -DQB1***

EXCLUDES *Class I and II low-resolution HLA typing for HLA-A, -B, -C, -DRB 1/3/4/5, and DQB1 (81370)*

0.00 0.00 FUD XXX A

AMA: 2020,OctSE,1; 2018,Nov,9; 2018,Jan,8; 2017,Jan,8; 2016,Aug,9; 2016,Jan,13; 2015,Jan,16

81376 **one locus *(eg, HLA-DRB1, -DRB3/4/5, -DQB1, -DQA1, -DPB1, or -DPA1)*, each**

INCLUDES Low-resolution typing, HLA-DRB1/3/4/5 reported as single locus

EXCLUDES *Low-resolution typing for HLA-DRB1/3/4/5 and -DQB1 (81375)*

0.00 0.00 FUD XXX A

AMA: 2020,OctSE,1; 2018,Nov,9; 2018,Jan,8; 2017,Jan,8; 2016,Aug,9; 2016,Jan,13; 2015,Jan,16

81377 **one antigen equivalent, each**

EXCLUDES *Testing for presence or absence more than two antigen equivalents at locus (81376)*

0.00 0.00 FUD XXX A

AMA: 2020,OctSE,1; 2018,Nov,9; 2018,Jan,8; 2017,Jan,8; 2016,Aug,9; 2016,Jan,13; 2015,Jan,16

81378 **HLA Class I and II typing, high resolution (ie, alleles or allele groups), *HLA-A, -B, -C, and -DRB1***

0.00 0.00 FUD XXX A

AMA: 2020,OctSE,1; 2018,Nov,9; 2018,Jan,8; 2017,Jan,8; 2016,Aug,9; 2016,Jan,13; 2015,Jan,16

81379 **HLA Class I typing, high resolution (ie, alleles or allele groups); complete (ie, *HLA-A, -B, and -C*)**

0.00 0.00 FUD XXX A

AMA: 2020,OctSE,1; 2018,Nov,9; 2018,Jan,8; 2017,Jan,8; 2016,Aug,9; 2016,Jan,13; 2015,Jan,16

81380 **one locus (eg, *HLA-A, -B, or -C*), each**

EXCLUDES *Complete Class I high-resolution typing for HLA-A, -B, and -C (81379)*

Testing for presence or absence single allele or allele group using high-resolution methodology (81381)

0.00 0.00 FUD XXX A

AMA: 2020,OctSE,1; 2018,Nov,9; 2018,Jan,8; 2017,Jan,8; 2016,Aug,9; 2016,Jan,13; 2015,Jan,16

81381 **one allele or allele group (eg, *B*57:01P*), each**

EXCLUDES *Testing for presence or absence more than two alleles or allele groups at locus, report for each locus (81380)*

0.00 0.00 FUD XXX A

AMA: 2020,OctSE,1; 2018,Nov,9; 2018,Jan,8; 2017,Jan,8; 2016,Aug,9; 2016,Jan,13; 2015,Jan,16

81382 **HLA Class II typing, high resolution (ie, alleles or allele groups); one locus (eg, *HLA-DRB1, -DRB3/4/5, -DQB1, -DQA1, -DPB1, or -DPA1*), each**

INCLUDES Typing one or all DRB3/4/5 genes regarded as one locus

EXCLUDES *Testing for just presence or absence single allele or allele group using high-resolution methodology (81383)*

0.00 0.00 FUD XXX A

AMA: 2020,OctSE,1; 2018,Nov,9; 2018,Jan,8; 2017,Jan,8; 2016,Jan,13; 2015,Jan,16

81383 **one allele or allele group (eg, *HLA-DQB1*06:02P*), each**

EXCLUDES *Testing for presence or absence more than two alleles or allele groups at locus, report for each locus (81382)*

0.00 0.00 FUD XXX A

AMA: 2020,OctSE,1; 2018,Nov,9; 2018,Jan,8; 2017,Jan,8; 2016,Jan,13; 2015,Jan,16

81400-81479 [81479] Molecular Pathology Tier 2 Procedures

INCLUDES All analytical procedures in evaluation:
- Amplification
- Cell lysis
- Detection
- Digestion
- Extraction
- Nucleic acid stabilization

Code selection based on specific gene being reviewed
Codes arranged by technical resource level and work involved
Evaluation gene variant presence using common gene variant name
Generally, all listed gene variants in code description tested (lists not all inclusive)
Genes described using Human Genome Organization (HUGO) approved names
Histocompatibility testing
Protein or disease examples in code description (lists not all inclusive)
Qualitative results unless otherwise stated
Specific analytes listed after code description for selecting appropriate molecular pathology procedure
Targeted genomic testing (81410-81471 [81448])
Testing for more rare diseases

EXCLUDES *Full gene sequencing using separate gene variant assessment codes unless specifically stated in code description*
In situ hybridization analyses (88271-88275, 88365-88368 [88364, 88373, 88374])
Microbial identification (87149-87153, 87471-87801 [87623, 87624, 87625], 87900-87904 [87906, 87910, 87912])
Other related gene variants not listed in code description
Tier 1 molecular pathology (81105-81254 [81161, 81162, 81163, 81164, 81165, 81166, 81167, 81173, 81174, 81184, 81185, 81186, 81187, 81188, 81189, 81190, 81200, 81201, 81202, 81203, 81204, 81205, 81206, 81207, 81208, 81209, 81210, 81219, 81227, 81230, 81231, 81233, 81234, 81238, 81239, 81245, 81246, 81250, 81257, 81258, 81259, 81265, 81266, 81267, 81268, 81269, 81284, 81285, 81286, 81289, 81361, 81362, 81363, 81364])
Unlisted molecular pathology procedures ([81479])

Code also modifier 26 when only interpretation and report performed
Code also services required before cell lysis

81400 **Molecular pathology procedure, Level 1 (eg, identification of single germline variant [eg, SNP] by techniques such as restriction enzyme digestion or melt curve analysis)**

ACADM (acyl-CoA dehydrogenase, C-4 to C-12 straight chain, MCAD) (eg, medium chain acyl dehydrogenase deficiency), K304E variant

ACE (angiotensin converting enzyme) (eg, hereditary blood pressure regulation), insertion/deletion variant

AGTR1 (angiotensin II receptor, type 1) (eg, essential hypertension), 1166A>C variant

BCKDHA (branched chain keto acid dehydrogenase E1, alpha polypeptide) (eg, maple syrup urine disease, type 1A), Y438N variant

CCR5 (chemokine C-C motif receptor 5) (eg, HIV resistance), 32-bp deletion mutation/794 825del32 deletion

CLRN1 (clarin 1) (eg, Usher syndrome, type 3), N48K variant

F2 (coagulation factor 2) (eg, hereditary hypercoagulability), 1199G>A variant

F5 (coagulation factor V) (eg, hereditary hypercoagulability), HR2 variant

F7 (coagulation factor VII [serum prothrombin conversion accelerator]) (eg, hereditary hypercoagulability), R353Q variant

F13B (coagulation factor XIII, B polypeptide) (eg, hereditary hypercoagulability), V34L variant

FGB (fibrinogen beta chain) (eg, hereditary ischemic heart disease), -455G>A variant

FGFR1 (fibroblast growth factor receptor 1) (eg, Pfeiffer syndrome type 1, craniosynostosis), P252R variant

FGFR3 (fibroblast growth factor receptor 3) (eg, Muenke syndrome), P250R variant

FKTN (fukutin) (eg, Fukuyama congenital muscular dystrophy), retrotransposon insertion variant

GNE (glucosamine [UDP-N-acetyl]-2 -epimerase/N-acetylmannosamine kinase) (eg, inclusion body myopathy 2 [IBM2], Nonaka myopathy), M712T variant

IVD (isovaleryl-CoA dehydrogenase) (eg, isovaleric acidemia), A282V variant

LCT (lactase-phlorizin hydrolase) (eg, lactose intolerance), 13910 C>T variant

NEB (nebulin) (eg, nemaline myopathy 2), exon 55 deletion variant

PCDH15 (protocadherin-related 15) (eg, Usher syndrome type 1F), R245X variant

SERPINE1 (serpine peptidase inhibitor clade E, member 1, plasminogen activator inhibitor -1, PAI-1) (eg, thrombophilia), 4G variant

SHOC2 (soc-2 suppressor of clear homolog) (eg, Noonan-like syndrome with loose anagen hair), S2G variant

SRY (sex determining region Y) (eg, 46,XX testicular disorder of sex development, gonadal dysgenesis), gene analysis

TOR1A (torsin family 1, member A [torsin A]) (eg, early-onset primary dystonia [DYT1]), 907_909delGAG (904_906delGAG) variant

0.00 0.00 **FUD** XXX A

AMA: 2020,OctSE,1; 2019,Jul,3; 2018,Nov,9; 2018,Jan,8; 2017,Jan,8; 2016,Aug,9; 2016,Jan,13; 2015,Jan,16; 2015,Jan,3

▲ **81401** **Molecular pathology procedure, Level 2 (eg, 2-10 SNPs, 1 methylated variant, or 1 somatic variant [typically using nonsequencing target variant analysis], or detection of a dynamic mutation disorder/triplet repeat)**

ABCC8 (ATP-binding cassette, sub-family C [CFTR/MRP], member 8) (eg, familial hyperinsulinism), common variants (eg, c.3898-9G>A [c.3992-9G>A], F1388del)

ABL1 (ABL proto oncogene 1, non-receptor tyrosine kinase) (eg, acquired imatinib resistance), T315I variant

ACADM (acyl-CoA dehydrogenase, C-4 to C-12 straight chain, MCAD) (eg, medium chain acyl dehydrogenase deficiency), common variants (eg, K304E, Y42H)

ADRB2 (adrenergic beta-2 receptor surface) (eg, drug metabolism), common variants (eg, G16R, Q27E)

APOB (apolipoprotein B) (eg, familial hypercholesterolemia type B), common variants (eg, R3500Q, R3500W)

*APOE (apolipoprotein E) (eg, hyperlipoproteinemia type III, cardiovascular disease, Alzheimer disease), common variants (eg, *2, *3, *4)*

CBFB/MYH11 (inv(16)) (eg, acute myeloid leukemia), qualitative, and quantitative, if performed

CBS (cystathionine-beta-synthase) (eg, homocystinuria, cystathionine beta-synthase deficiency), common variants (eg, I278T, G307S)

CFH/ARMS2 (complement factor H/age-related maculopathy susceptibility 2) (eg, macular degeneration), common variants (eg, Y402H [CFH], A69S [ARMS2])

DEK/NUP214 (t(6;9))(eg, acute myeloid leukemia), translocation analysis, qualitative, and quantitative, if performed

E2A/PBX1 (t(1;19)) (eg, acute lymphocytic leukemia), translocation analysis, qualitative, and quantitative, if performed

EML4/ALK (inv(2)) (eg, non-small cell lung cancer), translocation or inversion analysis

ETV6/RUNX1 (t(12;21)) (eg, acute lymphocytic leukemia), translocation analysis, qualitative and quantitative, if performed

EWSR1/ATF1 (t(12;22)) (eg, clear cell sarcoma), translocation analysis, qualitative, and quantitative, if performed

EWSR1/ERG (t(21;22)) (eg, Ewing sarcoma/peripheral neuroectodermal tumor), translocation analysis, qualitative and quantitative, if performed

EWSR1/FLI1 (t(11;22)) (eg, Ewing sarcoma/peripheral neuroectodermal tumor), translocation analysis, qualitative and quantitative, if performed

EWSR1/WT1 (t(11;22)) (eg, desmoplastic small round cell tumor), translocation analysis, qualitative and quantitative, if performed

F11 (coagulation factor XI) (eg, coagulation disorder), common variants (eg, E117X [Type II], F283L [Type III], IVS14del14, and IVS14+1G>A [Type I])

FGFR3 (fibroblast growth factor receptor 3) (eg, achondroplasia, hypochondroplasia), common variants (eg, 1138G>A, 1138G>C, 1620C>A, 1620C>G)

FIP1L1/PDGFRA (del[4q12]) (eg, imatinib-sensitive chronic eosinophilic leukemia), qualitative and quantitative, if performed

FLG (filaggrin) (eg, ichthyosis vulgaris), common variants (eg, R501X, 2282del4, R2447X, S3247X, 3702delG)

FOXO1/PAX3 (t(2;13)) (eg, alveolar rhabdomyosarcoma), translocation analysis, qualitative and quantitative, if performed

FOXO1/PAX7 (t(1;13)) (eg, alveolar rhabdomyosarcoma), translocation analysis, qualitative and quantitative, if performed

FUS/DDIT3 (t(12;16)) (eg, myxoid liposarcoma), translocation analysis, qualitative, and quantitative, if performed

GALC (galactosylceramidase) (eg, Krabbe disease), common variants (eg, c.857G>A, 30-kb deletion)

GALT (galactose-1-phosphate uridylyltransferase) (eg, galactosemia), common variants (eg, Q188R, S135L, K285N, T138M, L195P, Y209C, IVS2-2A>G, P171S, del5kb, N314D, L218L/N314D)

H19 (imprinted maternally expressed transcript [non-protein coding]) (eg, Beckwith-Wiedemann syndrome), methylation analysis

IGH@/BCL2 (t(14;18)) (eg, follicular lymphoma), translocation and analysis; single breakpoint (eg) major breakpoint region [MBR] or minor cluster region [mcr]), qualitative or quantitative

(When both MBR and mcr breakpoints are performed, report [81278])

KCNQ1OT1 (KCNQ1 overlapping transcript 1 [non-protein coding]) (e.g, Beckwith-Wiedemann syndrome), methylation analysis

LINC00518 (long intergenic non-protein coding RNA 518) (eg, melanoma), expression analysis

LRRK2 (leucine-rich repeat kinase 2) (eg, Parkinson disease), common variants (eg, R1441G, G2019S, I2020T)

MED12 (mediator complex subunit 12) (eg, FG syndrome type 1, Lujan syndrome), common variants (eg, R961W, N1007S)

MEG3/DLK1 (maternally expressed 3 [non-protein coding]/delta-like 1 homolog [Drosophila]) (eg, intrauterine growth retardation), methylation analysis

MLL/AFF1 (t(4;11)) (eg acute lymphoblastic leukemia), translocation analysis, qualitative and quantitative, if performed

MLL/MLLT3 (t(9;11)) (eg, acute myeloid leukemia) translocation analysis, qualitative and quantitative, if performed

MT-RNR1 (mitochondrially encoded 12S RNA) (eg, nonsyndromic hearing loss), common variants (eg, m.1555>G, m1494C>T)

MUTYH (mutY homolog [E.coli]) (eg, MYH-associated polyposis), common variants (eg, Y165C, G382D)

MT-ATP6 (mitochondrially encoded ATP synthase 6) (eg, neuropathy with ataxia and retinitis pigmentosa [NARP], Leigh syndrome), common variants (eg, m.8993T>G, m.8993T>C)

MT-ND4, MT-ND6 (mitochondrially encoded NADH dehydrogenase 4, mitochondrially encoded NADH dehydrogenase 6) (eg, Leber hereditary optic neuropathy [LHON]), common variants (eg m.11778G>A, m3460G>A, m14484T>C)

MT-ND5 (mitochondrially encoded tRNA leucine 1 [UUA/G], mitochondrially encoded NADH dehydrogenase 5) (eg, mitochondrial encephalopathy with lactic acidosis and stroke-like episodes [MELAS]), common variants (eg, m.3243A>G, m.3271T>C, m.3252A>G, m.13513G>A)

MT-TK (mitochondrially encoded tRNA lysine) (eg, myoclonic epilepsy with ragged-red fibers [MERRF]), common variants (eg, m8344A>G, m.8356T>C)

MT-TL1 (mitochondrially encoded tRNA leucine 1[UUA/G]) (eg, diabetes and hearing loss), common variants (eg, m.3243A>G, m.14709 T>C) MT-TL1

MT-TS1, MT-RNR1 (mitochondrially encoded tRNA serine 1 [UCN], mitochondrially encoded 12S RNA) (eg, nonsyndromic sensorineural deafness [including aminoglycoside-induced nonsyndromic deafness]) common variants (eg, m.7445A>G, m.1555A>G)

NOD2 (nucleotide-binding oligomerization domain containing 2) (eg, Crohn's disease, Blau syndrome), common variants (eg, SNP 8, SNP 12, SNP 13)

NPM/ALK (t(2;5)) (eg, anaplastic large cell lymphoma), translocation analysis

PAX8/PPARG (t(2;3) (q13;p25)) (eg, follicular thyroid carcinoma), translocation analysis

PRAME (preferentially expressed antigen in melanoma)(eg, melanoma), expression analysis

PRSS1 (protease, serine, 1 [trypsin 1]) (eg, hereditary pancreatitis), common variants (eg, N29I, A16V, R122H)

PYGM (phosphorylase, glycogen, muscle) (eg, glycogen storage disease type V, McArdle disease), common variants (eg, R50X, G205S)

RUNX1/RUNX1T1 (t(8;21)) (eg, acute myeloid leukemia) translocation analysis, qualitative and quantitative, if performed

SS18/SSX1 (t(X;18)) (eg, synovial sarcoma), translocation analysis, qualitative and quantitative, if performed

SS18/SSX2 (t(X;18)) (eg, synovial sarcoma), translocation analysis, qualitative and quantitative, if performed

VWF (von Willebrand factor) (eg, von Willebrand disease type 2N), common variants (eg, T791M, R816W, R854Q)

⚒ 0.00 ⚕ 0.00 **FUD** XXX [A] [□]

AMA: 2020,OctSE,1; 2019,Sep,7; 2019,Jul,3; 2018,Nov,9; 2018,Jan,8; 2017,Jan,8; 2016,Aug,9; 2016,Jan,13; 2015,Jan,16; 2015,Jan,3

▲ **81402** **Molecular pathology procedure, Level 3 (eg, >10 SNPs, 2-10 methylated variants, or 2-10 somatic variants [typically using non-sequencing target variant analysis], immunoglobulin and T-cell receptor gene rearrangements, duplication/deletion variants of 1 exon, loss of heterozygosity [LOH], uniparental disomy [UPD])**

Chromosome 1p-/19q- (eg, glial tumors), deletion analysis

Chromosome 18q- (eg, D18S55, D18S58, D18S61, D18S64, and D18S69) (eg, colon cancer), allelic imbalance assessment (ie, loss of heterozygosity)

COL1A1/PDGFB (t(17;22)) (eg, dermatofibrosarcoma protuberans), translocation analysis, multiple breakpoints, qualitative, and quantitative, if performed

CYP21A2 (cytochrome P450, family 21, subfamily A, polypeptide 2) (eg, congenital adrenal hyperplasia, 21-hydroxylase deficiency), common variants (eg, IVS2-13G, P30L, I172N, exon 6 mutation cluster [I235N, V236E, M238K], V281L, L307FfsX6, Q318X, R356W, P453S, G110VfsX21, 30-kb deletion variant)

ESR1/PGR (receptor 1/progesterone receptor) ratio (eg, breast cancer)

MEFV (Mediterranean fever) (eg, familial Mediterranean fever), common variants (eg, E148Q, P369S, F479L, M680I, I692del, M694V, M694I, K695R, V726A, A744S, R761H)

TRD@ (T cell antigen receptor, delta) (eg, leukemia and lymphoma), gene rearrangement analysis, evaluation to detect abnormal clonal population

Uniparental disomy (UPD) (eg, Russell-Silver syndrome, Prader-Willi/Angelman syndrome), short tandem repeat (STR) analysis

⚒ 0.00 ⚕ 0.00 **FUD** XXX [A] [□]

AMA: 2020,OctSE,1; 2018,Nov,9; 2018,Jan,8; 2017,Jan,8; 2016,Aug,9; 2016,Jan,13; 2015,Jan,16; 2015,Jan,3

▲ **81403** **Molecular pathology procedure, Level 4 (eg, analysis of single exon by DNA sequence analysis, analysis of >10 amplicons**

using multiplex PCR in 2 or more independent reactions, mutation scanning or duplication/deletion variants of 2-5 exons)

ANG (angiogenin, ribonuclease, RNase A family, 5) (eg, amyotrophic lateral sclerosis), full gene sequence

ARX (aristaless-related homeobox) (eg, X-linked lissencephaly with ambiguous genitalia, X-linked mental retardation), duplication/deletion analysis

CEL (carboxyl ester lipase [bile salt-stimulated lipase]) (eg, maturity-onset diabetes of the young [MODY]), targeted sequence analysis of exon 11 (eg, c.1785delC, c.1686delT)

CTNNB1 (catenin [cadherin-associated protein], beta 1, 88kDa) (eg, desmoid tumors), targeted sequence analysis (eg, exon 3)

DAZ/SRY (deleted in azoospermia and sex determining region Y) (eg, male infertility), common deletions (eg, AZFa, AZFb, AZFc, AZFd)

DNMT3A (DNA [cytosine-5-]-methyltransferase 3 alpha) (eg, acute myeloid leukemia), targeted sequence analysis (eg, exon 23)

EPCAM (epithelial cell adhesion molecule) (eg, Lynch syndrome), duplication/deletion analysis

F8 (coagulation factor VIII) (eg, hemophilia A), inversion analysis, intron 1 and intron 22A

F12 (coagulation factor XII [Hageman factor]) (eg, angioedema, hereditary, type III; factor XII deficiency), targeted sequence analysis of exon 9

FGFR3 (fibroblast growth factor receptor 3) (eg, isolated craniosynostosis), targeted sequence analysis (eg, exon 7)

(For targeted sequence analysis of multiple FGFR3 exons, use 81404) (81404)

GJB1 (gap junction protein, beta 1) (eg, Charcot-Marie-Tooth X-linked), full gene sequence

GNAQ (guanine nucleotide-binding protein G[q] subunit alpha) (eg, uveal melanoma), common variants (eg, R183, Q209)

HRAS (v-Ha-ras Harvey rat sarcoma viral oncogene homolog) (eg, Costello syndrome), exon 2 sequence

Human erythrocyte antigen gene analyses (eg, SLC14A1 [Kidd blood group], BCAM [Lutheran blood group], ICAM4 [Landsteiner-Wiener blood group], SLC4A1 [Diego blood group], AQP1 [Colton blood group], ERMAP [Scianna blood group], RHCE [Rh blood group, CcEe antigens], KEL [Kell blood group], DARC [Duffy blood group], GYPA, GYPB, GYPE [MNS blood group], ART4 [Dombrock blood group]) (eg, sickle-cell disease, thalassemia, hemolytic transfusion reactions, hemolytic disease of the fetus or newborn), common variants

KCNC3 (potassium voltage-gated channel, Shaw-related subfamily, member 3) (eg, spinocerebellar ataxia), targeted sequence analysis (eg, exon 2)

KCNJ2 (potassium inwardly-rectifying channel, subfamily J, member 2) (eg, Andersen-Tawil syndrome), full gene sequence

KCNJ11 (potassium inwardly-rectifying channel, subfamily J, member 11) (eg, familial hyperinsulinism), full gene sequence

Killer cell immunoglobulin-like receptor (KIR) gene family (eg, hematopoietic stem cell transplantation), genotyping of KIR family genes

Known familial variant, not otherwise specified, for gene listed in Tier 1 or Tier 2, or identified during a genomic sequencing procedure, DNA sequence analysis, each variant exon

(For a known familial variant that is considered a common variant, use specific common variant Tier 1 or Tier 2 code)

MC4R (melanocortin 4 receptor) (eg, obesity), full gene sequence

*MICA (MHC class I polypeptide-related sequence A) (eg, solid organ transplantation), common variants (eg, *001, *002)*

MT-RNR1 (mitochondrially encoded 12S RNA) (eg, nonsyndromic hearing loss), full gene sequence

[26]/[TC] **PC/TC Only**   [A2]-[Z3] **ASC Payment**   [50] **Bilateral**   ♂ **Male Only**   ♀ **Female Only**   ⚒ **Facility RVU**   ⚕ **Non-Facility RVU**   [□] **CCI**   [✖] **CLIA**
FUD Follow-up Days   **CMS: IOM**   **AMA: CPT Asst**   [A]-[Y] **OPPSI**   [80]/[80] **Surg Assist Allowed / w/Doc**   [■] **Lab Crosswalk**   [■] **Radiology Crosswalk**

MT-TS1 (mitochondrially encoded tRNA serine 1) (eg, nonsyndromic hearing loss), full gene sequence

NDP (Norrie disease [pseudoglioma]) (eg, Norrie disease), duplication/deletion analysis

NHLRC1 (NHL repeat containing 1) (eg, progressive myoclonus epilepsy), full gene sequence

PHOX2B (paired-like homeobox 2b) (eg, congenital central hypoventilation syndrome), duplication/deletion analysis

PLN (phospholamban) (eg, dilated cardiomyopathy, hypertrophic cardiomyopathy), full gene sequence

RHD (Rh blood group, D antigen) (eg, hemolytic disease of the fetus and newborn, Rh maternal/fetal compatibility), deletion analysis (eg, exons 4, 5, and 7, pseudogene)

RHD (Rh blood group, D antigen) (eg, hemolytic disease of the fetus and newborn, Rh maternal/fetal compatibility), deletion analysis (eg, exons 4, 5, and 7, pseudogene), performed on cell-free fetal DNA in maternal blood

(For human erythrocyte gene analysis of RHD, use a separate unit of 81403)

SH2D1A (SH2 domain containing 1A) (eg, X-linked lymphoproliferative syndrome), duplication/deletion analysis

TWIST1 (twist homolog 1 [Drosophila]) (eg, Saethre-Chotzen syndrome), duplication/deletion analysis

UBA1 (ubiquitin-like modifier activating enzyme 1) (eg, spinal muscular atrophy, X-linked), targeted sequence analysis (eg, exon 15)

VHL (von Hippel-Lindau tumor suppressor) (eg, von Hippel-Lindau familial cancer syndrome), deletion/duplication analysis

VWF (von Willebrand factor) (eg, von Willebrand disease types 2A, 2B, 2M), targeted sequence analysis (eg, exon 28)

0.00 0.00 **FUD** XXX A

AMA: 2020,OctSE,1; 2019,Jul,3; 2018,Nov,9; 2018,May,6; 2018,Jan,8; 2017,Jan,8; 2016,Aug,9; 2016,Jan,13; 2015,Jan,16; 2015,Jan,3

▲ **81404 Molecular pathology procedure, Level 5 (eg, analysis of 2-5 exons by DNA sequence analysis, mutation scanning or duplication/deletion variants of 6-10 exons, or characterization of a dynamic mutation disorder/triplet repeat by Southern blot analysis)**

ACADS (acyl-CoA dehydrogenase, C-2 to C-3 short chain) (eg, short chain acyl-CoA dehydrogenase deficiency), targeted sequence analysis (eg, exons 5 and 6)

AQP2 (aquaporin 2 [collecting duct]) (eg, nephrogenic diabetes insipidus), full gene sequence

ARX (aristaless related homeobox) (eg, X-linked lissencephaly with ambiguous genitalia, X-linked mental retardation), full gene sequence

AVPR2 (arginine vasopressin receptor 2) (eg, nephrogenic diabetes insipidus), full gene sequence

BBS10 (Bardet-Biedl syndrome 10) (eg, Bardet-Biedl syndrome), full gene sequence

BTD (biotinidase) (eg, biotinidase deficiency), full gene sequence

C10orf2 (chromosome 10 open reading frame 2) (eg, mitochondrial DNA depletion syndrome), full gene sequence

CAV3 (caveolin 3) (eg, CAV3-related distal myopathy, limb-girdle muscular dystrophy type 1C), full gene sequence

CD40LG (CD40 ligand) (eg, X-linked hyper IgM syndrome), full gene sequence

CDKN2A (cyclin-dependent kinase inhibitor 2A) (eg, CDKN2A-related cutaneous malignant melanoma, familial atypical mole-malignant melanoma syndrome), full gene sequence

CLRN1 (clarin 1) (eg, Usher syndrome, type 3), full gene sequence

COX6B1 (cytochrome c oxidase subunit VIb polypeptide 1) (eg, mitochondrial respiratory chain complex IV deficiency), full gene sequence

CPT2 (carnitine palmitoyltransferase 2) (eg, carnitine palmitoyltransferase II deficiency), full gene sequence

CRX (cone-rod homeobox) (eg, cone-rod dystrophy 2, Leber congenital amaurosis), full gene sequence

CYP1B1 (cytochrome P450, family 1, subfamily B, polypeptide 1) (eg, primary congenital glaucoma), full gene sequence

EGR2 (early growth response 2) (eg, Charcot-Marie-Tooth), full gene sequence

EMD (emerin) (eg, Emery-Dreifuss muscular dystrophy), duplication/deletion analysis

EPM2A (epilepsy, progressive myoclonus type 2A, Lafora disease [laforin]) (eg, progressive myoclonus epilepsy), full gene sequence

FGF23 (fibroblast growth factor 23) (eg, hypophosphatemic rickets), full gene sequence

FGFR2 (fibroblast growth factor receptor 2) (eg, craniosynostosis, Apert syndrome, Crouzon syndrome), targeted sequence analysis (eg, exons 8, 10)

FGFR3 (fibroblast growth factor receptor 3) (eg, achondroplasia, hypochondroplasia), targeted sequence analysis (eg, exons 8, 11, 12, 13)

FHL1 (four and a half LIM domains 1) (eg, Emery-Dreifuss muscular dystrophy), full gene sequence

FKRP (Fukutin related protein) (eg, congenital muscular dystrophy type 1C [MDC1C], limb-girdle muscular dystrophy [LGMD] type 2I), full gene sequence

FOXG1 (forkhead box G1) (eg, Rett syndrome), full gene sequence

FSHMD1A (facioscapulohumeral muscular dystrophy 1A) (eg, facioscapulohumeral muscular dystrophy), evaluation to detect abnormal (eg, deleted) alleles

FSHMD1A (facioscapulohumeral muscular dystrophy 1A) (eg, facioscapulohumeral muscular dystrophy), characterization of haplotype(s) (ie, chromosome 4A and 4B haplotypes)

GH1 (growth hormone 1) (eg, growth hormone deficiency), full gene sequence

GP1BB (glycoprotein Ib [platelet], beta polypeptide) (eg, Bernard-Soulier syndrome type B), full gene sequence

(For common deletion variants of alpha globin 1 and alpha globin 2 genes, use 81257)

HNF1B (HNF1 homeobox B) (eg, maturity-onset diabetes of the young [MODY]), duplication/deletion analysis

HRAS (v-Ha-ras Harvey rat sarcoma viral oncogene homolog) (eg, Costello syndrome), full gene sequence

HSD3B2 (hydroxy-delta-5-steroid dehydrogenase, 3 beta- and steroid delta-isomerase 2) (eg, 3-beta-hydroxysteroid dehydrogenase type II deficiency), full gene sequence

HSD11B2 (hydroxysteroid [11-beta] dehydrogenase 2) (eg, mineralocorticoid excess syndrome), full gene sequence

HSPB1 (heat shock 27kDa protein 1) (eg, Charcot-Marie-Tooth disease), full gene sequence

INS (insulin) (eg, diabetes mellitus), full gene sequence

KCNJ1 (potassium inwardly-rectifying channel, subfamily J, member 1) (eg, Bartter syndrome), full gene sequence

KCNJ10 (potassium inwardly-rectifying channel, subfamily J, member 10) (eg, SeSAME syndrome, EAST syndrome, sensorineural hearing loss), full gene sequence

LITAF (lipopolysaccharide-induced TNF factor) (eg, Charcot-Marie-Tooth), full gene sequence

MEFV (Mediterranean fever) (eg, familial Mediterranean fever), full gene sequence

MEN1 (multiple endocrine neoplasia I) (eg, multiple endocrine neoplasia type 1, Wermer syndrome), duplication/deletion analysis

MMACHC (methylmalonic aciduria [cobalamin deficiency] cblC type, with homocystinuria) (eg, methylmalonic acidemia and homocystinuria), full gene sequence

MPV17 (MpV17 mitochondrial inner membrane protein) (eg, mitochondrial DNA depletion syndrome), duplication/deletion analysis

NDP (Norrie disease [pseudoglioma]) (eg, Norrie disease), full gene sequence

NDUFA1 (NADH dehydrogenase [ubiquinone] 1 alpha subcomplex, 1, 7.5kDa) (eg, Leigh syndrome, mitochondrial complex I deficiency), full gene sequence

NDUFAF2 (NADH dehydrogenase [ubiquinone] 1 alpha subcomplex, assembly factor 2) (eg, Leigh syndrome, mitochondrial complex I deficiency), full gene sequence

NDUFS4 (NADH dehydrogenase [ubiquinone] Fe-S protein 4, 18kDa [NADH-coenzyme Q reductase]) (eg, Leigh syndrome, mitochondrial complex I deficiency), full gene sequence

NIPA1 (non-imprinted in Prader-Willi/Angelman syndrome 1) (eg, spastic paraplegia), full gene sequence

NLGN4X (neuroligin 4, X-linked) (eg, autism spectrum disorders), duplication/deletion analysis

NPC2 (Niemann-Pick disease, type C2 [epididymal secretory protein E1]) (eg, Niemann-Pick disease type C2), full gene sequence

NR0B1 (nuclear receptor subfamily 0, group B, member 1) (eg, congenital adrenal hypoplasia), full gene sequence

PDX1 (pancreatic and duodenal homeobox 1) (eg, maturity-onset diabetes of the young [MODY]), full gene sequence

PHOX2B (paired-like homeobox 2b) (eg, congenital central hypoventilation syndrome), full gene sequence

PIK3CA (phosphatidylinositol-4,5-bisphosphate 3-kinase, catalytic subunit alpha) (eg, colorectal cancer), targeted sequence analysis (eg, exons 9 and 20)

PLP1 (proteolipid protein 1) (eg, Pelizaeus-Merzbacher disease, spastic paraplegia), duplication/deletion analysis

PQBP1 (polyglutamine binding protein 1) (eg, Renpenning syndrome), duplication/deletion analysis

PRNP (prion protein) (eg, genetic prion disease), full gene sequence

PROP1 (PROP paired-like homeobox 1) (eg, combined pituitary hormone deficiency), full gene sequence

PRPH2 (peripherin 2 [retinal degeneration, slow]) (eg, retinitis pigmentosa), full gene sequence

PRSS1 (protease, serine, 1 [trypsin 1]) (eg, hereditary pancreatitis), full gene sequence

RAF1 (v-raf-1 murine leukemia viral oncogene homolog 1) (eg, LEOPARD syndrome), targeted sequence analysis (eg, exons 7, 12, 14, 17)

RET (ret proto-oncogene) (eg, multiple endocrine neoplasia, type 2B and familial medullary thyroid carcinoma), common variants (eg, M918T, 2647_2648delinsTT, A883F)

RHO (rhodopsin) (eg, retinitis pigmentosa), full gene sequence

RP1 (retinitis pigmentosa 1) (eg, retinitis pigmentosa), full gene sequence

SCN1B (sodium channel, voltage-gated, type I, beta) (eg, Brugada syndrome), full gene sequence

SCO2 (SCO cytochrome oxidase deficient homolog 2 [SCO1L]) (eg, mitochondrial respiratory chain complex IV deficiency), full gene sequence

SDHC (succinate dehydrogenase complex, subunit C, integral membrane protein, 15kDa) (eg, hereditary paraganglioma-pheochromocytoma syndrome), duplication/deletion analysis

SDHD (succinate dehydrogenase complex, subunit D, integral membrane protein) (eg, hereditary paraganglioma), full gene sequence

SGCG (sarcoglycan, gamma [35kDa dystrophin-associated glycoprotein]) (eg, limb-girdle muscular dystrophy), duplication/deletion analysis

SH2D1A (SH2 domain containing 1A) (eg, X-linked lymphoproliferative syndrome), full gene sequence

SLC16A2 (solute carrier family 16, member 2 [thyroid hormone transporter]) (eg, specific thyroid hormone cell transporter deficiency, Allan-Herndon-Dudley syndrome), duplication/deletion analysis

SLC25A20 (solute carrier family 25 [carnitine/acylcarnitine translocase], member 20) (eg, carnitine-acylcarnitine translocase deficiency), duplication/deletion analysis

SLC25A4 (solute carrier family 25 [mitochondrial carrier; adenine nucleotide translocation], member 4) (eg, progressive external ophthalmoplegia), full gene sequence

SOD1 (superoxide dismutase 1, soluble) (eg, amyotrophic lateral sclerosis), full gene sequence

SPINK1 (serine peptidase inhibitor, Kazal type 1) (eg, hereditary pancreatitis), full gene sequence

STK11 (serine/threonine kinase 11) (eg, Peutz-Jeghers syndrome), duplication/deletion analysis

TACO1 (translational activator of mitochondrial encoded cytochrome c oxidase I) (eg, mitochondrial respiratory chain complex IV deficiency), full gene sequence

THAP1 (THAP domain containing, apoptosis associated protein 1) (eg, torsion dystonia), full gene sequence

TOR1A (torsin family 1, member A [torsin A]) (eg, torsion dystonia), full gene sequence

TTPA (tocopherol [alpha] transfer protein) (eg, ataxia), full gene sequence

TTR (transthyretin) (eg, familial transthyretin amyloidosis), full gene sequence

TWIST1 (twist homolog 1 [Drosophila]) (eg, Saethre-Chotzen syndrome), full gene sequence

TYR (tyrosinase [oculocutaneous albinism IA]) (eg, oculocutaneous albinism IA), full gene sequence

UGT1A1 (UDP glucuronosyltransferase 1 family, polypeptide A1) (eg, hereditary unconjugated hyperbilirubinemia [Crigler-Najjar syndrome]) full gene sequence

USH1G (Usher syndrome 1G [autosomal recessive]) (eg, Usher syndrome, type 1), full gene sequence

VWF (von Willebrand factor) (eg, von Willebrand disease type 1C), targeted sequence analysis (eg, exons 26, 27, 37)

VHL (von Hippel-Lindau tumor suppressor) (eg, von Hippel-Lindau familial cancer syndrome), full gene sequence

ZEB2 (zinc finger E-box binding homeobox 2) (eg, Mowat-Wilson syndrome), duplication/deletion analysis

ZNF41 (zinc finger protein 41) (eg, X-linked mental retardation 89), full gene sequence

0.00 0.00 **FUD** XXX A

AMA: 2020,OctSE,1; 2020,Apr,9; 2019,Jul,3; 2018,Nov,9; 2018,May,6; 2018,Jan,8; 2017,Jan,8; 2016,Aug,9; 2016,Jan,13; 2015,Jan,3; 2015,Jan,16

▲ **81405 Molecular pathology procedure, Level 6 (eg, analysis of 6-10 exons by DNA sequence analysis, mutation scanning or duplication/deletion variants of 11-25 exons, regionally targeted cytogenomic array analysis)**

ABCD1 (ATP-binding cassette, sub-family D [ALD], member 1) (eg, adrenoleukodystrophy), full gene sequence

ACADS (acyl-CoA dehydrogenase, C-2 to C-3 short chain) (eg, short chain acyl-CoA dehydrogenase deficiency), full gene sequence

ACTA2 (actin, alpha 2, smooth muscle, aorta) (eg, thoracic aortic aneurysms and aortic dissections), full gene sequence

ACTC1 (actin, alpha, cardiac muscle 1) (eg, familial hypertrophic cardiomyopathy), full gene sequence

ANKRD1 (ankyrin repeat domain 1) (eg, dilated cardiomyopathy), full gene sequence

APTX (aprataxin) (eg, ataxia with oculomotor apraxia 1), full gene sequence

ARSA (arylsulfatase A) (eg, arylsulfatase A deficiency), full gene sequence

BCKDHA (branched chain keto acid dehydrogenase E1, alpha polypeptide) (eg, maple syrup urine disease, type 1A), full gene sequence

BCS1L (BCS1-like [S. cerevisiae]) (eg, Leigh syndrome, mitochondrial complex III deficiency, GRACILE syndrome), full gene sequence

BMPR2 (bone morphogenetic protein receptor, type II [serine/threonine kinase]) (eg, heritable pulmonary arterial hypertension), duplication/deletion analysis

CASQ2 (calsequestrin 2 [cardiac muscle]) (eg, catecholaminergic polymorphic ventricular tachycardia), full gene sequence

CASR (calcium-sensing receptor) (eg, hypocalcemia), full gene sequence

CDKL5 (cyclin-dependent kinase-like 5) (eg, early infantile epileptic encephalopathy), duplication/deletion analysis

CHRNA4 (cholinergic receptor, nicotinic, alpha 4) (eg, nocturnal frontal lobe epilepsy), full gene sequence

CHRNB2 (cholinergic receptor, nicotinic, beta 2 [neuronal]) (eg, nocturnal frontal lobe epilepsy), full gene sequence

COX10 (COX10 homolog, cytochrome c oxidase assembly protein) (eg, mitochondrial respiratory chain complex IV deficiency), full gene sequence

COX15 (COX15 homolog, cytochrome c oxidase assembly protein) (eg, mitochondrial respiratory chain complex IV deficiency), full gene sequence

CPOX (coproporphyrinogen oxidase) (eg, hereditary coproporphyria), full gene sequence

CTRC (chymotrypsin C) (eg, hereditary pancreatitis), full gene sequence

CYP11B1 (cytochrome P450, family 11, subfamily B, polypeptide 1) (eg, congenital adrenal hyperplasia), full gene sequence

CYP17A1 (cytochrome P450, family 17, subfamily A, polypeptide 1) (eg, congenital adrenal hyperplasia), full gene sequence

CYP21A2 (cytochrome P450, family 21, subfamily A, polypeptide2) (eg, steroid 21-hydroxylase isoform, congenital adrenal hyperplasia), full gene sequence

Cytogenomic constitutional targeted microarray analysis of chromosome 22q13 by interrogation of genomic regions for copy number and single nucleotide polymorphism (SNP) variants for chromosomal abnormalities

(When performing genome-wide cytogenomic constitutional microarray analysis, see 81228, 81229) (81228-81229)

(Do not report analyte-specific molecular pathology procedures separately when the specific analytes are included as part of the microarray analysis of chromosome 22q13)

(Do not report 88271 when performing cytogenomic microarray analysis)

DBT (dihydrolipoamide branched chain transacylase E2) (eg, maple syrup urine disease, type 2), duplication/deletion analysis

DCX (doublecortin) (eg, X-linked lissencephaly), full gene sequence

DES (desmin) (eg, myofibrillar myopathy), full gene sequence

DFNB59 (deafness, autosomal recessive 59) (eg, autosomal recessive nonsyndromic hearing impairment), full gene sequence

DGUOK (deoxyguanosine kinase) (eg, hepatocerebral mitochondrial DNA depletion syndrome), full gene sequence

DHCR7 (7-dehydrocholesterol reductase) (eg, Smith-Lemli-Opitz syndrome), full gene sequence

EIF2B2 (eukaryotic translation initiation factor 2B, subunit 2 beta, 39kDa) (eg, leukoencephalopathy with vanishing white matter), full gene sequence

EMD (emerin) (eg, Emery-Dreifuss muscular dystrophy), full gene sequence

ENG (endoglin) (eg, hereditary hemorrhagic telangiectasia, type 1), duplication/deletion analysis

EYA1 (eyes absent homolog 1 [Drosophila]) (eg, branchio-oto-renal [BOR] spectrum disorders), duplication/deletion analysis

FGFR1 (fibroblast growth factor receptor 1) (eg, Kallmann syndrome 2), full gene sequence

FH (fumarate hydratase) (eg, fumarate hydratase deficiency, hereditary leiomyomatosis with renal cell cancer), full gene sequence

FKTN (fukutin) (eg, limb-girdle muscular dystrophy [LGMD] type 2M or 2L), full gene sequence

FTSJ1 (FtsJ RNA methyltransferase homolog 1 [E. coli]) (eg, X-linked mental retardation 9), duplication/deletion analysis

GABRG2 (gamma-aminobutyric acid [GABA] A receptor, gamma 2) (eg, generalized epilepsy with febrile seizures), full gene sequence

GCH1 (GTP cyclohydrolase 1) (eg, autosomal dominant dopa-responsive dystonia), full gene sequence

GDAP1 (ganglioside-induced differentiation-associated protein 1) (eg, Charcot-Marie-Tooth disease), full gene sequence

GFAP (glial fibrillary acidic protein) (eg, Alexander disease), full gene sequence

GHR (growth hormone receptor) (eg, Laron syndrome), full gene sequence

GHRHR (growth hormone releasing hormone receptor) (eg, growth hormone deficiency), full gene sequence

GLA (galactosidase, alpha) (eg, Fabry disease), full gene sequence

HNF1A (HNF1 homeobox A) (eg, maturity-onset diabetes of the young [MODY]), full gene sequence

HNF1B (HNF1 homeobox B) (eg, maturity-onset diabetes of the young [MODY]), full gene sequence

HTRA1 (HtrA serine peptidase 1) (eg, macular degeneration), full gene sequence

IDS (iduronate 2-sulfatase) (eg, mucopolysaccharidosis, type II), full gene sequence

IL2RG (interleukin 2 receptor, gamma) (eg, X-linked severe combined immunodeficiency), full gene sequence

ISPD (isoprenoid synthase domain containing) (eg, muscle-eye-brain disease, Walker-Warburg syndrome), full gene sequence

KRAS (Kirsten rat sarcoma viral oncogene homolog) (eg, Noonan syndrome), full gene sequence

LAMP2 (lysosomal-associated membrane protein 2) (eg, Danon disease), full gene sequence

LDLR (low density lipoprotein receptor) (eg, familial hypercholesterolemia), duplication/deletion analysis

MEN1 (multiple endocrine neoplasia I) (eg, multiple endocrine neoplasia type 1, Wermer syndrome), full gene sequence

MMAA (methylmalonic aciduria [cobalamine deficiency] type A) (eg, MMAA-related methylmalonic acidemia), full gene sequence

MMAB (methylmalonic aciduria [cobalamine deficiency] type B) (eg, MMAA-related methylmalonic acidemia), full gene sequence

MPI (mannose phosphate isomerase) (eg, congenital disorder of glycosylation 1b), full gene sequence

Pathology and Laboratory

81405 — 81405

MPV17 (MpV17 mitochondrial inner membrane protein) (eg, mitochondrial DNA depletion syndrome), full gene sequence

MPZ (myelin protein zero) (eg, Charcot-Marie-Tooth), full gene sequence

MTM1 (myotubularin 1) (eg, X-linked centronuclear myopathy), duplication/deletion analysis

MYL2 (myosin, light chain 2, regulatory, cardiac, slow) (eg, familial hypertrophic cardiomyopathy), full gene sequence

MYL3 (myosin, light chain 3, alkali, ventricular, skeletal, slow) (eg, familial hypertrophic cardiomyopathy), full gene sequence

MYOT (myotilin) (eg, limb-girdle muscular dystrophy), full gene sequence

NDUFS7 (NADH dehydrogenase [ubiquinone] Fe-S protein 7, 20kDa [NADH-coenzyme Q reductase]) (eg, Leigh syndrome, mitochondrial complex I deficiency), full gene sequence

NDUFS8 (NADH dehydrogenase [ubiquinone] Fe-S protein 8, 23kDa [NADH-coenzyme Q reductase]) (eg, Leigh syndrome, mitochondrial complex I deficiency), full gene sequence

NDUFV1 (NADH dehydrogenase [ubiquinone] flavoprotein 1, 51kDa) (eg, Leigh syndrome, mitochondrial complex I deficiency), full gene sequence

NEFL (neurofilament, light polypeptide) (eg, Charcot-Marie-Tooth), full gene sequence

NF2 (neurofibromin 2 [merlin]) (eg, neurofibromatosis, type 2), duplication/deletion analysis

NLGN3 (neuroligin 3) (eg, autism spectrum disorders), full gene sequence

NLGN4X (neuroligin 4, X-linked) (eg, autism spectrum disorders), full gene sequence

NPHP1 (nephronophthisis 1 [juvenile]) (eg, Joubert syndrome), deletion analysis, and duplication analysis, if performed

NPHS2 (nephrosis 2, idiopathic, steroid-resistant [podocin]) (eg, steroid-resistant nephrotic syndrome), full gene sequence

NSD1 (nuclear receptor binding SET domain protein 1) (eg, Sotos syndrome), duplication/deletion analysis

OTC (ornithine carbamoyltransferase) (eg, ornithine transcarbamylase deficiency), full gene sequence

PAFAH1B1 (platelet-activating factor acetylhydrolase 1b, regulatory subunit 1 [45kDa]) (eg, lissencephaly, Miller-Dieker syndrome), duplication/deletion analysis

PARK2 (Parkinson protein 2, E3 ubiquitin protein ligase [parkin]) (eg, Parkinson disease), duplication/deletion analysis

PCCA (propionyl CoA carboxylase, alpha polypeptide) (eg, propionic acidemia, type 1), duplication/deletion analysis

PCDH19 (protocadherin 19) (eg, epileptic encephalopathy), full gene sequence

PDHA1 (pyruvate dehydrogenase [lipoamide] alpha 1) (eg, lactic acidosis), duplication/deletion analysis

PDHB (pyruvate dehydrogenase [lipoamide] beta) (eg, lactic acidosis), full gene sequence

PINK1 (PTEN induced putative kinase 1) (eg, Parkinson disease), full gene sequence

PKLR (pyruvate kinase, liver and RBC) (eg, pyruvate kinase deficiency), full gene sequence

PLP1 (proteolipid protein 1) (eg, Pelizaeus-Merzbacher disease, spastic paraplegia), full gene sequence

POU1F1 (POU class 1 homeobox 1) (eg, combined pituitary hormone deficiency), full gene sequence

PQBP1 (polyglutamine binding protein 1) (eg, Renpenning syndrome), full gene sequence

PRX (periaxin) (eg, Charcot-Marie-Tooth disease), full gene sequence

PSEN1 (presenilin 1) (eg, Alzheimer's disease), full gene sequence

RAB7A (RAB7A, member RAS oncogene family) (eg, Charcot-Marie-Tooth disease), full gene sequence

RAI1 (retinoic acid induced 1) (eg, Smith-Magenis syndrome), full gene sequence

REEP1 (receptor accessory protein 1) (eg, spastic paraplegia), full gene sequence

RET (ret proto-oncogene) (eg, multiple endocrine neoplasia, type 2A and familial medullary thyroid carcinoma), targeted sequence analysis (eg, exons 10, 11, 13-16)

RPS19 (ribosomal protein S19) (eg, Diamond-Blackfan anemia), full gene sequence

RRM2B (ribonucleotide reductase M2 B [TP53 inducible]) (eg, mitochondrial DNA depletion), full gene sequence

SCO1 (SCO cytochrome oxidase deficient homolog 1) (eg, mitochondrial respiratory chain complex IV deficiency), full gene sequence

SDHB (succinate dehydrogenase complex, subunit B, iron sulfur) (eg, hereditary paraganglioma), full gene sequence

SDHC (succinate dehydrogenase complex, subunit C, integral membrane protein, 15kDa) (eg, hereditary paraganglioma-pheochromocytoma syndrome), full gene sequence

SGCA (sarcoglycan, alpha [50kDa dystrophin-associated glycoprotein]) (eg, limb-girdle muscular dystrophy), full gene sequence

SGCB (sarcoglycan, beta [43kDa dystrophin-associated glycoprotein]) (eg, limb-girdle muscular dystrophy), full gene sequence

SGCD (sarcoglycan, delta [35kDa dystrophin-associated glycoprotein]) (eg, limb-girdle muscular dystrophy), full gene sequence

SGCE (sarcoglycan, epsilon) (eg, myoclonic dystonia), duplication/deletion analysis

SGCG (sarcoglycan, gamma [35kDa dystrophin-associated glycoprotein]) (eg, limb-girdle muscular dystrophy), full gene sequence

SHOC2 (soc-2 suppressor of clear homolog) (eg, Noonan-like syndrome with loose anagen hair), full gene sequence

SHOX (short stature homeobox) (eg, Langer mesomelic dysplasia), full gene sequence

SIL1 (SIL1 homolog, endoplasmic reticulum chaperone [S. cerevisiae]) (eg, ataxia), full gene sequence

SLC2A1 (solute carrier family 2 [facilitated glucose transporter], member 1) (eg, glucose transporter type 1 [GLUT 1] deficiency syndrome), full gene sequence

SLC16A2 (solute carrier family 16, member 2 [thyroid hormone transporter]) (eg, specific thyroid hormone cell transporter deficiency, Allan-Herndon-Dudley syndrome), full gene sequence

SLC22A5 (solute carrier family 22 [organic cation/carnitine transporter], member 5) (eg, systemic primary carnitine deficiency), full gene sequence

SLC25A20 (solute carrier family 25 [carnitine/acylcarnitine translocase], member 20) (eg, carnitine-acylcarnitine translocase deficiency), full gene sequence

SMAD4 (SMAD family member 4) (eg, hemorrhagic telangiectasia syndrome, juvenile polyposis), duplication/deletion analysis

SPAST (spastin) (eg, spastic paraplegia), duplication/deletion analysis

SPG7 (spastic paraplegia 7 [pure and complicated autosomal recessive]) (eg, spastic paraplegia), duplication/deletion analysis

SPRED1 (sprouty-related, EVH1 domain containing 1) (eg, Legius syndrome), full gene sequence

STAT3 (signal transducer and activator of transcription 3 [acute-phase response factor]) (eg, autosomal dominant hyper-IgE syndrome), targeted sequence analysis (eg, exons 12, 13, 14, 16, 17, 20, 21)

STK11 (serine/threonine kinase 11) (eg, Peutz-Jeghers syndrome), full gene sequence

SURF1 (surfeit 1) (eg, mitochondrial respiratory chain complex IV deficiency), full gene sequence

TARDBP (TAR DNA binding protein) (eg, amyotrophic lateral sclerosis), full gene sequence

TBX5 (T-box 5) (eg, Holt-Oram syndrome), full gene sequence

TCF4 (transcription factor 4) (eg, Pitt-Hopkins syndrome), duplication/deletion analysis

TGFBR1 (transforming growth factor, beta receptor 1) (eg, Marfan syndrome), full gene sequence

TGFBR2 (transforming growth factor, beta receptor 2) (eg, Marfan syndrome), full gene sequence

THRB (thyroid hormone receptor, beta) (eg, thyroid hormone resistance, thyroid hormone beta receptor deficiency), full gene sequence or targeted sequence analysis of >5 exons

TK2 (thymidine kinase 2, mitochondrial) (eg, mitochondrial DNA depletion syndrome), full gene sequence

TNNC1 (troponin C type 1 [slow]) (eg, hypertrophic cardiomyopathy or dilated cardiomyopathy), full gene sequence

TNNI3 (troponin 1, type 3 [cardiac]) (eg, familial hypertrophic cardiomyopathy), full gene sequence

TPM1 (tropomyosin 1 [alpha]) (eg, familial hypertrophic cardiomyopathy), full gene sequence

TSC1 (tuberous sclerosis 1) (eg, tuberous sclerosis), duplication/deletion analysis

TYMP (thymidine phosphorylase) (eg, mitochondrial DNA depletion syndrome), full gene sequence

VWF (von Willebrand factor) (eg, von Willebrand disease type 2N), targeted sequence analysis (eg, exons 18-20, 23-25)

WT1 (Wilms tumor 1) (eg, Denys-Drash syndrome, familial Wilms tumor), full gene sequence

ZEB2 (zinc finger E-box binding homeobox 2) (eg, Mowat-Wilson syndrome), full gene sequence

0.00 0.00 **FUD** XXX A

AMA: 2020,OctSE,1; 2019,Jul,3; 2018,Nov,9; 2018,Sep,14; 2018,May,6; 2018,Jan,8; 2017,Jan,8; 2016,Aug,9; 2016,Jan,13; 2015,Jan,3; 2015,Jan,16

81406 Molecular pathology procedure, Level 7 (eg, analysis of 11-25 exons by DNA sequence analysis, mutation scanning or duplication/deletion variants of 26-50 exons)

ACADVL (acyl-CoA dehydrogenase, very long chain) (eg, very long chain acyl-coenzyme A dehydrogenase deficiency), full gene sequence

ACTN4 (actinin, alpha 4) (eg, focal segmental glomerulosclerosis), full gene sequence

AFG3L2 (AFG3 ATPase family gene 3-like 2 [S. cerevisiae]) (eg, spinocerebellar ataxia), full gene sequence

AIRE (autoimmune regulator) (eg, autoimmune polyendocrinopathy syndrome type 1), full gene sequence

ALDH7A1 (aldehyde dehydrogenase 7 family, member A1) (eg, pyridoxine-dependent epilepsy), full gene sequence

ANO5 (anoctamin 5) (eg, limb-girdle muscular dystrophy), full gene sequence

ANOS1 (anosim-1) (eg, Kallmann syndrome 1), full gene sequence

APP (amyloid beta [A4] precursor protein) (eg, Alzheimer's disease), full gene sequence

ASS1 (argininosuccinate synthase 1) (eg, citrullinemia type I), full gene sequence

ATL1 (atlastin GTPase 1) (eg, spastic paraplegia), full gene sequence

ATP1A2 (ATPase, Na+/K+ transporting, alpha 2 polypeptide) (eg, familial hemiplegic migraine), full gene sequence

ATP7B (ATPase, Cu++ transporting, beta polypeptide) (eg, Wilson disease), full gene sequence

BBS1 (Bardet-Biedl syndrome 1) (eg, Bardet-Biedl syndrome), full gene sequence

BBS2 (Bardet-Biedl syndrome 2) (eg, Bardet-Biedl syndrome), full gene sequence

BCKDHB (branched-chain keto acid dehydrogenase E1, beta polypeptide) (eg, maple syrup urine disease, type 1B), full gene sequence

BEST1 (bestrophin 1) (eg, vitelliform macular dystrophy), full gene sequence

BMPR2 (bone morphogenetic protein receptor, type II [serine/threonine kinase]) (eg, heritable pulmonary arterial hypertension), full gene sequence

BRAF (B-Raf proto-oncogene, serine/threonine kinase) (eg, Noonan syndrome), full gene sequence

BSCL2 (Berardinelli-Seip congenital lipodystrophy 2 [seipin]) (eg, Berardinelli-Seip congenital lipodystrophy), full gene sequence

BTK (Bruton agammaglobulinemia tyrosine kinase) (eg, X-linked agammaglobulinemia), full gene sequence

CACNB2 (calcium channel, voltage-dependent, beta 2 subunit) (eg, Brugada syndrome), full gene sequence

CAPN3 (calpain 3) (eg, limb-girdle muscular dystrophy [LGMD] type 2A, calpainopathy), full gene sequence

CBS (cystathionine-beta-synthase) (eg, homocystinuria, cystathionine beta-synthase deficiency), full gene sequence

CDH1 (cadherin 1, type 1, E-cadherin [epithelial]) (eg, hereditary diffuse gastric cancer), full gene sequence

CDKL5 (cyclin-dependent kinase-like 5) (eg, early infantile epileptic encephalopathy), full gene sequence

CLCN1 (chloride channel 1, skeletal muscle) (eg, myotonia congenita), full gene sequence

CLCNKB (chloride channel, voltage-sensitive Kb) (eg, Bartter syndrome 3 and 4b), full gene sequence

CNTNAP2 (contactin-associated protein-like 2) (eg, Pitt-Hopkins-like syndrome 1), full gene sequence

COL6A2 (collagen, type VI, alpha 2) (eg, collagen type VI-related disorders), duplication/deletion analysis

CPT1A (carnitine palmitoyltransferase 1A [liver]) (eg, carnitine palmitoyltransferase 1A [CPT1A] deficiency), full gene sequence

CRB1 (crumbs homolog 1 [Drosophila]) (eg, Leber congenital amaurosis), full gene sequence

CREBBP (CREB binding protein) (eg, Rubinstein-Taybi syndrome), duplication/deletion analysis

DBT (dihydrolipoamide branched chain transacylase E2) (eg, maple syrup urine disease, type 2), full gene sequence

DLAT (dihydrolipoamide S-acetyltransferase) (eg, pyruvate dehydrogenase E2 deficiency), full gene sequence

DLD (dihydrolipoamide dehydrogenase) (eg, maple syrup urine disease, type III), full gene sequence

DSC2 (desmocollin) (eg, arrhythmogenic right ventricular dysplasia/cardiomyopathy 11), full gene sequence

DSG2 (desmoglein 2) (eg, arrhythmogenic right ventricular dysplasia/cardiomyopathy 10), full gene sequence

DSP (desmoplakin) (eg, arrhythmogenic right ventricular dysplasia/cardiomyopathy 8), full gene sequence

EFHC1 (EF-hand domain [C-terminal] containing 1) (eg, juvenile myoclonic epilepsy), full gene sequence

EIF2B3 (eukaryotic translation initiation factor 2B, subunit 3 gamma, 58kDa) (eg, leukoencephalopathy with vanishing white matter), full gene sequence

EIF2B4 (eukaryotic translation initiation factor 2B, subunit 4 delta, 67kDa) (eg, leukoencephalopathy with vanishing white matter), full gene sequence

EIF2B5 (eukaryotic translation initiation factor 2B, subunit 5 epsilon, 82kDa) (eg, childhood ataxia with central nervous system hypomyelination/vanishing white matter), full gene sequence

ENG (endoglin) (eg, hereditary hemorrhagic telangiectasia, type 1), full gene sequence

EYA1 (eyes absent homolog 1 [Drosophila]) (eg, branchio-oto-renal [BOR] spectrum disorders), full gene sequence

F8 (coagulation factor VIII) (eg, hemophilia A), duplication/deletion analysis

FAH (fumarylacetoacetate hydrolase [fumarylacetoacetase]) (eg, tyrosinemia, type 1), full gene sequence

FASTKD2 (FAST kinase domains 2) (eg, mitochondrial respiratory chain complex IV deficiency), full gene sequence

FIG4 (FIG4 homolog, SAC1 lipid phosphatase domain containing [S. cerevisiae]) (eg, Charcot-Marie-Tooth disease), full gene sequence

FTSJ1 (FtsJ RNA methyltransferase homolog 1 [E. coli]) (eg, X-linked mental retardation 9), full gene sequence

FUS (fused in sarcoma) (eg, amyotrophic lateral sclerosis), full gene sequence

GAA (glucosidase, alpha; acid) (eg, glycogen storage disease type II [Pompe disease]), full gene sequence

GALC (galactosylceramidase) (eg, Krabbe disease), full gene sequence

GALT (galactose-1-phosphate uridylyltransferase) (eg, galactosemia), full gene sequence

GARS (glycyl-tRNA synthetase) (eg, Charcot-Marie-Tooth disease), full gene sequence

GCDH (glutaryl-CoA dehydrogenase) (eg, glutaricacidemia type 1), full gene sequence

GCK (glucokinase [hexokinase 4]) (eg, maturity-onset diabetes of the young [MODY]), full gene sequence

GLUD1 (glutamate dehydrogenase 1) (eg, familial hyperinsulinism), full gene sequence

GNE (glucosamine [UDP-N-acetyl]-2-epimerase/N-acetylmannosamine kinase) (eg, inclusion body myopathy 2 [IBM2], Nonaka myopathy), full gene sequence

GRN (granulin) (eg, frontotemporal dementia), full gene sequence

HADHA (hydroxyacyl-CoA dehydrogenase/3-ketoacyl-CoA thiolase/enoyl-CoA hydratase [trifunctional protein] alpha subunit) (eg, long chain acyl-coenzyme A dehydrogenase deficiency), full gene sequence

HADHB (hydroxyacyl-CoA dehydrogenase/3-ketoacyl-CoA thiolase/enoyl-CoA hydratase [trifunctional protein], beta subunit) (eg, trifunctional protein deficiency), full gene sequence

HEXA (hexosaminidase A, alpha polypeptide) (eg, Tay-Sachs disease), full gene sequence

HLCS (HLCS holocarboxylase synthetase) (eg, holocarboxylase synthetase deficiency), full gene sequence

HMBS (hydroxymethylbilane synthase) (eg, acute intermittent porphyria), full gene sequence

HNF4A (hepatocyte nuclear factor 4, alpha) (eg, maturity-onset diabetes of the young [MODY]), full gene sequence

IDUA (iduronidase, alpha-L-) (eg, mucopolysaccharidosis type I), full gene sequence

INF2 (inverted formin, FH2 and WH2 domain containing) (eg, focal segmental glomerulosclerosis), full gene sequence

IVD (isovaleryl-CoA dehydrogenase) (eg, isovaleric acidemia), full gene sequence

JAG1 (jagged 1) (eg, Alagille syndrome), duplication/deletion analysis

JUP (junction plakoglobin) (eg, arrhythmogenic right ventricular dysplasia/cardiomyopathy 11), full gene sequence

KCNH2 (potassium voltage-gated channel, subfamily H [eag-related], member 2) (eg, short QT syndrome, long QT syndrome), full gene sequence

KCNQ1 (potassium voltage-gated channel, KQT-like subfamily, member 1) (eg, short QT syndrome, long QT syndrome), full gene sequence

KCNQ2 (potassium voltage-gated channel, KQT-like subfamily, member 2) (eg, epileptic encephalopathy), full gene sequence

LDB3 (LIM domain binding 3) (eg, familial dilated cardiomyopathy, myofibrillar myopathy), full gene sequence

LDLR (low density lipoprotein receptor) (eg, familial hypercholesterolemia), full gene sequence

LEPR (leptin receptor(eg, obesity with hypogonadism), full gene sequence

LHCGR (luteinizing hormone/choriogonadotropin receptor) (eg, precocious male puberty), full gene sequence

LMNA (lamin A/C) (eg, Emery-Dreifuss muscular dystrophy [EDMD1, 2 and 3] limb-girdle muscular dystrophy [LGMD] type 1B, dilated cardiomyopathy [CMD1A], familial partial lipodystrophy [FPLD2]), full gene sequence

LRP5 (low density lipoprotein receptor-related protein 5) (eg, osteopetrosis), full gene sequence

MAP2K1 (mitogen-activated protein kinase 1) (eg, cardiofaciocutaneous syndrome), full gene sequence

MAP2K2 (mitogen-activated protein kinase 2) (eg, cardiofaciocutaneous syndrome), full gene sequence

MAPT (microtubule-associated protein tau) (eg, frontotemporal dementia), full gene sequence

MCCC1 (methylcrotonoyl-CoA carboxylase 1 [alpha]) (eg, 3-methylcrotonyl-CoA carboxylase deficiency), full gene sequence

MCCC2 (methylcrotonoyl-CoA carboxylase 2 [beta]) (eg, 3-methylcrotonyl carboxylase deficiency), full gene sequence

MFN2 (mitofusin 2) (eg, Charcot-Marie-Tooth disease), full gene sequence

MTM1 (myotubularin 1) (eg, X-linked centronuclear myopathy), full gene sequence

MUT (methylmalonyl CoA mutase) (eg, methylmalonic acidemia), full gene sequence

MUTYH (mutY homolog [E. coli]) (eg, MYH-associated polyposis), full gene sequence

NDUFS1 (NADH dehydrogenase [ubiquinone] Fe-S protein 1, 75kDa [NADH-coenzyme Q reductase]) (eg, Leigh syndrome, mitochondrial complex I deficiency), full gene sequence

NF2 (neurofibromin 2 [merlin]) (eg, neurofibromatosis, type 2), full gene sequence

NOTCH3 (notch 3) (eg, cerebral autosomal dominant arteriopathy with subcortical infarcts and leukoencephalopathy [CADASIL]), targeted sequence analysis (eg, exons 1-23)

NPC1 (Niemann-Pick disease, type C1) (eg, Niemann-Pick disease), full gene sequence

NPHP1 (nephronophthisis 1 [juvenile]) (eg, Joubert syndrome), full gene sequence

NSD1 (nuclear receptor binding SET domain protein 1) (eg, Sotos syndrome), full gene sequence

OPA1 (optic atrophy 1) (eg, optic atrophy), duplication/deletion analysis

OPTN (optineurin) (eg, amyotrophic lateral sclerosis), full gene sequence

PAFAH1B1 (platelet-activating factor acetylhydrolase 1b, regulatory subunit 1 [45kDa]) (eg, lissencephaly, Miller-Dieker syndrome), full gene sequence

PAH (phenylalanine hydroxylase) (eg, phenylketonuria), full gene sequence

PALB2 (partner and localizer of BRCA2) (eg, breast and pancreatic cancer), full gene sequence

PARK2 (Parkinson protein 2, E3 ubiquitin protein ligase [parkin]) (eg, Parkinson disease), full gene sequence

PAX2 (paired box 2) (eg, renal coloboma syndrome), full gene sequence

PC (pyruvate carboxylase) (eg, pyruvate carboxylase deficiency), full gene sequence

PCCA (propionyl CoA carboxylase, alpha polypeptide) (eg, propionic acidemia, type 1), full gene sequence

PCCB (propionyl CoA carboxylase, beta polypeptide) (eg, propionic acidemia), full gene sequence

PCDH15 (protocadherin-related 15) (eg, Usher syndrome type 1F), duplication/deletion analysis

PCSK9 (proprotein convertase subtilisin/kexin type 9) (eg familial hypercholesterolemia), full gene sequence

PDHA1 (pyruvate dehydrogenase [lipoamide] alpha 1) (eg, lactic acidosis), full gene sequence

PDHX (pyruvate dehydrogenase complex, component X) (eg, lactic acidosis), full gene sequence

PHEX (phosphate-regulating endopeptidase homolog, X-linked) (eg, hypophosphatemic rickets), full gene sequence

PKD2 (polycystic kidney disease 2 [autosomal dominant]) (eg, polycystic kidney disease), full gene sequence

PKP2 (plakophilin 2) (eg, arrhythmogenic right ventricular dysplasia/cardiomyopathy 9), full gene sequence

PNKD (eg, paroxysmal nonkinesigenic dyskinesia), full gene sequence

POLG (polymerase [DNA directed], gamma) (eg, Alpers-Huttenlocher syndrome, autosomal dominant progressive external ophthalmoplegia), full gene sequence

POMGNT1 (protein O-linked mannose beta1, 2-N acetylglucosaminyltransferase) (eg, muscle-eye-brain disease, Walker-Warburg syndrome), full gene sequence

POMT1 (protein-O-mannosyltransferase 1) (eg, limb-girdle muscular dystrophy [LGMD] type 2K, Walker-Warburg syndrome), full gene sequence

POMT2 (protein-O-mannosyltransferase 2) (eg, limb-girdle muscular dystrophy [LGMD] type 2N, Walker-Warburg syndrome), full gene sequence

PPOX (protoporphyrinogen oxidase) (eg, variegate porphyria), full gene sequence

PRKAG2 (protein kinase, AMP-activated, gamma 2 non-catalytic subunit) (eg, familial hypertrophic cardiomyopathy with Wolff-Parkinson-White syndrome, lethal congenital glycogen storage disease of heart), full gene sequence

PRKCG (protein kinase C, gamma) (eg, spinocerebellar ataxia), full gene sequence

PSEN2 (presenilin 2[Alzheimer's disease 4]) (eg, Alzheimer's disease), full gene sequence

PTPN11 (protein tyrosine phosphatase, non-receptor type 11) (eg, Noonan syndrome, LEOPARD syndrome), full gene sequence

PYGM (phosphorylase, glycogen, muscle) (eg, glycogen storage disease type V, McArdle disease), full gene sequence

RAF1 (v-raf-1 murine leukemia viral oncogene homolog 1) (eg, LEOPARD syndrome), full gene sequence

RET (ret proto-oncogene) (eg, Hirschsprung disease), full gene sequence

RPE65 (retinal pigment epithelium-specific protein 65kDa) (eg, retinitis pigmentosa, Leber congenital amaurosis), full gene sequence

RYR1 (ryanodine receptor 1, skeletal) (eg, malignant hyperthermia), targeted sequence analysis of exons with functionally-confirmed mutations

SCN4A (sodium channel, voltage-gated, type IV, alpha subunit) (eg, hyperkalemic periodic paralysis), full gene sequence

SCNN1A (sodium channel, nonvoltage-gated 1 alpha) (eg, pseudohypoaldosteronism), full gene sequence

SCNN1B (sodium channel, nonvoltage-gated 1, beta) (eg, Liddle syndrome, pseudohypoaldosteronism), full gene sequence

SCNN1G (sodium channel, nonvoltage-gated 1, gamma) (eg, Liddle syndrome, pseudohypoaldosteronism), full gene sequence

SDHA (succinate dehydrogenase complex, subunit A, flavoprotein [Fp]) (eg, Leigh syndrome, mitochondrial complex II deficiency), full gene sequence

SETX (senataxin) (eg, ataxia), full gene sequence

SGCE (sarcoglycan, epsilon) (eg, myoclonic dystonia), full gene sequence

SH3TC2 (SH3 domain and tetratricopeptide repeats 2) (eg, Charcot-Marie-Tooth disease), full gene sequence

SLC9A6 (solute carrier family 9 [sodium/hydrogen exchanger], member 6) (eg, Christianson syndrome), full gene sequence

SLC26A4 (solute carrier family 26, member 4) (eg, Pendred syndrome), full gene sequence

SLC37A4 (solute carrier family 37 [glucose-6-phosphate transporter], member 4) (eg, glycogen storage disease type Ib), full gene sequence

SMAD4 (SMAD family member 4) (eg, hemorrhagic telangiectasia syndrome, juvenile polyposis), full gene sequence

SOS1 (son of sevenless homolog 1) (eg, Noonan syndrome, gingival fibromatosis), full gene sequence

SPAST (spastin) (eg, spastic paraplegia), full gene sequence

SPG7 (spastic paraplegia 7 [pure and complicated autosomal recessive]) (eg, spastic paraplegia), full gene sequence

STXBP1 (syntaxin-binding protein 1) (eg, epileptic encephalopathy), full gene sequence

TAZ (tafazzin) (eg, methylglutaconic aciduria type 2, Barth syndrome), full gene sequence

TCF4 (transcription factor 4) (eg, Pitt-Hopkins syndrome), full gene sequence

TH (tyrosine hydroxylase) (eg, Segawa syndrome), full gene sequence

TMEM43 (transmembrane protein 43) (eg, arrhythmogenic right ventricular cardiomyopathy), full gene sequence

TNNT2 (troponin T, type 2 [cardiac]) (eg, familial hypertrophic cardiomyopathy), full gene sequence

TRPC6 (transient receptor potential cation channel, subfamily C, member 6) (eg, focal segmental glomerulosclerosis), full gene sequence

TSC1 (tuberous sclerosis 1) (eg, tuberous sclerosis), full gene sequence

TSC2 (tuberous sclerosis 2) (eg, tuberous sclerosis), duplication/deletion analysis

UBE3A (ubiquitin protein ligase E3A) (eg, Angelman syndrome) full gene sequence

UMOD (uromodulin) (eg, glomerulocystic kidney disease with hyperuricemia and isosthenuria), full gene sequence

VWF (von Willebrand factor) (von Willebrand disease type 2A), extended targeted sequence analysis (eg, exons 11-16, 24-26, 51, 52)

WAS (Wiskott-Aldrich syndrome [eczema-thrombocytopenia]) (eg, Wiskott-Aldrich syndrome), full gene sequence

0.00 0.00 **FUD** XXX A

AMA: 2020,OctSE,1; 2020,Feb,10; 2018,Nov,9; 2018,May,6; 2018,Jan,8; 2017,Apr,9; 2017,Jan,8; 2016,Aug,9; 2016,Jan,13; 2015,Jan,3; 2015,Jan,16

81407 Molecular pathology procedure, Level 8 (eg, analysis of 26-50 exons by DNA sequence analysis, mutation scanning or duplication/deletion variants of >50 exons, sequence analysis of multiple genes on one platform)

ABCC8 (ATP-binding cassette, sub-family C [CFTR/MRP], member 8) (eg, familial hyperinsulinism), full gene sequence

AGL (amylo-alpha-1, 6-glucosidase, 4-alpha-glucanotransferase) (eg, glycogen storage disease type III), full gene sequence

AHI1 (Abelson helper integration site 1) (eg, Joubert syndrome), full gene sequence

APOB (apolipoprotein B) (eg, familial hypercholesterolemia type B) full gene sequence

ASPM (asp [abnormal spindle] homolog, microcephaly associated [Drosophila]) (eg, primary microcephaly), full gene sequence

CHD7 (chromodomain helicase DNA binding protein 7) (eg, CHARGE syndrome), full gene sequence

COL4A4 (collagen, type IV, alpha 4) (eg, Alport syndrome), full gene sequence

COL4A5 (collagen, type IV, alpha 5) (eg, Alport syndrome), duplication/deletion analysis

COL6A1 (collagen, type VI, alpha 1) (eg, collagen type VI-related disorders), full gene sequence

COL6A2 (collagen, type VI, alpha 2) (eg, collagen type VI-related disorders), full gene sequence

COL6A3 (collagen, type VI, alpha 3) (eg, collagen type VI-related disorders), full gene sequence

CREBBP (CREB binding protein) (eg, Rubinstein-Taybi syndrome), full gene sequence

F8 (coagulation factor VIII) (eg, hemophilia A), full gene sequence

JAG1 (jagged 1) (eg, Alagille syndrome), full gene sequence

KDM5C (lysine [K]-specific demethylase 5C) (eg, X-linked mental retardation), full gene sequence

KIAA0196 (KIAA0196) (eg, spastic paraplegia), full gene sequence

L1CAM (L1 cell adhesion molecule) (eg, MASA syndrome, X-linked hydrocephaly), full gene sequence

LAMB2 (laminin, beta 2 [laminin S]) (eg, Pierson syndrome), full gene sequence

MYBPC3 (myosin binding protein C, cardiac) (eg, familial hypertrophic cardiomyopathy), full gene sequence

MYH6 (myosin, heavy chain 6, cardiac muscle, alpha) (eg, familial dilated cardiomyopathy), full gene sequence

MYH7 (myosin, heavy chain 7, cardiac muscle, beta) (eg, familial hypertrophic cardiomyopathy, Liang distal myopathy), full gene sequence

MYO7A (myosin VIIA) (eg, Usher syndrome, type 1), full gene sequence

NOTCH1 (notch 1) (eg, aortic valve disease), full gene sequence

NPHS1 (nephrosis 1, congenital, Finnish type [nephrin]) (eg, congenital Finnish nephrosis), full gene sequence

OPA1 (optic atrophy 1) (eg, optic atrophy), full gene sequence

PCDH15 (protocadherin-related 15) (eg, Usher syndrome, type 1), full gene sequence

PKD1 (polycystic kidney disease 1 [autosomal dominant]) (eg, polycystic kidney disease), full gene sequence

PLCE1 (phospholipase C, epsilon 1) (eg, nephrotic syndrome type 3), full gene sequence

SCN1A (sodium channel, voltage-gated, type 1, alpha subunit) (eg, generalized epilepsy with febrile seizures), full gene sequence

SCN5A (sodium channel, voltage-gated, type V, alpha subunit) (eg, familial dilated cardiomyopathy), full gene sequence

SLC12A1 (solute carrier family 12 [sodium/potassium/chloride transporters], member 1) (eg, Bartter syndrome), full gene sequence

SLC12A3 (solute carrier family 12 [sodium/chloride transporters], member 3) (eg, Gitelman syndrome), full gene sequence

SPG11 (spastic paraplegia 11 [autosomal recessive]) (eg, spastic paraplegia), full gene sequence

SPTBN2 (spectrin, beta, non-erythrocytic 2) (eg, spinocerebellar ataxia), full gene sequence

TMEM67 (transmembrane protein 67) (eg, Joubert syndrome), full gene sequence

TSC2 (tuberous sclerosis 2) (eg, tuberous sclerosis), full gene sequence

USH1C (Usher syndrome 1C [autosomal recessive, severe]) (eg, Usher syndrome, type 1), full gene sequence

VPS13B (vacuolar protein sorting 13 homolog B [yeast]) (eg, Cohen syndrome), duplication/deletion analysis

WDR62 (WD repeat domain 62) (eg, primary autosomal recessive microcephaly), full gene sequence

0.00 0.00 **FUD** XXX A

AMA: 2020,OctSE,1; 2019,Jul,3; 2018,Nov,9; 2018,May,6; 2018,Jan,8; 2017,Jan,8; 2016,Aug,9; 2016,Jan,13; 2015,Jan,16; 2015,Jan,3

81408 Molecular pathology procedure, Level 9 (eg, analysis of >50 exons in a single gene by DNA sequence analysis)

ABCA4 (ATP-binding cassette, sub-family A [ABC1], member 4) (eg, Stargardt disease, age-related macular degeneration), full gene sequence

ATM (ataxia telangiectasia mutated) (eg, ataxia telangiectasia), full gene sequence

CDH23 (cadherin-related 23) (eg, Usher syndrome, type 1), full gene sequence

CEP290 (centrosomal protein 290kDa) (eg, Joubert syndrome), full gene sequence

COL1A1 (collagen, type I, alpha 1) (eg, osteogenesis imperfecta, type I), full gene sequence

COL1A2 (collagen, type I, alpha 2) (eg, osteogenesis imperfecta, type I), full gene sequence

COL4A1 (collagen, type IV, alpha 1) (eg, brain small-vessel disease with hemorrhage), full gene sequence

COL4A3 (collagen, type IV, alpha 3 [Goodpasture antigen]) (eg, Alport syndrome), full gene sequence

COL4A5 (collagen, type IV, alpha 5) (eg, Alport syndrome), full gene sequence

DMD (dystrophin) (eg, Duchenne/Becker muscular dystrophy), full gene sequence

DYSF (dysferlin, limb girdle muscular dystrophy 2B [autosomal recessive]) (eg, limb-girdle muscular dystrophy), full gene sequence

FBN1 (fibrillin 1) (eg, Marfan syndrome), full gene sequence

ITPR1 (inositol 1,4,5-trisphosphate receptor, type 1) (eg, spinocerebellar ataxia), full gene sequence

LAMA2 (laminin, alpha 2) (eg, congenital muscular dystrophy), full gene sequence

LRRK2 (leucine-rich repeat kinase 2) (eg, Parkinson disease), full gene sequence

MYH11 (myosin, heavy chain 11, smooth muscle) (eg, thoracic aortic aneurysms and aortic dissections), full gene sequence

NEB (nebulin) (eg, nemaline myopathy 2), full gene sequence

NF1 (neurofibromin 1) (eg, neurofibromatosis, type 1), full gene sequence

PKHD1 (polycystic kidney and hepatic disease 1) (eg, autosomal recessive polycystic kidney disease), full gene sequence

RYR1 (ryanodine receptor 1, skeletal) (eg, malignant hyperthermia), full gene sequence

RYR2 (ryanodine receptor 2 [cardiac]) (eg, catecholaminergic polymorphic ventricular tachycardia, arrhythmogenic right ventricular dysplasia), full gene sequence or targeted sequence analysis of > 50 exons

USH2A (Usher syndrome 2A [autosomal recessive, mild]) (eg, Usher syndrome, type 2), full gene sequence

VPS13B (vacuolar protein sorting 13 homolog B [yeast]) (eg, Cohen syndrome), full gene sequence

VWF (von Willebrand factor) (eg, von Willebrand disease types 1 and 3), full gene sequence

🖩 0.00   🔪 0.00   **FUD** XXX   A ▢

AMA: 2020,OctSE,1; 2018,Nov,9; 2018,May,6; 2018,Jan,8; 2017,Jan,8; 2016,Aug,9; 2016,Jan,13; 2015,Jan,16; 2015,Jan,3

**81479**   **Unlisted molecular pathology procedure**

🖩 0.00   🔪 0.00   **FUD** XXX   A ▢

AMA: 2019,Jun,11; 2019,May,5; 2018,Dec,10; 2018,Dec,10; 2018,Nov,9; 2018,Sep,14; 2018,Jun,8; 2018,May,6; 2018,Jan,8; 2017,Apr,9; 2017,Jan,8; 2016,Sep,9; 2016,Aug,9; 2016,Apr,4; 2016,Jan,13; 2015,Jan,3; 2015,Jan,16

81410-81479 [81419, 81443, 81448, 81479] Genomic Sequencing

EXCLUDES   *In situ hybridization analyses (88271-88275, 88365-88368 [88364, 88373, 88374])*

Microbial identification (87149-87153, 87471-87801 [87623, 87624, 87625], 87900-87904 [87906, 87910, 87912])

81410   **Aortic dysfunction or dilation (eg, Marfan syndrome, Loeys Dietz syndrome, Ehler Danlos syndrome type IV, arterial tortuosity syndrome); genomic sequence analysis panel, must include sequencing of at least 9 genes, including *FBN1, TGFBR1, TGFBR2, COL3A1, MYH11, ACTA2, SLC2A10, SMAD3,* and *MYLK***

🖩 0.00   🔪 0.00   **FUD** XXX   A ▢

AMA: 2018,Jan,8; 2017,Jan,8; 2016,Jan,13; 2015,Jan,3

81411   **duplication/deletion analysis panel, must include analyses for *TGFBR1, TGFBR2, MYH11,* and *COL3A1***

🖩 0.00   🔪 0.00   **FUD** XXX   A ▢

AMA: 2018,Jan,8; 2017,Jan,8; 2016,Jan,13; 2015,Jan,3

81412   **Ashkenazi Jewish associated disorders (eg, Bloom syndrome, Canavan disease, cystic fibrosis, familial dysautonomia, Fanconi anemia group C, Gaucher disease, Tay-Sachs disease), genomic sequence analysis panel, must include sequencing of at least 9 genes, including *ASPA, BLM, CFTR, FANCC, GBA, HEXA, IKBKAP, MCOLN1,* and *SMPD1***

🖩 0.00   🔪 0.00   **FUD** XXX   A ▢

AMA: 2018,Nov,9; 2018,Jan,8; 2017,Jan,8; 2016,Apr,4

81413   **Cardiac ion channelopathies (eg, Brugada syndrome, long QT syndrome, short QT syndrome, catecholaminergic polymorphic ventricular tachycardia); genomic sequence analysis panel, must include sequencing of at least 10 genes, including ANK2, CASQ2, CAV3, KCNE1, KCNE2, KCNH2, KCNJ2, KCNQ1, RYR2, and SCN5A**

EXCLUDES   *Evaluation cardiomyopathy (81439)*

🖩 0.00   🔪 0.00   **FUD** XXX   A ▢

AMA: 2018,Jan,8; 2017,Apr,3

81414   **duplication/deletion gene analysis panel, must include analysis of at least 2 genes, including KCNH2 and KCNQ1**

EXCLUDES   *Evaluation cardiomyopathy (81439)*

🖩 0.00   🔪 0.00   **FUD** XXX   A ▢

AMA: 2018,Jan,8; 2017,Apr,3

● **#**   **81419**   **Epilepsy genomic sequence analysis panel, must include analyses for *ALDH7A1, CACNA1A, CDKL5, CHD2, GABRG2, GRIN2A, KCNQ2, MECP2, PCDH19, POLG, PRRT2, SCN1A, SCN1B, SCN2A, SCN8A, SLC2A1, SLC9A6, STXBP1, SYNGAP1, TCF4, TPP1, TSC1, TSC2,* and *ZEB2***

🖩 0.00   🔪 0.00   **FUD** 000

81415   **Exome (eg, unexplained constitutional or heritable disorder or syndrome); sequence analysis**

🖩 0.00   🔪 0.00   **FUD** XXX   A ▢

AMA: 2018,Jan,8; 2017,Jan,8; 2016,Jan,13; 2015,Jan,3

+   **81416**   **sequence analysis, each comparator exome (eg, parents, siblings) (List separately in addition to code for primary procedure)**

Code first (81415)

🖩 0.00   🔪 0.00   **FUD** XXX   A ▢

AMA: 2018,Jan,8; 2017,Jan,8; 2016,Jan,13; 2015,Jan,3

81417   **re-evaluation of previously obtained exome sequence (eg, updated knowledge or unrelated condition/syndrome)**

EXCLUDES   *Incidental results*

Microarray assessment (81228-81229)

🖩 0.00   🔪 0.00   **FUD** XXX   A ▢

AMA: 2018,Jan,8; 2017,Jan,8; 2016,Jan,13; 2015,Jan,3

81419   **Resequenced code. See code following 81414.**

81420   **Fetal chromosomal aneuploidy (eg, trisomy 21, monosomy X) genomic sequence analysis panel, circulating cell-free fetal DNA in maternal blood, must include analysis of chromosomes 13, 18, and 21**   M

EXCLUDES   *Genome-wide microarray analysis (81228-81229)*

Molecular cytogenetics (88271)

🖩 0.00   🔪 0.00   **FUD** XXX   A ▢

AMA: 2018,Apr,10; 2018,Jan,8; 2017,Jan,8; 2016,Jan,13; 2015,Dec,18; 2015,Jan,3

81422   **Fetal chromosomal microdeletion(s) genomic sequence analysis (eg, DiGeorge syndrome, Cri-du-chat syndrome), circulating cell-free fetal DNA in maternal blood**

EXCLUDES   *Genome-wide microarray analysis (81228-81229)*

Molecular cytogenetics (88271)

🖩 0.00   🔪 0.00   **FUD** XXX   A ▢

AMA: 2018,Jan,8; 2017,Apr,3

**81443**   **Genetic testing for severe inherited conditions (eg, cystic fibrosis, Ashkenazi Jewish-associated disorders [eg, Bloom syndrome, Canavan disease, Fanconi anemia type C, mucolipidosis type VI, Gaucher disease, Tay-Sachs disease], beta hemoglobinopathies, phenylketonuria, galactosemia), genomic sequence analysis panel, must include sequencing of at least 15 genes (eg, *ACADM, ARSA, ASPA, ATP7B, BCKDHA, BCKDHB, BLM, CFTR, DHCR7, FANCC, G6PC, GAA, GALT, GBA, GBE1, HBB, HEXA, IKBKAP, MCOLN1, PAH*)**

EXCLUDES   *When performed separately:*

Ashkenazi Jewish-associated disorder analysis only (81412)

Fragile X mental retardation (FMR1) analysis (81243)

Hemoglobin A testing ([81257])

Spinal muscular atrophy (SMN1) analysis (81329)

🖩 0.00   🔪 0.00   **FUD** XXX   ▢

AMA: 2019,Jul,3; 2018,Nov,9

81425   **Genome (eg, unexplained constitutional or heritable disorder or syndrome); sequence analysis**

🖩 0.00   🔪 0.00   **FUD** XXX   A ▢

AMA: 2018,Jan,8; 2017,Jan,8; 2016,Jan,13; 2015,Jan,3

+   **81426**   **sequence analysis, each comparator genome (eg, parents, siblings) (List separately in addition to code for primary procedure)**

Code first (81425)

🖩 0.00   🔪 0.00   **FUD** XXX   A ▢

AMA: 2018,Jan,8; 2017,Jan,8; 2016,Jan,13; 2015,Jan,3

81427   **re-evaluation of previously obtained genome sequence (eg, updated knowledge or unrelated condition/syndrome)**

EXCLUDES   *Genome-wide microarray analysis (81228-81229)*

Incidental results

🖩 0.00   🔪 0.00   **FUD** XXX   A ▢

AMA: 2018,Jan,8; 2017,Jan,8; 2016,Jan,13; 2015,Jan,3

81408 — 81427

● New Code   ▲ Revised Code   ○ Reinstated   ● New Web Release   ▲ Revised Web Release   + Add-on   Unlisted   Not Covered   # Resequenced
🔟 Optum Mod 50 Exempt   🅢 AMA Mod 51 Exempt   🖰 Optum Mod 51 Exempt   🔂 Mod 63 Exempt   ⁄ Non-FDA Drug   ★ Telemedicine   M Maternity   A Age Edit

81430 **Hearing loss (eg, nonsyndromic hearing loss, Usher syndrome, Pendred syndrome); genomic sequence analysis panel, must include sequencing of at least 60 genes, including *CDH23, CLRN1, GJB2, GPR98, MTRNR1, MYO7A, MYO15A, PCDH15, OTOF, SLC26A4, TMC1, TMPRSS3, USH1C, USH1G, USH2A*, and *WFS1***

0.00 0.00 FUD XXX A

AMA: 2018,Jan,8; 2017,Jan,8; 2016,Jan,13; 2015,Jan,3

81431 **duplication/deletion analysis panel, must include copy number analyses for *STRC* and *DFNB1* deletions in *GJB2* and *GJB6* genes**

0.00 0.00 FUD XXX A

AMA: 2018,Jan,8; 2017,Jan,8; 2016,Jan,13; 2015,Jan,3

81432 **Hereditary breast cancer-related disorders (eg, hereditary breast cancer, hereditary ovarian cancer, hereditary endometrial cancer); genomic sequence analysis panel, must include sequencing of at least 10 genes, always including *BRCA1, BRCA2, CDH1, MLH1, MSH2, MSH6, PALB2, PTEN, STK11, and TP53***

0.00 0.00 FUD XXX A

AMA: 2019,May,5; 2018,Jan,8; 2017,Jan,8; 2016,Apr,4

81433 **duplication/deletion analysis panel, must include analyses for *BRCA1, BRCA2, MLH1, MSH2*, and *STK11***

0.00 0.00 FUD XXX A

AMA: 2018,Jan,8; 2017,Jan,8; 2016,Apr,4

81434 **Hereditary retinal disorders (eg, retinitis pigmentosa, Leber congenital amaurosis, cone-rod dystrophy), genomic sequence analysis panel, must include sequencing of at least 15 genes, including *ABCA4, CNGA1, CRB1, EYS, PDE6A, PDE6B, PRPF31, PRPH2, RDH12, RHO, RP1, RP2, RPE65, RPGR*, and *USH2A***

0.00 0.00 FUD XXX A

AMA: 2018,Jan,8; 2017,Jan,8; 2016,Apr,4

81435 **Hereditary colon cancer disorders (eg, Lynch syndrome, PTEN hamartoma syndrome, Cowden syndrome, familial adenomatosis polyposis); genomic sequence analysis panel, must include sequencing of at least 10 genes, including *APC, BMPR1A, CDH1, MLH1, MSH2, MSH6, MUTYH, PTEN, SMAD4*, and *STK11***

0.00 0.00 FUD XXX A

AMA: 2018,Jan,8; 2017,Jan,8; 2016,Apr,4; 2016,Jan,13; 2015,Jan,3

81436 **duplication/deletion analysis panel, must include analysis of at least 5 genes, including *MLH1, MSH2, EPCAM, SMAD4*, and *STK11***

0.00 0.00 FUD XXX A

AMA: 2018,Jan,8; 2017,Jan,8; 2016,Apr,4; 2016,Jan,13; 2015,Jan,3

81437 **Hereditary neuroendocrine tumor disorders (eg, medullary thyroid carcinoma, parathyroid carcinoma, malignant pheochromocytoma or paraganglioma); genomic sequence analysis panel, must include sequencing of at least 6 genes, including *MAX, SDHB, SDHC, SDHD, TMEM127*, and *VHL***

0.00 0.00 FUD XXX A

AMA: 2018,Jan,8; 2017,Jan,8; 2016,Apr,4

81438 **duplication/deletion analysis panel, must include analyses for *SDHB, SDHC, SDHD*, and *VHL***

0.00 0.00 FUD XXX A

AMA: 2018,Jan,8; 2017,Jan,8; 2016,Apr,4

81448 **Hereditary peripheral neuropathies (eg, Charcot-Marie-Tooth, spastic paraplegia), genomic sequence analysis panel, must include sequencing of at least 5 peripheral neuropathy-related genes (eg, *BSCL2, GJB1, MFN2, MPZ, REEP1, SPAST, SPG11, SPTLC1*)**

0.00 0.00 FUD XXX A

AMA: 2018,May,6

81439 **Hereditary cardiomyopathy (eg, hypertrophic cardiomyopathy, dilated cardiomyopathy, arrhythmogenic right ventricular cardiomyopathy), genomic sequence analysis panel, must include sequencing of at least 5 cardiomyopathy-related genes (eg, *DSG2, MYBPC3, MYH7, PKP2, TTN*)**

EXCLUDES *Genetic sequencing for cardiac ion channelopathies (81413-81414)*

0.00 0.00 FUD XXX A

AMA: 2018,Sep,14; 2018,Jan,8; 2017,Apr,3

81440 **Nuclear encoded mitochondrial genes (eg, neurologic or myopathic phenotypes), genomic sequence panel, must include analysis of at least 100 genes, including *BCS1L, C10orf2, COQ2, COX10, DGUOK, MPV17, OPA1, PDSS2, POLG, POLG2, RRM2B, SCO1, SCO2, SLC25A4, SUCLA2, SUCLG1, TAZ, TK2*, and *TYMP***

0.00 0.00 FUD XXX A

AMA: 2018,Jan,8; 2017,Jan,8; 2016,Jan,13; 2015,Jan,3

81442 **Noonan spectrum disorders (eg, Noonan syndrome, cardio-facio-cutaneous syndrome, Costello syndrome, LEOPARD syndrome, Noonan-like syndrome), genomic sequence analysis panel, must include sequencing of at least 12 genes, including *BRAF, CBL, HRAS, KRAS, MAP2K1, MAP2K2, NRAS, PTPN11, RAF1, RIT1, SHOC2*, and *SOS1***

0.00 0.00 FUD XXX A

AMA: 2018,Jan,8; 2017,Jan,8; 2016,Apr,4

81443 **Resequenced code. See code following 81422.**

81445 **Targeted genomic sequence analysis panel, solid organ neoplasm, DNA analysis, and RNA analysis when performed, 5-50 genes (eg, *ALK, BRAF, CDKN2A, EGFR, ERBB2, KIT, KRAS, NRAS, MET, PDGFRA, PDGFRB, PGR, PIK3CA, PTEN, RET*), interrogation for sequence variants and copy number variants or rearrangements, if performed**

EXCLUDES *Microarray copy number assessment (81406)*

0.00 0.00 FUD XXX A

AMA: 2018,Jan,8; 2017,Jan,8; 2016,Apr,4; 2016,Jan,13; 2015,Jan,3

81448 **Resequenced code. See code following 81438.**

81450 **Targeted genomic sequence analysis panel, hematolymphoid neoplasm or disorder, DNA analysis, and RNA analysis when performed, 5-50 genes (eg, *BRAF, CEBPA, DNMT3A, EZH2, FLT3, IDH1, IDH2, JAK2, KRAS, KIT, MLL, NRAS, NPM1, NOTCH1*), interrogation for sequence variants, and copy number variants or rearrangements, or isoform expression or mRNA expression levels, if performed**

EXCLUDES *Microarray copy number assessment (81406)*

0.00 0.00 FUD XXX A

AMA: 2018,Jan,8; 2017,Jan,8; 2016,Apr,4; 2016,Jan,13; 2015,Jan,3

81455 **Targeted genomic sequence analysis panel, solid organ or hematolymphoid neoplasm, DNA analysis, and RNA analysis when performed, 51 or greater genes (eg, *ALK, BRAF, CDKN2A, CEBPA, DNMT3A, EGFR, ERBB2, EZH2, FLT3, IDH1, IDH2, JAK2, KIT, KRAS, MLL, NPM1, NRAS, MET, NOTCH1, PDGFRA, PDGFRB, PGR, PIK3CA, PTEN, RET*), interrogation for sequence variants and copy number variants or rearrangements, if performed**

EXCLUDES *Microarray copy number assessment (81406)*

0.00 0.00 FUD XXX A

AMA: 2018,Jan,8; 2017,Jan,8; 2016,Apr,4; 2016,Jan,13; 2015,Jan,3

81460 **Whole mitochondrial genome (eg, Leigh syndrome, mitochondrial encephalomyopathy, lactic acidosis, and stroke-like episodes [MELAS], myoclonic epilepsy with ragged-red fibers [MERFF], neuropathy, ataxia, and retinitis pigmentosa [NARP], Leber hereditary optic neuropathy [LHON]), genomic sequence, must include sequence analysis of entire mitochondrial genome with heteroplasmy detection**

0.00 0.00 FUD XXX A

AMA: 2018,Jan,8; 2017,Jan,8; 2016,Jan,13; 2015,Jan,3

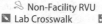

81465 Whole mitochondrial genome large deletion analysis panel (eg, Kearns-Sayre syndrome, chronic progressive external ophthalmoplegia), including heteroplasmy detection, if performed

0.00 0.00 FUD XXX A

AMA: 2018,Jan,8; 2017,Jan,8; 2016,Jan,13; 2015,Jan,3

81470 X-linked intellectual disability (XLID) (eg, syndromic and non-syndromic XLID); genomic sequence analysis panel, must include sequencing of at least 60 genes, including *ARX, ATRX, CDKL5, FGD1, FMR1, HUWE1, IL1RAPL, KDM5C, L1CAM, MECP2, MED12, MID1, OCRL, RPS6KA3,* and *SLC16A2*

0.00 0.00 FUD XXX A

AMA: 2018,Jan,8; 2017,Jan,8; 2016,Jan,13; 2015,Jan,3

81471 duplication/deletion gene analysis, must include analysis of at least 60 genes, including *ARX, ATRX, CDKL5, FGD1, FMR1, HUWE1, IL1RAPL, KDM5C, L1CAM, MECP2, MED12, MID1, OCRL, RPS6KA3,* and *SLC16A2*

0.00 0.00 FUD XXX A

AMA: 2018,Jan,8; 2017,Jan,8; 2016,Jan,13; 2015,Jan,3

***81479* Resequenced code. See code following 81408.**

81490-81599 [81500, 81503, 81504, 81522, 81540, 81546, 81595, 81596] Multianalyte Assays

INCLUDES Procedures using multiple assay panel results (eg, molecular pathology, fluorescent in situ hybridization, non-nucleic acid-based) and other patient information to perform algorithmic analysis

Required analytical services (eg, amplification, cell lysis, detection, digestion, extraction, hybridization, nucleic acid stabilization) and algorithmic analysis

EXCLUDES *Genomic resequencing tests (81410-81471 [81448])*

In situ hybridization analyses (88271-88275, 88365-88368 [88364, 88373, 88374])

Microbial identification (87149-87153, 87471-87801 [87623, 87624, 87625], 87900-87904 [87906, 87910, 87912])

Multianalyte assays with algorithmic analyses without a Category I code (0002M-0007M, 0011M-0013M)

Code also procedures performed prior to cell lysis (eg, microdissection) (88380-88381)

81490 Autoimmune (rheumatoid arthritis), analysis of 12 biomarkers using immunoassays, utilizing serum, prognostic algorithm reported as a disease activity score

EXCLUDES *C-reactive protein (86140)*

0.00 0.00 FUD XXX Q

 # 81595 Cardiology (heart transplant), mRNA, gene expression profiling by real-time quantitative PCR of 20 genes (11 content and 9 housekeeping), utilizing subfraction of peripheral blood, algorithm reported as a rejection risk score

0.00 0.00 FUD XXX A

AMA: 2019,Jun,11

81493 Coronary artery disease, mRNA, gene expression profiling by real-time RT-PCR of 23 genes, utilizing whole peripheral blood, algorithm reported as a risk score

0.00 0.00 FUD XXX A

***81500* Resequenced code. See code following 81538.**

***81503* Resequenced code. See code before 81539.**

***81504* Resequenced code. See code following resequenced code 81546.**

81506 Endocrinology (type 2 diabetes), biochemical assays of seven analytes (glucose, HbA1c, insulin, hs-CRP, adiponectin, ferritin, interleukin 2-receptor alpha), utilizing serum or plasma, algorithm reporting a risk score

EXCLUDES *C-reactive protein; high sensitivity (hsCRP) (86141)*

Ferritin (82728)

Glucose (82947)

Hemoglobin; glycosylated (A1C) (83036)

Immunoassay for analyte other than infectious agent antibody or infectious agent antigen (83520)

Insulin; total (83525)

Unlisted chemistry procedure (84999)

0.00 0.00 FUD XXX E

AMA: 2019,Jun,11; 2015,Jan,3

81507 Fetal aneuploidy (trisomy 21, 18, and 13) DNA sequence analysis of selected regions using maternal plasma, algorithm reported as a risk score for each trisomy ♀

EXCLUDES *Genome-wide microarray analysis (81228-81229)*

Molecular cytogenetics (88271)

0.00 0.00 FUD XXX A

AMA: 2019,Jun,11; 2018,Apr,10; 2015,Jan,3

81508 Fetal congenital abnormalities, biochemical assays of two proteins (PAPP-A, hCG [any form]), utilizing maternal serum, algorithm reported as a risk score ♀

EXCLUDES *Gonadotropin, chorionic (hCG) (84702)*

Pregnancy-associated plasma protein-A (PAPP-A) (84163)

0.00 0.00 FUD XXX E

AMA: 2019,Jun,11; 2015,Jan,3

81509 Fetal congenital abnormalities, biochemical assays of three proteins (PAPP-A, hCG [any form], DIA), utilizing maternal serum, algorithm reported as a risk score ♀

EXCLUDES *Gonadotropin, chorionic (hCG) (84702)*

Inhibin A (86336)

Pregnancy-associated plasma protein-A (PAPP-A) (84163)

0.00 0.00 FUD XXX E

AMA: 2019,Jun,11; 2015,Jan,3

81510 Fetal congenital abnormalities, biochemical assays of three analytes (AFP, uE3, hCG [any form]), utilizing maternal serum, algorithm reported as a risk score ♀

EXCLUDES *Alpha-fetoprotein (AFP) (82105)*

Estriol (82677)

Gonadotropin, chorionic (hCG) (84702)

0.00 0.00 FUD XXX E

AMA: 2019,Jun,11; 2015,Jan,3

81511 Fetal congenital abnormalities, biochemical assays of four analytes (AFP, uE3, hCG [any form], DIA) utilizing maternal serum, algorithm reported as a risk score (may include additional results from previous biochemical testing) ♀

EXCLUDES *Alpha-fetoprotein (AFP) (82105)*

Estriol (82677)

Gonadotropin, chorionic (hCG) (84702)

Inhibin A (86336)

0.00 0.00 FUD XXX E

AMA: 2019,Jun,11; 2015,Jan,3

81512 Fetal congenital abnormalities, biochemical assays of five analytes (AFP, uE3, total hCG, hyperglycosylated hCG, DIA) utilizing maternal serum, algorithm reported as a risk score ♀

EXCLUDES *Alpha-fetoprotein (AFP) (82105)*

Estriol (82677)

Gonadotropin, chorionic (hCG) (84702)

Inhibin A (86336)

0.00 0.00 FUD XXX E

AMA: 2019,Jun,11; 2015,Jan,3

● **81513** **Infectious disease, bacterial vaginosis, quantitative real-time amplification of RNA markers for Atopobium vaginae, Gardnerella vaginalis, and Lactobacillus species, utilizing vaginal-fluid specimens, algorithm reported as a positive or negative result for bacterial vaginosis**

● **81514** **Infectious disease, bacterial vaginosis and vaginitis, quantitative real-time amplification of DNA markers for Gardnerella vaginalis, Atopobium vaginae, Megasphaera type 1, Bacterial Vaginosis Associated Bacteria-2 (BVAB-2), and Lactobacillus species (L. crispatus and L. jensenii), utilizing vaginal-fluid specimens, algorithm reported as a positive or negative for high likelihood of bacterial vaginosis, includes separate detection of Trichomonas vaginalis and/or Candida species (C. albicans, C. tropicalis, C. parapsilosis, C. dubliniensis), Candida glabrata, Candida krusei, when reported**

EXCLUDES *Candida (87480-87482)*
Gardnerella vaginalis (87510-87512)
Trichomonas vaginalis (87660-87661)

\# **81596** **Infectious disease, chronic hepatitis C virus (HCV) infection, six biochemical assays (ALT, A2-macroglobulin, apolipoprotein A-1, total bilirubin, GGT, and haptoglobin) utilizing serum, prognostic algorithm reported as scores for fibrosis and necroinflammatory activity in liver**
0.00 0.00 FUD XXX
AMA: 2019,Jun,11; 2019,Jul,3

81518 **Oncology (breast), mRNA, gene expression profiling by real-time RT-PCR of 11 genes (7 content and 4 housekeeping), utilizing formalin-fixed paraffin-embedded tissue, algorithms reported as percentage risk for metastatic recurrence and likelihood of benefit from extended endocrine therapy**
0.00 0.00 FUD XXX
AMA: 2019,Jun,11; 2019,Jul,3

\# **81522** **Oncology (breast), mRNA, gene expression profiling by RT-PCR of 12 genes (8 content and 4 housekeeping), utilizing formalin-fixed paraffin-embedded tissue, algorithm reported as recurrence risk score**
0.00 0.00 FUD XXX

81519 **Oncology (breast), mRNA, gene expression profiling by real-time RT-PCR of 21 genes, utilizing formalin-fixed paraffin embedded tissue, algorithm reported as recurrence score**
0.00 0.00 FUD XXX A
AMA: 2019,Jun,11; 2018,Jan,8; 2017,Jan,8; 2016,Jan,13; 2015,Jan,3

81520 **Oncology (breast), mRNA gene expression profiling by hybrid capture of 58 genes (50 content and 8 housekeeping), utilizing formalin-fixed paraffin-embedded tissue, algorithm reported as a recurrence risk score**
0.00 0.00 FUD XXX A
AMA: 2019,Jun,11; 2018,Jun,8

81521 **Oncology (breast), mRNA, microarray gene expression profiling of 70 content genes and 465 housekeeping genes, utilizing fresh frozen or formalin-fixed paraffin-embedded tissue, algorithm reported as index related to risk of distant metastasis**
0.00 0.00 FUD XXX A
AMA: 2019,Jun,11; 2018,Jun,8

81522 **Resequenced code. See code following 81518.**

81525 **Oncology (colon), mRNA, gene expression profiling by real-time RT-PCR of 12 genes (7 content and 5 housekeeping), utilizing formalin-fixed paraffin-embedded tissue, algorithm reported as a recurrence score**
0.00 0.00 FUD XXX A
AMA: 2019,Jun,11

81528 **Oncology (colorectal) screening, quantitative real-time target and signal amplification of 10 DNA markers (*KRAS* mutations, promoter methylation of *NDRG4* and *BMP3*) and fecal hemoglobin, utilizing stool, algorithm reported as a positive or negative result**

EXCLUDES *Blood, occult, by fecal hemoglobin (82274)*
KRAS (Kirsten rat sarcoma viral oncogene homolog) (81275)

0.00 0.00 FUD XXX A
AMA: 2019,Jun,11

● **81529** **Oncology (cutaneous melanoma), mRNA, gene expression profiling by real-time RT-PCR of 31 genes (28 content and 3 housekeeping), utilizing formalin-fixed paraffin-embedded tissue, algorithm reported as recurrence risk, including likelihood of sentinel lymph node metastasis**

81535 **Oncology (gynecologic), live tumor cell culture and chemotherapeutic response by DAPI stain and morphology, predictive algorithm reported as a drug response score; first single drug or drug combination**
0.00 0.00 FUD XXX Q
AMA: 2019,Jun,11

\+ **81536** **each additional single drug or drug combination (List separately in addition to code for primary procedure)**
Code first (81535)
0.00 0.00 FUD XXX Q
AMA: 2019,Jun,11

81538 **Oncology (lung), mass spectrometric 8-protein signature, including amyloid A, utilizing serum, prognostic and predictive algorithm reported as good versus poor overall survival**
0.00 0.00 FUD XXX Q
AMA: 2019,Jun,11

\# **81500** **Oncology (ovarian), biochemical assays of two proteins (CA-125 and HE4), utilizing serum, with menopausal status, algorithm reported as a risk score** ♀

EXCLUDES *Human epididymis protein 4 (HE4) (86305)*
Immunoassay for tumor antigen, quantitative; CA 125 (86304)

0.00 0.00 FUD XXX E
AMA: 2019,Jun,11; 2015,Jan,3

\# **81503** **Oncology (ovarian), biochemical assays of five proteins (CA-125, apolipoprotein A1, beta-2 microglobulin, transferrin, and pre-albumin), utilizing serum, algorithm reported as a risk score** ♀

EXCLUDES *Apolipoprotein (82172)*
Beta-2 microglobulin (82232)
Immunoassay for tumor antigen, quantitative; CA 125 (86304)
Prealbumin (84134)
Transferrin (84466)

0.00 0.00 FUD XXX Q
AMA: 2019,Jun,11; 2015,Jan,3

81539 **Oncology (high-grade prostate cancer), biochemical assay of four proteins (Total PSA, Free PSA, Intact PSA, and human kallikrein-2 [hK2]), utilizing plasma or serum, prognostic algorithm reported as a probability score** ♂
0.00 0.00 FUD XXX Q
AMA: 2019,Jun,11; 2018,Jan,8; 2017,Apr,3

81540 **Resequenced code. See code before 81552.**

81541 **Oncology (prostate), mRNA gene expression profiling by real-time RT-PCR of 46 genes (31 content and 15 housekeeping), utilizing formalin-fixed paraffin-embedded tissue, algorithm reported as a disease-specific mortality risk score**
0.00 0.00 FUD XXX A
AMA: 2019,Jun,11; 2018,Aug,8

81542 Oncology (prostate), mRNA, microarray gene expression profiling of 22 content genes, utilizing formalin-fixed paraffin-embedded tissue, algorithm reported as metastasis risk score ♂
0.00 0.00 FUD XXX

~~**81545** Oncology (thyroid), gene expression analysis of 142 genes, utilizing fine needle aspirate, algorithm reported as a categorical result (eg, benign or suspicious)~~

81546 **Resequenced code. See code following 81551.**

81551 Oncology (prostate), promoter methylation profiling by real-time PCR of 3 genes (*GSTP1, APC, RASSF1*), utilizing formalin-fixed paraffin-embedded tissue, algorithm reported as a likelihood of prostate cancer detection on repeat biopsy
0.00 0.00 FUD XXX
AMA: 2019,Jun,11; 2018,Aug,8

● # **81546** Oncology (thyroid), mRNA, gene expression analysis of 10,196 genes, utilizing fine needle aspirate, algorithm reported as a categorical result (eg, benign or suspicious)
0.00 0.00 FUD 000

81504 Oncology (tissue of origin), microarray gene expression profiling of > 2000 genes, utilizing formalin-fixed paraffin-embedded tissue, algorithm reported as tissue similarity scores
0.00 0.00 FUD XXX
AMA: 2019,Jun,11; 2015,Jan,3

81540 Oncology (tumor of unknown origin), mRNA, gene expression profiling by real-time RT-PCR of 92 genes (87 content and 5 housekeeping) to classify tumor into main cancer type and subtype, utilizing formalin-fixed paraffin-embedded tissue, algorithm reported as a probability of a predicted main cancer type and subtype
0.00 0.00 FUD XXX
AMA: 2019,Jun,11

81552 Oncology (uveal melanoma), mRNA, gene expression profiling by real-time RT-PCR of 15 genes (12 content and 3 housekeeping), utilizing fine needle aspirate or formalin-fixed paraffin-embedded tissue, algorithm reported as risk of metastasis
0.00 0.00 FUD XXX
AMA: 2020,Jan,10

● **81554** Pulmonary disease (idiopathic pulmonary fibrosis [IPF]), mRNA, gene expression analysis of 190 genes, utilizing transbronchial biopsies, diagnostic algorithm reported as categorical result (eg, positive or negative for high probability of usual interstitial pneumonia [UIP])

81595 **Resequenced code. See code following 81490.**

81596 **Resequenced code. See code following 81514.**

81599 Unlisted multianalyte assay with algorithmic analysis
0.00 0.00 FUD XXX
AMA: 2019,Jun,11; 2018,Jun,8; 2018,Apr,10; 2015,Jan,3

82009-82030 Chemistry: Acetaldehyde—Adenosine

INCLUDES Clinical information not requested by ordering physician
Mathematically calculated results
Quantitative analysis unless otherwise specified
Specimens from any source unless otherwise specified

EXCLUDES *Analytes from nonrequested laboratory analysis*
Calculated results representing score or probability derived by algorithm
Drug testing ([80305, 80306, 80307], [80324, 80325, 80326, 80327, 80328, 80329, 80330, 80331, 80332, 80333, 80334, 80335, 80336, 80337, 80338, 80339, 80340, 80341, 80342, 80343, 80344, 80345, 80346, 80347, 80348, 80349, 80350, 80351, 80352, 80353, 80354, 80355, 80356, 80357, 80358, 80359, 80360, 80361, 80362, 80363, 80364, 80365, 80366, 80367, 80368, 80369, 80370, 80371, 80372, 80373, 80374, 80375, 80376, 80377, 83992])
Organ or disease panels (80048-80076 [80081])
Therapeutic drug assays (80150-80299 [80164, 80165, 80171])

82009 Ketone body(s) (eg, acetone, acetoacetic acid, beta-hydroxybutyrate); qualitative
0.00 0.00 FUD XXX
AMA: 2018,Jan,8; 2017,Jan,8; 2016,Jan,13; 2015,Jun,10; 2015,Apr,3; 2015,Jan,16

82010 quantitative
0.00 0.00 FUD XXX
AMA: 2018,Jan,8; 2017,Jan,8; 2016,Jan,13; 2015,Jun,10; 2015,Apr,3; 2015,Jan,16

82013 Acetylcholinesterase
EXCLUDES *Acid phosphatase (84060-84066)*
Gastric acid analysis (82930)
0.00 0.00 FUD XXX
AMA: 2015,Jun,10; 2015,Apr,3

82016 Acylcarnitines; qualitative, each specimen
0.00 0.00 FUD XXX
AMA: 2015,Jun,10; 2015,Apr,3

82017 quantitative, each specimen
EXCLUDES *Carnitine (82379)*
0.00 0.00 FUD XXX
AMA: 2015,Jun,10; 2015,Apr,3

82024 Adrenocorticotropic hormone (ACTH)
0.00 0.00 FUD XXX
AMA: 2015,Jun,10; 2015,Apr,3

82030 Adenosine, 5-monophosphate, cyclic (cyclic AMP)
0.00 0.00 FUD XXX
AMA: 2015,Jun,10; 2015,Apr,3

82040-82042 [82042] Chemistry: Albumin

INCLUDES Clinical information not requested by ordering physician
Mathematically calculated results
Quantitative analysis unless otherwise specified
Specimens from any other sources unless otherwise specified

EXCLUDES *Analytes from nonrequested laboratory analysis*
Calculated results representing score or probability derived by algorithm
Drug testing ([80305, 80306, 80307], [80324, 80325, 80326, 80327, 80328, 80329, 80330, 80331, 80332, 80333, 80334, 80335, 80336, 80337, 80338, 80339, 80340, 80341, 80342, 80343, 80344, 80345, 80346, 80347, 80348, 80349, 80350, 80351, 80352, 80353, 80354, 80355, 80356, 80357, 80358, 80359, 80360, 80361, 80362, 80363, 80364, 80365, 80366, 80367, 80368, 80369, 80370, 80371, 80372, 80373, 80374, 80375, 80376, 80377, 83992])
Organ or disease panels (80048-80076 [80081])
Therapeutic drug assays (80150-80299 [80164, 80165, 80171])

82040 Albumin; serum, plasma or whole blood
0.00 0.00 FUD XXX
AMA: 2018,Jan,8; 2017,Jan,8; 2016,Jan,13; 2015,Jun,10; 2015,Apr,3; 2015,Jan,16

82042 **Resequenced code. See code following 82045.**

82043 urine (eg, microalbumin), quantitative
0.00 0.00 FUD XXX
AMA: 2018,Jan,8; 2017,Jan,8; 2016,Jan,13; 2015,Jun,10; 2015,Apr,3; 2015,Jan,16

82044 **urine (eg, microalbumin), semiquantitative (eg, reagent strip assay)**

EXCLUDES *Prealbumin (84134)*

0.00 0.00 FUD XXX

AMA: 2018,Jan,8; 2017,Jan,8; 2016,Jan,13; 2015,Jun,10; 2015,Apr,3; 2015,Jan,16

82045 **ischemia modified**

0.00 0.00 FUD XXX

AMA: 2015,Jun,10; 2015,Apr,3

82042 **other source, quantitative, each specimen**

EXCLUDES *Total protein (84155-84157, 84160)*

0.00 0.00 FUD XXX

AMA: 2015,Jun,10; 2015,Apr,3

82075-82107 Chemistry: Alcohol—Alpha-fetoprotein (AFP)

INCLUDES Clinical information not requested by ordering physician
Mathematically calculated results
Quantitative analysis unless otherwise specified
Specimens from any source unless otherwise specified

EXCLUDES *Analytes from nonrequested laboratory analysis*
Calculated results representing score or probability derived by algorithm
Drug testing ([80305, 80306, 80307], [80324, 80325, 80326, 80327, 80328, 80329, 80330, 80331, 80332, 80333, 80334, 80335, 80336, 80337, 80338, 80339, 80340, 80341, 80342, 80343, 80344, 80345, 80346, 80347, 80348, 80349, 80350, 80351, 80352, 80353, 80354, 80355, 80356, 80357, 80358, 80359, 80360, 80361, 80362, 80363, 80364, 80365, 80366, 80367, 80368, 80369, 80370, 80371, 80372, 80373, 80374, 80375, 80376, 80377, 83992])
Organ or disease panels (80048-80076 [80081])
Therapeutic drug assays (80150-80299 [80164, 80165, 80171])

▲ 82075 **Alcohol (ethanol); breath**

0.00 0.00 FUD XXX

AMA: 2015,Jun,10; 2015,Apr,3

● 82077 **any specimen except urine and breath, immunoassay (eg, IA, EIA, ELISA, RIA, EMIT, FPIA) and enzymatic methods (eg, alcohol dehydrogenase)**

EXCLUDES *Alcohol (ethanol) confirmatory drug testing ([80320])*

82085 **Aldolase**

0.00 0.00 FUD XXX

AMA: 2015,Jun,10; 2015,Apr,3

82088 **Aldosterone**

EXCLUDES *Alkaline phosphatase (84075, 84080)*
Alphaketoglutarate (82009-82010)
Alphatocopherol (VitaminE) (84446)

0.00 0.00 FUD XXX

AMA: 2015,Jun,10; 2015,Apr,3

82103 **Alpha-1-antitrypsin; total**

0.00 0.00 FUD XXX

AMA: 2015,Jun,10; 2015,Apr,3

82104 **phenotype**

0.00 0.00 FUD XXX

AMA: 2015,Jun,10; 2015,Apr,3

82105 **Alpha-fetoprotein (AFP); serum**

0.00 0.00 FUD XXX

AMA: 2015,Jun,10; 2015,Apr,3

82106 **amniotic fluid** M

0.00 0.00 FUD XXX

AMA: 2015,Jun,10; 2015,Apr,3

82107 **AFP-L3 fraction isoform and total AFP (including ratio)**

0.00 0.00 FUD XXX

AMA: 2015,Jun,10; 2015,Apr,3

82108 Chemistry: Aluminum

CMS: 100-02,11,20.2 ESRD Laboratory Services

INCLUDES Clinical information not requested by ordering physician
Mathematically calculated results
Quantitative analysis unless otherwise specified
Specimens from any source unless otherwise specified

EXCLUDES *Analytes from nonrequested laboratory analysis*
Calculated results representing score or probability derived by algorithm
Drug testing ([80305, 80306, 80307], [80324, 80325, 80326, 80327, 80328, 80329, 80330, 80331, 80332, 80333, 80334, 80335, 80336, 80337, 80338, 80339, 80340, 80341, 80342, 80343, 80344, 80345, 80346, 80347, 80348, 80349, 80350, 80351, 80352, 80353, 80354, 80355, 80356, 80357, 80358, 80359, 80360, 80361, 80362, 80363, 80364, 80365, 80366, 80367, 80368, 80369, 80370, 80371, 80372, 80373, 80374, 80375, 80376, 80377, 83992])
Organ or disease panels (80048-80076 [80081])
Therapeutic drug assays (80150-80299 [80164, 80165, 80171])

82108 **Aluminum**

0.00 0.00 FUD XXX

AMA: 2015,Jun,10; 2015,Apr,3

82120-82261 Chemistry: Amines—Biotinidase

INCLUDES Clinical information not requested by ordering physician
Mathematically calculated results
Quantitative analysis unless otherwise specified
Specimens from any source unless otherwise specified

EXCLUDES *Analytes from nonrequested laboratory analysis*
Calculated results representing score or probability derived by algorithm
Drug testing ([80305, 80306, 80307], [80324, 80325, 80326, 80327, 80328, 80329, 80330, 80331, 80332, 80333, 80334, 80335, 80336, 80337, 80338, 80339, 80340, 80341, 80342, 80343, 80344, 80345, 80346, 80347, 80348, 80349, 80350, 80351, 80352, 80353, 80354, 80355, 80356, 80357, 80358, 80359, 80360, 80361, 80362, 80363, 80364, 80365, 80366, 80367, 80368, 80369, 80370, 80371, 80372, 80373, 80374, 80375, 80376, 80377, 83992])
Organ or disease panels (80048-80076 [80081])
Therapeutic drug assays (80150-80299 [80164, 80165, 80171])

82120 **Amines, vaginal fluid, qualitative** ♀

EXCLUDES *Combined pH and amines test for vaginitis (82120, 83986)*

0.00 0.00 FUD XXX

AMA: 2018,Jan,8; 2017,Jan,8; 2016,Jan,13; 2015,Jun,10; 2015,Apr,3; 2015,Jan,16

82127 **Amino acids; single, qualitative, each specimen**

0.00 0.00 FUD XXX

AMA: 2015,Jun,10; 2015,Apr,3

82128 **multiple, qualitative, each specimen**

0.00 0.00 FUD XXX

AMA: 2015,Jun,10; 2015,Apr,3

82131 **single, quantitative, each specimen**

INCLUDES Van Slyke method

0.00 0.00 FUD XXX

AMA: 2018,Jan,8; 2017,Jan,8; 2016,Jan,13; 2015,Jun,10; 2015,Apr,3; 2015,Jan,16

82135 **Aminolevulinic acid, delta (ALA)**

0.00 0.00 FUD XXX

AMA: 2015,Jun,10; 2015,Apr,3

82136 **Amino acids, 2 to 5 amino acids, quantitative, each specimen**

0.00 0.00 FUD XXX

AMA: 2015,Jun,10; 2015,Apr,3

82139 **Amino acids, 6 or more amino acids, quantitative, each specimen**

0.00 0.00 FUD XXX

AMA: 2015,Jun,10; 2015,Apr,3

82140 **Ammonia**

0.00 0.00 FUD XXX

AMA: 2015,Jun,10; 2015,Apr,3

82143 **Amniotic fluid scan (spectrophotometric)** M ♀

EXCLUDES *Amobarbital ([80345])*
L/S ratio (83661)

0.00 0.00 FUD XXX

AMA: 2015,Jun,10; 2015,Apr,3

82150 **Amylase**
0.00 0.00 FUD XXX
AMA: 2015,Jun,10; 2015,Apr,3

82154 **Androstanediol glucuronide**
0.00 0.00 FUD XXX
AMA: 2018,Jan,8; 2017,Jan,8; 2016,Jan,13; 2015,Jun,10; 2015,Apr,3; 2015,Jan,16

82157 **Androstenedione**
0.00 0.00 FUD XXX
AMA: 2015,Jun,10; 2015,Apr,3

82160 **Androsterone**
0.00 0.00 FUD XXX
AMA: 2015,Jun,10; 2015,Apr,3

82163 **Angiotensin II**
0.00 0.00 FUD XXX
AMA: 2015,Jun,10; 2015,Apr,3

82164 **Angiotensin I - converting enzyme (ACE)**
EXCLUDES *Antidiuretic hormone (ADH) (84588)*
Antimony (83015)
Antitrypsin, alpha-1- (82103-82104)
0.00 0.00 FUD XXX
AMA: 2015,Jun,10; 2015,Apr,3

82172 **Apolipoprotein, each**
0.00 0.00 FUD XXX
AMA: 2015,Jun,10; 2015,Apr,3

82175 **Arsenic**
EXCLUDES *Heavy metal screening (83015)*
0.00 0.00 FUD XXX
AMA: 2015,Jun,10; 2015,Apr,3

82180 **Ascorbic acid (Vitamin C), blood**
EXCLUDES *Aspirin (acetylsalicylic acid) ([80329, 80330, 80331])*
Atherogenic index, blood, ultracentrifugation, quantitative (83701)
Salicylate therapeutic drug assay ([80179])
0.00 0.00 FUD XXX
AMA: 2015,Jun,10; 2015,Apr,3

82190 **Atomic absorption spectroscopy, each analyte**
0.00 0.00 FUD XXX
AMA: 2015,Jun,10; 2015,Apr,3

82232 **Beta-2 microglobulin**
0.00 0.00 FUD XXX
AMA: 2015,Jun,10; 2015,Apr,3

82239 **Bile acids; total**
0.00 0.00 FUD XXX
AMA: 2015,Jun,10; 2015,Apr,3

82240 **cholylglycine**
EXCLUDES *Bile pigments, urine (81000-81005)*
0.00 0.00 FUD XXX
AMA: 2015,Jun,10; 2015,Apr,3

82247 **Bilirubin; total**
INCLUDES Van Den Bergh test
0.00 0.00 FUD XXX
AMA: 2018,Jan,8; 2017,Jan,8; 2016,Jan,13; 2015,Jun,10; 2015,Apr,3; 2015,Jan,16

82248 **direct**
0.00 0.00 FUD XXX
AMA: 2018,Jan,8; 2017,Jan,8; 2016,Jan,13; 2015,Jun,10; 2015,Apr,3; 2015,Jan,16

82252 **feces, qualitative**
0.00 0.00 FUD XXX
AMA: 2015,Jun,10; 2015,Apr,3

82261 **Biotinidase, each specimen**
0.00 0.00 FUD XXX
AMA: 2015,Jun,10; 2015,Apr,3

82270-82274 Chemistry: Occult Blood

CMS: 100-04,16,70.8 CLIA Waived Tests; 100-04,18,60 Colorectal Cancer Screening

INCLUDES Clinical information not requested by ordering physician
Mathematically calculated results
Quantitative analysis unless otherwise specified
Specimens from any source unless otherwise specified

EXCLUDES *Analytes from nonrequested laboratory analysis*
Calculated results representing score or probability derived by algorithm
Drug testing ([80305, 80306, 80307], [80324, 80325, 80326, 80327, 80328, 80329, 80330, 80331, 80332, 80333, 80334, 80335, 80336, 80337, 80338, 80339, 80340, 80341, 80342, 80343, 80344, 80345, 80346, 80347, 80348, 80349, 80350, 80351, 80352, 80353, 80354, 80355, 80356, 80357, 80358, 80359, 80360, 80361, 80362, 80363, 80364, 80365, 80366, 80367, 80368, 80369, 80370, 80371, 80372, 80373, 80374, 80375, 80376, 80377, 83992])
Organ or disease panels (80048-80076 [80081])
Therapeutic drug assays (80150-80299 [80164, 80165, 80171])

82270 **Blood, occult, by peroxidase activity (eg, guaiac), qualitative; feces, consecutive collected specimens with single determination, for colorectal neoplasm screening (ie, patient was provided 3 cards or single triple card for consecutive collection)**
INCLUDES Day test
0.00 0.00 FUD XXX
AMA: 2018,Jan,8; 2017,Jan,8; 2016,Jan,13; 2015,Jun,10; 2015,Apr,3; 2015,Jan,16

82271 **other sources**
0.00 0.00 FUD XXX
AMA: 2015,Jun,10; 2015,Apr,3

82272 **Blood, occult, by peroxidase activity (eg, guaiac), qualitative, feces, 1-3 simultaneous determinations, performed for other than colorectal neoplasm screening**
0.00 0.00 FUD XXX
AMA: 2018,Jan,8; 2017,Jan,8; 2016,Jan,13; 2015,Jun,10; 2015,Apr,3; 2015,Jan,16

82274 **Blood, occult, by fecal hemoglobin determination by immunoassay, qualitative, feces, 1-3 simultaneous determinations**
0.00 0.00 FUD XXX
AMA: 2015,Jun,10; 2015,Apr,3

82286-82308 [82652] Chemistry: Bradykinin—Calcitonin

INCLUDES Clinical information not requested by ordering physician
Mathematically calculated results
Quantitative analysis unless otherwise specified
Specimens from any source unless otherwise specified

EXCLUDES *Analytes from nonrequested laboratory analysis*
Calculated results representing score or probability derived by algorithm
Drug testing ([80305, 80306, 80307], [80324, 80325, 80326, 80327, 80328, 80329, 80330, 80331, 80332, 80333, 80334, 80335, 80336, 80337, 80338, 80339, 80340, 80341, 80342, 80343, 80344, 80345, 80346, 80347, 80348, 80349, 80350, 80351, 80352, 80353, 80354, 80355, 80356, 80357, 80358, 80359, 80360, 80361, 80362, 80363, 80364, 80365, 80366, 80367, 80368, 80369, 80370, 80371, 80372, 80373, 80374, 80375, 80376, 80377, 83992])
Organ or disease panels (80048-80076 [80081])
Therapeutic drug assays (80150-80299 [80164, 80165, 80171])

82286 **Bradykinin**
0.00 0.00 FUD XXX
AMA: 2015,Jun,10; 2015,Apr,3

82300 **Cadmium**
0.00 0.00 FUD XXX
AMA: 2015,Jun,10; 2015,Apr,3

82306 **Vitamin D; 25 hydroxy, includes fraction(s), if performed**
0.00 0.00 FUD XXX
AMA: 2015,Jun,10; 2015,Apr,3

82652 **1, 25 dihydroxy, includes fraction(s), if performed**
0.00 0.00 FUD XXX
AMA: 2015,Jun,10; 2015,Apr,3

82308 **Calcitonin**
0.00 0.00 FUD XXX
AMA: 2015,Jun,10; 2015,Apr,3

82310-82373 Chemistry: Calcium, total; Carbohydrate Deficient Transferrin

INCLUDES Clinical information not requested by ordering physician
Mathematically calculated results
Quantitative analysis unless otherwise specified
Specimens from any source unless otherwise specified

EXCLUDES Analytes from nonrequested laboratory analysis
Calculated results representing score or probability derived by algorithm
Drug testing ([80305, 80306, 80307], [80324, 80325, 80326, 80327, 80328, 80329, 80330, 80331, 80332, 80333, 80334, 80335, 80336, 80337, 80338, 80339, 80340, 80341, 80342, 80343, 80344, 80345, 80346, 80347, 80348, 80349, 80350, 80351, 80352, 80353, 80354, 80355, 80356, 80357, 80358, 80359, 80360, 80361, 80362, 80363, 80364, 80365, 80366, 80367, 80368, 80369, 80370, 80371, 80372, 80373, 80374, 80375, 80376, 80377, 83992])
Organ or disease panels (80048-80076 [80081])
Therapeutic drug assays (80150-80299 [80164, 80165, 80171])

82310 **Calcium; total**
🚑 0.00   ⚖ 0.00   **FUD** XXX   ☒ ▣ ▢
AMA: 2018,Jan,8; 2017,Jan,8; 2016,Jan,13; 2015,Jun,10; 2015,Apr,3; 2015,Jan,16

82330 **ionized**
🚑 0.00   ⚖ 0.00   **FUD** XXX   ☒ ▣ ▢
AMA: 2018,Jan,8; 2017,Jan,8; 2016,Jan,13; 2015,Jun,10; 2015,Apr,3; 2015,Jan,16

82331 **after calcium infusion test**
🚑 0.00   ⚖ 0.00   **FUD** XXX   ▣ ▢
AMA: 2015,Jun,10; 2015,Apr,3

82340 **urine quantitative, timed specimen**
🚑 0.00   ⚖ 0.00   **FUD** XXX   ▣ ▢
AMA: 2015,Jun,10; 2015,Apr,3

82355 **Calculus; qualitative analysis**
🚑 0.00   ⚖ 0.00   **FUD** XXX   ▣ ▢
AMA: 2015,Jun,10; 2015,Apr,3

82360 **quantitative analysis, chemical**
🚑 0.00   ⚖ 0.00   **FUD** XXX   ▣ ▢
AMA: 2015,Jun,10; 2015,Apr,3

82365 **infrared spectroscopy**
🚑 0.00   ⚖ 0.00   **FUD** XXX   ▣ ▢
AMA: 2015,Jun,10; 2015,Apr,3

82370 **X-ray diffraction**
🚑 0.00   ⚖ 0.00   **FUD** XXX   ▣ ▢
AMA: 2015,Jun,10; 2015,Apr,3

82373 **Carbohydrate deficient transferrin**
🚑 0.00   ⚖ 0.00   **FUD** XXX   ▣ ▢
AMA: 2015,Jun,10; 2015,Apr,3

82374 Chemistry: Carbon Dioxide

CMS: 100-02,11,20.2 ESRD Laboratory Services; 100-02,11,30.2.2 Automated Multi-Channel Chemistry (AMCC) Tests; 100-04,16,40.6.1 Automated Multi-Channel Chemistry (AMCC) Tests for ESRD Beneficiaries; 100-04,16,70.8 CLIA Waived Tests; 100-04,16,90.2 Organ or Disease Oriented Panels

INCLUDES Clinical information not requested by ordering physician
Mathematically calculated results
Quantitative analysis unless otherwise specified
Specimens from any source unless otherwise specified

EXCLUDES Analytes from nonrequested laboratory analysis
Calculated results representing score or probability derived by algorithm
Drug testing ([80305, 80306, 80307], [80324, 80325, 80326, 80327, 80328, 80329, 80330, 80331, 80332, 80333, 80334, 80335, 80336, 80337, 80338, 80339, 80340, 80341, 80342, 80343, 80344, 80345, 80346, 80347, 80348, 80349, 80350, 80351, 80352, 80353, 80354, 80355, 80356, 80357, 80358, 80359, 80360, 80361, 80362, 80363, 80364, 80365, 80366, 80367, 80368, 80369, 80370, 80371, 80372, 80373, 80374, 80375, 80376, 80377, 83992])
Organ or disease panels (80048-80076 [80081])
Therapeutic drug assays (80150-80299 [80164, 80165, 80171])

82374 **Carbon dioxide (bicarbonate)**
EXCLUDES Blood gases (82803)
🚑 0.00   ⚖ 0.00   **FUD** XXX   ☒ ▣ ▢
AMA: 2018,Jan,8; 2017,Jan,8; 2016,Jan,13; 2015,Jun,10; 2015,Apr,3; 2015,Jan,16

82375-82376 Chemistry: Carboxyhemoglobin (Carbon Monoxide)

INCLUDES Clinical information not requested by ordering physician
Mathematically calculated results
Specimens from any source unless otherwise specified

EXCLUDES Analytes from nonrequested laboratory analysis
Calculated results representing score or probability derived by algorithm
Drug testing ([80305, 80306, 80307], [80324, 80325, 80326, 80327, 80328, 80329, 80330, 80331, 80332, 80333, 80334, 80335, 80336, 80337, 80338, 80339, 80340, 80341, 80342, 80343, 80344, 80345, 80346, 80347, 80348, 80349, 80350, 80351, 80352, 80353, 80354, 80355, 80356, 80357, 80358, 80359, 80360, 80361, 80362, 80363, 80364, 80365, 80366, 80367, 80368, 80369, 80370, 80371, 80372, 80373, 80374, 80375, 80376, 80377, 83992])
Organ or disease panels (80048-80076 [80081])
Transcutaneous measurement of carboxyhemoglobin (88740)

82375 **Carboxyhemoglobin; quantitative**
🚑 0.00   ⚖ 0.00   **FUD** XXX   ▣ ▢
AMA: 2018,Jan,8; 2017,Jan,8; 2016,Jan,13; 2015,Jun,10; 2015,Apr,3; 2015,Jan,16

82376 **qualitative**
🚑 0.00   ⚖ 0.00   **FUD** XXX   ▣ ▢
AMA: 2015,Jun,10; 2015,Apr,3

82378 Chemistry: Carcinoembryonic Antigen (CEA)

CMS: 100-03,190.26 Carcinoembryonic Antigen (CEA)

INCLUDES Clinical information not requested by ordering physician

EXCLUDES Analytes from nonrequested laboratory analysis
Calculated results representing score or probability derived by algorithm

82378 **Carcinoembryonic antigen (CEA)**
🚑 0.00   ⚖ 0.00   **FUD** XXX   ▣ ▢
AMA: 2018,Jan,8; 2017,Jan,8; 2016,Jan,13; 2015,Jun,10; 2015,Apr,3; 2015,Jan,16

82379-82415 Chemistry: Carnitine—Chloramphenicol

INCLUDES Clinical information not requested by ordering physician
Mathematically calculated results
Quantitative analysis unless otherwise specified
Specimens from any source unless otherwise specified

EXCLUDES Analytes from nonrequested laboratory analysis
Calculated results representing score or probability derived by algorithm
Drug testing ([80305, 80306, 80307], [80324, 80325, 80326, 80327, 80328, 80329, 80330, 80331, 80332, 80333, 80334, 80335, 80336, 80337, 80338, 80339, 80340, 80341, 80342, 80343, 80344, 80345, 80346, 80347, 80348, 80349, 80350, 80351, 80352, 80353, 80354, 80355, 80356, 80357, 80358, 80359, 80360, 80361, 80362, 80363, 80364, 80365, 80366, 80367, 80368, 80369, 80370, 80371, 80372, 80373, 80374, 80375, 80376, 80377, 83992])
Organ or disease panels (80048-80076 [80081])
Therapeutic drug assays (80150-80299 [80164, 80165, 80171])

82379 **Carnitine (total and free), quantitative, each specimen**
EXCLUDES Acylcarnitine (82016-82017)
🚑 0.00   ⚖ 0.00   **FUD** XXX   ▣ ▢
AMA: 2015,Jun,10; 2015,Apr,3

82380 **Carotene**
🚑 0.00   ⚖ 0.00   **FUD** XXX   ▣ ▢
AMA: 2015,Jun,10; 2015,Apr,3

82382 **Catecholamines; total urine**
🚑 0.00   ⚖ 0.00   **FUD** XXX   ▣ ▢
AMA: 2015,Jun,10; 2015,Apr,3

82383 **blood**
🚑 0.00   ⚖ 0.00   **FUD** XXX   ▣ ▢
AMA: 2015,Jun,10; 2015,Apr,3

82384 **fractionated**
EXCLUDES Urine metabolites (83835, 84585)
🚑 0.00   ⚖ 0.00   **FUD** XXX   ▣ ▢
AMA: 2015,Jun,10; 2015,Apr,3

82387 **Cathepsin-D**
🚑 0.00   ⚖ 0.00   **FUD** XXX   ▣ ▢
AMA: 2015,Jun,10; 2015,Apr,3

82390 **Ceruloplasmin**
🚑 0.00   ⚖ 0.00   **FUD** XXX   ▣ ▢
AMA: 2015,Jun,10; 2015,Apr,3

26/TC PC/TC Only   A2-73 ASC Payment   50 Bilateral   ♂ Male Only   ♀ Female Only   🚑 Facility RVU   ⚖ Non-Facility RVU   ▢ CCI   ☒ CLIA
FUD Follow-up Days   CMS: IOM   AMA: CPT Asst   A-Y OPPSI   80/80 Surg Assist Allowed / w/Doc   ▣ Lab Crosswalk   ▤ Radiology Crosswalk

82397 **Chemiluminescent assay**
🚑 0.00 ⚕ 0.00 **FUD** XXX [Q][□]
AMA: 2018,Jan,8; 2017,Jan,8; 2016,Jan,13; 2015,Jun,10; 2015,Apr,3; 2015,Jan,16

82415 **Chloramphenicol**
🚑 0.00 ⚕ 0.00 **FUD** XXX [Q][□]
AMA: 2015,Jun,10; 2015,Apr,3

82435-82438 Chemistry: Chloride

INCLUDES Clinical information not requested by ordering physician
Mathematically calculated results
Quantitative analysis unless otherwise specified
Specimens from any source unless otherwise specified

EXCLUDES Analytes from nonrequested laboratory analysis
Calculated results representing score or probability derived by algorithm
Organ or disease panels (80048-80076 [80081])
Therapeutic drug assays (80150-80299 [80164, 80165, 80171])

82435 **Chloride; blood**
🚑 0.00 ⚕ 0.00 **FUD** XXX [X][Q][□]
AMA: 2018,Jan,8; 2017,Jan,8; 2016,Jan,13; 2015,Jun,10; 2015,Apr,3; 2015,Jan,16

82436 **urine**
🚑 0.00 ⚕ 0.00 **FUD** XXX [Q][□]
AMA: 2015,Jun,10; 2015,Apr,3

82438 **other source**
EXCLUDES Sweat collections by iontophoresis (89230)
🚑 0.00 ⚕ 0.00 **FUD** XXX [Q][□]
AMA: 2018,Jan,8; 2017,Jan,8; 2016,Jan,13; 2015,Jun,10; 2015,Apr,3; 2015,Jan,16

82441 Chemistry: Chlorinated Hydrocarbons

INCLUDES Clinical information not requested by ordering physician
Mathematically calculated results
Quantitative analysis unless otherwise specified
Specimens from any source unless otherwise specified

EXCLUDES Analytes from nonrequested laboratory analysis
Calculated results representing a score or probability derived by algorithm

82441 **Chlorinated hydrocarbons, screen**
EXCLUDES Cholecalciferol (Vitamin D) (82306)
🚑 0.00 ⚕ 0.00 **FUD** XXX [Q][□]
AMA: 2015,Jun,10; 2015,Apr,3

82465 Chemistry: Cholesterol, Total

CMS: 100-03,190.23 Lipid Testing; 100-04,16,40.6.1 Automated Multi-Channel Chemistry (AMCC) Tests for ESRD Beneficiaries; 100-04,16,70.8 CLIA Waived Tests; 100-04,16,90.2 Organ or Disease Oriented Panels

INCLUDES Clinical information not requested by ordering physician
Mathematically calculated results
Quantitative analysis unless otherwise specified

EXCLUDES Analytes from nonrequested laboratory analysis
Calculated results representing score or probability derived by algorithm
Organ or disease panels (80048-80076 [80081])

82465 **Cholesterol, serum or whole blood, total**
EXCLUDES High density lipoprotein (HDL) (83718)
🚑 0.00 ⚕ 0.00 **FUD** XXX [X][A][□]
AMA: 2018,Jan,8; 2017,Jan,8; 2016,Jan,13; 2015,Jun,10; 2015,Apr,3; 2015,Jan,16

82480-82507 Chemistry: Cholinesterase—Citrate

INCLUDES Clinical information not requested by ordering physician
Mathematically calculated results
Quantitative analysis unless otherwise specified
Specimens from any source unless otherwise specified

EXCLUDES Analytes from nonrequested laboratory analysis
Calculated results representing score or probability derived by algorithm
Drug testing ([80305, 80306, 80307], [80324, 80325, 80326, 80327, 80328, 80329, 80330, 80331, 80332, 80333, 80334, 80335, 80336, 80337, 80338, 80339, 80340, 80341, 80342, 80343, 80344, 80345, 80346, 80347, 80348, 80349, 80350, 80351, 80352, 80353, 80354, 80355, 80356, 80357, 80358, 80359, 80360, 80361, 80362, 80363, 80364, 80365, 80366, 80367, 80368, 80369, 80370, 80371, 80372, 80373, 80374, 80375, 80376, 80377, 83992])
Organ or disease panels (80048-80076 [80081])
Therapeutic drug assays (80150-80299 [80164, 80165, 80171])

82480 **Cholinesterase; serum**
🚑 0.00 ⚕ 0.00 **FUD** XXX [Q][□]
AMA: 2015,Jun,10; 2015,Apr,3

82482 **RBC**
🚑 0.00 ⚕ 0.00 **FUD** XXX [Q][□]
AMA: 2015,Jun,10; 2015,Apr,3

82485 **Chondroitin B sulfate, quantitative**
EXCLUDES Chorionic gonadotropin (84702-84703)
🚑 0.00 ⚕ 0.00 **FUD** XXX [Q][□]
AMA: 2015,Jun,10; 2015,Apr,3

82495 **Chromium**
🚑 0.00 ⚕ 0.00 **FUD** XXX [Q][□]
AMA: 2015,Jun,10; 2015,Apr,3

82507 **Citrate**
EXCLUDES Cocaine, qualitative analysis ([80353])
Codeine, qualitative analysis ([80361])
Complement (86160-86162)
🚑 0.00 ⚕ 0.00 **FUD** XXX [Q][□]
AMA: 2015,Jun,10; 2015,Apr,3

82523 Chemistry: Collagen Crosslinks, Any Method

CMS: 100-03,190.19 NCD for Collagen Crosslinks, Any Method; 100-04,16,70.8 CLIA Waived Tests

INCLUDES Clinical information not requested by ordering physician
Mathematically calculated results
Quantitative analysis unless otherwise specified
Specimens from any source unless otherwise specified

EXCLUDES Analytes from nonrequested laboratory analysis
Calculated results representing score or probability derived by algorithm
Organ or disease panels (80048-80076 [80081])
Therapeutic drug assays (80150-80299 [80164, 80165, 80171])

82523 **Collagen cross links, any method**
🚑 0.00 ⚕ 0.00 **FUD** XXX [X][Q][□]
AMA: 2015,Jun,10; 2015,Apr,3

82525-82735 [82652, 82681] Chemistry: Copper—Fluoride

INCLUDES Clinical information not requested by ordering physician
Mathematically calculated results
Quantitative analysis unless otherwise specified
Specimens from any source unless otherwise specified

EXCLUDES Analytes from nonrequested laboratory analysis
Calculated results representing score or probability derived by algorithm
Drug testing ([80305, 80306, 80307], [80324, 80325, 80326, 80327, 80328, 80329, 80330, 80331, 80332, 80333, 80334, 80335, 80336, 80337, 80338, 80339, 80340, 80341, 80342, 80343, 80344, 80345, 80346, 80347, 80348, 80349, 80350, 80351, 80352, 80353, 80354, 80355, 80356, 80357, 80358, 80359, 80360, 80361, 80362, 80363, 80364, 80365, 80366, 80367, 80368, 80369, 80370, 80371, 80372, 80373, 80374, 80375, 80376, 80377, 83992])
Organ or disease panels (80048-80076 [80081])
Therapeutic drug assays (80150-80299 [80164, 80165, 80171])

82525 **Copper**
EXCLUDES Coproporphyrin (84119-84120)
Corticosteroids (83491)
🚑 0.00 ⚕ 0.00 **FUD** XXX [Q][□]
AMA: 2015,Jun,10; 2015,Apr,3

82528 **Corticosterone**
INCLUDES Porter-Silber test
🚑 0.00 ⚕ 0.00 **FUD** XXX [Q][□]
AMA: 2015,Jun,10; 2015,Apr,3

82530 **Cortisol; free**
🚑 0.00 ⚕ 0.00 **FUD** XXX [Q][□]
AMA: 2018,Jan,8; 2017,Jan,8; 2016,Jan,13; 2015,Jun,10; 2015,Apr,3; 2015,Jan,16

82533 **total**
🚑 0.00 ⚕ 0.00 **FUD** XXX [Q][□]
AMA: 2018,Jan,8; 2017,Jan,8; 2016,Jan,13; 2015,Jun,10; 2015,Apr,3; 2015,Jan,16

82540 **Creatine**
🚑 0.00 ⚕ 0.00 **FUD** XXX [Q][□]
AMA: 2015,Jun,10; 2015,Apr,3

Pathology and Laboratory

82542 — 82681

82542 Column chromatography, includes mass spectrometry, if performed (eg, HPLC, LC, LC/MS, LC/MS-MS, GC, GC/MS-MS, GC/MS, HPLC/MS), non-drug analyte(s) not elsewhere specified, qualitative or quantitative, each specimen

EXCLUDES *Column chromatography/mass spectrometry drugs/substances ([80305, 80306, 80307], [80320, 80321, 80322, 80323, 80324, 80325, 80326, 80327, 80328, 80329, 80330, 80331, 80332, 80333, 80334, 80335, 80336, 80337, 80338, 80339, 80340, 80341, 80342, 80343, 80344, 80345, 80346, 80347, 80348, 80349, 80350, 80351, 80352, 80353, 80354, 80355, 80356, 80357, 80358, 80359, 80360, 80361, 80362, 80363, 80364, 80365, 80366, 80367, 80368, 80369, 80370, 80371, 80372, 80373, 80374, 80375, 80376, 80377, 83992])*

Procedure performed more than one time per specimen

🚑 0.00 ⚕ 0.00 **FUD** XXX 🔲🔳

AMA: 2018,Jan,8; 2017,Jan,8; 2016,Jan,13; 2015,Jun,10; 2015,Apr,3

82550 Creatine kinase (CK), (CPK); total

🚑 0.00 ⚕ 0.00 **FUD** XXX ❎🔲🔳

AMA: 2018,Jan,8; 2017,Jan,8; 2016,Jan,13; 2015,Jun,10; 2015,Apr,3; 2015,Jan,16

82552 isoenzymes

🚑 0.00 ⚕ 0.00 **FUD** XXX 🔲🔳

AMA: 2018,Jan,8; 2017,Jan,8; 2016,Jan,13; 2015,Jun,10; 2015,Apr,3; 2015,Jan,16

82553 MB fraction only

🚑 0.00 ⚕ 0.00 **FUD** XXX 🔲🔳

AMA: 2018,Jan,8; 2017,Jan,8; 2016,Jan,13; 2015,Jun,10; 2015,Apr,3; 2015,Jan,16

82554 isoforms

🚑 0.00 ⚕ 0.00 **FUD** XXX 🔲🔳

AMA: 2018,Jan,8; 2017,Jan,8; 2016,Jan,13; 2015,Jun,10; 2015,Apr,3; 2015,Jan,16

82565 Creatinine; blood

🚑 0.00 ⚕ 0.00 **FUD** XXX ❎🔲🔳

AMA: 2018,Jan,8; 2017,Jan,8; 2016,Jan,13; 2015,Jun,10; 2015,Apr,3; 2015,Jan,16

82570 other source

🚑 0.00 ⚕ 0.00 **FUD** XXX ❎🔲🔳

AMA: 2015,Jun,10; 2015,Apr,3

82575 clearance

INCLUDES Holten test

🚑 0.00 ⚕ 0.00 **FUD** XXX 🔲🔳

AMA: 2015,Jun,10; 2015,Apr,3

82585 Cryofibrinogen

🚑 0.00 ⚕ 0.00 **FUD** XXX 🔲🔳

AMA: 2015,Jun,10; 2015,Apr,3

82595 Cryoglobulin, qualitative or semi-quantitative (eg, cryocrit)

EXCLUDES *Crystals, pyrophosphate vs urate (89060)*
Quantitative, cryoglobulin (82784-82785)

🚑 0.00 ⚕ 0.00 **FUD** XXX 🔲🔳

AMA: 2015,Jun,10; 2015,Apr,3

82600 Cyanide

🚑 0.00 ⚕ 0.00 **FUD** XXX 🔲🔳

AMA: 2015,Jun,10; 2015,Apr,3

82607 Cyanocobalamin (Vitamin B-12);

EXCLUDES *Cyclic AMP (82030)*
Cyclosporine (80158)

🚑 0.00 ⚕ 0.00 **FUD** XXX 🔲🔳

AMA: 2015,Jun,10; 2015,Apr,3

82608 unsaturated binding capacity

EXCLUDES *Cyclic AMP (82030)*
Cyclosporine (80158)

🚑 0.00 ⚕ 0.00 **FUD** XXX 🔲🔳

AMA: 2015,Jun,10; 2015,Apr,3

82610 Cystatin C

🚑 0.00 ⚕ 0.00 **FUD** XXX 🔲🔳

AMA: 2018,Jan,8; 2017,Jan,8; 2016,Jan,13; 2015,Jun,10; 2015,Apr,3; 2015,Jan,16

82615 Cystine and homocystine, urine, qualitative

🚑 0.00 ⚕ 0.00 **FUD** XXX 🔲🔳

AMA: 2015,Jun,10; 2015,Apr,3

82626 Dehydroepiandrosterone (DHEA)

EXCLUDES *Anabolic steroids ([80327, 80328])*

🚑 0.00 ⚕ 0.00 **FUD** XXX 🔲🔳

AMA: 2018,Jan,8; 2017,Jan,8; 2016,Jan,13; 2015,Jun,10; 2015,Apr,3; 2015,Jan,16

82627 Dehydroepiandrosterone-sulfate (DHEA-S)

EXCLUDES *Delta-aminolevulinic acid (ALA) (82135)*

🚑 0.00 ⚕ 0.00 **FUD** XXX 🔲🔳

AMA: 2018,Jan,8; 2017,Jan,8; 2016,Jan,13; 2015,Jun,10; 2015,Apr,3; 2015,Jan,16

82633 Desoxycorticosterone, 11-

🚑 0.00 ⚕ 0.00 **FUD** XXX 🔲🔳

AMA: 2015,Jun,10; 2015,Apr,3

82634 Deoxycortisol, 11-

EXCLUDES *Dexamethasone suppression test (80420)*
Diastase, urine (82150)

🚑 0.00 ⚕ 0.00 **FUD** XXX 🔲🔳

AMA: 2015,Jun,10; 2015,Apr,3

82638 Dibucaine number

EXCLUDES *Dichloroethane (82441)*
Dichloromethane (82441)
Diethylether (84600)

🚑 0.00 ⚕ 0.00 **FUD** XXX 🔲🔳

AMA: 2015,Jun,10; 2015,Apr,3

82642 Dihydrotestosterone (DHT)

EXCLUDES *Anabolic drug testing analysis dihydrotestosterone ([80327, 80328])*
Dipropylacetic acid ([80164])
Dopamine (82382)
Duodenal contents, individual enzymes for intubation and collection (43756-43757)

🚑 0.00 ⚕ 0.00 **FUD** XXX 🔳

82652 Resequenced code. See code following 82306.

82656 Elastase, pancreatic (EL-1), fecal, qualitative or semi-quantitative

🚑 0.00 ⚕ 0.00 **FUD** XXX 🔲🔳

AMA: 2018,Jan,8; 2017,Jan,8; 2016,Jan,13; 2015,Jun,10; 2015,Apr,3; 2015,Jan,16

82657 Enzyme activity in blood cells, cultured cells, or tissue, not elsewhere specified; nonradioactive substrate, each specimen

🚑 0.00 ⚕ 0.00 **FUD** XXX 🔲🔳

AMA: 2015,Jun,10; 2015,Apr,3

82658 radioactive substrate, each specimen

🚑 0.00 ⚕ 0.00 **FUD** XXX 🔲🔳

AMA: 2015,Jun,10; 2015,Apr,3

82664 Electrophoretic technique, not elsewhere specified

EXCLUDES *Endocrine receptor assays (84233-84235)*

🚑 0.00 ⚕ 0.00 **FUD** XXX 🔲🔳

AMA: 2015,Jun,10; 2015,Apr,3

82668 Erythropoietin

🚑 0.00 ⚕ 0.00 **FUD** XXX 🔲🔳

AMA: 2015,Jun,10; 2015,Apr,3

▲ **82670** Estradiol; total

🚑 0.00 ⚕ 0.00 **FUD** XXX 🔲🔳

AMA: 2015,Jun,10; 2015,Apr,3

● # **82681** free, direct measurement (eg, equilibrium dialysis)

🚑 0.00 ⚕ 0.00 **FUD** 000

| 26/TC PC/TC Only | A2-Z3 ASC Payment | 50 Bilateral | ♂ Male Only | ♀ Female Only | 🚑 Facility RVU | ⚕ Non-Facility RVU | 🔲 CCI | ❎ CLIA |
| FUD Follow-up Days | CMS: IOM | AMA: CPT Asst | A-Y OPPSI | 80/80 Surg Assist Allowed / w/Doc | | 🔳 Lab Crosswalk | 🔲 Radiology Crosswalk | |

82671 **Estrogens; fractionated**
EXCLUDES *Estrogen receptor assay (84233)*
0.00 0.00 FUD XXX
AMA: 2015,Jun,10; 2015,Apr,3

82672 **total**
EXCLUDES *Estrogen receptor assay (84233)*
0.00 0.00 FUD XXX
AMA: 2015,Jun,10; 2015,Apr,3

82677 **Estriol**
0.00 0.00 FUD XXX
AMA: 2015,Jun,10; 2015,Apr,3

82679 **Estrone**
EXCLUDES *Alcohol (ethanol) definitive drug testing ([80320])*
Alcohol (ethanol) therapeutic drug assay (82077)
0.00 0.00 FUD XXX
AMA: 2015,Jun,10; 2015,Apr,3

82681 **Resequenced code. See code following 82670.**

82693 **Ethylene glycol**
0.00 0.00 FUD XXX
AMA: 2015,Jun,10; 2015,Apr,3

82696 **Etiocholanolone**
EXCLUDES *Fractionation ketosteroids (83593)*
0.00 0.00 FUD XXX
AMA: 2015,Jun,10; 2015,Apr,3

82705 **Fat or lipids, feces; qualitative**
0.00 0.00 FUD XXX
AMA: 2015,Jun,10; 2015,Apr,3

82710 **quantitative**
0.00 0.00 FUD XXX
AMA: 2015,Jun,10; 2015,Apr,3

82715 **Fat differential, feces, quantitative**
0.00 0.00 FUD XXX
AMA: 2015,Jun,10; 2015,Apr,3

82725 **Fatty acids, nonesterified**
0.00 0.00 FUD XXX
AMA: 2015,Jun,10; 2015,Apr,3

82726 **Very long chain fatty acids**
0.00 0.00 FUD XXX
AMA: 2015,Jun,10; 2015,Apr,3

82728 **Ferritin**
EXCLUDES *Fetal hemoglobin (83030, 83033, 85460)*
Fetoprotein, alpha-1 (82105-82106)
0.00 0.00 FUD XXX
AMA: 2015,Jun,10; 2015,Apr,3

82731 **Fetal fibronectin, cervicovaginal secretions, semi-quantitative** M ♀
0.00 0.00 FUD XXX
AMA: 2015,Jun,10; 2015,Apr,3

82735 **Fluoride**
EXCLUDES *Foam stability test (83662)*
0.00 0.00 FUD XXX
AMA: 2015,Jun,10; 2015,Apr,3

82746-82941 Chemistry: Folic Acid—Gastrin

INCLUDES Clinical information not requested by ordering physician
Mathematically calculated results
Quantitative analysis unless otherwise specified
Specimens from any source unless otherwise specified

EXCLUDES *Analytes from nonrequested laboratory analysis*
Calculated results representing score or probability derived by algorithm
Drug testing ([80305, 80306, 80307], [80324, 80325, 80326, 80327, 80328, 80329, 80330, 80331, 80332, 80333, 80334, 80335, 80336, 80337, 80338, 80339, 80340, 80341, 80342, 80343, 80344, 80345, 80346, 80347, 80348, 80349, 80350, 80351, 80352, 80353, 80354, 80355, 80356, 80357, 80358, 80359, 80360, 80361, 80362, 80363, 80364, 80365, 80366, 80367, 80368, 80369, 80370, 80371, 80372, 80373, 80374, 80375, 80376, 80377, 83992])
Organ or disease panels (80048-80076 [80081])
Therapeutic drug assays (80150-80299 [80164, 80165, 80171])

82746 **Folic acid; serum**
0.00 0.00 FUD XXX
AMA: 2015,Jun,10; 2015,Apr,3

82747 **RBC**
EXCLUDES *Follicle stimulating hormone (FSH) (83001)*
0.00 0.00 FUD XXX
AMA: 2015,Jun,10; 2015,Apr,3

82757 **Fructose, semen**
EXCLUDES *Fructosamine (82985)*
Fructose, TLC screen (84375)
0.00 0.00 FUD XXX
AMA: 2015,Jun,10; 2015,Apr,3

82759 **Galactokinase, RBC**
0.00 0.00 FUD XXX
AMA: 2015,Jun,10; 2015,Apr,3

82760 **Galactose**
0.00 0.00 FUD XXX
AMA: 2015,Jun,10; 2015,Apr,3

82775 **Galactose-1-phosphate uridyl transferase; quantitative**
0.00 0.00 FUD XXX
AMA: 2015,Jun,10; 2015,Apr,3

82776 **screen**
0.00 0.00 FUD XXX
AMA: 2015,Jun,10; 2015,Apr,3

82777 **Galectin-3**
0.00 0.00 FUD XXX
AMA: 2015,Jun,10; 2015,Apr,3

82784 **Gammaglobulin (immunoglobulin); IgA, IgD, IgG, IgM, each**
INCLUDES Farr test
0.00 0.00 FUD XXX
AMA: 2018,Jan,8; 2017,Jan,8; 2016,Jan,13; 2015,Jun,10; 2015,Apr,3; 2015,Jan,16

82785 **IgE**
INCLUDES Farr test
EXCLUDES *Allergen specific, IgE (86003, 86005)*
0.00 0.00 FUD XXX
AMA: 2018,Jan,8; 2017,Jan,8; 2016,Jan,13; 2015,Jun,10; 2015,Apr,3; 2015,Jan,16

82787 **immunoglobulin subclasses (eg, IgG1, 2, 3, or 4), each**
EXCLUDES *Gamma-glutamyltransferase (GGT) (82977)*
0.00 0.00 FUD XXX
AMA: 2015,Jun,10; 2015,Apr,3

82800 **Gases, blood, pH only**
0.00 0.00 FUD XXX
AMA: 2015,Jun,10; 2015,Apr,3

82803 **Gases, blood, any combination of pH, pCO2, pO2, CO2, HCO3 (including calculated O2 saturation);**
INCLUDES Two or more listed analytes
0.00 0.00 FUD XXX
AMA: 2015,Jun,10; 2015,Apr,3

82805 with O2 saturation, by direct measurement, except pulse oximetry
0.00 0.00 FUD XXX
AMA: 2015,Jun,10; 2015,Apr,3

82810 Gases, blood, O2 saturation only, by direct measurement, except pulse oximetry
EXCLUDES *Pulse oximetry (94760)*
0.00 0.00 FUD XXX
AMA: 2015,Jun,10; 2015,Apr,3

82820 Hemoglobin-oxygen affinity (pO2 for 50% hemoglobin saturation with oxygen)
EXCLUDES *Gastric acid analysis (82930)*
0.00 0.00 FUD XXX
AMA: 2015,Jun,10; 2015,Apr,3

82930 Gastric acid analysis, includes pH if performed, each specimen
0.00 0.00 FUD XXX
AMA: 2018,Jan,8; 2017,Jan,8; 2016,Jan,13; 2015,Jun,10; 2015,Apr,3; 2015,Jan,16

82938 Gastrin after secretin stimulation
0.00 0.00 FUD XXX
AMA: 2015,Jun,10; 2015,Apr,3

82941 Gastrin
EXCLUDES *Gentamicin (80170)*
GGT (82977)
Qualitative column chromatography report specific analyte or (82542)
0.00 0.00 FUD XXX
AMA: 2015,Jun,10; 2015,Apr,3

82943-82962 Chemistry: Glucagon—Glucose Testing

CMS: 100-03,190.20 Blood Glucose Testing
INCLUDES Clinical information not requested by ordering physician
Mathematically calculated results
Quantitative analysis unless otherwise specified
Specimens from any source unless otherwise specified
EXCLUDES *Analytes from nonrequested laboratory analysis*
Calculated results representing score or probability derived by algorithm
Organ or disease panels (80048-80076 [80081])
Therapeutic drug assays (80150-80299 [80164, 80165, 80171])
Code also glucose administration injection (96374)

82943 Glucagon
0.00 0.00 FUD XXX
AMA: 2015,Jun,10; 2015,Apr,3

82945 Glucose, body fluid, other than blood
0.00 0.00 FUD XXX
AMA: 2015,Jun,10; 2015,Apr,3

82946 Glucagon tolerance test
0.00 0.00 FUD XXX
AMA: 2015,Jun,10; 2015,Apr,3

82947 Glucose; quantitative, blood (except reagent strip)
0.00 0.00 FUD XXX
AMA: 2018,Jan,8; 2017,Jan,8; 2016,Jan,13; 2015,Jun,10; 2015,Apr,3; 2015,Jan,16

82948 blood, reagent strip
0.00 0.00 FUD XXX
AMA: 2018,Jan,8; 2017,Jan,8; 2016,Jan,13; 2015,Jun,10; 2015,Apr,3; 2015,Jan,16

82950 post glucose dose (includes glucose)
0.00 0.00 FUD XXX
AMA: 2018,Jan,8; 2017,Jan,8; 2016,Jan,13; 2015,Jun,10; 2015,Apr,3; 2015,Jan,16

82951 tolerance test (GTT), 3 specimens (includes glucose)
0.00 0.00 FUD XXX
AMA: 2018,Jan,8; 2017,Jan,8; 2016,Jan,13; 2015,Jun,10; 2015,Apr,3; 2015,Jan,16

+ **82952** tolerance test, each additional beyond 3 specimens (List separately in addition to code for primary procedure)
EXCLUDES *Insulin tolerance test (80434-80435)*
Leucine tolerance test (80428)
Semiquantitative urine glucose (81000, 81002, 81005, 81099)
Code first (82951)
0.00 0.00 FUD XXX
AMA: 2018,Jan,8; 2017,Jan,8; 2016,Jan,13; 2015,Jun,10; 2015,Apr,3; 2015,Jan,16

82955 Glucose-6-phosphate dehydrogenase (G6PD); quantitative
Code also glucose tolerance test with medication, when performed (96374)
0.00 0.00 FUD XXX
AMA: 2015,Jun,10; 2015,Apr,3

82960 screen
Code also glucose tolerance test with medication, when performed (96374)
0.00 0.00 FUD XXX
AMA: 2015,Jun,10; 2015,Apr,3

82962 Glucose, blood by glucose monitoring device(s) cleared by the FDA specifically for home use
0.00 0.00 FUD XXX
AMA: 2018,Jan,8; 2017,Jan,8; 2016,Jan,13; 2015,Jun,10; 2015,Apr,3; 2015,Jan,16

82963-83690 Chemistry: Glucosidase—Lipase

INCLUDES Clinical information not requested by ordering physician
Mathematically calculated results
Quantitative analysis unless otherwise specified
Specimens from any source unless otherwise specified
EXCLUDES *Analytes from nonrequested laboratory analysis*
Calculated results representing score or probability derived by algorithm
Drug testing ([80305, 80306, 80307], [80324, 80325, 80326, 80327, 80328, 80329, 80330, 80331, 80332, 80333, 80334, 80335, 80336, 80337, 80338, 80339, 80340, 80341, 80342, 80343, 80344, 80345, 80346, 80347, 80348, 80349, 80350, 80351, 80352, 80353, 80354, 80355, 80356, 80357, 80358, 80359, 80360, 80361, 80362, 80363, 80364, 80365, 80366, 80367, 80368, 80369, 80370, 80371, 80372, 80373, 80374, 80375, 80376, 80377, 83992])
Organ or disease panels (80048-80076 [80081])
Therapeutic drug assays (80150-80299 [80164, 80165, 80171])

82963 Glucosidase, beta
0.00 0.00 FUD XXX
AMA: 2015,Jun,10; 2015,Apr,3

82965 Glutamate dehydrogenase
0.00 0.00 FUD XXX
AMA: 2015,Jun,10; 2015,Apr,3

82977 Glutamyltransferase, gamma (GGT)
0.00 0.00 FUD XXX
AMA: 2018,Jan,8; 2017,Jan,8; 2016,Jan,13; 2015,Jun,10; 2015,Apr,3; 2015,Jan,16

82978 Glutathione
0.00 0.00 FUD XXX
AMA: 2015,Jun,10; 2015,Apr,3

82979 Glutathione reductase, RBC
EXCLUDES *Glycohemoglobin (83036)*
0.00 0.00 FUD XXX
AMA: 2015,Jun,10; 2015,Apr,3

82985 Glycated protein
EXCLUDES *Gonadotropin chorionic (hCG) (84702-84703)*
0.00 0.00 FUD XXX
AMA: 2018,Jan,8; 2017,Jan,8; 2016,Jan,13; 2015,Jun,10; 2015,Apr,3; 2015,Jan,16

83001 Gonadotropin; follicle stimulating hormone (FSH)
0.00 0.00 FUD XXX
AMA: 2015,Jun,10; 2015,Apr,3

83002 luteinizing hormone (LH)
EXCLUDES *Luteinizing releasing factor (LRH) (83727)*
0.00 0.00 FUD XXX
AMA: 2015,Jun,10; 2015,Apr,3

83003 Growth hormone, human (HGH) (somatotropin)

EXCLUDES *Antibody to human growth hormone (86277)*

0.00 0.00 FUD XXX

AMA: 2015,Jun,10; 2015,Apr,3

83006 Growth stimulation expressed gene 2 (ST2, Interleukin 1 receptor like-1)

0.00 0.00 FUD XXX

AMA: 2015,Jun,10; 2015,Apr,3

83009 Helicobacter pylori, blood test analysis for urease activity, non-radioactive isotope (eg, C-13)

EXCLUDES *H. pylori, breath test analysis for urease activity (83013-83014)*

0.00 0.00 FUD XXX

AMA: 2015,Jun,10; 2015,Apr,3

83010 Haptoglobin; quantitative

0.00 0.00 FUD XXX

AMA: 2015,Jun,10; 2015,Apr,3

83012 phenotypes

0.00 0.00 FUD XXX

AMA: 2015,Jun,10; 2015,Apr,3

83013 Helicobacter pylori; breath test analysis for urease activity, non-radioactive isotope (eg, C-13)

0.00 0.00 FUD XXX

AMA: 2020,OctSE,1; 2018,Jan,8; 2017,Jan,8; 2016,Jan,13; 2015,Jun,10; 2015,Apr,3; 2015,Jan,16

83014 drug administration

EXCLUDES *H. pylori:*
Blood test analysis for urease activity (83009)
Enzyme immunoassay (87339)
Liquid scintillation counter (78267-78268)
Stool (87338)

0.00 0.00 FUD XXX

AMA: 2020,OctSE,1; 2018,Jan,8; 2017,Jan,8; 2016,Jan,13; 2015,Jun,10; 2015,Apr,3; 2015,Jan,16

83015 Heavy metal (eg, arsenic, barium, beryllium, bismuth, antimony, mercury); qualitative, any number of analytes

INCLUDES Reinsch test

0.00 0.00 FUD XXX

AMA: 2015,Jun,10; 2015,Apr,3

83018 quantitative, each, not elsewhere specified

EXCLUDES *Evaluation known heavy metal with specific code*

0.00 0.00 FUD XXX

AMA: 2015,Jun,10; 2015,Apr,3

83020 Hemoglobin fractionation and quantitation; electrophoresis (eg, A2, S, C, and/or F)

0.00 0.00 FUD XXX

AMA: 2015,Jun,10; 2015,Apr,3

83021 chromatography (eg, A2, S, C, and/or F)

EXCLUDES *Analysis glycosylated (A1c) hemoglobin by chromatography or electrophoresis without identified hemoglobin variant (83036)*

0.00 0.00 FUD XXX

AMA: 2018,Jan,8; 2017,Jan,8; 2016,Jan,13; 2015,Jun,10; 2015,Apr,3; 2015,Jan,16

83026 Hemoglobin; by copper sulfate method, non-automated

0.00 0.00 FUD XXX

AMA: 2015,Jun,10; 2015,Apr,3

83030 F (fetal), chemical

0.00 0.00 FUD XXX

AMA: 2015,Jun,10; 2015,Apr,3

83033 F (fetal), qualitative

0.00 0.00 FUD XXX

AMA: 2015,Jun,10; 2015,Apr,3

83036 glycosylated (A1C)

EXCLUDES *Analysis glycosylated (A1c) hemoglobin by chromatography or electrophoresis without identified hemoglobin variant (83020-83021)*
Detection hemoglobin, fecal, by immunoassay (82274)

0.00 0.00 FUD XXX

AMA: 2018,Jan,8; 2017,Jan,8; 2016,Jan,13; 2015,Jun,10; 2015,Apr,3; 2015,Jan,16

83037 glycosylated (A1C) by device cleared by FDA for home use

0.00 0.00 FUD XXX

AMA: 2018,Jan,8; 2017,Jan,8; 2016,Jan,13; 2015,Jun,10; 2015,Apr,3; 2015,Jan,16

83045 methemoglobin, qualitative

0.00 0.00 FUD XXX

AMA: 2015,Jun,10; 2015,Apr,3

83050 methemoglobin, quantitative

EXCLUDES *Transcutaneous methemoglobin test (88741)*

0.00 0.00 FUD XXX

AMA: 2018,Jan,8; 2017,Jan,8; 2016,Jan,13; 2015,Jun,10; 2015,Apr,3; 2015,Jan,16

83051 plasma

0.00 0.00 FUD XXX

AMA: 2015,Jun,10; 2015,Apr,3

83060 sulfhemoglobin, quantitative

0.00 0.00 FUD XXX

AMA: 2015,Jun,10; 2015,Apr,3

83065 thermolabile

0.00 0.00 FUD XXX

AMA: 2015,Jun,10; 2015,Apr,3

83068 unstable, screen

0.00 0.00 FUD XXX

AMA: 2015,Jun,10; 2015,Apr,3

83069 urine

0.00 0.00 FUD XXX

AMA: 2015,Jun,10; 2015,Apr,3

83070 Hemosiderin, qualitative

EXCLUDES *HIAA (83497)*
Qualitative column chromatography report specific analyte or (82542)

0.00 0.00 FUD XXX

AMA: 2015,Jun,10; 2015,Apr,3

83080 b-Hexosaminidase, each assay

0.00 0.00 FUD XXX

AMA: 2015,Jun,10; 2015,Apr,3

83088 Histamine

EXCLUDES *Hollander test (43754-43755)*

0.00 0.00 FUD XXX

AMA: 2015,Jun,10; 2015,Apr,3

83090 Homocysteine

0.00 0.00 FUD XXX

AMA: 2018,Jan,8; 2017,Jan,8; 2016,Jan,13; 2015,Jun,10; 2015,Apr,3; 2015,Jan,16

83150 Homovanillic acid (HVA)

EXCLUDES *Hormone testing report from alphabetic list in Chemistry section*
Hydrogen/methane breath test (91065)

0.00 0.00 FUD XXX

AMA: 2015,Jun,10; 2015,Apr,3

83491 Hydroxycorticosteroids, 17- (17-OHCS)

EXCLUDES *Cortisol (82530, 82533)*
Deoxycortisol (82634)

0.00 0.00 FUD XXX

AMA: 2015,Jun,10; 2015,Apr,3

83497 Hydroxyindolacetic acid, 5-(HIAA)
EXCLUDES *5-Hydroxytryptamine (84260)*
Urine qualitative test (81005)
0.00 0.00 FUD XXX
AMA: 2015,Jun,10; 2015,Apr,3

83498 Hydroxyprogesterone, 17-d
0.00 0.00 FUD XXX
AMA: 2015,Jun,10; 2015,Apr,3

83500 Hydroxyproline; free
0.00 0.00 FUD XXX
AMA: 2015,Jun,10; 2015,Apr,3

83505 total
0.00 0.00 FUD XXX
AMA: 2015,Jun,10; 2015,Apr,3

83516 Immunoassay for analyte other than infectious agent antibody or infectious agent antigen; qualitative or semiquantitative, multiple step method
0.00 0.00 FUD XXX
AMA: 2020,OctSE,1; 2020,AugSE,1; 2020,AugSE,1; 2020,AugSE,1; 2015,Jun,10; 2015,Apr,3

83518 qualitative or semiquantitative, single step method (eg, reagent strip)
0.00 0.00 FUD XXX
AMA: 2020,OctSE,1; 2015,Jun,10; 2015,Apr,3

83519 quantitative, by radioimmunoassay (eg, RIA)
0.00 0.00 FUD XXX
AMA: 2020,OctSE,1; 2018,Jan,8; 2017,Jan,8; 2016,Jan,13; 2015,Jun,10; 2015,Apr,3; 2015,Jan,16

83520 quantitative, not otherwise specified
EXCLUDES *Immunoassays for antibodies to infectious agent antigen report specific analyte/method from Immunology*
Immunoassay of tumor antigens not elsewhere specified (86316)
Immunoglobulins (82784, 82785)
0.00 0.00 FUD XXX
AMA: 2020,OctSE,1; 2015,Jun,10; 2015,Apr,3

83525 Insulin; total
EXCLUDES *Proinsulin (84206)*
0.00 0.00 FUD XXX
AMA: 2015,Jun,10; 2015,Apr,3

83527 free
0.00 0.00 FUD XXX
AMA: 2018,Jan,8; 2017,Jan,8; 2016,Jan,13; 2015,Jun,10; 2015,Apr,3; 2015,Jan,16

83528 Intrinsic factor
EXCLUDES *Intrinsic factor antibodies (86340)*
0.00 0.00 FUD XXX
AMA: 2015,Jun,10; 2015,Apr,3

83540 Iron
0.00 0.00 FUD XXX
AMA: 2018,Jan,8; 2017,Jan,8; 2016,Jan,13; 2015,Jun,10; 2015,Apr,3; 2015,Jan,16

83550 Iron binding capacity
0.00 0.00 FUD XXX
AMA: 2015,Jun,10; 2015,Apr,3

83570 Isocitric dehydrogenase (IDH)
EXCLUDES *Isonicotinic acid hydrazide, INH, report specific method*
Isopropyl alcohol ([80320])
0.00 0.00 FUD XXX
AMA: 2015,Jun,10; 2015,Apr,3

83582 Ketogenic steroids, fractionation
EXCLUDES *Ketone bodies:*
Serum (82009, 82010)
Urine (81000-81003)
0.00 0.00 FUD XXX
AMA: 2015,Jun,10; 2015,Apr,3

83586 Ketosteroids, 17- (17-KS); total
0.00 0.00 FUD XXX
AMA: 2015,Jun,10; 2015,Apr,3

83593 fractionation
0.00 0.00 FUD XXX
AMA: 2015,Jun,10; 2015,Apr,3

83605 Lactate (lactic acid)
0.00 0.00 FUD XXX
AMA: 2015,Jun,10; 2015,Apr,3

83615 Lactate dehydrogenase (LD), (LDH);
0.00 0.00 FUD XXX
AMA: 2018,Jan,8; 2017,Jan,8; 2016,Jan,13; 2015,Jun,10; 2015,Apr,3; 2015,Jan,16

83625 isoenzymes, separation and quantitation
0.00 0.00 FUD XXX
AMA: 2018,Jan,8; 2017,Jan,8; 2016,Jan,13; 2015,Jun,10; 2015,Apr,3; 2015,Jan,16

83630 Lactoferrin, fecal; qualitative
0.00 0.00 FUD XXX
AMA: 2018,Jan,8; 2017,Jan,8; 2016,Jan,13; 2015,Jun,10; 2015,Apr,3; 2015,Jan,16

83631 quantitative
0.00 0.00 FUD XXX
AMA: 2018,Jan,8; 2017,Jan,8; 2016,Jan,13; 2015,Jun,10; 2015,Apr,3; 2015,Jan,16

83632 Lactogen, human placental (HPL) human chorionic somatomammotropin
0.00 0.00 FUD XXX
AMA: 2015,Jun,10; 2015,Apr,3

83633 Lactose, urine, qualitative
EXCLUDES *Lactase deficiency breath hydrogen/methane test (91065)*
Lactose tolerance test (82951, 82952)
0.00 0.00 FUD XXX
AMA: 2015,Jun,10; 2015,Apr,3

83655 Lead
0.00 0.00 FUD XXX
AMA: 2015,Jun,10; 2015,Apr,3

83661 Fetal lung maturity assessment; lecithin sphingomyelin (L/S) ratio
0.00 0.00 FUD XXX
AMA: 2018,Jan,8; 2017,Jan,8; 2016,Jan,13; 2015,Jun,10; 2015,Apr,3; 2015,Jan,16

83662 foam stability test
0.00 0.00 FUD XXX
AMA: 2015,Jun,10; 2015,Apr,3

83663 fluorescence polarization
0.00 0.00 FUD XXX
AMA: 2015,Jun,10; 2015,Apr,3

83664 lamellar body density
EXCLUDES *Phosphatidylglycerol (84081)*
0.00 0.00 FUD XXX
AMA: 2015,Jun,10; 2015,Apr,3

83670 Leucine aminopeptidase (LAP)
0.00 0.00 FUD XXX
AMA: 2015,Jun,10; 2015,Apr,3

83690 Lipase
0.00 0.00 FUD XXX
AMA: 2015,Jun,10; 2015,Apr,3

83695-83727 Chemistry: Lipoprotein—Luteinizing Releasing Factor

INCLUDES Clinical information not requested by ordering physician
Mathematically calculated results
Quantitative analysis unless otherwise specified
Specimens from any source unless otherwise specified

EXCLUDES *Analytes from nonrequested laboratory analysis*
Calculated results representing score or probability derived by algorithm
Organ or disease panels (80048-80076 [80081])
Therapeutic drug assays (80150-80299 [80164, 80165, 80171])

83695 Lipoprotein (a)
0.00 0.00 FUD XXX
AMA: 2018,Jan,8; 2017,Jan,8; 2016,Jan,13; 2015,Jun,10; 2015,Apr,3; 2015,Jan,16

83698 Lipoprotein-associated phospholipase A2 (Lp-PLA2)
EXCLUDES *Secretory type II phospholipase A2 (sPLA2-IIA) (0423T)*
0.00 0.00 FUD XXX
AMA: 2015,Jun,10; 2015,Apr,3

83700 Lipoprotein, blood; electrophoretic separation and quantitation
0.00 0.00 FUD XXX
AMA: 2018,Jan,8; 2017,Jan,8; 2016,Jan,13; 2015,Jun,10; 2015,Apr,3; 2015,Jan,16

83701 high resolution fractionation and quantitation of lipoproteins including lipoprotein subclasses when performed (eg, electrophoresis, ultracentrifugation)
0.00 0.00 FUD XXX
AMA: 2018,Jan,8; 2017,Jan,8; 2016,Jan,13; 2015,Jun,10; 2015,Apr,3; 2015,Jan,16

83704 quantitation of lipoprotein particle number(s) (eg, by nuclear magnetic resonance spectroscopy), includes lipoprotein particle subclass(es), when performed
0.00 0.00 FUD XXX
AMA: 2018,Jan,8; 2017,Jan,8; 2016,Jan,13; 2015,Jun,10; 2015,Apr,3; 2015,Jan,16

83718 Lipoprotein, direct measurement; high density cholesterol (HDL cholesterol)
0.00 0.00 FUD XXX
AMA: 2018,Jan,8; 2017,Jan,8; 2016,Jan,13; 2015,Jun,10; 2015,Apr,3; 2015,Jan,16

83719 VLDL cholesterol
0.00 0.00 FUD XXX
AMA: 2018,Jan,8; 2017,Jan,8; 2016,Jan,13; 2015,Jun,10; 2015,Apr,3; 2015,Jan,16

83721 LDL cholesterol
EXCLUDES *Fractionation by high resolution electrophoresis or ultracentrifugation (83701)*
Lipoprotein particle numbers and subclasses analysis by nuclear magnetic resonance spectroscopy (83704)
0.00 0.00 FUD XXX
AMA: 2018,Jan,8; 2017,Jan,8; 2016,Jan,13; 2015,Jun,10; 2015,Apr,3; 2015,Jan,16

83722 small dense LDL cholesterol
EXCLUDES *Fractionation by high resolution electrophoresis or ultracentrifugation (83701)*
Lipoprotein particle numbers/subclass analysis by nuclear magnetic resonance spectroscopy (83704)
0.00 0.00 FUD XXX

83727 Luteinizing releasing factor (LRH)
EXCLUDES *alpha-2-Macroglobulin (86329)*
Luteinizing hormone (LH) (83002)
0.00 0.00 FUD XXX
AMA: 2015,Jun,10; 2015,Apr,3

83735-83885 Chemistry: Magnesium—Nickel

INCLUDES Clinical information not requested by the ordering physician
Mathematically calculated results
Quantitative analysis unless otherwise specified
Specimens from any source unless otherwise specified

EXCLUDES *Analytes from nonrequested laboratory analysis*
Calculated results representing a score or probability derived by algorithm
Organ or disease panels (80048-80076 [80081])
Therapeutic drug assays (80150-80299 [80164, 80165, 80171])

83735 Magnesium
0.00 0.00 FUD XXX
AMA: 2015,Jun,10; 2015,Apr,3

83775 Malate dehydrogenase
EXCLUDES *Maltose tolerance (82951, 82952)*
Mammotropin (84146)
0.00 0.00 FUD XXX
AMA: 2015,Jun,10; 2015,Apr,3

83785 Manganese
0.00 0.00 FUD XXX
AMA: 2015,Jun,10; 2015,Apr,3

83789 Mass spectrometry and tandem mass spectrometry (eg, MS, MS/MS, MALDI, MS-TOF, QTOF), non-drug analyte(s) not elsewhere specified, qualitative or quantitative, each specimen
EXCLUDES *Column chromatography/mass spectrometry drugs or substances ([80305], [80306], [80307], [80320, 80321, 80322, 80323, 80324, 80325, 80326, 80327, 80328, 80329, 80330, 80331, 80332, 80333, 80334, 80335, 80336, 80337, 80338, 80339, 80340, 80341, 80342, 80343, 80344, 80345, 80346, 80347, 80348, 80349, 80350, 80351, 80352, 80353, 80354, 80355, 80356, 80357, 80358, 80359, 80360, 80361, 80362, 80363, 80364, 80365, 80366, 80367, 80368, 80369, 80370, 80371, 80372, 80373, 80374, 80375, 80376, 80377, 83992])*
Procedure performed more than one time per specimen
Report specific analyte testing with code(s) from Chemistry section
0.00 0.00 FUD XXX
AMA: 2015,Jun,10; 2015,Apr,3

83825 Mercury, quantitative
EXCLUDES *Mercury screen (83015)*
0.00 0.00 FUD XXX
AMA: 2015,Jun,10; 2015,Apr,3

83835 Metanephrines
EXCLUDES *Catecholamines (82382-82384)*
Methamphetamine ([80324], [80325], [80326])
Methane breath test (91065)
0.00 0.00 FUD XXX
AMA: 2015,Jun,10; 2015,Apr,3

83857 Methemalbumin
EXCLUDES *Methemoglobin (83045, 83050)*
Methyl alcohol ([80320])
Microalbumin
Quantitative (82043)
Semiquantitative (82044)
0.00 0.00 FUD XXX
AMA: 2015,Jun,10; 2015,Apr,3

83861 Microfluidic analysis utilizing an integrated collection and analysis device, tear osmolarity
EXCLUDES *beta-2 Microglobulin (82232)*
Code also when performed on both eyes 83861 X 2
0.00 0.00 FUD XXX
AMA: 2015,Jun,10; 2015,Apr,3

83864 Mucopolysaccharides, acid, quantitative
0.00 0.00 FUD XXX
AMA: 2015,Jun,10; 2015,Apr,3

83872 Mucin, synovial fluid (Ropes test)
0.00 0.00 FUD XXX
AMA: 2015,Jun,10; 2015,Apr,3

Pathology and Laboratory

83873 Myelin basic protein, cerebrospinal fluid
> EXCLUDES *Oligoclonal bands (83916)*
> 🔧 0.00 ⚕ 0.00 **FUD** XXX [Q][☐]
> **AMA:** 2015,Jun,10; 2015,Apr,3

83874 Myoglobin
> 🔧 0.00 ⚕ 0.00 **FUD** XXX [Q][☐]
> **AMA:** 2018,Jan,8; 2017,Jan,8; 2016,Jan,13; 2015,Jun,10; 2015,Apr,3; 2015,Jan,16

83876 Myeloperoxidase (MPO)
> 🔧 0.00 ⚕ 0.00 **FUD** XXX [Q][☐]
> **AMA:** 2015,Jun,10; 2015,Apr,3

83880 Natriuretic peptide
> 🔧 0.00 ⚕ 0.00 **FUD** XXX [X][Q][☐]
> **AMA:** 2018,Jan,8; 2017,Jan,8; 2016,Jan,13; 2015,Jun,10; 2015,Apr,3; 2015,Jan,16

83883 Nephelometry, each analyte not elsewhere specified
> 🔧 0.00 ⚕ 0.00 **FUD** XXX [Q][☐]
> **AMA:** 2015,Jun,10; 2015,Apr,3

83885 Nickel
> 🔧 0.00 ⚕ 0.00 **FUD** XXX [Q][☐]
> **AMA:** 2015,Jun,10; 2015,Apr,3

83915-84066 [83992] Chemistry: Nucleotidase 5'- —Phosphatase (Acid)

> INCLUDES Clinical information not requested by ordering physician
> Mathematically calculated results
> Quantitative analysis unless otherwise specified
> Specimens from any source unless otherwise specified
> EXCLUDES *Analytes from nonrequested laboratory analysis*
> *Calculated results representing score or probability derived by algorithm*
> *Drug testing ([80305, 80306, 80307], [80324, 80325, 80326, 80327, 80328, 80329, 80330, 80331, 80332, 80333, 80334, 80335, 80336, 80337, 80338, 80339, 80340, 80341, 80342, 80343, 80344, 80345, 80346, 80347, 80348, 80349, 80350, 80351, 80352, 80353, 80354, 80355, 80356, 80357, 80358, 80359, 80360, 80361, 80362, 80363, 80364, 80365, 80366, 80367, 80368, 80369, 80370, 80371, 80372, 80373, 80374, 80375, 80376, 80377, 83992])*
> *Organ or disease panels (80048-80076 [80081])*
> *Therapeutic drug assays (80150-80299 [80164, 80165, 80171])*

83915 Nucleotidase 5'-
> 🔧 0.00 ⚕ 0.00 **FUD** XXX [Q][☐]
> **AMA:** 2015,Jun,10; 2015,Apr,3

83916 Oligoclonal immune (oligoclonal bands)
> 🔧 0.00 ⚕ 0.00 **FUD** XXX [Q][☐]
> **AMA:** 2015,Jun,10; 2015,Apr,3

83918 Organic acids; total, quantitative, each specimen
> 🔧 0.00 ⚕ 0.00 **FUD** XXX [Q][☐]
> **AMA:** 2018,Jan,8; 2017,Jan,8; 2016,Jan,13; 2015,Jun,10; 2015,Apr,3; 2015,Jan,16

83919 qualitative, each specimen
> 🔧 0.00 ⚕ 0.00 **FUD** XXX [Q][☐]
> **AMA:** 2015,Jun,10; 2015,Apr,3

83921 Organic acid, single, quantitative
> 🔧 0.00 ⚕ 0.00 **FUD** XXX [Q][☐]
> **AMA:** 2015,Jun,10; 2015,Apr,3

83930 Osmolality; blood
> EXCLUDES *Tear osmolarity (83861)*
> 🔧 0.00 ⚕ 0.00 **FUD** XXX [Q][☐]
> **AMA:** 2015,Jun,10; 2015,Apr,3

83935 urine
> EXCLUDES *Tear osmolarity (83861)*
> 🔧 0.00 ⚕ 0.00 **FUD** XXX [Q][☐]
> **AMA:** 2015,Jun,10; 2015,Apr,3

83937 Osteocalcin (bone g1a protein)
> 🔧 0.00 ⚕ 0.00 **FUD** XXX [Q][☐]
> **AMA:** 2018,Jan,8; 2017,Jan,8; 2016,Jan,13; 2015,Jun,10; 2015,Apr,3; 2015,Jan,16

83945 Oxalate
> 🔧 0.00 ⚕ 0.00 **FUD** XXX [Q][☐]
> **AMA:** 2015,Jun,10; 2015,Apr,3

83950 Oncoprotein; HER-2/neu
> EXCLUDES *Tissue (88342, 88365)*
> 🔧 0.00 ⚕ 0.00 **FUD** XXX [Q][☐]
> **AMA:** 2015,Jun,10; 2015,Apr,3

83951 des-gamma-carboxy-prothrombin (DCP)
> 🔧 0.00 ⚕ 0.00 **FUD** XXX [Q][☐]
> **AMA:** 2015,Jun,10; 2015,Apr,3

83970 Parathormone (parathyroid hormone)
> EXCLUDES *Chlorinated hydrocarbon screen (82441)*
> *Quantitative pesticide report code for specific method*
> 🔧 0.00 ⚕ 0.00 **FUD** XXX [Q][☐]
> **AMA:** 2015,Jun,10; 2015,Apr,3

83986 pH; body fluid, not otherwise specified
> EXCLUDES *Blood pH (82800, 82803)*
> 🔧 0.00 ⚕ 0.00 **FUD** XXX [X][Q][☐]
> **AMA:** 2018,Jan,8; 2017,Jan,8; 2016,May,13; 2016,Jan,13; 2015,Jun,10; 2015,Apr,3; 2015,Jan,16

83987 exhaled breath condensate
> EXCLUDES *Blood pH (82800, 82803)*
> *Phenobarbital ([80345])*
> 🔧 0.00 ⚕ 0.00 **FUD** XXX [Q][☐]
> **AMA:** 2015,Jun,10; 2015,Apr,3

83992 Resequenced code. See code following resequenced code 80365.

83993 Calprotectin, fecal
> 🔧 0.00 ⚕ 0.00 **FUD** XXX [Q][☐]
> **AMA:** 2018,Jan,8; 2017,Jan,8; 2016,Jan,13; 2015,Jun,10; 2015,Apr,3; 2015,Jan,16

84030 Phenylalanine (PKU), blood
> INCLUDES Guthrie test
> EXCLUDES *Phenylalanine-tyrosine ratio (84030, 84510)*
> 🔧 0.00 ⚕ 0.00 **FUD** XXX [Q][☐]
> **AMA:** 2015,Jun,10; 2015,Apr,3

84035 Phenylketones, qualitative
> 🔧 0.00 ⚕ 0.00 **FUD** XXX [Q][☐]
> **AMA:** 2015,Jun,10; 2015,Apr,3

84060 Phosphatase, acid; total
> 🔧 0.00 ⚕ 0.00 **FUD** XXX [Q][☐]
> **AMA:** 2015,Jun,10; 2015,Apr,3

84066 prostatic
> 🔧 0.00 ⚕ 0.00 **FUD** XXX [Q][☐]
> **AMA:** 2015,Jun,10; 2015,Apr,3

84075-84080 Chemistry: Phosphatase (Alkaline)

> **CMS:** 100-03,160.17 Payment for L-Dopa /Associated Inpatient Hospital Services
> INCLUDES Clinical information not requested by ordering physician
> Mathematically calculated results
> Quantitative analysis unless otherwise specified
> Specimens from any source unless otherwise specified
> EXCLUDES *Analytes from nonrequested laboratory analysis*
> *Calculated results representing score or probability derived by algorithm*
> *Organ or disease panels (80048-80076 [80081])*

84075 Phosphatase, alkaline;
> 🔧 0.00 ⚕ 0.00 **FUD** XXX [X][Q][☐]
> **AMA:** 2018,Jan,8; 2017,Jan,8; 2016,Jan,13; 2015,Jun,10; 2015,Apr,3; 2015,Jan,16

84078 heat stable (total not included)
> 🔧 0.00 ⚕ 0.00 **FUD** XXX [Q][☐]
> **AMA:** 2015,Jun,10; 2015,Apr,3

84080 isoenzymes
> 🔧 0.00 ⚕ 0.00 **FUD** XXX [Q][☐]
> **AMA:** 2015,Jun,10; 2015,Apr,3

| 26/TC PC/TC Only | A2-Z3 ASC Payment | 50 Bilateral | ♂ Male Only | ♀ Female Only | 🔧 Facility RVU | ⚕ Non-Facility RVU | ☐ CCI | X CLIA |
| FUD Follow-up Days | CMS: IOM | AMA: CPT Asst | A-Y OPPSI | 80/80 Surg Assist Allowed / w/Doc | | Lab Crosswalk | Radiology Crosswalk | |

84081-84150 Chemistry: Phosphatidylglycerol—Prostaglandin

INCLUDES Clinical information not requested by ordering physician
Mathematically calculated results
Quantitative analysis unless otherwise specified
Specimens from any source unless otherwise specified

EXCLUDES *Analytes from nonrequested laboratory analysis*
Calculated results representing score or probability derived by algorithm
Organ or disease panels (80048-80076 [80081])
Therapeutic drug assays (80150-80299 [80164, 80165, 80171])

84081 Phosphatidylglycerol
EXCLUDES *Cholinesterase (82480, 82482)*
Inorganic phosphates (84100)
Organic phosphates, report code for specific method
0.00 0.00 FUD XXX
AMA: 2015,Jun,10; 2015,Apr,3

84085 Phosphogluconate, 6-, dehydrogenase, RBC
0.00 0.00 FUD XXX
AMA: 2015,Jun,10; 2015,Apr,3

84087 Phosphohexose isomerase
0.00 0.00 FUD XXX
AMA: 2015,Jun,10; 2015,Apr,3

84100 Phosphorus inorganic (phosphate);
0.00 0.00 FUD XXX
AMA: 2018,Jan,8; 2017,Jan,8; 2016,Jan,13; 2015,Jun,10; 2015,Apr,3; 2015,Jan,16

84105 urine
EXCLUDES *Pituitary gonadotropins (83001-83002)*
PKU (84030, 84035)
0.00 0.00 FUD XXX
AMA: 2015,Jun,10; 2015,Apr,3

84106 Porphobilinogen, urine; qualitative
0.00 0.00 FUD XXX
AMA: 2015,Jun,10; 2015,Apr,3

84110 quantitative
0.00 0.00 FUD XXX
AMA: 2015,Jun,10; 2015,Apr,3

84112 Evaluation of cervicovaginal fluid for specific amniotic fluid protein(s) (eg, placental alpha microglobulin-1 [PAMG-1], placental protein 12 [PP12], alpha-fetoprotein), qualitative, each specimen ♀
0.00 0.00 FUD XXX
AMA: 2015,Jun,10; 2015,Apr,3

84119 Porphyrins, urine; qualitative
0.00 0.00 FUD XXX
AMA: 2015,Jun,10; 2015,Apr,3

84120 quantitation and fractionation
0.00 0.00 FUD XXX
AMA: 2015,Jun,10; 2015,Apr,3

84126 Porphyrins, feces, quantitative
EXCLUDES *Porphyrin precursors (82135, 84106, 84110)*
Protoporphyrin, RBC (84202, 84203)
0.00 0.00 FUD XXX
AMA: 2015,Jun,10; 2015,Apr,3

84132 Potassium; serum, plasma or whole blood
0.00 0.00 FUD XXX
AMA: 2018,Jan,8; 2017,Jan,8; 2016,Jan,13; 2015,Jun,10; 2015,Apr,3; 2015,Jan,16

84133 urine
0.00 0.00 FUD XXX
AMA: 2015,Jun,10; 2015,Apr,3

84134 Prealbumin
EXCLUDES *Microalbumin (82043-82044)*
0.00 0.00 FUD XXX
AMA: 2015,Jun,10; 2015,Apr,3

84135 Pregnanediol ♀
0.00 0.00 FUD XXX
AMA: 2015,Jun,10; 2015,Apr,3

84138 Pregnanetriol ♀
0.00 0.00 FUD XXX
AMA: 2015,Jun,10; 2015,Apr,3

84140 Pregnenolone
0.00 0.00 FUD XXX
AMA: 2018,Jan,8; 2017,Jan,8; 2016,Jan,13; 2015,Jun,10; 2015,Apr,3; 2015,Jan,16

84143 17-hydroxypregnenolone
0.00 0.00 FUD XXX
AMA: 2018,Jan,8; 2017,Jan,8; 2016,Jan,13; 2015,Jun,10; 2015,Apr,3; 2015,Jan,16

84144 Progesterone
EXCLUDES *Progesterone receptor assay (84234)*
Proinsulin (84206)
0.00 0.00 FUD XXX
AMA: 2015,Jun,10; 2015,Apr,3

84145 Procalcitonin (PCT)
0.00 0.00 FUD XXX
AMA: 2015,Jun,10; 2015,Apr,3

84146 Prolactin
0.00 0.00 FUD XXX
AMA: 2015,Jun,10; 2015,Apr,3

84150 Prostaglandin, each
0.00 0.00 FUD XXX
AMA: 2015,Jun,10; 2015,Apr,3

84152-84154 Chemistry: Prostate Specific Antigen

CMS: 100-03,190.31 Prostate Specific Antigen (PSA); 100-03,210.1 Prostate Cancer Screening Tests

INCLUDES Clinical information not requested by ordering physician
Mathematically calculated results
Quantitative analysis unless otherwise specified

EXCLUDES *Analytes from nonrequested laboratory analysis*
Calculated results representing score or probability derived by algorithm

84152 Prostate specific antigen (PSA); complexed (direct measurement) ♂
0.00 0.00 FUD XXX
AMA: 2015,Jun,10; 2015,Apr,3

84153 total ♂
0.00 0.00 FUD XXX
AMA: 2018,Jan,8; 2017,Jan,8; 2016,Jan,13; 2015,Jun,10; 2015,Apr,3; 2015,Jan,16

84154 free ♂
0.00 0.00 FUD XXX
AMA: 2018,Jan,8; 2017,Jan,8; 2016,Jan,13; 2015,Jun,10; 2015,Apr,3; 2015,Jan,16

84155-84157 Chemistry: Protein, Total (Not by Refractometry)

INCLUDES Clinical information not requested by ordering physician
Mathematically calculated results

EXCLUDES *Analytes from nonrequested laboratory analysis*
Calculated results representing score or probability derived by algorithm
Organ or disease panels (80048-80076 [80081])

84155 Protein, total, except by refractometry; serum, plasma or whole blood
0.00 0.00 FUD XXX
AMA: 2018,Jan,8; 2017,Jan,8; 2016,Jan,13; 2015,Jun,10; 2015,Apr,3; 2015,Jan,16

84156 urine
0.00 0.00 FUD XXX
AMA: 2015,Jun,10; 2015,Apr,3

84157 other source (eg, synovial fluid, cerebrospinal fluid)
0.00 0.00 FUD XXX
AMA: 2015,Jun,10; 2015,Apr,3

84160-84432 Chemistry: Protein, Total (Refractometry)—Thyroglobulin

INCLUDES Clinical information not requested by ordering physician
Mathematically calculated results
Quantitative analysis unless otherwise specified
Specimens from any source unless otherwise specified

EXCLUDES *Analytes from nonrequested laboratory analysis*
Calculated results representing score or probability derived by algorithm
Drug testing ([80305, 80306, 80307], [80324, 80325, 80326, 80327, 80328, 80329, 80330, 80331, 80332, 80333, 80334, 80335, 80336, 80337, 80338, 80339, 80340, 80341, 80342, 80343, 80344, 80345, 80346, 80347, 80348, 80349, 80350, 80351, 80352, 80353, 80354, 80355, 80356, 80357, 80358, 80359, 80360, 80361, 80362, 80363, 80364, 80365, 80366, 80367, 80368, 80369, 80370, 80371, 80372, 80373, 80374, 80375, 80376, 80377, 83992])
Organ or disease panels (80048-80076 [80081])
Therapeutic drug assays (80150-80299 [80164, 80165, 80171])

84160 **Protein, total, by refractometry, any source**
EXCLUDES *Urine total protein, dipstick method (81000-81003)*
0.00 0.00 **FUD** XXX
AMA: 2015,Jun,10; 2015,Apr,3

84163 **Pregnancy-associated plasma protein-A (PAPP-A)** ♀
0.00 0.00 **FUD** XXX
AMA: 2015,Jun,10; 2015,Apr,3

84165 **Protein; electrophoretic fractionation and quantitation, serum**
0.00 0.00 **FUD** XXX
AMA: 2015,Jun,10; 2015,Apr,3

84166 **electrophoretic fractionation and quantitation, other fluids with concentration (eg, urine, CSF)**
0.00 0.00 **FUD** XXX
AMA: 2015,Jun,10; 2015,Apr,3

84181 **Western Blot, with interpretation and report, blood or other body fluid**
0.00 0.00 **FUD** XXX
AMA: 2015,Jun,10; 2015,Apr,3

84182 **Western Blot, with interpretation and report, blood or other body fluid, immunological probe for band identification, each**
EXCLUDES *Western Blot tissue analysis (88371)*
0.00 0.00 **FUD** XXX
AMA: 2015,Jun,10; 2015,Apr,3

84202 **Protoporphyrin, RBC; quantitative**
0.00 0.00 **FUD** XXX
AMA: 2015,Jun,10; 2015,Apr,3

84203 **screen**
0.00 0.00 **FUD** XXX
AMA: 2015,Jun,10; 2015,Apr,3

84206 **Proinsulin**
EXCLUDES *Pseudocholinesterase (82480)*
0.00 0.00 **FUD** XXX
AMA: 2015,Jun,10; 2015,Apr,3

84207 **Pyridoxal phosphate (Vitamin B-6)**
0.00 0.00 **FUD** XXX
AMA: 2015,Jun,10; 2015,Apr,3

84210 **Pyruvate**
0.00 0.00 **FUD** XXX
AMA: 2015,Jun,10; 2015,Apr,3

84220 **Pyruvate kinase**
0.00 0.00 **FUD** XXX
AMA: 2015,Jun,10; 2015,Apr,3

84228 **Quinine**
0.00 0.00 **FUD** XXX
AMA: 2018,Jan,8; 2017,Jan,8; 2016,Jan,13; 2015,Jun,10; 2015,Apr,3

84233 **Receptor assay; estrogen**
0.00 0.00 **FUD** XXX
AMA: 2015,Jun,10; 2015,Apr,3

84234 **progesterone**
0.00 0.00 **FUD** XXX
AMA: 2015,Jun,10; 2015,Apr,3

84235 **endocrine, other than estrogen or progesterone (specify hormone)**
0.00 0.00 **FUD** XXX
AMA: 2015,Jun,10; 2015,Apr,3

84238 **non-endocrine (specify receptor)**
0.00 0.00 **FUD** XXX
AMA: 2018,Jan,8; 2017,Jan,8; 2016,Jan,13; 2015,Jun,10; 2015,Apr,3; 2015,Jan,16

84244 **Renin**
0.00 0.00 **FUD** XXX
AMA: 2015,Jun,10; 2015,Apr,3

84252 **Riboflavin (Vitamin B-2)**
EXCLUDES *Salicylates ([80329], [80330], [80331])*
Salicylate therapeutic drug assay ([80179])
Secretin test reported with appropriate analyses (43756, 43757, 99070)
0.00 0.00 **FUD** XXX
AMA: 2015,Jun,10; 2015,Apr,3

84255 **Selenium**
0.00 0.00 **FUD** XXX
AMA: 2015,Jun,10; 2015,Apr,3

84260 **Serotonin**
EXCLUDES *Urine metabolites (HIAA) (83497)*
0.00 0.00 **FUD** XXX
AMA: 2015,Jun,10; 2015,Apr,3

84270 **Sex hormone binding globulin (SHBG)**
0.00 0.00 **FUD** XXX
AMA: 2018,Jan,8; 2017,Jan,8; 2016,Jan,13; 2015,Jun,10; 2015,Apr,3; 2015,Jan,16

84275 **Sialic acid**
EXCLUDES *Sickle hemoglobin (85660)*
0.00 0.00 **FUD** XXX
AMA: 2015,Jun,10; 2015,Apr,3

84285 **Silica**
0.00 0.00 **FUD** XXX
AMA: 2015,Jun,10; 2015,Apr,3

84295 **Sodium; serum, plasma or whole blood**
0.00 0.00 **FUD** XXX
AMA: 2018,Jan,8; 2017,Jan,8; 2016,Jan,13; 2015,Jun,10; 2015,Apr,3; 2015,Jan,16

84300 **urine**
0.00 0.00 **FUD** XXX
AMA: 2015,Jun,10; 2015,Apr,3

84302 **other source**
EXCLUDES *Somatomammotropin (83632)*
Somatotropin (83003)
0.00 0.00 **FUD** XXX
AMA: 2018,Jan,8; 2017,Jan,8; 2016,Jan,13; 2015,Jun,10; 2015,Apr,3; 2015,Jan,16

84305 **Somatomedin**
0.00 0.00 **FUD** XXX
AMA: 2018,Jan,8; 2017,Jan,8; 2016,Jan,13; 2015,Jun,10; 2015,Apr,3; 2015,Jan,16

84307 **Somatostatin**
0.00 0.00 **FUD** XXX
AMA: 2018,Jan,8; 2017,Jan,8; 2016,Jan,13; 2015,Jun,10; 2015,Apr,3; 2015,Jan,16

84311 **Spectrophotometry, analyte not elsewhere specified**
0.00 0.00 **FUD** XXX
AMA: 2015,Jun,10; 2015,Apr,3

84315 **Specific gravity (except urine)**
EXCLUDES *Stone analysis (82355-82370)*
Suppression of growth stimulation expressed gene 2 [ST2] testing (83006)
Urine specific gravity (81000-81003)
0.00 0.00 FUD XXX
AMA: 2015,Jun,10; 2015,Apr,3

84375 **Sugars, chromatographic, TLC or paper chromatography**
0.00 0.00 FUD XXX
AMA: 2015,Jun,10; 2015,Apr,3

84376 **Sugars (mono-, di-, and oligosaccharides); single qualitative, each specimen**
0.00 0.00 FUD XXX
AMA: 2018,Jan,8; 2017,Jan,8; 2016,Jan,13; 2015,Jun,10; 2015,Apr,3; 2015,Jan,16

84377 **multiple qualitative, each specimen**
0.00 0.00 FUD XXX
AMA: 2018,Jan,8; 2017,Jan,8; 2016,Jan,13; 2015,Jun,10; 2015,Apr,3; 2015,Jan,16

84378 **single quantitative, each specimen**
0.00 0.00 FUD XXX
AMA: 2015,Jun,10; 2015,Apr,3

84379 **multiple quantitative, each specimen**
0.00 0.00 FUD XXX
AMA: 2018,Jan,8; 2017,Jan,8; 2016,Jan,13; 2015,Jun,10; 2015,Apr,3; 2015,Jan,16

84392 **Sulfate, urine**
EXCLUDES *Sulfhemoglobin (83060)*
T-3 (84479-84481)
T-4 (84436-84439)
0.00 0.00 FUD XXX
AMA: 2015,Jun,10; 2015,Apr,3

84402 **Testosterone; free**
EXCLUDES *Anabolic steroids ([80327, 80328])*
0.00 0.00 FUD XXX
AMA: 2015,Jun,10; 2015,Apr,3

84403 **total**
EXCLUDES *Anabolic steroids ([80327, 80328])*
0.00 0.00 FUD XXX
AMA: 2015,Jun,10; 2015,Apr,3

84410 **bioavailable, direct measurement (eg, differential precipitation)**
0.00 0.00 FUD XXX

84425 **Thiamine (Vitamin B-1)**
0.00 0.00 FUD XXX
AMA: 2015,Jun,10; 2015,Apr,3

84430 **Thiocyanate**
0.00 0.00 FUD XXX
AMA: 2015,Jun,10; 2015,Apr,3

84431 **Thromboxane metabolite(s), including thromboxane if performed, urine**
Code also determination concurrent urine creatinine (82570)
0.00 0.00 FUD XXX
AMA: 2015,Jun,10; 2015,Apr,3

84432 **Thyroglobulin**
EXCLUDES *Thyroglobulin antibody (86800)*
Thyrotropin releasing hormone (TRH) (80438, 80439)
0.00 0.00 FUD XXX
AMA: 2018,Jan,8; 2017,Jan,8; 2016,Jan,13; 2015,Jun,10; 2015,Apr,3; 2015,Jan,16

84436-84445 Chemistry: Thyroid Tests

CMS: 100-03,190.22 Thyroid Testing

INCLUDES Clinical information not requested by the ordering physician
Mathematically calculated results
Quantitative analysis unless otherwise specified
Specimens from any source unless otherwise specified

EXCLUDES *Analytes from nonrequested laboratory analysis*
Calculated results representing a score or probability derived by algorithm
Organ or disease panels (80048-80076 [80081])
Therapeutic drug assays (80150-80299 [80164, 80165, 80171])

84436 **Thyroxine; total**
0.00 0.00 FUD XXX
AMA: 2018,Jan,8; 2017,Jan,8; 2016,Jan,13; 2015,Jun,10; 2015,Apr,3; 2015,Jan,16

84437 **requiring elution (eg, neonatal)**
0.00 0.00 FUD XXX
AMA: 2015,Jun,10; 2015,Apr,3

84439 **free**
0.00 0.00 FUD XXX
AMA: 2015,Jun,10; 2015,Apr,3

84442 **Thyroxine binding globulin (TBG)**
0.00 0.00 FUD XXX
AMA: 2015,Jun,10; 2015,Apr,3

84443 **Thyroid stimulating hormone (TSH)**
0.00 0.00 FUD XXX
AMA: 2015,Jun,10; 2015,Apr,3

84445 **Thyroid stimulating immune globulins (TSI)**
EXCLUDES *Tobramycin (80200)*
0.00 0.00 FUD XXX
AMA: 2018,Jan,8; 2017,Jan,8; 2016,Jan,13; 2015,Jun,10; 2015,Apr,3; 2015,Jan,16

84446-84449 Chemistry: Tocopherol Alpha—Transcortin

INCLUDES Clinical information not requested by ordering physician
Mathematically calculated results
Quantitative analysis unless otherwise specified
Specimens from any source unless otherwise specified

EXCLUDES *Analytes from nonrequested laboratory analysis*
Calculated results representing score or probability derived by algorithm
Organ or disease panels (80048-80076 [80081])
Therapeutic drug assays (80150-80299 [80164, 80165, 80171])

84446 **Tocopherol alpha (Vitamin E)**
0.00 0.00 FUD XXX
AMA: 2015,Jun,10; 2015,Apr,3

84449 **Transcortin (cortisol binding globulin)**
0.00 0.00 FUD XXX
AMA: 2018,Jan,8; 2017,Jan,8; 2016,Jan,13; 2015,Jun,10; 2015,Apr,3; 2015,Jan,16

84450-84460 Chemistry: Transferase

CMS: 100-02,11,30.2.2 Automated Multi-Channel Chemistry (AMCC) Tests; 100-03,160.17 Payment for L-Dopa /Associated Inpatient Hospital Services; 100-04,16,40.6.1 Automated Multi-Channel Chemistry (AMCC) Tests for ESRD Beneficiaries; 100-04,16,70.8 CLIA Waived Tests

INCLUDES Clinical information not requested by ordering physician
Mathematically calculated results
Quantitative analysis unless otherwise specified

EXCLUDES *Analytes from nonrequested laboratory analysis*
Calculated results representing score or probability derived by algorithm

84450 **Transferase; aspartate amino (AST) (SGOT)**
0.00 0.00 FUD XXX
AMA: 2018,Jan,8; 2017,Jan,8; 2016,Jan,13; 2015,Jun,10; 2015,Apr,3; 2015,Jan,16

84460 **alanine amino (ALT) (SGPT)**
0.00 0.00 FUD XXX
AMA: 2018,Jan,8; 2017,Jan,8; 2016,Jan,13; 2015,Jun,10; 2015,Apr,3; 2015,Jan,16

84466 Chemistry: Transferrin

CMS: 100-02,11,20.2 ESRD Laboratory Services; 100-03,190.18 Serum Iron Studies

INCLUDES Clinical information not requested by ordering physician
Mathematically calculated results
Quantitative analysis unless otherwise specified

EXCLUDES *Analytes from nonrequested laboratory analysis*
Calculated results representing score or probability derived by algorithm

84466   Transferrin

EXCLUDES *Iron binding capacity (83550)*

🖩 0.00   ⚕ 0.00   **FUD** XXX   ▣ ▢

AMA: 2018,Jan,8; 2017,Jan,8; 2016,Jan,13; 2015,Jun,10;
2015,Apr,3; 2015,Jan,16

84478 Chemistry: Triglycerides

CMS: 100-02,11,30.2.2 Automated Multi-Channel Chemistry (AMCC) Tests; 100-03,190.23 Lipid Testing;
100-04,16,70.8 CLIA Waived Tests; 100-04,16,90.2 Organ or Disease Oriented Panels

INCLUDES Clinical information not requested by ordering physician
Mathematically calculated results

EXCLUDES *Analytes from nonrequested laboratory analysis*
Calculated results representing score or probability derived by algorithm
Organ or disease panels (80048-80076 [80081])

84478   Triglycerides

🖩 0.00   ⚕ 0.00   **FUD** XXX   ☒ Ⓐ ▢

AMA: 2018,Jan,8; 2017,Jan,8; 2016,Jan,13; 2015,Jun,10;
2015,Apr,3; 2015,Jan,16

84479-84482 Chemistry: Thyroid Hormone—Triiodothyronine

CMS: 100-03,190.22 Thyroid Testing

INCLUDES Clinical information not requested by ordering physician
Mathematically calculated results
Quantitative analysis unless otherwise specified
Specimens from any source unless otherwise specified

EXCLUDES *Analytes from nonrequested laboratory analysis*
Calculated results representing score or probability derived by algorithm
Organ or disease panels (80048-80076 [80081])

84479   Thyroid hormone (T3 or T4) uptake or thyroid hormone binding ratio (THBR)

🖩 0.00   ⚕ 0.00   **FUD** XXX   ▣ ▢

AMA: 2018,Jan,8; 2017,Jan,8; 2016,Jan,13; 2015,Jun,10;
2015,Apr,3; 2015,Jan,16

84480   Triiodothyronine T3; total (TT-3)

🖩 0.00   ⚕ 0.00   **FUD** XXX   ▣ ▢

AMA: 2015,Jun,10; 2015,Apr,3

84481   free

🖩 0.00   ⚕ 0.00   **FUD** XXX   ▣ ▢

AMA: 2015,Jun,10; 2015,Apr,3

84482   reverse

🖩 0.00   ⚕ 0.00   **FUD** XXX   ▣ ▢

AMA: 2018,Jan,8; 2017,Jan,8; 2016,Jan,13; 2015,Jun,10;
2015,Apr,3; 2015,Jan,16

84484-84512 Chemistry: Troponin (Quantitative)—Troponin (Qualitative)

INCLUDES Clinical information not requested by ordering physician
Mathematically calculated results
Specimens from any source unless otherwise specified

EXCLUDES *Analytes from nonrequested laboratory analysis*
Calculated results representing score or probability derived by algorithm
Organ or disease panels

84484   Troponin, quantitative

EXCLUDES *Qualitative troponin assay (84512)*

🖩 0.00   ⚕ 0.00   **FUD** XXX   ▣ ▢

AMA: 2018,Jan,8; 2017,Jan,8; 2016,Jan,13; 2015,Jun,10;
2015,Apr,3; 2015,Jan,16

84485   Trypsin; duodenal fluid

🖩 0.00   ⚕ 0.00   **FUD** XXX   ▣ ▢

AMA: 2015,Jun,10; 2015,Apr,3

84488   feces, qualitative

🖩 0.00   ⚕ 0.00   **FUD** XXX   ▣ ▢

AMA: 2015,Jun,10; 2015,Apr,3

84490   feces, quantitative, 24-hour collection

🖩 0.00   ⚕ 0.00   **FUD** XXX   ▣ ▢

AMA: 2015,Jun,10; 2015,Apr,3

84510   Tyrosine

EXCLUDES *Urate crystal identification (89060)*

🖩 0.00   ⚕ 0.00   **FUD** XXX   ▣ ▢

AMA: 2015,Jun,10; 2015,Apr,3

84512   Troponin, qualitative

EXCLUDES *Quantitative troponin assay (84484)*

🖩 0.00   ⚕ 0.00   **FUD** XXX   ▣ ▢

AMA: 2018,Jan,8; 2017,Jan,8; 2016,Jan,13; 2015,Jun,10;
2015,Apr,3; 2015,Jan,16

84520-84525 Chemistry: Urea Nitrogen (Blood)

CMS: 100-03,160.17 Payment for L-Dopa /Associated Inpatient Hospital Services

INCLUDES Clinical information not requested by ordering physician
Mathematically calculated results

EXCLUDES *Analytes from nonrequested laboratory analysis*
Calculated results representing score or probability derived by algorithm
Organ or disease panels (80048-80076 [80081])

84520   Urea nitrogen; quantitative

🖩 0.00   ⚕ 0.00   **FUD** XXX   ☒ ▣ ▢

AMA: 2018,Jan,8; 2017,Jan,8; 2016,Jan,13; 2015,Jun,10;
2015,Apr,3; 2015,Jan,16

84525   semiquantitative (eg, reagent strip test)

INCLUDES Patterson's test

🖩 0.00   ⚕ 0.00   **FUD** XXX   ▣ ▢

AMA: 2018,Jan,8; 2017,Jan,8; 2016,Jan,13; 2015,Jun,10;
2015,Apr,3; 2015,Jan,16

84540-84630 Chemistry: Urea Nitrogen (Urine)—Zinc

INCLUDES Clinical information not requested by ordering physician
Mathematically calculated results
Quantitative analysis unless otherwise specified
Specimens from any source unless otherwise specified

EXCLUDES *Analytes from nonrequested laboratory analysis*
Calculated results representing score or probability derived by algorithm
Organ or disease panels (80048-80076 [80081])
Therapeutic drug assays (80150-80299 [80164, 80165, 80171])

84540   Urea nitrogen, urine

🖩 0.00   ⚕ 0.00   **FUD** XXX   ▣ ▢

AMA: 2015,Jun,10; 2015,Apr,3

84545   Urea nitrogen, clearance

🖩 0.00   ⚕ 0.00   **FUD** XXX   ▣ ▢

AMA: 2015,Jun,10; 2015,Apr,3

84550   Uric acid; blood

🖩 0.00   ⚕ 0.00   **FUD** XXX   ☒ ▣ ▢

AMA: 2018,Jan,8; 2017,Jan,8; 2016,Jan,13; 2015,Jun,10;
2015,Apr,3; 2015,Jan,16

84560   other source

🖩 0.00   ⚕ 0.00   **FUD** XXX   ▣ ▢

AMA: 2015,Jun,10; 2015,Apr,3

84577   Urobilinogen, feces, quantitative

🖩 0.00   ⚕ 0.00   **FUD** XXX   ▣ ▢

AMA: 2015,Jun,10; 2015,Apr,3

84578   Urobilinogen, urine; qualitative

🖩 0.00   ⚕ 0.00   **FUD** XXX   ▣ ▢

AMA: 2015,Jun,10; 2015,Apr,3

84580   quantitative, timed specimen

🖩 0.00   ⚕ 0.00   **FUD** XXX   ▣ ▢

AMA: 2015,Jun,10; 2015,Apr,3

84583   semiquantitative

EXCLUDES *Uroporphyrins (84120)*
Valproic acid (dipropylacetic acid) ([80164])

🖩 0.00   ⚕ 0.00   **FUD** XXX   ▣ ▢

AMA: 2015,Jun,10; 2015,Apr,3

84585   Vanillylmandelic acid (VMA), urine

🖩 0.00   ⚕ 0.00   **FUD** XXX   ▣ ▢

AMA: 2015,Jun,10; 2015,Apr,3

26/TC PC/TC Only   A2-Z3 ASC Payment   50 Bilateral   ♂ Male Only   ♀ Female Only   🖩 Facility RVU   ⚕ Non-Facility RVU   ▢ CCI   ☒ CLIA
FUD Follow-up Days   **CMS:** IOM   **AMA:** CPT Asst   Ⓐ-Ⓨ OPPSI   80/80 Surg Assist Allowed / w/Doc   ▣ Lab Crosswalk   ▣ Radiology Crosswalk

84586   Vasoactive intestinal peptide (VIP)
🔲 0.00   ⚕ 0.00   **FUD** XXX   Ⓠ▯
AMA: 2018,Jan,8; 2017,Jan,8; 2016,Jan,13; 2015,Jun,10; 2015,Apr,3; 2015,Jan,16

84588   Vasopressin (antidiuretic hormone, ADH)
🔲 0.00   ⚕ 0.00   **FUD** XXX   Ⓠ▯
AMA: 2018,Jan,7; 2015,Jun,10; 2015,Apr,3

84590   Vitamin A
EXCLUDES   *Vitamin B-1 (84425)*
            Vitamin B-2 (84252)
            Vitamin B-6 (84207)
            Vitamin B-12 (82607)
            Vitamin C (82180)
            Vitamin D (82306, [82652])
            Vitamin E (84446)
🔲 0.00   ⚕ 0.00   **FUD** XXX   Ⓠ▯
AMA: 2015,Jun,10; 2015,Apr,3

84591   Vitamin, not otherwise specified
🔲 0.00   ⚕ 0.00   **FUD** XXX   Ⓠ▯
AMA: 2015,Jun,10; 2015,Apr,3

84597   Vitamin K
EXCLUDES   *Vanillylmandelic acid (VMA) (84585)*
🔲 0.00   ⚕ 0.00   **FUD** XXX   Ⓠ▯
AMA: 2015,Jun,10; 2015,Apr,3

84600   Volatiles (eg, acetic anhydride, diethylether)
EXCLUDES   *Carbon tetrachloride, dichloroethane, dichloromethane (82441)*
            Isopropyl alcohol and methanol ([80320])
            Volume, blood, RISA, or Cr-51 (78110, 78111)
🔲 0.00   ⚕ 0.00   **FUD** XXX   Ⓠ▯
AMA: 2015,Jun,10; 2015,Apr,3

84620   Xylose absorption test, blood and/or urine
EXCLUDES   *Administration (99070)*
🔲 0.00   ⚕ 0.00   **FUD** XXX   Ⓠ▯
AMA: 2015,Jun,10; 2015,Apr,3

84630   Zinc
🔲 0.00   ⚕ 0.00   **FUD** XXX   Ⓠ▯
AMA: 2015,Jun,10; 2015,Apr,3

84681-84999 Other and Unlisted Chemistry Tests

INCLUDES   Clinical information not requested by ordering physician
            Mathematically calculated results
            Quantitative analysis unless otherwise specified
            Specimens from any source unless otherwise specified
EXCLUDES   *Analytes from nonrequested laboratory analysis*
            Calculated results representing score or probability derived by algorithm
            Confirmational testing, not otherwise specified drug ([80375, 80376, 80377], 80299)
            Organ or disease panels (80048-80076 [80081])

84681   C-peptide
🔲 0.00   ⚕ 0.00   **FUD** XXX   Ⓠ▯
AMA: 2015,Jun,10; 2015,Apr,3

84702   Gonadotropin, chorionic (hCG); quantitative
🔲 0.00   ⚕ 0.00   **FUD** XXX   Ⓠ▯
AMA: 2015,Jun,10; 2015,Apr,3

84703   qualitative
EXCLUDES   *Urine pregnancy test by visual color comparison (81025)*
🔲 0.00   ⚕ 0.00   **FUD** XXX   ☒Ⓠ▯
AMA: 2015,Jun,10; 2015,Apr,3

84704   free beta chain
🔲 0.00   ⚕ 0.00   **FUD** XXX   Ⓠ▯
AMA: 2018,Jan,8; 2017,Jan,8; 2016,Jan,13; 2015,Jun,10; 2015,Apr,3; 2015,Jan,16

84830   Ovulation tests, by visual color comparison methods for human luteinizing hormone   ♀
🔲 0.00   ⚕ 0.00   **FUD** XXX   ☒Ⓠ▯
AMA: 2018,Jan,8; 2017,Jan,8; 2016,Jan,13; 2015,Jun,10; 2015,Apr,3

84999   Unlisted chemistry procedure
EXCLUDES   *Definitive drug testing, not otherwise specified ([80375], [80376], [80377], 80299)*
🔲 0.00   ⚕ 0.00   **FUD** XXX   Ⓠ▯
AMA: 2018,Jan,8; 2017,Jan,8; 2016,Jan,13; 2015,Apr,3; 2015,Jan,16

85002 Bleeding Time Test

EXCLUDES   *Agglutinins (86000, 86156, 86157)*
            Antiplasmin (85410)
            Antithrombin III (85300, 85301)
            Blood banking procedures (86077-86079)

85002   Bleeding time
🔲 0.00   ⚕ 0.00   **FUD** XXX   Ⓠ▯
AMA: 2018,Jan,8; 2017,Jan,8; 2016,Jan,13; 2015,Jan,16

85004-85049 Blood Counts

CMS: 100-03,190.15 Blood Counts
EXCLUDES   *Agglutinins (86000, 86156-86157)*
            Antiplasmin (85410)
            Antithrombin III (85300-85301)
            Blood banking procedures (86850-86999)

85004   Blood count; automated differential WBC count
🔲 0.00   ⚕ 0.00   **FUD** XXX   Ⓠ▯
AMA: 2018,Jan,8; 2017,Jan,8; 2016,Jan,13; 2015,Jan,16

85007   blood smear, microscopic examination with manual differential WBC count
🔲 0.00   ⚕ 0.00   **FUD** XXX   Ⓠ▯
AMA: 2018,Jan,8; 2017,Jan,8; 2016,Jan,13; 2015,Jan,16

85008   blood smear, microscopic examination without manual differential WBC count
EXCLUDES   *Cell count other fluids (eg, CSF) (89050-89051)*
🔲 0.00   ⚕ 0.00   **FUD** XXX   Ⓠ▯
AMA: 2018,Jan,8; 2017,Jan,8; 2016,Jan,13; 2015,Jan,16

85009   manual differential WBC count, buffy coat
EXCLUDES   *Eosinophils, nasal smear (89190)*
🔲 0.00   ⚕ 0.00   **FUD** XXX   Ⓠ▯
AMA: 2018,Jan,8; 2017,Jan,8; 2016,Jan,13; 2015,Jan,16

85013   spun microhematocrit
🔲 0.00   ⚕ 0.00   **FUD** XXX   ☒Ⓠ▯
AMA: 2005,Aug,7-8; 2005,Jul,11-12

85014   hematocrit (Hct)
🔲 0.00   ⚕ 0.00   **FUD** XXX   ☒Ⓠ▯
AMA: 2018,Jan,8; 2017,Jan,8; 2016,Jan,13; 2015,Jan,16

85018   hemoglobin (Hgb)
EXCLUDES   *Immunoassay, hemoglobin, fecal (82274)*
            Other hemoglobin determination (83020-83069)
            Transcutaneous hemoglobin measurement (88738)
🔲 0.00   ⚕ 0.00   **FUD** XXX   ☒Ⓠ▯
AMA: 2018,Jan,8; 2017,Jan,8; 2016,Jan,13; 2015,Jan,16

85025   complete (CBC), automated (Hgb, Hct, RBC, WBC and platelet count) and automated differential WBC count
🔲 0.00   ⚕ 0.00   **FUD** XXX   ☒Ⓠ▯
AMA: 2018,Jan,8; 2017,Jan,8; 2016,Jan,13; 2015,Jan,16

85027   complete (CBC), automated (Hgb, Hct, RBC, WBC and platelet count)
🔲 0.00   ⚕ 0.00   **FUD** XXX   Ⓠ▯
AMA: 2018,Jan,8; 2017,Jan,8; 2016,Jan,13; 2015,Jan,16

85032   manual cell count (erythrocyte, leukocyte, or platelet) each
🔲 0.00   ⚕ 0.00   **FUD** XXX   Ⓠ▯
AMA: 2018,Jan,8; 2017,Jan,8; 2016,Jan,13; 2015,Jan,16

85041   red blood cell (RBC), automated
EXCLUDES   *Complete blood count (85025, 85027)*
🔲 0.00   ⚕ 0.00   **FUD** XXX   Ⓠ▯
AMA: 2018,Jan,8; 2017,Jan,8; 2016,Jan,13; 2015,Jan,16

85044   reticulocyte, manual
🔲 0.00   ⚕ 0.00   **FUD** XXX   Ⓠ▯
AMA: 2018,Jan,8; 2017,Jan,8; 2016,Jan,13; 2015,Jan,16

85045 **reticulocyte, automated**
0.00 0.00 FUD XXX
AMA: 2018,Jan,8; 2017,Jan,8; 2016,Jan,13; 2015,Jan,16

85046 **reticulocytes, automated, including 1 or more cellular parameters (eg, reticulocyte hemoglobin content [CHr], immature reticulocyte fraction [IRF], reticulocyte volume [MRV], RNA content), direct measurement**
0.00 0.00 FUD XXX
AMA: 2005,Aug,7-8; 2005,Jul,11-12

85048 **leukocyte (WBC), automated**
0.00 0.00 FUD XXX
AMA: 2018,Jan,8; 2017,Jan,8; 2016,Jan,13; 2015,Jan,16

85049 **platelet, automated**
0.00 0.00 FUD XXX
AMA: 2005,Aug,7-8; 2005,Jul,11-12

85055-85705 Coagulopathy Testing

EXCLUDES *Agglutinins (86000, 86156-86157)*
Antiplasmin (85410)
Antithrombin III (85300-85301)
Blood banking procedures (86850-86999)

85055 **Reticulated platelet assay**
0.00 0.00 FUD XXX
AMA: 2005,Aug,7-8; 2005,Jul,11-12

85060 **Blood smear, peripheral, interpretation by physician with written report**
0.70 0.70 FUD XXX B 80
AMA: 2005,Aug,7-8; 2005,Jul,11-12

85097 **Bone marrow, smear interpretation**
EXCLUDES *Bone biopsy (20220, 20225, 20240, 20245, 20250-20251)*
Special stains (88312-88313)
1.42 2.11 FUD XXX 02 80
AMA: 2018,Jan,8; 2017,Jan,8; 2016,Jan,13; 2015,Jan,16

85130 **Chromogenic substrate assay**
EXCLUDES *Circulating anticoagulant screen (mixing studies) (85611, 85732)*
0.00 0.00 FUD XXX
AMA: 2005,Aug,7-8; 2005,Jul,11-12

85170 **Clot retraction**
0.00 0.00 FUD XXX
AMA: 2005,Aug,7-8; 2005,Jul,11-12

85175 **Clot lysis time, whole blood dilution**
EXCLUDES *Clotting factor I (fibrinogen) (85384, 85385)*
0.00 0.00 FUD XXX
AMA: 2005,Aug,7-8; 2005,Jul,11-12

85210 **Clotting; factor II, prothrombin, specific**
EXCLUDES *Prothrombin time (85610-85611)*
Russell viper venom time (85612-85613)
0.00 0.00 FUD XXX
AMA: 2005,Aug,7-8; 2005,Jul,11-12

85220 **factor V (AcG or proaccelerin), labile factor**
0.00 0.00 FUD XXX
AMA: 2005,Aug,7-8; 2005,Jul,11-12

85230 **factor VII (proconvertin, stable factor)**
0.00 0.00 FUD XXX
AMA: 2005,Aug,7-8; 2005,Jul,11-12

85240 **factor VIII (AHG), 1-stage**
0.00 0.00 FUD XXX
AMA: 2005,Aug,7-8; 2005,Jul,11-12

85244 **factor VIII related antigen**
0.00 0.00 FUD XXX
AMA: 2005,Aug,7-8; 2005,Jul,11-12

85245 **factor VIII, VW factor, ristocetin cofactor**
0.00 0.00 FUD XXX
AMA: 2005,Aug,7-8; 2005,Jul,11-12

85246 **factor VIII, VW factor antigen**
0.00 0.00 FUD XXX
AMA: 2005,Aug,7-8; 2005,Jul,11-12

85247 **factor VIII, von Willebrand factor, multimetric analysis**
0.00 0.00 FUD XXX
AMA: 2005,Aug,7-8; 2005,Jul,11-12

85250 **factor IX (PTC or Christmas)**
0.00 0.00 FUD XXX
AMA: 2005,Aug,7-8; 2005,Jul,11-12

85260 **factor X (Stuart-Prower)**
0.00 0.00 FUD XXX
AMA: 2005,Aug,7-8; 2005,Jul,11-12

85270 **factor XI (PTA)**
0.00 0.00 FUD XXX
AMA: 2005,Aug,7-8; 2005,Jul,11-12

85280 **factor XII (Hageman)**
0.00 0.00 FUD XXX
AMA: 2005,Aug,7-8; 2005,Jul,11-12

85290 **factor XIII (fibrin stabilizing)**
0.00 0.00 FUD XXX
AMA: 2005,Aug,7-8; 2005,Jul,11-12

85291 **factor XIII (fibrin stabilizing), screen solubility**
0.00 0.00 FUD XXX
AMA: 2005,Aug,7-8; 2005,Jul,11-12

85292 **prekallikrein assay (Fletcher factor assay)**
0.00 0.00 FUD XXX
AMA: 2005,Aug,7-8; 2005,Jul,11-12

85293 **high molecular weight kininogen assay (Fitzgerald factor assay)**
0.00 0.00 FUD XXX
AMA: 2005,Aug,7-8; 2005,Jul,11-12

85300 **Clotting inhibitors or anticoagulants; antithrombin III, activity**
0.00 0.00 FUD XXX
AMA: 2005,Aug,7-8; 2005,Jul,11-12

85301 **antithrombin III, antigen assay**
0.00 0.00 FUD XXX
AMA: 2005,Aug,7-8; 2005,Jul,11-12

85302 **protein C, antigen**
0.00 0.00 FUD XXX
AMA: 2005,Aug,7-8; 2005,Jul,11-12

85303 **protein C, activity**
0.00 0.00 FUD XXX
AMA: 2005,Aug,7-8; 2005,Jul,11-12

85305 **protein S, total**
0.00 0.00 FUD XXX
AMA: 2005,Jul,11-12; 2005,Aug,7-8

85306 **protein S, free**
0.00 0.00 FUD XXX
AMA: 2005,Aug,7-8; 2005,Jul,11-12

85307 **Activated Protein C (APC) resistance assay**
0.00 0.00 FUD XXX
AMA: 2005,Aug,7-8; 2005,Jul,11-12

85335 **Factor inhibitor test**
0.00 0.00 FUD XXX
AMA: 2005,Aug,7-8; 2005,Jul,11-12

85337 **Thrombomodulin**
EXCLUDES *Mixing studies for inhibitors (85732)*
0.00 0.00 FUD XXX
AMA: 2005,Aug,7-8; 2005,Jul,11-12

85345 **Coagulation time; Lee and White**
0.00 0.00 FUD XXX
AMA: 2005,Aug,7-8; 2005,Jul,11-12

85347 **activated**
0.00 0.00 FUD XXX
AMA: 2019,Apr,10

85348 **other methods**
EXCLUDES *Differential count (85007-85009, 85025)*
Duke bleeding time (85002)
Eosinophils, nasal smear (89190)
0.00 0.00 FUD XXX
AMA: 2005,Aug,7-8; 2005,Jul,11-12

85360 **Euglobulin lysis**
EXCLUDES *Fetal hemoglobin (83030, 83033, 85460)*
0.00 0.00 FUD XXX
AMA: 2005,Aug,7-8; 2005,Jul,11-12

85362 **Fibrin(ogen) degradation (split) products (FDP) (FSP); agglutination slide, semiquantitative**
EXCLUDES *Immunoelectrophoresis (86320)*
0.00 0.00 FUD XXX
AMA: 2005,Aug,7-8; 2005,Jul,11-12

85366 **paracoagulation**
0.00 0.00 FUD XXX
AMA: 2005,Aug,7-8; 2005,Jul,11-12

85370 **quantitative**
0.00 0.00 FUD XXX
AMA: 2005,Aug,7-8; 2005,Jul,11-12

85378 **Fibrin degradation products, D-dimer; qualitative or semiquantitative**
0.00 0.00 FUD XXX
AMA: 2018,Jan,8; 2017,Jan,8; 2016,Jan,13; 2015,Jan,16

85379 **quantitative**
INCLUDES Ultrasensitive and standard sensitivity quantitative D-dimer (85379)
0.00 0.00 FUD XXX
AMA: 2005,Aug,7-8; 2005,Jul,11-12

85380 **ultrasensitive (eg, for evaluation for venous thromboembolism), qualitative or semiquantitative**
0.00 0.00 FUD XXX
AMA: 2018,Jan,8; 2017,Jan,8; 2016,Jan,13; 2015,Jan,16

85384 **Fibrinogen; activity**
0.00 0.00 FUD XXX
AMA: 2019,Apr,10

85385 **antigen**
0.00 0.00 FUD XXX
AMA: 2005,Jul,11-12; 2005,Aug,7-8

85390 **Fibrinolysins or coagulopathy screen, interpretation and report**
0.00 0.00 FUD XXX 80
AMA: 2019,Apr,10

85396 **Coagulation/fibrinolysis assay, whole blood (eg, viscoelastic clot assessment), including use of any pharmacologic additive(s), as indicated, including interpretation and written report, per day**
0.58 0.58 FUD XXX N 80
AMA: 2019,Apr,10

85397 **Coagulation and fibrinolysis, functional activity, not otherwise specified (eg, ADAMTS-13), each analyte**
0.00 0.00 FUD XXX

85400 **Fibrinolytic factors and inhibitors; plasmin**
0.00 0.00 FUD XXX
AMA: 2005,Aug,7-8; 2005,Jul,11-12

85410 **alpha-2 antiplasmin**
0.00 0.00 FUD XXX
AMA: 2005,Aug,7-8; 2005,Jul,11-12

85415 **plasminogen activator**
0.00 0.00 FUD XXX
AMA: 2005,Aug,7-8; 2005,Jul,11-12

85420 **plasminogen, except antigenic assay**
0.00 0.00 FUD XXX
AMA: 2005,Aug,7-8; 2005,Jul,11-12

85421 **plasminogen, antigenic assay**
EXCLUDES *Fragility, red blood cell (85547, 85555-85557)*
0.00 0.00 FUD XXX
AMA: 2005,Aug,7-8; 2005,Jul,11-12

85441 **Heinz bodies; direct**
0.00 0.00 FUD XXX
AMA: 2005,Aug,7-8; 2005,Jul,11-12

85445 **induced, acetyl phenylhydrazine**
EXCLUDES *Hematocrit (PCV) (85014, 85025, 85027)*
Hemoglobin (83020-83068, 85018, 85025, 85027)
0.00 0.00 FUD XXX
AMA: 2005,Aug,7-8; 2005,Jul,11-12

85460 **Hemoglobin or RBCs, fetal, for fetomaternal hemorrhage; differential lysis (Kleihauer-Betke)** M ♀
EXCLUDES *Hemoglobin F (83030, 83033)*
Hemolysins (86940-86941)
0.00 0.00 FUD XXX
AMA: 2018,Jan,8; 2017,Jan,8; 2016,Jan,13; 2015,Jan,16

85461 **rosette** M ♀
0.00 0.00 FUD XXX
AMA: 2005,Jul,11-12; 2005,Aug,7-8

85475 **Hemolysin, acid**
INCLUDES Ham test
EXCLUDES *Hemolysins and agglutinins (86940-86941)*
0.00 0.00 FUD XXX
AMA: 2005,Aug,7-8; 2005,Jul,11-12

85520 **Heparin assay**
0.00 0.00 FUD XXX
AMA: 2005,Aug,7-8; 2005,Jul,11-12

85525 **Heparin neutralization**
0.00 0.00 FUD XXX
AMA: 2018,Jan,8; 2017,Aug,9

85530 **Heparin-protamine tolerance test**
0.00 0.00 FUD XXX
AMA: 2005,Aug,7-8; 2005,Jul,11-12

85536 **Iron stain, peripheral blood**
EXCLUDES *Iron stains on bone marrow or other tissues with physician evaluation (88313)*
0.00 0.00 FUD XXX
AMA: 2005,Aug,7-8; 2005,Jul,11-12

85540 **Leukocyte alkaline phosphatase with count**
0.00 0.00 FUD XXX
AMA: 2005,Aug,7-8; 2005,Jul,11-12

85547 **Mechanical fragility, RBC**
0.00 0.00 FUD XXX
AMA: 2005,Aug,7-8; 2005,Jul,11-12

85549 **Muramidase**
EXCLUDES *Nitroblue tetrazolium dye test (86384)*
0.00 0.00 FUD XXX
AMA: 2005,Aug,7-8; 2005,Jul,11-12

85555 **Osmotic fragility, RBC; unincubated**
0.00 0.00 FUD XXX
AMA: 2005,Aug,7-8; 2005,Jul,11-12

85557 **incubated**
EXCLUDES *Packed cell volume (85013)*
Parasites, blood (eg, malaria smears) (87207)
Partial thromboplastin time (85730, 85732)
Plasmin (85400)
Plasminogen (85420)
Plasminogen activator (85415)
0.00 0.00 FUD XXX
AMA: 2005,Aug,7-8; 2005,Jul,11-12

85576 **Platelet, aggregation (in vitro), each agent**
EXCLUDES *Thromboxane metabolite(s), including thromboxane, when performed, in urine (84431)*
🚑 0.00 ⚕ 0.00 **FUD** XXX ☒ Ⓠ ⑧⓪ ▣
AMA: 2019,Apr,10; 2018,Jan,8; 2017,Jan,8; 2016,Jan,13; 2015,Jan,16

85597 **Phospholipid neutralization; platelet**
🚑 0.00 ⚕ 0.00 **FUD** XXX Ⓠ ▣
AMA: 2018,Jan,8; 2017,Jan,8; 2016,Jan,13; 2015,Jan,16

85598 **hexagonal phospholipid**
🚑 0.00 ⚕ 0.00 **FUD** XXX Ⓠ ▣
AMA: 2018,Jan,8; 2017,Jan,8; 2016,Jan,13; 2015,Jan,16

85610 **Prothrombin time;**
🚑 0.00 ⚕ 0.00 **FUD** XXX ☒ Ⓠ ▣
AMA: 2005,Aug,7-8; 2005,Jul,11-12

85611 **substitution, plasma fractions, each**
🚑 0.00 ⚕ 0.00 **FUD** XXX Ⓠ ▣
AMA: 2005,Aug,7-8; 2005,Jul,11-12

85612 **Russell viper venom time (includes venom); undiluted**
🚑 0.00 ⚕ 0.00 **FUD** XXX Ⓠ ▣
AMA: 2005,Aug,7-8; 2005,Jul,11-12

85613 **diluted**
EXCLUDES *Red blood cell count (85025, 85027, 85041)*
🚑 0.00 ⚕ 0.00 **FUD** XXX Ⓠ ▣
AMA: 2005,Aug,7-8; 2005,Jul,11-12

85635 **Reptilase test**
EXCLUDES *Reticulocyte count (85044-85045)*
🚑 0.00 ⚕ 0.00 **FUD** XXX Ⓠ ▣
AMA: 2005,Aug,7-8; 2005,Jul,11-12

85651 **Sedimentation rate, erythrocyte; non-automated**
🚑 0.00 ⚕ 0.00 **FUD** XXX ☒ Ⓠ ▣
AMA: 2005,Aug,7-8; 2005,Jul,11-12

85652 **automated**
INCLUDES *Westergren test*
🚑 0.00 ⚕ 0.00 **FUD** XXX Ⓠ ▣
AMA: 2005,Aug,7-8; 2005,Jul,11-12

85660 **Sickling of RBC, reduction**
EXCLUDES *Hemoglobin electrophoresis (83020)*
Smears (87207)
🚑 0.00 ⚕ 0.00 **FUD** XXX Ⓠ ▣
AMA: 2005,Aug,7-8; 2005,Jul,11-12

85670 **Thrombin time; plasma**
🚑 0.00 ⚕ 0.00 **FUD** XXX Ⓠ ▣
AMA: 2005,Jul,11-12; 2005,Aug,7-8

85675 **titer**
🚑 0.00 ⚕ 0.00 **FUD** XXX Ⓠ ▣
AMA: 2005,Jul,11-12; 2005,Aug,7-8

85705 **Thromboplastin inhibition, tissue**
EXCLUDES *Individual clotting factors (85245-85247)*
🚑 0.00 ⚕ 0.00 **FUD** XXX Ⓠ ▣
AMA: 2005,Aug,7-8; 2005,Jul,11-12

85730-85732 Partial Thromboplastin Time (PTT)

EXCLUDES *Agglutinins (86000, 86156-86157)*
Antiplasmin (85410)
Antithrombin III (85300-85301)
Blood banking procedures (86850-86999)

85730 **Thromboplastin time, partial (PTT); plasma or whole blood**
INCLUDES *Hicks-Pitney test*
🚑 0.00 ⚕ 0.00 **FUD** XXX Ⓠ ▣
AMA: 2005,Aug,7-8; 2005,Jul,11-12

85732 **substitution, plasma fractions, each**
🚑 0.00 ⚕ 0.00 **FUD** XXX Ⓠ ▣
AMA: 2018,Jan,8; 2017,Jan,8; 2016,Jan,13; 2015,Jan,16

85810-85999 Blood Viscosity and Unlisted Hematology Procedures

85810 **Viscosity**
EXCLUDES *von Willebrand factor assay (85245-85247)*
WBC count (85025, 85027, 85048, 89050)
🚑 0.00 ⚕ 0.00 **FUD** XXX Ⓠ ▣
AMA: 2018,Jan,8; 2017,Jan,8; 2016,Jan,13; 2015,Jan,16

85999 **Unlisted hematology and coagulation procedure**
🚑 0.00 ⚕ 0.00 **FUD** XXX Ⓠ ▣
AMA: 2018,Jan,8; 2017,Aug,9; 2017,Jan,8; 2016,Jan,13; 2015,Jan,16

86000-86063 Antibody Testing

86000 **Agglutinins, febrile (eg, Brucella, Francisella, Murine typhus, Q fever, Rocky Mountain spotted fever, scrub typhus), each antigen**
EXCLUDES *Infectious agent antibodies (86602-86804)*
🚑 0.00 ⚕ 0.00 **FUD** XXX Ⓠ ▣
AMA: 2018,Jan,8; 2017,Jan,8; 2016,Jan,13; 2015,Jan,16

86001 **Allergen specific IgG quantitative or semiquantitative, each allergen**
EXCLUDES *Agglutinins and autohemolysins (86940-86941)*
🚑 0.00 ⚕ 0.00 **FUD** XXX Ⓠ ▣
AMA: 2005,Aug,7-8; 2005,Jul,11-12

86003 **Allergen specific IgE; quantitative or semiquantitative, crude allergen extract, each**
EXCLUDES *Total quantitative IgE (82785)*
🚑 0.00 ⚕ 0.00 **FUD** XXX Ⓠ ▣
AMA: 2018,Jan,8; 2017,Jan,8; 2016,Jan,13; 2015,Jan,16

86005 **qualitative, multiallergen screen (eg, disk, sponge, card)**
EXCLUDES *Total qualitative IgE (83518)*
🚑 0.00 ⚕ 0.00 **FUD** XXX Ⓠ ▣
AMA: 2018,Jan,8; 2017,Jan,8; 2016,Jan,13; 2015,Jan,16

86008 **quantitative or semiquantitative, recombinant or purified component, each**
EXCLUDES *Alpha-1 antitrypsin (82103, 82104)*
Alpha-1 feto-protein (82105, 82106)
Anti-AChR (acetylcholine receptor) antibody titer (86255, 86256)
Anticardiolipin antibody (86147)
Anti-deoxyribonuclease titer (86215)
Anti-DNA (86225)
🚑 0.00 ⚕ 0.00 **FUD** XXX Ⓠ ▣

86021 **Antibody identification; leukocyte antibodies**
🚑 0.00 ⚕ 0.00 **FUD** XXX Ⓠ ▣
AMA: 2020,AugSE,1; 2020,AugSE,1; 2020,AugSE,1

86022 **platelet antibodies**
🚑 0.00 ⚕ 0.00 **FUD** XXX Ⓠ ▣
AMA: 2020,AugSE,1; 2020,AugSE,1; 2020,AugSE,1

86023 **platelet associated immunoglobulin assay**
🚑 0.00 ⚕ 0.00 **FUD** XXX Ⓠ ▣
AMA: 2020,AugSE,1; 2020,AugSE,1; 2020,AugSE,1

86038 **Antinuclear antibodies (ANA);**
🚑 0.00 ⚕ 0.00 **FUD** XXX Ⓠ ▣
AMA: 2005,Aug,7-8; 2005,Jul,11-12

86039 **titer**
EXCLUDES *Antistreptococcal antibody, ie, anti-DNAse (86215)*
Antistreptokinase titer (86590)
🚑 0.00 ⚕ 0.00 **FUD** XXX Ⓠ ▣
AMA: 2005,Aug,7-8; 2005,Jul,11-12

86060 **Antistreptolysin 0; titer**
EXCLUDES *Antibodies, infectious agents (86602-86804)*
🚑 0.00 ⚕ 0.00 **FUD** XXX Ⓠ ▣
AMA: 2005,Jul,11-12; 2005,Aug,7-8

🅰🅱/🆃🅲 PC/TC Only 🅰🅽-🆉🅱 ASC Payment 🅐🅞 Bilateral ♂ Male Only ♀ Female Only 🚑 Facility RVU ⚕ Non-Facility RVU ▣ CCI ☒ CLIA
FUD Follow-up Days **CMS:** IOM **AMA:** CPT Asst 🅐-🆈 OPPSI ⑧⓪/⑧⓪ Surg Assist Allowed / w/Doc ▣ Lab Crosswalk 🔖 Radiology Crosswalk

86063 **screen**

EXCLUDES *Antibodies to blastomyces (86612)*
Antibodies, infectious agents (86602-86804)

0.00 0.00 FUD XXX

AMA: 2005,Jul,11-12; 2005,Aug,7-8

86077-86079 Blood Bank Services

86077 **Blood bank physician services; difficult cross match and/or evaluation of irregular antibody(s), interpretation and written report**

1.46 1.57 FUD XXX

AMA: 2005,Aug,7-8; 2005,Jul,11-12

86078 **investigation of transfusion reaction including suspicion of transmissible disease, interpretation and written report**

1.46 1.57 FUD XXX

AMA: 2005,Aug,7-8; 2005,Jul,11-12

86079 **authorization for deviation from standard blood banking procedures (eg, use of outdated blood, transfusion of Rh incompatible units), with written report**

EXCLUDES *Brucella antibodies (86622)*
Candida antibodies (86628)
Candida skin test (86485)

1.46 1.56 FUD XXX

AMA: 2005,Aug,7-8; 2005,Jul,11-12

86140-86344 [86152, 86153, 86328] Diagnostic Immunology Testing

86140 **C-reactive protein;**

EXCLUDES *Candidiasis (86628)*

0.00 0.00 FUD XXX

AMA: 2005,Aug,7-8; 2005,Jul,11-12

86141 **high sensitivity (hsCRP)**

0.00 0.00 FUD XXX

AMA: 2005,Aug,7-8; 2005,Jul,11-12

86146 **Beta 2 Glycoprotein I antibody, each**

0.00 0.00 FUD XXX

AMA: 2005,Aug,7-8; 2005,Jul,11-12

86147 **Cardiolipin (phospholipid) antibody, each Ig class**

0.00 0.00 FUD XXX

AMA: 2005,Aug,7-8; 2005,Jul,11-12

\# **86152** **Cell enumeration using immunologic selection and identification in fluid specimen (eg, circulating tumor cells in blood);**

EXCLUDES *Flow cytometric immunophenotyping (88184-88189)*
Flow cytometric quantitation (86355-86357, 86359-86361, 86367)

Code also physician interpretation/report when performed ([86153])

0.00 0.00 FUD XXX

\# **86153** **physician interpretation and report, when required**

EXCLUDES *Flow cytometric immunophenotyping (88184-88189)*
Flow cytometric quantitation (86355-86357, 86359-86361, 86367)

Code first cell enumeration, when performed ([86152])

0.00 0.00 FUD 000

86148 **Anti-phosphatidylserine (phospholipid) antibody**

EXCLUDES *Antiprothrombin (phospholipid cofactor) antibody (86849)*

0.00 0.00 FUD XXX

AMA: 2018,Jan,8; 2017,Jan,8; 2016,Jan,13; 2015,Jan,16

86152 **Resequenced code. See code following 86147.**

86153 **Resequenced code. See code before 86148.**

86155 **Chemotaxis assay, specify method**

EXCLUDES *Antibodies, coccidioides (86635)*
Clostridium difficile toxin (87230)
Skin test, coccidioides (86490)

0.00 0.00 FUD XXX

AMA: 2005,Aug,7-8; 2005,Jul,11-12

86156 **Cold agglutinin; screen**

0.00 0.00 FUD XXX

AMA: 2005,Aug,7-8; 2005,Jul,11-12

86157 **titer**

0.00 0.00 FUD XXX

AMA: 2005,Aug,7-8; 2005,Jul,11-12

86160 **Complement; antigen, each component**

0.00 0.00 FUD XXX

AMA: 2005,Aug,7-8; 2005,Jul,11-12

86161 **functional activity, each component**

0.00 0.00 FUD XXX

AMA: 2005,Aug,7-8; 2005,Jul,11-12

86162 **total hemolytic (CH50)**

0.00 0.00 FUD XXX

AMA: 2005,Aug,7-8; 2005,Jul,11-12

86171 **Complement fixation tests, each antigen**

EXCLUDES *Coombs test*

0.00 0.00 FUD XXX

AMA: 2005,Aug,7-8; 2005,Jul,11-12

86200 **Cyclic citrullinated peptide (CCP), antibody**

0.00 0.00 FUD XXX

AMA: 2018,Jan,8; 2017,Jan,8; 2016,Jan,13; 2015,Jan,16

86215 **Deoxyribonuclease, antibody**

0.00 0.00 FUD XXX

AMA: 2005,Aug,7-8; 2005,Jul,11-12

86225 **Deoxyribonucleic acid (DNA) antibody; native or double stranded**

EXCLUDES *Echinococcus antibodies, report code for specific method*
HIV antibody tests (86701-86703)

0.00 0.00 FUD XXX

AMA: 2005,Aug,7-8; 2005,Jul,11-12

86226 **single stranded**

EXCLUDES *Anti D.S, DNA, IFA, eg, using C. Lucilae (86255-86256)*

0.00 0.00 FUD XXX

AMA: 2005,Aug,7-8; 2005,Jul,11-12

86235 **Extractable nuclear antigen, antibody to, any method (eg, nRNP, SS-A, SS-B, Sm, RNP, Sc170, J01), each antibody**

0.00 0.00 FUD XXX

AMA: 2005,Aug,7-8; 2005,Jul,11-12

86255 **Fluorescent noninfectious agent antibody; screen, each antibody**

0.00 0.00 FUD XXX

AMA: 2020,AugSE,1; 2020,AugSE,1; 2020,AugSE,1

86256 **titer, each antibody**

EXCLUDES *Fluorescent technique for antigen identification in tissue (88346, [88350])*
FTA (86780)
Gel (agar) diffusion tests (86331)
Indirect fluorescence (88346, [88350])

0.00 0.00 FUD XXX

AMA: 2020,AugSE,1; 2020,AugSE,1; 2020,AugSE,1

86277 **Growth hormone, human (HGH), antibody**

0.00 0.00 FUD XXX

AMA: 2005,Aug,7-8; 2005,Jul,11-12

86280 **Hemagglutination inhibition test (HAI)**

EXCLUDES *Antibodies to infectious agents (86602-86804)*
Rubella (86762)

0.00 0.00 FUD XXX

AMA: 2005,Aug,7-8; 2005,Jul,11-12

86294 **Immunoassay for tumor antigen, qualitative or semiquantitative (eg, bladder tumor antigen)**
EXCLUDES *Qualitative NMP22 protein (86386)*
0.00 0.00 FUD XXX
AMA: 2005,Aug,7-8; 2005,Jul,11-12

86300 **Immunoassay for tumor antigen, quantitative; CA 15-3 (27.29)**
0.00 0.00 FUD XXX
AMA: 2005,Aug,7-8; 2005,Jul,11-12

86301 **CA 19-9**
0.00 0.00 FUD XXX
AMA: 2005,Aug,7-8; 2005,Jul,11-12

86304 **CA 125**
EXCLUDES *Antibody, hepatitis delta agent (86692)*
Measurement serum HER-2/neu oncoprotein (83950)
0.00 0.00 FUD XXX
AMA: 2005,Aug,7-8; 2005,Jul,11-12

86305 **Human epididymis protein 4 (HE4)**
0.00 0.00 FUD XXX

86308 **Heterophile antibodies; screening**
EXCLUDES *Antibodies, infectious agents (86602-86804)*
0.00 0.00 FUD XXX
AMA: 2005,Jul,11-12; 2005,Aug,7-8

86309 **titer**
EXCLUDES *Antibodies, infectious agents (86602-86804)*
0.00 0.00 FUD XXX
AMA: 2005,Jul,11-12; 2005,Aug,7-8

86310 **titers after absorption with beef cells and guinea pig kidney**
EXCLUDES *Antibodies, infectious agents (86602-86804)*
Histoplasma antibodies (86698)
Histoplasmosis skin test (86510)
Human growth hormone antibody (86277)
0.00 0.00 FUD XXX
AMA: 2005,Jul,11-12; 2005,Aug,7-8

86316 **Immunoassay for tumor antigen, other antigen, quantitative (eg, CA 50, 72-4, 549), each**
0.00 0.00 FUD XXX
AMA: 2018,Jan,8; 2017,Jan,8; 2016,Jan,13; 2015,Jan,16

86317 **Immunoassay for infectious agent antibody, quantitative, not otherwise specified**
EXCLUDES *Immunoassay techniques for infectious antigens (87301-87451)*
Immunoassay techniques for noninfectious antigens (83516, 83518-83520)
Immunoassay techniques with direct/visual observation for infectious antigens (87802-87899 [87806, 87811])
Particle agglutination test (86403)
0.00 0.00 FUD XXX
AMA: 2020,OctSE,1

▲ **86318** **Immunoassay for infectious agent antibody(ies), qualitative or semiquantitative, single-step method (eg, reagent strip);**
0.00 0.00 FUD XXX
AMA: 2020,AugSE,1; 2020,AugSE,1; 2020,AugSE,1; 2018,Jan,8; 2017,Jan,8; 2016,Jan,13; 2015,Jan,16

● # **86328** **severe acute respiratory syndrome coronavirus 2 (SARS-CoV-2) (Coronavirus disease [COVID-19])**
INCLUDES Testing for antibodies only
EXCLUDES *Severe acute respiratory syndrome coronavirus 2 [SARS-CoV-2] [coronavirus disease {COVID-19}] testing via multiple-step method (86769)*
Testing for presence neutralizing antibodies that block cell infection ([86408, 86409])
0.00 0.00 FUD XXX
AMA: 2020,SepSE,1; 2020,AugSE,1; 2020,SepSE,1; 2020,AugSE,1; 2020,AugSE,1

86320 **Immunoelectrophoresis; serum**
0.00 0.00 FUD XXX
AMA: 2005,Jul,11-12; 2005,Aug,7-8

86325 **other fluids (eg, urine, cerebrospinal fluid) with concentration**
0.00 0.00 FUD XXX
AMA: 2005,Jul,11-12; 2005,Aug,7-8

86327 **crossed (2-dimensional assay)**
0.00 0.00 FUD XXX
AMA: 2005,Jul,11-12; 2005,Aug,7-8

86328 **Resequenced code. See code following 86318.**

86329 **Immunodiffusion; not elsewhere specified**
0.00 0.00 FUD XXX
AMA: 2018,Jan,8; 2017,Jan,8; 2016,Jan,13; 2015,Jan,16

86331 **gel diffusion, qualitative (Ouchterlony), each antigen or antibody**
0.00 0.00 FUD XXX
AMA: 2005,Aug,7-8; 2005,Jul,11-12

86332 **Immune complex assay**
0.00 0.00 FUD XXX
AMA: 2005,Aug,7-8; 2005,Jul,11-12

86334 **Immunofixation electrophoresis; serum**
0.00 0.00 FUD XXX
AMA: 2005,Jul,11-12; 2005,Aug,7-8

86335 **other fluids with concentration (eg, urine, CSF)**
0.00 0.00 FUD XXX
AMA: 2005,Aug,7-8; 2005,Jul,11-12

86336 **Inhibin A**
0.00 0.00 FUD XXX
AMA: 2005,Aug,7-8; 2005,Jul,11-12

86337 **Insulin antibodies**
0.00 0.00 FUD XXX
AMA: 2005,Aug,7-8; 2005,Jul,11-12

86340 **Intrinsic factor antibodies**
EXCLUDES *Antibodies, leptospira (86720)*
Leukoagglutinins (86021)
0.00 0.00 FUD XXX
AMA: 2005,Jul,11-12; 2005,Aug,7-8

86341 **Islet cell antibody**
0.00 0.00 FUD XXX
AMA: 2018,Jan,8; 2017,Jan,8; 2016,Jan,13; 2015,Jan,16

86343 **Leukocyte histamine release test (LHR)**
0.00 0.00 FUD XXX
AMA: 2005,Aug,7-8; 2005,Jul,11-12

86344 **Leukocyte phagocytosis**
0.00 0.00 FUD XXX
AMA: 2005,Aug,7-8; 2005,Jul,11-12

86352 Assay Cellular Function

86352 **Cellular function assay involving stimulation (eg, mitogen or antigen) and detection of biomarker (eg, ATP)**
0.00 0.00 FUD XXX

86353 Lymphocyte Mitogen Response Assay

CMS: 100-03,190.8 Lymphocyte Mitogen Response Assays

86353 **Lymphocyte transformation, mitogen (phytomitogen) or antigen induced blastogenesis**
EXCLUDES *Cellular function assay with stimulation and biomarker detection (86352)*
Malaria antibodies (86750)
0.00 0.00 FUD XXX
AMA: 2005,Aug,7-8; 2005,Jul,11-12

86355-86593 [86408, 86409, 86413] Additional Diagnostic Immunology Testing

86355 B cells, total count
EXCLUDES *Flow cytometry interpretation (88187-88189)*
0.00 0.00 FUD XXX
AMA: 2018,Jan,8; 2017,Jan,8; 2016,Jan,13; 2015,Jan,16

86356 Mononuclear cell antigen, quantitative (eg, flow cytometry), not otherwise specified, each antigen
EXCLUDES *Flow cytometry interpretation (88187-88189)*
0.00 0.00 FUD XXX
AMA: 2018,Jan,8; 2017,Jan,8; 2016,Jan,13; 2015,Jan,16

86357 Natural killer (NK) cells, total count
EXCLUDES *Flow cytometry interpretation (88187-88189)*
0.00 0.00 FUD XXX
AMA: 2018,Jan,8; 2017,Jan,8; 2016,Jan,13; 2015,Jan,16

86359 T cells; total count
EXCLUDES *Flow cytometry interpretation (88187-88189)*
0.00 0.00 FUD XXX
AMA: 2018,Jan,8; 2017,Jan,8; 2016,Jan,13; 2015,Jan,16

86360 absolute CD4 and CD8 count, including ratio
EXCLUDES *Flow cytometry interpretation (88187-88189)*
0.00 0.00 FUD XXX
AMA: 2018,Jan,8; 2017,Jan,8; 2016,Jan,13; 2015,Jan,16

86361 absolute CD4 count
EXCLUDES *Flow cytometry interpretation (88187-88189)*
0.00 0.00 FUD XXX
AMA: 2018,Jan,8; 2017,Jan,8; 2016,Jan,13; 2015,Jan,16

86367 Stem cells (ie, CD34), total count
EXCLUDES *Flow cytometric immunophenotyping, potential hematolymphoid neoplasia assessment (88184-88189)*
Flow cytometry interpretation (88187-88189)
0.00 0.00 FUD XXX
AMA: 2018,Jan,8; 2017,Jan,8; 2016,Jan,13; 2015,Jan,16

86376 Microsomal antibodies (eg, thyroid or liver-kidney), each
0.00 0.00 FUD XXX
AMA: 2020,AugSE,1; 2020,AugSE,1; 2020,AugSE,1

86382 Neutralization test, viral
0.00 0.00 FUD XXX
AMA: 2005,Aug,7-8; 2005,Jul,11-12

● # **86408 Neutralizing antibody, severe acute respiratory syndrome coronavirus 2 (SARS-CoV-2) (Coronavirus disease [COVID-19]); screen**
INCLUDES Testing for presence neutralizing antibodies that block cell infection
EXCLUDES *Testing for presence antibodies only ([86328])*
0.00 0.00 FUD 000
AMA: 2020,AugSE,1

● # **86409 titer**
INCLUDES Testing for presence neutralizing antibodies that block cell infection
EXCLUDES *Testing for presence antibodies only ([86328])*
0.00 0.00 FUD 000
AMA: 2020,AugSE,1

● # **86413 Severe acute respiratory syndrome coronavirus 2 (SARS-CoV-2) (Coronavirus disease [COVID-19]) antibody, quantitative**
INCLUDES Testing for presence and adaptive immune response to SARS-CoV-2
0.00 0.00 FUD 000
AMA: 2020,SepSE,1

86384 Nitroblue tetrazolium dye test (NTD)
0.00 0.00 FUD XXX
AMA: 2005,Aug,7-8; 2005,Jul,11-12

86386 Nuclear Matrix Protein 22 (NMP22), qualitative
EXCLUDES *Ouchterlony diffusion (86331)*
Platelet antibodies (86022, 86023)
0.00 0.00 FUD XXX

86403 Particle agglutination; screen, each antibody
0.00 0.00 FUD XXX
AMA: 2020,OctSE,1

86406 titer, each antibody
EXCLUDES *Pregnancy test (84702, 84703)*
Rapid plasma reagin test (RPR) (86592, 86593)
0.00 0.00 FUD XXX
AMA: 2005,Jul,11-12; 2005,Aug,7-8

86408 **Resequenced code. See code following 86382.**

86409 **Resequenced code. See code following 86382.**

86413 **Resequenced code. See code following resequenced code 86409.**

86430 Rheumatoid factor; qualitative
0.00 0.00 FUD XXX
AMA: 2005,Aug,7-8; 2005,Jul,11-12

86431 quantitative
EXCLUDES *Serologic syphilis testing (86592, 86593)*
0.00 0.00 FUD XXX
AMA: 2005,Aug,7-8; 2005,Jul,11-12

86480 Tuberculosis test, cell mediated immunity antigen response measurement; gamma interferon
0.00 0.00 FUD XXX
AMA: 2019,Dec,12; 2018,Jan,8; 2017,Jan,8; 2016,Jan,13; 2015,Jan,16

86481 enumeration of gamma interferon-producing T-cells in cell suspension
0.00 0.00 FUD XXX
AMA: 2019,Dec,12

86485 Skin test; candida
EXCLUDES *Candida antibody (86628)*
0.00 0.00 FUD XXX
AMA: 2005,Jul,11-12; 2005,Aug,7-8

86486 unlisted antigen, each
0.15 0.15 FUD XXX
AMA: 2008,Apr,5-7

86490 coccidioidomycosis
2.49 2.49 FUD XXX
AMA: 2005,Aug,7-8; 2005,Jul,11-12

86510 histoplasmosis
EXCLUDES *Histoplasma antibody (86698)*
0.19 0.19 FUD XXX
AMA: 2005,Aug,7-8; 2005,Jul,11-12

86580 tuberculosis, intradermal
INCLUDES Heaf test
Intradermal Mantoux test
EXCLUDES *Antibodies to sporothrix, report code for specific method*
Skin test for allergy (95012-95199)
Smooth muscle antibody (86255-86256)
Tuberculosis test, cell mediated immunity measurement gamma interferon antigen response (86480)
0.24 0.24 FUD XXX
AMA: 2005,Aug,7-8; 2005,Jul,11-12

86590 Streptokinase, antibody
EXCLUDES *Antibodies, infectious agents (86602-86804)*
Streptolysin O antibody, antistreptolysin O (86060, 86063)
0.00 0.00 FUD XXX
AMA: 2005,Jul,11-12; 2005,Aug,7-8

86592 **Syphilis test, non-treponemal antibody; qualitative (eg, VDRL, RPR, ART)**

INCLUDES Wasserman test

EXCLUDES *Antibodies to infectious agents (86602-86804)*

0.00 0.00 FUD XXX A

AMA: 2005,Jul,11-12; 2005,Aug,7-8

86593 **quantitative**

EXCLUDES *Antibodies, infectious agents (86602-86804)*
Tetanus antibody (86774)
Thyroglobulin (84432)
Thyroglobulin antibody (86800)
Thyroid microsomal antibody (86376)
Toxoplasma antibody (86777-86778)

0.00 0.00 FUD XXX A

AMA: 2005,Jul,11-12; 2005,Aug,7-8

86602-86698 Testing for Antibodies to Infectious Agents: Actinomyces—Histoplasma

INCLUDES Qualitative or semiquantitative immunoassays performed by multiple-step methods for detection, antibodies to infectious agents

EXCLUDES *Detection:*
Antibodies other than those to infectious agents, see specific antibody or method
Infectious agent/antigen (87260-87899 [87623, 87624, 87625, 87806])
Immunoassays by single-step method (86318, [86328])

86602 **Antibody; actinomyces**

0.00 0.00 FUD XXX Q

AMA: 2020,OctSE,1; 2020,AugSE,1; 2020,AugSE,1; 2020,AugSE,1; 2018,Jan,8; 2017,Jan,8; 2016,Jan,13; 2015,Jan,16

86603 **adenovirus**

0.00 0.00 FUD XXX Q

AMA: 2020,OctSE,1; 2020,AugSE,1; 2020,AugSE,1; 2020,AugSE,1

86606 **Aspergillus**

0.00 0.00 FUD XXX Q

AMA: 2020,OctSE,1; 2020,AugSE,1; 2020,AugSE,1; 2020,AugSE,1

86609 **bacterium, not elsewhere specified**

0.00 0.00 FUD XXX Q

AMA: 2020,OctSE,1; 2020,AugSE,1; 2020,AugSE,1; 2020,AugSE,1

86611 **Bartonella**

0.00 0.00 FUD XXX Q

AMA: 2020,OctSE,1; 2020,AugSE,1; 2020,AugSE,1; 2020,AugSE,1

86612 **Blastomyces**

0.00 0.00 FUD XXX Q

AMA: 2020,OctSE,1; 2020,AugSE,1; 2020,AugSE,1; 2020,AugSE,1

86615 **Bordetella**

0.00 0.00 FUD XXX Q

AMA: 2020,OctSE,1; 2020,AugSE,1; 2020,AugSE,1; 2020,AugSE,1

86617 **Borrelia burgdorferi (Lyme disease) confirmatory test (eg, Western Blot or immunoblot)**

0.00 0.00 FUD XXX Q

AMA: 2020,OctSE,1; 2020,AugSE,1; 2020,AugSE,1; 2020,AugSE,1

86618 **Borrelia burgdorferi (Lyme disease)**

0.00 0.00 FUD XXX Q

AMA: 2020,OctSE,1; 2020,AugSE,1; 2020,AugSE,1; 2020,AugSE,1

86619 **Borrelia (relapsing fever)**

0.00 0.00 FUD XXX Q

AMA: 2020,OctSE,1; 2020,AugSE,1; 2020,AugSE,1; 2020,AugSE,1

86622 **Brucella**

0.00 0.00 FUD XXX Q

AMA: 2020,OctSE,1; 2020,AugSE,1; 2020,AugSE,1; 2020,AugSE,1

86625 **Campylobacter**

0.00 0.00 FUD XXX Q

AMA: 2020,OctSE,1; 2020,AugSE,1; 2020,AugSE,1; 2020,AugSE,1

86628 **Candida**

EXCLUDES *Candida skin test (86485)*

0.00 0.00 FUD XXX Q

AMA: 2020,OctSE,1; 2020,AugSE,1; 2020,AugSE,1; 2020,AugSE,1

86631 **Chlamydia**

0.00 0.00 FUD XXX A

AMA: 2020,OctSE,1; 2020,AugSE,1; 2020,AugSE,1; 2020,AugSE,1

86632 **Chlamydia, IgM**

EXCLUDES *Chlamydia antigen (87270, 87320)*
Fluorescent antibody technique (86255-86256)

0.00 0.00 FUD XXX A

AMA: 2020,OctSE,1; 2020,AugSE,1; 2020,AugSE,1; 2020,AugSE,1

86635 **Coccidioides**

EXCLUDES *Severe Acute Respiratory Syndrome Coronavirus 2 [SARS-CoV-2] [Coronavirus disease {COVID-19}] antibody testing ([86328], 86769)*

0.00 0.00 FUD XXX Q

AMA: 2020,OctSE,1; 2020,AugSE,1; 2020,AugSE,1; 2020,AugSE,1

86638 **Coxiella burnetii (Q fever)**

0.00 0.00 FUD XXX Q

AMA: 2020,OctSE,1; 2020,AugSE,1; 2020,AugSE,1; 2020,AugSE,1

86641 **Cryptococcus**

0.00 0.00 FUD XXX Q

AMA: 2020,OctSE,1; 2020,AugSE,1; 2020,AugSE,1; 2020,AugSE,1

86644 **cytomegalovirus (CMV)**

0.00 0.00 FUD XXX Q

AMA: 2020,OctSE,1; 2020,AugSE,1; 2020,AugSE,1; 2020,AugSE,1

86645 **cytomegalovirus (CMV), IgM**

0.00 0.00 FUD XXX Q

AMA: 2020,OctSE,1; 2020,AugSE,1; 2020,AugSE,1; 2020,AugSE,1; 2018,Jan,8; 2017,Jan,8; 2016,Jan,13; 2015,Jan,16

86648 **Diphtheria**

0.00 0.00 FUD XXX Q

AMA: 2020,OctSE,1; 2020,AugSE,1; 2020,AugSE,1; 2020,AugSE,1

86651 **encephalitis, California (La Crosse)**

0.00 0.00 FUD XXX Q

AMA: 2020,OctSE,1; 2020,AugSE,1; 2020,AugSE,1; 2020,AugSE,1

86652 **encephalitis, Eastern equine**

0.00 0.00 FUD XXX Q

AMA: 2020,OctSE,1; 2020,AugSE,1; 2020,AugSE,1; 2020,AugSE,1

86653 **encephalitis, St. Louis**

0.00 0.00 FUD XXX Q

AMA: 2020,OctSE,1; 2020,AugSE,1; 2020,AugSE,1; 2020,AugSE,1

86654 **encephalitis, Western equine**

0.00 0.00 FUD XXX Q

AMA: 2020,OctSE,1; 2020,AugSE,1; 2020,AugSE,1; 2020,AugSE,1

86658 **enterovirus (eg, coxsackie, echo, polio)**

EXCLUDES *Antibodies to:*
Trichinella (86784)
Trypanosoma—see code for specific methodology
Tuberculosis (86580)
Viral—see code for specific methodology

0.00 0.00 FUD XXX Q

AMA: 2020,OctSE,1; 2020,AugSE,1; 2020,AugSE,1; 2020,AugSE,1

86663 **Epstein-Barr (EB) virus, early antigen (EA)**

0.00 0.00 FUD XXX Q

AMA: 2020,OctSE,1; 2020,AugSE,1; 2020,AugSE,1; 2020,AugSE,1

86664 **Epstein-Barr (EB) virus, nuclear antigen (EBNA)**

0.00 0.00 FUD XXX Q

AMA: 2020,OctSE,1; 2020,AugSE,1; 2020,AugSE,1; 2020,AugSE,1

86665 **Epstein-Barr (EB) virus, viral capsid (VCA)**

0.00 0.00 FUD XXX Q

AMA: 2020,OctSE,1; 2020,AugSE,1; 2020,AugSE,1; 2020,AugSE,1

86666 **Ehrlichia**

0.00 0.00 FUD XXX Q

AMA: 2020,OctSE,1; 2020,AugSE,1; 2020,AugSE,1; 2020,AugSE,1

86668 **Francisella tularensis**

0.00 0.00 FUD XXX Q

AMA: 2020,OctSE,1; 2020,AugSE,1; 2020,AugSE,1; 2020,AugSE,1

86671 **fungus, not elsewhere specified**
0.00 0.00 FUD XXX
AMA: 2020,OctSE,1; 2020,AugSE,1; 2020,AugSE,1; 2020,AugSE,1

86674 **Giardia lamblia**
0.00 0.00 FUD XXX
AMA: 2020,OctSE,1; 2020,AugSE,1; 2020,AugSE,1; 2020,AugSE,1

86677 **Helicobacter pylori**
0.00 0.00 FUD XXX
AMA: 2020,OctSE,1; 2020,AugSE,1; 2020,AugSE,1; 2020,AugSE,1; 2018,Jan,8; 2017,Jan,8; 2016,Jan,13; 2015,Jan,16

86682 **helminth, not elsewhere specified**
0.00 0.00 FUD XXX
AMA: 2020,OctSE,1; 2020,AugSE,1; 2020,AugSE,1; 2020,AugSE,1

86684 **Haemophilus influenza**
0.00 0.00 FUD XXX
AMA: 2020,OctSE,1; 2020,AugSE,1; 2020,AugSE,1; 2020,AugSE,1

86687 **HTLV-I**
0.00 0.00 FUD XXX
AMA: 2020,OctSE,1; 2020,AugSE,1; 2020,AugSE,1; 2020,AugSE,1

86688 **HTLV-II**
0.00 0.00 FUD XXX
AMA: 2020,OctSE,1; 2020,AugSE,1; 2020,AugSE,1; 2020,AugSE,1

86689 **HTLV or HIV antibody, confirmatory test (eg, Western Blot)**
0.00 0.00 FUD XXX
AMA: 2020,OctSE,1; 2020,AugSE,1; 2020,AugSE,1; 2020,AugSE,1; 2018,Jan,8; 2017,Jan,8; 2016,Jan,13; 2015,Jan,16

86692 **hepatitis, delta agent**
EXCLUDES *Hepatitis delta agent, antigen (87380)*
0.00 0.00 FUD XXX
AMA: 2020,OctSE,1; 2020,AugSE,1; 2020,AugSE,1; 2020,AugSE,1

86694 **herpes simplex, non-specific type test**
0.00 0.00 FUD XXX
AMA: 2020,OctSE,1; 2020,AugSE,1; 2020,AugSE,1; 2020,AugSE,1

86695 **herpes simplex, type 1**
0.00 0.00 FUD XXX
AMA: 2020,OctSE,1; 2020,AugSE,1; 2020,AugSE,1; 2020,AugSE,1; 2018,Jan,8; 2017,Jan,8; 2016,Jan,13; 2015,Jan,16

86696 **herpes simplex, type 2**
0.00 0.00 FUD XXX
AMA: 2020,OctSE,1; 2020,AugSE,1; 2020,AugSE,1; 2020,AugSE,1

86698 **histoplasma**
0.00 0.00 FUD XXX
AMA: 2020,OctSE,1; 2020,AugSE,1; 2020,AugSE,1; 2020,AugSE,1

86701-86703 Testing for HIV Antibodies

CMS: 100-03,190.14 Human Immunodeficiency Virus Testing (Diagnosis); 100-03,190.9 Serologic Testing for Acquired Immunodeficiency Syndrome (AIDS)

INCLUDES Qualitative or semiquantitative immunoassays performed by multiple-step methods for detection, antibodies to infectious agents

EXCLUDES *Confirmatory test for HIV antibody (86689)*
HIV-1 antigen (87390)
HIV-1 antigen(s) with HIV 1 and 2 antibodies, single result (87389)
HIV-2 antigen (87391)
Immunoassays by single-step method (86318)

Code also modifier 92 for test performed using kit or transportable instrument comprising (all or part) single-use, disposable analytical chamber

86701 **Antibody; HIV-1**
0.00 0.00 FUD XXX
AMA: 2020,OctSE,1; 2020,AugSE,1; 2020,AugSE,1; 2020,AugSE,1; 2018,Jan,8; 2017,Jan,8; 2016,Jan,13; 2015,Jan,16

86702 **HIV-2**
0.00 0.00 FUD XXX
AMA: 2020,OctSE,1; 2020,AugSE,1; 2020,AugSE,1; 2020,AugSE,1; 2018,Jan,8; 2017,Jan,8; 2016,Jan,13; 2015,Jan,16

86703 **HIV-1 and HIV-2, single result**
0.00 0.00 FUD XXX
AMA: 2020,OctSE,1; 2020,AugSE,1; 2020,AugSE,1; 2020,AugSE,1; 2018,Jan,8; 2017,Jan,8; 2016,Jan,13; 2015,Jan,16

86704-86804 Testing for Infectious Disease Antibodies: Hepatitis—Yersinia

INCLUDES Qualitative or semiquantitative immunoassays performed by multiple-step methods for detection, antibodies to infectious agents

EXCLUDES *Detection of:*
Antibodies other than those to infectious agents, see specific antibody or method
Infectious agent/antigen (87260-87899 [87623, 87624, 87625, 87806])
Immunoassays by single-step method (86318)

86704 **Hepatitis B core antibody (HBcAb); total**
0.00 0.00 FUD XXX
AMA: 2020,OctSE,1; 2020,AugSE,1; 2020,AugSE,1; 2020,AugSE,1; 2018,Jan,8; 2017,Jan,8; 2016,Jan,13; 2015,Jan,16

86705 **IgM antibody**
0.00 0.00 FUD XXX
AMA: 2020,OctSE,1; 2020,AugSE,1; 2020,AugSE,1; 2020,AugSE,1; 2018,Jan,8; 2017,Jan,8; 2016,Jan,13; 2015,Jan,16

86706 **Hepatitis B surface antibody (HBsAb)**
0.00 0.00 FUD XXX
AMA: 2020,OctSE,1; 2020,AugSE,1; 2020,AugSE,1; 2020,AugSE,1

86707 **Hepatitis Be antibody (HBeAb)**
0.00 0.00 FUD XXX
AMA: 2020,OctSE,1; 2020,AugSE,1; 2020,AugSE,1; 2020,AugSE,1

86708 **Hepatitis A antibody (HAAb)**
0.00 0.00 FUD XXX
AMA: 2020,OctSE,1; 2020,AugSE,1; 2020,AugSE,1; 2020,AugSE,1; 2018,Jan,8; 2017,Jan,8; 2016,Jan,13; 2015,Jan,16

86709 **Hepatitis A antibody (HAAb), IgM antibody**
0.00 0.00 FUD XXX
AMA: 2020,OctSE,1; 2020,AugSE,1; 2020,AugSE,1; 2020,AugSE,1; 2018,Jan,8; 2017,Jan,8; 2016,Jan,13; 2015,Jan,16

86710 **Antibody; influenza virus**
0.00 0.00 FUD XXX
AMA: 2020,OctSE,1; 2020,AugSE,1; 2020,AugSE,1; 2020,AugSE,1; 2018,Jan,8; 2017,Jan,8; 2016,Jan,13; 2015,Jan,16

86711 **JC (John Cunningham) virus**
0.00 0.00 FUD XXX
AMA: 2020,OctSE,1; 2020,AugSE,1; 2020,AugSE,1; 2020,AugSE,1

86713 **Legionella**
0.00 0.00 FUD XXX
AMA: 2020,OctSE,1; 2020,AugSE,1; 2020,AugSE,1; 2020,AugSE,1

86717 **Leishmania**
0.00 0.00 FUD XXX
AMA: 2020,OctSE,1; 2020,AugSE,1; 2020,AugSE,1; 2020,AugSE,1

86720 **Leptospira**
0.00 0.00 FUD XXX
AMA: 2020,OctSE,1; 2020,AugSE,1; 2020,AugSE,1; 2020,AugSE,1

86723 **Listeria monocytogenes**
0.00 0.00 FUD XXX
AMA: 2020,OctSE,1; 2020,AugSE,1; 2020,AugSE,1; 2020,AugSE,1

86727 **lymphocytic choriomeningitis**
0.00 0.00 FUD XXX
AMA: 2020,OctSE,1; 2020,AugSE,1; 2020,AugSE,1; 2020,AugSE,1

86732 **mucormycosis**
0.00 0.00 FUD XXX
AMA: 2020,OctSE,1; 2020,AugSE,1; 2020,AugSE,1; 2020,AugSE,1

86735 **mumps**
0.00 0.00 FUD XXX
AMA: 2020,OctSE,1; 2020,AugSE,1; 2020,AugSE,1; 2020,AugSE,1; 2018,Jan,8; 2017,Jan,8; 2016,Jan,13; 2015,Jan,16

86738 **mycoplasma**
0.00 0.00 FUD XXX
AMA: 2020,OctSE,1; 2020,AugSE,1; 2020,AugSE,1; 2020,AugSE,1

86741 **Neisseria meningitidis**
0.00 0.00 FUD XXX
AMA: 2020,OctSE,1; 2020,AugSE,1; 2020,AugSE,1; 2020,AugSE,1

86744 **Nocardia**
0.00 0.00 FUD XXX
AMA: 2020,OctSE,1; 2020,AugSE,1; 2020,AugSE,1; 2020,AugSE,1

86747 **parvovirus**
0.00 0.00 FUD XXX
AMA: 2020,OctSE,1; 2020,AugSE,1; 2020,AugSE,1; 2020,AugSE,1

86750 **Plasmodium (malaria)**
0.00 0.00 FUD XXX
AMA: 2020,OctSE,1; 2020,AugSE,1; 2020,AugSE,1; 2020,AugSE,1

86753 **protozoa, not elsewhere specified**
0.00 0.00 FUD XXX
AMA: 2020,OctSE,1; 2020,AugSE,1; 2020,AugSE,1; 2020,AugSE,1

86756 **respiratory syncytial virus**
0.00 0.00 FUD XXX
AMA: 2020,OctSE,1; 2020,AugSE,1; 2020,AugSE,1; 2020,AugSE,1

86757 **Rickettsia**
0.00 0.00 FUD XXX
AMA: 2020,OctSE,1; 2020,AugSE,1; 2020,AugSE,1; 2020,AugSE,1

86759 **rotavirus**
0.00 0.00 FUD XXX
AMA: 2020,OctSE,1; 2020,AugSE,1; 2020,AugSE,1; 2020,AugSE,1

86762 **rubella**
0.00 0.00 FUD XXX
AMA: 2020,OctSE,1; 2020,AugSE,1; 2020,AugSE,1; 2020,AugSE,1

86765 **rubeola**
0.00 0.00 FUD XXX
AMA: 2020,OctSE,1; 2020,AugSE,1; 2020,AugSE,1; 2020,AugSE,1

86768 **Salmonella**
0.00 0.00 FUD XXX
AMA: 2020,OctSE,1; 2020,AugSE,1; 2020,AugSE,1; 2020,AugSE,1

● **86769** **severe acute respiratory syndrome coronavirus 2 (SARS-CoV-2) (Coronavirus disease [COVID-19])**
EXCLUDES *Antibody, severe acute respiratory syndrome coronavirus 2 (SARS-CoV-2) (coronavirus disease [COVID-19]), includes titer(s) (0224U)*
Severe acute respiratory syndrome coronavirus 2 (SARS-CoV-2) (coronavirus disease [COVID-19]) antibody testing via single-step method ([86328])
AMA: 2020,SepSE,1; 2020,OctSE,1; 2020,AugSE,1; 2020,SepSE,1; 2020,AugSE,1; 2020,AugSE,1; 2020,May,3; 2020,JuneSE,1

86771 **Shigella**
0.00 0.00 FUD XXX
AMA: 2020,OctSE,1; 2020,AugSE,1; 2020,AugSE,1; 2020,AugSE,1

86774 **tetanus**
0.00 0.00 FUD XXX
AMA: 2020,OctSE,1; 2020,AugSE,1; 2020,AugSE,1; 2020,AugSE,1

86777 **Toxoplasma**
0.00 0.00 FUD XXX
AMA: 2020,OctSE,1; 2020,AugSE,1; 2020,AugSE,1; 2020,AugSE,1

86778 **Toxoplasma, IgM**
0.00 0.00 FUD XXX
AMA: 2020,OctSE,1; 2020,AugSE,1; 2020,AugSE,1; 2020,AugSE,1

86780 **Treponema pallidum**
EXCLUDES *Nontreponemal antibody analysis syphilis testing (86592-86593)*
0.00 0.00 FUD XXX
AMA: 2020,OctSE,1; 2020,AugSE,1; 2020,AugSE,1; 2020,AugSE,1

86784 **Trichinella**
0.00 0.00 FUD XXX
AMA: 2020,OctSE,1; 2020,AugSE,1; 2020,AugSE,1; 2020,AugSE,1

86787 **varicella-zoster**
0.00 0.00 FUD XXX
AMA: 2020,OctSE,1; 2020,AugSE,1; 2020,AugSE,1; 2020,AugSE,1

86788 **West Nile virus, IgM**
0.00 0.00 FUD XXX
AMA: 2020,OctSE,1; 2020,AugSE,1; 2020,AugSE,1; 2020,AugSE,1

86789 **West Nile virus**
0.00 0.00 FUD XXX
AMA: 2020,OctSE,1; 2020,AugSE,1; 2020,AugSE,1; 2020,AugSE,1

86790 **virus, not elsewhere specified**
0.00 0.00 FUD XXX
AMA: 2020,OctSE,1; 2020,AugSE,1; 2020,AugSE,1; 2020,AugSE,1

86793 **Yersinia**
0.00 0.00 FUD XXX
AMA: 2020,OctSE,1; 2020,AugSE,1; 2020,AugSE,1; 2020,AugSE,1

86794 **Zika virus, IgM**
0.00 0.00 FUD XXX
AMA: 2020,OctSE,1; 2020,AugSE,1; 2020,AugSE,1; 2020,AugSE,1

86800 **Thyroglobulin antibody**
EXCLUDES *Thyroglobulin (84432)*
0.00 0.00 FUD XXX
AMA: 2020,OctSE,1; 2020,AugSE,1; 2020,AugSE,1; 2020,AugSE,1

86803 **Hepatitis C antibody;**
0.00 0.00 FUD XXX
AMA: 2020,OctSE,1; 2020,AugSE,1; 2020,AugSE,1; 2020,AugSE,1

86804 **confirmatory test (eg, immunoblot)**
0.00 0.00 FUD XXX
AMA: 2020,OctSE,1; 2020,AugSE,1; 2020,AugSE,1; 2020,AugSE,1; 2018,Jan,8; 2017,Jan,8; 2016,Jan,13; 2015,Jan,16

86805-86808 Pre-Transplant Antibody Cross Matching

86805 **Lymphocytotoxicity assay, visual crossmatch; with titration**
0.00 0.00 FUD XXX
AMA: 2018,Jan,8; 2017,Jan,8; 2016,Jan,13; 2015,Jan,16

86806 **without titration**
0.00 0.00 FUD XXX
AMA: 2005,Aug,7-8; 2005,Jul,11-12

86807 **Serum screening for cytotoxic percent reactive antibody (PRA); standard method**
0.00 0.00 FUD XXX
AMA: 2018,Jan,8; 2017,Jan,8; 2016,Jan,13; 2015,Jan,16

86808 **quick method**
0.00 0.00 FUD XXX
AMA: 2018,Jan,8; 2017,Jan,8; 2016,Jan,13; 2015,Jan,16

86812-86826 Histocompatibility Testing

CMS: 100-03,110.23 Stem Cell Transplantation; 100-03,190.1 Histocompatibility Testing; 100-04,3,90.3 Stem Cell Transplantation; 100-04,3,90.3.1 Allogeneic Stem Cell Transplantation; 100-04,3,90.3.3 Billing for Allogeneic Stem Cell Transplants; 100-04,32,90 Billing for Stem Cell Transplantation; 100-04,4,231.11 Billing for Allogeneic Stem Cell Transplants

EXCLUDES *HLA typing by molecular pathology techniques (81370-81383)*

86812 **HLA typing; A, B, or C (eg, A10, B7, B27), single antigen**
0.00 0.00 FUD XXX
AMA: 2018,Jan,8; 2017,Jan,8; 2016,Jan,13; 2015,Jan,16

86813 **A, B, or C, multiple antigens**
0.00 0.00 FUD XXX
AMA: 2018,Jan,8; 2017,Jan,8; 2016,Jan,13; 2015,Jan,16

86816 **DR/DQ, single antigen**
0.00 0.00 FUD XXX
AMA: 2018,Jan,8; 2017,Jan,8; 2016,Jan,13; 2015,Jan,16

86817 **DR/DQ, multiple antigens**
0.00 0.00 FUD XXX
AMA: 2018,Jan,8; 2017,Jan,8; 2016,Jan,13; 2015,Jan,16

86821 **lymphocyte culture, mixed (MLC)**
0.00 0.00 FUD XXX
AMA: 2018,Jan,8; 2017,Jan,8; 2016,Jan,13; 2015,Jan,16

86825 **Human leukocyte antigen (HLA) crossmatch, non-cytotoxic (eg, using flow cytometry); first serum sample or dilution**

INCLUDES Autologous HLA crossmatch

EXCLUDES *B cells (86355)*
Flow cytometry (88184-88189)
Lymphocytotoxicity visual crossmatch (86805-86806)
T cells (86359)

0.00 0.00 **FUD** XXX Q

AMA: 2020,Aug,14

\+ **86826** **each additional serum sample or sample dilution (List separately in addition to primary procedure)**

INCLUDES Autologous HLA crossmatch

EXCLUDES *B cells (86355)*
Flow cytometry (88184-88189)
Lymphocytotoxicity visual crossmatch (86805-86806)
T cells (86359)

Code first (86825)

0.00 0.00 **FUD** XXX Q

AMA: 2020,Aug,14

86828-86849 HLA Antibodies

86828 **Antibody to human leukocyte antigens (HLA), solid phase assays (eg, microspheres or beads, ELISA, flow cytometry); qualitative assessment of the presence or absence of antibody(ies) to HLA Class I and Class II HLA antigens**

Code also solid phase testing, untreated and treated specimens, either class of HLA after treatment (86828-86833)

0.00 0.00 **FUD** XXX Q

86829 **qualitative assessment of the presence or absence of antibody(ies) to HLA Class I or Class II HLA antigens**

Code also solid phase testing, untreated and treated specimens, either class of HLA after treatment (86828-86833)

0.00 0.00 **FUD** XXX Q

86830 **antibody identification by qualitative panel using complete HLA phenotypes, HLA Class I**

Code also solid phase testing, untreated and treated specimens, either class of HLA after treatment (86828-86833)

0.00 0.00 **FUD** XXX Q

86831 **antibody identification by qualitative panel using complete HLA phenotypes, HLA Class II**

Code also solid phase testing, untreated and treated specimens, either class of HLA after treatment (86828-86833)

0.00 0.00 **FUD** XXX Q

86832 **high definition qualitative panel for identification of antibody specificities (eg, individual antigen per bead methodology), HLA Class I**

Code also solid phase testing, untreated and treated specimens, either class of HLA after treatment (86828-86833)

0.00 0.00 **FUD** XXX Q

86833 **high definition qualitative panel for identification of antibody specificities (eg, individual antigen per bead methodology), HLA Class II**

Code also solid phase testing, untreated and treated specimens, either class of HLA after treatment (86828-86833)

0.00 0.00 **FUD** XXX Q

86834 **semi-quantitative panel (eg, titer), HLA Class I**

0.00 0.00 **FUD** XXX Q

86835 **semi-quantitative panel (eg, titer), HLA Class II**

0.00 0.00 **FUD** XXX Q

86849 **Unlisted immunology procedure**

0.00 0.00 **FUD** XXX N

AMA: 2019,Dec,12; 2018,Jan,8; 2017,Jan,8; 2016,Jan,13; 2015,Jan,16

86850-86999 Transfusion Services

EXCLUDES *Apheresis (36511-36512)*
Therapeutic phlebotomy (99195)

86850 **Antibody screen, RBC, each serum technique**

0.00 0.00 **FUD** XXX Q1

AMA: 2020,AugSE,1; 2020,AugSE,1; 2020,AugSE,1; 2018,Jan,8; 2017,Jan,8; 2016,Jan,13; 2015,Jan,16

86860 **Antibody elution (RBC), each elution**

0.00 0.00 **FUD** XXX Q1

AMA: 2020,AugSE,1; 2020,AugSE,1; 2020,AugSE,1

86870 **Antibody identification, RBC antibodies, each panel for each serum technique**

0.00 0.00 **FUD** XXX Q2

AMA: 2020,AugSE,1; 2020,AugSE,1; 2020,AugSE,1; 2018,Jan,8; 2017,Jan,8; 2016,Jan,13; 2015,Jan,16

86880 **Antihuman globulin test (Coombs test); direct, each antiserum**

0.00 0.00 **FUD** XXX Q1

AMA: 2005,Aug,7-8; 2005,Jul,11-12

86885 **indirect, qualitative, each reagent red cell**

0.00 0.00 **FUD** XXX Q1

AMA: 2018,Jan,8; 2017,Jan,8; 2016,Jan,13; 2015,Jan,16

86886 **indirect, each antibody titer**

EXCLUDES *Indirect antihuman globulin (Coombs) test for RBC antibody identification using reagent red cell panels (86870)*
Indirect antihuman globulin (Coombs) test for RBC antibody screening (86850)

0.00 0.00 **FUD** XXX Q1

AMA: 2018,Jan,8; 2017,Jan,8; 2016,Jan,13; 2015,Jan,16

86890 **Autologous blood or component, collection processing and storage; predeposited**

0.00 0.00 **FUD** XXX Q1

AMA: 2018,Jan,8; 2017,Jan,8; 2016,Jan,13; 2015,Jan,16

86891 **intra- or postoperative salvage**

0.00 0.00 **FUD** XXX Q1

AMA: 2005,Aug,7-8; 2005,Jul,11-12

86900 **Blood typing, serologic; ABO**

0.00 0.00 **FUD** XXX Q1

AMA: 2005,Jul,11-12; 2005,Aug,7-8

86901 **Rh (D)**

0.00 0.00 **FUD** XXX Q1

AMA: 2018,Jan,8; 2017,Jan,8; 2016,Jan,13; 2015,Jan,16

86902 **antigen testing of donor blood using reagent serum, each antigen test**

Code also one time for each antigen, each unit blood, when multiple units tested for same antigen

0.00 0.00 **FUD** XXX Q1

AMA: 2010,Dec,7-10

86904 **antigen screening for compatible unit using patient serum, per unit screened**

0.00 0.00 **FUD** XXX Q1

AMA: 2005,Aug,7-8; 2005,Jul,11-12

86905 **RBC antigens, other than ABO or Rh (D), each**

0.00 0.00 **FUD** XXX Q1

AMA: 2005,Jul,11-12; 2005,Aug,7-8

86906 **Rh phenotyping, complete**

EXCLUDES *Reporting molecular pathology procedures for human erythrocyte antigen typing (81403)*

0.00 0.00 **FUD** XXX Q1

AMA: 2005,Jul,11-12; 2005,Aug,7-8

86910 **Blood typing, for paternity testing, per individual; ABO, Rh and MN**

0.00 0.00 **FUD** XXX E

AMA: 2005,Jul,11-12; 2005,Aug,7-8

86911 **each additional antigen system**
0.00 0.00 FUD XXX E
AMA: 2005,Jul,11-12; 2005,Aug,7-8

86920 **Compatibility test each unit; immediate spin technique**
0.00 0.00 FUD XXX Q1
AMA: 2018,Jan,8; 2017,Jan,8; 2016,Jan,13; 2015,Jan,16

86921 **incubation technique**
0.00 0.00 FUD XXX Q1
AMA: 2018,Jan,8; 2017,Jan,8; 2016,Jan,13; 2015,Jan,16

86922 **antiglobulin technique**
0.00 0.00 FUD XXX Q1
AMA: 2018,Jan,8; 2017,Jan,8; 2016,Jan,13; 2015,Jan,16

86923 **electronic**
EXCLUDES *Other compatibility test techniques (86920-86922)*
0.00 0.00 FUD XXX Q1
AMA: 2018,Jan,8; 2017,Jan,8; 2016,Jan,13; 2015,Jan,16

86927 **Fresh frozen plasma, thawing, each unit**
0.00 0.00 FUD XXX S
AMA: 2005,Aug,7-8; 2005,Jul,11-12

86930 **Frozen blood, each unit; freezing (includes preparation)**
0.00 0.00 FUD XXX Q1
AMA: 2018,Jan,8; 2017,Jan,8; 2016,Jan,13; 2015,Jan,16

86931 **thawing**
0.00 0.00 FUD XXX Q1
AMA: 2018,Jan,8; 2017,Jan,8; 2016,Jan,13; 2015,Jan,16

86932 **freezing (includes preparation) and thawing**
0.00 0.00 FUD XXX Q1
AMA: 2018,Jan,8; 2017,Jan,8; 2016,Jan,13; 2015,Jan,16

86940 **Hemolysins and agglutinins; auto, screen, each**
0.00 0.00 FUD XXX Q
AMA: 2005,Aug,7-8; 2005,Jul,11-12

86941 **incubated**
0.00 0.00 FUD XXX Q
AMA: 2005,Jul,11-12; 2005,Aug,7-8

86945 **Irradiation of blood product, each unit**
0.00 0.00 FUD XXX Q1
AMA: 2018,Jan,8; 2017,Jan,8; 2016,Jan,13; 2015,Jan,16

86950 **Leukocyte transfusion**
EXCLUDES *Infusion allogeneic lymphocytes (38242)*
Leukapheresis (36511)
0.00 0.00 FUD XXX Q1
AMA: 2018,Jan,8; 2017,Jan,8; 2016,Jan,13; 2015,Jan,16

86960 **Volume reduction of blood or blood product (eg, red blood cells or platelets), each unit**
0.00 0.00 FUD XXX Q1
AMA: 2018,Jan,8; 2017,Jan,8; 2016,Jan,13; 2015,Jan,16

86965 **Pooling of platelets or other blood products**
EXCLUDES *Autologous WBC injection (0481T)*
Injection platelet rich plasma (0232T)
0.00 0.00 FUD XXX Q1
AMA: 2018,Jan,8; 2017,Jan,8; 2016,Jan,13; 2015,Jan,16

86970 **Pretreatment of RBCs for use in RBC antibody detection, identification, and/or compatibility testing; incubation with chemical agents or drugs, each**
0.00 0.00 FUD XXX Q1
AMA: 2005,Jul,11-12; 2005,Aug,7-8

86971 **incubation with enzymes, each**
0.00 0.00 FUD XXX Q1
AMA: 2005,Jul,11-12; 2005,Aug,7-8

86972 **by density gradient separation**
0.00 0.00 FUD XXX Q1
AMA: 2005,Jul,11-12; 2005,Aug,7-8

86975 **Pretreatment of serum for use in RBC antibody identification; incubation with drugs, each**
0.00 0.00 FUD XXX Q1
AMA: 2005,Jul,11-12; 2005,Aug,7-8

86976 **by dilution**
0.00 0.00 FUD XXX Q1
AMA: 2005,Jul,11-12; 2005,Aug,7-8

86977 **incubation with inhibitors, each**
0.00 0.00 FUD XXX Q1
AMA: 2005,Jul,11-12; 2005,Aug,7-8

86978 **by differential red cell absorption using patient RBCs or RBCs of known phenotype, each absorption**
0.00 0.00 FUD XXX Q1
AMA: 2005,Jul,11-12; 2005,Aug,7-8

86985 **Splitting of blood or blood products, each unit**
0.00 0.00 FUD XXX Q1
AMA: 2018,Jan,8; 2017,Jan,8; 2016,Jan,13; 2015,Jan,16

86999 **Unlisted transfusion medicine procedure**
0.00 0.00 FUD XXX Q1
AMA: 2018,Jan,8; 2017,Jan,8; 2016,Jan,13; 2015,Jan,16

87003-87118 Identification of Microorganisms

INCLUDES Bacteriology, mycology, parasitology, and virology
EXCLUDES *Additional tests using molecular probes, chromatography, nucleic acid resequencing, or immunologic techniques (87140-87158)*
Code also modifier 59 for multiple specimens or sites
Code also modifier 91 for repeat procedures performed on same day

87003 **Animal inoculation, small animal, with observation and dissection**
0.00 0.00 FUD XXX Q
AMA: 2005,Aug,7-8; 2005,Jul,11-12

87015 **Concentration (any type), for infectious agents**
EXCLUDES *Direct smear for ova and parasites (87177)*
0.00 0.00 FUD XXX Q
AMA: 2005,Aug,7-8; 2005,Jul,11-12

87040 **Culture, bacterial; blood, aerobic, with isolation and presumptive identification of isolates (includes anaerobic culture, if appropriate)**
0.00 0.00 FUD XXX Q
AMA: 2018,Jan,8; 2017,Jan,8; 2016,Jan,13; 2015,Jan,16

87045 **stool, aerobic, with isolation and preliminary examination (eg, KIA, LIA), Salmonella and Shigella species**
0.00 0.00 FUD XXX Q
AMA: 2005,Aug,7-8; 2005,Jul,11-12

87046 **stool, aerobic, additional pathogens, isolation and presumptive identification of isolates, each plate**
0.00 0.00 FUD XXX Q
AMA: 2018,Jan,8; 2017,Jan,8; 2016,Jan,13; 2015,Jan,16

87070 **any other source except urine, blood or stool, aerobic, with isolation and presumptive identification of isolates**
EXCLUDES *Urine (87088)*
0.00 0.00 FUD XXX Q
AMA: 2018,Jan,8; 2017,Jan,8; 2016,Jan,13; 2015,Jan,16

87071 **quantitative, aerobic with isolation and presumptive identification of isolates, any source except urine, blood or stool**
EXCLUDES *Urine (87088)*
0.00 0.00 FUD XXX Q
AMA: 2018,Jan,8; 2017,Jan,8; 2016,Jan,13; 2015,Jan,16

87073 **quantitative, anaerobic with isolation and presumptive identification of isolates, any source except urine, blood or stool**
EXCLUDES *Definitive identification isolates (87076, 87077)*
Typing isolates (87140-87158)
0.00 0.00 FUD XXX Q
AMA: 2018,Jan,8; 2017,Jan,8; 2016,Jan,13; 2015,Jan,16

87075 any source, except blood, anaerobic with isolation and presumptive identification of isolates
🔧 0.00 ⚗ 0.00 **FUD** XXX [Q][▣]
AMA: 2005,Aug,7-8; 2005,Jul,11-12

87076 anaerobic isolate, additional methods required for definitive identification, each isolate
🔧 0.00 ⚗ 0.00 **FUD** XXX [Q][▣]
AMA: 2018,Jan,8; 2017,Jan,8; 2016,Jan,13; 2015,Jan,16

87077 aerobic isolate, additional methods required for definitive identification, each isolate
🔧 0.00 ⚗ 0.00 **FUD** XXX [X][Q][▣]
AMA: 2018,Jan,8; 2017,Jan,8; 2016,Jan,13; 2015,Jan,16

87081 Culture, presumptive, pathogenic organisms, screening only;
🔧 0.00 ⚗ 0.00 **FUD** XXX [Q][▣]
AMA: 2018,Jan,8; 2017,Jan,8; 2016,Jan,13; 2015,Jan,16

87084 with colony estimation from density chart
🔧 0.00 ⚗ 0.00 **FUD** XXX [Q][▣]
AMA: 2005,Aug,7-8; 2005,Jul,11-12

87086 Culture, bacterial; quantitative colony count, urine
🔧 0.00 ⚗ 0.00 **FUD** XXX [Q][▣]
AMA: 2018,Jan,8; 2017,Jan,8; 2016,Jan,13; 2015,Jan,16

87088 with isolation and presumptive identification of each isolate, urine
🔧 0.00 ⚗ 0.00 **FUD** XXX [Q][▣]
AMA: 2018,Jan,8; 2017,Jan,8; 2016,Jan,13; 2015,Jan,16

87101 Culture, fungi (mold or yeast) isolation, with presumptive identification of isolates; skin, hair, or nail
🔧 0.00 ⚗ 0.00 **FUD** XXX [Q][▣]
AMA: 2018,Jan,8; 2017,Jan,8; 2016,Jan,13; 2015,Jan,16

87102 other source (except blood)
🔧 0.00 ⚗ 0.00 **FUD** XXX [Q][▣]
AMA: 2005,Aug,7-8; 2005,Jul,11-12

87103 blood
🔧 0.00 ⚗ 0.00 **FUD** XXX [Q][▣]
AMA: 2005,Aug,7-8; 2005,Jul,11-12

87106 Culture, fungi, definitive identification, each organism; yeast
🔧 0.00 ⚗ 0.00 **FUD** XXX [Q][▣]
AMA: 2005,Aug,7-8; 2005,Jul,11-12

87107 mold
🔧 0.00 ⚗ 0.00 **FUD** XXX [Q][▣]
AMA: 2005,Aug,7-8; 2005,Jul,11-12

87109 Culture, mycoplasma, any source
🔧 0.00 ⚗ 0.00 **FUD** XXX [Q][▣]
AMA: 2005,Aug,7-8; 2005,Jul,11-12

87110 Culture, chlamydia, any source
EXCLUDES Immunofluorescence staining shell vials (87140)
🔧 0.00 ⚗ 0.00 **FUD** XXX [A][▣]
AMA: 2005,Aug,7-8; 2005,Jul,11-12

87116 Culture, tubercle or other acid-fast bacilli (eg, TB, AFB, mycobacteria) any source, with isolation and presumptive identification of isolates
EXCLUDES Concentration (87015)
🔧 0.00 ⚗ 0.00 **FUD** XXX [Q][▣]
AMA: 2005,Aug,7-8; 2005,Jul,11-12

87118 Culture, mycobacterial, definitive identification, each isolate
🔧 0.00 ⚗ 0.00 **FUD** XXX [Q][▣]
AMA: 2005,Aug,7-8; 2005,Jul,11-12

87140-87158 Additional Culture Typing Techniques

INCLUDES Bacteriology, mycology, parasitology, and virology
EXCLUDES *Reporting molecular procedure codes as substitute for codes in this range (81105-81183 [81173, 81174, 81200, 81201, 81202, 81203, 81204], 81400-81408, [81479])*
Code also definitive identification
Code also modifier 59 for multiple specimens or sites
Code also modifier 91 for repeat procedures performed on same day

87140 Culture, typing; immunofluorescent method, each antiserum
🔧 0.00 ⚗ 0.00 **FUD** XXX [Q][▣]
AMA: 2020,OctSE,1; 2018,Jan,8; 2017,Jan,8; 2016,Jan,13; 2015,Jan,16

87143 gas liquid chromatography (GLC) or high pressure liquid chromatography (HPLC) method
🔧 0.00 ⚗ 0.00 **FUD** XXX [Q][▣]
AMA: 2020,OctSE,1

87147 immunologic method, other than immunofluorescence (eg, agglutination grouping), per antiserum
🔧 0.00 ⚗ 0.00 **FUD** XXX [Q][▣]
AMA: 2020,OctSE,1; 2018,Jan,8; 2017,Jan,8; 2016,Jan,13; 2015,Jan,16

87149 identification by nucleic acid (DNA or RNA) probe, direct probe technique, per culture or isolate, each organism probed
🔧 0.00 ⚗ 0.00 **FUD** XXX [Q][▣]
AMA: 2020,OctSE,1; 2018,Jan,8; 2017,Jan,8; 2016,Jan,13; 2015,Jan,16

87150 identification by nucleic acid (DNA or RNA) probe, amplified probe technique, per culture or isolate, each organism probed
🔧 0.00 ⚗ 0.00 **FUD** XXX [Q][▣]
AMA: 2020,OctSE,1; 2018,Jan,8; 2017,Jan,8; 2016,Jan,13; 2015,Jan,16

87152 identification by pulse field gel typing
🔧 0.00 ⚗ 0.00 **FUD** XXX [Q][▣]
AMA: 2020,OctSE,1; 2018,Jan,8; 2017,Jan,8; 2016,Jan,13; 2015,Jan,16

87153 identification by nucleic acid sequencing method, each isolate (eg, sequencing of the 16S rRNA gene)
🔧 0.00 ⚗ 0.00 **FUD** XXX [Q][▣]
AMA: 2020,OctSE,1; 2018,Jan,8; 2017,Jan,8; 2016,Jan,13; 2015,Jan,16

87158 other methods
🔧 0.00 ⚗ 0.00 **FUD** XXX [Q][▣]
AMA: 2020,OctSE,1; 2018,Jan,8; 2017,Jan,8; 2016,Jan,13; 2015,Jan,16

87164-87255 Identification of Organism from Primary Source and Sensitivity Studies

INCLUDES Bacteriology, mycology, parasitology, and virology
EXCLUDES *Additional tests using molecular probes, chromatography, or immunologic techniques (87140-87158)*
Code also modifier 59 for multiple specimens or sites
Code also modifier 91 for repeat procedures performed on same day

87164 Dark field examination, any source (eg, penile, vaginal, oral, skin); includes specimen collection
🔧 0.00 ⚗ 0.00 **FUD** XXX [Q][80][▣]
AMA: 2005,Jul,11-12; 2005,Aug,7-8

87166 without collection
🔧 0.00 ⚗ 0.00 **FUD** XXX [Q][▣]
AMA: 2005,Aug,7-8; 2005,Jul,11-12

87168 Macroscopic examination; arthropod
🔧 0.00 ⚗ 0.00 **FUD** XXX [Q][▣]
AMA: 2005,Aug,7-8; 2005,Jul,11-12

87169 parasite
🔧 0.00 ⚗ 0.00 **FUD** XXX [Q][▣]
AMA: 2005,Aug,7-8; 2005,Jul,11-12

● New Code ▲ Revised Code ○ Reinstated ● New Web Release ▲ Revised Web Release + Add-on Unlisted Not Covered # Resequenced
50 Optum Mod 50 Exempt ⊘ AMA Mod 51 Exempt 51 Optum Mod 51 Exempt 63 Mod 63 Exempt ⁄ Non-FDA Drug ★ Telemedicine M Maternity A Age Edit

87172 **Pinworm exam (eg, cellophane tape prep)**
0.00 0.00 FUD XXX
AMA: 2005,Aug,7-8; 2005,Jul,11-12

87176 **Homogenization, tissue, for culture**
0.00 0.00 FUD XXX
AMA: 2005,Aug,7-8; 2005,Jul,11-12

87177 **Ova and parasites, direct smears, concentration and identification**
EXCLUDES *Coccidia or microsporidia exam (87207)*
Complex special stain (trichrome, iron hematoxylin) (87209)
Concentration for infectious agents (87015)
Direct smears from primary source (87207)
Nucleic acid probes in cytologic material (88365)
0.00 0.00 FUD XXX
AMA: 2018,Jan,8; 2017,Jan,8; 2016,Jan,13; 2015,Jan,16

87181 **Susceptibility studies, antimicrobial agent; agar dilution method, per agent (eg, antibiotic gradient strip)**
0.00 0.00 FUD XXX
AMA: 2018,Jan,8; 2017,Jan,8; 2016,Jan,13; 2015,Jan,16

87184 **disk method, per plate (12 or fewer agents)**
0.00 0.00 FUD XXX
AMA: 2018,Jan,8; 2017,Jan,8; 2016,Jan,13; 2015,Jan,16

87185 **enzyme detection (eg, beta lactamase), per enzyme**
0.00 0.00 FUD XXX
AMA: 2018,Jan,8; 2017,Jan,8; 2016,Jan,13; 2015,Jan,16

87186 **microdilution or agar dilution (minimum inhibitory concentration [MIC] or breakpoint), each multi-antimicrobial, per plate**
0.00 0.00 FUD XXX
AMA: 2018,Jan,8; 2017,Jan,8; 2016,Jan,13; 2015,Jan,16

\+ **87187** **microdilution or agar dilution, minimum lethal concentration (MLC), each plate (List separately in addition to code for primary procedure)**
Code first (87186, 87188)
0.00 0.00 FUD XXX
AMA: 2018,Jan,8; 2017,Jan,8; 2016,Jan,13; 2015,Jan,16

87188 **macrobroth dilution method, each agent**
0.00 0.00 FUD XXX
AMA: 2018,Jan,8; 2017,Jan,8; 2016,Jan,13; 2015,Jan,16

87190 **mycobacteria, proportion method, each agent**
EXCLUDES *Other mycobacterial susceptibility studies (87181, 87184, 87186, 87188)*
0.00 0.00 FUD XXX
AMA: 2005,Aug,7-8; 2005,Jul,11-12

87197 **Serum bactericidal titer (Schlichter test)**
0.00 0.00 FUD XXX
AMA: 2005,Aug,7-8; 2005,Jul,11-12

87205 **Smear, primary source with interpretation; Gram or Giemsa stain for bacteria, fungi, or cell types**
0.00 0.00 FUD XXX
AMA: 2018,Jan,8; 2017,Jan,8; 2016,Jan,13; 2015,Jan,16

87206 **fluorescent and/or acid fast stain for bacteria, fungi, parasites, viruses or cell types**
0.00 0.00 FUD XXX
AMA: 2005,Aug,7-8; 2005,Jul,11-12

87207 **special stain for inclusion bodies or parasites (eg, malaria, coccidia, microsporidia, trypanosomes, herpes viruses)**
EXCLUDES *Direct smears with concentration and identification (87177)*
Fat, fibers, meat, nasal eosinophils, starch (89049-89240)
Thick smear preparation (87015)
0.00 0.00 FUD XXX 80
AMA: 2018,Jan,8; 2017,Jan,8; 2016,Jan,13; 2015,Jan,16

87209 **complex special stain (eg, trichrome, iron hemotoxylin) for ova and parasites**
0.00 0.00 FUD XXX
AMA: 2018,Jan,8; 2017,Jan,8; 2016,Jan,13; 2015,Jan,16

87210 **wet mount for infectious agents (eg, saline, India ink, KOH preps)**
EXCLUDES *KOH evaluation skin, hair, or nails (87220)*
0.00 0.00 FUD XXX
AMA: 2018,Jan,8; 2017,Jan,8; 2016,May,13

87220 **Tissue examination by KOH slide of samples from skin, hair, or nails for fungi or ectoparasite ova or mites (eg, scabies)**
0.00 0.00 FUD XXX
AMA: 2005,Aug,7-8; 2005,Jul,11-12

87230 **Toxin or antitoxin assay, tissue culture (eg, Clostridium difficile toxin)**
0.00 0.00 FUD XXX
AMA: 2005,Aug,7-8; 2005,Jul,11-12

87250 **Virus isolation; inoculation of embryonated eggs, or small animal, includes observation and dissection**
0.00 0.00 FUD XXX
AMA: 2020,OctSE,1

87252 **tissue culture inoculation, observation, and presumptive identification by cytopathic effect**
0.00 0.00 FUD XXX
AMA: 2005,Aug,7-8; 2005,Jul,11-12

87253 **tissue culture, additional studies or definitive identification (eg, hemabsorption, neutralization, immunofluorescence stain), each isolate**
EXCLUDES *Electron microscopy (88348)*
Inclusion bodies in:
Fluids (88106)
Smears (87207-87210)
Tissue sections (88304-88309)
0.00 0.00 FUD XXX
AMA: 2005,Aug,7-8; 2005,Jul,11-12

87254 **centrifuge enhanced (shell vial) technique, includes identification with immunofluorescence stain, each virus**
Code also (87252)
0.00 0.00 FUD XXX
AMA: 2018,Jan,8; 2017,Jan,8; 2016,Jan,13; 2015,Jan,16

87255 **including identification by non-immunologic method, other than by cytopathic effect (eg, virus specific enzymatic activity)**
0.00 0.00 FUD XXX
AMA: 2020,OctSE,1; 2018,Jan,8; 2017,Jan,8; 2016,Jan,13; 2015,Jan,16

87260-87300 Fluorescence Microscopy by Organism

INCLUDES Primary source only
EXCLUDES *Comparable tests on culture material (87140-87158)*
Identification antibodies (86602-86804)
Immunoassay techniques with direct/visual observation for infectious antigens (87260-87300)
Microscopic identification infectious agents via direct/indirect immunofluorescent assay (IFA) techniques (87301-87451, 87802-87899 [87806, 87811])
Nonspecific agent detection (87299, 87449, 87797-87799, 87899)
Code also modifier 59 for different species or strains reported by same code

87260 **Infectious agent antigen detection by immunofluorescent technique; adenovirus**
0.00 0.00 FUD XXX
AMA: 2020,OctSE,1; 2020,AugSE,1; 2020,AugSE,1; 2020,AugSE,1

87265 **Bordetella pertussis/parapertussis**
0.00 0.00 FUD XXX
AMA: 2020,OctSE,1; 2020,AugSE,1; 2020,AugSE,1; 2020,AugSE,1

87267 **Enterovirus, direct fluorescent antibody (DFA)**
0.00 0.00 FUD XXX
AMA: 2020,OctSE,1; 2020,AugSE,1; 2020,AugSE,1; 2020,AugSE,1; 2018,Jan,8; 2017,Jan,8; 2016,Jan,13; 2015,Jan,16

87269 **giardia**
0.00 0.00 **FUD** XXX
AMA: 2020,OctSE,1; 2020,AugSE,1; 2020,AugSE,1; 2020,AugSE,1

87270 **Chlamydia trachomatis**
0.00 0.00 **FUD** XXX
AMA: 2020,OctSE,1; 2020,AugSE,1; 2020,AugSE,1; 2020,AugSE,1

87271 **Cytomegalovirus, direct fluorescent antibody (DFA)**
0.00 0.00 **FUD** XXX
AMA: 2020,OctSE,1; 2020,AugSE,1; 2020,AugSE,1; 2020,AugSE,1; 2018,Jan,8; 2017,Jan,8; 2016,Jan,13; 2015,Jan,16

87272 **cryptosporidium**
0.00 0.00 **FUD** XXX
AMA: 2020,OctSE,1; 2020,AugSE,1; 2020,AugSE,1; 2020,AugSE,1

87273 **Herpes simplex virus type 2**
0.00 0.00 **FUD** XXX
AMA: 2020,OctSE,1; 2020,AugSE,1; 2020,AugSE,1; 2020,AugSE,1

87274 **Herpes simplex virus type 1**
0.00 0.00 **FUD** XXX
AMA: 2020,OctSE,1; 2020,AugSE,1; 2020,AugSE,1; 2020,AugSE,1

87275 **influenza B virus**
0.00 0.00 **FUD** XXX
AMA: 2020,OctSE,1; 2020,AugSE,1; 2020,AugSE,1; 2020,AugSE,1; 2018,Jan,8; 2017,Jan,8; 2016,Jan,13; 2015,Jan,16

87276 **influenza A virus**
0.00 0.00 **FUD** XXX
AMA: 2020,OctSE,1; 2020,AugSE,1; 2020,AugSE,1; 2020,AugSE,1; 2018,Jan,8; 2017,Jan,8; 2016,Jan,13; 2015,Jan,16

87278 **Legionella pneumophila**
0.00 0.00 **FUD** XXX
AMA: 2020,OctSE,1; 2020,AugSE,1; 2020,AugSE,1; 2020,AugSE,1

87279 **Parainfluenza virus, each type**
0.00 0.00 **FUD** XXX
AMA: 2020,OctSE,1; 2020,AugSE,1; 2020,AugSE,1; 2020,AugSE,1

87280 **respiratory syncytial virus**
0.00 0.00 **FUD** XXX
AMA: 2020,OctSE,1; 2020,AugSE,1; 2020,AugSE,1; 2020,AugSE,1

87281 **Pneumocystis carinii**
0.00 0.00 **FUD** XXX
AMA: 2020,OctSE,1; 2020,AugSE,1; 2020,AugSE,1; 2020,AugSE,1

87283 **Rubeola**
0.00 0.00 **FUD** XXX
AMA: 2020,OctSE,1; 2020,AugSE,1; 2020,AugSE,1; 2020,AugSE,1

87285 **Treponema pallidum**
0.00 0.00 **FUD** XXX
AMA: 2020,OctSE,1; 2020,AugSE,1; 2020,AugSE,1; 2020,AugSE,1

87290 **Varicella zoster virus**
0.00 0.00 **FUD** XXX
AMA: 2020,OctSE,1; 2020,AugSE,1; 2020,AugSE,1; 2020,AugSE,1

87299 **not otherwise specified, each organism**
0.00 0.00 **FUD** XXX
AMA: 2020,OctSE,1; 2020,AugSE,1; 2020,AugSE,1; 2020,AugSE,1; 2018,Jan,8; 2017,Jan,8; 2016,Jan,13; 2015,Jan,16

87300 **Infectious agent antigen detection by immunofluorescent technique, polyvalent for multiple organisms, each polyvalent antiserum**
EXCLUDES *Physician evaluation infectious disease agents by immunofluorescence (88346)*
0.00 0.00 **FUD** XXX
AMA: 2020,OctSE,1; 2020,AugSE,1; 2020,AugSE,1; 2020,AugSE,1

87301-87451 Enzyme Immunoassay Technique by Organism

INCLUDES Primary source only
EXCLUDES *Comparable tests on culture material (87140-87158)*
Identification antibodies (86602-86804)
Nonspecific agent detection (87449, 87797-87799, 87899)
Code also modifier 59 for different species or strains reported by same code

▲ **87301** **Infectious agent antigen detection by immunoassay technique, (eg, enzyme immunoassay [EIA], enzyme-linked immunosorbent assay [ELISA], fluorescence immunoassay [FIA], immunochemiluminometric assay [IMCA]) qualitative or semiquantitative; adenovirus enteric types 40/41**
0.00 0.00 **FUD** XXX
AMA: 2020,OctSE,1; 2020,AugSE,1; 2020,AugSE,1; 2020,AugSE,1; 2020,May,3; 2020,JuneSE,1; 2018,Jan,8; 2017,Jan,8; 2016,Jan,13; 2015,Jan,16

▲ **87305** **Aspergillus**
0.00 0.00 **FUD** XXX
AMA: 2020,OctSE,1; 2020,AugSE,1; 2020,AugSE,1; 2020,AugSE,1

▲ **87320** **Chlamydia trachomatis**
0.00 0.00 **FUD** XXX
AMA: 2020,OctSE,1; 2020,AugSE,1; 2020,AugSE,1; 2020,AugSE,1

▲ **87324** **Clostridium difficile toxin(s)**
0.00 0.00 **FUD** XXX
AMA: 2020,OctSE,1; 2020,AugSE,1; 2020,AugSE,1; 2020,AugSE,1

▲ **87327** **Cryptococcus neoformans**
EXCLUDES *Cryptococcus latex agglutination (86403)*
0.00 0.00 **FUD** XXX
AMA: 2020,OctSE,1; 2020,AugSE,1; 2020,AugSE,1; 2020,AugSE,1

▲ **87328** **cryptosporidium**
0.00 0.00 **FUD** XXX
AMA: 2020,OctSE,1; 2020,AugSE,1; 2020,AugSE,1; 2020,AugSE,1

▲ **87329** **giardia**
0.00 0.00 **FUD** XXX
AMA: 2020,OctSE,1; 2020,AugSE,1; 2020,AugSE,1; 2020,AugSE,1

▲ **87332** **cytomegalovirus**
0.00 0.00 **FUD** XXX
AMA: 2020,OctSE,1; 2020,AugSE,1; 2020,AugSE,1; 2020,AugSE,1

▲ **87335** **Escherichia coli 0157**
EXCLUDES *Giardia antigen (87329)*
0.00 0.00 **FUD** XXX
AMA: 2020,OctSE,1; 2020,AugSE,1; 2020,AugSE,1; 2020,AugSE,1

▲ **87336** **Entamoeba histolytica dispar group**
0.00 0.00 **FUD** XXX
AMA: 2020,OctSE,1; 2020,AugSE,1; 2020,AugSE,1; 2020,AugSE,1

▲ **87337** **Entamoeba histolytica group**
0.00 0.00 **FUD** XXX
AMA: 2020,OctSE,1; 2020,AugSE,1; 2020,AugSE,1; 2020,AugSE,1

▲ **87338** **Helicobacter pylori, stool**
0.00 0.00 **FUD** XXX
AMA: 2020,OctSE,1; 2020,AugSE,1; 2020,AugSE,1; 2020,AugSE,1; 2018,Jan,8; 2017,Jan,8; 2016,Jan,13; 2015,Jan,16

▲ **87339** **Helicobacter pylori**
EXCLUDES *H. pylori:*
Breath and blood by mass spectrometry (83013-83014)
Liquid scintillation counter (78267-78268)
Stool (87338)
0.00 0.00 **FUD** XXX
AMA: 2020,OctSE,1; 2020,AugSE,1; 2020,AugSE,1; 2020,AugSE,1

▲ **87340** **hepatitis B surface antigen (HBsAg)**
0.00 0.00 **FUD** XXX
AMA: 2020,OctSE,1; 2020,AugSE,1; 2020,AugSE,1; 2020,AugSE,1; 2018,Jan,8; 2017,Jan,8; 2016,Jan,13; 2015,Jan,16

▲ **87341** **hepatitis B surface antigen (HBsAg) neutralization**
0.00 0.00 FUD XXX
AMA: 2020,OctSE,1; 2020,AugSE,1; 2020,AugSE,1; 2020,AugSE,1

87350 **hepatitis Be antigen (HBeAg)**
0.00 0.00 FUD XXX
AMA: 2020,OctSE,1; 2020,AugSE,1; 2020,AugSE,1; 2020,AugSE,1

▲ **87380** **hepatitis, delta agent**
0.00 0.00 FUD XXX
AMA: 2020,OctSE,1; 2020,AugSE,1; 2020,AugSE,1; 2020,AugSE,1

▲ **87385** **Histoplasma capsulatum**
0.00 0.00 FUD XXX
AMA: 2020,OctSE,1; 2020,AugSE,1; 2020,AugSE,1; 2020,AugSE,1

▲ **87389** **HIV-1 antigen(s), with HIV-1 and HIV-2 antibodies, single result**
Code also modifier 92 for test performed using kit or transportable instrument comprising (all or part) single-use, disposable analytical chamber
0.00 0.00 FUD XXX
AMA: 2020,OctSE,1; 2020,AugSE,1; 2020,AugSE,1; 2020,AugSE,1

▲ **87390** **HIV-1**
0.00 0.00 FUD XXX
AMA: 2020,OctSE,1; 2020,AugSE,1; 2020,AugSE,1; 2020,AugSE,1

▲ **87391** **HIV-2**
0.00 0.00 FUD XXX
AMA: 2020,OctSE,1; 2020,AugSE,1; 2020,AugSE,1; 2020,AugSE,1

▲ **87400** **Influenza, A or B, each**
0.00 0.00 FUD XXX
AMA: 2020,OctSE,1; 2020,AugSE,1; 2020,AugSE,1; 2020,AugSE,1; 2018,Jan,8; 2017,Jan,8; 2016,Jan,13; 2015,Jan,16

▲ **87420** **respiratory syncytial virus**
0.00 0.00 FUD XXX
AMA: 2020,OctSE,1; 2020,AugSE,1; 2020,AugSE,1; 2020,AugSE,1

▲ **87425** **rotavirus**
0.00 0.00 FUD XXX
AMA: 2020,OctSE,1; 2020,AugSE,1; 2020,AugSE,1; 2020,AugSE,1

▲ **87426** **severe acute respiratory syndrome coronavirus (eg, SARS-CoV, SARS-CoV-2 [COVID-19])**
AMA: 2020,OctSE,1; 2020,AugSE,1; 2020,AugSE,1; 2020,AugSE,1

▲ **87427** **Shiga-like toxin**
0.00 0.00 FUD XXX
AMA: 2020,OctSE,1; 2020,AugSE,1; 2020,AugSE,1; 2020,AugSE,1

▲ **87430** **Streptococcus, group A**
0.00 0.00 FUD XXX
AMA: 2020,OctSE,1; 2020,AugSE,1; 2020,AugSE,1; 2020,AugSE,1; 2018,Jan,8; 2017,Jan,8; 2016,Jan,13; 2015,Jan,16

▲ **87449** **not otherwise specified, each organism**
0.00 0.00 FUD XXX
AMA: 2020,OctSE,1; 2020,AugSE,1; 2020,AugSE,1; 2020,AugSE,1; 2018,Jan,8; 2017,Jan,8; 2016,Jan,13; 2015,Jan,16

87450 ~~**single step method, not otherwise specified, each organism**~~
To report, see (87301-87451, 87802-87899 [87806, 87811])

▲ **87451** **polyvalent for multiple organisms, each polyvalent antiserum**
0.00 0.00 FUD XXX
AMA: 2020,OctSE,1; 2020,AugSE,1; 2020,AugSE,1; 2020,AugSE,1

87471-87801 [87623, 87624, 87625] Detection Infectious Agent by Probe Techniques

INCLUDES Primary source only

EXCLUDES *Comparable tests on culture material (87140-87158)*
Identification antibodies (86602-86804)
Nonspecific agent detection (87299, 87449, 87797-87799, 87899)
Reporting molecular procedure codes as substitute for codes in this range (81161-81408 [81105, 81106, 81107, 81108, 81109, 81110, 81111, 81112, 81120, 81121, 81161, 81162, 81230, 81231, 81238, 81269, 81283, 81287, 81288, 81334])

Code also modifier 59 for different species or strains reported by same code

87471 **Infectious agent detection by nucleic acid (DNA or RNA); Bartonella henselae and Bartonella quintana, amplified probe technique**
0.00 0.00 FUD XXX
AMA: 2020,OctSE,1; 2020,AugSE,1; 2020,AugSE,1; 2020,AugSE,1; 2018,Jan,8; 2017,Jan,8; 2016,Jan,13; 2015,Jan,16

87472 **Bartonella henselae and Bartonella quintana, quantification**
0.00 0.00 FUD XXX
AMA: 2020,OctSE,1; 2020,AugSE,1; 2020,AugSE,1; 2020,AugSE,1; 2018,Jan,8; 2017,Jan,8; 2016,Jan,13; 2015,Jan,16

87475 **Borrelia burgdorferi, direct probe technique**
0.00 0.00 FUD XXX
AMA: 2020,OctSE,1; 2020,AugSE,1; 2020,AugSE,1; 2020,AugSE,1; 2018,Jan,8; 2017,Jan,8; 2016,Jan,13; 2015,Jan,16

87476 **Borrelia burgdorferi, amplified probe technique**
0.00 0.00 FUD XXX
AMA: 2020,OctSE,1; 2020,AugSE,1; 2020,AugSE,1; 2020,AugSE,1; 2018,Jan,8; 2017,Jan,8; 2016,Jan,13; 2015,Jan,16

87480 **Candida species, direct probe technique**
0.00 0.00 FUD XXX
AMA: 2020,OctSE,1; 2020,AugSE,1; 2020,AugSE,1; 2020,AugSE,1; 2018,Jan,8; 2017,Jan,8; 2016,Jan,13; 2015,Jan,16

87481 **Candida species, amplified probe technique**
0.00 0.00 FUD XXX
AMA: 2020,OctSE,1; 2020,AugSE,1; 2020,AugSE,1; 2020,AugSE,1; 2018,Jan,8; 2017,Jan,8; 2016,Jan,13; 2015,Jan,16

87482 **Candida species, quantification**
0.00 0.00 FUD XXX
AMA: 2020,OctSE,1; 2020,AugSE,1; 2020,AugSE,1; 2020,AugSE,1; 2018,Jan,8; 2017,Jan,8; 2016,Jan,13; 2015,Jan,16

87483 **central nervous system pathogen (eg, Neisseria meningitidis, Streptococcus pneumoniae, Listeria, Haemophilus influenzae, E. coli, Streptococcus agalactiae, enterovirus, human parechovirus, herpes simplex virus type 1 and 2, human herpesvirus 6, cytomegalovirus, varicella zoster virus, Cryptococcus), includes multiplex reverse transcription, when performed, and multiplex amplified probe technique, multiple types or subtypes, 12-25 targets**
0.00 0.00 FUD XXX
AMA: 2020,OctSE,1; 2020,AugSE,1; 2020,AugSE,1; 2020,AugSE,1

87485 **Chlamydia pneumoniae, direct probe technique**
0.00 0.00 FUD XXX
AMA: 2020,OctSE,1; 2020,AugSE,1; 2020,AugSE,1; 2020,AugSE,1; 2018,Jan,8; 2017,Jan,8; 2016,Jan,13; 2015,Jan,16

87486 **Chlamydia pneumoniae, amplified probe technique**
0.00 0.00 FUD XXX
AMA: 2020,OctSE,1; 2020,AugSE,1; 2020,AugSE,1; 2020,AugSE,1; 2018,Jan,8; 2017,Jan,8; 2016,Jan,13; 2015,Jan,16

87487 **Chlamydia pneumoniae, quantification**
0.00 0.00 FUD XXX
AMA: 2020,OctSE,1; 2020,AugSE,1; 2020,AugSE,1; 2020,AugSE,1; 2018,Jan,8; 2017,Jan,8; 2016,Jan,13; 2015,Jan,16

87490 **Chlamydia trachomatis, direct probe technique**
0.00 0.00 FUD XXX
AMA: 2020,OctSE,1; 2020,AugSE,1; 2020,AugSE,1; 2020,AugSE,1; 2018,Jan,8; 2017,Jan,8; 2016,Jan,13; 2015,Jan,16

87491 **Chlamydia trachomatis, amplified probe technique**
0.00 0.00 FUD XXX
AMA: 2020,OctSE,1; 2020,AugSE,1; 2020,AugSE,1; 2020,AugSE,1; 2018,Jan,8; 2017,Jan,8; 2016,Jan,13; 2015,Jan,16

87492 **Chlamydia trachomatis, quantification**
0.00 0.00 FUD XXX
AMA: 2020,OctSE,1; 2020,AugSE,1; 2020,AugSE,1; 2020,AugSE,1; 2018,Jan,8; 2017,Jan,8; 2016,Jan,13; 2015,Jan,16

87493 **Clostridium difficile, toxin gene(s), amplified probe technique**
0.00 0.00 FUD XXX
AMA: 2020,OctSE,1; 2020,AugSE,1; 2020,AugSE,1; 2020,AugSE,1; 2018,Jan,8; 2017,Jan,8; 2016,Jan,13; 2015,Jan,16

87495 **cytomegalovirus, direct probe technique**
0.00 0.00 FUD XXX
AMA: 2020,OctSE,1; 2020,AugSE,1; 2020,AugSE,1; 2020,AugSE,1; 2018,Jan,8; 2017,Jan,8; 2016,Jan,13; 2015,Jan,16

87496 **cytomegalovirus, amplified probe technique**
0.00 0.00 FUD XXX
AMA: 2020,OctSE,1; 2020,AugSE,1; 2020,AugSE,1; 2020,AugSE,1; 2018,Jan,8; 2017,Jan,8; 2016,Jan,13; 2015,Jan,16

87497 **cytomegalovirus, quantification**
0.00 0.00 FUD XXX
AMA: 2020,OctSE,1; 2020,AugSE,1; 2020,AugSE,1; 2020,AugSE,1; 2018,Jan,8; 2017,Jan,8; 2016,Jan,13; 2015,Jan,16

87498 **enterovirus, amplified probe technique, includes reverse transcription when performed**
0.00 0.00 FUD XXX
AMA: 2020,OctSE,1; 2020,AugSE,1; 2020,AugSE,1; 2020,AugSE,1; 2018,Jan,8; 2017,Jan,8; 2016,Jan,13; 2015,Jan,16

87500 **vancomycin resistance (eg, enterococcus species van A, van B), amplified probe technique**
0.00 0.00 FUD XXX
AMA: 2020,OctSE,1; 2020,AugSE,1; 2020,AugSE,1; 2020,AugSE,1; 2018,Jan,8; 2017,Jan,8; 2016,Jan,13; 2015,Jan,16

87501 **influenza virus, includes reverse transcription, when performed, and amplified probe technique, each type or subtype**
0.00 0.00 FUD XXX
AMA: 2020,OctSE,1; 2020,AugSE,1; 2020,AugSE,1; 2020,AugSE,1; 2018,Jan,8; 2017,Jan,8; 2016,Jan,13; 2015,Jan,16

87502 **influenza virus, for multiple types or sub-types, includes multiplex reverse transcription, when performed, and multiplex amplified probe technique, first 2 types or sub-types**
0.00 0.00 FUD XXX
AMA: 2020,OctSE,1; 2020,AugSE,1; 2020,AugSE,1; 2020,AugSE,1; 2018,Jan,8; 2017,Jan,8; 2016,Jan,13; 2015,Jan,16

+ **87503** **influenza virus, for multiple types or sub-types, includes multiplex reverse transcription, when performed, and multiplex amplified probe technique, each additional influenza virus type or sub-type beyond 2 (List separately in addition to code for primary procedure)**
Code first (87502)
0.00 0.00 FUD XXX
AMA: 2020,OctSE,1; 2020,AugSE,1; 2020,AugSE,1; 2020,AugSE,1; 2018,Jan,8; 2017,Jan,8; 2016,Jan,13; 2015,Jan,16

87505 **gastrointestinal pathogen (eg, Clostridium difficile, E. coli, Salmonella, Shigella, norovirus, Giardia), includes multiplex reverse transcription, when performed, and multiplex amplified probe technique, multiple types or subtypes, 3-5 targets**
0.00 0.00 FUD XXX
AMA: 2020,OctSE,1; 2020,AugSE,1; 2020,AugSE,1; 2020,AugSE,1

87506 **gastrointestinal pathogen (eg, Clostridium difficile, E. coli, Salmonella, Shigella, norovirus, Giardia), includes multiplex reverse transcription, when performed, and multiplex amplified probe technique, multiple types or subtypes, 6-11 targets**
0.00 0.00 FUD XXX
AMA: 2020,OctSE,1; 2020,AugSE,1; 2020,AugSE,1; 2020,AugSE,1

87507 **gastrointestinal pathogen (eg, Clostridium difficile, E. coli, Salmonella, Shigella, norovirus, Giardia), includes multiplex reverse transcription, when performed, and multiplex amplified probe technique, multiple types or subtypes, 12-25 targets**
0.00 0.00 FUD XXX
AMA: 2020,OctSE,1; 2020,AugSE,1; 2020,AugSE,1; 2020,AugSE,1

87510 **Gardnerella vaginalis, direct probe technique**
0.00 0.00 FUD XXX
AMA: 2020,OctSE,1; 2020,AugSE,1; 2020,AugSE,1; 2020,AugSE,1; 2018,Jan,8; 2017,Jan,8; 2016,Jan,13; 2015,Jan,16

87511 **Gardnerella vaginalis, amplified probe technique**
0.00 0.00 FUD XXX
AMA: 2020,OctSE,1; 2020,AugSE,1; 2020,AugSE,1; 2020,AugSE,1; 2018,Jan,8; 2017,Jan,8; 2016,Jan,13; 2015,Jan,16

87512 **Gardnerella vaginalis, quantification**
0.00 0.00 FUD XXX
AMA: 2020,OctSE,1; 2020,AugSE,1; 2020,AugSE,1; 2020,AugSE,1; 2018,Jan,8; 2017,Jan,8; 2016,Jan,13; 2015,Jan,16

87516 **hepatitis B virus, amplified probe technique**
0.00 0.00 FUD XXX
AMA: 2020,OctSE,1; 2020,AugSE,1; 2020,AugSE,1; 2020,AugSE,1; 2018,Jan,8; 2017,Jan,8; 2016,Jan,13; 2015,Jan,16

87517 **hepatitis B virus, quantification**
0.00 0.00 FUD XXX
AMA: 2020,OctSE,1; 2020,AugSE,1; 2020,AugSE,1; 2020,AugSE,1; 2018,Jan,8; 2017,Jan,8; 2016,Jan,13; 2015,Jan,16

87520 **hepatitis C, direct probe technique**
0.00 0.00 FUD XXX
AMA: 2020,OctSE,1; 2020,AugSE,1; 2020,AugSE,1; 2020,AugSE,1; 2018,Jan,8; 2017,Jan,8; 2016,Jan,13; 2015,Jan,16

87521 **hepatitis C, amplified probe technique, includes reverse transcription when performed**
0.00 0.00 FUD XXX
AMA: 2020,OctSE,1; 2020,AugSE,1; 2020,AugSE,1; 2020,AugSE,1; 2018,Jan,8; 2017,Jan,8; 2016,Jan,13; 2015,Jan,16

87522 **hepatitis C, quantification, includes reverse transcription when performed**
0.00 0.00 FUD XXX
AMA: 2020,OctSE,1; 2020,AugSE,1; 2020,AugSE,1; 2020,AugSE,1; 2018,Jan,8; 2017,Jan,8; 2016,Jan,13; 2015,Jan,16

87525 **hepatitis G, direct probe technique**
0.00 0.00 FUD XXX
AMA: 2020,OctSE,1; 2020,AugSE,1; 2020,AugSE,1; 2020,AugSE,1; 2018,Jan,8; 2017,Jan,8; 2016,Jan,13; 2015,Jan,16

87526 **hepatitis G, amplified probe technique**
0.00 0.00 FUD XXX
AMA: 2020,OctSE,1; 2020,AugSE,1; 2020,AugSE,1; 2020,AugSE,1; 2018,Jan,8; 2017,Jan,8; 2016,Jan,13; 2015,Jan,16

87527 **hepatitis G, quantification**
0.00 0.00 FUD XXX
AMA: 2020,OctSE,1; 2020,AugSE,1; 2020,AugSE,1; 2020,AugSE,1; 2018,Jan,8; 2017,Jan,8; 2016,Jan,13; 2015,Jan,16

87528 **Herpes simplex virus, direct probe technique**
0.00 0.00 FUD XXX
AMA: 2020,OctSE,1; 2020,AugSE,1; 2020,AugSE,1; 2020,AugSE,1; 2018,Jan,8; 2017,Jan,8; 2016,Jan,13; 2015,Jan,16

87529 **Herpes simplex virus, amplified probe technique**
0.00 0.00 FUD XXX
AMA: 2020,OctSE,1; 2020,AugSE,1; 2020,AugSE,1; 2020,AugSE,1; 2018,Jan,8; 2017,Jan,8; 2016,Jan,13; 2015,Jan,16

87530 Herpes simplex virus, quantification
0.00 0.00 FUD XXX
AMA: 2020,OctSE,1; 2020,AugSE,1; 2020,AugSE,1; 2020,AugSE,1; 2018,Jan,8; 2017,Jan,8; 2016,Jan,13; 2015,Jan,16

87531 Herpes virus-6, direct probe technique
0.00 0.00 FUD XXX
AMA: 2020,OctSE,1; 2020,AugSE,1; 2020,AugSE,1; 2020,AugSE,1; 2018,Jan,8; 2017,Jan,8; 2016,Jan,13; 2015,Jan,16

87532 Herpes virus-6, amplified probe technique
0.00 0.00 FUD XXX
AMA: 2020,OctSE,1; 2020,AugSE,1; 2020,AugSE,1; 2020,AugSE,1; 2018,Jan,8; 2017,Jan,8; 2016,Jan,13; 2015,Jan,16

87533 Herpes virus-6, quantification
0.00 0.00 FUD XXX
AMA: 2020,OctSE,1; 2020,AugSE,1; 2020,AugSE,1; 2020,AugSE,1; 2018,Jan,8; 2017,Jan,8; 2016,Jan,13; 2015,Jan,16

87534 HIV-1, direct probe technique
0.00 0.00 FUD XXX
AMA: 2020,OctSE,1; 2020,AugSE,1; 2020,AugSE,1; 2020,AugSE,1; 2018,Jan,8; 2017,Jan,8; 2016,Jan,13; 2015,Jan,16

87535 HIV-1, amplified probe technique, includes reverse transcription when performed
0.00 0.00 FUD XXX
AMA: 2020,OctSE,1; 2020,AugSE,1; 2020,AugSE,1; 2020,AugSE,1; 2018,Jan,8; 2017,Jan,8; 2016,Jan,13; 2015,Jan,16

87536 HIV-1, quantification, includes reverse transcription when performed
0.00 0.00 FUD XXX
AMA: 2020,OctSE,1; 2020,AugSE,1; 2020,AugSE,1; 2020,AugSE,1; 2018,Jan,8; 2017,Jan,8; 2016,Jan,13; 2015,Jan,16

87537 HIV-2, direct probe technique
0.00 0.00 FUD XXX
AMA: 2020,OctSE,1; 2020,AugSE,1; 2020,AugSE,1; 2020,AugSE,1; 2018,Jan,8; 2017,Jan,8; 2016,Jan,13; 2015,Jan,16

87538 HIV-2, amplified probe technique, includes reverse transcription when performed
0.00 0.00 FUD XXX
AMA: 2020,OctSE,1; 2020,AugSE,1; 2020,AugSE,1; 2020,AugSE,1; 2018,Jan,8; 2017,Jan,8; 2016,Jan,13; 2015,Jan,16

87539 HIV-2, quantification, includes reverse transcription when performed
0.00 0.00 FUD XXX
AMA: 2020,OctSE,1; 2020,AugSE,1; 2020,AugSE,1; 2020,AugSE,1; 2018,Jan,8; 2017,Jan,8; 2016,Jan,13; 2015,Jan,16

87623 Human Papillomavirus (HPV), low-risk types (eg, 6, 11, 42, 43, 44)
0.00 0.00 FUD XXX
AMA: 2020,OctSE,1; 2020,AugSE,1; 2020,AugSE,1; 2020,AugSE,1

87624 Human Papillomavirus (HPV), high-risk types (eg, 16, 18, 31, 33, 35, 39, 45, 51, 52, 56, 58, 59, 68)
INCLUDES Low- and high-risk types in one assay
0.00 0.00 FUD XXX
AMA: 2020,OctSE,1; 2020,AugSE,1; 2020,AugSE,1; 2020,AugSE,1; 2018,Jan,8; 2017,Jan,8; 2016,Jan,13; 2015,Oct,9

87625 Human Papillomavirus (HPV), types 16 and 18 only, includes type 45, if performed
EXCLUDES *HPV detection (genotyping) (0500T)*
0.00 0.00 FUD XXX
AMA: 2020,OctSE,1; 2020,AugSE,1; 2020,AugSE,1; 2020,AugSE,1; 2018,Jan,8; 2017,Jan,8; 2016,Jan,13; 2015,Oct,9; 2015,Jun,10

87540 Legionella pneumophila, direct probe technique
0.00 0.00 FUD XXX
AMA: 2020,OctSE,1; 2020,AugSE,1; 2020,AugSE,1; 2020,AugSE,1; 2018,Jan,8; 2017,Jan,8; 2016,Jan,13; 2015,Jan,16

87541 Legionella pneumophila, amplified probe technique
0.00 0.00 FUD XXX
AMA: 2020,OctSE,1; 2020,AugSE,1; 2020,AugSE,1; 2020,AugSE,1; 2018,Jan,8; 2017,Jan,8; 2016,Jan,13; 2015,Jan,16

87542 Legionella pneumophila, quantification
0.00 0.00 FUD XXX
AMA: 2020,OctSE,1; 2020,AugSE,1; 2020,AugSE,1; 2020,AugSE,1; 2018,Jan,8; 2017,Jan,8; 2016,Jan,13; 2015,Jan,16

87550 Mycobacteria species, direct probe technique
0.00 0.00 FUD XXX
AMA: 2020,OctSE,1; 2020,AugSE,1; 2020,AugSE,1; 2020,AugSE,1; 2018,Jan,8; 2017,Jan,8; 2016,Jan,13; 2015,Jan,16

87551 Mycobacteria species, amplified probe technique
0.00 0.00 FUD XXX
AMA: 2020,OctSE,1; 2020,AugSE,1; 2020,AugSE,1; 2020,AugSE,1; 2018,Jan,8; 2017,Jan,8; 2016,Jan,13; 2015,Jan,16

87552 Mycobacteria species, quantification
0.00 0.00 FUD XXX
AMA: 2020,OctSE,1; 2020,AugSE,1; 2020,AugSE,1; 2020,AugSE,1; 2018,Jan,8; 2017,Jan,8; 2016,Jan,13; 2015,Jan,16

87555 Mycobacteria tuberculosis, direct probe technique
0.00 0.00 FUD XXX
AMA: 2020,OctSE,1; 2020,AugSE,1; 2020,AugSE,1; 2020,AugSE,1; 2018,Jan,8; 2017,Jan,8; 2016,Jan,13; 2015,Jan,16

87556 Mycobacteria tuberculosis, amplified probe technique
0.00 0.00 FUD XXX
AMA: 2020,OctSE,1; 2020,AugSE,1; 2020,AugSE,1; 2020,AugSE,1; 2018,Jan,8; 2017,Jan,8; 2016,Jan,13; 2015,Jan,16

87557 Mycobacteria tuberculosis, quantification
0.00 0.00 FUD XXX
AMA: 2020,OctSE,1; 2020,AugSE,1; 2020,AugSE,1; 2020,AugSE,1; 2018,Jan,8; 2017,Jan,8; 2016,Jan,13; 2015,Jan,16

87560 Mycobacteria avium-intracellulare, direct probe technique
0.00 0.00 FUD XXX
AMA: 2020,OctSE,1; 2020,AugSE,1; 2020,AugSE,1; 2020,AugSE,1; 2018,Jan,8; 2017,Jan,8; 2016,Jan,13; 2015,Jan,16

87561 Mycobacteria avium-intracellulare, amplified probe technique
0.00 0.00 FUD XXX
AMA: 2020,OctSE,1; 2020,AugSE,1; 2020,AugSE,1; 2020,AugSE,1; 2018,Jan,8; 2017,Jan,8; 2016,Jan,13; 2015,Jan,16

87562 Mycobacteria avium-intracellulare, quantification
0.00 0.00 FUD XXX
AMA: 2020,OctSE,1; 2020,AugSE,1; 2020,AugSE,1; 2020,AugSE,1; 2018,Jan,8; 2017,Jan,8; 2016,Jan,13; 2015,Jan,16

87563 Mycoplasma genitalium, amplified probe technique
0.00 0.00 FUD XXX
AMA: 2020,OctSE,1; 2020,AugSE,1; 2020,AugSE,1; 2020,AugSE,1

87580 Mycoplasma pneumoniae, direct probe technique
0.00 0.00 FUD XXX
AMA: 2020,OctSE,1; 2020,AugSE,1; 2020,AugSE,1; 2020,AugSE,1; 2018,Jan,8; 2017,Jan,8; 2016,Jan,13; 2015,Jan,16

87581 Mycoplasma pneumoniae, amplified probe technique
0.00 0.00 FUD XXX
AMA: 2020,OctSE,1; 2020,AugSE,1; 2020,AugSE,1; 2020,AugSE,1; 2018,Jan,8; 2017,Jan,8; 2016,Jan,13; 2015,Jan,16

87582 Mycoplasma pneumoniae, quantification
0.00 0.00 FUD XXX
AMA: 2020,OctSE,1; 2020,AugSE,1; 2020,AugSE,1; 2020,AugSE,1; 2018,Jan,8; 2017,Jan,8; 2016,Jan,13; 2015,Jan,16

87590 Neisseria gonorrhoeae, direct probe technique
0.00 0.00 FUD XXX
AMA: 2020,OctSE,1; 2020,AugSE,1; 2020,AugSE,1; 2020,AugSE,1; 2018,Jan,8; 2017,Jan,8; 2016,Jan,13; 2015,Jan,16

87591 **Neisseria gonorrhoeae, amplified probe technique**
0.00 0.00 FUD XXX
AMA: 2020,OctSE,1; 2020,AugSE,1; 2020,AugSE,1; 2020,AugSE,1; 2018,Jan,8; 2017,Jan,8; 2016,Jan,13; 2015,Jan,16

87592 **Neisseria gonorrhoeae, quantification**
0.00 0.00 FUD XXX
AMA: 2020,OctSE,1; 2020,AugSE,1; 2020,AugSE,1; 2020,AugSE,1; 2018,Jan,8; 2017,Jan,8; 2016,Jan,13; 2015,Jan,16

87623 **Resequenced code. See code following 87539.**

87624 **Resequenced code. See code following 87539.**

87625 **Resequenced code. See code before 87540.**

87631 **respiratory virus (eg, adenovirus, influenza virus, coronavirus, metapneumovirus, parainfluenza virus, respiratory syncytial virus, rhinovirus), includes multiplex reverse transcription, when performed, and multiplex amplified probe technique, multiple types or subtypes, 3-5 targets**
INCLUDES Detection multiple respiratory viruses with one test
EXCLUDES *Assay for severe acute respiratory syndrome coronavirus 2 (SARS-CoV-2) (Coronavirus disease) (COVID-19) (87635)*
Assays for typing or subtyping influenza viruses only (87501-87503)
Single test for detection multiple infectious organisms (87800-87801)
0.00 0.00 FUD XXX
AMA: 2020,OctSE,1; 2020,AugSE,1; 2020,AugSE,1; 2020,AugSE,1; 2020,Apr,3; 2020,Mar,3; 2018,Jan,8; 2017,Jan,8; 2016,Jan,13; 2015,Jan,16

87632 **respiratory virus (eg, adenovirus, influenza virus, coronavirus, metapneumovirus, parainfluenza virus, respiratory syncytial virus, rhinovirus), includes multiplex reverse transcription, when performed, and multiplex amplified probe technique, multiple types or subtypes, 6-11 targets**
INCLUDES Detection multiple respiratory viruses with one test
EXCLUDES *Assay for severe acute respiratory syndrome coronavirus 2 (SARS-CoV-2) (Coronavirus disease) (COVID-19) (87635)*
Assays for typing or subtyping influenza viruses only (87501-87503)
Single test to detect multiple infectious organisms (87800-87801)
0.00 0.00 FUD XXX
AMA: 2020,OctSE,1; 2020,AugSE,1; 2020,AugSE,1; 2020,AugSE,1; 2020,Apr,3; 2020,Mar,3; 2018,Jan,8; 2017,Jan,8; 2016,Jan,13; 2015,Jan,16

87633 **respiratory virus (eg, adenovirus, influenza virus, coronavirus, metapneumovirus, parainfluenza virus, respiratory syncytial virus, rhinovirus), includes multiplex reverse transcription, when performed, and multiplex amplified probe technique, multiple types or subtypes, 12-25 targets**
INCLUDES Detection multiple respiratory viruses with one test
EXCLUDES *Assay for severe acute respiratory syndrome coronavirus 2 (SARS-CoV-2) (Coronavirus disease) (COVID-19) (87635)*
Assays for typing or subtyping influenza viruses only (87501-87503)
Single test to detect multiple infectious organisms (87800-87801)
0.00 0.00 FUD XXX
AMA: 2020,OctSE,1; 2020,AugSE,1; 2020,AugSE,1; 2020,AugSE,1; 2020,Apr,3; 2020,Mar,3; 2018,Jan,8; 2017,Jan,8; 2016,Jan,13; 2015,Jan,16

87634 **respiratory syncytial virus, amplified probe technique**
EXCLUDES *Assays for RSV with other respiratory viruses (87631-87633)*
0.00 0.00 FUD XXX
AMA: 2020,OctSE,1; 2020,AugSE,1; 2020,AugSE,1; 2020,AugSE,1

● **87635** **severe acute respiratory syndrome coronavirus 2 (SARS-CoV-2) (Coronavirus disease [COVID-19]), amplified probe technique**
EXCLUDES *HCPCS codes for reporting coronavirus testing (U0001-U0002)*
Proprietary Laboratory Analyses (PLA) used to detect multiple types or subtypes of respiratory pathogens (0098U-0100U)
Single procedure nucleic acid assays to detect multiple respiratory viruses by multiplex reaction (87631-87633)
Code also code 87635, with modifier 59, for assays performed on specimens from different anatomic locations, when performed
AMA: 2020,OctSE,1; 2020,AugSE,1; 2020,AugSE,1; 2020,AugSE,1; 2020,Apr,3; 2020,Mar,3

● **87636** **severe acute respiratory syndrome coronavirus 2 (SARS-CoV-2) (Coronavirus disease [COVID-19]) and influenza virus types A and B, multiplex amplified probe technique**
EXCLUDES *Nucleic acid detection multiple respiratory infectious agents (87631-87633):*
including Severe Acute Respiratory Syndrome coronavirus 2 (SARS-CoV-2) (Coronavirus disease) (COVID-19) with additional agents beyond influenza A and B and respiratory syncytial virus
not including Severe Acute Respiratory Syndrome coronavirus 2 (SARS-CoV-2) (Coronavirus disease) (COVID-19)

● **87637** **severe acute respiratory syndrome coronavirus 2 (SARS-CoV-2) (Coronavirus disease [COVID-19]), influenza virus types A and B, and respiratory syncytial virus, multiplex amplified probe technique**
EXCLUDES *Nucleic acid detection multiple respiratory infectious agents (87631-87633):*
Including severe acute respiratory syndrome coronavirus 2 (SARS-CoV-2) (coronavirus disease) (COVID-19) with additional agents beyond influenza A and B and respiratory syncytial virus
Not including severe acute respiratory syndrome coronavirus 2 (SARS-CoV-2) (coronavirus disease) (COVID-19)

87640 **Staphylococcus aureus, amplified probe technique**
0.00 0.00 FUD XXX
AMA: 2020,OctSE,1; 2020,AugSE,1; 2020,AugSE,1; 2020,AugSE,1; 2018,Jan,8; 2017,Jan,8; 2016,Jan,13; 2015,Jan,16

87641 **Staphylococcus aureus, methicillin resistant, amplified probe technique**
EXCLUDES *Assays that detect methicillin resistance and identify Staphylococcus aureus using single nucleic acid sequence (87641)*
0.00 0.00 FUD XXX
AMA: 2020,OctSE,1; 2020,AugSE,1; 2020,AugSE,1; 2020,AugSE,1; 2018,Jan,8; 2017,Jan,8; 2016,Jan,13; 2015,Jan,16

87650 **Streptococcus, group A, direct probe technique**
0.00 0.00 FUD XXX
AMA: 2020,OctSE,1; 2020,AugSE,1; 2020,AugSE,1; 2020,AugSE,1; 2018,Jan,8; 2017,Jan,8; 2016,Jan,13; 2015,Jan,16

87651 **Streptococcus, group A, amplified probe technique**
0.00 0.00 FUD XXX
AMA: 2020,OctSE,1; 2020,AugSE,1; 2020,AugSE,1; 2020,AugSE,1; 2018,Jan,8; 2017,Jan,8; 2016,Jan,13; 2015,Jan,16

87652 **Streptococcus, group A, quantification**
0.00 0.00 FUD XXX
AMA: 2020,OctSE,1; 2020,AugSE,1; 2020,AugSE,1; 2020,AugSE,1; 2018,Jan,8; 2017,Jan,8; 2016,Jan,13; 2015,Jan,16

87653 **Streptococcus, group B, amplified probe technique**
0.00 0.00 FUD XXX
AMA: 2020,OctSE,1; 2020,AugSE,1; 2020,AugSE,1; 2020,AugSE,1; 2018,Jan,8; 2017,Jan,8; 2016,Jan,13; 2015,Jan,16

87660 **Trichomonas vaginalis, direct probe technique**
0.00 0.00 FUD XXX
AMA: 2020,OctSE,1; 2020,AugSE,1; 2020,AugSE,1; 2020,AugSE,1; 2018,Jan,8; 2017,Jan,8; 2016,Jan,13; 2015,Jan,16

87661 **Trichomonas vaginalis, amplified probe technique**
0.00 0.00 FUD XXX
AMA: 2020,OctSE,1; 2020,AugSE,1; 2020,AugSE,1; 2020,AugSE,1

87662 **Zika virus, amplified probe technique**
0.00 0.00 FUD XXX
AMA: 2020,OctSE,1; 2020,AugSE,1; 2020,AugSE,1; 2020,AugSE,1

87797 **Infectious agent detection by nucleic acid (DNA or RNA), not otherwise specified; direct probe technique, each organism**
0.00 0.00 FUD XXX
AMA: 2020,OctSE,1; 2020,AugSE,1; 2020,AugSE,1; 2020,AugSE,1; 2018,Jan,8; 2017,Jan,8; 2016,Aug,9; 2016,Jan,13; 2015,Jan,16

87798 **amplified probe technique, each organism**
0.00 0.00 FUD XXX
AMA: 2020,OctSE,1; 2020,AugSE,1; 2020,AugSE,1; 2020,AugSE,1; 2018,Jan,8; 2017,Jan,8; 2016,Jan,13; 2015,Jan,16

87799 **quantification, each organism**
0.00 0.00 FUD XXX
AMA: 2020,OctSE,1; 2020,AugSE,1; 2020,AugSE,1; 2020,AugSE,1; 2018,Jan,8; 2017,Jan,8; 2016,Jan,13; 2015,Jan,16

87800 **Infectious agent detection by nucleic acid (DNA or RNA), multiple organisms; direct probe(s) technique**
INCLUDES Single test to detect multiple infectious organisms
EXCLUDES *Detection specific infectious agents not otherwise specified (87797-87799)*
Each specific organism nucleic acid detection from primary source (87471-87660 [87623, 87624, 87625])
0.00 0.00 FUD XXX
AMA: 2020,OctSE,1; 2020,AugSE,1; 2020,AugSE,1; 2020,AugSE,1; 2018,Jan,8; 2017,Jan,8; 2016,Aug,9; 2016,Jan,13; 2015,Jan,16

87801 **amplified probe(s) technique**
INCLUDES Single test to detect multiple infectious organisms
EXCLUDES *Detection multiple respiratory viruses with one test (87631-87633)*
Detection specific infectious agents not otherwise specified (87797-87799)
Each specific organism nucleic acid detection from primary source (87471-87660 [87623, 87624, 87625])
0.00 0.00 FUD XXX
AMA: 2020,OctSE,1; 2020,AugSE,1; 2020,AugSE,1; 2020,AugSE,1; 2018,Jan,8; 2017,Jan,8; 2016,Jan,13; 2015,Jan,16

87802-87899 [87806, 87811] Detection Infectious Agent by Immunoassay with Direct Optical Observation

▲ **87802** **Infectious agent antigen detection by immunoassay with direct optical (ie, visual) observation; Streptococcus, group B**
0.00 0.00 FUD XXX
AMA: 2020,OctSE,1; 2020,AugSE,1; 2020,AugSE,1; 2020,AugSE,1

▲ **87803** **Clostridium difficile toxin A**
0.00 0.00 FUD XXX
AMA: 2020,OctSE,1; 2020,AugSE,1; 2020,AugSE,1; 2020,AugSE,1

▲ # **87806** **HIV-1 antigen(s), with HIV-1 and HIV-2 antibodies**
0.00 0.00 FUD XXX
AMA: 2020,OctSE,1; 2020,AugSE,1; 2020,AugSE,1; 2020,AugSE,1

▲ **87804** **Influenza**
0.00 0.00 FUD XXX
AMA: 2020,OctSE,1; 2020,AugSE,1; 2020,AugSE,1; 2020,AugSE,1; 2018,Jan,8; 2017,Jan,8; 2016,Jan,13; 2015,Jan,16

87806 **Resequenced code. See code following 87803.**

▲ **87807** **respiratory syncytial virus**
0.00 0.00 FUD XXX
AMA: 2020,OctSE,1; 2020,AugSE,1; 2020,AugSE,1; 2020,AugSE,1

● # **87811** **severe acute respiratory syndrome coronavirus 2 (SARS-CoV-2) (Coronavirus disease [COVID-19])**

▲ **87808** **Trichomonas vaginalis**
0.00 0.00 FUD XXX
AMA: 2020,OctSE,1; 2020,AugSE,1; 2020,AugSE,1; 2020,AugSE,1

▲ **87809** **adenovirus**
0.00 0.00 FUD XXX
AMA: 2020,OctSE,1; 2020,AugSE,1; 2020,AugSE,1; 2020,AugSE,1; 2018,Jan,8; 2017,Jan,8; 2016,Jan,13; 2015,Jan,16

▲ **87810** **Chlamydia trachomatis**
0.00 0.00 FUD XXX
AMA: 2020,OctSE,1; 2020,AugSE,1; 2020,AugSE,1; 2020,AugSE,1; 2018,Jan,8; 2017,Jan,8; 2016,Jan,13; 2015,Jan,16

87811 **Resequenced code. See code following 87807.**

▲ **87850** **Neisseria gonorrhoeae**
0.00 0.00 FUD XXX
AMA: 2020,OctSE,1; 2020,AugSE,1; 2020,AugSE,1; 2020,AugSE,1; 2018,Jan,8; 2017,Jan,8; 2016,Jan,13; 2015,Jan,16

▲ **87880** **Streptococcus, group A**
0.00 0.00 FUD XXX
AMA: 2020,OctSE,1; 2020,AugSE,1; 2020,AugSE,1; 2020,AugSE,1; 2018,Jan,8; 2017,Jan,8; 2016,Jan,13; 2015,Jan,16

▲ **87899** **not otherwise specified**
0.00 0.00 FUD XXX
AMA: 2020,OctSE,1; 2020,AugSE,1; 2020,AugSE,1; 2020,AugSE,1; 2018,Jan,8; 2017,Jan,8; 2016,Jan,13; 2015,Jan,16

87900-87999 [87906, 87910, 87912] Drug Sensitivity Genotype/Phenotype

87900 **Infectious agent drug susceptibility phenotype prediction using regularly updated genotypic bioinformatics**
0.00 0.00 FUD XXX
AMA: 2020,OctSE,1; 2018,Jan,8; 2017,Jan,8; 2016,Jan,13; 2015,Dec,18; 2015,Jan,16

87910 **Infectious agent genotype analysis by nucleic acid (DNA or RNA); cytomegalovirus**
EXCLUDES *HPV detection (genotyping) (0500T)*
HIV-1 infectious agent phenotype prediction (87900)
0.00 0.00 FUD XXX
AMA: 2018,Jan,8; 2017,Jan,8; 2016,Jan,13; 2015,Jan,16

87901 **HIV-1, reverse transcriptase and protease regions**
EXCLUDES *Infectious agent drug susceptibility phenotype prediction for HIV-1 (87900)*
0.00 0.00 FUD XXX
AMA: 2020,OctSE,1; 2018,Jan,8; 2017,Jan,8; 2016,Jan,13; 2015,Jan,16

87906 **HIV-1, other region (eg, integrase, fusion)**
EXCLUDES *HIV-1 infectious agent phenotype prediction (87900)*
0.00 0.00 FUD XXX
AMA: 2018,Jan,8; 2017,Jan,8; 2016,Jan,13; 2015,Jan,16

87912 **Hepatitis B virus**
0.00 0.00 FUD XXX
AMA: 2018,Jan,8; 2017,Jan,8; 2016,Jan,13; 2015,Jan,16

87902 **Hepatitis C virus**
0.00 0.00 FUD XXX
AMA: 2020,OctSE,1; 2018,Jan,8; 2017,Jan,8; 2016,Jan,13; 2015,Dec,18; 2015,Nov,10; 2015,Jan,16

87903 **Infectious agent phenotype analysis by nucleic acid (DNA or RNA) with drug resistance tissue culture analysis, HIV 1; first through 10 drugs tested**
0.00 0.00 FUD XXX
AMA: 2020,OctSE,1; 2018,Jan,8; 2017,Jan,8; 2016,Jan,13; 2015,Jan,16

+ **87904** **each additional drug tested (List separately in addition to code for primary procedure)**
Code first (87903)
0.00 0.00 FUD XXX
AMA: 2018,Jan,8; 2017,Jan,8; 2016,Jan,13; 2015,Jan,16

87905 **Infectious agent enzymatic activity other than virus (eg, sialidase activity in vaginal fluid)**
EXCLUDES *Virus isolation identified by nonimmunologic method, and by noncytopathic effect (87255)*
0.00 0.00 FUD XXX

87906 **Resequenced code. See code following 87901.**

87910 **Resequenced code. See code following 87900.**

87912 **Resequenced code. See code before 87902.**

87999 **Unlisted microbiology procedure**
0.00 0.00 FUD XXX
AMA: 2018,Jan,8; 2017,Jan,8; 2016,Jan,13; 2015,Jan,16

88000-88099 Autopsy Services

CMS: 100-02,15,80.1 Payment for Clinical Laboratory Services
INCLUDES Services for physicians only

88000 **Necropsy (autopsy), gross examination only; without CNS**
0.00 0.00 FUD XXX
AMA: 2018,Jan,8; 2017,Jan,8; 2016,Jan,13; 2015,Jan,16

88005 **with brain**
0.00 0.00 FUD XXX
AMA: 2005,Jul,11-12; 2005,Aug,7-8

88007 **with brain and spinal cord**
0.00 0.00 FUD XXX
AMA: 2005,Jul,11-12; 2005,Aug,7-8

88012 **infant with brain**
0.00 0.00 FUD XXX
AMA: 2005,Jul,11-12; 2005,Aug,7-8

88014 **stillborn or newborn with brain**
0.00 0.00 FUD XXX
AMA: 2005,Jul,11-12; 2005,Aug,7-8

88016 **macerated stillborn**
0.00 0.00 FUD XXX
AMA: 2005,Jul,11-12; 2005,Aug,7-8

88020 **Necropsy (autopsy), gross and microscopic; without CNS**
0.00 0.00 FUD XXX
AMA: 2005,Jul,11-12; 2005,Aug,7-8

88025 **with brain**
0.00 0.00 FUD XXX
AMA: 2005,Jul,11-12; 2005,Aug,7-8

88027 **with brain and spinal cord**
0.00 0.00 FUD XXX
AMA: 2005,Jul,11-12; 2005,Aug,7-8

88028 **infant with brain**
0.00 0.00 FUD XXX
AMA: 2005,Jul,11-12; 2005,Aug,7-8

88029 **stillborn or newborn with brain**
0.00 0.00 FUD XXX
AMA: 2005,Jul,11-12; 2005,Aug,7-8

88036 **Necropsy (autopsy), limited, gross and/or microscopic; regional**
0.00 0.00 FUD XXX
AMA: 2005,Jul,11-12; 2005,Aug,7-8

88037 **single organ**
0.00 0.00 FUD XXX
AMA: 2005,Jul,11-12; 2005,Aug,7-8

88040 **Necropsy (autopsy); forensic examination**
0.00 0.00 FUD XXX
AMA: 2005,Jul,11-12; 2005,Aug,7-8

88045 **coroner's call**
0.00 0.00 FUD XXX
AMA: 2005,Jul,11-12; 2005,Aug,7-8

88099 **Unlisted necropsy (autopsy) procedure**
0.00 0.00 FUD XXX
AMA: 2018,Jan,8; 2017,Jan,8; 2016,Jan,13; 2015,Jan,16

88104-88140 Cytopathology: Other Than Cervical/Vaginal

88104 **Cytopathology, fluids, washings or brushings, except cervical or vaginal; smears with interpretation**
1.93 1.93 FUD XXX
AMA: 2018,Jan,8; 2017,Jan,8; 2016,Jan,13; 2015,Jan,16

88106 **simple filter method with interpretation**
EXCLUDES *Cytopathology smears with interpretation (88104)*
Selective cellular enhancement (nongynecological) including filter transfer techniques (88112)
1.81 1.81 FUD XXX
AMA: 2018,Jan,8; 2017,Jan,8; 2016,Jan,13; 2015,Jan,16

88108 **Cytopathology, concentration technique, smears and interpretation (eg, Saccomanno technique)**
EXCLUDES *Cervical or vaginal smears (88150-88155)*
Gastric intubation with lavage (43754-43755)
(74340)
1.71 1.71 FUD XXX
AMA: 2018,Jan,8; 2017,Jan,8; 2016,Jan,13; 2015,Jan,16

88112 **Cytopathology, selective cellular enhancement technique with interpretation (eg, liquid based slide preparation method), except cervical or vaginal**
EXCLUDES *Cytopathology cellular enhancement technique (88108)*
1.90 1.90 FUD XXX
AMA: 2005,Aug,7-8; 2005,Jul,11-12

88120 **Cytopathology, in situ hybridization (eg, FISH), urinary tract specimen with morphometric analysis, 3-5 molecular probes, each specimen; manual**
EXCLUDES *More than five probes (88399)*
Morphometric in situ hybridization on specimens other than urinary tract (88367-88368 [88373, 88374])
16.3 16.3 FUD XXX
AMA: 2010,Dec,7-10

88121 **using computer-assisted technology**
EXCLUDES *More than five probes (88399)*
Morphometric in situ hybridization on specimens other than urinary tract (88367-88368 [88373, 88374])
12.4 12.4 FUD XXX
AMA: 2010,Dec,7-10

88125 **Cytopathology, forensic (eg, sperm)**
0.75 0.75 FUD XXX
AMA: 2005,Aug,7-8; 2005,Jul,11-12

88130 **Sex chromatin identification; Barr bodies**
0.00 0.00 FUD XXX
AMA: 2005,Aug,7-8; 2005,Jul,11-12

88140 **peripheral blood smear, polymorphonuclear drumsticks**
EXCLUDES *Guard stain (88313)*
0.00 0.00 FUD XXX
AMA: 2018,Jan,8; 2017,Jan,8; 2016,Jan,13; 2015,Jan,16

88141-88155 Pap Smears

CMS: 100-03,210.2 Screening Pap Smears/Pelvic Examinations for Early Cancer Detection
EXCLUDES *Non-Bethesda method (88150-88153)*

88141 **Cytopathology, cervical or vaginal (any reporting system), requiring interpretation by physician** ♀
Code also (88142-88153, 88164-88167, 88174-88175)
0.90 0.90 FUD XXX
AMA: 2018,Jan,8; 2017,Jan,8; 2016,Jan,13; 2015,Jan,16

88142 **Cytopathology, cervical or vaginal (any reporting system), collected in preservative fluid, automated thin layer preparation; manual screening under physician supervision** ♀

INCLUDES Bethesda or non-Bethesda method

0.00 0.00 FUD XXX

AMA: 2018,Jan,8; 2017,Jan,8; 2016,Jan,13; 2015,Jan,16

88143 **with manual screening and rescreening under physician supervision** ♀

INCLUDES Bethesda or non-Bethesda method

EXCLUDES *Automated screening automated thin layer preparation (88174-88175)*

0.00 0.00 FUD XXX

AMA: 2018,Jan,8; 2017,Jan,8; 2016,Jan,13; 2015,Jan,16

88147 **Cytopathology smears, cervical or vaginal; screening by automated system under physician supervision** ♀

0.00 0.00 FUD XXX

AMA: 2018,Jan,8; 2017,Jan,8; 2016,Jan,13; 2015,Jan,16

88148 **screening by automated system with manual rescreening under physician supervision** ♀

0.00 0.00 FUD XXX

AMA: 2018,Jan,8; 2017,Jan,8; 2016,Jan,13; 2015,Jan,16

88150 **Cytopathology, slides, cervical or vaginal; manual screening under physician supervision** ♀

EXCLUDES *Bethesda method Pap smears (88164-88167)*

0.00 0.00 FUD XXX

AMA: 2018,Jan,8; 2017,Jan,8; 2016,Jan,13; 2015,Jan,16

88152 **with manual screening and computer-assisted rescreening under physician supervision**

EXCLUDES *Bethesda method Pap smears (88164-88167)*

0.00 0.00 FUD XXX

AMA: 2018,Jan,8; 2017,Jan,8; 2016,Jan,13; 2015,Jan,16

88153 **with manual screening and rescreening under physician supervision** ♀

EXCLUDES *Bethesda method Pap smears (88164-88167)*

0.00 0.00 FUD XXX

AMA: 2018,Jan,8; 2017,Jan,8; 2016,Jan,13; 2015,Jan,16

\+ **88155** **Cytopathology, slides, cervical or vaginal, definitive hormonal evaluation (eg, maturation index, karyopyknotic index, estrogenic index) (List separately in addition to code[s] for other technical and interpretation services)** ♀

Code first (88142-88153, 88164-88167, 88174-88175)

0.00 0.00 FUD XXX

AMA: 2018,Jan,8; 2017,Jan,8; 2016,Jan,13; 2015,Jan,16

88160-88162 Cytopathology Smears (Other Than Pap)

88160 **Cytopathology, smears, any other source; screening and interpretation**

2.01 2.01 FUD XXX

AMA: 2006,Dec,10-12; 2005,Jul,11-12

88161 **preparation, screening and interpretation**

1.87 1.87 FUD XXX

AMA: 2018,Jan,8; 2017,Jan,8; 2016,Jan,13; 2015,Jan,16

88162 **extended study involving over 5 slides and/or multiple stains**

EXCLUDES *Aerosol collection sputum (89220)*
Special stains (88312-88314)

2.80 2.80 FUD XXX

AMA: 2005,Aug,7-8; 2005,Jul,11-12

88164-88167 Pap Smears: Bethesda System

CMS: 100-03,210.2 Screening Pap Smears/Pelvic Examinations for Early Cancer Detection

EXCLUDES *Non-Bethesda method (88150-88153)*

88164 **Cytopathology, slides, cervical or vaginal (the Bethesda System); manual screening under physician supervision** ♀

0.00 0.00 FUD XXX

AMA: 2018,Jan,8; 2017,Jan,8; 2016,Jan,13; 2015,Jan,16

88165 **with manual screening and rescreening under physician supervision** ♀

0.00 0.00 FUD XXX

AMA: 2018,Jan,8; 2017,Jan,8; 2016,Jan,13; 2015,Jan,16

88166 **with manual screening and computer-assisted rescreening under physician supervision** ♀

0.00 0.00 FUD XXX

AMA: 2018,Jan,8; 2017,Jan,8; 2016,Jan,13; 2015,Jan,16

88167 **with manual screening and computer-assisted rescreening using cell selection and review under physician supervision** ♀

EXCLUDES *Fine needle aspiration ([10004, 10005, 10006, 10007, 10008, 10009, 10010, 10011, 10012])*

0.00 0.00 FUD XXX

AMA: 2018,Jan,8; 2017,Jan,8; 2016,Jan,13; 2015,Jan,16

88172-88177 [88177] Cytopathology of Needle Biopsy

EXCLUDES *Fine needle aspiration (10021, [10004, 10005, 10006, 10007, 10008, 10009, 10010, 10011, 10012])*

88172 **Cytopathology, evaluation of fine needle aspirate; immediate cytohistologic study to determine adequacy for diagnosis, first evaluation episode, each site**

INCLUDES Submission complete set cytologic material for evaluation no matter how many needle passes performed or slides prepared from each site

EXCLUDES *Cytologic examination during intraoperative pathology consultation (88333-88334)*

1.58 1.58 FUD XXX

AMA: 2019,Feb,8; 2019,Apr,4; 2018,Jan,8; 2017,Jan,8; 2016,Jan,13; 2016,Jan,11; 2015,Jan,16

88173 **interpretation and report**

INCLUDES Interpretation and report from each anatomical site no matter how many passes or evaluation episodes performed during aspiration

EXCLUDES *Cytologic examination during intraoperative pathology consultation (88333-88334)*

4.32 4.32 FUD XXX

AMA: 2019,Feb,8; 2019,Apr,4; 2018,Jan,8; 2017,Jan,8; 2016,Jan,13; 2015,Jan,16

\+ # **88177** **immediate cytohistologic study to determine adequacy for diagnosis, each separate additional evaluation episode, same site (List separately in addition to code for primary procedure)**

Code also each additional immediate repeat evaluation episode(s) required from same site (i.e., previous sample inadequate)

Code first (88172)

0.84 0.84 FUD ZZZ

AMA: 2019,Apr,4; 2018,Jan,8; 2017,Jan,8; 2016,Jan,11

88174-88177 [88177] Pap Smears: Automated Screening

EXCLUDES *Non-Bethesda method (88150-88153)*

88174 **Cytopathology, cervical or vaginal (any reporting system), collected in preservative fluid, automated thin layer preparation; screening by automated system, under physician supervision** ♀

INCLUDES Bethesda or non-Bethesda method

0.00 0.00 FUD XXX

AMA: 2018,Jan,8; 2017,Jan,8; 2016,Jan,13; 2015,Jan,16

88175 **with screening by automated system and manual rescreening or review, under physician supervision** ♀

INCLUDES Bethesda or non-Bethesda method

EXCLUDES *Manual screening (88142-88143)*

0.00 0.00 FUD XXX

AMA: 2018,Jan,8; 2017,Jan,8; 2016,Jan,13; 2015,Jan,16

88177 **Resequenced code. See code following 88173.**

88182-88199 Cytopathology Using the Fluorescence-Activated Cell Sorter

88182 Flow cytometry, cell cycle or DNA analysis

EXCLUDES *DNA ploidy analysis by morphometric technique (88358)*

3.79 3.79 FUD XXX Q2 80

AMA: 2018,Jan,8; 2017,Jan,8; 2016,Jan,13; 2015,Jan,16

88184 Flow cytometry, cell surface, cytoplasmic, or nuclear marker, technical component only; first marker

1.88 1.88 FUD XXX Q2 80 TC

AMA: 2018,Jan,8; 2017,Jan,8; 2016,Jan,13; 2015,Jan,16

\+ **88185 each additional marker (List separately in addition to code for first marker)**

Code first (88184)

0.62 0.62 FUD ZZZ N 80 TC

AMA: 2018,Jan,8; 2017,Jan,8; 2016,Jan,13; 2015,Jan,16

88187 Flow cytometry, interpretation; 2 to 8 markers

EXCLUDES *Antibody assessment by flow cytometry (83516-83520, 86000-86849 [86152, 86153])*
Cell enumeration by immunologic selection and identification ([86152, 86153])
Interpretation (86355-86357, 86359-86361, 86367)

1.08 1.08 FUD XXX B 80 26

AMA: 2018,Jan,8; 2017,Jan,8; 2016,Jan,13; 2015,Jan,16

88188 9 to 15 markers

EXCLUDES *Antibody assessment by flow cytometry (83516-83520, 86000-86849 [86152, 86153])*
Cell enumeration by immunologic selection and identification ([86152, 86153])
Interpretation (86355-86357, 86359-86361, 86367)

1.83 1.83 FUD XXX B 80 26

AMA: 2018,Jan,8; 2017,Jan,8; 2016,Jan,13; 2015,Jan,16

88189 16 or more markers

EXCLUDES *Antibody assessment by flow cytometry (83516-83520, 86000-86849 [86152, 86153])*
Cell enumeration using immunologic selection and identification in fluid sample ([86152, 86153])
Interpretation (86355-86357, 86359-86361, 86367)

2.45 2.45 FUD XXX B 80 26

AMA: 2018,Jan,8; 2017,Jan,8; 2016,Jan,13; 2015,Jan,16

88199 Unlisted cytopathology procedure

EXCLUDES *Electron microscopy (88348)*

0.00 0.00 FUD XXX Q1 80

AMA: 2018,Jan,8; 2017,Jan,8; 2016,Jan,13; 2015,Jan,16

88230-88299 Cytogenic Studies

CMS: 100-03,190.3 Cytogenic Studies

EXCLUDES *Acetylcholinesterase (82013)*
Alpha-fetoprotein (amniotic fluid or serum) (82105-82106)
Microdissection (88380)
Molecular pathology codes (81105-81383 [81105, 81106, 81107, 81108, 81109, 81110, 81111, 81112, 81120, 81121, 81161, 81162, 81163, 81164, 81165, 81166, 81167, 81173, 81174, 81184, 81185, 81186, 81187, 81188, 81189, 81190, 81200, 81201, 81202, 81203, 81204, 81205, 81206, 81207, 81208, 81209, 81210, 81219, 81227, 81230, 81231, 81233, 81234, 81238, 81239, 81245, 81246, 81250, 81257, 81258, 81259, 81261, 81262, 81263, 81264, 81265, 81266, 81267, 81268, 81269, 81271, 81274, 81283, 81284, 81285, 81286, 81287, 81288, 81289, 81291, 81292, 81293, 81294, 81295, 81301, 81302, 81303, 81304, 81306, 81312, 81320, 81324, 81325, 81326, 81332, 81334, 81336, 81337, 81343, 81344, 81345, 81361, 81362, 81363, 81364], 81400-81408, [81479], 81410-81471 [81448], 81500-81512, 81599)

88230 Tissue culture for non-neoplastic disorders; lymphocyte

0.00 0.00 FUD XXX Q

AMA: 2018,Jan,8; 2017,Jan,8; 2016,Jan,13; 2015,Jan,16

88233 skin or other solid tissue biopsy

0.00 0.00 FUD XXX Q

AMA: 2018,Jan,8; 2017,Jan,8; 2016,Jan,13; 2015,Jan,16

88235 amniotic fluid or chorionic villus cells M

0.00 0.00 FUD XXX Q

AMA: 2018,Jan,8; 2017,Jan,8; 2016,Jan,13; 2015,Jan,16

88237 Tissue culture for neoplastic disorders; bone marrow, blood cells

0.00 0.00 FUD XXX Q

AMA: 2018,Jan,8; 2017,Jan,8; 2016,Jan,13; 2015,Jan,16

88239 solid tumor

0.00 0.00 FUD XXX Q

AMA: 2018,Jan,8; 2017,Jan,8; 2016,Jan,13; 2015,Jan,16

88240 Cryopreservation, freezing and storage of cells, each cell line

EXCLUDES *Therapeutic cryopreservation and storage (38207)*

0.00 0.00 FUD XXX Q

AMA: 2018,Jan,8; 2017,Jan,8; 2016,Jan,13; 2015,Jan,16

88241 Thawing and expansion of frozen cells, each aliquot

EXCLUDES *Therapeutic thawing of prior harvest (38208)*

0.00 0.00 FUD XXX Q

AMA: 2018,Jan,8; 2017,Jan,8; 2016,Jan,13; 2015,Jan,16

88245 Chromosome analysis for breakage syndromes; baseline Sister Chromatid Exchange (SCE), 20-25 cells

0.00 0.00 FUD XXX Q

AMA: 2018,Jan,8; 2017,Jan,8; 2016,Jan,13; 2015,Jan,16

88248 baseline breakage, score 50-100 cells, count 20 cells, 2 karyotypes (eg, for ataxia telangiectasia, Fanconi anemia, fragile X)

0.00 0.00 FUD XXX Q

AMA: 2018,Jan,8; 2017,Jan,8; 2016,Jan,13; 2015,Jan,16

88249 score 100 cells, clastogen stress (eg, diepoxybutane, mitomycin C, ionizing radiation, UV radiation)

0.00 0.00 FUD XXX Q

AMA: 2018,Jan,8; 2017,Jan,8; 2016,Jan,13; 2015,Jan,16

88261 Chromosome analysis; count 5 cells, 1 karyotype, with banding

0.00 0.00 FUD XXX Q

AMA: 2018,Jan,8; 2017,Jan,8; 2016,Jan,13; 2015,Jan,16

88262 count 15-20 cells, 2 karyotypes, with banding

0.00 0.00 FUD XXX Q

AMA: 2019,Aug,10; 2018,Jan,8; 2017,Jan,8; 2016,Jan,13; 2015,Jan,16

88263 count 45 cells for mosaicism, 2 karyotypes, with banding

0.00 0.00 FUD XXX Q

AMA: 2018,Jan,8; 2017,Jan,8; 2016,Jan,13; 2015,Jan,16

88264 analyze 20-25 cells

0.00 0.00 FUD XXX Q

AMA: 2019,Aug,10; 2018,Jan,8; 2017,Jan,8; 2016,Jan,13; 2015,Jan,16

88267 Chromosome analysis, amniotic fluid or chorionic villus, count 15 cells, 1 karyotype, with banding M ♀

0.00 0.00 FUD XXX Q

AMA: 2018,Jan,8; 2017,Jan,8; 2016,Jan,13; 2015,Jan,16

88269 Chromosome analysis, in situ for amniotic fluid cells, count cells from 6-12 colonies, 1 karyotype, with banding M ♀

0.00 0.00 FUD XXX Q

AMA: 2018,Jan,8; 2017,Jan,8; 2016,Jan,13; 2015,Jan,16

88271 Molecular cytogenetics; DNA probe, each (eg, FISH)

EXCLUDES *Cytogenomic microarray analysis (81228-81229, 81405-81406, [81479])*
Fetal chromosome analysis using maternal blood (81420-81422)

0.00 0.00 FUD XXX Q

AMA: 2020,Feb,10; 2018,Jan,8; 2017,Apr,3; 2017,Jan,8; 2016,Jan,13; 2015,Jan,16

88272 chromosomal in situ hybridization, analyze 3-5 cells (eg, for derivatives and markers)

0.00 0.00 FUD XXX Q

AMA: 2018,Jan,8; 2017,Jan,8; 2016,Jan,13; 2015,Jan,16

88273 **chromosomal in situ hybridization, analyze 10-30 cells (eg, for microdeletions)**
0.00 0.00 FUD XXX Q
AMA: 2018,Jan,8; 2017,Jan,8; 2016,Jan,13; 2015,Jan,16

88274 **interphase in situ hybridization, analyze 25-99 cells**
0.00 0.00 FUD XXX Q
AMA: 2018,Jan,8; 2017,Jan,8; 2016,Jan,13; 2015,Jan,16

88275 **interphase in situ hybridization, analyze 100-300 cells**
0.00 0.00 FUD XXX Q
AMA: 2018,Jan,8; 2017,Jan,8; 2016,Jan,13; 2015,Jan,16

88280 **Chromosome analysis; additional karyotypes, each study**
0.00 0.00 FUD XXX Q
AMA: 2018,Jan,8; 2017,Jan,8; 2016,Jan,13; 2015,Jan,16

88283 **additional specialized banding technique (eg, NOR, C-banding)**
0.00 0.00 FUD XXX Q
AMA: 2018,Jan,8; 2017,Jan,8; 2016,Jan,13; 2015,Jan,16

88285 **additional cells counted, each study**
0.00 0.00 FUD XXX Q
AMA: 2018,Jan,8; 2017,Jan,8; 2016,Jan,13; 2015,Jan,16

88289 **additional high resolution study**
0.00 0.00 FUD XXX Q
AMA: 2018,Jan,8; 2017,Jan,8; 2016,Jan,13; 2015,Jan,16

88291 **Cytogenetics and molecular cytogenetics, interpretation and report**
0.94 0.94 FUD XXX M 80 26
AMA: 2018,Jan,8; 2017,Jan,8; 2016,Jan,13; 2015,Jan,16

88299 **Unlisted cytogenetic study**
0.00 0.00 FUD XXX Q1 80
AMA: 2018,Jan,8; 2017,Jan,8; 2016,Jan,13; 2015,Jan,16

88300 Evaluation of Surgical Specimen: Gross Anatomy

CMS: 100-02,15,80.1 Payment for Clinical Laboratory Services

INCLUDES Attainment, examination, and reporting
Unit of service is the specimen

EXCLUDES *Additional procedures (88311-88365 [88341, 88350], 88399)*
Microscopic exam (88302-88309)

88300 **Level I - Surgical pathology, gross examination only**
0.44 0.44 FUD XXX Q1 80
AMA: 2018,Jan,8; 2017,Jan,8; 2016,Jan,13; 2015,Jan,16

88302-88309 Evaluation of Surgical Specimens: Gross and Microscopic Anatomy

CMS: 100-02,15,80.1 Payment for Clinical Laboratory Services

INCLUDES Attainment, examination, and reporting
Unit of service is the specimen

EXCLUDES *Additional procedures (88311-88365 [88341, 88350], 88399)*
Mohs surgery (17311-17315)

88302 **Level II - Surgical pathology, gross and microscopic examination**

INCLUDES Confirming identification and disease absence:
- Appendix, incidental
- Fallopian tube, sterilization
- Fingers or toes traumatic amputation
- Foreskin, newborn
- Hernia sac, any site
- Hydrocele sac
- Nerve
- Skin, plastic repair
- Sympathetic ganglion
- Testis, castration
- Vaginal mucosa, incidental
- Vas deferens, sterilization

0.87 0.87 FUD XXX Q1 80
AMA: 2018,Jan,8; 2017,Jan,8; 2016,Jan,13; 2015,Jan,16

88304 **Level III - Surgical pathology, gross and microscopic examination**

INCLUDES
- Abortion, induced
- Abscess
- Anal tag
- Aneurysm-atrial/ventricular
- Appendix, other than incidental
- Artery, atheromatous plaque
- Bartholin's gland cyst
- Bone fragment(s), other than pathologic fracture
- Bursa/ synovial cyst
- Carpal tunnel tissue
- Cartilage, shavings
- Cholesteatoma
- Colon, colostomy stoma
- Conjunctiva-biopsy/pterygium
- Cornea
- Diverticulum-esophagus/small intestine
- Dupuytren's contracture tissue
- Femoral head, other than fracture
- Fissure/fistula
- Foreskin, other than newborn
- Gallbladder
- Ganglion cyst
- Hematoma
- Hemorrhoids
- Hydatid of Morgagni
- Intervertebral disc
- Joint, loose body
- Meniscus
- Mucocele, salivary
- Neuroma-Morton's/traumatic
- Pilonidal cyst/sinus
- Polyps, inflammatory-nasal/sinusoidal
- Skin-cyst/tag/debridement
- Soft tissue, debridement
- Soft tissue, lipoma
- Spermatocele
- Tendon/tendon sheath
- Testicular appendage
- Thrombus or embolus
- Tonsil and/or adenoids
- Varicocele
- Vas deferens, other than sterilization
- Vein, varicosity

1.16 1.16 FUD XXX Q1 80
AMA: 2018,Jan,8; 2017,Jan,8; 2016,Jan,13; 2015,Jan,16

88305 **Level IV - Surgical pathology, gross and microscopic examination**

INCLUDES
- Abortion, spontaneous/missed
- Artery, biopsy
- Bone exostosis
- Bone marrow, biopsy
- Brain/meninges, other than for tumor resection
- Breast biopsy without microscopic assessment of surgical margin
- Breast reduction mammoplasty
- Bronchus, biopsy
- Cell block, any source
- Cervix, biopsy
- Colon, biopsy
- Duodenum, biopsy
- Endocervix, curettings/biopsy
- Endometrium, curettings/biopsy
- Esophagus, biopsy
- Extremity, amputation, traumatic
- Fallopian tube, biopsy
- Fallopian tube, ectopic pregnancy
- Femoral head, fracture
- Finger/toes, amputation, nontraumatic
- Gingiva/oral mucosa, biopsy
- Heart valve
- Joint resection
- Kidney biopsy
- Larynx biopsy

Leiomyoma(s), uterine myomectomy-without uterus
Lip, biopsy/wedge resection
Lung, transbronchial biopsy
Lymph node, biopsy
Muscle, biopsy
Nasal mucosa, biopsy
Nasopharynx/oropharynx, biopsy
Nerve biopsy
Odontogenic/dental cyst
Omentum, biopsy
Ovary, biopsy/wedge resection
Ovary with or without tube, nonneoplastic
Parathyroid gland
Peritoneum, biopsy
Pituitary tumor
Placenta, other than third trimester
Pleura/pericardium-biopsy/tissue
Polyp:
- Cervical/endometrial
- Colorectal
- Stomach/small intestine

Prostate:
- Needle biopsy
- TUR

Salivary gland, biopsy
Sinus, paranasal biopsy
Skin, other than cyst/tag/debridement/plastic repair
Small intestine, biopsy
Soft tissue, other than tumor/mas/lipoma/debridement
Spleen
Stomach biopsy
Synovium
Testis, other than tumor/biopsy, castration
Thyroglossal duct/brachial cleft cyst
Tongue, biopsy
Tonsil, biopsy
Trachea biopsy
Ureter, biopsy
Urethra, biopsy
Urinary bladder, biopsy
Uterus, with or without tubes and ovaries, for prolapse
Vagina biopsy
Vulva/labial biopsy

1.98 1.98 **FUD** XXX 01 80
AMA: 2018,May,3; 2018,Jan,8; 2017,Jan,8; 2016,Jan,13; 2015,Jan,16

88307 Level V - Surgical pathology, gross and microscopic examination

INCLUDES Adrenal resection
Bone, biopsy/curettings
Bone fragment(s), pathologic fractures
Brain, biopsy
Brain meninges, tumor resection
Breast, excision of lesion, requiring microscopic evaluation of surgical margins
Breast, mastectomy-partial/simple
Cervix, conization
Colon, segmental resection, other than for tumor
Extremity, amputation, nontraumatic
Eye, enucleation
Kidney, partial/total nephrectomy
Larynx, partial/total resection
Liver
- Biopsy, needle/wedge
- Partial resection

Lung, wedge biopsy
Lymph nodes, regional resection
Mediastinum, mass
Myocardium, biopsy
Odontogenic tumor
Ovary with or without tube, neoplastic
Pancreas, biopsy
Placenta, third trimester
Prostate, except radical resection
Salivary gland
Sentinel lymph node
Small intestine, resection, other than for tumor
Soft tissue mass (except lipoma)-biopsy/simple excision
Stomach-subtotal/total resection, other than for tumor
Testis, biopsy
Thymus, tumor
Thyroid, total/lobe
Ureter, resection
Urinary bladder, TUR
Uterus, with or without tubes and ovaries, other than neoplastic/prolapse

7.59 7.59 **FUD** XXX 02 80
AMA: 2018,Jan,8; 2017,Jan,8; 2016,Jan,13; 2015,Jan,16

88309 Level VI - Surgical pathology, gross and microscopic examination

INCLUDES Bone resection
Breast, mastectomy-with regional lymph nodes
Colon:
- Segmental resection for tumor
- Total resection

Esophagus, partial/total resection
Extremity, disarticulation
Fetus, with dissection
Larynx, partial/total resection-with regional lymph nodes
Lung-total/lobe/segment resection
Pancreas, total/subtotal resection
Prostate, radical resection
Small intestine, resection for tumor
Soft tissue tumor, extensive resection
Stomach, subtotal/total resection for tumor
Testis, tumor
Tongue/tonsil, resection for tumor
Urinary bladder, partial/total resection
Uterus, with or without tubes and ovaries, neoplastic
Vulva, total/subtotal resection

EXCLUDES *Evaluation fine needle aspirate (88172-88173)*
Fine needle aspiration (10021, [10004, 10005, 10006, 10007, 10008, 10009, 10010, 10011, 10012])

11.8 11.8 **FUD** XXX 02 80
AMA: 2018,Jan,8; 2017,Jan,8; 2016,Jan,13; 2015,Jan,16

88311-88399 [88341, 88350, 88364, 88373, 88374, 88377] Additional Surgical Pathology Services

CMS: 100-02,15,80.1 Payment for Clinical Laboratory Services

\+ **88311** **Decalcification procedure (List separately in addition to code for surgical pathology examination)**
Code first surgical pathology exam (88302-88309)
0.61 0.61 FUD XXX N 80
AMA: 2018,Jan,8; 2017,Jan,8; 2016,Jan,13; 2015,Jan,16

88312 **Special stain including interpretation and report; Group I for microorganisms (eg, acid fast, methenamine silver)**
INCLUDES Reporting one unit for each special stain performed on surgical pathology block, cytologic sample, or hematologic smear
2.97 2.97 FUD XXX Q1 80
AMA: 2018,Jan,8; 2017,Jan,8; 2016,Jan,13; 2015,Jan,16

88313 **Group II, all other (eg, iron, trichrome), except stain for microorganisms, stains for enzyme constituents, or immunocytochemistry and immunohistochemistry**
INCLUDES Reporting one unit for each special stain performed on surgical pathology block, cytologic sample, or hematologic smear
EXCLUDES *Immunocytochemistry and immunohistochemistry (88342)*
2.05 2.05 FUD XXX Q1 80
AMA: 2018,Jan,8; 2017,Jan,8; 2016,Jan,13; 2015,Jan,16

\+ **88314** **histochemical stain on frozen tissue block (List separately in addition to code for primary procedure)**
INCLUDES Reporting one unit for each special stain on each frozen surgical pathology block
EXCLUDES *Routine frozen section stain during Mohs surgery (17311-17315)*
Special stain performed on frozen tissue section specimen to identify enzyme constituents (88319)
Code also modifier 59 for nonroutine histochemical stain on frozen section during Mohs surgery
Code first (17311-17315, 88302-88309, 88331-88332)
2.73 2.73 FUD XXX N 80
AMA: 2018,Jan,8; 2017,Jan,8; 2016,Jan,13; 2015,Jan,16

88319 **Group III, for enzyme constituents**
INCLUDES Reporting one unit for each special stain on each frozen surgical pathology block
EXCLUDES *Detection of enzyme constituents by immunohistochemical or immunocytochemical methodology (88342)*
2.74 2.74 FUD XXX Q2 80
AMA: 2018,Jan,8; 2017,Jan,8; 2016,Jan,13; 2015,Jan,16

88321 **Consultation and report on referred slides prepared elsewhere**
2.44 2.84 FUD XXX Q1 80
AMA: 2018,Jan,8; 2017,Jan,8; 2016,Jan,13; 2015,Jan,16

88323 **Consultation and report on referred material requiring preparation of slides**
3.28 3.28 FUD XXX Q1 80
AMA: 2018,Jan,8; 2017,Jan,8; 2016,Jan,13; 2015,Jan,16

88325 **Consultation, comprehensive, with review of records and specimens, with report on referred material**
4.29 5.12 FUD XXX Q1 80
AMA: 2018,Jan,8; 2017,Jan,8; 2016,Jan,13; 2015,Jan,16

88329 **Pathology consultation during surgery;**
1.04 1.47 FUD XXX Q1 80
AMA: 2018,Jan,8; 2017,Jan,8; 2016,Jan,13; 2015,Jan,16

88331 **first tissue block, with frozen section(s), single specimen**
Code also cytologic evaluation performed at same time (88334)
2.75 2.75 FUD XXX Q1 80
AMA: 2018,Jan,8; 2017,Jan,8; 2016,Jan,13; 2015,Jan,16

\+ **88332** **each additional tissue block with frozen section(s) (List separately in addition to code for primary procedure)**
Code first (88331)
1.54 1.54 FUD XXX N 80
AMA: 2018,Jan,8; 2017,Jan,8; 2016,Jan,13; 2015,Jan,16

88333 **cytologic examination (eg, touch prep, squash prep), initial site**
EXCLUDES *Intraprocedural cytologic evaluation fine needle aspirate (88172)*
Nonintraoperative cytologic examination (88160-88162)
2.53 2.53 FUD XXX Q2 80
AMA: 2018,Jan,8; 2017,Jan,8; 2016,Jan,13; 2015,Jan,16

\+ **88334** **cytologic examination (eg, touch prep, squash prep), each additional site (List separately in addition to code for primary procedure)**
EXCLUDES *Intraprocedural cytologic evaluation fine needle aspirate (88172)*
Nonintraoperative cytologic examination (88160-88162)
Percutaneous needle biopsy requiring intraprocedural cytologic examination (88333)
Code first (88331, 88333)
1.58 1.58 FUD ZZZ N 80
AMA: 2018,Jan,8; 2017,Jan,8; 2016,Jan,13; 2015,Jan,16

88341 **Resequenced code. See code following 88342.**

88342 **Immunohistochemistry or immunocytochemistry, per specimen; initial single antibody stain procedure**
EXCLUDES *Morphometric analysis, tumor immunohistochemistry, on same antibody (88360-88361)*
Multiplex antibody stain (88344)
Reporting code more than one time for each specific antibody
3.01 3.01 FUD XXX Q2 80
AMA: 2018,Jan,8; 2017,Jan,8; 2016,Jan,13; 2015,Jun,10; 2015,Jan,16

\+ # **88341** **each additional single antibody stain procedure (List separately in addition to code for primary procedure)**
EXCLUDES *Morphometric analysis (88360-88361)*
Multiplex antibody stain (88344)
Reporting code more than one time for each specific antibody
Code first (88342)
2.62 2.62 FUD ZZZ N 80
AMA: 2018,Jan,8; 2017,Jan,8; 2016,Jan,13; 2015,Jun,10

88344 **each multiplex antibody stain procedure**
INCLUDES Staining with multiple antibodies on same slide
EXCLUDES *Morphometric analysis, tumor immunohistochemistry, on same antibody (88360-88361)*
Reporting code more than one time for each specific antibody
4.86 4.86 FUD XXX Q1 80
AMA: 2018,Jan,8; 2017,Jan,8; 2016,Jan,13; 2015,Jun,10

88346 **Immunofluorescence, per specimen; initial single antibody stain procedure**
EXCLUDES *Fluorescent in situ hybridization studies (88364-88369 [88364, 88373, 88374, 88377])*
Multiple immunofluorescence analysis (88399)
3.11 3.11 FUD XXX Q2 80
AMA: 2018,Jan,8; 2017,Jan,8; 2016,Jan,13; 2015,Jan,16

\+ # **88350** **each additional single antibody stain procedure (List separately in addition to code for primary procedure)**
EXCLUDES *Fluorescent in situ hybridization studies (88364-88369 [88364, 88373, 88374, 88377])*
Multiple immunofluorescence analysis (88399)
Code first (88346)
2.18 2.18 FUD ZZZ N 80

88348 **Electron microscopy, diagnostic**
10.9 10.9 FUD XXX Q2 80
AMA: 2011,Dec,14-18; 2005,Jul,11-12

88350 **Resequenced code. See code following 88346.**

88355 Morphometric analysis; skeletal muscle
3.88 3.88 FUD XXX
AMA: 2018,Jan,8; 2017,Jan,8; 2016,Jan,13; 2015,Jan,16

88356 nerve
6.34 6.34 FUD XXX
AMA: 2018,Jan,8; 2017,Jan,8; 2016,Jan,13; 2015,Jan,16

88358 tumor (eg, DNA ploidy)
EXCLUDES *Special stain, Group II (88313)*
3.61 3.61 FUD XXX
AMA: 2018,Jan,8; 2017,Jan,8; 2016,Jan,13; 2015,Jan,16

88360 Morphometric analysis, tumor immunohistochemistry (eg, Her-2/neu, estrogen receptor/progesterone receptor), quantitative or semiquantitative, per specimen, each single antibody stain procedure; manual
EXCLUDES *Additional stain procedures unless each test for different antibody (88341, 88342, 88344)*
Morphometric analysis using in situ hybridization techniques (88367-88368 [88373, 88374])
3.60 3.60 FUD XXX
AMA: 2018,Jan,8; 2017,Jan,8; 2016,Jan,13; 2015,Jun,10; 2015,Jan,16

88361 using computer-assisted technology
EXCLUDES *Additional stain procedures unless each test for different antibody (88341, 88342, 88344)*
Morphometric analysis using in situ hybridization techniques (88367-88368 [88373, 88374])
3.58 3.58 FUD XXX
AMA: 2018,Jan,8; 2017,Jan,8; 2016,Jan,13; 2015,Jun,10; 2015,Jan,16

88362 Nerve teasing preparations
5.92 5.92 FUD XXX
AMA: 2018,Jan,8; 2017,Jan,8; 2016,Jan,13; 2015,Jan,16

88363 Examination and selection of retrieved archival (ie, previously diagnosed) tissue(s) for molecular analysis (eg, KRAS mutational analysis)
INCLUDES Archival retrieval only
0.57 0.67 FUD XXX
AMA: 2018,Jan,8; 2017,Jan,8; 2016,Jan,13; 2015,Jan,16

88364 **Resequenced code. See code following 88365.**

88365 In situ hybridization (eg, FISH), per specimen; initial single probe stain procedure
EXCLUDES *Morphometric analysis probe stain procedures with same probe (88367, [88374], 88368, [88377])*
5.10 5.10 FUD XXX
AMA: 2018,Nov,11; 2018,Jan,8; 2017,Jan,8; 2016,Jan,13; 2015,Jan,16

+ # **88364 each additional single probe stain procedure (List separately in addition to code for primary procedure)**
Code first (88365)
3.74 3.74 FUD ZZZ

88366 each multiplex probe stain procedure
EXCLUDES *Morphometric analysis probe stain procedures (88367, [88374], 88368, [88377])*
7.80 7.80 FUD XXX

88367 Morphometric analysis, in situ hybridization (quantitative or semi-quantitative), using computer-assisted technology, per specimen; initial single probe stain procedure
EXCLUDES *In situ hybridization probe stain procedures for same probe (88365, 88366, 88368, [88377])*
Morphometric in situ hybridization evaluation urinary tract cytologic specimens (88120-88121)
3.08 3.08 FUD XXX
AMA: 2018,Jan,8; 2017,Jan,8; 2016,Jan,13; 2015,Jan,16

+ # **88373 each additional single probe stain procedure (List separately in addition to code for primary procedure)**
Code first (88367)
2.11 2.11 FUD ZZZ

88374 each multiplex probe stain procedure
EXCLUDES *In situ hybridization probe stain procedures for same probe (88365, 88366, 88368, [88377])*
9.65 9.65 FUD XXX

88368 Morphometric analysis, in situ hybridization (quantitative or semi-quantitative), manual, per specimen; initial single probe stain procedure
EXCLUDES *In situ hybridization probe stain procedures for same probe (88365, 88366-88367, [88374])*
Morphometric in situ hybridization evaluation urinary tract cytologic specimens (88120-88121)
3.59 3.59 FUD XXX
AMA: 2018,Jan,8; 2017,Jan,8; 2016,Jan,13; 2015,Jan,16

+ **88369 each additional single probe stain procedure (List separately in addition to code for primary procedure)**
Code first (88368)
3.23 3.23 FUD ZZZ

88377 each multiplex probe stain procedure
EXCLUDES *In situ hybridization probe stain procedures for same probe (88365, 88366-88367, [88374])*
Morphometric in situ hybridization evaluation, urinary tract cytologic specimens (88120-88121)
11.4 11.4 FUD XXX

88371 Protein analysis of tissue by Western Blot, with interpretation and report;
0.00 0.00 FUD XXX
AMA: 2018,Jan,8; 2017,Jan,8; 2016,Jan,13; 2015,Dec,18; 2015,Jan,16

88372 immunological probe for band identification, each
0.00 0.00 FUD XXX
AMA: 2018,Jan,8; 2017,Jan,8; 2016,Jan,13; 2015,Jan,16

88373 **Resequenced code. See code following 88367.**

88374 **Resequenced code. See code following 88367.**

88375 Optical endomicroscopic image(s), interpretation and report, real-time or referred, each endoscopic session
EXCLUDES *Endoscopic procedures that include optical endomicroscopy (43206, 43252, 0397T)*
1.42 1.42 FUD XXX
AMA: 2018,Jan,8; 2017,Jan,8; 2016,Jan,13; 2015,Jan,16

88377 **Resequenced code. See code following 88369.**

88380 Microdissection (ie, sample preparation of microscopically identified target); laser capture
EXCLUDES *Microdissection, manual procedure (88381)*
3.78 3.78 FUD XXX
AMA: 2018,Aug,3; 2018,Jan,8; 2017,Jan,8; 2016,Jan,13; 2015,Jan,16

88381 manual
EXCLUDES *Microdissection, laser capture procedure (88380)*
4.34 4.34 FUD XXX
AMA: 2018,Aug,3; 2018,Jan,8; 2017,Jan,8; 2016,Jan,13; 2015,Jan,16

88387 Macroscopic examination, dissection, and preparation of tissue for non-microscopic analytical studies (eg, nucleic acid-based molecular studies); each tissue preparation (eg, a single lymph node)
EXCLUDES *Pathology consultation during surgery (88329-88334, 88388)*
Tissue preparation for microbiologic cultures or flow cytometric studies
1.00 1.00 FUD XXX
AMA: 2018,Jan,8; 2017,Jan,8; 2016,Jan,13; 2015,Jan,16

+ **88388** **in conjunction with a touch imprint, intraoperative consultation, or frozen section, each tissue preparation (eg, a single lymph node) (List separately in addition to code for primary procedure)**

> EXCLUDES *Tissue preparation for microbiologic cultures or flow cytometric studies*

Code first (88329-88334)

🚗 1.00 ⚕ 1.00 **FUD** XXX N 80 ▭

AMA: 2018,Jan,8; 2017,Jan,8; 2016,Jan,13; 2015,Jan,16

88399 **Unlisted surgical pathology procedure**

🚗 0.00 ⚕ 0.00 **FUD** XXX Q1 80 ▭

AMA: 2018,Jan,8; 2017,Jan,8; 2016,Jan,13; 2015,Jan,16

88720-88749 Transcutaneous Procedures

> EXCLUDES *Transcutaneous oxyhemoglobin measurement (0493T)*
> *Wavelength fluorescent spectroscopy advanced glycation end products (skin) (88749)*

88720 **Bilirubin, total, transcutaneous**

> EXCLUDES *Transdermal oxygen saturation testing (94760-94762)*

🚗 0.00 ⚕ 0.00 **FUD** XXX Q ▭

AMA: 2020,May,13; 2018,Jan,8; 2017,Jan,8; 2016,Jan,13; 2015,Jan,16

88738 **Hemoglobin (Hgb), quantitative, transcutaneous**

> EXCLUDES *In vitro hemoglobin measurement (85018)*

🚗 0.00 ⚕ 0.00 **FUD** XXX Q ▭

AMA: 2018,Jan,8; 2017,Jan,8; 2016,Jan,13; 2015,Jan,16

88740 **Hemoglobin, quantitative, transcutaneous, per day; carboxyhemoglobin**

> EXCLUDES *In vitro carboxyhemoglobin measurement (82375)*

🚗 0.00 ⚕ 0.00 **FUD** XXX Q ▭

AMA: 2018,Jan,8; 2017,Jan,8; 2016,Jan,13; 2015,Jan,16

88741 **methemoglobin**

> EXCLUDES *In vitro quantitative methemoglobin measurement (83050)*

🚗 0.00 ⚕ 0.00 **FUD** XXX Q ▭

AMA: 2018,Jan,8; 2017,Jan,8; 2016,Jan,13; 2015,Jan,16

88749 **Unlisted in vivo (eg, transcutaneous) laboratory service**

> INCLUDES *All in vivo measurements not specifically listed*

🚗 0.00 ⚕ 0.00 **FUD** XXX Q ▭

AMA: 2010,Dec,7-10

89049-89240 Other Pathology Services

89049 **Caffeine halothane contracture test (CHCT) for malignant hyperthermia susceptibility, including interpretation and report**

🚗 1.77 ⚕ 7.06 **FUD** XXX Q1 80 ▭

AMA: 2018,Jan,8; 2017,Jan,8; 2016,Jan,13; 2015,Jan,16

89050 **Cell count, miscellaneous body fluids (eg, cerebrospinal fluid, joint fluid), except blood;**

🚗 0.00 ⚕ 0.00 **FUD** XXX Q ▭

AMA: 2018,Jan,8; 2017,Jan,8; 2016,Jan,13; 2015,Jan,16

89051 **with differential count**

🚗 0.00 ⚕ 0.00 **FUD** XXX Q ▭

AMA: 2018,Jan,8; 2017,Jan,8; 2016,Jan,13; 2015,Jan,16

89055 **Leukocyte assessment, fecal, qualitative or semiquantitative**

🚗 0.00 ⚕ 0.00 **FUD** XXX Q ▭

AMA: 2018,Jan,8; 2017,Jan,8; 2016,Jan,13; 2015,Jan,16

89060 **Crystal identification by light microscopy with or without polarizing lens analysis, tissue or any body fluid (except urine)**

> EXCLUDES *Crystal identification on paraffin embedded tissue*

🚗 0.00 ⚕ 0.00 **FUD** XXX Q 80 ▭

AMA: 2018,Jan,8; 2017,Jan,8; 2016,Jan,13; 2015,Jan,16

89125 **Fat stain, feces, urine, or respiratory secretions**

🚗 0.00 ⚕ 0.00 **FUD** XXX Q ▭

AMA: 2018,Jan,8; 2017,Jan,8; 2016,Jan,13; 2015,Jan,16

89160 **Meat fibers, feces**

🚗 0.00 ⚕ 0.00 **FUD** XXX Q ▭

AMA: 2018,Jan,8; 2017,Jan,8; 2016,Jan,13; 2015,Jan,16

89190 **Nasal smear for eosinophils**

> EXCLUDES *Occult blood feces (82270)*
> *Paternity tests (86910)*

🚗 0.00 ⚕ 0.00 **FUD** XXX Q ▭

AMA: 2018,Jan,8; 2017,Jan,8; 2016,Jan,13; 2015,Jan,16

89220 **Sputum, obtaining specimen, aerosol induced technique (separate procedure)**

🚗 0.46 ⚕ 0.46 **FUD** XXX Q1 80 TC ▭

AMA: 2018,Jan,8; 2017,Jan,8; 2016,Jan,13; 2015,Jan,16

89230 **Sweat collection by iontophoresis**

🚗 0.07 ⚕ 0.07 **FUD** XXX Q1 80 TC ▭

AMA: 2018,Jan,8; 2017,Jan,8; 2016,Jan,13; 2015,Jan,16

89240 **Unlisted miscellaneous pathology test**

🚗 0.00 ⚕ 0.00 **FUD** XXX Q1 80 ▭

AMA: 2018,Jan,8; 2017,Jan,8; 2016,Jan,13; 2015,Jan,16

89250-89398 Infertility Treatment Services

CMS: 100-02,1,100 Treatment for Infertility

89250 **Culture of oocyte(s)/embryo(s), less than 4 days;**

🚗 0.00 ⚕ 0.00 **FUD** XXX Q1 ▭

AMA: 2018,Jan,8; 2017,Jan,8; 2016,Jan,13; 2015,Jan,16

89251 **with co-culture of oocyte(s)/embryos**

> EXCLUDES *Extended culture oocyte(s)/embryo(s) (89272)*

🚗 0.00 ⚕ 0.00 **FUD** XXX Q2 ▭

AMA: 2018,Jan,8; 2017,Jan,8; 2016,Jan,13; 2015,Jan,16

89253 **Assisted embryo hatching, microtechniques (any method)**

🚗 0.00 ⚕ 0.00 **FUD** XXX Q1 ▭

AMA: 2018,Jan,8; 2017,Jan,8; 2016,Jan,13; 2015,Jan,16

89254 **Oocyte identification from follicular fluid**

🚗 0.00 ⚕ 0.00 **FUD** XXX Q1 ▭

AMA: 2018,Jan,8; 2017,Jan,8; 2016,Jan,13; 2015,Jan,16

89255 **Preparation of embryo for transfer (any method)**

🚗 0.00 ⚕ 0.00 **FUD** XXX Q1 ▭

AMA: 2018,Jan,8; 2017,Jan,8; 2016,Jan,13; 2015,Jan,16

89257 **Sperm identification from aspiration (other than seminal fluid)**

> EXCLUDES *Semen analysis (89300-89320)*
> *Sperm identification from testis tissue (89264)*

🚗 0.00 ⚕ 0.00 **FUD** XXX Q1 ▭

AMA: 2018,Jan,8; 2017,Jan,8; 2016,Jan,13; 2015,Jan,16

89258 **Cryopreservation; embryo(s)**

🚗 0.00 ⚕ 0.00 **FUD** XXX Q2 ▭

AMA: 2018,Jan,8; 2017,Jan,8; 2016,Jan,13; 2015,Jan,16

89259 **sperm**

> EXCLUDES *Cryopreservation testicular reproductive tissue (89335)*

🚗 0.00 ⚕ 0.00 **FUD** XXX Q1 ▭

AMA: 2018,Jan,8; 2017,Jan,8; 2016,Jan,13; 2015,Jan,16

89260 **Sperm isolation; simple prep (eg, sperm wash and swim-up) for insemination or diagnosis with semen analysis**

🚗 0.00 ⚕ 0.00 **FUD** XXX Q1 ▭

AMA: 2018,Jan,8; 2017,Jan,8; 2016,Jan,13; 2015,Jan,16

89261 **complex prep (eg, Percoll gradient, albumin gradient) for insemination or diagnosis with semen analysis**

> EXCLUDES *Semen analysis without sperm wash or swim-up (89320)*

🚗 0.00 ⚕ 0.00 **FUD** XXX Q1 ▭

AMA: 2018,Jan,8; 2017,Jan,8; 2016,Jan,13; 2015,Jan,16

89264 **Sperm identification from testis tissue, fresh or cryopreserved** ♂

> EXCLUDES *Biopsy testis (54500, 54505)*
> *Semen analysis (89300-89320)*
> *Sperm identification from aspiration (89257)*

🚗 0.00 ⚕ 0.00 **FUD** XXX Q1 ▭

AMA: 2018,Jan,8; 2017,Jan,8; 2016,Jan,13; 2015,Jan,16

26/TC PC/TC Only	A2-Z3 ASC Payment	50 Bilateral	♂ Male Only	♀ Female Only	🚗 Facility RVU	⚕ Non-Facility RVU	▭ CCI	✖ CLIA
FUD Follow-up Days	CMS: IOM	AMA: CPT Asst	A-Y OPPSI	80/80 Surg Assist Allowed / w/Doc	◼ Lab Crosswalk	◼ Radiology Crosswalk

89268 **Insemination of oocytes**
0.00 0.00 FUD XXX [Q1]
AMA: 2018,Jan,8; 2017,Jan,8; 2016,Jan,13; 2015,Jan,16

89272 **Extended culture of oocyte(s)/embryo(s), 4-7 days**
0.00 0.00 FUD XXX [Q2]
AMA: 2018,Jan,8; 2017,Jan,8; 2016,Jan,13; 2015,Jan,16

89280 **Assisted oocyte fertilization, microtechnique; less than or equal to 10 oocytes**
0.00 0.00 FUD XXX [Q2]
AMA: 2018,Jan,8; 2017,Jan,8; 2016,Jan,13; 2015,Jan,16

89281 **greater than 10 oocytes**
0.00 0.00 FUD XXX [Q1]
AMA: 2018,Jan,8; 2017,Jan,8; 2016,Jan,13; 2015,Jan,16

89290 **Biopsy, oocyte polar body or embryo blastomere, microtechnique (for pre-implantation genetic diagnosis); less than or equal to 5 embryos**
0.00 0.00 FUD XXX [Q1]
AMA: 2018,Jan,8; 2017,Jan,8; 2016,Jan,13; 2015,Jan,16

89291 **greater than 5 embryos**
0.00 0.00 FUD XXX [Q1]
AMA: 2018,Jan,8; 2017,Jan,8; 2016,Jan,13; 2015,Jan,16

89300 **Semen analysis; presence and/or motility of sperm including Huhner test (post coital)**
0.00 0.00 FUD XXX [X] [Q]
AMA: 2018,Jan,8; 2017,Jan,8; 2016,Jan,13; 2015,Jan,16

89310 **motility and count (not including Huhner test)** ♂
0.00 0.00 FUD XXX [Q]
AMA: 2018,Jan,8; 2017,Jan,8; 2016,Jan,13; 2015,Jan,16

89320 **volume, count, motility, and differential** ♂
EXCLUDES *Skin testing (86485-86580, 95012-95199)*
0.00 0.00 FUD XXX [Q]
AMA: 2018,Jan,8; 2017,Jan,8; 2016,Jan,13; 2015,Jan,16

89321 **sperm presence and motility of sperm, if performed** ♂
EXCLUDES *Hyaluronan binding assay (HBA) (89398)*
0.00 0.00 FUD XXX [X] [Q]
AMA: 2018,Jan,8; 2017,Jan,8; 2016,Jan,13; 2015,Jan,16

89322 **volume, count, motility, and differential using strict morphologic criteria (eg, Kruger)** ♂
0.00 0.00 FUD XXX [Q]
AMA: 2018,Jan,8; 2017,Jan,8; 2016,Jan,13; 2015,Jan,16

89325 **Sperm antibodies** ♂
EXCLUDES *Medicolegal identification sperm (88125)*
0.00 0.00 FUD XXX [Q]
AMA: 2018,Jan,8; 2017,Jan,8; 2016,Jan,13; 2015,Jan,16

89329 **Sperm evaluation; hamster penetration test** ♂
0.00 0.00 FUD XXX [Q]
AMA: 2018,Jan,8; 2017,Jan,8; 2016,Jan,13; 2015,Jan,16

89330 **cervical mucus penetration test, with or without spinnbarkeit test** ♂
0.00 0.00 FUD XXX [Q]
AMA: 2018,Jan,8; 2017,Jan,8; 2016,Jan,13; 2015,Jan,16

89331 **Sperm evaluation, for retrograde ejaculation, urine (sperm concentration, motility, and morphology, as indicated)** ♂
EXCLUDES *Detection sperm in urine (81015)*
Code also semen analysis on concurrent sperm specimen (89300-89322)
0.00 0.00 FUD XXX [Q]
AMA: 2018,Jan,8; 2017,Jan,8; 2016,Jan,13; 2015,Jan,16

89335 **Cryopreservation, reproductive tissue, testicular**
EXCLUDES *Cryopreservation:*
- *Embryo(s) (89258)*
- *Immature oocyte(s) (89398)*
- *Mature oocytes (89337)*
- *Ovarian reproductive tissue (89398)*
- *Sperm (89259)*

0.00 0.00 FUD XXX [Q1]
AMA: 2018,Jan,8; 2017,Jan,8; 2016,Jan,13; 2015,Jan,16

89337 **Cryopreservation, mature oocyte(s)** ♀
EXCLUDES *Cryopreservation immature oocyte[s] (89398)*
0.00 0.00 FUD XXX [Q1]
AMA: 2018,Jan,8; 2017,Jan,8; 2016,Jan,13; 2015,Jan,16

89342 **Storage (per year); embryo(s)**
0.00 0.00 FUD XXX [Q1]
AMA: 2018,Jan,8; 2017,Jan,8; 2016,Jan,13; 2015,Jan,16

89343 **sperm/semen**
0.00 0.00 FUD XXX [Q1]
AMA: 2018,Jan,8; 2017,Jan,8; 2016,Jan,13; 2015,Jan,16

89344 **reproductive tissue, testicular/ovarian**
0.00 0.00 FUD XXX [Q1]
AMA: 2018,Jan,8; 2017,Jan,8; 2016,Jan,13; 2015,Jan,16

89346 **oocyte(s)**
0.00 0.00 FUD XXX [Q2]
AMA: 2018,Jan,8; 2017,Jan,8; 2016,Jan,13; 2015,Jan,16

89352 **Thawing of cryopreserved; embryo(s)**
0.00 0.00 FUD XXX [Q1]
AMA: 2018,Jan,8; 2017,Jan,8; 2016,Jan,13; 2015,Jan,16

89353 **sperm/semen, each aliquot**
0.00 0.00 FUD XXX [Q1]
AMA: 2018,Jan,8; 2017,Jan,8; 2016,Jan,13; 2015,Jan,16

89354 **reproductive tissue, testicular/ovarian**
0.00 0.00 FUD XXX [Q1]
AMA: 2018,Jan,8; 2017,Jan,8; 2016,Jan,13; 2015,Jan,16

89356 **oocytes, each aliquot**
0.00 0.00 FUD XXX [Q1]
AMA: 2018,Jan,8; 2017,Jan,8; 2016,Jan,13; 2015,Jan,16

89398 **Unlisted reproductive medicine laboratory procedure**
INCLUDES Cryopreservation:
- immature oocytes
- ovarian reproductive tissue

Hyaluronan binding assay (HBA)
0.00 0.00 FUD XXX [Q1]

0001U-0241U Proprietary Laboratory Analysis (PLA)

In response to the Protecting Access to Medicare Act of 2014 (PAMA), which focuses on payment and coding of clinical laboratory studies paid for under the Medicare Clinical Laboratory Fee Schedule (CLFS), the AMA has developed a new category of CPT codes known as Proprietary Laboratory Analyses (PLA), which will be released on a quarterly basis. These alphanumeric codes will appear at the end of the Pathology and Laboratory chapter of the CPT book and will include a wide range of tests. Codes in this section can also be found in Appendix L along with the procedure's proprietary name and clinical laboratory or manufacturer. When multiple codes have identical code descriptors and can only be distinguished by a proprietary test name, instructional notes are provided to help ensure accurate code assignment.

INCLUDES All necessary investigative services
PLA codes take priority over other CPT codes

EXCLUDES *Additional procedures necessary before cell lysis (88380-88381)*

0001U **Red blood cell antigen typing, DNA, human erythrocyte antigen gene analysis of 35 antigens from 11 blood groups, utilizing whole blood, common RBC alleles reported**
INCLUDES PreciseType® HEA Test, Immucor, Inc
0.00 0.00 FUD 000 [A]
AMA: 2019,Jun,11

0002U **Oncology (colorectal), quantitative assessment of three urine metabolites (ascorbic acid, succinic acid and carnitine) by liquid chromatography with tandem mass spectrometry (LC-MS/MS) using multiple reaction monitoring acquisition, algorithm reported as likelihood of adenomatous polyps**
INCLUDES PolypDX™, Atlantic Diagnostic Laboratories, LLC, Metabolomic Technologies Inc
0.00 0.00 FUD 000 [Q]
AMA: 2018,Aug,3

0003U Oncology (ovarian) biochemical assays of five proteins (apolipoprotein A-1, CA 125 II, follicle stimulating hormone, human epididymis protein 4, transferrin), utilizing serum, algorithm reported as a likelihood score

INCLUDES Overa (OVA1 Next Generation), Aspira Labs, Inc, Vermillion, Inc

0.00 0.00 FUD 000 Q

0005U Oncology (prostate) gene expression profile by real-time RT-PCR of 3 genes (*ERG, PCA3,* and *SPDEF*), urine, algorithm reported as risk score

INCLUDES ExosomeDx® Prostate (IntelliScore), Exosome Diagnostics, Inc, Exosome Diagnostics, Inc

0.00 0.00 FUD 000 Q

0006U ~~**Detection of interacting medications, substances, supplements and foods, 120 or more analytes, definitive chromatography with mass spectrometry, urine, description and severity of each interaction identified, per date of service**~~

0007U Drug test(s), presumptive, with definitive confirmation of positive results, any number of drug classes, urine, includes specimen verification including DNA authentication in comparison to buccal DNA, per date of service

INCLUDES ToxProtect, Genotox Laboratories Ltd

0.00 0.00 FUD 000 Q

AMA: 2018,Jan,6

0008U Helicobacter pylori detection and antibiotic resistance, DNA, 16S and 23S rRNA, gyrA, pbp1, rdxA and rpoB, next-generation sequencing, formalin-fixed paraffin-embedded or fresh tissue or fecal sample, predictive, reported as positive or negative for resistance to clarithromycin, fluoroquinolones, metronidazole, amoxicillin, tetracycline, and rifabutin

INCLUDES AmHPR® H. pylori Antibiotic Resistance Panel, American Molecular Laboratories, Inc

0.00 0.00 FUD 000 A

0009U Oncology (breast cancer), ERBB2 (HER2) copy number by FISH, tumor cells from formalin fixed paraffin embedded tissue isolated using image-based dielectrophoresis (DEP) sorting, reported as ERBB2 gene amplified or non-amplified

INCLUDES DEPArray™ HER2, PacificDx

0.00 0.00 FUD 000 Q

0010U Infectious disease (bacterial), strain typing by whole genome sequencing, phylogenetic-based report of strain relatedness, per submitted isolate

INCLUDES Bacterial Typing by Whole Genome Sequencing, Mayo Clinic

0.00 0.00 FUD 000 A

0011U Prescription drug monitoring, evaluation of drugs present by LC-MS/MS, using oral fluid, reported as a comparison to an estimated steady-state range, per date of service including all drug compounds and metabolites

INCLUDES Cordant CORE™, Cordant Health Solutions

0.00 0.00 FUD 000 Q

0012U Germline disorders, gene rearrangement detection by whole genome next-generation sequencing, DNA, whole blood, report of specific gene rearrangement(s)

INCLUDES MatePair Targeted Rearrangements, Congenital, Mayo Clinic

0.00 0.00 FUD 000 A

0013U Oncology (solid organ neoplasia), gene rearrangement detection by whole genome next-generation sequencing, DNA, fresh or frozen tissue or cells, report of specific gene rearrangement(s)

INCLUDES MatePair Targeted Rearrangements, Oncology, Mayo Clinic

0.00 0.00 FUD 000 A

0014U Hematology (hematolymphoid neoplasia), gene rearrangement detection by whole genome next-generation sequencing, DNA, whole blood or bone marrow, report of specific gene rearrangement(s)

INCLUDES MatePair Targeted Rearrangements, Hematologic, Mayo Clinic

0.00 0.00 FUD 000 A

0016U Oncology (hematolymphoid neoplasia), RNA, *BCR/ABL1* major and minor breakpoint fusion transcripts, quantitative PCR amplification, blood or bone marrow, report of fusion not detected or detected with quantitation

INCLUDES BCR-ABL1 major and minor breakpoint fusion transcripts, University of Iowa, Department of Pathology, Asuragen

0.00 0.00 FUD 000 A

0017U Oncology (hematolymphoid neoplasia), *JAK2* mutation, DNA, PCR amplification of exons 12-14 and sequence analysis, blood or bone marrow, report of *JAK2* mutation not detected or detected

INCLUDES *JAK2* Mutation, University of Iowa, Department of Pathology

0.00 0.00 FUD 000 A

0018U Oncology (thyroid), microRNA profiling by RT-PCR of 10 microRNA sequences, utilizing fine needle aspirate, algorithm reported as a positive or negative result for moderate to high risk of malignancy

INCLUDES ThyraMIR™, Interpace Diagnostics

0.00 0.00 FUD 000 A

0019U Oncology, RNA, gene expression by whole transcriptome sequencing, formalin-fixed paraffin embedded tissue or fresh frozen tissue, predictive algorithm reported as potential targets for therapeutic agents

INCLUDES OncoTarget/OncoTreat, Columbia University Department of Pathology and Cell Biology, Darwin Health

0.00 0.00 FUD 000 A

0021U Oncology (prostate), detection of 8 autoantibodies (ARF 6, NKX3-1, 5'-UTR-BMI1, CEP 164, 3'-UTR-Ropporin, Desmocollin, AURKAIP-1, CSNK2A2), multiplexed immunoassay and flow cytometry serum, algorithm reported as risk score

INCLUDES Apifiny®, Armune BioScience, Inc

0.00 0.00 FUD 000 Q

0022U Targeted genomic sequence analysis panel, non-small cell lung neoplasia, DNA and RNA analysis, 23 genes, interrogation for sequence variants and rearrangements, reported as presence/absence of variants and associated therapy(ies) to consider

INCLUDES Oncomine™ Dx Target Test, Thermo Fisher Scientific

0.00 0.00 FUD 000 A

0023U Oncology (acute myelogenous leukemia), DNA, genotyping of internal tandem duplication, p.D835, p.I836, using mononuclear cells, reported as detection or non-detection of *FLT3* mutation and indication for or against the use of midostaurin

INCLUDES LeukoStrat® CDx *FLT3* Mutation Assay, LabPMM LLC, an Invivoscribe Technologies, Inc Company, Invivoscribe Technologies, Inc

0.00 0.00 FUD 000 A

0024U Glycosylated acute phase proteins (GlycA), nuclear magnetic resonance spectroscopy, quantitative

INCLUDES GlycA, Laboratory Corporation of America, Laboratory Corporation of America

0.00 0.00 FUD 000 Q

0025U Tenofovir, by liquid chromatography with tandem mass spectrometry (LC-MS/MS), urine, quantitative

INCLUDES UrSure Tenofovir Quantification Test, Synergy Medical Laboratories, UrSure Inc

0.00 0.00 FUD 000 Q

0026U Oncology (thyroid), DNA and mRNA of 112 genes, next-generation sequencing, fine needle aspirate of thyroid nodule, algorithmic analysis reported as a categorical result ("Positive, high probability of malignancy" or "Negative, low probability of malignancy")

INCLUDES Thyroseq Genomic Classifier, CBLPath, Inc, University of Pittsburgh Medical Center

0.00 0.00 FUD 000

0027U *JAK2 (Janus kinase 2)* (eg, myeloproliferative disorder) gene analysis, targeted sequence analysis exons 12-15

INCLUDES *JAK2* Exons 12 to 15 Sequencing, Mayo Clinic, Mayo Clinic

0.00 0.00 FUD 000

0029U Drug metabolism (adverse drug reactions and drug response), targeted sequence analysis (ie, *CYP1A2, CYP2C19, CYP2C9, CYP2D6, CYP3A4, CYP3A5, CYP4F2, SLCO1B1, VKORC1* and rs12777823)

INCLUDES Focused Pharmacogenomics Panel, Mayo Clinic, Mayo Clinic

0.00 0.00 FUD 000

0030U Drug metabolism (warfarin drug response), targeted sequence analysis (ie, *CYP2C9, CYP4F2, VKORC1*, rs12777823)

INCLUDES Warfarin Response Genotype, Mayo Clinic, Mayo Clinic

0.00 0.00 FUD 000

0031U *CYP1A2 (cytochrome P450 family 1, subfamily A, member 2)*(eg, drug metabolism) gene analysis, common variants (ie, *1F, *1K, *6, *7)

INCLUDES Cytochrome P450 1A2 Genotype, Mayo Clinic, Mayo Clinic

0.00 0.00 FUD 000

0032U *COMT (catechol-O-methyltransferase)(drug metabolism)* gene analysis, c.472G>A (rs4680) variant

INCLUDES Catechol-O-Methyltransferase (*COMT*) Genotype, Mayo Clinic, Mayo Clinic

0.00 0.00 FUD 000

0033U *HTR2A (5-hydroxytryptamine receptor 2A), HTR2C (5-hydroxytryptamine receptor 2C)* (eg, citalopram metabolism) gene analysis, common variants (ie, *HTR2A* rs7997012 [c.614-2211T>C], *HTR2C* rs3813929 [c.-759C>T] and rs1414334 [c.551-3008C>G])

INCLUDES Serotonin Receptor Genotype (*HTR2A* and *HTR2C*), Mayo Clinic, Mayo Clinic

0.00 0.00 FUD 000

0034U *TPMT (thiopurine S-methyltransferase), NUDT15 (nudix hydroxylase 15)(eg, thiopurine metabolism)*, gene analysis, common variants (ie, *TPMT* *2, *3A, *3B, *3C, *4, *5, *6, *8, *12; *NUDT15* *3, *4, *5)

INCLUDES Thiopurine Methyltransferase (*TPMT*) and Nudix Hydrolase (*NUDT15*) Genotyping, Mayo Clinic, Mayo Clinic

0.00 0.00 FUD 000

0035U Neurology (prion disease), cerebrospinal fluid, detection of prion protein by quaking-induced conformational conversion, qualitative

INCLUDES Real-time quaking-induced conversion for prion detection (RT-QuIC), National Prion Disease Pathology Surveillance Center

0.00 0.00 FUD 000

0036U Exome (ie, somatic mutations), paired formalin-fixed paraffin-embedded tumor tissue and normal specimen, sequence analyses

INCLUDES EXaCT-1 Whole Exome Testing, Lab of Oncology-Molecular Detection, Weill Cornell Medicine-Clinical Genomics Laboratory

0.00 0.00 FUD 000

0037U Targeted genomic sequence analysis, solid organ neoplasm, DNA analysis of 324 genes, interrogation for sequence variants, gene copy number amplifications, gene rearrangements, microsatellite instability and tumor mutational burden

INCLUDES FoundationOne CDx™ (F1CDx), Foundation Medicine, Inc, Foundation Medicine, Inc

0.00 0.00 FUD 000

0038U Vitamin D, 25 hydroxy D2 and D3, by LC-MS/MS, serum microsample, quantitative

INCLUDES Sensieva™ Droplet 25OH Vitamin D2/D3 Microvolume LC/MS Assay, InSource Diagnostics, InSource Diagnostics

0.00 0.00 FUD 000

0039U Deoxyribonucleic acid (DNA) antibody, double stranded, high avidity

INCLUDES Anti-dsDNA, High Salt/Avidity, University of Washington, Department of Laboratory Medicine, Bio-Rad

0.00 0.00 FUD 000

0040U *BCR/ABL1 (t(9;22))* (eg, chronic myelogenous leukemia) translocation analysis, major breakpoint, quantitative

INCLUDES MRDx BCR-ABL Test, MolecularMD, MolecularMD

0.00 0.00 FUD 000

0041U Borrelia burgdorferi, antibody detection of 5 recombinant protein groups, by immunoblot, IgM

INCLUDES Lyme ImmunoBlot IgM, IGeneX Inc, ID-FISH Technology Inc. (ASR) (Lyme ImmunoBlot IgM Strips Only)

0.00 0.00 FUD 000

0042U Borrelia burgdorferi, antibody detection of 12 recombinant protein groups, by immunoblot, IgG

INCLUDES Lyme ImmunoBlot IgG, IGeneX Inc, ID-FISH Technology Inc (ASR) (Lyme ImmunoBlot IgG Strips Only)

0.00 0.00 FUD 000

0043U Tick-borne relapsing fever Borrelia group, antibody detection to 4 recombinant protein groups, by immunoblot, IgM

INCLUDES Tick-Borne Relapsing Fever (TBRF) Borrelia ImmunoBlots IgM Test, IGeneX Inc, ID-FISH Technology Inc (Provides TBRF ImmunoBlot IgM Strips)

0.00 0.00 FUD 000

0044U Tick-borne relapsing fever Borrelia group, antibody detection to 4 recombinant protein groups, by immunoblot, IgG

INCLUDES Tick-Borne Relapsing Fever (TBRF) Borrelia ImmunoBlots IgG Test, IGeneX Inc, ID-FISH Technology Inc (Provides TBRF ImmunoBlot IgG Strips)

0.00 0.00 FUD 000

0045U Oncology (breast ductal carcinoma in situ), mRNA, gene expression profiling by real-time RT-PCR of 12 genes (7 content and 5 housekeeping), utilizing formalin-fixed paraffin-embedded tissue, algorithm reported as recurrence score

INCLUDES The Oncotype DX® Breast DCIS Score™ Test, Genomic Health, Inc, Genomic Health, Inc

0.00 0.00 FUD 000

0046U *FLT3* (fms-related tyrosine kinase 3) (eg, acute myeloid leukemia) internal tandem duplication (ITD) variants, quantitative

INCLUDES FLT3 ITD MRD by NGS, LabPMM LLC, an Invivoscribe Technologies, Inc Company

0.00 0.00 FUD 000

Pathology and Laboratory

0026U — 0046U

● New Code ▲ Revised Code ○ Reinstated ● New Web Release ▲ Revised Web Release + Add-on Unlisted Not Covered # Resequenced
⑤⓪ Optum Mod 50 Exempt ⊘ AMA Mod 51 Exempt ⑤① Optum Mod 51 Exempt ⑥③ Mod 63 Exempt ✓ Non-FDA Drug ★ Telemedicine M Maternity A Age Edit

0047U Oncology (prostate), mRNA, gene expression profiling by real-time RT-PCR of 17 genes (12 content and 5 housekeeping), utilizing formalin-fixed paraffin-embedded tissue, algorithm reported as a risk score

INCLUDES Oncotype DX Genomic Prostate Score, Genomic Health, Inc, Genomic Health, Inc

0.00 0.00 FUD 000

0048U Oncology (solid organ neoplasia), DNA, targeted sequencing of protein-coding exons of 468 cancer-associated genes, including interrogation for somatic mutations and microsatellite instability, matched with normal specimens, utilizing formalin-fixed paraffin-embedded tumor tissue, report of clinically significant mutation(s)

INCLUDES MSK-IMPACT (Integrated Mutation Profiling of Actionable Cancer Targets), Memorial Sloan Kettering Cancer Center

0.00 0.00 FUD 000

0049U NPM1 (nucleophosmin) (eg, acute myeloid leukemia) gene analysis, quantitative

INCLUDES *NPM1* MRD by NGS, LabPMM LLC, an Invivoscribe Technologies, Inc Company

0.00 0.00 FUD 000

0050U Targeted genomic sequence analysis panel, acute myelogenous leukemia, DNA analysis, 194 genes, interrogation for sequence variants, copy number variants or rearrangements

INCLUDES MyAML NGS Panel, LabPMM LLC, an Invivoscribe Technologies, Inc Company

0.00 0.00 FUD 000

0051U Prescription drug monitoring, evaluation of drugs present by LC-MS/MS, urine, 31 drug panel, reported as quantitative results, detected or not detected, per date of service

INCLUDES UCompliDx, Elite Medical Laboratory Solutions, LLC, Elite Medical Laboratory Solutions, LLC (LDT)

0.00 0.00 FUD 000

0052U Lipoprotein, blood, high resolution fractionation and quantitation of lipoproteins, including all five major lipoprotein classes and subclasses of HDL, LDL, and VLDL by vertical auto profile ultracentrifugation

INCLUDES VAP Cholesterol Test, VAP Diagnostics Laboratory, Inc, VAP Diagnostics Laboratory, Inc

0.00 0.00 FUD 000

0053U Oncology (prostate cancer), FISH analysis of 4 genes (*ASAP1, HDAC9, CHD1* and *PTEN*), needle biopsy specimen, algorithm reported as probability of higher tumor grade

INCLUDES Prostate Cancer Risk Panel, Mayo Clinic, Laboratory Developed Test

0.00 0.00 FUD 000

0054U Prescription drug monitoring, 14 or more classes of drugs and substances, definitive tandem mass spectrometry with chromatography, capillary blood, quantitative report with therapeutic and toxic ranges, including steady-state range for the prescribed dose when detected, per date of service

INCLUDES AssuranceRx Micro Serum, Firstox Laboratories, LLC, Firstox Laboratories, LLC

0.00 0.00 FUD 000

0055U Cardiology (heart transplant), cell-free DNA, PCR assay of 96 DNA target sequences (94 single nucleotide polymorphism targets and two control targets), plasma

INCLUDES myTAIHEART, TAI Diagnostics, Inc, TAI Diagnostics, Inc

0.00 0.00 FUD 000

0056U Hematology (acute myelogenous leukemia), DNA, whole genome next-generation sequencing to detect gene rearrangement(s), blood or bone marrow, report of specific gene rearrangement(s)

INCLUDES MatePair Acute Myeloid Leukemia Panel, Mayo Clinic, Laboratory Developed Test

0.00 0.00 FUD 000

0057U ~~Oncology (solid organ neoplasia), mRNA, gene expression profiling by massively parallel sequencing for analysis of 51 genes, utilizing formalin-fixed paraffin-embedded tissue, algorithm reported as a normalized percentile rank~~

0058U Oncology (Merkel cell carcinoma), detection of antibodies to the Merkel cell polyoma virus oncoprotein (small T antigen), serum, quantitative

INCLUDES Merkel SmT Oncoprotein Antibody Titer, University of Washington, Department of Laboratory Medicine

0.00 0.00 FUD 000

0059U Oncology (Merkel cell carcinoma), detection of antibodies to the Merkel cell polyoma virus capsid protein (VP1), serum, reported as positive or negative

INCLUDES Merkel Virus VP1 Capsid Antibody, University of Washington, Department of Laboratory Medicine

0.00 0.00 FUD 000

0060U Twin zygosity, genomic targeted sequence analysis of chromosome 2, using circulating cell-free fetal DNA in maternal blood

INCLUDES Twins Zygosity PLA, Natera, Inc, Natera, Inc

0.00 0.00 FUD 000

0061U Transcutaneous measurement of five biomarkers (tissue oxygenation [StO2], oxyhemoglobin [ctHbO2], deoxyhemoglobin [ctHbR], papillary and reticular dermal hemoglobin concentrations [ctHb1 and ctHb2]), using spatial frequency domain imaging (SFDI) and multi-spectral analysis

INCLUDES Transcutaneous multispectral measurement of tissue oxygenation and hemoglobin using spatial frequency domain imaging (SFDI), Modulated Imaging, Inc, Modulated Imaging, Inc

0.00 0.00 FUD 000

0062U Autoimmune (systemic lupus erythematosus), IgG and IgM analysis of 80 biomarkers, utilizing serum, algorithm reported with a risk score

INCLUDES SLE-key® Rule Out, Veracis Inc, Veracis Inc

0.00 0.00 FUD 000

0063U Neurology (autism), 32 amines by LC-MS/MS, using plasma, algorithm reported as metabolic signature associated with autism spectrum disorder

INCLUDES NPDX ASD ADM Panel I, Stemina Biomarker Discovery, Inc, Stemina Biomarker Discovery, Inc d/b/a NeuroPointDX

0.00 0.00 FUD 000

0064U Antibody, Treponema pallidum, total and rapid plasma reagin (RPR), immunoassay, qualitative

INCLUDES BioPlex 2200 Syphilis Total & RPR Assay, Bio-Rad Laboratories, Bio-Rad Laboratories

0.00 0.00 FUD 000

0065U Syphilis test, non-treponemal antibody, immunoassay, qualitative (RPR)

INCLUDES BioPlex 2200 RPR Assay, Bio-Rad Laboratories, Bio-Rad Laboratories

0.00 0.00 FUD 000

0066U Placental alpha-micro globulin-1 (PAMG-1), immunoassay with direct optical observation, cervico-vaginal fluid, each specimen

INCLUDES PartoSure™ Test, Parsagen Diagnostics, Inc, Parsagen Diagnostics, Inc, a QIAGEN Company

0.00 0.00 FUD 000

0067U **Oncology (breast), immunohistochemistry, protein expression profiling of 4 biomarkers (matrix metalloproteinase-1 [MMP-1], carcinoembryonic antigen-related cell adhesion molecule 6 [CEACAM6], hyaluronoglucosaminidase [HYAL1], highly expressed in cancer protein [HEC1]), formalin-fixed paraffin-embedded precancerous breast tissue, algorithm reported as carcinoma risk score**

INCLUDES BBDRisk Dx™, Silbiotech, Inc, Silbiotech, Inc

0.00 0.00 FUD 000

0068U **Candida species panel (*C. albicans, C. glabrata, C. parapsilosis, C. kruseii, C tropicalis, and C. auris*), amplified probe technique with qualitative report of the presence or absence of each species**

INCLUDES MYCODART-PCR™ Dual Amplification Real Time PCR Panel for 6 Candida species, RealTime Laboratories, Inc/MycoDART, Inc, RealTime Laboratories, Inc

0.00 0.00 FUD 000

0069U **Oncology (colorectal), microRNA, RT-PCR expression profiling of miR-31-3p, formalin-fixed paraffin-embedded tissue, algorithm reported as an expression score**

INCLUDES miR-31*now*™, GoPath Laboratories, GoPath Laboratories

0.00 0.00 FUD 000

0070U ***CYP2D6 (cytochrome P450, family 2, subfamily D, polypeptide 6)* (eg, drug metabolism) gene analysis, common and select rare variants (ie, *2, *3, *4, *4N, *5, *6, *7, *8, *9, *10, *11, *12, *13, *14A, *14B, *15, *17, *29, *35, *36, *41, *57, *61, *63, *68, *83, *xN)**

INCLUDES *CYP2D6* Common Variants and Copy Number, Mayo Clinic, Laboratory Developed Test

0.00 0.00 FUD 000

\+ **0071U** ***CYP2D6 (cytochrome P450, family 2, subfamily D, polypeptide 6)* (eg, drug metabolism) gene analysis, full gene sequence (List separately in addition to code for primary procedure)**

INCLUDES *CYP2D6* Full Gene Sequencing, Mayo Clinic, Laboratory Developed Test

Code first (0070U)

0.00 0.00 FUD 000

\+ **0072U** ***CYP2D6 (cytochrome P450, family 2, subfamily D, polypeptide 6)* (eg, drug metabolism) gene analysis, targeted sequence analysis (ie, CYP2D6-2D7 hybrid gene) (List separately in addition to code for primary procedure)**

INCLUDES *CYP2D6-2D7* Hybrid Gene Targeted Sequence Analysis, Mayo Clinic, Laboratory Developed Test

Code first (0070U)

0.00 0.00 FUD 000

\+ **0073U** ***CYP2D6 (cytochrome P450, family 2, subfamily D, polypeptide 6)* (eg, drug metabolism) gene analysis, targeted sequence analysis (ie, CYP2D7-2D6 hybrid gene) (List separately in addition to code for primary procedure)**

INCLUDES *CYP2D7-2D6* Hybrid Gene Targeted Sequence Analysis, Mayo Clinic, Laboratory Developed Test

Code first (0070U)

0.00 0.00 FUD 000

\+ **0074U** ***CYP2D6 (cytochrome P450, family 2, subfamily D, polypeptide 6)* (eg, drug metabolism) gene analysis, targeted sequence analysis (ie, non-duplicated gene when duplication/multiplication is trans) (List separately in addition to code for primary procedure)**

INCLUDES *CYP2D6* trans-duplication/multiplication non-duplicated gene targeted sequence analysis, Mayo Clinic, Laboratory Developed Test

Code first (0070U)

0.00 0.00 FUD 000

\+ **0075U** ***CYP2D6 (cytochrome P450, family 2, subfamily D, polypeptide 6)* (eg, drug metabolism) gene analysis, targeted sequence analysis (ie, 5' gene duplication/multiplication) (List separately in addition to code for primary procedure)**

INCLUDES *CYP2D6* 5' gene duplication/multiplication targeted sequence analysis, Mayo Clinic, Laboratory Developed Test

Code first (0070U)

0.00 0.00 FUD 000

\+ **0076U** ***CYP2D6 (cytochrome P450, family 2, subfamily D, polypeptide 6)* (eg, drug metabolism) gene analysis, targeted sequence analysis (ie, 3' gene duplication/ multiplication) (List separately in addition to code for primary procedure)**

INCLUDES *CYP2D6* 3' gene duplication/multiplication targeted sequence analysis, Mayo Clinic, Laboratory Developed Test

Code first (0070U)

0.00 0.00 FUD 000

0077U **Immunoglobulin paraprotein (M-protein), qualitative, immunoprecipitation and mass spectrometry, blood or urine, including isotype**

INCLUDES M-Protein Detection and Isotyping by MALDI-TOF Mass Spectrometry, Mayo Clinic, Laboratory Developed Test

0.00 0.00 FUD 000

0078U **Pain management (opioid-use disorder) genotyping panel, 16 common variants (ie, *ABCB1, COMT, DAT1, DBH, DOR, DRD1, DRD2, DRD4, GABA, GAL, HTR2A, HTTLPR, MTHFR, MUOR, OPRK1, OPRM1*), buccal swab or other germline tissue sample, algorithm reported as positive or negative risk of opioid-use disorder**

INCLUDES INFINITI® Neural Response Panel, PersonalizeDx Labs, AutoGenomics Inc

0.00 0.00 FUD 000

0079U **Comparative DNA analysis using multiple selected single-nucleotide polymorphisms (SNPs), urine and buccal DNA, for specimen identity verification**

INCLUDES ToxLok™, InSource Diagnostics, InSource Diagnostics

0.00 0.00 FUD 000

0080U **Oncology (lung), mass spectrometric analysis of galectin-3-binding protein and scavenger receptor cysteine-rich type 1 protein M130, with five clinical risk factors (age, smoking status, nodule diameter, nodule-spiculation status and nodule location), utilizing plasma, algorithm reported as a categorical probability of malignancy**

INCLUDES BDX-XL2, Biodesix®, Inc, Biodesix®, Inc

0.00 0.00 FUD 000

0082U **Drug test(s), definitive, 90 or more drugs or substances, definitive chromatography with mass spectrometry, and presumptive, any number of drug classes, by instrument chemistry analyzer (utilizing immunoassay), urine, report of presence or absence of each drug, drug metabolite or substance with description and severity of significant interactions per date of service**

INCLUDES NextGen Precision™ Testing, Precision Diagnostics, Precision Diagnostics LBN Precision Toxicology, LLC

0.00 0.00 FUD 000

0083U **Oncology, response to chemotherapy drugs using motility contrast tomography, fresh or frozen tissue, reported as likelihood of sensitivity or resistance to drugs or drug combinations**

INCLUDES Onco4D™, Animated Dynamics, Inc, Animated Dynamics, Inc

0.00 0.00 FUD 000

0084U **Red blood cell antigen typing, DNA, genotyping of 10 blood groups with phenotype prediction of 37 red blood cell antigens**

INCLUDES BLOODchip® ID CORE XT™, Grifols Diagnostic Solutions Inc

0.00 0.00 FUD 000

0086U **Infectious disease (bacterial and fungal), organism identification, blood culture, using rRNA FISH, 6 or more organism targets, reported as positive or negative with phenotypic minimum inhibitory concentration (MIC)-based antimicrobial susceptibility**

INCLUDES Accelerate PhenoTest™ BC kit, Accelerate Diagnostics, Inc

0.00 0.00 FUD 000

0087U **Cardiology (heart transplant), mRNA gene expression profiling by microarray of 1283 genes, transplant biopsy tissue, allograft rejection and injury algorithm reported as a probability score**

INCLUDES Molecular Microscope® MMDx—Heart, Kashi Clinical Laboratories

0.00 0.00 FUD 000

0088U **Transplantation medicine (kidney allograft rejection), microarray gene expression profiling of 1494 genes, utilizing transplant biopsy tissue, algorithm reported as a probability score for rejection**

INCLUDES Molecular Microscope® MMDx—Kidney, Kashi Clinical Laboratories

0.00 0.00 FUD 000

0089U **Oncology (melanoma), gene expression profiling by RTqPCR, *PRAME* and *LINC00518*, superficial collection using adhesive patch(es)**

INCLUDES Pigmented Lesion Assay (PLA), DermTech

0.00 0.00 FUD 000

0090U **Oncology (cutaneous melanoma), mRNA gene expression profiling by RT-PCR of 23 genes (14 content and 9 housekeeping), utilizing formalin-fixed paraffin-embedded tissue, algorithm reported as a categorical result (ie, benign, indeterminate, malignant)**

INCLUDES myPath® Melanoma, Myriad Genetic Laboratories

0.00 0.00 FUD 000

0091U **Oncology (colorectal) screening, cell enumeration of circulating tumor cells, utilizing whole blood, algorithm, for the presence of adenoma or cancer, reported as a positive or negative result**

INCLUDES FirstSightCRC™, CellMax Life

0.00 0.00 FUD 000

0092U **Oncology (lung), three protein biomarkers, immunoassay using magnetic nanosensor technology, plasma, algorithm reported as risk score for likelihood of malignancy**

INCLUDES REVEAL Lung Nodule Characterization, MagArray, Inc

0.00 0.00 FUD 000

0093U **Prescription drug monitoring, evaluation of 65 common drugs by LC-MS/MS, urine, each drug reported detected or not detected**

INCLUDES ComplyRX, Claro Labs

0.00 0.00 FUD 000

0094U **Genome (eg, unexplained constitutional or heritable disorder or syndrome), rapid sequence analysis**

INCLUDES RCIGM Rapid Whole Genome Sequencing, Rady Children's Institute for Genomic Medicine (RCIGM)

0.00 0.00 FUD 000

0095U **Inflammation (eosinophilic esophagitis), ELISA analysis of eotaxin-3 *(CCL26 [C-C motif chemokine ligand 26])* and major basic protein *(PRG2 [proteoglycan 2, pro eosinophil major basic protein])*, specimen obtained by swallowed nylon string, algorithm reported as predictive probability index for active eosinophilic esophagitis**

INCLUDES Esophageal String Test™ (EST), Cambridge Biomedical, Inc

0.00 0.00 FUD 000

0096U **Human papillomavirus (HPV), high-risk types (ie, 16, 18, 31, 33, 35, 39, 45, 51, 52, 56, 58, 59, 66, 68), male urine**

INCLUDES HPV, High-Risk, Male Urine, Molecular Testing Labs

0.00 0.00 FUD 000

0097U **Gastrointestinal pathogen, multiplex reverse transcription and multiplex amplified probe technique, multiple types or subtypes, 22 targets (Campylobacter [C. jejuni/C. coli/C. upsaliensis], Clostridium difficile [C. difficile] toxin A/B, Plesiomonas shigelloides, Salmonella, Vibrio [V. parahaemolyticus/V. vulnificus/V. cholerae], including specific identification of Vibrio cholerae, Yersinia enterocolitica, Enteroaggregative Escherichia coli [EAEC], Enteropathogenic Escherichia coli [EPEC], Enterotoxigenic Escherichia coli [ETEC] lt/st, Shiga-like toxin-producing Escherichia coli [STEC] stx1/stx2 [including specific identification of the E. coli O157 serogroup within STEC], Shigella/Enteroinvasive Escherichia coli [EIEC], Cryptosporidium, Cyclospora cayetanensis, Entamoeba histolytica, Giardia lamblia [also known as G. intestinalis and G. duodenalis], adenovirus F 40/41, astrovirus, norovirus GI/GII, rotavirus A, sapovirus [Genogroups I, II, IV, and V])**

INCLUDES BioFire® FilmArray® Gastrointestinal (GI) Panel, BioFire® Diagnostics

0.00 0.00 FUD 000

0098U **Respiratory pathogen, multiplex reverse transcription and multiplex amplified probe technique, multiple types or subtypes, 14 targets (adenovirus, coronavirus, human metapneumovirus, influenza A, influenza A subtype H1, influenza A subtype H3, influenza A subtype H1-2009, influenza B, parainfluenza virus, human rhinovirus/enterovirus, respiratory syncytial virus, Bordetella pertussis, Chlamydophila pneumoniae, Mycoplasma pneumoniae)**

INCLUDES BioFire® FilmArray® Respiratory Panel (RP) EZ, BioFire® Diagnostics

0.00 0.00 FUD 000

AMA: 2020,Apr,3; 2020,Mar,3

0099U **Respiratory pathogen, multiplex reverse transcription and multiplex amplified probe technique, multiple types or subtypes, 20 targets (adenovirus, coronavirus 229E, coronavirus HKU1, coronavirus, coronavirus OC43, human metapneumovirus, influenza A, influenza A subtype, influenza A subtype H3, influenza A subtype H1-2009, influenza, parainfluenza virus, parainfluenza virus 2, parainfluenza virus 3, parainfluenza virus 4, human rhinovirus/enterovirus, respiratory syncytial virus, Bordetella pertussis, Chlamydophila pneumonia, Mycoplasma pneumoniae)**

INCLUDES BioFire® FilmArray® Respiratory Panel (RP), BioFire® Diagnostics

EXCLUDES *Assay for severe acute respiratory syndrome coronavirus 2 (SARS-CoV-2) (Coronavirus disease) (COVID-19) (87635)*

0.00 0.00 FUD 000

AMA: 2020,Apr,3; 2020,Mar,3

0100U **Respiratory pathogen, multiplex reverse transcription and multiplex amplified probe technique, multiple types or subtypes, 21 targets (adenovirus, coronavirus 229E, coronavirus HKU1, coronavirus NL63, coronavirus OC43, human metapneumovirus, human rhinovirus/enterovirus, influenza A, including subtypes H1, H1-2009, and H3, influenza B, parainfluenza virus 1, parainfluenza virus 2, parainfluenza virus 3, parainfluenza virus 4, respiratory syncytial virus, Bordetella parapertussis [IS1001], Bordetella pertussis [ptxP], Chlamydia pneumoniae, Mycoplasma pneumoniae)**

INCLUDES BioFire® FilmArray® Respiratory Panel 2 (RP2), BioFire® Diagnostics

0.00 0.00 FUD 000

AMA: 2020,Apr,3; 2020,Mar,3

0101U **Hereditary colon cancer disorders (eg, Lynch syndrome, *PTEN* hamartoma syndrome, Cowden syndrome, familial adenomatosis polyposis), genomic sequence analysis panel utilizing a combination of NGS, Sanger, MLPA, and array CGH, with MRNA analytics to resolve variants of unknown significance when indicated (15 genes [sequencing and deletion/duplication], *EPCAM* and *GREM1* [deletion/duplication only])**

INCLUDES ColoNext®, Ambry Genetics®, Ambry Genetics®

0.00 0.00 FUD 000

0102U **Hereditary breast cancer-related disorders (eg, hereditary breast cancer, hereditary ovarian cancer, hereditary endometrial cancer), genomic sequence analysis panel utilizing a combination of NGS, Sanger, MLPA, and array CGH, with mRNA analytics to resolve variants of unknown significance when indicated (17 genes [sequencing and deletion/duplication])**

INCLUDES BreastNext®, Ambry Genetics®, Ambry Genetics®

0.00 0.00 FUD 000

0103U **Hereditary ovarian cancer (eg, hereditary ovarian cancer, hereditary endometrial cancer), genomic sequence analysis panel utilizing a combination of NGS, Sanger, MLPA, and array CGH, with MRNA analytics to resolve variants of unknown significance when indicated (24 genes [sequencing and deletion/duplication], *EPCAM* [deletion/duplication only])**

INCLUDES OvaNext®, Ambry Genetics®, Ambry Genetics®

0.00 0.00 FUD 000

0105U **Nephrology (chronic kidney disease), multiplex electrochemiluminescent immunoassay (ECLIA) of tumor necrosis factor receptor 1A, receptor superfamily 2 *(TNFR1, TNFR2)*, and kidney injury molecule-1 (KIM-1) combined with longitudinal clinical data, including *APOL1* genotype if available, and plasma (isolated fresh or frozen), algorithm reported as probability score for rapid kidney function decline (RKFD)**

INCLUDES KidneyIntelXT™, RenalytixAI, RenalytixAI

0.00 0.00 FUD 000

0106U **Gastric emptying, serial collection of 7 timed breath specimens, non-radioisotope carbon-13 (^{13}C) spirulina substrate, analysis of each specimen by gas isotope ratio mass spectrometry, reported as rate of $^{13}CO_2$ excretion**

INCLUDES 13C-Spirulina Gastric Emptying Breath Test (GEBT), Cairn Diagnostics d/b/a Advanced Breath Diagnostics, LLC, Cairn Diagnostics d/b/a Advanced Breath Diagnostics, LLC

0.00 0.00 FUD 000

0107U **Clostridium difficile toxin(s) antigen detection by immunoassay technique, stool, qualitative, multiple-step method**

INCLUDES Singulex Clarity C. diff toxins A/B assay, Singulex

0.00 0.00 FUD 000

0108U **Gastroenterology (Barrett's esophagus), whole slide-digital imaging, including morphometric analysis, computer-assisted quantitative immunolabeling of 9 protein biomarkers (p16, AMACR, p53, CD68, COX-2, CD45RO, HIF1a, HER-2, K20) and morphology, formalin-fixed paraffin-embedded tissue, algorithm reported as risk of progression to high-grade dysplasia or cancer**

INCLUDES TissueCypher® Barrett's Esophagus Assay, Cernostics, Cernostics

0.00 0.00 FUD 000

0109U **Infectious disease (Aspergillus species), real-time PCR for detection of DNA from 4 species *(A. fumigatus, A. terreus, A. niger*, and *A. flavus*), blood, lavage fluid, or tissue, qualitative reporting of presence or absence of each species**

INCLUDES MYCODART-PCR™ Dual Amplification Real Time PCR Panel for 4 Aspergillus species, RealTime Laboratories, Inc/MycoDART, Inc

0.00 0.00 FUD 000

0110U **Prescription drug monitoring, one or more oral oncology drug(s) and substances, definitive tandem mass spectrometry with chromatography, serum or plasma from capillary blood or venous blood, quantitative report with steady-state range for the prescribed drug(s) when detected**

INCLUDES Oral OncolyticAssuranceRX, Firstox Laboratories, LLC, Firstox Laboratories, LLC

0.00 0.00 FUD 000

0111U **Oncology (colon cancer), targeted *KRAS* (codons 12, 13, and 61) and *NRAS* (codons 12, 13, and 61) gene analysis utilizing formalin-fixed paraffin-embedded tissue**

INCLUDES Praxis(™) Extended RAS Panel, Illumina, Illumina

0.00 0.00 FUD 000

0112U **Infectious agent detection and identification, targeted sequence analysis (16S and 18S rRNA genes) with drug-resistance gene**

INCLUDES MicroGenDX qPCR & NGS For Infection, MicroGenDX, MicroGenDX

0.00 0.00 FUD 000

0113U **Oncology (prostate), measurement of *PCA3* and *TMPRSS2-ERG* in urine and PSA in serum following prostatic massage, by RNA amplification and fluorescence-based detection, algorithm reported as risk score**

INCLUDES MiPS (Mi-Prostate Score), MLabs, Mlabs

0.00 0.00 FUD 000

0114U **Gastroenterology (Barrett's esophagus), *VIM* and *CCNA1* methylation analysis, esophageal cells, algorithm reported as likelihood for Barrett's esophagus**

INCLUDES EsoGuard™, Lucid Diagnostics, Lucid Diagnostics

0.00 0.00 FUD 000

0115U **Respiratory infectious agent detection by nucleic acid (DNA and RNA), 18 viral types and subtypes and 2 bacterial targets, amplified probe technique, including multiplex reverse transcription for RNA targets, each analyte reported as detected or not detected**

INCLUDES ePlex Respiratory Pathogen (RP) Panel, GenMark Diagnostics, Inc, GenMark Diagnostics, Inc

0.00 0.00 FUD 000

AMA: 2020,Apr,3

0116U **Prescription drug monitoring, enzyme immunoassay of 35 or more drugs confirmed with LC-MS/MS, oral fluid, algorithm results reported as a patient-compliance measurement with risk of drug to drug interactions for prescribed medications**

INCLUDES Snapshot Oral Fluid Compliance, Ethos Laboratories

0.00 0.00 FUD 000

Pathology and Laboratory

0100U — 0116U

0117U Pain management, analysis of 11 endogenous analytes (methylmalonic acid, xanthurenic acid, homocysteine, pyroglutamic acid, vanilmandelate, 5-hydroxyindoleacetic acid, hydroxymethylglutarate, ethylmalonate, 3-hydroxypropyl mercapturic acid (3-HPMA), quinolinic acid, kynurenic acid), LC-MS/MS, urine, algorithm reported as a pain-index score with likelihood of atypical biochemical function associated with pain

INCLUDES Foundation PI[SM], Ethos Laboratories

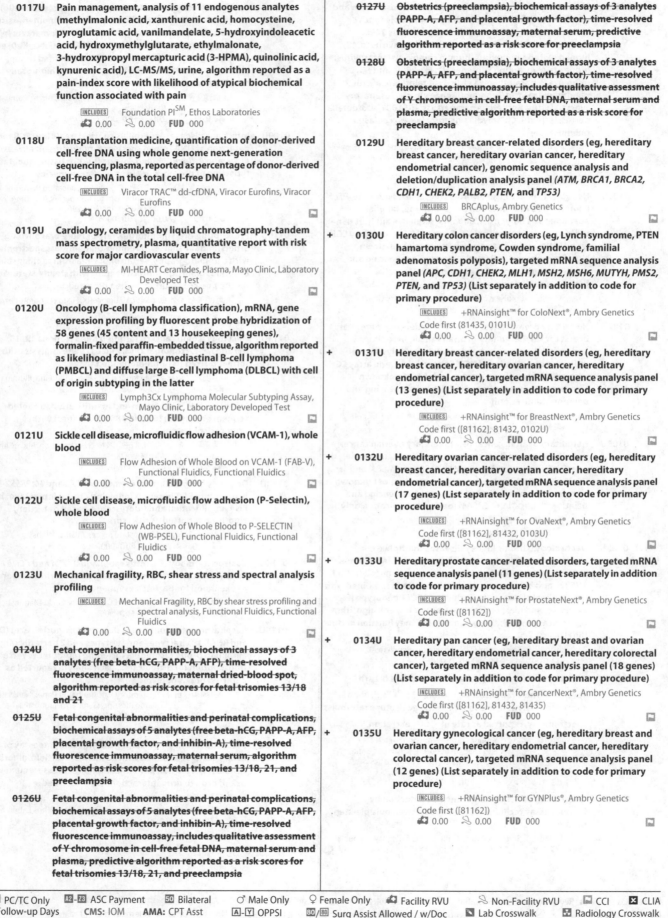

0.00 0.00 FUD 000

0118U Transplantation medicine, quantification of donor-derived cell-free DNA using whole genome next-generation sequencing, plasma, reported as percentage of donor-derived cell-free DNA in the total cell-free DNA

INCLUDES Viracor TRAC™ dd-cfDNA, Viracor Eurofins, Viracor Eurofins

0.00 0.00 FUD 000

0119U Cardiology, ceramides by liquid chromatography-tandem mass spectrometry, plasma, quantitative report with risk score for major cardiovascular events

INCLUDES MI-HEART Ceramides, Plasma, Mayo Clinic, Laboratory Developed Test

0.00 0.00 FUD 000

0120U Oncology (B-cell lymphoma classification), mRNA, gene expression profiling by fluorescent probe hybridization of 58 genes (45 content and 13 housekeeping genes), formalin-fixed paraffin-embedded tissue, algorithm reported as likelihood for primary mediastinal B-cell lymphoma (PMBCL) and diffuse large B-cell lymphoma (DLBCL) with cell of origin subtyping in the latter

INCLUDES Lymph3Cx Lymphoma Molecular Subtyping Assay, Mayo Clinic, Laboratory Developed Test

0.00 0.00 FUD 000

0121U Sickle cell disease, microfluidic flow adhesion (VCAM-1), whole blood

INCLUDES Flow Adhesion of Whole Blood on VCAM-1 (FAB-V), Functional Fluidics, Functional Fluidics

0.00 0.00 FUD 000

0122U Sickle cell disease, microfluidic flow adhesion (P-Selectin), whole blood

INCLUDES Flow Adhesion of Whole Blood to P-SELECTIN (WB-PSEL), Functional Fluidics, Functional Fluidics

0.00 0.00 FUD 000

0123U Mechanical fragility, RBC, shear stress and spectral analysis profiling

INCLUDES Mechanical Fragility, RBC by shear stress profiling and spectral analysis, Functional Fluidics, Functional Fluidics

0.00 0.00 FUD 000

0124U ~~**Fetal congenital abnormalities, biochemical assays of 3 analytes (free beta-hCG, PAPP-A, AFP), time-resolved fluorescence immunoassay, maternal dried-blood spot, algorithm reported as risk scores for fetal trisomies 13/18 and 21**~~

0125U ~~**Fetal congenital abnormalities and perinatal complications, biochemical assays of 5 analytes (free beta-hCG, PAPP-A, AFP, placental growth factor, and inhibin-A), time-resolved fluorescence immunoassay, maternal serum, algorithm reported as risk scores for fetal trisomies 13/18, 21, and preeclampsia**~~

0126U ~~**Fetal congenital abnormalities and perinatal complications, biochemical assays of 5 analytes (free beta-hCG, PAPP-A, AFP, placental growth factor, and inhibin-A), time-resolved fluorescence immunoassay, includes qualitative assessment of Y chromosome in cell-free fetal DNA, maternal serum and plasma, predictive algorithm reported as a risk scores for fetal trisomies 13/18, 21, and preeclampsia**~~

0127U ~~**Obstetrics (preeclampsia), biochemical assays of 3 analytes (PAPP-A, AFP, and placental growth factor), time-resolved fluorescence immunoassay, maternal serum, predictive algorithm reported as a risk score for preeclampsia**~~

0128U ~~**Obstetrics (preeclampsia), biochemical assays of 3 analytes (PAPP-A, AFP, and placental growth factor), time-resolved fluorescence immunoassay, includes qualitative assessment of Y chromosome in cell-free fetal DNA, maternal serum and plasma, predictive algorithm reported as a risk score for preeclampsia**~~

0129U Hereditary breast cancer-related disorders (eg, hereditary breast cancer, hereditary ovarian cancer, hereditary endometrial cancer), genomic sequence analysis and deletion/duplication analysis panel *(ATM, BRCA1, BRCA2, CDH1, CHEK2, PALB2, PTEN, and TP53)*

INCLUDES BRCAplus, Ambry Genetics

0.00 0.00 FUD 000

+ **0130U Hereditary colon cancer disorders (eg, Lynch syndrome, PTEN hamartoma syndrome, Cowden syndrome, familial adenomatosis polyposis), targeted mRNA sequence analysis panel *(APC, CDH1, CHEK2, MLH1, MSH2, MSH6, MUTYH, PMS2, PTEN, and TP53)* (List separately in addition to code for primary procedure)**

INCLUDES +RNAinsight™ for ColoNext®, Ambry Genetics

Code first (81435, 0101U)

0.00 0.00 FUD 000

+ **0131U Hereditary breast cancer-related disorders (eg, hereditary breast cancer, hereditary ovarian cancer, hereditary endometrial cancer), targeted mRNA sequence analysis panel (13 genes) (List separately in addition to code for primary procedure)**

INCLUDES +RNAinsight™ for BreastNext®, Ambry Genetics

Code first ([81162], 81432, 0102U)

0.00 0.00 FUD 000

+ **0132U Hereditary ovarian cancer-related disorders (eg, hereditary breast cancer, hereditary ovarian cancer, hereditary endometrial cancer), targeted mRNA sequence analysis panel (17 genes) (List separately in addition to code for primary procedure)**

INCLUDES +RNAinsight™ for OvaNext®, Ambry Genetics

Code first ([81162], 81432, 0103U)

0.00 0.00 FUD 000

+ **0133U Hereditary prostate cancer-related disorders, targeted mRNA sequence analysis panel (11 genes) (List separately in addition to code for primary procedure)**

INCLUDES +RNAinsight™ for ProstateNext®, Ambry Genetics

Code first ([81162])

0.00 0.00 FUD 000

+ **0134U Hereditary pan cancer (eg, hereditary breast and ovarian cancer, hereditary endometrial cancer, hereditary colorectal cancer), targeted mRNA sequence analysis panel (18 genes) (List separately in addition to code for primary procedure)**

INCLUDES +RNAinsight™ for CancerNext®, Ambry Genetics

Code first ([81162], 81432, 81435)

0.00 0.00 FUD 000

+ **0135U Hereditary gynecological cancer (eg, hereditary breast and ovarian cancer, hereditary endometrial cancer, hereditary colorectal cancer), targeted mRNA sequence analysis panel (12 genes) (List separately in addition to code for primary procedure)**

INCLUDES +RNAinsight™ for GYNPlus®, Ambry Genetics

Code first ([81162])

0.00 0.00 FUD 000

+ **0136U** ***ATM (ataxia telangiectasia mutated)*** **(eg, ataxia telangiectasia) mRNA sequence analysis (List separately in addition to code for primary procedure)**

INCLUDES +RNAinsight™ for *ATM*, Ambry Genetics

Code first (81408)

0.00 0.00 FUD 000

+ **0137U** ***PALB2 (partner and localizer of BRCA2)*** **(eg, breast and pancreatic cancer) mRNA sequence analysis (List separately in addition to code for ...**

INCLUDES +RNAinsight™ for *PALB2*, Ambry Genetics

Code first (81406)

0.00 0.00 FUD 000

+ **0138U** ***BRCA1 (BRCA1, DNA repair associated), BRCA2 (BRCA2, DNA repair associated)*** **(eg, hereditary breast and ovarian cancer) mRNA sequence analysis (List separately in addition to code for primary procedure)**

INCLUDES +RNAinsight™ for *BRCA1/2*, Ambry Genetics

Code first ([81162])

0.00 0.00 FUD 000

● **0139U** **Neurology (autism spectrum disorder [ASD]), quantitative measurements of 6 central carbon metabolites (ie, α-ketoglutarate, alanine, lactate, phenylalanine, pyruvate, and succinate), LC-MS/MS, plasma, algorithmic analysis with result reported as negative or positive (with metabolic subtypes of ASD)**

NPDX ASD Energy Metabolism, Stemina Biomarker Discovery, Inc, Stemina Biomarker Discovery, Inc.

● **0140U** **Infectious disease (fungi), fungal pathogen identification, DNA (15 fungal targets), blood culture, amplified probe technique, each target reported as detected or not detected**

INCLUDES ePlex® BCID Fungal Pathogens Panel, GenMark Diagnostics, Inc, GenMark Diagnostics, Inc

● **0141U** **Infectious disease (bacteria and fungi), gram-positive organism identification and drug resistance element detection, DNA (20 gram-positive bacterial targets, 4 resistance genes, 1 pan gram-negative bacterial target, 1 pan Candida target), blood culture, amplified probe technique, each target reported as detected or not detected**

INCLUDES ePlex® BCID Gram-Positive Panel, GenMark Diagnostics, Inc, GenMark Diagnostics, Inc

● **0142U** **Infectious disease (bacteria and fungi), gram-negative bacterial identification and drug resistance element detection, DNA (21 gram-negative bacterial targets, 6 resistance genes, 1 pan gram-positive bacterial target, 1 pan Candida target), amplified probe technique, each target reported as detected or not detected**

INCLUDES ePlex® BCID Gram-Negative Panel, GenMark Diagnostics, Inc, GenMark Diagnostics, Inc

● **0143U** **Drug assay, definitive, 120 or more drugs or metabolites, urine, quantitative liquid chromatography with tandem mass spectrometry (LC-MS/MS) using multiple reaction monitoring (MRM), with drug or metabolite description, comments including sample validation, per date of service**

INCLUDES CareViewRx, Newstar Medical Laboratories, LLC, Newstar Medical Laboratories, LLC

EXCLUDES *PsychViewRx Plus analysis by Newstar Medical Laboratories, LLC. To report, see (0150U)*

● **0144U** **Drug assay, definitive, 160 or more drugs or metabolites, urine, quantitative liquid chromatography with tandem mass spectrometry (LC-MS/MS) using multiple reaction monitoring (MRM), with drug or metabolite description, comments including sample validation, per date of service**

INCLUDES CareViewRx Plus, Newstar Medical Laboratories, LLC, Newstar Medical Laboratories, LLC

● **0145U** **Drug assay, definitive, 65 or more drugs or metabolites, urine, quantitative liquid chromatography with tandem mass spectrometry (LC-MS/MS) using multiple reaction monitoring (MRM), with drug or metabolite description, comments including sample validation, per date of service**

INCLUDES PainViewRx, Newstar Medical Laboratories, LLC, Newstar Medical Laboratories, LLC

● **0146U** **Drug assay, definitive, 80 or more drugs or metabolites, urine, by quantitative liquid chromatography with tandem mass spectrometry (LC-MS/MS) using multiple reaction monitoring (MRM), with drug or metabolite description, comments including sample validation, per date of service**

INCLUDES PainViewRx Plus, Newstar Medical Laboratories, LLC, Newstar Medical Laboratories, LLC

● **0147U** **Drug assay, definitive, 85 or more drugs or metabolites, urine, quantitative liquid chromatography with tandem mass spectrometry (LC-MS/MS) using multiple reaction monitoring (MRM), with drug or metabolite description, comments including sample validation, per date of service**

INCLUDES RiskViewRx, Newstar Medical Laboratories, LLC, Newstar Medical Laboratories, LLC

● **0148U** **Drug assay, definitive, 100 or more drugs or metabolites, urine, quantitative liquid chromatography with tandem mass spectrometry (LC-MS/MS) using multiple reaction monitoring (MRM), with drug or metabolite description, comments including sample validation, per date of service**

INCLUDES RiskViewRx Plus, Newstar Medical Laboratories, LLC, Newstar Medical Laboratories, LLC

● **0149U** **Drug assay, definitive, 60 or more drugs or metabolites, urine, quantitative liquid chromatography with tandem mass spectrometry (LC-MS/MS) using multiple reaction monitoring (MRM), with drug or metabolite description, comments including sample validation, per date of service**

INCLUDES PsychViewRx, Newstar Medical Laboratories, LLC, Newstar Medical Laboratories, LLC

● **0150U** **Drug assay, definitive, 120 or more drugs or metabolites, urine, quantitative liquid chromatography with tandem mass spectrometry (LC-MS/MS) using multiple reaction monitoring (MRM), with drug or metabolite description, comments including sample validation, per date of service**

INCLUDES PsychViewRx Plus, Newstar Medical Laboratories, LLC, Newstar Medical Laboratories, LLC

EXCLUDES *CareViewRx analysis by Newstar Medical Laboratories, LLC. To report, see (0143U)*

● **0151U** **Infectious disease (bacterial or viral respiratory tract infection), pathogen specific nucleic acid (DNA or RNA), 33 targets, real-time semi-quantitative PCR, bronchoalveolar lavage, sputum, or endotracheal aspirate, detection of 33 organismal and antibiotic resistance genes with limited semi-quantitative results**

INCLUDES BioFire® FilmArray® Pneumonia Panel, BioFire® Diagnostics, BioFire® Diagnostics

AMA: 2020,Apr,3

▲ **0152U** **Infectious disease (bacteria, fungi, parasites, and DNA viruses), microbial cell-free DNA, plasma, untargeted next-generation sequencing, report for significant positive pathogens**

INCLUDES Karius® Test, Karius Inc, Karius Inc

● **0153U** **Oncology (breast), mRNA, gene expression profiling by next-generation sequencing of 101 genes, utilizing formalin-fixed paraffin-embedded tissue, algorithm reported as a triple negative breast cancer clinical subtype(s) with information on immune cell involvement**

INCLUDES Insight TNBCtype™, Insight Molecular Labs

▲ **0154U** **Oncology (urothelial cancer), RNA, analysis by real-time RT-PCR of the *FGFR3 (fibroblast growth factor receptor3)* gene analysis (ie, p.R248C [c.742C>T], p.S249C [c.746C>G], p.G370C [c.1108G>T], p.Y373C [c.1118A>G], FGFR3-TACC3v1, and FGFR3-TACC3v3) utilizing formalin-fixed paraffin-embedded urothelial cancer tumor tissue, reported as *FGFR* gene alteration status**

INCLUDES therascreen® *FGFR* RGQ RT-PCR Kit, QIAGEN, QIAGEN GmbH

AMA: 2020,Jun,11

▲ **0155U** **Oncology (breast cancer), DNA, *PIK3CA (phosphatidylinositol-4,5-bisphosphate 3-kinase, catalytic subunit alpha)* (eg, breast cancer) gene analysis (ie, p.C420R, p.E542K, p.E545A, p.E545D [g.1635G>T only], p.E545G, p.E545K, p.Q546E, p.Q546R, p.H1047L, p.H1047R, p.H1047Y), utilizing formalin-fixed paraffin-embedded breast tumor tissue, reported as *PIK3CA* gene mutation status**

INCLUDES therascreen® *PIK3CA* RGQ PCR Kit, QIAGEN, QIAGEN GmbH

AMA: 2020,Jun,11

● **0156U** **Copy number (eg, intellectual disability, dysmorphology), sequence analysis**

INCLUDES SMASH™, New York Genome Center, Marvel Genomics™

● + **0157U** ***APC (APC regulator of WNT signaling pathway)* (eg, familial adenomatosis polyposis [FAP]) mRNA sequence analysis (List separately in addition to code for primary procedure)**

INCLUDES CustomNext + RNA: *APC*, Ambry Genetics®, Ambry Genetics®

Code first ([81201])

Facility RVU 0.00 Non-Facility RVU 0.00 **FUD** 000

● + **0158U** ***MLH1 (mutL homolog 1)* (eg, hereditary non-polyposis colorectal cancer, Lynch syndrome) mRNA sequence analysis (List separately in addition to code for primary procedure)**

INCLUDES CustomNext + RNA: *MLH1*, Ambry Genetics®, Ambry Genetics®

Code first ([81292])

Facility RVU 0.00 Non-Facility RVU 0.00 **FUD** 000

● + **0159U** ***MSH2 (mutS homolog 2)* (eg, hereditary colon cancer, Lynch syndrome) mRNA sequence analysis (List separately in addition to code for primary procedure)**

INCLUDES CustomNext + RNA: *MSH2*, Ambry Genetics®, Ambry Genetics®

Code first ([81295])

Facility RVU 0.00 Non-Facility RVU 0.00 **FUD** 000

● + **0160U** ***MSH6 (mutS homolog 6)* (eg, hereditary colon cancer, Lynch syndrome) mRNA sequence analysis (List separately in addition to code for primary procedure)**

INCLUDES CustomNext + RNA: *MSH6*, Ambry Genetics®, Ambry Genetics®

Code first (81298)

Facility RVU 0.00 Non-Facility RVU 0.00 **FUD** 000

● + **0161U** ***PMS2 (PMS1 homolog 2, mismatch repair system component)* (eg, hereditary non-polyposis colorectal cancer, Lynch syndrome) mRNA sequence analysis (List separately in addition to code for primary procedure)**

INCLUDES CustomNext + RNA: *PMS2*, Ambry Genetics®, Ambry Genetics®

Code first (81317)

Facility RVU 0.00 Non-Facility RVU 0.00 **FUD** 000

● + **0162U** **Hereditary colon cancer (Lynch syndrome), targeted mRNA sequence analysis panel *(MLH1, MSH2, MSH6, PMS2)* (List separately in addition to code for primary procedure)**

INCLUDES CustomNext + RNA: Lynch *(MLH1, MSH2, MSH6, PMS2)*, Ambry Genetics®, Ambry Genetics®

Code first ([81292], [81295], 81298, 81317, 81435)

Facility RVU 0.00 Non-Facility RVU 0.00 **FUD** 000

● **0163U** **Oncology (colorectal) screening, biochemical enzyme-linked immunosorbent assay (ELISA) of 3 plasma or serum proteins (teratocarcinoma derived growth factor-1 [TDGF-1, Cripto-1], carcinoembryonic antigen [CEA], extracellular matrix protein [ECM]), with demographic data (age, gender, CRC-screening compliance) using a proprietary algorithm and reported as likelihood of CRC or advanced adenomas**

INCLUDES BeScreened™-CRC, Beacon Biomedical Inc, Beacon Biomedical Inc

AMA: 2020,Jun,11

● **0164U** **Gastroenterology (irritable bowel syndrome [IBS]), immunoassay for anti-CdtB and anti-vinculin antibodies, utilizing plasma, algorithm for elevated or not elevated qualitative results**

INCLUDES ibs-smart™, Gemelli Biotech, Gemelli Biotech

AMA: 2020,Jun,11

▲ **0165U** **Peanut allergen-specific quantitative assessment of multiple epitopes using enzyme-linked immunosorbent assay (ELISA), blood, individual epitope results and probability of peanut allergy**

INCLUDES VeriMAP™ Peanut Dx – Bead-based Epitope Assay, AllerGenis™ Clinical Laboratory, AllerGenis™ LLC

AMA: 2020,Jun,11

● **0166U** **Liver disease, 10 biochemical assays (α2-macroglobulin, haptoglobin, apolipoprotein A1, bilirubin, GGT, ALT, AST, triglycerides, cholesterol, fasting glucose) and biometric and demographic data, utilizing serum, algorithm reported as scores for fibrosis, necroinflammatory activity, and steatosis with a summary interpretation**

INCLUDES LiverFASt™, Fibronostics, Fibronostics

AMA: 2020,Jun,11

● **0167U** **Gonadotropin, chorionic (hCG), immunoassay with direct optical observation, blood**

INCLUDES ADEXUSDx hCG Test, NOWDiagnostics, NOWDiagnostics

AMA: 2020,Jun,11

● **0168U** **Fetal aneuploidy (trisomy 21, 18, and 13) DNA sequence analysis of selected regions using maternal plasma without fetal fraction cutoff, algorithm reported as a risk score for each trisomy**

INCLUDES Vanadis® NIPT, PerkinElmer, Inc, PerkinElmer Genomics

AMA: 2020,Jun,11

● **0169U** ***NUDT15 (nudix hydrolase 15)* and *TPMT (thiopurine S-methyltransferase)* (eg, drug metabolism) gene analysis, common variants**

INCLUDES NT *(NUDT15* and *TPMT)* genotyping panel, RPRD Diagnostics

AMA: 2020,Jun,11

● **0170U** **Neurology (autism spectrum disorder [ASD]), RNA, next-generation sequencing, saliva, algorithmic analysis, and results reported as predictive probability of ASD diagnosis**

INCLUDES Clarifi™, Quadrant Biosciences, Inc, Quadrant Biosciences, Inc

AMA: 2020,Jun,11

● **0171U** **Targeted genomic sequence analysis panel, acute myeloid leukemia, myelodysplastic syndrome, and myeloproliferative neoplasms, DNA analysis, 23 genes, interrogation for sequence variants, rearrangements and minimal residual disease, reported as presence/absence**

INCLUDES MyMRD® NGS Panel, Laboratory for Personalized Molecular Medicine, Laboratory for Personalized Molecular Medicine

AMA: 2020,Jun,11

● **0172U** **Oncology (solid tumor as indicated by the label), somatic mutation analysis of *BRCA1 (BRCA1, DNA repair associated)*, *BRCA2 (BRCA2, DNA repair associated)* and analysis of homologous recombination deficiency pathways, DNA, formalin-fixed paraffin-embedded tissue, algorithm quantifying tumor genomic instability score**

INCLUDES myChoice® CDx, Myriad Genetics Laboratories, Inc, Myriad Genetics Laboratories, Inc

● **0173U** **Psychiatry (ie, depression, anxiety), genomic analysis panel, includes variant analysis of 14 genes**

INCLUDES Psych HealthPGx Panel, RPRD Diagnostics, RPRD Diagnostics

● **0174U** **Oncology (solid tumor), mass spectrometric 30 protein targets, formalin-fixed paraffin-embedded tissue, prognostic and predictive algorithm reported as likely, unlikely, or uncertain benefit of 39 chemotherapy and targeted therapeutic oncology agents**

INCLUDES LC-MS/MS Targeted Proteomic Assay, OncoOmicDx Laboratory, LDT

● **0175U** **Psychiatry (eg, depression, anxiety), genomic analysis panel, variant analysis of 15 genes**

INCLUDES Genomind® Professional PGx Express™ CORE, Genomind, Inc, Genomind, Inc

● **0176U** **Cytolethal distending toxin B (CdtB) and vinculin IgG antibodies by immunoassay (ie, ELISA)**

INCLUDES IBS*Schek*®, Commonwealth Diagnostics International, Inc, Commonwealth Diagnostics International, Inc

● **0177U** **Oncology (breast cancer), DNA, *PIK3CA (phosphatidylinositol-4,5-bisphosphate 3-kinase catalytic subunit alpha)* gene analysis of 11 gene variants utilizing plasma, reported as *PIK3CA* gene mutation status**

INCLUDES therascreen® *PIK3CA* RGQ PCR Kit, QIAGEN, QIAGEN GmbH

● **0178U** **Peanut allergen-specific quantitative assessment of multiple epitopes using enzyme-linked immunosorbent assay (ELISA), blood, report of minimum eliciting exposure for a clinical reaction**

INCLUDES VeriMAP™ Peanut Sensitivity - Bead Based Epitope Assay, AllerGenis™ Clinical Laboratory, AllerGenis™ LLC

● **0179U** **Oncology (non-small cell lung cancer), cell-free DNA, targeted sequence analysis of 23 genes (single nucleotide variations, insertions and deletions, fusions without prior knowledge of partner/breakpoint, copy number variations), with report of significant mutation(s)**

INCLUDES Resolution ctDx Lung™, Resolution Bioscience, Resolution Bioscience, Inc

● **0180U** **Red cell antigen (ABO blood group) genotyping (ABO), gene analysis Sanger/chain termination/conventional sequencing, *ABO (ABO, alpha 1-3-N-acetylgalactosaminyltransferase and alpha 1-3-galactosyltransferase)* gene, including subtyping, 7 exons**

INCLUDES Navigator ABO Sequencing, Grifols Immunohematology Center, Grifols Immunohematology Center

● **0181U** **Red cell antigen (Colton blood group) genotyping (CO), gene analysis, *AQP1 (aquaporin 1 [Colton blood group])* exon 1**

INCLUDES Navigator CO Sequencing, Grifols Immunohematology Center, Grifols Immunohematology Center

● **0182U** **Red cell antigen (Cromer blood group) genotyping (CROM), gene analysis, *CD55 (CD55 molecule [Cromer blood group])* exons 1-10**

INCLUDES Navigator CROM Sequencing, Grifols Immunohematology Center, Grifols Immunohematology Center

● **0183U** **Red cell antigen (Diego blood group) genotyping (DI), gene analysis, *SLC4A1 (solute carrier family 4 member 1 [Diego blood group])* exon 19**

INCLUDES Navigator DI Sequencing, Grifols Immunohematology Center, Grifols Immunohematology Center

● **0184U** **Red cell antigen (Dombrock blood group) genotyping (DO), gene analysis, *ART4 (ADP-ribosyltransferase 4 [Dombrock blood group])* exon 2**

INCLUDES Navigator DO Sequencing, Grifols Immunohematology Center, Grifols Immunohematology Center

● **0185U** **Red cell antigen (H blood group) genotyping (FUT1), gene analysis, *FUT1 (fucosyltransferase 1 [H blood group])* exon 4**

INCLUDES Navigator FUT1 Sequencing, Grifols Immunohematology Center, Grifols Immunohematology Center

● **0186U** **Red cell antigen (H blood group) genotyping (FUT2), gene analysis, *FUT2 (fucosyltransferase 2)* exon 2**

INCLUDES Navigator FUT2 Sequencing, Grifols Immunohematology Center, Grifols Immunohematology Center

● **0187U** **Red cell antigen (Duffy blood group) genotyping (FY), gene analysis, *ACKR1 (atypical chemokine receptor 1 [Duffy blood group])* exons 1-2**

INCLUDES Navigator FY Sequencing, Grifols Immunohematology Center, Grifols Immunohematology Center

● **0188U** **Red cell antigen (Gerbich blood group) genotyping (GE), gene analysis, *GYPC (glycophorin C [Gerbich blood group])* exons 1-4**

INCLUDES Navigator GE Sequencing, Grifols Immunohematology Center, Grifols Immunohematology Center

● **0189U** **Red cell antigen (MNS blood group) genotyping (GYPA), gene analysis, *GYPA (glycophorin A [MNS blood group])* introns 1, 5, exon 2**

INCLUDES Navigator GYPA Sequencing, Grifols Immunohematology Center, Grifols Immunohematology Center

● **0190U** **Red cell antigen (MNS blood group) genotyping (GYPB), gene analysis, *GYPB (glycophorin B [MNS blood group])* introns 1, 5, pseudoexon 3**

INCLUDES Navigator GYPB Sequencing, Grifols Immunohematology Center, Grifols Immunohematology Center

● **0191U** **Red cell antigen (Indian blood group) genotyping (IN), gene analysis, *CD44 (CD44 molecule [Indian blood group])* exons 2, 3, 6**

INCLUDES Navigator IN Sequencing, Grifols Immunohematology Center, Grifols Immunohematology Center

● **0192U** **Red cell antigen (Kidd blood group) genotyping (JK), gene analysis, *SLC14A1 (solute carrier family 14 member 1 [Kidd blood group])* gene promoter, exon 9**

INCLUDES Navigator JK Sequencing, Grifols Immunohematology Center, Grifols Immunohematology Center

● **0193U** **Red cell antigen (JR blood group) genotyping (JR), gene analysis, *ABCG2 (ATP binding cassette subfamily G member 2 [Junior blood group])* exons 2-26**

INCLUDES Navigator JR Sequencing, Grifols Immunohematology Center, Grifols Immunohematology Center

● **0194U** **Red cell antigen (Kell blood group) genotyping (KEL), gene analysis, *KEL (Kell metallo-endopeptidase [Kell blood group])* exon 8**

INCLUDES Navigator KEL Sequencing, Grifols Immunohematology Center, Grifols Immunohematology Center

● **0195U** ***KLF1 (Kruppel-like factor 1)*, targeted sequencing (ie, exon 13)**

INCLUDES Navigator *KLF1* Sequencing, Grifols Immunohematology Center, Grifols Immunohematology Center

● **0196U Red cell antigen (Lutheran blood group) genotyping (LU), gene analysis, *BCAM (basal cell adhesion molecule [Lutheran blood group])* exon 3**

INCLUDES Navigator LU Sequencing, Grifols Immunohematology Center, Grifols Immunohematology Center

● **0197U Red cell antigen (Landsteiner-Wiener blood group) genotyping (LW), gene analysis, *ICAM4 (intercellular adhesion molecule 4 [Landsteiner-Wiener blood group])* exon 1**

INCLUDES Navigator LW Sequencing, Grifols Immunohematology Center, Grifols Immunohematology Center

● **0198U Red cell antigen (RH blood group) genotyping (RHD and RHCE), gene analysis Sanger/chain termination/conventional sequencing, *RHD (Rh blood group D antigen)* exons 1-10 and *RHCE (Rh blood group CcEe antigens)* exon 5**

INCLUDES Navigator RHD/CE Sequencing, Grifols Immunohematology Center, Grifols Immunohematology Center

● **0199U Red cell antigen (Scianna blood group) genotyping (SC), gene analysis, *ERMAP (erythroblast membrane associated protein [Scianna blood group])* exons 4, 12**

INCLUDES Navigator SC Sequencing, Grifols Immunohematology Center, Grifols Immunohematology Center

● **0200U Red cell antigen (Kx blood group) genotyping (XK), gene analysis, *XK (X-linked Kx blood group)* exons 1-3**

INCLUDES Navigator XK Sequencing, Grifols Immunohematology Center, Grifols Immunohematology Center

● **0201U Red cell antigen (Yt blood group) genotyping (YT), gene analysis, *ACHE (acetylcholinesterase [Cartwright blood group])* exon 2**

INCLUDES Navigator YT Sequencing, Grifols Immunohematology Center, Grifols Immunohematology Center

● **0202U Infectious disease (bacterial or viral respiratory tract infection), pathogen-specific nucleic acid (DNA or RNA), 22 targets including severe acute respiratory syndrome coronavirus 2 (SARS-CoV-2), qualitative RT-PCR, nasopharyngeal swab, each pathogen reported as detected or not detected**

INCLUDES BioFire® Respiratory Panel 2.1 (RP2.1), BioFire® Diagnostics, BioFire® Diagnostics, LLC

EXCLUDES *QIAstat-Dx Respiratory SARS CoV-2 Panel, QIAGEN Sciences, QIAGEN GmbH. To report, see (0223U)*

AMA: 2020,AugSE,1; 2020,AugSE,1; 2020,AugSE,1; 2020,MaySE,1; 2020,May,3; 2020,JuneSE,1

● **0203U Autoimmune (inflammatory bowel disease), mRNA, gene expression profiling by quantitative RT-PCR, 17 genes (15 target and 2 reference genes), whole blood, reported as a continuous risk score and classification of inflammatory bowel disease aggressiveness**

INCLUDES PredictSURE IBD™ Test, KSL Diagnostics, PredictImmune Ltd

● **0204U Oncology (thyroid), mRNA, gene expression analysis of 593 genes (including *BRAF, RAS, RET, PAX8,* and *NTRK*) for sequence variants and rearrangements, utilizing fine needle aspirate, reported as detected or not detected**

INCLUDES Afirma Xpression Atlas, Veracyte, Inc, Veracyte, Inc

● **0205U Ophthalmology (age-related macular degeneration), analysis of 3 gene variants (2 *CFH* gene, 1 *ARMS2* gene), using PCR and MALDI-TOF, buccal swab, reported as positive or negative for neovascular age-related macular-degeneration risk associated with zinc supplements**

INCLUDES Vita Risk®, Arctic Medical Laboratories, Arctic Medical Laboratories

● **0206U Neurology (Alzheimer disease); cell aggregation using morphometric imaging and protein kinase C-epsilon (PKCe) concentration in response to amylospheroid treatment by ELISA, cultured skin fibroblasts, each reported as positive or negative for Alzheimer disease**

INCLUDES DISCERN™ , NeuroDiagnostics, NeuroDiagnostics

● + **0207U quantitative imaging of phosphorylated *ERK1* and *ERK2* in response to bradykinin treatment by in situ immunofluorescence, using cultured skin fibroblasts, reported as a probability index for Alzheimer disease (List separately in addition to code for primary procedure)**

INCLUDES DISCERN™ , NeuroDiagnostics, NeuroDiagnostics

Code first (0206U)

Facility RVU 0.00 Non-Facility RVU 0.00 **FUD** 000

● **0208U Oncology (medullary thyroid carcinoma), mRNA, gene expression analysis of 108 genes, utilizing fine needle aspirate, algorithm reported as positive or negative for medullary thyroid carcinoma**

INCLUDES Afirma Medullary Thyroid Carcinoma (MTC) Classifier, Veracyte, Inc, Veracyte, Inc

● **0209U Cytogenomic constitutional (genome-wide) analysis, interrogation of genomic regions for copy number, structural changes and areas of homozygosity for chromosomal abnormalities**

INCLUDES CNGnome™, PerkinElmer Genomics, PerkinElmer Genomics

● **0210U Syphilis test, non-treponemal antibody, immunoassay, quantitative (RPR)**

INCLUDES BioPlex 2200 RPR Assay - Quantitative, Bio-Rad Laboratories, Bio-Rad Laboratories

● **0211U Oncology (pan-tumor), DNA and RNA by next-generation sequencing, utilizing formalin-fixed paraffin-embedded tissue, interpretative report for single nucleotide variants, copy number alterations, tumor mutational burden, and microsatellite instability, with therapy association**

INCLUDES MI Cancer Seek™ - NGS Analysis, Caris MPI d/b/a Caris Life Sciences, Caris MPI d/b/a Caris Life Sciences

● **0212U Rare diseases (constitutional/heritable disorders), whole genome and mitochondrial DNA sequence analysis, including small sequence changes, deletions, duplications, short tandem repeat gene expansions, and variants in non-uniquely mappable regions, blood or saliva, identification and categorization of genetic variants, proband**

INCLUDES Genomic Unity® Whole Genome Analysis – Proband, Variantyx Inc, Variantyx Inc

EXCLUDES *Genome (e.g., unexplained constitutional or heritable disorder or syndrome); sequence analysis (81425)*

● **0213U Rare diseases (constitutional/heritable disorders), whole genome and mitochondrial DNA sequence analysis, including small sequence changes, deletions, duplications, short tandem repeat gene expansions, and variants in non-uniquely mappable regions, blood or saliva, identification and categorization of genetic variants, each comparator genome (eg, parent, sibling)**

INCLUDES Genomic Unity® Whole Genome Analysis - Comparator, Variantyx Inc, Variantyx Inc

EXCLUDES *Genome (e.g., unexplained constitutional or heritable disorder or syndrome); sequence analysis, each comparator genome (e.g., parents, siblings) (81426)*

● **0214U Rare diseases (constitutional/heritable disorders), whole exome and mitochondrial DNA sequence analysis, including small sequence changes, deletions, duplications, short tandem repeat gene expansions, and variants in non-uniquely mappable regions, blood or saliva, identification and categorization of genetic variants, proband**

INCLUDES Genomic Unity® Exome Plus Analysis - Proband, Variantyx Inc, Variantyx Inc

EXCLUDES *Exome (e.g., unexplained constitutional or heritable disorder or syndrome); sequence analysis (81415)*

● **0215U** **Rare diseases (constitutional/heritable disorders), whole exome and mitochondrial DNA sequence analysis, including small sequence changes, deletions, duplications, short tandem repeat gene expansions, and variants in non-uniquely mappable regions, blood or saliva, identification and categorization of genetic variants, each comparator exome (eg, parent, sibling)**

INCLUDES Genomic Unity® Exome Plus Analysis - Comparator, Variantyx Inc, Variantyx Inc

EXCLUDES *Exome (e.g., unexplained constitutional or heritable disorder or syndrome); sequence analysis, each comparator exome (e.g., parents, siblings) (81416)*

● **0216U** **Neurology (inherited ataxias), genomic DNA sequence analysis of 12 common genes including small sequence changes, deletions, duplications, short tandem repeat gene expansions, and variants in non-uniquely mappable regions, blood or saliva, identification and categorization of genetic variants**

INCLUDES Genomic Unity® Ataxia Repeat Expansion and Sequence Analysis, Variantyx Inc, Variantyx Inc

● **0217U** **Neurology (inherited ataxias), genomic DNA sequence analysis of 51 genes including small sequence changes, deletions, duplications, short tandem repeat gene expansions, and variants in non-uniquely mappable regions, blood or saliva, identification and categorization of genetic variants**

INCLUDES Genomic Unity® Comprehensive Ataxia Repeat Expansion and Sequence Analysis, Variantyx Inc, Variantyx Inc

● **0218U** **Neurology (muscular dystrophy), *DMD* gene sequence analysis, including small sequence changes, deletions, duplications, and variants in non-uniquely mappable regions, blood or saliva, identification and characterization of genetic variants**

INCLUDES Genomic Unity® DMD Analysis, Variantyx Inc, Variantyx Inc

● **0219U** **Infectious agent (human immunodeficiency virus), targeted viral next-generation sequence analysis (ie, protease [PR], reverse transcriptase [RT], integrase [INT]), algorithm reported as prediction of antiviral drug susceptibility**

INCLUDES *Sentosa*® SQ HIV-1 Genotyping Assay, Vela Diagnostics USA, Inc, Vela Operations Singapore Pte Ltd

● **0220U** **Oncology (breast cancer), image analysis with artificial intelligence assessment of 12 histologic and immunohistochemical features, reported as a recurrence score**

INCLUDES PreciseDx™ Breast Cancer Test, PreciseDx, PreciseDx

● **0221U** **Red cell antigen (ABO blood group) genotyping (ABO), gene analysis, next-generation sequencing, *ABO (ABO, alpha 1-3-N-acetylgalactosaminyltransferase and alpha 1-3-galactosyltransferase)* gene**

INCLUDES Navigator ABO Blood Group NGS, Grifols Immunohematology Center, Grifols Immunohematology Center

● **0222U** **Red cell antigen (RH blood group) genotyping (RHD and RHCE), gene analysis, next-generation sequencing, RH proximal promoter, exons 1-10, portions of introns 2-3**

INCLUDES Navigator Rh Blood Group NGS, Grifols Immunohematology Center, Grifols Immunohematology Center

● **0223U** **Infectious disease (bacterial or viral respiratory tract infection), pathogen-specific nucleic acid (DNA or RNA), 22 targets including severe acute respiratory syndrome coronavirus 2 (SARS-CoV-2), qualitative RT-PCR, nasopharyngeal swab, each pathogen reported as detected or not detected**

INCLUDES QIAstat-Dx Respiratory SARS CoV-2 Panel, QIAGEN Sciences, QIAGEN GmbH

EXCLUDES *BioFire® Respiratory Panel 2.1 (RP2.1), BioFire® Diagnostics, BioFire® Diagnostics, LLC. To report, see (0202U)*

AMA: 2020,AugSE,1; 2020,AugSE,1; 2020,AugSE,1

● **0224U** **Antibody, severe acute respiratory syndrome coronavirus 2 (SARS-CoV-2) (Coronavirus disease [COVID-19]), includes titer(s), when performed**

INCLUDES COVID-19 Antibody Test, Mt Sinai, Mount Sinai Laboratory

EXCLUDES *Antibody; severe acute respiratory syndrome coronavirus 2 (SARS-CoV-2) (coronavirus disease [COVID-19]) (86769)*

AMA: 2020,AugSE,1; 2020,AugSE,1; 2020,AugSE,1

● **0225U** **Infectious disease (bacterial or viral respiratory tract infection) pathogen-specific DNA and RNA, 21 targets, including severe acute respiratory syndrome coronavirus 2 (SARS-CoV-2), amplified probe technique, including multiplex reverse transcription for RNA targets, each analyte reported as detected or not detected**

INCLUDES ePlex® Respiratory Pathogen Panel 2, GenMark Dx, GenMark Diagnostics, Inc

AMA: 2020,AugSE,1

● **0226U** **Surrogate viral neutralization test (sVNT), severe acute respiratory syndrome coronavirus 2 (SARS-CoV-2) (Coronavirus disease [COVID-19]), ELISA, plasma, serum**

INCLUDES Tru-Immune™, Ethos Laboratories, GenScript® USA Inc

AMA: 2020,AugSE,1

● **0227U** **Drug assay, presumptive, 30 or more drugs or metabolites, urine, liquid chromatography with tandem mass spectrometry (LC-MS/MS) using multiple reaction monitoring (MRM), with drug or metabolite description, includes sample validation**

INCLUDES Comprehensive Screen, Aspenti Health

● **0228U** **Oncology (prostate), multianalyte molecular profile by photometric detection of macromolecules adsorbed on nanosponge array slides with machine learning, utilizing first morning voided urine, algorithm reported as likelihood of prostate cancer**

INCLUDES PanGIA Prostate, Genetics Institute of America, Entopsis, LLC

● **0229U** ***BCAT1 (Branched chain amino acid transaminase 1)* or *IKZF1 (IKAROS family zinc finger 1)* (eg, colorectal cancer) promoter methylation analysis**

INCLUDES Colvera®, Clinical Genomics Pathology Inc

● **0230U** ***AR (androgen receptor)* (eg, spinal and bulbar muscular atrophy, Kennedy disease, X chromosome inactivation), full sequence analysis, including small sequence changes in exonic and intronic regions, deletions, duplications, short tandem repeat (STR) expansions, mobile element insertions, and variants in non-uniquely mappable regions**

INCLUDES Genomic Unity® AR Analysis, Variantyx Inc, Variantyx Inc

● **0231U** ***CACNA1A (calcium voltage-gated channel subunit alpha 1A)* (eg, spinocerebellar ataxia), full gene analysis, including small sequence changes in exonic and intronic regions, deletions, duplications, short tandem repeat (STR) gene expansions, mobile element insertions, and variants in non-uniquely mappable regions**

INCLUDES Genomic Unity® CACNA1A Analysis, Variantyx Inc, Variantyx Inc

● **0232U** ***CSTB (cystatin B)*** **(eg, progressive myoclonic epilepsy type 1A, Unverricht-Lundborg disease), full gene analysis, including small sequence changes in exonic and intronic regions, deletions, duplications, short tandem repeat (STR) expansions, mobile element insertions, and variants in non-uniquely mappable regions**

INCLUDES Genomic Unity® CSTB Analysis, Variantyx Inc, Variantyx Inc

● **0233U** ***FXN (frataxin)*** **(eg, Friedreich ataxia), gene analysis, including small sequence changes in exonic and intronic regions, deletions, duplications, short tandem repeat (STR) expansions, mobile element insertions, and variants in non-uniquely mappable regions**

INCLUDES Genomic Unity® FXN Analysis, Variantyx Inc, Variantyx Inc

● **0234U** ***MECP2 (methyl CpG binding protein 2)*** **(eg, Rett syndrome), full gene analysis, including small sequence changes in exonic and intronic regions, deletions, duplications, mobile element insertions, and variants in non-uniquely mappable regions**

INCLUDES Genomic Unity® MECP2 Analysis, Variantyx Inc, Variantyx Inc

● **0235U** ***PTEN (phosphatase and tensin homolog)*** **(eg, Cowden syndrome, PTEN hamartoma tumor syndrome), full gene analysis, including small sequence changes in exonic and intronic regions, deletions, duplications, mobile element insertions, and variants in non-uniquely mappable regions**

INCLUDES Genomic Unity® PTEN Analysis, Variantyx Inc, Variantyx Inc

● **0236U** ***SMN1 (survival of motor neuron 1, telomeric)*** **and** ***SMN2 (survival of motor neuron 2, centromeric)*** **(eg, spinal muscular atrophy) full gene analysis, including small sequence changes in exonic and intronic regions, duplications and deletions, and mobile element insertions**

INCLUDES Genomic Unity® SMN1/2 Analysis, Variantyx Inc, Variantyx Inc

● **0237U** **Cardiac ion channelopathies (eg, Brugada syndrome, long QT syndrome, short QT syndrome, catecholaminergic polymorphic ventricular tachycardia), genomic sequence analysis panel including** ***ANK2, CASQ2, CAV3, KCNE1, KCNE2, KCNH2, KCNJ2, KCNQ1, RYR2,*** **and** ***SCN5A,*** **including small sequence changes in exonic and intronic regions, deletions, duplications, mobile element insertions, and variants in non-uniquely mappable regions**

INCLUDES Genomic Unity® Cardiac Ion Channelopathies Analysis, Variantyx Inc, Variantyx Inc

● **0238U** **Oncology (Lynch syndrome), genomic DNA sequence analysis of** ***MLH1, MSH2, MSH6, PMS2,*** **and** ***EPCAM,*** **including small sequence changes in exonic and intronic regions, deletions, duplications, mobile element insertions, and variants in non-uniquely mappable regions**

INCLUDES Genomic Unity® Lynch Syndrome Analysis, Variantyx Inc, Variantyx Inc

● **0239U** **Targeted genomic sequence analysis panel, solid organ neoplasm, cell-free DNA, analysis of 311 or more genes, interrogation for sequence variants, including substitutions, insertions, deletions, select rearrangements, and copy number variations**

INCLUDES FoundationOne® Liquid CDx, FOUNDATION MEDICINE, INC, FOUNDATION MEDICINE, INC

● **0240U** **Infectious disease (viral respiratory tract infection), pathogen-specific RNA, 3 targets (severe acute respiratory syndrome coronavirus 2 [SARS-CoV-2], influenza A, influenza B), upper respiratory specimen, each pathogen reported as detected or not detected**

INCLUDES Xpert® Xpress SARS-CoV-2/Flu/RSV (SARS-CoV-2 & Flu targets only), Cepheid

● **0241U** **Infectious disease (viral respiratory tract infection), pathogen-specific RNA, 4 targets (severe acute respiratory syndrome coronavirus 2 [SARS-CoV-2], influenza A, influenza B, respiratory syncytial virus [RSV]), upper respiratory specimen, each pathogen reported as detected or not detected**

INCLUDES Xpert® Xpress SARS-CoV-2/Flu/RSV (all targets), Cepheid

90281-90399 Immunoglobulin Products

INCLUDES Immune globulin product only
Anti-infectives
Antitoxins
Isoantibodies
Monoclonal antibodies

Code also (96365-96372, 96374-96375)

90281 Immune globulin (Ig), human, for intramuscular use
INCLUDES Gamastan
0.00 0.00 FUD XXX
AMA: 2020,Jan,11; 2018,Jan,8; 2017,Jan,8; 2016,Jan,13; 2015,Jan,16

90283 Immune globulin (IgIV), human, for intravenous use
0.00 0.00 FUD XXX
AMA: 2020,Jan,11; 2018,Jan,8; 2017,Jan,8; 2016,Jan,13; 2015,Jan,16

90284 Immune globulin (SCIg), human, for use in subcutaneous infusions, 100 mg, each
0.00 0.00 FUD XXX
AMA: 2020,Jan,11; 2018,Jan,8; 2017,Jan,8; 2016,Jan,13; 2015,Jan,16

90287 Botulinum antitoxin, equine, any route
0.00 0.00 FUD XXX
AMA: 2020,Jan,11; 2018,Jan,8; 2017,Jan,8; 2016,Jan,13; 2015,Jan,16

90288 Botulism immune globulin, human, for intravenous use
0.00 0.00 FUD XXX
AMA: 2020,Jan,11; 2018,Jan,8; 2017,Jan,8; 2016,Jan,13; 2015,Jan,16

90291 Cytomegalovirus immune globulin (CMV-IgIV), human, for intravenous use
INCLUDES Cytogram
0.00 0.00 FUD XXX
AMA: 2020,Jan,11; 2018,Jan,8; 2017,Jan,8; 2016,Jan,13; 2015,Jan,16

90296 Diphtheria antitoxin, equine, any route
0.00 0.00 FUD XXX
AMA: 2020,Jan,11; 2018,Jan,8; 2017,Jan,8; 2016,Jan,13; 2015,Jan,16

90371 Hepatitis B immune globulin (HBIg), human, for intramuscular use
INCLUDES HBIG
0.00 0.00 FUD XXX
AMA: 2020,Jan,11; 2018,Jan,8; 2017,Jan,8; 2016,Jan,13; 2015,Jan,16

90375 Rabies immune globulin (RIg), human, for intramuscular and/or subcutaneous use
INCLUDES HyperRAB
0.00 0.00 FUD XXX
AMA: 2020,Jan,11; 2018,Jan,8; 2017,Jan,8; 2016,Jan,13; 2015,Jan,16

90376 Rabies immune globulin, heat-treated (RIg-HT), human, for intramuscular and/or subcutaneous use
0.00 0.00 FUD XXX
AMA: 2020,Jan,11; 2018,Jan,8; 2017,Jan,8; 2016,Jan,13; 2015,Jan,16

● **90377 Rabies immune globulin, heat- and solvent/detergent-treated (RIg-HT S/D), human, for intramuscular and/or subcutaneous use**
0.00 0.00 FUD 000

90378 Respiratory syncytial virus, monoclonal antibody, recombinant, for intramuscular use, 50 mg, each
INCLUDES Synagis
0.00 0.00 FUD XXX
AMA: 2020,Jan,11; 2018,Jan,8; 2017,Jan,8; 2016,Jan,13; 2015,Jan,16

90384 Rho(D) immune globulin (RhIg), human, full-dose, for intramuscular use
0.00 0.00 FUD XXX
AMA: 2020,Jan,11; 2018,Jan,8; 2017,Jan,8; 2016,Jan,13; 2015,Jan,16

90385 Rho(D) immune globulin (RhIg), human, mini-dose, for intramuscular use
0.00 0.00 FUD XXX
AMA: 2020,Jan,11; 2018,Jan,8; 2017,Jan,8; 2016,Jan,13; 2015,Jan,16

90386 Rho(D) immune globulin (RhIgIV), human, for intravenous use
0.00 0.00 FUD XXX
AMA: 2020,Jan,11; 2018,Jan,8; 2017,Jan,8; 2016,Jan,13; 2015,Jan,16

90389 Tetanus immune globulin (TIg), human, for intramuscular use
INCLUDES HyperTET S/D (Tetanus Immune Globulin)
0.00 0.00 FUD XXX
AMA: 2020,Jan,11; 2018,Jan,8; 2017,Jan,8; 2016,Jan,13; 2015,Jan,16

90393 Vaccinia immune globulin, human, for intramuscular use
0.00 0.00 FUD XXX
AMA: 2020,Jan,11; 2018,Jan,8; 2017,Jan,8; 2016,Jan,13; 2015,Jan,16

90396 Varicella-zoster immune globulin, human, for intramuscular use
INCLUDES VariZIG
0.00 0.00 FUD XXX
AMA: 2020,Jan,11; 2018,Jan,8; 2017,Jan,8; 2016,Jan,13; 2015,Jan,16

90399 Unlisted immune globulin
0.00 0.00 FUD XXX
AMA: 2020,Jan,11; 2018,Jan,8; 2017,Jan,8; 2016,Jan,13; 2015,Jan,16

90460-90461 Injections Provided with Counseling

INCLUDES All components influenza vaccine, report one time only
Combination vaccines which comprise multiple vaccine components
Components (all antigens) in vaccines to prevent disease due to specific organisms
Counseling by physician or other qualified health care professional
Multivalent antigens or multiple antigen serotypes against single organisms considered one component
Patient/family face-to-face counseling by doctor or qualified health care professional for patients age 18 years and younger

EXCLUDES *Administration influenza and pneumococcal vaccine for Medicare patients (G0008-G0009)*
Allergy testing (95004-95028)
Bacterial/viral/fungal skin tests (86485-86580)
Diagnostic or therapeutic injections (96365-96371, 96372-96379)
Vaccines provided without face-to-face counseling from physician or qualified health care professional or to patients age 18 years and older (90471-90474)

Code also significant, separately identifiable E/M service when appropriate
Code also toxoid/vaccine (90476-90749 [90620, 90621, 90625, 90630, 90644, 90672, 90673, 90674, 90750, 90756])

90460 Immunization administration through 18 years of age via any route of administration, with counseling by physician or other qualified health care professional; first or only component of each vaccine or toxoid administered
Code also each additional component in vaccine (e.g., 5-year-old receives DtaP-IPV IM administration, and MMR/Varicella vaccines SQ administration. Report initial component two times, and additional components six times)
0.47 0.47 FUD XXX
AMA: 2020,Jul,11; 2020,Jan,11; 2018,Nov,7; 2018,Jan,8; 2017,Jan,8; 2016,Oct,6; 2016,Jan,13; 2015,May,6; 2015,Apr,10; 2015,Apr,9; 2015,Jan,16

\+ **90461** **each additional vaccine or toxoid component administered (List separately in addition to code for primary procedure)** A

Code also each additional component in vaccine (e.g., 5-year-old receives DtaP-IPV IM administration, and MMR/Varicella vaccines SQ administration. Report initial component two times, and additional components six times)

Code first initial component in each vaccine provided (90460)

0.36 0.36 FUD ZZZ B 80

AMA: 2020,Jul,11; 2020,Jan,11; 2018,Nov,7; 2018,Jan,8; 2017,Jan,8; 2016,Oct,6; 2016,Jan,13; 2015,May,6; 2015,Apr,10; 2015,Jan,16

90471-90474 Injections and Other Routes of Administration Without Physician Counseling

CMS: 100-04,18,10.4 CWF Edits for Influenza Virus and Pneumococcal Vaccinations

EXCLUDES *Administration influenza and pneumococcal vaccine for Medicare patients (G0008-G0009)*
Administration vaccine with counseling (90460-90461)
Allergy testing (95004-95028)
Bacterial/viral/fungal skin tests (86485-86580)
Diagnostic or therapeutic injections (96365-96371, 96374)
Patient/family face-to-face counseling

Code also significant separately identifiable E/M service when appropriate

Code also toxoid/vaccine (90476-90749 [90620, 90621, 90625, 90630, 90644, 90672, 90673, 90674, 90750, 90756])

90471 **Immunization administration (includes percutaneous, intradermal, subcutaneous, or intramuscular injections); 1 vaccine (single or combination vaccine/toxoid)**

EXCLUDES *Intranasal/oral administration (90473)*

0.40 0.40 FUD XXX Q1 80

AMA: 2020,Jul,11; 2020,Jan,11; 2019,Jun,11; 2018,Nov,7; 2018,Jan,8; 2017,Jan,8; 2016,Oct,6; 2016,Jan,13; 2015,May,6; 2015,Apr,9; 2015,Apr,10; 2015,Jan,16

\+ **90472** **each additional vaccine (single or combination vaccine/toxoid) (List separately in addition to code for primary procedure)**

EXCLUDES *BCG vaccine, intravesical administration (51720, 90586)*
Immune globulin administration (96365-96371, 96374)
Immune globulin product (90281-90399)

Code first initial vaccine (90460, 90471, 90473)

0.36 0.36 FUD ZZZ N 80

AMA: 2020,Jul,11; 2020,Jan,11; 2018,Nov,7; 2018,Jan,8; 2017,Jan,8; 2016,Oct,6; 2016,Jan,13; 2015,May,6; 2015,Apr,9; 2015,Apr,10; 2015,Jan,16

90473 **Immunization administration by intranasal or oral route; 1 vaccine (single or combination vaccine/toxoid)**

EXCLUDES *Administration by injection (90471)*

0.47 0.47 FUD XXX Q1 80

AMA: 2020,Jan,11; 2018,Nov,7; 2018,Jan,8; 2017,Jan,8; 2016,Jan,13; 2015,May,6; 2015,Jan,16

\+ **90474** **each additional vaccine (single or combination vaccine/toxoid) (List separately in addition to code for primary procedure)**

Code first initial vaccine (90460, 90471, 90473)

0.36 0.36 FUD ZZZ N 80

AMA: 2018,Nov,7; 2018,Jan,8; 2017,Jan,8; 2016,Jan,13; 2015,May,6; 2015,Apr,9; 2015,Jan,16

90476-90756 [90619, 90620, 90621, 90625, 90630, 90644, 90672, 90673, 90674, 90694, 90750, 90756] Vaccination Products

INCLUDES Patient's age for reporting purposes, not for product license
Vaccine product only

EXCLUDES *Immune globulins and administration (90281-90399, 96365-96375)*
Reporting each combination vaccine component individually

Code also administration vaccine (90460-90474)

Code also significant separately identifiable E/M service when appropriate

90476 **Adenovirus vaccine, type 4, live, for oral use**

INCLUDES Adeno-4

0.00 0.00 FUD XXX 51 N N1

AMA: 2018,Jan,8; 2017,Jan,8; 2016,Jan,13; 2015,May,6; 2015,Jan,16

90477 **Adenovirus vaccine, type 7, live, for oral use**

INCLUDES Adeno-7

0.00 0.00 FUD XXX 51 M

AMA: 2018,Jan,8; 2017,Jan,8; 2016,Jan,13; 2015,May,6; 2015,Jan,16

90581 **Anthrax vaccine, for subcutaneous or intramuscular use**

INCLUDES BioThrax

0.00 0.00 FUD XXX 51 E

AMA: 2018,Jan,8; 2017,Jan,8; 2016,Jan,13; 2015,May,6; 2015,Jan,16

90585 **Bacillus Calmette-Guerin vaccine (BCG) for tuberculosis, live, for percutaneous use**

INCLUDES Mycobax

0.00 0.00 FUD XXX 51 M

AMA: 2018,Jan,8; 2017,Jan,8; 2016,Jan,13; 2015,May,6; 2015,Jan,16

90586 **Bacillus Calmette-Guerin vaccine (BCG) for bladder cancer, live, for intravesical use**

INCLUDES TheraCys
TICE BCG

0.00 0.00 FUD XXX 51 B

AMA: 2020,Jan,11; 2018,Jan,8; 2017,Jan,8; 2016,Jan,13; 2015,May,6; 2015,Jan,16

90587 **Dengue vaccine, quadrivalent, live, 3 dose schedule, for subcutaneous use**

0.00 0.00 FUD XXX 51 E

AMA: 2018,Nov,7; 2018,Jan,8

90619 **Resequenced code. See code following 90734.**

90620 **Resequenced code. See code following 90734.**

90621 **Resequenced code. See code following 90734.**

90625 **Resequenced code. See code following 90723.**

90630 **Resequenced code. See code following 90654.**

90632 **Hepatitis A vaccine (HepA), adult dosage, for intramuscular use** A

INCLUDES Havrix
Vaqta

0.00 0.00 FUD XXX 51 N N1

AMA: 2018,Jan,8; 2017,Jan,8; 2016,Jan,13; 2015,May,6; 2015,Jan,16

90633 **Hepatitis A vaccine (HepA), pediatric/adolescent dosage-2 dose schedule, for intramuscular use** A

INCLUDES Havrix
Vaqta

0.00 0.00 FUD XXX 51 N N1

AMA: 2018,Jan,8; 2017,Jan,8; 2016,Jan,13; 2015,May,6; 2015,Jan,16

90634 **Hepatitis A vaccine (HepA), pediatric/adolescent dosage-3 dose schedule, for intramuscular use** A

INCLUDES Havrix

0.00 0.00 FUD XXX 51 N N1

AMA: 2018,Jan,8; 2017,Jan,8; 2016,Jan,13; 2015,May,6; 2015,Jan,16

90636 **Hepatitis A and hepatitis B vaccine (HepA-HepB), adult dosage, for intramuscular use** A

INCLUDES Twinrix

0.00 0.00 FUD XXX 51 N N1

AMA: 2018,Jan,8; 2017,Jan,8; 2016,Jan,13; 2015,May,6; 2015,Jan,16

90644 **Resequenced code. See code following 90732.**

90647 **Haemophilus influenzae type b vaccine (Hib), PRP-OMP conjugate, 3 dose schedule, for intramuscular use**

INCLUDES PedvaxHIB

0.00 0.00 FUD XXX 51 N N1

AMA: 2018,Jan,8; 2017,Jan,8; 2016,Jan,13; 2015,May,6; 2015,Jan,16

90648 Haemophilus influenzae type b vaccine (Hib), PRP-T conjugate, 4 dose schedule, for intramuscular use

INCLUDES ActHIB
Hiberix
OmniHIB

0.00 0.00 FUD XXX

AMA: 2018,Jan,8; 2017,Jan,8; 2016,Jan,13; 2015,May,6; 2015,Jan,16

90649 Human Papillomavirus vaccine, types 6, 11, 16, 18, quadrivalent (4vHPV), 3 dose schedule, for intramuscular use

INCLUDES Gardasil

0.00 0.00 FUD XXX

AMA: 2018,Jan,8; 2017,Jan,8; 2016,Jan,13; 2015,May,6; 2015,Jan,16

90650 Human Papillomavirus vaccine, types 16, 18, bivalent (2vHPV), 3 dose schedule, for intramuscular use

INCLUDES Cervarix

0.00 0.00 FUD XXX

AMA: 2018,Jan,8; 2017,Jan,8; 2016,Jan,13; 2015,May,6; 2015,Jan,16

90651 Human Papillomavirus vaccine types 6, 11, 16, 18, 31, 33, 45, 52, 58, nonavalent (9vHPV), 2 or 3 dose schedule, for intramuscular use

INCLUDES GARDASIL 9

0.00 0.00 FUD XXX

AMA: 2018,Nov,7; 2018,Jan,8; 2017,Jan,8; 2016,Jan,13; 2015,May,6; 2015,Jan,16

90653 Influenza vaccine, inactivated (IIV), subunit, adjuvanted, for intramuscular use

INCLUDES Fluad

0.00 0.00 FUD XXX

AMA: 2019,Jun,11; 2018,Jan,8; 2017,Jan,8; 2016,Oct,6; 2016,Jan,13; 2015,May,6; 2015,Jan,16

90654 Influenza virus vaccine, trivalent (IIV3), split virus, preservative-free, for intradermal use

INCLUDES Fluzone intradermal

0.00 0.00 FUD XXX

AMA: 2018,Jan,8; 2017,Jan,8; 2016,Jan,13; 2015,May,6; 2015,Apr,9; 2015,Jan,16

\# **90630 Influenza virus vaccine, quadrivalent (IIV4), split virus, preservative free, for intradermal use**

INCLUDES Fluzone Intradermal Quadrivalent

0.00 0.00 FUD XXX

AMA: 2018,Jan,8; 2017,Jan,8; 2016,Jan,13; 2015,May,6; 2015,Jan,16

90655 Influenza virus vaccine, trivalent (IIV3), split virus, preservative free, 0.25 mL dosage, for intramuscular use

INCLUDES Afluria
Fluzone, no preservative, pediatric dose

0.00 0.00 FUD XXX

AMA: 2018,Jan,8; 2017,Jan,8; 2016,Oct,6; 2016,May,9; 2016,Jan,13; 2015,May,6; 2015,Jan,16

90656 Influenza virus vaccine, trivalent (IIV3), split virus, preservative free, 0.5 mL dosage, for intramuscular use

INCLUDES Afluria

0.00 0.00 FUD XXX

AMA: 2018,Jan,8; 2017,Jan,8; 2016,Oct,6; 2016,May,9; 2016,Jan,13; 2015,May,6; 2015,Jan,16

90657 Influenza virus vaccine, trivalent (IIV3), split virus, 0.25 mL dosage, for intramuscular use

INCLUDES Afluria
Flulaval
Fluvirin
Fluzone (5 ml vial [0.25ml dose])

0.00 0.00 FUD XXX

AMA: 2018,Jan,8; 2017,Jan,8; 2016,Oct,6; 2016,May,9; 2016,Jan,13; 2015,May,6; 2015,Jan,16

90658 Influenza virus vaccine, trivalent (IIV3), split virus, 0.5 mL dosage, for intramuscular use

INCLUDES Afluria
Flulaval
Fluvirin
Fluzone

0.00 0.00 FUD XXX

AMA: 2018,Jan,8; 2017,Jan,8; 2016,Oct,6; 2016,May,9; 2016,Jan,13; 2015,May,6; 2015,Jan,16

90660 Influenza virus vaccine, trivalent, live (LAIV3), for intranasal use

INCLUDES FluMist

0.00 0.00 FUD XXX

AMA: 2018,Jan,8; 2017,Jan,8; 2016,Jan,13; 2015,May,6; 2015,Jan,16

\# **90672 Influenza virus vaccine, quadrivalent, live (LAIV4), for intranasal use**

INCLUDES FluMist Quadrivalent

0.00 0.00 FUD XXX

AMA: 2018,Jan,8; 2017,Jan,8; 2016,Jan,13; 2015,May,6; 2015,Jan,16

90661 Influenza virus vaccine (ccIIV3), derived from cell cultures, subunit, preservative and antibiotic free, for intramuscular use

INCLUDES Flucelvax

0.00 0.00 FUD XXX

AMA: 2018,Jan,8; 2017,Jan,8; 2016,Oct,6; 2016,Jan,13; 2015,May,6; 2015,Jan,16

\# **90674 Influenza virus vaccine, quadrivalent (ccIIV4), derived from cell cultures, subunit, preservative and antibiotic free, 0.5 mL dosage, for intramuscular use**

INCLUDES Flucelvax Quadrivalent

0.00 0.00 FUD XXX

AMA: 2018,Jan,8; 2017,Jan,8; 2016,Oct,6

\# **90756 Influenza virus vaccine, quadrivalent (ccIIV4), derived from cell cultures, subunit, antibiotic free, 0.5mL dosage, for intramuscular use**

INCLUDES Flucelvax Quadrivalent

0.00 0.00 FUD XXX

AMA: 2018,Nov,7

\# **90673 Influenza virus vaccine, trivalent (RIV3), derived from recombinant DNA, hemagglutinin (HA) protein only, preservative and antibiotic free, for intramuscular use**

0.00 0.00 FUD XXX

AMA: 2018,Jan,8; 2017,Jan,8; 2016,Jan,13; 2015,May,6; 2015,Jan,16

90662 Influenza virus vaccine (IIV), split virus, preservative free, enhanced immunogenicity via increased antigen content, for intramuscular use

INCLUDES Fluzone high-dose Quadribalent

0.00 0.00 FUD XXX

AMA: 2018,Jan,8; 2017,Jan,8; 2016,Jan,13; 2015,May,6; 2015,Jan,16

90664 Influenza virus vaccine, live (LAIV), pandemic formulation, for intranasal use

0.00 0.00 FUD XXX

AMA: 2018,Jan,8; 2017,Jan,8; 2016,Jan,13; 2015,May,6; 2015,Jan,16

90666 Influenza virus vaccine (IIV), pandemic formulation, split virus, preservative free, for intramuscular use
0.00 0.00 FUD XXX
AMA: 2018,Jan,8; 2017,Jan,8; 2016,Jan,13; 2015,May,6; 2015,Jan,16

90667 Influenza virus vaccine (IIV), pandemic formulation, split virus, adjuvanted, for intramuscular use
0.00 0.00 FUD XXX
AMA: 2018,Jan,8; 2017,Jan,8; 2016,Jan,13; 2015,May,6; 2015,Jan,16

90668 Influenza virus vaccine (IIV), pandemic formulation, split virus, for intramuscular use
0.00 0.00 FUD XXX
AMA: 2018,Jan,8; 2017,Jan,8; 2016,Jan,13; 2015,May,6; 2015,Jan,16

90670 Pneumococcal conjugate vaccine, 13 valent (PCV13), for intramuscular use
INCLUDES Prevnar 13
0.00 0.00 FUD XXX
AMA: 2018,Jan,8; 2017,Jan,8; 2016,Jan,13; 2015,May,6; 2015,Jan,16

90672 **Resequenced code. See code following 90660.**

90673 **Resequenced code. See code before 90662.**

90674 **Resequenced code. See code following 90661.**

90675 Rabies vaccine, for intramuscular use
INCLUDES Imovax
RabAvert
0.00 0.00 FUD XXX
AMA: 2018,Jan,8; 2017,Jan,8; 2016,Jan,13; 2015,May,6; 2015,Jan,16

90676 Rabies vaccine, for intradermal use
0.00 0.00 FUD XXX
AMA: 2018,Jan,8; 2017,Jan,8; 2016,Jan,13; 2015,May,6; 2015,Jan,16

90680 Rotavirus vaccine, pentavalent (RV5), 3 dose schedule, live, for oral use
INCLUDES RotaTeq
0.00 0.00 FUD XXX
AMA: 2018,Jan,8; 2017,Jan,8; 2016,Jan,13; 2015,May,6; 2015,Jan,16

90681 Rotavirus vaccine, human, attenuated (RV1), 2 dose schedule, live, for oral use
INCLUDES Rotarix
0.00 0.00 FUD XXX
AMA: 2018,Jan,8; 2017,Jan,8; 2016,Jan,13; 2015,May,6; 2015,Jan,16

90682 Influenza virus vaccine, quadrivalent (RIV4), derived from recombinant DNA, hemagglutinin (HA) protein only, preservative and antibiotic free, for intramuscular use
INCLUDES Flublok Quadrivalent
0.00 0.00 FUD XXX
AMA: 2018,Nov,7; 2018,Jan,8; 2017,Jan,8

90685 Influenza virus vaccine, quadrivalent (IIV4), split virus, preservative free, 0.25 mL, for intramuscular use A
INCLUDES Afluria Quadrivalent
Fluzone Quadrivalent
0.00 0.00 FUD XXX
AMA: 2018,Jan,8; 2017,Jan,8; 2016,Oct,6; 2016,May,9; 2016,Jan,13; 2015,May,6; 2015,Jan,16

90686 Influenza virus vaccine, quadrivalent (IIV4), split virus, preservative free, 0.5 mL dosage, for intramuscular use A
INCLUDES Afluria Quadrivalent
Fluarix Quadrivalent
FluLaval Quadrivalent
Fluzone Quadrivalent
0.00 0.00 FUD XXX
AMA: 2018,Jan,8; 2017,Jan,8; 2016,Oct,6; 2016,May,9; 2016,Jan,13; 2015,May,6; 2015,Jan,16

90687 Influenza virus vaccine, quadrivalent (IIV4), split virus, 0.25 mL dosage, for intramuscular use A
INCLUDES Afluria Quadrivalent
Fluzone Quadrivalent
0.00 0.00 FUD XXX
AMA: 2018,Jan,8; 2017,Jan,8; 2016,Oct,6; 2016,May,9; 2016,Jan,13; 2015,May,6; 2015,Jan,16

90688 Influenza virus vaccine, quadrivalent (IIV4), split virus, 0.5 mL dosage, for intramuscular use A
INCLUDES Afluria Quadrivalent
Flulaval Quadrivalent
Fluzone Quadrivalent
0.00 0.00 FUD XXX
AMA: 2020,Jul,11; 2018,Jan,8; 2017,Jan,8; 2016,Oct,6; 2016,May,9; 2016,Jan,13; 2015,May,6; 2015,Jan,16

90689 Influenza virus vaccine quadrivalent (IIV4), inactivated, adjuvanted, preservative free, 0.25 mL dosage, for intramuscular use
0.00 0.00 FUD XXX
AMA: 2020,Jul,11; 2019,Jul,10; 2018,Nov,7

90694 Influenza virus vaccine, quadrivalent (aIIV4), inactivated, adjuvanted, preservative free, 0.5 mL dosage, for intramuscular use
INCLUDES Fluad Quadrivalent
0.00 0.00 FUD XXX
AMA: 2020,Jul,11

90690 Typhoid vaccine, live, oral
INCLUDES Vivotif
0.00 0.00 FUD XXX
AMA: 2020,Jul,11; 2018,Jan,8; 2017,Jan,8; 2016,Jan,13; 2015,May,6; 2015,Jan,16

90691 Typhoid vaccine, Vi capsular polysaccharide (ViCPs), for intramuscular use
INCLUDES Typhim Vi
0.00 0.00 FUD XXX
AMA: 2020,Jul,11; 2018,Jan,8; 2017,Jan,8; 2016,Jan,13; 2015,May,6; 2015,Jan,16

90694 **Resequenced code. See code following 90689.**

90696 Diphtheria, tetanus toxoids, acellular pertussis vaccine and inactivated poliovirus vaccine (DTaP-IPV), when administered to children 4 through 6 years of age, for intramuscular use A
INCLUDES KINRIX
Quadracel
0.00 0.00 FUD XXX
AMA: 2018,Jan,8; 2017,Jan,8; 2016,Jan,13; 2015,May,6; 2015,Jan,16

90697 Diphtheria, tetanus toxoids, acellular pertussis vaccine, inactivated poliovirus vaccine, Haemophilus influenzae type b PRP-OMP conjugate vaccine, and hepatitis B vaccine (DTaP-IPV-Hib-HepB), for intramuscular use
0.00 0.00 FUD XXX
AMA: 2018,Jan,8; 2017,Jan,8; 2016,Jan,13; 2015,May,6; 2015,Jan,16

90698 Diphtheria, tetanus toxoids, acellular pertussis vaccine, Haemophilus influenzae type b, and inactivated poliovirus vaccine, (DTaP-IPV/Hib), for intramuscular use
INCLUDES Pentacel
0.00 0.00 FUD XXX
AMA: 2018,Jan,8; 2017,Jan,8; 2016,Jan,13; 2015,May,6; 2015,Jan,16

90700 Diphtheria, tetanus toxoids, and acellular pertussis vaccine (DTaP), when administered to individuals younger than 7 years, for intramuscular use
INCLUDES Daptacel
Infanrix
0.00 0.00 FUD XXX
AMA: 2018,Jan,8; 2017,Jan,8; 2016,Jan,13; 2015,May,6; 2015,Jan,16

90702 Diphtheria and tetanus toxoids adsorbed (DT) when administered to individuals younger than 7 years, for intramuscular use
INCLUDES Diphtheria and Tetanus Toxoids Adsorbed USP (For Pediatric Use)
0.00 0.00 FUD XXX
AMA: 2018,Jan,8; 2017,Jan,8; 2016,Jan,13; 2015,May,6; 2015,Jan,16

90707 Measles, mumps and rubella virus vaccine (MMR), live, for subcutaneous use
INCLUDES M-M-R II
0.00 0.00 FUD XXX
AMA: 2018,Jan,8; 2017,Jan,8; 2016,Jan,13; 2015,May,6; 2015,Jan,16

90710 Measles, mumps, rubella, and varicella vaccine (MMRV), live, for subcutaneous use
INCLUDES ProQuad
0.00 0.00 FUD XXX
AMA: 2018,Jan,8; 2017,Jan,8; 2016,Jan,13; 2015,May,6; 2015,Jan,16

90713 Poliovirus vaccine, inactivated (IPV), for subcutaneous or intramuscular use
INCLUDES IPOL
0.00 0.00 FUD XXX
AMA: 2018,Jan,8; 2017,Jan,8; 2016,Jan,13; 2015,May,6; 2015,Jan,16

90714 Tetanus and diphtheria toxoids adsorbed (Td), preservative free, when administered to individuals 7 years or older, for intramuscular use
INCLUDES Tenivac
Tetanus-diphtheria toxoids absorbed
0.00 0.00 FUD XXX
AMA: 2018,Jan,8; 2017,Jan,8; 2016,Jan,13; 2015,May,6; 2015,Jan,16

90715 Tetanus, diphtheria toxoids and acellular pertussis vaccine (Tdap), when administered to individuals 7 years or older, for intramuscular use
INCLUDES Adacel
Boostrix
0.00 0.00 FUD XXX
AMA: 2018,Jan,8; 2017,Jan,8; 2016,Jan,13; 2015,May,6; 2015,Jan,16

90716 Varicella virus vaccine (VAR), live, for subcutaneous use
INCLUDES Varivax
0.00 0.00 FUD XXX
AMA: 2018,Jan,8; 2017,Jan,8; 2016,Jan,13; 2015,May,6; 2015,Mar,3; 2015,Jan,16

90717 Yellow fever vaccine, live, for subcutaneous use
INCLUDES YF-VAX
0.00 0.00 FUD XXX
AMA: 2018,Jan,8; 2017,Jan,8; 2016,Jan,13; 2015,May,6; 2015,Jan,16

90723 Diphtheria, tetanus toxoids, acellular pertussis vaccine, hepatitis B, and inactivated poliovirus vaccine (DTaP-HepB-IPV), for intramuscular use
INCLUDES PEDIARIX
0.00 0.00 FUD XXX
AMA: 2018,Jan,8; 2017,Jan,8; 2016,Jan,13; 2015,May,6; 2015,Jan,16

90625 Cholera vaccine, live, adult dosage, 1 dose schedule, for oral use
0.00 0.00 FUD XXX
AMA: 2018,Jan,8; 2017,Jan,8; 2016,Oct,6; 2016,Jan,13

90732 Pneumococcal polysaccharide vaccine, 23-valent (PPSV23), adult or immunosuppressed patient dosage, when administered to individuals 2 years or older, for subcutaneous or intramuscular use
INCLUDES Pneumovax 23
0.00 0.00 FUD XXX
AMA: 2018,Jan,8; 2017,Jan,8; 2016,Jan,13; 2015,May,6; 2015,Jan,16

90644 Meningococcal conjugate vaccine, serogroups C & Y and Haemophilus influenzae type b vaccine (Hib-MenCY), 4 dose schedule, when administered to children 6 weeks-18 months of age, for intramuscular use
INCLUDES MenHibrix
0.00 0.00 FUD XXX
AMA: 2018,Jan,8; 2017,Jan,8; 2016,Jan,13; 2015,May,6; 2015,Jan,16

90733 Meningococcal polysaccharide vaccine, serogroups A, C, Y, W-135, quadrivalent (MPSV4), for subcutaneous use
INCLUDES Menomune-A/C/Y/W-135
0.00 0.00 FUD XXX
AMA: 2018,Jan,8; 2017,Jan,8; 2016,Jan,13; 2015,May,6; 2015,Jan,16

90734 Meningococcal conjugate vaccine, serogroups A, C, W, Y, quadrivalent, diphtheria toxoid carrier (MenACWY-D) or CRM197 carrier (MenACWY-CRM), for intramuscular use
INCLUDES Menactra
Menveo
0.00 0.00 FUD XXX
AMA: 2020,Jan,11; 2018,Jan,8; 2017,Jan,8; 2016,Oct,6; 2016,Jan,13; 2015,May,6; 2015,Jan,16

90619 Meningococcal conjugate vaccine, serogroups A, C, W, Y, quadrivalent, tetanus toxoid carrier (MenACWY-TT), for intramuscular use
0.00 0.00 FUD XXX
AMA: 2020,Jan,11

90620 Meningococcal recombinant protein and outer membrane vesicle vaccine, serogroup B (MenB-4C), 2 dose schedule, for intramuscular use
INCLUDES Bexsero
0.00 0.00 FUD XXX
AMA: 2018,Nov,7; 2018,Jan,8; 2017,Jan,8; 2016,Jan,13; 2015,May,6; 2015,Jan,16

90621 Meningococcal recombinant lipoprotein vaccine, serogroup B (MenB-FHbp), 2 or 3 dose schedule, for intramuscular use
INCLUDES Trumenba
0.00 0.00 FUD XXX
AMA: 2018,Nov,7; 2018,Jan,8; 2017,Jan,8; 2016,Jan,13; 2015,May,6; 2015,Jan,16

90736 Zoster (shingles) vaccine (HZV), live, for subcutaneous injection
INCLUDES Zostavax
0.00 0.00 FUD XXX
AMA: 2018,Nov,7; 2018,Jan,8; 2017,Jan,8; 2016,Jan,13; 2015,May,6; 2015,Jan,16

90750 **Zoster (shingles) vaccine (HZV), recombinant, subunit, adjuvanted, for intramuscular use**

0.00 0.00 FUD XXX

AMA: 2018,Nov,7

90738 **Japanese encephalitis virus vaccine, inactivated, for intramuscular use**

INCLUDES Ixiaro

0.00 0.00 FUD XXX

AMA: 2018,Jan,8; 2017,Jan,8; 2016,Jan,13; 2015,May,6; 2015,Jan,16

90739 **Hepatitis B vaccine (HepB), adult dosage, 2 dose schedule, for intramuscular use**

0.00 0.00 FUD XXX

AMA: 2018,Nov,7; 2018,Jan,8; 2017,Jan,8; 2016,Jan,13; 2015,May,6; 2015,Jan,16

90740 **Hepatitis B vaccine (HepB), dialysis or immunosuppressed patient dosage, 3 dose schedule, for intramuscular use**

INCLUDES Recombivax HB

0.00 0.00 FUD XXX

AMA: 2018,Jan,8; 2017,Jan,8; 2016,Jan,13; 2015,May,6; 2015,Jan,16

90743 **Hepatitis B vaccine (HepB), adolescent, 2 dose schedule, for intramuscular use**

INCLUDES Energix-B
Recombivax HB

0.00 0.00 FUD XXX

AMA: 2018,Jan,8; 2017,Jan,8; 2016,Jan,13; 2015,May,6; 2015,Jan,16

90744 **Hepatitis B vaccine (HepB), pediatric/adolescent dosage, 3 dose schedule, for intramuscular use**

INCLUDES Energix-B
Flucelvax Quadrivalent
Recombivax HB

0.00 0.00 FUD XXX

AMA: 2018,Jan,8; 2017,Jan,8; 2016,Jan,13; 2015,May,6; 2015,Jan,16

90746 **Hepatitis B vaccine (HepB), adult dosage, 3 dose schedule, for intramuscular use**

INCLUDES Energix-B
Recombivax HB

0.00 0.00 FUD XXX

AMA: 2018,Jan,8; 2017,Jan,8; 2016,Jan,13; 2015,May,6; 2015,Jan,16

90747 **Hepatitis B vaccine (HepB), dialysis or immunosuppressed patient dosage, 4 dose schedule, for intramuscular use**

INCLUDES Energix-B
RECOMBIVAX dialysis

0.00 0.00 FUD XXX

AMA: 2018,Jan,8; 2017,Jan,8; 2016,Jan,13; 2015,May,6; 2015,Jan,16

90748 **Hepatitis B and Haemophilus influenzae type b vaccine (Hib-HepB), for intramuscular use**

INCLUDES COMVAX

0.00 0.00 FUD XXX

AMA: 2018,Jan,8; 2017,Jan,8; 2016,Jan,13; 2015,May,6; 2015,Jan,16

90749 **Unlisted vaccine/toxoid**

0.00 0.00 FUD XXX

AMA: 2018,Jan,8; 2017,Jan,8; 2016,Jan,13; 2015,May,6; 2015,Jan,16

90750 **Resequenced code. See code following 90736.**

90756 **Resequenced code. See code following 90661.**

90785 Complex Interactive Encounter

CMS: 100-02,15,160 Clinical Psychologist Services; 100-02,15,170 Clinical Social Worker (CSW) Services; 100-03,10.3 Inpatient Pain Rehabilitation Programs; 100-03,10.4 Outpatient Hospital Pain Rehabilitation Programs; 100-03,130.1 Inpatient Stays for Alcoholism Treatment; 100-04,12,100 Teaching Physician Services; 100-04,4,260.1 Special Partial Hospitalization Billing Requirements forHospitals, Community Mental Health Centers, and Critical Access Hospitals; 100-04,4,260.1.1 Bill Review for Partial Hospitalization Services Provided in Community Mental Health Centers (CMHC)

INCLUDES Complicated communication issues affecting psychiatric service
Involved communication with:
- Emotionally charged or dissonant family members
- Patients wanting others present during visit (e.g., family member, translator)
- Patients with impaired or undeveloped verbal skills
- Patients with third parties responsible for their care (e.g., parents, guardians)
- Third-party involvement (e.g., schools, probation and parole officers, child protective agencies)

One or more following activity:
- Discussion sentinel event demanding third-party involvement (i.e., abuse or neglect reported to state agency)
- Interference by caregiver's behavior or emotional state to understand and assist in treatment plan
- Managing discordant communication complicating care among participating members (e.g., arguing, reactivity)
- Nonverbal communication methods (e.g., toys, other devices, or translator) to eliminate communication barriers

EXCLUDES *Adaptive behavior assessment/treatment ([97151, 97152, 97153, 97154, 97155, 97156, 97157, 97158], 0362T, 0373T)*
Crisis psychotherapy (90839-90840)

\+ **90785** **Interactive complexity (List separately in addition to the code for primary procedure)**

Code first, when performed (99202-99255 [99224, 99225, 99226], 99304-99337, 99341-99350, 90791-90792, 90832-90834, 90836-90838, 90853)

0.39 0.42 FUD ZZZ

AMA: 2020,Aug,3; 2018,Nov,3; 2018,Jul,12; 2018,Apr,9; 2018,Jan,8; 2017,Jan,8; 2016,Dec,11; 2016,Jan,13; 2015,Jan,16

90791-90792 Psychiatric Evaluations

CMS: 100-02,15,170 Clinical Social Worker (CSW) Services; 100-03,10.3 Inpatient Pain Rehabilitation Programs; 100-03,130.1 Inpatient Stays for Alcoholism Treatment; 100-03,130.2 Outpatient Hospital Services for Alcoholism; 100-04,12,100 Teaching Physician Services; 100-04,12,190.3 List of Telehealth Services; 100-04,12,190.6 Payment Methodology for Physician/Practitioner at the Distant Site ; 100-04,12,190.6.1 Submission of Telehealth Claims for Distant Site Practitioners; 100-04,12,190.7 Contractor Editing of Telehealth Claims; 100-04,4,260.1 Special Partial Hospitalization Billing Requirements forHospitals, Community Mental Health Centers, and Critical Access Hospitals; 100-04,4,260.1.1 Bill Review for Partial Hospitalization Services Provided in Community Mental Health Centers (CMHC)

INCLUDES Diagnostic assessment or reassessment without psychotherapy services

EXCLUDES *Adaptive behavior assessment/treatment ([97151, 97152, 97153, 97154, 97155, 97156, 97157, 97158], 0362T, 0373T)*
Crisis psychotherapy (90839-90840)
E/M services (99202-99337 [99224, 99225, 99226], 99341-99350, 99366-99368, 99401-99443 [99415, 99416, 99417, 99421, 99422, 99423, 99439])

Code also interactive complexity services when applicable (90785)

90791 **Psychiatric diagnostic evaluation**

3.54 3.89 FUD XXX ★ 03

AMA: 2020,Aug,3; 2018,Nov,3; 2018,Jul,12; 2018,Apr,9; 2018,Jan,8; 2017,Nov,3; 2017,Jan,8; 2016,Jan,13; 2015,Jan,16

90792 **Psychiatric diagnostic evaluation with medical services**

4.01 4.37 FUD XXX ★ 03

AMA: 2020,Aug,3; 2019,Dec,14; 2018,Nov,3; 2018,Jul,12; 2018,Apr,9; 2018,Jan,8; 2017,Nov,3; 2017,Jan,8; 2016,Jan,13; 2015,Jan,16

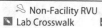

90832-90838 Psychotherapy Services

CMS: 100-02,15,160 Clinical Psychologist Services; 100-02,15,170 Clinical Social Worker (CSW) Services; 100-03,130.1 Inpatient Stays for Alcoholism Treatment; 100-03,130.2 Outpatient Hospital Services for Alcoholism; 100-03,130.3 Chemical Aversion Therapy for Treatment of Alcoholism; 100-04,12,100 Teaching Physician Services; 100-04,12,160 Independent Psychologist Services; 100-04,12,170 Clinical Psychologist Services; 100-04,12,190.3 List of Telehealth Services; 100-04,12,190.6 Payment Methodology for Physician/Practitioner at the Distant Site ; 100-04,12,190.6.1 Submission of Telehealth Claims for Distant Site Practitioners; 100-04,12,190.7 Contractor Editing of Telehealth Claims

INCLUDES Face-to-face time with patient (family, other informers may also be present)
Pharmacologic management in time allocated to psychotherapy service codes
Psychotherapy only (90832, 90834, 90837)
Psychotherapy with separately identifiable medical E/M services includes add-on codes (90833, 90836, 90838)
Service times no less than 16 minutes
Services provided in all settings
Therapeutic communication to:
  Ameliorate patient's mental and behavioral symptoms
  Modify behavior
  Support and encourage personality growth and development
Treatment for:
  Behavior disturbances
  Mental illness

EXCLUDES *Adaptive behavior assessment/treatment ([97151, 97152, 97153, 97154, 97155, 97156, 97157, 97158], 0362T, 0373T)*
Crisis psychotherapy (90839-90840)
Family psychotherapy (90846-90847)
Code also interactive complexity services with time provider spends performing service reflected in time for appropriate psychotherapy code (90785)

90832 **Psychotherapy, 30 minutes with patient**
  🔧 1.76   ⚖ 1.90   **FUD** XXX   ★ 03 💬

  AMA: 2020,Aug,3; 2018,Nov,3; 2018,Jul,12; 2018,Jan,8; 2017,Nov,3; 2017,Sep,11; 2017,Jan,8; 2016,Dec,11; 2016,Jan,13; 2015,Oct,9; 2015,Jan,16

+ **90833** **Psychotherapy, 30 minutes with patient when performed with an evaluation and management service (List separately in addition to the code for primary procedure)**
  Code first (99202-99255 [99224, 99225, 99226], 99304-99337, 99341-99350)
  🔧 1.84   ⚖ 1.97   **FUD** ZZZ   ★ N 💬

  AMA: 2020,Aug,3; 2018,Nov,3; 2018,Jul,12; 2018,Jan,8; 2017,Nov,3; 2017,Jan,8; 2016,Dec,11; 2016,Jan,13; 2015,Oct,9; 2015,Jan,16

90834 **Psychotherapy, 45 minutes with patient**
  🔧 2.35   ⚖ 2.53   **FUD** XXX   ★ 03 💬

  AMA: 2020,Aug,3; 2018,Nov,3; 2018,Jul,12; 2018,Jan,8; 2017,Nov,3; 2017,Jan,8; 2016,Dec,11; 2016,Jan,13; 2015,Oct,9; 2015,Jan,16

+ **90836** **Psychotherapy, 45 minutes with patient when performed with an evaluation and management service (List separately in addition to the code for primary procedure)**
  Code first (99202-99255 [99224, 99225, 99226], 99304-99337, 99341-99350)
  🔧 2.33   ⚖ 2.49   **FUD** ZZZ   ★ N 💬

  AMA: 2020,Aug,3; 2018,Nov,3; 2018,Jul,12; 2018,Jan,8; 2017,Nov,3; 2017,Jan,8; 2016,Dec,11; 2016,Jan,13; 2015,Oct,9; 2015,Jan,16

90837 **Psychotherapy, 60 minutes with patient**
  Code also prolonged service for psychotherapy performed without E/M service face-to-face with patient lasting 90 minutes or longer (99354-99357)
  🔧 3.53   ⚖ 3.80   **FUD** XXX   ★ 03 💬

  AMA: 2020,Sep,3; 2020,Aug,3; 2018,Nov,3; 2018,Jul,12; 2018,Jan,8; 2017,Nov,3; 2017,Jan,8; 2016,Dec,11; 2016,Jan,13; 2015,Oct,3; 2015,Oct,9; 2015,Jan,16

+ **90838** **Psychotherapy, 60 minutes with patient when performed with an evaluation and management service (List separately in addition to the code for primary procedure)**
  Code first (99202-99255 [99224, 99225, 99226], 99304-99337, 99341-99350)
  🔧 3.08   ⚖ 3.29   **FUD** ZZZ   ★ N 💬

  AMA: 2020,Aug,3; 2018,Nov,3; 2018,Jul,12; 2018,Jan,8; 2017,Nov,3; 2017,Jan,8; 2016,Dec,11; 2016,Jan,13; 2015,Oct,9; 2015,Jan,16

90839-90840 Services for Patients in Crisis

CMS: 100-02,15,170 Clinical Social Worker (CSW) Services; 100-03,130.1 Inpatient Stays for Alcoholism Treatment; 100-03,130.3 Chemical Aversion Therapy for Treatment of Alcoholism; 100-04,12,100 Teaching Physician Services; 100-04,12,160 Independent Psychologist Services; 100-04,12,160.1 Payment of Independent Psychologist Services; 100-04,12,170 Clinical Psychologist Services

INCLUDES 30 minutes or more face-to-face time with patient (for all or part service) and/or family providing crisis psychotherapy
All time spent exclusively with patient (for all or part service) and/or family, even if time not continuous
Emergent care to patient in severe distress (e.g., life threatening or complex)
Institute interventions to minimize psychological trauma
Measures to ease crisis and reestablish safety
Psychotherapy

EXCLUDES *Adaptive behavior assessment/treatment ([97151, 97152, 97153, 97154, 97155, 97156, 97157, 97158], 0362T, 0373T)*
Other psychiatric services (90785-90899)

90839 **Psychotherapy for crisis; first 60 minutes**
  INCLUDES First 30-74 minutes crisis psychotherapy per day
  EXCLUDES *Reporting code more than one time per day, even when service not continuous on that date*
  🔧 3.69   ⚖ 3.96   **FUD** XXX   03 80 💬

  AMA: 2020,Aug,3; 2018,Nov,3; 2018,Jul,12; 2018,Jan,8; 2017,Nov,3; 2017,Jan,8; 2016,Jan,13; 2015,Oct,9; 2015,Jan,16

+ **90840** **each additional 30 minutes (List separately in addition to code for primary service)**
  INCLUDES Up to 30 minutes time beyond initial 74 minutes
  Code first (90839)
  🔧 1.76   ⚖ 1.90   **FUD** ZZZ   N 80 💬

  AMA: 2020,Aug,3; 2018,Nov,3; 2018,Jul,12; 2018,Jan,8; 2017,Nov,3; 2017,Jan,8; 2016,Jan,13; 2015,Oct,9; 2015,Jan,16

90845-90863 Additional Psychotherapy Services

CMS: 100-02,15,170 Clinical Social Worker (CSW) Services; 100-03,10.3 Inpatient Pain Rehabilitation Programs; 100-03,10.4 Outpatient Hospital Pain Rehabilitation Programs

EXCLUDES *Adaptive behavior assessment/treatment ([97151, 97152, 97153, 97154, 97155, 97156, 97157, 97158], 0362T, 0373T)*
Analysis/programming neurostimulators for vagus nerve stimulation therapy (95970, 95976-95977)
Crisis psychotherapy (90839-90840)

90845 **Psychoanalysis**
  🔧 2.53   ⚖ 2.78   **FUD** XXX   ★ 03 80 💬

  AMA: 2020,Aug,3; 2018,Nov,3; 2018,Jul,12; 2018,Jan,8; 2017,Jan,8; 2016,Jan,13; 2015,Oct,9; 2015,Jan,16

90846 **Family psychotherapy (without the patient present), 50 minutes**
  EXCLUDES *Service times less than 26 minutes*
  🔧 2.85   ⚖ 2.87   **FUD** XXX   ★ 03 80 💬

  AMA: 2020,Aug,3; 2018,Nov,3; 2018,Jul,12; 2018,Jan,8; 2017,Nov,3; 2017,Mar,10; 2017,Jan,8; 2016,Dec,11; 2016,Jan,13; 2015,Oct,9; 2015,Jan,16

90847 **Family psychotherapy (conjoint psychotherapy) (with patient present), 50 minutes**
  EXCLUDES *Service times less than 26 minutes*
  Service times more than 80 minutes, see prolonged services (99354-99357)
  🔧 2.96   ⚖ 3.18   **FUD** XXX   ★ 03 80 💬

  AMA: 2020,Sep,3; 2020,Aug,3; 2018,Nov,3; 2018,Jul,12; 2018,Jan,8; 2017,Nov,3; 2017,Jan,8; 2016,Dec,11; 2016,Jan,13; 2015,Oct,9; 2015,Jan,16

● New Code   ▲ Revised Code   ○ Reinstated   ● New Web Release   ▲ Revised Web Release   + Add-on   Unlisted   Not Covered   # Resequenced
50 Optum Mod 50 Exempt   ⊘ AMA Mod 51 Exempt   51 Optum Mod 51 Exempt   63 Mod 63 Exempt   ⁄ Non-FDA Drug   ★ Telemedicine   M Maternity   ⚠ Age Edit

90849 **Multiple-family group psychotherapy**
0.87 1.17 FUD XXX 03 80
AMA: 2020,Aug,3; 2018,Nov,3; 2018,Jul,12; 2018,Jan,8; 2017,Nov,3; 2017,Jan,8; 2016,Jan,13; 2015,Oct,9; 2015,Jan,16

90853 **Group psychotherapy (other than of a multiple-family group)**
Code also group psychotherapy with interactive complexity (90785)
0.70 0.76 FUD XXX 03 80
AMA: 2020,Aug,3; 2018,Nov,3; 2018,Jul,12; 2018,Jan,8; 2017,Nov,3; 2017,Mar,10; 2017,Jan,8; 2016,Jan,13; 2015,Oct,9; 2015,Jan,16

+ **90863** **Pharmacologic management, including prescription and review of medication, when performed with psychotherapy services (List separately in addition to the code for primary procedure)**
INCLUDES Pharmacologic management in time allocated to psychotherapy service codes
Code first (90832, 90834, 90837)
0.70 0.74 FUD XXX ★ E
AMA: 2020,Aug,3; 2018,Nov,3; 2018,Jul,12; 2018,Jan,8; 2017,Jan,8; 2016,Jan,13; 2015,Jan,16

90865-90870 Other Psychiatric Treatment

EXCLUDES *Adaptive behavior assessment/treatment ([97151, 97152, 97153, 97154, 97155, 97156, 97157, 97158], 0362T, 0373T)*
Analysis/programming neurostimulators for vagus nerve stimulation therapy (95970, 95976-95977)
Crisis psychotherapy (90839-90840)

90865 **Narcosynthesis for psychiatric diagnostic and therapeutic purposes (eg, sodium amobarbital (Amytal) interview)**
3.59 4.79 FUD XXX 03 80
AMA: 2020,Aug,3; 2018,Nov,3; 2018,Jul,12; 2018,Jan,8; 2017,Jan,8; 2016,Jan,13; 2015,Jan,16

90867 **Therapeutic repetitive transcranial magnetic stimulation (TMS) treatment; initial, including cortical mapping, motor threshold determination, delivery and management**
INCLUDES E/M services related directly to:
Cortical mapping
Delivery and management TMS services
Motor threshold determination
EXCLUDES *Electromyography (95860, 95870)*
Evoked potential studies (95928, 95929, [95939])
Medication management
Reporting code more than one time for each treatment course
Significant, separately identifiable E/M service
Significant, separately identifiable psychotherapy service
Subsequent transcranial magnetic stimulation (TMS) treatment:
Delivery and management (90868)
Motor threshold redetermination (90869)
0.00 0.00 FUD 000 S
AMA: 2020,Aug,3; 2018,Nov,3; 2018,Jul,12

90868 **subsequent delivery and management, per session**
INCLUDES E/M services related directly to:
Cortical mapping
Delivery and management TMS services
Motor threshold determination
EXCLUDES *Medication management*
Significant, separately identifiable E/M service
Significant, separately identifiable psychotherapy service
0.00 0.00 FUD 000 S
AMA: 2020,Aug,3; 2018,Nov,3; 2018,Jul,12

90869 **subsequent motor threshold re-determination with delivery and management**
INCLUDES E/M services related directly to:
Cortical mapping
Delivery and management TMS services
Motor threshold determination
EXCLUDES *Electromyography (95860, 95870)*
Evoked potential studies (95928-95929, [95939])
Medication management
Significant, separately identifiable E/M service
Significant, separately identifiable psychotherapy service
Transcranial magnetic stimulation (TMS) treatment:
Initial (90867)
Subsequent delivery and managment (90868)
0.00 0.00 FUD 000 S
AMA: 2020,Aug,3; 2018,Nov,3; 2018,Jul,12

90870 **Electroconvulsive therapy (includes necessary monitoring)**
3.12 4.96 FUD 000 S 80
AMA: 2020,Aug,3; 2018,Nov,3; 2018,Jul,12; 2018,Jan,8; 2017,Jan,8; 2016,Jan,13; 2015,Jan,16

90875-90880 Psychiatric Therapy with Biofeedback or Hypnosis

CMS: 100-02,15,170 Clinical Social Worker (CSW) Services; 100-04,12,160 Independent Psychologist Services; 100-04,12,160.1 Payment of Independent Psychologist Services; 100-04,12,170 Clinical Psychologist Services

EXCLUDES *Adaptive behavior assessment/treatment ([97151, 97152, 97153, 97154, 97155, 97156, 97157, 97158], 0362T, 0373T)*
Analysis/programming neurostimulators for vagus nerve stimulation therapy (95970, 95976-95977)
Crisis psychotherapy (90839-90840)

90875 **Individual psychophysiological therapy incorporating biofeedback training by any modality (face-to-face with the patient), with psychotherapy (eg, insight oriented, behavior modifying or supportive psychotherapy); 30 minutes**
1.73 1.80 FUD XXX E
AMA: 2020,Aug,3; 2018,Nov,3; 2018,Jul,12; 2018,Jan,8; 2017,Jan,8; 2016,Jan,13; 2015,Jan,16

90876 **45 minutes**
2.74 3.05 FUD XXX E
AMA: 2020,Aug,3; 2018,Nov,3; 2018,Jul,12; 2018,Jan,8; 2017,Jan,8; 2016,Jan,13; 2015,Jan,16

90880 **Hypnotherapy**
2.58 2.98 FUD XXX 03 80
AMA: 2020,Aug,3; 2018,Nov,3; 2018,Jul,12; 2018,Jan,8; 2017,Jan,8; 2016,Jan,13; 2015,Jan,16

90882-90899 Psychiatric Services without Patient Face-to-Face Contact

CMS: 100-04,12,160 Independent Psychologist Services; 100-04,12,160.1 Payment of Independent Psychologist Services

EXCLUDES *Analysis/programming neurostimulators for vagus nerve stimulation therapy (95970, 95976-95977)*
Crisis psychotherapy (90839-90840)

90882 **Environmental intervention for medical management purposes on a psychiatric patient's behalf with agencies, employers, or institutions**
0.00 0.00 FUD XXX E
AMA: 2020,Aug,3; 2018,Nov,3; 2018,Jul,12; 2018,Jan,8; 2017,Jan,8; 2016,Jan,13; 2015,Jan,16

90885 **Psychiatric evaluation of hospital records, other psychiatric reports, psychometric and/or projective tests, and other accumulated data for medical diagnostic purposes**
1.43 1.43 FUD XXX N
AMA: 2020,Aug,3; 2018,Nov,3; 2018,Jul,12; 2018,Jan,8; 2017,Jan,8; 2016,Jan,13; 2015,Jan,16

90887 **Interpretation or explanation of results of psychiatric, other medical examinations and procedures, or other accumulated data to family or other responsible persons, or advising them how to assist patient**

EXCLUDES *Adaptive behavior assessment/treatment ([97151, 97152, 97153, 97154, 97155, 97156, 97157, 97158], 0362T, 0373T)*

2.14 2.48 FUD XXX N

AMA: 2020,Aug,3; 2018,Nov,3; 2018,Jul,12; 2018,Jan,8; 2017,Jan,8; 2016,Jan,13; 2015,Jan,16

90889 **Preparation of report of patient's psychiatric status, history, treatment, or progress (other than for legal or consultative purposes) for other individuals, agencies, or insurance carriers**

0.00 0.00 FUD XXX N

AMA: 2020,Aug,3; 2018,Nov,3; 2018,Jul,12; 2018,Jan,8; 2017,Jan,8; 2016,Jan,13; 2015,Jan,16

90899 **Unlisted psychiatric service or procedure**

0.00 0.00 FUD XXX Q3 80

AMA: 2020,Aug,3; 2018,Nov,3; 2018,Jul,12; 2018,Jan,8; 2017,Jan,8; 2016,Jan,13; 2015,Jan,16

90901-90913 Biofeedback Therapy

EXCLUDES *Psychophysiological therapy utilizing biofeedback training (90875-90876)*

90901 **Biofeedback training by any modality**

0.57 1.13 FUD 000 A 80

AMA: 2020,Jun,13; 2018,Jan,8; 2017,Jan,8; 2016,Jan,13; 2015,Jan,16

90912 **Biofeedback training, perineal muscles, anorectal or urethral sphincter, including EMG and/or manometry, when performed; initial 15 minutes of one-on-one physician or other qualified health care professional contact with the patient**

EXCLUDES *Incontinence treatment using pulsed magnetic neuromodulation (53899)*
Testing rectal sensation, tone, and compliance (91120)

1.26 2.27 FUD 000 80

AMA: 2020,Jun,13

\+ **90913** **each additional 15 minutes of one-on-one physician or other qualified health care professional contact with the patient (List separately in addition to code for primary procedure)**

EXCLUDES *Incontinence treatment using pulsed magnetic neuromodulation (53899)*
Testing rectal sensation, tone, and compliance (91120)

Code first (90912)

0.70 0.92 FUD ZZZ 80

AMA: 2020,Jun,13

90935-90940 Hemodialysis Services: Inpatient ESRD and Outpatient Non-ESRD

CMS: 100-02,11,20 Renal Dialysis Items and Services ; 100-04,3,100.6 Inpatient Renal Services

EXCLUDES *Attendance by physician or other qualified health care provider for prolonged period of time (99354-99360 [99415, 99416])*
Blood specimen collection from partial/complete implantable venous access device (36591)
Declotting cannula (36831, 36833, 36860-36861)
Hemodialysis home visit by non-physician health care professional (99512)
Therapeutic apheresis procedures (36511-36516)
Thrombolytic agent declotting implanted vascular access device/catheter (36593)

Code also significant separately identifiable E/M service not related to dialysis procedure or renal failure with modifier 25 (99202-99215, 99217-99223 [99224, 99225, 99226], 99231-99239, 99241-99245, 99281-99285, 99291-99292, 99304-99318, 99324-99337, 99341-99350, 99466-99467, 99468-99472, 99475-99480)

90935 **Hemodialysis procedure with single evaluation by a physician or other qualified health care professional**

INCLUDES All E/M services related to patient's renal disease rendered on day dialysis performed
Inpatient ESRD and non-ESRD procedures
Only one patient evaluation related to hemodialysis procedure
Outpatient non-ESRD dialysis

2.07 2.07 FUD 000 S 80

AMA: 2018,Jan,8; 2017,Jan,8; 2016,Jan,13; 2015,Jan,16

90937 **Hemodialysis procedure requiring repeated evaluation(s) with or without substantial revision of dialysis prescription**

INCLUDES All E/M services related to patient's renal disease rendered on day dialysis performed
Inpatient ESRD and non-ESRD procedures
Outpatient non-ESRD dialysis
Re-evaluation patient during hemodialysis procedure

2.95 2.95 FUD 000 B 80

AMA: 2018,Jan,8; 2017,Jan,8; 2016,Jan,13; 2015,Jan,16

90940 **Hemodialysis access flow study to determine blood flow in grafts and arteriovenous fistulae by an indicator method**

EXCLUDES *Hemodialysis access duplex scan (93990)*

0.00 0.00 FUD XXX N

AMA: 2018,Jan,8; 2017,Jan,8; 2016,Jan,13; 2015,Jan,16

90945-90947 Dialysis Techniques Other Than Hemodialysis

CMS: 100-04,12,40.3 Global Surgery Review; 100-04,3,100.6 Inpatient Renal Services

INCLUDES All E/M services related to patient's renal disease rendered on day dialysis performed
Procedures other than hemodialysis:
Continuous renal replacement therapies
Hemofiltration
Peritoneal dialysis

EXCLUDES *Attendance by physician or other qualified health care provider for prolonged time period (99354-99360 [99415, 99416])*
Hemodialysis
Tunneled intraperitoneal catheter insertion
Open (49421)
Percutaneous (49418)

Code also significant, separately identifiable E/M service not related to dialysis procedure or renal failure with modifier 25 (99202-99215, 99217-99223 [99224, 99225, 99226], 99231-99239, 99241-99245, 99281-99285, 99291-99292, 99304-99318, 99324-99337, 99341-99350, 99466-99467, 99468-99472, 99475-99480)

90945 **Dialysis procedure other than hemodialysis (eg, peritoneal dialysis, hemofiltration, or other continuous renal replacement therapies), with single evaluation by a physician or other qualified health care professional**

INCLUDES Only one patient evaluation related to procedure

EXCLUDES *Peritoneal dialysis home infusion (99601, 99602)*

2.42 2.42 FUD 000 V 80

AMA: 2018,Jan,8; 2017,Jan,8; 2016,Jan,13; 2015,Jan,16

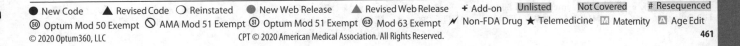

90947 **Dialysis procedure other than hemodialysis (eg, peritoneal dialysis, hemofiltration, or other continuous renal replacement therapies) requiring repeated evaluations by a physician or other qualified health care professional, with or without substantial revision of dialysis prescription**

EXCLUDES *Re-evaluation during procedure*

3.51 3.51 FUD 000 B 80

AMA: 2018,Jan,8; 2017,Jan,8; 2016,Jan,13; 2015,Jan,16

90951-90962 End-stage Renal Disease Monthly Outpatient Services

CMS: 100-02,11,20 Renal Dialysis Items and Services ; 100-04,12,190.3 List of Telehealth Services; 100-04,12,190.3.4 ESRD-Related Services as a Telehealth Service; 100-04,8,140.1 ESRD-Related Services Under the Monthly Capitation Payment

INCLUDES Establishing dialyzing cycle
Management dialysis visits
Outpatient E/M dialysis visits
Patient management during dialysis for month
Telephone calls

EXCLUDES *ESRD/non-ESRD dialysis services performed in inpatient setting (90935-90937, 90945-90947)*
Non-ESRD dialysis services performed in outpatient setting (90935-90937, 90945-90947)
Non-ESRD related E/M services that cannot be performed during dialysis session
Services provided in same month with:
Chronic care management ([99439, 99490, 99491])
Complex chronic care management (99487-99489)

90951 **End-stage renal disease (ESRD) related services monthly, for patients younger than 2 years of age to include monitoring for the adequacy of nutrition, assessment of growth and development, and counseling of parents; with 4 or more face-to-face visits by a physician or other qualified health care professional per month** A

26.6 26.6 FUD XXX ★ M 80

AMA: 2018,Feb,11; 2018,Jan,8; 2017,Jan,8; 2016,Jan,13; 2015,Jan,16

90952 **with 2-3 face-to-face visits by a physician or other qualified health care professional per month** A

0.00 0.00 FUD XXX ★ M 80

AMA: 2018,Feb,11; 2018,Jan,8; 2017,Jan,8; 2016,Jan,13; 2015,Jan,16

90953 **with 1 face-to-face visit by a physician or other qualified health care professional per month** A

0.00 0.00 FUD XXX M 80

AMA: 2018,Feb,11; 2018,Jan,8; 2017,Jan,8; 2016,Jan,13; 2015,Jan,16

90954 **End-stage renal disease (ESRD) related services monthly, for patients 2-11 years of age to include monitoring for the adequacy of nutrition, assessment of growth and development, and counseling of parents; with 4 or more face-to-face visits by a physician or other qualified health care professional per month** A

22.9 22.9 FUD XXX ★ M 80

AMA: 2018,Feb,11; 2018,Jan,8; 2017,Jan,8; 2016,Jan,13; 2015,Jan,16

90955 **with 2-3 face-to-face visits by a physician or other qualified health care professional per month** A

12.9 12.9 FUD XXX ★ M 80

AMA: 2018,Feb,11; 2018,Jan,8; 2017,Jan,8; 2016,Jan,13; 2015,Jan,16

90956 **with 1 face-to-face visit by a physician or other qualified health care professional per month** A

9.00 9.00 FUD XXX M 80

AMA: 2018,Feb,11; 2018,Jan,8; 2017,Jan,8; 2016,Jan,13; 2015,Jan,16

90957 **End-stage renal disease (ESRD) related services monthly, for patients 12-19 years of age to include monitoring for the adequacy of nutrition, assessment of growth and development, and counseling of parents; with 4 or more face-to-face visits by a physician or other qualified health care professional per month** A

18.3 18.3 FUD XXX ★ M 80

AMA: 2018,Feb,11; 2018,Jan,8; 2017,Jan,8; 2016,Jan,13; 2015,Jan,16

90958 **with 2-3 face-to-face visits by a physician or other qualified health care professional per month** A

12.3 12.3 FUD XXX ★ M 80

AMA: 2018,Feb,11; 2018,Jan,8; 2017,Jan,8; 2016,Jan,13; 2015,Jan,16

90959 **with 1 face-to-face visit by a physician or other qualified health care professional per month** A

8.41 8.41 FUD XXX M 80

AMA: 2018,Feb,11; 2018,Jan,8; 2017,Jan,8; 2016,Jan,13; 2015,Jan,16

90960 **End-stage renal disease (ESRD) related services monthly, for patients 20 years of age and older; with 4 or more face-to-face visits by a physician or other qualified health care professional per month** A

8.07 8.07 FUD XXX ★ M 80

AMA: 2018,Feb,11; 2018,Jan,8; 2017,Jan,8; 2016,Jan,13; 2015,Jan,16

90961 **with 2-3 face-to-face visits by a physician or other qualified health care professional per month** A

6.74 6.74 FUD XXX ★ M 80

AMA: 2018,Feb,11; 2018,Jan,8; 2017,Jan,8; 2016,Jan,13; 2015,Jan,16

90962 **with 1 face-to-face visit by a physician or other qualified health care professional per month** A

5.21 5.21 FUD XXX M 80

AMA: 2018,Feb,11; 2018,Jan,8; 2017,Jan,8; 2016,Jan,13; 2015,Jan,16

90963-90966 End-stage Renal Disease Monthly Home Dialysis Services

CMS: 100-02,11,20 Renal Dialysis Items and Services ; 100-04,12,190.3.4 ESRD-Related Services as a Telehealth Service; 100-04,8,140.1 ESRD-Related Services Under the Monthly Capitation Payment; 100-04,8,140.1.1 Payment for Managing Patients on Home Dialysis

INCLUDES ESRD services for home dialysis patients
Services provided for full month

EXCLUDES *Services provided in same month with:*
Chronic care management ([99439, 99490, 99491])
Complex chronic care management (99487-99489)

90963 **End-stage renal disease (ESRD) related services for home dialysis per full month, for patients younger than 2 years of age to include monitoring for the adequacy of nutrition, assessment of growth and development, and counseling of parents** A

15.4 15.4 FUD XXX M 80

AMA: 2018,Feb,11; 2018,Jan,8; 2017,Jan,8; 2016,Jan,13; 2015,Jan,16

90964 **End-stage renal disease (ESRD) related services for home dialysis per full month, for patients 2-11 years of age to include monitoring for the adequacy of nutrition, assessment of growth and development, and counseling of parents** A

13.5 13.5 FUD XXX M 80

AMA: 2018,Feb,11; 2018,Jan,8; 2017,Jan,8; 2016,Jan,13; 2015,Jan,16

90965 **End-stage renal disease (ESRD) related services for home dialysis per full month, for patients 12-19 years of age to include monitoring for the adequacy of nutrition, assessment of growth and development, and counseling of parents** A

12.9 12.9 FUD XXX M 80

AMA: 2018,Feb,11; 2018,Jan,8; 2017,Jan,8; 2016,Jan,13; 2015,Jan,16

90966 **End-stage renal disease (ESRD) related services for home dialysis per full month, for patients 20 years of age and older** A

6.72 6.72 FUD XXX M 80

AMA: 2018,Feb,11; 2018,Jan,8; 2017,Jan,8; 2016,Jan,13; 2015,Jan,16

90967-90970 End-stage Renal Disease Services: Partial Month

CMS: 100-02,11,20 Renal Dialysis Items and Services

INCLUDES ESRD services for less than full month, such as:
- Outpatient ESRD-related services initiated prior to assessment completion
- Patient spending partial month as hospital inpatient
- Patient who is transient, dies, recovers, or undergoes kidney transplant

Services reported on daily basis, less hospitalization days

EXCLUDES *Services provided in same month with:*
- *Chronic care management ([99439, 99490, 99491])*
- *Complex chronic care management (99487-99489)*

90967 **End-stage renal disease (ESRD) related services for dialysis less than a full month of service, per day; for patients younger than 2 years of age** A

0.51 0.51 FUD XXX M 80

AMA: 2018,Feb,11; 2018,Jan,8; 2017,Jan,8; 2016,Jan,13; 2015,Jan,16

90968 **for patients 2-11 years of age** A

0.45 0.45 FUD XXX M 80

AMA: 2018,Feb,11; 2018,Jan,8; 2017,Jan,8; 2016,Jan,13; 2015,Jan,16

90969 **for patients 12-19 years of age** A

0.43 0.43 FUD XXX M 80

AMA: 2018,Feb,11; 2018,Jan,8; 2017,Jan,8; 2016,Jan,13; 2015,Jan,16

90970 **for patients 20 years of age and older** A

0.22 0.22 FUD XXX M 80

AMA: 2018,Feb,11; 2018,Jan,8; 2017,Jan,8; 2016,Jan,13; 2015,Jan,16

90989-90993 Dialysis Training Services

CMS: 100-04,3,100.6 Inpatient Renal Services

90989 **Dialysis training, patient, including helper where applicable, any mode, completed course**

0.00 0.00 FUD XXX B

AMA: 2018,Feb,11; 2018,Jan,8; 2017,Jan,8; 2016,Jan,13; 2015,Jan,16

90993 **Dialysis training, patient, including helper where applicable, any mode, course not completed, per training session**

0.00 0.00 FUD XXX B

AMA: 2018,Feb,11; 2018,Jan,8; 2017,Jan,8; 2016,Jan,13; 2015,Jan,16

90997-90999 Hemoperfusion and Unlisted Dialysis Procedures

CMS: 100-04,3,100.6 Inpatient Renal Services

90997 **Hemoperfusion (eg, with activated charcoal or resin)**

2.53 2.53 FUD 000 B 80

AMA: 2018,Feb,11

90999 **Unlisted dialysis procedure, inpatient or outpatient**

0.00 0.00 FUD XXX B 80

AMA: 2018,Feb,11

91010-91022 Esophageal Manometry

91010 **Esophageal motility (manometric study of the esophagus and/or gastroesophageal junction) study with interpretation and report;**

EXCLUDES *Esophageal motility studies with high-resolution esophageal pressure topography (91299)*

Code also for esophageal motility studies with stimulant or perfusion (91013)

5.38 5.38 FUD 000 S 80

AMA: 2018,Feb,11

+ **91013** **with stimulation or perfusion (eg, stimulant, acid or alkali perfusion) (List separately in addition to code for primary procedure)**

EXCLUDES *Esophageal motility studies with high-resolution esophageal pressure topography (91299)*

Reporting code more than one time for each session

Code first (91010)

0.73 0.73 FUD ZZZ N 80

AMA: 2018,Feb,11

91020 **Gastric motility (manometric) studies**

EXCLUDES *Gastrointestinal imaging by wireless capsule (91112)*

7.01 7.01 FUD 000 S 80

AMA: 2018,Feb,11; 2018,Jan,8; 2017,Jan,8; 2016,Jan,13; 2015,Jan,16

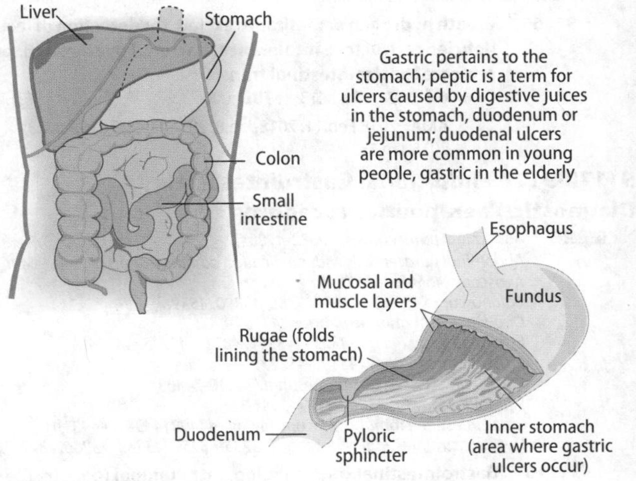

91022 **Duodenal motility (manometric) study**

EXCLUDES *Fluoroscopy (76000)*
Gastric motility study (91020)
Gastrointestinal imaging by wireless capsule (91112)

4.77 4.77 FUD 000 S 80

AMA: 2018,Feb,11; 2018,Jan,8; 2017,Jan,8; 2016,Jan,13; 2015,Jan,16

91030-91040 Esophageal Reflux Tests

EXCLUDES *Duodenal intubation/aspiration (43756-43757)*
Esophagoscopy (43180-43233 [43211, 43212, 43213, 43214])
Insertion:
- *Esophageal tamponade tube (43460)*
- *Insertion long gastrointestinal tube (44500)*

Radiologic services, gastrointestinal (74210-74363)
Upper gastrointestinal endoscopy (43235-43259 [43233, 43266, 43270])

91030 **Esophagus, acid perfusion (Bernstein) test for esophagitis**

3.91 3.91 FUD 000 S 80

AMA: 2018,Feb,11

91034 **Esophagus, gastroesophageal reflux test; with nasal catheter pH electrode(s) placement, recording, analysis and interpretation**

5.41 5.41 FUD 000 S 80

AMA: 2018,Feb,11; 2018,Jan,8; 2017,Jan,8; 2016,Jan,13; 2015,Jan,16

91035 **with mucosal attached telemetry pH electrode placement, recording, analysis and interpretation**

INCLUDES Endoscopy only to place device

13.6 13.6 FUD 000 S Z2 80

AMA: 2018,Feb,11; 2018,Jan,8; 2017,Jan,8; 2016,Jan,13; 2015,Jan,16

91037 **Esophageal function test, gastroesophageal reflux test with nasal catheter intraluminal impedance electrode(s) placement, recording, analysis and interpretation;**

4.66 4.66 FUD 000 S 80

AMA: 2018,Feb,11

91038 **prolonged (greater than 1 hour, up to 24 hours)**

12.4 12.4 FUD 000 S 80

AMA: 2018,Feb,11; 2018,Jan,8; 2017,Jan,8; 2016,Jan,13; 2015,Jan,16

91040 **Esophageal balloon distension study, diagnostic, with provocation when performed**

EXCLUDES *Reporting code more than one time for each session*

13.5 13.5 FUD 000 S 80

AMA: 2018,Feb,11; 2018,Jan,8; 2017,Jan,6

91065 Breath Analysis

CMS: 100-03,100.5 Diagnostic Breath Analysis

EXCLUDES *H. pylori breath test analysis, radioactive (C-14) or nonradioactive (C-13) (78268, 83013)*

Code also each challenge administered

91065 **Breath hydrogen or methane test (eg, for detection of lactase deficiency, fructose intolerance, bacterial overgrowth, or oro-cecal gastrointestinal transit)**

2.13 2.13 FUD 000 S 80

AMA: 2018,Feb,11; 2018,Jan,8; 2017,Jan,8; 2016,Jan,13; 2015,Jan,16

91110-91299 Additional Gastrointestinal Diagnostic/Therapeutic Procedures

EXCLUDES
Abdominal paracentesis (49082-49084)
Abdominal paracentesis with medication administration (96440, 96446)
Anoscopy (46600-46615)
Colonoscopy (45378-45393 [45388, 45390, 45398])
Duodenal intubation/aspiration (43756-43757)
Esophagoscopy (43180-43233 [43211, 43212, 43213, 43214])
Proctosigmoidoscopy (45300-45327)
Radiologic services, gastrointestinal (74210-74363)
Sigmoidoscopy (45330-45350 [45346])
Small intestine/stomal endoscopy (44360-44408 [44381, 44401])
Upper gastrointestinal endoscopy (43235-43259 [43233, 43266, 43270])

91110 **Gastrointestinal tract imaging, intraluminal (eg, capsule endoscopy), esophagus through ileum, with interpretation and report**

EXCLUDES
Imaging colon (0355T)
Imaging esophagus through ileum (91111)

Code also modifier 52 when ileum not visualized

24.9 24.9 FUD XXX T 80

AMA: 2018,Feb,11; 2018,Jan,8; 2017,Jan,8; 2016,Jan,13; 2015,Jan,16

91111 **Gastrointestinal tract imaging, intraluminal (eg, capsule endoscopy), esophagus with interpretation and report**

EXCLUDES
Imaging colon (0355T)
Imaging esophagus through ileum (91111)
Wireless capsule to measure transit times or pressure in gastrointestinal tract (91112)

24.4 24.4 FUD XXX T 80

AMA: 2018,Feb,11; 2018,Jan,8; 2017,Jan,8; 2016,Jan,13; 2015,Jan,16

91112 **Gastrointestinal transit and pressure measurement, stomach through colon, wireless capsule, with interpretation and report**

EXCLUDES
Colon motility study (91117)
Duodenal motility study (91022)
Gastric motility studies (91020)
pH body fluid (83986)

40.9 40.9 FUD XXX T 80

AMA: 2018,Feb,11; 2018,Jan,8; 2017,Jan,8; 2016,Jan,13; 2015,Jan,16

91117 **Colon motility (manometric) study, minimum 6 hours continuous recording (including provocation tests, eg, meal, intracolonic balloon distension, pharmacologic agents, if performed), with interpretation and report**

EXCLUDES
Anal manometry (91122)
Rectal sensation, tone and compliance testing (91120)
Reporting code more than one time no matter how many provocations
Wireless capsule to measure transit times or pressure in gastrointestinal tract (91112)

3.96 3.96 FUD 000 T 80

AMA: 2018,Feb,11; 2018,Jan,8; 2017,Jan,8; 2016,Jan,13; 2015,Jan,16

91120 **Rectal sensation, tone, and compliance test (ie, response to graded balloon distention)**

EXCLUDES
Anorectal manometry (91122)
Biofeedback training (90912, 90913)
Colon motility study (91117)

13.7 13.7 FUD XXX S 80

AMA: 2020,Jun,13; 2018,Feb,11; 2018,Jan,8; 2017,Jan,8; 2016,Jan,13; 2015,Jan,16

91122 **Anorectal manometry**

EXCLUDES *Colon motility study (91117)*

7.13 7.13 FUD 000 T 80

AMA: 2018,Feb,11

91132 **Electrogastrography, diagnostic, transcutaneous;**

6.80 6.80 FUD XXX S 80

AMA: 2018,Feb,11

91133 **with provocative testing**

9.82 9.82 FUD XXX Q1 80

AMA: 2018,Feb,11

91200 **Liver elastography, mechanically induced shear wave (eg, vibration), without imaging, with interpretation and report**

EXCLUDES *Ultrasound elastography parenchyma (76981-76983)*

1.05 1.05 FUD XXX Q1 80

AMA: 2019,Aug,3; 2018,Feb,11; 2018,Jan,8; 2017,Oct,9

91299 **Unlisted diagnostic gastroenterology procedure**

0.00 0.00 FUD XXX S 80

AMA: 2018,Feb,11; 2018,Jan,8; 2017,Jan,8; 2016,Jan,13; 2015,Jan,16

92002-92014 Ophthalmic Medical Services

CMS: 100-02,15,30.4 Optometrist's Services

[INCLUDES] Routine ophthalmoscopy

Services provided to established patients who have received professional services from physician or other qualified health care provider or another physician or other qualified health care professional within same group practice/exact same specialty and subspecialty within past three years

Services provided to new patients who have received no professional services from physician or other qualified health care provider or another physician or other qualified health care professional within same group practice/exact same specialty and subspecialty within past three years

[EXCLUDES] *Retinal polarization scan (0469T)*
Surgical procedures on eye/ocular adnexa (65091-68899 [66987, 66988, 67810])
Visual screening tests (99173-99174 [99177])

92002 **Ophthalmological services: medical examination and evaluation with initiation of diagnostic and treatment program; intermediate, new patient**

[INCLUDES] Evaluation new/existing condition complicated by new diagnostic or management problem
Integrated services where medical decision making cannot be separated from examination methods
Intermediate services:
  External ocular/adnexal examination
  General medical observation
  History
Other diagnostic procedures:
  Biomicroscopy
  Mydriasis
  Ophthalmoscopy
  Tonometry
Problems not related to primary diagnosis

🚗 1.36 ⚕ 2.37 **FUD** XXX   [V] [80] 🖵

AMA: 2018,Feb,11; 2018,Feb,3; 2018,Jan,8; 2017,Sep,14; 2017,Jan,8; 2016,Jan,13; 2015,Jan,16

92004 **comprehensive, new patient, 1 or more visits**

[INCLUDES] Comprehensive services:
  Basic sensorimotor examination
  Biomicroscopy
  Dilation (cycloplegia)
  External examinations
  General medical observation
  Gross visual fields
  History
  Initiation diagnostic/treatment programs
  Mydriasis
  Ophthalmoscopic examinations
  Other diagnostic procedures
  Prescription medication
  Special diagnostic/treatment services
  Tonometry
General evaluation complete visual system
Integrated services where medical decision making cannot be separated from examination methods
Single service that need not be performed at one session

🚗 2.77 ⚕ 4.23 **FUD** XXX   [V] [80] 🖵

AMA: 2018,Feb,11; 2018,Feb,3; 2018,Jan,8; 2017,Sep,14; 2017,Jan,8; 2016,Nov,9; 2016,Jan,13; 2015,Jan,16

92012 **Ophthalmological services: medical examination and evaluation, with initiation or continuation of diagnostic and treatment program; intermediate, established patient**

[INCLUDES] Evaluation new/existing condition complicated by new diagnostic or management problem
Integrated services where medical decision making cannot be separated from examination methods
Problems not related to primary diagnosis
Intermediate services:
  External ocular/adnexal examination
  General medical observation
  History
Other diagnostic procedures:
  Biomicroscopy
  Mydriasis
  Ophthalmoscopy
  Tonometry

🚗 1.49 ⚕ 2.49 **FUD** XXX   [V] [80] 🖵

AMA: 2018,Feb,11; 2018,Feb,3; 2018,Jan,8; 2017,Sep,14; 2017,Jan,8; 2016,Jan,13; 2015,Jan,16

92014 **comprehensive, established patient, 1 or more visits**

[INCLUDES] General evaluation complete visual system
Integrated services where medical decision making cannot be separated from examination methods
Single service that need not be performed at one session
Comprehensive services:
  Basic sensorimotor examination
  Biomicroscopy
  Dilation (cycloplegia)
  External examinations
  General medical observation
  Gross visual fields
  History
  Initiation diagnostic/treatment programs
  Mydriasis
  Ophthalmoscopic examinations
  Other diagnostic procedures
  Prescription medication
  Special diagnostic/treatment services
  Tonometry

🚗 2.23 ⚕ 3.55 **FUD** XXX   [V] [80] 🖵

AMA: 2018,Feb,11; 2018,Feb,3; 2018,Jan,8; 2017,Sep,14; 2017,Jan,8; 2016,Nov,9; 2016,Jan,13; 2015,Jan,16

92015-92145 Ophthalmic Special Services

[INCLUDES] Routine ophthalmoscopy

[EXCLUDES] *Surgical procedures on eye/ocular adnexa (65091-68899 [66987, 66988, 67810])*

Code also E/M services, when performed
Code also general ophthalmological services, when performed (92002-92014)

92015 **Determination of refractive state**

[INCLUDES] Lens prescription:
  Absorptive factor
  Axis
  Impact resistance
  Lens power
  Prism
Specification lens type:
  Bifocal
  Monofocal

[EXCLUDES] *Ocular screening, instrument based (99173-99174 [99177])*

🚗 0.55 ⚕ 0.56 **FUD** XXX   [E] 🖵

AMA: 2018,Feb,11; 2018,Jan,8; 2017,Jan,8; 2016,Mar,10; 2016,Jan,13; 2015,Jan,16

92018 **Ophthalmological examination and evaluation, under general anesthesia, with or without manipulation of globe for passive range of motion or other manipulation to facilitate diagnostic examination; complete**

🚗 4.13 ⚕ 4.13 **FUD** XXX   [J] [80] 🖵

AMA: 2018,Feb,11; 2018,Jan,8; 2017,Jan,8; 2016,Jan,13; 2015,Jan,16

● New Code ▲ Revised Code ○ Reinstated ● New Web Release ▲ Revised Web Release + Add-on Unlisted Not Covered # Resequenced
⑤⓪ Optum Mod 50 Exempt ⊘ AMA Mod 51 Exempt ⑤① Optum Mod 51 Exempt ⑥③ Mod 63 Exempt ⁄ Non-FDA Drug ★ Telemedicine Ⓜ Maternity Ⓐ Age Edit

92019 limited

Facility RVU 2.05 Non-Facility RVU 2.05 FUD XXX J 80

AMA: 2018,Feb,11; 2018,Jan,8; 2017,Jan,8; 2016,Jan,13; 2015,Jan,16

92020 Gonioscopy (separate procedure)

EXCLUDES *Gonioscopy under general anesthesia (92018)*
Laser trabeculostomy ab interno (0621T-0622T)

Facility RVU 0.60 Non-Facility RVU 0.78 FUD XXX Q1 80

AMA: 2018,Feb,11; 2018,Jan,8; 2017,Jan,8; 2016,Jan,13; 2015,Jan,16

92025 Computerized corneal topography, unilateral or bilateral, with interpretation and report

EXCLUDES *Corneal transplant procedures (65710-65771)*
Manual keratoscopy

Facility RVU 1.07 Non-Facility RVU 1.07 FUD XXX Q1 80

AMA: 2018,Feb,11; 2018,Jan,8; 2017,Jan,8; 2016,Jan,13; 2015,Jan,16

92060 Sensorimotor examination with multiple measurements of ocular deviation (eg, restrictive or paretic muscle with diplopia) with interpretation and report (separate procedure)

Facility RVU 1.79 Non-Facility RVU 1.79 FUD XXX Q1 80

AMA: 2018,Feb,11; 2018,Jan,8; 2017,Jan,8; 2016,Jan,13; 2015,Jan,16

92065 Orthoptic and/or pleoptic training, with continuing medical direction and evaluation

Facility RVU 1.49 Non-Facility RVU 1.49 FUD XXX Q1 80

AMA: 2018,Feb,11; 2018,Jan,8; 2017,Jan,8; 2016,Jan,13; 2015,Jan,16

92071 Fitting of contact lens for treatment of ocular surface disease

EXCLUDES *Contact lens service for keratoconus (92072)*

Code also lens supply with appropriate supply code or (99070)

Facility RVU 0.95 Non-Facility RVU 1.07 FUD XXX N 80 50

AMA: 2018,Feb,11

92072 Fitting of contact lens for management of keratoconus, initial fitting

EXCLUDES *Contact lens service for disease ocular surface (92071)*
Subsequent fittings (99211-99215, 92012-92014)

Code also lens supply with appropriate supply code or (99070)

Facility RVU 2.84 Non-Facility RVU 3.72 FUD XXX N 80

AMA: 2018,Feb,11; 2018,Jan,8; 2017,Sep,14; 2017,Jan,8; 2016,Jan,13; 2015,Jan,16

92081 Visual field examination, unilateral or bilateral, with interpretation and report; limited examination (eg, tangent screen, Autoplot, arc perimeter, or single stimulus level automated test, such as Octopus 3 or 7 equivalent)

INCLUDES Gross visual testing/confrontation testing

Facility RVU 0.96 Non-Facility RVU 0.96 FUD XXX Q1 80

AMA: 2018,Feb,11; 2018,Jan,8; 2017,Jan,8; 2016,Jan,13; 2015,Jan,16

92082 intermediate examination (eg, at least 2 isopters on Goldmann perimeter, or semiquantitative, automated suprathreshold screening program, Humphrey suprathreshold automatic diagnostic test, Octopus program 33)

INCLUDES Gross visual testing/confrontation testing

Facility RVU 1.34 Non-Facility RVU 1.34 FUD XXX Q1 80

AMA: 2018,Feb,11; 2018,Jan,8; 2017,Jan,8; 2016,Jan,13; 2015,Jan,16

92083 extended examination (eg, Goldmann visual fields with at least 3 isopters plotted and static determination within the central 30°, or quantitative, automated threshold perimetry, Octopus program G-1, 32 or 42, Humphrey visual field analyzer full threshold programs 30-2, 24-2, or 30/60-2)

INCLUDES Gross visual field testing/confrontation testing

EXCLUDES *Assessment visual field, by data transmission, by patient to surveillance center (0378T-0379T)*

Facility RVU 1.78 Non-Facility RVU 1.78 FUD XXX Q1 80

AMA: 2018,Feb,11; 2018,Jan,8; 2017,Jan,8; 2016,Jan,13; 2015,Jan,16

92100 Serial tonometry (separate procedure) with multiple measurements of intraocular pressure over an extended time period with interpretation and report, same day (eg, diurnal curve or medical treatment of acute elevation of intraocular pressure)

EXCLUDES *Intraocular pressure monitoring for 24 hours or more (0329T)*
Ocular blood flow measurements (0198T)
Single-episode tonometry (99202-99215, 92002-92004)

Facility RVU 0.96 Non-Facility RVU 2.32 FUD XXX N 80

AMA: 2018,Feb,11; 2018,Jan,8; 2017,Jan,8; 2016,Jan,13; 2015,Jan,16

92132 Scanning computerized ophthalmic diagnostic imaging, anterior segment, with interpretation and report, unilateral or bilateral

EXCLUDES *Imaging anterior segment with specular microscopy and endothelial cell analysis (92286)*
Scanning computerized ophthalmic diagnostic imaging optic nerve and retina (92133-92134)
Tear film imaging (0330T)

Facility RVU 0.89 Non-Facility RVU 0.89 FUD XXX Q1 80

AMA: 2018,Feb,11; 2018,Jan,8; 2017,Jan,8; 2016,Jan,13; 2015,Jan,16

92133 Scanning computerized ophthalmic diagnostic imaging, posterior segment, with interpretation and report, unilateral or bilateral; optic nerve

EXCLUDES *Remote imaging for retinal disease (92227-92228)*
Scanning computerized ophthalmic imaging retina same visit (92134)

Facility RVU 1.05 Non-Facility RVU 1.05 FUD XXX Q1 80

AMA: 2018,Feb,11; 2018,Jan,8; 2017,Jan,8; 2016,Jan,13; 2015,Jan,16

92134 retina

EXCLUDES *Remote imaging for retinal disease (92227-92228)*
Scanning computerized ophthalmic imaging retina same visit (92134)

Facility RVU 1.15 Non-Facility RVU 1.15 FUD XXX Q1 80

AMA: 2018,Feb,11; 2018,Jan,8; 2017,Jan,8; 2016,Jan,13; 2015,Jan,16

92136 Ophthalmic biometry by partial coherence interferometry with intraocular lens power calculation

EXCLUDES *Tear film imaging (0330T)*

Facility RVU 1.76 Non-Facility RVU 1.76 FUD XXX Q1 80

AMA: 2018,Feb,11; 2018,Jan,8; 2017,Jan,8; 2016,Jan,13; 2015,Jan,16

92145 Corneal hysteresis determination, by air impulse stimulation, unilateral or bilateral, with interpretation and report

Facility RVU 0.42 Non-Facility RVU 0.42 FUD XXX Q1 80

AMA: 2018,Feb,11

92201-92287 Other Ophthalmology Services

EXCLUDES *Ophthalmological exam under anesthesia (92018)*
Prescription, fitting, and/or medical supervision ocular prosthesis adaptation by physician (99202-99215, 99241-99245, 92002-92014)
Surgical procedures on eye/ocular adnexa (65091-68899 [66987, 66988, 67810])

92201 Ophthalmoscopy, extended; with retinal drawing and scleral depression of peripheral retinal disease (eg, for retinal tear, retinal detachment, retinal tumor) with interpretation and report, unilateral or bilateral
EXCLUDES *Fundus photography with interpretation and report (92250)*
0.65 0.71 FUD XXX 80
AMA: 2019,Dec,3

92202 with drawing of optic nerve or macula (eg, for glaucoma, macular pathology, tumor) with interpretation and report, unilateral or bilateral
EXCLUDES *Fundus photography with interpretation and report (92250)*
0.42 0.45 FUD XXX 80
AMA: 2019,Dec,3

▲ **92227 Imaging of retina for detection or monitoring of disease; with remote clinical staff review and report, unilateral or bilateral**
EXCLUDES *Fundus photography with interpretation and report (92250)*
Imaging for retinal disease:
Point of care automated analysis and report (92229)
Remote interpretation and report (92228)
Scanning computerized ophthalmic imaging:
Optic nerve (92133)
Retina (92134)
0.40 0.40 FUD XXX ★ Q1 80 TC
AMA: 2019,Aug,10; 2018,Feb,11; 2018,Jan,8; 2017,Jan,8; 2016,Jul,8; 2016,Jan,13; 2015,Jan,16

▲ **92228 with remote physician or other qualified health care professional interpretation and report, unilateral or bilateral**
EXCLUDES *Fundus photography with interpretation and report (92250)*
Imaging for retinal disease:
Point of care automated analysis and report (92229)
Remote clinical staff review and report (92227)
Scanning computerized ophthalmic imaging:
Optic nerve (92133)
Retina (92134)
0.96 0.96 FUD XXX ★ Q1 80
AMA: 2018,Feb,11; 2018,Jan,8; 2017,Jan,8; 2016,Jan,13; 2015,Jan,16

● **92229 point-of-care automated analysis and report, unilateral or bilateral**
EXCLUDES *Fundus photography with interpretation and report (92250)*
Remote imaging for retinal disease (92227-92228)
Scanning computerized ophthalmic imaging:
Optic nerve (92133)
Retina (92134)

92230 Fluorescein angioscopy with interpretation and report
0.95 1.83 FUD XXX Q1 80
AMA: 2018,Feb,11; 2018,Jan,8; 2017,Jan,8; 2016,Jan,13; 2015,Jan,16

92235 Fluorescein angiography (includes multiframe imaging) with interpretation and report, unilateral or bilateral
EXCLUDES *Fluorescein and indocyanine-green angiography (92242)*
2.59 2.59 FUD XXX S 80
AMA: 2018,Feb,11; 2018,Jan,8; 2017,Jun,8; 2017,Jan,8; 2016,Jan,13; 2015,Jan,16

92240 Indocyanine-green angiography (includes multiframe imaging) with interpretation and report, unilateral or bilateral
EXCLUDES *Fluorescein and indocyanine-green angiography (92242)*
5.69 5.69 FUD XXX S 80
AMA: 2018,Feb,11; 2018,Jan,8; 2017,Jun,8; 2017,Jan,8; 2016,Jan,13; 2015,Jan,16

92242 Fluorescein angiography and indocyanine-green angiography (includes multiframe imaging) performed at the same patient encounter with interpretation and report, unilateral or bilateral
6.71 6.71 FUD XXX S 80
AMA: 2018,Feb,11; 2018,Jan,8; 2017,Jun,8

92250 Fundus photography with interpretation and report
1.27 1.27 FUD XXX Q1 80
AMA: 2019,Dec,3; 2018,Feb,11; 2018,Jan,8; 2017,Jan,8; 2016,Jul,8; 2016,Jan,13; 2015,May,9; 2015,Jan,16

92260 Ophthalmodynamometry
0.31 0.55 FUD XXX Q1 80
AMA: 2018,Feb,11; 2018,Jan,8; 2017,Jan,8; 2016,Jan,13; 2015,Jan,16

92265 Needle oculoelectromyography, 1 or more extraocular muscles, 1 or both eyes, with interpretation and report
2.48 2.48 FUD XXX Q1 80
AMA: 2018,Feb,11; 2018,Jan,8; 2017,Jan,8; 2016,Jan,13; 2015,Jan,16

92270 Electro-oculography with interpretation and report
EXCLUDES *Recording saccadic eye movement (92700)*
Vestibular function testing (92537-92538, 92540-92542, 92544-92549)
2.73 2.73 FUD XXX Q1 80
AMA: 2020,Apr,7; 2018,Feb,11; 2018,Jan,8; 2017,Jan,8; 2016,Jan,13; 2015,Sep,7; 2015,Jan,16

92273 Electroretinography (ERG), with interpretation and report; full field (ie, ffERG, flash ERG, Ganzfeld ERG)
EXCLUDES *Pattern electroretinography (PERG) (0509T)*
3.78 3.78 FUD XXX 80
AMA: 2019,Jan,12

92274 multifocal (mfERG)
EXCLUDES *Pattern electroretinography (PERG) (0509T)*
2.56 2.56 FUD XXX 80
AMA: 2019,Jan,12

92283 Color vision examination, extended, eg, anomaloscope or equivalent
1.52 1.52 FUD XXX Q1 80
AMA: 2018,Feb,11; 2018,Jan,8; 2017,Jan,8; 2016,Jan,13; 2015,Jan,16

92284 Dark adaptation examination with interpretation and report
1.74 1.74 FUD XXX Q1 80
AMA: 2018,Feb,11; 2018,Jan,8; 2017,Jan,8; 2016,Jan,13; 2015,Jan,16

92285 External ocular photography with interpretation and report for documentation of medical progress (eg, close-up photography, slit lamp photography, goniophotography, stereo-photography)
0.61 0.61 FUD XXX Q1 80
AMA: 2018,Feb,11; 2018,Jan,8; 2017,Jan,8; 2016,Jan,13; 2015,Jan,16

92286 Anterior segment imaging with interpretation and report; with specular microscopy and endothelial cell analysis
1.10 1.10 FUD XXX Q1 80
AMA: 2018,Feb,11; 2018,Jan,8; 2017,Jan,8; 2016,Jan,13; 2015,Jan,16

92287 **with fluorescein angiography**
Facility RVU 4.46 Non-Facility RVU 4.46 FUD XXX Q1 80 CCI
AMA: 2018,Feb,11; 2018,Jan,8; 2017,Jan,8; 2016,Jan,13; 2015,Jan,16

92310-92326 Services Related to Contact Lenses

CMS: 100-02,15,30.4 Optometrist's Services

INCLUDES Incidental revision lens during training period
Patient training/instruction
Specification optical/physical characteristics:
Curvature
Flexibility
Gas-permeability
Power
Size

EXCLUDES *Extended wear lenses follow up (92012-92014)*
General ophthalmological services
Therapeutic/surgical use contact lens (68340, 92071-92072)

92310 **Prescription of optical and physical characteristics of and fitting of contact lens, with medical supervision of adaptation; corneal lens, both eyes, except for aphakia**
Code also modifier 52 for prescription and fitting only one eye
Facility RVU 1.71 Non-Facility RVU 2.86 FUD XXX E CCI
AMA: 2018,Feb,11; 2018,Jan,8; 2017,Jan,8; 2016,Jan,13; 2015,Jan,16

92311 **corneal lens for aphakia, 1 eye**
Facility RVU 1.54 Non-Facility RVU 2.95 FUD XXX Q1 80 CCI
AMA: 2018,Feb,11; 2018,Jan,8; 2017,Jan,8; 2016,Jan,13; 2015,Jan,16

92312 **corneal lens for aphakia, both eyes**
Facility RVU 1.77 Non-Facility RVU 3.42 FUD XXX Q1 80 CCI
AMA: 2018,Feb,11; 2018,Jan,8; 2017,Jan,8; 2016,Jan,13; 2015,Jan,16

92313 **corneoscleral lens**
Facility RVU 1.31 Non-Facility RVU 2.78 FUD XXX Q1 80 CCI
AMA: 2018,Feb,11; 2018,Jan,8; 2017,Jan,8; 2016,Jan,13; 2015,Jan,16

92314 **Prescription of optical and physical characteristics of contact lens, with medical supervision of adaptation and direction of fitting by independent technician; corneal lens, both eyes except for aphakia**
Code also modifier 52 for prescription and fitting only one eye
Facility RVU 1.02 Non-Facility RVU 2.43 FUD XXX E CCI
AMA: 2018,Feb,11; 2018,Jan,8; 2017,Jan,8; 2016,Jan,13; 2015,Jan,16

92315 **corneal lens for aphakia, 1 eye**
Facility RVU 0.62 Non-Facility RVU 2.19 FUD XXX Q1 80 CCI
AMA: 2018,Feb,11; 2018,Jan,8; 2017,Jan,8; 2016,Jan,13; 2015,Jan,16

92316 **corneal lens for aphakia, both eyes**
Facility RVU 0.93 Non-Facility RVU 2.72 FUD XXX Q1 80 CCI
AMA: 2018,Feb,11; 2018,Jan,8; 2017,Jan,8; 2016,Jan,13; 2015,Jan,16

92317 **corneoscleral lens**
Facility RVU 0.62 Non-Facility RVU 2.29 FUD XXX Q1 80 CCI
AMA: 2018,Feb,11; 2018,Jan,8; 2017,Jan,8; 2016,Jan,13; 2015,Jan,16

92325 **Modification of contact lens (separate procedure), with medical supervision of adaptation**
Facility RVU 1.24 Non-Facility RVU 1.24 FUD XXX Q1 80 CCI
AMA: 2018,Feb,11; 2018,Jan,8; 2017,Jan,8; 2016,Jan,13; 2015,Jan,16

92326 **Replacement of contact lens**
Facility RVU 1.05 Non-Facility RVU 1.05 FUD XXX Q1 80 CCI
AMA: 2018,Feb,11; 2018,Jan,8; 2017,Jan,8; 2016,Jan,13; 2015,Jan,16

92340-92499 Services Related to Eyeglasses

CMS: 100-02,15,30.4 Optometrist's Services

INCLUDES Anatomical facial characteristics measurement
Final adjustment of spectacles to visual axes/anatomical topography
Written laboratory specifications

EXCLUDES *Materials supply*

92340 **Fitting of spectacles, except for aphakia; monofocal**
Facility RVU 0.53 Non-Facility RVU 0.99 FUD XXX E CCI
AMA: 2018,Feb,11; 2018,Jan,8; 2017,Jan,8; 2016,Jan,13; 2015,Jan,16

92341 **bifocal**
Facility RVU 0.70 Non-Facility RVU 1.15 FUD XXX E CCI
AMA: 2018,Feb,11; 2018,Jan,8; 2017,Jan,8; 2016,Jan,13; 2015,Jan,16

92342 **multifocal, other than bifocal**
Facility RVU 0.77 Non-Facility RVU 1.23 FUD XXX E CCI
AMA: 2018,Feb,11; 2018,Jan,8; 2017,Jan,8; 2016,Jan,13; 2015,Jan,16

92352 **Fitting of spectacle prosthesis for aphakia; monofocal**
Facility RVU 0.53 Non-Facility RVU 1.17 FUD XXX Q1 CCI
AMA: 2018,Feb,11; 2018,Jan,8; 2017,Jan,8; 2016,Jan,13; 2015,Jan,16

92353 **multifocal**
Facility RVU 0.72 Non-Facility RVU 1.36 FUD XXX Q1 CCI
AMA: 2018,Feb,11; 2018,Jan,8; 2017,Jan,8; 2016,Jan,13; 2015,Jan,16

92354 **Fitting of spectacle mounted low vision aid; single element system**
Facility RVU 0.38 Non-Facility RVU 0.38 FUD XXX Q1 CCI
AMA: 2018,Feb,11; 2018,Jan,8; 2017,Jan,8; 2016,Jan,13; 2015,Jan,16

92355 **telescopic or other compound lens system**
Facility RVU 0.58 Non-Facility RVU 0.58 FUD XXX Q1 CCI
AMA: 2018,Feb,11; 2018,Jan,8; 2017,Jan,8; 2016,Jan,13; 2015,Jan,16

92358 **Prosthesis service for aphakia, temporary (disposable or loan, including materials)**
Facility RVU 0.32 Non-Facility RVU 0.32 FUD XXX Q1 CCI
AMA: 2018,Feb,11; 2018,Jan,8; 2017,Jan,8; 2016,Jan,13; 2015,Jan,16

92370 **Repair and refitting spectacles; except for aphakia**
Facility RVU 0.46 Non-Facility RVU 0.88 FUD XXX E CCI
AMA: 2018,Feb,11; 2018,Jan,8; 2017,Jan,8; 2016,Jan,13; 2015,Jan,16

92371 **spectacle prosthesis for aphakia**
Facility RVU 0.33 Non-Facility RVU 0.33 FUD XXX Q1 CCI
AMA: 2018,Feb,11; 2018,Jan,8; 2017,Jan,8; 2016,Jan,13; 2015,Jan,16

92499 **Unlisted ophthalmological service or procedure**
Facility RVU 0.00 Non-Facility RVU 0.00 FUD XXX Q1 80 CCI
AMA: 2020,Aug,14; 2019,Jan,12; 2018,Jul,3; 2018,Feb,11; 2018,Jan,8; 2017,Jan,8; 2016,Jan,13; 2015,Jan,16

92502-92526 [92517, 92518, 92519] Special Procedures of the Ears/Nose/Throat

INCLUDES Anterior rhinoscopy, tuning fork testing, otoscopy, or removal non-impacted cerumen
Diagnostic/treatment services not generally included in E/M service

EXCLUDES *Laryngoscopy with stroboscopy (31579)*

92502 **Otolaryngologic examination under general anesthesia**
Facility RVU 2.73 Non-Facility RVU 2.73 FUD 000 T 80 CCI
AMA: 2018,Feb,11; 2018,Jan,8; 2017,Jan,8; 2016,Sep,6

92504 **Binocular microscopy (separate diagnostic procedure)**
Facility RVU 0.27 Non-Facility RVU 0.83 FUD XXX N 80 CCI
AMA: 2018,Feb,11; 2018,Jan,8; 2017,Jan,8; 2016,Sep,6; 2016,Jan,13; 2015,Jan,16

92507 **Treatment of speech, language, voice, communication, and/or auditory processing disorder; individual**

EXCLUDES *Adaptive behavior treatment ([97153], [97155])*
Auditory rehabilitation:
Postlingual hearing loss (92633)
Prelingual hearing loss (92630)
Programming cochlear implant (92601-92604)

2.25 2.25 FUD XXX A 80

AMA: 2018,Dec,7; 2018,Dec,7; 2018,Nov,3; 2018,Feb,11; 2018,Jan,8; 2017,Jan,8; 2016,Sep,6; 2016,Jan,13; 2015,Jan,16

92508 **group, 2 or more individuals**

EXCLUDES *Adaptive behavior treatment ([97154], [97158])*
Auditory rehabilitation:
Postlingual hearing loss (92633)
Prelingual hearing loss (92630)
Programming cochlear implant (92601-92604)

0.67 0.67 FUD XXX A 80

AMA: 2018,Nov,3; 2018,Feb,11; 2018,Jan,8; 2017,Jan,8; 2016,Sep,6; 2016,Jan,13; 2015,Jan,16

92511 **Nasopharyngoscopy with endoscope (separate procedure)**

EXCLUDES *Diagnostic flexible laryngoscopy (31575)*
Nasopharyngoscopic dilation eustachian tube (69705-69706)
Transnasal esophagoscopy (43197-43198)

1.08 3.15 FUD 000 T 80

AMA: 2018,Feb,11; 2018,Jan,8; 2017,Jul,7; 2017,Jan,8; 2016,Dec,13; 2016,Sep,6

92512 **Nasal function studies (eg, rhinomanometry)**

0.80 1.68 FUD XXX S 80

AMA: 2018,Feb,11; 2018,Jan,8; 2017,Jan,8; 2016,Sep,6

92516 **Facial nerve function studies (eg, electroneuronography)**

0.65 1.94 FUD XXX S 80

AMA: 2018,Feb,11; 2018,Jan,8; 2017,Jan,8; 2016,Sep,6

92517 **Resequenced code. See code following 92549.**

92518 **Resequenced code. See code following 92549.**

92519 **Resequenced code. See code following 92549.**

92520 **Laryngeal function studies (ie, aerodynamic testing and acoustic testing)**

EXCLUDES *Other laryngeal function testing (92700)*
Swallowing/laryngeal sensory testing with flexible fiberoptic endoscope (92611-92617)

Code also modifier 52 for single test

1.17 2.28 FUD XXX Q1 80

AMA: 2018,Feb,11; 2018,Jan,8; 2017,Jan,8; 2016,Sep,6; 2016,Jan,13; 2015,Jan,16

92521 **Evaluation of speech fluency (eg, stuttering, cluttering)**

INCLUDES Ability to execute motor movements needed for speech
Comprehension written and verbal expression
Determination patient's ability to create and communicate expressive thought
Evaluation ability to produce speech sound

3.21 3.21 FUD XXX A 80

AMA: 2018,Feb,11; 2018,Jan,8; 2017,Jan,8; 2016,Sep,6; 2016,Jan,13; 2015,Jan,16

92522 **Evaluation of speech sound production (eg, articulation, phonological process, apraxia, dysarthria);**

INCLUDES Ability to execute motor movements needed for speech
Comprehension written and verbal expression
Determination patient's ability to create and communicate expressive thought
Evaluation ability to produce speech sound

2.60 2.60 FUD XXX A 80

AMA: 2018,Feb,11; 2018,Jan,8; 2017,Jan,8; 2016,Sep,6; 2016,Jan,13; 2015,Jan,16

92523 **with evaluation of language comprehension and expression (eg, receptive and expressive language)**

INCLUDES Ability to execute motor movements needed for speech
Comprehension written and verbal expression
Determination patient's ability to create and communicate expressive thought
Evaluation ability to produce speech sound

5.54 5.54 FUD XXX A 80

AMA: 2018,Feb,11; 2018,Jan,8; 2017,Jan,8; 2016,Sep,6; 2016,Jan,13; 2015,Jan,16

92524 **Behavioral and qualitative analysis of voice and resonance**

INCLUDES Ability to execute motor movements needed for speech
Comprehension written and verbal expression
Determination patient's ability to create and communicate expressive thought
Evaluation ability to produce speech sound

2.51 2.51 FUD XXX A 80

AMA: 2018,Feb,11; 2018,Jan,8; 2017,Jan,8; 2016,Sep,6; 2016,Jan,13; 2015,Jan,16

92526 **Treatment of swallowing dysfunction and/or oral function for feeding**

2.48 2.48 FUD XXX A 80

AMA: 2018,Feb,11; 2018,Jan,8; 2017,Jan,8; 2016,Sep,6

92531-92519 [92517, 92518, 92519] Vestibular Function Tests

92531 **Spontaneous nystagmus, including gaze**

EXCLUDES *When performed with E/M services (99202-99215, 99218-99223 [99224, 99225, 99226], 99231-99236, 99241-99245, 99304-99318, 99324-99337)*

0.00 0.00 FUD XXX N

AMA: 2020,Aug,14; 2018,Feb,11

92532 **Positional nystagmus test**

EXCLUDES *When performed with E/M services (99202-99215, 99218-99223 [99224, 99225, 99226], 99231-99236, 99241-99245, 99304-99318, 99324-99337)*

0.00 0.00 FUD XXX N

AMA: 2020,Aug,14; 2018,Feb,11

92533 **Caloric vestibular test, each irrigation (binaural, bithermal stimulation constitutes 4 tests)**

INCLUDES Barany caloric test

0.00 0.00 FUD XXX N

AMA: 2020,Aug,14; 2018,Feb,11; 2018,Jan,8; 2017,Jan,8; 2016,Jan,13; 2015,Jan,16

92534 **Optokinetic nystagmus test**

0.00 0.00 FUD XXX N

AMA: 2020,Aug,14; 2018,Feb,11

92537 **Caloric vestibular test with recording, bilateral; bithermal (ie, one warm and one cool irrigation in each ear for a total of four irrigations)**

EXCLUDES *Electro-oculography (92270)*
Monothermal caloric vestibular test (92538)

Code also modifier 52 when only three irrigations performed

1.18 1.18 FUD XXX S 80

AMA: 2020,Aug,14; 2018,Feb,11; 2015,Sep,7

92538 **monothermal (ie, one irrigation in each ear for a total of two irrigations)**

EXCLUDES *Bithermal caloric vestibular test (92537)*
Electro-oculography (92270)

Code also modifier 52 only one irrigation performed

0.64 0.64 FUD XXX S 80

AMA: 2020,Aug,14; 2018,Feb,11; 2015,Sep,7

92540 Basic vestibular evaluation, includes spontaneous nystagmus test with eccentric gaze fixation nystagmus, with recording, positional nystagmus test, minimum of 4 positions, with recording, optokinetic nystagmus test, bidirectional foveal and peripheral stimulation, with recording, and oscillating tracking test, with recording

EXCLUDES *Vestibular function tests (92270, 92541-92542, 92544-92545)*

3.04 3.04 FUD XXX S 80

AMA: 2020,Aug,14; 2018,Feb,11; 2018,Jan,8; 2017,Jan,8; 2016,Jan,13; 2015,Sep,7

92541 Spontaneous nystagmus test, including gaze and fixation nystagmus, with recording

EXCLUDES *Vestibular function tests (92270, 92540, 92542, 92544-92545)*

0.71 0.71 FUD XXX Q1 80

AMA: 2020,Aug,14; 2019,Jan,12; 2018,Feb,11; 2018,Jan,8; 2017,Jan,8; 2016,Jan,13; 2015,Sep,7; 2015,Jan,16

92542 Positional nystagmus test, minimum of 4 positions, with recording

EXCLUDES *Vestibular function tests (92270, 92540-92541, 92544-92545)*

0.84 0.84 FUD XXX Q1 80

AMA: 2020,Aug,14; 2018,Feb,11; 2018,Jan,8; 2017,Jan,8; 2016,Jan,13; 2015,Sep,7; 2015,Jan,16

92544 Optokinetic nystagmus test, bidirectional, foveal or peripheral stimulation, with recording

EXCLUDES *Vestibular function tests (92270, 92540-92542, 92545)*

0.49 0.49 FUD XXX S 80

AMA: 2020,Aug,14; 2018,Feb,11; 2018,Jan,8; 2017,Jan,8; 2016,Jan,13; 2015,Sep,7; 2015,Jan,16

92545 Oscillating tracking test, with recording

EXCLUDES *Vestibular function tests (92270, 92540-92542, 92544)*

0.47 0.47 FUD XXX S 80

AMA: 2020,Aug,14; 2018,Feb,11; 2018,Jan,8; 2017,Jan,8; 2016,Jan,13; 2015,Sep,7; 2015,Jan,16

92546 Sinusoidal vertical axis rotational testing

EXCLUDES *Electro-oculography (92270)*

2.95 2.95 FUD XXX S 80

AMA: 2020,Aug,14; 2018,Feb,11; 2018,Jan,8; 2017,Jan,8; 2016,Jan,13; 2015,Sep,7; 2015,Jan,16

\+ **92547 Use of vertical electrodes (List separately in addition to code for primary procedure)**

EXCLUDES *Electro-oculography (92270)*
Unlisted vestibular tests (92700)

Code first (92540-92546)

0.21 0.21 FUD ZZZ N 80 TC

AMA: 2020,Aug,14; 2018,Feb,11; 2018,Jan,8; 2017,Jan,8; 2016,Jan,13; 2015,Sep,7; 2015,Jan,16

92548 Computerized dynamic posturography sensory organization test (CDP-SOT), 6 conditions (ie, eyes open, eyes closed, visual sway, platform sway, eyes closed platform sway, platform and visual sway), including interpretation and report;

EXCLUDES *Electro-oculography (92270)*

1.41 1.41 FUD XXX Q1 80

AMA: 2020,Aug,14; 2020,Apr,7; 2018,Feb,11; 2018,Jan,8; 2017,Jan,8; 2016,Jan,13; 2015,Sep,7; 2015,Jan,16

92549 with motor control test (MCT) and adaptation test (ADT)

EXCLUDES *Electro-oculography (92270)*

1.80 1.80 FUD XXX 80

AMA: 2020,Aug,14; 2020,Apr,7

● # **92517 Vestibular evoked myogenic potential (VEMP) testing, with interpretation and report; cervical (cVEMP)**

EXCLUDES *Electro-oculography (92270)*
Vestibular evoked myogenic potential testing:
Cervical and ocular ([92519])
Ocular ([92518])

0.00 0.00 FUD 000

● # **92518 ocular (oVEMP)**

EXCLUDES *Electro-oculography (92270)*
Vestibular evoked myogenic potential testing:
Cervical ([92517])
Cervical and ocular ([92519])

0.00 0.00 FUD 000

● # **92519 cervical (cVEMP) and ocular (oVEMP)**

EXCLUDES *Electro-oculography (92270)*
Vestibular evoked myogenic potential testing:
Cervical only ([92517])
Ocular only ([92518])

0.00 0.00 FUD 000

92550-92597 [92558, 92597, 92650, 92651, 92652, 92653] Hearing and Speech Tests

INCLUDES Calibrated electronic equipment, recording results, and report with interpretation
Diagnostic/treatment services not generally included in comprehensive otorhinolaryngologic evaluation or office visit
Testing both ears
Tuning fork and whisper tests

EXCLUDES *Evaluation speech/language/hearing problems using performance observation/assessment (92521-92524)*

Code also modifier 52 for unilateral testing

92550 Tympanometry and reflex threshold measurements

INCLUDES Tympanometry, acoustic reflex testing individual codes (92567-92568)

0.62 0.62 FUD XXX Q1 80

AMA: 2018,Feb,11; 2018,Jan,8; 2017,Jan,8; 2016,Jan,13; 2015,Jan,16

92551 Screening test, pure tone, air only

0.33 0.33 FUD XXX E

AMA: 2018,Feb,11; 2018,Jan,8; 2017,Jan,8; 2016,Jan,13; 2015,Jan,16

92552 Pure tone audiometry (threshold); air only

EXCLUDES *Automated test (0208T)*

0.89 0.89 FUD XXX Q1 80 TC

AMA: 2018,Feb,11; 2018,Jan,8; 2017,Jan,8; 2016,Jan,13; 2015,Jan,16

92553 air and bone

EXCLUDES *Automated test (0209T)*

1.08 1.08 FUD XXX Q1 80 TC

AMA: 2018,Feb,11; 2018,Jan,8; 2017,Jan,8; 2016,Jan,13; 2015,Jan,16

92555 Speech audiometry threshold;

EXCLUDES *Automated test (0210T)*

0.68 0.68 FUD XXX Q1 80 TC

AMA: 2018,Feb,11; 2018,Jan,8; 2017,Jan,8; 2016,Jan,13; 2015,Jan,16

92556 with speech recognition

EXCLUDES *Automated test (0211T)*

1.07 1.07 FUD XXX Q1 80 TC

AMA: 2018,Feb,11; 2018,Jan,8; 2017,Jan,8; 2016,Jan,13; 2015,Jan,16

92557 Comprehensive audiometry threshold evaluation and speech recognition (92553 and 92556 combined)

EXCLUDES *Automated test (0208T-0212T)*
Evaluation/selection hearing aid (92590-92595)

0.93 1.08 FUD XXX Q1 80

AMA: 2018,Feb,11; 2018,Jan,8; 2017,Jan,8; 2016,Jan,13; 2015,Jan,16

92558 **Resequenced code. See code before 92587.**

92559 Audiometric testing of groups

INCLUDES For group testing, indicate tests performed

0.00 0.00 FUD XXX E

AMA: 2018,Feb,11; 2018,Jan,8; 2017,Jan,8; 2016,Jan,13; 2015,Jan,16

92560 Bekesy audiometry; screening
0.00 0.00 FUD XXX E
AMA: 2018,Feb,11; 2018,Jan,8; 2017,Jan,8; 2016,Jan,13; 2015,Jan,16

92561 diagnostic
1.10 1.10 FUD XXX Q1 80 TC
AMA: 2018,Feb,11; 2018,Jan,8; 2017,Jan,8; 2016,Jan,13; 2015,Jan,16

92562 Loudness balance test, alternate binaural or monaural
INCLUDES ABLB test
1.28 1.28 FUD XXX Q1 80 TC
AMA: 2018,Feb,11; 2018,Jan,8; 2017,Jan,8; 2016,Jan,13; 2015,Jan,16

92563 Tone decay test
0.87 0.87 FUD XXX Q1 80 TC
AMA: 2018,Feb,11; 2018,Jan,8; 2017,Jan,8; 2016,Jan,13; 2015,Jan,16

92564 Short increment sensitivity index (SISI)
0.71 0.71 FUD XXX Q1 80 TC
AMA: 2018,Feb,11; 2018,Jan,8; 2017,Jan,8; 2016,Jan,13; 2015,Jan,16

92565 Stenger test, pure tone
0.44 0.44 FUD XXX Q1 80 TC
AMA: 2018,Feb,11; 2018,Jan,8; 2017,Jan,8; 2016,Jan,13; 2015,Jan,16

92567 Tympanometry (impedance testing)
0.31 0.43 FUD XXX Q1 80
AMA: 2018,Feb,11; 2018,Jan,8; 2017,Jan,8; 2016,Jan,13; 2015,Jan,16

92568 Acoustic reflex testing, threshold
0.44 0.45 FUD XXX Q1 80
AMA: 2018,Feb,11; 2018,Jan,8; 2017,Jan,8; 2016,Jan,13; 2015,Jan,16

92570 Acoustic immittance testing, includes tympanometry (impedance testing), acoustic reflex threshold testing, and acoustic reflex decay testing
INCLUDES Tympanometry, acoustic reflex testing individual codes (92567-92568)
0.85 0.94 FUD XXX Q1 80
AMA: 2018,Feb,11; 2018,Jan,8; 2017,Jan,8; 2016,Jan,13; 2015,Jan,16

92571 Filtered speech test
0.76 0.76 FUD XXX Q1 80 TC
AMA: 2018,Feb,11; 2018,Jan,8; 2017,Jan,8; 2016,Jan,13; 2015,Jan,16

92572 Staggered spondaic word test
1.21 1.21 FUD XXX Q1 80 TC
AMA: 2018,Feb,11; 2018,Jan,8; 2017,Jan,8; 2016,Jan,13; 2015,Jan,16

92575 Sensorineural acuity level test
1.79 1.79 FUD XXX Q1 80 TC
AMA: 2018,Feb,11; 2018,Jan,8; 2017,Jan,8; 2016,Jan,13; 2015,Jan,16

92576 Synthetic sentence identification test
1.02 1.02 FUD XXX Q1 80 TC
AMA: 2018,Feb,11; 2018,Jan,8; 2017,Jan,8; 2016,Jan,13; 2015,Jan,16

92577 Stenger test, speech
0.39 0.39 FUD XXX Q1 80 TC
AMA: 2018,Feb,11; 2018,Jan,8; 2017,Jan,8; 2016,Jan,13; 2015,Jan,16

92579 Visual reinforcement audiometry (VRA)
1.09 1.31 FUD XXX Q1 80
AMA: 2018,Feb,11; 2018,Jan,8; 2017,Jan,8; 2016,Jan,13; 2015,Jan,16

92582 Conditioning play audiometry
2.06 2.06 FUD XXX Q1 80 TC
AMA: 2018,Feb,11; 2018,Jan,8; 2017,Jan,8; 2016,Jan,13; 2015,Jan,16

92583 Select picture audiometry
1.35 1.35 FUD XXX Q1 80 TC
AMA: 2018,Feb,11; 2018,Jan,8; 2017,Jan,8; 2016,Jan,13; 2015,Jan,16

92584 Electrocochleography
2.09 2.09 FUD XXX S 80 TC
AMA: 2018,Feb,11; 2018,Jan,8; 2017,Jan,8; 2016,Jan,13; 2015,Jan,16

92585 ~~Auditory evoked potentials for evoked response audiometry and/or testing of the central nervous system; comprehensive~~
To report, see ([92652], [92653])

92586 ~~limited~~
To report, see ([92650], [92651])

● # **92650 Auditory evoked potentials; screening of auditory potential with broadband stimuli, automated analysis**
0.00 0.00 FUD 000

● # **92651 for hearing status determination, broadband stimuli, with interpretation and report**
0.00 0.00 FUD 000

● # **92652 for threshold estimation at multiple frequencies, with interpretation and report**
EXCLUDES *Hearing status determination ([92651])*
0.00 0.00 FUD 000

● # **92653 neurodiagnostic, with interpretation and report**
0.00 0.00 FUD 000

92558 Evoked otoacoustic emissions, screening (qualitative measurement of distortion product or transient evoked otoacoustic emissions), automated analysis
0.25 0.28 FUD XXX E
AMA: 2018,Feb,11; 2018,Jan,8; 2017,Jan,8; 2016,Jan,13; 2015,Jan,16

92587 Distortion product evoked otoacoustic emissions; limited evaluation (to confirm the presence or absence of hearing disorder, 3-6 frequencies) or transient evoked otoacoustic emissions, with interpretation and report
0.63 0.63 FUD XXX S 80
AMA: 2018,Feb,11; 2018,Jan,8; 2017,Jan,8; 2016,Jan,13; 2015,Jan,16

92588 comprehensive diagnostic evaluation (quantitative analysis of outer hair cell function by cochlear mapping, minimum of 12 frequencies), with interpretation and report
EXCLUDES *Evaluation central auditory function (92620-92621)*
0.96 0.96 FUD XXX S 80
AMA: 2018,Feb,11; 2018,Jan,8; 2017,Jan,8; 2016,Jan,13; 2015,Jan,16

92590 Hearing aid examination and selection; monaural
0.00 0.00 FUD XXX E
AMA: 2020,Jul,3; 2018,Feb,11; 2018,Jan,8; 2017,Jan,8; 2016,Jan,13; 2015,Jan,16

92591 binaural
0.00 0.00 FUD XXX E
AMA: 2020,Jul,3; 2018,Feb,11; 2018,Jan,8; 2017,Jan,8; 2016,Jan,13; 2015,Jan,16

92592 Hearing aid check; monaural
0.00 0.00 FUD XXX E
AMA: 2020,Jul,3; 2018,Feb,11; 2018,Jan,8; 2017,Jan,8; 2016,Jan,13; 2015,Jan,16

92593 binaural
0.00 0.00 FUD XXX E
AMA: 2020,Jul,3; 2018,Feb,11; 2018,Jan,8; 2017,Jan,8; 2016,Jan,13; 2015,Jan,16

92594 **Electroacoustic evaluation for hearing aid; monaural**
0.00 0.00 FUD XXX E
AMA: 2020,Jul,3; 2018,Feb,11; 2018,Jan,8; 2017,Jan,8; 2016,Jan,13; 2015,Jan,16

92595 **binaural**
0.00 0.00 FUD XXX E
AMA: 2020,Jul,3; 2018,Feb,11; 2018,Jan,8; 2017,Jan,8; 2016,Jan,13; 2015,Jan,16

92596 **Ear protector attenuation measurements**
1.89 1.89 FUD XXX Q1 80 TC
AMA: 2018,Feb,11; 2018,Jan,8; 2017,Jan,8; 2016,Jan,13; 2015,Jan,16

92597 **Resequenced code. See code following 92604.**

92601-92609 [92597, 92618] Services Related to Hearing and Speech Devices

INCLUDES Diagnostic/treatment services not generally included in comprehensive otorhinolaryngologic evaluation or office visit

92601 **Diagnostic analysis of cochlear implant, patient younger than 7 years of age; with programming** A
INCLUDES Connection to cochlear implant
Postoperative analysis/fitting previously placed external devices
Stimulator programming
EXCLUDES *Cochlear implant placement (69930)*
3.57 4.68 FUD XXX S 80
AMA: 2020,Jul,3; 2018,Feb,11; 2018,Jan,8; 2017,Jan,8; 2016,Sep,6; 2016,Jan,13; 2015,Jan,16

92602 **subsequent reprogramming** A
INCLUDES Internal stimulator re-programming
Subsequent sessions for external transmitter measurements/adjustment
EXCLUDES *Analysis with programming (92601)*
Aural rehabilitation services after cochlear implant (92626-92627, 92630-92633)
Cochlear implant placement (69930)
2.02 2.92 FUD XXX S 80
AMA: 2020,Jul,3; 2018,Feb,11; 2018,Jan,8; 2017,Jan,8; 2016,Sep,6; 2016,Jan,13; 2015,Jan,16

92603 **Diagnostic analysis of cochlear implant, age 7 years or older; with programming** A
INCLUDES Connection to cochlear implant
Postoperative analysis/fitting previously placed external devices
Stimulator programming
EXCLUDES *Cochlear implant placement (69930)*
3.47 4.37 FUD XXX S 80
AMA: 2020,Jul,3; 2018,Feb,11; 2018,Jan,8; 2017,Jan,8; 2016,Sep,6; 2016,Jan,13; 2015,Jan,16

92604 **subsequent reprogramming** A
INCLUDES Internal stimulator reprogramming
Subsequent sessions for external transmitter measurements/adjustment
EXCLUDES *Analysis with programming (92603)*
Cochlear implant placement (69930)
1.94 2.60 FUD XXX S 80
AMA: 2020,Jul,3; 2018,Feb,11; 2018,Jan,8; 2017,Jan,8; 2016,Sep,6; 2016,Jan,13; 2015,Jan,16

92597 **Evaluation for use and/or fitting of voice prosthetic device to supplement oral speech**
EXCLUDES *Augmentative or alternative communication device services (92605, [92618], 92607-92608)*
2.06 2.06 FUD XXX A 80
AMA: 2018,Feb,11; 2018,Jan,8; 2017,Jan,8; 2016,Jan,13; 2015,Jan,16

92605 **Evaluation for prescription of non-speech-generating augmentative and alternative communication device, face-to-face with the patient; first hour**
EXCLUDES *Prosthetic voice device fitting or use evaluation (92597)*
2.53 2.65 FUD XXX A
AMA: 2018,Feb,11; 2018,Jan,8; 2017,Jan,8; 2016,Jan,13; 2015,Jan,16

+ # **92618** **each additional 30 minutes (List separately in addition to code for primary procedure)**
Code first (92605)
0.94 0.96 FUD ZZZ A
AMA: 2018,Feb,11

92606 **Therapeutic service(s) for the use of non-speech-generating device, including programming and modification**
2.02 2.35 FUD XXX A
AMA: 2018,Feb,11; 2018,Jan,8; 2017,Jan,8; 2016,Jan,13; 2015,Jan,16

92607 **Evaluation for prescription for speech-generating augmentative and alternative communication device, face-to-face with the patient; first hour**
EXCLUDES *Evaluation for prescription non-speech generating device (92605)*
Evaluation for use/fitting voice prosthetic (92597)
3.69 3.69 FUD XXX A 80
AMA: 2018,Feb,11; 2018,Jan,8; 2017,Jan,8; 2016,Jan,13; 2015,Jan,16

+ **92608** **each additional 30 minutes (List separately in addition to code for primary procedure)**
Code first initial hour (92607)
1.47 1.47 FUD ZZZ A 80
AMA: 2018,Feb,11; 2018,Jan,8; 2017,Jan,8; 2016,Jan,13; 2015,Jan,16

92609 **Therapeutic services for the use of speech-generating device, including programming and modification**
EXCLUDES *Therapeutic services for use non-speech generating device (92606)*
3.08 3.08 FUD XXX A 80
AMA: 2018,Feb,11; 2018,Jan,8; 2017,Jan,8; 2016,Jan,13; 2015,Jan,16

92610-92618 [92618] Swallowing Evaluations

92610 **Evaluation of oral and pharyngeal swallowing function**
EXCLUDES *Evaluation with flexible endoscope (92612-92617)*
Motion fluoroscopic evaluation swallowing function (92611)
2.06 2.45 FUD XXX A 80
AMA: 2018,Feb,11; 2018,Jan,8; 2017,Apr,8; 2017,Jan,8; 2016,Jan,13; 2015,Jan,16

92611 **Motion fluoroscopic evaluation of swallowing function by cine or video recording**
EXCLUDES *Diagnostic flexible laryngoscopy (31575)*
Evaluation oral/pharyngeal swallowing function (92610)
(74230)
2.55 2.55 FUD XXX A 80
AMA: 2020,Aug,9; 2018,Feb,11; 2018,Jan,8; 2017,Apr,8; 2017,Jan,8; 2016,Sep,6; 2016,Jan,13; 2015,Jan,16

92612 **Flexible endoscopic evaluation of swallowing by cine or video recording;**
EXCLUDES *Diagnostic flexible fiberoptic laryngoscopy (31575)*
Flexible endoscopic examination/testing without cine or video recording (92700)
1.94 5.42 FUD XXX A 80
AMA: 2018,Feb,11; 2018,Jan,8; 2017,Jul,7; 2017,Apr,8; 2017,Jan,8; 2016,Dec,13; 2016,Sep,6; 2016,Jan,13; 2015,Jan,16

92613 **interpretation and report only**

EXCLUDES *Diagnostic flexible laryngoscopy (31575)*
Oral/pharyngeal swallowing function examination (92610)
Swallowing function motion fluoroscopic examination (92611)

1.07 1.07 FUD XXX B 80

AMA: 2018,Feb,11; 2018,Jan,8; 2017,Jul,7; 2017,Apr,8; 2017,Jan,8; 2016,Dec,13; 2016,Sep,6; 2016,Jan,13; 2015,Jan,16

92614 **Flexible endoscopic evaluation, laryngeal sensory testing by cine or video recording;**

EXCLUDES *Diagnostic flexible laryngoscopy (31575)*
Flexible endoscopic examination/testing without cine or video recording (92700)

1.90 4.03 FUD XXX A 80

AMA: 2018,Feb,11; 2018,Jan,8; 2017,Jul,7; 2017,Apr,8; 2017,Jan,8; 2016,Dec,13; 2016,Sep,6; 2016,Jan,13; 2015,Jan,16

92615 **interpretation and report only**

EXCLUDES *Diagnostic flexible laryngoscopy (31575)*

0.94 0.94 FUD XXX E 80

AMA: 2018,Feb,11; 2018,Jan,8; 2017,Jul,7; 2017,Apr,8; 2017,Jan,8; 2016,Dec,13; 2016,Sep,6; 2016,Jan,13; 2015,Jan,16

92616 **Flexible endoscopic evaluation of swallowing and laryngeal sensory testing by cine or video recording;**

EXCLUDES *Diagnostic flexible fiberoptic laryngoscopy (31575)*
Flexible endoscopic examination/testing without cine or video recording (92700)

2.84 5.85 FUD XXX A 80

AMA: 2018,Feb,11; 2018,Jan,8; 2017,Jul,7; 2017,Apr,8; 2017,Jan,8; 2016,Dec,13; 2016,Sep,6; 2016,Jan,13; 2015,Jan,16

92617 **interpretation and report only**

EXCLUDES *Diagnostic flexible laryngoscopy (31575)*

1.18 1.18 FUD XXX E 80

AMA: 2018,Feb,11; 2018,Jan,8; 2017,Jul,7; 2017,Apr,8; 2017,Jan,8; 2016,Dec,13; 2016,Sep,6; 2016,Jan,13; 2015,Jan,16

92618 **Resequenced code. See code following 92605.**

92620-92700 [92650, 92651, 92652, 92653] Diagnostic Hearing Evaluations and Rehabilitation

INCLUDES Diagnostic/treatment services not generally included in comprehensive otorhinolaryngologic evaluation or office visit

92620 **Evaluation of central auditory function, with report; initial 60 minutes**

EXCLUDES *Voice analysis (92521-92524)*

2.32 2.67 FUD XXX Q1 80

AMA: 2018,Feb,11; 2018,Jan,8; 2017,Jan,8; 2016,Jan,13; 2015,Jan,16

+ **92621** **each additional 15 minutes (List separately in addition to code for primary procedure)**

EXCLUDES *Voice analysis (92521-92524)*

Code first (92620)

0.54 0.64 FUD ZZZ N 80

AMA: 2018,Feb,11; 2018,Jan,8; 2017,Jan,8; 2016,Jan,13; 2015,Jan,16

92625 **Assessment of tinnitus (includes pitch, loudness matching, and masking)**

EXCLUDES *Loudness test (92562)*

Code also modifier 52 for unilateral procedure

1.78 1.99 FUD XXX Q1 80

AMA: 2018,Feb,11; 2018,Jan,8; 2017,Jan,8; 2016,Jan,13; 2015,Jan,16

92626 **Evaluation of auditory function for surgically implanted device(s) candidacy or postoperative status of a surgically implanted device(s); first hour**

INCLUDES Assessment to determine patient's proficiency in remaining hearing to identify speech
Face-to-face time spent with patient or family

EXCLUDES *Hearing aid evaluation, fitting, follow-up, or selection (92590-92591, 92592-92593, 92594-92595)*

2.16 2.55 FUD XXX Q1 80

AMA: 2020,Jul,3; 2018,Feb,11; 2018,Jan,8; 2017,Jan,8; 2016,Sep,6; 2016,Jan,13; 2015,Jan,16

+ **92627** **each additional 15 minutes (List separately in addition to code for primary procedure)**

INCLUDES Assessment to determine patient's proficiency in remaining hearing to identify speech
Face-to-face time spent with patient or family

EXCLUDES *Hearing aid evaluation, fitting, follow-up, or selection (92590-92591, 92592-92593, 92594-92595)*

Code first initial hour (92626)

0.51 0.64 FUD ZZZ N 80

AMA: 2020,Jul,3; 2018,Feb,11; 2018,Jan,8; 2017,Jan,8; 2016,Sep,6; 2016,Jan,13; 2015,Jan,16

92630 **Auditory rehabilitation; prelingual hearing loss**

0.00 0.00 FUD XXX E

AMA: 2018,Feb,11; 2018,Jan,8; 2017,Jan,8; 2016,Sep,6; 2016,Jan,13; 2015,Jan,16

92633 **postlingual hearing loss**

0.00 0.00 FUD XXX E

AMA: 2018,Feb,11; 2018,Jan,8; 2017,Jan,8; 2016,Sep,6; 2016,Jan,13; 2015,Jan,16

92640 **Diagnostic analysis with programming of auditory brainstem implant, per hour**

EXCLUDES *Nonprogramming services (cardiac monitoring)*

2.73 3.25 FUD XXX S 80

AMA: 2018,Feb,11

92650 **Resequenced code. See code following 92584.**

92651 **Resequenced code. See code following 92584.**

92652 **Resequenced code. See code following 92584.**

92653 **Resequenced code. See code following 92584.**

92700 **Unlisted otorhinolaryngological service or procedure**

INCLUDES Lombard test

0.00 0.00 FUD XXX Q1 80

AMA: 2018,Feb,11; 2018,Jan,8; 2017,Apr,8; 2017,Jan,8; 2016,Sep,6; 2016,Jan,13; 2015,Sep,7; 2015,Sep,12; 2015,Jan,16

92920-92953 [92920, 92921, 92924, 92925, 92928, 92929, 92933, 92934, 92937, 92938, 92941, 92943, 92944] Emergency Cardiac Procedures

92920 **Resequenced code. See code following 92998.**

92921 **Resequenced code. See code following 92998.**

92924 **Resequenced code. See code following 92998.**

92925 **Resequenced code. See code following 92998.**

92928 **Resequenced code. See code following 92998.**

92929 **Resequenced code. See code following 92998.**

92933 **Resequenced code. See code following 92998.**

92934 **Resequenced code. See code following 92998.**

92937 **Resequenced code. See code following 92998.**

92938 **Resequenced code. See code following 92998.**

92941 **Resequenced code. See code following 92998.**

92943 **Resequenced code. See code following 92998.**

92944 **Resequenced code. See code following 92998.**

92950 **Cardiopulmonary resuscitation (eg, in cardiac arrest)**
INCLUDES Cardiac defibrillation
EXCLUDES *Critical care services (99291-99292)*
5.35 8.92 FUD 000 S 80
AMA: 2018,Feb,11; 2018,Jan,8; 2017,Jan,8; 2016,Jan,13; 2015,Jan,16

92953 **Temporary transcutaneous pacing**
EXCLUDES *Direction ambulance/rescue personnel by physician or other qualified health care professional (99288)*
0.03 0.03 FUD 000 03 80
AMA: 2019,Aug,8; 2018,Feb,11; 2018,Jan,8; 2017,Jan,8; 2016,Jan,13; 2015,Jan,16

92960-92961 Cardioversion

92960 **Cardioversion, elective, electrical conversion of arrhythmia; external**
3.13 4.51 FUD 000 S 80
AMA: 2018,Feb,11; 2018,Jan,8; 2017,Jan,8; 2016,Jan,13; 2015,Jan,16

92961 **internal (separate procedure)**
EXCLUDES *Device evaluation for implantable defibrillator/multi-lead pacemaker system (93282-93284, 93287, 93289, 93295-93296)*
Electrophysiological studies (93618-93624, 93631, 93640-93642)
Intracardiac ablation (93650-93657, 93662)
7.23 7.23 FUD 000 S
AMA: 2018,Feb,11; 2018,Jan,8; 2017,Jan,8; 2016,Jan,13; 2015,Feb,3; 2015,Jan,16

92970-92979 [92973, 92974, 92975, 92977, 92978, 92979] Circulatory Assist: External/Internal

EXCLUDES *Atrial septostomy, any method (33741)*
Catheter placement for use in circulatory assist devices (intra-aortic balloon pump) (33970)

92970 **Cardioassist-method of circulatory assist; internal**
5.52 5.52 FUD 000 C 80
AMA: 2018,Feb,11

92971 **external**
2.91 2.91 FUD 000 C 80
AMA: 2018,Feb,11

92973 **Resequenced code. See code following 92998.**

92974 **Resequenced code. See code following 92998.**

92975 **Resequenced code. See code following 92998.**

92977 **Resequenced code. See code following 92998.**

92978 **Resequenced code. See code following 92998.**

92979 **Resequenced code. See code following 92998.**

92986-92993 Percutaneous Procedures of Heart Valves and Septum

EXCLUDES *Atrial septostomy, any method (33741)*

92986 **Percutaneous balloon valvuloplasty; aortic valve**
38.3 38.3 FUD 090 J 80
AMA: 2018,Feb,11; 2018,Jan,8; 2017,Jan,8; 2016,Jan,13; 2015,Feb,3; 2015,Jan,16

92987 **mitral valve**
39.3 39.3 FUD 090 J 80
AMA: 2018,Feb,11; 2018,Jan,8; 2017,Jan,8; 2016,Jan,13; 2015,Feb,3

92990 **pulmonary valve**
31.4 31.4 FUD 090 J 80
AMA: 2018,Feb,11; 2018,Jan,8; 2017,Jan,8; 2016,Jan,13; 2015,Jul,10; 2015,Feb,3

92992 ~~**Atrial septectomy or septostomy; transvenous method, balloon (eg, Rashkind type) (includes cardiac catheterization)**~~

92993 ~~**blade method (Park septostomy) (includes cardiac catheterization)**~~

92997-92998 Percutaneous Angioplasty: Pulmonary Artery

92997 **Percutaneous transluminal pulmonary artery balloon angioplasty; single vessel**
18.4 18.4 FUD 000 J 80
AMA: 2018,Feb,11; 2018,Jan,8; 2017,Jul,3; 2017,Jan,8; 2016,Mar,5; 2016,Jan,13; 2015,Feb,3

\+ **92998** **each additional vessel (List separately in addition to code for primary procedure)**
Code first single vessel (92997)
9.44 9.44 FUD ZZZ N 80
AMA: 2018,Feb,11; 2018,Jan,8; 2017,Jul,3; 2017,Jan,8; 2016,Mar,5; 2016,Jan,13; 2015,Feb,3

92920-92944 [92920, 92921, 92924, 92925, 92928, 92929, 92933, 92934, 92937, 92938, 92941, 92943, 92944] Intravascular Coronary Procedures

INCLUDES Accessing vessel
- Additional procedures performed in third branch, major coronary artery
- All procedures performed in all branch segments, coronary arteries
  - Branches left anterior descending (diagonals), left circumflex (marginals), and right (posterior descending, posterolaterals)
  - Distal, proximal, and mid segments
- All procedures performed in all segments, major coronary arteries through native vessels:
  - Distal, proximal, and mid segments
  - Left main, left anterior descending, left circumflex, right, and ramus intermedius arteries
- All procedures performed in major coronary arteries or recognized coronary artery branches through coronary artery bypass graft
  - Sequential bypass graft with more than single distal anastomosis as one graft
  - Branching bypass grafts (e.g., "Y" grafts) include coronary vessel for primary graft, with each branch off primary graft making up an additional coronary vessel
  - Each coronary artery bypass graft denotes single coronary vessel
  - Embolic protection devices when used
- Arteriotomy closure through access sheath
- Atherectomy (e.g., directional, laser, rotational)
- Balloon angioplasty (e.g., cryoplasty, cutting balloon, wired balloons)
- Cardiac catheterization and related procedures when included in coronary revascularization service (93454-93461, 93563-93564)
- Imaging once procedure complete
- Percutaneous coronary interventions (PCI) for coronary vessel disease, native and bypass grafts
- Procedures in left main and ramus intermedius coronary artery branches as they are unrecognized for individual code assignment
- Radiological supervision and interpretation intervention(s)
- Reporting most comprehensive treatment in given vessel according to intensity hierarchy for base and add-on codes:
  - Add-on codes: 92944 = 92938 > 92934 > 92925 > 92929 > 92921
  - Base codes (report only one): 92943 = 92941 = 92933 > 92924 > 92937 = 92928 > 92920
- Revascularization achieved with single procedure when single lesion continues from one target vessel (major artery, branch, or bypass graft) to another target vessel
- Selective vessel catheterization
- Stenting (e.g., balloon expandable, bare metal, covered, drug eluting, self-expanding)
- Traversing lesion

EXCLUDES *Application intravascular radioelements (77770-77772)*
Insertion device for coronary intravascular brachytherapy (92974)
Reduction septum (e.g., alcohol ablation) (93799)

Code also add-on codes for procedures performed during same session in additional recognized target vessel branches
Code also diagnostic angiography during interventional procedure when:
- No previous catheter-based coronary angiography study available, and full diagnostic study performed, with decision to perform intervention based on that study
- Previous study available, but documentation states patient's condition changed since previous study or target area visualization inadequate, or change occurs during procedure warranting additional evaluation outside current target area

Code also diagnostic angiography performed at session separate from interventional procedure
Code also individual base codes for treatment major native coronary artery segment and another segment same artery requiring treatment through bypass graft when performed at same time
Code also procedures for both vessels for bifurcation lesion
Code also procedures performed in second branch major coronary artery
Code also treatment arterial segment requiring access through bypass graft

\# **92920** **Percutaneous transluminal coronary angioplasty; single major coronary artery or branch**
15.4 15.4 FUD 000 J J8 80
AMA: 2018,Feb,11; 2018,Jan,8; 2017,Jul,3; 2017,Jan,8; 2016,Jan,13; 2015,Jan,16

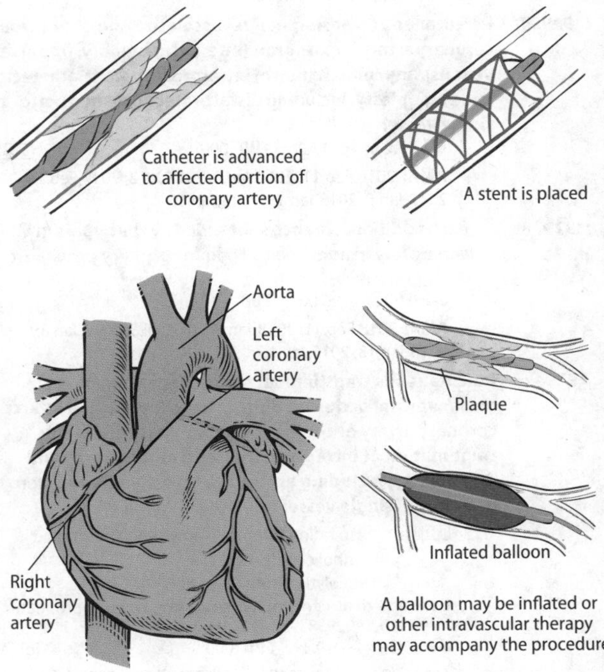
Catheter is advanced to affected portion of coronary artery
A stent is placed
Aorta
Left coronary artery
Plaque
Inflated balloon
Right coronary artery
A balloon may be inflated or other intravascular therapy may accompany the procedure

\+ # **92921** **each additional branch of a major coronary artery (List separately in addition to code for primary procedure)**
Code first (92920, 92924, 92928, 92933, 92937, 92941, 92943)
0.00 0.00 FUD ZZZ N N1
AMA: 2018,Feb,11; 2018,Jan,8; 2017,Jul,3; 2017,Jan,8; 2016,Jan,13; 2015,Jan,16

\# **92924** **Percutaneous transluminal coronary atherectomy, with coronary angioplasty when performed; single major coronary artery or branch**
18.4 18.4 FUD 000 J 80
AMA: 2018,Feb,11; 2018,Jan,8; 2017,Jul,3; 2017,Jan,8; 2016,Jan,13; 2015,Jan,16

\+ # **92925** **each additional branch of a major coronary artery (List separately in addition to code for primary procedure)**
Code first (92924, 92928, 92933, 92937, 92941, 92943)
0.00 0.00 FUD ZZZ N
AMA: 2018,Feb,11; 2018,Jan,8; 2017,Jul,3; 2017,Jan,8; 2016,Jan,13; 2015,Jan,16

\# **92928** **Percutaneous transcatheter placement of intracoronary stent(s), with coronary angioplasty when performed; single major coronary artery or branch**
17.2 17.2 FUD 000 J J8 80
AMA: 2018,Feb,11; 2018,Jan,8; 2017,Jul,3; 2017,Feb,14; 2017,Jan,8; 2017,Jan,6; 2016,Jan,13; 2015,Jan,16

\+ # **92929** **each additional branch of a major coronary artery (List separately in addition to code for primary procedure)**
Code first (92928, 92933, 92937, 92941, 92943)
0.00 0.00 FUD ZZZ N N1
AMA: 2018,Feb,11; 2018,Jan,8; 2017,Jul,3; 2017,Jan,8; 2017,Jan,6; 2016,Jan,13; 2015,Jan,16

\# **92933** **Percutaneous transluminal coronary atherectomy, with intracoronary stent, with coronary angioplasty when performed; single major coronary artery or branch**
19.3 19.3 FUD 000 J 80
AMA: 2018,Feb,11; 2018,Jan,8; 2017,Jul,3; 2017,Jan,8; 2016,Jan,13; 2015,Jan,16

+ # **92934** **each additional branch of a major coronary artery (List separately in addition to code for primary procedure)**

Code first (92933, 92937, 92941, 92943)

Facility RVU 0.00 Non-Facility RVU 0.00 FUD ZZZ N CCI

AMA: 2018,Feb,11; 2018,Jan,8; 2017,Jul,3; 2017,Jan,8; 2016,Jan,13; 2015,Jan,16

92937 **Percutaneous transluminal revascularization of or through coronary artery bypass graft (internal mammary, free arterial, venous), any combination of intracoronary stent, atherectomy and angioplasty, including distal protection when performed; single vessel**

Facility RVU 17.2 Non-Facility RVU 17.2 FUD 000 J 80 CCI

AMA: 2018,Feb,11; 2018,Jan,8; 2017,Jul,3; 2017,Feb,14; 2017,Jan,8; 2016,Jan,13; 2015,Jan,16

+ # **92938** **each additional branch subtended by the bypass graft (List separately in addition to code for primary procedure)**

Code first (92937)

Facility RVU 0.00 Non-Facility RVU 0.00 FUD ZZZ N CCI

AMA: 2018,Feb,11; 2018,Jan,8; 2017,Jul,3; 2017,Jan,8; 2016,Jan,13; 2015,Jan,16

92941 **Percutaneous transluminal revascularization of acute total/subtotal occlusion during acute myocardial infarction, coronary artery or coronary artery bypass graft, any combination of intracoronary stent, atherectomy and angioplasty, including aspiration thrombectomy when performed, single vessel**

INCLUDES Aspiration thrombectomy, when performed
Embolic protection
Rheolytic thrombectomy

Code also treatment additional vessels, when appropriate (92920-92938, 92943-92944)

Facility RVU 19.3 Non-Facility RVU 19.3 FUD 000 C 80 CCI

AMA: 2020,Jul,13; 2018,Feb,11; 2018,Jan,8; 2017,Jul,3; 2017,Feb,14; 2017,Jan,8; 2016,Jan,13; 2015,Jan,16

92943 **Percutaneous transluminal revascularization of chronic total occlusion, coronary artery, coronary artery branch, or coronary artery bypass graft, any combination of intracoronary stent, atherectomy and angioplasty; single vessel**

INCLUDES Antegrade flow deficiency with angiography and clinical criteria indicating chronic total occlusion

Facility RVU 19.3 Non-Facility RVU 19.3 FUD 000 J 80 CCI

AMA: 2018,Feb,11; 2018,Jan,8; 2017,Jul,3; 2017,Jan,8; 2016,Jan,13; 2015,Jan,16

+ # **92944** **each additional coronary artery, coronary artery branch, or bypass graft (List separately in addition to code for primary procedure)**

EXCLUDES *Application intravascular radioelements (77770-77772)*

Code first (92924, 92928, 92933, 92937, 92941, 92943)

Facility RVU 0.00 Non-Facility RVU 0.00 FUD ZZZ N CCI

AMA: 2018,Feb,11; 2018,Jan,8; 2017,Jul,3; 2017,Jan,8; 2016,Jan,13; 2015,Jan,16

92973-92979 [92973, 92974, 92975, 92977, 92978, 92979] Additional Coronary Artery Procedures

+ # **92973** **Percutaneous transluminal coronary thrombectomy mechanical (List separately in addition to code for primary procedure)**

EXCLUDES *Aspiration thrombectomy*

Code first (92920, 92924, 92928, 92933, 92937, 92941, 92943, 92975, 93454-93461, 93563-93564)

Facility RVU 5.15 Non-Facility RVU 5.15 FUD ZZZ N 80 CCI

AMA: 2020,Jul,13; 2018,Feb,11; 2018,Jan,8; 2017,Feb,14; 2017,Jan,8; 2016,Jan,13; 2015,Jan,16

+ # **92974** **Transcatheter placement of radiation delivery device for subsequent coronary intravascular brachytherapy (List separately in addition to code for primary procedure)**

EXCLUDES *Application intravascular radioelements (77770-77772)*

Code first (92920, 92924, 92928, 92933, 92937, 92941, 92943, 93454-93461)

Facility RVU 4.68 Non-Facility RVU 4.68 FUD ZZZ N 80 CCI

AMA: 2018,Feb,11; 2018,Jan,8; 2017,Feb,14; 2017,Jan,8; 2016,Jan,13; 2015,Jan,16

92975 **Thrombolysis, coronary; by intracoronary infusion, including selective coronary angiography**

EXCLUDES *Thrombolysis, cerebral (37195)*
Thrombolysis other than coronary ([37211, 37212, 37213, 37214])

Facility RVU 10.9 Non-Facility RVU 10.9 FUD 000 C 80 CCI

AMA: 2018,Feb,11

92977 **by intravenous infusion**

EXCLUDES *Thrombolysis, cerebral (37195)*
Thrombolysis other than coronary ([37211, 37212, 37213, 37214])

Facility RVU 1.51 Non-Facility RVU 1.51 FUD XXX T 80 CCI

AMA: 2018,Feb,11

+ # **92978** **Endoluminal imaging of coronary vessel or graft using intravascular ultrasound (IVUS) or optical coherence tomography (OCT) during diagnostic evaluation and/or therapeutic intervention including imaging supervision, interpretation and report; initial vessel (List separately in addition to code for primary procedure)**

Code first primary procedure (92920, 92924, 92928, 92933, 92937, 92941, 92943, 92975, 93454-93461, 93563-93564)

Facility RVU 0.00 Non-Facility RVU 0.00 FUD ZZZ N 80 CCI

AMA: 2018,Feb,11; 2018,Jan,8; 2017,Jan,8; 2016,Jan,13; 2015,Jan,16

+ # **92979** **each additional vessel (List separately in addition to code for primary procedure)**

INCLUDES Transducer manipulations/repositioning in vessel examined, before and after therapeutic intervention

EXCLUDES *Intravascular spectroscopy (93799)*

Code first initial vessel (92978)

Facility RVU 0.00 Non-Facility RVU 0.00 FUD ZZZ N 80 CCI

AMA: 2018,Feb,11; 2018,Jan,8; 2017,Jan,8; 2016,Jan,13; 2015,Jan,16

93000-93010 Electrocardiographic Services

INCLUDES Specific order for service, separate written and signed report, and documentation medical necessity

EXCLUDES *Acoustic cardiography (93799)*
Echocardiography (93303-93350)
Intracardiac ischemia monitoring system (0525T-0532T)
Reporting codes for telemetry monitoring strip review

93000 **Electrocardiogram, routine ECG with at least 12 leads; with interpretation and report**

Facility RVU 0.48 Non-Facility RVU 0.48 FUD XXX M 80 CCI

AMA: 2018,Feb,11; 2018,Jan,8; 2017,Oct,3; 2017,Jan,8; 2016,Jan,13; 2015,Jan,16

93005 **tracing only, without interpretation and report**

Facility RVU 0.24 Non-Facility RVU 0.24 FUD XXX Q1 80 TC CCI

AMA: 2018,Feb,11; 2018,Jan,8; 2017,Oct,3; 2017,Jan,8; 2016,Apr,8; 2016,Jan,13; 2015,Jan,16

93010 **interpretation and report only**
0.24 0.24 FUD XXX B 80 26
AMA: 2018,Feb,11; 2018,Jan,8; 2017,Oct,3; 2017,Jan,8; 2016,Apr,8; 2016,Jan,13; 2015,Jan,16

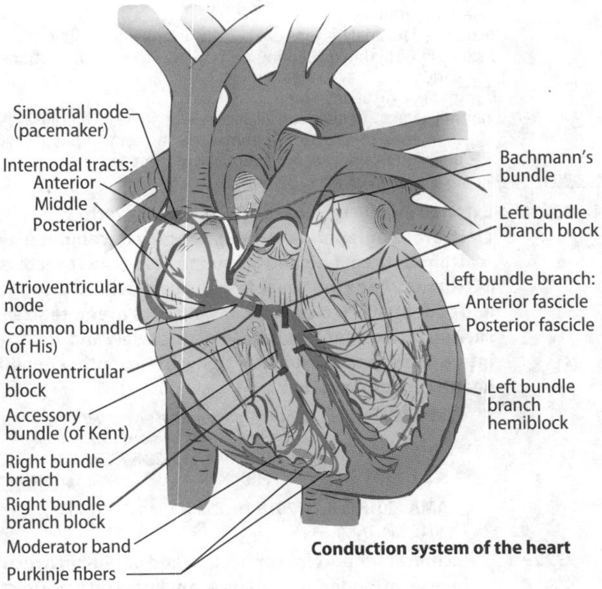

Conduction system of the heart

93015-93018 Stress Test

93015 **Cardiovascular stress test using maximal or submaximal treadmill or bicycle exercise, continuous electrocardiographic monitoring, and/or pharmacological stress; with supervision, interpretation and report**
2.01 2.01 FUD XXX B 80
AMA: 2020,Jul,5; 2018,Feb,11; 2018,Jan,8; 2017,Oct,3; 2017,Jan,8; 2016,Jan,13; 2015,Jan,16

93016 **supervision only, without interpretation and report**
0.63 0.63 FUD XXX B 80 26
AMA: 2020,Jul,5; 2018,Feb,11; 2018,Jan,8; 2017,Oct,3; 2017,Jan,8; 2016,Jan,13; 2015,Jan,16

93017 **tracing only, without interpretation and report**
0.95 0.95 FUD XXX Q1 80 TC
AMA: 2020,Jul,5; 2018,Feb,11; 2018,Jan,8; 2017,Oct,3; 2017,Jan,8; 2016,Jan,13; 2015,Jan,16

93018 **interpretation and report only**
0.42 0.42 FUD XXX B 80 26
AMA: 2020,Jul,5; 2018,Feb,11; 2018,Jan,8; 2017,Oct,3; 2017,Jan,8; 2016,Jan,13; 2015,Jan,16

93024 Provocation Test for Coronary Vasospasm

93024 **Ergonovine provocation test**
3.10 3.10 FUD XXX Q1 80
AMA: 2018,Feb,11

93025 Microvolt T-Wave Alternans

CMS: 100-03,20.30 Microvolt T-Wave Alternans (MTWA); 100-04,32,370 Microvolt T-wave Alternans; 100-04,32,370.1 Coding and Claims Processing for MTWA; 100-04,32,370.2 Messaging for MTWA

INCLUDES Specific order for service, separate written and signed report, and documentation medical necessity

EXCLUDES *Echocardiography (93303-93350)*
Reporting codes for telemetry monitoring strip review

93025 **Microvolt T-wave alternans for assessment of ventricular arrhythmias**
4.23 4.23 FUD XXX S 80
AMA: 2018,Feb,11; 2018,Jan,8; 2017,Jan,8; 2016,Jan,13; 2015,Jan,16

93040-93042 Rhythm Strips

INCLUDES Specific order for service, separate written and signed report, and documentation medical necessity

EXCLUDES *Device evaluation ([93261], 93279-93289 [93260], 93291-93296, 93298)*
Echocardiography (93303-93350)
Reporting codes for telemetry monitoring strip review

93040 **Rhythm ECG, 1-3 leads; with interpretation and report**
0.36 0.36 FUD XXX B 80
AMA: 2020,Sep,7; 2018,Feb,11; 2018,Jan,8; 2017,Oct,3; 2017,Jan,8; 2016,Jan,13; 2015,Jan,16

93041 **tracing only without interpretation and report**
0.16 0.16 FUD XXX Q1 80 TC
AMA: 2018,Feb,11; 2018,Jan,8; 2017,Oct,3; 2017,Jan,8; 2016,Jan,13; 2015,Jan,16

93042 **interpretation and report only**
0.20 0.20 FUD XXX B 80 26
AMA: 2018,Feb,11; 2018,Jan,8; 2017,Oct,3; 2017,Jan,8; 2016,Jan,13; 2015,Jan,16

93050 Arterial Waveform Analysis

EXCLUDES *Reporting code with any intra-arterial diagnostic or interventional procedure*

93050 **Arterial pressure waveform analysis for assessment of central arterial pressures, includes obtaining waveform(s), digitization and application of nonlinear mathematical transformations to determine central arterial pressures and augmentation index, with interpretation and report, upper extremity artery, non-invasive**
0.46 0.46 FUD XXX Q1 80
AMA: 2018,Feb,11

93224-93227 Holter Monitor

INCLUDES Cardiac monitoring using in-person as well as remote technology for electrocardiographic data assessment
Up to 48 hours recording on continuous basis

EXCLUDES *Echocardiography (93303-93355 [93356])*
Implantable patient activated cardiac event recorders (93285, 93291, 93297-93298)
More than 48 hours monitoring ([93241, 93242, 93243, 93244, 93245, 93246, 93247, 93248])

Code also modifier 52 when less than 12 hours continuous recording provided

93224 **External electrocardiographic recording up to 48 hours by continuous rhythm recording and storage; includes recording, scanning analysis with report, review and interpretation by a physician or other qualified health care professional**
2.51 2.51 FUD XXX M 80
AMA: 2018,Feb,11; 2018,Jan,8; 2017,Jan,8; 2016,Jan,13; 2015,Jan,16

93225 **recording (includes connection, recording, and disconnection)**
0.72 0.72 FUD XXX Q1 80 TC
AMA: 2018,Feb,11; 2018,Jan,8; 2017,Jan,8; 2016,Jan,13; 2015,Jan,16

93226 **scanning analysis with report**
1.03 1.03 FUD XXX Q1 80 TC
AMA: 2018,Feb,11; 2018,Jan,8; 2017,Jan,8; 2016,Jan,13; 2015,Jan,16

93227 **review and interpretation by a physician or other qualified health care professional**
0.75 0.75 FUD XXX M 80 26
AMA: 2018,Mar,5; 2018,Feb,11; 2018,Jan,8; 2017,Jan,8; 2016,Jan,13; 2015,Jan,16

93241 — 93268

93241-93248 [93241, 93242, 93243, 93244, 93245, 93246, 93247, 93248] External Electrocardiographic Recording

INCLUDES Cardiac monitoring using in-person as well as remote technology for electrocardiographic data assessment

EXCLUDES *During same monitoring period:*
External ECG event recording up to 30 days (93268-93272)
External ECG event recording without 24 hour attended monitoring (0497T-0498T)
Remote physiological monitoring, collection and interpretation ([99453, 99454], [99091])
Echocardiography (93303-93355 [93356])
Implantable patient activated cardiac event recorders (93285, 93291, 93297-93298)
Less than 48 hours monitoring (93224-93227)

● # **93241** **External electrocardiographic recording for more than 48 hours up to 7 days by continuous rhythm recording and storage; includes recording, scanning analysis with report, review and interpretation**

    EXCLUDES *More than 7 days and up to 15 days monitoring ([93245, 93246, 93247, 93248])*

    🚑 0.00   ⚕ 0.00 **FUD** 000

● # **93242** **recording (includes connection and initial recording)**

    EXCLUDES *More than 7 days and up to 15 days monitoring ([93245, 93246, 93247, 93248])*

    🚑 0.00   ⚕ 0.00 **FUD** 000

● # **93243** **scanning analysis with report**

    EXCLUDES *More than 7 days and up to 15 days monitoring ([93245, 93246, 93247, 93248])*

    🚑 0.00   ⚕ 0.00 **FUD** 000

● # **93244** **review and interpretation**

    EXCLUDES *More than 7 days and up to 15 days monitoring ([93245, 93246, 93247, 93248])*

    🚑 0.00   ⚕ 0.00 **FUD** 000

● # **93245** **External electrocardiographic recording for more than 7 days up to 15 days by continuous rhythm recording and storage; includes recording, scanning analysis with report, review and interpretation**

    EXCLUDES *More than 48 hours up to 7 days monitoring ([93241, 93242, 93243, 93244])*

    🚑 0.00   ⚕ 0.00 **FUD** 000

● # **93246** **recording (includes connection and initial recording)**

    EXCLUDES *More than 48 hours up to 7 days monitoring ([93241, 93242, 93243, 93244])*

    🚑 0.00   ⚕ 0.00 **FUD** 000

● # **93247** **scanning analysis with report**

    EXCLUDES *More than 48 hours up to 7 days monitoring ([93241, 93242, 93243, 93244])*

    🚑 0.00   ⚕ 0.00 **FUD** 000

● # **93248** **review and interpretation**

    EXCLUDES *More than 48 hours up to 7 days monitoring ([93241, 93242, 93243, 93244])*

    🚑 0.00   ⚕ 0.00 **FUD** 000

93228-93248 [93241, 93242, 93243, 93244, 93245, 93246, 93247, 93248] Remote Cardiovascular Telemetry

INCLUDES Cardiac monitoring using in-person as well as remote technology for electrocardiographic data assessment
Mobile telemetry monitors with capacity to:
Detect arrhythmias
Real-time data analysis for signal quality evaluation quality
Records ECG rhythm on continuous basis using external electrodes on patient
Transmit tracing at any time
Transmit data to attended surveillance center where technician available to respond to device or rhythm alerts and contact physician or qualified health care professional when needed

EXCLUDES *Reporting code more than one time in 30-day period*

  93228 **External mobile cardiovascular telemetry with electrocardiographic recording, concurrent computerized real time data analysis and greater than 24 hours of accessible ECG data storage (retrievable with query) with ECG triggered and patient selected events transmitted to a remote attended surveillance center for up to 30 days; review and interpretation with report by a physician or other qualified health care professional**

    EXCLUDES *Cardiovascular monitors that do not perform automatic ECG triggered transmissions to attended surveillance center (93224-93227, 93268-93272)*

    🚑 0.74   ⚕ 0.74 **FUD** XXX ★ M 80 26 □

    AMA: 2018,Feb,11; 2018,Jan,8; 2017,Jan,8; 2016,Jan,13; 2015,Jan,16

  93229 **technical support for connection and patient instructions for use, attended surveillance, analysis and transmission of daily and emergent data reports as prescribed by a physician or other qualified health care professional**

    🚑 19.9   ⚕ 19.9 **FUD** XXX ★ S 80 TC □

    AMA: 2018,Feb,11; 2018,Jan,8; 2017,Jan,8; 2016,Jan,13; 2015,Jan,16

  93241 **Resequenced code. See code following 93227.**

  93242 **Resequenced code. See code following 93227.**

  93243 **Resequenced code. See code following 93227.**

  93244 **Resequenced code. See code following 93227.**

  93245 **Resequenced code. See code following 93227.**

  93246 **Resequenced code. See code following 93227.**

  93247 **Resequenced code. See code following 93227.**

  93248 **Resequenced code. See code following 93227.**

93260-93272 [93260, 93261, 93264] Event Monitors

INCLUDES ECG rhythm derived elements, which differ from physiologic data and include heart rhythm, rate, ST analysis, heart rate variability, T-wave alternans, among others
Event monitors that:
Record ECGs in response to patient activation or automatic detection algorithm (or both)
Require attended surveillance
Transmit data upon request (although not immediately when activated)

EXCLUDES *Monitoring cardiovascular devices (93279-93289 [93260], 93291-93296, 93298)*

  93260 **Resequenced code. See code following 93284.**

  93261 **Resequenced code. See code following 93289.**

  93264 **Resequenced code. See code before 93278.**

  93268 **External patient and, when performed, auto activated electrocardiographic rhythm derived event recording with symptom-related memory loop with remote download capability up to 30 days, 24-hour attended monitoring; includes transmission, review and interpretation by a physician or other qualified health care professional**

    EXCLUDES *Implantable patient activated cardiac event recorders (93285, 93291, 93298)*
Subcutaneous cardiac rhythm monitor (33285)

    🚑 5.70   ⚕ 5.70 **FUD** XXX ★ M 80 □

    AMA: 2018,Feb,11; 2018,Jan,8; 2017,Jan,8; 2016,Jan,13; 2015,Jan,16

26/TC PC/TC Only A2-Z3 ASC Payment 50 Bilateral ♂ Male Only ♀ Female Only 🚑 Facility RVU ⚕ Non-Facility RVU □ CCI ❌ CLIA
FUD Follow-up Days **CMS:** IOM **AMA:** CPT Asst A-Y OPPSI 80/80 Surg Assist Allowed / w/Doc Lab Crosswalk Radiology Crosswalk

93270 **recording (includes connection, recording, and disconnection)**

0.26 0.26 FUD XXX ★ Q1 80 TC

AMA: 2018,Feb,11; 2018,Jan,8; 2017,Jan,8; 2016,Jan,13; 2015,Jan,16

93271 **transmission and analysis**

4.72 4.72 FUD XXX ★ S 80 TC

AMA: 2018,Feb,11; 2018,Jan,8; 2017,Jan,8; 2016,Jan,13; 2015,Jan,16

93272 **review and interpretation by a physician or other qualified health care professional**

EXCLUDES *Implantable patient activated cardiac event recorders (93285, 93291, 93298)*

Subcutaneous cardiac rhythm monitor (33285)

0.72 0.72 FUD XXX ★ M 80 26

AMA: 2018,Mar,5; 2018,Feb,11; 2018,Jan,8; 2017,Jan,8; 2016,Jan,13; 2015,Jan,16

93278 Signal-averaged Electrocardiography

EXCLUDES *Echocardiography (93303-93355)*

Code also modifier 26 for interpretation and report only

93278 **Signal-averaged electrocardiography (SAECG), with or without ECG**

0.87 0.87 FUD XXX Q1 80

AMA: 2018,Feb,11; 2018,Jan,8; 2017,Jan,8; 2016,Jan,13; 2015,Jan,16

93264 [93264] Wireless Pulmonary Artery Pressure Sensor Monitoring

INCLUDES Data collection from internal sensor in pulmonary artery

Downloads, interpretation, analysis, and report that must occur at least one time per week

Transmission and storage of data

EXCLUDES *Reporting code wehn monitoring for less than 30-day period*

Reporting code more than one time in 30 days

\# 93264 **Remote monitoring of a wireless pulmonary artery pressure sensor for up to 30 days, including at least weekly downloads of pulmonary artery pressure recordings, interpretation(s), trend analysis, and report(s) by a physician or other qualified health care professional**

1.03 1.43 FUD XXX 80

AMA: 2020,Feb,7; 2019,Oct,3; 2019,Jun,3

93279-93298 [93260, 93261] Monitoring of Cardiovascular Devices

INCLUDES Implantable cardiovascular monitor (ICM) interrogation:

- Analysis at least one recorded physiologic cardiovascular data element from either internal or external sensors
- Programmed parameters

Implantable defibrillator interrogation:

- Battery
- Capture and sensing functions
- Leads
- Presence or absence therapy for ventricular tachyarrhythmias
- Programmed parameters
- Underlying heart rhythm

Implantable loop recorder (ILR) interrogation:

- Heart rate and rhythm during recorded episodes from both patient-initiated and device detected events
- Programmed parameters

In-person interrogation/device evaluation (93288)

In-person periprocedural device evaluation/programming device system parameters (93286)

Interrogation evaluation device

Pacemaker interrogation:

- Battery
- Capture and sensing functions
- Heart rhythm
- Leads
- Programmed parameters

Time period established by initiation remote monitoring or 91st day implantable defibrillator/pacemaker monitoring or 31st day ILR monitoring and extending for succeeding 30- or 90-day period

EXCLUDES *Wearable device monitoring (93224-93272)*

93279 **Programming device evaluation (in person) with iterative adjustment of the implantable device to test the function of the device and select optimal permanent programmed values with analysis, review and report by a physician or other qualified health care professional; single lead pacemaker system or leadless pacemaker system in one cardiac chamber**

EXCLUDES *External ECG event recording up to 30 days (93268-93272)*

Peri-procedural and interrogation device evaluation (93286, 93288)

Rhythm strips (93040-93042)

1.72 1.72 FUD XXX Q1 80

AMA: 2019,Oct,3; 2019,Mar,6; 2018,Feb,11; 2018,Jan,8; 2017,Jan,8; 2016,Aug,5; 2016,May,5; 2016,Jan,13; 2015,Jan,16

93280 **dual lead pacemaker system**

EXCLUDES *External ECG event recording up to 30 days (93268-93272)*

Peri-procedural and interrogation device evaluation (93286, 93288)

Rhythm strips (93040-93042)

1.83 1.83 FUD XXX Q1 80

AMA: 2019,Oct,3; 2018,Feb,11; 2018,Jan,8; 2017,Jan,8; 2016,Aug,5; 2016,May,5; 2016,Jan,13; 2015,Jan,16

93281 **multiple lead pacemaker system**

EXCLUDES *External ECG event recording up to 30 days (93268-93272)*

Peri-procedural and interrogation device evaluation (93286, 93288)

Rhythm strips (93040-93042)

2.17 2.17 FUD XXX Q1 80

AMA: 2019,Oct,3; 2018,Feb,11; 2018,Jan,8; 2017,Jan,8; 2016,Aug,5; 2016,May,5; 2016,Jan,13; 2015,Jan,16

Medicine

93270 — 93281

93282 **single lead transvenous implantable defibrillator system**

EXCLUDES *Device evaluation subcutaneous lead defibrillator system (93260)*
External ECG event recording up to 30 days (93268-93272)
Peri-procedural and interrogation device evaluation (93287, 93289)
Rhythm strips (93040-93042)
Wearable cardio-defibrillator system services (93745)

2.08 2.08 FUD XXX Q1 80

AMA: 2019,Oct,3; 2018,Feb,11; 2018,Jan,8; 2017,Jan,8; 2016,Aug,5; 2016,Jan,13; 2015,Jan,16

93283 **dual lead transvenous implantable defibrillator system**

EXCLUDES *External ECG event recording up to 30 days (93268-93272)*
Peri-procedural and interrogation device evaluation (93287, 93289)
Rhythm strips (93040-93042)

2.60 2.60 FUD XXX Q1 80

AMA: 2019,Oct,3; 2018,Feb,11; 2018,Jan,8; 2017,Jan,8; 2016,Aug,5; 2016,Jan,13; 2015,Jan,16

93284 **multiple lead transvenous implantable defibrillator system**

EXCLUDES *External ECG event recording up to 30 days (93268-93272)*
Peri-procedural and interrogation device evaluation (93287, 93289)
Rhythm strips (93040-93042)

2.81 2.81 FUD XXX Q1 80

AMA: 2019,Oct,3; 2018,Feb,11; 2018,Jan,8; 2017,Jan,8; 2016,Aug,5; 2016,Jan,13; 2015,Jan,16

93260 **implantable subcutaneous lead defibrillator system**

EXCLUDES *Device evaluation (93261, 93282, 93287)*
External ECG event recording up to 30 days (93268-93272)
Insertion/removal/replacement implantable defibrillator (33240, 33241, [33262], [33270, 33271, 33272, 33273])
Rhythm strips (93040-93042)

2.04 2.04 FUD XXX Q1 80

AMA: 2019,Oct,3; 2018,Feb,11; 2018,Jan,8; 2017,Jan,8; 2016,Aug,5; 2016,Jan,13; 2015,Jan,16

93285 **subcutaneous cardiac rhythm monitor system**

EXCLUDES *Device evaluation (93279-93284, 93291)*
External ECG event recording up to 30 days (93268-93272)
Insertion subcutaneous cardiac rhythm monitor (33285)
Rhythm strips (93040-93042)

1.52 1.52 FUD XXX Q1 80

AMA: 2019,Oct,3; 2019,Apr,3; 2018,Feb,11; 2018,Jan,8; 2017,Jan,8; 2016,Aug,5; 2016,Jan,13; 2015,Jan,16

93286 **Peri-procedural device evaluation (in person) and programming of device system parameters before or after a surgery, procedure, or test with analysis, review and report by a physician or other qualified health care professional; single, dual, or multiple lead pacemaker system, or leadless pacemaker system**

INCLUDES One evaluation and programming (if performed once before and once after, report as two units)

EXCLUDES *Device evaluation (93279-93281, 93288)*
External ECG event recording up to 30 days (93268-93272)
Rhythm strips (93040-93042)
Services related to cardiac contractility modulation systems (0408T-0411T, 0414T-0415T)
Subcutaneous implantable defibrillator peri-procedural device evaluation and programming (93260, 93261)

0.99 0.99 FUD XXX N 80

AMA: 2019,Oct,3; 2019,Mar,6; 2018,Feb,11; 2018,Jan,8; 2017,Jan,8; 2016,Aug,5; 2016,May,5; 2016,Jan,13; 2015,Jan,16

93287 **single, dual, or multiple lead implantable defibrillator system**

INCLUDES One evaluation and programming (if performed once before and once after, report as two units)

EXCLUDES *Device evaluation (93282-93284, 93289)*
External ECG event recording up to 30 days (93268-93272)
Rhythm strips (93040-93042)
Services related to cardiac contractility modulation systems (0408T-0411T, 0414T-0415T)
Subcutaneous implantable defibrillator peri-procedural device evaluation and programming (93260, 93261)

1.36 1.36 FUD XXX N 80

AMA: 2019,Oct,3; 2018,Feb,11; 2018,Jan,8; 2017,Jan,8; 2016,Aug,5; 2016,May,5; 2016,Jan,13; 2015,Jan,16

93288 **Interrogation device evaluation (in person) with analysis, review and report by a physician or other qualified health care professional, includes connection, recording and disconnection per patient encounter; single, dual, or multiple lead pacemaker system, or leadless pacemaker system**

EXCLUDES *Device evaluation (93279-93281, 93286, 93294-93295)*
External ECG event recording up to 30 days (93268-93272)
Rhythm strips (93040-93042)

1.25 1.25 FUD XXX Q1 80

AMA: 2019,Oct,3; 2019,Mar,6; 2018,Feb,11; 2018,Jan,8; 2017,Jan,8; 2016,Aug,5; 2016,May,5; 2016,Jan,13; 2015,Jan,16

93289 **single, dual, or multiple lead transvenous implantable defibrillator system, including analysis of heart rhythm derived data elements**

EXCLUDES *Monitoring physiologic cardiovascular data elements derived from implantable defibrillator (93290)*
Device evaluation (93261, 93282-93284, 93287, 93295-93296)
External ECG event recording up to 30 days (93268-93272)
Rhythm strips (93040-93042)

1.70 1.70 FUD XXX Q1 80

AMA: 2019,Oct,3; 2018,Feb,11; 2018,Jan,8; 2017,Jan,8; 2016,Aug,5; 2016,May,5; 2016,Jan,13; 2015,Jan,16

93261 **implantable subcutaneous lead defibrillator system**

EXCLUDES *Device evaluation (93260, 93287, 93289)*
External ECG event recording up to 30 days (93268-93272)
Insertion/removal/replacement implantable defibrillator (33240, 33241, [33262], [33270, 33271, 33272, 33273])
Rhythm strips (93040-93042)

1.87 1.87 FUD XXX Q1 80

AMA: 2019,Oct,3; 2018,Feb,11; 2018,Jan,8; 2017,Jan,8; 2016,Aug,5; 2016,Jan,13; 2015,Jan,16

93290 **implantable cardiovascular physiologic monitor system, including analysis of 1 or more recorded physiologic cardiovascular data elements from all internal and external sensors**

EXCLUDES *Device evaluation (93297)*
Heart rhythm derived data (93289)

1.19 1.19 FUD XXX Q1 80

AMA: 2020,Feb,7; 2019,Oct,3; 2018,Feb,11; 2018,Jan,8; 2017,Jan,8; 2016,Aug,5; 2016,Jan,13; 2015,Jan,16

93291 **subcutaneous cardiac rhythm monitor system, including heart rhythm derived data analysis**

EXCLUDES *Device evaluation (93288-93290 [93261], 93298)*
External ECG event recording up to 30 days (93268-93272)
Insertion subcutaneous cardiac rhythm monitor (33285)
Rhythm strips (93040-93042)

1.22 1.22 FUD XXX Q1 80

AMA: 2019,Oct,3; 2019,Apr,3; 2018,Feb,11; 2018,Jan,8; 2017,Jan,8; 2016,Aug,5; 2016,Jan,13; 2015,Jan,16

93292 **wearable defibrillator system**

EXCLUDES *External ECG event recording up to 30 days (93268-93272)*
Rhythm strips (93040-93042)
Wearable cardioverter-defibrillator system (93745)

1.27 1.27 FUD XXX Q1 80

AMA: 2019,Oct,3; 2018,Feb,11; 2018,Jan,8; 2017,Jan,8; 2016,Aug,5; 2016,Jan,13; 2015,Jan,16

93293 **Transtelephonic rhythm strip pacemaker evaluation(s) single, dual, or multiple lead pacemaker system, includes recording with and without magnet application with analysis, review and report(s) by a physician or other qualified health care professional, up to 90 days**

EXCLUDES *Device evaluation (93294)*
External ECG event recording up to 30 days (93268-93272)
Rhythm strips (93040-93042)
Reporting code more than one time in 90-day period
Reporting code when monitoring period less than 30 days

1.48 1.48 FUD XXX Q1 80

AMA: 2019,Oct,3; 2018,Feb,11; 2018,Jan,8; 2017,Jan,8; 2016,Aug,5; 2016,Jan,13; 2015,Jan,16

93294 **Interrogation device evaluation(s) (remote), up to 90 days; single, dual, or multiple lead pacemaker system, or leadless pacemaker system with interim analysis, review(s) and report(s) by a physician or other qualified health care professional**

EXCLUDES *Device evaluation (93288, 93293)*
External ECG event recording up to 30 days (93268-93272)
Rhythm strips (93040-93042)
Reporting code more than one time in 90-day period
Reporting code when monitoring period less than 30 days

0.87 0.87 FUD XXX M 80 26

AMA: 2019,Oct,3; 2019,Mar,6; 2018,Feb,11; 2018,Jan,8; 2017,Jan,8; 2016,Aug,5; 2016,Jan,13; 2015,Jan,16

93295 **single, dual, or multiple lead implantable defibrillator system with interim analysis, review(s) and report(s) by a physician or other qualified health care professional**

EXCLUDES *Device evaluation (93289)*
External ECG event recording up to 30 days (93268-93272)
Remote interrogation device evaluation implantable cardioverter-defibrillator with substernal lead (0578T, 0579T)
Remote monitoring physiological cardiovascular data (93297)
Rhythm strips (93040-93042)
Reporting code more than one time in 90-day period
Reporting code when monitoring period less than 30 days

1.09 1.09 FUD XXX M 80 26

AMA: 2019,Oct,3; 2018,Feb,11; 2018,Jan,8; 2017,Jan,8; 2016,Aug,5; 2016,Jan,13; 2015,Jan,16

93296 **single, dual, or multiple lead pacemaker system, leadless pacemaker system, or implantable defibrillator system, remote data acquisition(s), receipt of transmissions and technician review, technical support and distribution of results**

EXCLUDES *Device evaluation (93288-93289)*
External ECG event recording up to 30 days (93268-93272)
Remote interrogation device evaluation implantable cardioverter-defibrillator with substernal lead (0578T, 0579T)
Rhythm strips (93040-93042)
Reporting code more than one time in 90-day period
Reporting code when monitoring period less than 30 days

0.72 0.72 FUD XXX Q1 80 TC

AMA: 2019,Oct,3; 2019,Mar,6; 2019,Jan,6; 2018,Feb,11; 2018,Jan,8; 2017,Jan,8; 2016,Aug,5; 2016,Jan,13; 2015,Jan,16

93297 **Interrogation device evaluation(s), (remote) up to 30 days; implantable cardiovascular physiologic monitor system, including analysis of 1 or more recorded physiologic cardiovascular data elements from all internal and external sensors, analysis, review(s) and report(s) by a physician or other qualified health care professional**

EXCLUDES *Collection and interpretation physiologic data digitally stored and/or transmitted ([99091])*
Device evaluation (93290, 93298)
Heart rhythm derived data (93295)
Remote monitoring physiologic parameter(s) with daily recording(s) or programmed alert(s) ([99454])
Remote monitoring wireless pulmonary artery pressure sensor (93264)
Reporting code more than one time in 30-day period
Reporting code when monitoring period less than 10 days

0.75 0.75 FUD XXX M 80 26

AMA: 2020,Feb,12; 2019,Oct,3; 2018,Feb,11; 2018,Jan,8; 2017,Jan,8; 2016,Aug,5; 2016,Jan,13; 2015,Jan,16

93298 **subcutaneous cardiac rhythm monitor system, including analysis of recorded heart rhythm data, analysis, review(s) and report(s) by a physician or other qualified health care professional**

EXCLUDES *Collection and interpretation physiologic data digitally stored and/or transmitted ([99091])*
Device evaluation (93291, 93297)
External ECG event recording up to 30 days (93268-93272)
Implantation patient-activated cardiac event recorder (33285)
Remote monitoring physiologic parameter(s) with daily recording(s) or programmed alert(s) ([99454])
Reporting code more than one time in 30-day period
Reporting code when monitoring period less than 10 days
Rhythm strips (93040-93042)

0.75 0.75 FUD XXX M 80 26

AMA: 2020,Feb,12; 2019,Oct,3; 2019,Apr,3; 2018,Feb,11; 2018,Jan,8; 2017,Jan,8; 2016,Aug,5; 2016,Jan,13; 2015,Jan,16

93303-93356 [93356] Echocardiography

INCLUDES Interpretation and report
Obtaining ultrasonic signals from heart/great arteries
Report study including:
Description recognized abnormalities
Documentation all clinically relevant findings including obtained quantitative measurements
Interpretation all information obtained
Two-dimensional image/doppler ultrasonic signal documentation
Ultrasound exam:
Adjacent great vessels
Cardiac chambers/valves
Pericardium

EXCLUDES *Contrast agents and/or drugs used for pharmacological stress*
Echocardiography, fetal (76825-76828)
Ultrasound with thorough examination organ(s) or anatomic region/documentation image/final written report

93303 **Transthoracic echocardiography for congenital cardiac anomalies; complete**
6.65 6.65 FUD XXX S 80
AMA: 2020,Jul,12; 2020,Apr,10; 2020,Jan,7; 2018,Feb,11; 2018,Jan,8; 2017,Jan,8; 2016,Jan,13; 2015,May,10; 2015,Jan,16

93304 **follow-up or limited study**
4.53 4.53 FUD XXX S 80
AMA: 2020,Jul,12; 2020,Jan,7; 2018,Feb,11; 2018,Jan,8; 2017,Jan,8; 2016,Jan,13; 2015,May,10; 2015,Jan,16

93306 **Echocardiography, transthoracic, real-time with image documentation (2D), includes M-mode recording, when performed, complete, with spectral Doppler echocardiography, and with color flow Doppler echocardiography**
INCLUDES Doppler and color flow
Two-dimensional and M-mode
EXCLUDES *Transthoracic without spectral and color doppler (93307)*
5.84 5.84 FUD XXX S 80
AMA: 2020,Jul,12; 2020,May,12; 2020,Jan,7; 2018,Dec,10; 2018,Dec,10; 2018,Feb,11; 2018,Jan,8; 2017,Jan,8; 2016,Apr,8; 2016,Jan,13; 2015,May,10; 2015,Jan,16

93307 **Echocardiography, transthoracic, real-time with image documentation (2D), includes M-mode recording, when performed, complete, without spectral or color Doppler echocardiography**
INCLUDES Additional structures that may be viewed such as pulmonary vein or artery, pulmonic valve, inferior vena cava
Obtaining/recording appropriate measurements
Two-dimensional/selected M-mode exam:
Adjacent portions aorta
Aortic/mitral/tricuspid valves
Left/right atria
Left/right ventricles
Pericardium
Using multiple views as required to obtain complete functional/anatomic evaluation
EXCLUDES *Doppler echocardiography (93320-93321, 93325)*
3.97 3.97 FUD XXX S 80
AMA: 2020,Jul,12; 2020,May,12; 2020,Jan,7; 2018,Feb,11; 2018,Jan,8; 2017,Jan,8; 2016,Apr,8; 2016,Jan,13; 2015,May,10; 2015,Jan,16

93308 **Echocardiography, transthoracic, real-time with image documentation (2D), includes M-mode recording, when performed, follow-up or limited study**
INCLUDES Exam that does not evaluate/document attempt to evaluate all structures comprising complete echocardiographic exam
2.79 2.79 FUD XXX S 80
AMA: 2020,Jul,12; 2020,May,12; 2020,Jan,7; 2018,Dec,10; 2018,Dec,10; 2018,Feb,11; 2018,Jan,8; 2017,Jan,8; 2016,Apr,8; 2016,Jan,13; 2015,May,10; 2015,Jan,16

93312 **Echocardiography, transesophageal, real-time with image documentation (2D) (with or without M-mode recording); including probe placement, image acquisition, interpretation and report**
EXCLUDES *Transesophageal echocardiography (93355)*
6.97 6.97 FUD XXX S 80
AMA: 2020,Jan,7; 2018,Feb,11; 2018,Jan,8; 2017,Jan,8; 2016,Jan,13; 2015,Jan,16

93313 **placement of transesophageal probe only**
EXCLUDES *Procedure when performed by same person performing transesophageal echocardiography (93355)*
0.33 0.33 FUD XXX S 80
AMA: 2020,Jan,7; 2018,Feb,11; 2018,Jan,8; 2017,Jan,8; 2016,Jan,13; 2015,Jan,16

93314 **image acquisition, interpretation and report only**
EXCLUDES *Transesophageal echocardiography (93355)*
6.73 6.73 FUD XXX N 80
AMA: 2020,Jan,7; 2018,Feb,11; 2018,Jan,8; 2017,Jan,8; 2016,Jan,13; 2015,Jan,16

93315 **Transesophageal echocardiography for congenital cardiac anomalies; including probe placement, image acquisition, interpretation and report**
EXCLUDES *Transesophageal echocardiography (93355)*
0.00 0.00 FUD XXX S 80
AMA: 2020,Jan,7; 2018,Feb,11; 2018,Jan,8; 2017,Jan,8; 2016,Jan,13; 2015,Jan,16

93316 **placement of transesophageal probe only**
EXCLUDES *Transesophageal echocardiography (93355)*
0.79 0.79 FUD XXX S 80
AMA: 2020,Jan,7; 2018,Feb,11; 2018,Jan,8; 2017,Jan,8; 2016,Jan,13; 2015,Jan,16

93317 **image acquisition, interpretation and report only**
EXCLUDES *Transesophageal echocardiography (93355)*
0.00 0.00 FUD XXX N 80
AMA: 2020,Jan,7; 2018,Feb,11; 2018,Jan,8; 2017,Jan,8; 2016,Jan,13; 2015,Jan,16

93318 **Echocardiography, transesophageal (TEE) for monitoring purposes, including probe placement, real time 2-dimensional image acquisition and interpretation leading to ongoing (continuous) assessment of (dynamically changing) cardiac pumping function and to therapeutic measures on an immediate time basis**
EXCLUDES *Transesophageal echocardiography (93355)*
0.00 0.00 FUD XXX S 80
AMA: 2020,Jan,7; 2018,Feb,11; 2018,Jan,8; 2017,Jan,8; 2016,Jan,13; 2015,Jan,16

\+ **93320** **Doppler echocardiography, pulsed wave and/or continuous wave with spectral display (List separately in addition to codes for echocardiographic imaging); complete**
EXCLUDES *Transesophageal echocardiography (93355)*
Code first (93303-93304, 93312, 93314-93315, 93317, 93350-93351)
1.51 1.51 FUD ZZZ N 80
AMA: 2020,May,12; 2020,Jan,7; 2018,Feb,11; 2018,Jan,8; 2017,Jan,8; 2016,Jan,13; 2015,Jan,16

\+ **93321** **follow-up or limited study (List separately in addition to codes for echocardiographic imaging)**
EXCLUDES *Transesophageal echocardiography (93355)*
Code first (93303-93304, 93308, 93312, 93314-93315, 93317, 93350-93351)
0.76 0.76 FUD ZZZ N 80
AMA: 2020,Jan,7; 2018,Feb,11; 2018,Jan,8; 2017,Jan,8; 2016,Jan,13; 2015,Jan,16

\+ 93325 **Doppler echocardiography color flow velocity mapping (List separately in addition to codes for echocardiography)**

EXCLUDES *Transesophageal echocardiography (93355)*

Code first (76825-76828, 93303-93304, 93308, 93312, 93314-93315, 93317, 93350-93351)

0.70 0.70 FUD ZZZ N 80

AMA: 2020,May,12; 2020,Jan,7; 2018,Feb,11; 2018,Jan,8; 2017,Jan,8; 2016,Jul,8; 2016,Jan,13; 2015,Jan,16

93350 **Echocardiography, transthoracic, real-time with image documentation (2D), includes M-mode recording, when performed, during rest and cardiovascular stress test using treadmill, bicycle exercise and/or pharmacologically induced stress, with interpretation and report;**

EXCLUDES *Cardiovascular stress test, complete procedure (93015)*

Code also exercise stress testing (93016-93018)

5.31 5.31 FUD XXX S 80

AMA: 2020,Jul,12; 2018,Feb,11; 2018,Jan,8; 2017,Jan,8; 2016,Apr,8; 2016,Jan,13; 2015,Jan,16

93351 **including performance of continuous electrocardiographic monitoring, with supervision by a physician or other qualified health care professional**

INCLUDES Stress echocardiogram performed with complete cardiovascular stress test

EXCLUDES *Cardiovascular stress test (93015-93018)*
Echocardiography (93350)
Professional only components complete stress test and stress echocardiogram performed in facility by same physician, append modifier 26
Reporting code for professional component (modifier 26 appended) with (93016, 93018, 93350)

Code also components cardiovascular stress test when professional services not performed by same physician performing stress echocardiogram (93016-93018)

6.63 6.63 FUD XXX S

AMA: 2020,Jul,12; 2018,Feb,11; 2018,Jan,8; 2017,Jan,8; 2016,Apr,8; 2016,Jan,13; 2015,Jan,16

\+ # 93356 **Myocardial strain imaging using speckle tracking-derived assessment of myocardial mechanics (List separately in addition to codes for echocardiography imaging)**

EXCLUDES *Reporting code more than one time for each session*

Code first (93303-93304, 93306, 93307, 93308, 93350-93351)

0.34 1.13 FUD ZZZ 80

AMA: 2020,Jul,12; 2020,Apr,10

\+ 93352 **Use of echocardiographic contrast agent during stress echocardiography (List separately in addition to code for primary procedure)**

EXCLUDES *Reporting code more than one time for each stress echocardiogram*

Code first (93350, 93351)

0.95 0.95 FUD ZZZ M 80

AMA: 2018,Feb,11; 2018,Jan,8; 2017,Jan,8; 2016,Jan,13; 2015,Jan,16

93355 **Echocardiography, transesophageal (TEE) for guidance of a transcatheter intracardiac or great vessel(s) structural intervention(s) (eg,TAVR, transcatheter pulmonary valve replacement, mitral valve repair, paravalvular regurgitation repair, left atrial appendage occlusion/closure, ventricular septal defect closure) (peri-and intra-procedural), real-time image acquisition and documentation, guidance with quantitative measurements, probe manipulation, interpretation, and report, including diagnostic transesophageal echocardiography and, when performed, administration of ultrasound contrast, Doppler, color flow, and 3D**

EXCLUDES *3D rendering (76376-76377)*
Doppler echocardiography (93320-93321, 93325)
Transesophageal echocardiography (93312-93318)
Transesophageal probe positioning by different provider (93313)

6.57 6.57 FUD XXX N 80

AMA: 2018,Feb,11

93356 **Resequenced code. See code following 93351.**

93451-93505 Heart Catheterization

INCLUDES Access site imaging and placement closure device
Catheter insertion and positioning
Contrast injection (except as listed below)
Imaging and insertion closure device
Radiology supervision and interpretation
Roadmapping angiography

EXCLUDES *Congenital cardiac cath procedures (93530-93533)*

Code also separately identifiable:
Aortography (93567)
Noncardiac angiography (see radiology and vascular codes)
Pulmonary angiography (93568)
Right ventricular or atrial injection (93566)

93451 **Right heart catheterization including measurement(s) of oxygen saturation and cardiac output, when performed**

INCLUDES Cardiac output review
Insertion catheter into one or more right cardiac chambers or areas
Obtaining samples for blood gas

EXCLUDES *Catheterization procedures including right side heart (93453, 93456-93457, 93460-93461)*
Implantation wireless pulmonary artery pressure sensor (33289)
Indicator dilution studies (93561-93562)
Percutaneous repair congenital interatrial defect (93580)
Swan-Ganz catheter insertion (93503)
Transcatheter implantation interatrial septal shunt device, percutaneous approach (0613T)
Transcatheter ultrasound ablation nerves innervating pulmonary arteries, percutaneous approach (0632T)
Valve repair or annulus reconstruction (33418, 0345T, 0483T, 0484T, 0544T, 0545T)

Code also administration medication or exercise to repeat assessment hemodynamic measurement (93463-93464)

22.1 22.1 FUD 000 J 62 80

AMA: 2019,Jun,3; 2019,Mar,6; 2018,Dec,10; 2018,Dec,10; 2018,Feb,11; 2018,Jan,8; 2017,Dec,13; 2017,Jul,3; 2017,Jan,8; 2016,Mar,5; 2016,Jan,13; 2015,Sep,3; 2015,Jan,16

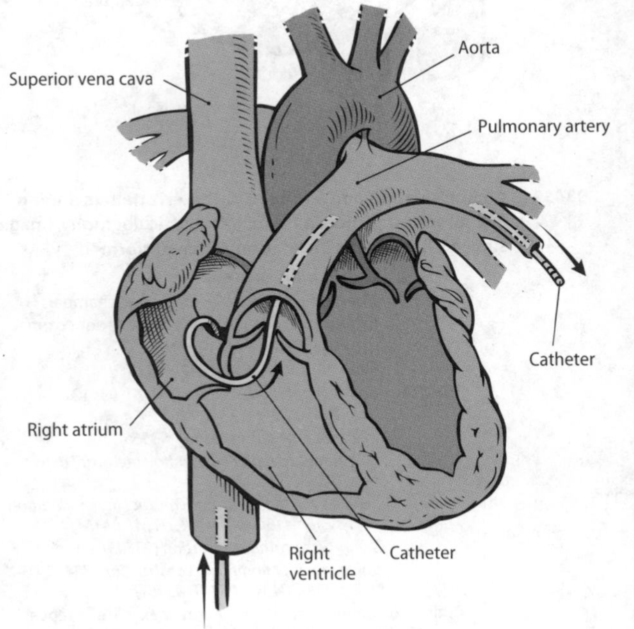

93452 Left heart catheterization including intraprocedural injection(s) for left ventriculography, imaging supervision and interpretation, when performed

INCLUDES Insertion catheter into left cardiac chambers

EXCLUDES *Catheterization procedures including injections for left ventriculography (93453, 93458-93461)*
Injection procedures (93561-93565)
Percutaneous repair congenital interatrial defect (93580)
Services related to cardiac contractility modulation systems (0408T-0411T, 0414T-0415T)
Swan-Ganz catheter insertion (93503)
Valve repair or annulus reconstruction (33418, 0345T, 0483T, 0484T, 0544T, 0545T)

Code also administration medication or exercise to repeat assessment hemodynamic measurement (93463-93464)
Code also transapical or transseptal puncture (93462)

25.9 25.9 **FUD** 000 J G2 80

AMA: 2018,Feb,11; 2018,Jan,8; 2017,Jul,3; 2017,Jan,8; 2016,Jan,13; 2015,Jan,16

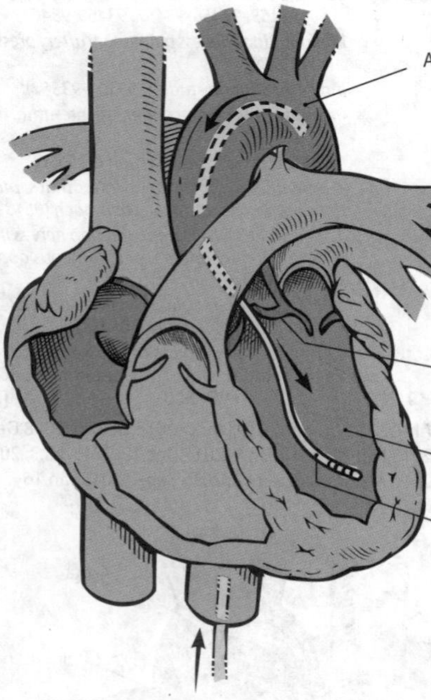

93453 Combined right and left heart catheterization including intraprocedural injection(s) for left ventriculography, imaging supervision and interpretation, when performed

INCLUDES Cardiac output review
Insertion catheter into left cardiac chambers
Insertion catheter into one or more right cardiac chambers or areas
Obtaining samples for blood gas

EXCLUDES *Catheterization procedures (93451-93452, 93456-93461)*
Injection procedures (93561-93565)
Percutaneous repair congenital interatrial defect (93580)
Services related to cardiac contractility modulation systems (0408T-0411T, 0414T-0415T)
Swan-Ganz catheter insertion (93503)
Valve repair or annulus reconstruction (33418, 0345T, 0483T, 0484T, 0544T, 0545T)

Code also administration medication or exercise to repeat assessment hemodynamic measurement (93463-93464)
Code also transapical or transseptal puncture (93462)

33.3 33.3 **FUD** 000 J G2 80

AMA: 2019,Jun,3; 2019,Mar,6; 2018,Feb,11; 2018,Jan,8; 2017,Jul,3; 2017,Jan,8; 2016,Mar,5; 2016,Jan,13; 2015,Sep,3; 2015,Jan,16

93454 Catheter placement in coronary artery(s) for coronary angiography, including intraprocedural injection(s) for coronary angiography, imaging supervision and interpretation;

EXCLUDES *Injection procedures (93561-93565)*
Swan-Ganz catheter insertion (93503)
Valve repair or annulus reconstruction (33418, 0345T, 0483T, 0484T, 0544T, 0545T)

25.9 25.9 **FUD** 000 J G2 80

AMA: 2018,Feb,11; 2018,Jan,8; 2017,Feb,14; 2017,Jan,8; 2016,Mar,5; 2016,Jan,13; 2015,Jan,16

93455 with catheter placement(s) in bypass graft(s) (internal mammary, free arterial, venous grafts) including intraprocedural injection(s) for bypass graft angiography

EXCLUDES *Injection procedures (93561-93565)*
Percutaneous repair congenital interatrial defect (93580)
Swan-Ganz catheter insertion (93503)
Valve repair or annulus reconstruction (33418, 0345T, 0483T, 0484T, 0544T, 0545T)

29.5 29.5 **FUD** 000 J G2 80

AMA: 2018,Feb,11; 2018,Jan,8; 2017,Jan,8; 2016,Mar,5; 2016,Jan,13; 2015,Jan,16

93456 with right heart catheterization

INCLUDES Cardiac output review
Insertion catheter into one or more right cardiac chambers or areas
Obtaining samples for blood gas

EXCLUDES *Injection procedures (93561-93565)*
Percutaneous repair congenital interatrial defect (93580)
Swan-Ganz catheter insertion (93503)
Valve repair or annulus reconstruction (33418, 0345T, 0483T, 0484T, 0544T, 0545T)

Code also administration medication or exercise to repeat assessment hemodynamic measurement (93463-93464)

31.4 31.4 **FUD** 000 J G2 80

AMA: 2019,Jun,3; 2019,Mar,6; 2018,Feb,11; 2018,Jan,8; 2017,Jul,3; 2017,Jan,8; 2016,Mar,5; 2016,Jan,13; 2015,Sep,3; 2015,Jan,16

93457 with catheter placement(s) in bypass graft(s) (internal mammary, free arterial, venous grafts) including intraprocedural injection(s) for bypass graft angiography and right heart catheterization

INCLUDES Cardiac output review
Insertion catheter into one more right cardiac chambers or areas
Obtaining samples for blood gas

EXCLUDES *Injection procedures (93561-93565)*
Percutaneous repair congenital interatrial defect (93580)
Swan-Ganz catheter insertion (93503)
Valve repair or annulus reconstruction (33418, 0345T, 0483T, 0484T, 0544T, 0545T)

Code also administration medication or exercise to repeat assessment hemodynamic measurement (93463-93464)

36.4 36.4 **FUD** 000 J G2 80

AMA: 2019,Jun,3; 2019,Mar,6; 2018,Feb,11; 2018,Jan,8; 2017,Jan,8; 2016,Mar,5; 2016,Jan,13; 2015,Sep,3; 2015,Jan,16

93458 with left heart catheterization including intraprocedural injection(s) for left ventriculography, when performed

INCLUDES Insertion catheter into left cardiac chambers

EXCLUDES *Injection procedures (93561-93565)*

Percutaneous repair congenital interatrial defect (93580)

Services related to cardiac contractility modulation systems (0408T-0411T, 0414T-0415T)

Swan-Ganz catheter insertion (93503)

Valve repair or annulus reconstruction (33418, 0345T, 0483T, 0484T, 0544T, 0545T)

Code also administration medication or exercise to repeat assessment hemodynamic measurement (93463-93464)

Code also transapical or transseptal puncture (93462)

🚑 30.4   ⚕ 30.4   **FUD** 000   [J] [G2] [80] ▭

AMA: 2018,Feb,11; 2018,Jan,8; 2017,Jul,3; 2017,Jan,8; 2016,Mar,5; 2016,Jan,13; 2015,Sep,3; 2015,Jan,16

93459 with left heart catheterization including intraprocedural injection(s) for left ventriculography, when performed, catheter placement(s) in bypass graft(s) (internal mammary, free arterial, venous grafts) with bypass graft angiography

INCLUDES Insertion catheter into left cardiac chambers

EXCLUDES *Injection procedures (93561-93565)*

Percutaneous repair congenital interatrial defect (93580)

Services related to cardiac contractility modulation systems (0408T-0411T, 0414T-0415T)

Swan-Ganz catheter insertion (93503)

Valve repair or annulus reconstruction (33418, 0345T, 0483T, 0484T, 0544T, 0545T)

Code also administration medication or exercise to repeat assessment hemodynamic measurement (93463-93464)

Code also transapical or transseptal puncture (93462)

🚑 32.4   ⚕ 32.4   **FUD** 000   [J] [G2] [80] ▭

AMA: 2018,Feb,11; 2018,Jan,8; 2017,Jul,3; 2017,Jan,8; 2016,Mar,5; 2016,Jan,13; 2015,Sep,3; 2015,Jan,16

93460 with right and left heart catheterization including intraprocedural injection(s) for left ventriculography, when performed

INCLUDES Cardiac output review

Insertion catheter into left cardiac chambers

Insertion catheter into one or more right cardiac chambers or areas

Obtaining samples for blood gas

EXCLUDES *Injection procedures (93561-93565)*

Percutaneous repair congenital interatrial defect (93580)

Services related to cardiac contractility modulation systems (0408T-0411T, 0414T-0415T)

Swan-Ganz catheter insertion (93503)

Valve repair or annulus reconstruction (33418, 0345T, 0483T, 0484T, 0544T, 0545T)

Code also administration medication or exercise to repeat assessment hemodynamic measurement (93463-93464)

Code also transapical or transseptal puncture (93462)

🚑 35.4   ⚕ 35.4   **FUD** 000   [J] [G2] [80] ▭

AMA: 2019,Jun,3; 2019,Mar,6; 2018,Feb,11; 2018,Jan,8; 2017,Jul,3; 2017,Jan,8; 2016,Mar,5; 2016,Jan,13; 2015,Sep,3; 2015,Jan,16

93461 with right and left heart catheterization including intraprocedural injection(s) for left ventriculography, when performed, catheter placement(s) in bypass graft(s) (internal mammary, free arterial, venous grafts) with bypass graft angiography

INCLUDES Cardiac output review

Insertion catheter into left cardiac chambers

Insertion catheter into one or more right cardiac chambers or areas

Obtaining samples for blood gas

EXCLUDES *Injection procedures (93561-93565)*

Percutaneous repair congenital interatrial defect (93580)

Services related to cardiac contractility modulation systems (0408T-0411T, 0414T-0415T)

Swan-Ganz catheter insertion (93503)

Valve repair or annulus reconstruction (33418, 0345T, 0483T, 0484T, 0544T, 0545T)

Code also administration medication or exercise to repeat assessment hemodynamic measurement (93463-93464)

Code also transapical or transseptal puncture (93462)

🚑 40.0   ⚕ 40.0   **FUD** 000   [J] [G2] [80] ▭

AMA: 2019,Jun,3; 2019,Mar,6; 2018,Feb,11; 2018,Jan,8; 2017,Jul,3; 2017,Jan,8; 2016,Mar,5; 2016,Jan,13; 2015,Sep,3; 2015,Jan,16

+ 93462 Left heart catheterization by transseptal puncture through intact septum or by transapical puncture (List separately in addition to code for primary procedure)

INCLUDES Insertion catheter into left cardiac chambers

EXCLUDES *Comprehensive electrophysiologic evaluation (93656)*

Transseptal approach for percutaneous closure paravalvular leak (93590)

Valve repair or annulus reconstruction unless performed with transapical puncture (0345T, 0544T)

Code also percutaneous closure paravalvular leak when transapical puncture performed (93590-93591)

Code first (33477, 93452-93453, 93458-93461, 93582, 93653-93654)

🚑 6.11   ⚕ 6.11   **FUD** ZZZ   [N] [N1] [80] ▭

AMA: 2018,Feb,11; 2018,Jan,8; 2017,Sep,3; 2017,Jul,3; 2017,Jan,8; 2016,Jan,13; 2015,Sep,3; 2015,Jan,16

+ 93463 Pharmacologic agent administration (eg, inhaled nitric oxide, intravenous infusion of nitroprusside, dobutamine, milrinone, or other agent) including assessing hemodynamic measurements before, during, after and repeat pharmacologic agent administration, when performed (List separately in addition to code for primary procedure)

EXCLUDES *Coronary interventional procedures (92920-92944, 92975, 92977)*

Reporting code more than one time per catheterization

Code first (33477, 93451-93453, 93456-93461, 93530-93533, 93580-93581)

🚑 2.82   ⚕ 2.82   **FUD** ZZZ   [N] [80] ▭

AMA: 2018,Feb,11; 2018,Jan,8; 2017,Jan,8; 2016,Jan,13; 2015,Jan,16

+ 93464 Physiologic exercise study (eg, bicycle or arm ergometry) including assessing hemodynamic measurements before and after (List separately in addition to code for primary procedure)

EXCLUDES *Administration of pharmacologic agent (93463)*

Bundle of His recording (93600)

Reporting code more than one time per catheterization

Code first (33477, 93451-93453, 93456-93461, 93530-93533)

🚑 7.04   ⚕ 7.04   **FUD** ZZZ   [N] [80] ▭

AMA: 2018,Feb,11; 2018,Jan,8; 2017,Jan,8; 2016,Jan,13; 2015,Jan,16

● New Code   ▲ Revised Code   ○ Reinstated   ● New Web Release   ▲ Revised Web Release   + Add-on   Unlisted   Not Covered   # Resequenced

㊿ Optum Mod 50 Exempt   ⊘ AMA Mod 51 Exempt   ⑤① Optum Mod 51 Exempt   ⑥③ Mod 63 Exempt   ⁄ Non-FDA Drug   ★ Telemedicine   [M] Maternity   [A] Age Edit

Medicine

93503 Insertion and placement of flow directed catheter (eg, Swan-Ganz) for monitoring purposes

EXCLUDES *Diagnostic cardiac catheterization (93451-93461, 93530-93533)*
Subsequent monitoring (99356-99357)
Transcatheter ultrasound ablation nerves innervating pulmonary arteries, percutaneous approach (0632T)

2.55 2.55 **FUD** 000 T 80

AMA: 2018,Feb,11; 2018,Jan,8; 2017,Jan,8; 2016,Jan,13; 2015,Jan,16

93505 Endomyocardial biopsy

EXCLUDES *Intravascular brachytherapy radionuclide insertion (77770-77772)*
Transcatheter insertion brachytherapy delivery device (92974)

20.1 20.1 **FUD** 000 T 80

AMA: 2018,Feb,11; 2018,Jan,8; 2017,Dec,13; 2017,Jan,8; 2016,Jan,13; 2015,Jan,16

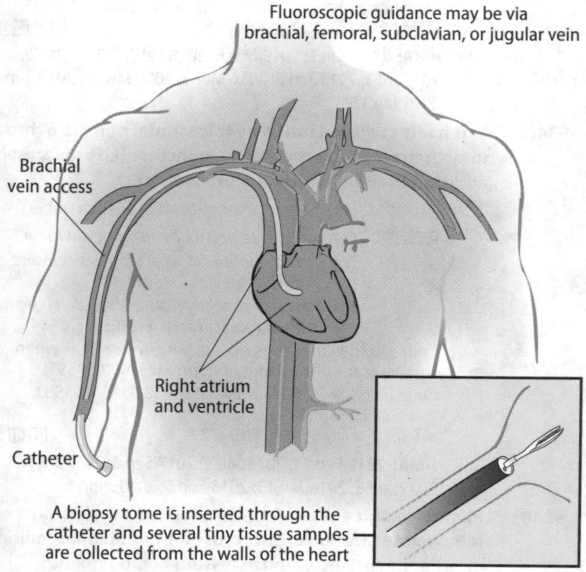
Fluoroscopic guidance may be via brachial, femoral, subclavian, or jugular vein
Brachial vein access
Right atrium and ventricle
Catheter
A biopsy tome is inserted through the catheter and several tiny tissue samples are collected from the walls of the heart

93530-93533 Congenital Heart Defect Catheterization

INCLUDES Access site imaging and placement closure device
Cardiac output review
Insertion catheter into one or more right cardiac chambers or areas
Obtaining samples for blood gas
Radiology supervision and interpretation
Roadmapping angiography

EXCLUDES *Cardiac cath on noncongenital heart (93451-93453, 93456-93461)*
Percutaneous repair congenital interatrial defect (93580)
Swan-Ganz catheter insertion (93503)

Code also (93563-93568)

93530 Right heart catheterization, for congenital cardiac anomalies

0.00 0.00 **FUD** 000 J 80

AMA: 2019,Jun,3; 2019,Mar,6; 2018,Feb,11; 2018,Jan,8; 2017,Jul,3; 2017,Jan,8; 2016,Mar,5; 2016,Jan,13; 2015,Sep,3; 2015,Jan,16

93531 Combined right heart catheterization and retrograde left heart catheterization, for congenital cardiac anomalies

0.00 0.00 **FUD** 000 J 80

AMA: 2019,Jun,3; 2019,Mar,6; 2018,Feb,11; 2018,Jan,8; 2017,Jul,3; 2017,Jan,8; 2016,Mar,5; 2016,Jan,13; 2015,Sep,3; 2015,Jan,16

93532 Combined right heart catheterization and transseptal left heart catheterization through intact septum with or without retrograde left heart catheterization, for congenital cardiac anomalies

0.00 0.00 **FUD** 000 J 80

AMA: 2019,Jun,3; 2019,Mar,6; 2018,Feb,11; 2018,Jan,8; 2017,Jul,3; 2017,Jan,8; 2016,Mar,5; 2016,Jan,13; 2015,Sep,3; 2015,Jan,16

93533 Combined right heart catheterization and transseptal left heart catheterization through existing septal opening, with or without retrograde left heart catheterization, for congenital cardiac anomalies

0.00 0.00 **FUD** 000 J 80

AMA: 2019,Jun,3; 2019,Mar,6; 2018,Feb,11; 2018,Jan,8; 2017,Jul,3; 2017,Jan,8; 2016,Mar,5; 2016,Jan,13; 2015,Sep,3; 2015,Jan,16

93561-93568 Injection Procedures

INCLUDES Automatic power injector
Catheter repositioning
Radiology supervision and interpretation

93561 Indicator dilution studies such as dye or thermodilution, including arterial and/or venous catheterization; with cardiac output measurement (separate procedure)

EXCLUDES *Cardiac output, radioisotope method (78472-78473, 78481)*
Catheterization procedures (93451-93462)
Percutaneous closure patent ductus arteriosus (93582)

0.00 0.00 **FUD** ZZZ N 80

AMA: 2019,Aug,8; 2018,Feb,11; 2018,Jan,8; 2017,Jan,8; 2016,Jan,13; 2015,Jan,16

93562 subsequent measurement of cardiac output

EXCLUDES *Cardiac output, radioisotope method (78472-78473, 78481)*
Catheterization procedures (93451-93462)
Percutaneous closure patent ductus arteriosus (93582)

0.00 0.00 **FUD** ZZZ N 80

AMA: 2019,Aug,8; 2018,Feb,11; 2018,Jan,8; 2017,Jan,8; 2016,Jan,13; 2015,Jan,16

+ **93563 Injection procedure during cardiac catheterization including imaging supervision, interpretation, and report; for selective coronary angiography during congenital heart catheterization (List separately in addition to code for primary procedure)**

EXCLUDES *Catheterization procedures (93452-93461)*
Valve repair or annulus reconstruction (33418, 0345T, 0483T, 0484T, 0544T, 0545T)

Code first (93530-93533)

1.69 1.69 **FUD** ZZZ N 80

AMA: 2018,Feb,11; 2018,Jan,8; 2017,Jan,8; 2016,Mar,5; 2016,Jan,13; 2015,Jan,16

+ **93564 for selective opacification of aortocoronary venous or arterial bypass graft(s) (eg, aortocoronary saphenous vein, free radial artery, or free mammary artery graft) to one or more coronary arteries and in situ arterial conduits (eg, internal mammary), whether native or used for bypass to one or more coronary arteries during congenital heart catheterization, when performed (List separately in addition to code for primary procedure)**

EXCLUDES *Catheterization procedures (93452-93461)*
Percutaneous repair congenital interatrial defect (93580)
Valve repair or annulus reconstruction (33418, 0345T, 0483T, 0484T, 0544T, 0545T)

Code first (93530-93533)

1.79 1.79 **FUD** ZZZ N 80

AMA: 2018,Feb,11; 2018,Jan,8; 2017,Jan,8; 2016,Mar,5; 2016,Jan,13; 2015,Jan,16

+ **93565** **for selective left ventricular or left atrial angiography (List separately in addition to code for primary procedure)**

EXCLUDES *Catheterization procedures (93452-93461)*
Percutaneous repair congenital interatrial defect (93580)

Code first (93530-93533)

1.31 1.31 FUD ZZZ N 80

AMA: 2018,Feb,11; 2018,Jan,8; 2017,Jan,8; 2016,Jan,13; 2015,Jan,16

+ **93566** **for selective right ventricular or right atrial angiography (List separately in addition to code for primary procedure)**

EXCLUDES *Annulus reconstruction (0545T)*
Percutaneous repair congenital interatrial defect (93580)
Right ventriculography when performed during insertion leadless pacemaker ([33274])

Code first (93451, 93453, 93456-93457, 93460-93461, 93530-93533)

1.35 4.38 FUD ZZZ N N1 80

AMA: 2019,Mar,6; 2018,Feb,11; 2018,Jan,8; 2017,Jan,8; 2016,Aug,5; 2016,May,5; 2016,Mar,5; 2016,Jan,13; 2015,May,3; 2015,Jan,16

+ **93567** **for supravalvular aortography (List separately in addition to code for primary procedure)**

EXCLUDES *Abdominal aortography or non-supravalvular thoracic aortography at same time as cardiac catheterization (36221, 75600-75630)*

Code first (93451-93461, 93530-93533)

1.53 3.71 FUD ZZZ N N1 80

AMA: 2018,Feb,11; 2018,Jan,8; 2017,Jan,8; 2016,Mar,5; 2016,Jan,13; 2015,Jan,16

+ **93568** **for pulmonary angiography (List separately in addition to code for primary procedure)**

EXCLUDES *Transcatheter ultrasound ablation nerves innervating pulmonary arteries, percutaneous approach (0632T)*

Code first (93451, 93453, 93456-93457, 93460-93461, 93530-93533, 93582-93583)

1.38 3.97 FUD ZZZ N N1 80

AMA: 2019,Jun,3; 2019,Apr,10; 2018,Feb,11; 2018,Jan,8; 2017,Jan,8; 2016,Mar,5; 2016,Jan,13; 2015,Jan,16

93571-93572 Coronary Artery Doppler Studies

INCLUDES Doppler transducer manipulations/repositioning within vessel examined, during coronary angiography/therapeutic intervention (angioplasty)

EXCLUDES *Intraprocedural coronary fractional flow reserve (FFR) ([0523T])*

+ **93571** **Intravascular Doppler velocity and/or pressure derived coronary flow reserve measurement (coronary vessel or graft) during coronary angiography including pharmacologically induced stress; initial vessel (List separately in addition to code for primary procedure)**

Code first (92920, 92924, 92928, 92933, 92937, 92941, 92943, 92975, 93454-93461, 93563-93564)

0.00 0.00 FUD ZZZ N N1 80

AMA: 2018,Feb,11; 2018,Jan,8; 2017,Jan,8; 2016,Jan,13; 2015,Dec,18; 2015,May,10; 2015,Jan,16

+ **93572** **each additional vessel (List separately in addition to code for primary procedure)**

Code first initial vessel (93571)

0.00 0.00 FUD ZZZ N N1 80

AMA: 2018,Feb,11; 2018,Jan,8; 2017,Jan,8; 2016,Jan,13; 2015,Dec,18; 2015,May,10; 2015,Jan,16

93580-93583 Percutaneous Repair of Congenital Heart Defects

93580 **Percutaneous transcatheter closure of congenital interatrial communication (ie, Fontan fenestration, atrial septal defect) with implant**

INCLUDES Injection contrast for right heart atrial/ventricular angiograms (93564-93566)
Right heart catheterization (93451, 93453, 93456-93457, 93460-93461, 93530-93533)

EXCLUDES *Bypass graft angiography (93455)*
Injection contrast for left heart atrial/ventricular angiograms (93458-93459)
Left heart catheterization (93452, 93458-93459)

Code also echocardiography, when performed (93303-93317, 93662)

28.2 28.2 FUD 000 J 80

AMA: 2018,Feb,11; 2018,Jan,8; 2017,Jan,8; 2016,Jan,13; 2015,Jan,16

93581 **Percutaneous transcatheter closure of a congenital ventricular septal defect with implant**

INCLUDES Injection contrast for right heart atrial/ventricular angiograms (93564-93566)
Right heart catheterization (93451, 93453, 93456-93457, 93460-93461, 93530-93533)

EXCLUDES *Bypass graft angiography (93455)*
Injection contrast for left heart atrial/ventricular angiograms (93458-93459)
Left heart catheterization (93452, 93458-93459)

Code also echocardiography, when performed (93303-93317, 93662)

38.7 38.7 FUD 000 J 80

AMA: 2018,Feb,11; 2018,Jan,8; 2017,Jan,8; 2016,Jan,13; 2015,Jan,16

93582 **Percutaneous transcatheter closure of patent ductus arteriosus**

INCLUDES Aorta catheter placement (36200)
Aortography (75600-75605, 93567)
Heart catheterization (93451-93461, 93530-93533)

EXCLUDES *Catheterization pulmonary artery (36013-36014)*
Intracardiac echocardiographic services (93662)
Left heart catheterization performed via transapical puncture or transseptal puncture through intact septum (93462)
Ligation repair (33820, 33822, 33824)
Other cardiac angiographic procedures (93563-93566, 93568)
Other echocardiographic services by different provider (93315-93317)

19.4 19.4 FUD 000 J 80

AMA: 2019,Apr,10; 2018,Feb,11; 2018,Jan,8; 2017,Jan,8; 2016,Jan,13; 2015,Jan,16

Medicine

93583 — 93613

93583 **Percutaneous transcatheter septal reduction therapy (eg, alcohol septal ablation) including temporary pacemaker insertion when performed**

INCLUDES Alcohol injection (93463)
Coronary angiography during procedure to roadmap, guide intervention, measure vessel, and complete angiography (93454-93461, 93531-93533, 93563, 93563, 93565)
Left heart catheterization (93452-93453, 93458-93461, 93531-93533)
Temporary pacemaker insertion (33210)

EXCLUDES *Intracardiac echocardiographic services when performed (93662)*
Myectomy (surgical ventriculomyotomy) to treat idiopathic hypertrophic subaortic stenosis (33416)
Other echocardiographic services rendered by different provider (93312-93317)

Code also diagnostic cardiac catheterization procedures if patient's condition (clinical indication) changed since intervention or prior study, no available prior catheter-based diagnostic study in treatment zone, or prior study not adequate (93451, 93454-93457, 93530, 93563-93564, 93566-93568)

21.6 21.6 **FUD** 000 C 80

AMA: 2018,Feb,11

93590-93592 Percutaneous Repair Paravalvular Leak

INCLUDES Access with insertion and positioning of device
Angiography
Fluoroscopy (76000)
Imaging guidance
Left heart catheterization (93452-93453, 93459-93461, 93531-93533)

Code also diagnostic right heart catheterization and angiography performed:
Previous study available but documentation states patient's condition changed since previous study; visualization insufficient; or change necessitates re-evaluation; append modifier 59
When no previous study available and complete diagnostic study performed; append modifier 59

93590 **Percutaneous transcatheter closure of paravalvular leak; initial occlusion device, mitral valve**

INCLUDES Transseptal puncture (93462)

Code also for transapical puncture (93462)

31.0 31.0 **FUD** 000 J 80

AMA: 2018,Feb,11; 2018,Jan,8; 2017,Sep,3

93591 **initial occlusion device, aortic valve**

EXCLUDES *Transapical or transseptal puncture (93462)*

25.8 25.8 **FUD** 000 J 80

AMA: 2018,Feb,11; 2018,Jan,8; 2017,Sep,3

\+ **93592** **each additional occlusion device (List separately in addition to code for primary procedure)**

Code first (93590-93591)

11.3 11.3 **FUD** ZZZ N 80

AMA: 2018,Feb,11; 2018,Jan,8; 2017,Sep,3

93600-93603 Recording of Intracardiac Electrograms

INCLUDES Unusual situations in which there may be recording/pacing/attempt at arrhythmia induction from only one side heart

EXCLUDES *Comprehensive electrophysiological studies (93619-93620, 93653-93654, 93656)*

93600 **Bundle of His recording**

0.00 0.00 **FUD** 000 J 80

AMA: 2018,Feb,11; 2018,Jan,8; 2017,Jan,8; 2016,Jan,13; 2015,Jan,16

93602 **Intra-atrial recording**

0.00 0.00 **FUD** 000 J 80

AMA: 2018,Feb,11; 2018,Jan,8; 2017,Jan,8; 2016,Jan,13; 2015,Jan,16

93603 **Right ventricular recording**

0.00 0.00 **FUD** 000 J 80

AMA: 2018,Feb,11; 2018,Jan,8; 2017,Jan,8; 2016,Jan,13; 2015,Jan,16

93609-93613 Intracardiac Mapping and Pacing

\+ **93609** **Intraventricular and/or intra-atrial mapping of tachycardia site(s) with catheter manipulation to record from multiple sites to identify origin of tachycardia (List separately in addition to code for primary procedure)**

EXCLUDES *Intracardiac 3D mapping (93613)*
Intracardiac ablation with 3D mapping (93654)

Code first (93620, 93653, 93656)

0.00 0.00 **FUD** ZZZ N 80

AMA: 2018,Feb,11; 2018,Jan,8; 2017,Jan,8; 2016,Jan,13; 2015,Jan,16

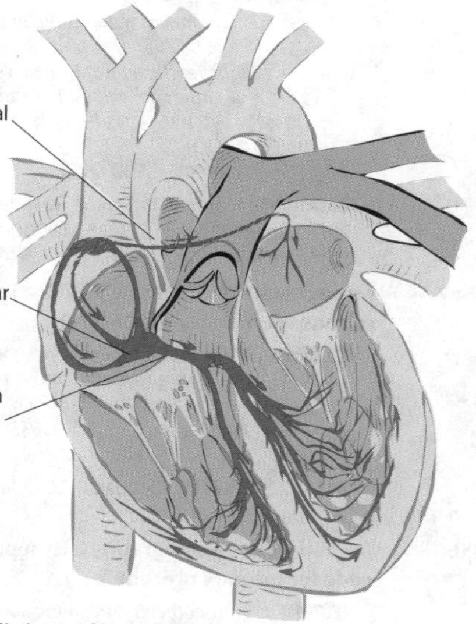

Tachycardia is rapid heartbeat

93610 **Intra-atrial pacing**

INCLUDES Unusual situations in which there may be recording/pacing/attempt at arrhythmia induction from only one side heart

EXCLUDES *Comprehensive electrophysiological studies (93619-93620)*
Intracardiac ablation (93653-93654, 93656)

0.00 0.00 **FUD** 000 J 80

AMA: 2018,Feb,11; 2018,Jan,8; 2017,Jan,8; 2016,Jan,13; 2015,Jan,16

93612 **Intraventricular pacing**

INCLUDES Unusual situations in which there may be recording/pacing/attempt at arrhythmia induction from only one side heart

EXCLUDES *Comprehensive electrophysiological studies (93619-93622)*
Intracardiac ablation (93653-93654, 93656)

0.00 0.00 **FUD** 000 J 80

AMA: 2018,Feb,11; 2018,Jan,8; 2017,Jan,8; 2016,Jan,13; 2015,Jan,16

\+ **93613** **Intracardiac electrophysiologic 3-dimensional mapping (List separately in addition to code for primary procedure)**

EXCLUDES *Intracardiac ablation with 3D mapping (93654)*
Mapping tachycardia site (93609)

Code first (93620, 93653, 93656)

8.63 8.63 **FUD** ZZZ N 80

AMA: 2018,Feb,11; 2018,Jan,8; 2017,Jan,8; 2016,Jan,13; 2015,Jan,16

26/TC PC/TC Only A2-Z3 ASC Payment 50 Bilateral ♂ Male Only ♀ Female Only Facility RVU Non-Facility RVU CCI CLIA
FUD Follow-up Days **CMS:** IOM **AMA:** CPT Asst A-Y OPPSI 80/80 Surg Assist Allowed / w/Doc Lab Crosswalk Radiology Crosswalk

93615-93616 Recording and Pacing via Esophagus

93615 Esophageal recording of atrial electrogram with or without ventricular electrogram(s);
0.00 0.00 FUD 000
AMA: 2018,Feb,11; 2018,Jan,8; 2017,Jan,8; 2016,Jan,13; 2015,Jan,16

93616 with pacing
0.00 0.00 FUD 000
AMA: 2018,Feb,11; 2018,Jan,8; 2017,Jan,8; 2016,Jan,13; 2015,Jan,16

93618 Pacing to Produce an Arrhythmia

CMS: 100-03,20.12 Diagnostic Endocardial Electrical Stimulation (Pacing)

INCLUDES Unusual situations in which there may be recording/pacing/attempt at arrhythmia induction from only one side heart

EXCLUDES *Comprehensive electrophysiological studies (93619-93622)*
Intracardiac ablation (93653-93654, 93656)
Intracardiac phonocardiogram (93799)

93618 Induction of arrhythmia by electrical pacing
0.00 0.00 FUD 000
AMA: 2018,Feb,11; 2018,Jan,8; 2017,Jan,8; 2016,Jan,13; 2015,Jan,16

93619-93623 Comprehensive Electrophysiological Studies

CMS: 100-03,20.12 Diagnostic Endocardial Electrical Stimulation (Pacing)

93619 Comprehensive electrophysiologic evaluation with right atrial pacing and recording, right ventricular pacing and recording, His bundle recording, including insertion and repositioning of multiple electrode catheters, without induction or attempted induction of arrhythmia

INCLUDES Evaluation sinus node/atrioventricular node/His-Purkinje conduction system without arrhythmia induction

EXCLUDES *Comprehensive electrophysiological studies (93620-93622)*
Intracardiac ablation (93653-93657)
Intracardiac pacing (93610, 93612, 93618)
Recording intracardiac electrograms (93600-93603)

0.00 0.00 FUD 000
AMA: 2018,Feb,11; 2018,Jan,8; 2017,Jan,8; 2016,Jan,13; 2015,Jan,16

93620 Comprehensive electrophysiologic evaluation including insertion and repositioning of multiple electrode catheters with induction or attempted induction of arrhythmia; with right atrial pacing and recording, right ventricular pacing and recording, His bundle recording

INCLUDES Recording/pacing/attempted arrhythmia induction from one or more site(s) in heart

EXCLUDES *Comprehensive electrophysiological study without induction/attempted induction arrhythmia (93619)*
Intracardiac ablation (93653-93657)
Intracardiac pacing (93610, 93612, 93618)
Recording intracardiac electrograms (93600-93603)

0.00 0.00 FUD 000
AMA: 2018,Feb,11; 2018,Jan,8; 2017,Jan,8; 2016,Jan,13; 2015,Jan,16

\+ **93621 with left atrial pacing and recording from coronary sinus or left atrium (List separately in addition to code for primary procedure)**

INCLUDES Recording/pacing/attempted arrhythmia induction from one or more site(s) in heart

EXCLUDES *Intracardiac ablation (93656)*

Code first (93620, 93653-93654)
0.00 0.00 FUD ZZZ
AMA: 2018,Feb,11; 2018,Jan,8; 2017,Jan,8; 2016,Jan,13; 2015,Jan,16

\+ **93622 with left ventricular pacing and recording (List separately in addition to code for primary procedure)**

EXCLUDES *Intracardiac ablation (93654)*

Code first (93620, 93653, 93656)
0.00 0.00 FUD ZZZ
AMA: 2018,Feb,11; 2018,Jan,8; 2017,Jan,8; 2016,Jan,13; 2015,Jan,16

\+ **93623 Programmed stimulation and pacing after intravenous drug infusion (List separately in addition to code for primary procedure)**

INCLUDES Recording/pacing/attempted arrhythmia induction from one or more site(s) in heart

EXCLUDES *Reporting code more than one time per day*

Code first comprehensive electrophysiologic evaluation (93610, 93612, 93619-93620, 93653-93654, 93656)
0.00 0.00 FUD ZZZ
AMA: 2018,Feb,11; 2018,Jan,8; 2017,Jan,8; 2016,Jan,13; 2015,Jan,16

93624-93631 Followup and Intraoperative Electrophysiologic Studies

CMS: 100-03,20.12 Diagnostic Endocardial Electrical Stimulation (Pacing)

93624 Electrophysiologic follow-up study with pacing and recording to test effectiveness of therapy, including induction or attempted induction of arrhythmia

INCLUDES Recording/pacing/attempted arrhythmia induction from one or more site(s) in heart

0.00 0.00 FUD 000
AMA: 2018,Feb,11; 2018,Jan,8; 2017,Jan,8; 2016,Jan,13; 2015,Jan,16

93631 Intra-operative epicardial and endocardial pacing and mapping to localize the site of tachycardia or zone of slow conduction for surgical correction

EXCLUDES *Operative ablation arrhythmogenic focus or pathway by separate provider (33250-33261)*

0.00 0.00 FUD 000
AMA: 2018,Feb,11; 2018,Jan,8; 2017,Jan,8; 2016,Jan,13; 2015,Jan,16

93640-93644 Electrophysiologic Studies of Cardioverter-Defibrillators

INCLUDES Recording/pacing/attempted arrhythmia induction from one or more site(s) in heart

93640 Electrophysiologic evaluation of single or dual chamber pacing cardioverter-defibrillator leads including defibrillation threshold evaluation (induction of arrhythmia, evaluation of sensing and pacing for arrhythmia termination) at time of initial implantation or replacement;
0.00 0.00 FUD 000
AMA: 2018,Feb,11; 2018,Jan,8; 2017,Jan,8; 2016,Jan,13; 2015,Jan,16

93641 with testing of single or dual chamber pacing cardioverter-defibrillator pulse generator

EXCLUDES *Single/dual chamber pacing cardioverter-defibrillators reprogramming/electronic analysis, subsequent/periodic (93282-93283, 93289, 93292, 93295, 93642)*

0.00 0.00 FUD 000
AMA: 2018,Feb,11; 2018,Jan,8; 2017,Jan,8; 2016,Jan,13; 2015,Jan,16

93642 Electrophysiologic evaluation of single or dual chamber transvenous pacing cardioverter-defibrillator (includes defibrillation threshold evaluation, induction of arrhythmia, evaluation of sensing and pacing for arrhythmia termination, and programming or reprogramming of sensing or therapeutic parameters)
9.71 9.71 FUD 000
AMA: 2018,Feb,11; 2018,Jan,8; 2017,Jan,8; 2016,Jan,13; 2015,Jan,16

93644 **Electrophysiologic evaluation of subcutaneous implantable defibrillator (includes defibrillation threshold evaluation, induction of arrhythmia, evaluation of sensing for arrhythmia termination, and programming or reprogramming of sensing or therapeutic parameters)**

EXCLUDES *Electrophysiological evaluation subcutaneous implantable defibrillator system with substernal electrode (0577T)*
Insertion/replacement subcutaneous implantable defibrillator ([33270])
Subcutaneous cardioverter-defibrillator electrophysiologic evaluation, subsequent/periodic (93260-93261)

5.65 5.65 **FUD** 000 N 80

AMA: 2018,Feb,11

93650-93657 Intracardiac Ablation

INCLUDES Ablation services include selective delivery cryo-energy or radiofrequency to targeted tissue
Electrophysiologic studies performed in same session with ablation

93650 **Intracardiac catheter ablation of atrioventricular node function, atrioventricular conduction for creation of complete heart block, with or without temporary pacemaker placement**

17.2 17.2 **FUD** 000 J 80

AMA: 2018,Feb,11; 2018,Jan,8; 2017,Jan,8; 2016,Jan,13; 2015,Jan,16

93653 **Comprehensive electrophysiologic evaluation including insertion and repositioning of multiple electrode catheters with induction or attempted induction of an arrhythmia with right atrial pacing and recording, right ventricular pacing and recording (when necessary), and His bundle recording (when necessary) with intracardiac catheter ablation of arrhythmogenic focus; with treatment of supraventricular tachycardia by ablation of fast or slow atrioventricular pathway, accessory atrioventricular connection, cavo-tricuspid isthmus or other single atrial focus or source of atrial re-entry**

EXCLUDES *Comprehensive electrophysiological studies (93619-93620)*
Electrophysiologic evaluation pacing cardioverter defibrillator (93642)
Intracardiac ablation with transseptal catheterization (93656)
Intracardiac ablation with treatment ventricular arrhythmia (93654)
Intracardiac pacing (93610, 93612, 93618)
Recording intracardiac electrograms (93600-93603)

24.3 24.3 **FUD** 000 J 80

AMA: 2018,Feb,11; 2018,Jan,8; 2017,Jan,8; 2016,Jan,13; 2015,Jan,16

93654 **with treatment of ventricular tachycardia or focus of ventricular ectopy including intracardiac electrophysiologic 3D mapping, when performed, and left ventricular pacing and recording, when performed**

EXCLUDES *Comprehensive electrophysiological studies (93619-93620, 93622)*
Device evaluation (93279-93284, 93286-93289)
Electrophysiologic evaluation pacing cardioverter defibrillator (93642)
Intracardiac ablation with transseptal catheterization (93656)
Intracardiac ablation with treatment supraventricular tachycardia (93653)
Intracardiac pacing (93609-93613, 93618)
Recording intracardiac electrograms (93600-93603)

32.6 32.6 **FUD** 000 J 80

AMA: 2018,Feb,11; 2018,Jan,8; 2017,Jan,8; 2016,Jan,13; 2015,Jan,16

\+ **93655** **Intracardiac catheter ablation of a discrete mechanism of arrhythmia which is distinct from the primary ablated mechanism, including repeat diagnostic maneuvers, to treat a spontaneous or induced arrhythmia (List separately in addition to code for primary procedure)**

Code first (93653-93654, 93656)

12.4 12.4 **FUD** ZZZ N 80

AMA: 2018,Feb,11; 2018,Jan,8; 2017,Jan,8; 2016,Jan,13; 2015,Jan,16

93656 **Comprehensive electrophysiologic evaluation including transseptal catheterizations, insertion and repositioning of multiple electrode catheters with induction or attempted induction of an arrhythmia including left or right atrial pacing/recording when necessary, right ventricular pacing/recording when necessary, and His bundle recording when necessary with intracardiac catheter ablation of atrial fibrillation by pulmonary vein isolation**

INCLUDES His bundle recording when indicated
Left atrial pacing/recording
Right ventricular pacing/recording

EXCLUDES *Comprehensive electrophysiological studies (93619-93621)*
Device evaluation (93279-93284, 93286-93289)
Electrophysiologic evaluation with treatment ventricular tachycardia (93654)
Intracardiac ablation with treatment supraventricular tachycardia (93653)
Intracardiac pacing (93610, 93612, 93618)
Left heart catheterization by transseptal puncture (93462)
Recording intracardiac electrograms (93600-93603)

32.7 32.7 **FUD** 000 J 80

AMA: 2019,Sep,10; 2018,Feb,11; 2018,Jan,8; 2017,Jan,8; 2016,Jan,13; 2015,Jan,16

\+ **93657** **Additional linear or focal intracardiac catheter ablation of the left or right atrium for treatment of atrial fibrillation remaining after completion of pulmonary vein isolation (List separately in addition to code for primary procedure)**

Code first (93656)

12.3 12.3 **FUD** ZZZ N 80

AMA: 2019,Sep,10; 2018,Feb,11; 2018,Jan,8; 2017,Jan,8; 2016,Jan,13; 2015,Jan,16

93660-93662 Other Tests for Cardiac Function

93660 **Evaluation of cardiovascular function with tilt table evaluation, with continuous ECG monitoring and intermittent blood pressure monitoring, with or without pharmacological intervention**

EXCLUDES *Autonomic nervous system function testing (95921, 95924, [95943])*

4.50 4.50 **FUD** 000 S 80

AMA: 2018,Feb,11; 2018,Jan,8; 2017,Jan,8; 2016,Jan,13; 2015,Jan,16

\+ **93662** **Intracardiac echocardiography during therapeutic/diagnostic intervention, including imaging supervision and interpretation (List separately in addition to code for primary procedure)**

EXCLUDES *Internal cardioversion (92961)*
Transcatheter implantation interatrial septal shunt device, percutaneous approach (0613T)
Transcatheter tricuspid valve repair with prosthesis, percutaneous approach (0569T-0570T)

Code first (as appropriate) (92987, 93453, 93460-93462, 93532, 93580-93583, 93620-93622, 93653-93654, 93656)

0.00 0.00 **FUD** ZZZ N 80

AMA: 2018,Feb,11; 2018,Jan,8; 2017,Jan,8; 2016,Jan,13; 2015,Jan,16

93668 Rehabilitation Services: Peripheral Arterial Disease

CMS: 100-03,1,20.35 Supervised Exercise Therapy (SET) for Symptomatic Peripheral Artery Disease (PAD)(Effective May 25, 2017; 100-04,32,390 Supervised exercise therapy (SET) Symptomatic Peripheral Artery Disease; 100-04,32,390.1 General Billing Requirements for Supervised exercise therapy (SET) for PAD; 100-04,32,390.2 Coding Requirements for SET for PAD; 100-04,32,390.3 Special Billing Requirements for Professional Claims; 100-04,32,390.4 Special Billing Requirements for Institutional Claims; 100-04,32,390.5 Common Working File (CWF) Requirements; 100-04,32,390.6 Applicable Medicare Summary Notice (MSN), Remittance Advice Remark Codes (RARCs), and Claim Adjustment Reason Code (CARC) Messaging

INCLUDES Monitoring:
- Other cardiovascular limitations for workload adjustment
- Patient's claudication threshold

Motorized treadmill or track
Sessions lasting 45-60 minutes
Supervision by exercise physiologist/nurse

Code also appropriate E/M service, when performed

93668 **Peripheral arterial disease (PAD) rehabilitation, per session**
0.50 0.50 **FUD** XXX S 80 TC
AMA: 2018,Feb,11

93701-93702 Thoracic Electrical Bioimpedance

EXCLUDES *Bioelectrical impedance analysis whole body (0358T)*
Indirect measurement left ventricular filling pressure by computerized calibration arterial waveform response to Valsalva (93799)

93701 **Bioimpedance-derived physiologic cardiovascular analysis**
0.71 0.71 **FUD** XXX Q1 80 TC
AMA: 2018,Feb,11; 2018,Jan,8; 2017,Jan,8; 2016,Jan,13; 2015,Jan,16

93702 **Bioimpedance spectroscopy (BIS), extracellular fluid analysis for lymphedema assessment(s)**
3.57 3.57 **FUD** XXX S 80 TC
AMA: 2018,Feb,11

93724 Electronic Analysis of Pacemaker Function

93724 **Electronic analysis of antitachycardia pacemaker system (includes electrocardiographic recording, programming of device, induction and termination of tachycardia via implanted pacemaker, and interpretation of recordings)**
8.04 8.04 **FUD** 000 S 80
AMA: 2018,Feb,11; 2018,Jan,8; 2017,Jan,8; 2016,Jan,13; 2015,Jan,16

93740 Temperature Gradient Assessment

93740 **Temperature gradient studies**
0.23 0.23 **FUD** XXX Q1
AMA: 2018,Feb,11

93745 Wearable Cardioverter-Defibrillator System Services

EXCLUDES *Device evaluation (93282, 93292)*

93745 **Initial set-up and programming by a physician or other qualified health care professional of wearable cardioverter-defibrillator includes initial programming of system, establishing baseline electronic ECG, transmission of data to data repository, patient instruction in wearing system and patient reporting of problems or events**
0.00 0.00 **FUD** XXX S 80
AMA: 2018,Feb,11

93750 Ventricular Assist Device (VAD) Interrogation

CMS: 100-03,20.9 Artificial Hearts and Related Devices; 100-03,20.9.1 Ventricular Assist Devices; 100-04,32,320.1 Artificial Hearts Prior to May 1, 2008; 100-04,32,320.2 Coding for Artificial Hearts After May 1, 2008; 100-04,32,320.3 Ventricular Assist Devices; 100-04,32,320.3.1 Post-cardiotomy; 100-04,32,320.3.2 Bridge- to -Transplantation

EXCLUDES *Insertion ventricular assist device (33975-33976, 33979)*
Removal/replacement ventricular assist device (33981-33983)

93750 **Interrogation of ventricular assist device (VAD), in person, with physician or other qualified health care professional analysis of device parameters (eg, drivelines, alarms, power surges), review of device function (eg, flow and volume status, septum status, recovery), with programming, if performed, and report**
1.32 1.58 **FUD** XXX S 80
AMA: 2018,Dec,10; 2018,Dec,10; 2018,Feb,11; 2018,Jan,8; 2017,Jan,8; 2016,Jan,13; 2015,Jan,16

93770 Peripheral Venous Blood Pressure Assessment

CMS: 100-03,20.19 Ambulatory Blood Pressure Monitoring (20.19)

EXCLUDES *Cannulization, central venous (36500, 36555-36556)*

93770 **Determination of venous pressure**
0.23 0.23 **FUD** XXX N
AMA: 2018,Feb,11

93784-93790 Ambulatory Blood Pressure Monitoring

CMS: 100-03,20.19 Ambulatory Blood Pressure Monitoring (20.19); 100-04,32,10.1 Ambulatory Blood Pressure Monitoring Billing Requirements

EXCLUDES *Self-measured blood pressure monitoring ([99473, 99474])*

93784 **Ambulatory blood pressure monitoring, utilizing report-generating software, automated, worn continuously for 24 hours or longer; including recording, scanning analysis, interpretation and report**
1.51 1.51 **FUD** XXX B 80
AMA: 2020,Apr,5; 2018,Feb,11

93786 **recording only**
0.83 0.83 **FUD** XXX Q1 80 TC
AMA: 2020,Apr,5; 2018,Feb,11

93788 **scanning analysis with report**
0.14 0.14 **FUD** XXX Q1 80 TC
AMA: 2020,Apr,5; 2018,Feb,11

93790 **review with interpretation and report**
0.53 0.53 **FUD** XXX M 80 26
AMA: 2020,Apr,5; 2018,Feb,11

93792-93793 INR Monitoring

CMS: 100-03,190.11 Home PT/INR Monitoring for Anticoagulation Management; 100-04,32,60.4.1 Anticoagulation Management: Covered Diagnosis Codes

EXCLUDES *Chronic care management services provided during same month ([99439, 99490, 99491])*
Complex chronic care management services provided during same month (99487-99489)
Online digital assessment and management services by nonphysician healthcare professional (98970-98972)
Online digital evaluation and management services by physician or other qualified health care professional ([99421, 99422, 99423])
Telephone assessment and management service by nonphysician healthcare professional (98966-98968)
Telephone evaluation and management service by physician or other qualified healthcare professional (99441-99443)

93792 **Patient/caregiver training for initiation of home international normalized ratio (INR) monitoring under the direction of a physician or other qualified health care professional, face-to-face, including use and care of the INR monitor, obtaining blood sample, instructions for reporting home INR test results, and documentation of patient's/caregiver's ability to perform testing and report results**

Code also INR home monitoring equipment with appropriate supply code or (99070)

Code also significantly separately identifiable E/M service on same date service using modifier 25

1.84 1.84 **FUD** XXX B 80 TC
AMA: 2018,Mar,7; 2018,Feb,11

93793 **Anticoagulant management for a patient taking warfarin, must include review and interpretation of a new home, office, or lab international normalized ratio (INR) test result, patient instructions, dosage adjustment (as needed), and scheduling of additional test(s), when performed**

EXCLUDES *E/M services performed same date (99202-99215, 99241-99245)*

Reporting code more than one time per day

0.33 0.33 **FUD** XXX B 80 26

AMA: 2020,Feb,7; 2018,Mar,7; 2018,Feb,11; 2018,Jan,8; 2017,Nov,10

93797-93799 Cardiac Rehabilitation

CMS: 100-02,15,232 Cardiac Rehabilitation (CR) and Intensive Cardiac Rehabilitation (ICR) Services Furnished On or After January 1, 2010; 100-04,32,140.2 Cardiac Rehabilitation On or After January 1, 2010; 100-04,32,140.2.1 Coding Cardiac Rehabilitation Services On or After January 1, 2010; 100-04,32,140.2.2.2 Institutional Claims for CR and ICR Services; 100-04,32,140.2.2.4 CR Services Exceeding 36 Sessions; 100-04,32,140.3 Intensive Cardiac Rehabilitation Program Services Furnished On or After January 1, 2010; 100-08,15,4.2.8 Cardiac Rehabilitation (CR) and Intensive Cardiac Rehabilitation (ICR)

93797 **Physician or other qualified health care professional services for outpatient cardiac rehabilitation; without continuous ECG monitoring (per session)**

0.25 0.46 **FUD** 000 S 80

AMA: 2018,Feb,11

93798 **with continuous ECG monitoring (per session)**

0.40 0.72 **FUD** 000 S 80

AMA: 2018,Feb,11

93799 **Unlisted cardiovascular service or procedure**

0.00 0.00 **FUD** XXX S 80

AMA: 2018,Dec,10; 2018,Dec,10; 2018,Sep,10; 2018,Aug,10; 2018,Feb,11; 2018,Jan,8; 2017,Jan,8; 2016,May,5; 2016,Jan,13; 2015,Jan,16

93880-93895 Noninvasive Tests Extracranial/Intracranial Arteries

INCLUDES Patient care required to perform/supervise studies and interpret results

EXCLUDES *Hand-held Dopplers that do not provide hard copy or vascular flow bidirectional analysis (see E/M codes)*

93880 **Duplex scan of extracranial arteries; complete bilateral study**

EXCLUDES *Common carotid intima-media thickness (IMT) studies (93895)*

5.64 5.64 **FUD** XXX S 80

AMA: 2018,Feb,11; 2018,Jan,8; 2017,Jan,8; 2016,Jan,13; 2015,Jan,16

93882 **unilateral or limited study**

EXCLUDES *Common carotid intima-media thickness (IMT) studies (93895)*

3.64 3.64 **FUD** XXX S 80

AMA: 2018,Feb,11; 2018,Jan,8; 2017,Jan,8; 2016,Jan,13; 2015,Jan,16

93886 **Transcranial Doppler study of the intracranial arteries; complete study**

INCLUDES Complete transcranial doppler (TCD) study

Ultrasound evaluation right/left anterior circulation territories and posterior circulation territory

7.70 7.70 **FUD** XXX S 80

AMA: 2018,Feb,11; 2018,Jan,8; 2017,Jan,8; 2016,Jan,13; 2015,Jan,16

93888 **limited study**

INCLUDES Limited TCD study

Ultrasound examination two or fewer territories (right/left anterior circulation, posterior circulation)

4.47 4.47 **FUD** XXX S 80

AMA: 2018,Feb,11; 2018,Jan,8; 2017,Jan,8; 2016,Jan,13; 2015,Jan,16

93890 **vasoreactivity study**

EXCLUDES *Limited TCD study (93888)*

7.82 7.82 **FUD** XXX Q1 80

AMA: 2018,Feb,11; 2018,Jan,8; 2017,Jan,8; 2016,Jan,13; 2015,Jan,16

93892 **emboli detection without intravenous microbubble injection**

EXCLUDES *Limited TCD study (93888)*

8.81 8.81 **FUD** XXX Q1 80

AMA: 2018,Feb,11; 2018,Jan,8; 2017,Jan,8; 2016,Jan,13; 2015,Jan,16

93893 **emboli detection with intravenous microbubble injection**

EXCLUDES *Limited TCD study (93888)*

9.81 9.81 **FUD** XXX Q1 80

AMA: 2018,Feb,11; 2018,Jan,8; 2017,Jan,8; 2016,Jan,13; 2015,Jan,16

93895 **Quantitative carotid intima media thickness and carotid atheroma evaluation, bilateral**

EXCLUDES *Complete and limited duplex studies (93880, 93882)*

0.00 0.00 **FUD** XXX E 80

AMA: 2018,Feb,11

93922-93971 Noninvasive Vascular Studies: Extremities

CMS: 100-04,8,180 Noninvasive Studies for ESRD Patients

INCLUDES Patient care required to perform/supervise studies and interpret results

EXCLUDES *Hand-held dopplers that do not provide hard copy or vascular flow bidirectional analysis (see E/M codes)*

93922 Limited bilateral noninvasive physiologic studies of upper or lower extremity arteries, (eg, for lower extremity: ankle/brachial indices at distal posterior tibial and anterior tibial/dorsalis pedis arteries plus bidirectional, Doppler waveform recording and analysis at 1-2 levels, or ankle/brachial indices at distal posterior tibial and anterior tibial/dorsalis pedis arteries plus volume plethysmography at 1-2 levels, or ankle/brachial indices at distal posterior tibial and anterior tibial/dorsalis pedis arteries with, transcutaneous oxygen tension measurement at 1-2 levels)

INCLUDES Evaluation:
- Doppler analysis bidirectional blood flow
- Nonimaging physiologic recordings pressure
- Oxygen tension measurements and/or plethysmography

Lower extremity (potential levels include high thigh, low thigh, calf, ankle, metatarsal and toes) limited study includes either:
- Ankle/brachial indices distal posterior tibial and anterior tibial/dorsalis pedis arteries plus bidirectional Doppler waveform recording and analysis 1-2 levels; OR
- Ankle/brachial indices distal posterior tibial and anterior tibial/dorsalis pedis arteries plus volume plethysmography 1-2 levels; OR
- Ankle/brachial indices distal posterior tibial and anterior tibial/dorsalis pedis arteries with transcutaneous oxygen tension measurements 1-2 levels

Unilateral provocative functional measurement

Unilateral study 3 or move levels

Upper extremity (potential levels include arm, forearm, wrist, and digits) limited study includes:
- Doppler-determined systolic pressures and bidirectional waveform recording with analysis 1-2 levels; OR
- Doppler-determined systolic pressures and transcutaneous oxygen tension measurements 1-2 levels; OR
- Doppler-determined systolic pressures and volume plethysmography 1-2 levels

EXCLUDES *Reporting code more than one time for lower extremity(ies)*

Reporting code more than one time for upper extremity(ies)

Transcutaneous oxyhemoglobin, deoxyhemoglobin and tissue oxygenation measurement (0631T)

Transcutaneous oxyhemoglobin measurement (0493T)

Code also modifier 52 for unilateral study 1-2 levels

Code also twice for upper and lower extremity study and append modifier 59

2.40 2.40 **FUD** XXX 01 80

AMA: 2019,Oct,8; 2018,Feb,11; 2018,Jan,8; 2017,Jan,8; 2016,Jan,13; 2015,Jan,16

93923 Complete bilateral noninvasive physiologic studies of upper or lower extremity arteries, 3 or more levels (eg, for lower extremity: ankle/brachial indices at distal posterior tibial and anterior tibial/dorsalis pedis arteries plus segmental blood pressure measurements with bidirectional Doppler waveform recording and analysis, at 3 or more levels, or ankle/brachial indices at distal posterior tibial and anterior tibial/dorsalis pedis arteries plus segmental volume plethysmography at 3 or more levels, or ankle/brachial indices at distal posterior tibial and anterior tibial/dorsalis pedis arteries plus segmental transcutaneous oxygen tension measurements at 3 or more levels), or single level study with provocative functional maneuvers (eg, measurements with postural provocative tests, or measurements with reactive hyperemia)

INCLUDES Evaluation:
- Doppler analysis bidirectional blood flow
- Nonimaging physiologic recordings pressures
- Oxygen tension measurements

Lower extremity:
- Ankle/brachial indices distal posterior tibial and anterior tibial/dorsalis pedis arteries plus bidirectional Doppler waveform recording and analysis 3 or more levels; OR
- Ankle/brachial indices distal posterior tibial and anterior tibial/dorsalis pedis arteries with transcutaneous oxygen tension measurements 3 or more levels; OR
- Ankle/brachial indices distal posterior tibial and anterior tibial/dorsalis pedis arteries plus volume plethysmography 3 or more levels; OR

Provocative functional maneuvers and measurement single level

Upper extremity complete study:
- Doppler-determined systolic pressures and bidirectional waveform recording with analysis 3 or more levels; OR
- Doppler-determined systolic pressures and transcutaneous oxygen tension measurements 3 or more levels; OR
- Doppler-determined systolic pressures and volume plethysmography 3 or more levels; OR

EXCLUDES *Reporting code more than one time for lower extremity(ies)*

Reporting coe more than one time for upper extremity(ies)

Transcutaneous oxyhemoglobin, deoxyhemoglobin and tissue oxygenation measurement (0631T)

Unilateral study 3 or more levels (93922)

Code also twice for upper and lower extremity study and append modifier 59

3.78 3.78 **FUD** XXX S 80

AMA: 2020,Sep,14; 2019,Oct,8; 2018,Feb,11; 2018,Jan,8; 2017,Jan,8; 2016,Jan,13; 2015,Jan,16

93924 Noninvasive physiologic studies of lower extremity arteries, at rest and following treadmill stress testing, (ie, bidirectional Doppler waveform or volume plethysmography recording and analysis at rest with ankle/brachial indices immediately after and at timed intervals following performance of a standardized protocol on a motorized treadmill plus recording of time of onset of claudication or other symptoms, maximal walking time, and time to recovery) complete bilateral study

INCLUDES Evaluation:
- Doppler analysis bidirectional blood flow
- Nonimaging physiologic recordings pressures
- Oxygen tension measurements
- Plethysmography

EXCLUDES *Noninvasive vascular studies extremities (93922-93923)*

Other types exercise

4.62 4.62 **FUD** XXX S 80

AMA: 2019,Oct,8; 2018,Feb,11; 2018,Jan,8; 2017,Jan,8; 2016,Jan,13; 2015,Jan,16

93925 **Duplex scan of lower extremity arteries or arterial bypass grafts; complete bilateral study**

EXCLUDES *Preoperative arterial inflow and venous outflow duplex scan for creation hemodialysis access, same extremities (93985)*

7.25 7.25 FUD XXX S 80

AMA: 2019,Oct,8; 2018,Feb,11; 2018,Jan,8; 2017,Jan,8; 2016,Sep,9; 2016,Jan,13; 2015,Jan,16

93926 **unilateral or limited study**

EXCLUDES *Preoperative arterial inflow and venous outflow duplex scan for creation hemodialysis access, same extremity (93986)*

4.24 4.24 FUD XXX S 80

AMA: 2019,Oct,8; 2018,Feb,11; 2018,Jan,8; 2017,Jan,8; 2016,Sep,9; 2016,Jan,13; 2015,Jan,16

93930 **Duplex scan of upper extremity arteries or arterial bypass grafts; complete bilateral study**

EXCLUDES *Preoperative arterial inflow and venous outflow duplex scan for creation hemodialysis access, same extremity(ies) (93985-93986)*

5.83 5.83 FUD XXX S 80

AMA: 2019,Oct,8; 2018,Feb,11; 2018,Jan,8; 2017,Jan,8; 2016,Sep,9; 2016,Jan,13; 2015,Jan,16

93931 **unilateral or limited study**

EXCLUDES *Preoperative arterial inflow and venous outflow duplex scan for creation hemodialysis access, same extremity (93985-93986)*

3.63 3.63 FUD XXX S 80

AMA: 2019,Oct,8; 2018,Feb,11; 2018,Jan,8; 2017,Jan,8; 2016,Sep,9; 2016,Jan,13; 2015,Jan,16

93970 **Duplex scan of extremity veins including responses to compression and other maneuvers; complete bilateral study**

EXCLUDES *Endovenous ablation (36475-36476, 36478-36479)*
Preoperative arterial inflow and venous outflow duplex scan for creation hemodialysis access, same extremity(ies) (93985-93986)

5.52 5.52 FUD XXX S 80

AMA: 2019,Oct,8; 2018,Mar,3; 2018,Feb,11; 2018,Jan,8; 2017,Jan,8; 2016,Nov,3; 2016,Sep,9; 2016,Jan,13; 2015,Jan,16

93971 **unilateral or limited study**

EXCLUDES *Endovenous ablation (36475-36476, 36478-36479)*
Preoperative arterial inflow and venous outflow duplex scan for creation hemodialysis access, same extremity (93985-93986)

3.44 3.44 FUD XXX S 80

AMA: 2019,Oct,8; 2018,Mar,3; 2018,Feb,11; 2018,Jan,8; 2017,Jan,8; 2016,Nov,3; 2016,Sep,9; 2016,Jan,13; 2015,Aug,8; 2015,Jan,16

93975-93981 Noninvasive Vascular Studies: Abdomen/Chest/Pelvis

93975 **Duplex scan of arterial inflow and venous outflow of abdominal, pelvic, scrotal contents and/or retroperitoneal organs; complete study**

7.83 7.83 FUD XXX S 80

AMA: 2018,Feb,11; 2018,Jan,8; 2017,Jan,8; 2016,Aug,9; 2016,Jan,13; 2015,Mar,9; 2015,Jan,16

93976 **limited study**

4.64 4.64 FUD XXX S 80

AMA: 2018,Feb,11; 2018,Jan,8; 2017,Jan,8; 2016,Aug,9; 2016,Jan,13; 2015,Mar,9; 2015,Jan,16

93978 **Duplex scan of aorta, inferior vena cava, iliac vasculature, or bypass grafts; complete study**

EXCLUDES *Ultrasound screening for abdominal aortic aneurysm (76706)*

5.34 5.34 FUD XXX S 80

AMA: 2018,Feb,11; 2018,Jan,8; 2017,Jan,8; 2016,Jan,13; 2015,Jan,16

93979 **unilateral or limited study**

EXCLUDES *Ultrasound screening for abdominal aortic aneurysm (76706)*

3.40 3.40 FUD XXX Q1 80

AMA: 2018,Feb,11; 2018,Jan,8; 2017,Jan,8; 2016,Jan,13; 2015,Jan,16

93980 **Duplex scan of arterial inflow and venous outflow of penile vessels; complete study**

3.53 3.53 FUD XXX S 80

AMA: 2018,Feb,11; 2018,Jan,8; 2017,Jan,8; 2016,Jan,13; 2015,Jan,16

93981 **follow-up or limited study**

2.15 2.15 FUD XXX S 80

AMA: 2018,Feb,11; 2018,Jan,8; 2017,Jan,8; 2016,Jan,13; 2015,Jan,16

93985-93998 Noninvasive Vascular Studies: Hemodialysis Access

93985 **Duplex scan of arterial inflow and venous outflow for preoperative vessel assessment prior to creation of hemodialysis access; complete bilateral study**

EXCLUDES *Duplex scan extremity arteries only, same extremity(ies) (93925, 93930)*
Duplex scan extremity veins only, same extremity(ies) (93970)
Duplex scan hemodialysis access, arterial inflow, and venous outflow, same extremity(ies) (93990)
Physiologic arterial evaluation extremities (93922-93924)

7.53 7.53 FUD XXX P2 80

93986 **complete unilateral study**

EXCLUDES *Duplex scan extremity arteries only, same extremity (93926, 93931)*
Duplex scan extremity veins only, same extremity (93971)
Duplex scan hemodialysis access, arterial inflow and venous outflow, same extremity (93990)
Physiologic arterial evaluation extremities (93922-93924)

4.37 4.37 FUD XXX P2 80

93990 **Duplex scan of hemodialysis access (including arterial inflow, body of access and venous outflow)**

EXCLUDES *Hemodialysis access flow measurement by indicator method (90940)*

4.39 4.39 FUD XXX Q1 80

AMA: 2019,Oct,8; 2018,Feb,11; 2018,Jan,8; 2017,Jan,8; 2016,Jan,13; 2015,Jan,16

93998 **Unlisted noninvasive vascular diagnostic study**

0.00 0.00 FUD XXX Q1 80

AMA: 2018,Feb,11; 2018,Jan,8; 2017,Jan,8; 2016,Jan,13; 2015,Jan,16

94002-94005 Ventilator Management Services

94002 **Ventilation assist and management, initiation of pressure or volume preset ventilators for assisted or controlled breathing; hospital inpatient/observation, initial day**

EXCLUDES *E/M services*

2.63 2.63 FUD XXX Q3 80

AMA: 2019,Aug,8; 2018,Feb,11; 2018,Jan,8; 2017,Jan,8; 2016,Jan,13; 2015,Jan,16

94003 **hospital inpatient/observation, each subsequent day**

EXCLUDES *E/M services*

1.90 1.90 FUD XXX Q3 80

AMA: 2019,Aug,8; 2018,Feb,11; 2018,Jan,8; 2017,Jan,8; 2016,Jan,13; 2015,Jan,16

94004 **nursing facility, per day**

EXCLUDES *E/M services*

1.40 1.40 FUD XXX B 80

AMA: 2019,Aug,8; 2018,Feb,11; 2018,Jan,8; 2017,Jan,8; 2016,Jan,13; 2015,Jan,16

94005 **Home ventilator management care plan oversight of a patient (patient not present) in home, domiciliary or rest home (eg, assisted living) requiring review of status, review of laboratories and other studies and revision of orders and respiratory care plan (as appropriate), within a calendar month, 30 minutes or more**

Code also when different provider reports care plan oversight in same 30 days (99339-99340, 99374-99378)

2.61 2.61 FUD XXX M

AMA: 2018,Feb,11; 2018,Jan,8; 2017,Jan,8; 2016,Jan,13; 2015,Jan,16

94010-94799 [94619] Respiratory Services: Diagnostic and Therapeutic

INCLUDES Laboratory procedure(s)
Test results interpretation

EXCLUDES *Separately identifiable E/M service*

94010 **Spirometry, including graphic record, total and timed vital capacity, expiratory flow rate measurement(s), with or without maximal voluntary ventilation**

INCLUDES Measurement expiratory airflow and volumes

EXCLUDES *Diffusing capacity (94729)*
Other respiratory function services (94150, 94200, 94375, 94728)

1.00 1.00 FUD XXX Q1 80

AMA: 2019,May,10; 2019,Mar,10; 2019,Apr,10; 2018,Feb,11; 2018,Jan,8; 2017,Jan,8; 2016,Jan,13; 2015,Sep,9; 2015,Jan,16

94011 **Measurement of spirometric forced expiratory flows in an infant or child through 2 years of age**

2.46 2.46 FUD XXX Q1 80

AMA: 2019,Mar,10; 2018,Feb,11; 2018,Jan,8; 2017,Jan,8; 2016,Jan,13; 2015,Jan,16

94012 **Measurement of spirometric forced expiratory flows, before and after bronchodilator, in an infant or child through 2 years of age**

4.02 4.02 FUD XXX Q1 80

AMA: 2019,Mar,10; 2018,Feb,11; 2018,Jan,8; 2017,Jan,8; 2016,Jan,13; 2015,Jan,16

94013 **Measurement of lung volumes (ie, functional residual capacity [FRC], forced vital capacity [FVC], and expiratory reserve volume [ERV]) in an infant or child through 2 years of age**

0.55 0.55 FUD XXX S 80

AMA: 2019,Mar,10; 2018,Feb,11; 2018,Jan,8; 2017,Jan,8; 2016,Jan,13; 2015,Jan,16

94014 **Patient-initiated spirometric recording per 30-day period of time; includes reinforced education, transmission of spirometric tracing, data capture, analysis of transmitted data, periodic recalibration and review and interpretation by a physician or other qualified health care professional**

1.58 1.58 FUD XXX Q1 80

AMA: 2019,Mar,10; 2018,Feb,11; 2018,Jan,8; 2017,Jan,8; 2016,Jan,13; 2015,Jan,16

94015 **recording (includes hook-up, reinforced education, data transmission, data capture, trend analysis, and periodic recalibration)**

0.86 0.86 FUD XXX Q1 80 TC

AMA: 2019,Mar,10; 2018,Feb,11; 2018,Jan,8; 2017,Jan,8; 2016,Jan,13; 2015,Jan,16

94016 **review and interpretation only by a physician or other qualified health care professional**

0.72 0.72 FUD XXX A 80 26

AMA: 2019,Mar,10; 2018,Feb,11; 2018,Jan,8; 2017,Jan,8; 2016,Jan,13; 2015,Jan,16

94060 **Bronchodilation responsiveness, spirometry as in 94010, pre- and post-bronchodilator administration**

INCLUDES Spirometry performed prior to and after bronchodilator has been administered

EXCLUDES *Bronchospasm prolonged exercise test with pre- and post-spirometry (94617, [94619])*
Diffusing capacity (94729)
Other respiratory function services (94150, 94200, 94375, 94640, 94728)

Code also bronchodilator supply with appropriate supply code or (99070)

1.68 1.68 FUD XXX S 80

AMA: 2019,Mar,10; 2019,Apr,10; 2018,Feb,11; 2018,Jan,8; 2017,Jan,8; 2016,Jan,13; 2015,Sep,9; 2015,Jan,16

94070 **Bronchospasm provocation evaluation, multiple spirometric determinations as in 94010, with administered agents (eg, antigen[s], cold air, methacholine)**

EXCLUDES *Diffusing capacity (94729)*
Inhalation treatment (diagnostic or therapeutic) (94640)

Code also antigen(s) administration with appropriate supply code or (99070)

1.67 1.67 FUD XXX S 80

AMA: 2019,Mar,10; 2018,Feb,11; 2018,Jan,8; 2017,Jan,8; 2016,Jan,13; 2015,Sep,9; 2015,Jan,16

94150 **Vital capacity, total (separate procedure)**

EXCLUDES *Other respiratory function services (94010, 94060, 94728)*
Thoracic gas volumes (94726-94727)

0.71 0.71 FUD XXX Q1

AMA: 2019,Mar,10; 2018,Sep,14; 2018,Feb,11; 2018,Jan,8; 2017,Jan,8; 2016,Jan,13; 2015,Jan,16

94200 **Maximum breathing capacity, maximal voluntary ventilation**

EXCLUDES *Other respiratory function services (94010, 94060)*

0.78 0.78 FUD XXX Q1 80

AMA: 2019,Mar,10; 2018,Feb,11; 2018,Jan,8; 2017,Jan,8; 2016,Jan,13; 2015,Jan,16

94250 ~~**Expired gas collection, quantitative, single procedure (separate procedure)**~~

94375 **Respiratory flow volume loop**

INCLUDES Obstruction pattern identification in central or peripheral airways (inspiratory and/or expiratory)

EXCLUDES *Diffusing capacity (94729)*
Other respiratory function services (94010, 94060, 94728)

1.10 1.10 FUD XXX Q1 80

AMA: 2019,Mar,10; 2018,Feb,11; 2018,Jan,8; 2017,Jan,8; 2016,Jan,13; 2015,Jan,16

94400 ~~**Breathing response to CO2 (CO2 response curve)**~~

94450 **Breathing response to hypoxia (hypoxia response curve)**

EXCLUDES *HAST - high altitude simulation test (94452, 94453)*

1.88 1.88 FUD XXX Q1 80

AMA: 2019,Mar,10; 2018,Feb,11; 2018,Jan,8; 2017,Jan,8; 2016,Jan,13; 2015,Jan,16

94452 **High altitude simulation test (HAST), with interpretation and report by a physician or other qualified health care professional;**

EXCLUDES *HAST test with supplemental oxygen titration (94453)*
Noninvasive pulse oximetry (94760-94761)
Obtaining arterial blood gases (36600)

1.48 1.48 FUD XXX Q1 80

AMA: 2019,Mar,10; 2018,Feb,11; 2018,Jan,8; 2017,Jan,8; 2016,Jan,13; 2015,Jan,16

94453 with supplemental oxygen titration

EXCLUDES *HAST test without supplemental oxygen titration (94452)*
Noninvasive pulse oximetry (94760-94761)
Obtaining arterial blood gases (36600)

2.03 2.03 FUD XXX Q1 80

AMA: 2019,Mar,10; 2018,Feb,11; 2018,Jan,8; 2017,Jan,8; 2016,Jan,13; 2015,Jan,16

94610 Intrapulmonary surfactant administration by a physician or other qualified health care professional through endotracheal tube

INCLUDES Reporting once per dosing episode

EXCLUDES *Intubation, endotracheal (31500)*
Neonatal critical care (99468-99472)

1.59 1.59 FUD XXX Q1 80

AMA: 2019,Mar,10; 2018,Feb,11; 2018,Jan,8; 2017,Jan,8; 2016,Jan,13; 2015,Jan,16

▲ **94617 Exercise test for bronchospasm, including pre- and post-spirometry and pulse oximetry; with electrocardiographic recording(s)**

EXCLUDES *Cardiovascular stress test (93015-93018)*
ECG monitoring (93000-93010, 93040-93042)
Pulse oximetry (94760-94761)

2.66 2.66 FUD XXX Q1 80

AMA: 2019,May,10; 2019,Mar,10; 2018,Feb,11; 2018,Jan,8; 2017,Oct,3

● # **94619 without electrocardiographic recording(s)**

EXCLUDES *Cardiovascular stress test (93015-93018)*
ECG monitoring (93000-93010, 93040-93042)
Pulse oximetry (94760-94761)

0.00 0.00 FUD 000

94618 Pulmonary stress testing (eg, 6-minute walk test), including measurement of heart rate, oximetry, and oxygen titration, when performed

EXCLUDES *Pulse oximetry (94760-94761)*

0.95 0.95 FUD XXX Q1 80

AMA: 2019,May,10; 2019,Mar,10; 2018,Feb,11; 2018,Jan,8; 2017,Oct,3

94619 **Resequenced code. See code following 94617.**

94621 Cardiopulmonary exercise testing, including measurements of minute ventilation, CO2 production, O2 uptake, and electrocardiographic recordings

EXCLUDES *Cardiovascular stress test (93015-93018)*
ECG monitoring (93000-93010, 93040-93042)
Oxygen uptake expired gas analysis (94680-94690)
Pulse oximetry (94760-94761)

4.50 4.50 FUD XXX S 80

AMA: 2019,May,10; 2019,Mar,10; 2018,Feb,11; 2018,Jan,8; 2017,Oct,3; 2017,Jan,8; 2016,Jan,13; 2015,Jan,16

94640 Pressurized or nonpressurized inhalation treatment for acute airway obstruction for therapeutic purposes and/or for diagnostic purposes such as sputum induction with an aerosol generator, nebulizer, metered dose inhaler or intermittent positive pressure breathing (IPPB) device

EXCLUDES *One hour or more continuous inhalation treatment (94644, 94645)*
Other respiratory function services (94060, 94070)

Code also modifier 76 when more than one inhalation treatment performed on same date

0.51 0.51 FUD XXX Q1 80

AMA: 2019,Mar,10; 2018,Feb,11; 2018,Jan,8; 2017,Jan,8; 2016,Jan,13; 2015,Sep,9; 2015,Jan,16

94642 Aerosol inhalation of pentamidine for pneumocystis carinii pneumonia treatment or prophylaxis

0.00 0.00 FUD XXX Q1 80

AMA: 2019,Mar,10; 2018,Feb,11; 2018,Jan,8; 2017,Jan,8; 2016,Jan,13; 2015,Jan,16

94644 Continuous inhalation treatment with aerosol medication for acute airway obstruction; first hour

EXCLUDES *Services less than one hour (94640)*

1.51 1.51 FUD XXX Q1 80

AMA: 2019,Mar,10; 2018,Feb,11; 2018,Jan,8; 2017,Jan,8; 2016,Jan,13; 2015,Sep,9; 2015,Jan,16

\+ **94645 each additional hour (List separately in addition to code for primary procedure)**

Code first initial hour (94644)

0.47 0.47 FUD XXX N 80

AMA: 2019,Mar,10; 2018,Feb,11; 2018,Jan,8; 2017,Jan,8; 2016,Jan,13; 2015,Sep,9; 2015,Jan,16

94660 Continuous positive airway pressure ventilation (CPAP), initiation and management

1.09 1.81 FUD XXX Q1 80

AMA: 2019,Aug,8; 2019,Mar,10; 2018,Feb,11; 2018,Jan,8; 2017,Jan,8; 2016,Jan,13; 2015,Jan,16

94662 Continuous negative pressure ventilation (CNP), initiation and management

1.03 1.03 FUD XXX Q3 80

AMA: 2019,Aug,8; 2019,Mar,10; 2018,Feb,11; 2018,Jan,8; 2017,Jan,8; 2016,Jan,13; 2015,Jan,16

94664 Demonstration and/or evaluation of patient utilization of an aerosol generator, nebulizer, metered dose inhaler or IPPB device

INCLUDES Reporting only one time per day

0.48 0.48 FUD XXX Q1 80

AMA: 2019,Mar,10; 2018,Feb,11; 2018,Jan,8; 2017,Jan,8; 2016,Jan,13; 2015,Jan,16

94667 Manipulation chest wall, such as cupping, percussing, and vibration to facilitate lung function; initial demonstration and/or evaluation

0.71 0.71 FUD XXX Q1 80

AMA: 2019,Mar,10; 2018,Feb,11; 2018,Jan,8; 2017,Jan,8; 2016,Jan,13; 2015,Sep,9; 2015,Jan,16

94668 subsequent

0.92 0.92 FUD XXX Q1 80

AMA: 2019,Mar,10; 2018,Feb,11; 2018,Jan,8; 2017,Jan,8; 2016,Jan,13; 2015,Sep,9; 2015,Jan,16

94669 Mechanical chest wall oscillation to facilitate lung function, per session

INCLUDES Application external wrap or vest to provide mechanical oscillation

0.90 0.90 FUD XXX Q1 80

AMA: 2019,Mar,10; 2018,Feb,11; 2018,Jan,8; 2017,Jan,8; 2016,Jan,13; 2015,Jan,16

94680 Oxygen uptake, expired gas analysis; rest and exercise, direct, simple

EXCLUDES *Cardiopulmonary stress testing (94621)*

1.51 1.51 FUD XXX Q1 80

AMA: 2019,Mar,10; 2018,Feb,11; 2018,Jan,8; 2017,Oct,3; 2017,Jan,8; 2016,Jan,13; 2015,Jan,16

94681 including CO2 output, percentage oxygen extracted

EXCLUDES *Cardiopulmonary stress testing (94621)*

1.49 1.49 FUD XXX Q1 80

AMA: 2019,Mar,10; 2018,Feb,11; 2018,Jan,8; 2017,Oct,3; 2017,Jan,8; 2016,Jan,13; 2015,Jan,16

94690 rest, indirect (separate procedure)

EXCLUDES *Arterial puncture (36600)*
Cardiopulmonary stress testing (94621)

1.49 1.49 FUD XXX Q1 80

AMA: 2019,Mar,10; 2018,Feb,11; 2018,Jan,8; 2017,Oct,3; 2017,Jan,8; 2016,Jan,13; 2015,Jan,16

94726 Plethysmography for determination of lung volumes and, when performed, airway resistance

INCLUDES Airway resistance
Determination:
Functional residual capacity
Residual volume
Total lung capacity

EXCLUDES *Airway resistance by oscillometry (94728)*
Bronchial provocation (94070)
Diffusing capacity (94729)
Gas dilution or washout (94727)
Spirometry (94010, 94060)

1.52 1.52 FUD XXX Q1 80

AMA: 2019,Mar,10; 2018,Feb,11; 2018,Jan,8; 2017,Jan,8; 2016,Jan,13; 2015,Jan,16

94727 Gas dilution or washout for determination of lung volumes and, when performed, distribution of ventilation and closing volumes

INCLUDES Closing volume
Lung volume measurement
Ventilation distribution

EXCLUDES *Bronchial provocation (94070)*
Diffusing capacity (94729)
Plethysmography for lung volume/airway resistance (94726)
Spirometry (94010, 94060)

1.23 1.23 FUD XXX Q1 80

AMA: 2019,Mar,10; 2018,Feb,11; 2018,Jan,8; 2017,Jan,8; 2016,Jan,13; 2015,Jan,16

94728 Airway resistance by oscillometry

EXCLUDES *Diffusing capacity (94729)*
Gas dilution techniques
Other respiratory function services (94010, 94060, 94070, 94375, 94726)

1.15 1.15 FUD XXX Q1 80

AMA: 2019,Mar,10; 2018,Feb,11; 2018,Jan,8; 2017,Jan,8; 2016,Jan,13; 2015,Jan,16

+ **94729 Diffusing capacity (eg, carbon monoxide, membrane) (List separately in addition to code for primary procedure)**

Code first (94010, 94060, 94070, 94375, 94726-94728)

1.56 1.56 FUD ZZZ N 80

AMA: 2019,Mar,10; 2018,Feb,11; 2018,Jan,8; 2017,Jan,8; 2016,Jan,13; 2015,Jan,16

94750 ~~**Pulmonary compliance study (eg, plethysmography, volume and pressure measurements)**~~

94760 Noninvasive ear or pulse oximetry for oxygen saturation; single determination

EXCLUDES *Blood gases (82803-82810)*
Cardiopulmonary stress testing (94621)
Exercise test for bronchospasm (94617)
Pulmonary stress testing (94618)

0.07 0.07 FUD XXX N 80 TC

AMA: 2019,Aug,8; 2019,Mar,10; 2019,Jan,6; 2018,Feb,11; 2018,Jan,8; 2017,Oct,3; 2017,Jan,8; 2016,Jan,13; 2015,Jan,16

94761 multiple determinations (eg, during exercise)

EXCLUDES *Cardiopulmonary stress testing (94621)*
Exercise test for bronchospasm (94617, [94619])
Pulmonary stress testing (94618)

0.11 0.11 FUD XXX N 80 TC

AMA: 2019,Aug,8; 2019,Mar,10; 2018,Feb,11; 2018,Jan,8; 2017,Oct,3; 2017,Jan,8; 2016,Jan,13; 2015,Jan,16

94762 by continuous overnight monitoring (separate procedure)

0.71 0.71 FUD XXX Q3 80 TC

AMA: 2019,Aug,8; 2019,Mar,10; 2018,Feb,11; 2018,Jan,8; 2017,Jan,8; 2016,Jan,13; 2015,Jan,16

94770 ~~**Carbon dioxide, expired gas determination by infrared analyzer**~~

94772 Circadian respiratory pattern recording (pediatric pneumogram), 12-24 hour continuous recording, infant A

EXCLUDES *Electromyograms/EEG/ECG/respiration recordings*

0.00 0.00 FUD XXX S 80

AMA: 2019,Mar,10; 2018,Feb,11; 2018,Jan,8; 2017,Jan,8; 2016,Jan,13; 2015,Jan,16

94774 Pediatric home apnea monitoring event recording including respiratory rate, pattern and heart rate per 30-day period of time; includes monitor attachment, download of data, review, interpretation, and preparation of a report by a physician or other qualified health care professional A

INCLUDES Oxygen saturation monitoring

EXCLUDES *Event monitors (93268-93272)*
Holter monitor (93224-93227)
Pediatric home apnea services (94775-94777)
Remote cardiovascular telemetry (93228-93229)
Sleep testing (95805-95811 [95800, 95801])

0.00 0.00 FUD YYY B 80

AMA: 2019,Mar,10; 2018,Feb,11; 2018,Jan,8; 2017,Jan,8; 2016,Jan,13; 2015,Jan,16

94775 monitor attachment only (includes hook-up, initiation of recording and disconnection) A

INCLUDES Oxygen saturation monitoring

EXCLUDES *Event monitors (93268-93272)*
Holter monitor (93224-93227)
Remote cardiovascular telemetry (93228-93229)
Sleep testing (95805-95811 [95800, 95801])

0.00 0.00 FUD YYY S 80 TC

AMA: 2019,Mar,10; 2018,Feb,11; 2018,Jan,8; 2017,Jan,8; 2016,Jan,13; 2015,Jan,16

94776 monitoring, download of information, receipt of transmission(s) and analyses by computer only A

INCLUDES Oxygen saturation monitoring

EXCLUDES *Event monitors (93268-93272)*
Holter monitor (93224-93227)
Remote cardiovascular telemetry (93228-93229)
Sleep testing (95805-95811 [95800, 95801])

0.00 0.00 FUD YYY S 80 TC

AMA: 2019,Mar,10; 2018,Feb,11; 2018,Jan,8; 2017,Jan,8; 2016,Jan,13; 2015,Jan,16

94777 review, interpretation and preparation of report only by a physician or other qualified health care professional A

INCLUDES Oxygen saturation monitoring

EXCLUDES *Event monitors (93268-93272)*
Holter monitor (93224-93227)
Remote cardiovascular telemetry (93228-93229)
Sleep testing (95805-95811 [95800, 95801])

0.00 0.00 FUD YYY B 80 26

AMA: 2019,Mar,10; 2018,Feb,11; 2018,Jan,8; 2017,Jan,8; 2016,Jan,13; 2015,Jan,16

94780 Car seat/bed testing for airway integrity, for infants through 12 months of age, with continual clinical staff observation and continuous recording of pulse oximetry, heart rate and respiratory rate, with interpretation and report; 60 minutes A

EXCLUDES *Pediatric and neonatal critical care services (99468-99476, 99477-99480)*
Pulse oximetry (94760-94761)
Reporting code for service less than 60 minutes
Rhythm strips (93040-93042)

0.68 1.45 FUD XXX Q1

AMA: 2019,Mar,10; 2018,Feb,11; 2018,Jan,8; 2017,Jan,8; 2016,Jan,13; 2015,May,10; 2015,Jan,16

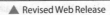

+ **94781** **each additional full 30 minutes (List separately in addition to code for primary procedure)** A

Code first (94780)

0.24 0.57 FUD ZZZ N

AMA: 2019,Mar,10; 2018,Feb,11; 2018,Jan,8; 2017,Jan,8; 2016,Jan,13; 2015,May,10; 2015,Jan,16

94799 **Unlisted pulmonary service or procedure**

0.00 0.00 FUD XXX Q1 80

AMA: 2019,Mar,10; 2018,Sep,14; 2018,Feb,11; 2018,Jan,8; 2017,Jan,8; 2016,Jan,13; 2015,Dec,16; 2015,May,10; 2015,Jan,16

95004-95071 Allergy Tests

EXCLUDES *Drugs administered for intractable/severe allergic reaction (eg, antihistamines, epinephrine, steroids) (96372)*
E/M services when reporting test interpretation/report
Laboratory tests for allergies (86000-86999 [86152, 86153])

Code also medical conferences regarding equipment use (eg, air filters, humidifiers, dehumidifiers), climate therapy, physical, occupational, and recreation therapy using appropriate E/M codes

Code also significant, separately identifiable E/M services using modifier 25, when performed (99202-99215, 99217-99223 [99224, 99225, 99226], 99231-99233, 99241-99255, 99281-99285, 99304-99318, 99324-99337, 99341-99350, 99381-99429 [99415, 99416, 99417, 99421, 99422, 99423])

95004 **Percutaneous tests (scratch, puncture, prick) with allergenic extracts, immediate type reaction, including test interpretation and report, specify number of tests**

0.12 0.12 FUD XXX Q1 80

AMA: 2018,Feb,11; 2018,Jan,8; 2017,Jan,8; 2016,Jan,13; 2015,Jan,16

95012 **Nitric oxide expired gas determination**

0.56 0.56 FUD XXX Q1 80

AMA: 2018,Feb,11; 2018,Jan,8; 2017,Jan,8; 2016,Jan,13; 2015,Jan,16

95017 **Allergy testing, any combination of percutaneous (scratch, puncture, prick) and intracutaneous (intradermal), sequential and incremental, with venoms, immediate type reaction, including test interpretation and report, specify number of tests**

0.11 0.23 FUD XXX Q1 80

AMA: 2018,Feb,11; 2018,Jan,8; 2017,Jan,8; 2016,Jan,13; 2015,Jul,9; 2015,Jan,16

95018 **Allergy testing, any combination of percutaneous (scratch, puncture, prick) and intracutaneous (intradermal), sequential and incremental, with drugs or biologicals, immediate type reaction, including test interpretation and report, specify number of tests**

0.21 0.61 FUD XXX Q1 80

AMA: 2018,Feb,11; 2018,Jan,8; 2017,Jan,8; 2016,Jan,13; 2015,Jul,9; 2015,Jan,16

95024 **Intracutaneous (intradermal) tests with allergenic extracts, immediate type reaction, including test interpretation and report, specify number of tests**

0.03 0.23 FUD XXX Q1 80

AMA: 2018,Feb,11; 2018,Jan,8; 2017,Jan,8; 2016,Jan,13; 2015,Jan,16

95027 **Intracutaneous (intradermal) tests, sequential and incremental, with allergenic extracts for airborne allergens, immediate type reaction, including test interpretation and report, specify number of tests**

0.14 0.14 FUD XXX Q1 80

AMA: 2018,Feb,11; 2018,Jan,8; 2017,Jan,8; 2016,Jan,13; 2015,Jan,16

95028 **Intracutaneous (intradermal) tests with allergenic extracts, delayed type reaction, including reading, specify number of tests**

0.37 0.37 FUD XXX Q1 80 TC

AMA: 2018,Feb,11; 2018,Jan,8; 2017,Jan,8; 2016,Jan,13; 2015,Jan,16

95044 **Patch or application test(s) (specify number of tests)**

0.16 0.16 FUD XXX Q1 80

AMA: 2018,Feb,11; 2018,Jan,8; 2017,Jan,8; 2016,Jan,13; 2015,Jan,16

95052 **Photo patch test(s) (specify number of tests)**

0.18 0.18 FUD XXX Q1 80

AMA: 2018,Feb,11; 2018,Jan,8; 2017,Jan,8; 2016,Jan,13; 2015,Jan,16

95056 **Photo tests**

1.31 1.31 FUD XXX Q1 80

AMA: 2018,Feb,11; 2018,Jan,8; 2017,Jan,8; 2016,Jan,13; 2015,Jan,16

95060 **Ophthalmic mucous membrane tests**

0.99 0.99 FUD XXX Q1 80 TC

AMA: 2018,Feb,11; 2018,Jan,8; 2017,Jan,8; 2016,Jan,13; 2015,Jan,16

95065 **Direct nasal mucous membrane test**

0.73 0.73 FUD XXX Q1 80 TC

AMA: 2018,Feb,11; 2018,Jan,8; 2017,Jan,8; 2016,Jan,13; 2015,Jan,16

▲ **95070** **Inhalation bronchial challenge testing (not including necessary pulmonary function tests), with histamine, methacholine, or similar compounds**

EXCLUDES *Pulmonary function tests (94060, 94070)*

0.90 0.90 FUD XXX S 80 TC

AMA: 2018,Feb,11; 2018,Jan,8; 2017,Jan,8; 2016,Jan,13; 2015,Jan,16

~~**95071** **with antigens or gases, specify**~~

95076-95079 Challenge Ingestion Testing

CMS: 100-03,110.12 Challenge Ingestion Food Testing

INCLUDES Assessment and monitoring for allergic reactions (eg, blood pressure, peak flow meter)
Testing time until test ends or to point E/M service needed

EXCLUDES *Reporting code for testing time less than 61 minutes, such as positive challenge resulting in ending test (report E/M codes as appropriate)*

Code also interventions when appropriate (eg, injection of epinephrine or steroid)

95076 **Ingestion challenge test (sequential and incremental ingestion of test items, eg, food, drug or other substance); initial 120 minutes of testing**

INCLUDES First 120 minutes testing time (not face-to-face time with physician)

2.15 3.43 FUD XXX S 80

AMA: 2018,Feb,11; 2018,Jan,8; 2017,Jan,8; 2016,Jan,13; 2015,Jan,16

+ **95079** **each additional 60 minutes of testing (List separately in addition to code for primary procedure)**

INCLUDES Includes each 60 minutes additional testing time (not face-to-face time with physician)

Code first (95076)

1.97 2.42 FUD ZZZ N 80

AMA: 2018,Feb,11; 2018,Jan,8; 2017,Jan,8; 2016,Jan,13; 2015,Jan,16

95115-95199 Allergy Immunotherapy

CMS: 100-03,110.9 Antigens Prepared for Sublingual Administration

INCLUDES Allergen immunotherapy professional services

EXCLUDES *Bacterial/viral/fungal extracts skin testing (86485-86580, 95028)*
Procedures for testing: (see Pathology/Immunology section or code:) (95199)
Leukocyte histamine release (LHR)
Lymphocytic transformation test (LTT)
Mast cell degranulation test (MCDT)
Migration inhibitory factor test (MIF)
Nitroblue tetrazolium dye test (NTD)
Radioallergosorbent testing (RAST)
Rat mast cell technique (RMCT)
Transfer factor test (TFT)
Special reports for allergy patients (99080)

Code also significant separately identifiable E/M services, when performed

95115 **Professional services for allergen immunotherapy not including provision of allergenic extracts; single injection**
0.26 0.26 FUD XXX Q1 80
AMA: 2020,Sep,14; 2019,Jun,14; 2018,Feb,11; 2018,Jan,8; 2017,Jan,8; 2016,Jan,13; 2015,Jan,16

95117 **2 or more injections**
0.30 0.30 FUD XXX Q1 80
AMA: 2020,Sep,14; 2019,Jun,14; 2018,Feb,11; 2018,Jan,8; 2017,Jan,8; 2016,Jan,13; 2015,Jan,16

95120 **Professional services for allergen immunotherapy in the office or institution of the prescribing physician or other qualified health care professional, including provision of allergenic extract; single injection**
0.00 0.00 FUD XXX E
AMA: 2018,Feb,11; 2018,Jan,8; 2017,Jan,8; 2016,Jan,13; 2015,Jan,16

95125 **2 or more injections**
0.00 0.00 FUD XXX E
AMA: 2018,Feb,11; 2018,Jan,8; 2017,Jan,8; 2016,Jan,13; 2015,Jan,16

95130 **single stinging insect venom**
0.00 0.00 FUD XXX E
AMA: 2018,Feb,11; 2018,Jan,8; 2017,Jan,8; 2016,Jan,13; 2015,Jan,16

95131 **2 stinging insect venoms**
0.00 0.00 FUD XXX E
AMA: 2018,Feb,11; 2018,Jan,8; 2017,Jan,8; 2016,Jan,13; 2015,Jan,16

95132 **3 stinging insect venoms**
0.00 0.00 FUD XXX E
AMA: 2018,Feb,11; 2018,Jan,8; 2017,Jan,8; 2016,Jan,13; 2015,Jan,16

95133 **4 stinging insect venoms**
0.00 0.00 FUD XXX E
AMA: 2018,Feb,11; 2018,Jan,8; 2017,Jan,8; 2016,Jan,13; 2015,Jan,16

95134 **5 stinging insect venoms**
0.00 0.00 FUD XXX E
AMA: 2018,Feb,11; 2018,Jan,8; 2017,Jan,8; 2016,Jan,13; 2015,Jan,16

95144 **Professional services for the supervision of preparation and provision of antigens for allergen immunotherapy, single dose vial(s) (specify number of vials)**
INCLUDES Single dose vial/single dose of antigen administered in one injection
0.09 0.41 FUD XXX Q1 80
AMA: 2018,Feb,11; 2018,Jan,8; 2017,Jan,8; 2016,Jan,13; 2015,Jan,16

95145 **Professional services for the supervision of preparation and provision of antigens for allergen immunotherapy (specify number of doses); single stinging insect venom**
0.09 0.81 FUD XXX Q1 80
AMA: 2018,Feb,11; 2018,Jan,8; 2017,Jan,8; 2016,Jan,13; 2015,Jan,16

95146 **2 single stinging insect venoms**
0.09 1.50 FUD XXX Q1 80
AMA: 2018,Feb,11; 2018,Jan,8; 2017,Jan,8; 2016,Jan,13; 2015,Jan,16

95147 **3 single stinging insect venoms**
0.09 1.55 FUD XXX Q1 80
AMA: 2018,Feb,11; 2018,Jan,8; 2017,Jan,8; 2016,Jan,13; 2015,Jan,16

95148 **4 single stinging insect venoms**
0.09 2.23 FUD XXX Q1 80
AMA: 2018,Feb,11; 2018,Jan,8; 2017,Jan,8; 2016,Jan,13; 2015,Jan,16

95149 **5 single stinging insect venoms**
0.09 3.12 FUD XXX Q1 80
AMA: 2018,Feb,11; 2018,Jan,8; 2017,Jan,8; 2016,Jan,13; 2015,Jan,16

95165 **Professional services for the supervision of preparation and provision of antigens for allergen immunotherapy; single or multiple antigens (specify number of doses)**
0.09 0.40 FUD XXX Q1 80
AMA: 2018,Feb,11; 2018,Jan,8; 2017,Jan,8; 2016,Jan,13; 2015,Jan,16

95170 **whole body extract of biting insect or other arthropod (specify number of doses)**
INCLUDES Dose which is amount of antigen(s) administered in single injection from multiple dose vial
0.09 0.31 FUD XXX Q1 80
AMA: 2018,Feb,11; 2018,Jan,8; 2017,Jan,8; 2016,Jan,13; 2015,Jan,16

95180 **Rapid desensitization procedure, each hour (eg, insulin, penicillin, equine serum)**
2.96 3.92 FUD XXX Q1 80
AMA: 2019,Jun,14; 2018,Feb,11; 2018,Jan,8; 2017,Jan,8; 2016,Jan,13; 2015,Jan,16

95199 **Unlisted allergy/clinical immunologic service or procedure**
0.00 0.00 FUD XXX Q1 80
AMA: 2018,Feb,11; 2018,Jan,8; 2017,Jan,8; 2016,Jan,13; 2015,Jan,16

95249-95251 [95249] Glucose Monitoring By Subcutaneous Device

EXCLUDES *Physiologic data collection/interpretation (99091)*

Code also when data receiver owned by patient for sensor placement, hook-up, monitor calibration, training, and printout (95999)

95249 **Resequenced code. See code following 95250.**

95250 **Ambulatory continuous glucose monitoring of interstitial tissue fluid via a subcutaneous sensor for a minimum of 72 hours; physician or other qualified health care professional (office) provided equipment, sensor placement, hook-up, calibration of monitor, patient training, removal of sensor, and printout of recording**
EXCLUDES *Reporting code more than one time per month*
Subcutaneous pocket with insertion interstitial glucose monitor (0446T)
4.23 4.23 FUD XXX V 80 TC
AMA: 2019,Jan,6; 2018,Jun,6; 2018,Mar,5; 2018,Feb,11; 2018,Jan,8; 2017,Jan,8; 2016,Jan,13; 2015,Jan,16

\# **95249** **patient-provided equipment, sensor placement, hook-up, calibration of monitor, patient training, and printout of recording**
INCLUDES Performing complete collection initial data in provider's office
EXCLUDES *Reporting code more than one time during period patient owns data receiver*
Subcutaneous pocket with insertion interstitial glucose monitor (0446T)
1.54 1.54 FUD XXX S 80 TC
AMA: 2018,Jun,6; 2018,Feb,11

95251 **analysis, interpretation and report**

EXCLUDES *Reporting code more than one time per month*

1.02 1.02 **FUD** XXX B 80 26

AMA: 2018,Jun,6; 2018,Mar,5; 2018,Feb,11; 2018,Jan,8; 2017,Jan,8; 2016,Jan,13; 2015,Jan,16

95700-95783 [95700, 95705, 95706, 95707, 95708, 95709, 95710, 95711, 95712, 95713, 95714, 95715, 95716, 95717, 95718, 95719, 95720, 95721, 95722, 95723, 95724, 95725, 95726, 95782, 95783, 95800, 95801] Sleep Studies

INCLUDES Assessment sleep disorders in adults and children
Continuous and simultaneous monitoring and recording physiological sleep parameters six hours or more
Evaluation patient's response to therapies
Physician:
- Interpretation
- Recording
- Report

Portable and in-laboratory technology
Recording sessions may be:
- Attended studies that include technologist or qualified health care professional presence to respond to patient needs or technical issues at bedside
- Remote without technologist or qualified health professional presence
- Unattended without technologist or qualified health care professional presence

Testing parameters include:
- Actigraphy: Noninvasive portable device to record gross motor movements to approximate sleep and wakeful periods
- Electrooculogram (EOG): Records electrical activity associated with eye movements
- Maintenance of wakefulness test (MWT): Attended study to determine patient's ability to stay awake
- Multiple sleep latency test (MSLT): Attended study to determine patient tendency to fall asleep
- Peripheral arterial tonometry (PAT): Pulsatile volume changes in digit measured to determine activity in sympathetic nervous system for respiratory analysis
- Polysomnography: Attended continuous, simultaneous recording physiological sleep parameters for at least six hours in sleep laboratory setting that also includes four or more:
  1. Airflow-oral and/or nasal
  2. Bilateral anterior tibialis EMG
  3. Electrocardiogram (ECG)
  4. Oxyhemoglobin saturation, SpO2
  5. Respiratory effort
- Positive airway pressure (PAP): Noninvasive devices to treat sleep-related disorders
- Respiratory airflow (ventilation): Assessment air movement during inhalation and exhalation as measured by nasal pressure sensors and thermistor
- Respiratory analysis: Assessment respiration components obtained by other methods such as airflow or peripheral arterial tone
- Respiratory effort: Diaphragm and/or intercostal muscle contraction for airflow measured using transducers to estimate thoracic and abdominal motion
- Respiratory movement: Measures chest and abdomen movement during respiration
- Sleep latency: Pertains to time it takes to get to sleep
- Sleep staging: Determining separate sleep levels according to physiological measurements
- Total sleep time: Determined by actigraphy and other methods

EXCLUDES *E/M services*

95700 **Resequenced code. See code following 95967.**
95705 **Resequenced code. See code following 95967.**
95706 **Resequenced code. See code following 95967.**
95707 **Resequenced code. See code following 95967.**
95708 **Resequenced code. See code following 95967.**
95709 **Resequenced code. See code following 95967.**
95710 **Resequenced code. See code following 95967.**
95711 **Resequenced code. See code following 95967.**
95712 **Resequenced code. See code following 95967.**
95713 **Resequenced code. See code following 95967.**
95714 **Resequenced code. See code following 95967.**
95715 **Resequenced code. See code following 95967.**
95716 **Resequenced code. See code following 95967.**
95717 **Resequenced code. See code following 95967.**
95718 **Resequenced code. See code following 95967.**
95719 **Resequenced code. See code following 95967.**
95720 **Resequenced code. See code following 95967.**
95721 **Resequenced code. See code following 95967.**
95722 **Resequenced code. See code following 95967.**
95723 **Resequenced code. See code following 95967.**
95724 **Resequenced code. See code following 95967.**
95725 **Resequenced code. See code following 95967.**
95726 **Resequenced code. See code following 95967.**
95782 **Resequenced code. See code following 95811.**
95783 **Resequenced code. See code following 95811.**
95800 **Resequenced code. See code following 95806.**
95801 **Resequenced code. See code following 95806.**

95803 **Actigraphy testing, recording, analysis, interpretation, and report (minimum of 72 hours to 14 consecutive days of recording)**

EXCLUDES *Reporting code more than one time in 14-day period*
Sleep studies (95806-95811 [95800, 95801])

4.22 4.22 **FUD** XXX 01 80

AMA: 2018,Feb,11; 2018,Jan,8; 2017,Jan,8; 2016,Jan,13; 2015,Jan,16

95805 **Multiple sleep latency or maintenance of wakefulness testing, recording, analysis and interpretation of physiological measurements of sleep during multiple trials to assess sleepiness**

INCLUDES Physiological sleep parameters as measured by:
- Frontal, central, and occipital EEG leads (three leads)
- Left and right EOG
- Submental EMG lead

EXCLUDES *Polysomnography (95808-95811)*
Sleep study, not attended (95806)

Code also modifier 52 when less than four nap opportunities recorded

11.7 11.7 **FUD** XXX S 80

AMA: 2018,Feb,11; 2018,Jan,8; 2017,Jan,8; 2016,Jan,13; 2015,Jan,16

95806 **Sleep study, unattended, simultaneous recording of, heart rate, oxygen saturation, respiratory airflow, and respiratory effort (eg, thoracoabdominal movement)**

EXCLUDES *Arterial waveform analysis (93050)*
Event monitors (93268-93272)
Holter monitor (93224-93227)
Remote cardiovascular telemetry (93228-93229)
Rhythm strips (93041-93042)
Unattended sleep study with minimum heart rate, oxygen saturation, and respiratory analysis measurement ([95801])
Unattended sleep study with heart rate, oxygen saturation, respiratory analysis, and sleep time measurement ([95800])

Code also modifier 52 for fewer than six hours recording

3.90 3.90 **FUD** XXX S 80

AMA: 2018,Feb,11; 2018,Jan,8; 2017,Jan,8; 2016,Jan,13; 2015,Jan,16

95800 **Sleep study, unattended, simultaneous recording; heart rate, oxygen saturation, respiratory analysis (eg, by airflow or peripheral arterial tone), and sleep time**

EXCLUDES *Actigraphy testing (95803)*
Arterial waveform analysis (93050)
Event monitors (93268-93272)
Holter monitor (93224-93227)
Remote cardiovascular telemetry (93228-93229)
Rhythm strips (93041-93042)
Unattended sleep study with heart rate, oxygen saturation, respiratory airflow and respiratory effort measurement (95806)
Unattended sleep study with minimum heart rate, oxygen saturation, and respiratory analysis measurement ([95801])

Code also modifier 52 for fewer than 6 hours recording
4.68 4.68 **FUD** XXX S 80
AMA: 2018,Feb,11; 2018,Jan,8; 2017,Jan,8; 2016,Jan,13; 2015,Jan,16

95801 **minimum of heart rate, oxygen saturation, and respiratory analysis (eg, by airflow or peripheral arterial tone)**

EXCLUDES *Arterial waveform analysis (93050)*
Event monitors (93268-93272)
Holter monitor (93224-93227)
Remote cardiovascular telemetry (93228-93229)
Rhythm strips (93041-93042)
Unattended sleep study with heart rate, oxygen saturation, respiratory airflow and respiratory effort measurement (95806)
Unattended sleep study with heart rate, oxygen saturation, respiratory analysis, and sleep time measurement ([95800])

Code also modifier 52 for fewer than 6 hours recording
2.57 2.57 **FUD** XXX Q1 80
AMA: 2018,Feb,11; 2018,Jan,8; 2017,Jan,8; 2016,Jan,13; 2015,Jan,16

95807 **Sleep study, simultaneous recording of ventilation, respiratory effort, ECG or heart rate, and oxygen saturation, attended by a technologist**

EXCLUDES *Polysomnography (95808-95811)*
Sleep study, not attended (95806)

Code also modifier 52 for fewer than six hours recording
11.4 11.4 **FUD** XXX S 80
AMA: 2018,Feb,11; 2018,Jan,8; 2017,Jan,8; 2016,Jan,13; 2015,Jan,16

95808 **Polysomnography; any age, sleep staging with 1-3 additional parameters of sleep, attended by a technologist**

EXCLUDES *Sleep study, not attended (95806)*
18.4 18.4 **FUD** XXX S 80
AMA: 2018,Feb,11; 2018,Jan,8; 2017,Jan,8; 2016,Jan,13; 2015,Jan,16

95810 **age 6 years or older, sleep staging with 4 or more additional parameters of sleep, attended by a technologist** A

EXCLUDES *Sleep study, not attended (95806)*

Code also modifier 52 for fewer than six hours recording
17.2 17.2 **FUD** XXX S 80
AMA: 2018,Feb,11; 2018,Jan,8; 2017,Jan,8; 2016,Jan,13; 2015,Jan,16

95811 **age 6 years or older, sleep staging with 4 or more additional parameters of sleep, with initiation of continuous positive airway pressure therapy or bilevel ventilation, attended by a technologist** A

EXCLUDES *Sleep study, not attended (95806)*

Code also modifier 52 for fewer than six hours recording
17.9 17.9 **FUD** XXX S 80
AMA: 2018,Feb,11; 2018,Jan,8; 2017,Jan,8; 2016,Jan,13; 2015,Jan,16

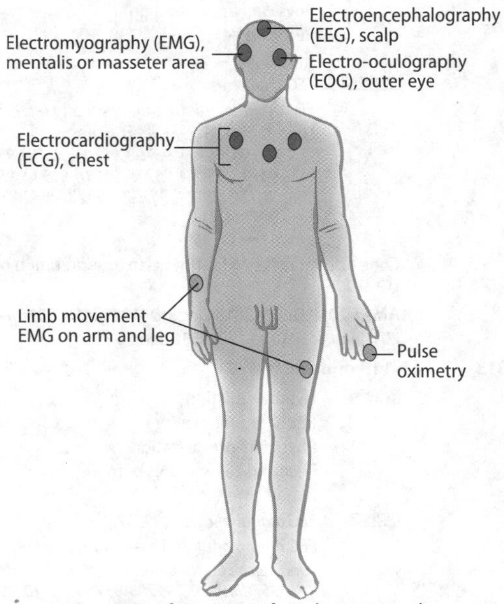

Core areas of monitoring for polysomnography

95782 **younger than 6 years, sleep staging with 4 or more additional parameters of sleep, attended by a technologist** A

Code also modifier 52 for fewer than 7 hours recording
25.4 25.4 **FUD** XXX S 80
AMA: 2018,Feb,11; 2018,Jan,8; 2017,Jan,8; 2016,Jan,13; 2015,Jan,16

95783 **younger than 6 years, sleep staging with 4 or more additional parameters of sleep, with initiation of continuous positive airway pressure therapy or bi-level ventilation, attended by a technologist** A

Code also modifier 52 for fewer than seven hours recording
27.1 27.1 **FUD** XXX S 80
AMA: 2018,Feb,11; 2018,Jan,8; 2017,Jan,8; 2016,Jan,13; 2015,Jan,16

95812-95830 [95829] Evaluation of Brain Activity by Electroencephalogram

INCLUDES Only time when time is recorded, data collected, and does not include set-up and take-down

EXCLUDES *E/M services*

95812 Electroencephalogram (EEG) extended monitoring; 41-60 minutes

INCLUDES Hyperventilation
Photic stimulation
Physician interpretation
Recording 41-60 minutes
Report

EXCLUDES *EEG digital analysis (95957)*
EEG during nonintracranial surgery (95955)
Long-term EEG (two hours or more) ([95700, 95705, 95706, 95707, 95708, 95709, 95710, 95711, 95712, 95713, 95714, 95715, 95716, 95717, 95718, 95719, 95720, 95721, 95722, 95723, 95724, 95725, 95726])
Wada test (95958)

Code also modifier 26 for physician interpretation only

9.29 9.29 **FUD** XXX S 80

AMA: 2018,Dec,3; 2018,Dec,3; 2018,Feb,11; 2018,Jan,8; 2017,Jan,8; 2016,Jan,13; 2015,Jan,16

95813 61-119 minutes

INCLUDES Hyperventilation
Photic stimulation
Physician interpretation
Recording 61 minutes or more
Report

EXCLUDES *EEG digital analysis (95957)*
EEG during nonintracranial surgery (95955)
Long-term EEG (two hours or more) ([95700, 95705, 95706, 95707, 95708, 95709, 95710, 95711, 95712, 95713, 95714, 95715, 95716, 95717, 95718, 95719, 95720, 95721, 95722, 95723, 95724, 95725, 95726])
Wada test (95958)

Code also modifier 26 for physician interpretation only

11.4 11.4 **FUD** XXX S 80

AMA: 2018,Dec,3; 2018,Dec,3; 2018,Feb,11; 2018,Jan,8; 2017,Jan,8; 2016,Jan,13; 2015,Jan,16

95816 Electroencephalogram (EEG); including recording awake and drowsy

INCLUDES Photic stimulation
Physician interpretation
Recording 20-40 minutes
Report

EXCLUDES *EEG digital analysis (95957)*
EEG during nonintracranial surgery (95955)
Long-term EEG (two hours or more) ([95700, 95705, 95706, 95707, 95708, 95709, 95710, 95711, 95712, 95713, 95714, 95715, 95716, 95717, 95718, 95719, 95720, 95721, 95722, 95723, 95724, 95725, 95726])
Wada test (95958)

Code also modifier 26 for physician interpretation only

10.2 10.2 **FUD** XXX S 80

AMA: 2018,Dec,3; 2018,Dec,3; 2018,Feb,11; 2018,Jan,8; 2017,Jan,8; 2016,Jan,13; 2015,Dec,16; 2015,Jan,16

95819 including recording awake and asleep

INCLUDES Hyperventilation
Photic stimulation
Physician interpretation
Recording 20-40 minutes
Report

EXCLUDES *EEG digital analysis (95957)*
EEG during nonintracranial surgery (95955)
Long-term EEG (two hours or more) ([95700, 95705, 95706, 95707, 95708, 95709, 95710, 95711, 95712, 95713, 95714, 95715, 95716, 95717, 95718, 95719, 95720, 95721, 95722, 95723, 95724, 95725, 95726])
Wada test (95958)

Code also modifier 26 for interpretation only

12.0 12.0 **FUD** XXX S 80

AMA: 2018,Dec,3; 2018,Dec,3; 2018,Feb,11; 2018,Jan,8; 2017,Jan,8; 2016,Jan,13; 2015,Dec,16; 2015,Jan,16

95822 recording in coma or sleep only

INCLUDES Hyperventilation
Photic stimulation
Physician interpretation
Recording 20-40 minutes
Report

EXCLUDES *EEG digital analysis (95957)*
EEG during nonintracranial surgery (95955)
Long-term EEG (two hours or more) ([95700, 95705, 95706, 95707, 95708, 95709, 95710, 95711, 95712, 95713, 95714, 95715, 95716, 95717, 95718, 95719, 95720, 95721, 95722, 95723, 95724, 95725, 95726])
Wada test (95958)

Code also modifier 26 for interpretation only

10.9 10.9 **FUD** XXX S 80

AMA: 2018,Dec,3; 2018,Dec,3; 2018,Feb,11; 2018,Jan,8; 2017,Jan,8; 2016,Jan,13; 2015,Jan,16

95824 cerebral death evaluation only

INCLUDES Physician interpretation
Recording
Report

EXCLUDES *EEG digital analysis (95957)*
EEG during nonintracranial surgery (95955)
Long-term EEG (two hours or more) ([95700, 95705, 95706, 95707, 95708, 95709, 95710, 95711, 95712, 95713, 95714, 95715, 95716, 95717, 95718, 95719, 95720, 95721, 95722, 95723, 95724, 95725, 95726])
Wada test (95958)

Code also modifier 26 for physician interpretation only

0.00 0.00 **FUD** XXX S 80

AMA: 2018,Feb,11

95829 **Resequenced code. See code following 95830.**

95830 Insertion by physician or other qualified health care professional of sphenoidal electrodes for electroencephalographic (EEG) recording

2.64 10.9 **FUD** XXX B 80

AMA: 2018,Feb,11

95829-95836 [95829, 95836] Evaluation of Brain Activity by Electrocorticography

95829 Electrocorticogram at surgery (separate procedure)

INCLUDES EEG recording from electrodes placed in or on brain
Interpretation and review during surgical procedure

Code also modifier 26 for interpretation only

52.9 52.9 **FUD** XXX N 80

AMA: 2018,Dec,3; 2018,Dec,3; 2018,Feb,11

\# **95836 Electrocorticogram from an implanted brain neurostimulator pulse generator/transmitter, including recording, with interpretation and written report, up to 30 days**

INCLUDES Intracranial recordings up to 30 days (unattended) with storage for later review

EXCLUDES *EEG digital analysis (95957)*

Programming neurostimulator during 30-day period ([95983, 95984])

Reporting code more than one time for documented 30-day period

3.19 3.19 FUD XXX [80]

AMA: 2018,Dec,3; 2018,Dec,3

95836-95857 [95836] Evaluation of Muscles and Range of Motion

95836 **Resequenced code. See code following 95830.**

95851 Range of motion measurements and report (separate procedure); each extremity (excluding hand) or each trunk section (spine)

0.22 0.59 FUD XXX [A] [80]

AMA: 2018,Feb,11; 2018,Jan,8; 2017,Jan,8; 2016,Dec,16; 2016,Jan,13; 2015,Jan,16

95852 hand, with or without comparison with normal side

0.17 0.53 FUD XXX [A] [80]

AMA: 2018,Feb,11; 2018,Jan,8; 2017,Jan,8; 2016,Jan,13; 2015,Jan,16

95857 Cholinesterase inhibitor challenge test for myasthenia gravis

0.85 1.54 FUD XXX [S] [80]

AMA: 2018,Feb,11; 2018,Jan,8; 2017,Jan,8; 2016,Jan,13; 2015,Jan,16

95860-95887 [95885, 95886, 95887] Evaluation of Nerve and Muscle Function: EMGs with/without Nerve Conduction Studies

INCLUDES Physician interpretation

Recording

Report

EXCLUDES *E/M services*

95860 Needle electromyography; 1 extremity with or without related paraspinal areas

INCLUDES Testing five or more muscles per extremity

EXCLUDES *Dynamic electromyography during motion analysis studies (96002-96003)*

Guidance for chemodenervation (95873-95874)

Code also modifier 26 for interpretation only

3.43 3.43 FUD XXX [Q1] [80]

AMA: 2018,Feb,11; 2018,Jan,8; 2017,Jan,8; 2016,Jan,13; 2015,Mar,6; 2015,Jan,16

95861 2 extremities with or without related paraspinal areas

INCLUDES Testing five or more muscles per extremity

EXCLUDES *Dynamic electromyography during motion analysis studies (96002-96003)*

Guidance for chemodenervation (95873-95874)

Code also modifier 26 for interpretation only

4.90 4.90 FUD XXX [Q1] [80]

AMA: 2018,Feb,11; 2018,Jan,8; 2017,Jan,8; 2016,Jan,13; 2015,Mar,6; 2015,Jan,16

95863 3 extremities with or without related paraspinal areas

INCLUDES Testing five or more muscles per extremity

EXCLUDES *Dynamic electromyography during motion analysis studies (96002-96003)*

Guidance for chemodenervation (95873-95874)

Code also modifier 26 for interpretation only

6.15 6.15 FUD XXX [S] [80]

AMA: 2018,Feb,11; 2018,Jan,8; 2017,Jan,8; 2016,Jan,13; 2015,Mar,6; 2015,Jan,16

95864 4 extremities with or without related paraspinal areas

INCLUDES Testing five or more muscles per extremity

EXCLUDES *Dynamic electromyography during motion analysis studies (96002-96003)*

Guidance for chemodenervation (95873-95874)

Code also modifier 26 for interpretation only

7.07 7.07 FUD XXX [S] [80]

AMA: 2018,Feb,11; 2018,Jan,8; 2017,Jan,8; 2016,Jan,13; 2015,Mar,6; 2015,Jan,16

95865 larynx

EXCLUDES *Dynamic electromyography during motion analysis studies (96002-96003)*

Guidance for chemodenervation (95873-95874)

Code also modifier 26 for interpretation only

Code also modifier 52 for unilateral procedure

4.34 4.34 FUD XXX [Q1] [80]

AMA: 2018,Feb,11; 2018,Jan,8; 2017,Jan,8; 2016,Jan,13; 2015,Mar,6; 2015,Jan,16

95866 hemidiaphragm

EXCLUDES *Dynamic electromyography during motion analysis studies (96002-96003)*

Guidance for chemodenervation (95873-95874)

Code also modifier 26 for interpretation only

3.90 3.90 FUD XXX [Q1] [80]

AMA: 2018,Feb,11; 2018,Jan,8; 2017,Jan,8; 2016,Jan,13; 2015,Mar,6; 2015,Jan,16

95867 cranial nerve supplied muscle(s), unilateral

EXCLUDES *Guidance for chemodenervation (95873-95874)*

Code also modifier 26 for interpretation only

3.05 3.05 FUD XXX [S] [80]

AMA: 2018,Feb,11; 2018,Jan,8; 2017,Jan,8; 2016,Jan,13; 2015,Mar,6; 2015,Jan,16

95868 cranial nerve supplied muscles, bilateral

EXCLUDES *Guidance for chemodenervation (95873-95874)*

3.93 3.93 FUD XXX [S] [80]

AMA: 2018,Feb,11; 2018,Jan,8; 2017,Jan,8; 2016,Jan,13; 2015,Mar,6; 2015,Jan,16

95869 thoracic paraspinal muscles (excluding T1 or T12)

EXCLUDES *Dynamic electromyography during motion analysis studies (96002-96003)*

Guidance for chemodenervation (95873-95874)

2.67 2.67 FUD XXX [Q1] [80]

AMA: 2018,Feb,11; 2018,Jan,8; 2017,Jan,8; 2016,Jan,13; 2015,Mar,6; 2015,Jan,16

95870 limited study of muscles in 1 extremity or non-limb (axial) muscles (unilateral or bilateral), other than thoracic paraspinal, cranial nerve supplied muscles, or sphincters

INCLUDES Adson test

Testing four or less muscles per extremity

EXCLUDES *Anal/urethral sphincter/detrusor/urethra/perineum musculature (51785-51792)*

Complete study extremities (95860-95864)

Dynamic electromyography during motion analysis studies (96002-96003)

Eye muscles (92265)

Guidance for chemodenervation (95873-95874)

2.56 2.56 FUD XXX [Q1] [80]

AMA: 2018,Feb,11; 2018,Jan,8; 2017,Jan,8; 2016,Jan,13; 2015,Mar,6; 2015,Jan,16

95872 Needle electromyography using single fiber electrode, with quantitative measurement of jitter, blocking and/or fiber density, any/all sites of each muscle studied

EXCLUDES *Dynamic electromyography during motion analysis studies (96002-96003)*

5.66 5.66 FUD XXX [S] [80]

AMA: 2018,Feb,11; 2018,Jan,8; 2017,Jan,8; 2016,Jan,13; 2015,Mar,6; 2015,Jan,16

+ # 95885 Needle electromyography, each extremity, with related paraspinal areas, when performed, done with nerve conduction, amplitude and latency/velocity study; limited (List separately in addition to code for primary procedure)

INCLUDES Testing four or less muscles per extremity

EXCLUDES *Dynamic electromyography during motion analysis studies (96002-96003)*
Motor and sensory nerve conduction (95905)
Needle electromyography extremities (95860-95864, 95870)
Reporting code more than one time per extremity

Code also, when applicable, for combined maximum total four units per patient when all four extremities tested ([95886])

Code first nerve conduction tests (95907-95913)

1.77 1.77 **FUD** ZZZ N 80

AMA: 2018,Feb,11; 2018,Jan,8; 2017,Jul,10; 2017,Jan,8; 2016,Jan,13; 2015,Mar,6; 2015,Jan,16

+ # 95886 complete, five or more muscles studied, innervated by three or more nerves or four or more spinal levels (List separately in addition to code for primary procedure)

INCLUDES Testing five or more muscles per extremity

EXCLUDES *Dynamic electromyography during motion analysis studies (96002-96003)*
Motor and sensory nerve conduction (95905)
Needle electromyography extremities (95860-95864, 95870)
Reporting code more than one time per extremity

Code also, when applicable, for combined maximum total four units per patient when all four extremities tested ([95885])

Code first nerve conduction tests (95907-95913)

2.68 2.68 **FUD** ZZZ N 80

AMA: 2018,Feb,11; 2018,Jan,8; 2017,Jul,10; 2017,Jan,8; 2016,Jan,13; 2015,Mar,6; 2015,Jan,16

+ # 95887 Needle electromyography, non-extremity (cranial nerve supplied or axial) muscle(s) done with nerve conduction, amplitude and latency/velocity study (List separately in addition to code for primary procedure)

INCLUDES Nerve study unilateral cranial nerve innervated muscles

EXCLUDES *Dynamic electromyography during motion analysis studies (96002-96003)*
Guidance for chemodenervation (95874)
Motor and sensory nerve conduction (95905)
Needle electromyography cranial nerve supplied muscles (95867-95868)
Needle electromyography except for thoracic paraspinal, cranial nerve supplied muscles, or sphincters (95870)
Nerve study extra-ocular or laryngeal nerves
Reporting code more than once per anatomic site

Code also twice when performed bilaterally

Code first nerve conduction tests (95907-95913)

2.40 2.40 **FUD** ZZZ N 80

AMA: 2018,Feb,11; 2018,Jan,8; 2017,Jul,10; 2017,Jan,8; 2016,Jan,13; 2015,Mar,6; 2015,Jan,16

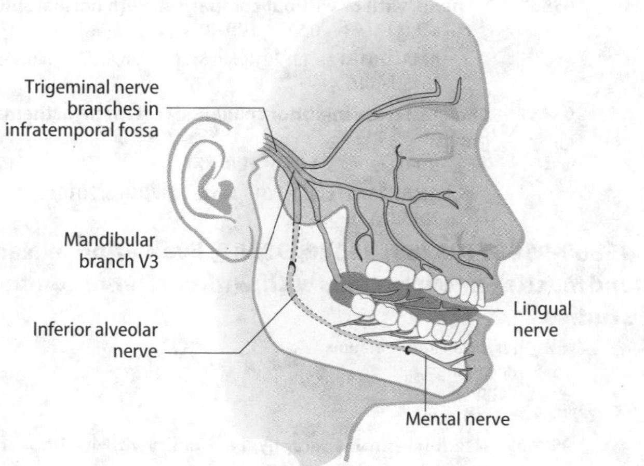

Cranial nerves: trigeminal branches of lower face and select facial nerves

Needle EMG is performed to determine conduction, amplitude, and latency/velocity

+ 95873 Electrical stimulation for guidance in conjunction with chemodenervation (List separately in addition to code for primary procedure)

EXCLUDES *Chemodenervation larynx (64617)*
Injection anesthetic or steroid, sacroiliac joint (64451)
Needle electromyography (95860-95870)
Needle electromyography guidance for chemodenervation (95874)
Radiofrequency ablation, sacroiliac joint ([64625])
Reporting more than one guidance code for each chemodenervation code

Code first chemodenervation (64612, 64615-64616, 64642-64647)

2.17 2.17 **FUD** ZZZ N 80

AMA: 2019,Dec,8; 2019,Apr,9; 2018,Feb,11; 2018,Jan,8; 2017,Jan,8; 2016,Jan,13; 2015,Mar,6; 2015,Jan,16

+ **95874 Needle electromyography for guidance in conjunction with chemodenervation (List separately in addition to code for primary procedure)**

EXCLUDES *Chemodenervation larynx (64617)*
Injection anesthetic or steroid, sacroiliac joint (64451)
Needle electromyography (95860-95870)
Needle electromyography guidance for chemodenervation (95873)
Radiofrequency ablation, sacroiliac joint ([64625])
Reporting more than one guidance code for each chemodenervation code

Code first chemodenervation (64612, 64615-64616, 64642-64647)

2.23 2.23 FUD ZZZ N 80

AMA: 2019,Dec,8; 2019,Apr,9; 2018,Feb,11; 2018,Jan,8; 2017,Jan,8; 2016,Jan,13; 2015,Mar,6; 2015,Jan,16

95875 Ischemic limb exercise test with serial specimen(s) acquisition for muscle(s) metabolite(s)

3.75 3.75 FUD XXX S 80

AMA: 2018,Feb,11; 2018,Jan,8; 2017,Jan,8; 2016,Jan,13; 2015,Mar,6; 2015,Jan,16

95885 **Resequenced code. See code following 95872.**

95886 **Resequenced code. See code following 95872.**

95887 **Resequenced code. See code before 95873.**

95905-95913 Evaluation of Nerve Function: Nerve Conduction Studies

INCLUDES Conduction studies motor and sensory nerves
Reports from on-site examiner including interpretation results using established methodologies, calculations, comparisons to normal studies, and interpretation by physician or other qualified health care professional
Single conduction study comprising sensory and motor conduction test with/without F or H wave testing, and all orthodromic and antidromic impulses
Total number tests performed indicate appropriate code

EXCLUDES *Reporting code for more than one study when multiple sites on same nerve tested*

Code also electromyography performed with nerve conduction studies, as appropriate ([95885, 95886, 95887])

95905 Motor and/or sensory nerve conduction, using preconfigured electrode array(s), amplitude and latency/velocity study, each limb, includes F-wave study when performed, with interpretation and report

INCLUDES Study with preconfigured electrodes that are customized to a specific body location

EXCLUDES *Needle electromyography ([95885, 95886])*
Nerve conduction studies (95907-95913)
Reporting code more than one time for each limb studied

1.80 1.80 FUD XXX ⊘ Q1 80

AMA: 2018,Feb,11; 2018,Jan,8; 2017,Jan,8; 2016,Jan,13; 2015,Jan,16

95907 Nerve conduction studies; 1-2 studies

2.71 2.71 FUD XXX S 80

AMA: 2018,Aug,10; 2018,Feb,11; 2018,Jan,8; 2017,Dec,14; 2017,Jan,8; 2016,Jan,13; 2015,Jan,16

95908 3-4 studies

3.44 3.44 FUD XXX S 80

AMA: 2018,Aug,10; 2018,Feb,11; 2018,Jan,8; 2017,Jan,8; 2016,Jan,13; 2015,Mar,6; 2015,Jan,16

95909 5-6 studies

4.20 4.20 FUD XXX S 80

AMA: 2018,Aug,10; 2018,Feb,11; 2018,Jan,8; 2017,Jan,8; 2016,Jan,13; 2015,Jan,16

95910 7-8 studies

5.42 5.42 FUD XXX S 80

AMA: 2018,Aug,10; 2018,Feb,11; 2018,Jan,8; 2017,Jan,8; 2016,Jan,13; 2015,Jan,16

95911 9-10 studies

6.49 6.49 FUD XXX S 80

AMA: 2018,Aug,10; 2018,Feb,11; 2018,Jan,8; 2017,Jan,8; 2016,Jan,13; 2015,Jan,16

95912 11-12 studies

7.43 7.43 FUD XXX S 80

AMA: 2018,Aug,10; 2018,Feb,11; 2018,Jan,8; 2017,Jan,8; 2016,Jan,13; 2015,Jan,16

95913 13 or more studies

8.60 8.60 FUD XXX S 80

AMA: 2018,Aug,10; 2018,Feb,11; 2018,Jan,8; 2017,Jan,8; 2016,Jan,13; 2015,Jan,16

95940-95941 [95940, 95941] Intraoperative Neurophysiological Monitoring

INCLUDES Monitoring, testing, and data evaluation during surgical procedures by monitoring professional dedicated only to performing necessary testing and monitoring
Monitoring services provided by anesthesiologist or surgeon separately

EXCLUDES *Baseline neurophysiologic monitoring*
EEG during nonintracranial surgery (95955)
Electrocorticography ([95829])
Intraoperative cortical and subcortical mapping (95961-95962)
Neurostimulator programming/analysis (95971-95972, 95976-95977, [95983, 95984])
Time required for set-up, recording, interpretation, and electrode removal

Code also baseline studies (eg, EMGs, NCVs), no more than one time per operative session
Code also services provided after midnight using date when monitoring started and total monitoring time
Code also standby time prior to procedure (99360)
Code first ([92653], 95822, 95860-95870, 95907-95913, 95925-95937 [95938, 95939])

+ # **95940 Continuous intraoperative neurophysiology monitoring in the operating room, one on one monitoring requiring personal attendance, each 15 minutes (List separately in addition to code for primary procedure)**

INCLUDES 15 minute increments monitoring service
Based on time spent monitoring, despite number tests or parameters monitored
Continuous intraoperative neurophysiologic monitoring by dedicated monitoring professional in operating room providing one-on-one patient care
Monitoring time distinct from baseline neurophysiologic study time(s) or other services (e.g., mapping)
Monitoring time may begin prior to incision
Total all monitoring time for procedures overlapping midnight

EXCLUDES *Time spent in executing or interpreting baseline neurophysiologic study or studies*

Code also monitoring from outside operative room, when applicable ([95941])

0.93 0.93 FUD XXX N 80

AMA: 2018,Feb,11; 2018,Jan,8; 2017,Aug,8; 2017,Jan,8; 2016,Jan,13; 2015,Jan,16

+ # **95941 Continuous intraoperative neurophysiology monitoring, from outside the operating room (remote or nearby) or for monitoring of more than one case while in the operating room, per hour (List separately in addition to code for primary procedure)**

INCLUDES Based on time spent monitoring, despite number tests or parameters monitored
Monitoring time distinct from baseline neurophysiologic study time(s) or other services (e.g., mapping)
One hour increments monitoring service

0.00 0.00 FUD XXX N

AMA: 2018,Feb,11; 2018,Jan,8; 2017,Aug,8; 2017,Jan,8; 2016,Jan,13; 2015,Jan,16

95921-95943 [95943] Evaluation of Autonomic Nervous System

INCLUDES Physician interpretation
Recording
Report
Testing for autonomic dysfunction including site and autonomic subsystems

95921 **Testing of autonomic nervous system function; cardiovagal innervation (parasympathetic function), including 2 or more of the following: heart rate response to deep breathing with recorded R-R interval, Valsalva ratio, and 30:15 ratio**

INCLUDES Data storage for waveform analysis
Display on monitor
Minimum two elements performed:
Cardiovascular function indicated by 30:15 ration (R/R interval at beat 30)/(R-R interval at beat 15)
Heart rate response to deep breathing obtained by visual quantitative recording analysis with patient taking five to six breaths per minute
Valsalva ratio (at least two) obtained by dividing highest heart rate by lowest
Monitoring heart rate by electrocardiography; rate obtained from time between two successive R waves (R-R interval)
Testing most usually in prone position
Tilt table testing, when performed

EXCLUDES *Autonomic nervous system testing with sympathetic adrenergic function testing (95922, 95924)*
Simultaneous measures parasympathetic and sympathetic function ([95943])

2.36 2.36 FUD XXX S 80

AMA: 2020,Sep,7; 2018,Feb,11; 2018,Jan,8; 2017,Jan,8; 2016,Jan,13; 2015,Jan,16

95922 **vasomotor adrenergic innervation (sympathetic adrenergic function), including beat-to-beat blood pressure and R-R interval changes during Valsalva maneuver and at least 5 minutes of passive tilt**

EXCLUDES *Autonomic nervous system testing with parasympathetic function (95921, 95924)*
Simultaneous measures parasympathetic and sympathetic function ([95943])

2.79 2.79 FUD XXX Q1 80

AMA: 2020,Sep,7; 2018,Feb,11; 2018,Jan,8; 2017,Jan,8; 2016,Jan,13; 2015,Jan,16

95923 **sudomotor, including 1 or more of the following: quantitative sudomotor axon reflex test (QSART), silastic sweat imprint, thermoregulatory sweat test, and changes in sympathetic skin potential**

3.64 3.64 FUD XXX Q1 80

AMA: 2020,Sep,7; 2018,Feb,11; 2018,Jan,8; 2017,Jan,8; 2016,Jan,13; 2015,Jan,16

95924 **combined parasympathetic and sympathetic adrenergic function testing with at least 5 minutes of passive tilt**

INCLUDES Tilt table testing adrenergic and parasympathetic function

EXCLUDES *Autonomic nervous system testing with parasympathetic function (95921-95922)*
Simultaneous measures parasympathetic and sympathetic function ([95943])

4.25 4.25 FUD XXX S 80

AMA: 2020,Sep,7; 2018,Feb,11; 2018,Jan,8; 2017,Jan,8; 2016,Jan,13; 2015,Jan,16

95943 **Simultaneous, independent, quantitative measures of both parasympathetic function and sympathetic function, based on time-frequency analysis of heart rate variability concurrent with time-frequency analysis of continuous respiratory activity, with mean heart rate and blood pressure measures, during rest, paced (deep) breathing, Valsalva maneuvers, and head-up postural change**

EXCLUDES *Autonomic nervous system testing (95921-95922, 95924)*
Rhythm ECG (93040)

0.00 0.00 FUD XXX S 80

AMA: 2020,Sep,7; 2018,Feb,11; 2018,Jan,8; 2017,Jan,8; 2016,Jan,13; 2015,Jan,16

95925-95943 [95938, 95939, 95940, 95941, 95943] Neurotransmission Studies

95925 **Short-latency somatosensory evoked potential study, stimulation of any/all peripheral nerves or skin sites, recording from the central nervous system; in upper limbs**

EXCLUDES *Auditory evoked potentials ([92653])*
Evoked potential study both upper and lower limbs ([95938])
Evoked potential study lower limbs (95926)

3.95 3.95 FUD XXX S 80

AMA: 2018,Feb,11; 2018,Jan,8; 2017,Jan,8; 2016,Jan,13; 2015,Jan,16

95926 **in lower limbs**

EXCLUDES *Auditory evoked potentials ([92653])*
Evoked potential study both upper and lower limbs ([95938])
Evoked potential study upper limbs (95925)

3.76 3.76 FUD XXX S 80

AMA: 2018,Feb,11; 2018,Jan,8; 2017,Jan,8; 2016,Jan,13; 2015,Jan,16

95938 **in upper and lower limbs**

9.79 9.79 FUD XXX S 80

AMA: 2018,Feb,11; 2018,Jan,8; 2017,Jan,8; 2016,Jan,13; 2015,Jan,16

95927 **in the trunk or head**

EXCLUDES *Auditory evoked potentials ([92653])*
Code also modifier 52 for unilateral test

3.74 3.74 FUD XXX S 80

AMA: 2018,Feb,11; 2018,Jan,8; 2017,Jan,8; 2016,Jan,13; 2015,Jan,16

95928 **Central motor evoked potential study (transcranial motor stimulation); upper limbs**

EXCLUDES *Central motor evoked potential study lower limbs (95929)*

6.38 6.38 FUD XXX S 80

AMA: 2018,Feb,11; 2018,Jan,8; 2017,Jan,8; 2016,Jan,13; 2015,Jan,16

95929 **lower limbs**

EXCLUDES *Central motor evoked potential study upper limbs (95928)*

6.57 6.57 FUD XXX S 80

AMA: 2018,Feb,11; 2018,Jan,8; 2017,Jan,8; 2016,Jan,13; 2015,Jan,16

95939 **in upper and lower limbs**

EXCLUDES *Central motor evoked potential study either lower or upper limbs (95928-95929)*

14.5 14.5 FUD XXX S 80

AMA: 2018,Feb,11; 2018,Jan,8; 2017,Jan,8; 2016,Jan,13; 2015,Jan,16

95930 Visual evoked potential (VEP) checkerboard or flash testing, central nervous system except glaucoma, with interpretation and report

EXCLUDES *Visual acuity screening using automated visual evoked potential devices (0333T)*
Visual evoked glaucoma testing ([0464T])

1.88 1.88 FUD XXX S 80

AMA: 2018,Feb,11; 2018,Feb,3; 2018,Jan,8; 2017,Jan,8; 2016,Jan,13; 2015,Jan,16

95933 Orbicularis oculi (blink) reflex, by electrodiagnostic testing

2.30 2.30 FUD XXX 01 80

AMA: 2018,Feb,11; 2018,Jan,8; 2017,Jul,10; 2017,Jan,8; 2016,Jan,13; 2015,Jan,16

95937 Neuromuscular junction testing (repetitive stimulation, paired stimuli), each nerve, any 1 method

2.48 2.48 FUD XXX S 80

AMA: 2020,Aug,14; 2018,Feb,11; 2018,Jan,8; 2017,Jan,8; 2016,Feb,13; 2016,Jan,13; 2015,Jan,16

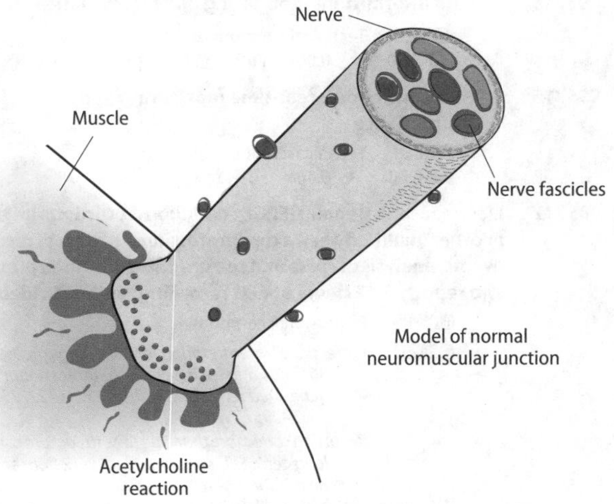

A selected neuromusular junction is repeatedly stimulated.
The test is useful to demonstrate reduced muscle action potential from fatigue

95938 **Resequenced code. See code following 95926.**

95939 **Resequenced code. See code following 95929.**

95940 **Resequenced code. See code following 95913.**

95941 **Resequenced code. See code following 95913.**

95943 **Resequenced code. See code following 95924.**

95954-95962 Electroencephalography For Seizure Monitoring/Intraoperative Use

EXCLUDES *E/M services*

95954 Pharmacological or physical activation requiring physician or other qualified health care professional attendance during EEG recording of activation phase (eg, thiopental activation test)

11.0 11.0 FUD XXX S 80

AMA: 2018,Feb,11; 2018,Jan,8; 2017,Jan,8; 2016,Jan,13; 2015,Jan,16

95955 Electroencephalogram (EEG) during nonintracranial surgery (eg, carotid surgery)

5.94 5.94 FUD XXX N 80

AMA: 2018,Feb,11; 2018,Jan,8; 2017,Jan,8; 2016,Jan,13; 2015,Jan,16

95957 Digital analysis of electroencephalogram (EEG) (eg, for epileptic spike analysis)

EXCLUDES *Use of automated spike and seizure detection/trending software, when performed ([95700, 95705, 95706, 95707, 95708, 95709, 95710, 95711, 95712, 95713, 95714, 95715, 95716, 95717, 95718, 95719, 95720, 95721, 95722, 95723, 95724, 95725, 95726])*

7.62 7.62 FUD XXX N 80

AMA: 2018,Dec,3; 2018,Dec,3; 2018,Feb,11; 2018,Jan,8; 2017,Jan,8; 2016,Jan,13; 2015,Jan,16

95958 Wada activation test for hemispheric function, including electroencephalographic (EEG) monitoring

16.3 16.3 FUD XXX S 80

AMA: 2018,Feb,11

95961 Functional cortical and subcortical mapping by stimulation and/or recording of electrodes on brain surface, or of depth electrodes, to provoke seizures or identify vital brain structures; initial hour of attendance by a physician or other qualified health care professional

INCLUDES One hour attendance by physician or other qualified health care professional

Code also each additional hour attendance by physician or other qualified health care professional, when appropriate (95962)

Code also long-term EEG (two hours or more), when performed ([95700, 95705, 95706, 95707, 95708, 95709, 95710, 95711, 95712, 95713, 95714, 95715, 95716, 95717, 95718, 95719, 95720, 95721, 95722, 95723, 95724, 95725, 95726])

Code also modifier 52 for 30 minutes or less attendance by physician or other qualified health care professional

8.79 8.79 FUD XXX S 80

AMA: 2018,Dec,3; 2018,Dec,3; 2018,Feb,11; 2018,Jan,8; 2017,Jan,8; 2016,Jan,13; 2015,Jan,16

\+ **95962 each additional hour of attendance by a physician or other qualified health care professional (List separately in addition to code for primary procedure)**

INCLUDES One hour attendance by physician or other qualified health care professional

Code also long-term EEG (two hours or more), when performed ([95700, 95705, 95706, 95707, 95708, 95709, 95710, 95711, 95712, 95713, 95714, 95715, 95716, 95717, 95718, 95719, 95720, 95721, 95722, 95723, 95724, 95725, 95726])

Code first initial hour (95961)

7.46 7.46 FUD ZZZ N 80

AMA: 2018,Feb,11; 2018,Jan,8; 2017,Jan,8; 2016,Jan,13; 2015,Jan,16

95965-95967 Magnetoencephalography

INCLUDES Physician interpretation
Recording
Report

EXCLUDES *CT provided with magnetoencephalography (70450-70470, 70496)*
Electroencephalography provided with magnetoencephalography (95812-95824)
E/M services
MRI provided with magnetoencephalography (70551-70553)
Somatosensory evoked potentials/auditory evoked potentials/visual evoked potentials provided with magnetic evoked field responses ([92653], 95925, 95926, 95930)

95965 Magnetoencephalography (MEG), recording and analysis; for spontaneous brain magnetic activity (eg, epileptic cerebral cortex localization)

0.00 0.00 FUD XXX S 80

AMA: 2018,Feb,11

95966 for evoked magnetic fields, single modality (eg, sensory, motor, language, or visual cortex localization)

0.00 0.00 FUD XXX S 80

AMA: 2018,Feb,11

\+ **95967 for evoked magnetic fields, each additional modality (eg, sensory, motor, language, or visual cortex localization) (List separately in addition to code for primary procedure)**

Code first single modality (95966)

0.00 0.00 FUD ZZZ N 80

AMA: 2018,Feb,11

95700-95726 [95700, 95705, 95706, 95707, 95708, 95709, 95710, 95711, 95712, 95713, 95714, 95715, 95716, 95717, 95718, 95719, 95720, 95721, 95722, 95723, 95724, 95725, 95726] Electronencephalogram (EEG)

INCLUDES Automated spike and seizure detection/trending software, when performed
Determination:
Eligibility for epilepsy surgery
Location and type seizures
Differentiation seizures from other conditions
Monitoring:
Seizure treatment
Status epilepticus

EXCLUDES *Diagnostic EEG recording time less than two hours*
Routine EEG (95812-95813, 95816, 95819, 95822)

Code also cortical or subcortical mapping, when performed (95961-95962)

95700 **Electroencephalogram (EEG) continuous recording, with video when performed, setup, patient education, and takedown when performed, administered in person by EEG technologist, minimum of 8 channels**
INCLUDES Technical component
EXCLUDES *EEG performed using patient-placed electrodes, performed by non-EEG technologist, or remote supervision by EEG technologist (95999)*
Reporting code more than one time each session
0.00 0.00 FUD XXX 80

95705 **Electroencephalogram (EEG), without video, review of data, technical description by EEG technologist, 2-12 hours; unmonitored**
INCLUDES Technical component
EXCLUDES *Reporting code more than one time to capture complete long-term EEG session or final 2-12 hour segment past 26 hours*
0.00 0.00 FUD XXX 80

95706 **with intermittent monitoring and maintenance**
INCLUDES Technical component
EXCLUDES *Reporting code more than one time to capture complete long-term EEG session or final 2-12 hour segment past 26 hours*
0.00 0.00 FUD XXX 80

95707 **with continuous, real-time monitoring and maintenance**
INCLUDES Technical component
EXCLUDES *Reporting code more than one time to capture complete long-term EEG session or final 2-12 hour segment past 26 hours*
0.00 0.00 FUD XXX 80

95708 **Electroencephalogram (EEG), without video, review of data, technical description by EEG technologist, each increment of 12-26 hours; unmonitored**
INCLUDES Technical component
0.00 0.00 FUD XXX 80

95709 **with intermittent monitoring and maintenance**
INCLUDES Technical component
0.00 0.00 FUD XXX 80

95710 **with continuous, real-time monitoring and maintenance**
INCLUDES Technical component
0.00 0.00 FUD XXX 80

95711 **Electroencephalogram with video (VEEG), review of data, technical description by EEG technologist, 2-12 hours; unmonitored**
INCLUDES Technical component
EXCLUDES *Reporting code more than one time to capture complete long-term EEG session or final 2-12 hour segment past 26 hours*
0.00 0.00 FUD XXX 80

95712 **with intermittent monitoring and maintenance**
INCLUDES Technical component
EXCLUDES *Reporting code more than one time to capture complete long-term EEG session or final 2-12 hour segment past 26 hours*
0.00 0.00 FUD XXX 80

95713 **with continuous, real-time monitoring and maintenance**
INCLUDES Technical component
EXCLUDES *Reporting code more than one time to capture complete long-term EEG session or final 2-12 hour segment past 26 hours*
0.00 0.00 FUD XXX 80

95714 **Electroencephalogram with video (VEEG), review of data, technical description by EEG technologist, each increment of 12-26 hours; unmonitored**
INCLUDES Technical component
0.00 0.00 FUD XXX 80

95715 **with intermittent monitoring and maintenance**
INCLUDES Technical component
0.00 0.00 FUD XXX 80

95716 **with continuous, real-time monitoring and maintenance**
INCLUDES Technical component
0.00 0.00 FUD XXX 80

95717 **Electroencephalogram (EEG), continuous recording, physician or other qualified health care professional review of recorded events, analysis of spike and seizure detection, interpretation and report, 2-12 hours of EEG recording; without video**
INCLUDES Professional component
EXCLUDES *Professional interpretation for recordings greater than 36 hours and for which entire professional report generated retroactively ([95721, 95722, 95723, 95724, 95725, 95726])*
Reporting code more than one time to capture complete long-term EEG session or final 2-12 hour segment past 24 hours
2.90 2.94 FUD XXX 80

95718 **with video (VEEG)**
INCLUDES Professional component
EXCLUDES *Professional interpretation for recordings greater than 36 hours and for which entire professional report generated retroactively ([95721, 95722, 95723, 95724, 95725, 95726])*
Reporting code more than one time to capture complete long-term EEG session or final 2-12 hour segment past 24 hours
3.81 3.87 FUD XXX 80

95719 **Electroencephalogram (EEG), continuous recording, physician or other qualified health care professional review of recorded events, analysis of spike and seizure detection, each increment of greater than 12 hours, up to 26 hours of EEG recording, interpretation and report after each 24-hour period; without video**
INCLUDES Professional component
Single report or multiple reports during 26-hour reporting period
EXCLUDES *Professional interpretation for recordings greater than 36 hours and for which entire professional report generated retroactively ([95721, 95722, 95723, 95724, 95725, 95726])*
Reporting code more than once for multiple day studies after each 24-hour period during extended EEG recording time ([95719, 95720])
Reporting code more than one time to capture between 12-26 hours
Code also EEG, 2-12 hours for studies longer than 26 hours ([95717, 95718])
4.50 4.55 FUD XXX 80

26/TC PC/TC Only · A2-Z3 ASC Payment · 50 Bilateral · ♂ Male Only · ♀ Female Only · Facility RVU · Non-Facility RVU · CCI · CLIA
FUD Follow-up Days · CMS: IOM · AMA: CPT Asst · A-Y OPPSI · 80/80 Surg Assist Allowed / w/Doc · Lab Crosswalk · Radiology Crosswalk

95720 **with video (VEEG)**

INCLUDES Professional component
Single report or multiple reports during 26-hour reporting period

EXCLUDES *Professional interpretation for recordings greater than 36 hours and for which entire professional report generated retroactively ([95721, 95722, 95723, 95724, 95725, 95726])*
Reporting code more than one time to capture between 12-26 hours
Reporting code more than once for multiple day studies after each 24-hour period during extended EEG recording time ([95719, 95720])

Code also EEG, 2-12 hours for studies longer than 26 hours ([95717, 95718])

5.90 5.99 FUD XXX 80

95721 **Electroencephalogram (EEG), continuous recording, physician or other qualified health care professional review of recorded events, analysis of spike and seizure detection, interpretation, and summary report, complete study; greater than 36 hours, up to 60 hours of EEG recording, without video**

INCLUDES Professional interpretation for recordings greater than 36 hours and for which entire professional report generated retroactively

EXCLUDES *EEG, continuous recording, less than 36 hours ([95717, 95718, 95719, 95720])*

5.92 6.04 FUD XXX 80

95722 **greater than 36 hours, up to 60 hours of EEG recording, with video (VEEG)**

INCLUDES Professional interpretation for recordings greater than 36 hours and for which entire professional report generated retroactively

EXCLUDES *EEG, continuous recording, less than 36 hours ([95717, 95718, 95719, 95720])*

7.20 7.33 FUD XXX 80

95723 **greater than 60 hours, up to 84 hours of EEG recording, without video**

INCLUDES Professional interpretation for recordings greater than 36 hours and for which entire professional report generated retroactively

EXCLUDES *EEG, continuous recording, less than 36 hours ([95717, 95718, 95719, 95720])*

7.33 7.49 FUD XXX 80

95724 **greater than 60 hours, up to 84 hours of EEG recording, with video (VEEG)**

INCLUDES Professional interpretation for recordings greater than 36 hours and for which entire professional report generated retroactively

EXCLUDES *EEG, continuous recording, less than 36 hours ([95717, 95718, 95719, 95720])*

9.18 9.36 FUD XXX 80

95725 **greater than 84 hours of EEG recording, without video**

INCLUDES Professional interpretation for recordings greater than 36 hours and for which entire professional report generated retroactively

EXCLUDES *EEG, continuous recording, less than 36 hours ([95717, 95718, 95719, 95720])*

8.34 8.55 FUD XXX 80

AMA: 2011,Jan,11; 2009,Jan,11-31

95726 **greater than 84 hours of EEG recording, with video (VEEG)**

INCLUDES Professional interpretation for recordings greater than 36 hours and for which entire professional report generated retroactively

EXCLUDES *EEG, continuous recording, less than 36 hours ([95717, 95718, 95719, 95720])*

11.6 11.8 FUD XXX 80

95970-95984 [95983, 95984] Evaluation of Implanted Neurostimulator with/without Programming

INCLUDES Documentation settings, electrode impedances system parameters before programming
Insertion electrode array(s) into target area (permanent or trial)
Multiple adjustments to parameters necessary during programming session
Neurostimulators distinguished by nervous system area stimulated:
- Brain: Deep brain stimulation or cortical stimulation (brain surface)
- Cranial nerves: Includes12 pairs cranial nerves, branches, divisions, intracranial and extracranial segments
- Spinal cord and peripheral nerves: Nerves originating in spinal cord and nerves and ganglia outside spinal cord.

Parameters (vary by system) include:
- Amplitude
- Burst
- Cycling on/off
- Detection algorithms
- Dose lockout
- Frequency
- Pulse width
- Responsive neurostimulation

EXCLUDES *Implantation/replacement neurostimulator electrodes (43647, 43881, 61850-61868, 63650-63655, 64553-64581)*
Neurostimulation system, posterior tibial nerve (0587T-0590T)
Neurostimulator pulse generator/receiver:
- *Insertion (61885-61886, 63685, 64568, 64590)*
- *Revision/removal (61888, 63688, 64569, 64570, 64595)*

Revision/removal neurostimulator electrodes (43648, 43882, 61880, 63661-63664, 64569-64570, 64585)

95970 **Electronic analysis of implanted neurostimulator pulse generator/transmitter (eg, contact group[s], interleaving, amplitude, pulse width, frequency [Hz], on/off cycling, burst, magnet mode, dose lockout, patient selectable parameters, responsive neurostimulation, detection algorithms, closed loop parameters, and passive parameters) by physician or other qualified health care professional; with brain, cranial nerve, spinal cord, peripheral nerve, or sacral nerve, neurostimulator pulse generator/transmitter, without programming**

INCLUDES Analysis implanted neurostimulator without programming

EXCLUDES *Programming with analysis (95971-95972, 95976-95977, [95983, 95984])*

0.54 0.55 FUD XXX 01 80

AMA: 2019,Feb,6; 2018,Oct,8; 2018,Feb,11; 2018,Jan,8; 2017,Jan,8; 2016,Jul,7; 2016,Jan,13; 2015,Jan,16

95971 **with simple spinal cord or peripheral nerve (eg, sacral nerve) neurostimulator pulse generator/transmitter programming by physician or other qualified health care professional**

EXCLUDES *Programming neurostimulator for complex spinal cord or peripheral nerve (95972)*

1.17 1.44 FUD XXX S 80

AMA: 2019,Feb,6; 2018,Oct,8; 2018,Feb,11; 2018,Jan,8; 2017,Jan,8; 2016,Jul,7; 2016,Jan,13; 2015,Jan,16

95972 **with complex spinal cord or peripheral nerve (eg, sacral nerve) neurostimulator pulse generator/transmitter programming by physician or other qualified health care professional**

1.19 1.62 FUD XXX S 80

AMA: 2019,Feb,6; 2018,Oct,8; 2018,Feb,11; 2018,Jan,8; 2017,Jan,8; 2016,Jul,7; 2016,Jan,13; 2015,Jan,16

95976 **with simple cranial nerve neurostimulator pulse generator/transmitter programming by physician or other qualified health care professional**

EXCLUDES *Programming neurostimulator for complex cranial nerve (95977)*

1.16 1.18 FUD XXX 80

AMA: 2019,Feb,6

95977 **with complex cranial nerve neurostimulator pulse generator/transmitter programming by physician or other qualified health care professional**
1.52 1.54 FUD XXX 80
AMA: 2019,Feb,6

\# **95983** **with brain neurostimulator pulse generator/transmitter programming, first 15 minutes face-to-face time with physician or other qualified health care professional**
1.44 1.46 FUD XXX 80
AMA: 2019,Feb,6; 2018,Dec,3; 2018,Dec,3

\+ # **95984** **with brain neurostimulator pulse generator/transmitter programming, each additional 15 minutes face-to-face time with physician or other qualified health care professional (List separately in addition to code for primary procedure)**
Code first ([95983])
1.26 1.27 FUD ZZZ 80
AMA: 2019,Feb,6; 2018,Dec,3; 2018,Dec,3

95980 **Electronic analysis of implanted neurostimulator pulse generator system (eg, rate, pulse amplitude and duration, configuration of wave form, battery status, electrode selectability, output modulation, cycling, impedance and patient measurements) gastric neurostimulator pulse generator/transmitter; intraoperative, with programming**
INCLUDES Gastric neurostimulator lesser curvature
EXCLUDES *Analysis, with programming when performed, vagus nerve trunk stimulator for morbid obesity (0312T, 0317T)*
1.32 1.32 FUD XXX N 80
AMA: 2018,Feb,11; 2018,Jan,8; 2017,Jan,8; 2016,Jul,7; 2016,Jan,13; 2015,Jan,16

95981 **subsequent, without reprogramming**
EXCLUDES *Analysis, with programming when performed, vagus nerve trunk stimulator for morbid obesity (0312T, 0317T)*
0.51 1.01 FUD XXX Q1 80
AMA: 2018,Feb,11; 2018,Jan,8; 2017,Jan,8; 2016,Jul,7; 2016,Jan,13; 2015,Jan,16

95982 **subsequent, with reprogramming**
EXCLUDES *Analysis, with programming when performed, vagus nerve trunk stimulator for morbid obesity (0312T, 0317T)*
1.06 1.61 FUD XXX Q1 80
AMA: 2018,Feb,11; 2018,Jan,8; 2017,Jan,8; 2016,Jul,7; 2016,Jan,13; 2015,Jan,16

95983 **Resequenced code. See code following 95977.**

95984 **Resequenced code. See code following 95977.**

95990-95991 Refill/Upkeep of Implanted Drug Delivery Pump to Central Nervous System

EXCLUDES *Analysis/reprogramming implanted pump for infusion (62367-62370)*
E/M services

95990 **Refilling and maintenance of implantable pump or reservoir for drug delivery, spinal (intrathecal, epidural) or brain (intraventricular), includes electronic analysis of pump, when performed;**
2.55 2.55 FUD XXX S 80
AMA: 2018,Feb,11; 2018,Jan,8; 2017,Jan,8; 2016,Jan,13; 2015,Jan,16

95991 **requiring skill of a physician or other qualified health care professional**
1.14 3.30 FUD XXX T 80
AMA: 2018,Feb,11; 2018,Jan,8; 2017,Jan,8; 2016,Jan,13; 2015,Jan,16

95992-95999 Other and Unlisted Neurological Procedures

95992 **Canalith repositioning procedure(s) (eg, Epley maneuver, Semont maneuver), per day**
EXCLUDES *Nystagmus testing (92531-92532)*
1.08 1.27 FUD XXX A 80
AMA: 2018,Feb,11; 2018,Jan,8; 2017,Jan,8; 2016,Jan,13; 2015,Jan,16

95999 **Unlisted neurological or neuromuscular diagnostic procedure**
0.00 0.00 FUD XXX Q1 80
AMA: 2018,Aug,10; 2018,Feb,11; 2018,Jan,8; 2017,Jan,8; 2016,Jan,13; 2015,Aug,8; 2015,Jan,16

96000-96004 Motion Analysis Studies

CMS: 100-02,15,230.4 Services By a Physical/Occupational Therapist in Private Practice
INCLUDES Services provided as part major therapeutic/diagnostic decision making
Services provided in dedicated motion analysis department with these capabilities:
3D kinetics/dynamic electromyography
Computerized 3D kinematics
Videotaping from front/back/both sides
EXCLUDES *E/M services*
Gait training (97116)
Needle electromyography (95860-95872 [95885, 95886, 95887])

96000 **Comprehensive computer-based motion analysis by video-taping and 3D kinematics;**
2.72 2.72 FUD XXX S 80
AMA: 2018,Feb,11; 2018,Jan,8; 2017,Jan,8; 2016,Jan,13; 2015,Jan,16

96001 **with dynamic plantar pressure measurements during walking**
3.65 3.65 FUD XXX S 80
AMA: 2018,Feb,11; 2018,Jan,8; 2017,Jan,8; 2016,Jan,13; 2015,Jan,16

96002 **Dynamic surface electromyography, during walking or other functional activities, 1-12 muscles**
0.63 0.63 FUD XXX S 80
AMA: 2018,Feb,11; 2018,Jan,8; 2017,Jan,8; 2016,Jan,13; 2015,Aug,8; 2015,Jan,16

96003 **Dynamic fine wire electromyography, during walking or other functional activities, 1 muscle**
0.49 0.49 FUD XXX Q1 80
AMA: 2018,Feb,11; 2018,Jan,8; 2017,Jan,8; 2016,Jan,13; 2015,Jan,16

96004 **Review and interpretation by physician or other qualified health care professional of comprehensive computer-based motion analysis, dynamic plantar pressure measurements, dynamic surface electromyography during walking or other functional activities, and dynamic fine wire electromyography, with written report**
3.24 3.24 FUD XXX B 80 26
AMA: 2018,Feb,11; 2018,Jan,8; 2017,Jan,8; 2016,Jan,13; 2015,Aug,8; 2015,Jan,16

96020 Neurofunctional Brain Testing

INCLUDES Selection/administration, testing:
- Cognition
- Determining validity neurofunctional testing relative to separately interpreted functional magnetic resonance images
- Functional neuroimaging
- Language
- Memory
- Monitoring performance of testing
- Movement
- Other neurological functions
- Sensation

EXCLUDES *Clinical depression treatment by repetitive transcranial magnetic stimulation (90867-90868)*
Developmental test administration (96112-96113)
E/M services on same date
MRI brain (70554-70555)
Neurobehavioral status examination (96116, 96121)
Neuropsychological testing (96132-96133)
Psychological testing (96130-96131)

96020 Neurofunctional testing selection and administration during noninvasive imaging functional brain mapping, with test administered entirely by a physician or other qualified health care professional (ie, psychologist), with review of test results and report

0.00 0.00 FUD XXX N 80

AMA: 2018,Feb,11; 2018,Jan,8; 2017,Jan,8; 2016,Jan,13; 2015,Jan,16

96040 Genetic Counseling Services

INCLUDES Analysis for genetic risk assessment
- Counseling patient/family
- Counseling services
- Face-to-face interviews
- Obtaining structured family genetic history
- Pedigree construction
- Review medical data/family information
- Services provided by trained genetic counselor
- Services provided during one or more sessions
- Thirty minutes face-to-face time, reported one time for each 16-30 minutes service

EXCLUDES *Education/genetic counseling by physician or other qualified health care provider to group (99078)*
Education/genetic counseling by physician or other qualified health care provider to individual; report appropriate E/M code
Education regarding genetic risks by nonphysician to group (98961, 98962)
Genetic counseling and/or risk factor reduction intervention from physician or other qualified health care provider provided to patients without symptoms/diagnosis (99401-99412)
Reporting code when 15 minutes or less face-to-face time provided

96040 Medical genetics and genetic counseling services, each 30 minutes face-to-face with patient/family

1.30 1.30 FUD XXX ★ B

AMA: 2018,Feb,11; 2018,Jan,8; 2017,Jan,8; 2016,Jan,13; 2015,Jan,16

97151-97158 [97151, 97152, 97153, 97154, 97155, 97156, 97157, 97158] Adaptive Behavior Assessments and Treatments

INCLUDES Adaptive behavior deficits (e.g., impairment in social, communication, self care skills)
Assessment and treatment that focuses on:
- Maladaptive behaviors (e.g., repetitive movements, risk harm to self, others, property)
- Secondary functional impairment due to consequences deficient adaptive and maladaptive behaviors (e.g., communication, play, leisure, social interactions)
- Treatment determined based on goals and targets identified in assessments

 # 97151 Behavior identification assessment, administered by a physician or other qualified health care professional, each 15 minutes of the physician's or other qualified health care professional's time face-to-face with patient and/or guardian(s)/caregiver(s) administering assessments and discussing findings and recommendations, and non-face-to-face analyzing past data, scoring/interpreting the assessment, and preparing the report/treatment plan

EXCLUDES *Health and behavior assessment and intervention (96156, 96158-96159, [96164, 96165], [96167, 96168], [96170, 96171])*
Medical team conference (99366-99368)
Neurobehavioral status examination (96116, 96121)
Neuropsychological testing (96132-96133, 96136-96139, 96146)
Psychiatric diagnostic evaluation (90791-90792)
Speech evaluations (92521-92524)

Code also more than one time on same or different days until assessment complete

Code also supporting assessment depending on time patient spends face-to-face with one or more technicians (counting only time spent by one technician) ([97152], 0362T)

0.00 0.00 FUD XXX 80

AMA: 2018,Nov,3

 # 97152 Behavior identification-supporting assessment, administered by one technician under the direction of a physician or other qualified health care professional, face-to-face with the patient, each 15 minutes

EXCLUDES *Health and behavior assessment and intervention (96156, 96158-96159, [96164, 96165], [96167, 96168], [96170, 96171])*
Medical team conference (99366-99368)
Neurobehavioral status examination (96116, 96121)
Neuropsychological testing (96132-96133, 96136-96139, 96146)
Psychiatric diagnostic evaluation (90791-90792)
Speech evaluations (92521-92524)

Code also more than one time on same or different days until assessment complete

Code also supporting assessment depending on time patient spends face-to-face with one or more technicians (counting only time spent by one technician) ([97152], 0362T)

0.00 0.00 FUD XXX 80

AMA: 2018,Nov,3

\# **97153 Adaptive behavior treatment by protocol, administered by technician under the direction of a physician or other qualified health care professional, face-to-face with one patient, each 15 minutes**

INCLUDES Face-to-face service with one patient only
Provided by technician under physician/other qualified healthcare professional direction

EXCLUDES *Aphasia and cognitive performance testing (96105, [96125])*
Behavioral/developmental screening/testing (96110-96113 [96127])
Health and behavior assessment and intervention (96156, 96158-96159, [96164, 96165], [96167, 96168], [96170, 96171])
Health risk assessment (96160-96161)
Neurobehavioral status examination (96116, 96121)
Psychiatric services (90785-90899)
Testing administration with scoring (96136-96139, 96146)
Testing evaluation (96130-96133)
Therapeutic procedure(s), individual patient (97129)
Treatment speech disorders (individual) (92507)

0.00 0.00 **FUD** XXX 80

AMA: 2020,Jul,10; 2018,Nov,3

\# **97154 Group adaptive behavior treatment by protocol, administered by technician under the direction of a physician or other qualified health care professional, face-to-face with two or more patients, each 15 minutes**

INCLUDES Face-to-face service with one patient only
Provided by technician under physician/other qualified healthcare professional direction

EXCLUDES *Aphasia and cognitive performance testing (96105, [96125])*
Behavioral/developmental screening/testing (96110-96113, [96127])
Health and behavior assessment and intervention (96156, 96158-96159, [96164, 96165], [96167, 96168], [96170, 96171])
Neurobehavioral status examination (96116, 96121)
Psychiatric services (90785-90899)
Testing administration with scoring (96136-96139, 96146)
Testing evaluation (96130-96133)
Therapeutic procedure(s) group, two or more patients (97150)
Treatment speech disorders (group) (92508)

0.00 0.00 **FUD** XXX 80

AMA: 2018,Nov,3

\# **97155 Adaptive behavior treatment with protocol modification, administered by physician or other qualified health care professional, which may include simultaneous direction of technician, face-to-face with one patient, each 15 minutes**

INCLUDES Face-to-face service with one patient only
Provided by technician under physician/other qualified healthcare professional direction

EXCLUDES *Aphasia and cognitive performance testing (96105, [96125])*
Behavioral/developmental screening/testing (96110-96113, [96127])
Health and behavior assessment and intervention (96156, 96158-96159, [96164, 96165], [96167, 96168], [96170, 96171])
Neurobehavioral status examination (96116, 96121)
Psychiatric services (90785-90899)
Testing administration with scoring (96136-96139, 96146)
Testing evaluation (96130-96133)
Therapeutic procedure(s), individual patient (97129)
Treatment speech disorders (individual) (92507)

0.00 0.00 **FUD** XXX 80

AMA: 2020,Jul,10; 2018,Nov,3

\# **97156 Family adaptive behavior treatment guidance, administered by physician or other qualified health care professional (with or without the patient present), face-to-face with guardian(s)/caregiver(s), each 15 minutes**

INCLUDES Provided by physician/other qualified healthcare professional
Without patient presence

EXCLUDES *Aphasia and cognitive performance testing (96105, [96125])*
Behavioral/developmental screening/testing (96110-96113 [96127])
Health and behavior assessment and intervention (96156, 96158-96159, [96164, 96165], [96167, 96168], [96170, 96171])
Neurobehavioral status examination (96116, 96121)
Psychiatric services (90785-90899)
Testing administration with scoring (96136-96139, 96146)
Testing evaluation (96130-96133)

0.00 0.00 **FUD** XXX 80

AMA: 2018,Nov,3

\# **97157 Multiple-family group adaptive behavior treatment guidance, administered by physician or other qualified health care professional (without the patient present), face-to-face with multiple sets of guardians/caregivers, each 15 minutes**

INCLUDES Provided by physician/other qualified healthcare professional
Without patient presence

EXCLUDES *Aphasia and cognitive performance testing (96105, [96125])*
Behavioral/developmental screening/testing (96110-96113 [96127])
Groups more than eight families
Health and behavior assessment and intervention (96156, 96158-96159, [96164, 96165], [96167, 96168], [96170, 96171])
Neurobehavioral status examination (96116, 96121)
Psychiatric services (90785-90899)
Testing administration with scoring (96136-96139, 96146)
Testing evaluation (96130-96133)

0.00 0.00 **FUD** XXX 80

AMA: 2018,Nov,3

\# **97158 Group adaptive behavior treatment with protocol modification, administered by physician or other qualified health care professional, face-to-face with multiple patients, each 15 minutes**

INCLUDES Face-to-face service with one patient only
Provided by technician under physician/other qualified healthcare professional direction

EXCLUDES *Aphasia and cognitive performance testing (96105, [96125])*
Behavioral/developmental screening/testing (96110-96113 [96127])
Groups more than eight families
Health and behavior assessment and intervention (96156, 96158-96159, [96164, 96165], [96167, 96168], [96170, 96171])
Neurobehavioral status examination (96116, 96121)
Psychiatric services (90785-90899)
Testing administration with scoring (96136-96139, 96146)
Testing evaluation (96130-96133)
Therapeutic procedure(s) group of two or more patients (97150)
Treatment speech disorders (group) (92508)

0.00 0.00 **FUD** XXX 80

AMA: 2018,Nov,3

96105-96146 [96125, 96127] Testing Services

INCLUDES Interpretation and report when performed by qualified healthcare professional
Results when automatically generated

EXCLUDES Adaptive behavior assessments and treatments ([97151, 97152, 97153, 97154, 97155, 97156, 97157, 97158], 0362T, 0373T)
Cognitive skills development (97129, 97533)

96105 **Assessment of aphasia (includes assessment of expressive and receptive speech and language function, language comprehension, speech production ability, reading, spelling, writing, eg, by Boston Diagnostic Aphasia Examination) with interpretation and report, per hour**

> EXCLUDES Reporting code for less than 31 minutes
> 🚑 2.96 ⚖ 2.96 **FUD** XXX   A 80 💻
>
> **AMA:** 2018,Nov,3; 2018,Oct,5; 2018,Feb,11; 2018,Jan,8; 2017,Jan,8; 2016,Jan,13; 2015,Aug,5; 2015,Jan,16

\# **96125** **Standardized cognitive performance testing (eg, Ross Information Processing Assessment) per hour of a qualified health care professional's time, both face-to-face time administering tests to the patient and time interpreting these test results and preparing the report**

> EXCLUDES Neuropsychological testing (96132-96139, 96146)
> 🚑 3.10 ⚖ 3.10 **FUD** XXX   A 80 💻
>
> **AMA:** 2018,Nov,3; 2018,Oct,5; 2018,Feb,11; 2018,Jan,8; 2017,Jan,8; 2016,Jan,13; 2015,Aug,5; 2015,Jan,16

96110 **Developmental screening (eg, developmental milestone survey, speech and language delay screen), with scoring and documentation, per standardized instrument**

> EXCLUDES Emotional/behavioral assessment ([96127])
> 🚑 0.28 ⚖ 0.28 **FUD** XXX   E 💻
>
> **AMA:** 2018,Nov,3; 2018,Feb,11; 2018,Jan,8; 2017,Feb,14; 2017,Jan,8; 2016,Jan,13; 2015,Aug,5; 2015,Jan,16

96112 **Developmental test administration (including assessment of fine and/or gross motor, language, cognitive level, social, memory and/or executive functions by standardized developmental instruments when performed), by physician or other qualified health care professional, with interpretation and report; first hour**

> EXCLUDES Reporting code for less than 31 minutes
> 🚑 3.61 ⚖ 3.83 **FUD** XXX   80 💻
>
> **AMA:** 2018,Nov,3

\+ **96113** **each additional 30 minutes (List separately in addition to code for primary procedure)**

> EXCLUDES Reporting code for less than 16 minutes
> 🚑 1.65 ⚖ 1.74 **FUD** ZZZ   80 💻
>
> **AMA:** 2018,Nov,3

\# **96127** **Brief emotional/behavioral assessment (eg, depression inventory, attention-deficit/hyperactivity disorder [ADHD] scale), with scoring and documentation, per standardized instrument**

> 🚑 0.15 ⚖ 0.15 **FUD** XXX   Q1 80 TC 💻
>
> **AMA:** 2018,Nov,3; 2018,Oct,5; 2018,Apr,9; 2018,Feb,11; 2018,Jan,8; 2017,Feb,14; 2017,Jan,8; 2016,Jan,13; 2015,Aug,5

96116 **Neurobehavioral status exam (clinical assessment of thinking, reasoning and judgment, [eg, acquired knowledge, attention, language, memory, planning and problem solving, and visual spatial abilities]), by physician or other qualified health care professional, both face-to-face time with the patient and time interpreting test results and preparing the report; first hour**

> EXCLUDES Neuropsychological testing (96132-96139, 96146)
> Reporting code for less than 31 minutes
> 🚑 2.41 ⚖ 2.70 **FUD** XXX   ★ 03 80 💻
>
> **AMA:** 2018,Nov,3; 2018,Oct,5; 2018,Feb,11; 2018,Jan,8; 2017,Jan,8; 2016,Jan,13; 2015,Aug,5; 2015,Jan,16

\+ **96121** **each additional hour (List separately in addition to code for primary procedure)**

> EXCLUDES Reporting code for less than 31 minutes
> Code first (96116)
> 🚑 2.22 ⚖ 2.39 **FUD** ZZZ   80 💻
>
> **AMA:** 2018,Nov,3

96125 Resequenced code. See code following 96105.

96127 Resequenced code. See code following 96113.

96130 **Psychological testing evaluation services by physician or other qualified health care professional, including integration of patient data, interpretation of standardized test results and clinical data, clinical decision making, treatment planning and report, and interactive feedback to the patient, family member(s) or caregiver(s), when performed; first hour**

> EXCLUDES Reporting code for less than 31 minutes
> 🚑 3.08 ⚖ 3.38 **FUD** XXX   80 💻
>
> **AMA:** 2019,Dec,14; 2019,Sep,10; 2018,Nov,3

\+ **96131** **each additional hour (List separately in addition to code for primary procedure)**

> EXCLUDES Reporting code for less than 31 minutes
> 🚑 2.37 ⚖ 2.60 **FUD** ZZZ   80 💻
>
> **AMA:** 2019,Dec,14; 2019,Sep,10; 2018,Nov,3

96132 **Neuropsychological testing evaluation services by physician or other qualified health care professional, including integration of patient data, interpretation of standardized test results and clinical data, clinical decision making, treatment planning and report, and interactive feedback to the patient, family member(s) or caregiver(s), when performed; first hour**

> EXCLUDES Reporting code for less than 31 minutes
> 🚑 3.04 ⚖ 3.78 **FUD** XXX   80 💻
>
> **AMA:** 2019,Dec,14; 2019,Sep,10; 2018,Nov,3

\+ **96133** **each additional hour (List separately in addition to code for primary procedure)**

> EXCLUDES Reporting code for less than 16 minutes
> 🚑 2.34 ⚖ 2.84 **FUD** ZZZ   80 💻
>
> **AMA:** 2019,Dec,14; 2019,Sep,10; 2018,Nov,3

96136 **Psychological or neuropsychological test administration and scoring by physician or other qualified health care professional, two or more tests, any method; first 30 minutes**

> EXCLUDES Reporting code for less than 16 minutes
> Code also testing evaluation on same or different days (96130-96133)
> 🚑 0.70 ⚖ 1.33 **FUD** XXX   80 💻
>
> **AMA:** 2020,Aug,3; 2019,Dec,14; 2019,Sep,10; 2018,Nov,3

\+ **96137** **each additional 30 minutes (List separately in addition to code for primary procedure)**

> EXCLUDES Reporting code for less than 16 minutes
> Code also testing evaluation on same or different days (96130-96133)
> 🚑 0.55 ⚖ 1.22 **FUD** ZZZ   80 💻
>
> **AMA:** 2020,Aug,3; 2019,Dec,14; 2019,Sep,10; 2018,Nov,3

96138 **Psychological or neuropsychological test administration and scoring by technician, two or more tests, any method; first 30 minutes**

> EXCLUDES Reporting code for less than 16 minutes
> Code also testing evaluation on same or different days (96130-96133)
> 🚑 1.07 ⚖ 1.07 **FUD** XXX   80 💻
>
> **AMA:** 2018,Nov,3

\+ **96139** **each additional 30 minutes (List separately in addition to code for primary procedure)**

> EXCLUDES Reporting code for less than 16 minutes
> Code also testing evaluation on same or different days (96130-96133)
> 🚑 1.07 ⚖ 1.07 **FUD** ZZZ   80 💻
>
> **AMA:** 2018,Nov,3

● New Code ▲ Revised Code ○ Reinstated ● New Web Release ▲ Revised Web Release + Add-on Unlisted Not Covered # Resequenced
50 Optum Mod 50 Exempt ⊘ AMA Mod 51 Exempt 51 Optum Mod 51 Exempt 63 Mod 63 Exempt ✗ Non-FDA Drug ★ Telemedicine M Maternity A Age Edit

96146 **Psychological or neuropsychological test administration, with single automated, standardized instrument via electronic platform, with automated result only**

EXCLUDES *Testing provided by physician, other qualified healthcare professional, or technician ([96127], 96136-96139)*

0.06 0.06 FUD XXX 80

AMA: 2018,Nov,3

96156-96171 [96164, 96165, 96167, 96168, 96170, 96171] Biopsychosocial Assessment/Intervention

INCLUDES Services for patients that have primary physical illnesses/diagnoses/symptoms who may benefit from assessments/interventions that focus on biopsychosocial factors related to patient's health status

Services used to identify factors important to prevention/treatment/management physical health problems:

Behavioral
Cognitive
Emotional
Psychological
Social

EXCLUDES *Adaptive behavior services ([97151, 97152, 97153, 97154, 97155, 97156, 97157, 97158], 0362T, 0373T)*
E/M services same date
Health and behavior assessment and intervention (96156, 96158-96159)
Preventive medicine counseling services (99401-99412)

96156 **Health behavior assessment, or re-assessment (ie, health-focused clinical interview, behavioral observations, clinical decision making)**

EXCLUDES *Psychotherapy services (90785-90899)*

2.51 2.77 FUD XXX 80

AMA: 2020,Aug,3; 2020,Jul,7

96158 **Health behavior intervention, individual, face-to-face; initial 30 minutes**

EXCLUDES *Psychotherapy services (90785-90899)*

1.71 1.89 FUD XXX 80

AMA: 2020,Aug,3; 2020,Jul,7

\+ **96159** **each additional 15 minutes (List separately in addition to code for primary service)**

EXCLUDES *Psychotherapy services (90785-90899)*

Code first (96158)

0.59 0.66 FUD ZZZ 80

AMA: 2020,Aug,3; 2020,Jul,7

96164 **Health behavior intervention, group (2 or more patients), face-to-face; initial 30 minutes**

EXCLUDES *Psychotherapy services (90785-90899)*

0.25 0.28 FUD XXX 80

AMA: 2020,Aug,3; 2020,Jul,7

\+ # **96165** **each additional 15 minutes (List separately in addition to code for primary service)**

EXCLUDES *Psychotherapy services (90785-90899)*

Code first ([96164])

0.11 0.13 FUD ZZZ 80

AMA: 2020,Aug,3; 2020,Jul,7

96167 **Health behavior intervention, family (with the patient present), face-to-face; initial 30 minutes**

EXCLUDES *Psychotherapy services (90785-90899)*

1.83 2.03 FUD XXX 80

AMA: 2020,Aug,3

\+ # **96168** **each additional 15 minutes (List separately in addition to code for primary service)**

EXCLUDES *Psychotherapy services (90785-90899)*

Code first ([96167])

0.65 0.72 FUD ZZZ 80

AMA: 2020,Aug,3

96170 **Health behavior intervention, family (without the patient present), face-to-face; initial 30 minutes**

EXCLUDES *Psychotherapy services (90785-90899)*

2.19 2.30 FUD XXX

AMA: 2020,Aug,3

\+ # **96171** **each additional 15 minutes (List separately in addition to code for primary service)**

EXCLUDES *Psychotherapy services (90785-90899)*

Code first ([96170])

0.80 0.84 FUD ZZZ

AMA: 2020,Aug,3

96160-96171 [96164, 96165, 96167, 96168, 96170, 96171] Health Risk Assessments

96160 **Administration of patient-focused health risk assessment instrument (eg, health hazard appraisal) with scoring and documentation, per standardized instrument**

0.11 0.11 FUD ZZZ S

AMA: 2020,Aug,3; 2018,Feb,11; 2018,Jan,8; 2017,Feb,14; 2017,Jan,8; 2016,Nov,5

96161 **Administration of caregiver-focused health risk assessment instrument (eg, depression inventory) for the benefit of the patient, with scoring and documentation, per standardized instrument**

0.09 0.09 FUD ZZZ S

AMA: 2020,Aug,3; 2018,Feb,11; 2018,Jan,8; 2017,Feb,14; 2017,Jan,8; 2016,Nov,5

96164 **Resequenced code. See code following 96159.**

96165 **Resequenced code. See code following 96159.**

96167 **Resequenced code. See code following 96159.**

96168 **Resequenced code. See code following 96159.**

96170 **Resequenced code. See code following 96159.**

96171 **Resequenced code. See code following 96159.**

96360-96361 Intravenous Fluid Infusion for Hydration (Nonchemotherapy)

CMS: 100-04,4,230.2 OPPS Drug Administration

INCLUDES Administration prepackaged fluids and electrolytes
Coding hierarchy rules for facility reporting only:
Chemotherapy services primary to diagnostic, prophylactic, and therapeutic services
Diagnostic, prophylactic, and therapeutic services primary to hydration services
Infusions primary to pushes
Pushes primary to injections
Constant observance/attendance by person administering drug or substance
Infusion 15 minutes or less
Direct supervision by physician or other qualified health care provider:
Direction personnel
Minimal supervision for:
Consent
Safety oversight
Supervision personnel
If done to facilitate injection/infusion:
Flush at infusion end
Indwelling IV, subcutaneous catheter/port access
Local anesthesia
Start IV
Supplies/tubing/syringes
Report initial code for primary reason for visit despite order infusions or injections given
Treatment plan verification

EXCLUDES *Catheter/port declotting (36593)*
Drugs/other substances
Minimal infusion to keep vein open or during other therapeutic infusions
Reporting code for hydration infusion 31 minutes or less
Reporting code for second initial service on same date for accessing multilumen catheter, restarting IV, or when two IV lines are needed to meet infusion rate
Services provided by physicians or other qualified health care providers in facility settings
Significant separately identifiable E/M service, when performed

96360 **Intravenous infusion, hydration; initial, 31 minutes to 1 hour**

EXCLUDES *Reporting code when service performed as concurrent infusion*

1.07 1.07 **FUD** XXX S 80

AMA: 2019,Jun,5; 2018,Feb,11; 2018,Jan,8; 2017,Jan,8; 2016,Jan,13; 2015,Jan,16

\+ **96361** **each additional hour (List separately in addition to code for primary procedure)**

INCLUDES Hydration infusion of more than 30 minutes beyond 1 hour
Hydration provided as secondary or subsequent service after different initial service via same IV access site

Code first (96360)

0.38 0.38 **FUD** ZZZ S 80

AMA: 2019,Jun,5; 2018,Feb,11; 2018,Jan,8; 2017,Jan,8; 2016,Jan,13; 2015,Jan,16

96365-96371 Infusions: Diagnostic/Preventive/Therapeutic

CMS: 100-04,4,230.2 OPPS Drug Administration

INCLUDES Administration fluid
Administration substances/drugs
Coding hierarchy rules for facility reporting:
Chemotherapy services primary to diagnostic, prophylactic, and therapeutic services
Diagnostic, prophylactic, and therapeutic services primary to hydration services
Infusions primary to pushes
Pushes primary to injections
Constant presence by health care professional administering substance/drug
Direct supervision by physician or other qualified health care provider:
Consent
Direction personnel
Patient assessment
Safety oversight
Supervision personnel
If done to facilitate injection/infusion:
Flush at infusion end
Indwelling IV, subcutaneous catheter/port access
Local anesthesia
Start IV
Supplies/tubing/syringes
Infusion 16 minutes or more
Training to assess patient and monitor vital signs
Training to prepare/dose/dispose
Treatment plan verification

EXCLUDES *Catheter/port declotting (36593)*
Services provided by physicians or other qualified health care providers in facility settings
Significant separately identifiable E/M service, when performed
Reporting code for second initial service on same date for accessing multilumen catheter, restarting IV, or when two IV lines needed to meet infusion rate
Reporting code with other procedures where IV push or infusion is integral to procedure

Code also drugs/materials

96365 **Intravenous infusion, for therapy, prophylaxis, or diagnosis (specify substance or drug); initial, up to 1 hour**

Code also second initial service with modifier 59 when patient's condition or drug protocol mandates use of two IV lines

2.00 2.00 **FUD** XXX S 80

AMA: 2020,Jan,11; 2018,Dec,8; 2018,Dec,8; 2018,Sep,14; 2018,May,10; 2018,Feb,11; 2018,Jan,8; 2017,Jan,8; 2016,Jan,13; 2015,Jan,16

\+ **96366** **each additional hour (List separately in addition to code for primary procedure)**

INCLUDES Additional hours sequential infusion
Infusion intervals more than 30 minutes beyond one hour
Second and subsequent infusions same drug or substance

Code also additional infusion, when appropriate (96367)
Code first (96365)

0.61 0.61 **FUD** ZZZ S 80

AMA: 2020,Jan,11; 2018,Sep,14; 2018,Feb,11; 2018,Jan,8; 2017,Jan,8; 2016,Jan,13; 2015,Jan,16

\+ **96367** **additional sequential infusion of a new drug/substance, up to 1 hour (List separately in addition to code for primary procedure)**

INCLUDES Secondary or subsequent service with new drug or substance after different initial service via same IV access

EXCLUDES *Reporting code more than one time per sequential infusion same mix*

Code first (96365, 96374, 96409, 96413)

0.87 0.87 **FUD** ZZZ S 80

AMA: 2020,Jan,11; 2018,Feb,11; 2018,Jan,8; 2017,Jan,8; 2016,Jan,13; 2015,Jan,16

\+ **96368** **concurrent infusion (List separately in addition to code for primary procedure)**

EXCLUDES *Reporting code more than one time per service date*

Code first (96365, 96366, 96413, 96415, 96416)

0.59 0.59 **FUD** ZZZ N 80

AMA: 2020,Jan,11; 2018,Feb,11; 2018,Jan,8; 2017,Jan,8; 2016,Jan,13; 2015,Jan,16

96369 **Subcutaneous infusion for therapy or prophylaxis (specify substance or drug); initial, up to 1 hour, including pump set-up and establishment of subcutaneous infusion site(s)**

EXCLUDES *Infusions 15 minutes or less (96372)*

Reporting code more than one time per encounter

4.69 4.69 **FUD** XXX S 80

AMA: 2020,Jan,11; 2018,Feb,11; 2018,Jan,8; 2017,Jan,8; 2016,Jan,13; 2015,Jan,16

\+ **96370** **each additional hour (List separately in addition to code for primary procedure)**

INCLUDES Infusions more than 30 minutes beyond one hour

Code first (96369)

0.44 0.44 **FUD** ZZZ S 80

AMA: 2020,Jan,11; 2018,Feb,11; 2018,Jan,8; 2017,Jan,8; 2016,Jan,13; 2015,Jan,16

\+ **96371** **additional pump set-up with establishment of new subcutaneous infusion site(s) (List separately in addition to code for primary procedure)**

EXCLUDES *Reporting code more than one time per encounter*

Code first (96369)

1.84 1.84 **FUD** ZZZ Q1 80

AMA: 2020,Jan,11; 2018,Feb,11; 2018,Jan,8; 2017,Jan,8; 2016,Jan,13; 2015,Jan,16

96372-96379 Injections: Diagnostic/Preventive/Therapeutic

CMS: 100-04,4,230.2 OPPS Drug Administration

INCLUDES Administration fluid
Administration substances/drugs
Coding hierarchy rules for facility reporting:
- Chemotherapy services primary to diagnostic, prophylactic, and therapeutic services
- Diagnostic, prophylactic, and therapeutic services primary to hydration services
- Infusions primary to pushes
- Pushes primary to injections

Constant presence by health care professional administering substance/drug
Direct supervision by physician or other qualified health care provider:
- Consent
- Direction personnel
- Patient assessment
- Safety oversight
- Supervision personnel

If done to facilitate injection/infusion:
- Flush at infusion end
- Indwelling IV, subcutaneous catheter/port access
- Local anesthesia
- Start IV
- Supplies/tubing/syringes

Infusion 15 minutes or less
Training to assess patient and monitor vital signs
Training to prepare/dose/dispose
Treatment plan verification

EXCLUDES *Catheter/port declotting (36593)*
Reporting code for second initial service on same date for accessing multilumen catheter, restarting IV, or when two IV lines needed to meet infusion rate
Reporting code with other procedures where IV push or infusion is integral to procedure
Services provided by physicians or other qualified health care providers in facility settings
Significant separately identifiable E/M service, when performed

Code also drugs/materials

96372 **Therapeutic, prophylactic, or diagnostic injection (specify substance or drug); subcutaneous or intramuscular**

INCLUDES Direct supervision by physician or other qualified health care provider when reported by physician/other qualified health care provider. When reported by hospital, physician/other qualified health care provider need not be present
Hormonal therapy injections (non-antineoplastic) (96372)

EXCLUDES *Administration vaccines/toxoids (90460-90474)*
Allergen immunotherapy injections (95115-95117)
Antineoplastic hormonal injections (96402)
Antineoplastic nonhormonal injections (96401)
Injections administered without direct supervision by physician or other qualified health care provider (99211)

0.40 0.40 **FUD** XXX Q1 80

AMA: 2018,Dec,10; 2018,Dec,10; 2018,Feb,11; 2018,Jan,8; 2017,Jan,8; 2016,Oct,9; 2016,Jan,13; 2015,Jan,16

96373 **intra-arterial**

0.53 0.53 **FUD** XXX S 80

AMA: 2018,Feb,11; 2018,Jan,8; 2017,Jan,8; 2016,Jan,13; 2015,Jan,16

96374 **intravenous push, single or initial substance/drug**

1.10 1.10 **FUD** XXX S 80

AMA: 2020,Jan,11; 2019,Sep,5; 2019,Jun,9; 2018,Feb,11; 2018,Jan,8; 2017,Jan,8; 2016,Jan,13; 2015,Nov,3; 2015,Jan,16

\+ **96375** **each additional sequential intravenous push of a new substance/drug (List separately in addition to code for primary procedure)**

INCLUDES IV push new substance/drug provided as secondary or subsequent service after different initial service via same IV access site

Code first (96365, 96374, 96409, 96413)

0.47 0.47 **FUD** ZZZ S 80

AMA: 2019,Sep,5; 2018,Feb,11; 2018,Jan,8; 2017,Jan,8; 2016,Jan,13; 2015,Nov,3; 2015,Jan,16

+ **96376** **each additional sequential intravenous push of the same substance/drug provided in a facility (List separately in addition to code for primary procedure)**

INCLUDES Facilities only

EXCLUDES *IV push performed within 30 minutes push same substance or drug*

Services performed by any nonfacilty provider

Code first (96365, 96374, 96409, 96413)

0.00 0.00 FUD ZZZ N

AMA: 2018,Dec,8; 2018,Dec,8; 2018,Feb,11; 2018,Jan,8; 2017,Jan,8; 2016,Jan,13; 2015,Jan,16

96377 **Application of on-body injector (includes cannula insertion) for timed subcutaneous injection**

0.56 0.56 FUD XXX Q1 80

AMA: 2018,Feb,11; 2018,Jan,8; 2017,Jan,8; 2016,Oct,9

96379 **Unlisted therapeutic, prophylactic, or diagnostic intravenous or intra-arterial injection or infusion**

0.00 0.00 FUD XXX Q1 80

AMA: 2018,Feb,11; 2018,Jan,8; 2017,Jan,8; 2016,Jan,13; 2015,Jan,16

96401-96411 Chemotherapy and Other Complex Drugs, Biologicals: Injection and IV Push

CMS: 100-03,110.2 Certain Drugs Distributed by the National Cancer Institute; 100-03,110.6 Scalp Hypothermia During Chemotherapy, to Prevent Hair Loss; 100-04,4,230.2 OPPS Drug Administration

INCLUDES Highly complex services that require direct supervision for:
- Consent
- Patient assessment
- Safety oversight
- Supervision

More intense work and monitoring clinical staff by physician or other qualified health care provider due to greater risk severe patient reactions

Parenteral administration:
- Anti-neoplastic agents for noncancer diagnoses
- Monoclonal antibody agents
- Nonradionuclide antineoplastic drugs
- Other biologic response modifiers

EXCLUDES *Reporting code for second initial service on same date for accessing multilumen catheter, restarting IV, or when two IV lines needed to meet infusion rate*

96401 **Chemotherapy administration, subcutaneous or intramuscular; non-hormonal anti-neoplastic**

EXCLUDES *Services performed by physicians or other qualified health care providers in facility settings*

2.22 2.22 FUD XXX Q1 80

AMA: 2018,Feb,11; 2018,Jan,8; 2017,Jan,8; 2016,Jan,13; 2015,Jan,16

96402 **hormonal anti-neoplastic**

EXCLUDES *Services performed by physicians or other qualified health care providers in facility settings*

0.87 0.87 FUD XXX Q1 80

AMA: 2018,Feb,11; 2018,Jan,8; 2017,Jan,8; 2016,Jan,13; 2015,Jan,16

96405 **Chemotherapy administration; intralesional, up to and including 7 lesions**

0.84 2.31 FUD 000 Q1

AMA: 2018,Feb,11; 2018,Jan,8; 2017,Jan,8; 2016,Jan,13; 2015,Jan,16

96406 **intralesional, more than 7 lesions**

1.31 3.46 FUD 000 S

AMA: 2018,Feb,11; 2018,Jan,8; 2017,Jan,8; 2016,Jan,13; 2015,Jan,16

96409 **intravenous, push technique, single or initial substance/drug**

INCLUDES Push technique includes:
- Administration injection directly into vessel or access line by health care professional; or
- Infusion less than or equal to 15 minutes

EXCLUDES *Insertion arterial and venous cannula(s) for extracorpororeal circulation (36823)*

Services performed by physicians or other qualified health care providers in facility settings

3.05 3.05 FUD XXX S 80

AMA: 2018,Feb,11; 2018,Jan,8; 2017,Jan,8; 2016,Jan,13; 2015,Jan,16

+ **96411** **intravenous, push technique, each additional substance/drug (List separately in addition to code for primary procedure)**

INCLUDES Push technique includes:
- Administration injection directly into vessel or access line by health care professional; or
- Infusion less than or equal to 15 minutes

EXCLUDES *Insertion arterial and venous cannula(s) for extracorpororeal circulation (36823)*

Services performed by physicians or other qualified health care providers in facility settings

Code first initial substance/drug (96409, 96413)

1.65 1.65 FUD ZZZ S 80

AMA: 2018,Feb,11; 2018,Jan,8; 2017,Jan,8; 2016,Jan,13; 2015,Jan,16

96413-96417 Chemotherapy and Complex Drugs, Biologicals: Intravenous Infusion

CMS: 100-03,110.2 Certain Drugs Distributed by the National Cancer Institute; 100-03,110.6 Scalp Hypothermia During Chemotherapy, to Prevent Hair Loss; 100-04,4,230.2 OPPS Drug Administration

INCLUDES Administration:
- Access to IV/catheter/port
- Drug preparation
- Flushing at infusion completion
- Hydration fluid
- Local anesthesia
- Routine tubing/syringe/supplies
- Starting IV

Highly complex services that require direct supervision for:
- Consent
- Patient assessment
- Safety oversight
- Supervision

More intense work and monitoring clinical staff by physician or other qualified health care provider due to greater risk severe patient reactions

Parenteral administration:
- Antineoplastic agents for noncancer diagnoses
- Monoclonal antibody agents
- Nonradionuclide antineoplastic drugs
- Other biologic response modifiers

EXCLUDES *Administration nonchemotherapy agents such as antibiotics/steroids/analgesics*
Declotting catheter/port (36593)
Home infusion (99601-99602)
Insertion arterial and venous cannula(s) for extracorpororeal circulation (36823)
Reporting code for second initial service on same date for accessing multilumen catheter, restarting IV, or when two IV lines needed to meet infusion rate
Services provided by physicians or other qualified health care providers in facility settings

Code also drug or substance
Code also significant separately identifiable E/M service, when performed

96413 Chemotherapy administration, intravenous infusion technique; up to 1 hour, single or initial substance/drug

INCLUDES Push technique includes:
- Administration injection directly into vessel or access line by health care professional; or
- Infusion less than or equal to 15 minutes

EXCLUDES *Hydration administered as secondary or subsequent service via same IV access site (96361)*
Therapeutic/prophylactic/diagnostic drug infusion/injection through the same intravenous access (96366, 96367, 96375)

Code also second initial service with modifier 59 when patient's condition or drug protocol mandates use of two IV lines

Facility RVU 3.97 Non-Facility RVU 3.97 **FUD** XXX S 80

AMA: 2018,Feb,11; 2018,Jan,8; 2017,Jan,8; 2016,Jan,13; 2015,Jan,16

\+ **96415 each additional hour (List separately in addition to code for primary procedure)**

INCLUDES Infusion intervals more than 30 minutes past 1-hour increments

Code first initial hour (96413)

Facility RVU 0.86 Non-Facility RVU 0.86 **FUD** ZZZ S 80

AMA: 2018,Feb,11; 2018,Jan,8; 2017,Jan,8; 2016,Jan,13; 2015,Jan,16

96416 initiation of prolonged chemotherapy infusion (more than 8 hours), requiring use of a portable or implantable pump

EXCLUDES *Portable or implantable infusion pump/reservoir refilling/maintenance for drug delivery (96521-96523)*

Facility RVU 3.98 Non-Facility RVU 3.98 **FUD** XXX S 80

AMA: 2018,Feb,11; 2018,Jan,8; 2017,Jan,8; 2016,Jan,13; 2015,Jan,16

\+ **96417 each additional sequential infusion (different substance/drug), up to 1 hour (List separately in addition to code for primary procedure)**

INCLUDES Push technique includes:
- Administration injection directly into vessel or access line by health care professional; or
- Infusion less than or equal to 15 minutes

EXCLUDES *Additional hour(s) sequential infusion (96415)*
Reporting code more than one time per sequential infusion

Code first initial substance/drug (96413)

Facility RVU 1.92 Non-Facility RVU 1.92 **FUD** ZZZ S 80

AMA: 2018,Feb,11; 2018,Jan,8; 2017,Jan,8; 2016,Jan,13; 2015,Jan,16

96420-96425 Chemotherapy and Complex Drugs, Biologicals: Intra-arterial

CMS: 100-03,110.2 Certain Drugs Distributed by the National Cancer Institute; 100-03,110.6 Scalp Hypothermia During Chemotherapy, to Prevent Hair Loss; 100-04,4,230.2 OPPS Drug Administration

INCLUDES Administration:
- Access to IV/catheter/port
- Drug preparation
- Flushing at infusion completion
- Hydration fluid
- Local anesthesia
- Routine tubing/syringe/supplies
- Starting IV

Highly complex services that require direct supervision for:
- Consent
- Patient assessment
- Safety oversight
- Supervision

More intense work and monitoring clinical staff by physician or other qualified health care provider due to greater risk severe patient reactions

Parenteral administration:
- Antineoplastic agents for noncancer diagnoses
- Monoclonal antibody agents
- Nonradionuclide antineoplastic drugs
- Other biologic response modifiers

EXCLUDES *Administration nonchemotherapy agents such as antibiotics/steroids/analgesics*
Declotting catheter/port (36593)
Home infusion (99601-99602)
Reporting code for second initial service on same date for accessing multilumen catheter, restarting IV, or when two IV lines needed to meet an infusion rate
Services provided by physicians or other qualified health care providers in facility settings

Code also drug or substance
Code also significant separately identifiable E/M service, when performed

96420 Chemotherapy administration, intra-arterial; push technique

INCLUDES Push technique includes:
- Administration injection directly into vessel or access line by health care professional; or
- Infusion less than or equal to 15 minutes

Regional chemotherapy perfusion

EXCLUDES *Insertion arterial and venous cannula(s) for extracorpororeal circulation (36823)*
Placement intra-arterial catheter

Facility RVU 2.95 Non-Facility RVU 2.95 **FUD** XXX S 80

AMA: 2018,Feb,11; 2018,Jan,8; 2017,Jan,8; 2016,Mar,3; 2016,Jan,13; 2015,Nov,3; 2015,Jan,16

96422 infusion technique, up to 1 hour

INCLUDES Push technique includes:
- Administration injection directly into vessel or access line by health care professional; or
- Infusion less than or equal to 15 minutes

Regional chemotherapy perfusion

EXCLUDES *Insertion arterial and venous cannula(s) for extracorpororeal circulation (36823)*
Placement intra-arterial catheter

Facility RVU 4.85 Non-Facility RVU 4.85 **FUD** XXX S 80

AMA: 2018,Feb,11; 2018,Jan,8; 2017,Jan,8; 2016,Mar,3; 2016,Jan,13; 2015,Nov,3; 2015,Jan,16

+ **96423** **infusion technique, each additional hour (List separately in addition to code for primary procedure)**

INCLUDES Infusion intervals more than 30 minutes past 1-hour increments
Regional chemotherapy perfusion

EXCLUDES *Insertion arterial and venous cannula(s) for extracorpororeal circulation (36823)*
Placement intra-arterial catheter

Code first initial hour (96422)

2.24 2.24 **FUD** ZZZ S 80

AMA: 2018,Feb,11; 2018,Jan,8; 2017,Jan,8; 2016,Mar,3; 2016,Jan,13; 2015,Nov,3; 2015,Jan,16

96425 **infusion technique, initiation of prolonged infusion (more than 8 hours), requiring the use of a portable or implantable pump**

INCLUDES Regional chemotherapy perfusion

EXCLUDES *Insertion arterial and venous cannula(s) for extracorpororeal circulation (36823)*
Placement intra-arterial catheter
Portable or implantable infusion pump/reservoir refilling/maintenance for drug delivery (96521-96523)

5.14 5.14 **FUD** XXX S 80

AMA: 2018,Feb,11; 2018,Jan,8; 2017,Jan,8; 2016,Mar,3; 2016,Jan,13; 2015,Nov,3; 2015,Jan,16

96440-96450 Chemotherapy Administration: Intrathecal/Peritoneal Cavity/Pleural Cavity

CMS: 100-03,110.2 Certain Drugs Distributed by the National Cancer Institute; 100-04,4,230.2 OPPS Drug Administration

96440 **Chemotherapy administration into pleural cavity, requiring and including thoracentesis**

3.57 23.6 **FUD** 000 S 80

AMA: 2018,Feb,11; 2018,Jan,8; 2017,Jan,8; 2016,Jan,13; 2015,Jan,16

96446 **Chemotherapy administration into the peritoneal cavity via indwelling port or catheter**

0.79 5.78 **FUD** XXX S 80

AMA: 2018,Feb,11; 2018,Jan,8; 2017,Jan,8; 2016,Jan,13; 2015,Jan,16

96450 **Chemotherapy administration, into CNS (eg, intrathecal), requiring and including spinal puncture**

EXCLUDES *Chemotherapy administration, intravesical/bladder (51720)*
Fluoroscopy (77003)
Insertion catheter/reservoir:
Intraventricular (61210, 61215)
Subarachnoid (62350-62351, 62360-62362)

2.27 5.13 **FUD** 000 S 80

AMA: 2018,Feb,11; 2018,Jan,8; 2017,Jan,8; 2016,Jan,13; 2015,Jan,16

96521-96523 Refill/Upkeep of Drug Delivery Device

CMS: 100-04,4,230.2 OPPS Drug Administration

INCLUDES Administration:
- Access to IV/catheter/port
- Drug preparation
- Flushing at infusion completion
- Hydration fluid
- Local anesthesia
- Routine tubing/syringe/supplies
- Starting IV

Highly complex services that require direct supervision for:
- Consent
- Patient assessment
- Safety oversight
- Supervision

Parenteral administration:
- Antineoplastic agents for noncancer diagnoses
- Monoclonal antibody agents
- Nonradionuclide antineoplastic drugs
- Other biologic response modifiers

Therapeutic drugs other than chemotherapy

EXCLUDES *Administration nonchemotherapy agents such as antibiotics/steroids/analgesics*
Blood specimen collection from completely implantable venous access device (36591)
Declotting catheter/port (36593)
Home infusion (99601-99602)
Services provided by physicians or other qualified health care providers in facility settings

Code also drug or substance
Code also significant separately identifiable E/M service, when performed

96521 **Refilling and maintenance of portable pump**

4.13 4.13 **FUD** XXX S 80

AMA: 2018,Feb,11; 2018,Jan,8; 2017,Jan,8; 2016,Jan,13; 2015,Jan,16

96522 **Refilling and maintenance of implantable pump or reservoir for drug delivery, systemic (eg, intravenous, intra-arterial)**

EXCLUDES *Implantable infusion pump refilling/maintenance for spinal/brain drug delivery (95990-95991)*

3.45 3.45 **FUD** XXX S 80

AMA: 2018,Feb,11; 2018,Jan,8; 2017,Jan,8; 2016,Jan,13; 2015,Jan,16

96523 **Irrigation of implanted venous access device for drug delivery systems**

EXCLUDES *Direct supervision by physician or other qualified health care provider in facility settings*
Reporting code with any other services on same service date

0.77 0.77 **FUD** XXX Q1 80

AMA: 2018,Feb,11; 2018,Jan,8; 2017,Jan,8; 2016,Jan,13; 2015,Jan,16

96542-96549 Chemotherapy Injection Into Brain

CMS: 100-04,4,230.2 OPPS Drug Administration

INCLUDES Administration:
- Access to IV/catheter/port
- Drug preparation
- Flushing at infusion completion
- Hydration fluid
- Local anesthesia
- Routine tubing/syringe/supplies
- Starting IV

Highly complex services that require direct supervision for:
- Consent
- Patient assessment
- Safety oversight
- Supervision

Parenteral administration:
- Antineoplastic agents for noncancer diagnoses
- Monoclonal antibody agents
- Nonradionuclide antineoplastic drugs
- Other biologic response modifiers

EXCLUDES *Administration nonchemotherapy agents such as antibiotics/steroids/analgesics*
Blood specimen collection from completely implantable venous access device (36591)
Declotting catheter/port (36593)
Home infusion (99601-99602)

Code also drug or substance
Code also significant separately identifiable E/M service, when performed

96542 **Chemotherapy injection, subarachnoid or intraventricular via subcutaneous reservoir, single or multiple agents**

EXCLUDES *Oral radioactive isotope therapy (79005)*

1.19 | 3.77 | FUD XXX | S 80

AMA: 2018,Feb,11; 2018,Jan,8; 2017,Jan,8; 2016,Jan,13; 2015,Jan,16

96549 **Unlisted chemotherapy procedure**

0.00 | 0.00 | FUD XXX | Q1 80

AMA: 2018,Feb,11; 2018,Jan,8; 2017,Jan,8; 2016,Jan,13; 2015,Jan,16

96567-96574 Destruction of Lesions: Photodynamic Therapy

EXCLUDES *Ocular photodynamic therapy (67221)*

96567 **Photodynamic therapy by external application of light to destroy premalignant lesions of the skin and adjacent mucosa with application and illumination/activation of photosensitive drug(s), per day**

INCLUDES Services provided without direct participation by physician or other qualified healthcare professional

3.50 | 3.50 | FUD XXX | Q1 80

AMA: 2018,Jul,14; 2018,Feb,10; 2018,Feb,11; 2018,Jan,8; 2017,Jan,8; 2016,Jan,13; 2015,Jan,16

+ **96570** **Photodynamic therapy by endoscopic application of light to ablate abnormal tissue via activation of photosensitive drug(s); first 30 minutes (List separately in addition to code for endoscopy or bronchoscopy procedures of lung and gastrointestinal tract)**

Code also for 38-52 minutes (96571)
Code also modifier 52 when services with report less than 23 minutes
Code first (31641, 43229)

1.48 | 1.48 | FUD ZZZ | N

AMA: 2018,Feb,11; 2018,Jan,8; 2017,Jan,8; 2016,Jan,13; 2015,Jan,16

+ **96571** **each additional 15 minutes (List separately in addition to code for endoscopy or bronchoscopy procedures of lung and gastrointestinal tract)**

EXCLUDES *23-37 minutes service (96570)*

Code first (96570)
Code first when appropriate (31641, 43229)

0.83 | 0.83 | FUD ZZZ | N

AMA: 2018,Feb,11; 2018,Jan,8; 2017,Jan,8; 2016,Jan,13; 2015,Jan,16

96573 **Photodynamic therapy by external application of light to destroy premalignant lesions of the skin and adjacent mucosa with application and illumination/activation of photosensitizing drug(s) provided by a physician or other qualified health care professional, per day**

INCLUDES Application photosensitizer to lesions at anatomical site
Debridement, when performed
Light to activate photosensitizer for destruction premalignant lesions

EXCLUDES *Debridement lesion with photodynamic therapy provided by physician or other qualified healthcare professional (96574)*
Photodynamic therapy by external application light to same anatomical site (96567)
Services provided to same area on same date as photodynamic therapy:
- *Biopsy (11102-11107)*
- *Debridement (11000-11001, 11004-11005)*
- *Excision lesion (11400-11471)*
- *Shaving lesion (11300-11313)*

6.03 | 6.03 | FUD 000 | Q1 80

AMA: 2018,Jul,14; 2018,Feb,11; 2018,Feb,10

96574 **Debridement of premalignant hyperkeratotic lesion(s) (ie, targeted curettage, abrasion) followed with photodynamic therapy by external application of light to destroy premalignant lesions of the skin and adjacent mucosa with application and illumination/activation of photosensitizing drug(s) provided by a physician or other qualified health care professional, per day**

INCLUDES Application photosensitizer to lesions at anatomical site
Debridement, when performed
Light to activate photosensitizer for destruction premalignant lesions

EXCLUDES *Photodynamic therapy by external application light for destruction premalignant lesions (96573)*
Photodynamic therapy by external application light to same anatomical site (96567)
Services provided to same area on same as photodynamic therapy:
- *Biopsy (11102-11107)*
- *Debridement (11000-11001, 11004-11005)*
- *Excision lesion (11400-11471)*
- *Shaving lesion (11300-11313)*

7.25 | 7.25 | FUD 000 | Q1 80

AMA: 2018,Feb,10; 2018,Feb,11

96900-96999 Diagnostic/Therapeutic Skin Procedures

EXCLUDES *E/M services*
Injection, intralesional (11900-11901)

96900 **Actinotherapy (ultraviolet light)**

EXCLUDES *Rhinophototherapy (30999)*

(88160-88161)

0.61 | 0.61 | FUD XXX | Q1 80

AMA: 2018,Feb,11; 2018,Jan,8; 2017,Jan,8; 2016,Nov,9; 2016,Sep,3; 2016,Jan,13; 2015,Jan,16

96902 **Microscopic examination of hairs plucked or clipped by the examiner (excluding hair collected by the patient) to determine telogen and anagen counts, or structural hair shaft abnormality**

(88160-88161)

0.59 | 0.62 | FUD XXX | N

AMA: 2018,Feb,11

96904 **Whole body integumentary photography, for monitoring of high risk patients with dysplastic nevus syndrome or a history of dysplastic nevi, or patients with a personal or familial history of melanoma**

(88160-88161)

1.82 | 1.82 | FUD XXX | N 80

AMA: 2018,Feb,11

96910 **Photochemotherapy; tar and ultraviolet B (Goeckerman treatment) or petrolatum and ultraviolet B**
(88160-88161)
3.28 3.28 FUD XXX Q1 80
AMA: 2018,Feb,11; 2018,Jan,8; 2017,Jan,8; 2016,Sep,3; 2016,Jan,13; 2015,Jan,16

96912 **psoralens and ultraviolet A (PUVA)**
(88160-88161)
2.80 2.80 FUD XXX Q1 80
AMA: 2018,Feb,11; 2018,Jan,8; 2017,Jan,8; 2016,Sep,3; 2016,Jan,13; 2015,Jan,16

96913 **Photochemotherapy (Goeckerman and/or PUVA) for severe photoresponsive dermatoses requiring at least 4-8 hours of care under direct supervision of the physician (includes application of medication and dressings)**
(88160-88161)
4.06 4.06 FUD XXX T 80
AMA: 2018,Feb,11; 2018,Jan,8; 2017,Jan,8; 2016,Sep,3

96920 **Laser treatment for inflammatory skin disease (psoriasis); total area less than 250 sq cm**
EXCLUDES *Destruction by laser:*
Benign lesions (17110-17111)
Cutaneous vascular proliferative lesions (17106-17108)
Malignant lesions (17260-17286)
Premalignant lesions (17000-17004)
(88160-88161)
1.90 4.64 FUD 000 Q1
AMA: 2020,Jul,13; 2018,Feb,11; 2018,Jan,8; 2017,Jan,8; 2016,Sep,3; 2016,Jan,13; 2015,Jan,16

96921 **250 sq cm to 500 sq cm**
EXCLUDES *Destruction by laser:*
Benign lesions (17110-17111)
Cutaneous vascular proliferative lesions (17106-17108)
Malignant lesions (17260-17286)
Premalignant lesions (17000-17004)
(88160-88161)
2.14 5.09 FUD 000 Q1
AMA: 2020,Jul,13; 2018,Feb,11; 2018,Jan,8; 2017,Jan,8; 2016,Sep,3; 2016,Jan,13; 2015,Jan,16

96922 **over 500 sq cm**
EXCLUDES *Destruction by laser:*
Benign lesions (17110-17111)
Cutaneous vascular proliferative lesions (17106-17108)
Malignant lesions (17260-17286)
Premalignant lesions (17000-17004)
(88160-88161)
3.43 6.91 FUD 000 Q1
AMA: 2020,Jul,13; 2018,Feb,11; 2018,Jan,8; 2017,Jan,8; 2016,Sep,3; 2016,Jan,13; 2015,Jan,16

96931 **Reflectance confocal microscopy (RCM) for cellular and sub-cellular imaging of skin; image acquisition and interpretation and report, first lesion**
EXCLUDES *Optical coherence tomography for skin imaging (0470T-0471T)*
Reflectance confocal microscopy examination without generated mosaic images (96999)
4.78 4.78 FUD XXX M 80
AMA: 2018,Feb,11; 2018,Jan,8; 2017,Sep,9

96932 **image acquisition only, first lesion**
EXCLUDES *Optical coherence tomography for skin imaging (0470T-0471T)*
Reflectance confocal microscopy examination without generated mosaic images (96999)
3.47 3.47 FUD XXX Q1 80 TC
AMA: 2018,Feb,11; 2018,Jan,8; 2017,Sep,9

96933 **interpretation and report only, first lesion**
EXCLUDES *Optical coherence tomography for skin imaging (0470T-0471T)*
Reflectance confocal microscopy examination without generated mosaic images (96999)
1.32 1.32 FUD XXX B 80 26
AMA: 2018,Feb,11; 2018,Jan,8; 2017,Sep,9

+ **96934** **image acquisition and interpretation and report, each additional lesion (List separately in addition to code for primary procedure)**
EXCLUDES *Optical coherence tomography for skin imaging (0470T-0471T)*
Reflectance confocal microscopy examination without generated mosaic images (96999)
Code first (96931)
2.10 2.10 FUD ZZZ N 80
AMA: 2018,Feb,11; 2018,Jan,8; 2017,Sep,9

+ **96935** **image acquisition only, each additional lesion (List separately in addition to code for primary procedure)**
EXCLUDES *Optical coherence tomography for skin imaging (0470T-0471T)*
Reflectance confocal microscopy examination without generated mosaic images (96999)
Code first (96932)
0.99 0.99 FUD ZZZ N 80 TC
AMA: 2018,Feb,11; 2018,Jan,8; 2017,Sep,9

+ **96936** **interpretation and report only, each additional lesion (List separately in addition to code for primary procedure)**
EXCLUDES *Optical coherence tomography for skin imaging (0470T-0471T)*
Reflectance confocal microscopy examination without generated mosaic images (96999)
Code first (96933)
1.11 1.11 FUD ZZZ N 80 26
AMA: 2018,Feb,11; 2018,Jan,8; 2017,Sep,9

96999 **Unlisted special dermatological service or procedure**
0.00 0.00 FUD XXX Q1 80
AMA: 2020,Jul,13; 2018,Feb,11; 2018,Jan,8; 2017,Sep,9; 2017,Jan,8; 2016,Sep,3; 2016,Jan,13; 2015,Jan,16

97161-97164 [97161, 97162, 97163, 97164] Assessment: Physical Therapy

CMS: 100-02,15,220 Coverage of Outpatient Rehabilitation Therapy Services; 100-02,15,220.4 Functional Reporting; 100-02,15,230 Practice of Physical Therapy, Occupational Therapy, and Speech-Language Pathology; 100-02,15,230.1 Practice of Physical Therapy; 100-02,15,230.4 Services By a Physical/Occupational Therapist in Private Practice; 100-04,5,10.3.2 Therapy Cap Exceptions; 100-04,5,10.3.3 Use of the KX Modifier; 100-04,5,10.6 Functional Reporting; 100-04,5,20.2 Reporting Units of Service

INCLUDES Care plan creation
Evaluation body systems as defined in 1997 E/M documentation guidelines:
Cardiovascular system: Vital signs, edema extremities
Integumentary system: Inspection for skin abnormalities
Mental status: Orientation, judgment, thought processes
Musculoskeletal system: Evaluation gait and station, motion range, muscle strength, height, and weight
Neuromuscular evaluation: Balance, abnormal movements

EXCLUDES *Biofeedback traning via EMG (90901)*
Joint motion range (95851-95852)
Transcutaneous nerve stimulation (TENS) (97014, 97032)

97161 **Physical therapy evaluation: low complexity, requiring these components: A history with no personal factors and/or comorbidities that impact the plan of care; An examination of body system(s) using standardized tests and measures addressing 1-2 elements from any of the following: body structures and functions, activity limitations, and/or participation restrictions; A clinical presentation with stable and/or uncomplicated characteristics; and Clinical decision making of low complexity using standardized patient assessment instrument and/or measurable assessment of functional outcome. Typically, 20 minutes are spent face-to-face with the patient and/or family.**
2.38 2.38 FUD XXX 51 A 80
AMA: 2018,May,5; 2018,Feb,11; 2018,Jan,8; 2017,Aug,3; 2017,Jun,6; 2017,Jan,8

Medicine

96910 — 97161

97162 **Physical therapy evaluation: moderate complexity, requiring these components: A history of present problem with 1-2 personal factors and/or comorbidities that impact the plan of care; An examination of body systems using standardized tests and measures in addressing a total of 3 or more elements from any of the following: body structures and functions, activity limitations, and/or participation restrictions; An evolving clinical presentation with changing characteristics; and Clinical decision making of moderate complexity using standardized patient assessment instrument and/or measurable assessment of functional outcome. Typically, 30 minutes are spent face-to-face with the patient and/or family.**

2.38 2.38 FUD XXX (51) A 80

AMA: 2018,May,5; 2018,Feb,11; 2018,Jan,8; 2017,Aug,3; 2017,Jun,6; 2017,Jan,8

97163 **Physical therapy evaluation: high complexity, requiring these components: A history of present problem with 3 or more personal factors and/or comorbidities that impact the plan of care; An examination of body systems using standardized tests and measures addressing a total of 4 or more elements from any of the following: body structures and functions, activity limitations, and/or participation restrictions; A clinical presentation with unstable and unpredictable characteristics; and Clinical decision making of high complexity using standardized patient assessment instrument and/or measurable assessment of functional outcome. Typically, 45 minutes are spent face-to-face with the patient and/or family.**

2.40 2.40 FUD XXX (51) A 80

AMA: 2018,May,5; 2018,Feb,11; 2018,Jan,8; 2017,Aug,3; 2017,Jun,6; 2017,Jan,8

97164 **Re-evaluation of physical therapy established plan of care, requiring these components: An examination including a review of history and use of standardized tests and measures is required; and Revised plan of care using a standardized patient assessment instrument and/or measurable assessment of functional outcome Typically, 20 minutes are spent face-to-face with the patient and/or family.**

1.63 1.63 FUD XXX (51) A 80

AMA: 2018,May,5; 2018,Feb,11; 2018,Jan,8; 2017,Aug,3; 2017,Jun,6; 2017,Jan,8

97165-97168 [97165, 97166, 97167, 97168] Assessment: Occupational Therapy

CMS: 100-02,15,220 Coverage of Outpatient Rehabilitation Therapy Services; 100-02,15,220.4 Functional Reporting; 100-02,15,230 Practice of Physical Therapy, Occupational Therapy, and Speech-Language Pathology; 100-02,15,230.1 Practice of Physical Therapy; 100-02,15,230.2 Practice of Occupational Therapy; 100-02,15,230.4 Services By a Physical/Occupational Therapist in Private Practice; 100-04,5,10.3.2 Exceptions Process; 100-04,5,10.3.3 Use of the KX Modifier; 100-04,5,10.6 Functional Reporting; 100-04,5,20.2 Reporting Units of Service

INCLUDES Care plan creation
Evaluations as appropriate
Medical history
Occupational status
Past therapy history

97165 **Occupational therapy evaluation, low complexity, requiring these components: An occupational profile and medical and therapy history, which includes a brief history including review of medical and/or therapy records relating to the presenting problem; An assessment(s) that identifies 1-3 performance deficits (ie, relating to physical, cognitive, or psychosocial skills) that result in activity limitations and/or participation restrictions; and Clinical decision making of low complexity, which includes an analysis of the occupational profile, analysis of data from problem-focused assessment(s), and consideration of a limited number of treatment options. Patient presents with no comorbidities that affect occupational performance. Modification of tasks or assistance (eg, physical or verbal) with assessment(s) is not necessary to enable completion of evaluation component. Typically, 30 minutes are spent face-to-face with the patient and/or family.**

2.57 2.57 FUD XXX (51) A 80

AMA: 2018,May,5; 2018,Feb,11; 2018,Jan,8; 2017,Jun,6; 2017,Feb,3; 2017,Jan,8

97166 **Occupational therapy evaluation, moderate complexity, requiring these components: An occupational profile and medical and therapy history, which includes an expanded review of medical and/or therapy records and additional review of physical, cognitive, or psychosocial history related to current functional performance; An assessment(s) that identifies 3-5 performance deficits (ie, relating to physical, cognitive, or psychosocial skills) that result in activity limitations and/or participation restrictions; and Clinical decision making of moderate analytic complexity, which includes an analysis of the occupational profile, analysis of data from detailed assessment(s), and consideration of several treatment options. Patient may present with comorbidities that affect occupational performance. Minimal to moderate modification of tasks or assistance (eg, physical or verbal) with assessment(s) is necessary to enable patient to complete evaluation component. Typically, 45 minutes are spent face-to-face with the patient and/or family.**

2.58 2.58 FUD XXX (51) A 80

AMA: 2018,May,5; 2018,Feb,11; 2018,Jan,8; 2017,Jun,6; 2017,Feb,3; 2017,Jan,8

97167 Occupational therapy evaluation, high complexity, requiring these components: An occupational profile and medical and therapy history, which includes review of medical and/or therapy records and extensive additional review of physical, cognitive, or psychosocial history related to current functional performance; An assessment(s) that identifies 5 or more performance deficits (ie, relating to physical, cognitive, or psychosocial skills) that result in activity limitations and/or participation restrictions; and Clinical decision making of high analytic complexity, which includes an analysis of the patient profile, analysis of data from comprehensive assessment(s), and consideration of multiple treatment options. Patient presents with comorbidities that affect occupational performance. Significant modification of tasks or assistance (eg, physical or verbal) with assessment(s) is necessary to enable patient to complete evaluation component. Typically, 60 minutes are spent face-to-face with the patient and/or family.

2.57 2.57 FUD XXX

AMA: 2018,May,5; 2018,Feb,11; 2018,Jan,8; 2017,Jun,6; 2017,Feb,3; 2017,Jan,8

97168 Re-evaluation of occupational therapy established plan of care, requiring these components: An assessment of changes in patient functional or medical status with revised plan of care; An update to the initial occupational profile to reflect changes in condition or environment that affect future interventions and/or goals; and A revised plan of care. A formal reevaluation is performed when there is a documented change in functional status or a significant change to the plan of care is required. Typically, 30 minutes are spent face-to-face with the patient and/or family.

1.75 1.75 FUD XXX

AMA: 2018,May,5; 2018,Feb,11; 2018,Jan,8; 2017,Jun,6; 2017,Feb,3; 2017,Jan,8

97169-97172 [97169, 97170, 97171, 97172] Assessment: Athletic Training

CMS: 100-02,15,220 Coverage of Outpatient Rehabilitation Therapy Services; 100-02,15,230 Practice of Physical Therapy, Occupational Therapy, and Speech-Language Pathology; 100-02,15,230.1 Practice of Physical Therapy

INCLUDES Care plan creation
Evaluation body systems as defined in 1997 E/M documentation guidelines:
- Cardiovascular system: Vital signs, edema extremities
- Integumentary system: Inspection for skin abnormalities
- Musculoskeletal system: Evaluation gait and station, motion range, muscle strength, height, and weight
- Neuromuscular evaluation: Balance, abnormal movements

97169 Athletic training evaluation, low complexity, requiring these components: A history and physical activity profile with no comorbidities that affect physical activity; An examination of affected body area and other symptomatic or related systems addressing 1-2 elements from any of the following: body structures, physical activity, and/or participation deficiencies; and Clinical decision making of low complexity using standardized patient assessment instrument and/or measurable assessment of functional outcome. Typically, 15 minutes are spent face-to-face with the patient and/or family.

0.00 0.00 FUD XXX

AMA: 2018,May,5; 2018,Feb,11; 2018,Jan,8; 2017,Jun,6; 2017,Jan,8

97170 Athletic training evaluation, moderate complexity, requiring these components: A medical history and physical activity profile with 1-2 comorbidities that affect physical activity; An examination of affected body area and other symptomatic or related systems addressing a total of 3 or more elements from any of the following: body structures, physical activity, and/or participation deficiencies; and Clinical decision making of moderate complexity using standardized patient assessment instrument and/or measurable assessment of functional outcome. Typically, 30 minutes are spent face-to-face with the patient and/or family.

0.00 0.00 FUD XXX

AMA: 2018,May,5; 2018,Feb,11; 2018,Jan,8; 2017,Jun,6; 2017,Jan,8

97171 Athletic training evaluation, high complexity, requiring these components: A medical history and physical activity profile, with 3 or more comorbidities that affect physical activity; A comprehensive examination of body systems using standardized tests and measures addressing a total of 4 or more elements from any of the following: body structures, physical activity, and/or participation deficiencies; Clinical presentation with unstable and unpredictable characteristics; and Clinical decision making of high complexity using standardized patient assessment instrument and/or measurable assessment of functional outcome. Typically, 45 minutes are spent face-to-face with the patient and/or family.

0.00 0.00 FUD XXX

AMA: 2018,May,5; 2018,Feb,11; 2018,Jan,8; 2017,Jun,6; 2017,Jan,8

97172 Re-evaluation of athletic training established plan of care requiring these components: An assessment of patient's current functional status when there is a documented change; and A revised plan of care using a standardized patient assessment instrument and/or measurable assessment of functional outcome with an update in management options, goals, and interventions. Typically, 20 minutes are spent face-to-face with the patient and/or family.

0.00 0.00 FUD XXX

AMA: 2018,May,5; 2018,Feb,11; 2018,Jan,8; 2017,Jun,6; 2017,Jan,8

97010-97028 Physical Therapy Treatment Modalities: Supervised

CMS: 100-02,15,220 Coverage of Outpatient Rehabilitation Therapy Services; 100-02,15,220.4 Functional Reporting; 100-02,15,230 Practice of Physical Therapy, Occupational Therapy, and Speech-Language Pathology; 100-02,15,230.1 Practice of Physical Therapy; 100-02,15,230.2 Practice of Occupational Therapy; 100-02,15,230.4 Services By a Physical/Occupational Therapist in Private Practice; 100-03,10.3 Inpatient Pain Rehabilitation Programs; 100-03,10.4 Outpatient Hospital Pain Rehabilitation Programs; 100-03,160.17 Payment for L-Dopa /Associated Inpatient Hospital Services; 100-04,5,10 Part B Outpatient Rehabilitation and Comprehensive Outpatient Rehabilitation Facility (CORF) Services - General; 100-04,5,10.3.2 Exceptions Process; 100-04,5,10.3.3 Use of the KX Modifier; 100-04,5,20.2 Reporting Units of Service

INCLUDES Adding incremental treatment time intervals for same visit to calculate total service time

EXCLUDES
Direct patient contact by provider
Electromyography (95860-95872 [95885, 95886, 95887])
EMG biofeedback training (90901)
Muscle and motion range tests ([97161, 97162, 97163, 97164, 97165, 97166, 97167, 97168, 97169, 97170, 97171, 97172])
Nerve conduction studies (95905-95913)

97010 Application of a modality to 1 or more areas; hot or cold packs

0.18 0.18 FUD XXX

AMA: 2018,May,5; 2018,Feb,11; 2018,Jan,8; 2017,Jan,8; 2016,Jun,8; 2016,Jan,13; 2015,Jan,16

97012 traction, mechanical

0.42 0.42 FUD XXX

AMA: 2020,Jul,13; 2018,May,5; 2018,Feb,11; 2018,Jan,8; 2017,Jan,8; 2016,Jun,8; 2016,Jan,13; 2015,Jan,16

97014 **electrical stimulation (unattended)**

EXCLUDES *Acupuncture with electrical stimulation (97813, 97814)*

0.42 0.42 FUD XXX

AMA: 2019,Jul,10; 2018,Oct,11; 2018,Oct,8; 2018,May,5; 2018,Feb,11; 2018,Jan,8; 2017,Jan,8; 2016,Jan,13; 2015,Jan,16

97016 **vasopneumatic devices**

0.36 0.36 FUD XXX

AMA: 2018,May,5; 2018,Feb,11; 2018,Jan,8; 2017,Jan,8; 2016,Jan,13; 2015,Jan,16

97018 **paraffin bath**

0.20 0.20 FUD XXX

AMA: 2018,May,5; 2018,Feb,11; 2018,Jan,8; 2017,Jan,8; 2016,Jan,13; 2015,Jan,16

97022 **whirlpool**

0.51 0.51 FUD XXX

AMA: 2018,May,5; 2018,Feb,11; 2018,Jan,8; 2017,Jan,8; 2016,Jan,13; 2015,Jan,16

97024 **diathermy (eg, microwave)**

0.20 0.20 FUD XXX

AMA: 2018,May,5; 2018,Feb,11; 2018,Jan,8; 2017,Jan,8; 2016,Jan,13; 2015,Jan,16

97026 **infrared**

0.18 0.18 FUD XXX

AMA: 2018,May,5; 2018,Feb,11; 2018,Jan,8; 2017,Jan,8; 2016,Jan,13; 2015,Jan,16

97028 **ultraviolet**

0.23 0.23 FUD XXX

AMA: 2018,May,5; 2018,Feb,11; 2018,Jan,8; 2017,Jan,8; 2016,Jan,13; 2015,Jan,16

97032-97039 Physical Therapy Treatment Modalities: Constant Attendance

CMS: 100-02,15,220 Coverage of Outpatient Rehabilitation Therapy Services; 100-02,15,220.4 Functional Reporting; 100-02,15,230 Practice of Physical Therapy, Occupational Therapy, and Speech-Language Pathology; 100-02,15,230.1 Practice of Physical Therapy; 100-02,15,230.2 Practice of Occupational Therapy; 100-02,15,230.4 Services By a Physical/Occupational Therapist in Private Practice; 100-03,10.3 Inpatient Pain Rehabilitation Programs; 100-03,10.4 Outpatient Hospital Pain Rehabilitation Programs; 100-03,160.17 Payment for L-Dopa /Associated Inpatient Hospital Services; 100-04,5,10 Part B Outpatient Rehabilitation and Comprehensive Outpatient Rehabilitation Facility (CORF) Services - General; 100-04,5,10.3.2 Exceptions Process; 100-04,5,10.3.3 Use of the KX Modifier; 100-04,5,20.2 Reporting Units of Service

INCLUDES Adding incremental treatment time intervals for same visit to calculate total service time
Direct patient contact by provider

EXCLUDES *Electromyography (95860-95872 [95885, 95886, 95887])*
EMG biofeedback training (90901)
Muscle and motion range tests ([97161, 97162, 97163, 97164, 97165, 97166, 97167, 97168, 97169, 97170, 97171, 97172])
Nerve conduction studies (95905-95913)

97032 **Application of a modality to 1 or more areas; electrical stimulation (manual), each 15 minutes**

EXCLUDES *Transcutaneous electrical modulation pain reprocessing (TEMPR) (scrambler therapy) (0278T)*

0.42 0.42 FUD XXX

AMA: 2019,Jul,10; 2018,Oct,11; 2018,Oct,8; 2018,May,5; 2018,Feb,11; 2018,Jan,8; 2017,Jan,8; 2016,Jan,13; 2015,Jan,16

97033 **iontophoresis, each 15 minutes**

0.59 0.59 FUD XXX

AMA: 2018,May,5; 2018,Feb,11; 2018,Jan,8; 2017,Jan,8; 2016,Jan,13; 2015,Jan,16

97034 **contrast baths, each 15 minutes**

0.43 0.43 FUD XXX

AMA: 2018,May,5; 2018,Feb,11; 2018,Jan,8; 2017,Jan,8; 2016,Jan,13; 2015,Jan,16

97035 **ultrasound, each 15 minutes**

0.39 0.39 FUD XXX

AMA: 2018,May,5; 2018,Feb,11; 2018,Jan,8; 2017,Jan,8; 2016,Jan,13; 2015,Jan,16

97036 **Hubbard tank, each 15 minutes**

0.99 0.99 FUD XXX

AMA: 2018,May,5; 2018,Feb,11; 2018,Jan,8; 2017,Jan,8; 2016,Jan,13; 2015,Jan,16

97039 **Unlisted modality (specify type and time if constant attendance)**

0.00 0.00 FUD XXX

AMA: 2020,Jul,13; 2018,May,5; 2018,Feb,11; 2018,Jan,8; 2017,Jan,8; 2016,Nov,9; 2016,Jun,8; 2016,Jan,13; 2015,Jan,16

97110-97546 [97151, 97152, 97153, 97154, 97155, 97156, 97157, 97158, 97161, 97162, 97163, 97164, 97165, 97166, 97167, 97168, 97169, 97170, 97171, 97172] Other Therapeutic Techniques With Direct Patient Contact

CMS: 100-02,15,220 Coverage of Outpatient Rehabilitation Therapy Services; 100-02,15,230 Practice of Physical Therapy, Occupational Therapy, and Speech-Language Pathology; 100-02,15,230.1 Practice of Physical Therapy; 100-02,15,230.2 Practice of Occupational Therapy; 100-02,15,230.4 Services By a Physical/Occupational Therapist in Private Practice; 100-03,10.3 Inpatient Pain Rehabilitation Programs; 100-03,10.4 Outpatient Hospital Pain Rehabilitation Programs; 100-04,5,10 Part B Outpatient Rehabilitation and Comprehensive Outpatient Rehabilitation Facility (CORF) Services - General; 100-04,5,20.2 Reporting Units of Service

INCLUDES Application clinical skills/services to improve function
Direct patient contact by provider

EXCLUDES *Electromyography (95860-95872 [95885, 95886, 95887])*
EMG biofeedback training (90901)
Muscle and motion range tests ([97161, 97162, 97163, 97164, 97165, 97166, 97167, 97168, 97169, 97170, 97171, 97172])
Nerve conduction studies (95905-95913)

97110 **Therapeutic procedure, 1 or more areas, each 15 minutes; therapeutic exercises to develop strength and endurance, range of motion and flexibility**

0.87 0.87 FUD XXX

AMA: 2019,Jun,14; 2018,Dec,7; 2018,Dec,7; 2018,May,5; 2018,Feb,11; 2018,Jan,8; 2017,Dec,14; 2017,Jan,8; 2016,Jun,8; 2016,Jan,13; 2015,Jan,16

97112 **neuromuscular reeducation of movement, balance, coordination, kinesthetic sense, posture, and/or proprioception for sitting and/or standing activities**

0.99 0.99 FUD XXX

AMA: 2018,May,5; 2018,Feb,11; 2018,Jan,8; 2017,Jan,8; 2016,Jan,13; 2015,Jan,16

97113 **aquatic therapy with therapeutic exercises**

1.10 1.10 FUD XXX

AMA: 2018,May,5; 2018,Feb,11; 2018,Jan,8; 2017,Jan,8; 2016,Jan,13; 2015,Jan,16

97116 **gait training (includes stair climbing)**

EXCLUDES *Comprehensive gait/motion analysis (96000-96003)*

0.86 0.86 FUD XXX

AMA: 2018,May,5; 2018,Feb,11; 2018,Jan,8; 2017,Jan,8; 2016,Jan,13; 2015,Jan,16

97124 **massage, including effleurage, petrissage and/or tapotement (stroking, compression, percussion)**

EXCLUDES *Myofascial release (97140)*

0.81 0.81 FUD XXX

AMA: 2020,Jul,10; 2019,Jun,14; 2018,May,5; 2018,Feb,11; 2018,Jan,8; 2017,Jan,8; 2016,Jun,8; 2016,Jan,13; 2015,Jan,16

97129 **Therapeutic interventions that focus on cognitive function (eg, attention, memory, reasoning, executive function, problem solving, and/or pragmatic functioning) and compensatory strategies to manage the performance of an activity (eg, managing time or schedules, initiating, organizing, and sequencing tasks), direct (one-on-one) patient contact; initial 15 minutes**

EXCLUDES *Adaptive behavior treatment ([97153], [97155])*
Reporting code more than one time per day

0.67 0.68 FUD XXX

AMA: 2020,Jul,10

+ **97130** **each additional 15 minutes (List separately in addition to code for primary procedure)**

    EXCLUDES *Adaptive behavior treatment ([97153], [97155])*
    Code first (97129)
    📇 0.65   ✂ 0.65   **FUD** ZZZ   Ⓢ⁵¹ 80 ▱
    AMA: 2020,Jul,10

97139 **Unlisted therapeutic procedure (specify)**
    📇 0.00   ✂ 0.00   **FUD** XXX   A 80 ▱
    AMA: 2018,May,5; 2018,Feb,11; 2018,Jan,8; 2017,Jan,8;
    2016,Jan,13; 2015,Jan,16

97140 **Manual therapy techniques (eg, mobilization/manipulation, manual lymphatic drainage, manual traction), 1 or more regions, each 15 minutes**
    EXCLUDES *Insertion needle without injection ([20560, 20561])*
    📇 0.80   ✂ 0.80   **FUD** XXX   Ⓢ⁵¹ A 80 ▱
    AMA: 2020,Jul,10; 2020,Feb,9; 2019,Jun,14; 2018,May,5;
    2018,Feb,11; 2018,Jan,8; 2017,Jan,8; 2016,Nov,9; 2016,Sep,9;
    2016,Aug,3; 2016,Jan,13; 2015,Mar,9; 2015,Jan,16

97150 **Therapeutic procedure(s), group (2 or more individuals)**
    INCLUDES Constant attendance by physician/therapist
    Reporting this procedure for each group member
    EXCLUDES *Adaptive behavior services ([97154], [97158])*
    Osteopathic manipulative treatment (98925-98929)
    📇 0.52   ✂ 0.52   **FUD** XXX   Ⓢ⁵¹ A 80 ▱
    AMA: 2020,Jul,7; 2018,Nov,3; 2018,May,5; 2018,Feb,11;
    2018,Jan,8; 2017,Jan,8; 2016,Jan,13; 2015,Jan,16

97151 Resequenced code. See code following 96040.

97152 Resequenced code. See code following 96040.

97153 Resequenced code. See code following 96040.

97154 Resequenced code. See code following 96040.

97155 Resequenced code. See code following 96040.

97156 Resequenced code. See code following 96040.

97157 Resequenced code. See code following 96040.

97158 Resequenced code. See code following 96040.

97161 Resequenced code. See code before 97010.

97162 Resequenced code. See code before 97010.

97163 Resequenced code. See code before 97010.

97164 Resequenced code. See code before 97010.

97165 Resequenced code. See code before 97010.

97166 Resequenced code. See code before 97010.

97167 Resequenced code. See code before 97010.

97168 Resequenced code. See code before 97010.

97169 Resequenced code. See code before 97010.

97170 Resequenced code. See code before 97010.

97171 Resequenced code. See code before 97010.

97172 Resequenced code. See code before 97010.

97530 **Therapeutic activities, direct (one-on-one) patient contact (use of dynamic activities to improve functional performance), each 15 minutes**
    📇 1.13   ✂ 1.13   **FUD** XXX   Ⓢ⁵¹ A 80 ▱
    AMA: 2018,Dec,7; 2018,Dec,7; 2018,May,5; 2018,Feb,11;
    2018,Jan,8; 2017,Jan,8; 2016,Jan,13; 2015,Jan,16

97533 **Sensory integrative techniques to enhance sensory processing and promote adaptive responses to environmental demands, direct (one-on-one) patient contact, each 15 minutes**
    📇 1.47   ✂ 1.47   **FUD** XXX   Ⓢ⁵¹ A 80 ▱
    AMA: 2018,May,5; 2018,Feb,11; 2018,Jan,8; 2017,Jan,8;
    2016,Jan,13; 2015,Jan,16

97535 **Self-care/home management training (eg, activities of daily living (ADL) and compensatory training, meal preparation, safety procedures, and instructions in use of assistive technology devices/adaptive equipment) direct one-on-one contact, each 15 minutes**
    📇 0.97   ✂ 0.97   **FUD** XXX   Ⓢ A 80 ▱
    AMA: 2018,May,5; 2018,Feb,11; 2018,Jan,8; 2017,Jan,8;
    2016,Aug,3; 2016,Jan,13; 2015,Jun,10; 2015,Mar,9; 2015,Jan,16

97537 **Community/work reintegration training (eg, shopping, transportation, money management, avocational activities and/or work environment/modification analysis, work task analysis, use of assistive technology device/adaptive equipment), direct one-on-one contact, each 15 minutes**
    EXCLUDES *Wheelchair management/propulsion training (97542)*
    📇 0.93   ✂ 0.93   **FUD** XXX   Ⓢ A 80 ▱
    AMA: 2018,May,5; 2018,Feb,11; 2018,Jan,8; 2017,Jan,8;
    2016,Jan,13; 2015,Jan,16

97542 **Wheelchair management (eg, assessment, fitting, training), each 15 minutes**
    📇 0.94   ✂ 0.94   **FUD** XXX   Ⓢ A 80 ▱
    AMA: 2018,May,5; 2018,Feb,11; 2018,Jan,8; 2017,Jan,8;
    2016,Jan,13; 2015,Jun,10; 2015,Jan,16

97545 **Work hardening/conditioning; initial 2 hours**
    📇 0.00   ✂ 0.00   **FUD** XXX   Ⓢ A 80 ▱
    AMA: 2018,May,5; 2018,Feb,11; 2018,Jan,8; 2017,Jan,8;
    2016,Jan,13; 2015,Jan,16

+ **97546** **each additional hour (List separately in addition to code for primary procedure)**
    Code first initial two hours (97545)
    📇 0.00   ✂ 0.00   **FUD** ZZZ   Ⓢ A 80 ▱
    AMA: 2018,May,5; 2018,Feb,11; 2018,Jan,8; 2017,Jan,8;
    2016,Jan,13; 2015,Jan,16

● New Code   ▲ Revised Code   ○ Reinstated   ● New Web Release   ▲ Revised Web Release   + Add-on   Unlisted   Not Covered   # Resequenced
⑤⁰ Optum Mod 50 Exempt   ⊘ AMA Mod 51 Exempt   Ⓢ⁵¹ Optum Mod 51 Exempt   ⑥³ Mod 63 Exempt   ✗ Non-FDA Drug   ★ Telemedicine   Ⓜ Maternity   A Age Edit

97597-97610 Treatment of Wounds

CMS: 100-02,15,220.4 Functional Reporting; 100-02,15,230.4 Services By a Physical/Occupational Therapist in Private Practice; 100-03,270.3 Blood-derived Products for Chronic Nonhealing Wounds; 100-04,4,200.9 Billing for "Sometimes Therapy" Services that May be Paid as Non-Therapy Services; 100-04,5,10 Part B Outpatient Rehabilitation and Comprehensive Outpatient Rehabilitation Facility (CORF) Services - General; 100-04,5,10.3.2 Exceptions Process; 100-04,5,10.3.3 Use of the KX Modifier

INCLUDES Direct patient contact
Removing devitalized/necrotic tissue and promoting healing

EXCLUDES *Burn wound debridement (16020-16030)*

97597 **Debridement (eg, high pressure waterjet with/without suction, sharp selective debridement with scissors, scalpel and forceps), open wound, (eg, fibrin, devitalized epidermis and/or dermis, exudate, debris, biofilm), including topical application(s), wound assessment, use of a whirlpool, when performed and instruction(s) for ongoing care, per session, total wound(s) surface area; first 20 sq cm or less**

INCLUDES Chemical cauterization (17250)

0.68 2.52 **FUD** 000 (51) T 80

AMA: 2018,May,5; 2018,Feb,11; 2018,Jan,8; 2017,Jan,8; 2016,Oct,3; 2016,Aug,9; 2016,Jan,13; 2015,Jan,16

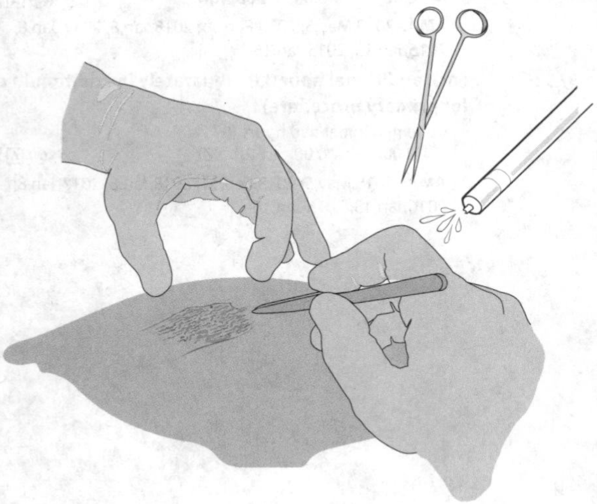

Wound may be washed, addressed with scissors, and/or tweezers and scalpel

\+ **97598** **each additional 20 sq cm, or part thereof (List separately in addition to code for primary procedure)**

INCLUDES Chemical cauterization (17250)

Code first (97597)

0.74 1.31 **FUD** ZZZ (51) N 80

AMA: 2018,May,5; 2018,Feb,11; 2018,Jan,8; 2017,Jan,8; 2016,Oct,3; 2016,Aug,9; 2016,Jan,13; 2015,Jan,16

97602 **Removal of devitalized tissue from wound(s), non-selective debridement, without anesthesia (eg, wet-to-moist dressings, enzymatic, abrasion, larval therapy), including topical application(s), wound assessment, and instruction(s) for ongoing care, per session**

INCLUDES Chemical cauterization (17250)

0.00 0.00 **FUD** XXX (51) Q1

AMA: 2018,May,5; 2018,Feb,11; 2018,Jan,8; 2017,Jan,8; 2016,Oct,3; 2016,Jan,13; 2015,Jan,16

97605 **Negative pressure wound therapy (eg, vacuum assisted drainage collection), utilizing durable medical equipment (DME), including topical application(s), wound assessment, and instruction(s) for ongoing care, per session; total wound(s) surface area less than or equal to 50 square centimeters**

EXCLUDES *Negative pressure wound therapy using disposable medical equipment (97607-97608)*

0.74 1.24 **FUD** XXX (51) Q1 80

AMA: 2018,May,5; 2018,Feb,11; 2018,Jan,8; 2017,Jan,8; 2016,Feb,13; 2016,Jan,13; 2015,Jan,16

97606 **total wound(s) surface area greater than 50 square centimeters**

EXCLUDES *Negative pressure wound therapy using disposable medical equipment (97607-97608)*

0.80 1.46 **FUD** XXX (51) Q1 80

AMA: 2018,May,5; 2018,Feb,11; 2018,Jan,8; 2017,Jan,8; 2016,Feb,13; 2016,Jan,13; 2015,Jan,16

97607 **Negative pressure wound therapy, (eg, vacuum assisted drainage collection), utilizing disposable, non-durable medical equipment including provision of exudate management collection system, topical application(s), wound assessment, and instructions for ongoing care, per session; total wound(s) surface area less than or equal to 50 square centimeters**

EXCLUDES *Negative pressure wound therapy using durable medical equipment (97605-97606)*

0.00 0.00 **FUD** XXX (51) T 80

AMA: 2018,May,5; 2018,Feb,11; 2018,Jan,8; 2017,Jan,8; 2016,Jan,13; 2015,Jan,16

97608 **total wound(s) surface area greater than 50 square centimeters**

EXCLUDES *Negative pressure wound therapy using durable medical equipment (97605-97606)*

0.00 0.00 **FUD** XXX (51) T 80

AMA: 2018,May,5; 2018,Feb,11; 2018,Jan,8; 2017,Jan,8; 2016,Jan,13; 2015,Jan,16

97610 **Low frequency, non-contact, non-thermal ultrasound, including topical application(s), when performed, wound assessment, and instruction(s) for ongoing care, per day**

0.48 6.39 **FUD** XXX (51) Q1 80

AMA: 2018,May,5; 2018,Feb,11; 2018,Jan,8; 2017,Jan,8; 2016,Jan,13; 2015,Jan,16

97750-97799 Assessments and Training

CMS: 100-02,15,220 Coverage of Outpatient Rehabilitation Therapy Services; 100-02,15,220.4 Functional Reporting; 100-02,15,230 Practice of Physical Therapy, Occupational Therapy, and Speech-Language Pathology; 100-02,15,230.1 Practice of Physical Therapy; 100-02,15,230.2 Practice of Occupational Therapy; 100-02,15,230.4 Services By a Physical/Occupational Therapist in Private Practice; 100-04,5,10 Part B Outpatient Rehabilitation and Comprehensive Outpatient Rehabilitation Facility (CORF) Services - General; 100-04,5,10.3.2 Therapy Cap Exceptions; 100-04,5,10.3.3 Use of the KX Modifier

97750 **Physical performance test or measurement (eg, musculoskeletal, functional capacity), with written report, each 15 minutes**

INCLUDES Direct patient contact

EXCLUDES *Electromyography (95860-95872, [95885, 95886, 95887])*
Joint motion range (95851-95852)
Nerve velocity determination (95905, 95907-95913)

0.99 0.99 **FUD** XXX (51) A 80

AMA: 2018,May,5; 2018,Feb,11; 2018,Jan,8; 2017,Jan,8; 2016,Jan,13; 2015,Jan,16

97755 **Assistive technology assessment (eg, to restore, augment or compensate for existing function, optimize functional tasks and/or maximize environmental accessibility), direct one-on-one contact, with written report, each 15 minutes**

INCLUDES Direct patient contact

EXCLUDES *Augmentative/alternative communication device (92605, 92607)*
Electromyography (95860-95872, [95885, 95886, 95887])
Joint motion range (95851-95852)
Nerve velocity determination (95905, 95907-95913)

1.09 1.09 FUD XXX ⑤① A 80

AMA: 2018,May,5; 2018,Feb,11

97760 **Orthotic(s) management and training (including assessment and fitting when not otherwise reported), upper extremity(ies), lower extremity(ies) and/or trunk, initial orthotic(s) encounter, each 15 minutes**

EXCLUDES *Gait training, when performed on same extremity (97116)*

1.40 1.40 FUD XXX ⑤① A 80

AMA: 2018,May,5; 2018,Feb,11; 2018,Jan,8; 2017,Jan,8; 2016,Jan,13; 2015,Jan,16

97761 **Prosthetic(s) training, upper and/or lower extremity(ies), initial prosthetic(s) encounter, each 15 minutes**

1.16 1.16 FUD XXX ⑤① A 80

AMA: 2018,May,5; 2018,Feb,11; 2018,Jan,8; 2017,Jan,8; 2016,Jan,13; 2015,Jan,16

97763 **Orthotic(s)/prosthetic(s) management and/or training, upper extremity(ies), lower extremity(ies), and/or trunk, subsequent orthotic(s)/prosthetic(s) encounter, each 15 minutes**

EXCLUDES *Initial encounter for orthotics and prosthetics management and training (97760-97761)*

1.50 1.50 FUD XXX ⑤① A 80

AMA: 2018,May,5; 2018,Feb,11

97799 **Unlisted physical medicine/rehabilitation service or procedure**

0.00 0.00 FUD XXX A 80

AMA: 2018,May,5; 2018,Feb,11; 2018,Jan,8; 2017,Jan,8; 2016,Nov,9; 2016,Jan,13; 2015,Jan,16

97802-97804 Medical Nutrition Therapy Services

CMS: 100-02,13,220 Preventive Health Services; 100-03,180.1 Medical Nutrition Therapy; 100-04,12,190.3 List of Telehealth Services; 100-04,12,190.6 Payment Methodology for Physician/Practitioner at the Distant Site ; 100-04,12,190.6.1 Submission of Telehealth Claims for Distant Site Practitioners; 100-04,12,190.7 Contractor Editing of Telehealth Claims; 100-04,4,300 Medical Nutrition Therapy Services; 100-04,4,300.6 CWF Edits for MNT/DSMT

EXCLUDES *Medical nutrition therapy assessment/intervention provided by physician or other qualified health care provider; report appropriate E/M codes*

97802 **Medical nutrition therapy; initial assessment and intervention, individual, face-to-face with the patient, each 15 minutes**

0.96 1.05 FUD XXX ★ A 80

AMA: 2020,Jul,7; 2018,Feb,11; 2018,Jan,8; 2017,Jan,8; 2016,Jan,13; 2015,Jan,16

97803 **re-assessment and intervention, individual, face-to-face with the patient, each 15 minutes**

0.81 0.92 FUD XXX ★ A 80

AMA: 2020,Jul,7; 2018,Feb,11; 2018,Jan,8; 2017,Jan,8; 2016,Jan,13; 2015,Jan,16

97804 **group (2 or more individual(s)), each 30 minutes**

0.45 0.48 FUD XXX ★ A 80

AMA: 2020,Jul,7; 2018,Feb,11; 2018,Jan,8; 2017,Jan,8; 2016,Jan,13; 2015,Jan,16

97810-97814 Acupuncture

CMS: 100-03,10.3 Inpatient Pain Rehabilitation Programs; 100-03,10.4 Outpatient Hospital Pain Rehabilitation Programs; 100-03,30.3 Acupuncture; 100-03,30.3.1 Acupuncture for Fibromyalgia; 100-03,30.3.2 Acupuncture for Osteoarthritis

INCLUDES 15 minute increments face-to-face contact with patient
Reporting only one code for each 15 minute increment

EXCLUDES *Insertion needle without injection ([20560, 20561])*

Code also significant separately identifiable E/M service with modifier 25, when performed

97810 **Acupuncture, 1 or more needles; without electrical stimulation, initial 15 minutes of personal one-on-one contact with the patient**

EXCLUDES *Treatment with electrical stimulation (97813-97814)*

0.87 1.03 FUD XXX E

AMA: 2020,Feb,9; 2018,Feb,11; 2018,Jan,8; 2017,Jan,8; 2016,Jan,13; 2015,Jan,16

+ 97811 **without electrical stimulation, each additional 15 minutes of personal one-on-one contact with the patient, with re-insertion of needle(s) (List separately in addition to code for primary procedure)**

EXCLUDES *Treatment with electrical stimulation (97813-97814)*

Code first initial 15 minutes (97810)

0.72 0.78 FUD ZZZ E

AMA: 2020,Feb,9; 2018,Feb,11; 2018,Jan,8; 2017,Jan,8; 2016,Jan,13; 2015,Jan,16

97813 **with electrical stimulation, initial 15 minutes of personal one-on-one contact with the patient**

EXCLUDES *Treatment without electrical stimulation (97813-97814)*

0.94 1.13 FUD XXX E

AMA: 2020,Feb,9; 2018,Feb,11; 2018,Jan,8; 2017,Jan,8; 2016,Jan,13; 2015,Jan,16

+ 97814 **with electrical stimulation, each additional 15 minutes of personal one-on-one contact with the patient, with re-insertion of needle(s) (List separately in addition to code for primary procedure)**

EXCLUDES *Treatment without electrical stimulation (97813-97814)*

Code first initial 15 minutes (97813)

0.79 0.91 FUD ZZZ E

AMA: 2020,Feb,9; 2018,Feb,11; 2018,Jan,8; 2017,Jan,8; 2016,Jan,13; 2015,Jan,16

98925-98929 Osteopathic Manipulation

CMS: 100-03,150.1 Manipulation

INCLUDES Body regions:
- Abdomen/visceral region
- Cervical region
- Head region
- Lower extremities
- Lumbar region
- Pelvic region
- Rib cage region
- Sacral region
- Thoracic region
- Upper extremities

Physician applied manual treatment done to eliminate/alleviate somatic dysfunction and related disorders with multiple techniques

Code also significant separately identifiable E/M service with modifier 25, when performed

98925 **Osteopathic manipulative treatment (OMT); 1-2 body regions involved**

0.68 0.89 FUD 000 01 80

AMA: 2018,Aug,9; 2018,Feb,11; 2018,Jan,8; 2017,Dec,14; 2017,Jan,8; 2016,Jan,13; 2015,Jan,16

98926 **3-4 body regions involved**

1.03 1.29 FUD 000 01 80

AMA: 2018,Aug,9; 2018,Feb,11; 2018,Jan,8; 2017,Jan,8; 2016,Jan,13; 2015,Jan,16

98927 **5-6 body regions involved**

1.35 1.68 FUD 000 01 80

AMA: 2018,Aug,9; 2018,Feb,11; 2018,Jan,8; 2017,Jan,8; 2016,Jan,13; 2015,Jan,16

98928 **7-8 body regions involved**
Facility RVU 1.69 Non-Facility RVU 2.05 **FUD** 000 Q1 80
AMA: 2018,Aug,9; 2018,Feb,11; 2018,Jan,8; 2017,Jan,8; 2016,Jan,13; 2015,Jan,16

98929 **9-10 body regions involved**
Facility RVU 2.07 Non-Facility RVU 2.45 **FUD** 000 Q1 80
AMA: 2018,Aug,9; 2018,Feb,11; 2018,Jan,8; 2017,Jan,8; 2016,Jan,13; 2015,Jan,16

98940-98943 Chiropractic Manipulation

CMS: 100-01,5,70.6 Chiropractors; 100-02,15,240 Chiropractic Services - General; 100-02,15,240.1.3 Necessity for Treatment; 100-02,15,30.5 Chiropractor's Services; 100-03,150.1 Manipulation

INCLUDES Five extraspinal regions:
- Abdomen
- Head, including temporomandibular joint, excluding atlanto-occipital region
- Lower extremities
- Rib cage, not including costotransverse/costovertebral joints
- Upper extremities

Five spinal regions:
- Cervical region (atlanto-occipital joint)
- Lumbar region
- Pelvic region (sacro-iliac joint)
- Sacral region
- Thoracic region (costovertebral/costotransverse joints)

Manual treatment performed to influence joint/neurophysical function

Code also significant separately identifiable E/M service with modifier 25, when performed

98940 **Chiropractic manipulative treatment (CMT); spinal, 1-2 regions**
Facility RVU 0.64 Non-Facility RVU 0.80 **FUD** 000 Q1 80
AMA: 2018,Nov,11; 2018,Feb,11; 2018,Jan,8; 2017,Jan,8; 2016,Jan,13; 2015,Jan,16

98941 **spinal, 3-4 regions**
Facility RVU 0.98 Non-Facility RVU 1.15 **FUD** 000 Q1 80
AMA: 2018,Nov,11; 2018,Feb,11; 2018,Jan,8; 2017,Jan,8; 2016,Jan,13; 2015,Jan,16

98942 **spinal, 5 regions**
Facility RVU 1.33 Non-Facility RVU 1.50 **FUD** 000 Q1 80
AMA: 2018,Nov,11; 2018,Feb,11; 2018,Jan,8; 2017,Jan,8; 2016,Jan,13; 2015,Jan,16

98943 **extraspinal, 1 or more regions**
Facility RVU 0.67 Non-Facility RVU 0.77 **FUD** XXX E
AMA: 2018,Nov,11; 2018,Feb,11; 2018,Jan,8; 2017,Jan,8; 2016,Jan,13; 2015,Jan,16

98960-98962 Self-Management Training

INCLUDES Education/training services:
- Prescribed by physician or other qualified health care professional
- Provided by qualified nonphysician health care provider

Standardized curriculum that may be modified as necessary for:
- Clinical needs
- Cultural norms
- Health literacy

Teaching patient how to manage illness/delay comorbidity(s)

EXCLUDES *Collection/interpretation physiologic data ([99091])*
Complex chronic care management (99487, 99489)
Counseling/education to group (99078)
Counseling/risk factor reduction without symptoms/established disease (99401-99412)
Genetic counseling education services (96040, 98961-98962)
Health and behavior assessment and intervention (96156, 96158-96159, [96164, 96165], [96167, 96168], [96170, 96171])
Medical nutrition therapy (97802-97804)
Physician supervision in home, domiciliary, or rest home (99339, 99340, 99374-99375, 99379-99380)
Services provided in which time would be reported with other services
Services provided with cumulative time of less than 5 minutes
Supervision hospice patient (99377-99378)
Transitional care management (99495, 99496)

98960 **Education and training for patient self-management by a qualified, nonphysician health care professional using a standardized curriculum, face-to-face with the patient (could include caregiver/family) each 30 minutes; individual patient**
Facility RVU 0.77 Non-Facility RVU 0.77 **FUD** XXX ★ E
AMA: 2020,Jul,7; 2018,Aug,6; 2018,Feb,11; 2018,Jan,8; 2017,Jan,8; 2016,Jan,13; 2015,Jan,16

98961 **2-4 patients**
INCLUDES Group education regarding genetic risks
Facility RVU 0.37 Non-Facility RVU 0.37 **FUD** XXX ★ E
AMA: 2020,Jul,7; 2018,Aug,6; 2018,Feb,11; 2018,Jan,8; 2017,Jan,8; 2016,Jan,13; 2015,Jan,16

98962 **5-8 patients**
INCLUDES Group education regarding genetic risks
Facility RVU 0.27 Non-Facility RVU 0.27 **FUD** XXX ★ E
AMA: 2020,Jul,7; 2018,Aug,6; 2018,Feb,11; 2018,Jan,8; 2017,Jan,8; 2016,Jan,13; 2015,Jan,16

98966-98968 Nonphysician Telephone Services

INCLUDES Assessment and management services provided by telephone by qualified health care professional
Care episodes initiated by established patient or his/her guardian

EXCLUDES *Call initiated by qualified health care professional*
Calls during postoperative period
Decision to see patient at next available urgent care appointment
Decision to see patient within 24 hours from patient call
Monitoring INR (93792-93793)
Patient management services during same time frame as ([99439, 99490, 99491], 99487-99489)
Reporting codes when same codes billed within past seven days
Telephone services considered previous or subsequent service component
Telephone services provided by physician (99441-99443)

98966 **Telephone assessment and management service provided by a qualified nonphysician health care professional to an established patient, parent, or guardian not originating from a related assessment and management service provided within the previous 7 days nor leading to an assessment and management service or procedure within the next 24 hours or soonest available appointment; 5-10 minutes of medical discussion**
Facility RVU 0.36 Non-Facility RVU 0.39 **FUD** XXX E 80
AMA: 2018,Mar,7; 2018,Feb,11; 2018,Jan,8; 2017,Jan,8; 2016,Jan,13; 2015,Jan,16

98967 **11-20 minutes of medical discussion**
Facility RVU 0.72 Non-Facility RVU 0.76 **FUD** XXX E 80
AMA: 2018,Mar,7; 2018,Feb,11; 2018,Jan,8; 2017,Jan,8; 2016,Jan,13; 2015,Jan,16

98968 **21-30 minutes of medical discussion**
    📖 1.08   ✂ 1.12   **FUD** XXX   E 80 💬
    AMA: 2018,Mar,7; 2018,Feb,11; 2018,Jan,8; 2017,Jan,8; 2016,Jan,13; 2015,Jan,16

98970-98972 Nonphysician Online Service

Timely reply to patient as well as:
    Ordering laboratory services
    Permanent service record; either hard copy or electronic
    Providing prescription
    Related telephone calls

EXCLUDES   *Monitoring INR (93792-93793)*
    Online digital assessment and management service provided by qualified health care professional ([99421, 99422, 99423])
    Online evaluation service:
       Provided during postoperative period
       Provided more than once in seven day period
       Related to service provided in previous seven days
       Provided with cumulative time less than 5 minutes
       Where time would be reported as another service
    Patient management services during same time frame as:
       Chronic care management ([99439, 99490, 99491])
       Collection/interpretation physiologic data ([99091])
       Complex chronic care management (99487-99489)
       Physician supervision in home, domiciliary, or rest home (99339-99340, 99374-99375, 99379-99380)
       Supervision hospice patient (99377-99378)

98970 **Qualified nonphysician health care professional online digital assessment and management, for an established patient, for up to 7 days, cumulative time during the 7 days; 5-10 minutes**
    📖 0.00   ✂ 0.00   **FUD** XXX   💬
    AMA: 2020,Jan,3

98971 **11-20 minutes**
    📖 0.00   ✂ 0.00   **FUD** XXX   💬
    AMA: 2020,Jan,3

98972 **21 or more minutes**
    📖 0.00   ✂ 0.00   **FUD** XXX   💬
    AMA: 2020,Jan,3

99000-99091 [99091] Supplemental Services and Supplies

INCLUDES   Supplemental reporting for services adjunct to basic service provided

99000 **Handling and/or conveyance of specimen for transfer from the office to a laboratory**
    📖 0.00   ✂ 0.00   **FUD** XXX   E 💬
    AMA: 2018,Dec,10; 2018,Dec,10; 2018,Feb,11; 2018,Jan,8; 2017,Jan,8; 2016,Jan,13; 2015,Jan,16

99001 **Handling and/or conveyance of specimen for transfer from the patient in other than an office to a laboratory (distance may be indicated)**
    📖 0.00   ✂ 0.00   **FUD** XXX   E 💬
    AMA: 2018,Dec,10; 2018,Dec,10; 2018,Feb,11; 2018,Jan,8; 2017,Jan,8; 2016,Jan,13; 2015,Jan,16

99002 **Handling, conveyance, and/or any other service in connection with the implementation of an order involving devices (eg, designing, fitting, packaging, handling, delivery or mailing) when devices such as orthotics, protectives, prosthetics are fabricated by an outside laboratory or shop but which items have been designed, and are to be fitted and adjusted by the attending physician or other qualified health care professional**
    EXCLUDES   *Venous blood routine collection (36415)*
    📖 0.00   ✂ 0.00   **FUD** XXX   B 💬
    AMA: 2018,Dec,10; 2018,Dec,10; 2018,Feb,11; 2018,Jan,8; 2017,Jan,8; 2016,Jan,13; 2015,Jan,16

99024 **Postoperative follow-up visit, normally included in the surgical package, to indicate that an evaluation and management service was performed during a postoperative period for a reason(s) related to the original procedure**
    📖 0.00   ✂ 0.00   **FUD** XXX   B 💬
    AMA: 2018,Dec,10; 2018,Dec,10; 2018,Feb,11; 2018,Jan,8; 2017,Jul,9; 2017,Jan,3; 2017,Jan,8; 2016,Jan,13; 2015,Mar,3; 2015,Jan,16

99026 **Hospital mandated on call service; in-hospital, each hour**
    EXCLUDES   *Physician stand-by services with prolonged physician attendance (99360)*
       Time spent providing procedures or services that may be separately reported
    📖 0.00   ✂ 0.00   **FUD** XXX   E 💬
    AMA: 2018,Dec,10; 2018,Dec,10; 2018,Feb,11; 2018,Jan,8; 2017,Jan,8; 2016,Jan,13; 2015,Jan,16

99027 **out-of-hospital, each hour**
    EXCLUDES   *Physician stand-by services with prolonged physician attendance (99360)*
       Time spent providing procedures or services that may be separately reported
    📖 0.00   ✂ 0.00   **FUD** XXX   E 💬
    AMA: 2018,Dec,10; 2018,Dec,10; 2018,Feb,11; 2018,Jan,8; 2017,Jan,8; 2016,Jan,13; 2015,Jan,16

99050 **Services provided in the office at times other than regularly scheduled office hours, or days when the office is normally closed (eg, holidays, Saturday or Sunday), in addition to basic service**
    Code also more than one adjunct code per encounter when appropriate
    Code first basic service provided
    📖 0.00   ✂ 0.00   **FUD** XXX   51 B 💬
    AMA: 2018,Dec,10; 2018,Dec,10; 2018,Feb,11; 2018,Jan,8; 2017,Jan,8; 2016,Jan,13; 2015,Jan,16

99051 **Service(s) provided in the office during regularly scheduled evening, weekend, or holiday office hours, in addition to basic service**
    Code also more than one adjunct code per encounter when appropriate
    Code first basic service provided
    📖 0.00   ✂ 0.00   **FUD** XXX   51 B 💬
    AMA: 2018,Dec,10; 2018,Dec,10; 2018,Feb,11; 2018,Jan,8; 2017,Jan,8; 2016,Jan,13; 2015,Jan,16

99053 **Service(s) provided between 10:00 PM and 8:00 AM at 24-hour facility, in addition to basic service**
    Code also more than one adjunct code per encounter when appropriate
    Code first basic service provided
    📖 0.00   ✂ 0.00   **FUD** XXX   51 B 💬
    AMA: 2018,Dec,10; 2018,Dec,10; 2018,Feb,11; 2018,Jan,8; 2017,Jan,8; 2016,Jan,13; 2015,Jan,16

99056 **Service(s) typically provided in the office, provided out of the office at request of patient, in addition to basic service**
    Code also more than one adjunct code per encounter when appropriate
    Code first basic service provided
    📖 0.00   ✂ 0.00   **FUD** XXX   51 B 💬
    AMA: 2018,Dec,10; 2018,Dec,10; 2018,Feb,11; 2018,Jan,8; 2017,Jan,8; 2016,Jan,13; 2015,Jan,16

99058 **Service(s) provided on an emergency basis in the office, which disrupts other scheduled office services, in addition to basic service**
    Code also more than one adjunct code per encounter when appropriate
    Code first basic service provided
    📖 0.00   ✂ 0.00   **FUD** XXX   51 B 💬
    AMA: 2018,Dec,10; 2018,Dec,10; 2018,Feb,11; 2018,Jan,8; 2017,Jan,8; 2016,Jan,13; 2015,Jan,16

99060 **Service(s) provided on an emergency basis, out of the office, which disrupts other scheduled office services, in addition to basic service**
    Code also more than one adjunct code per encounter when appropriate
    Code first basic service provided
    📖 0.00   ✂ 0.00   **FUD** XXX   51 B 💬
    AMA: 2018,Dec,10; 2018,Dec,10; 2018,Feb,11; 2018,Jan,8; 2017,Jan,8; 2016,Jan,13; 2015,Jan,16

● New Code   ▲ Revised Code   ○ Reinstated   ● New Web Release   ▲ Revised Web Release   + Add-on   Unlisted   Not Covered   # Resequenced
50 Optum Mod 50 Exempt   ⊘ AMA Mod 51 Exempt   51 Optum Mod 51 Exempt   63 Mod 63 Exempt   ✗ Non-FDA Drug   ★ Telemedicine   M Maternity   A Age Edit

99070 Supplies and materials (except spectacles), provided by the physician or other qualified health care professional over and above those usually included with the office visit or other services rendered (list drugs, trays, supplies, or materials provided)

EXCLUDES *Additional supplies, materials, and clinical staff time required for patient symptom review, personal protective equipment (PPE) use, and heightened cleaning processes due to respiratory-transmitted infectious disease during a declared public health emergency (PHE), as defined by law (99072)*

Spectacles supply

0.00 0.00 FUD XXX B

AMA: 2020,SepSE,1; 2020,SepSE,1; 2019,Apr,10; 2019,Feb,10; 2018,Dec,10; 2018,Dec,10; 2018,Jun,11; 2018,Mar,7; 2018,Jan,3; 2018,Jan,8; 2017,Sep,14; 2017,Jan,8; 2017,Jan,6; 2016,Jan,13; 2015,Jan,16

99071 Educational supplies, such as books, tapes, and pamphlets, for the patient's education at cost to physician or other qualified health care professional

0.00 0.00 FUD XXX B

AMA: 2018,Dec,10; 2018,Dec,10; 2018,Jan,8; 2017,Jan,8; 2016,Jan,13; 2015,Jan,16

● **99072 Additional supplies, materials, and clinical staff time over and above those usually included in an office visit or other nonfacility service(s), when performed during a Public Health Emergency, as defined by law, due to respiratory-transmitted infectious disease**

INCLUDES Additional supplies, materials, and clinical staff time required for patient symptom review, personal protective equipment (PPE) use, and heightened cleaning processes due to respiratory-transmitted infectious disease during a declared public health emergency (PHE), as defined by law

EXCLUDES *Reporting more than one time per encounter, despite number services provided during encounter*

Supplies and materials provided, above those normally included in the encounter, unrelated to a declared PHE (99070)

AMA: 2020,SepSE,1

99075 Medical testimony

0.00 0.00 FUD XXX E

AMA: 2018,Dec,10; 2018,Dec,10; 2018,Jan,8; 2017,Jan,8; 2016,Jan,13; 2015,Jan,16

99078 Physician or other qualified health care professional qualified by education, training, licensure/regulation (when applicable) educational services rendered to patients in a group setting (eg, prenatal, obesity, or diabetic instructions)

0.00 0.00 FUD XXX N

AMA: 2018,Dec,10; 2018,Dec,10; 2018,Jan,8; 2017,Jan,8; 2016,Jan,13; 2015,Jan,16

99080 Special reports such as insurance forms, more than the information conveyed in the usual medical communications or standard reporting form

EXCLUDES *Completion workmen's compensation forms (99455-99456)*

0.00 0.00 FUD XXX B

AMA: 2018,Dec,10; 2018,Dec,10; 2018,Jan,8; 2017,Jan,8; 2016,Jan,13; 2015,Jan,16

99082 Unusual travel (eg, transportation and escort of patient)

0.00 0.00 FUD XXX B 80

AMA: 2018,Dec,10; 2018,Dec,10; 2018,Jan,8; 2017,Jan,8; 2016,Jan,13; 2015,Jan,16

99091 **Resequenced code. See code following resequenced code 99454.**

99100-99140 Modifying Factors for Anesthesia Services

CMS: 100-04,12,140.3 Payment for Qualified Nonphysician Anesthetists; 100-04,12,140.3.3 Billing Modifiers; 100-04,12,140.3.4 General Billing Instructions; 100-04,12,140.4.1 Anesthesiologist/Qualified Nonphysican Anesthetist; 100-04,12,140.4.2 Anesthetist and Anesthesiologist in a Single Procedure; 100-04,12,140.4.4 Conversion Factors for Anesthesia Services; 100-04,4,250.3.2 Anesthesia in a Hospital Outpatient Setting

Code first primary anesthesia procedure

+ **99100 Anesthesia for patient of extreme age, younger than 1 year and older than 70 (List separately in addition to code for primary anesthesia procedure)** A

EXCLUDES *Anesthesia services for infants one year old or less (00326, 00561, 00834, 00836)*

0.00 0.00 FUD ZZZ B

AMA: 2019,Oct,10; 2018,Jan,8; 2017,Dec,8; 2017,Jan,8; 2016,Jan,13; 2015,Jan,16

+ **99116 Anesthesia complicated by utilization of total body hypothermia (List separately in addition to code for primary anesthesia procedure)**

EXCLUDES *Anesthesia for procedures on heart/pericardial sac/great vessels chest with pump oxygenator (00561)*

0.00 0.00 FUD ZZZ B

AMA: 2019,Oct,10; 2018,Jan,8; 2017,Dec,8; 2017,Jan,8; 2016,Jan,13; 2015,Jan,16

+ **99135 Anesthesia complicated by utilization of controlled hypotension (List separately in addition to code for primary anesthesia procedure)**

EXCLUDES *Anesthesia for procedures on heart/pericardial sac/great vessels chest with pump oxygenator (00561)*

0.00 0.00 FUD ZZZ B

AMA: 2019,Oct,10; 2018,Jan,8; 2017,Dec,8; 2017,Jan,8; 2016,Jan,13; 2015,Jan,16

+ **99140 Anesthesia complicated by emergency conditions (specify) (List separately in addition to code for primary anesthesia procedure)**

INCLUDES Conditions where treatment delay could be dangerous to life or health

0.00 0.00 FUD ZZZ B

AMA: 2019,Oct,10; 2018,Jan,8; 2017,Dec,8; 2017,Jan,8; 2016,Jan,13; 2015,Jan,16

99151-99157 Moderate Sedation Services

INCLUDES Intraservice work that begins with sedation administration and ends when procedure complete

Monitoring:

- Patient response to drugs
- Vital signs

Ordering and providing drug to patient (first and subsequent)

Pre- and postservice procedures

99151 Moderate sedation services provided by the same physician or other qualified health care professional performing the diagnostic or therapeutic service that the sedation supports, requiring the presence of an independent trained observer to assist in the monitoring of the patient's level of consciousness and physiological status; initial 15 minutes of intraservice time, patient younger than 5 years of age

INCLUDES First 15 minutes intraservice time for patients under age 5

Services provided to patients by same service provider for which moderate sedation necessary with monitoring by trained observer

0.70 2.20 FUD XXX N

AMA: 2019,Feb,10; 2018,Jan,8; 2017,Sep,11; 2017,Jun,3; 2017,Jan,3

99152 initial 15 minutes of intraservice time, patient age 5 years or older

INCLUDES First 15 minutes intraservice time for patients age 5 and over

Services provided to patients by same service provider for which moderate sedation necessary with monitoring by trained observer

0.35 1.44 FUD XXX N

AMA: 2019,May,10; 2019,Feb,10; 2018,Jan,8; 2017,Sep,11; 2017,Jun,3; 2017,Jan,3

\+ **99153** **each additional 15 minutes intraservice time (List separately in addition to code for primary service)**

INCLUDES Services provided to patients by same service provider for which moderate sedation necessary with monitoring by trained observer (99155-99157)

EXCLUDES *Services provided to patients by physician/other qualified health care professional other than provider rendering service*

Code first (99151-99152)

0.31 0.31 FUD ZZZ N TC

AMA: 2019,May,10; 2019,Feb,10; 2018,Jan,8; 2017,Sep,11; 2017,Jun,3; 2017,Jan,3

99155 **Moderate sedation services provided by a physician or other qualified health care professional other than the physician or other qualified health care professional performing the diagnostic or therapeutic service that the sedation supports; initial 15 minutes of intraservice time, patient younger than 5 years of age**

INCLUDES First 15 minutes intraservice time for patients under age 5
Services provided to patients by physician/other qualified health care professional other than provider rendering service for which moderate sedation necessary

2.54 2.54 FUD XXX N

AMA: 2019,Feb,10; 2018,Jan,8; 2017,Sep,11; 2017,Jun,3; 2017,Jan,3

99156 **initial 15 minutes of intraservice time, patient age 5 years or older**

INCLUDES First 15 minutes intraservice time for patients age 5 and over
Services provided to patients by physician/other qualified health care professional other than provider rendering service for which moderate sedation necessary

2.24 2.24 FUD XXX N

AMA: 2019,Feb,10; 2018,Jan,8; 2017,Sep,11; 2017,Jun,3; 2017,Jan,3

\+ **99157** **each additional 15 minutes intraservice time (List separately in addition to code for primary service)**

INCLUDES Each subsequent 15 minutes services
Services provided to patients by physician/other qualified health care professional other than provider rendering service for which moderate sedation necessary (99151-99152)

EXCLUDES *Services provided to patients by same service provider for which moderate sedation necessary with monitoring by trained observer (99151-99152)*

Code first (99155-99156)

1.64 1.64 FUD ZZZ N

AMA: 2019,Feb,10; 2018,Jan,8; 2017,Sep,11; 2017,Jun,3; 2017,Jan,3

99170 Specialized Examination of Child

EXCLUDES *Moderate sedation (99151-99157)*

99170 **Anogenital examination, magnified, in childhood for suspected trauma, including image recording when performed** A

2.47 4.48 FUD 000 T

AMA: 2018,Jan,8; 2017,Jan,8; 2016,Jan,13; 2015,Jan,16

99172-99173 Visual Acuity Screening Tests

INCLUDES Graduated visual acuity stimuli that allow quantitative determination/estimation visual acuity

EXCLUDES *General ophthalmological or E/M services*

99172 **Visual function screening, automated or semi-automated bilateral quantitative determination of visual acuity, ocular alignment, color vision by pseudoisochromatic plates, and field of vision (may include all or some screening of the determination[s] for contrast sensitivity, vision under glare)**

EXCLUDES *Screening for visual acuity, amblyogenic factors, retinal polarization scan (99173, 99174 [99177], 0469T)*

0.00 0.00 FUD XXX E

AMA: 2018,Jan,8; 2017,Jan,8; 2016,Jan,13; 2015,Jan,16

99173 **Screening test of visual acuity, quantitative, bilateral**

EXCLUDES *Screening for visual function, amblyogenic factors (99172, 99174, [99177])*

0.08 0.08 FUD XXX E

AMA: 2018,Jan,8; 2017,Jan,8; 2016,Jan,13; 2015,Jan,16

99174-99177 [99177] Screening For Amblyogenic Factors

EXCLUDES *General ophthalmological services (92002-92014)*
Screening for visual acuity (99172-99173, [99177])

99174 **Instrument-based ocular screening (eg, photoscreening, automated-refraction), bilateral; with remote analysis and report**

EXCLUDES *Ocular screening on-site analysis ([99177])*

0.16 0.16 FUD XXX E

AMA: 2018,Feb,3; 2018,Jan,8; 2017,Jan,8; 2016,Mar,10; 2016,Jan,13; 2015,Jan,16

\# **99177** **with on-site analysis**

EXCLUDES *Remote ocular screening (99174)*
Retinal polarization scan (0469T)

0.14 0.14 FUD XXX E

AMA: 2018,Feb,3; 2018,Jan,8; 2017,Jan,8; 2016,Mar,10

99175-99177 [99177] Drug Administration to Induce Vomiting

EXCLUDES *Diagnostic gastric lavage (43754-43755)*
Diagnostic gastric intubation (43754-43755)

99175 **Ipecac or similar administration for individual emesis and continued observation until stomach adequately emptied of poison**

0.73 0.73 FUD XXX N 80

AMA: 1997,Nov,1

99177 **Resequenced code. See code following 99174.**

99183-99184 Hyperbaric Oxygen Therapy

CMS: 100-03,20.29 Hyperbaric Oxygen Therapy; 100-04,32,30.1 HBO Therapy for Lower Extremity Diabetic Wounds

EXCLUDES *E/M services, when performed*
Other procedures such as wound debridement, when performed

99183 **Physician or other qualified health care professional attendance and supervision of hyperbaric oxygen therapy, per session**

3.12 3.12 FUD XXX B 80 26

AMA: 2018,Jan,8; 2017,Jan,8; 2016,Jan,13; 2015,Jan,16

99184 **Initiation of selective head or total body hypothermia in the critically ill neonate, includes appropriate patient selection by review of clinical, imaging and laboratory data, confirmation of esophageal temperature probe location, evaluation of amplitude EEG, supervision of controlled hypothermia, and assessment of patient tolerance of cooling** A

EXCLUDES *Reporting code more than one time per hospitalization*

6.33 6.33 FUD XXX C 80

AMA: 2018,Jan,8; 2017,Jan,8; 2016,Jan,13; 2015,Oct,8

99188 Topical Fluoride Application

99188 **Application of topical fluoride varnish by a physician or other qualified health care professional**
0.29 0.35 FUD XXX E 80

99190-99192 Assemble and Manage Pump with Oxygenator/Heat Exchange

99190 **Assembly and operation of pump with oxygenator or heat exchanger (with or without ECG and/or pressure monitoring); each hour**
0.00 0.00 FUD XXX C
AMA: 1997,Nov,1

99191 **45 minutes**
0.00 0.00 FUD XXX C
AMA: 1997,Nov,1

99192 **30 minutes**
0.00 0.00 FUD XXX C
AMA: 1997,Nov,1

99195-99199 Therapeutic Phlebotomy and Unlisted Procedures

99195 **Phlebotomy, therapeutic (separate procedure)**
2.86 2.86 FUD XXX Q1 80
AMA: 2018,Jan,8; 2017,Jan,8; 2016,Jan,13; 2015,Jan,16

99199 **Unlisted special service, procedure or report**
0.00 0.00 FUD XXX B 80
AMA: 2018,Jan,8; 2017,Jan,8; 2016,Jan,13; 2015,Jan,16

99500-99602 Home Visit By Non-Physician Professionals

INCLUDES Services performed by non-physician providers
Services provided in patient's:
- Assisted living apartment
- Custodial care facility
- Group home
- Nontraditional private home
- Residence
- School

EXCLUDES *Home visits performed by physicians (99341-99350)*
Other services/procedures provided by physicians to patients at home

Code also home visit E/M codes when health care provider authorized to report (99341-99350)
Code also significant separately identifiable E/M service, when performed

99500 **Home visit for prenatal monitoring and assessment to include fetal heart rate, non-stress test, uterine monitoring, and gestational diabetes monitoring** M ♀
0.00 0.00 FUD XXX E
AMA: 2018,Jan,8; 2017,Jan,8; 2016,Jan,13; 2015,Jan,16

99501 **Home visit for postnatal assessment and follow-up care** M ♀
0.00 0.00 FUD XXX E
AMA: 2018,Jan,8; 2017,Jan,8; 2016,Jan,13; 2015,Jan,16

99502 **Home visit for newborn care and assessment** A
0.00 0.00 FUD XXX E
AMA: 2018,Jan,8; 2017,Jan,8; 2016,Jan,13; 2015,Jan,16

99503 **Home visit for respiratory therapy care (eg, bronchodilator, oxygen therapy, respiratory assessment, apnea evaluation)**
0.00 0.00 FUD XXX E
AMA: 2018,Jan,8; 2017,Jan,8; 2016,Jan,13; 2015,Jan,16

99504 **Home visit for mechanical ventilation care**
0.00 0.00 FUD XXX E
AMA: 2018,Jan,8; 2017,Jan,8; 2016,Jan,13; 2015,Jan,16

99505 **Home visit for stoma care and maintenance including colostomy and cystostomy**
0.00 0.00 FUD XXX E
AMA: 2018,Jan,8; 2017,Jan,8; 2016,Jan,13; 2015,Jan,16

99506 **Home visit for intramuscular injections**
0.00 0.00 FUD XXX E
AMA: 2018,Jan,8; 2017,Jan,8; 2016,Jan,13; 2015,Jan,16

99507 **Home visit for care and maintenance of catheter(s) (eg, urinary, drainage, and enteral)**
0.00 0.00 FUD XXX E
AMA: 2018,Jan,8; 2017,Jan,8; 2016,Jan,13; 2015,Jan,16

99509 **Home visit for assistance with activities of daily living and personal care**
EXCLUDES *Medical nutrition therapy/assessment home services (97802-97804)*
Self-care/home management training (97535)
Speech therapy home services (92507-92508)
0.00 0.00 FUD XXX E
AMA: 2018,Jan,8; 2017,Jan,8; 2016,Jan,13; 2015,Jan,16

99510 **Home visit for individual, family, or marriage counseling**
0.00 0.00 FUD XXX E
AMA: 2018,Jan,8; 2017,Jan,8; 2016,Jan,13; 2015,Jan,16

99511 **Home visit for fecal impaction management and enema administration**
0.00 0.00 FUD XXX E
AMA: 2018,Jan,8; 2017,Jan,8; 2016,Jan,13; 2015,Jan,16

99512 **Home visit for hemodialysis**
EXCLUDES *Peritoneal dialysis home infusion (99601-99602)*
0.00 0.00 FUD XXX E
AMA: 2018,Jan,8; 2017,Jan,8; 2016,Jan,13; 2015,Jan,16

99600 **Unlisted home visit service or procedure**
0.00 0.00 FUD XXX E
AMA: 2018,Jan,8; 2017,Jan,8; 2016,Jan,13; 2015,Jan,16

99601 **Home infusion/specialty drug administration, per visit (up to 2 hours);**
0.00 0.00 FUD XXX E
AMA: 2005,Nov,1-9; 2003,Oct,7

+ **99602** **each additional hour (List separately in addition to code for primary procedure)**
Code first (99601)
0.00 0.00 FUD XXX E
AMA: 2005,Nov,1-9; 2003,Oct,7

99605-99607 Medication Management By Pharmacist

INCLUDES Direct (face-to-face) assessment and intervention by pharmacist:
- Managing medication complications and/or interactions
- Maximizing patient's response to drug therapy

Documenting required elements:
- Advice given regarding improvement treatment compliance and outcomes
- Medication profile (prescription and nonprescription)
- Review applicable patient history

EXCLUDES *Routine tasks associated with dispensing and related activities (e.g., providing product information)*

99605 **Medication therapy management service(s) provided by a pharmacist, individual, face-to-face with patient, with assessment and intervention if provided; initial 15 minutes, new patient**
0.00 0.00 FUD XXX E
AMA: 2018,Apr,9; 2018,Jan,8; 2017,Jan,8; 2016,Jan,13; 2015,Jan,16

99606 **initial 15 minutes, established patient**
0.00 0.00 FUD XXX E
AMA: 2018,Apr,9; 2018,Jan,8; 2017,Jan,8; 2016,Jan,13; 2015,Jan,16

+ **99607** **each additional 15 minutes (List separately in addition to code for primary service)**
Code first (99605, 99606)
0.00 0.00 FUD XXX E
AMA: 2018,Apr,9; 2018,Jan,8; 2017,Jan,8; 2016,Jan,13; 2015,Jan,16

Evaluation and Management (E/M) Services Guidelines

Information unique to this section is defined or identified below.

For additional information about evaluation and management services, see Appendix C: Evaluation and Management Extended Guidelines. This appendix includes comprehensive explanations and instructions for the correct selection of an E&M service code based on federal documentation standards.

Classification of Evaluation and Management (E/M) Services

The E/M section is divided into broad categories such as office visits, hospital visits, and consultations. Most of the categories are further divided into two or more subcategories of E/M services. For example, there are two subcategories of office visits (new patient and established patient) and there are two subcategories of hospital visits (initial and subsequent). The subcategories of E/M services are further classified into levels of E/M services that are identified by specific codes.

The basic format of the levels of E/M services is the same for most categories. First, a unique code number is listed. Second, the place and/or type of service is specified, eg, office consultation. Third, the content of the service is defined. Fourth, time is specified. (A detailed discussion of time is provided following the Decision Tree for New vs Established Patients.)

Definitions of Commonly Used Terms

Certain key words and phrases are used throughout the E/M section. The following definitions are intended to reduce the potential for differing interpretations and to increase the consistency of reporting by physicians and other qualified health care professionals. The definitions in the E/M section are provided solely for the basis of code selection.

Some definitions are common to all categories of services, and others are specific to one or more categories only.

New and Established Patient

Solely for the purposes of distinguishing between new and established patients, professional services are those face-to-face services rendered by physicians and other qualified health care professionals who may report E/M services with a specific CPT® code or codes. A new patient is one who has not received any professional services from the physician/qualified health care professional or another physician/qualified health care professional of the exact same specialty and subspecialty who belongs to the same group practice, within the past three years.

An established patient is one who has received professional services from the physician/qualified health care professional or another physician/qualified health care professional of the exact same specialty and subspecialty who belongs to the same group practice, within the past three years. See the decision tree at right.

When a physician/qualified health care professional is on call or covering for another physician/qualified health care professional, the patient's encounter is classified as it would have been by the physician/qualified health care professional who is not available. When advanced practice nurses and physician assistants are working with physicians, they are considered as working in the exact same specialty and exact same subspecialties as the physician.

No distinction is made between new and established patients in the emergency department. E/M services in the emergency department category may be reported for any new or established patient who presents for treatment in the emergency department.

The decision tree in the next column is provided to aid in determining whether to report the E/M service provided as a new or an established patient encounter.

Time

The inclusion of time in the definitions of levels of E/M services has been implicit in prior editions of the CPT codebook. The inclusion of time as an explicit factor beginning in CPT 1992 was done to assist in selecting the most appropriate level of E/M services. Beginning with CPT 2021, except for 99211, time alone may be used to select the appropriate code level for the office or other outpatient E/M services codes (99202, 99203, 99204, 99205, 99212, 99213, 99214, 99215). Different categories of services use time differently. It is important to review the instructions for each category.

Time is **not** a descriptive component for the emergency department levels of E/M services because emergency department services are typically provided on a variable intensity basis, often involving multiple encounters with several patients over an extended period of time. Therefore, it is often difficult to provide accurate estimates of the time spent face-to-face with the patient.

Time may be used to select a code level in office or other outpatient services whether or not counseling and/or coordination of care dominates the service. Time may only be used for selecting the level of the ***other*** E/M services when counseling and/or coordination of care dominates the service.

When time is used for reporting E/M services codes, the time defined in the service descriptors is used for selecting the appropriate level of services. The E/M services for which these guidelines apply require a face-to-face encounter with the physician or other qualified health care professional. For office or other outpatient services, if the physician's or other qualified health care professional's time is spent in the supervision of clinical staff who perform the face-to-face services of the encounter, use 99211.

A shared or split visit is defined as a visit in which a physician and other qualified health care professional(s) jointly provide the face-to-face and non-face-to-face work related to the visit. When time is being used to select the appropriate level of services for which time-based reporting of shared or split visits is allowed, the time personally spent by the physician and other qualified health care professional(s) assessing and managing the patient on the date of the encounter is summed to define total time. Only distinct time should be summed for shared or split visits (ie, when two or more individuals jointly meet with or discuss the patient, only the time of one individual should be counted).

When prolonged time occurs, the appropriate prolonged services code may be reported. The appropriate time should be documented in the medical record when it is used as the basis for code selection.

Face-to-face time (outpatient consultations [99241, 99242, 99243, 99244, 99245], domiciliary, rest home, or custodial services [99324, 99325, 99326, 99327, 99328, 99334, 99335, 99336, 99337], home services [99341, 99342, 99343, 99344, 99345, 99347, 99348, 99349, 99350], cognitive assessment and care plan services [99483]): For coding purposes, face-to-face time for these services is defined as only that time spent face-to-face with the patient and/or family. This includes the time spent performing such tasks as obtaining a history, examination, and counseling the patient.

Unit/floor time (hospital observation services [99218, 99219, 99220, 99224, 99225, 99226, 99234, 99235, 99236], hospital inpatient services [99221, 99222, 99223, 99231, 99232, 99233], inpatient consultations [99251, 99252, 99253, 99254, 99255], nursing facility services [99304, 99305, 99306, 99307, 99308, 99309, 99310, 99315, 99316, 99318]): For coding purposes, time for these services is defined as unit/floor time, which includes the time present on the patient's hospital unit and at the bedside rendering services for that patient. This includes the time to establish and/or review the patient's chart, examine the patient, write notes, and communicate with other professionals and the patient's family.

Total time on the date of the encounter (office or other outpatient services [99202, 99203, 99204, 99205, 99212, 99213, 99214, 99215]): For coding purposes, time for these services is the total time on the date of the encounter. It includes both the face-to-face and non-face-to-face time personally spent by the physician and/or other qualified health care professional(s) on the day of the encounter (includes time in activities that require the physician or other qualified health care professional and does not include time in activities normally performed by clinical staff).

Physician/other qualified health care professional time includes the following activities, when performed:

- Preparing to see the patient (e.g., review of tests)

- Obtaining and/or reviewing separately obtained history
- Performing a medically appropriate examination and/or evaluation
- Counseling and educating the patient/family/caregiver
- Ordering medications, tests, or procedures
- Referring and communicating with other health care professionals (when not separately reported)
- Documenting clinical information in the electronic or other health record
- Independently interpreting results (not separately reported) and communicating results to the patient/family/caregiver
- Care coordination (not separately reported)

Concurrent Care and Transfer of Care

Concurrent care is the provision of similar services (e.g., hospital visits) to the same patient by more than one physician or other qualified health care professional on the same day. When concurrent care is provided, no special reporting is required. Transfer of care is the process whereby a physician or other qualified health care professional who is managing some or all of a patient's problems relinquishes this responsibility to another physician or other qualified health care professional who explicitly agrees to accept this responsibility and who, from the initial encounter, is not providing consultative services. The physician or other qualified health care professional transferring care is then no longer providing care for these problems though he or she may continue providing care for other conditions when appropriate. Consultation codes should not be reported by the physician or other qualified health care professional who has agreed to accept transfer of care before an initial evaluation, but they are appropriate to report if the decision to accept transfer of care cannot be made until after the initial consultation evaluation, regardless of site of service.

Decision Tree for New vs Established Patients

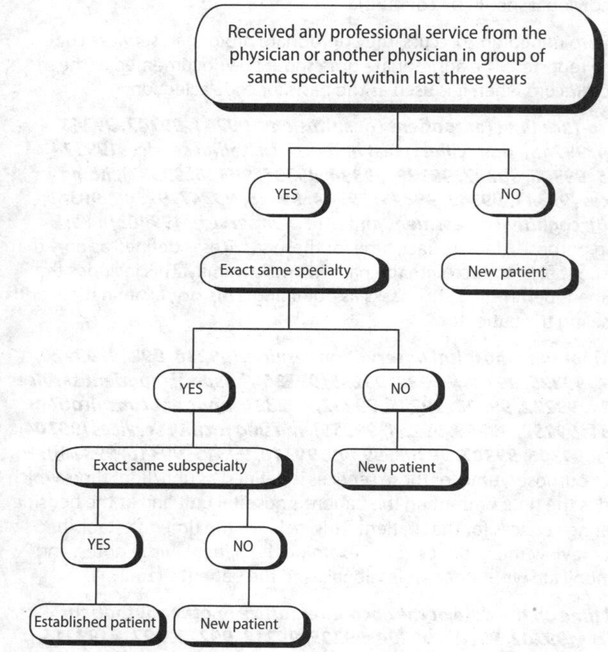

Counseling

Counseling is a discussion with a patient and/or family concerning one or more of the following areas:

- Diagnostic results, impressions, and/or recommended diagnostic studies
- Prognosis
- Risks and benefits of management (treatment) options
- Instructions for management (treatment) and/or follow-up
- Importance of compliance with chosen management (treatment) options
- Risk factor reduction
- Patient and family education

(For psychotherapy, see 90832–90834, 90836–90840)

Services Reported Separately

Any specifically identifiable procedure or service (ie, identified with a specific CPT code) performed on the date of E/M services may be reported separately.

The actual performance and/or interpretation of diagnostic tests/studies during a patient encounter are not included in determining the levels of E/M services when reported separately. Physician performance of diagnostic tests/studies for which specific CPT codes are available may be reported separately, in addition to the appropriate E/M code. The physician's interpretation of the results of diagnostic tests/studies (ie, professional component) with preparation of a separation distinctly identifiable signed written report may also be reported separately, using the appropriate CPT code and, if required, with modifier 26 appended. If a test/study is independently interpreted in order to manage the patient as part of the E/M service, but is not separately reported, it is part of MDM.

The physician or other qualified health care professional may need to indicate that on the day a procedure or service identified by a CPT code was performed, the patient's condition required a significant separately identifiable E/M service. The E/M service may be caused or prompted by the symptoms or condition for which the procedure and/or service was provided. This circumstance may be reported by adding modifier 25 to the appropriate level of E/M service. As such, different diagnoses are not required for reporting of the procedure and the E/M services on the same date.

Levels of E/M Services

Within each category or subcategory of E/M service, there are three to five levels of E/M services available for reporting purposes. Levels of E/M services are **not** interchangeable among the different categories or subcategories of service. For example, the first level of E/M services in the subcategory of office visit, new patient, does not have the same definition as the first level of E/M services in the subcategory of office visit, established patient. Each level of E/M services may be used by all physicians or other qualified health care professionals.

The levels of E/M services include examinations, evaluations, treatments, conferences with or concerning patients, preventive pediatric and adult health supervision, and similar medical services, such as the determination of the need and/or location for appropriate care. Medical screening includes the history, examination, and medical decision-making required to determine the need and/or location for appropriate care and treatment of the patient (eg, office and other outpatient setting, emergency department, nursing facility). The levels of E/M services encompass the wide variations in skill, effort, time, responsibility, and medical knowledge required for the prevention or diagnosis and treatment of illness or injury and the promotion of optimal health. Each level of E/M services may be used by all physicians or other qualified health care professionals.

The descriptors for the levels of E/M services recognize seven components, six of which are used in defining the levels of E/M services. These components are:

- History
- Examination
- Medical decision making
- Counseling
- Coordination of care
- Nature of presenting problem
- Time

The first three of these components (history, examination, and medical decision making) are considered the **key** components in selecting a level of E/M services. (See "Determine the Extent of History Obtained.")

The next three components (counseling, coordination of care, and the nature of the presenting problem) are considered **contributory** factors in the majority of encounters. Although the first two of these contributory factors are important E/M services, it is not required that these services be provided at every patient encounter.

Coordination of care with other physicians, other qualified health care professionals, or agencies without a patient encounter on that day is reported using the case management codes.

The final component, time, is discussed in detail before the Decision Tree for New vs Established Patients.

Chief Complaint
A chief complaint is a concise statement describing the symptom, problem, condition, diagnosis, or other factor that is the reason for the encounter, usually stated in the patient's words.

History of Present Illness
A chronological description of the development of the patient's present illness from the first sign and/or symptom to the present. This includes a description of location, quality, severity, timing, context, modifying factors, and associated signs and symptoms significantly related to the presenting problem.

Nature of Presenting Problem
A presenting problem is a disease, condition, illness, injury, symptom, sign, finding, complaint, or other reason for encounter, with or without a diagnosis being established at the time of the encounter. The E/M codes recognize five types of presenting problems that are defined as follows:

Minimal: A problem that may not require the presence of the physician or other qualified health care professional, but service is provided under the physician's or other qualified health care professional's supervision.

Self-limited or minor: A problem that runs a definite and prescribed course, is transient in nature, and is not likely to permanently alter health status.

Low severity: A problem where the risk of morbidity without treatment is low; there is little to no risk of mortality without treatment; full recovery without functional impairment is expected.

Moderate severity: A problem where the risk of morbidity without treatment is moderate; there is moderate risk of mortality without treatment; uncertain prognosis OR increased probability of prolonged functional impairment.

High severity: A problem where the risk of morbidity without treatment is high to extreme; there is a moderate to high risk of mortality without treatment OR high probability of severe, prolonged functional impairment.

Past History
A review of the patient's past experiences with illnesses, injuries, and treatments that includes significant information about:

- Prior major illnesses and injuries
- Prior operations
- Prior hospitalizations
- Current medications
- Allergies (eg, drug, food)
- Age appropriate immunization status
- Age appropriate feeding/dietary status

Family History
A review of medical events in the patient's family that includes significant information about:

- The health status of cause of death of parents, siblings, and children
- Specific diseases related to problems identified in the Chief Complaint or History of the Present Illness, and/or System Review
- Diseases of family members that may be hereditary or place the patient at risk

Social History
An age appropriate review of past and current activities that includes significant information about:

- Marital status and/or living arrangements
- Current employment
- Occupational history
- Military history
- Use of drugs, alcohol, and tobacco
- Level of education
- Sexual history
- Other relevant social factors

System Review (Review of Systems)
An inventory of body systems obtained through a series of questions seeking to identify signs and/or symptoms that the patient may be experiencing or has experienced. For the purposes of the CPT codebook the following elements of a system review have been identified:

- Constitutional symptoms (fever, weight loss, etc)
- Eyes
- Ears, nose, mouth, throat
- Cardiovascular
- Respiratory
- Gastrointestinal
- Genitourinary
- Musculoskeletal
- Integumentary (skin and/or breast)
- Neurological
- Psychiatric
- Endocrine
- Hematologic/lymphatic
- Allergic/immunologic

The review of systems helps define the problem, clarify the differential diagnosis, identify needed testing, or serves as baseline data on other systems that might be affected by any possible management options.

Instructions for Selecting a Level of E/M Service

Review the Reporting Instructions for the Selected Category or Subcategory
Most of the categories and many of the subcategories of service have special guidelines or instructions unique to that category or subcategory. Where these are indicated, eg, "Inpatient Hospital Care," special instructions will be presented preceding the levels of E/M services.

Review the Level of E/M Service Descriptors and Examples in the Selected Category or Subcategory
The descriptors for the levels of E/M services recognize seven components, six of which are used in defining the levels of E/M services. These components are:

- History
- Examination
- Medical decision making
- Counseling
- Coordination of care
- Nature of presenting problem
- Time

The first three of these components (ie, history, examination, and medical decision making) should be considered the **key** components in selecting the level of E/M services. An exception to this rule is in the case of visits that consist predominantly of counseling or coordination of care.

The nature of the presenting problem and time are provided in some levels to assist the physician in determining the appropriate level of E/M service.

Determine the Extent of History Obtained

The extent of the history is dependent upon clinical judgment and on the nature of the presenting problem(s). The levels of E/M services recognize four types of history that are defined as follows:

Problem focused: Chief complaint; brief history of present illness or problem.

Expanded problem focused: Chief complaint; brief history of present illness; problem pertinent system review.

Detailed: Chief complaint; extended history of present illness; problem pertinent system review extended to include a review of a limited number of additional systems; pertinent past, family, and/or social history directly related to the patient's problems.

Comprehensive: Chief complaint; extended history of present illness; review of systems that is directly related to the problem(s) identified in the history of the present illness plus a review of all additional body systems; **complete** past, family, and social history.

The comprehensive history obtained as part of the preventive medicine E/M service is not problem-oriented and does not involve a chief complaint or present illness. It does, however, include a comprehensive system review and comprehensive or interval past, family, and social history as well as a comprehensive assessment/history of pertinent risk factors.

Determine the Extent of Examination Performed

The extent of the examination performed is dependent on clinical judgment and on the nature of the presenting problem(s). The levels of E/M services recognize four types of examination that are defined as follows:

Problem focused: A limited examination of the affected body area or organ system.

Expanded problem focused: A limited examination of the affected body area or organ system and other symptomatic or related organ system(s).

Detailed: An extended examination of the affected body area(s) and other symptomatic or related organ system(s).

Comprehensive: A general multisystem examination or a complete examination of a single organ system. **Note:** The comprehensive examination performed as part of the preventive medicine E/M service is multisystem, but its extent is based on age and risk factors identified.

For the purposes of these CPT definitions, the following body areas are recognized:

- Head, including the face
- Neck
- Chest, including breasts and axilla
- Abdomen
- Genitalia, groin, buttocks
- Back
- Each extremity

For the purposes of these CPT definitions, the following organ systems are recognized:

- Eyes
- Ears, nose, mouth, and throat
- Cardiovascular
- Respiratory
- Gastrointestinal
- Genitourinary
- Musculoskeletal
- Skin
- Neurologic
- Psychiatric
- Hematologic/lymphatic/immunologic

Determine the Complexity of Medical Decision Making

Medical decision making refers to the complexity of establishing a diagnosis and/or selecting a management option as measured by:

- The number of possible diagnoses and/or the number of management options that must be considered
- The amount and/or complexity of medical records, diagnostic tests, and/or other information that must be obtained, reviewed, and analyzed
- The risk of significant complications, morbidity, and/or mortality, as well as comorbidities associated with the patient's presenting problem(s), the diagnostic procedure(s), and/or the possible management options

Four types of medical decision making are recognized: straightforward, low complexity, moderate complexity, and high complexity. To qualify for a given type of decision making, two of the three elements in Table 1 must be met or exceeded.

Comorbidities and underlying diseases, in and of themselves, are not considered in selecting a level of E/M services unless their presence significantly increases the complexity of the medical decision making.

Select the Appropriate Level of E/M Services Based on the Following

For the following categories/subcategories, **all of the key components**, ie, history, examination, and medical decision making, must meet or exceed the stated requirements to qualify for a particular level of E/M service: initial observation care; initial hospital care; observation or inpatient hospital care (including admission and discharge services); office or other outpatient consultations; inpatient consultations; emergency department services; initial nursing facility care; other nursing facility services; domiciliary care, new patient; and home services, new patient.

For the following categories/subcategories, **two of the three key components** (ie, history, examination, and medical decision making) must meet or exceed the stated requirements to qualify for a particular level of E/M services: subsequent observation care; subsequent hospital care; subsequent nursing facility care; domiciliary care, established patient; and home services, established patient.

When counseling and/or coordination of care dominates (more than 50 percent) the encounter with the patient and/or family (face-to-face time in the office or other outpatient setting or floor/unit time in the hospital or nursing facility), then **time** shall be considered the key or controlling factor to qualify for a particular level of E/M services. This includes time spent with parties who have assumed responsibility for the care of the patient or decision making whether or not they are family members (e.g., foster parents, person acting in loco parentis, legal guardian). The extent of counseling and/or coordination of care must be documented in the medical record.

CONSULTATION CODES AND MEDICARE REIMBURSEMENT

The Centers for Medicare and Medicaid Services (CMS) no longer provides benefits for CPT consultation codes. CMS has, however, redistributed the value of the consultation codes across the other E/M codes for services which are covered by Medicare. CMS has retained codes 99241 - 99251 in the Medicare Physician Fee Schedule for those private payers that use this data for reimbursement. Note that private payers may choose to follow CMS or CPT guidelines, and the use of consultation codes should be verified with individual payers.

Table 1

Complexity of Medical Decision Making

Number of Diagnoses or Management Options	*Amount and/or Complexity of Data to Be Reviewed*	*Risk of Complications and/or Morbidity or Mortality*	*Type of Decision Making*
minimal	minimal or none	minimal	**straightforward**
limited	limited	low	**low complexity**
multiple	moderate	moderate	**moderate complexity**
extensive	extensive	high	**high complexity**

Guidelines for Office or Other Outpatient E/M Services

History and/or Examination

Office or other outpatient services include a medically appropriate history and/or physical examination, when performed. The nature and extent of the history and/or physical examination are determined by the treating physician or other qualified health care professional reporting the service. The care team may collect information and the patient or caregiver may supply information directly (eg, by electronic health record [EHR] portal or questionnaire) that is reviewed by the reporting physician or other qualified health care professional. The extent of history and physical examination is not an element in selection of the level of office or other outpatient code.

Number and Complexity of Problems Addressed at the Encounter

One element used in selecting the level of office or other outpatient services is the number and complexity of the problems that are addressed at an encounter. Multiple new or established conditions may be addressed at the same time and may affect MDM. Symptoms may cluster around a specific diagnosis and each symptom is not necessarily a unique condition. Comorbidities/underlying diseases, in and of themselves, are not considered in selecting a level of E/M services **unless** they are addressed, and their presence increases the amount and/or complexity of data to be reviewed and analyzed or the risk of complications and/or morbidity or mortality of patient management. The final diagnosis for a condition does not, in and of itself, determine the complexity or risk, as extensive evaluation may be required to reach the conclusion that the signs or symptoms do not represent a highly morbid condition. Multiple problems of a lower severity may, in the aggregate, create higher risk due to interaction. Definitions for the elements of MDM (see Table 2, Levels of Medical Decision Making) for other office or other outpatient services are:

Problem: A problem is a disease, condition, illness, injury, symptom, sign, finding, complaint, or other matter addressed at the encounter, with or without a diagnosis being established at the time of the encounter.

Problem addressed: A problem is addressed or managed when it is evaluated or treated at the encounter by the physician or other qualified health care professional reporting the service. This includes consideration of further testing or treatment that may not be elected by virtue of risk/benefit analysis or patient/parent/guardian/surrogate choice. Notation in the patient's medical record that another professional is managing the problem without additional assessment or care coordination documented does not qualify as being addressed or managed by the physician or other qualified health care professional reporting the service. Referral without evaluation (by history, examination, or diagnostic study[ies]) or consideration of treatment does not qualify as being addressed or managed by the physician or other qualified health care professional reporting the service.

Minimal problem: A problem that may not require the presence of the physician or other qualified health care professional, but the service is provided under the physician's or other qualified health care professional's supervision (see 99211).

Self-limited or minor problem: A problem that runs a definite and prescribed course, is transient in nature, and is not likely to permanently alter health status.

Stable, chronic illness: A problem with an expected duration of at least one year or until the death of the patient. For the purpose of defining chronicity, conditions are treated as chronic whether or not stage or severity changes (eg, uncontrolled diabetes and controlled diabetes are a single chronic condition). "Stable" for the purposes of categorizing MDM is defined by the specific treatment goals for an individual patient. A patient who is not at his or her treatment goal is not stable, even if the condition has not changed and there is no short\term threat to life or function. For example, in a patient with persistently poorly controlled blood pressure for whom better control is a goal is not stable, even if the pressures are not changing and the patient is asymptomatic, the risk of morbidity **without** treatment is significant. Examples may include well-controlled hypertension, non-insulin dependent diabetes, cataract, or benign prostatic hyperplasia.

Acute, uncomplicated illness or injury: A recent or new short-term problem with low risk of morbidity for which treatment is considered. There is little to no risk of mortality with treatment, and full recovery without functional impairment is expected. A problem that is normally self-limited or minor but is not resolving consistent with a definite and prescribed course is an acute, uncomplicated illness. Examples may include cystitis, allergic rhinitis, or a simple sprain.

Chronic illness with exacerbation, progression, or side effects of treatment: A chronic illness that is acutely worsening, poorly controlled, or progressing with an intent to control progression and requiring additional supportive care or requiring attention to treatment for side effects but that does not require consideration of hospital level of care.

Undiagnosed new problem with uncertain prognosis: A problem in the differential diagnosis that represents a condition likely to result in a high risk of morbidity without treatment. An example may be a lump in the breast.

Acute illness with systemic symptoms: An illness that causes systemic symptoms and has a high risk of morbidity without treatment. For systemic general symptoms, such as fever, body aches, or fatigue in a minor illness that may be treated to alleviate symptoms, shorten the course of illness, or to prevent complications, see the definitions for self-limited or minor problem or acute, uncomplicated illness or injury. Systemic symptoms may not be general but may be single system. Examples may include pyelonephritis, pneumonitis, or colitis.

Acute, complicated injury: An injury which requires treatment that includes evaluation of body systems that are not directly part of the injured organ, the injury is extensive, or the treatment options are multiple and/or associated with risk of morbidity. An example may be a head injury with brief loss of consciousness.

Chronic illness with severe exacerbation, progression, or side effects of treatment: The severe exacerbation or progression of a chronic illness or severe side effects of treatment that have significant risk of morbidity and may require hospital level of care.

Acute or chronic illness or injury that poses a threat to life or bodily function: An acute illness with systemic symptoms, an acute complicated injury, or a chronic illness or injury with exacerbation and/or progression or side effects of treatment, that poses a threat to life or bodily function in the near term without treatment. Examples may include acute myocardial infarction, pulmonary embolus, severe respiratory distress, progressive severe rheumatoid arthritis, psychiatric illness with potential threat to self or others, peritonitis, acute renal failure, or an abrupt change in neurologic status.

Test: Tests are imaging, laboratory, psychometric, or physiologic data. A clinical laboratory panel (eg, basic metabolic panel [80047]) is a single test. The differentiation between single or multiple unique tests is defined in accordance with the CPT code set.

External: External records, communications and/or test results are from an external physician, other qualified health care professional, facility, or health care organization.

External physician or other qualified health care professional: An external physician or other qualified health care professional who is not in the same group practice or is of a different specialty or subspecialty. This includes licensed professionals who are practicing independently. The individual may also be a facility or organizational provider such as from a hospital, nursing facility, or home health care agency.

Independent historian(s): An individual (eg, parent, guardian, surrogate, spouse, witness) who provides a history in addition to a history provided by the patient who is unable to provide a complete or reliable history (eg, due to developmental stage, dementia, or psychosis) or because a confirmatory history is judged to be necessary. In the case where there may be conflict or poor communication between multiple historians and more than one historian is needed, the independent historian requirement is met.

Independent interpretation: The interpretation of a test for which there is a CPT code and an interpretation or report is customary. This does not apply when the physician or other qualified health care professional is reporting the service or has previously report the service for the patient. A form of interpretation should be documented but need not conform to the usual standards of a complete report for the test.

Appropriate source: For the purpose of the **discussion of management** data element (see Table 2, Levels of Medical Decision Making), an appropriate source includes professionals who are not health care professionals but may be involved in the management of the patient (eg, lawyer, parole officer, case manager, teacher). It does not include discussion with family or informal caregivers.

Risk: The probability and/or consequences of an event. The assessment of the level of risk is affected by the nature of the event under consideration. For example, a low probability of death may be high risk, whereas a high chance of a minor, self-limited adverse effect of treatment may be low risk. Definitions of risk are based upon the usual behavior and thought processes of a physician or other qualified health care professional in the same specialty. Trained clinicians apply common language usage meanings to terms such as high, medium, low, or minimal risk and do not require quantification for these definitions (though quantification may be provided when evidence-based medicine has established probabilities). For the purposes of MDM, level of risk is based upon consequences of the problem(s) addressed at the encounter when appropriately treated. Risk also includes MDM related to the need to initiate or forego further testing, treatment, and/or hospitalization.

Morbidity: A state of illness or functional impairment that is expected to be of substantial duration during which function is limited, quality of life is impaired, or there is organ damage that may not be transient despite treatment.

Social determinants of health: Economic and social conditions that influence the health of people and communities. Examples may include food and housing insecurity.

Drug therapy requiring intensive monitoring for toxicity: A drug that requires intensive monitoring is a therapeutic agent that has the potential to cause serious morbidity or death., The monitoring is performed for assessment of these adverse effects and not primarily for assessment of therapeutic efficacy. The monitoring should be that which is generally accepted practice for the agent but may be patient-specific in some cases. Intensive monitoring may be long-term or short-term. Long-term intensive monitoring is not performed less than quarterly. The monitoring may be performed with a laboratory test, a physiologic test, or imaging. Monitoring by history or examination does not qualify. The monitoring affects the level of MDM in an encounter in which it is considered in the management of the patient. Examples may include monitoring for cytopenia in the use of an antineoplastic agent between dose cycles or the short-term intensive monitoring of electrolytes and renal function in a patient who is undergoing diuresis. Examples of monitoring that do not qualify include monitoring glucose levels during insulin therapy, as the primary reason is the therapeutic effect (even if hypoglycemia is a concern) or annual electrolytes and renal function for a patient on a diuretic, as the frequency does not meet the threshold.

Instructions for Selecting a Level of Office or Other Outpatient E/M Services

Select the appropriate level of E/M services based on the following:

1. The level of the MDM as defined for each service, or
2. The total time for E/M services performed on the date of the encounter.

Medical Decision Making

MDM includes establishing diagnoses, assessing the status of a condition, and/or selecting a management option. MDM in the office or other outpatient services codes is defined by three elements:

- The number and complexity of problem(s) that are addressed during the encounter.
- The amount and/or complexity of data to be reviewed and analyzed. These data include medical records, tests, and/or other information that must be obtained, ordered, reviewed, and analyzed for the encounter. This includes information obtained from multiple sources or interprofessional communications that are not reported separately and interpretation of tests that are not reported separately. Ordering a test is included in the category of test result(s) and the review of the test result is part of the encounter and not a subsequent encounter. Data are divided into three categories:
  - Tests, documents, orders, or independent historian(s). (Each unique test, order, or document is counted to meet a threshold number.)
  - Independent interpretation of tests.
  - Discussion of management or test interpretation with external physician or other qualified health care professional or appropriate source.
- The risk of complications and/or morbidity or mortality of patient management decisions made at the visit, associated with the patient's problem(s), the diagnostic procedure(s), treatment(s). This includes the possible management options selected and those considered but not selected, after shared MDM with the patient and/or family. For example, a decision about hospitalization includes consideration of alternative levels of care. Examples may include a psychiatric patient with a sufficient degree of support in the outpatient setting or the decision to not hospitalize a patient with advanced dementia with an acute condition that would generally warrant in patient care, but for whom the goal is palliative treatment.

Four types of MDM are recognized: straightforward, low, moderate, and high. The concept of the level of MDM does not apply to 99211. Shared MDM involves eliciting patient and/or family preferences, patient and/or family education, and explaining risks and benefits of management options. MDM may be impacted by role and management responsibility.

When the physician or other qualified health care professional is reporting a separate CPT code that includes interpretation and/or report, the interpretation and/or report should not count toward the MDM when selecting a level of office or other outpatient services. When the physician or other qualified health care professional is reporting a separate service for discussion of management with a physician or another qualified health care professional, the discussion is not counted toward the MDM when selecting a level of office or other outpatient services.

The Levels of Medical Decision Making (MDM) table (Table2) is a guide to assist in selecting the level of MDM for reporting an office or other outpatient E/M services code. The table includes the four levels of MDM (ie, straightforward, low, moderate, high) and the three elements of MDM (ie, number and complexity of problems addressed at the encounter, amount and/or complexity of data reviewed and analyzed, and risk of complications and/or morbidity or mortality of patient management). To qualify for a particular level of MDM, two of the three elements for that level of MDM must be met or exceeded. See Table 2: Levels of Medical Decision Making (MDM) below.

Table 2: Levels of Medical Decision Making (MDM)

		Elements of Medical Decision Making		
Code	**Level of MDM (Based on 2 out of 3 Elements of MDM)**	**Number and Complexity of Problems Addressed**	**Amount and/or Complexity of Data to be Reviewed and Analyzed**	**Risk of Complications and/or Morbidity or Mortality of Patient Management**
99211	N/A	N/A	N/A	N/A
99202 **99212**	**Straightforward**	**Minimal** • **1** self-limited or minor problem	**Minimal or none**	**Minimal risk of morbidity from additional diagnostic testing or treatment**
99203 **99213**	**Low**	**Low** • **2** or more self-limited or minor problems; **or** • stable chronic illness; **or** • **1** acute, uncomplicated illness or injury	**Limited** *(Must meet the requirements of at least 1 of the 2 categories)* **Category 1: Tests and documents** • Any combination of 2 from the following: - Review of prior external note(s) from each unique source*; - review of the result(s) of each unique test*; - ordering of each unique test* **or** **Category 2: Assessment requiring an independent historian(s)** *(For the categories of independent interpretation of tests and discussion of management or test interpretation, see moderate or high)*	**Low risk of morbidity from additional diagnostic testing or treatment**

**Each unique test, order, or document contributes to the combination of 2 or combination of 3 in Category 1 below.*

Elements of Medical Decision Making				
Code	**Level of MDM (Based on 2 out of 3 Elements of MDM)**	**Number and Complexity of Problems Addressed**	**Amount and/or Complexity of Data to be Reviewed and Analyzed**	**Risk of Complications and/or Morbidity or Mortality of Patient Management**
99204 **99214**	**Moderate**	**Moderate** • **1** or more chronic illnesses with exacerbation, progression, or side effects of treatment; **or** • **2** or more stable chronic illnesses; **or** • **1** undiagnosed new problem with uncertain prognosis; **or** • **1** acute illness with systemic symptoms; **or** • **1** acute complicated injury	**Moderate** *(Must meet the requirements of at least 1 out of 3 categories)* **Category 1: Tests, documents, or independent historian(s)** • Any combination of 3 from the following: - Review of prior external note(s) from each unique source*; - Review of the result(s) of each unique test*; - Ordering of each unique test*; - Assessment requiring an independent historian(s) **or** **Category 2: Independent interpretation of tests** • Independent interpretation of a test performed by another physician/other qualified health care professional (not separately reported); **or** **Category 3: Discussion of management or test interpretation** Discussion of management or test interpretation with external physician/other qualified health care professional\appropriate source (not separately reported)	**Moderate risk of morbidity from additional diagnostic testing or treatment** *Examples only:* • Prescription drug management • Decision regarding minor surgery with identified patient or procedure risk factors • Decision regarding elective major surgery without identified patient or procedure risk factors Diagnosis or treatment significantly limited by social determinants of health
99205 **99215**	**High**	**High** • **1** or more chronic illnesses with severe exacerbation, progression, or side effects of treatment; **or** • **1** acute or chronic illness or injury that poses a threat to life or bodily function	**Extensive** *(Must meet the requirements of at least 2 out of 3 categories)* **Category 1: Tests, documents, or independent historian(s)** • **Any combination of 3 from the following:** - Review of prior external note(s) from each unique source*; - Review of the result(s) of each unique test*; - Ordering of each unique test*; - Assessment requiring an independent historian(s) **or** **Category 2: Independent interpretation of tests** • **Independent interpretation of a test performed by another physician/other qualified health care professional (not separately reported);** **or** **Category 3: Discussion of management or test interpretation** • Discussion of management or test interpretation with external physician/other qualified health care professional/appropriate source (not separately reported)	**High risk of morbidity from additional diagnostic testing or treatment** *Examples only:* • Drug therapy requiring intensive monitoring for toxicity • Decision regarding elective major surgery with identified patient or procedure risk factors • Decision regarding emergency major surgery • Decision regarding hospitalization • Decision not to resuscitate or to de-escalate care because of poor prognosis

**Each unique test, order, or document contributes to the combination of 2 or combination of 3 in Category 1 below.*

Time

For instructions on using time to select the level of office or other outpatient E/M services code, see the ***Time*** subsection in the ***Guidelines Common to All E/M Services.***

Unlisted Service

An E/M service may be provided that is not listed in this section of the CPT codebook. When reporting such a service, the appropriate unlisted code may be used to indicate the service, identifying it by "Special Report," as discussed in the following paragraph. The "Unlisted Services" and accompanying codes for the E/M section are as follows:

99429 **Unlisted preventive** medicine service

99499 **Unlisted evaluation and management** service

Special Report

An unlisted service or one that is unusual, variable, or new may require a special report demonstrating the medical appropriateness of the service. Pertinent information should include an adequate definition or description of the nature, extent, and need for the procedure and the time, effort, and equipment necessary to provide the service. Additional items that may be included are complexity of symptoms, final diagnosis, pertinent physical findings, diagnostic and therapeutic procedures, concurrent problems, and follow-up care.

Clinical Examples

Clinical examples of the codes for E/M services are provided to assist in understanding the meaning of the descriptors and selecting the correct code. The clinical examples are listed in Appendix C. Each example was developed by the specialties shown. The same problem, when seen by different specialties, may involve different amounts of work. Therefore, the appropriate level of encounter should be reported using the descriptors rather than the examples.

99201-99215 Outpatient and Other Visits

CMS: 100-04,11,40.1.3 Independent Attending Physician Services; 100-04,12,190.3 List of Telehealth Services; 100-04,12,190.6 Payment Methodology for Physician/Practitioner at the Distant Site ; 100-04,12,190.6.1 Submission of Telehealth Claims for Distant Site Practitioners; 100-04,12,190.7 Contractor Editing of Telehealth Claims; 100-04,12,230 Primary Care Incentive Payment Program; 100-04,12,230.1 Definition of Primary Care Practitioners and Services; 100-04,12,230.2 Coordination with Other Payments; 100-04,12,230.3 Claims Processing and Payment; 100-04,12,30.6.10 Consultation Services; 100-04,12,30.6.15.1 Prolonged Services With Direct Face-to-Face Patient Contact; 100-04,12,30.6.4 Services Furnished Incident to Physician's Service; 100-04,12,30.6.7 Payment for Office or Other Outpatient E&M Visits; 100-04,12,40.3 Global Surgery Review; 100-04,18,80.2 Contractor Billing Requirements; 100-04,32,12.1 Counseling to Prevent Tobacco Use HCPCS and Diagnosis Coding; 100-04,32,130.1 Billing and Payment of External counterpulsation (ECP)

INCLUDES Established patients: received prior professional services from physician or qualified health care professional or another physician or qualified health care professional in exact same specialty practice and subspecialty in previous three years (99211-99215)
New patients: have not received professional services from physician or qualified health care professional or any other physician or qualified health care professional in same practice in exact same specialty and subspecialty in previous three years (99202-99205)
Office visits
Outpatient services (including services prior to formal admission to facility)

EXCLUDES *Services provided in:*
Emergency department (99281-99285)
Hospital observation (99217-99220 [99224, 99225, 99226])
Hospital observation or inpatient with same day admission and discharge (99234-99236)

~~**99201 Office or other outpatient visit for the evaluation and management of a new patient, which requires these 3 key components: A problem focused history; A problem focused examination; Straightforward medical decision making. Counseling and/or coordination of care with other physicians, other qualified health care professionals, or agencies are provided consistent with the nature of the problem(s) and the patient's and/or family's needs. Usually, the presenting problem(s) are self limited or minor. Typically, 10 minutes are spent face-to-face with the patient and/or family.**~~

To report, see (99202)

▲ **99202 Office or other outpatient visit for the evaluation and management of a new patient, which requires a medically appropriate history and/or examination and straightforward medical decision making. When using time for code selection, 15-29 minutes of total time is spent on the date of the encounter.**

1.43 2.15 **FUD** XXX ★ B 80

AMA: 2020,Sep,14; 2020,Sep,3; 2020,Jun,3; 2020,May,3; 2020,Feb,3; 2020,Jan,3; 2019,Oct,10; 2019,Feb,3; 2019,Jan,3; 2018,Sep,14; 2018,Apr,10; 2018,Apr,9; 2018,Mar,7; 2018,Jan,8; 2017,Aug,3; 2017,Jun,6; 2017,Jan,8; 2016,Dec,11; 2016,Sep,6; 2016,Mar,10; 2016,Jan,13; 2016,Jan,7; 2015,Dec,3; 2015,Oct,3; 2015,Jan,16; 2015,Jan,12

▲ **99203 Office or other outpatient visit for the evaluation and management of a new patient, which requires a medically appropriate history and/or examination and low level of medical decision making. When using time for code selection, 30-44 minutes of total time is spent on the date of the encounter.**

2.15 3.05 **FUD** XXX ★ B 80

AMA: 2020,Sep,3; 2020,Sep,14; 2020,Jun,3; 2020,May,3; 2020,Feb,3; 2020,Jan,3; 2019,Oct,10; 2019,Feb,3; 2019,Jan,3; 2018,Sep,14; 2018,Apr,9; 2018,Apr,10; 2018,Mar,7; 2018,Jan,8; 2017,Aug,3; 2017,Jun,6; 2017,Jan,8; 2016,Dec,11; 2016,Sep,6; 2016,Mar,10; 2016,Jan,7; 2016,Jan,13; 2015,Dec,3; 2015,Oct,3; 2015,Jan,12; 2015,Jan,16

▲ **99204 Office or other outpatient visit for the evaluation and management of a new patient, which requires a medically appropriate history and/or examination and moderate level of medical decision making. When using time for code selection, 45-59 minutes of total time is spent on the date of the encounter.**

3.64 4.63 **FUD** XXX ★ B 80

AMA: 2020,Sep,3; 2020,Sep,14; 2020,Jun,3; 2020,May,3; 2020,Feb,3; 2020,Jan,3; 2019,Oct,10; 2019,Feb,3; 2019,Jan,3; 2018,Sep,14; 2018,Apr,9; 2018,Apr,10; 2018,Mar,7; 2018,Jan,8; 2017,Aug,3; 2017,Jun,6; 2017,Jan,8; 2016,Dec,11; 2016,Sep,6; 2016,Mar,10; 2016,Jan,7; 2016,Jan,13; 2015,Dec,3; 2015,Oct,3; 2015,Jan,12; 2015,Jan,16

▲ **99205 Office or other outpatient visit for the evaluation and management of a new patient, which requires a medically appropriate history and/or examination and high level of medical decision making. When using time for code selection, 60-74 minutes of total time is spent on the date of the encounter.**

Prolonged services (lasting 75 minutes or more) ([99417])

4.75 5.82 **FUD** XXX ★ B 80

AMA: 2020,Sep,3; 2020,Sep,14; 2020,Jun,3; 2020,May,3; 2020,Feb,3; 2020,Jan,3; 2019,Oct,10; 2019,Feb,3; 2019,Jan,3; 2018,Sep,14; 2018,Apr,9; 2018,Apr,10; 2018,Mar,7; 2018,Jan,8; 2017,Aug,3; 2017,Jun,6; 2017,Jan,8; 2016,Dec,11; 2016,Sep,6; 2016,Mar,10; 2016,Jan,7; 2016,Jan,13; 2015,Dec,3; 2015,Oct,3; 2015,Jan,12; 2015,Jan,16

▲ **99211 Office or other outpatient visit for the evaluation and management of an established patient, that may not require the presence of a physician or other qualified health care professional. Usually, the presenting problem(s) are minimal.**

0.26 0.65 **FUD** XXX B 80

AMA: 2020,Sep,3; 2020,Sep,14; 2020,Jun,3; 2020,May,3; 2020,Feb,3; 2020,Jan,3; 2019,Oct,10; 2019,Feb,3; 2019,Jan,3; 2018,Sep,14; 2018,Apr,10; 2018,Apr,9; 2018,Mar,7; 2018,Jan,8; 2017,Aug,3; 2017,Jun,6; 2017,Mar,10; 2017,Jan,8; 2016,Dec,11; 2016,Sep,6; 2016,Mar,10; 2016,Jan,13; 2016,Jan,7; 2015,Dec,3; 2015,Oct,3; 2015,Jan,16; 2015,Jan,12

▲ **99212 Office or other outpatient visit for the evaluation and management of an established patient, which requires a medically appropriate history and/or examination and straightforward medical decision making. When using time for code selection, 10-19 minutes of total time is spent on the date of the encounter.**

0.73 1.28 **FUD** XXX ★ B 80

AMA: 2020,Sep,3; 2020,Sep,14; 2020,Jun,3; 2020,May,3; 2020,Feb,3; 2020,Jan,3; 2019,Oct,10; 2019,Feb,3; 2019,Jan,3; 2018,Sep,14; 2018,Apr,9; 2018,Apr,10; 2018,Mar,7; 2018,Jan,8; 2017,Oct,5; 2017,Aug,3; 2017,Jun,6; 2017,Jan,8; 2016,Dec,11; 2016,Sep,6; 2016,Mar,10; 2016,Jan,7; 2016,Jan,13; 2015,Dec,3; 2015,Oct,3; 2015,Jan,12; 2015,Jan,16

▲ **99213 Office or other outpatient visit for the evaluation and management of an established patient, which requires a medically appropriate history and/or examination and low level of medical decision making. When using time for code selection, 20-29 minutes of total time is spent on the date of the encounter.**

1.45 2.11 **FUD** XXX ★ B 80

AMA: 2020,Sep,3; 2020,Sep,14; 2020,Jun,3; 2020,May,3; 2020,Feb,3; 2020,Jan,3; 2019,Oct,10; 2019,Feb,3; 2019,Jan,3; 2018,Sep,14; 2018,Apr,9; 2018,Apr,10; 2018,Mar,7; 2018,Jan,8; 2017,Aug,3; 2017,Jun,6; 2017,Jan,8; 2016,Dec,11; 2016,Sep,6; 2016,Mar,10; 2016,Jan,13; 2016,Jan,7; 2015,Dec,3; 2015,Oct,3; 2015,Jan,12; 2015,Jan,16

▲ **99214** **Office or other outpatient visit for the evaluation and management of an established patient, which requires a medically appropriate history and/or examination and moderate level of medical decision making. When using time for code selection, 30-39 minutes of total time is spent on the date of the encounter.**

2.22 3.06 **FUD** XXX ★ B 80

AMA: 2020,Sep,3; 2020,Sep,14; 2020,Jun,3; 2020,May,3; 2020,Feb,3; 2020,Jan,3; 2019,Oct,10; 2019,Feb,3; 2019,Jan,3; 2018,Sep,14; 2018,Apr,9; 2018,Apr,10; 2018,Mar,7; 2018,Jan,8; 2017,Aug,3; 2017,Jun,6; 2017,Jan,8; 2016,Dec,11; 2016,Sep,6; 2016,Mar,10; 2016,Jan,13; 2016,Jan,7; 2015,Dec,3; 2015,Oct,3; 2015,Jan,16; 2015,Jan,12

▲ **99215** **Office or other outpatient visit for the evaluation and management of an established patient, which requires a medically appropriate history and/or examination and high level of medical decision making. When using time for code selection, 40-54 minutes of total time is spent on the date of the encounter.**

EXCLUDES *Prolonged services (lasting 55 minutes or more) ([99417])*

3.13 4.10 **FUD** XXX ★ B 80

AMA: 2020,Sep,3; 2020,Sep,14; 2020,Jun,3; 2020,May,3; 2020,Feb,3; 2020,Jan,3; 2019,Oct,10; 2019,Feb,3; 2019,Jan,3; 2018,Sep,14; 2018,Apr,9; 2018,Apr,10; 2018,Mar,7; 2018,Jan,8; 2017,Aug,3; 2017,Jun,6; 2017,Jan,8; 2016,Dec,11; 2016,Sep,6; 2016,Mar,10; 2016,Jan,13; 2016,Jan,7; 2015,Dec,3; 2015,Oct,3; 2015,Jan,16; 2015,Jan,12

99217-99220 Facility Observation Visits: Initial and Discharge

CMS: 100-04,11,40.1.3 Independent Attending Physician Services; 100-04,12,30.6.4 Services Furnished Incident to Physician's Service; 100-04,12,30.6.8 Payment for Hospital Observation Services; 100-04,12,40.3 Global Surgery Review; 100-04,32,130.1 Billing and Payment of External counterpulsation (ECP)

INCLUDES Services provided on same date in other settings or departments associated with observation status admission (99202-99215, 99281-99285, 99304-99318, 99324-99337, 99341-99350, 99381-99429 [99415, 99416, 99417, 99421, 99422, 99423])
Services provided to new and established patients admitted to hospital specifically for observation (not required to be designated hospital area)

EXCLUDES *Services provided by physicians or another qualified health care professional other than admitting physician ([99224, 99225, 99226], 99241-99245)*
Services provided to patient admitted and discharged from observation status on same date (99234-99236)
Services provided to patient admitted to hospital following observation status (99221-99223)
Services provided to patient discharged from inpatient care (99238-99239)

99217 **Observation care discharge day management (This code is to be utilized to report all services provided to a patient on discharge from outpatient hospital "observation status" if the discharge is on other than the initial date of "observation status." To report services to a patient designated as "observation status" or "inpatient status" and discharged on the same date, use the codes for Observation or Inpatient Care Services [including Admission and Discharge Services, 99234-99236 as appropriate.])**

INCLUDES Discussing observation admission with patient
Final patient evaluation:
Discharge instructions
Sign off on discharge medical records

2.06 2.06 **FUD** XXX B 80

AMA: 2019,Jul,10; 2018,Jan,8; 2017,Aug,3; 2017,Jun,6; 2017,Jan,8; 2016,Dec,11; 2016,Jan,13; 2016,Jan,7; 2015,Dec,3; 2015,Jan,16

99218 **Initial observation care, per day, for the evaluation and management of a patient which requires these 3 key components: A detailed or comprehensive history; A detailed or comprehensive examination; and Medical decision making that is straightforward or of low complexity. Counseling and/or coordination of care with other physicians, other qualified health care professionals, or agencies are provided consistent with the nature of the problem(s) and the patient's and/or family's needs. Usually, the problem(s) requiring admission to outpatient hospital "observation status" are of low severity. Typically, 30 minutes are spent at the bedside and on the patient's hospital floor or unit.**

2.81 2.81 **FUD** XXX B 80

AMA: 2020,Sep,3; 2019,Jul,10; 2018,Dec,8; 2018,Dec,8; 2018,Jan,8; 2017,Aug,3; 2017,Jun,6; 2017,Jan,8; 2016,Dec,11; 2016,Jan,7; 2016,Jan,13; 2015,Dec,3; 2015,Jul,3; 2015,Mar,3; 2015,Jan,16

99219 **Initial observation care, per day, for the evaluation and management of a patient, which requires these 3 key components: A comprehensive history; A comprehensive examination; and Medical decision making of moderate complexity. Counseling and/or coordination of care with other physicians, other qualified health care professionals, or agencies are provided consistent with the nature of the problem(s) and the patient's and/or family's needs. Usually, the problem(s) requiring admission to outpatient hospital "observation status" are of moderate severity. Typically, 50 minutes are spent at the bedside and on the patient's hospital floor or unit.**

3.83 3.83 **FUD** XXX B 80

AMA: 2020,Sep,3; 2019,Jul,10; 2018,Dec,8; 2018,Dec,8; 2018,Jan,8; 2017,Aug,3; 2017,Jun,6; 2017,Jan,8; 2016,Dec,11; 2016,Jan,13; 2016,Jan,7; 2015,Dec,3; 2015,Jul,3; 2015,Jan,16

99220 **Initial observation care, per day, for the evaluation and management of a patient, which requires these 3 key components: A comprehensive history; A comprehensive examination; and Medical decision making of high complexity. Counseling and/or coordination of care with other physicians, other qualified health care professionals, or agencies are provided consistent with the nature of the problem(s) and the patient's and/or family's needs. Usually, the problem(s) requiring admission to outpatient hospital "observation status" are of high severity. Typically, 70 minutes are spent at the bedside and on the patient's hospital floor or unit.**

5.22 5.22 **FUD** XXX B 80

AMA: 2020,Sep,3; 2019,Jul,10; 2018,Dec,8; 2018,Dec,8; 2018,Jan,8; 2017,Aug,3; 2017,Jun,6; 2017,Jan,8; 2016,Dec,11; 2016,Jan,13; 2016,Jan,7; 2015,Dec,3; 2015,Jul,3; 2015,Jan,16

99224-99226 [99224, 99225, 99226] Facility Observation Visits: Subsequent

CMS: 100-04,11,40.1.3 Independent Attending Physician Services; 100-04,12,30.6.4 Services Furnished Incident to Physician's Service; 100-04,12,30.6.8 Payment for Hospital Observation Services; 100-04,12,30.6.9.1 Initial Hospital Care and Observation or Inpatient Care Services

INCLUDES Changes in patient's status (e.g., physical condition, history; response to medical management)
Medical record review
Review diagnostic test results
Services provided on same date in other settings or departments associated with observation status admission (99202-99215, 99281-99285, 99304-99318, 99324-99337, 99341-99350, 99381-99429 [99415, 99416, 99417, 99421, 99422, 99423])

EXCLUDES *Observation admission and discharge on same day (99234-99236)*

99224 **Subsequent observation care, per day, for the evaluation and management of a patient, which requires at least 2 of these 3 key components: Problem focused interval history; Problem focused examination; Medical decision making that is straightforward or of low complexity. Counseling and/or coordination of care with other physicians, other qualified health care professionals, or agencies are provided consistent with the nature of the problem(s) and the patient's and/or family's needs. Usually, the patient is stable, recovering, or improving. Typically, 15 minutes are spent at the bedside and on the patient's hospital floor or unit.**

1.12 1.12 FUD XXX B 80

AMA: 2020,Sep,3; 2019,Jul,10; 2018,Jan,8; 2017,Aug,3; 2017,Jun,6; 2017,Jan,8; 2016,Dec,11; 2016,Jan,7; 2016,Jan,13; 2015,Dec,3; 2015,Jan,16

99225 **Subsequent observation care, per day, for the evaluation and management of a patient, which requires at least 2 of these 3 key components: An expanded problem focused interval history; An expanded problem focused examination; Medical decision making of moderate complexity. Counseling and/or coordination of care with other physicians, other qualified health care professionals, or agencies are provided consistent with the nature of the problem(s) and the patient's and/or family's needs. Usually, the patient is responding inadequately to therapy or has developed a minor complication. Typically, 25 minutes are spent at the bedside and on the patient's hospital floor or unit.**

2.06 2.06 FUD XXX B 80

AMA: 2020,Sep,3; 2019,Jul,10; 2018,Jan,8; 2017,Aug,3; 2017,Jun,6; 2017,Jan,8; 2016,Dec,11; 2016,Jan,7; 2016,Jan,13; 2015,Dec,3; 2015,Jan,16

99226 **Subsequent observation care, per day, for the evaluation and management of a patient, which requires at least 2 of these 3 key components: A detailed interval history; A detailed examination; Medical decision making of high complexity. Counseling and/or coordination of care with other physicians, other qualified health care professionals, or agencies are provided consistent with the nature of the problem(s) and the patient's and/or family's needs. Usually, the patient is unstable or has developed a significant complication or a significant new problem. Typically, 35 minutes are spent at the bedside and on the patient's hospital floor or unit.**

2.95 2.95 FUD XXX B 80

AMA: 2020,Sep,3; 2019,Jul,10; 2018,Jan,8; 2017,Aug,3; 2017,Jun,6; 2017,Jan,8; 2016,Dec,11; 2016,Jan,7; 2016,Jan,13; 2015,Dec,3; 2015,Jan,16

99221-99233 [99224, 99225, 99226] Inpatient Hospital Visits: Initial and Subsequent

CMS: 100-04,11,40.1.3 Independent Attending Physician Services; 100-04,12,30.6.10 Consultation Services; 100-04,12,30.6.15.1 Prolonged Services With Direct Face-to-Face Patient Contact; 100-04,12,30.6.4 Services Furnished Incident to Physician's Service; 100-04,12,30.6.9 Hospital Visit and Critical Care on Same Day

INCLUDES Initial physician services provided to patient in hospital or "partial" hospital settings (99221-99223)
Services provided on admission date in other settings or departments associated with observation status admission (99202-99215, 99281-99285, 99304-99318, 99324-99337, 99341-99350, 99381-99397)
Services provided to new or established patient

EXCLUDES *Inpatient admission and discharge on same date (99234-99236)*
Inpatient E/M services provided by other than admitting physician

99221 **Initial hospital care, per day, for the evaluation and management of a patient, which requires these 3 key components: A detailed or comprehensive history; A detailed or comprehensive examination; and Medical decision making that is straightforward or of low complexity. Counseling and/or coordination of care with other physicians, other qualified health care professionals, or agencies are provided consistent with the nature of the problem(s) and the patient's and/or family's needs. Usually, the problem(s) requiring admission are of low severity. Typically, 30 minutes are spent at the bedside and on the patient's hospital floor or unit.**

2.86 2.86 FUD XXX B 80

AMA: 2020,Sep,3; 2018,Dec,8; 2018,Dec,8; 2018,Jan,8; 2017,Aug,3; 2017,Jun,6; 2017,Jan,8; 2016,Dec,11; 2016,Mar,10; 2016,Jan,13; 2016,Jan,7; 2015,Dec,3; 2015,Dec,18; 2015,Jul,3; 2015,Jan,16

99222 **Initial hospital care, per day, for the evaluation and management of a patient, which requires these 3 key components: A comprehensive history; A comprehensive examination; and Medical decision making of moderate complexity. Counseling and/or coordination of care with other physicians, other qualified health care professionals, or agencies are provided consistent with the nature of the problem(s) and the patient's and/or family's needs. Usually, the problem(s) requiring admission are of moderate severity. Typically, 50 minutes are spent at the bedside and on the patient's hospital floor or unit.**

3.86 3.86 FUD XXX B 80

AMA: 2020,Sep,3; 2018,Dec,8; 2018,Dec,8; 2018,Jan,8; 2017,Aug,3; 2017,Jun,6; 2017,Jan,8; 2016,Dec,11; 2016,Mar,10; 2016,Jan,13; 2016,Jan,7; 2015,Dec,3; 2015,Dec,18; 2015,Jul,3; 2015,Mar,3; 2015,Jan,16

99223 **Initial hospital care, per day, for the evaluation and management of a patient, which requires these 3 key components: A comprehensive history; A comprehensive examination; and Medical decision making of high complexity. Counseling and/or coordination of care with other physicians, other qualified health care professionals, or agencies are provided consistent with the nature of the problem(s) and the patient's and/or family's needs. Usually, the problem(s) requiring admission are of high severity. Typically, 70 minutes are spent at the bedside and on the patient's hospital floor or unit.**

5.71 5.71 FUD XXX B 80

AMA: 2020,Sep,3; 2018,Dec,8; 2018,Dec,8; 2018,Jan,8; 2017,Aug,3; 2017,Jun,6; 2017,Jan,8; 2016,Dec,11; 2016,Mar,10; 2016,Jan,13; 2016,Jan,7; 2015,Dec,3; 2015,Dec,18; 2015,Jul,3; 2015,Jan,16

99224 **Resequenced code. See code following 99220.**

99225 **Resequenced code. See code following 99220.**

99226 **Resequenced code. See code following 99220.**

99231 **Subsequent hospital care, per day, for the evaluation and management of a patient, which requires at least 2 of these 3 key components: A problem focused interval history; A problem focused examination; Medical decision making that is straightforward or of low complexity. Counseling and/or coordination of care with other physicians, other qualified health care professionals, or agencies are provided consistent with the nature of the problem(s) and the patient's and/or family's needs. Usually, the patient is stable, recovering or improving. Typically, 15 minutes are spent at the bedside and on the patient's hospital floor or unit.**

1.11 1.11 **FUD** XXX ★ B 80

AMA: 2020,Sep,3; 2018,Dec,8; 2018,Dec,8; 2018,Jan,8; 2017,Aug,3; 2017,Jun,6; 2017,Jan,8; 2016,Dec,11; 2016,Jan,13; 2016,Jan,7; 2015,Dec,3; 2015,Jul,3; 2015,Jan,16

99232 **Subsequent hospital care, per day, for the evaluation and management of a patient, which requires at least 2 of these 3 key components: An expanded problem focused interval history; An expanded problem focused examination; Medical decision making of moderate complexity. Counseling and/or coordination of care with other physicians, other qualified health care professionals, or agencies are provided consistent with the nature of the problem(s) and the patient's and/or family's needs. Usually, the patient is responding inadequately to therapy or has developed a minor complication. Typically, 25 minutes are spent at the bedside and on the patient's hospital floor or unit.**

2.05 2.05 **FUD** XXX ★ B 80

AMA: 2020,Sep,3; 2018,Dec,8; 2018,Dec,8; 2018,Jan,8; 2017,Aug,3; 2017,Jun,6; 2017,Jan,8; 2016,Dec,11; 2016,Oct,8; 2016,Jan,13; 2016,Jan,7; 2015,Dec,3; 2015,Jul,3; 2015,Jan,16

99233 **Subsequent hospital care, per day, for the evaluation and management of a patient, which requires at least 2 of these 3 key components: A detailed interval history; A detailed examination; Medical decision making of high complexity. Counseling and/or coordination of care with other physicians, other qualified health care professionals, or agencies are provided consistent with the nature of the problem(s) and the patient's and/or family's needs. Usually, the patient is unstable or has developed a significant complication or a significant new problem. Typically, 35 minutes are spent at the bedside and on the patient's hospital floor or unit.**

2.93 2.93 **FUD** XXX ★ B 80

AMA: 2020,Sep,3; 2018,Dec,8; 2018,Dec,8; 2018,Jan,8; 2017,Aug,3; 2017,Jun,6; 2017,Jan,8; 2016,Dec,11; 2016,Oct,8; 2016,Jan,13; 2016,Jan,7; 2015,Dec,3; 2015,Jul,3; 2015,Jan,16

99234-99236 Observation/Inpatient Visits: Admitted/Discharged on Same Date

CMS: 100-04,11,40.1.3 Independent Attending Physician Services; 100-04,12,30.6.4 Services Furnished Incident to Physician's Service; 100-04,12,30.6.8 Payment for Hospital Observation Services; 100-04,12,30.6.9 Payment for Inpatient Hospital Visits - General; 100-04,12,30.6.9.1 Initial Hospital Care and Observation or Inpatient Care Services; 100-04,12,30.6.9.2 Subsequent Hospital Visit and Discharge Management; 100-04,12,40.3 Global Surgery Review

INCLUDES Admission and discharge services on same date in observation or inpatient setting

All services provided by admitting physician or other qualified health care professional on same date, even when initiated in another setting (e.g., emergency department, nursing facility, office)

EXCLUDES *Services provided to patients admitted to observation and discharged on different date (99217-99220, [99224, 99225, 99226])*

99234 **Observation or inpatient hospital care, for the evaluation and management of a patient including admission and discharge on the same date, which requires these 3 key components: A detailed or comprehensive history; A detailed or comprehensive examination; and Medical decision making that is straightforward or of low complexity. Counseling and/or coordination of care with other physicians, other qualified health care professionals, or agencies are provided consistent with the nature of the problem(s) and the patient's and/or family's needs. Usually the presenting problem(s) requiring admission are of low severity. Typically, 40 minutes are spent at the bedside and on the patient's hospital floor or unit.**

3.75 3.75 **FUD** XXX B 80

AMA: 2020,Sep,3; 2018,Dec,8; 2018,Dec,8; 2018,Apr,10; 2018,Jan,8; 2017,Aug,3; 2017,Jun,6; 2017,Jan,8; 2016,Dec,11; 2016,Jan,13; 2015,Jul,3; 2015,Jan,16

99235 **Observation or inpatient hospital care, for the evaluation and management of a patient including admission and discharge on the same date, which requires these 3 key components: A comprehensive history; A comprehensive examination; and Medical decision making of moderate complexity. Counseling and/or coordination of care with other physicians, other qualified health care professionals, or agencies are provided consistent with the nature of the problem(s) and the patient's and/or family's needs. Usually the presenting problem(s) requiring admission are of moderate severity. Typically, 50 minutes are spent at the bedside and on the patient's hospital floor or unit.**

4.77 4.77 **FUD** XXX B 80

AMA: 2020,Sep,3; 2018,Dec,8; 2018,Dec,8; 2018,Apr,10; 2018,Jan,8; 2017,Aug,3; 2017,Jun,6; 2017,Jan,8; 2016,Dec,11; 2016,Jan,13; 2015,Jul,3; 2015,Jan,16

99236 **Observation or inpatient hospital care, for the evaluation and management of a patient including admission and discharge on the same date, which requires these 3 key components: A comprehensive history; A comprehensive examination; and Medical decision making of high complexity. Counseling and/or coordination of care with other physicians, other qualified health care professionals, or agencies are provided consistent with the nature of the problem(s) and the patient's and/or family's needs. Usually the presenting problem(s) requiring admission are of high severity. Typically, 55 minutes are spent at the bedside and on the patient's hospital floor or unit.**

6.14 6.14 **FUD** XXX B 80

AMA: 2020,Sep,3; 2018,Dec,8; 2018,Dec,8; 2018,Apr,10; 2018,Jan,8; 2017,Aug,3; 2017,Jun,6; 2017,Jan,8; 2016,Dec,11; 2016,Jan,13; 2015,Jul,3; 2015,Jan,16

99238-99239 Inpatient Hospital Discharge Services

CMS: 100-04,11,40.1.3 Independent Attending Physician Services; 100-04,12,30.6.4 Services Furnished Incident to Physician's Service; 100-04,12,30.6.9 Swing Bed Visits; 100-04,12,30.6.9.1 Initial Hospital Care and Observation or Inpatient Care Services; 100-04,12,30.6.9.2 Subsequent Hospital Visit and Discharge Management; 100-04,12,40.3 Global Surgery Review

INCLUDES All services on discharge day when discharge and admission are not on same day
Discharge instructions
Final patient evaluation
Final preparation patient's medical records
Provision prescriptions/referrals, as needed
Review inpatient admission

EXCLUDES *Admission/discharge on same date (99234-99236)*
Discharge from observation (99217)
Discharge from nursing facility (99315-99316)
Healthy newborn evaluated and discharged on same date (99463)
Services provided by other than attending physician or other qualified health care professional on discharge date (99231-99233)

99238 Hospital discharge day management; 30 minutes or less

2.06 2.06 **FUD** XXX B 80

AMA: 2018,Dec,8; 2018,Dec,8; 2018,Jan,8; 2017,Aug,3; 2017,Jun,6; 2017,Jan,8; 2016,Dec,11; 2016,Jan,13; 2015,Jan,16

99239 more than 30 minutes

3.02 3.02 **FUD** XXX B 80

AMA: 2018,Dec,8; 2018,Dec,8; 2018,Jan,8; 2017,Aug,3; 2017,Jun,6; 2017,Jan,8; 2016,Dec,11; 2016,Jan,13; 2015,Jan,16

99241-99245 Consultations: Office and Outpatient

CMS: 100-04,11,40.1.3 Independent Attending Physician Services; 100-04,12,190.6 Payment Methodology for Physician/Practitioner at the Distant Site ; 100-04,12,190.6.1 Submission of Telehealth Claims for Distant Site Practitioners; 100-04,12,190.7 Contractor Editing of Telehealth Claims; 100-04,12,30.6.10 Consultation Services; 100-04,12,30.6.15.1 Prolonged Services With Direct Face-to-Face Patient Contact; 100-04,12,30.6.4 Services Furnished Incident to Physician's Service; 100-04,12,30.6.9.1 Initial Hospital Care and Observation or Inpatient Care Services; 100-04,12,40.3 Global Surgery Review; 100-04,32,130.1 Billing and Payment of External counterpulsation (ECP); 100-04,4,160 Clinic and Emergency Visits Under OPPS

INCLUDES All outpatient consultations provided in office, outpatient or other ambulatory facility, domiciliary/rest home, emergency department, patient's home, and hospital observation
Documentation consultation request from appropriate source
Documentation need for consultation in patient's medical record
One consultation per consultant
Provision by physician or qualified nonphysician practitioner whose advice, opinion, recommendation, suggestion, direction, or counsel, etc., requested for evaluating/treating patient since that individual's specific medical expertise beyond requesting physician knowledge
Provision written report, findings/recommendations from consultant to referring physician
Third-party mandated consultation; append modifier 32

EXCLUDES *Another appropriately requested and documented consultation pertaining to same/new problem; repeat consultation code reporting*
Any distinctly recognizable procedure/service provided on or following consultation
Care assumption (all or partial); report subsequent codes as appropriate for place of service (99211-99215, 99334-99337, 99347-99350)
Consultation prompted by patient/family; report codes for office, domiciliary/rest home, or home visits instead (99202-99215, 99324-99337, 99341-99350)
Services provided to Medicare patients; E/M code as appropriate for place of service or HCPCS code (99202-99215, 99221-99223, 99231-99233, G0406-G0408, G0425-G0427)

99241 Office consultation for a new or established patient, which requires these 3 key components: A problem focused history; A problem focused examination; and Straightforward medical decision making. Counseling and/or coordination of care with other physicians, other qualified health care professionals, or agencies are provided consistent with the nature of the problem(s) and the patient's and/or family's needs. Usually, the presenting problem(s) are self limited or minor. Typically, 15 minutes are spent face-to-face with the patient and/or family.

0.92 1.34 **FUD** XXX ★ E

AMA: 2020,Sep,3; 2018,Apr,9; 2018,Apr,10; 2018,Mar,7; 2018,Jan,8; 2017,Aug,3; 2017,Jun,6; 2017,Jan,8; 2016,Dec,11; 2016,Sep,6; 2016,Jan,13; 2016,Jan,7; 2015,Jan,12; 2015,Jan,16

99242 Office consultation for a new or established patient, which requires these 3 key components: An expanded problem focused history; An expanded problem focused examination; and Straightforward medical decision making. Counseling and/or coordination of care with other physicians, other qualified health care professionals, or agencies are provided consistent with the nature of the problem(s) and the patient's and/or family's needs. Usually, the presenting problem(s) are of low severity. Typically, 30 minutes are spent face-to-face with the patient and/or family.

1.93 2.52 **FUD** XXX ★ E

AMA: 2020,Sep,3; 2018,Apr,9; 2018,Apr,10; 2018,Mar,7; 2018,Jan,8; 2017,Aug,3; 2017,Jun,6; 2017,Jun,8; 2017,Jan,8; 2016,Dec,11; 2016,Sep,6; 2016,Jan,7; 2016,Jan,13; 2015,Jan,12; 2015,Jan,16

99243 Office consultation for a new or established patient, which requires these 3 key components: A detailed history; A detailed examination; and Medical decision making of low complexity. Counseling and/or coordination of care with other physicians, other qualified health care professionals, or agencies are provided consistent with the nature of the problem(s) and the patient's and/or family's needs. Usually, the presenting problem(s) are of moderate severity. Typically, 40 minutes are spent face-to-face with the patient and/or family.

2.74 3.49 **FUD** XXX ★ E

AMA: 2020,Sep,3; 2018,Apr,9; 2018,Apr,10; 2018,Mar,7; 2018,Jan,8; 2017,Aug,3; 2017,Jun,6; 2017,Jan,8; 2016,Dec,11; 2016,Sep,6; 2016,Jan,7; 2016,Jan,13; 2015,Jan,12; 2015,Jan,16

99244 Office consultation for a new or established patient, which requires these 3 key components: A comprehensive history; A comprehensive examination; and Medical decision making of moderate complexity. Counseling and/or coordination of care with other physicians, other qualified health care professionals, or agencies are provided consistent with the nature of the problem(s) and the patient's and/or family's needs. Usually, the presenting problem(s) are of moderate to high severity. Typically, 60 minutes are spent face-to-face with the patient and/or family.

4.41 5.23 **FUD** XXX ★ E

AMA: 2020,Sep,3; 2018,Apr,9; 2018,Apr,10; 2018,Mar,7; 2018,Jan,8; 2017,Aug,3; 2017,Jun,6; 2017,Jan,8; 2016,Dec,11; 2016,Sep,6; 2016,Jan,7; 2016,Jan,13; 2015,Jan,16; 2015,Jan,12

99245 Office consultation for a new or established patient, which requires these 3 key components: A comprehensive history; A comprehensive examination; and Medical decision making of high complexity. Counseling and/or coordination of care with other physicians, other qualified health care professionals, or agencies are provided consistent with the nature of the problem(s) and the patient's and/or family's needs. Usually, the presenting problem(s) are of moderate to high severity. Typically, 80 minutes are spent face-to-face with the patient and/or family.

5.37 6.29 **FUD** XXX ★ E

AMA: 2020,Sep,3; 2018,Apr,9; 2018,Apr,10; 2018,Mar,7; 2018,Jan,8; 2017,Aug,3; 2017,Jun,6; 2017,Jan,8; 2016,Dec,11; 2016,Sep,6; 2016,Jan,7; 2016,Jan,13; 2015,Jan,12; 2015,Jan,16

99251-99255 Consultations: Inpatient

CMS: 100-04,11,40.1.3 Independent Attending Physician Services; 100-04,12,190.6 Payment Methodology for Physician/Practitioner at the Distant Site ; 100-04,12,190.6.1 Submission of Telehealth Claims for Distant Site Practitioners; 100-04,12,190.7 Contractor Editing of Telehealth Claims; 100-04,12,30.6.10 Consultation Services; 100-04,12,30.6.15.1 Prolonged Services With Direct Face-to-Face Patient Contact; 100-04,12,30.6.4 Services Furnished Incident to Physician's Service; 100-04,12,30.6.9.1 Initial Hospital Care and Observation or Inpatient Care Services; 100-04,12,40.3 Global Surgery Review

INCLUDES All outpatient consultations provided in office, outpatient or other ambulatory facility, domiciliary/rest home, emergency department, patient's home, and hospital observation
Documentation consultation request from appropriate source
Documentation need for consultation in patient's medical record
One consultation per consultant
Provision by physician or qualified nonphysician practitioner whose advice, opinion, recommendation, suggestion, direction, or counsel, etc., requested for evaluating/treating patient since that individual's specific medical expertise beyond requesting physician knowledge
Provision written report, findings/recommendations from consultant to referring physician
Third-party mandated consultation; append modifier 32

EXCLUDES *Another appropriately requested and documented consultation pertaining to same/new problem; repeat consultation code reporting*
Any distinctly recognizable procedure/service provided on or following consultation
Care assumption (all or partial); report subsequent codes as appropriate for place of service (99231-99233, 99307-99310)
Consultation prompted by patient/family; report codes for office, domiciliary/rest home, or home visits instead (99202-99215, 99234-99337, 99341-99350)
Services provided to Medicare patients; E/M code as appropriate for place of service or HCPCS code (99202-99215, 99324-99337, 99341-99350)

99251 **Inpatient consultation for a new or established patient, which requires these 3 key components: A problem focused history; A problem focused examination; and Straightforward medical decision making. Counseling and/or coordination of care with other physicians, other qualified health care professionals, or agencies are provided consistent with the nature of the problem(s) and the patient's and/or family's needs. Usually, the presenting problem(s) are self limited or minor. Typically, 20 minutes are spent at the bedside and on the patient's hospital floor or unit.**

1.38 1.38 **FUD** XXX ★ E

AMA: 2020,Sep,3; 2018,Jan,8; 2017,Aug,3; 2017,Jun,6; 2017,Jan,8; 2016,Dec,11; 2016,Jan,7; 2016,Jan,13; 2015,Jan,16

99252 **Inpatient consultation for a new or established patient, which requires these 3 key components: An expanded problem focused history; An expanded problem focused examination; and Straightforward medical decision making. Counseling and/or coordination of care with other physicians, other qualified health care professionals, or agencies are provided consistent with the nature of the problem(s) and the patient's and/or family's needs. Usually, the presenting problem(s) are of low severity. Typically, 40 minutes are spent at the bedside and on the patient's hospital floor or unit.**

2.13 2.13 **FUD** XXX ★ E

AMA: 2020,Sep,3; 2018,Jan,8; 2017,Aug,3; 2017,Jun,6; 2017,Jan,8; 2016,Dec,11; 2016,Jan,13; 2016,Jan,7; 2015,Jan,16

99253 **Inpatient consultation for a new or established patient, which requires these 3 key components: A detailed history; A detailed examination; and Medical decision making of low complexity. Counseling and/or coordination of care with other physicians, other qualified health care professionals, or agencies are provided consistent with the nature of the problem(s) and the patient's and/or family's needs. Usually, the presenting problem(s) are of moderate severity. Typically, 55 minutes are spent at the bedside and on the patient's hospital floor or unit.**

3.25 3.25 **FUD** XXX ★ E

AMA: 2020,Sep,3; 2018,Jan,8; 2017,Aug,3; 2017,Jun,6; 2017,Jan,8; 2016,Dec,11; 2016,Jan,13; 2016,Jan,7; 2015,Jan,16

99254 **Inpatient consultation for a new or established patient, which requires these 3 key components: A comprehensive history; A comprehensive examination; and Medical decision making of moderate complexity. Counseling and/or coordination of care with other physicians, other qualified health care professionals, or agencies are provided consistent with the nature of the problem(s) and the patient's and/or family's needs. Usually, the presenting problem(s) are of moderate to high severity. Typically, 80 minutes are spent at the bedside and on the patient's hospital floor or unit.**

4.72 4.72 **FUD** XXX ★ E

AMA: 2020,Sep,3; 2018,Jan,8; 2017,Aug,3; 2017,Jun,6; 2017,Jan,8; 2016,Dec,11; 2016,Jan,7; 2016,Jan,13; 2015,Jan,16

99255 **Inpatient consultation for a new or established patient, which requires these 3 key components: A comprehensive history; A comprehensive examination; and Medical decision making of high complexity. Counseling and/or coordination of care with other physicians, other qualified health care professionals, or agencies are provided consistent with the nature of the problem(s) and the patient's and/or family's needs. Usually, the presenting problem(s) are of moderate to high severity. Typically, 110 minutes are spent at the bedside and on the patient's hospital floor or unit.**

5.76 5.76 **FUD** XXX ★ E

AMA: 2020,Sep,3; 2018,Jan,8; 2017,Aug,3; 2017,Jun,6; 2017,Jan,8; 2016,Dec,11; 2016,Jan,7; 2016,Jan,13; 2015,Jan,16

99281-99288 Emergency Department Visits

CMS: 100-04,11,40.1.3 Independent Attending Physician Services; 100-04,12,30.6.11 Emergency Department Visits; 100-04,4,160 Clinic and Emergency Visits Under OPPS

INCLUDES Any time spent with patient, which usually involves multiple encounters while patient in emergency department
Care provided to new and established patients

EXCLUDES *Critical care services (99291-99292)*
Observation services (99217-99220, 99234-99236)

99281 **Emergency department visit for the evaluation and management of a patient, which requires these 3 key components: A problem focused history; A problem focused examination; and Straightforward medical decision making. Counseling and/or coordination of care with other physicians, other qualified health care professionals, or agencies are provided consistent with the nature of the problem(s) and the patient's and/or family's needs. Usually, the presenting problem(s) are self limited or minor.**

0.60 0.60 **FUD** XXX J 80

AMA: 2020,Jul,13; 2019,Jul,10; 2018,Jan,8; 2017,Aug,3; 2017,Jun,6; 2017,Jan,8; 2016,Jan,13; 2016,Jan,7; 2015,Jan,16; 2015,Jan,12

99282 **Emergency department visit for the evaluation and management of a patient, which requires these 3 key components: An expanded problem focused history; An expanded problem focused examination; and Medical decision making of low complexity. Counseling and/or coordination of care with other physicians, other qualified health care professionals, or agencies are provided consistent with the nature of the problem(s) and the patient's and/or family's needs. Usually, the presenting problem(s) are of low to moderate severity.**

1.17 1.17 **FUD** XXX J 80

AMA: 2020,Jul,13; 2019,Jul,10; 2018,Jan,8; 2017,Aug,3; 2017,Jun,6; 2017,Jan,8; 2016,Jan,7; 2016,Jan,13; 2015,Jan,12; 2015,Jan,16

99283 **Emergency department visit for the evaluation and management of a patient, which requires these 3 key components: An expanded problem focused history; An expanded problem focused examination; and Medical decision making of moderate complexity. Counseling and/or coordination of care with other physicians, other qualified health care professionals, or agencies are provided consistent with the nature of the problem(s) and the patient's and/or family's needs. Usually, the presenting problem(s) are of moderate severity.**

1.84 1.84 **FUD** XXX J 80

AMA: 2020,Jul,13; 2019,Jul,10; 2018,Jan,8; 2017,Aug,3; 2017,Jun,6; 2017,Jan,8; 2016,Jan,7; 2016,Jan,13; 2015,Jan,16; 2015,Jan,12

99284 **Emergency department visit for the evaluation and management of a patient, which requires these 3 key components: A detailed history; A detailed examination; and Medical decision making of moderate complexity. Counseling and/or coordination of care with other physicians, other qualified health care professionals, or agencies are provided consistent with the nature of the problem(s) and the patient's and/or family's needs. Usually, the presenting problem(s) are of high severity, and require urgent evaluation by the physician, or other qualified health care professionals but do not pose an immediate significant threat to life or physiologic function.**

3.38 3.38 **FUD** XXX J 80

AMA: 2020,Jul,13; 2019,Jul,10; 2018,Jan,8; 2017,Aug,3; 2017,Jun,6; 2017,Jan,8; 2016,Jan,13; 2016,Jan,7; 2015,Jan,16; 2015,Jan,12

99285 **Emergency department visit for the evaluation and management of a patient, which requires these 3 key components within the constraints imposed by the urgency of the patient's clinical condition and/or mental status: A comprehensive history; A comprehensive examination; and Medical decision making of high complexity. Counseling and/or coordination of care with other physicians, other qualified health care professionals, or agencies are provided consistent with the nature of the problem(s) and the patient's and/or family's needs. Usually, the presenting problem(s) are of high severity and pose an immediate significant threat to life or physiologic function.**

4.89 4.89 **FUD** XXX J 80

AMA: 2020,Jul,13; 2020,Jan,12; 2019,Jul,10; 2018,Jan,8; 2017,Aug,3; 2017,Jun,6; 2017,Jan,8; 2016,Jan,7; 2016,Jan,13; 2015,Jan,12; 2015,Jan,16

99288 **Physician or other qualified health care professional direction of emergency medical systems (EMS) emergency care, advanced life support**

INCLUDES Management provided by emergency/intensive care based physician or other qualified health care professional via voice contact to ambulance/rescue staff for services such as heart monitoring and drug administration

0.00 0.00 **FUD** XXX B

AMA: 2018,Jan,8; 2017,Aug,3; 2017,Jun,6; 2017,Jan,8; 2016,Jan,13; 2015,Jan,16

99291-99292 Critical Care Visits: Patients 72 Months of Age and Older

CMS: 100-04,11,40.1.3 Independent Attending Physician Services; 100-04,12,30.6.4 Services Furnished Incident to Physician's Service; 100-04,12,30.6.9 Swing Bed Visits; 100-04,12,40.3 Global Surgery Review; 100-04,4,160 Clinic and Emergency Visits Under OPPS; 100-04,4,160.1 Critical Care Services

INCLUDES
- 30 minutes or more direct care provided by physician or other qualified health care professional to critically ill or injured patient, any location
- All activities performed outside unit or off floor
- All time spent exclusively with patient/family/caregivers on nursing unit or elsewhere
- Outpatient critical care provided to neonates and pediatric patients age 71 months or younger
- Physician or other qualified health care professional presence during interfacility transfer for critically ill/injured patients age 24 months or older
- Professional services for interpretation:
  - Blood gases
  - Chest films (71045-71046)
  - Measurement cardiac output (93561-93562)
  - Other computer stored information
  - Pulse oximetry (94760-94762)
- Professional services:
  - Gastric intubation (43752-43753)
  - Transcutaneous pacing, temporary (92953)
  - Venous access, arterial puncture (36000, 36410, 36415, 36591, 36600)
  - Ventilation assistance and management, includes CPAP, CNP (94002-94004, 94660, 94662)

EXCLUDES
- *All services less than 30 minutes; report appropriate E/M code*
- *Inpatient critical care services provided to child age 2 through 5 years old (99475-99476)*
- *Inpatient critical care services provided to infants age 29 days through 24 months old (99471-99472)*
- *Inpatient critical care services provided to neonates age 28 days or younger (99468-99469)*
- *Other procedures not listed as included performed by physician or other qualified health care professional rendering critical care*
- *Patients not critically ill but in critical care department (report appropriate E/M code)*
- *Physician or other qualified health care professional presence during interfacility transfer for critically ill/injured patients age 24 months or younger (99466-99467)*
- *Supervisory services control physician during interfacility transfer for critically ill/injured patients age 24 months or younger ([99485, 99486])*

99291 **Critical care, evaluation and management of the critically ill or critically injured patient; first 30-74 minutes**

6.28 7.89 **FUD** XXX J 80

AMA: 2020,Feb,7; 2020,Jan,12; 2019,Dec,14; 2019,Aug,8; 2019,Jul,10; 2018,Dec,8; 2018,Dec,8; 2018,Jun,9; 2018,Jan,8; 2017,Aug,3; 2017,Jun,6; 2017,Jan,8; 2016,Oct,8; 2016,Aug,9; 2016,May,3; 2016,Jan,13; 2015,Jul,3; 2015,Feb,10; 2015,Jan,16

\+ **99292** **each additional 30 minutes (List separately in addition to code for primary service)**

Code first (99291)

3.16 3.49 **FUD** ZZZ N 80

AMA: 2020,Feb,7; 2019,Dec,14; 2019,Aug,8; 2019,Jul,10; 2018,Dec,8; 2018,Dec,8; 2018,Jun,9; 2018,Jan,8; 2017,Aug,3; 2017,Jun,6; 2017,Jan,8; 2016,Aug,9; 2016,May,3; 2016,Jan,13; 2015,Jul,3; 2015,Feb,10; 2015,Jan,16

99304-99310 Nursing Facility Visits

CMS: 100-04,11,40.1.3 Independent Attending Physician Services; 100-04,12,230 Primary Care Incentive Payment Program; 100-04,12,230.1 Definition of Primary Care Practitioners and Services; 100-04,12,230.2 Coordination with Other Payments; 100-04,12,230.3 Claims Processing and Payment; 100-04,12,30.6.10 Consultation Services; 100-04,12,30.6.13 Nursing Facility Visits; 100-04,12,30.6.15.1 Prolonged Services With Direct Face-to-Face Patient Contact; 100-04,12,30.6.4 Services Furnished Incident to Physician's Service; 100-04,12,30.6.9 Swing Bed Visits

INCLUDES All E/M services provided by admitting physician on nursing facility admission date in other locations (e.g., office, emergency department)
Initial care, subsequent care, discharge, and yearly assessments
Initial services include patient assessment and physician participation in developing plan of care (99304-99306)
Services provided in psychiatric residential treatment center
Services provided to new and established patients in nursing facility (skilled, intermediate, and long-term care facilities)
Subsequent services include physician review medical records, reassessment, and review test results (99307-99310)

EXCLUDES *Care plan oversight services (99379-99380)*

Code also hospital discharge services on same admission or readmission date to nursing home (99217, 99234-99236, 99238-99239)

99304 **Initial nursing facility care, per day, for the evaluation and management of a patient, which requires these 3 key components: A detailed or comprehensive history; A detailed or comprehensive examination; and Medical decision making that is straightforward or of low complexity. Counseling and/or coordination of care with other physicians, other qualified health care professionals, or agencies are provided consistent with the nature of the problem(s) and the patient's and/or family's needs. Usually, the problem(s) requiring admission are of low severity. Typically, 25 minutes are spent at the bedside and on the patient's facility floor or unit.**

2.55 2.55 **FUD** XXX B 80

AMA: 2020,Sep,3; 2018,Jan,8; 2017,Aug,3; 2017,Jun,6; 2017,Jan,8; 2016,Dec,11; 2016,Jan,13; 2016,Jan,7; 2015,Jan,16

99305 **Initial nursing facility care, per day, for the evaluation and management of a patient, which requires these 3 key components: A comprehensive history; A comprehensive examination; and Medical decision making of moderate complexity. Counseling and/or coordination of care with other physicians, other qualified health care professionals, or agencies are provided consistent with the nature of the problem(s) and the patient's and/or family's needs. Usually, the problem(s) requiring admission are of moderate severity. Typically, 35 minutes are spent at the bedside and on the patient's facility floor or unit.**

3.65 3.65 **FUD** XXX B 80

AMA: 2020,Sep,3; 2018,Jan,8; 2017,Aug,3; 2017,Jun,6; 2017,Jan,8; 2016,Dec,11; 2016,Jan,13; 2016,Jan,7; 2015,Jan,16

99306 **Initial nursing facility care, per day, for the evaluation and management of a patient, which requires these 3 key components: A comprehensive history; A comprehensive examination; and Medical decision making of high complexity. Counseling and/or coordination of care with other physicians, other qualified health care professionals, or agencies are provided consistent with the nature of the problem(s) and the patient's and/or family's needs. Usually, the problem(s) requiring admission are of high severity. Typically, 45 minutes are spent at the bedside and on the patient's facility floor or unit.**

4.71 4.71 **FUD** XXX B 80

AMA: 2020,Sep,3; 2018,Jan,8; 2017,Aug,3; 2017,Jun,6; 2017,Jan,8; 2016,Dec,11; 2016,Jan,13; 2016,Jan,7; 2015,Jan,16

99307 **Subsequent nursing facility care, per day, for the evaluation and management of a patient, which requires at least 2 of these 3 key components: A problem focused interval history; A problem focused examination; Straightforward medical decision making. Counseling and/or coordination of care with other physicians, other qualified health care professionals, or agencies are provided consistent with the nature of the problem(s) and the patient's and/or family's needs. Usually, the patient is stable, recovering, or improving. Typically, 10 minutes are spent at the bedside and on the patient's facility floor or unit.**

1.24 1.24 **FUD** XXX ★ B 80

AMA: 2020,Sep,3; 2018,Jan,8; 2017,Aug,3; 2017,Jun,6; 2017,Jan,8; 2016,Dec,11; 2016,Jan,13; 2016,Jan,7; 2015,Jan,16

99308 **Subsequent nursing facility care, per day, for the evaluation and management of a patient, which requires at least 2 of these 3 key components: An expanded problem focused interval history; An expanded problem focused examination; Medical decision making of low complexity. Counseling and/or coordination of care with other physicians, other qualified health care professionals, or agencies are provided consistent with the nature of the problem(s) and the patient's and/or family's needs. Usually, the patient is responding inadequately to therapy or has developed a minor complication. Typically, 15 minutes are spent at the bedside and on the patient's facility floor or unit.**

1.94 1.94 **FUD** XXX ★ B 80

AMA: 2020,Sep,3; 2018,Jan,8; 2017,Aug,3; 2017,Jun,6; 2017,Jan,8; 2016,Dec,11; 2016,Jan,13; 2016,Jan,7; 2015,Jan,16

99309 **Subsequent nursing facility care, per day, for the evaluation and management of a patient, which requires at least 2 of these 3 key components: A detailed interval history; A detailed examination; Medical decision making of moderate complexity. Counseling and/or coordination of care with other physicians, other qualified health care professionals, or agencies are provided consistent with the nature of the problem(s) and the patient's and/or family's needs. Usually, the patient has developed a significant complication or a significant new problem. Typically, 25 minutes are spent at the bedside and on the patient's facility floor or unit.**

2.57 2.57 **FUD** XXX ★ B 80

AMA: 2020,Sep,3; 2018,Jan,8; 2017,Aug,3; 2017,Jun,6; 2017,Jan,8; 2016,Dec,11; 2016,Jan,13; 2016,Jan,7; 2015,Jan,16

99310 **Subsequent nursing facility care, per day, for the evaluation and management of a patient, which requires at least 2 of these 3 key components: A comprehensive interval history; A comprehensive examination; Medical decision making of high complexity. Counseling and/or coordination of care with other physicians, other qualified health care professionals, or agencies are provided consistent with the nature of the problem(s) and the patient's and/or family's needs. The patient may be unstable or may have developed a significant new problem requiring immediate physician attention. Typically, 35 minutes are spent at the bedside and on the patient's facility floor or unit.**

3.79 3.79 **FUD** XXX ★ B 80

AMA: 2020,Sep,3; 2018,Jan,8; 2017,Aug,3; 2017,Jun,6; 2017,Jan,8; 2016,Dec,11; 2016,Jan,13; 2016,Jan,7; 2015,Jan,16

99315-99316 Nursing Home Discharge

CMS: 100-04,11,40.1.3 Independent Attending Physician Services; 100-04,12,230 Primary Care Incentive Payment Program; 100-04,12,230.1 Definition of Primary Care Practitioners and Services; 100-04,12,230.2 Coordination with Other Payments; 100-04,12,230.3 Claims Processing and Payment; 100-04,12,30.6.13 Nursing Facility Visits; 100-04,12,30.6.4 Services Furnished Incident to Physician's Service; 100-04,12,40.3 Global Surgery Review

INCLUDES Discharge services include all time spent by physician or other qualified health care professional:
- Completion discharge records
- Discharge instructions for patient and caregivers
- Discussion regarding stay in facility
- Final patient examination
- Provide prescriptions and referrals as appropriate

99315 Nursing facility discharge day management; 30 minutes or less

2.07 2.07 **FUD** XXX B 80

AMA: 2018,Jan,8; 2017,Aug,3; 2017,Jun,6; 2017,Jan,8; 2016,Dec,11; 2016,Jan,13; 2016,Jan,7; 2015,Jan,16

99316 more than 30 minutes

2.97 2.97 **FUD** XXX B 80

AMA: 2018,Jan,8; 2017,Aug,3; 2017,Jun,6; 2017,Jan,8; 2016,Dec,11; 2016,Jan,13; 2016,Jan,7; 2015,Jan,16

99318 Annual Nursing Home Assessment

CMS: 100-04,11,40.1.3 Independent Attending Physician Services; 100-04,12,230 Primary Care Incentive Payment Program; 100-04,12,230.1 Definition of Primary Care Practitioners and Services; 100-04,12,230.2 Coordination with Other Payments; 100-04,12,230.3 Claims Processing and Payment; 100-04,12,30.6.13 Nursing Facility Visits; 100-04,12,30.6.15.1 Prolonged Services With Direct Face-to-Face Patient Contact; 100-04,12,30.6.4 Services Furnished Incident to Physician's Service; 100-04,12,30.6.9 Swing Bed Visits

INCLUDES Includes nursing facility visits on same date as (99304-99316)

99318 Evaluation and management of a patient involving an annual nursing facility assessment, which requires these 3 key components: A detailed interval history; A comprehensive examination; and Medical decision making that is of low to moderate complexity. Counseling and/or coordination of care with other physicians, other qualified health care professionals, or agencies are provided consistent with the nature of the problem(s) and the patient's and/or family's needs. Usually, the patient is stable, recovering, or improving. Typically, 30 minutes are spent at the bedside and on the patient's facility floor or unit.

2.70 2.70 **FUD** XXX B 80

AMA: 2018,Jan,8; 2017,Aug,3; 2017,Jun,6; 2017,Jan,8; 2016,Dec,11; 2016,Jan,7; 2016,Jan,13; 2015,Jan,16

99324-99337 Domiciliary Care, Rest Home, Assisted Living Visits

CMS: 100-04,12,230 Primary Care Incentive Payment Program; 100-04,12,230.1 Definition of Primary Care Practitioners and Services; 100-04,12,230.2 Coordination with Other Payments; 100-04,12,230.3 Claims Processing and Payment; 100-04,12,30.6.14 Domiciliary Care, Rest Home, Assisted Living Visits; 100-04,12,30.6.15.1 Prolonged Services With Direct Face-to-Face Patient Contact; 100-04,12,30.6.4 Services Furnished Incident to Physician's Service

INCLUDES E/M services for patients residing in assisted living, domiciliary care, and rest homes where medical care not included

Services provided to new patients or established patients (99324-99328, 99334-99337)

EXCLUDES *Care plan oversight services provided to patient in rest home under home health agency care (99374-99375)*

Care plan oversight services provided to patient under hospice agency care (99377-99378)

99324 Domiciliary or rest home visit for the evaluation and management of a new patient, which requires these 3 key components: A problem focused history; A problem focused examination; and Straightforward medical decision making. Counseling and/or coordination of care with other physicians, other qualified health care professionals, or agencies are provided consistent with the nature of the problem(s) and the patient's and/or family's needs. Usually, the presenting problem(s) are of low severity. Typically, 20 minutes are spent with the patient and/or family or caregiver.

1.54 1.54 **FUD** XXX B 80

AMA: 2020,Sep,3; 2018,Apr,9; 2018,Jan,8; 2017,Aug,3; 2017,Jun,6; 2017,Jan,8; 2016,Dec,11; 2016,Jan,7; 2016,Jan,13; 2015,Jan,16

99325 Domiciliary or rest home visit for the evaluation and management of a new patient, which requires these 3 key components: An expanded problem focused history; An expanded problem focused examination; and Medical decision making of low complexity. Counseling and/or coordination of care with other physicians, other qualified health care professionals, or agencies are provided consistent with the nature of the problem(s) and the patient's and/or family's needs. Usually, the presenting problem(s) are of moderate severity. Typically, 30 minutes are spent with the patient and/or family or caregiver.

2.26 2.26 **FUD** XXX B 80

AMA: 2020,Sep,3; 2018,Apr,9; 2018,Jan,8; 2017,Aug,3; 2017,Jun,6; 2017,Jan,8; 2016,Dec,11; 2016,Jan,7; 2016,Jan,13; 2015,Jan,16

99326 Domiciliary or rest home visit for the evaluation and management of a new patient, which requires these 3 key components: A detailed history; A detailed examination; and Medical decision making of moderate complexity. Counseling and/or coordination of care with other physicians, other qualified health care professionals, or agencies are provided consistent with the nature of the problem(s) and the patient's and/or family's needs. Usually, the presenting problem(s) are of moderate to high severity. Typically, 45 minutes are spent with the patient and/or family or caregiver.

3.92 3.92 **FUD** XXX B 80

AMA: 2020,Sep,3; 2018,Apr,9; 2018,Jan,8; 2017,Aug,3; 2017,Jun,6; 2017,Jan,8; 2016,Dec,11; 2016,Jan,7; 2016,Jan,13; 2015,Jan,16

99327 **Domiciliary or rest home visit for the evaluation and management of a new patient, which requires these 3 key components: A comprehensive history; A comprehensive examination; and Medical decision making of moderate complexity. Counseling and/or coordination of care with other physicians, other qualified health care professionals, or agencies are provided consistent with the nature of the problem(s) and the patient's and/or family's needs. Usually, the presenting problem(s) are of high severity. Typically, 60 minutes are spent with the patient and/or family or caregiver.**

5.26 5.26 FUD XXX B 80

AMA: 2020,Sep,3; 2018,Apr,9; 2018,Jan,8; 2017,Aug,3; 2017,Jun,6; 2017,Jan,8; 2016,Dec,11; 2016,Jan,7; 2016,Jan,13; 2015,Jan,16

99328 **Domiciliary or rest home visit for the evaluation and management of a new patient, which requires these 3 key components: A comprehensive history; A comprehensive examination; and Medical decision making of high complexity. Counseling and/or coordination of care with other physicians, other qualified health care professionals, or agencies are provided consistent with the nature of the problem(s) and the patient's and/or family's needs. Usually, the patient is unstable or has developed a significant new problem requiring immediate physician attention. Typically, 75 minutes are spent with the patient and/or family or caregiver.**

6.20 6.20 FUD XXX B 80

AMA: 2020,Sep,3; 2018,Apr,9; 2018,Jan,8; 2017,Aug,3; 2017,Jun,6; 2017,Jan,8; 2016,Dec,11; 2016,Jan,7; 2016,Jan,13; 2015,Jan,16

99334 **Domiciliary or rest home visit for the evaluation and management of an established patient, which requires at least 2 of these 3 key components: A problem focused interval history; A problem focused examination; Straightforward medical decision making. Counseling and/or coordination of care with other physicians, other qualified health care professionals, or agencies are provided consistent with the nature of the problem(s) and the patient's and/or family's needs. Usually, the presenting problem(s) are self-limited or minor. Typically, 15 minutes are spent with the patient and/or family or caregiver.**

1.70 1.70 FUD XXX B 80

AMA: 2020,Sep,3; 2018,Apr,9; 2018,Jan,8; 2017,Aug,3; 2017,Jun,6; 2017,Jan,8; 2016,Dec,11; 2016,Jan,7; 2016,Jan,13; 2015,Jan,16

99335 **Domiciliary or rest home visit for the evaluation and management of an established patient, which requires at least 2 of these 3 key components: An expanded problem focused interval history; An expanded problem focused examination; Medical decision making of low complexity. Counseling and/or coordination of care with other physicians, other qualified health care professionals, or agencies are provided consistent with the nature of the problem(s) and the patient's and/or family's needs. Usually, the presenting problem(s) are of low to moderate severity. Typically, 25 minutes are spent with the patient and/or family or caregiver.**

2.68 2.68 FUD XXX B 80

AMA: 2020,Sep,3; 2018,Apr,9; 2018,Jan,8; 2017,Aug,3; 2017,Jun,6; 2017,Jan,8; 2016,Dec,11; 2016,Jan,7; 2016,Jan,13; 2015,Jan,16

99336 **Domiciliary or rest home visit for the evaluation and management of an established patient, which requires at least 2 of these 3 key components: A detailed interval history; A detailed examination; Medical decision making of moderate complexity. Counseling and/or coordination of care with other physicians, other qualified health care professionals, or agencies are provided consistent with the nature of the problem(s) and the patient's and/or family's needs. Usually, the presenting problem(s) are of moderate to high severity. Typically, 40 minutes are spent with the patient and/or family or caregiver.**

3.80 3.80 FUD XXX B 80

AMA: 2020,Sep,3; 2018,Apr,9; 2018,Jan,8; 2017,Aug,3; 2017,Jun,6; 2017,Jan,8; 2016,Dec,11; 2016,Jan,7; 2016,Jan,13; 2015,Jan,16

99337 **Domiciliary or rest home visit for the evaluation and management of an established patient, which requires at least 2 of these 3 key components: A comprehensive interval history; A comprehensive examination; Medical decision making of moderate to high complexity. Counseling and/or coordination of care with other physicians, other qualified health care professionals, or agencies are provided consistent with the nature of the problem(s) and the patient's and/or family's needs. Usually, the presenting problem(s) are of moderate to high severity. The patient may be unstable or may have developed a significant new problem requiring immediate physician attention. Typically, 60 minutes are spent with the patient and/or family or caregiver.**

5.47 5.47 FUD XXX B 80

AMA: 2020,Sep,3; 2018,Apr,9; 2018,Jan,8; 2017,Aug,3; 2017,Jun,6; 2017,Jan,8; 2016,Dec,11; 2016,Jan,7; 2016,Jan,13; 2015,Jan,16

99339-99340 Care Plan Oversight: Rest Home, Domiciliary Care, Assisted Living, and Home

CMS: 100-04,12,180 Payment of Care Plan Oversight (CPO); 100-04,12,180.1 Billing for Care Plan Oversight (CPO); 100-04,12,230 Primary Care Incentive Payment Program; 100-04,12,230.1 Definition of Primary Care Practitioners and Services; 100-04,12,230.2 Coordination with Other Payments; 100-04,12,230.3 Claims Processing and Payment; 100-04,12,30.6.14 Domiciliary Care, Rest Home, Assisted Living Visits; 100-04,12,30.6.4 Services Furnished Incident to Physician's Service

INCLUDES Care plan oversight for patients residing in assisted living, domiciliary care, private residences, and rest homes

Patient management services during same time frame as ([99421, 99422, 99423], 99441-99443, 98966-98968)

EXCLUDES *Care plan oversight services furnished under home health agency, nursing facility, or hospice (99374-99380)*

99339 **Individual physician supervision of a patient (patient not present) in home, domiciliary or rest home (eg, assisted living facility) requiring complex and multidisciplinary care modalities involving regular physician development and/or revision of care plans, review of subsequent reports of patient status, review of related laboratory and other studies, communication (including telephone calls) for purposes of assessment or care decisions with health care professional(s), family member(s), surrogate decision maker(s) (eg, legal guardian) and/or key caregiver(s) involved in patient's care, integration of new information into the medical treatment plan and/or adjustment of medical therapy, within a calendar month; 15-29 minutes**

2.17 2.17 FUD XXX B

AMA: 2019,Jan,6; 2018,Oct,9; 2018,Jan,8; 2017,Aug,3; 2017,Jun,6; 2017,Jan,8; 2016,Jan,13; 2015,Jan,16

99340 **30 minutes or more**

3.05 3.05 FUD XXX B

AMA: 2019,Jan,6; 2018,Oct,9; 2018,Jan,8; 2017,Aug,3; 2017,Jun,6; 2017,Jan,8; 2016,Jan,13; 2015,Jan,16

99341-99350 Home Visits

CMS: 100-04,11,40.1.3 Independent Attending Physician Services; 100-04,12,230 Primary Care Incentive Payment Program; 100-04,12,230.1 Definition of Primary Care Practitioners and Services; 100-04,12,230.2 Coordination with Other Payments; 100-04,12,230.3 Claims Processing and Payment; 100-04,12,30.6.14 Domiciliary Care, Rest Home, Assisted Living Visits; 100-04,12,30.6.14.1 Home Visits; 100-04,12,30.6.15.1 Prolonged Services With Direct Face-to-Face Patient Contact; 100-04,12,30.6.4 Services Furnished Incident to Physician's Service; 100-04,12,40.3 Global Surgery Review; 100-04,30.6.14.1 Home Services (Codes 99341 - 99350)

INCLUDES Services for new or established patient (99341-99345, 99347-99350)
Services provided to patient in private home (e.g., private residence, temporary or short-term housing such as campground, cruise ship, hostel, or hotel)

EXCLUDES *Services provided to patients under home health agency or hospice care (99374-99378)*

99341 **Home visit for the evaluation and management of a new patient, which requires these 3 key components: A problem focused history; A problem focused examination; and Straightforward medical decision making. Counseling and/or coordination of care with other physicians, other qualified health care professionals, or agencies are provided consistent with the nature of the problem(s) and the patient's and/or family's needs. Usually, the presenting problem(s) are of low severity. Typically, 20 minutes are spent face-to-face with the patient and/or family.**

1.56 1.56 **FUD** XXX B 80

AMA: 2020,Sep,3; 2018,Apr,9; 2018,Jan,8; 2017,Aug,3; 2017,Jun,6; 2017,Jan,8; 2016,Dec,11; 2016,Jan,7; 2016,Jan,13; 2015,Jan,16

99342 **Home visit for the evaluation and management of a new patient, which requires these 3 key components: An expanded problem focused history; An expanded problem focused examination; and Medical decision making of low complexity. Counseling and/or coordination of care with other physicians, other qualified health care professionals, or agencies are provided consistent with the nature of the problem(s) and the patient's and/or family's needs. Usually, the presenting problem(s) are of moderate severity. Typically, 30 minutes are spent face-to-face with the patient and/or family.**

2.25 2.25 **FUD** XXX B 80

AMA: 2020,Sep,3; 2018,Apr,9; 2018,Jan,8; 2017,Aug,3; 2017,Jun,6; 2017,Jan,8; 2016,Dec,11; 2016,Jan,7; 2016,Jan,13; 2015,Jan,16

99343 **Home visit for the evaluation and management of a new patient, which requires these 3 key components: A detailed history; A detailed examination; and Medical decision making of moderate complexity. Counseling and/or coordination of care with other physicians, other qualified health care professionals, or agencies are provided consistent with the nature of the problem(s) and the patient's and/or family's needs. Usually, the presenting problem(s) are of moderate to high severity. Typically, 45 minutes are spent face-to-face with the patient and/or family.**

3.67 3.67 **FUD** XXX B 80

AMA: 2020,Sep,3; 2018,Apr,9; 2018,Jan,8; 2017,Aug,3; 2017,Jun,6; 2017,Jan,8; 2016,Dec,11; 2016,Jan,7; 2016,Jan,13; 2015,Jan,16

99344 **Home visit for the evaluation and management of a new patient, which requires these 3 key components: A comprehensive history; A comprehensive examination; and Medical decision making of moderate complexity. Counseling and/or coordination of care with other physicians, other qualified health care professionals, or agencies are provided consistent with the nature of the problem(s) and the patient's and/or family's needs. Usually, the presenting problem(s) are of high severity. Typically, 60 minutes are spent face-to-face with the patient and/or family.**

5.14 5.14 **FUD** XXX B 80

AMA: 2020,Sep,3; 2018,Apr,9; 2018,Jan,8; 2017,Aug,3; 2017,Jun,6; 2017,Jan,8; 2016,Dec,11; 2016,Jan,7; 2016,Jan,13; 2015,Jan,16

99345 **Home visit for the evaluation and management of a new patient, which requires these 3 key components: A comprehensive history; A comprehensive examination; and Medical decision making of high complexity. Counseling and/or coordination of care with other physicians, other qualified health care professionals, or agencies are provided consistent with the nature of the problem(s) and the patient's and/or family's needs. Usually, the patient is unstable or has developed a significant new problem requiring immediate physician attention. Typically, 75 minutes are spent face-to-face with the patient and/or family.**

6.27 6.27 **FUD** XXX B 80

AMA: 2020,Sep,3; 2018,Apr,9; 2018,Jan,8; 2017,Aug,3; 2017,Jun,6; 2017,Jan,8; 2016,Dec,11; 2016,Jan,7; 2016,Jan,13; 2015,Jan,16

99347 **Home visit for the evaluation and management of an established patient, which requires at least 2 of these 3 key components: A problem focused interval history; A problem focused examination; Straightforward medical decision making. Counseling and/or coordination of care with other physicians, other qualified health care professionals, or agencies are provided consistent with the nature of the problem(s) and the patient's and/or family's needs. Usually, the presenting problem(s) are self limited or minor. Typically, 15 minutes are spent face-to-face with the patient and/or family.**

1.56 1.56 **FUD** XXX B 80

AMA: 2020,Sep,3; 2018,Apr,9; 2018,Jan,8; 2017,Aug,3; 2017,Jun,6; 2017,Jan,8; 2016,Dec,11; 2016,Jan,7; 2016,Jan,13; 2015,Jan,16

99348 **Home visit for the evaluation and management of an established patient, which requires at least 2 of these 3 key components: An expanded problem focused interval history; An expanded problem focused examination; Medical decision making of low complexity. Counseling and/or coordination of care with other physicians, other qualified health care professionals, or agencies are provided consistent with the nature of the problem(s) and the patient's and/or family's needs. Usually, the presenting problem(s) are of low to moderate severity. Typically, 25 minutes are spent face-to-face with the patient and/or family.**

2.37 2.37 **FUD** XXX B 80

AMA: 2020,Sep,3; 2018,Apr,9; 2018,Jan,8; 2017,Aug,3; 2017,Jun,6; 2017,Jan,8; 2016,Dec,11; 2016,Jan,7; 2016,Jan,13; 2015,Jan,16

99349 **Home visit for the evaluation and management of an established patient, which requires at least 2 of these 3 key components: A detailed interval history; A detailed examination; Medical decision making of moderate complexity. Counseling and/or coordination of care with other physicians, other qualified health care professionals, or agencies are provided consistent with the nature of the problem(s) and the patient's and/or family's needs. Usually, the presenting problem(s) are moderate to high severity. Typically, 40 minutes are spent face-to-face with the patient and/or family.**

3.64 3.64 **FUD** XXX B 80

AMA: 2020,Sep,3; 2018,Apr,9; 2018,Jan,8; 2017,Aug,3; 2017,Jun,6; 2017,Jan,8; 2016,Dec,11; 2016,Jan,7; 2016,Jan,13; 2015,Jan,16

99350 Home visit for the evaluation and management of an established patient, which requires at least 2 of these 3 key components: A comprehensive interval history; A comprehensive examination; Medical decision making of moderate to high complexity. Counseling and/or coordination of care with other physicians, other qualified health care professionals, or agencies are provided consistent with the nature of the problem(s) and the patient's and/or family's needs. Usually, the presenting problem(s) are of moderate to high severity. The patient may be unstable or may have developed a significant new problem requiring immediate physician attention. Typically, 60 minutes are spent face-to-face with the patient and/or family.

🚑 5.05   ⚕ 5.05   **FUD** XXX   B 80 🖵

AMA: 2020,Sep,3; 2018,Apr,9; 2018,Jan,8; 2017,Aug,3; 2017,Jun,6; 2017,Jan,8; 2016,Dec,11; 2016,Jan,7; 2016,Jan,13; 2015,Jan,16

99354-99357 Prolonged Services Direct Contact

CMS: 100-04,11,40.1.3 Independent Attending Physician Services; 100-04,12,30.6.15.1 Prolonged Services With Direct Face-to-Face Patient Contact; 100-04,12,30.6.4 Services Furnished Incident to Physician's Service

INCLUDES   Personal contact with patient by physician or other qualified health professional
Services extending beyond customary service provided in inpatient, observation, or outpatient setting
Time spent providing additional indirect contact services on floor, hospital unit, or nursing facility during same session as direct contact
Time spent providing prolonged services on service date, even when time not continuous

EXCLUDES   *Services less than 30 minutes, less than15 minutes after first hour, or after final 30 minutes*
Services provided independent from personal contact date with patient (99358-99359)
Code first E/M service code, as appropriate

▲ + **99354** Prolonged service(s) in the outpatient setting requiring direct patient contact beyond the time of the usual service; first hour (List separately in addition to code for outpatient Evaluation and Management or psychotherapy service, except with office or other outpatient services [99202, 99203, 99204, 99205, 99212, 99213, 99214, 99215])

EXCLUDES   *Office or other outpatient visit (99202-99205, 99212-99215)*
Prolonged office/outpatient services ([99417])
Prolonged service provided by clinical staff under supervision ([99415, 99416])
Reporting code more than one time per service date
Code first (99241-99245, 99324-99337, 99341-99350, 90837, 90847)

🚑 3.44   ⚕ 3.67   **FUD** ZZZ   ★ N 80 🖵

AMA: 2020,Sep,3; 2020,Feb,3; 2019,Oct,10; 2019,Jun,7; 2018,Jan,8; 2017,Jan,8; 2016,Dec,11; 2016,Jan,13; 2015,Oct,9; 2015,Oct,3; 2015,Jan,16

▲ + **99355** each additional 30 minutes (List separately in addition to code for prolonged service)

EXCLUDES   *Office or other outpatient visit (99202-99205, 99212-99215)*
Prolonged office/outpatient services ([99417])
Prolonged service provided by clinical staff under supervision ([99415, 99416])
Code first (99354)

🚑 2.60   ⚕ 2.80   **FUD** ZZZ   ★ N 80 🖵

AMA: 2020,Sep,3; 2020,Feb,3; 2019,Oct,10; 2019,Jun,7; 2018,Jan,8; 2017,Jan,8; 2016,Dec,11; 2016,Jan,13; 2015,Oct,9; 2015,Oct,3; 2015,Jan,16

▲ + **99356** Prolonged service in the inpatient or observation setting, requiring unit/floor time beyond the usual service; first hour (List separately in addition to code for inpatient or observation Evaluation and Management service)

EXCLUDES   *Reporting code more than one time per service date*
Code first (99218-99223 [99224, 99225, 99226], 99231-99236, 99251-99255, 99304-99310, 90837, 90847)

🚑 2.60   ⚕ 2.60   **FUD** ZZZ   C 80 🖵

AMA: 2020,Sep,3; 2019,Jun,7; 2018,Jan,8; 2017,Jan,8; 2016,Dec,11; 2016,Jan,13; 2015,Oct,3; 2015,Oct,9; 2015,Jan,16

+ **99357** each additional 30 minutes (List separately in addition to code for prolonged service)

Code first (99356)

🚑 2.61   ⚕ 2.61   **FUD** ZZZ   C 80 🖵

AMA: 2020,Sep,3; 2019,Jun,7; 2018,Jan,8; 2017,Jan,8; 2016,Dec,11; 2016,Jan,13; 2015,Oct,3; 2015,Oct,9; 2015,Jan,16

99358-99359 Prolonged Services Indirect Contact

CMS: 100-04,11,40.1.3 Independent Attending Physician Services; 100-04,12,30.6.15.2 Prolonged Services Without Face to Face Service; 100-04,12,30.6.4 Services Furnished Incident to Physician's Service

INCLUDES   Services extending beyond customary service
Time spent providing indirect contact services by physician or other qualified health care professional in relation to patient management where face-to-face services have or will occur on different date
Time spent providing prolonged services on service date, even when time not continuous

EXCLUDES   *Any additional unit or floor time in hospital or nursing facility during same evaluation and management session*
Behavioral health integration care management services (99484)
Time without direct patient contact for other services:
Care plan oversight (99339-99340, 99374-99380)
Chronic care management services provided during same month ([99491])
INR monitoring services (93792-93793)
Medical team conference (99366-99368)
Online and telephone consultative services (99446-99452 [99451, 99452])
Online medical services ([99421, 99422, 99423])
Patient management services during same time frame as (99487-99489, 99495-99496)
Psychiatric collaborative care management services during same month (99492-99494)
Reporting code more than one time per service date
Services less than 30 minutes, less than15 minutes after first hour, or after final 30 minutes
Code also E/M or other services provided, excluding (99202-99205, 99212-99215, 99217)

99358 Prolonged evaluation and management service before and/or after direct patient care; first hour

EXCLUDES   *Use of code more than one time per date of service*

🚑 3.15   ⚕ 3.15   **FUD** XXX   N 80 🖵

AMA: 2020,Sep,3; 2020,Feb,3; 2019,Jun,7; 2019,Jan,13; 2018,Oct,9; 2018,Jan,8; 2017,Jan,8; 2016,Jan,13; 2015,Jan,16

+ **99359** each additional 30 minutes (List separately in addition to code for prolonged service)

Code first (99358)

🚑 1.52   ⚕ 1.52   **FUD** ZZZ   N 80 🖵

AMA: 2020,Sep,3; 2020,Feb,3; 2019,Jun,7; 2019,Jan,13; 2018,Oct,9; 2018,Jan,8; 2017,Jan,8; 2016,Jan,13; 2015,Jan,16

99415-99417 [99415, 99416, 99417] Prolonged Clinical Staff Services Under Supervision

INCLUDES   Time spent by clinical staff providing prolonged face-to-face services extending beyond customary service under physician or other qualified health professional supervision
Time spent by clinical staff providing prolonged services on service date, even when time not continuous

EXCLUDES   *Prolonged service provided by physician or other qualified health care professional (99354-99355, [99417])*

▲ + # **99415** Prolonged clinical staff service (the service beyond the highest time in the range of total time of the service) during an evaluation and management service in the office or outpatient setting, direct patient contact with physician supervision; first hour (List separately in addition to code for outpatient Evaluation and Management service)

EXCLUDES   *Reporting code more than one time per service date*
Reporting code with ([99417])
Services less than 30 minutes
Services provided to more than two patients at same time
Code first (99202-99205, 99212-99215)

🚑 0.28   ⚕ 0.28   **FUD** ZZZ   N 80 TC 🖵

AMA: 2020,Sep,3; 2020,Feb,3; 2019,Oct,10; 2018,Jan,8; 2017,Jan,8; 2016,Mar,8; 2016,Feb,13; 2016,Jan,13; 2015,Oct,3

● New Code   ▲ Revised Code   ○ Reinstated   ● New Web Release   ▲ Revised Web Release   + Add-on   Unlisted   Not Covered   # Resequenced
50 Optum Mod 50 Exempt   ⊘ AMA Mod 51 Exempt   51 Optum Mod 51 Exempt   63 Mod 63 Exempt   ⊿ Non-FDA Drug   ★ Telemedicine   M Maternity   A Age Edit

▲ + # 99416

each additional 30 minutes (List separately in addition to code for prolonged service)

EXCLUDES *Reporting code with ([99417])*
Services less than 30 minutes, less than 15 minutes after first hour, or after final 30 minutes
Services provided to more than two patients at same time

Code first ([99415])

⚕ 0.13   ⚘ 0.13   **FUD** ZZZ   N 80 TC

AMA: 2020,Sep,3; 2020,Feb,3; 2019,Oct,10; 2018,Jan,8; 2017,Jan,8; 2016,Mar,8; 2016,Feb,13; 2016,Jan,13; 2015,Oct,3

● + # 99417

Prolonged office or other outpatient evaluation and management service(s) beyond the minimum required time of the primary procedure which has been selected using total time, requiring total time with or without direct patient contact beyond the usual service, on the date of the primary service, each 15 minutes of total time (List separately in addition to codes 99205, 99215 for office or other outpatient Evaluation and Management services)

INCLUDES *Total time prolonged services provided same date with both direct and indirect patient contact by physician or QHCP*

EXCLUDES *Services less than 15 minutes*

Code first (99205 or 99215)

⚕ 0.00   ⚘ 0.00   **FUD** 000   ★

99360 Standby Services

CMS: 100-04,11,40.1.3 Independent Attending Physician Services; 100-04,12,30.6.15.3 Standby Services; 100-04,12,30.6.4 Services Furnished Incident to Physician's Service

INCLUDES Services requested by physician or qualified health care professional that involve no direct patient contact
Total standby time for day

EXCLUDES *Delivery attendance (99464)*
Less than 30 minutes standby time
On-call services mandated by hospital (99026-99027)

Code also as appropriate (99460, 99465)

99360

Standby service, requiring prolonged attendance, each 30 minutes (eg, operative standby, standby for frozen section, for cesarean/high risk delivery, for monitoring EEG)

⚕ 1.75   ⚘ 1.75   **FUD** XXX   B ▫

AMA: 2018,Jan,8; 2017,Jan,8; 2016,Jan,13; 2015,Jan,16

99366-99368 Interdisciplinary Conferences

CMS: 100-04,11,40.1.3 Independent Attending Physician Services

INCLUDES Documentation conference participation, contribution, and recommendations
Face-to-face participation by minimum of three qualified people from different specialties or disciplines
Individual patient review from start to conclusion
Only participants who have performed face-to-face evaluations or direct treatment to patient within previous 60 days
Team conferences 30 minutes or more

EXCLUDES *Conferences less than 30 minutes (not reportable)*
More than one individual from same specialty at same encounter
Patient management services during same month as ([99439, 99490, 99491], 99487-99489)
Time spent record keeping or writing report

99366

Medical team conference with interdisciplinary team of health care professionals, face-to-face with patient and/or family, 30 minutes or more, participation by nonphysician qualified health care professional

EXCLUDES *Team conferences by physician with patient or family present, see appropriate E/M service code*

⚕ 1.19   ⚘ 1.21   **FUD** XXX   N ▫

AMA: 2018,Apr,9; 2018,Jan,8; 2017,Jan,8; 2016,Jan,13; 2015,Jan,16

99367

Medical team conference with interdisciplinary team of health care professionals, patient and/or family not present, 30 minutes or more; participation by physician

⚕ 1.60   ⚘ 1.60   **FUD** XXX   N ▫

AMA: 2019,Dec,14; 2018,Apr,9; 2018,Jan,8; 2017,Jan,8; 2016,Jan,13; 2015,Jan,16

99368

participation by nonphysician qualified health care professional

⚕ 1.04   ⚘ 1.04   **FUD** XXX   N ▫

AMA: 2018,Apr,9; 2018,Jan,8; 2017,Jan,8; 2016,Jan,13; 2015,Jan,16

99374-99380 Care Plan Oversight: Patient Under Care of HHA, Hospice, or Nursing Facility

CMS: 100-04,11,40.1.3 Independent Attending Physician Services; 100-04,12,180 Payment of Care Plan Oversight (CPO); 100-04,12,180.1 Billing for Care Plan Oversight (CPO); 100-04,12,30.6.4 Services Furnished Incident to Physician's Service

INCLUDES Analysis reports, diagnostic tests, treatment plans
Discussions with other health care providers, outside practice, involved in patient's care
Establishment and revisions to care plans within 30-day period
Payment to one physician per month for covered care plan oversight services (must be same one who signed plan of care)

EXCLUDES *Care plan oversight services provided in hospice agency (99377-99378)*
Care plan oversight services provided in assisted living, domiciliary care, or private residence, not under home health agency or hospice care (99339-99340)
Patient management services during same time frame as ([99421, 99422, 99423], 99441-99443, 98966-98968)
Routine postoperative care provided during global surgery period
Time discussing treatment with patient and/or caregivers

Code also office/outpatient visits, hospital, home, nursing facility, domiciliary, or non-face-to-face services

99374

Supervision of a patient under care of home health agency (patient not present) in home, domiciliary or equivalent environment (eg, Alzheimer's facility) requiring complex and multidisciplinary care modalities involving regular development and/or revision of care plans by that individual, review of subsequent reports of patient status, review of related laboratory and other studies, communication (including telephone calls) for purposes of assessment or care decisions with health care professional(s), family member(s), surrogate decision maker(s) (eg, legal guardian) and/or key caregiver(s) involved in patient's care, integration of new information into the medical treatment plan and/or adjustment of medical therapy, within a calendar month; 15-29 minutes

⚕ 1.60   ⚘ 1.96   **FUD** XXX   B ▫

AMA: 2019,Jan,6; 2018,Jan,8; 2017,Jan,8; 2016,Jan,13; 2015,Jan,16

99375

30 minutes or more

⚕ 2.53   ⚘ 2.96   **FUD** XXX   E ▫

AMA: 2019,Jan,6; 2018,Jan,8; 2017,Jan,8; 2016,Jan,13; 2015,Jan,16

99377

Supervision of a hospice patient (patient not present) requiring complex and multidisciplinary care modalities involving regular development and/or revision of care plans by that individual, review of subsequent reports of patient status, review of related laboratory and other studies, communication (including telephone calls) for purposes of assessment or care decisions with health care professional(s), family member(s), surrogate decision maker(s) (eg, legal guardian) and/or key caregiver(s) involved in patient's care, integration of new information into the medical treatment plan and/or adjustment of medical therapy, within a calendar month; 15-29 minutes

⚕ 1.60   ⚘ 1.96   **FUD** XXX   B ▫

AMA: 2019,Jan,6; 2018,Jan,8; 2017,Jan,8; 2016,Jan,13; 2015,Jan,16

99378

30 minutes or more

⚕ 2.50   ⚘ 2.94   **FUD** XXX   E ▫

AMA: 2019,Jan,6; 2018,Jan,8; 2017,Jan,8; 2016,Jan,13; 2015,Jan,16

26/TC PC/TC Only   A2-Z3 ASC Payment   50 Bilateral   ♂ Male Only   ♀ Female Only   ⚕ Facility RVU   ⚘ Non-Facility RVU   ▫ CCI   ✖ CLIA
FUD Follow-up Days   **CMS:** IOM   **AMA:** CPT Asst   A-Y OPPSI   80/80 Surg Assist Allowed / w/Doc   ▪ Lab Crosswalk   ▪ Radiology Crosswalk

99379 **Supervision of a nursing facility patient (patient not present) requiring complex and multidisciplinary care modalities involving regular development and/or revision of care plans by that individual, review of subsequent reports of patient status, review of related laboratory and other studies, communication (including telephone calls) for purposes of assessment or care decisions with health care professional(s), family member(s), surrogate decision maker(s) (eg, legal guardian) and/or key caregiver(s) involved in patient's care, integration of new information into the medical treatment plan and/or adjustment of medical therapy, within a calendar month; 15-29 minutes**
1.60 1.96 **FUD** XXX B
AMA: 2019,Jan,6; 2018,Jan,8; 2017,Jan,8; 2016,Jan,13; 2015,Jan,16

99380 **30 minutes or more**
2.53 2.96 **FUD** XXX B
AMA: 2019,Jan,6; 2018,Jan,8; 2017,Jan,8; 2016,Jan,13; 2015,Jan,16

99381-99397 Preventive Medicine Visits

CMS: 100-04,11,40.1.3 Independent Attending Physician Services; 100-04,12,30.6.2 Medically Necessary and Preventive Medicine Service on Same Date; 100-04,12,30.6.4 Services Furnished Incident to Physician's Service

INCLUDES Care for small problem or pre-existing condition that requires no extra work
New patients or established patients (99381-99387, 99391-99397)
Regular preventive care (e.g., well-child exams) for all age groups

EXCLUDES *Behavioral change interventions (99406-99409)*
Counseling/risk factor reduction interventions not provided with preventive medical examination (99401-99412)
Diagnostic tests and other procedures

Code also immunization counseling, administration, and product (90460-90461, 90471-90474, 90476-90749 [90620, 90621, 90625, 90630, 90644, 90672, 90673, 90674, 90750, 90756])
Code also significant, separately identifiable E/M service on same date for substantial problems requiring additional work using modifier 25 and (99202-99215)

99381 **Initial comprehensive preventive medicine evaluation and management of an individual including an age and gender appropriate history, examination, counseling/anticipatory guidance/risk factor reduction interventions, and the ordering of laboratory/diagnostic procedures, new patient; infant (age younger than 1 year)** A
2.19 3.13 **FUD** XXX E
AMA: 2018,Jan,8; 2017,Jan,8; 2016,Mar,8; 2016,Jan,13; 2015,Jan,16

99382 **early childhood (age 1 through 4 years)** A
2.32 3.28 **FUD** XXX E
AMA: 2018,Jan,8; 2017,Jan,8; 2016,Mar,8; 2016,Jan,13; 2015,Jan,16

99383 **late childhood (age 5 through 11 years)** A
2.46 3.41 **FUD** XXX E
AMA: 2018,Jan,8; 2017,Jan,8; 2016,Mar,8; 2016,Jan,13; 2015,Jan,16

99384 **adolescent (age 12 through 17 years)** A
2.88 3.85 **FUD** XXX E
AMA: 2018,Jan,8; 2017,Jan,8; 2016,Mar,8; 2016,Jan,13; 2015,Jan,12; 2015,Jan,16

99385 **18-39 years** A
2.76 3.72 **FUD** XXX E
AMA: 2018,Jan,8; 2017,Jan,8; 2016,Mar,8; 2016,Jan,13; 2015,Jan,12; 2015,Jan,16

99386 **40-64 years** A
3.36 4.32 **FUD** XXX E
AMA: 2018,Jan,8; 2017,Jan,8; 2016,Mar,8; 2016,Jan,13; 2015,Jan,12; 2015,Jan,16

99387 **65 years and older** A
3.67 4.72 **FUD** XXX E
AMA: 2018,Jan,8; 2017,Jan,8; 2016,Mar,8; 2016,Jan,13; 2015,Jan,16

99391 **Periodic comprehensive preventive medicine reevaluation and management of an individual including an age and gender appropriate history, examination, counseling/anticipatory guidance/risk factor reduction interventions, and the ordering of laboratory/diagnostic procedures, established patient; infant (age younger than 1 year)** A
1.98 2.82 **FUD** XXX E
AMA: 2018,Jan,8; 2017,Jan,8; 2016,Mar,8; 2016,Jan,13; 2015,Jan,16

99392 **early childhood (age 1 through 4 years)** A
2.17 3.01 **FUD** XXX E
AMA: 2018,Jan,8; 2017,Jan,8; 2016,Mar,8; 2016,Jan,13; 2015,Jan,16

99393 **late childhood (age 5 through 11 years)** A
2.17 3.00 **FUD** XXX E
AMA: 2018,Jan,8; 2017,Jan,8; 2016,Mar,8; 2016,Jan,13; 2015,Jan,16

99394 **adolescent (age 12 through 17 years)** A
2.46 3.29 **FUD** XXX E
AMA: 2018,Jan,8; 2017,Jan,8; 2016,Mar,8; 2016,Jan,13; 2015,Jan,12; 2015,Jan,16

99395 **18-39 years** A
2.53 3.36 **FUD** XXX E
AMA: 2018,Jan,8; 2017,Jan,8; 2016,Mar,8; 2016,Jan,13; 2015,Jan,16; 2015,Jan,12

99396 **40-64 years** A
2.74 3.58 **FUD** XXX E
AMA: 2018,Jan,8; 2017,Sep,11; 2017,Jan,8; 2016,Mar,8; 2016,Jan,13; 2015,Jan,12; 2015,Jan,16

99397 **65 years and older** A
2.93 3.87 **FUD** XXX E
AMA: 2018,Jan,8; 2017,Jan,8; 2016,Mar,8; 2016,Jan,13; 2015,Jan,16

99401-99423 [99415, 99416, 99417, 99421, 99422, 99423] Counseling Services: Risk Factor and Behavioral Change Modification

INCLUDES Face-to-face services for new and established patients based on 15- to 60-minute time increments
Health and behavioral services provided on same day (96156-96159 [96164, 96165, 96167, 96168, 96170, 96171])
Issues such as healthy diet, exercise, alcohol, and drug abuse
Services provided by physician or other qualified healthcare professional for promoting health and reducing illness and injury

EXCLUDES *Counseling and risk factor reduction interventions included in preventive medicine services (99381-99397)*
Counseling services provided to patient groups with existing symptoms or illness (99078)

Code also significant, separately identifiable E/M services when performed and append modifier 25 to service

99401 **Preventive medicine counseling and/or risk factor reduction intervention(s) provided to an individual (separate procedure); approximately 15 minutes**
0.70 1.10 **FUD** XXX E
AMA: 2020,Aug,3; 2018,Jan,8; 2017,Jan,8; 2016,Mar,8; 2016,Jan,13; 2015,Jan,16

99402 **approximately 30 minutes**
1.42 1.81 **FUD** XXX E
AMA: 2020,Aug,3; 2018,Jan,8; 2017,Jan,8; 2016,Mar,8; 2016,Jan,13; 2015,Jan,16

99403 **approximately 45 minutes**
2.12 2.51 **FUD** XXX E
AMA: 2020,Aug,3; 2018,Jan,8; 2017,Jan,8; 2016,Mar,8; 2016,Jan,13; 2015,Jan,16

99404 **approximately 60 minutes**
2.81 3.21 **FUD** XXX E
AMA: 2020,Aug,3; 2018,Jan,8; 2017,Jan,8; 2016,Mar,8; 2016,Jan,13; 2015,Jan,16

99406 **Smoking and tobacco use cessation counseling visit; intermediate, greater than 3 minutes up to 10 minutes**
Facility RVU 0.35 Non-Facility RVU 0.43 FUD XXX ★ S 80
AMA: 2020,Sep,14; 2020,Aug,3; 2018,Jan,8; 2017,Nov,3; 2017,Jan,8; 2016,Mar,8; 2016,Jan,13; 2015,Jan,16

99407 **intensive, greater than 10 minutes**
INCLUDES Services 11-14 minutes
Facility RVU 0.73 Non-Facility RVU 0.80 FUD XXX ★ S 80
AMA: 2020,Aug,3; 2018,Jan,8; 2017,Nov,3; 2017,Jan,8; 2016,Mar,8; 2016,Jan,13; 2015,Jan,16

99408 **Alcohol and/or substance (other than tobacco) abuse structured screening (eg, AUDIT, DAST), and brief intervention (SBI) services; 15 to 30 minutes**
INCLUDES Health risk assessment (96160-96161)
Services 15 minutes or more
Only initial screening and brief intervention
Facility RVU 0.94 Non-Facility RVU 1.01 FUD XXX ★ E
AMA: 2020,Aug,3; 2018,Jan,8; 2017,Nov,3; 2017,Jan,8; 2016,Nov,5; 2016,Mar,8; 2016,Jan,13; 2015,Jan,16

99409 **greater than 30 minutes**
INCLUDES Health risk assessment (96160-96161)
Only initial screening and brief intervention
Services 31 minutes or more
Facility RVU 1.88 Non-Facility RVU 1.95 FUD XXX ★ E
AMA: 2020,Aug,3; 2018,Jan,8; 2017,Nov,3; 2017,Jan,8; 2016,Nov,5; 2016,Mar,8; 2016,Jan,13; 2015,Jan,16

99411 **Preventive medicine counseling and/or risk factor reduction intervention(s) provided to individuals in a group setting (separate procedure); approximately 30 minutes**
Facility RVU 0.22 Non-Facility RVU 0.55 FUD XXX E
AMA: 2020,Aug,3; 2018,Jan,8; 2017,Jan,8; 2016,Mar,8; 2016,Jan,13; 2015,Jan,16

99412 **approximately 60 minutes**
Facility RVU 0.36 Non-Facility RVU 0.69 FUD XXX E
AMA: 2020,Aug,3; 2018,Jan,8; 2017,Jan,8; 2016,Mar,8; 2016,Jan,13; 2015,Jan,16

99415 **Resequenced code. See code following 99359.**

99416 **Resequenced code. See code following 99359.**

99421 **Resequenced code. See code following 99443.**

99422 **Resequenced code. See code following 99443.**

99423 **Resequenced code. See code following 99443.**

99429-99439 [99439] Other Preventive Medicine

99429 **Unlisted preventive medicine service**
Facility RVU 0.00 Non-Facility RVU 0.00 FUD XXX E
AMA: 2018,Jan,8; 2017,Jan,8; 2016,Mar,8; 2016,Jan,13; 2015,Jan,16

99439 **Resequenced code. See code following resequenced code 99490.**

99441-99443 Telephone Calls for Patient Management

CMS: 100-04,11,40.1.3 Independent Attending Physician Services

INCLUDES Care initiated by established patient or patient's guardian
Non-face-to-face E/M services provided by physician or other health care provider qualified to report E/M services
Related E/M services provided within:
Postoperative period
Seven days prior to service

EXCLUDES *Patient management services during same time frame as (99339-99340, 99374-99380, 99487-99489, 99495-99496, 93792-93793)*
Reporting codes more than one time for telephone and online services when reported within 7-day time period by same provider
Services provided by qualified nonphysician health care professional unable to report E/M codes (98966-98968)

99441 **Telephone evaluation and management service by a physician or other qualified health care professional who may report evaluation and management services provided to an established patient, parent, or guardian not originating from a related E/M service provided within the previous 7 days nor leading to an E/M service or procedure within the next 24 hours or soonest available appointment; 5-10 minutes of medical discussion**
Facility RVU 0.36 Non-Facility RVU 0.39 FUD XXX E 80
AMA: 2020,JulBULL,1; 2019,Mar,8; 2018,Mar,7; 2018,Jan,8; 2017,Jan,8; 2016,Jan,13; 2015,Jan,16

99442 **11-20 minutes of medical discussion**
Facility RVU 0.72 Non-Facility RVU 0.76 FUD XXX E 80
AMA: 2020,JulBULL,1; 2019,Mar,8; 2018,Mar,7; 2018,Jan,8; 2017,Jan,8; 2016,Jan,13; 2015,Jan,16

99443 **21-30 minutes of medical discussion**
Facility RVU 1.08 Non-Facility RVU 1.12 FUD XXX E 80
AMA: 2020,JulBULL,1; 2019,Mar,8; 2018,Mar,7; 2018,Jan,8; 2017,Jan,8; 2016,Jan,13; 2015,Jan,16

99421-99423 [99421, 99422, 99423] Digital Evaluation and Management Services

CMS: 100-04,11,40.1.3 Independent Attending Physician Services

INCLUDES Cumulative service time within seven-day time frame needed to evaluate, assess, and manage the patient:
Ordering tests
Prescription generation
Separate digital inquiry for new and unrelated problem
Subsequent communication digitally supported (i.e., email, online, telephone)
Digital service initiated by established patient

EXCLUDES *Clinical staff time*
Digital evaluation by qualified nonphysician health care professional (98970-98972)
Digital evaluation peformed with separately reportable E/M services during same time frame for new or established patient:
Inquiries related to previously completed procedure and within postoperative period
INR monitoring (93792-93793)
Office consultation (99241-99245)
Office or other outpatient visit (99202-99205, 99212-99215)
Patient management services (99339-99340, 99374-99380, [99091], 99487-99489)
Digital service less than 5 minutes
Reporting code more than one time in 7 days

\# **99421** **Online digital evaluation and management service, for an established patient, for up to 7 days, cumulative time during the 7 days; 5-10 minutes**
Facility RVU 0.37 Non-Facility RVU 0.43 FUD XXX 80
AMA: 2020,Jan,3

\# **99422** **11-20 minutes**
Facility RVU 0.76 Non-Facility RVU 0.86 FUD XXX 80
AMA: 2020,Jan,3

\# **99423** **21 or more minutes**
Facility RVU 1.21 Non-Facility RVU 1.39 FUD XXX 80
AMA: 2020,Jan,3

99446-99452 [99451, 99452] Online and Telephone Consultative Services

INCLUDES Multiple telephone and/or internet contact needed to complete consultation (e.g., test result(s) follow-up)
New or established patient with new problem or exacerbation existing problem and not seen within last 14 days
Review pertinent lab, imaging and/or pathology studies, medical records, medications

EXCLUDES *Any service less than 5 minutes*
Communication with family with or without patient present ([99421, 99422, 99423], 99441-99443, 98966-98967)
Transfer care only

99446 **Interprofessional telephone/Internet/electronic health record assessment and management service provided by a consultative physician, including a verbal and written report to the patient's treating/requesting physician or other qualified health care professional; 5-10 minutes of medical consultative discussion and review**

INCLUDES Verbal and written reports from consultant to requesting provider
EXCLUDES *Prolonged services without direct patient contact (99358-99359)*
Reporting code more than one time in 7 days
0.51 0.51 FUD XXX E 80
AMA: 2019,Jun,7; 2019,Jan,3; 2018,Jan,8; 2017,Jan,8; 2016,Jan,13; 2015,Jan,16

99447 **11-20 minutes of medical consultative discussion and review**

INCLUDES Verbal and written reports from consultant to requesting provider
EXCLUDES *Prolonged services without direct patient contact (99358-99359)*
Reporting code more than one time in 7 days
1.01 1.01 FUD XXX E 80
AMA: 2019,Jun,7; 2019,Jan,3; 2018,Jan,8; 2017,Jan,8; 2016,Jan,13; 2015,Jan,16

99448 **21-30 minutes of medical consultative discussion and review**

INCLUDES Verbal and written reports from consultant to requesting provider
EXCLUDES *Prolonged services without direct patient contact (99358-99359)*
Reporting code more than one time in 7 days
1.52 1.52 FUD XXX E 80
AMA: 2019,Jun,7; 2019,Jan,3; 2018,Jan,8; 2017,Jan,8; 2016,Jan,13; 2015,Jan,16

99449 **31 minutes or more of medical consultative discussion and review**

INCLUDES Verbal and written reports from consultant to requesting provider
EXCLUDES *Prolonged services without direct patient contact (99358-99359)*
Reporting code more than one time in 7 days
2.02 2.02 FUD XXX E 80
AMA: 2019,Jun,7; 2019,Jan,3; 2018,Jan,8; 2017,Jan,8; 2016,Jan,13; 2015,Jan,16

99451 **Interprofessional telephone/Internet/electronic health record assessment and management service provided by a consultative physician, including a written report to the patient's treating/requesting physician or other qualified health care professional, 5 minutes or more of medical consultative time**

INCLUDES Verbal and written reports from consultant to requesting provider
EXCLUDES *Prolonged services without direct patient contact (99358-99359)*
Reporting code more than one time in 7 days
1.04 1.04 FUD XXX 80
AMA: 2019,Jun,7; 2019,Jan,3

99452 **Interprofessional telephone/Internet/electronic health record referral service(s) provided by a treating/requesting physician or other qualified health care professional, 30 minutes**

INCLUDES Time preparing for referral, 16 to 30 minutes
EXCLUDES *Requesting physician's time 30 minutes over typical E/M service, patient not on site (99358-99359)*
Requesting physician's time 30 minutes over typical E/M service, patient on site (99354-99357)
Reporting code more than one time every 14 days
1.04 1.04 FUD XXX 80
AMA: 2020,Jun,3; 2019,Jun,7; 2019,Jan,3

99453-99474 [99091, 99453, 99454, 99473, 99474] Remote Monitoring/Collection Biological Data

99453 **Remote monitoring of physiologic parameter(s) (eg, weight, blood pressure, pulse oximetry, respiratory flow rate), initial; set-up and patient education on use of equipment**

INCLUDES 30-day period physiologic monitoring parameters such as weight, blood pressure, pulse oximetry
Services ordered by physician or other qualified healthcare professional
Services provided for each care episode (starts when monitoring begins and ends when treatment goals achieved)
Set-up and instructions for use
Treatment with device approved by FDA
EXCLUDES *Monitoring less than 16 days*
Reporting codes when services included in other monitoring services (e.g., 93296, 94760, 95250)
0.52 0.52 FUD XXX 80
AMA: 2020,Apr,5; 2019,Mar,10; 2019,Jan,3; 2019,Jan,6

99454 **device(s) supply with daily recording(s) or programmed alert(s) transmission, each 30 days**

INCLUDES 30-day period physiologic monitoring parameters such as weight, blood pressure, pulse oximetry
Service ordered by physician or other qualified healthcare professional
Supplying device
Treatment with device approved by FDA
EXCLUDES *Monitoring less than 16 days*
Remote monitoring treatment management
Reporting codes when services included in other monitoring services (e.g., 93296, 94760, 95250)
Self-measured blood pressure monitoring ([99473, 99474])
1.73 1.73 FUD XXX 80
AMA: 2020,Apr,5; 2019,Oct,3; 2019,Mar,10; 2019,Jan,3; 2019,Jan,6

99091 **Collection and interpretation of physiologic data (eg, ECG, blood pressure, glucose monitoring) digitally stored and/or transmitted by the patient and/or caregiver to the physician or other qualified health care professional, qualified by education, training, licensure/regulation (when applicable) requiring a minimum of 30 minutes of time, each 30 days**

INCLUDES E/M services provided on same service date
EXCLUDES *Care plan oversight services within same calendar month (99339-99340, 99374-99380)*
Chronic care management services within same calendar month ([99491])
Data transfer/interpretation from clinical lab or hospital computers
Remote physiologic monitoring treatment management within same calendar month ([99457])
Reporting code more than one time in 30 days
Reporting codes when services included in other monitoring services such as (93227, 93272, 95250)
Services for which more specific codes exist, such as:
Ambulatory continuous glucose monitoring (95250)
Electrocardiographic services (93227, 93272)
1.62 1.62 FUD XXX N 80
AMA: 2020,Apr,5; 2020,Feb,7; 2019,Oct,3; 2019,Jun,3; 2019,Jan,6; 2018,Dec,10; 2018,Dec,10; 2018,Jun,6; 2018,Mar,5; 2018,Feb,7; 2018,Jan,8; 2017,Jan,8; 2016,Jan,13; 2015,Jan,16

99473 **Self-measured blood pressure using a device validated for clinical accuracy; patient education/training and device calibration**

EXCLUDES *Reporting code more than once per device*
Reporting codes when services included in same calendar month as:
Ambulatory blood pressure monitoring (93784-93790)
Chronic care management service ([99439, 99490, 99491], 99487-99489)
Remote physiologic monitoring, collection and interpretation ([99453, 99454], [99091], [99457])

0.31 0.31 FUD XXX 80

AMA: 2020,Apr,5; 2020,Feb,7; 2020,Jan,3

99474 **separate self-measurements of two readings one minute apart, twice daily over a 30-day period (minimum of 12 readings), collection of data reported by the patient and/or caregiver to the physician or other qualified health care professional, with report of average systolic and diastolic pressures and subsequent communication of a treatment plan to the patient**

EXCLUDES *Reporting code more than once per device*
Reporting codes when services included in same calendar month as:
Ambulatory blood pressure monitoring (93784-93790)
Chronic care management services ([99439, 99490, 99491], 99487-99489)
Remote physiologic monitoring, collection and interpretation services ([99453, 99454], [99091], [99457])

0.25 0.42 FUD XXX 80

AMA: 2020,Apr,5; 2020,Feb,7; 2020,Jan,3

99457-99458 [99457, 99458] Remote Monitoring Management

CMS: 100-04,11,40.1.3 Independent Attending Physician Services

INCLUDES Interactive live communication with patient at least 20 minutes per month
Remote monitoring results used for patient management
Reporting code each 30 days no matter number parameters monitored
Service ordered by physician or other qualified healthcare professional
Time managing care when more specific service codes not available
Treatment with device approved by FDA

EXCLUDES *Reporting code for services lasting less than 20 mintues*
Reporting code on same service date as E/M services (99202-99215, 99221-99223, 99231-99233, 99251-99255, 99324-99328, 99334-99337, 99341-99350)

Code also, when appropriate:
Behavioral health integration services ([99484], 99492-99494)
Chronic care management services ([99439], [99490], [99491], 99487, 99489)
Transitional care management services (99495-99496)

99457 **Remote physiologic monitoring treatment management services, clinical staff/physician/other qualified health care professional time in a calendar month requiring interactive communication with the patient/caregiver during the month; first 20 minutes**

EXCLUDES *Collection and interpretation physiologic data ([99091])*

0.90 1.43 FUD XXX 80

AMA: 2020,Apr,5; 2020,Feb,7; 2019,Jun,3; 2019,Jan,3; 2019,Jan,6

+ # 99458 **each additional 20 minutes (List separately in addition to code for primary procedure)**

EXCLUDES *Reporting code when 20 minutes additional treatment time not obtained ([99457])*

Code first ([99457])

0.91 1.17 FUD ZZZ 80

AMA: 2020,Feb,7

99450-99458 [99451, 99452, 99453, 99454, 99457, 99458] Life/Disability Insurance Eligibility Visits

INCLUDES Assessment services for insurance eligibility and work-related disability without medical management of the patient's illness/injury
Services provided to new/established patients at any site of service

EXCLUDES *Any additional E&M services or procedures performed on the same date of service: report with appropriate code*

99450 **Basic life and/or disability examination that includes: Measurement of height, weight, and blood pressure; Completion of a medical history following a life insurance pro forma; Collection of blood sample and/or urinalysis complying with "chain of custody" protocols; and Completion of necessary documentation/certificates.**

0.00 0.00 FUD XXX E

AMA: 2019,Jun,7; 2018,Jan,8; 2017,Jan,8; 2016,Jan,13; 2015,Jan,16

99451 **Resequenced code. See code following 99449.**

99452 **Resequenced code. See code following 99449.**

99453 **Resequenced code. See code following 99449.**

99454 **Resequenced code. See code following 99449.**

99455 **Work related or medical disability examination by the treating physician that includes: Completion of a medical history commensurate with the patient's condition; Performance of an examination commensurate with the patient's condition; Formulation of a diagnosis, assessment of capabilities and stability, and calculation of impairment; Development of future medical treatment plan; and Completion of necessary documentation/certificates and report.**

INCLUDES Special reports (99080)

0.00 0.00 FUD XXX B 80

AMA: 2018,Jan,8; 2017,Jan,8; 2016,Jan,13; 2015,Jan,16

99456 **Work related or medical disability examination by other than the treating physician that includes: Completion of a medical history commensurate with the patient's condition; Performance of an examination commensurate with the patient's condition; Formulation of a diagnosis, assessment of capabilities and stability, and calculation of impairment; Development of future medical treatment plan; and Completion of necessary documentation/certificates and report.**

INCLUDES Special reports (99080)

0.00 0.00 FUD XXX B 80

AMA: 2018,Jan,8; 2017,Jan,8; 2016,Jan,13; 2015,Jan,16

99457 **Resequenced code. See code before resequenced code 99474.**

99458 **Resequenced code. See code before 99450.**

99460-99463 Evaluation and Management Services for Age 28 Days or Less

CMS: 100-04,12,30.6.4 Services Furnished Incident to Physician's Service

INCLUDES Family consultation
Healthy newborn history and physical
Medical record documentation
Ordering diagnostic test and treatments
Services provided to healthy newborns age 28 days or younger

EXCLUDES *Neonatal intensive and critical care services (99466-99469 [99485, 99486], 99477-99480)*
Newborn follow-up services in office or outpatient setting (99202-99215, 99381, 99391)
Newborn hospital discharge services when provided on date subsequent to admission (99238-99239)
Nonroutine neonatal inpatient evaluation and management services (99221-99233)

Code also attendance at delivery (99464)
Code also circumcision (54150)
Code also emergency resuscitation services (99465)

99460 **Initial hospital or birthing center care, per day, for evaluation and management of normal newborn infant** A

2.70 2.70 FUD XXX V 80

AMA: 2018,Jan,8; 2017,Jan,8; 2016,Jan,13; 2015,Jan,16

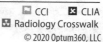

99461 **Initial care, per day, for evaluation and management of normal newborn infant seen in other than hospital or birthing center** Ⓐ
1.78 2.57 FUD XXX M 80
AMA: 2018,Jan,8; 2017,Jan,8; 2016,Jan,13; 2015,Jan,16

99462 **Subsequent hospital care, per day, for evaluation and management of normal newborn** Ⓐ
1.19 1.19 FUD XXX C 80
AMA: 2018,Jan,8; 2017,Jan,8; 2016,Jan,13; 2015,Jan,16

99463 **Initial hospital or birthing center care, per day, for evaluation and management of normal newborn infant admitted and discharged on the same date** Ⓐ
3.13 3.13 FUD XXX V 80
AMA: 2018,Jan,8; 2017,Jan,8; 2016,Jan,13; 2015,Jan,16

99464-99465 Newborn Delivery Attendance/Resuscitation

CMS: 100-04,12,30.6.4 Services Furnished Incident to Physician's Service

99464 **Attendance at delivery (when requested by the delivering physician or other qualified health care professional) and initial stabilization of newborn** Ⓐ
EXCLUDES *Resuscitation at delivery (99465)*
2.12 2.12 FUD XXX N 80
AMA: 2018,Jan,8; 2017,Jan,8; 2016,Jan,13; 2015,Jan,16

99465 **Delivery/birthing room resuscitation, provision of positive pressure ventilation and/or chest compressions in the presence of acute inadequate ventilation and/or cardiac output** Ⓐ
EXCLUDES *Attendance at delivery (99464)*
Code also any necessary procedures performed as resuscitation component
4.13 4.13 FUD XXX S 80
AMA: 2018,Jan,8; 2017,Jan,8; 2016,Jan,13; 2015,Jan,16

99466-99467 Critical Care Transport Age 24 Months or Younger

CMS: 100-04,12,30.6.4 Services Furnished Incident to Physician's Service

INCLUDES Face-to-face care starting when physician assumes patient responsibility at referring facility until receiving facility accepts patient
Physician presence during interfacility transfer critically ill/injured patient age 24 months or younger
Services provided by physician during transport:
- Blood gases
- Chest x-rays (71045-71046)
- Data stored in computers (e.g., ECGs, blood pressures, hematologic data)
- Gastric intubation (43752-43753)
- Interpretation cardiac output measurements (93562)
- Pulse oximetry (94760-94762)
- Routine monitoring:
  - Heart rate
  - Respiratory rate
- Temporary transcutaneous pacing (92953)
- Vascular access procedures (36000, 36400, 36405-36406, 36415, 36591, 36600)
- Ventilatory management (94002-94003, 94660, 94662)

EXCLUDES *Neonatal hypothermia (99184)*
Patient critical care transport services with personal patient contact less than 30 minutes
Physician directed emergency care via two-way voice communication with transporting staff (99288, [99485, 99486])
Physician services directing transport (control physician) ([99485, 99486])
Services less than 30 minutes in duration (see E/M codes)

Code also any services not designated as included in critical care transport service

99466 **Critical care face-to-face services, during an interfacility transport of critically ill or critically injured pediatric patient, 24 months of age or younger; first 30-74 minutes of hands-on care during transport** Ⓐ
6.75 6.75 FUD XXX N 80
AMA: 2018,Jun,9; 2018,Jan,8; 2017,Jan,8; 2016,Jan,13; 2015,Jan,16

\+ **99467** **each additional 30 minutes (List separately in addition to code for primary service)** Ⓐ
Code first (99466)
3.38 3.38 FUD ZZZ N 80
AMA: 2018,Jun,9; 2018,Jan,8; 2017,Jan,8; 2016,Jan,13; 2015,Jan,16

99485-99486 [99485, 99486] Critical Care Transport Supervision Age 24 Months or Younger

INCLUDES Advice for treatment to transport team from control physician
Non face-to-face care starts with first contact by control physician with transport team and ends when patient responsibility assumed by receiving facility

EXCLUDES *Emergency systems physician direction for pediatric patient older than 24 months (99288)*
Services less than 15 minutes
Services performed by control physician for same time period
Services performed by same physician providing critical care transport (99466-99467)
Services provided by transport team

\# **99485** **Supervision by a control physician of interfacility transport care of the critically ill or critically injured pediatric patient, 24 months of age or younger, includes two-way communication with transport team before transport, at the referring facility and during the transport, including data interpretation and report; first 30 minutes** Ⓐ
2.17 2.17 FUD XXX B
AMA: 2018,Jun,9; 2018,Jan,8; 2017,Jan,8; 2016,Jan,13; 2015,Jan,16

\+ # **99486** **each additional 30 minutes (List separately in addition to code for primary procedure)** Ⓐ
Code first ([99485])
1.88 1.88 FUD XXX B
AMA: 2018,Jun,9; 2018,Jan,8; 2017,Jan,8; 2016,Jan,13; 2015,Jan,16

Evaluation and Management
99461 — 99486

99468-99476 [99473, 99474] Critical Care Age 5 Years or Younger

CMS: 100-04,12,30.6.4 Services Furnished Incident to Physician's Service

INCLUDES All services included in codes 99291-99292 as well as (which may be reported by facilities only):
- Administration blood/blood components (36430, 36440)
- Administration intravenous fluids (96360-96361)
- Administration surfactant (94610)
- Bladder aspiration, suprapubic (51100)
- Bladder catheterization (51701, 51702)
- Car seat evaluation (94780-94781)
- Catheterization umbilical artery (36660)
- Catheterization umbilical vein (36510)
- Central venous catheter, centrally inserted (36555)
- Endotracheal intubation (31500)
- Lumbar puncture (62270)
- Oral or nasogastric tube placement (43752)
- Pulmonary function testing, performed at bedside (94375)
- Pulse or ear oximetry (94760-94762)
- Vascular access, arteries (36140, 36620)
- Vascular access, venous (36400-36406, 36420, 36600)
- Ventilatory management (94002-94004, 94660)

Initial and subsequent care provided to critically ill infant or child
Other hospital care or intensive care services by same group or individual done on same day patient transferred to initial neonatal/pediatric critical care
Readmission to critical unit on same day or during same stay (subsequent care)

EXCLUDES *Critical care services for patients age six years or older (99291-99292)*
Critical care services provided by second physician or different physician specialty (99291-99292)
Interfacility transport services by same or different individual, same or different specialty or group, on same service date (99466-99467, [99485, 99486])
Neonatal hypothermia (99184)
Services performed by individual in another group receiving patient transferred to lower care level (99231-99233, 99478-99480)
Services performed by individual transferring patient to lower care level (99231-99233, 99291-99292)
Services performed by same or different individual in same group on same day (99291-99292)
Services performed by transferring individual prior to patient transfer to individual in different group (99221-99233, 99291-99292, 99460-99462, 99477-99480)

Code also normal newborn care when done on same day by same group or individual providing critical care. Report modifier 25 with initial critical care code (99460-99462)

99468 **Initial inpatient neonatal critical care, per day, for the evaluation and management of a critically ill neonate, 28 days of age or younger** A
26.0 26.0 FUD XXX C 80
AMA: 2018,Dec,8; 2018,Dec,8; 2018,Jun,9; 2018,Jan,8; 2017,Jan,8; 2016,May,3; 2016,Jan,13; 2015,Oct,8; 2015,Jul,3; 2015,Feb,10; 2015,Jan,16

99469 **Subsequent inpatient neonatal critical care, per day, for the evaluation and management of a critically ill neonate, 28 days of age or younger** A
11.2 11.2 FUD XXX C 80
AMA: 2018,Dec,8; 2018,Dec,8; 2018,Jun,9; 2018,Jan,8; 2017,Jan,8; 2016,May,3; 2016,Jan,13; 2015,Oct,8; 2015,Jul,3; 2015,Feb,10; 2015,Jan,16

99471 **Initial inpatient pediatric critical care, per day, for the evaluation and management of a critically ill infant or young child, 29 days through 24 months of age** A
22.5 22.5 FUD XXX C 80
AMA: 2018,Dec,8; 2018,Dec,8; 2018,Jun,9; 2018,Jan,8; 2017,Jan,8; 2016,May,3; 2016,Jan,13; 2015,Jul,3; 2015,Feb,10; 2015,Jan,16

99472 **Subsequent inpatient pediatric critical care, per day, for the evaluation and management of a critically ill infant or young child, 29 days through 24 months of age** A
11.5 11.5 FUD XXX C 80
AMA: 2018,Dec,8; 2018,Dec,8; 2018,Jun,9; 2018,Jan,8; 2017,Jan,8; 2016,May,3; 2016,Jan,13; 2015,Jul,3; 2015,Feb,10; 2015,Jan,16

99473 **Resequenced code. See code before 99450.**

99474 **Resequenced code. See code before 99450.**

99475 **Initial inpatient pediatric critical care, per day, for the evaluation and management of a critically ill infant or young child, 2 through 5 years of age** A
15.8 15.8 FUD XXX C 80
AMA: 2018,Dec,8; 2018,Dec,8; 2018,Jun,9; 2018,Jan,8; 2017,Jan,8; 2016,May,3; 2016,Jan,13; 2015,Jul,3; 2015,Feb,10; 2015,Jan,16

99476 **Subsequent inpatient pediatric critical care, per day, for the evaluation and management of a critically ill infant or young child, 2 through 5 years of age** A
9.86 9.86 FUD XXX C 80
AMA: 2018,Dec,8; 2018,Dec,8; 2018,Jun,9; 2018,Jan,8; 2017,Jan,8; 2016,May,3; 2016,Jan,13; 2015,Jul,3; 2015,Feb,10; 2015,Jan,16

99477-99480 Initial Inpatient Neonatal Intensive Care and Other Services

CMS: 100-04,12,30.6.4 Services Furnished Incident to Physician's Service

INCLUDES All services included in codes 99291-99292 as well as (which may be reported by facilities only):
- Adjustments to enteral and/or parenteral nutrition
- Airway and ventilator management (31500, 94002-94004, 94375, 94610, 94660)
- Bladder catheterization (51701-51702)
- Blood transfusion (36430, 36440)
- Car seat evaluation (94780-94781)
- Constant and/or frequent monitoring vital signs
- Continuous observation by the healthcare team
- Heat maintenance
- Intensive cardiac or respiratory monitoring
- Oral or nasogastric tube insertion (43752)
- Oxygen saturation (94760-94762)
- Spinal puncture (62270)
- Suprapubic catheterization (51100)
- Vascular access procedures (36000, 36140, 36400, 36405-36406, 36420, 36510, 36555, 36600, 36620, 36660)

EXCLUDES *Critical care services for patient transferred after initial or subsequent intensive care provided (99291-99292)*
Initial day intensive care provided by transferring individual same day neonate/infant transferred to lower care level (99477)
Inpatient neonatal/pediatric critical care services received on same day (99468-99476)
Necessary resuscitation services done as delivery care component prior to admission
Neonatal hypothermia (99184)
Services provided by receiving individual when patient transferred for critical care (99468-99476)
Services for receiving provider when patient improves after initial day and transferred to lower care level (99231-99233, 99478-99480)
Subsequent care sick neonate, under age 28 days, more than 5000 grams, not requiring critical or intensive care services (99231-99233)

Code also care provided by receiving individual when patient transferred to individual in different group (99231-99233, 99462)
Code also initial neonatal intensive care service when physician or other qualified health care professional present for delivery and/or neonate requires resuscitation (99464-99465); append modifier 25 to (99477)

99477 **Initial hospital care, per day, for the evaluation and management of the neonate, 28 days of age or younger, who requires intensive observation, frequent interventions, and other intensive care services** A
EXCLUDES *Initiation care critically ill neonate (99468)*
Initiation inpatient care normal newborn (99460)
9.85 9.85 FUD XXX C 80
AMA: 2018,Dec,8; 2018,Dec,8; 2018,Jan,8; 2017,Jan,8; 2016,Jan,13; 2015,Jul,3; 2015,Jan,16

99478 **Subsequent intensive care, per day, for the evaluation and management of the recovering very low birth weight infant (present body weight less than 1500 grams)** A
3.87 3.87 FUD XXX C 80
AMA: 2018,Dec,8; 2018,Dec,8; 2018,Jun,11; 2018,Jan,8; 2017,Jan,8; 2016,Jan,13; 2015,Jul,3; 2015,Jan,16

99479 **Subsequent intensive care, per day, for the evaluation and management of the recovering low birth weight infant (present body weight of 1500-2500 grams)** A

3.52 3.52 FUD XXX C 80

AMA: 2018,Dec,8; 2018,Dec,8; 2018,Jun,11; 2018,Jan,8; 2017,Jan,8; 2016,Jan,13; 2015,Jul,3; 2015,Jan,16

99480 **Subsequent intensive care, per day, for the evaluation and management of the recovering infant (present body weight of 2501-5000 grams)** A

3.37 3.37 FUD XXX C 80

AMA: 2018,Dec,8; 2018,Dec,8; 2018,Jun,11; 2018,Jan,8; 2017,Jan,8; 2016,Jan,13; 2015,Jul,3; 2015,Jan,16

99483-99486 [99484, 99485, 99486] Cognitive Impairment Services

INCLUDES Assessment and care plan services during same time frame as:
- E/M services (99202-99215, 99241-99245, 99324-99337, 99341-99350, 99366-99368, 99497-99498)
- Medication management (99605-99607)
- Need for services evaluation (e.g., legal, financial, meals, personal care)
- Patient and caregiver focused risk assessment (96160-96161)
- Psychiatric and psychological services (90785, 90791-90792, [96127])
- Psychological or neuropsychological tests (96146)

Consideration other conditions that may cause cognitive impairment (e.g., infection, hydrocephalus, stroke, medications)

Evaluation and care plans for new or existing patients with cognitive impairment symptoms

EXCLUDES *Reporting code more than one time per 180-day period*

99483 **Assessment of and care planning for a patient with cognitive impairment, requiring an independent historian, in the office or other outpatient, home or domiciliary or rest home, with all of the following required elements: Cognition-focused evaluation including a pertinent history and examination; Medical decision making of moderate or high complexity; Functional assessment (eg, basic and instrumental activities of daily living), including decision-making capacity; Use of standardized instruments for staging of dementia (eg, functional assessment staging test [FAST], clinical dementia rating [CDR]); Medication reconciliation and review for high-risk medications; Evaluation for neuropsychiatric and behavioral symptoms, including depression, including use of standardized screening instrument(s); Evaluation of safety (eg, home), including motor vehicle operation; Identification of caregiver(s), caregiver knowledge, caregiver needs, social supports, and the willingness of caregiver to take on caregiving tasks; Development, updating or revision, or review of an Advance Care Plan; Creation of a written care plan, including initial plans to address any neuropsychiatric symptoms, neuro-cognitive symptoms, functional limitations, and referral to community resources as needed (eg, rehabilitation services, adult day programs, support groups) shared with the patient and/or caregiver with initial education and support. Typically, 50 minutes are spent face-to-face with the patient and/or family or caregiver.**

5.12 7.35 FUD XXX S 80

AMA: 2020,Sep,3; 2018,Jul,12; 2018,Apr,9; 2018,Jan,8

99484 **Resequenced code. See code before 99450.**

99485 **Resequenced code. See code following 99467.**

99486 **Resequenced code. See code following 99467.**

99490-99491 [99439, 99490, 99491] Coordination of Services for Chronic Care

CMS: 100-02,13,230.2 Chronic Care Management and General Behavioral Health Integration Services; 100-04,11,40.1.3 Independent Attending Physician Services

INCLUDES Case management services provided to patients that:
- Have two or more conditions anticipated to endure more than 12 months or until patient's death
- High risk that conditions will result in decompensation, deterioration, or death
- Require at least 20 minutes staff time monthly

EXCLUDES *Patient management services during same time frame as (99339-99340, 99374-99380, 99487-99489, 90951-90970, 99605-99607)*

Service time reported with (99358-99359, 99366-99368, [99421, 99422, 99423], 99441-99443, [99091], [99484], 99492-99494, 93792-93793, 98960-98962, 98966-98968, 99071, 99078, 99080)

▲ # **99490** **Chronic care management services with the following required elements: multiple (two or more) chronic conditions expected to last at least 12 months, or until the death of the patient, chronic conditions place the patient at significant risk of death, acute exacerbation/decompensation, or functional decline, comprehensive care plan established, implemented, revised, or monitored; first 20 minutes of clinical staff time directed by a physician or other qualified health care professional, per calendar month.**

EXCLUDES *Chronic care management provided personally by physician or other qualified health care professional ([99491])*

Reporting code more than once per calendar month

Qualified nonphysician health care professional online digital assessment and management (98970-98972)

0.90 1.17 FUD XXX S 80

AMA: 2020,Apr,5; 2020,Feb,7; 2019,Jan,6; 2018,Oct,9; 2018,Jul,12; 2018,Apr,9; 2018,Mar,7; 2018,Mar,5; 2018,Feb,7; 2018,Jan,8; 2017,Jan,8; 2016,Jan,13; 2015,Feb,3; 2015,Jan,16

● + # **99439** **Chronic care management services with the following required elements: multiple (two or more) chronic conditions expected to last at least 12 months, or until the death of the patient, chronic conditions place the patient at significant risk of death, acute exacerbation/decompensation, or functional decline, comprehensive care plan established, implemented, revised, or monitored; each additional 20 minutes of clinical staff time directed by a physician or other qualified health care professional, per calendar month (List separately in addition to code for primary procedure)**

EXCLUDES *Reporting code more than twice per calendar month*

Qualified nonphysician health care professional online digital assessment and management (98970-98972)

Code first ([99490])

0.00 0.00 FUD 000

99491 **Chronic care management services, provided personally by a physician or other qualified health care professional, at least 30 minutes of physician or other qualified health care professional time, per calendar month, with the following required elements: multiple (two or more) chronic conditions expected to last at least 12 months, or until the death of the patient; chronic conditions place the patient at significant risk of death, acute exacerbation/decompensation, or functional decline; comprehensive care plan established, implemented, revised, or monitored**

EXCLUDES *Chronic care management provided by medically directed clinical staff only ([99439], [99490])*

Reporting code more than once per calendar month

Transitional care management services (99495-99496)

2.33 2.33 FUD XXX 80

AMA: 2020,Apr,5

99487-99491 [99490, 99491] Coordination of Complex Services for Chronic Care

INCLUDES All clinical non-face-to-face time with patient, family, and caregivers
Only services given by physician or other qualified health caregiver who has care coordination role for patient for month
Patient management services during same time frame as (99339-99340, 99374-99380, [99439, 99490, 99491], 90951-90970, 99605-99607)
Service time reported with (99358-99359, 99366-99368, [99421, 99422, 99423], 99441-99443, [99091], 93792-93793, 98960-98962, 98966-98972, 99071, 99078, 99080, 99605-99607)
Services provided to patients in rest home, domiciliary, assisted living facility, or at home including:
Caregiver education to family or patient, addressing independent living and self-management
Communication with patient and all caregivers and professionals regarding care
Determining which community and health resources benefit patient
Developing and maintaining care plan
Facilitation services and care
Health outcomes data and registry documentation
Providing communication with home health and other patient utilized services
Support for treatment and medication adherence
Services that address activities daily living, psychosocial, and medical needs

EXCLUDES *E/M services by same/different individual during care management services time frame*
Psychiatric collaborative care management (99484, 99492-99494)

▲ **99487** **Complex chronic care management services with the following required elements: multiple (two or more) chronic conditions expected to last at least 12 months, or until the death of the patient, chronic conditions place the patient at significant risk of death, acute exacerbation/decompensation, or functional decline, comprehensive care plan established, implemented, revised, or monitored, moderate or high complexity medical decision making; first 60 minutes of clinical staff time directed by a physician or other qualified health care professional, per calendar month.**

INCLUDES Clinical services, 60 to 74 minutes, during calendar month
1.47 2.58 **FUD** XXX S 80
AMA: 2020,Apr,5; 2020,Feb,7; 2019,Jan,6; 2018,Oct,9; 2018,Jul,12; 2018,Apr,9; 2018,Mar,7; 2018,Mar,5; 2018,Feb,7; 2018,Jan,8; 2017,Apr,9; 2017,Jan,8; 2016,Jan,13; 2015,Jan,16

▲ + **99489** **each additional 30 minutes of clinical staff time directed by a physician or other qualified health care professional, per calendar month (List separately in addition to code for primary procedure)**

EXCLUDES *Clinical services less than 30 minutes beyond initial 60 minutes, per calendar month*
Code first (99487)
0.74 1.29 **FUD** ZZZ N 80
AMA: 2020,Apr,5; 2020,Feb,7; 2019,Jan,6; 2018,Oct,9; 2018,Jul,12; 2018,Apr,9; 2018,Mar,7; 2018,Mar,5; 2018,Feb,7; 2018,Jan,8; 2017,Apr,9; 2017,Jan,8; 2016,Jan,13; 2015,Jan,16

99490 **Resequenced code. See code before 99487.**

99491 **Resequenced code. See code before 99487.**

99492-99494 Psychiatric Collaborative Care

CMS: 100-02,13,230.2 Chronic Care Management and General Behavioral Health Integration Services

INCLUDES Services provided during calendar month by physician or other qualified healthcare profession for patients with psychiatric diagnosis
Assessment behavioral health status
Creation and care plan revision
Treatment provided during care episode during which goals may be met, not achieved, or lack of services during six-month period

EXCLUDES *Additional services provided by behavioral health care manager during same calendar month period (do not count as time for 99492-99494):*
Psychiatric evaluation (90791-90792)
Psychotherapy (99406-99407, 99408-99409, 90832-90834, 90836-90838, 90839-90840, 90846-90847, 90849, 90853)
Services provided by psychiatric consultant (do not count as time for 99492-99494): (E/M services) and psychiatric evaluation (90791-90792)

99492 **Initial psychiatric collaborative care management, first 70 minutes in the first calendar month of behavioral health care manager activities, in consultation with a psychiatric consultant, and directed by the treating physician or other qualified health care professional, with the following required elements: outreach to and engagement in treatment of a patient directed by the treating physician or other qualified health care professional; initial assessment of the patient, including administration of validated rating scales, with the development of an individualized treatment plan; review by the psychiatric consultant with modifications of the plan if recommended; entering patient in a registry and tracking patient follow-up and progress using the registry, with appropriate documentation, and participation in weekly caseload consultation with the psychiatric consultant; and provision of brief interventions using evidence-based techniques such as behavioral activation, motivational interviewing, and other focused treatment strategies.**

EXCLUDES *Services less than 36 minutes*
Subsequent collaborative care managment in same calendar month (99493)
2.50 4.35 **FUD** XXX S 80
AMA: 2020,Feb,7; 2019,Jan,6; 2018,Jul,12; 2018,Mar,5; 2018,Feb,7; 2018,Jan,8; 2017,Nov,3

99493 **Subsequent psychiatric collaborative care management, first 60 minutes in a subsequent month of behavioral health care manager activities, in consultation with a psychiatric consultant, and directed by the treating physician or other qualified health care professional, with the following required elements: tracking patient follow-up and progress using the registry, with appropriate documentation; participation in weekly caseload consultation with the psychiatric consultant; ongoing collaboration with and coordination of the patient's mental health care with the treating physician or other qualified health care professional and any other treating mental health providers; additional review of progress and recommendations for changes in treatment, as indicated, including medications, based on recommendations provided by the psychiatric consultant; provision of brief interventions using evidence-based techniques such as behavioral activation, motivational interviewing, and other focused treatment strategies; monitoring of patient outcomes using validated rating scales; and relapse prevention planning with patients as they achieve remission of symptoms and/or other treatment goals and are prepared for discharge from active treatment.**

EXCLUDES *Initial collaborative care managment in same calendar month (99492)*
2.25 3.50 **FUD** XXX S 80
AMA: 2020,Feb,7; 2019,Jan,6; 2018,Jul,12; 2018,Mar,5; 2018,Feb,7; 2018,Jan,8; 2017,Nov,3

\+ **99494** **Initial or subsequent psychiatric collaborative care management, each additional 30 minutes in a calendar month of behavioral health care manager activities, in consultation with a psychiatric consultant, and directed by the treating physician or other qualified health care professional (List separately in addition to code for primary procedure)**

INCLUDES Coordination care with emergency department staff

Code first (99492, 99493)

1.20 1.77 **FUD** ZZZ N 80

AMA: 2020,Feb,7; 2019,Jan,6; 2018,Jul,12; 2018,Mar,5; 2018,Feb,7; 2018,Jan,8; 2017,Nov,3

99495-99496 Management of Transitional Care Services

CMS: 100-02,13,230.1 Transitional Care Management Services; 100-04,11,40.1.3 Independent Attending Physician Services; 100-04,12,190.3 List of Telehealth Services

INCLUDES First interaction (face-to-face, by telephone, or electronic) with patient or his/her caregiver and must be done within two working days from discharge
- Initial face-to-face; must be done within code time frame and include medication management
- New or established patient with moderate to high complexity medical decision making needs during care transitions
- Patient management services during same time frame as (99339-99340, 99358-99359, 99366-99368, 99374-99380, 99441-99443, [99091], 99487-99489, 90951-90970, 93792-93793, 98960-98962, 98966-98968, 99071, 99078, 99080, 99605-99607)
- Services from discharge day up to 29 days post discharge
- Subsequent discharge within 30 days
- Without face-to-face patient care given by physician or other qualified health care professional includes:
  - Contacting qualified health care professionals for specific patient problems
  - Discharge information review
  - Follow-up and referral arrangements with community resources and providers
  - Need for follow-up care review based on tests and treatments
  - Patient, family, and caregiver education
- Without face-to-face patient care given by staff under physician guidance or other qualified health care professional includes:
  - Caregiver education to family or patient, addressing independent living and self-management
  - Communication with patient and all caregivers and professionals regarding care
  - Determining which community and health resources benefit patient
  - Facilitation services and care
  - Providing communication with home health and other patient utilized services
  - Support for treatment and medication adherence

EXCLUDES *E/M services after first face-to-face visit*

99495 **Transitional Care Management Services with the following required elements: Communication (direct contact, telephone, electronic) with the patient and/or caregiver within 2 business days of discharge Medical decision making of at least moderate complexity during the service period Face-to-face visit, within 14 calendar days of discharge**

3.11 4.62 **FUD** XXX ★ V 80

AMA: 2020,Feb,7; 2020,Jan,3; 2019,Jan,6; 2018,Jul,12; 2018,Apr,9; 2018,Mar,5; 2018,Mar,7; 2018,Feb,7; 2018,Jan,8; 2017,Jan,8; 2016,Jan,13; 2015,Jan,16

99496 **Transitional Care Management Services with the following required elements: Communication (direct contact, telephone, electronic) with the patient and/or caregiver within 2 business days of discharge Medical decision making of high complexity during the service period Face-to-face visit, within 7 calendar days of discharge**

4.51 6.52 **FUD** XXX ★ V 80

AMA: 2020,Feb,7; 2020,Jan,3; 2019,Jan,6; 2018,Jul,12; 2018,Apr,9; 2018,Mar,5; 2018,Mar,7; 2018,Feb,7; 2018,Jan,8; 2017,Jan,8; 2016,Jan,13; 2015,Jan,16

99497-99498 Advance Directive Guidance

CMS: 100-02,15,280.5.1 Advance Care Planning with an Annual Wellness Visit; 100-04,11,40.1.3 Independent Attending Physician Services; 100-04,18,140.8 Advance Care Planning with an Annual Wellness Visit (AWV); 100-04,4,200.11 Advance Care Planning as an Optional Element of an Annual Wellness Visit

EXCLUDES *Critical care services (99291-99292, 99468-99469, 99471-99472, 99475-99476, 99477-99480)*
- *Services for cognitive care (99483)*
- *Treatment/management for active problem (see appropriate E/M service)*

99497 **Advance care planning including the explanation and discussion of advance directives such as standard forms (with completion of such forms, when performed), by the physician or other qualified health care professional; first 30 minutes, face-to-face with the patient, family member(s), and/or surrogate**

2.23 2.40 **FUD** XXX Q1 80

AMA: 2018,Apr,9; 2018,Jan,8; 2017,Jan,8; 2016,Feb,7; 2016,Jan,13; 2015,Jan,16

\+ **99498** **each additional 30 minutes (List separately in addition to code for primary procedure)**

Code first (99497)

2.10 2.11 **FUD** ZZZ N 80

AMA: 2018,Apr,9; 2018,Jan,8; 2017,Jan,8; 2016,Feb,7; 2016,Jan,13; 2015,Jan,16

99484 [99484] Behavioral Health Integration Care

CMS: 100-02,13,230.2 Chronic Care Management and General Behavioral Health Integration Services

INCLUDES Care management services requiring 20 minutes or more per calendar month
- Coordination of care with emergency department staff
- Face to face services when necessary
- Provided as outpatient service
- Provision services by clinical staff and reported by supervising physician or other qualified healthcare professional
- Provision services to patients with ongoing relationship
- Treatment plan and specific service components

EXCLUDES *Other services for which time or activities associated with service not used to meet requirements for 99484:*
- *Behavioral health integration care in same month ([99484])*
- *Chronic care management ([99439], [99490], 99487-99489)*
- *Psychiatric collaborative care in same calendar month (99492-99494)*
- *Psychotherapy services (90785-90899)*
- *Transitional care management (99495-99496)*

\# **99484** **Care management services for behavioral health conditions, at least 20 minutes of clinical staff time, directed by a physician or other qualified health care professional, per calendar month, with the following required elements: initial assessment or follow-up monitoring, including the use of applicable validated rating scales; behavioral health care planning in relation to behavioral/psychiatric health problems, including revision for patients who are not progressing or whose status changes; facilitating and coordinating treatment such as psychotherapy, pharmacotherapy, counseling and/or psychiatric consultation; and continuity of care with a designated member of the care team.**

0.91 1.33 **FUD** XXX S 80

AMA: 2020,Feb,7; 2019,Jan,6; 2018,Jul,12; 2018,Mar,5; 2018,Feb,7; 2018,Jan,8

99499 Unlisted Evaluation and Management Services

CMS: 100-04,12,30.6.10 Consultation Services; 100-04,12,30.6.4 Services Furnished Incident to Physician's Service; 100-04,12,30.6.9.1 Initial Hospital Care and Observation or Inpatient Care Services

99499 **Unlisted evaluation and management service**

0.00 0.00 **FUD** XXX B 80

AMA: 2019,Aug,8; 2018,Jan,8; 2017,Jan,8; 2016,Jan,13; 2015,Jan,16

[illegible]

[illegible] Cr[illegible]

[illegible]

[illegible]

[illegible]

[illegible]

[illegible] and [illegible] Services

[illegible]

0001F-0015F Quality Measures with Multiple Components

INCLUDES Several measures grouped within single code descriptor to make possible reporting for clinical conditions when all components have been met

0001F **Heart failure assessed (includes assessment of all the following components) (CAD): Blood pressure measured (2000F) Level of activity assessed (1003F) Clinical symptoms of volume overload (excess) assessed (1004F) Weight, recorded (2001F) Clinical signs of volume overload (excess) assessed (2002F)**

INCLUDES Blood pressure measured (2000F)
Clinical signs volume overload (excess) assessed (2002F)
Clinical symptoms volume overload (excess) assessed (1004F)
Level activity assessed (1003F)
Weight recorded (2001F)

0.00 0.00 FUD XXX E

AMA: 2018,Jan,8; 2017,Jan,8; 2016,Jan,13; 2015,Jan,16

0005F **Osteoarthritis assessed (OA) Includes assessment of all the following components: Osteoarthritis symptoms and functional status assessed (1006F) Use of anti-inflammatory or over-the-counter (OTC) analgesic medications assessed (1007F) Initial examination of the involved joint(s) (includes visual inspection, palpation, range of motion) (2004F)**

INCLUDES Anti-inflammatory or over-the-counter (OTC) analgesic medication usage assessed (1007F)
Initial examination involved joint(s) (includes visual inspection/palpation/range) (2004F)
Osteoarthritis symptoms and functional status assessed (1006F)

0.00 0.00 FUD XXX E

AMA: 2005,Oct,1-5

0012F **Community-acquired bacterial pneumonia assessment (includes all of the following components) (CAP): Co-morbid conditions assessed (1026F) Vital signs recorded (2010F) Mental status assessed (2014F) Hydration status assessed (2018F)**

INCLUDES Co-morbid conditions assessed (1026F)
Hydration status assessed (2018F)
Mental status assessed (2014F)
Vital signs recorded (2010F)

0.00 0.00 FUD XXX E

0014F **Comprehensive preoperative assessment performed for cataract surgery with intraocular lens (IOL) placement (includes assessment of all of the following components) (EC): Dilated fundus evaluation performed within 12 months prior to cataract surgery (2020F) Pre-surgical (cataract) axial length, corneal power measurement and method of intraocular lens power calculation documented (must be performed within 12 months prior to surgery) (3073F) Preoperative assessment of functional or medical indication(s) for surgery prior to the cataract surgery with intraocular lens placement (must be performed within 12 months prior to cataract surgery) (3325F)**

INCLUDES Evaluation dilated fundus done within 12 months prior to surgery (2020F)
Preoperative assessment functional or medical indications done within 12 months prior to surgery (3325F)
Presurgical measurement axial length, corneal power, and IOL power calculation performed within 12 months prior to surgery (3073F)

0.00 0.00 FUD XXX E

AMA: 2008,Mar,8-12

0015F **Melanoma follow up completed (includes assessment of all of the following components) (ML): History obtained regarding new or changing moles (1050F) Complete physical skin exam performed (2029F) Patient counseled to perform a monthly self skin examination (5005F)**

INCLUDES Complete physical skin exam (2029F)
Counseling to perform monthly skin self-examination (5005F)
History obtained new or changing moles (1050F)

0.00 0.00 FUD XXX E

AMA: 2008,Mar,8-12

0500F-0584F Care Provided According to Prevailing Guidelines

INCLUDES Utilization measures or patient care provided for certain clinical purposes

0500F **Initial prenatal care visit (report at first prenatal encounter with health care professional providing obstetrical care. Report also date of visit and, in a separate field, the date of the last menstrual period [LMP]) (Prenatal)** M ♀

0.00 0.00 FUD XXX E

AMA: 2018,Jan,8; 2017,Jan,8; 2016,Jan,13; 2015,Jan,16

0501F **Prenatal flow sheet documented in medical record by first prenatal visit (documentation includes at minimum blood pressure, weight, urine protein, uterine size, fetal heart tones, and estimated date of delivery). Report also: date of visit and, in a separate field, the date of the last menstrual period [LMP] (Note: If reporting 0501F Prenatal flow sheet, it is not necessary to report 0500F Initial prenatal care visit) (Prenatal)** M ♀

0.00 0.00 FUD XXX E

AMA: 2004,Nov,1

0502F **Subsequent prenatal care visit (Prenatal) [Excludes: patients who are seen for a condition unrelated to pregnancy or prenatal care (eg, an upper respiratory infection; patients seen for consultation only, not for continuing care)]** M ♀

EXCLUDES *Patients seen for unrelated pregnancy/prenatal care condition (e.g., upper respiratory infection; patients seen for consultation only, not for continuing care)*

0.00 0.00 FUD XXX E

AMA: 2004,Nov,1

0503F **Postpartum care visit (Prenatal)** M ♀

0.00 0.00 FUD XXX E

AMA: 2004,Nov,1

0505F **Hemodialysis plan of care documented (ESRD, P-ESRD)**

0.00 0.00 FUD XXX E

AMA: 2008,Mar,8-12

0507F **Peritoneal dialysis plan of care documented (ESRD)**

0.00 0.00 FUD XXX E

AMA: 2008,Mar,8-12

0509F **Urinary incontinence plan of care documented (GER)**

0.00 0.00 FUD XXX M

0513F **Elevated blood pressure plan of care documented (CKD)**

0.00 0.00 FUD XXX M

AMA: 2008,Mar,8-12

0514F **Plan of care for elevated hemoglobin level documented for patient receiving Erythropoiesis-Stimulating Agent therapy (ESA) (CKD)**

0.00 0.00 FUD XXX E

AMA: 2008,Mar,8-12

0516F **Anemia plan of care documented (ESRD)**

0.00 0.00 FUD XXX E

AMA: 2008,Mar,8-12

0517F **Glaucoma plan of care documented (EC)**

0.00 0.00 FUD XXX M

AMA: 2008,Mar,8-12

0518F **Falls plan of care documented (GER)**
Facility RVU 0.00 Non-Facility RVU 0.00 **FUD** XXX M
AMA: 2008,Mar,8-12

0519F **Planned chemotherapy regimen, including at a minimum: drug(s) prescribed, dose, and duration, documented prior to initiation of a new treatment regimen (ONC)**
Facility RVU 0.00 Non-Facility RVU 0.00 **FUD** XXX E
AMA: 2008,Mar,8-12

0520F **Radiation dose limits to normal tissues established prior to the initiation of a course of 3D conformal radiation for a minimum of 2 tissue/organ (ONC)**
Facility RVU 0.00 Non-Facility RVU 0.00 **FUD** XXX M
AMA: 2008,Mar,8-12

0521F **Plan of care to address pain documented (COA) (ONC)**
Facility RVU 0.00 Non-Facility RVU 0.00 **FUD** XXX M
AMA: 2008,Mar,8-12

0525F **Initial visit for episode (BkP)**
Facility RVU 0.00 Non-Facility RVU 0.00 **FUD** XXX E
AMA: 2008,Mar,8-12

0526F **Subsequent visit for episode (BkP)**
Facility RVU 0.00 Non-Facility RVU 0.00 **FUD** XXX M
AMA: 2008,Mar,8-12

0528F **Recommended follow-up interval for repeat colonoscopy of at least 10 years documented in colonoscopy report (End/Polyp)**
Facility RVU 0.00 Non-Facility RVU 0.00 **FUD** XXX M

0529F **Interval of 3 or more years since patient's last colonoscopy, documented (End/Polyp)**
Facility RVU 0.00 Non-Facility RVU 0.00 **FUD** XXX M

0535F **Dyspnea management plan of care, documented (Pall Cr)**
Facility RVU 0.00 Non-Facility RVU 0.00 **FUD** XXX E

0540F **Glucorticoid Management Plan Documented (RA)**
Facility RVU 0.00 Non-Facility RVU 0.00 **FUD** XXX M

0545F **Plan for follow-up care for major depressive disorder, documented (MDD ADOL)**
Facility RVU 0.00 Non-Facility RVU 0.00 **FUD** XXX E

0550F **Cytopathology report on routine nongynecologic specimen finalized within two working days of accession date (PATH)**
Facility RVU 0.00 Non-Facility RVU 0.00 **FUD** XXX E

0551F **Cytopathology report on nongynecologic specimen with documentation that the specimen was non-routine (PATH)**
Facility RVU 0.00 Non-Facility RVU 0.00 **FUD** XXX E

0555F **Symptom management plan of care documented (HF)**
Facility RVU 0.00 Non-Facility RVU 0.00 **FUD** XXX E

0556F **Plan of care to achieve lipid control documented (CAD)**
Facility RVU 0.00 Non-Facility RVU 0.00 **FUD** XXX E

0557F **Plan of care to manage anginal symptoms documented (CAD)**
Facility RVU 0.00 Non-Facility RVU 0.00 **FUD** XXX E

0575F **HIV RNA control plan of care, documented (HIV)**
Facility RVU 0.00 Non-Facility RVU 0.00 **FUD** XXX E

0580F **Multidisciplinary care plan developed or updated (ALS)**
Facility RVU 0.00 Non-Facility RVU 0.00 **FUD** XXX E

0581F **Patient transferred directly from anesthetizing location to critical care unit (Peri2)**
Facility RVU 0.00 Non-Facility RVU 0.00 **FUD** XXX M

0582F **Patient not transferred directly from anesthetizing location to critical care unit (Peri2)**
Facility RVU 0.00 Non-Facility RVU 0.00 **FUD** XXX E

0583F **Transfer of care checklist used (Peri2)**
Facility RVU 0.00 Non-Facility RVU 0.00 **FUD** XXX M

0584F **Transfer of care checklist not used (Peri2)**
Facility RVU 0.00 Non-Facility RVU 0.00 **FUD** XXX E

1000F-1505F Elements of History/Review of Systems

INCLUDES Measures for specific aspects patient history or systems review

1000F **Tobacco use assessed (CAD, CAP, COPD, PV) (DM)**
Facility RVU 0.00 Non-Facility RVU 0.00 **FUD** XXX E
AMA: 2018,Jan,8; 2017,Jan,8; 2016,Jan,13; 2015,Jan,16

1002F **Anginal symptoms and level of activity assessed (NMA-No Measure Associated)**
Facility RVU 0.00 Non-Facility RVU 0.00 **FUD** XXX E
AMA: 2004,Nov,1

1003F **Level of activity assessed (NMA-No Measure Associated)**
Facility RVU 0.00 Non-Facility RVU 0.00 **FUD** XXX E
AMA: 2006,Dec,10-12

1004F **Clinical symptoms of volume overload (excess) assessed (NMA-No Measure Associated)**
Facility RVU 0.00 Non-Facility RVU 0.00 **FUD** XXX E
AMA: 2006,Dec,10-12

1005F **Asthma symptoms evaluated (includes documentation of numeric frequency of symptoms or patient completion of an asthma assessment tool/survey/questionnaire) (NMA-No Measure Associated)**
Facility RVU 0.00 Non-Facility RVU 0.00 **FUD** XXX E

1006F **Osteoarthritis symptoms and functional status assessed (may include the use of a standardized scale or the completion of an assessment questionnaire, such as the SF-36, AAOS Hip & Knee Questionnaire) (OA) [Instructions: Report when osteoarthritis is addressed during the patient encounter]**
INCLUDES Osteoarthritis when addressed during patient encounter
Facility RVU 0.00 Non-Facility RVU 0.00 **FUD** XXX M

1007F **Use of anti-inflammatory or analgesic over-the-counter (OTC) medications for symptom relief assessed (OA)**
Facility RVU 0.00 Non-Facility RVU 0.00 **FUD** XXX E

1008F **Gastrointestinal and renal risk factors assessed for patients on prescribed or OTC non-steroidal anti-inflammatory drug (NSAID) (OA)**
Facility RVU 0.00 Non-Facility RVU 0.00 **FUD** XXX E

1010F **Severity of angina assessed by level of activity (CAD)**
Facility RVU 0.00 Non-Facility RVU 0.00 **FUD** XXX E

1011F **Angina present (CAD)**
Facility RVU 0.00 Non-Facility RVU 0.00 **FUD** XXX E

1012F **Angina absent (CAD)**
Facility RVU 0.00 Non-Facility RVU 0.00 **FUD** XXX E

1015F **Chronic obstructive pulmonary disease (COPD) symptoms assessed (Includes assessment of at least 1 of the following: dyspnea, cough/sputum, wheezing), or respiratory symptom assessment tool completed (COPD)**
Facility RVU 0.00 Non-Facility RVU 0.00 **FUD** XXX E

1018F **Dyspnea assessed, not present (COPD)**
Facility RVU 0.00 Non-Facility RVU 0.00 **FUD** XXX E

1019F **Dyspnea assessed, present (COPD)**
Facility RVU 0.00 Non-Facility RVU 0.00 **FUD** XXX E

1022F **Pneumococcus immunization status assessed (CAP, COPD)**
Facility RVU 0.00 Non-Facility RVU 0.00 **FUD** XXX E
AMA: 2010,Jul,3-5; 2008,Mar,8-12

1026F **Co-morbid conditions assessed (eg, includes assessment for presence or absence of: malignancy, liver disease, congestive heart failure, cerebrovascular disease, renal disease, chronic obstructive pulmonary disease, asthma, diabetes, other co-morbid conditions) (CAP)**
Facility RVU 0.00 Non-Facility RVU 0.00 **FUD** XXX E

1030F **Influenza immunization status assessed (CAP)**
Facility RVU 0.00 Non-Facility RVU 0.00 **FUD** XXX E
AMA: 2008,Mar,8-12

1031F **Smoking status and exposure to second hand smoke in the home assessed (Asthma)**
0.00 0.00 FUD XXX E

1032F **Current tobacco smoker or currently exposed to secondhand smoke (Asthma)**
0.00 0.00 FUD XXX E

1033F **Current tobacco non-smoker and not currently exposed to secondhand smoke (Asthma)**
0.00 0.00 FUD XXX E

1034F **Current tobacco smoker (CAD, CAP, COPD, PV) (DM)**
0.00 0.00 FUD XXX E
AMA: 2008,Mar,8-12

1035F **Current smokeless tobacco user (eg, chew, snuff) (PV)**
0.00 0.00 FUD XXX E
AMA: 2008,Mar,8-12

1036F **Current tobacco non-user (CAD, CAP, COPD, PV) (DM) (IBD)**
0.00 0.00 FUD XXX M
AMA: 2008,Mar,8-12

1038F **Persistent asthma (mild, moderate or severe) (Asthma)**
0.00 0.00 FUD XXX M
AMA: 2018,Jan,8; 2017,Jan,8; 2016,Jan,13; 2015,Jan,16

1039F **Intermittent asthma (Asthma)**
0.00 0.00 FUD XXX M
AMA: 2018,Jan,8; 2017,Jan,8; 2016,Jan,13; 2015,Jan,16

1040F **DSM-5 criteria for major depressive disorder documented at the initial evaluation (MDD, MDD ADOL)**
0.00 0.00 FUD XXX E
AMA: 2008,Mar,8-12

1050F **History obtained regarding new or changing moles (ML)**
0.00 0.00 FUD XXX E
AMA: 2008,Mar,8-12

1052F **Type, anatomic location, and activity all assessed (IBD)**
0.00 0.00 FUD XXX E

1055F **Visual functional status assessed (EC)**
0.00 0.00 FUD XXX E

1060F **Documentation of permanent or persistent or paroxysmal atrial fibrillation (STR)**
0.00 0.00 FUD XXX E

1061F **Documentation of absence of permanent and persistent and paroxysmal atrial fibrillation (STR)**
0.00 0.00 FUD XXX E

1065F **Ischemic stroke symptom onset of less than 3 hours prior to arrival (STR)**
0.00 0.00 FUD XXX E

1066F **Ischemic stroke symptom onset greater than or equal to 3 hours prior to arrival (STR)**
0.00 0.00 FUD XXX E

1070F **Alarm symptoms (involuntary weight loss, dysphagia, or gastrointestinal bleeding) assessed; none present (GERD)**
0.00 0.00 FUD XXX E

1071F **1 or more present (GERD)**
0.00 0.00 FUD XXX E

1090F **Presence or absence of urinary incontinence assessed (GER)**
0.00 0.00 FUD XXX M

1091F **Urinary incontinence characterized (eg, frequency, volume, timing, type of symptoms, how bothersome) (GER)**
0.00 0.00 FUD XXX E

1100F **Patient screened for future fall risk; documentation of 2 or more falls in the past year or any fall with injury in the past year (GER)**
0.00 0.00 FUD XXX M
AMA: 2008,Mar,8-12

1101F **documentation of no falls in the past year or only 1 fall without injury in the past year (GER)**
0.00 0.00 FUD XXX M
AMA: 2008,Mar,8-12

1110F **Patient discharged from an inpatient facility (eg, hospital, skilled nursing facility, or rehabilitation facility) within the last 60 days (GER)**
0.00 0.00 FUD XXX E

1111F **Discharge medications reconciled with the current medication list in outpatient medical record (COA) (GER)**
0.00 0.00 FUD XXX M

1116F **Auricular or periauricular pain assessed (AOE)**
0.00 0.00 FUD XXX E
AMA: 2008,Mar,8-12

1118F **GERD symptoms assessed after 12 months of therapy (GERD)**
0.00 0.00 FUD XXX E
AMA: 2008,Mar,8-12

1119F **Initial evaluation for condition (HEP C)(EPI, DSP)**
0.00 0.00 FUD XXX E
AMA: 2008,Mar,8-12

1121F **Subsequent evaluation for condition (HEP C)(EPI)**
0.00 0.00 FUD XXX E
AMA: 2008,Mar,8-12

1123F **Advance Care Planning discussed and documented advance care plan or surrogate decision maker documented in the medical record (DEM) (GER, Pall Cr)**
0.00 0.00 FUD XXX M
AMA: 2008,Mar,8-12

1124F **Advance Care Planning discussed and documented in the medical record, patient did not wish or was not able to name a surrogate decision maker or provide an advance care plan (DEM) (GER, Pall Cr)**
0.00 0.00 FUD XXX M
AMA: 2008,Mar,8-12

1125F **Pain severity quantified; pain present (COA) (ONC)**
0.00 0.00 FUD XXX M
AMA: 2008,Mar,8-12

1126F **no pain present (COA) (ONC)**
0.00 0.00 FUD XXX M
AMA: 2008,Mar,8-12

1127F **New episode for condition (NMA-No Measure Associated)**
0.00 0.00 FUD XXX E
AMA: 2008,Mar,8-12

1128F **Subsequent episode for condition (NMA-No Measure Associated)**
0.00 0.00 FUD XXX E
AMA: 2008,Mar,8-12

1130F **Back pain and function assessed, including all of the following: Pain assessment and functional status and patient history, including notation of presence or absence of "red flags" (warning signs) and assessment of prior treatment and response, and employment status (BkP)**
0.00 0.00 FUD XXX E
AMA: 2008,Mar,8-12

1134F **Episode of back pain lasting 6 weeks or less (BkP)**
0.00 0.00 FUD XXX E
AMA: 2008,Mar,8-12

1135F **Episode of back pain lasting longer than 6 weeks (BkP)**
0.00 0.00 FUD XXX E
AMA: 2008,Mar,8-12

1136F **Episode of back pain lasting 12 weeks or less (BkP)**
0.00 0.00 FUD XXX E
AMA: 2008,Mar,8-12

Category II Codes

1031F — 1136F

1137F Episode of back pain lasting longer than 12 weeks (BkP)
0.00 0.00 FUD XXX E
AMA: 2008,Mar,8-12

1150F Documentation that a patient has a substantial risk of death within 1 year (Pall Cr)
0.00 0.00 FUD XXX E

1151F Documentation that a patient does not have a substantial risk of death within one year (Pall Cr)
0.00 0.00 FUD XXX E

1152F Documentation of advanced disease diagnosis, goals of care prioritize comfort (Pall Cr)
0.00 0.00 FUD XXX E

1153F Documentation of advanced disease diagnosis, goals of care do not prioritize comfort (Pall Cr)
0.00 0.00 FUD XXX E

1157F Advance care plan or similar legal document present in the medical record (COA)
0.00 0.00 FUD XXX E

1158F Advance care planning discussion documented in the medical record (COA)
0.00 0.00 FUD XXX M

1159F Medication list documented in medical record (COA)
0.00 0.00 FUD XXX E

1160F Review of all medications by a prescribing practitioner or clinical pharmacist (such as, prescriptions, OTCs, herbal therapies and supplements) documented in the medical record (COA)
0.00 0.00 FUD XXX E

1170F Functional status assessed (COA) (RA)
0.00 0.00 FUD XXX M

1175F Functional status for dementia assessed and results reviewed (DEM)
0.00 0.00 FUD XXX E

1180F All specified thromboembolic risk factors assessed (AFIB)
0.00 0.00 FUD XXX E

1181F Neuropsychiatric symptoms assessed and results reviewed (DEM)
0.00 0.00 FUD XXX E

1182F Neuropsychiatric symptoms, one or more present (DEM)
0.00 0.00 FUD XXX E

1183F Neuropsychiatric symptoms, absent (DEM)
0.00 0.00 FUD XXX E

1200F Seizure type(s) and current seizure frequency(ies) documented (EPI)
0.00 0.00 FUD XXX E

1205F Etiology of epilepsy or epilepsy syndrome(s) reviewed and documented (EPI)
0.00 0.00 FUD XXX E

1220F Patient screened for depression (SUD)
0.00 0.00 FUD XXX E

1400F Parkinson's disease diagnosis reviewed (Prkns)
0.00 0.00 FUD XXX E

1450F Symptoms improved or remained consistent with treatment goals since last assessment (HF)
0.00 0.00 FUD XXX E

1451F Symptoms demonstrated clinically important deterioration since last assessment (HF)
0.00 0.00 FUD XXX E

1460F Qualifying cardiac event/diagnosis in previous 12 months (CAD)
0.00 0.00 FUD XXX M

1461F No qualifying cardiac event/diagnosis in previous 12 months (CAD)
0.00 0.00 FUD XXX M

1490F Dementia severity classified, mild (DEM)
0.00 0.00 FUD XXX E

1491F Dementia severity classified, moderate (DEM)
0.00 0.00 FUD XXX E

1493F Dementia severity classified, severe (DEM)
0.00 0.00 FUD XXX E

1494F Cognition assessed and reviewed (DEM)
0.00 0.00 FUD XXX E

1500F Symptoms and signs of distal symmetric polyneuropathy reviewed and documented (DSP)
0.00 0.00 FUD XXX E

1501F Not initial evaluation for condition (DSP)
0.00 0.00 FUD XXX E

1502F Patient queried about pain and pain interference with function using a valid and reliable instrument (DSP)
0.00 0.00 FUD XXX E

1503F Patient queried about symptoms of respiratory insufficiency (ALS)
0.00 0.00 FUD XXX E

1504F Patient has respiratory insufficiency (ALS)
0.00 0.00 FUD XXX E

1505F Patient does not have respiratory insufficiency (ALS)
0.00 0.00 FUD XXX E

2000F-2060F [2033F] Elements of Examination

INCLUDES Components clinical assessment or physical exam

2000F Blood pressure measured (CKD)(DM)
0.00 0.00 FUD XXX M
AMA: 2018,Jan,8; 2017,Jan,8; 2016,Jan,13; 2015,Jan,16

2001F Weight recorded (PAG)
0.00 0.00 FUD XXX E
AMA: 2006,Dec,10-12

2002F Clinical signs of volume overload (excess) assessed (NMA-No Measure Associated)
0.00 0.00 FUD XXX E
AMA: 2006,Dec,10-12

2004F Initial examination of the involved joint(s) (includes visual inspection, palpation, range of motion) (OA) [Instructions: Report only for initial osteoarthritis visit or for visits for new joint involvement]
INCLUDES Visits for initial osteoarthritis examination or new joint involvement
0.00 0.00 FUD XXX E
AMA: 2004,Feb,3; 2003,Aug,1

2010F Vital signs (temperature, pulse, respiratory rate, and blood pressure) documented and reviewed (CAP) (EM)
0.00 0.00 FUD XXX E

2014F Mental status assessed (CAP) (EM)
0.00 0.00 FUD XXX E

2015F Asthma impairment assessed (Asthma)
0.00 0.00 FUD XXX E

2016F Asthma risk assessed (Asthma)
0.00 0.00 FUD XXX E

2018F Hydration status assessed (normal/mildly dehydrated/severely dehydrated) (CAP)
0.00 0.00 FUD XXX E

2019F Dilated macular exam performed, including documentation of the presence or absence of macular thickening or hemorrhage and the level of macular degeneration severity (EC)
0.00 0.00 FUD XXX E

2020F **Dilated fundus evaluation performed within 12 months prior to cataract surgery (EC)**
0.00 0.00 FUD XXX E
AMA: 2008,Mar,8-12

2021F **Dilated macular or fundus exam performed, including documentation of the presence or absence of macular edema and level of severity of retinopathy (EC)**
0.00 0.00 FUD XXX E

2022F **Dilated retinal eye exam with interpretation by an ophthalmologist or optometrist documented and reviewed; with evidence of retinopathy (DM)**
0.00 0.00 FUD XXX M
AMA: 2008,Mar,8-12

2023F **without evidence of retinopathy (DM)**
0.00 0.00 FUD XXX

2024F **7 standard field stereoscopic retinal photos with interpretation by an ophthalmologist or optometrist documented and reviewed; with evidence of retinopathy (DM)**
0.00 0.00 FUD XXX M
AMA: 2008,Mar,8-12

2025F **without evidence of retinopathy (DM)**
0.00 0.00 FUD XXX

2026F **Eye imaging validated to match diagnosis from 7 standard field stereoscopic retinal photos results documented and reviewed; with evidence of retinopathy (DM)**
0.00 0.00 FUD XXX M
AMA: 2008,Mar,8-12

\# **2033F** **without evidence of retinopathy (DM)**
0.00 0.00 FUD XXX

2027F **Optic nerve head evaluation performed (EC)**
0.00 0.00 FUD XXX M

2028F **Foot examination performed (includes examination through visual inspection, sensory exam with monofilament, and pulse exam - report when any of the 3 components are completed) (DM)**
0.00 0.00 FUD XXX E

2029F **Complete physical skin exam performed (ML)**
0.00 0.00 FUD XXX E
AMA: 2008,Mar,8-12

2030F **Hydration status documented, normally hydrated (PAG)**
0.00 0.00 FUD XXX E

2031F **Hydration status documented, dehydrated (PAG)**
0.00 0.00 FUD XXX E

2033F **Resequenced code. See code following 2026F.**

2035F **Tympanic membrane mobility assessed with pneumatic otoscopy or tympanometry (OME)**
0.00 0.00 FUD XXX E
AMA: 2008,Mar,8-12

2040F **Physical examination on the date of the initial visit for low back pain performed, in accordance with specifications (BkP)**
0.00 0.00 FUD XXX E
AMA: 2008,Mar,8-12

2044F **Documentation of mental health assessment prior to intervention (back surgery or epidural steroid injection) or for back pain episode lasting longer than 6 weeks (BkP)**
0.00 0.00 FUD XXX E
AMA: 2008,Mar,8-12

2050F **Wound characteristics including size and nature of wound base tissue and amount of drainage prior to debridement documented (CWC)**
0.00 0.00 FUD XXX E

2060F **Patient interviewed directly on or before date of diagnosis of major depressive disorder (MDD ADOL)**
0.00 0.00 FUD XXX E

3006F-3776F [3051F, 3052F] Findings from Diagnostic or Screening Tests

INCLUDES Results and medical decision making with regards to ordered tests:
- Clinical laboratory tests
- Other examination procedures
- Radiological examinations

3006F **Chest X-ray results documented and reviewed (CAP)**
0.00 0.00 FUD XXX E
AMA: 2018,Jan,8; 2017,Jan,8; 2016,Jan,13; 2015,Jan,16

3008F **Body Mass Index (BMI), documented (PV)**
0.00 0.00 FUD XXX E

3011F **Lipid panel results documented and reviewed (must include total cholesterol, HDL-C, triglycerides and calculated LDL-C) (CAD)**
0.00 0.00 FUD XXX E

3014F **Screening mammography results documented and reviewed (PV)**
0.00 0.00 FUD XXX E
AMA: 2008,Mar,8-12

3015F **Cervical cancer screening results documented and reviewed (PV)** ♀
0.00 0.00 FUD XXX E

3016F **Patient screened for unhealthy alcohol use using a systematic screening method (PV) (DSP)**
0.00 0.00 FUD XXX E

3017F **Colorectal cancer screening results documented and reviewed (PV)**
0.00 0.00 FUD XXX M
AMA: 2008,Mar,8-12

3018F **Pre-procedure risk assessment and depth of insertion and quality of the bowel prep and complete description of polyp(s) found, including location of each polyp, size, number and gross morphology and recommendations for follow-up in final colonoscopy report documented (End/Polyp)**
0.00 0.00 FUD XXX E

3019F **Left ventricular ejection fraction (LVEF) assessment planned post discharge (HF)**
0.00 0.00 FUD XXX E

3020F **Left ventricular function (LVF) assessment (eg, echocardiography, nuclear test, or ventriculography) documented in the medical record (Includes quantitative or qualitative assessment results) (NMA-No Measure Associated)**
0.00 0.00 FUD XXX E
AMA: 2006,Dec,10-12

3021F **Left ventricular ejection fraction (LVEF) less than 40% or documentation of moderately or severely depressed left ventricular systolic function (CAD, HF)**
0.00 0.00 FUD XXX M

3022F **Left ventricular ejection fraction (LVEF) greater than or equal to 40% or documentation as normal or mildly depressed left ventricular systolic function (CAD, HF)**
0.00 0.00 FUD XXX M

3023F **Spirometry results documented and reviewed (COPD)**
0.00 0.00 FUD XXX M

3025F **Spirometry test results demonstrate FEV1/FVC less than 70% with COPD symptoms (eg, dyspnea, cough/sputum, wheezing) (CAP, COPD)**
0.00 0.00 FUD XXX E

3027F **Spirometry test results demonstrate FEV1/FVC greater than or equal to 70% or patient does not have COPD symptoms (COPD)**
0.00 0.00 FUD XXX E

3028F **Oxygen saturation results documented and reviewed (includes assessment through pulse oximetry or arterial blood gas measurement) (CAP, COPD) (EM)**
0.00 0.00 FUD XXX E

3035F **Oxygen saturation less than or equal to 88% or a PaO2 less than or equal to 55 mm Hg (COPD)**
0.00 0.00 FUD XXX E

3037F **Oxygen saturation greater than 88% or PaO2 greater than 55 mm Hg (COPD)**
0.00 0.00 FUD XXX E

3038F **Pulmonary function test performed within 12 months prior to surgery (Lung/Esop Cx)**
0.00 0.00 FUD XXX E

3040F **Functional expiratory volume (FEV1) less than 40% of predicted value (COPD)**
0.00 0.00 FUD XXX E

3042F **Functional expiratory volume (FEV1) greater than or equal to 40% of predicted value (COPD)**
0.00 0.00 FUD XXX E

3044F **Most recent hemoglobin A1c (HbA1c) level less than 7.0% (DM)**
0.00 0.00 FUD XXX M

\# **3051F** **Most recent hemoglobin A1c (HbA1c) level greater than or equal to 7.0% and less than 8.0% (DM)**
0.00 0.00 FUD XXX

\# **3052F** **Most recent hemoglobin A1c (HbA1c) level greater than or equal to 8.0% and less than or equal to 9.0% (DM)**
0.00 0.00 FUD XXX

3046F **Most recent hemoglobin A1c level greater than 9.0% (DM)**
EXCLUDES *Hemoglobin A1c less than or equal to 9.0% (3044F, [3051F], [3052F])*
0.00 0.00 FUD XXX M

3048F **Most recent LDL-C less than 100 mg/dL (CAD) (DM)**
0.00 0.00 FUD XXX E

3049F **Most recent LDL-C 100-129 mg/dL (CAD) (DM)**
0.00 0.00 FUD XXX E

3050F **Most recent LDL-C greater than or equal to 130 mg/dL (CAD) (DM)**
0.00 0.00 FUD XXX E

3051F **Resequenced code. See code following 3044F.**

3052F **Resequenced code. See code before 3046F.**

3055F **Left ventricular ejection fraction (LVEF) less than or equal to 35% (HF)**
0.00 0.00 FUD XXX E

3056F **Left ventricular ejection fraction (LVEF) greater than 35% or no LVEF result available (HF)**
0.00 0.00 FUD XXX E

3060F **Positive microalbuminuria test result documented and reviewed (DM)**
0.00 0.00 FUD XXX M

3061F **Negative microalbuminuria test result documented and reviewed (DM)**
0.00 0.00 FUD XXX M

3062F **Positive macroalbuminuria test result documented and reviewed (DM)**
0.00 0.00 FUD XXX M

3066F **Documentation of treatment for nephropathy (eg, patient receiving dialysis, patient being treated for ESRD, CRF, ARF, or renal insufficiency, any visit to a nephrologist) (DM)**
0.00 0.00 FUD XXX M

3072F **Low risk for retinopathy (no evidence of retinopathy in the prior year) (DM)**
0.00 0.00 FUD XXX M
AMA: 2008,Mar,8-12

3073F **Pre-surgical (cataract) axial length, corneal power measurement and method of intraocular lens power calculation documented within 12 months prior to surgery (EC)**
0.00 0.00 FUD XXX E
AMA: 2008,Mar,8-12

3074F **Most recent systolic blood pressure less than 130 mm Hg (DM), (HTN, CKD, CAD)**
0.00 0.00 FUD XXX E
AMA: 2008,Mar,8-12

3075F **Most recent systolic blood pressure 130-139 mm Hg (DM) (HTN, CKD, CAD)**
0.00 0.00 FUD XXX E
AMA: 2008,Mar,8-12

3077F **Most recent systolic blood pressure greater than or equal to 140 mm Hg (HTN, CKD, CAD) (DM)**
0.00 0.00 FUD XXX E
AMA: 2008,Mar,8-12

3078F **Most recent diastolic blood pressure less than 80 mm Hg (HTN, CKD, CAD) (DM)**
0.00 0.00 FUD XXX E
AMA: 2008,Mar,8-12

3079F **Most recent diastolic blood pressure 80-89 mm Hg (HTN, CKD, CAD) (DM)**
0.00 0.00 FUD XXX E
AMA: 2008,Mar,8-12

3080F **Most recent diastolic blood pressure greater than or equal to 90 mm Hg (HTN, CKD, CAD) (DM)**
0.00 0.00 FUD XXX E
AMA: 2008,Mar,8-12

3082F **Kt/V less than 1.2 (Clearance of urea [Kt]/volume [V]) (ESRD, P-ESRD)**
0.00 0.00 FUD XXX E
AMA: 2008,Mar,8-12

3083F **Kt/V equal to or greater than 1.2 and less than 1.7 (Clearance of urea [Kt]/volume [V]) (ESRD, P-ESRD)**
0.00 0.00 FUD XXX E
AMA: 2008,Mar,8-12

3084F **Kt/V greater than or equal to 1.7 (Clearance of urea [Kt]/volume [V]) (ESRD, P-ESRD)**
0.00 0.00 FUD XXX E
AMA: 2008,Mar,8-12

3085F **Suicide risk assessed (MDD, MDD ADOL)**
0.00 0.00 FUD XXX E

3088F **Major depressive disorder, mild (MDD)**
0.00 0.00 FUD XXX E

3089F **Major depressive disorder, moderate (MDD)**
0.00 0.00 FUD XXX E

3090F **Major depressive disorder, severe without psychotic features (MDD)**
0.00 0.00 FUD XXX E

3091F **Major depressive disorder, severe with psychotic features (MDD)**
0.00 0.00 FUD XXX E

3092F **Major depressive disorder, in remission (MDD)**
0.00 0.00 FUD XXX E

3093F **Documentation of new diagnosis of initial or recurrent episode of major depressive disorder (MDD)**
0.00 0.00 FUD XXX E
AMA: 2008,Mar,8-12

3095F **Central dual-energy X-ray absorptiometry (DXA) results documented (OP)(IBD)**
0.00 0.00 FUD XXX M

3096F **Central dual-energy X-ray absorptiometry (DXA) ordered (OP)(IBD)**
0.00 0.00 FUD XXX E

3100F **Carotid imaging study report (includes direct or indirect reference to measurements of distal internal carotid diameter as the denominator for stenosis measurement) (STR, RAD)**
0.00 0.00 FUD XXX M
AMA: 2008,Mar,8-12

3110F **Documentation in final CT or MRI report of presence or absence of hemorrhage and mass lesion and acute infarction (STR)**
0.00 0.00 FUD XXX E

3111F **CT or MRI of the brain performed in the hospital within 24 hours of arrival or performed in an outpatient imaging center, to confirm initial diagnosis of stroke, TIA or intracranial hemorrhage (STR)**
0.00 0.00 FUD XXX E

3112F **CT or MRI of the brain performed greater than 24 hours after arrival to the hospital or performed in an outpatient imaging center for purpose other than confirmation of initial diagnosis of stroke, TIA, or intracranial hemorrhage (STR)**
0.00 0.00 FUD XXX E

3115F **Quantitative results of an evaluation of current level of activity and clinical symptoms (HF)**
0.00 0.00 FUD XXX E

3117F **Heart failure disease specific structured assessment tool completed (HF)**
0.00 0.00 FUD XXX E

3118F **New York Heart Association (NYHA) Class documented (HF)**
0.00 0.00 FUD XXX E

3119F **No evaluation of level of activity or clinical symptoms (HF)**
0.00 0.00 FUD XXX E

3120F **12-Lead ECG Performed (EM)**
0.00 0.00 FUD XXX E

3126F **Esophageal biopsy report with a statement about dysplasia (present, absent, or indefinite, and if present, contains appropriate grading) (PATH)**
0.00 0.00 FUD XXX M

3130F **Upper gastrointestinal endoscopy performed (GERD)**
0.00 0.00 FUD XXX E

3132F **Documentation of referral for upper gastrointestinal endoscopy (GERD)**
0.00 0.00 FUD XXX E

3140F **Upper gastrointestinal endoscopy report indicates suspicion of Barrett's esophagus (GERD)**
0.00 0.00 FUD XXX E

3141F **Upper gastrointestinal endoscopy report indicates no suspicion of Barrett's esophagus (GERD)**
0.00 0.00 FUD XXX E

3142F **Barium swallow test ordered (GERD)**
INCLUDES Documentation barium swallow test
0.00 0.00 FUD XXX E

3150F **Forceps esophageal biopsy performed (GERD)**
0.00 0.00 FUD XXX E

3155F **Cytogenetic testing performed on bone marrow at time of diagnosis or prior to initiating treatment (HEM)**
0.00 0.00 FUD XXX M
AMA: 2008,Mar,8-12

3160F **Documentation of iron stores prior to initiating erythropoietin therapy (HEM)**
0.00 0.00 FUD XXX M
AMA: 2008,Mar,8-12

▲ **3170F** **Baseline flow cytometry studies performed at time of diagnosis or prior to initiating treatment (HEM)**
0.00 0.00 FUD XXX M
AMA: 2008,Mar,8-12

3200F **Barium swallow test not ordered (GERD)**
0.00 0.00 FUD XXX E

3210F **Group A Strep Test Performed (PHAR)**
0.00 0.00 FUD XXX M
AMA: 2008,Mar,8-12

3215F **Patient has documented immunity to Hepatitis A (HEP-C)**
0.00 0.00 FUD XXX E
AMA: 2008,Mar,8-12

3216F **Patient has documented immunity to Hepatitis B (HEP-C)(IBD)**
0.00 0.00 FUD XXX E
AMA: 2008,Mar,8-12

3218F **RNA testing for Hepatitis C documented as performed within 6 months prior to initiation of antiviral treatment for Hepatitis C (HEP-C)**
0.00 0.00 FUD XXX E
AMA: 2008,Mar,8-12

3220F **Hepatitis C quantitative RNA testing documented as performed at 12 weeks from initiation of antiviral treatment (HEP-C)**
0.00 0.00 FUD XXX E
AMA: 2008,Mar,8-12

3230F **Documentation that hearing test was performed within 6 months prior to tympanostomy tube insertion (OME)**
0.00 0.00 FUD XXX E
AMA: 2008,Mar,8-12

3250F **Specimen site other than anatomic location of primary tumor (PATH)**
0.00 0.00 FUD XXX M

3260F **pT category (primary tumor), pN category (regional lymph nodes), and histologic grade documented in pathology report (PATH)**
0.00 0.00 FUD XXX M
AMA: 2008,Mar,8-12

3265F **Ribonucleic acid (RNA) testing for Hepatitis C viremia ordered or results documented (HEP C)**
0.00 0.00 FUD XXX E
AMA: 2008,Mar,8-12

3266F **Hepatitis C genotype testing documented as performed prior to initiation of antiviral treatment for Hepatitis C (HEP C)**
0.00 0.00 FUD XXX E
AMA: 2008,Mar,8-12

3267F **Pathology report includes pT category, pN category, Gleason score, and statement about margin status (PATH)**
0.00 0.00 FUD XXX M

3268F **Prostate-specific antigen (PSA), and primary tumor (T) stage, and Gleason score documented prior to initiation of treatment (PRCA)**
0.00 0.00 FUD XXX E
AMA: 2008,Mar,8-12

Category II Codes

3093F — 3268F

3269F **Bone scan performed prior to initiation of treatment or at any time since diagnosis of prostate cancer (PRCA)**
0.00 0.00 FUD XXX M
AMA: 2008,Mar,8-12

3270F **Bone scan not performed prior to initiation of treatment nor at any time since diagnosis of prostate cancer (PRCA)**
0.00 0.00 FUD XXX M
AMA: 2008,Mar,8-12

3271F **Low risk of recurrence, prostate cancer (PRCA)**
0.00 0.00 FUD XXX E
AMA: 2008,Mar,8-12

3272F **Intermediate risk of recurrence, prostate cancer (PRCA)**
0.00 0.00 FUD XXX E
AMA: 2008,Mar,8-12

3273F **High risk of recurrence, prostate cancer (PRCA)**
0.00 0.00 FUD XXX E
AMA: 2008,Mar,8-12

3274F **Prostate cancer risk of recurrence not determined or neither low, intermediate nor high (PRCA)**
0.00 0.00 FUD XXX E
AMA: 2008,Mar,8-12

3278F **Serum levels of calcium, phosphorus, intact Parathyroid Hormone (PTH) and lipid profile ordered (CKD)**
0.00 0.00 FUD XXX E
AMA: 2008,Mar,8-12

3279F **Hemoglobin level greater than or equal to 13 g/dL (CKD, ESRD)**
0.00 0.00 FUD XXX E
AMA: 2008,Mar,8-12

3280F **Hemoglobin level 11 g/dL to 12.9 g/dL (CKD, ESRD)**
0.00 0.00 FUD XXX E
AMA: 2008,Mar,8-12

3281F **Hemoglobin level less than 11 g/dL (CKD, ESRD)**
0.00 0.00 FUD XXX E
AMA: 2008,Mar,8-12

3284F **Intraocular pressure (IOP) reduced by a value of greater than or equal to 15% from the pre-intervention level (EC)**
0.00 0.00 FUD XXX M
AMA: 2008,Mar,8-12

3285F **Intraocular pressure (IOP) reduced by a value less than 15% from the pre-intervention level (EC)**
0.00 0.00 FUD XXX M
AMA: 2008,Mar,8-12

3288F **Falls risk assessment documented (GER)**
0.00 0.00 FUD XXX M
AMA: 2008,Mar,8-12

3290F **Patient is D (Rh) negative and unsensitized (Pre-Cr)**
0.00 0.00 FUD XXX E
AMA: 2008,Mar,8-12

3291F **Patient is D (Rh) positive or sensitized (Pre-Cr)**
0.00 0.00 FUD XXX E
AMA: 2008,Mar,8-12

3292F **HIV testing ordered or documented and reviewed during the first or second prenatal visit (Pre-Cr)**
0.00 0.00 FUD XXX E

3293F **ABO and Rh blood typing documented as performed (Pre-Cr)**
0.00 0.00 FUD XXX E

3294F **Group B Streptococcus (GBS) screening documented as performed during week 35-37 gestation (Pre-Cr)**
0.00 0.00 FUD XXX E

3300F **American Joint Committee on Cancer (AJCC) stage documented and reviewed (ONC)**
0.00 0.00 FUD XXX M
AMA: 2008,Mar,8-12

3301F **Cancer stage documented in medical record as metastatic and reviewed (ONC)**
EXCLUDES *Cancer staging measures (3321F-3390F)*
0.00 0.00 FUD XXX M
AMA: 2008,Mar,8-12

3315F **Estrogen receptor (ER) or progesterone receptor (PR) positive breast cancer (ONC)**
0.00 0.00 FUD XXX E
AMA: 2008,Mar,8-12

3316F **Estrogen receptor (ER) and progesterone receptor (PR) negative breast cancer (ONC)**
0.00 0.00 FUD XXX E
AMA: 2008,Mar,8-12

3317F **Pathology report confirming malignancy documented in the medical record and reviewed prior to the initiation of chemotherapy (ONC)**
0.00 0.00 FUD XXX E
AMA: 2008,Mar,8-12

3318F **Pathology report confirming malignancy documented in the medical record and reviewed prior to the initiation of radiation therapy (ONC)**
0.00 0.00 FUD XXX E
AMA: 2008,Mar,8-12

3319F **1 of the following diagnostic imaging studies ordered: chest x-ray, CT, Ultrasound, MRI, PET, or nuclear medicine scans (ML)**
0.00 0.00 FUD XXX M
AMA: 2008,Mar,8-12

3320F **None of the following diagnostic imaging studies ordered: chest X-ray, CT, Ultrasound, MRI, PET, or nuclear medicine scans (ML)**
0.00 0.00 FUD XXX M
AMA: 2008,Mar,8-12

3321F **AJCC Cancer Stage 0 or IA Melanoma, documented (ML)**
0.00 0.00 FUD XXX M

3322F **Melanoma greater than AJCC Stage 0 or IA (ML)**
0.00 0.00 FUD XXX M

3323F **Clinical tumor, node and metastases (TNM) staging documented and reviewed prior to surgery (Lung/Esop Cx)**
0.00 0.00 FUD XXX E

3324F **MRI or CT scan ordered, reviewed or requested (EPI)**
0.00 0.00 FUD XXX E

3325F **Preoperative assessment of functional or medical indication(s) for surgery prior to the cataract surgery with intraocular lens placement (must be performed within 12 months prior to cataract surgery) (EC)**
0.00 0.00 FUD XXX E
AMA: 2008,Mar,8-12

3328F **Performance status documented and reviewed within 2 weeks prior to surgery (Lung/Esop Cx)**
0.00 0.00 FUD XXX E

3330F **Imaging study ordered (BkP)**
0.00 0.00 FUD XXX E
AMA: 2008,Mar,8-12

3331F **Imaging study not ordered (BkP)**
0.00 0.00 FUD XXX E
AMA: 2008,Mar,8-12

3340F **Mammogram assessment category of "incomplete: need additional imaging evaluation" documented (RAD)**
0.00 0.00 FUD XXX M
AMA: 2008,Mar,8-12

3341F **Mammogram assessment category of "negative," documented (RAD)**
0.00 0.00 FUD XXX M
AMA: 2008,Mar,8-12

3342F Mammogram assessment category of "benign," documented (RAD)
0.00 0.00 FUD XXX M
AMA: 2008,Mar,8-12

3343F Mammogram assessment category of "probably benign," documented (RAD)
0.00 0.00 FUD XXX M
AMA: 2008,Mar,8-12

3344F Mammogram assessment category of "suspicious," documented (RAD)
0.00 0.00 FUD XXX M
AMA: 2008,Mar,8-12

3345F Mammogram assessment category of "highly suggestive of malignancy," documented (RAD)
0.00 0.00 FUD XXX M
AMA: 2008,Mar,8-12

3350F Mammogram assessment category of "known biopsy proven malignancy," documented (RAD)
0.00 0.00 FUD XXX M
AMA: 2008,Mar,8-12

3351F Negative screen for depressive symptoms as categorized by using a standardized depression screening/assessment tool (MDD)
0.00 0.00 FUD XXX E

3352F No significant depressive symptoms as categorized by using a standardized depression assessment tool (MDD)
0.00 0.00 FUD XXX E

3353F Mild to moderate depressive symptoms as categorized by using a standardized depression screening/assessment tool (MDD)
0.00 0.00 FUD XXX E

3354F Clinically significant depressive symptoms as categorized by using a standardized depression screening/assessment tool (MDD)
0.00 0.00 FUD XXX E

3370F AJCC Breast Cancer Stage 0 documented (ONC)
0.00 0.00 FUD XXX E

3372F AJCC Breast Cancer Stage I: T1mic, T1a or T1b (tumor size ≤ 1 cm) documented (ONC)
0.00 0.00 FUD XXX E

3374F AJCC Breast Cancer Stage I: T1c (tumor size > 1 cm to 2 cm) documented (ONC)
0.00 0.00 FUD XXX E

3376F AJCC Breast Cancer Stage II documented (ONC)
0.00 0.00 FUD XXX E

3378F AJCC Breast Cancer Stage III documented (ONC)
0.00 0.00 FUD XXX E

3380F AJCC Breast Cancer Stage IV documented (ONC)
0.00 0.00 FUD XXX E

3382F AJCC colon cancer, Stage 0 documented (ONC)
0.00 0.00 FUD XXX E

3384F AJCC colon cancer, Stage I documented (ONC)
0.00 0.00 FUD XXX E

3386F AJCC colon cancer, Stage II documented (ONC)
0.00 0.00 FUD XXX E

3388F AJCC colon cancer, Stage III documented (ONC)
0.00 0.00 FUD XXX E

3390F AJCC colon cancer, Stage IV documented (ONC)
0.00 0.00 FUD XXX E

3394F Quantitative HER2 immunohistochemistry (IHC) evaluation of breast cancer consistent with the scoring system defined in the ASCO/CAP guidelines (PATH)
0.00 0.00 FUD XXX M

3395F Quantitative non-HER2 immunohistochemistry (IHC) evaluation of breast cancer (eg, testing for estrogen or progesterone receptors [ER/PR]) performed (PATH)
0.00 0.00 FUD XXX M

3450F Dyspnea screened, no dyspnea or mild dyspnea (Pall Cr)
0.00 0.00 FUD XXX E

3451F Dyspnea screened, moderate or severe dyspnea (Pall Cr)
0.00 0.00 FUD XXX E

3452F Dyspnea not screened (Pall Cr)
0.00 0.00 FUD XXX E

3455F TB screening performed and results interpreted within six months prior to initiation of first-time biologic disease modifying anti-rheumatic drug therapy for RA (RA)
0.00 0.00 FUD XXX M

3470F Rheumatoid arthritis (RA) disease activity, low (RA)
0.00 0.00 FUD XXX M

3471F Rheumatoid arthritis (RA) disease activity, moderate (RA)
0.00 0.00 FUD XXX M

3472F Rheumatoid arthritis (RA) disease activity, high (RA)
0.00 0.00 FUD XXX M

3475F Disease prognosis for rheumatoid arthritis assessed, poor prognosis documented (RA)
0.00 0.00 FUD XXX M

3476F Disease prognosis for rheumatoid arthritis assessed, good prognosis documented (RA)
0.00 0.00 FUD XXX M

3490F History of AIDS-defining condition (HIV)
0.00 0.00 FUD XXX E

3491F HIV indeterminate (infants of undetermined HIV status born of HIV-infected mothers) (HIV)
0.00 0.00 FUD XXX E

3492F History of nadir CD4+ cell count <350 cells/mm3 (HIV)
0.00 0.00 FUD XXX E

3493F No history of nadir CD4+ cell count <350 cells/mm3 and no history of AIDS-defining condition (HIV)
0.00 0.00 FUD XXX E

3494F CD4+ cell count <200 cells/mm3 (HIV)
0.00 0.00 FUD XXX E

3495F CD4+ cell count 200 - 499 cells/mm3 (HIV)
0.00 0.00 FUD XXX E

3496F CD4+ cell count ≥ 500 cells/mm3 (HIV)
0.00 0.00 FUD XXX E

3497F CD4+ cell percentage <15% (HIV)
0.00 0.00 FUD XXX E

3498F CD4+ cell percentage ≥ 15% (HIV)
0.00 0.00 FUD XXX E

3500F CD4+ cell count or CD4+ cell percentage documented as performed (HIV)
0.00 0.00 FUD XXX E

3502F HIV RNA viral load below limits of quantification (HIV)
0.00 0.00 FUD XXX E

3503F HIV RNA viral load not below limits of quantification (HIV)
0.00 0.00 FUD XXX E

3510F Documentation that tuberculosis (TB) screening test performed and results interpreted (HIV) (IBD)
0.00 0.00 FUD XXX E

3511F Chlamydia and gonorrhea screenings documented as performed (HIV)
0.00 0.00 FUD XXX E

3512F Syphilis screening documented as performed (HIV)
0.00 0.00 FUD XXX E

3513F **Hepatitis B screening documented as performed (HIV)**
0.00 0.00 FUD XXX E

3514F **Hepatitis C screening documented as performed (HIV)**
0.00 0.00 FUD XXX E

3515F **Patient has documented immunity to Hepatitis C (HIV)**
0.00 0.00 FUD XXX E

3517F **Hepatitis B Virus (HBV) status assessed and results interpreted within one year prior to receiving a first course of anti-TNF (tumor necrosis factor) therapy (IBD)**
0.00 0.00 FUD XXX E

3520F **Clostridium difficile testing performed (IBD)**
0.00 0.00 FUD XXX E

3550F **Low risk for thromboembolism (AFIB)**
0.00 0.00 FUD XXX E

3551F **Intermediate risk for thromboembolism (AFIB)**
0.00 0.00 FUD XXX E

3552F **High risk for thromboembolism (AFIB)**
0.00 0.00 FUD XXX E

3555F **Patient had International Normalized Ratio (INR) measurement performed (AFIB)**
0.00 0.00 FUD XXX E
AMA: 2010,Jul,3-5

3570F **Final report for bone scintigraphy study includes correlation with existing relevant imaging studies (eg, X-ray, MRI, CT) corresponding to the same anatomical region in question (NUC_MED)**
0.00 0.00 FUD XXX M

3572F **Patient considered to be potentially at risk for fracture in a weight-bearing site (NUC_MED)**
0.00 0.00 FUD XXX E

3573F **Patient not considered to be potentially at risk for fracture in a weight-bearing site (NUC_MED)**
0.00 0.00 FUD XXX E

3650F **Electroencephalogram (EEG) ordered, reviewed or requested (EPI)**
0.00 0.00 FUD XXX E

3700F **Psychiatric disorders or disturbances assessed (Prkns)**
0.00 0.00 FUD XXX E

3720F **Cognitive impairment or dysfunction assessed (Prkns)**
0.00 0.00 FUD XXX M

3725F **Screening for depression performed (DEM)**
0.00 0.00 FUD XXX M

3750F **Patient not receiving dose of corticosteroids greater than or equal to 10mg/day for 60 or greater consecutive days (IBD)**
0.00 0.00 FUD XXX E

3751F **Electrodiagnostic studies for distal symmetric polyneuropathy conducted (or requested), documented, and reviewed within 6 months of initial evaluation for condition (DSP)**
0.00 0.00 FUD XXX E

3752F **Electrodiagnostic studies for distal symmetric polyneuropathy not conducted (or requested), documented, or reviewed within 6 months of initial evaluation for condition (DSP)**
0.00 0.00 FUD XXX E

3753F **Patient has clear clinical symptoms and signs that are highly suggestive of neuropathy AND cannot be attributed to another condition, AND has an obvious cause for the neuropathy (DSP)**
0.00 0.00 FUD XXX E

3754F **Screening tests for diabetes mellitus reviewed, requested, or ordered (DSP)**
0.00 0.00 FUD XXX E

3755F **Cognitive and behavioral impairment screening performed (ALS)**
0.00 0.00 FUD XXX E

3756F **Patient has pseudobulbar affect, sialorrhea, or ALS-related symptoms (ALS)**
0.00 0.00 FUD XXX E

3757F **Patient does not have pseudobulbar affect, sialorrhea, or ALS-related symptoms (ALS)**
0.00 0.00 FUD XXX E

3758F **Patient referred for pulmonary function testing or peak cough expiratory flow (ALS)**
0.00 0.00 FUD XXX E

3759F **Patient screened for dysphagia, weight loss, and impaired nutrition, and results documented (ALS)**
0.00 0.00 FUD XXX E

3760F **Patient exhibits dysphagia, weight loss, or impaired nutrition (ALS)**
0.00 0.00 FUD XXX E

3761F **Patient does not exhibit dysphagia, weight loss, or impaired nutrition (ALS)**
0.00 0.00 FUD XXX E

3762F **Patient is dysarthric (ALS)**
0.00 0.00 FUD XXX E

3763F **Patient is not dysarthric (ALS)**
0.00 0.00 FUD XXX E

3775F **Adenoma(s) or other neoplasm detected during screening colonoscopy (SCADR)**
0.00 0.00 FUD XXX E

3776F **Adenoma(s) or other neoplasm not detected during screening colonoscopy (SCADR)**
0.00 0.00 FUD XXX E

4000F-4563F Therapies Provided (Includes Preventive Services)

INCLUDES Behavioral/pharmacologic/procedural therapies
Preventive services including patient education/counseling

4000F **Tobacco use cessation intervention, counseling (COPD, CAP, CAD, Asthma) (DM) (PV)**
0.00 0.00 FUD XXX E
AMA: 2018,Jan,8; 2017,Jan,8; 2016,Jan,13; 2015,Jan,16

4001F **Tobacco use cessation intervention, pharmacologic therapy (COPD, CAD, CAP, PV, Asthma) (DM) (PV)**
0.00 0.00 FUD XXX E
AMA: 2008,Mar,8-12; 2004,Nov,1

4003F **Patient education, written/oral, appropriate for patients with heart failure, performed (NMA-No Measure Associated)**
0.00 0.00 FUD XXX E
AMA: 2004,Nov,1

4004F **Patient screened for tobacco use and received tobacco cessation intervention (counseling, pharmacotherapy, or both), if identified as a tobacco user (PV, CAD)**
0.00 0.00 FUD XXX M

4005F **Pharmacologic therapy (other than minerals/vitamins) for osteoporosis prescribed (OP) (IBD)**
0.00 0.00 FUD XXX E

4008F **Beta-blocker therapy prescribed or currently being taken (CAD,HF)**
0.00 0.00 FUD XXX M

4010F **Angiotensin Converting Enzyme (ACE) Inhibitor or Angiotensin Receptor Blocker (ARB) therapy prescribed or currently being taken (CAD, CKD, HF) (DM)**
0.00 0.00 FUD XXX M

4011F **Oral antiplatelet therapy prescribed (CAD)**
0.00 0.00 FUD XXX E
AMA: 2004,Nov,1

4012F **Warfarin therapy prescribed (NMA-No Measure Associated)**
0.00 0.00 FUD XXX E

4013F **Statin therapy prescribed or currently being taken (CAD)**
0.00 0.00 FUD XXX E

4014F **Written discharge instructions provided to heart failure patients discharged home (Instructions include all of the following components: activity level, diet, discharge medications, follow-up appointment, weight monitoring, what to do if symptoms worsen) (NMA-No Measure Associated)**
0.00 0.00 FUD XXX E

4015F **Persistent asthma, preferred long term control medication or an acceptable alternative treatment, prescribed (NMA-No Measure Associated)**
EXCLUDES *Reporting code with modifier 1P*
Code also modifier 2P for patient reasons for not prescribing
0.00 0.00 FUD XXX E

4016F **Anti-inflammatory/analgesic agent prescribed (OA) (Use for prescribed or continued medication[s], including over-the-counter medication[s])**
INCLUDES Over-the-counter medication(s)
Prescribed/continued medication(s)
0.00 0.00 FUD XXX E

4017F **Gastrointestinal prophylaxis for NSAID use prescribed (OA)**
0.00 0.00 FUD XXX E

4018F **Therapeutic exercise for the involved joint(s) instructed or physical or occupational therapy prescribed (OA)**
0.00 0.00 FUD XXX E

4019F **Documentation of receipt of counseling on exercise and either both calcium and vitamin D use or counseling regarding both calcium and vitamin D use (OP)**
0.00 0.00 FUD XXX E

4025F **Inhaled bronchodilator prescribed (COPD)**
0.00 0.00 FUD XXX E

4030F **Long-term oxygen therapy prescribed (more than 15 hours per day) (COPD)**
0.00 0.00 FUD XXX E

4033F **Pulmonary rehabilitation exercise training recommended (COPD)**
Code also dyspnea assessed, present (1019F)
0.00 0.00 FUD XXX E

4035F **Influenza immunization recommended (COPD) (IBD)**
0.00 0.00 FUD XXX E
AMA: 2008,Mar,8-12

4037F **Influenza immunization ordered or administered (COPD, PV, CKD, ESRD)(IBD)**
0.00 0.00 FUD XXX E
AMA: 2008,Mar,8-12

4040F **Pneumococcal vaccine administered or previously received (COPD) (PV), (IBD)**
0.00 0.00 FUD XXX M
AMA: 2008,Mar,8-12

4041F **Documentation of order for cefazolin OR cefuroxime for antimicrobial prophylaxis (PERI 2)**
0.00 0.00 FUD XXX E

4042F **Documentation that prophylactic antibiotics were neither given within 4 hours prior to surgical incision nor given intraoperatively (PERI 2)**
0.00 0.00 FUD XXX E

4043F **Documentation that an order was given to discontinue prophylactic antibiotics within 48 hours of surgical end time, cardiac procedures (PERI 2)**
0.00 0.00 FUD XXX E

4044F **Documentation that an order was given for venous thromboembolism (VTE) prophylaxis to be given within 24 hours prior to incision time or 24 hours after surgery end time (PERI 2)**
0.00 0.00 FUD XXX M

4045F **Appropriate empiric antibiotic prescribed (CAP), (EM)**
0.00 0.00 FUD XXX E

4046F **Documentation that prophylactic antibiotics were given within 4 hours prior to surgical incision or given intraoperatively (PERI 2)**
0.00 0.00 FUD XXX E

4047F **Documentation of order for prophylactic parenteral antibiotics to be given within 1 hour (if fluoroquinolone or vancomycin, 2 hours) prior to surgical incision (or start of procedure when no incision is required) (PERI 2)**
0.00 0.00 FUD XXX E

4048F **Documentation that administration of prophylactic parenteral antibiotic was initiated within 1 hour (if fluoroquinolone or vancomycin, 2 hours) prior to surgical incision (or start of procedure when no incision is required) as ordered (PERI 2)**
0.00 0.00 FUD XXX E

4049F **Documentation that order was given to discontinue prophylactic antibiotics within 24 hours of surgical end time, non-cardiac procedure (PERI 2)**
0.00 0.00 FUD XXX E

4050F **Hypertension plan of care documented as appropriate (NMA-No Measure Associated)**
0.00 0.00 FUD XXX E

4051F **Referred for an arteriovenous (AV) fistula (ESRD, CKD)**
0.00 0.00 FUD XXX E
AMA: 2008,Mar,8-12

4052F **Hemodialysis via functioning arteriovenous (AV) fistula (ESRD)**
0.00 0.00 FUD XXX E
AMA: 2008,Mar,8-12

4053F **Hemodialysis via functioning arteriovenous (AV) graft (ESRD)**
0.00 0.00 FUD XXX E
AMA: 2008,Mar,8-12

4054F **Hemodialysis via catheter (ESRD)**
0.00 0.00 FUD XXX E
AMA: 2008,Mar,8-12

4055F **Patient receiving peritoneal dialysis (ESRD)**
0.00 0.00 FUD XXX E
AMA: 2008,Mar,8-12

4056F **Appropriate oral rehydration solution recommended (PAG)**
0.00 0.00 FUD XXX E

4058F **Pediatric gastroenteritis education provided to caregiver (PAG)**
0.00 0.00 FUD XXX E

4060F **Psychotherapy services provided (MDD, MDD ADOL)**
0.00 0.00 FUD XXX E

4062F **Patient referral for psychotherapy documented (MDD, MDD ADOL)**
0.00 0.00 FUD XXX E

4063F **Antidepressant pharmacotherapy considered and not prescribed (MDD ADOL)**
0.00 0.00 FUD XXX E

4064F **Antidepressant pharmacotherapy prescribed (MDD, MDD ADOL)**
0.00 0.00 FUD XXX E

4065F **Antipsychotic pharmacotherapy prescribed (MDD)**
0.00 0.00 FUD XXX E

4066F **Electroconvulsive therapy (ECT) provided (MDD)**
0.00 0.00 FUD XXX E

4067F **Patient referral for electroconvulsive therapy (ECT) documented (MDD)**
0.00 0.00 FUD XXX E

4069F **Venous thromboembolism (VTE) prophylaxis received (IBD)**
0.00 0.00 FUD XXX E

4070F **Deep vein thrombosis (DVT) prophylaxis received by end of hospital day 2 (STR)**
0.00 0.00 FUD XXX E

4073F **Oral antiplatelet therapy prescribed at discharge (STR)**
0.00 0.00 FUD XXX E

4075F **Anticoagulant therapy prescribed at discharge (STR)**
0.00 0.00 FUD XXX E

4077F **Documentation that tissue plasminogen activator (t-PA) administration was considered (STR)**
0.00 0.00 FUD XXX E

4079F **Documentation that rehabilitation services were considered (STR)**
0.00 0.00 FUD XXX E

4084F **Aspirin received within 24 hours before emergency department arrival or during emergency department stay (EM)**
0.00 0.00 FUD XXX E

4086F **Aspirin or clopidogrel prescribed or currently being taken (CAD)**
0.00 0.00 FUD XXX M

4090F **Patient receiving erythropoietin therapy (HEM)**
0.00 0.00 FUD XXX M
AMA: 2008,Mar,8-12

4095F **Patient not receiving erythropoietin therapy (HEM)**
0.00 0.00 FUD XXX E
AMA: 2008,Mar,8-12

4100F **Bisphosphonate therapy, intravenous, ordered or received (HEM)**
0.00 0.00 FUD XXX M
AMA: 2008,Mar,8-12

4110F **Internal mammary artery graft performed for primary, isolated coronary artery bypass graft procedure (CABG)**
0.00 0.00 FUD XXX M

4115F **Beta blocker administered within 24 hours prior to surgical incision (CABG)**
0.00 0.00 FUD XXX M

4120F **Antibiotic prescribed or dispensed (URI, PHAR), (A-BRONCH)**
0.00 0.00 FUD XXX M
AMA: 2008,Mar,8-12

4124F **Antibiotic neither prescribed nor dispensed (URI, PHAR), (A-BRONCH)**
0.00 0.00 FUD XXX M
AMA: 2008,Mar,8-12

4130F **Topical preparations (including OTC) prescribed for acute otitis externa (AOE)**
0.00 0.00 FUD XXX M
AMA: 2010,Jan,6-7; 2008,Mar,8-12

4131F **Systemic antimicrobial therapy prescribed (AOE)**
0.00 0.00 FUD XXX M
AMA: 2008,Mar,8-12

4132F **Systemic antimicrobial therapy not prescribed (AOE)**
0.00 0.00 FUD XXX M
AMA: 2008,Mar,8-12

4133F **Antihistamines or decongestants prescribed or recommended (OME)**
0.00 0.00 FUD XXX E
AMA: 2008,Mar,8-12

4134F **Antihistamines or decongestants neither prescribed nor recommended (OME)**
0.00 0.00 FUD XXX E
AMA: 2008,Mar,8-12

4135F **Systemic corticosteroids prescribed (OME)**
0.00 0.00 FUD XXX E
AMA: 2008,Mar,8-12

4136F **Systemic corticosteroids not prescribed (OME)**
0.00 0.00 FUD XXX E
AMA: 2008,Mar,8-12

4140F **Inhaled corticosteroids prescribed (Asthma)**
0.00 0.00 FUD XXX E

4142F **Corticosteroid sparing therapy prescribed (IBD)**
0.00 0.00 FUD XXX E

4144F **Alternative long-term control medication prescribed (Asthma)**
0.00 0.00 FUD XXX E

4145F **Two or more anti-hypertensive agents prescribed or currently being taken (CAD, HTN)**
0.00 0.00 FUD XXX E

4148F **Hepatitis A vaccine injection administered or previously received (HEP-C)**
0.00 0.00 FUD XXX E

4149F **Hepatitis B vaccine injection administered or previously received (HEP-C, HIV) (IBD)**
0.00 0.00 FUD XXX E

4150F **Patient receiving antiviral treatment for Hepatitis C (HEP-C)**
0.00 0.00 FUD XXX E
AMA: 2008,Mar,8-12

4151F **Patient did not start or is not receiving antiviral treatment for Hepatitis C during the measurement period (HEP-C)**
0.00 0.00 FUD XXX E
AMA: 2008,Mar,8-12

4153F **Combination peginterferon and ribavirin therapy prescribed (HEP-C)**
0.00 0.00 FUD XXX E
AMA: 2008,Mar,8-12

4155F **Hepatitis A vaccine series previously received (HEP-C)**
0.00 0.00 FUD XXX E
AMA: 2008,Mar,8-12

4157F **Hepatitis B vaccine series previously received (HEP-C)**
0.00 0.00 FUD XXX E
AMA: 2008,Mar,8-12

4158F **Patient counseled about risks of alcohol use (HEP-C)**
0.00 0.00 FUD XXX E
AMA: 2008,Mar,8-12

4159F **Counseling regarding contraception received prior to initiation of antiviral treatment (HEP-C)**
0.00 0.00 FUD XXX E
AMA: 2008,Mar,8-12

4163F **Patient counseling at a minimum on all of the following treatment options for clinically localized prostate cancer: active surveillance, and interstitial prostate brachytherapy, and external beam radiotherapy, and radical prostatectomy, provided prior to initiation of treatment (PRCA)**
0.00 0.00 FUD XXX E
AMA: 2008,Mar,8-12

4164F **Adjuvant (ie, in combination with external beam radiotherapy to the prostate for prostate cancer) hormonal therapy (gonadotropin-releasing hormone [GnRH] agonist or antagonist) prescribed/administered (PRCA)**
0.00 0.00 FUD XXX E
AMA: 2008,Mar,8-12

4165F **3-dimensional conformal radiotherapy (3D-CRT) or intensity modulated radiation therapy (IMRT) received (PRCA)**
0.00 0.00 FUD XXX E
AMA: 2008,Mar,8-12

4167F **Head of bed elevation (30-45 degrees) on first ventilator day ordered (CRIT)**
0.00 0.00 FUD XXX E
AMA: 2008,Mar,8-12

4168F **Patient receiving care in the intensive care unit (ICU) and receiving mechanical ventilation, 24 hours or less (CRIT)**
0.00 0.00 FUD XXX E
AMA: 2008,Mar,8-12

4169F **Patient either not receiving care in the intensive care unit (ICU) OR not receiving mechanical ventilation OR receiving mechanical ventilation greater than 24 hours (CRIT)**
0.00 0.00 FUD XXX E
AMA: 2008,Mar,8-12

4171F **Patient receiving erythropoiesis-stimulating agents (ESA) therapy (CKD)**
0.00 0.00 FUD XXX E
AMA: 2008,Mar,8-12

4172F **Patient not receiving erythropoiesis-stimulating agents (ESA) therapy (CKD)**
0.00 0.00 FUD XXX E
AMA: 2008,Mar,8-12

4174F **Counseling about the potential impact of glaucoma on visual functioning and quality of life, and importance of treatment adherence provided to patient and/or caregiver(s) (EC)**
0.00 0.00 FUD XXX E
AMA: 2008,Mar,8-12

4175F **Best-corrected visual acuity of 20/40 or better (distance or near) achieved within the 90 days following cataract surgery (EC)**
0.00 0.00 FUD XXX M
AMA: 2008,Mar,8-12

4176F **Counseling about value of protection from UV light and lack of proven efficacy of nutritional supplements in prevention or progression of cataract development provided to patient and/or caregiver(s) (NMA-No Measure Associated)**
0.00 0.00 FUD XXX E

4177F **Counseling about the benefits and/or risks of the Age-Related Eye Disease Study (AREDS) formulation for preventing progression of age-related macular degeneration (AMD) provided to patient and/or caregiver(s) (EC)**
0.00 0.00 FUD XXX M
AMA: 2008,Mar,8-12

4178F **Anti-D immune globulin received between 26 and 30 weeks gestation (Pre-Cr)** M
0.00 0.00 FUD XXX E
AMA: 2008,Mar,8-12

4179F **Tamoxifen or aromatase inhibitor (AI) prescribed (ONC)**
0.00 0.00 FUD XXX E
AMA: 2008,Mar,8-12

4180F **Adjuvant chemotherapy referred, prescribed, or previously received for Stage III colon cancer (ONC)**
0.00 0.00 FUD XXX E
AMA: 2008,Mar,8-12

4181F **Conformal radiation therapy received (NMA-No Measure Associated)**
0.00 0.00 FUD XXX E

4182F **Conformal radiation therapy not received (NMA-No Measure Associated)**
0.00 0.00 FUD XXX E

4185F **Continuous (12-months) therapy with proton pump inhibitor (PPI) or histamine H2 receptor antagonist (H2RA) received (GERD)**
0.00 0.00 FUD XXX E
AMA: 2008,Mar,8-12

4186F **No continuous (12-months) therapy with either proton pump inhibitor (PPI) or histamine H2 receptor antagonist (H2RA) received (GERD)**
0.00 0.00 FUD XXX E
AMA: 2008,Mar,8-12

4187F **Disease modifying anti-rheumatic drug therapy prescribed or dispensed (RA)**
0.00 0.00 FUD XXX E

4188F **Appropriate angiotensin converting enzyme (ACE)/angiotensin receptor blockers (ARB) therapeutic monitoring test ordered or performed (AM)**
0.00 0.00 FUD XXX E
AMA: 2008,Mar,8-12

4189F **Appropriate digoxin therapeutic monitoring test ordered or performed (AM)**
0.00 0.00 FUD XXX E
AMA: 2008,Mar,8-12

4190F **Appropriate diuretic therapeutic monitoring test ordered or performed (AM)**
0.00 0.00 FUD XXX E
AMA: 2008,Mar,8-12

4191F **Appropriate anticonvulsant therapeutic monitoring test ordered or performed (AM)**
0.00 0.00 FUD XXX E
AMA: 2008,Mar,8-12

4192F **Patient not receiving glucocorticoid therapy (RA)**
0.00 0.00 FUD XXX M

4193F **Patient receiving <10 mg daily prednisone (or equivalent), or RA activity is worsening, or glucocorticoid use is for less than 6 months (RA)**
0.00 0.00 FUD XXX M

4194F **Patient receiving ≥10 mg daily prednisone (or equivalent) for longer than 6 months, and improvement or no change in disease activity (RA)**
0.00 0.00 FUD XXX M

4195F **Patient receiving first-time biologic disease modifying anti-rheumatic drug therapy for rheumatoid arthritis (RA)**
0.00 0.00 FUD XXX M

4196F **Patient not receiving first-time biologic disease modifying anti-rheumatic drug therapy for rheumatoid arthritis (RA)**
0.00 0.00 FUD XXX M

4200F **External beam radiotherapy as primary therapy to prostate with or without nodal irradiation (PRCA)**
0.00 0.00 FUD XXX E
AMA: 2008,Mar,8-12

4201F **External beam radiotherapy with or without nodal irradiation as adjuvant or salvage therapy for prostate cancer patient (PRCA)**
0.00 0.00 FUD XXX E
AMA: 2008,Mar,8-12

4210F **Angiotensin converting enzyme (ACE) or angiotensin receptor blockers (ARB) medication therapy for 6 months or more (MM)**
0.00 0.00 FUD XXX E
AMA: 2008,Mar,8-12

4220F Digoxin medication therapy for 6 months or more (MM)
🏢 0.00 ⚕ 0.00 **FUD** XXX ⬛ E
AMA: 2008,Mar,8-12

4221F Diuretic medication therapy for 6 months or more (MM)
🏢 0.00 ⚕ 0.00 **FUD** XXX ⬛ E
AMA: 2008,Mar,8-12

4230F Anticonvulsant medication therapy for 6 months or more (MM)
🏢 0.00 ⚕ 0.00 **FUD** XXX ⬛ E
AMA: 2008,Mar,8-12

4240F Instruction in therapeutic exercise with follow-up provided to patients during episode of back pain lasting longer than 12 weeks (BkP)
🏢 0.00 ⚕ 0.00 **FUD** XXX ⬛ E
AMA: 2008,Mar,8-12

4242F Counseling for supervised exercise program provided to patients during episode of back pain lasting longer than 12 weeks (BkP)
🏢 0.00 ⚕ 0.00 **FUD** XXX ⬛ E
AMA: 2008,Mar,8-12

4245F Patient counseled during the initial visit to maintain or resume normal activities (BkP)
🏢 0.00 ⚕ 0.00 **FUD** XXX ⬛ E
AMA: 2008,Mar,8-12

4248F Patient counseled during the initial visit for an episode of back pain against bed rest lasting 4 days or longer (BkP)
🏢 0.00 ⚕ 0.00 **FUD** XXX ⬛ E
AMA: 2008,Mar,8-12

4250F Active warming used intraoperatively for the purpose of maintaining normothermia, or at least 1 body temperature equal to or greater than 36 degrees Centigrade (or 96.8 degrees Fahrenheit) recorded within the 30 minutes immediately before or the 15 minutes immediately after anesthesia end time (CRIT)
🏢 0.00 ⚕ 0.00 **FUD** XXX ⬛ E
AMA: 2008,Mar,8-12

4255F Duration of general or neuraxial anesthesia 60 minutes or longer, as documented in the anesthesia record (CRIT) (Peri2)
🏢 0.00 ⚕ 0.00 **FUD** XXX ⬛ M

4256F Duration of general or neuraxial anesthesia less than 60 minutes, as documented in the anesthesia record (CRIT) (Peri2)
🏢 0.00 ⚕ 0.00 **FUD** XXX ⬛ E

4260F Wound surface culture technique used (CWC)
🏢 0.00 ⚕ 0.00 **FUD** XXX ⬛ E

4261F Technique other than surface culture of the wound exudate used (eg, Levine/deep swab technique, semi-quantitative or quantitative swab technique) or wound surface culture technique not used (CWC)
🏢 0.00 ⚕ 0.00 **FUD** XXX ⬛ E

4265F Use of wet to dry dressings prescribed or recommended (CWC)
🏢 0.00 ⚕ 0.00 **FUD** XXX ⬛ E

4266F Use of wet to dry dressings neither prescribed nor recommended (CWC)
🏢 0.00 ⚕ 0.00 **FUD** XXX ⬛ E

4267F Compression therapy prescribed (CWC)
🏢 0.00 ⚕ 0.00 **FUD** XXX ⬛ E

4268F Patient education regarding the need for long term compression therapy including interval replacement of compression stockings received (CWC)
🏢 0.00 ⚕ 0.00 **FUD** XXX ⬛ E

4269F Appropriate method of offloading (pressure relief) prescribed (CWC)
🏢 0.00 ⚕ 0.00 **FUD** XXX ⬛ E

4270F Patient receiving potent antiretroviral therapy for 6 months or longer (HIV)
🏢 0.00 ⚕ 0.00 **FUD** XXX ⬛ E

4271F Patient receiving potent antiretroviral therapy for less than 6 months or not receiving potent antiretroviral therapy (HIV)
🏢 0.00 ⚕ 0.00 **FUD** XXX ⬛ E

4274F Influenza immunization administered or previously received (HIV) (P-ESRD)
🏢 0.00 ⚕ 0.00 **FUD** XXX ⬛ E

4276F Potent antiretroviral therapy prescribed (HIV)
🏢 0.00 ⚕ 0.00 **FUD** XXX ⬛ E

4279F Pneumocystis jiroveci pneumonia prophylaxis prescribed (HIV)
🏢 0.00 ⚕ 0.00 **FUD** XXX ⬛ E

4280F Pneumocystis jiroveci pneumonia prophylaxis prescribed within 3 months of low CD4+ cell count or percentage (HIV)
🏢 0.00 ⚕ 0.00 **FUD** XXX ⬛ E

4290F Patient screened for injection drug use (HIV)
🏢 0.00 ⚕ 0.00 **FUD** XXX ⬛ E

4293F Patient screened for high-risk sexual behavior (HIV)
🏢 0.00 ⚕ 0.00 **FUD** XXX ⬛ E

4300F Patient receiving warfarin therapy for nonvalvular atrial fibrillation or atrial flutter (AFIB)
🏢 0.00 ⚕ 0.00 **FUD** XXX ⬛ E

4301F Patient not receiving warfarin therapy for nonvalvular atrial fibrillation or atrial flutter (AFIB)
🏢 0.00 ⚕ 0.00 **FUD** XXX ⬛ E

4305F Patient education regarding appropriate foot care and daily inspection of the feet received (CWC)
🏢 0.00 ⚕ 0.00 **FUD** XXX ⬛ E

4306F Patient counseled regarding psychosocial and pharmacologic treatment options for opioid addiction (SUD)
🏢 0.00 ⚕ 0.00 **FUD** XXX ⬛ E

4320F Patient counseled regarding psychosocial and pharmacologic treatment options for alcohol dependence (SUD)
🏢 0.00 ⚕ 0.00 **FUD** XXX ⬛ E

4322F Caregiver provided with education and referred to additional resources for support (DEM)
🏢 0.00 ⚕ 0.00 **FUD** XXX ⬛ M

4324F Patient (or caregiver) queried about Parkinson's disease medication related motor complications (Prkns)
🏢 0.00 ⚕ 0.00 **FUD** XXX ⬛ E

4325F Medical and surgical treatment options reviewed with patient (or caregiver) (Prkns)
🏢 0.00 ⚕ 0.00 **FUD** XXX ⬛ M

4326F Patient (or caregiver) queried about symptoms of autonomic dysfunction (Prkns)
🏢 0.00 ⚕ 0.00 **FUD** XXX ⬛ E

4328F Patient (or caregiver) queried about sleep disturbances (Prkns)
🏢 0.00 ⚕ 0.00 **FUD** XXX ⬛ E

4330F Counseling about epilepsy specific safety issues provided to patient (or caregiver(s)) (EPI)
🏢 0.00 ⚕ 0.00 **FUD** XXX ⬛ E

4340F Counseling for women of childbearing potential with epilepsy (EPI)
🏢 0.00 ⚕ 0.00 **FUD** XXX ⬛ M

26/TC PC/TC Only	A2-Z3 ASC Payment	50 Bilateral	♂ Male Only	♀ Female Only	🏢 Facility RVU	⚕ Non-Facility RVU	⬜ CCI	✖ CLIA
FUD Follow-up Days	**CMS:** IOM	**AMA:** CPT Asst	A-Y OPPSI	80/81 Surg Assist Allowed / w/Doc	Lab Crosswalk	Radiology Crosswalk

4350F **Counseling provided on symptom management, end of life decisions, and palliation (DEM)**
0.00 0.00 FUD XXX E

4400F **Rehabilitative therapy options discussed with patient (or caregiver) (Prkns)**
0.00 0.00 FUD XXX M

4450F **Self-care education provided to patient (HF)**
0.00 0.00 FUD XXX E

4470F **Implantable cardioverter-defibrillator (ICD) counseling provided (HF)**
0.00 0.00 FUD XXX E

4480F **Patient receiving ACE inhibitor/ARB therapy and beta-blocker therapy for 3 months or longer (HF)**
0.00 0.00 FUD XXX E

4481F **Patient receiving ACE inhibitor/ARB therapy and beta-blocker therapy for less than 3 months or patient not receiving ACE inhibitor/ARB therapy and beta-blocker therapy (HF)**
0.00 0.00 FUD XXX E

4500F **Referred to an outpatient cardiac rehabilitation program (CAD)**
0.00 0.00 FUD XXX M

4510F **Previous cardiac rehabilitation for qualifying cardiac event completed (CAD)**
0.00 0.00 FUD XXX M

4525F **Neuropsychiatric intervention ordered (DEM)**
0.00 0.00 FUD XXX E

4526F **Neuropsychiatric intervention received (DEM)**
0.00 0.00 FUD XXX E

4540F **Disease modifying pharmacotherapy discussed (ALS)**
0.00 0.00 FUD XXX E

4541F **Patient offered treatment for pseudobulbar affect, sialorrhea, or ALS-related symptoms (ALS)**
0.00 0.00 FUD XXX E

4550F **Options for noninvasive respiratory support discussed with patient (ALS)**
0.00 0.00 FUD XXX E

4551F **Nutritional support offered (ALS)**
0.00 0.00 FUD XXX E

4552F **Patient offered referral to a speech language pathologist (ALS)**
0.00 0.00 FUD XXX E

4553F **Patient offered assistance in planning for end of life issues (ALS)**
0.00 0.00 FUD XXX E

4554F **Patient received inhalational anesthetic agent (Peri2)**
0.00 0.00 FUD XXX M

4555F **Patient did not receive inhalational anesthetic agent (Peri2)**
0.00 0.00 FUD XXX E

4556F **Patient exhibits 3 or more risk factors for post-operative nausea and vomiting (Peri2)**
0.00 0.00 FUD XXX M

4557F **Patient does not exhibit 3 or more risk factors for post-operative nausea and vomiting (Peri2)**
0.00 0.00 FUD XXX E

4558F **Patient received at least 2 prophylactic pharmacologic anti-emetic agents of different classes preoperatively and intraoperatively (Peri2)**
0.00 0.00 FUD XXX E

4559F **At least 1 body temperature measurement equal to or greater than 35.5 degrees Celsius (or 95.9 degrees Fahrenheit) recorded within the 30 minutes immediately before or the 15 minutes immediately after anesthesia end time (Peri2)**
0.00 0.00 FUD XXX E

4560F **Anesthesia technique did not involve general or neuraxial anesthesia (Peri2)**
0.00 0.00 FUD XXX E

4561F **Patient has a coronary artery stent (Peri2)**
0.00 0.00 FUD XXX E

4562F **Patient does not have a coronary artery stent (Peri2)**
0.00 0.00 FUD XXX E

4563F **Patient received aspirin within 24 hours prior to anesthesia start time (Peri2)**
0.00 0.00 FUD XXX E

5005F-5250F Results Conveyed and Documented

INCLUDES Patient's:
- Functional status
- Morbidity/mortality
- Satisfaction/experience with care

Review/communication test results to patients

5005F **Patient counseled on self-examination for new or changing moles (ML)**
0.00 0.00 FUD XXX E
AMA: 2008,Mar,8-12

5010F **Findings of dilated macular or fundus exam communicated to the physician or other qualified health care professional managing the diabetes care (EC)**
0.00 0.00 FUD XXX M

5015F **Documentation of communication that a fracture occurred and that the patient was or should be tested or treated for osteoporosis (OP)**
0.00 0.00 FUD XXX M

5020F **Treatment summary report communicated to physician(s) or other qualified health care professional(s) managing continuing care and to the patient within 1 month of completing treatment (ONC)**
0.00 0.00 FUD XXX E
AMA: 2008,Mar,8-12

5050F **Treatment plan communicated to provider(s) managing continuing care within 1 month of diagnosis (ML)**
0.00 0.00 FUD XXX M
AMA: 2008,Mar,8-12

5060F **Findings from diagnostic mammogram communicated to practice managing patient's on-going care within 3 business days of exam interpretation (RAD)**
0.00 0.00 FUD XXX E
AMA: 2008,Mar,8-12

5062F **Findings from diagnostic mammogram communicated to the patient within 5 days of exam interpretation (RAD)**
0.00 0.00 FUD XXX E
AMA: 2008,Mar,8-12

5100F **Potential risk for fracture communicated to the referring physician or other qualified health care professional within 24 hours of completion of the imaging study (NUC_MED)**
0.00 0.00 FUD XXX E

5200F **Consideration of referral for a neurological evaluation of appropriateness for surgical therapy for intractable epilepsy within the past 3 years (EPI)**
0.00 0.00 FUD XXX E

5250F **Asthma discharge plan provided to patient (Asthma)**
0.00 0.00 FUD XXX E

6005F-6150F Elements Related to Patient Safety Processes

INCLUDES Patient safety practices

6005F Rationale (eg, severity of illness and safety) for level of care (eg, home, hospital) documented (CAP)
0.00 0.00 FUD XXX E
AMA: 2018,Jan,8; 2017,Jan,8; 2016,Jan,13; 2015,Jan,16

6010F Dysphagia screening conducted prior to order for or receipt of any foods, fluids, or medication by mouth (STR)
0.00 0.00 FUD XXX E

6015F Patient receiving or eligible to receive foods, fluids, or medication by mouth (STR)
0.00 0.00 FUD XXX E

6020F NPO (nothing by mouth) ordered (STR)
0.00 0.00 FUD XXX E

6030F All elements of maximal sterile barrier technique, hand hygiene, skin preparation and, if ultrasound is used, sterile ultrasound techniques followed (CRIT)
0.00 0.00 FUD XXX M
AMA: 2008,Mar,8-12

6040F Use of appropriate radiation dose reduction devices OR manual techniques for appropriate moderation of exposure, documented (RAD)
0.00 0.00 FUD XXX E

6045F Radiation exposure or exposure time in final report for procedure using fluoroscopy, documented (RAD)
0.00 0.00 FUD XXX E
AMA: 2008,Mar,8-12

6070F Patient queried and counseled about anti-epileptic drug (AED) side effects (EPI)
0.00 0.00 FUD XXX E

6080F Patient (or caregiver) queried about falls (Prkns, DSP)
0.00 0.00 FUD XXX E

6090F Patient (or caregiver) counseled about safety issues appropriate to patient's stage of disease (Prkns)
0.00 0.00 FUD XXX E

6100F Timeout to verify correct patient, correct site, and correct procedure, documented (PATH)
0.00 0.00 FUD XXX E

6101F Safety counseling for dementia provided (DEM)
0.00 0.00 FUD XXX E

6102F Safety counseling for dementia ordered (DEM)
0.00 0.00 FUD XXX E

6110F Counseling provided regarding risks of driving and the alternatives to driving (DEM)
0.00 0.00 FUD XXX E

6150F Patient not receiving a first course of anti-TNF (tumor necrosis factor) therapy (IBD)
0.00 0.00 FUD XXX E

7010F-7025F Recall/Reminder System in Place

INCLUDES Provider capabilities
Measures that address setting or care system provided

7010F Patient information entered into a recall system that includes: target date for the next exam specified and a process to follow up with patients regarding missed or unscheduled appointments (ML)
0.00 0.00 FUD XXX M
AMA: 2008,Mar,8-12

7020F Mammogram assessment category (eg, Mammography Quality Standards Act [MQSA], Breast Imaging Reporting and Data System [BI-RADS], or FDA approved equivalent categories) entered into an internal database to allow for analysis of abnormal interpretation (recall) rate (RAD)
0.00 0.00 FUD XXX E
AMA: 2008,Mar,8-12

7025F Patient information entered into a reminder system with a target due date for the next mammogram (RAD)
0.00 0.00 FUD XXX M
AMA: 2008,Mar,8-12

9001F-9007F No Measure Associated

INCLUDES Care aspects not associated with measures at current time

9001F Aortic aneurysm less than 5.0 cm maximum diameter on centerline formatted CT or minor diameter on axial formatted CT (NMA-No Measure Associated)
0.00 0.00 FUD XXX E

9002F Aortic aneurysm 5.0 - 5.4 cm maximum diameter on centerline formatted CT or minor diameter on axial formatted CT (NMA-No Measure Associated)
0.00 0.00 FUD XXX E

9003F Aortic aneurysm 5.5 - 5.9 cm maximum diameter on centerline formatted CT or minor diameter on axial formatted CT (NMA-No Measure Associated)
0.00 0.00 FUD XXX M

9004F Aortic aneurysm 6.0 cm or greater maximum diameter on centerline formatted CT or minor diameter on axial formatted CT (NMA-No Measure Associated)
0.00 0.00 FUD XXX M

9005F Asymptomatic carotid stenosis: No history of any transient ischemic attack or stroke in any carotid or vertebrobasilar territory (NMA-No Measure Associated)
0.00 0.00 FUD XXX E

9006F Symptomatic carotid stenosis: Ipsilateral carotid territory TIA or stroke less than 120 days prior to procedure (NMA-No Measure Associated)
0.00 0.00 FUD XXX M

9007F Other carotid stenosis: Ipsilateral TIA or stroke 120 days or greater prior to procedure or any prior contralateral carotid territory or vertebrobasilar TIA or stroke (NMA-No Measure Associated)
0.00 0.00 FUD XXX M

0042T

0042T **Cerebral perfusion analysis using computed tomography with contrast administration, including post-processing of parametric maps with determination of cerebral blood flow, cerebral blood volume, and mean transit time**
0.00 0.00 FUD XXX N 80
AMA: 2003,Nov,5

0054T-0055T

+ **0054T** **Computer-assisted musculoskeletal surgical navigational orthopedic procedure, with image-guidance based on fluoroscopic images (List separately in addition to code for primary procedure)**
Code first primary procedure
0.00 0.00 FUD XXX N 80
AMA: 2018,Jan,8; 2017,Jan,8; 2016,Jan,13; 2015,Jan,16

+ **0055T** **Computer-assisted musculoskeletal surgical navigational orthopedic procedure, with image-guidance based on CT/MRI images (List separately in addition to code for primary procedure)**
INCLUDES Performance both CT and MRI in same session (one unit)
Code first primary procedure
0.00 0.00 FUD XXX N 80
AMA: 2018,Jan,8; 2017,Jan,8; 2016,Jan,13; 2015,Jan,16

0058T

EXCLUDES *Cryopreservation:*
Embryos (89258)
Oocyte(s), immature (89398)
Oocyte(s), mature (89337)
Sperm (89259)
Testicular reproductive tissue (89335)

~~**0058T**~~ ~~**Cryopreservation; reproductive tissue, ovarian**~~
To report, see (89398)

0071T-0072T

EXCLUDES *Insertion bladder catheter (51702)*
MRI guidance for parenchymal tissue ablation (77022)

0071T **Focused ultrasound ablation of uterine leiomyomata, including MR guidance; total leiomyomata volume less than 200 cc of tissue** ♀
0.00 0.00 FUD XXX J 80
AMA: 2005,Mar,1-6; 2005,Dec,3-6

0072T **total leiomyomata volume greater or equal to 200 cc of tissue** ♀
0.00 0.00 FUD XXX J 80
AMA: 2005,Mar,1-6; 2005,Dec,3-6

0075T-0076T

INCLUDES All diagnostic services for stenting
Ipsilateral extracranial vertebral selective catheterization when confirming need for stenting
EXCLUDES *Selective catheterization and imaging when stenting not required (report only selective catheterization codes)*

0075T **Transcatheter placement of extracranial vertebral artery stent(s), including radiologic supervision and interpretation, open or percutaneous; initial vessel**
0.00 0.00 FUD XXX C 80
AMA: 2018,Jan,8; 2017,Jan,8; 2016,Jan,13; 2015,Jan,16

+ **0076T** **each additional vessel (List separately in addition to code for primary procedure)**
Code first (0075T)
0.00 0.00 FUD XXX C 80
AMA: 2018,Jan,8; 2017,Jan,8; 2016,Jan,13; 2015,Jan,16

0085T

~~**0085T**~~ ~~**Breath test for heart transplant rejection**~~
To report, see (84999)

0095T-0098T

INCLUDES Fluoroscopy

+ **0095T** **Removal of total disc arthroplasty (artificial disc), anterior approach, each additional interspace, cervical (List separately in addition to code for primary procedure)**
EXCLUDES *Lumbar disc (0164T)*
Revision total disc arthroplasty, cervical (22861)
Revision total disc arthroplasty, lumbar (22862)
Code first (22864)
0.00 0.00 FUD XXX C 80
AMA: 2006,Feb,1-6; 2005,Jun,6-8

+ **0098T** **Revision including replacement of total disc arthroplasty (artificial disc), anterior approach, each additional interspace, cervical (List separately in addition to code for primary procedure)**
EXCLUDES *Application intervertebral biomechanical device(s) at same level (22853-22854, [22859])*
Removal total disc arthroplasty (0095T)
Spinal cord decompression (63001-63048)
Code first (22861)
0.00 0.00 FUD XXX C 80
AMA: 2006,Feb,1-6; 2005,Jun,6-8

0100T

0100T **Placement of a subconjunctival retinal prosthesis receiver and pulse generator, and implantation of intra-ocular retinal electrode array, with vitrectomy**
EXCLUDES *Evaluation and initial programming implantable retinal electrode array device (0472T)*
0.00 0.00 FUD XXX T J8 80
AMA: 2018,Feb,3; 2018,Jan,8; 2017,Jan,8; 2016,Jan,13; 2015,Jan,16

0101T-0513T [0512T, 0513T]

0101T **Extracorporeal shock wave involving musculoskeletal system, not otherwise specified, high energy**
EXCLUDES *Extracorporeal shock wave therapy integumentary system not otherwise specified ([0512T, 0513T])*
0.00 0.00 FUD XXX J G2 80
AMA: 2018,Dec,5; 2018,Dec,5; 2018,Jan,8; 2017,Jan,8; 2016,Jan,13; 2015,Jan,16

0102T **Extracorporeal shock wave, high energy, performed by a physician, requiring anesthesia other than local, involving lateral humeral epicondyle**
0.00 0.00 FUD XXX J G2 80
AMA: 2019,Jun,11; 2018,Dec,5; 2018,Dec,5; 2018,Jan,8; 2017,Jan,8; 2016,Jan,13; 2015,Jan,16

0512T **Extracorporeal shock wave for integumentary wound healing, high energy, including topical application and dressing care; initial wound**
0.00 0.00 FUD YYY R2 80
AMA: 2018,Dec,5; 2018,Dec,5

+ # **0513T** **each additional wound (List separately in addition to code for primary procedure)**
Code first ([0512T])
0.00 0.00 FUD ZZZ N1 80
AMA: 2018,Dec,5; 2018,Dec,5

0106T-0110T

0106T **Quantitative sensory testing (QST), testing and interpretation per extremity; using touch pressure stimuli to assess large diameter sensation**
0.00 0.00 FUD XXX Q1 80
AMA: 2018,Jan,8; 2017,Jan,8; 2016,Jan,13; 2015,Jan,16

0107T **using vibration stimuli to assess large diameter fiber sensation**
0.00 0.00 FUD XXX Q1 80
AMA: 2018,Jan,8; 2017,Jan,8; 2016,Jan,13; 2015,Jan,16

0108T **using cooling stimuli to assess small nerve fiber sensation and hyperalgesia**
0.00 0.00 FUD XXX Q1 80
AMA: 2018,Jan,8; 2017,Jan,8; 2016,Jan,13; 2015,Jan,16

0109T **using heat-pain stimuli to assess small nerve fiber sensation and hyperalgesia**
0.00 0.00 FUD XXX Q1 80
AMA: 2018,Jan,8; 2017,Jan,8; 2016,Jan,13; 2015,Jan,16

0110T **using other stimuli to assess sensation**
0.00 0.00 FUD XXX Q1 80
AMA: 2018,Jan,8; 2017,Jan,8; 2016,Jan,13; 2015,Jan,16

0111T-0126T

0111T ~~**Long-chain (C20-22) omega-3 fatty acids in red blood cell (RBC) membranes**~~
To report, see (82726)

0126T ~~**Common carotid intima-media thickness (IMT) study for evaluation of atherosclerotic burden or coronary heart disease risk factor assessment**~~
To report, see (93998)

0163T-0165T

CMS: 100-03,150.10 Lumbar Artificial Disc Replacement (LADR)

INCLUDES Fluoroscopy

EXCLUDES *Application intervertebral biomechanical device(s) at same level (22853-22854, [22859])*
Cervical disc procedures (22856)
Decompression (63001-63048)
Exploration retroperitoneal area at same level (49010)

\+ **0163T** **Total disc arthroplasty (artificial disc), anterior approach, including discectomy to prepare interspace (other than for decompression), each additional interspace, lumbar (List separately in addition to code for primary procedure)**
Code first (22857)
0.00 0.00 FUD YYY C 80
AMA: 2018,Jan,8; 2017,Jan,8; 2016,Jan,13; 2015,Jan,16

\+ **0164T** **Removal of total disc arthroplasty, (artificial disc), anterior approach, each additional interspace, lumbar (List separately in addition to code for primary procedure)**
Code first (22865)
0.00 0.00 FUD YYY C 80
AMA: 2018,Jan,8; 2017,Jan,8; 2016,Jan,13; 2015,Jan,16

\+ **0165T** **Revision including replacement of total disc arthroplasty (artificial disc), anterior approach, each additional interspace, lumbar (List separately in addition to code for primary procedure)**
Code first (22862)
0.00 0.00 FUD YYY C 80
AMA: 2018,Jan,8; 2017,Jan,8; 2016,Jan,13; 2015,Jan,16

0174T-0175T

\+ **0174T** **Computer-aided detection (CAD) (computer algorithm analysis of digital image data for lesion detection) with further physician review for interpretation and report, with or without digitization of film radiographic images, chest radiograph(s), performed concurrent with primary interpretation (List separately in addition to code for primary procedure)**
Code first (71045-71048)
0.00 0.00 FUD XXX N 80
AMA: 2018,Apr,7

0175T **Computer-aided detection (CAD) (computer algorithm analysis of digital image data for lesion detection) with further physician review for interpretation and report, with or without digitization of film radiographic images, chest radiograph(s), performed remote from primary interpretation**
INCLUDES Chest x-rays (71045-71048)
0.00 0.00 FUD XXX N 80
AMA: 2018,Apr,7

0184T

0184T **Excision of rectal tumor, transanal endoscopic microsurgical approach (ie, TEMS), including muscularis propria (ie, full thickness)**

INCLUDES Operating microscope (66990)
Proctosigmoidoscopy (45300, 45308-45309, 45315, 45317, 45320)

EXCLUDES *Nonendoscopic excision rectal tumor (45160, 45171-45172)*

0.00 0.00 FUD XXX J 80
AMA: 2018,Feb,11; 2018,Jan,8; 2017,Jan,8; 2016,Feb,12; 2016,Jan,13; 2015,Jan,16

0191T-0253T [0253T, 0376T]

0191T **Insertion of anterior segment aqueous drainage device, without extraocular reservoir, internal approach, into the trabecular meshwork; initial insertion**
0.00 0.00 FUD XXX J J8 80
AMA: 2018,Jul,3; 2018,Feb,3; 2018,Jan,8; 2017,Jan,8; 2016,Jan,13; 2015,Jan,16

\+ # **0376T** **each additional device insertion (List separately in addition to code for primary procedure)**
Code first (0191T)
0.00 0.00 FUD XXX N N1 80
AMA: 2018,Jul,3; 2018,Feb,3

\# **0253T** **Insertion of anterior segment aqueous drainage device, without extraocular reservoir, internal approach, into the suprachoroidal space**

EXCLUDES *Insertion aqueous drainage device, external approach (66183)*

0.00 0.00 FUD YYY J J8 80
AMA: 2018,Jul,3

0198T

0198T **Measurement of ocular blood flow by repetitive intraocular pressure sampling, with interpretation and report**
0.00 0.00 FUD XXX Q1 80
AMA: 2018,Jan,8; 2017,Jan,8; 2016,Jan,13; 2015,Jan,16

0200T-0201T

INCLUDES Deep bone biopsy (20225)

0200T **Percutaneous sacral augmentation (sacroplasty), unilateral injection(s), including the use of a balloon or mechanical device, when used, 1 or more needles, includes imaging guidance and bone biopsy, when performed**
0.00 0.00 FUD XXX J J8 80 50
AMA: 2018,Jan,8; 2017,Jan,8; 2016,Jan,13; 2015,Dec,18; 2015,Apr,8; 2015,Jan,8

0201T **Percutaneous sacral augmentation (sacroplasty), bilateral injections, including the use of a balloon or mechanical device, when used, 2 or more needles, includes imaging guidance and bone biopsy, when performed**
0.00 0.00 FUD XXX J G2 80
AMA: 2018,Jan,8; 2017,Jan,8; 2016,Jan,13; 2015,Dec,18; 2015,Apr,8; 2015,Jan,8

0202T-0563T [0563T]

0202T **Posterior vertebral joint(s) arthroplasty (eg, facet joint[s] replacement), including facetectomy, laminectomy, foraminotomy, and vertebral column fixation, injection of bone cement, when performed, including fluoroscopy, single level, lumbar spine**

INCLUDES Instrumentation (22840, 22853-22854, [22859])
Laminectomy (63005, 63012, 63017, 63047)
Laminotomy (63030, 63042)
Lumbar arthroplasty (22857)
Percutaneous lumbar vertebral augmentation (22514)
Percutaneous vertebroplasty (22511)
Spinal cord decompression (63056)

0.00 0.00 FUD XXX C 80

0207T **Evacuation of meibomian glands, automated, using heat and intermittent pressure, unilateral**

EXCLUDES *Evacuation using:*
Heat through wearable device ([0563T])
Manual expression only, report appropriate E/M code

0.00 0.00 FUD XXX Q1 80

AMA: 2018,Jan,8; 2017,Jan,8; 2016,Jan,13; 2015,Jan,16

0563T **Evacuation of meibomian glands, using heat delivered through wearable, open-eye eyelid treatment devices and manual gland expression, bilateral**

EXCLUDES *Evacuation using:*
Heat and intermittent pressure (0207T)
Manual expression only, report appropriate E/M code

0.00 0.00 FUD YYY 80

0208T-0212T

EXCLUDES *Manual audiometric testing by qualified health care professional, using audiometers (92551-92557)*

0208T **Pure tone audiometry (threshold), automated; air only**

0.00 0.00 FUD XXX Q1 80 TC

AMA: 2018,Jan,8; 2017,Jan,8; 2016,Jan,13; 2015,Jan,16

0209T **air and bone**

0.00 0.00 FUD XXX Q1 80 TC

AMA: 2018,Jan,8; 2017,Jan,8; 2016,Jan,13; 2015,Jan,16

0210T **Speech audiometry threshold, automated;**

0.00 0.00 FUD XXX Q1 80 TC

AMA: 2014,Aug,3

0211T **with speech recognition**

0.00 0.00 FUD XXX Q1 80 TC

AMA: 2018,Jan,8; 2017,Jan,8; 2016,Jan,13; 2015,Jan,16

0212T **Comprehensive audiometry threshold evaluation and speech recognition (0209T, 0211T combined), automated**

0.00 0.00 FUD XXX Q1 80 TC

AMA: 2018,Jan,8; 2017,Jan,8; 2016,Jan,13; 2015,Jan,16

0213T-0215T

INCLUDES Ultrasound guidance (76942)

0213T **Injection(s), diagnostic or therapeutic agent, paravertebral facet (zygapophyseal) joint (or nerves innervating that joint) with ultrasound guidance, cervical or thoracic; single level**

0.00 0.00 FUD XXX T R2 80 50

AMA: 2018,Jan,8; 2017,Jan,8; 2016,Jan,13; 2015,Jan,16

\+ 0214T **second level (List separately in addition to code for primary procedure)**

EXCLUDES *Reporting with modifier 50. Report once for each side when performed bilaterally*

Code first (0213T)

0.00 0.00 FUD ZZZ N N1 80 50

AMA: 2018,Jan,8; 2017,Jan,8; 2016,Jan,13; 2015,Jan,16

\+ 0215T **third and any additional level(s) (List separately in addition to code for primary procedure)**

EXCLUDES *Reporting code more than one time per service date*
Reporting with modifier 50. Report once for each side when performed bilaterally

Code first (0213T-0214T)

0.00 0.00 FUD ZZZ N N1 80 50

AMA: 2018,Jan,8; 2017,Jan,8; 2016,Jan,13; 2015,Jan,16

0216T-0218T

INCLUDES Ultrasound guidance (76942)

EXCLUDES *Injection with CT or fluoroscopic guidance (64490-64495)*

0216T **Injection(s), diagnostic or therapeutic agent, paravertebral facet (zygapophyseal) joint (or nerves innervating that joint) with ultrasound guidance, lumbar or sacral; single level**

0.00 0.00 FUD XXX T R2 80 50

AMA: 2018,Jan,8; 2017,Jan,8; 2016,Jan,13; 2015,Jan,16

\+ 0217T **second level (List separately in addition to code for primary procedure)**

EXCLUDES *Reporting with modifier 50. Report once for each side when performed bilaterally*

Code first (0216T)

0.00 0.00 FUD ZZZ N N1 80 50

AMA: 2018,Jan,8; 2017,Jan,8; 2016,Jan,13; 2015,Jan,16

\+ 0218T **third and any additional level(s) (List separately in addition to code for primary procedure)**

EXCLUDES *Reporting code more than one time per service date*
Reporting with modifier 50. Report once for each side when performed bilaterally

Code first (0216T-0217T)

0.00 0.00 FUD ZZZ N N1 80 50

AMA: 2018,Jan,8; 2017,Jan,8; 2016,Jan,13; 2015,Jan,16

0219T-0222T

INCLUDES Allografts at same level (20930-20931)
Application intervertebral biomechanical device(s) at same level (22853-22854, [22859])
Arthrodesis at same level (22600-22614)
Instrumentation at same level (22840)
Radiologic services

0219T **Placement of a posterior intrafacet implant(s), unilateral or bilateral, including imaging and placement of bone graft(s) or synthetic device(s), single level; cervical**

0.00 0.00 FUD XXX C 80

AMA: 2018,Jan,8; 2017,Jan,8; 2016,Jan,13; 2015,Jan,16

0220T **thoracic**

0.00 0.00 FUD XXX C 80

AMA: 2018,Jan,8; 2017,Jan,8; 2016,Jan,13; 2015,Jan,16

0221T **lumbar**

0.00 0.00 FUD XXX J 80

AMA: 2018,Jan,8; 2017,Jan,8; 2016,Jan,13; 2015,Jan,16

\+ 0222T **each additional vertebral segment (List separately in addition to code for primary procedure)**

Code first (0219T-0221T)

0.00 0.00 FUD ZZZ N 80

AMA: 2018,Jan,8; 2017,Jan,8; 2016,Jan,13; 2015,Jan,16

0228T-0231T

0228T ~~**Injection(s), anesthetic agent and/or steroid, transforaminal epidural, with ultrasound guidance, cervical or thoracic; single level**~~

To report, see (64999)

0229T ~~**each additional level (List separately in addition to code for primary procedure)**~~

To report, see (64999)

0230T ~~**Injection(s), anesthetic agent and/or steroid, transforaminal epidural, with ultrasound guidance, lumbar or sacral; single level**~~

To report, see (64999)

0231T ~~**each additional level (List separately in addition to code for primary procedure)**~~

To report, see (64999)

0232T

INCLUDES Arthrocentesis (20600-20611)
Blood collection (36415, 36592)
Fat and other soft tissue grafts ([15769], 15771-15774)
Imaging guidance (76942, 77002, 77012, 77021)
Injections (20550-20551)
Platelet/blood product pooling (86965)

EXCLUDES *Aspiration bone marrow for grafting, biopsy, harvesting for transplant (38220-38221, 38230)*
Injections white cell concentrate (0481T)

0232T **Injection(s), platelet rich plasma, any site, including image guidance, harvesting and preparation when performed**

0.00 0.00 FUD XXX Q1 N1

AMA: 2019,Oct,5; 2019,Apr,10; 2018,May,3; 2018,Jan,8; 2017,Jan,8; 2016,Jan,13; 2015,Jan,16

0234T-0253T [0253T]

INCLUDES Atherectomy by any technique in arteries above inguinal ligaments
Radiology supervision and interpretation

EXCLUDES *Accessing and catheterization vessel*
Atherectomy performed below inguinal ligaments (37225, 37227, 37229, 37231, 37233, 37235)
Closure arteriotomy by any technique
Negotiating lesion
Other interventions to same or different vessels
Protection from embolism

0234T Transluminal peripheral atherectomy, open or percutaneous, including radiological supervision and interpretation; renal artery
0.00 0.00 FUD YYY J 80
AMA: 2018,Jan,8; 2017,Jan,8; 2016,Jan,13; 2015,Jan,16

0235T visceral artery (except renal), each vessel
0.00 0.00 FUD YYY C 80
AMA: 2018,Jan,8; 2017,Jan,8; 2016,Jan,13; 2015,Jan,16

0236T abdominal aorta
0.00 0.00 FUD YYY J 80
AMA: 2018,Jan,8; 2017,Jan,8; 2016,Jan,13; 2015,Jan,16

0237T brachiocephalic trunk and branches, each vessel
0.00 0.00 FUD YYY J 80
AMA: 2018,Jan,8; 2017,Jan,8; 2016,Jan,13; 2015,Jan,16

0238T iliac artery, each vessel
0.00 0.00 FUD YYY J J8 80
AMA: 2018,Jan,8; 2017,Jan,8; 2016,Jan,13; 2015,Jan,16

0253T **Resequenced code. See code before 0198T.**

0263T-0265T

EXCLUDES *Bone marrow and stem cell services (38204-38242 [38243])*

0263T Intramuscular autologous bone marrow cell therapy, with preparation of harvested cells, multiple injections, one leg, including ultrasound guidance, if performed; complete procedure including unilateral or bilateral bone marrow harvest
INCLUDES Duplex scan (93925-93926)
Ultrasound guidance (76942)
0.00 0.00 FUD XXX S G2 80

0264T complete procedure excluding bone marrow harvest
INCLUDES Bone marrow harvest only (0265T)
Duplex scan (93925-93926)
Ultrasound guidance (76942)
0.00 0.00 FUD XXX S G2 80

0265T unilateral or bilateral bone marrow harvest only for intramuscular autologous bone marrow cell therapy
EXCLUDES *Complete procedure (0263T-0264T)*
0.00 0.00 FUD XXX S G2 80

0266T-0273T

0266T Implantation or replacement of carotid sinus baroreflex activation device; total system (includes generator placement, unilateral or bilateral lead placement, intra-operative interrogation, programming, and repositioning, when performed)
INCLUDES Components complete procedure (0267T-0268T)
0.00 0.00 FUD YYY C 80

0267T lead only, unilateral (includes intra-operative interrogation, programming, and repositioning, when performed)
EXCLUDES *Complete procedure (0266T)*
Device interrogation (0272T-0273T)
Removal/revision device or components (0269T-0271T)
0.00 0.00 FUD YYY T 80

0268T pulse generator only (includes intra-operative interrogation, programming, and repositioning, when performed)
EXCLUDES *Complete procedure (0266T)*
Device interrogation (0272T-0273T)
Removal/revision device or components (0269T-0271T)
0.00 0.00 FUD YYY J 80

0269T Revision or removal of carotid sinus baroreflex activation device; total system (includes generator placement, unilateral or bilateral lead placement, intra-operative interrogation, programming, and repositioning, when performed)
EXCLUDES *Device interrogation (0272T-0273T)*
Implantation/replacement device and/or components (0266T-0268T)
Removal/revision device or components (0270T-0271T)
0.00 0.00 FUD XXX Q2 G2 80

0270T lead only, unilateral (includes intra-operative interrogation, programming, and repositioning, when performed)
EXCLUDES *Device interrogation (0272T-0273T)*
Implantation/replacement device and/or components (0266T-0269T)
Removal/revision device or components (0271T)
0.00 0.00 FUD XXX Q2 G2 80

0271T pulse generator only (includes intra-operative interrogation, programming, and repositioning, when performed)
EXCLUDES *Device interrogation (0272T-0273T)*
Implantation/replacement device and/or components (0266T-0268T)
Removal/revision device or components (0271T-0273T)
0.00 0.00 FUD XXX Q2 G2 80

0272T Interrogation device evaluation (in person), carotid sinus baroreflex activation system, including telemetric iterative communication with the implantable device to monitor device diagnostics and programmed therapy values, with interpretation and report (eg, battery status, lead impedance, pulse amplitude, pulse width, therapy frequency, pathway mode, burst mode, therapy start/stop times each day);
EXCLUDES *Device interrogation (0273T)*
Implantation/replacement device and/or components (0266T-0268T)
Removal/revision device or components (0269T-0271T)
0.00 0.00 FUD XXX S 80

0273T with programming
EXCLUDES *Device interrogation (0272T)*
Implantation/replacement device and/or components (0266T-0268T)
Removal/revision device or components (0269T-0271T)
0.00 0.00 FUD XXX S 80

0274T-0275T

EXCLUDES *Laminotomy/hemilaminectomy by open and endoscopically assisted approach (63020-63035)*
Percutaneous decompression nucleus pulposus intervertebral disc by needle-based technique (62287)

0274T Percutaneous laminotomy/laminectomy (interlaminar approach) for decompression of neural elements, (with or without ligamentous resection, discectomy, facetectomy and/or foraminotomy), any method, under indirect image guidance (eg, fluoroscopic, CT), single or multiple levels, unilateral or bilateral; cervical or thoracic
0.00 0.00 FUD YYY J G2 80
AMA: 2018,Jan,8; 2017,Feb,12; 2017,Jan,8; 2016,Jan,13; 2015,Jan,16

0275T lumbar
0.00 0.00 FUD YYY J G2 80
AMA: 2018,Jan,8; 2017,Feb,12; 2017,Jan,8; 2016,Jan,13; 2015,Jan,16

0278T

0278T **Transcutaneous electrical modulation pain reprocessing (eg, scrambler therapy), each treatment session (includes placement of electrodes)**
0.00 0.00 FUD XXX Q1 N1 80

0290T

+ 0290T **Corneal incisions in the recipient cornea created using a laser, in preparation for penetrating or lamellar keratoplasty (List separately in addition to code for primary procedure)**
Code first (65710, 65730, 65750, 65755)
0.00 0.00 FUD ZZZ N N1 80
AMA: 2018,Jan,8; 2017,Jan,8; 2016,Jan,13; 2015,Jan,16

0295T-0298T

~~0295T~~ ~~**External electrocardiographic recording for more than 48 hours up to 21 days by continuous rhythm recording and storage; includes recording, scanning analysis with report, review and interpretation**~~
To report, see ([93241, 93242, 93243, 93244, 93245, 93246, 93247, 93248])

~~0296T~~ ~~**recording (includes connection and initial recording)**~~
To report, see ([93241, 93242, 93243, 93244, 93245, 93246, 93247, 93248])

~~0297T~~ ~~**scanning analysis with report**~~
To report, see ([93241, 93242, 93243, 93244, 93245, 93246, 93247, 93248])

~~0298T~~ ~~**review and interpretation**~~
To report, see ([93241, 93242, 93243, 93244, 93245, 93246, 93247, 93248])

0308T

0308T **Insertion of ocular telescope prosthesis including removal of crystalline lens or intraocular lens prosthesis**
INCLUDES Injection procedures (66020, 66030)
Iridectomy when performed (66600-66635, 66761)
Operating microscope (69990)
Repositioning intraocular lens (66825)
EXCLUDES *Cataract extraction (66982-66986)*
0.00 0.00 FUD YYY J J8 50
AMA: 2019,Dec,6; 2018,Jan,8; 2017,Jan,8; 2016,Jan,13; 2015,Jan,16

0312T-0317T

EXCLUDES *Analysis and/or programming (or reprogramming) vagus nerve stimulator (95970, 95976-95977)*
Implantation, replacement, removal, and/or revision vagus nerve neurostimulator (electrode array and/or pulse generator) for stimulation vagus nerve other than at esophagogastric junction (64568-64570)

0312T **Vagus nerve blocking therapy (morbid obesity); laparoscopic implantation of neurostimulator electrode array, anterior and posterior vagal trunks adjacent to esophagogastric junction (EGJ), with implantation of pulse generator, includes programming**
0.00 0.00 FUD XXX J 80
AMA: 2018,Jan,8; 2017,Jan,8; 2016,Jan,13; 2015,Jan,16

0313T **laparoscopic revision or replacement of vagal trunk neurostimulator electrode array, including connection to existing pulse generator**
0.00 0.00 FUD XXX T J8 80
AMA: 2018,Jan,8; 2017,Jan,8; 2016,Jan,13; 2015,Jan,16

0314T **laparoscopic removal of vagal trunk neurostimulator electrode array and pulse generator**
0.00 0.00 FUD XXX Q2 G2 80
AMA: 2018,Jan,8; 2017,Jan,8; 2016,Jan,13; 2015,Jan,16

0315T **removal of pulse generator**
EXCLUDES *Removal with replacement pulse generator (0316T)*
0.00 0.00 FUD XXX Q2 G2 80
AMA: 2018,Jan,8; 2017,Jan,8; 2016,Jan,13; 2015,Jan,16

0316T **replacement of pulse generator**
EXCLUDES *Removal without replacement pulse generator (0315T)*
0.00 0.00 FUD XXX J J8 80
AMA: 2018,Jan,8; 2017,Jan,8; 2016,Jan,13; 2015,Jan,16

0317T **neurostimulator pulse generator electronic analysis, includes reprogramming when performed**
EXCLUDES *Analysis and/or programming (or reprogramming) vagus nerve stimulator (95970, 95976-95977)*
0.00 0.00 FUD XXX Q1 80
AMA: 2018,Jan,8; 2017,Jan,8; 2016,Jan,13; 2015,Jan,16

0329T-0330T

0329T **Monitoring of intraocular pressure for 24 hours or longer, unilateral or bilateral, with interpretation and report**
0.00 0.00 FUD YYY E
AMA: 2018,Jan,8; 2017,Jan,8; 2016,Jan,13; 2015,Jan,16

0330T **Tear film imaging, unilateral or bilateral, with interpretation and report**
0.00 0.00 FUD YYY Q1 N1
AMA: 2018,Jan,8; 2017,Jan,8; 2016,Jan,13; 2015,Jan,16

0331T-0332T

EXCLUDES *Myocardial infarction avid imaging (78466, 78468, 78469)*

0331T **Myocardial sympathetic innervation imaging, planar qualitative and quantitative assessment;**
0.00 0.00 FUD YYY S Z2
AMA: 2018,Jan,8; 2017,Jan,8; 2016,Jan,13; 2015,Jan,16

0332T **with tomographic SPECT**
0.00 0.00 FUD YYY S Z2
AMA: 2018,Jan,8; 2017,Jan,8; 2016,Jan,13; 2015,Jan,16

0333T-0464T [0464T]

0333T **Visual evoked potential, screening of visual acuity, automated, with report**
EXCLUDES *Visual evoked potential testing for glaucoma ([0464T])*
0.00 0.00 FUD YYY E
AMA: 2018,Feb,3; 2018,Jan,8; 2017,Jan,8; 2016,Jan,13; 2015,Jan,16

0464T **Visual evoked potential, testing for glaucoma, with interpretation and report**
EXCLUDES *Visual evoked potential for visual acuity (0333T)*
0.00 0.00 FUD YYY S
AMA: 2018,Feb,3

0335T-0511T [0510T, 0511T]

0335T **Insertion of sinus tarsi implant**
EXCLUDES *Arthroscopic subtalar arthrodesis (29907)*
Open talotarsal joint dislocation repair (28585)
Subtalar arthrodesis (28725)
0.00 0.00 FUD YYY J J8

0510T **Removal of sinus tarsi implant**
0.00 0.00 FUD YYY G2 50

0511T **Removal and reinsertion of sinus tarsi implant**
0.00 0.00 FUD YYY J8 50

0338T-0339T

INCLUDES Selective catheter placement renal arteries (36251-36254)

0338T **Transcatheter renal sympathetic denervation, percutaneous approach including arterial puncture, selective catheter placement(s) renal artery(ies), fluoroscopy, contrast injection(s), intraprocedural roadmapping and radiological supervision and interpretation, including pressure gradient measurements, flush aortogram and diagnostic renal angiography when performed; unilateral**
0.00 0.00 FUD YYY J G2

0339T **bilateral**
0.00 0.00 FUD YYY J G2

0342T

0342T Therapeutic apheresis with selective HDL delipidation and plasma reinfusion

0.00 0.00 FUD YYY S G2

0345T

0345T Transcatheter mitral valve repair percutaneous approach via the coronary sinus

INCLUDES Coronary angiography (93563-93564)

EXCLUDES *Diagnostic cardiac catheterization procedures integral to valve procedure (93451-93461, 93530-93533, 93563-93564)*

Repair mitral valve including transseptal puncture (33418-33419)

Transcatheter implantation/replacement mitral valve (TMVI) (0483T-0484T)

Transcatheter mitral valve annulus reconstruction (0544T)

Code also transvascular ventricular support, when performed:
Balloon pump insertion (33967, 33970, 33973)
Ventricular assist device ([33995], 33990-33993, [33997])

0.00 0.00 FUD YYY C

AMA: 2018,Jan,8; 2017,Jan,8; 2016,Jan,13; 2015,Sep,3

0347T

0347T Placement of interstitial device(s) in bone for radiostereometric analysis (RSA)

0.00 0.00 FUD YYY Q1 N1

AMA: 2018,Jan,8; 2017,Jan,8; 2016,Jan,13; 2015,Jun,8

0348T-0350T

0348T Radiologic examination, radiostereometric analysis (RSA); spine, (includes cervical, thoracic and lumbosacral, when performed)

0.00 0.00 FUD YYY Q1 N1

AMA: 2018,Jan,8; 2017,Jan,8; 2016,Jan,13; 2015,Jun,8

0349T upper extremity(ies), (includes shoulder, elbow, and wrist, when performed)

0.00 0.00 FUD YYY Q1 N1

AMA: 2018,Jan,8; 2017,Jan,8; 2016,Jan,13; 2015,Jun,8

0350T lower extremity(ies), (includes hip, proximal femur, knee, and ankle, when performed)

0.00 0.00 FUD YYY Q1 N1

AMA: 2018,Jan,8; 2017,Jan,8; 2016,Jan,13; 2015,Jun,8

0351T-0354T

0351T Optical coherence tomography of breast or axillary lymph node, excised tissue, each specimen; real-time intraoperative

INCLUDES Interpretation and report (0352T)

0.00 0.00 FUD YYY N N1

AMA: 2018,Jan,8; 2017,Jan,8; 2016,Jan,13; 2015,Apr,6

0352T interpretation and report, real-time or referred

INCLUDES Interpretation and report (0351T)

0.00 0.00 FUD YYY B

AMA: 2018,Jan,8; 2017,Jan,8; 2016,Jan,13; 2015,Apr,6

0353T Optical coherence tomography of breast, surgical cavity; real-time intraoperative

INCLUDES Interpretation and report (0354T)

EXCLUDES *Reporting code more than one time per session*

0.00 0.00 FUD YYY N N1

AMA: 2018,Jan,8; 2017,Jan,8; 2016,Jan,13; 2015,Apr,6

0354T interpretation and report, real time or referred

0.00 0.00 FUD YYY B

AMA: 2018,Jan,8; 2017,Jan,8; 2016,Jan,13; 2015,Apr,6

0355T-0358T

0355T Gastrointestinal tract imaging, intraluminal (eg, capsule endoscopy), colon, with interpretation and report

INCLUDES Distal ileum imaging when performed

EXCLUDES *Capsule endoscopy esophagus only (91111)*

Capsule endoscopy esophagus through ileum (91110)

0.00 0.00 FUD YYY J

0356T Insertion of drug-eluting implant (including punctal dilation and implant removal when performed) into lacrimal canaliculus, each

EXCLUDES *Drug-eluting ocular insert (0444T-0445T)*

0.00 0.00 FUD YYY Q1 N1

AMA: 2018,Jan,8; 2017,Aug,7

0358T Bioelectrical impedance analysis whole body composition assessment, with interpretation and report

0.00 0.00 FUD YYY Q1

0362T-0376T [0376T]

INCLUDES Only one technician time when more than one technician in attendance
Provided by physician/other qualified healthcare professional while on-site (immediately available during procedure), but does not need to be face-to-face
Provided in environment appropriate for patient
Provided to patients with destructive behaviors

EXCLUDES *Adaptive behavior services ([97153, 97154, 97155, 97156, 97157, 97158])*
Aphasia assessment (96105)
Behavioral/developmental screening/testing (96110-96113, [96127])
Behavior/health assessment (96156-96159 [96164, 96165, 96167, 96168, 96170, 96171])
Cognitive testing ([96125])
Neurobehavioral testing (96116-96121)
Psychiatric evaluations/psychotherapy/interactive complexity (90785-90899)
Psychological/neuropsychological evaluation/testing (96130-96146)

0362T Behavior identification supporting assessment, each 15 minutes of technicians' time face-to-face with a patient, requiring the following components: administration by the physician or other qualified health care professional who is on site; with the assistance of two or more technicians; for a patient who exhibits destructive behavior; completion in an environment that is customized to the patient's behavior.

INCLUDES Comprises:
Functional analysis and behavioral assessment
Procedures and instruments to assess functional impairment and behavior levels
Structured observation with data collection not including direct patient involvement

EXCLUDES *Conferences by medical team (99366-99368)*
Occupational therapy evaluation ([97165, 97166, 97167, 97168])
Speech evaluation (92521-92524)

Code also when performed on different days until behavioral and supporting assessments complete

0.00 0.00 FUD YYY S

AMA: 2018,Nov,3; 2018,Jan,8; 2017,Jan,8; 2016,Jan,13; 2015,Jan,16

0373T Adaptive behavior treatment with protocol modification, each 15 minutes of technicians' time face-to-face with a patient, requiring the following components: administration by the physician or other qualified health care professional who is on site; with the assistance of two or more technicians; for a patient who exhibits destructive behavior; completion in an environment that is customized to the patient's behavior.

0.00 0.00 FUD YYY S

AMA: 2018,Nov,3; 2018,Jan,8; 2017,Jan,8; 2016,Jan,13; 2015,Jan,16

0376T **Resequenced code. See code following 0191T.**

0378T-0379T

0378T Visual field assessment, with concurrent real time data analysis and accessible data storage with patient initiated data transmitted to a remote surveillance center for up to 30 days; review and interpretation with report by a physician or other qualified health care professional

0.00 0.00 FUD XXX B 80

AMA: 2018,Jan,8; 2017,Jan,8; 2016,Jan,13; 2015,Jan,10

0379T technical support and patient instructions, surveillance, analysis and transmission of daily and emergent data reports as prescribed by a physician or other qualified health care professional

0.00 0.00 FUD XXX Q1 N1 80

AMA: 2018,Jan,8; 2017,Jan,8; 2016,Jan,13; 2015,Jan,10

0381T-0386T

~~0381T External heart rate and 3-axis accelerometer data recording up to 14 days to assess changes in heart rate and to monitor motion analysis for the purposes of diagnosing nocturnal epilepsy seizure events; includes report, scanning analysis with report, review and interpretation by a physician or other qualified health care professional~~

To report, see (95999)

~~0382T review and interpretation only~~

To report, see (95999)

~~0383T External heart rate and 3-axis accelerometer data recording from 15 to 30 days to assess changes in heart rate and to monitor motion analysis for the purposes of diagnosing nocturnal epilepsy seizure events; includes report, scanning analysis with report, review and interpretation by a physician or other qualified health care professional~~

To report, see (95999)

~~0384T review and interpretation only~~

To report, see (95999)

~~0385T External heart rate and 3-axis accelerometer data recording more than 30 days to assess changes in heart rate and to monitor motion analysis for the purposes of diagnosing nocturnal epilepsy seizure events; includes report, scanning analysis with report, review and interpretation by a physician or other qualified health care professional~~

To report, see (95999)

~~0386T review and interpretation only~~

To report, see (95999)

0394T-0395T

EXCLUDES *Radiation oncology procedures (77261-77263, 77300, 77306-77307, 77316-77318, 77332-77334, 77336, 77427-77499, 77761-77772, 77778, 77789)*

0394T High dose rate electronic brachytherapy, skin surface application, per fraction, includes basic dosimetry, when performed

EXCLUDES *Superficial non-brachytherapy radiation (77401)*

0.00 0.00 FUD XXX S Z2 80

0395T High dose rate electronic brachytherapy, interstitial or intracavitary treatment, per fraction, includes basic dosimetry, when performed

EXCLUDES *High dose rate skin surface application (0394T)*

0.00 0.00 FUD XXX S Z2 80

0396T-0398T

~~0396T Intra-operative use of kinetic balance sensor for implant stability during knee replacement arthroplasty (List separately in addition to code for primary procedure)~~

To report, see (27599)

\+ **0397T Endoscopic retrograde cholangiopancreatography (ERCP), with optical endomicroscopy (List separately in addition to code for primary procedure)**

INCLUDES Optical endomicroscopic image(s) (88375)

EXCLUDES *Reporting code more than one time per operative session*

Code first (43260-43265, [43274], [43275], [43276], [43277], [43278])

0.00 0.00 FUD XXX N N1 80

0398T Magnetic resonance image guided high intensity focused ultrasound (MRgFUS), stereotactic ablation lesion, intracranial for movement disorder including stereotactic navigation and frame placement when performed

INCLUDES Application stereotactic headframe (61800)
Stereotactic computer-assisted navigation (61781)

0.00 0.00 FUD XXX S 80

0400T-0401T

~~0400T Multi-spectral digital skin lesion analysis of clinically atypical cutaneous pigmented lesions for detection of melanomas and high risk melanocytic atypia; one to five lesions~~

To report, see (96999)

~~0401T six or more lesions~~

To report, see (96999)

0402T

0402T Collagen cross-linking of cornea, including removal of the corneal epithelium and intraoperative pachymetry, when performed (Report medication separately)

INCLUDES Corneal epithelium removal (65435)
Corneal pachymetry (76514)
Operating microscope (69990)

0.00 0.00 FUD XXX J R2 80

AMA: 2018,Jun,11; 2018,Jan,8; 2017,Jan,8; 2016,Feb,12

0403T-0488T [0488T]

INCLUDES Intensive behavioral counseling by trained lifestyle coach
Standardized course with emphasis on weight, exercise, stress management, and nutrition

0403T Preventive behavior change, intensive program of prevention of diabetes using a standardized diabetes prevention program curriculum, provided to individuals in a group setting, minimum 60 minutes, per day

EXCLUDES *Online/electronic diabetes prevention program ([0488T])*
Self-management training and education by nonphysician health care professional (98960-98962)

0.00 0.00 FUD XXX E 80

AMA: 2020,Jul,7; 2018,Aug,6; 2015,Aug,4

\# **0488T Preventive behavior change, online/electronic structured intensive program for prevention of diabetes using a standardized diabetes prevention program curriculum, provided to an individual, per 30 days**

INCLUDES In person elements when appropriate

EXCLUDES *Group diabetes prevention program (0403T)*
Self-management training and education by nonphysician health care professional (98960-98962)

0.00 0.00 FUD XXX E

AMA: 2020,Jul,7; 2018,Aug,6

0404T-0405T

0404T Transcervical uterine fibroid(s) ablation with ultrasound guidance, radiofrequency ♀

0.00 0.00 FUD XXX J 80

~~0405T Oversight of the care of an extracorporeal liver assist system patient requiring review of status, review of laboratories and other studies, and revision of orders and liver assist care plan (as appropriate), within a calendar month, 30 minutes or more of non-face-to-face time~~

To report, see (99499)

0408T-0418T

0408T **Insertion or replacement of permanent cardiac contractility modulation system, including contractility evaluation when performed, and programming of sensing and therapeutic parameters; pulse generator with transvenous electrodes**

INCLUDES Device evaluation (93286-93287, 0415T, 0417T-0418T)
Insertion or replacement entire system

EXCLUDES *Cardiac catheterization (93452-93453, 93456-93461)*

Code also removal each electrode when pulse generator and electrodes removed and replaced (0410T-0411T)

0.00 0.00 FUD XXX J J8 80

0409T **pulse generator only**

INCLUDES Device evaluation (93286-93287, 0415T, 0417T-0418T)

EXCLUDES *Cardiac catheterization (93452-93453, 93456-93461)*

0.00 0.00 FUD XXX J J8 80

0410T **atrial electrode only**

INCLUDES Device evaluation (93286-93287, 0415T, 0417T-0418T)
Each atrial electrode inserted or replaced

EXCLUDES *Cardiac catheterization (93452-93453, 93456-93461)*

0.00 0.00 FUD XXX J J8 80

0411T **ventricular electrode only**

INCLUDES Device evaluation (93286-93287, 0415T, 0417T-0418T)
Each ventricular electrode inserted or replaced

EXCLUDES *Cardiac catheterization (93452-93453, 93456-93461)*
Insertion or replacement complete CCM system (0408T)

0.00 0.00 FUD XXX J J8 80

0412T **Removal of permanent cardiac contractility modulation system; pulse generator only**

EXCLUDES *Device evaluation (0417T-0418T)*
Insertion or replacement complete CCM system (0408T)

0.00 0.00 FUD XXX Q2 G2 80

0413T **transvenous electrode (atrial or ventricular)**

INCLUDES Each electrode removed

EXCLUDES *Device evaluation (0417T-0418T)*
Insertion or replacement complete CCM system (0408T)

Code also removal and replacement electrode(s), as appropriate (0410T-0411T)

Code also removal pulse generator when leads also removed (0412T)

0.00 0.00 FUD XXX Q2 G2 80

0414T **Removal and replacement of permanent cardiac contractility modulation system pulse generator only**

INCLUDES Device evaluation (93286-93287, 0417T-0418T)

EXCLUDES *Cardiac catheterization (93452-93453, 93456-93461)*

Code also replacement pulse generator when leads also removed and replaced (0408T, 0412T-0413T)

0.00 0.00 FUD XXX J J8 80

0415T **Repositioning of previously implanted cardiac contractility modulation transvenous electrode, (atrial or ventricular lead)**

INCLUDES Device evaluation (93286-93287, 0417T-0418T)

EXCLUDES *Cardiac catheterization (93452-93453, 93456-93461)*
Insertion or replacement entire system or components (0408T-0411T)

0.00 0.00 FUD XXX T G2 80

0416T **Relocation of skin pocket for implanted cardiac contractility modulation pulse generator**

0.00 0.00 FUD XXX T G2 80

0417T **Programming device evaluation (in person) with iterative adjustment of the implantable device to test the function of the device and select optimal permanent programmed values with analysis, including review and report, implantable cardiac contractility modulation system**

EXCLUDES *Insertion/replacement/removal/repositioning device or components (0408T-0415T, 0418T)*

0.00 0.00 FUD XXX Q1 80

0418T **Interrogation device evaluation (in person) with analysis, review and report, includes connection, recording and disconnection per patient encounter, implantable cardiac contractility modulation system**

EXCLUDES *Insertion/replacement/removal/repositioning device or components (0408T-0415T, 0417T)*

0.00 0.00 FUD XXX Q1 80

0419T-0420T

EXCLUDES *Neurofibroma excision (64792)*
Reporting code more than one time per session

0419T **Destruction of neurofibroma, extensive (cutaneous, dermal extending into subcutaneous); face, head and neck, greater than 50 neurofibromas**

0.00 0.00 FUD XXX T R2 80

AMA: 2018,Jan,8; 2017,Jan,8; 2016,Apr,3

0420T **trunk and extremities, extensive, greater than 100 neurofibromas**

0.00 0.00 FUD XXX T R2 80

AMA: 2018,Jan,8; 2017,Jan,8; 2016,Apr,3

0421T-0423T

0421T **Transurethral waterjet ablation of prostate, including control of post-operative bleeding, including ultrasound guidance, complete (vasectomy, meatotomy, cystourethroscopy, urethral calibration and/or dilation, and internal urethrotomy are included when performed)** ♂

EXCLUDES *Transrectal ultrasound (76872)*
Transurethral prostate resection (52500, 52630)

0.00 0.00 FUD XXX J G2 80

AMA: 2020,Aug,6

0422T **Tactile breast imaging by computer-aided tactile sensors, unilateral or bilateral**

0.00 0.00 FUD XXX Q1 Z2 80

0423T **Secretory type II phospholipase A2 (sPLA2-IIA)**

EXCLUDES *Lipoprotein-associated phospholipase A2 [LpPLA2] (83698)*

0.00 0.00 FUD XXX A

0424T-0436T

INCLUDES Phrenic nerve stimulation system includes:
Pulse generator
Sensing lead (placed in azygos vein)
Stimulation lead (placed into right brachiocephalic vein or left pericardiophrenic vein)

0424T **Insertion or replacement of neurostimulator system for treatment of central sleep apnea; complete system (transvenous placement of right or left stimulation lead, sensing lead, implantable pulse generator)**

INCLUDES Device evaluation (0434T-0436T)
Insertion or replacement system components (0425T-0427T)
Repositioning leads (0432T-0433T)

Code also when pulse generator and all leads removed and replaced (0428T-0430T)

0.00 0.00 FUD XXX J J8 80

0425T **sensing lead only**

EXCLUDES *Device evaluation (0434T-0436T)*
Insertion/replacement complete system (0424T)
Repositioning leads (0432T-0433T)

0.00 0.00 FUD XXX J G2 80

0426T **stimulation lead only**

EXCLUDES *Device evaluation (0434T-0436T)*
Insertion/replacement complete system (0424T)
Repositioning leads (0432T-0433T)

0.00 0.00 FUD XXX J G2 80

26/TC PC/TC Only · A2-Z3 ASC Payment · 50 Bilateral · ♂ Male Only · ♀ Female Only · Facility RVU · Non-Facility RVU · CCI · CLIA
FUD Follow-up Days · CMS: IOM · AMA: CPT Asst · A-Y OPPSI · 80/80 Surg Assist Allowed / w/Doc · Lab Crosswalk · Radiology Crosswalk

0427T **pulse generator only**

EXCLUDES *Device evaluation (0434T-0436T)*
Insertion/replacement complete system (0424T)
Repositioning leads (0432T-0433T)

0.00 0.00 **FUD** XXX J G2 80

0428T **Removal of neurostimulator system for treatment of central sleep apnea; pulse generator only**

EXCLUDES *Device evaluation (0434T-0436T)*
Removal with replacement of pulse generator and all leads (0424T, 0429T-0430T)
Repositioning leads (0432T-0433T)

Code also when lead removed (0429T-0430T)

0.00 0.00 **FUD** XXX Q2 G2 80

0429T **sensing lead only**

INCLUDES Removal one sensing lead

EXCLUDES *Device evaluation (0434T-0436T)*

0.00 0.00 **FUD** XXX Q2 G2 80

0430T **stimulation lead only**

INCLUDES Removal one stimulation lead

EXCLUDES *Device evaluation (0434T-0436T)*

0.00 0.00 **FUD** XXX Q2 G2 80

AMA: 2015,Aug,4

0431T **Removal and replacement of neurostimulator system for treatment of central sleep apnea, pulse generator only**

EXCLUDES *Device evaluation (0434T-0436T)*
Removal with replacement generator and all three leads (0424T, 0428T-0430T)

0.00 0.00 **FUD** XXX J J8 80

0432T **Repositioning of neurostimulator system for treatment of central sleep apnea; stimulation lead only**

EXCLUDES *Device evaluation (0434T-0436T)*
Insertion/replacement complete system or components (0424T-0427T)

0.00 0.00 **FUD** XXX T G2 80

0433T **sensing lead only**

EXCLUDES *Device evaluation (0434T-0436T)*
Insertion/replacement complete system or components (0424T-0427T)

0.00 0.00 **FUD** XXX T G2 80

0434T **Interrogation device evaluation implanted neurostimulator pulse generator system for central sleep apnea**

EXCLUDES *Insertion/replacement complete system or components (0424T-0427T)*
Removal system or components (0428T-0431T)
Repositioning leads (0432T-0433T)

0.00 0.00 **FUD** XXX S G2 80

0435T **Programming device evaluation of implanted neurostimulator pulse generator system for central sleep apnea; single session**

EXCLUDES *Device evaluation (0436T)*
Insertion/replacement complete system or components (0424T-0427T)
Removal system or components (0428T-0431T)
Repositioning leads (0432T-0433T)

0.00 0.00 **FUD** XXX S 80

0436T **during sleep study**

EXCLUDES *Device evaluation (0435T)*
Insertion/replacement complete system or components (0424T-0427T)
Removal system or components (0428T-0431T)
Reporting code more than one time for each sleep study
Repositioning leads (0432T-0433T)

0.00 0.00 **FUD** XXX S 80

0437T-0439T

+ **0437T** **Implantation of non-biologic or synthetic implant (eg, polypropylene) for fascial reinforcement of the abdominal wall (List separately in addition to code for primary procedure)**

EXCLUDES *Implantation mesh, other material for repair incisional or ventral hernia (49560-49561, 49565-49566, 49568)*
Insertion mesh, other material for closure wound caused by necrotizing soft tissue infection (11004-11006, 49568)

0.00 0.00 **FUD** ZZZ N N1 80

+ **0439T** **Myocardial contrast perfusion echocardiography, at rest or with stress, for assessment of myocardial ischemia or viability (List separately in addition to code for primary procedure)**

Code first (93306-93308, 93350-93351)

0.00 0.00 **FUD** ZZZ N N1 80

AMA: 2018,Jan,8; 2017,Jan,8; 2016,Apr,8

0440T-0442T

0440T **Ablation, percutaneous, cryoablation, includes imaging guidance; upper extremity distal/peripheral nerve**

0.00 0.00 **FUD** YYY J G2 80

AMA: 2019,Apr,9; 2018,Jan,8

0441T **lower extremity distal/peripheral nerve**

0.00 0.00 **FUD** YYY J G2 80

AMA: 2019,Apr,9; 2018,Jan,8

0442T **nerve plexus or other truncal nerve (eg, brachial plexus, pudendal nerve)**

0.00 0.00 **FUD** YYY J J8 80

AMA: 2019,Apr,9; 2018,Jan,8

0443T

+ **0443T** **Real-time spectral analysis of prostate tissue by fluorescence spectroscopy, including imaging guidance (List separately in addition to code for primary procedure)** ♂

EXCLUDES *Reporting code more than one time for each session*

Code also (55700)

0.00 0.00 **FUD** ZZZ N N1 80

0444T-0445T

EXCLUDES *Insertion/removal drug-eluting stent into canaliculus (0356T)*

0444T **Initial placement of a drug-eluting ocular insert under one or more eyelids, including fitting, training, and insertion, unilateral or bilateral**

0.00 0.00 **FUD** YYY N N1 80

AMA: 2018,Jan,8; 2017,Aug,7

0445T **Subsequent placement of a drug-eluting ocular insert under one or more eyelids, including re-training, and removal of existing insert, unilateral or bilateral**

0.00 0.00 **FUD** YYY N N1 80

AMA: 2018,Jan,8; 2017,Aug,7

0446T-0448T

EXCLUDES *Placement non-implantable interstitial glucose sensor without pocket (95250)*

0446T **Creation of subcutaneous pocket with insertion of implantable interstitial glucose sensor, including system activation and patient training**

EXCLUDES *Interpretation/report ambulatory glucose monitoring interstitial tissue (95251)*
Removal interstitial glucose sensor (0447T-0448T)

0.00 0.00 **FUD** YYY T G2

AMA: 2018,Jun,6

0447T **Removal of implantable interstitial glucose sensor from subcutaneous pocket via incision**

0.00 0.00 **FUD** YYY Q2 G2

0448T **Removal of implantable interstitial glucose sensor with creation of subcutaneous pocket at different anatomic site and insertion of new implantable sensor, including system activation**

EXCLUDES *Initial insertion sensor (0446T)*
Removal sensor (0447T)

0.00 0.00 FUD YYY T G2

0449T-0450T

EXCLUDES *Removal by internal approach aqueous drainage device without extraocular reservoir in subconjunctival space (92499)*

0449T **Insertion of aqueous drainage device, without extraocular reservoir, internal approach, into the subconjunctival space; initial device**

0.00 0.00 FUD YYY J J8

AMA: 2018,Sep,3; 2018,Jul,3

+ **0450T** **each additional device (List separately in addition to code for primary procedure)**

Code first (0449T)

0.00 0.00 FUD YYY N N1

AMA: 2018,Jul,3

0451T-0463T

INCLUDES Access procedures (36000-36010)
Catheterization vessel (36200-36228)
Diagnostic angiography (75600-75774)
Imaging guidance (76000, 76936-76937, 77001-77002, 77011-77012, 77021)
Injection procedures (93561-93572)
Radiological supervision and interpretation

EXCLUDES *Cardiac catheterization (93451-93533)*

0451T **Insertion or replacement of a permanently implantable aortic counterpulsation ventricular assist system, endovascular approach, and programming of sensing and therapeutic parameters; complete system (counterpulsation device, vascular graft, implantable vascular hemostatic seal, mechano-electrical skin interface and subcutaneous electrodes)**

EXCLUDES *Aortic counterpulsation ventricular assist system procedures (0452T-0458T)*
Insertion intra-aortic balloon assist device (33967, 33970, 33973)
Insertion/removal percutaneous ventricular assist device ([33995], 33990-33991, [33997])
Insertion/replacement extracorporeal ventricular assist device (33975-33976, 33981)
Insertion/replacement intracorporeal ventricular assist device (33979, 33982-33983)

0.00 0.00 FUD YYY C

AMA: 2017,Dec,3

0452T **aortic counterpulsation device and vascular hemostatic seal**

EXCLUDES *Insertion intra-aortic balloon assist device (33973)*
Insertion intracorporeal ventricular assist device (33979, 33982-33983)
Insertion/removal percutaneous ventricular assist device ([33995], 33990-33991, [33997])
Insertion/replacement counterpulsation ventricular assist system procedures (0451T)
Removal counterpulsation ventricular assist system (0455T-0456T)

0.00 0.00 FUD YYY C

AMA: 2017,Dec,3

0453T **mechano-electrical skin interface**

EXCLUDES *Insertion intra-aortic balloon assist device (33973)*
Insertion intracorporeal ventricular assist device (33979, 33982-33983)
Insertion/removal percutaneous ventricular assist device ([33995], 33990-33991, [33997])
Insertion/replacement counterpulsation ventricular assist system procedures (0451T)
Removal counterpulsation ventricular assist system (0455T, 0457T)

0.00 0.00 FUD YYY J

0454T **subcutaneous electrode**

INCLUDES Each electrode inserted or replaced

EXCLUDES *Insertion intra-aortic balloon assist device (33973, 33982-33983)*
Insertion/removal percutaneous ventricular assist device ([33995], 33990-33991, [33997])
Insertion/replacement counterpulsation ventricular assist system (0451T)
Insertion/replacement intracorporeal ventricular assist device (33979, 33982-33983)
Removal device or component (0455T, 0458T)

0.00 0.00 FUD YYY J

0455T **Removal of permanently implantable aortic counterpulsation ventricular assist system; complete system (aortic counterpulsation device, vascular hemostatic seal, mechano-electrical skin interface and electrodes)**

EXCLUDES *Insertion/replacement system or component (0451T-0454T)*
Removal:
Extracorporeal ventricular assist device (33977-33978)
Intra-aortic balloon assist device (33968, 33971, 33974)
Intracorporeal ventricular assist device (33980)
Percutaneous ventricular assist device (33992)
System or component (0456T-0458T)

0.00 0.00 FUD YYY C

AMA: 2017,Dec,3

0456T **aortic counterpulsation device and vascular hemostatic seal**

EXCLUDES *Insertion/replacement system or component (0451T-0452T)*
Removal:
Aortic counterpulsation ventricular assist system (0455T)
Intra-aortic balloon assist device (33974)
Intracorporeal ventricular assist device (33980)
Percutaneous ventricular assist device (33992)

0.00 0.00 FUD YYY C

AMA: 2017,Dec,3

0457T **mechano-electrical skin interface**

EXCLUDES *Insertion/replacement system or component (0451T, 0453T)*
Removal:
Aortic counterpulsation ventricular assist system (0455T)
Intra-aortic balloon assist device (33974)
Intracorporeal ventricular assist device (33980)
Percutaneous ventricular assist device (33992)

0.00 0.00 FUD YYY Q2

0458T **subcutaneous electrode**

INCLUDES Each electrode removed

EXCLUDES *Insertion/replacement system or component (0451T, 0454T)*
Removal:
Aortic counterpulsation ventricular assist system (0455T)
Intra-aortic balloon assist device (33974)
Intracorporeal ventricular assist device (33980)
Percutaneous ventricular assist device (33992)

0.00 0.00 FUD YYY Q2

0459T **Relocation of skin pocket with replacement of implanted aortic counterpulsation ventricular assist device, mechano-electrical skin interface and electrodes**

EXCLUDES *Repositioning percutaneous ventricular assist device (33993)*

0.00 0.00 FUD YYY C

0460T **Repositioning of previously implanted aortic counterpulsation ventricular assist device; subcutaneous electrode**
INCLUDES Repositioning each electrode
EXCLUDES *Insertion/replacement system or component (0451T, 0454T)*
Repositioning percutaneous ventricular assist device (33993)
0.00 0.00 FUD YYY T

0461T **aortic counterpulsation device**
EXCLUDES *Repositioning percutaneous ventricular assist device (33993)*
0.00 0.00 FUD YYY C

0462T **Programming device evaluation (in person) with iterative adjustment of the implantable mechano-electrical skin interface and/or external driver to test the function of the device and select optimal permanent programmed values with analysis, including review and report, implantable aortic counterpulsation ventricular assist system, per day**
EXCLUDES *Device evaluation (0463T)*
Insertion/replacement system or component (0451T-0454T)
Relocation pocket (0459T)
Removal system or component (0455T-0458T)
Repositioning device (0460T-0461T)
0.00 0.00 FUD YYY S

0463T **Interrogation device evaluation (in person) with analysis, review and report, includes connection, recording and disconnection per patient encounter, implantable aortic counterpulsation ventricular assist system, per day**
EXCLUDES *Device evaluation (0462T)*
Insertion/replacement system or component (0451T-0454T)
Relocation pocket (0459T)
Removal system or component (0455T-0458T)
Repositioning device (0460T-0461T)
0.00 0.00 FUD YYY S

0464T [0464T]

0464T **Resequenced code. See code following 0333T.**

0465T-0469T

EXCLUDES *Replacement/revision cranial nerve neurostimulator electrode array (64569)*

0465T **Suprachoroidal injection of a pharmacologic agent (does not include supply of medication)**
EXCLUDES *Intravitreal implantation or injection (67025-67028)*
0.00 0.00 FUD YYY T R2
AMA: 2018,Feb,3

+ **0466T** **Insertion of chest wall respiratory sensor electrode or electrode array, including connection to pulse generator (List separately in addition to code for primary procedure)**
EXCLUDES *Revision/removal chest wall respiratory sensor electrode or array (0467T-0468T)*
Code first (64568)
0.00 0.00 FUD YYY N N1
AMA: 2018,Mar,9; 2018,Jan,8; 2017,Jan,8; 2016,Nov,6

0467T **Revision or replacement of chest wall respiratory sensor electrode or electrode array, including connection to existing pulse generator**
EXCLUDES *Insertion/removal chest wall respiratory sensor electrode or array (0466T, 0468T)*
Replacement/revision cranial nerve neurostimulator electrode array (64569)
0.00 0.00 FUD YYY Q2 G2
AMA: 2018,Mar,9; 2018,Jan,8; 2017,Jan,8; 2016,Nov,6

0468T **Removal of chest wall respiratory sensor electrode or electrode array**
EXCLUDES *Insertion/removal chest wall respiratory sensor electrode or array (0466T-0467T)*
Removal cranial neurostimulator electrode array (64570)
0.00 0.00 FUD YYY Q2 G2
AMA: 2018,Mar,9; 2018,Jan,8; 2017,Jan,8; 2016,Nov,6

0469T **Retinal polarization scan, ocular screening with on-site automated results, bilateral**
INCLUDES Ophthalmic medical services (92002-92014)
EXCLUDES *Ocular screening (99174, [99177])*
0.00 0.00 FUD XXX E
AMA: 2018,Feb,3

0470T-0471T

EXCLUDES *Optical coherence tomography coronary vessel or graft (92978-92979)*
Reflectance confocal microscopy (RCM) for cellular and subcellular skin imaging (96931-96936)

0470T **Optical coherence tomography (OCT) for microstructural and morphological imaging of skin, image acquisition, interpretation, and report; first lesion**
0.00 0.00 FUD XXX M

+ **0471T** **each additional lesion (List separately in addition to code for primary procedure)**
Code first (0470T)
0.00 0.00 FUD XXX N N1

0472T-0474T

0472T **Device evaluation, interrogation, and initial programming of intraocular retinal electrode array (eg, retinal prosthesis), in person, with iterative adjustment of the implantable device to test functionality, select optimal permanent programmed values with analysis, including visual training, with review and report by a qualified health care professional**
0.00 0.00 FUD XXX Q1
AMA: 2018,Feb,3

0473T **Device evaluation and interrogation of intraocular retinal electrode array (eg, retinal prosthesis), in person, including reprogramming and visual training, when performed, with review and report by a qualified health care professional**
INCLUDES Reprogramming device (0473T)
EXCLUDES *Placement intraocular retinal electrode display (0100T)*
0.00 0.00 FUD XXX Q1
AMA: 2018,Feb,3

0474T **Insertion of anterior segment aqueous drainage device, with creation of intraocular reservoir, internal approach, into the supraciliary space**
0.00 0.00 FUD XXX J
AMA: 2018,Dec,8; 2018,Dec,8; 2018,Jul,3; 2018,Feb,3

0475T-0478T

0475T **Recording of fetal magnetic cardiac signal using at least 3 channels; patient recording and storage, data scanning with signal extraction, technical analysis and result, as well as supervision, review, and interpretation of report by a physician or other qualified health care professional**
0.00 0.00 FUD XXX M

0476T **patient recording, data scanning, with raw electronic signal transfer of data and storage**
0.00 0.00 FUD XXX Q1

0477T **signal extraction, technical analysis, and result**
0.00 0.00 FUD XXX Q1

0478T **review, interpretation, report by physician or other qualified health care professional**
0.00 0.00 FUD XXX M

0479T-0480T

EXCLUDES *Ablative laser treatment for additional square cm open wound (0492T)*
Cicatricial lesion excision (11400-11446)
Reporting code more than one time per day

0479T **Fractional ablative laser fenestration of burn and traumatic scars for functional improvement; first 100 cm2 or part thereof, or 1% of body surface area of infants and children**
Facility RVU 0.00 Non-Facility RVU 0.00 FUD 000 T G2
AMA: 2018,Jan,8; 2017,Dec,13

\+ **0480T** **each additional 100 cm2, or each additional 1% of body surface area of infants and children, or part thereof (List separately in addition to code for primary procedure)**
Code first (0479T)
Facility RVU 0.00 Non-Facility RVU 0.00 FUD ZZZ N N1
AMA: 2018,Jan,8; 2017,Dec,13

0481T

0481T **Injection(s), autologous white blood cell concentrate (autologous protein solution), any site, including image guidance, harvesting and preparation, when performed**
INCLUDES Radiologic guidance (76942, 77002, 77012, 77021)
EXCLUDES *Blood collection (36415, 36592)*
Bone marrow procedures (38220-38222, 38230)
Injection platelet rich plasma (0232T)
Injections to tendon, ligament, or fascia (20550-20551)
Joint aspiration or injection (20600-20611)
Other tissue grafts ([15769], 15771-15774)
Pooling platelets (86965)
Facility RVU 0.00 Non-Facility RVU 0.00 FUD 000 Q1
AMA: 2019,Oct,5

0483T-0484T

INCLUDES Access and closure
Angiography
Balloon valvuloplasty
Contrast injections
Fluoroscopy
Radiological supervision and interpretation
Valve deployment and repositioning
Ventriculography
EXCLUDES *Diagnostic heart catheterization (93451-93453, 93456-93461, 93530-93533)*
Transcatheter mitral valve annulus reconstruction (0544T)
Transcatheter mitral valve repair through coronary sinus (0345T)
Transcatheter mitral valve repair with transseptal puncture, when performed (33418-33419)
Transcatheter tricuspid valve annulus reconstruction (0545T)
Code also cardiopulmonary bypass when provided (33367-33369)
Code also diagnostic cardiac catheterization procedures when no previous study available and append modifier 59 when:
Patient condition has changed
Previous study inadequate

0483T **Transcatheter mitral valve implantation/replacement (TMVI) with prosthetic valve; percutaneous approach, including transseptal puncture, when performed**
Facility RVU 0.00 Non-Facility RVU 0.00 FUD 000 C 80

0484T **transthoracic exposure (eg, thoracotomy, transapical)**
Facility RVU 0.00 Non-Facility RVU 0.00 FUD 000 C 80

0485T-0486T

0485T **Optical coherence tomography (OCT) of middle ear, with interpretation and report; unilateral**
Facility RVU 0.00 Non-Facility RVU 0.00 FUD XXX Q1 50

0486T **bilateral**
Facility RVU 0.00 Non-Facility RVU 0.00 FUD XXX Q1

0487T-0488T [0488T]

0487T **Biomechanical mapping, transvaginal, with report**
Facility RVU 0.00 Non-Facility RVU 0.00 FUD XXX Q1 N1

0488T **Resequenced code. See code following 0403T.**

0489T-0490T

EXCLUDES *Joint injection/aspiration (20600, 20604)*
Liposuction procedures (15876-15879)
Tissue grafts ([15769], 15771-15774)
Code also for complete procedure report both codes (0489T-0490T)

0489T **Autologous adipose-derived regenerative cell therapy for scleroderma in the hands; adipose tissue harvesting, isolation and preparation of harvested cells including incubation with cell dissociation enzymes, removal of non-viable cells and debris, determination of concentration and dilution of regenerative cells**
Facility RVU 0.00 Non-Facility RVU 0.00 FUD 000 E
AMA: 2019,Oct,5; 2018,Sep,12

0490T **multiple injections in one or both hands**
EXCLUDES *Single injections*
Facility RVU 0.00 Non-Facility RVU 0.00 FUD 000 E
AMA: 2019,Oct,5; 2018,Sep,12

0491T-0493T

0491T **Ablative laser treatment, non-contact, full field and fractional ablation, open wound, per day, total treatment surface area; first 20 sq cm or less**
Facility RVU 0.00 Non-Facility RVU 0.00 FUD 000 T G2

\+ **0492T** **each additional 20 sq cm, or part thereof (List separately in addition to code for primary procedure)**
EXCLUDES *Laser fenestration scars (0479T-0480T)*
Code first (0491T)
Facility RVU 0.00 Non-Facility RVU 0.00 FUD ZZZ N N1

0493T **Near-infrared spectroscopy studies of lower extremity wounds (eg, for oxyhemoglobin measurement)**
Facility RVU 0.00 Non-Facility RVU 0.00 FUD XXX N N1

0494T-0496T

0494T **Surgical preparation and cannulation of marginal (extended) cadaver donor lung(s) to ex vivo organ perfusion system, including decannulation, separation from the perfusion system, and cold preservation of the allograft prior to implantation, when performed**
Facility RVU 0.00 Non-Facility RVU 0.00 FUD XXX C 80

0495T **Initiation and monitoring marginal (extended) cadaver donor lung(s) organ perfusion system by physician or qualified health care professional, including physiological and laboratory assessment (eg, pulmonary artery flow, pulmonary artery pressure, left atrial pressure, pulmonary vascular resistance, mean/peak and plateau airway pressure, dynamic compliance and perfusate gas analysis), including bronchoscopy and X ray when performed; first two hours in sterile field**
Facility RVU 0.00 Non-Facility RVU 0.00 FUD XXX C

\+ **0496T** **each additional hour (List separately in addition to code for primary procedure)**
Code first (0495T)
Facility RVU 0.00 Non-Facility RVU 0.00 FUD ZZZ C

0497T-0498T

EXCLUDES *ECG event monitoring (93268, 93271-93272)*
ECG rhythm strips (93040-93042)
Remote telemetry (93228-93229)

0497T **External patient-activated, physician- or other qualified health care professional-prescribed, electrocardiographic rhythm derived event recorder without 24 hour attended monitoring; in-office connection**
Facility RVU 0.00 Non-Facility RVU 0.00 FUD XXX Q1 TC

0498T **review and interpretation by a physician or other qualified health care professional per 30 days with at least one patient-generated triggered event**
Facility RVU 0.00 Non-Facility RVU 0.00 FUD XXX M 26

0499T-0500T

0499T **Cystourethroscopy, with mechanical dilation and urethral therapeutic drug delivery for urethral stricture or stenosis, including fluoroscopy, when performed**

EXCLUDES *Cystourethroscopy for stricture (52281, 52283)*

0.00 0.00 FUD 000 E

0500T **Infectious agent detection by nucleic acid (DNA or RNA), human papillomavirus (HPV) for five or more separately reported high-risk HPV types (eg, 16, 18, 31, 33, 35, 39, 45, 51, 52, 56, 58, 59, 68) (ie, genotyping)**

EXCLUDES *Less than five high-risk HPV types ([87624, 87625])*

0.00 0.00 FUD XXX A

0501T-0523T [0523T, 0623T, 0624T, 0625T, 0626T]

EXCLUDES *Reporting code more than one time for each CT angiogram*

0501T **Noninvasive estimated coronary fractional flow reserve (FFR) derived from coronary computed tomography angiography data using computation fluid dynamics physiologic simulation software analysis of functional data to assess the severity of coronary artery disease; data preparation and transmission, analysis of fluid dynamics and simulated maximal coronary hyperemia, generation of estimated FFR model, with anatomical data review in comparison with estimated FFR model to reconcile discordant data, interpretation and report**

INCLUDES All complete test components (0501T-0504T)

EXCLUDES *Automated coronary plaque characterization/quantification using coronary CT angiography data ([0623T, 0624T, 0625T, 0626T])*

0.00 0.00 FUD XXX M

AMA: 2018,Sep,10

0502T **data preparation and transmission**

EXCLUDES *Automated coronary plaque characterization/quantification using coronary CT angiography data ([0623T, 0624T, 0625T, 0626T])*

0.00 0.00 FUD XXX N NI TC

AMA: 2018,Sep,10

0503T **analysis of fluid dynamics and simulated maximal coronary hyperemia, and generation of estimated FFR model**

EXCLUDES *Automated coronary plaque characterization/quantification using coronary CT angiography data ([0623T, 0624T, 0625T, 0626T])*

0.00 0.00 FUD XXX S NI TC

AMA: 2018,Sep,10

0504T **anatomical data review in comparison with estimated FFR model to reconcile discordant data, interpretation and report**

EXCLUDES *Automated coronary plaque characterization/quantification using coronary CT angiography data ([0623T, 0624T, 0625T, 0626T])*

0.00 0.00 FUD XXX M 26

AMA: 2018,Sep,10

● # **0623T** **Automated quantification and characterization of coronary atherosclerotic plaque to assess severity of coronary disease, using data from coronary computed tomographic angiography; data preparation and transmission, computerized analysis of data, with review of computerized analysis output to reconcile discordant data, interpretation and report**

INCLUDES All complete test components ([0623T, 0624T, 0625T, 0626T])

EXCLUDES *3D rendering (76376-76377)*

Noninvasive estimated coronary fractional flow reserve (FFR) (0501T-0504T)

0.00 0.00 FUD 000

● # **0624T** **data preparation and transmission**

EXCLUDES *3D rendering (76376-76377)*

Noninvasive estimated coronary fractional flow reserve (FFR) (0501T-0504T)

0.00 0.00 FUD 000

● # **0625T** **computerized analysis of data from coronary computed tomographic angiography**

EXCLUDES *3D rendering (76376-76377)*

Noninvasive estimated coronary fractional flow reserve (FFR) (0501T-0504T)

0.00 0.00 FUD 000

● # **0626T** **review of computerized analysis output to reconcile discordant data, interpretation and report**

EXCLUDES *3D rendering (76376-76377)*

Noninvasive estimated coronary fractional flow reserve (FFR) (0501T-0504T)

0.00 0.00 FUD 000

\+ # **0523T** **Intraprocedural coronary fractional flow reserve (FFR) with 3D functional mapping of color-coded FFR values for the coronary tree, derived from coronary angiogram data, for real-time review and interpretation of possible atherosclerotic stenosis(es) intervention (List separately in addition to code for primary procedure)**

EXCLUDES *3D rendering (76376-76377)*

Coronary artery doppler studies (93571-93572)

Noninvasive estimated coronary fractional flow reserve (FFR) (0501T-0504T)

Procedure reported more than one time each session

Code first (93454-93461)

0.00 0.00 FUD ZZZ NI 80

0505T-0514T [0510T, 0511T, 0512T, 0513T, 0620T]

0505T **Endovenous femoral-popliteal arterial revascularization, with transcatheter placement of intravascular stent graft(s) and closure by any method, including percutaneous or open vascular access, ultrasound guidance for vascular access when performed, all catheterization(s) and intraprocedural roadmapping and imaging guidance necessary to complete the intervention, all associated radiological supervision and interpretation, when performed, with crossing of the occlusive lesion in an extraluminal fashion**

INCLUDES All procedures performed on same side:

- Catheterization (arterial and venous)
- Diagnostic imaging for arteriography
- Radiologic supervision and interpretation

Ultrasound guidance (76937)

EXCLUDES *Balloon angioplasty arteries other than dialysis circuit ([37248, 37249])*

Revascularization femoral or popliteal artery (37224-37227)

Venous stenting (37238-37239)

0.00 0.00 FUD YYY 80

● # **0620T** **Endovascular venous arterialization, tibial or peroneal vein, with transcatheter placement of intravascular stent graft(s) and closure by any method, including percutaneous or open vascular access, ultrasound guidance for vascular access when performed, all catheterization(s) and intraprocedural roadmapping and imaging guidance necessary to complete the intervention, all associated radiological supervision and interpretation, when performed**

INCLUDES All procedures performed on same side:

- Catheterization (arterial and venous)
- Diagnostic imaging for arteriography
- Radiologic supervision and interpretation

EXCLUDES *When performed within tibial-peroneal segment:*

- *Endovascular revascularization procedures (37228-37231)*
- *Transcatheter intravascular stent placement (37238-37239)*
- *Transluminal balloon angioplasty ([37248, 37249])*

0.00 0.00 FUD 000

0506T **Macular pigment optical density measurement by heterochromatic flicker photometry, unilateral or bilateral, with interpretation and report**

0.00 0.00 FUD XXX 80

AMA: 2018,Dec,6; 2018,Dec,6

0507T **Near-infrared dual imaging (ie, simultaneous reflective and trans-illuminated light) of meibomian glands, unilateral or bilateral, with interpretation and report**

EXCLUDES *External ocular photography (92285)*
Tear film imaging (0330T)

0.00 0.00 FUD XXX 80

0508T **Pulse-echo ultrasound bone density measurement resulting in indicator of axial bone mineral density, tibia**

0.00 0.00 FUD XXX Z2 80

0509T **Electroretinography (ERG) with interpretation and report, pattern (PERG)**

EXCLUDES *Full field ERG (92273)*
Multifocal ERG (92274)

2.24 2.24 FUD XXX 80

AMA: 2019,Jan,12

0510T **Resequenced code. See code following 0335T.**

0511T **Resequenced code. See code following 0335T.**

0512T **Resequenced code. See code following 0102T.**

0513T **Resequenced code. See code following 0102T.**

\+ **0514T** **Intraoperative visual axis identification using patient fixation (List separately in addition to code for primary procedure)**

Code first (66982, 66984)

0.00 0.00 FUD ZZZ N1

AMA: 2018,Dec,6; 2018,Dec,6

0515T-0523T [0523T]

INCLUDES Complete system with two components
Pulse generator including battery and transmitter
Wireless endocardial left ventricular electrode

0515T **Insertion of wireless cardiac stimulator for left ventricular pacing, including device interrogation and programming, and imaging supervision and interpretation, when performed; complete system (includes electrode and generator [transmitter and battery])**

INCLUDES Catheterization (93452-93453, 93458-93461, 93531-93533)
Creation pockets
Electrode insertion
Imaging guidance (76000, 76998, 93303-93355)
Insertion complete wireless cardiac stimulator system
Interrogation device (0521T)
Programming device (0522T)
Pulse generator (battery and transmitter) (0517T)
Revision and repositioning

EXCLUDES *Insertion electrode as separate procedure (0516T)*
Removal/replacement device or components (0518T-0520T)

0.00 0.00 FUD YYY

0516T **electrode only**

INCLUDES Catheterization (93452-93453, 93458-93461, 93531-93533)
Imaging guidance (76000, 76998, 93303-93355)
Interrogation device (0521T)
Programming device (0522T)

EXCLUDES *Removal/replacement device or components (0518T-0520T)*

0.00 0.00 FUD YYY

0517T **pulse generator component(s) (battery and/or transmitter) only**

INCLUDES Catheterization (93452-93453, 93458-93461, 93531-93533)
Imaging guidance (76000, 76998, 93303-93355)
Interrogation device (0521T)
Programming device (0522T)

EXCLUDES *Removal/replacement device or components (0518T-0520T)*

0.00 0.00 FUD YYY

0518T **Removal of only pulse generator component(s) (battery and/or transmitter) of wireless cardiac stimulator for left ventricular pacing**

INCLUDES Catheterization (93452-93453, 93458-93461, 93531-93533)
Imaging guidance (76000, 76998, 93303-93355)
Interrogation device (0521T)
Programming device (0522T)
Pulse generator (battery and transmitter) (0517T)

EXCLUDES *Complete procedure (0515T)*
Insertion electrode only (0516T)
Removal/replacement device or components (0519T-0520T)

0.00 0.00 FUD YYY

0519T **Removal and replacement of wireless cardiac stimulator for left ventricular pacing; pulse generator component(s) (battery and/or transmitter)**

INCLUDES Catheterization (93452-93453, 93458-93461, 93531-93533)
Imaging guidance (76000, 76998, 93303-93355)
Interrogation device (0521T)
Programming device (0522T)
Pulse generator (battery and transmitter) (0517T)

EXCLUDES *Complete procedure (0515T)*
Insertion electrode only (0516T)
Removal/replacement device or components (0518T)

0.00 0.00 FUD YYY

0520T **pulse generator component(s) (battery and/or transmitter), including placement of a new electrode**

INCLUDES Catheterization (93452-93453, 93458-93461, 93531-93533)
Imaging guidance (76000, 76998, 93303-93355)
Interrogation device (0521T)
Programming device (0522T)
Pulse generator (battery and transmitter) (0517T)

EXCLUDES *Complete procedure (0515T)*
Insertion electrode only (0516T)
Removal only device or components (0518T)

0.00 0.00 FUD YYY

0521T **Interrogation device evaluation (in person) with analysis, review and report, includes connection, recording, and disconnection per patient encounter, wireless cardiac stimulator for left ventricular pacing**

INCLUDES Programming device (0522T)
Pulse generator (battery and transmitter) (0517T)

EXCLUDES *Complete procedure (0515T)*
Insertion electrode only (0516T)
Removal/replacement device or components (0518T-0520T)

0.00 0.00 FUD XXX

0522T Programming device evaluation (in person) with iterative adjustment of the implantable device to test the function of the device and select optimal permanent programmed values with analysis, including review and report, wireless cardiac stimulator for left ventricular pacing

    INCLUDES Interrogation device (0521T)
           Pulse generator (battery and transmitter) (0517T)
    EXCLUDES *Complete procedure (0515T)*
           Insertion electrode only (0516T)
           Removal/replacement device or components (0518T-0520T)

    📷 0.00   ✂ 0.00   **FUD** XXX

0523T Resequenced code. See code before 0505T.

0524T

0524T Endovenous catheter directed chemical ablation with balloon isolation of incompetent extremity vein, open or percutaneous, including all vascular access, catheter manipulation, diagnostic imaging, imaging guidance and monitoring

    📷 0.00   ✂ 0.00   **FUD** YYY   G2 50

0525T-0532T

0525T Insertion or replacement of intracardiac ischemia monitoring system, including testing of the lead and monitor, initial system programming, and imaging supervision and interpretation; complete system (electrode and implantable monitor)

    INCLUDES Electrocardiography (93000, 93005, 93010)
           Interrogation device (0529T)
           Programming device (0528T)
    EXCLUDES *Removal intracardiac ischemia monitor or components (0530T-0532T)*

    📷 0.00   ✂ 0.00   **FUD** YYY   J8

0526T electrode only

    INCLUDES Electrocardiography (93000, 93005, 93010)
           Interrogation device (0529T)
           Programming device (0528T)
    EXCLUDES *Removal intracardiac ischemia monitor or components (0530T-0532T)*

    📷 0.00   ✂ 0.00   **FUD** YYY   J8

0527T implantable monitor only

    INCLUDES Electrocardiography (93000, 93005, 93010)
           Interrogation device (0529T)
           Programming device (0528T)
    EXCLUDES *Removal intracardiac ischemia monitor or components (0530T-0532T)*

    📷 0.00   ✂ 0.00   **FUD** YYY   J8

0528T Programming device evaluation (in person) of intracardiac ischemia monitoring system with iterative adjustment of programmed values, with analysis, review, and report

    INCLUDES Electrocardiography (93000, 93005, 93010)
    EXCLUDES *Insertion/replacement intracardiac ischemia monitor or components (0525T-0527T)*
           Interrogation device (0529T)
           Removal intracardiac ischemia monitor or components (0530T-0532T)

    📷 0.00   ✂ 0.00   **FUD** XXX

0529T Interrogation device evaluation (in person) of intracardiac ischemia monitoring system with analysis, review, and report

    INCLUDES Electrocardiography (93000, 93005, 93010)
    EXCLUDES *Insertion/replacement electrode only (0526T)*
           Insertion/replacement intracardiac ischemia monitor or components (0525T-0527T)
           Programming device (0528T)
           Removal intracardiac ischemia monitor or components (0530T-0532T)

    📷 0.00   ✂ 0.00   **FUD** XXX

0530T Removal of intracardiac ischemia monitoring system, including all imaging supervision and interpretation; complete system (electrode and implantable monitor)

    EXCLUDES *Interrogation device (0529T)*
           Programming device (0528T)

    📷 0.00   ✂ 0.00   **FUD** YYY   G2

0531T electrode only

    EXCLUDES *Interrogation device (0529T)*
           Programming device (0528T)

    📷 0.00   ✂ 0.00   **FUD** YYY   G2

0532T implantable monitor only

    EXCLUDES *Interrogation device (0529T)*
           Programming device (0528T)

    📷 0.00   ✂ 0.00   **FUD** YYY   G2

0533T-0536T

0533T Continuous recording of movement disorder symptoms, including bradykinesia, dyskinesia, and tremor for 6 days up to 10 days; includes set-up, patient training, configuration of monitor, data upload, analysis and initial report configuration, download review, interpretation and report

    📷 0.00   ✂ 0.00   **FUD** XXX

0534T set-up, patient training, configuration of monitor
    📷 0.00   ✂ 0.00   **FUD** XXX

0535T data upload, analysis and initial report configuration
    📷 0.00   ✂ 0.00   **FUD** XXX

0536T download review, interpretation and report
    📷 0.00   ✂ 0.00   **FUD** XXX

0537T-0540T

    INCLUDES Administration genetically modified cells for treatment serious diseases (e.g., cancer)
           Evaluation prior to, during, and after CAR-T cell administration
           Infusion fluids and supportive medications provided with administration
           Management clinical staff
           Management untoward events (e.g., nausea)
           Physician certification, processing cells
           Physician presence during cell administration
Code also care provided not directly related to CAR-T cell administration (e.g., other medical problems) may be reported separately using appropriate E/M code and modifier 25

0537T Chimeric antigen receptor T-cell (CAR-T) therapy; harvesting of blood-derived T lymphocytes for development of genetically modified autologous CAR-T cells, per day

    EXCLUDES *Reporting more than one time per day despite times cells are collected*

    📷 0.00   ✂ 0.00   **FUD** XXX
    AMA: 2019,Jun,5

0538T preparation of blood-derived T lymphocytes for transportation (eg, cryopreservation, storage)
    📷 0.00   ✂ 0.00   **FUD** XXX
    AMA: 2019,Jun,5

0539T receipt and preparation of CAR-T cells for administration
    📷 0.00   ✂ 0.00   **FUD** XXX
    AMA: 2019,Jun,5

0540T CAR-T cell administration, autologous
    EXCLUDES *Reporting more than one time per day despite units administered*
    📷 0.00   ✂ 0.00   **FUD** YYY
    AMA: 2019,Jun,5

0541T-0542T

0541T Myocardial imaging by magnetocardiography (MCG) for detection of cardiac ischemia, by signal acquisition using minimum 36 channel grid, generation of magnetic-field time-series images, quantitative analysis of magnetic dipoles, machine learning-derived clinical scoring, and automated report generation, single study;

    📷 0.00   ✂ 0.00   **FUD** XXX   TC

● New Code   ▲ Revised Code   ○ Reinstated   ● New Web Release   ▲ Revised Web Release   + Add-on   Unlisted   Not Covered   # Resequenced
50 Optum Mod 50 Exempt   ⊘ AMA Mod 51 Exempt   51 Optum Mod 51 Exempt   63 Mod 63 Exempt   ✗ Non-FDA Drug   ★ Telemedicine   Ⓜ Maternity   Ⓐ Age Edit

0542T **interpretation and report**
0.00 0.00 FUD XXX 26

0543T

EXCLUDES *Transesophageal echocardiography (93355)*

0543T **Transapical mitral valve repair, including transthoracic echocardiography, when performed, with placement of artificial chordae tendineae**
0.00 0.00 FUD YYY 80

0544T-0545T

INCLUDES Adjustment/deployment reconstruction device
Catheterization
Insertion temporary pacemaker
Vascular access and closure

EXCLUDES *Fluoroscopic guidance (76000)*
Percutaneous mitral valve repair

Code also diagnostic angiography or catheterization and append modifier 59, when:
Prior study available but inadequate or patient's condition has changed
Prior study not available and full diagnostic study performed
Code also transcatheter implantation/replacement mitral valve (0483T)
Code also when performed:
Balloon pump insertion (33967, 33970, 33973)
Central bypass (33369)
Peripheral bypass (33367-33368)
Ventricular assist device (33990-33993)

0544T **Transcatheter mitral valve annulus reconstruction, with implantation of adjustable annulus reconstruction device, percutaneous approach including transseptal puncture**
EXCLUDES *Transcatheter mitral valve repair (33418-33419)*
Transcatheter mitral valve repair via coronary sinus (0345T)
0.00 0.00 FUD YYY 80

0545T **Transcatheter tricuspid valve annulus reconstruction with implantation of adjustable annulus reconstruction device, percutaneous approach**
EXCLUDES *Repositioning/plication tricuspid valve (33468)*
0.00 0.00 FUD YYY 80

0546T

EXCLUDES *Reporting code for re-excision of site*
Reporting code more than one time per partial mastectomy site

0546T **Radiofrequency spectroscopy, real time, intraoperative margin assessment, at the time of partial mastectomy, with report**
0.00 0.00 FUD YYY 80
AMA: 2020,May,9

0547T

0547T **Bone-material quality testing by microindentation(s) of the tibia(s), with results reported as a score**
0.00 0.00 FUD XXX 80

0548T-0551T

0548T **Transperineal periurethral balloon continence device; bilateral placement, including cystoscopy and fluoroscopy**
0.00 0.00 FUD YYY J8 80
AMA: 2020,Aug,6

0549T **unilateral placement, including cystoscopy and fluoroscopy**
0.00 0.00 FUD YYY J8 80
AMA: 2020,Aug,6

0550T **removal, each balloon**
0.00 0.00 FUD YYY G2 80
AMA: 2020,Aug,6

0551T **adjustment of balloon(s) fluid volume**
EXCLUDES *Insertion or removal periurethral balloon continence device (0548T-0550T)*
0.00 0.00 FUD YYY R2 80
AMA: 2020,Aug,6

0552T

0552T **Low-level laser therapy, dynamic photonic and dynamic thermokinetic energies, provided by a physician or other qualified health care professional**
0.00 0.00 FUD YYY 80

0553T

EXCLUDES *Angiography extremity (75710)*
Endovascular revascularization (37220-37221, 37224, 37226, 37238)
Injection for venography (36005)
Insertion catheter/needle, upper or lower extremity artery (36140)
Selective catheter placement (36011-36012, 36245-36246)
Transluminal balloon angioplasty ([37248])
Venography (75820)

0553T **Percutaneous transcatheter placement of iliac arteriovenous anastomosis implant, inclusive of all radiological supervision and interpretation, intraprocedural roadmapping, and imaging guidance necessary to complete the intervention**
0.00 0.00 FUD YYY 80

0554T-0557T

0554T **Bone strength and fracture risk using finite element analysis of functional data, and bone-mineral density, utilizing data from a computed tomography scan; retrieval and transmission of the scan data, assessment of bone strength and fracture risk and bone mineral density, interpretation and report**
INCLUDES Assessment, interpretation and report, and retrieval and transmission of data (0555T-0557T)
0.00 0.00 FUD XXX 80
AMA: 2020,Sep,11

0555T **retrieval and transmission of the scan data**
0.00 0.00 FUD XXX 80
AMA: 2020,Sep,11

0556T **assessment of bone strength and fracture risk and bone mineral density**
0.00 0.00 FUD XXX 80
AMA: 2020,Sep,11

0557T **interpretation and report**
0.00 0.00 FUD XXX 80
AMA: 2020,Sep,11

0558T

EXCLUDES *Computed tomography:*
abdominal aorta (75635)
abdomen/pelvis (72191-72194, 74150-74178)
chest/thorax (71250-71270, 71275)
colonography (74261-74263)
heart (75571-75574)
spine (72125-72133)
whole body (78816)

0558T **Computed tomography scan taken for the purpose of biomechanical computed tomography analysis**
0.00 0.00 FUD XXX Z2 80
AMA: 2020,Sep,11

0559T-0562T

EXCLUDES *3D rendering (76376-76377)*

0559T **Anatomic model 3D-printed from image data set(s); first individually prepared and processed component of an anatomic structure**
INCLUDES 3D printed anatomical model production
0.00 0.00 FUD XXX 80

\+ **0560T** **each additional individually prepared and processed component of an anatomic structure (List separately in addition to code for primary procedure)**
INCLUDES 3D printed anatomical model production
Code first (0559T)
0.00 0.00 FUD ZZZ 80

0561T   Anatomic guide 3D-printed and designed from image data set(s); first anatomic guide

     INCLUDES   3D printed cutting or drilling guides for use during surgery

     🚑 0.00   ✂ 0.00   **FUD** XXX   80 ▢

+   **0562T**   each additional anatomic guide (List separately in addition to code for primary procedure)

     INCLUDES   3D printed cutting or drilling guides for use during surgery

     Code first (0561T)

     🚑 0.00   ✂ 0.00   **FUD** ZZZ   80 ▢

0563T-0564T [0563T]

0563T   **Resequenced code. See code before code 0208T.**

0564T   Oncology, chemotherapeutic drug cytotoxicity assay of cancer stem cells (CSCs), from cultured CSCs and primary tumor cells, categorical drug response reported based on percent of cytotoxicity observed, a minimum of 14 drugs or drug combinations

     🚑 0.00   ✂ 0.00   **FUD** YYY   80

0565T-0566T

0565T   Autologous cellular implant derived from adipose tissue for the treatment of osteoarthritis of the knees; tissue harvesting and cellular implant creation

     EXCLUDES   *Other tissue grafts ([15769], 15771-15774)*

     🚑 0.00   ✂ 0.00   **FUD** YYY   80 ▢

0566T   injection of cellular implant into knee joint including ultrasound guidance, unilateral

     INCLUDES   Guidance for needle placement:

         Fluoroscopy (77002)

         Ultrasound (76942)

     EXCLUDES   *Arthrocentesis, with or without imaging guidance (20610-20611)*

     🚑 0.00   ✂ 0.00   **FUD** YYY   R2 80 ▢

0567T-0568T

0567T   Permanent fallopian tube occlusion with degradable biopolymer implant, transcervical approach, including transvaginal ultrasound   ♀

     INCLUDES   Transvaginal ultrasound (76830)

     EXCLUDES   *Catheter insertion and introduction saline/contrast for sonohysterography or hysterosalpingography (58340)*

         Hysterosalpingography (74740)

         Nonobstetric pelvic ultrasound (76856-76857)

         Surgical hysteroscopy with bilateral occlusion fallopian tube (58565)

         Transcervical catheterization fallopian tube (74742)

     🚑 0.00   ✂ 0.00   **FUD** YYY   80 ▢

0568T   Introduction of mixture of saline and air for sonosalpingography to confirm occlusion of fallopian tubes, transcervical approach, including transvaginal ultrasound and pelvic ultrasound   ♀

     INCLUDES   Transvaginal ultrasound (76830)

     EXCLUDES   *Catheter insertion and introduction saline/contrast for sonohysterography or hysterosalpingography (58340)*

         Hysterosalpingography (74740)

         Nonobstetric pelvic ultrasound (76856-76857)

         Sonohysterography (SIS) (76831)

         Surgical hysteroscopy with bilateral occlusion fallopian tube (58565)

         Transcervical catheterization fallopian tube (74742)

     🚑 0.00   ✂ 0.00   **FUD** YYY   80 ▢

0569T-0570T

     INCLUDES   Adjustment/deployment prosthetic device

         Catheterization

         Fluoroscopic guidance (76000)

         Intracardiac echocardiography (93662)

         Vascular access and closure

     EXCLUDES   *Open tricuspid valve procedures (33460, 33463-33465, 33468)*

Code also diagnostic angiography or catheterization and append modifier 59, when:

     Prior study available but inadequate or patient's condition has changed

     Prior study not available and full diagnostic study performed

Code also when performed:

     Balloon pump insertion (33967, 33970, 33973)

     Central bypass (33369)

     Peripheral bypass (33367-33368)

     Ventricular assist device (33990-33993)

     TEE, when done by different operator (93355)

0569T   Transcatheter tricuspid valve repair, percutaneous approach; initial prosthesis

     EXCLUDES   *Reporting code more than once per session*

     🚑 0.00   ✂ 0.00   **FUD** YYY   80 ▢

+   **0570T**   each additional prosthesis during same session (List separately in addition to code for primary procedure)

     Code first (0569T)

     🚑 0.00   ✂ 0.00   **FUD** ZZZ   80 ▢

0571T-0614T [0614T]

     EXCLUDES   *Defibrillator or pacemaker device evaluations (93279-93284, 93285-93289, 93290-93298)*

         Implantable defibrillator procedures (33215-33220, 33223-33226, 33240-33249 [33230, 33231, 33262, 33263, 33264])

         Pacemaker procedures (33202-33220 [33221], 33222-33226, 33233-33238 [33227, 33228, 33229])

         Subcutaneous implantable defibrillator system procedures:

            Electrophysiological evaluation (93644)

            Insertion electrode ([33271])

            Insertion/replacement entire system ([33270])

            Interrogation ([93261])

            Programming ([93260])

            Removal electrode ([33272])

            Repositioning electrode ([33273])

         Transcatheter permanent leadless pacemaker procedures:

            Insertion or replacement ([33274])

0571T   Insertion or replacement of implantable cardioverter-defibrillator system with substernal electrode(s), including all imaging guidance and electrophysiological evaluation (includes defibrillation threshold evaluation, induction of arrhythmia, evaluation of sensing for arrhythmia termination, and programming or reprogramming of sensing or therapeutic parameters), when performed

     INCLUDES   Imaging guidance

         Programming, interrogation, and electrophysiological evaluations (0575T-0577T)

     EXCLUDES   *Substernal electrode insertion only (0572T)*

Code also removal implantable cardioverter-defibrillator generator and substernal electrode(s), when total system replaced:

     Electrode(s) (0573T)

     Generator (0580T)

     🚑 0.00   ✂ 0.00   **FUD** YYY   80 ▢

0572T   Insertion of substernal implantable defibrillator electrode

     INCLUDES   Imaging guidance

     EXCLUDES   *Insertion generator and electrode (0571T)*

         Programming, interrogation, and electrophysiological evaluations (0575T-0577T)

         Removal generator only (0580T)

     🚑 0.00   ✂ 0.00   **FUD** YYY   80 ▢

● New Code   ▲ Revised Code   ○ Reinstated   ● New Web Release   ▲ Revised Web Release   + Add-on   Unlisted   Not Covered   # Resequenced

50 Optum Mod 50 Exempt   ⊘ AMA Mod 51 Exempt   51 Optum Mod 51 Exempt   63 Mod 63 Exempt   ✎ Non-FDA Drug   ★ Telemedicine   M Maternity   A Age Edit

0573T Removal of substernal implantable defibrillator electrode

INCLUDES Imaging guidance

EXCLUDES *Programming, interrogation, and electrophysiological evaluations (0575T-0577T)*

Code also removal implantable cardioverter-defibrillator generator and insertion new generator/electrode, when total system replaced:

Insertion new system (0571T)

Removal generator (0580T)

Code also removal generator when system not replaced (0580T)

0.00 0.00 FUD YYY 80

0574T Repositioning of previously implanted substernal implantable defibrillator-pacing electrode

INCLUDES Imaging guidance

EXCLUDES *Programming, interrogation, and electrophysiological evaluations (0575T-0577T)*

Substernal electrode insertion only (0572T)

0.00 0.00 FUD YYY 80

0575T Programming device evaluation (in person) of implantable cardioverter-defibrillator system with substernal electrode, with iterative adjustment of the implantable device to test the function of the device and select optimal permanent programmed values with analysis, review and report by a physician or other qualified health care professional

EXCLUDES *Interrogation and programming device (93260 [93260], 93282, 93287, 0576T)*

Programming during:

Electrode insertion (0572T)

Electrode removal (0573T)

Electrode repositioning (0574T)

Generator removal (0580T)

Insertion/replacement entire system (0571T)

Removal and replacement generator ([0614T])

0.00 0.00 FUD YYY 80

0576T Interrogation device evaluation (in person) of implantable cardioverter-defibrillator system with substernal electrode, with analysis, review and report by a physician or other qualified health care professional, includes connection, recording and disconnection per patient encounter

EXCLUDES *Interrogation and programming device (93261 [93261], 93289, 0575T)*

Interrogation during:

Electrode insertion (0572T)

Electrode removal (0573T)

Electrode repositioning (0574T)

Generator removal (0580T)

Insertion/replacement entire system (0571T)

Removal and replacement generator ([0614T])

0.00 0.00 FUD YYY 80

0577T Electrophysiologic evaluation of implantable cardioverter-defibrillator system with substernal electrode (includes defibrillation threshold evaluation, induction of arrhythmia, evaluation of sensing for arrhythmia termination, and programming or reprogramming of sensing or therapeutic parameters)

EXCLUDES *Electrophysiologic evaluation during:*

Electrode insertion (0572T)

Electrode removal (0573T)

Electrode repositioning (0574T)

Generator removal (0580T)

Insertion/replacement entire system (0571T)

Removal and replacement generator ([0614T])

Electrophysiologic evaluation of subcutaneous implantable defibrillator (93644)

0.00 0.00 FUD YYY 80

0578T Interrogation device evaluation(s) (remote), up to 90 days, substernal lead implantable cardioverter-defibrillator system with interim analysis, review(s) and report(s) by a physician or other qualified health care professional

EXCLUDES *In person device interrogation (0576T)*

Reporting code more than once per 90 days

0.00 0.00 FUD YYY 80

0579T Interrogation device evaluation(s) (remote), up to 90 days, substernal lead implantable cardioverter-defibrillator system, remote data acquisition(s), receipt of transmissions and technician review, technical support and distribution of results

EXCLUDES *In person device interrogation (0576T)*

Reporting code more than once per 90 days

0.00 0.00 FUD YYY 80

0580T Removal of substernal implantable defibrillator pulse generator only

INCLUDES Removal generator when system not replaced

EXCLUDES *Programming, interrogation, and electrophysiological evaluations (0575T-0577T)*

Removal and replacement generator ([33262])

Code also removal substernal electrode and insertion new generator/electrode, when total system replaced:

Insertion new system (0571T)

0.00 0.00 FUD YYY 80

● # **0614T Removal and replacement of substernal implantable defibrillator pulse generator**

EXCLUDES *Electrode insertion (0572T)*

Insertion/replacement entire system (0571T)

Programming, interrogation, and electrophysiological evaluations (0575T-0577T)

Removal generator only (0580T)

Removal/replacement single lead system ([33262])

0.00 0.00 FUD YYY J8 80

0581T-0582T

0581T Ablation, malignant breast tumor(s), percutaneous, cryotherapy, including imaging guidance when performed, unilateral

INCLUDES Ultrasound for:

Breast imaging (76641-76642)

Monitoring tissue ablation (76940)

Needle placement (76942)

EXCLUDES *Cryoablation for breast fibroadenoma(s) (19105)*

Reporting code more than once per treated breast

0.00 0.00 FUD YYY 80

0582T Transurethral ablation of malignant prostate tissue by high-energy water vapor thermotherapy, including intraoperative imaging and needle guidance ♂

INCLUDES 3D rendering (76376-76377)

Cystourethroscopy (52000)

MRI pelvis (72195-72197)

Radiologic guidance for:

Needle placement (76942, 77021)

Tissue ablation monitoring (76940, 77022)

Transrectal ultrasound (76872)

EXCLUDES *Destruction by radiofrequency-generated water vapor thermotherapy for benign prostatic hypertrophy (BPH) (53854)*

0.00 0.00 FUD YYY 80

0583T

0583T Tympanostomy (requiring insertion of ventilating tube), using an automated tube delivery system, iontophoresis local anesthesia

INCLUDES Binocular microscopy (92504)
Iontophoresis (97033)
Operating microscope (69990)

EXCLUDES *Myringotomy (69420-69421)*
Removal impacted cerumen (69209-69210)
Tympanostomy without automated delivery system (69433, 69436)

0.00 0.00 FUD YYY 80

0584T-0586T

0584T Islet cell transplant, includes portal vein catheterization and infusion, including all imaging, including guidance, and radiological supervision and interpretation, when performed; percutaneous

0.00 0.00 FUD YYY 80

0585T laparoscopic

0.00 0.00 FUD YYY 80

0586T open

0.00 0.00 FUD YYY 80

0587T-0590T

0587T Percutaneous implantation or replacement of integrated single device neurostimulation system including electrode array and receiver or pulse generator, including analysis, programming, and imaging guidance when performed, posterior tibial nerve

INCLUDES Electronic analysis (95970-95972, 0589T-0590T)

EXCLUDES *Insertion other neurostimulator devices (64555, 64566, 64575, 64590)*
Revision or removal integrated neurostimulation system (0588T)

0.00 0.00 FUD YYY J8 80

0588T Revision or removal of integrated single device neurostimulation system including electrode array and receiver or pulse generator, including analysis, programming, and imaging guidance when performed, posterior tibial nerve

INCLUDES Electronic analysis (95970-95972, 0589T-0590T)

EXCLUDES *Initial insertion or replacement integrated neurostimulation system (0587T)*
Insertion other neurostimulator devices (64555, 64566, 64575, 64590)

0.00 0.00 FUD YYY R2 80

0589T Electronic analysis with simple programming of implanted integrated neurostimulation system (eg, electrode array and receiver), including contact group(s), amplitude, pulse width, frequency (Hz), on/off cycling, burst, dose lockout, patient-selectable parameters, responsive neurostimulation, detection algorithms, closed-loop parameters, and passive parameters, when performed by physician or other qualified health care professional, posterior tibial nerve, 1-3 parameters

EXCLUDES *Electronic analysis other implanted neurostimulators (95970-95977, [95983, 95984])*
Electronic analysis with complex programming (0590T)
Reporting code during insertion, replacement, revision, or removal integrated neurostimulation system (0587T-0588T)
Reporting code during insertion, replacement, revision, or removal other neurostimulator device (generator and/or electrode) (43647-43648, 43881-43882, 61850-61888, 63650, 63655, 63661-63688, 64553-64595)

0.00 0.00 FUD YYY 80

0590T Electronic analysis with complex programming of implanted integrated neurostimulation system (eg, electrode array and receiver), including contact group(s), amplitude, pulse width, frequency (Hz), on/off cycling, burst, dose lockout, patient-selectable parameters, responsive neurostimulation, detection algorithms, closed-loop parameters, and passive parameters, when performed by physician or other qualified health care professional, posterior tibial nerve, 4 or more parameters

EXCLUDES *Electronic analysis other implanted neurostimulators (95970-95977, [95983, 95984])*
Electronic analysis with simple programming (0589T)
Reporting code during insertion, replacement, revision, or removal integrated neurostimulation system (0587T-0588T)
Reporting code during insertion, replacement, revision, or removal other neurostimulator device (generator and/or electrode) (43647-43648, 43881-43882, 61850-61888, 63650, 63655, 63661-63688, 64553-64595)

0.00 0.00 FUD YYY 80

0591T-0593T

INCLUDES Nonphysician health care professional coach trained to assist patients in obtaining improved health and well-being goals through:
Accountability
Active learning processes
Self-discovery

0591T Health and well-being coaching face-to-face; individual, initial assessment

EXCLUDES *Health and well-being coaching, follow-up session (0592T)*
Health and well-being coaching, group session (0593T)

0.00 0.00 FUD YYY 80

AMA: 2020,Jul,7

0592T individual, follow-up session, at least 30 minutes

EXCLUDES *Diabetic preventative behavior change program ([0488T])*
Education/training for self-management (98960)
Health and well-being coaching, group session (0593T)
Health and well-being coaching, initial session (0591T)
Health behavior assessment/intervention (96156-96159)
Medical nutrition therapy (97802-97804)

0.00 0.00 FUD YYY 80

AMA: 2020,Jul,7

0593T group (2 or more individuals), at least 30 minutes

EXCLUDES *Diabetic preventative behavior change program (0403T)*
Education/training for self-management (98961-98962)
Group therapy procedure (97150)
Health and well-being coaching, individual (0591T-0592T)
Health behavior assessment/intervention ([96164, 96165])

0.00 0.00 FUD YYY 80

AMA: 2020,Jul,7

0594T

● **0594T Osteotomy, humerus, with insertion of an externally controlled intramedullary lengthening device, including intraoperative imaging, initial and subsequent alignment assessments, computations of adjustment schedules, and management of the intramedullary lengthening device**

EXCLUDES *Application multiplane external fixation device (20696)*
Osteoplasty, humerus (24420)
Osteotomy, humerus (24400-24410)
Revision externally controlled intramedullary lengthening device (24999)
Treatment humeral shaft fracture (24516)

0.00 0.00 FUD YYY J8 80

Category III Codes

0596T — 0615T

0596T-0597T

EXCLUDES *Bladder irrigation (51700)*
Change cystostomy tube (51705)
Injection retrograde urethrocystography (51610)
Insertion bladder catheter (51701-51703)

● **0596T** **Temporary female intraurethral valve-pump (ie, voiding prosthesis); initial insertion, including urethral measurement** ♀
0.00 0.00 FUD YYY P2 80

● **0597T** **replacement** ♀
0.00 0.00 FUD YYY P2 80

0598T-0599T

● **0598T** **Noncontact real-time fluorescence wound imaging, for bacterial presence, location, and load, per session; first anatomic site (eg, lower extremity)**
0.00 0.00 FUD YYY Z2 80

● + **0599T** **each additional anatomic site (eg, upper extremity) (List separately in addition to code for primary procedure)**
Code first (0598T)
0.00 0.00 FUD YYY N1 80

0600T-0601T

● **0600T** **Ablation, irreversible electroporation; 1 or more tumors per organ, including imaging guidance, when performed, percutaneous**
INCLUDES Radiological guidance (76940, 77002, 77013, 77022)
0.00 0.00 FUD YYY J8 80

● **0601T** **1 or more tumors, including fluoroscopic and ultrasound guidance, when performed, open**
INCLUDES Fluoroscopic guidance (76940)
Ultrasound guidance (77002)
0.00 0.00 FUD YYY J8 80

0602T-0603T

● **0602T** **Glomerular filtration rate (GFR) measurement(s), transdermal, including sensor placement and administration of a single dose of fluorescent pyrazine agent**
EXCLUDES *Glomerular filtration rate (GFR) monitoring (0603T)*
0.00 0.00 FUD YYY 80

● **0603T** **Glomerular filtration rate (GFR) monitoring, transdermal, including sensor placement and administration of more than one dose of fluorescent pyrazine agent, each 24 hours**
EXCLUDES *Glomerular filtration rate (GFR) measurement(s) (0602T)*
0.00 0.00 FUD YYY 80

0604T-0606T

EXCLUDES *Remote physiologic monitoring treament management services ([99457], [99458])*

● **0604T** **Optical coherence tomography (OCT) of retina, remote, patient-initiated image capture and transmission to a remote surveillance center unilateral or bilateral; initial device provision, set-up and patient education on use of equipment**
0.00 0.00 FUD YYY 80

● **0605T** **remote surveillance center technical support, data analyses and reports, with a minimum of 8 daily recordings, each 30 days**
0.00 0.00 FUD YYY 80

● **0606T** **review, interpretation and report by the prescribing physician or other qualified health care professional of remote surveillance center data analyses, each 30 days**
0.00 0.00 FUD YYY 80

0607T-0608T

EXCLUDES *During same monitoring period:*
Cardiac event monitor (93268-93272)
External mobile cardiovascular telemetry (93228-93229)
Holter monitor procedures (93224-93227)
Interrogation cardiovasular physiologic monitoring system (93297)
Remote monitoring pulmonary artery pressure sensor ([93264])

● **0607T** **Remote monitoring of an external continuous pulmonary fluid monitoring system, including measurement of radiofrequency-derived pulmonary fluid levels, heart rate, respiration rate, activity, posture, and cardiovascular rhythm (eg, ECG data), transmitted to a remote 24-hour attended surveillance center; set-up and patient education on use of equipment**
EXCLUDES *Remote monitoring physiologic parameters, initial during same monitoring period ([99453])*
0.00 0.00 FUD YYY 80

● **0608T** **analysis of data received and transmission of reports to the physician or other qualified health care professional**
EXCLUDES *Remote monitoring physiologic parameters, each 30 days, during same monitoring period ([99454])*
Reporting more than once per 30 days
0.00 0.00 FUD YYY 80

0609T-0612T

EXCLUDES *Magnetic resonance angiography, spine (72159)*
Magnetic resonance imaging, spine (72141-72158)
Other magnetic spectroscopy (76390)

● **0609T** **Magnetic resonance spectroscopy, determination and localization of discogenic pain (cervical, thoracic, or lumbar); acquisition of single voxel data, per disc, on biomarkers (ie, lactic acid, carbohydrate, alanine, laal, propionic acid, proteoglycan, and collagen) in at least 3 discs**
0.00 0.00 FUD YYY 80

● **0610T** **transmission of biomarker data for software analysis**
0.00 0.00 FUD YYY 80

● **0611T** **postprocessing for algorithmic analysis of biomarker data for determination of relative chemical differences between discs**
0.00 0.00 FUD YYY 80

● **0612T** **interpretation and report**
0.00 0.00 FUD YYY 80

0613T

EXCLUDES *Heart catheterization (93451-93453, 93456-93462)*
Heart catheterization for congenital defect(s) (93530-93533)
Intracardiac echocardiography (93662)
Transcatheter/transvenous procedures atrial septectomy/septostomy (33741-33746)
Transesophageal echocardiography procedures (93313-93314, 93318, 93355)
Ultrasound guidance (76937)

● **0613T** **Percutaneous transcatheter implantation of interatrial septal shunt device, including right and left heart catheterization, intracardiac echocardiography, and imaging guidance by the proceduralist, when performed**
0.00 0.00 FUD YYY 80

0614T-0615T [0614T]

0614T **Resequenced code. See code following code 0580T.**

● **0615T** **Eye-movement analysis without spatial calibration, with interpretation and report**
EXCLUDES *Vestibular function tests (92540-92542, 92544-92547)*
0.00 0.00 FUD YYY 80

0616T-0618T

EXCLUDES *Iridectomy (66600)*
Repair/suture iris (66680, 66682)

● 0616T **Insertion of iris prosthesis, including suture fixation and repair or removal of iris, when performed; without removal of crystalline lens or intraocular lens, without insertion of intraocular lens**
0.00 0.00 FUD YYY J8 80

● 0617T **with removal of crystalline lens and insertion of intraocular lens**
EXCLUDES *Cataract extraction/removal:*
Extracapsular (66982, 66984)
Intracapsular (66983)
0.00 0.00 FUD YYY J8 80

● 0618T **with secondary intraocular lens placement or intraocular lens exchange**
EXCLUDES *Intraocular lens:*
Exchange (66986)
Insertion, secondary implant (66985)
0.00 0.00 FUD YYY J8 80

0619T

INCLUDES Cystourethroscopy (separate procedure) (52000)
EXCLUDES *Cystourethroscopy:*
with insertion transprostatic implant (52441-52442)
with mechanical dilation/drug delivery (0499T)
Laser:
Coagulation (52647)
Enucleation (52649)
Vaporization (52648)
Prostate, transurethral:
Destruction (53850-53854)
Incision (52450)
Resection (52500, 52601, 52630, 52640)
Transrectal ultrasound (76872)

● 0619T **Cystourethroscopy with transurethral anterior prostate commissurotomy and drug delivery, including transrectal ultrasound and fluoroscopy, when performed** ♂
0.00 0.00 FUD YYY J8 80

0620T-0622T [0620T]

0620T **Resequenced code. See code following 0505T.**

● 0621T **Trabeculostomy ab interno by laser**
EXCLUDES *Gonioscopy (92020)*

● 0622T **with use of ophthalmic endoscope**
EXCLUDES *Gonioscopy (92020)*

0623T-0626T [0623T, 0624T, 0625T, 0626T]

0623T **Resequenced code. See code following 0504T.**
0624T **Resequenced code. See code following 0504T.**
0625T **Resequenced code. See code following 0504T.**
0626T **Resequenced code. See code following 0504T.**

0627T-0630T

● 0627T **Percutaneous injection of allogeneic cellular and/or tissue-based product, intervertebral disc, unilateral or bilateral injection, with fluoroscopic guidance, lumbar; first level**
INCLUDES Fluoroscopic guidance (77003)

● + 0628T **each additional level (List separately in addition to code for primary procedure)**
EXCLUDES *Fluoroscopic guidance (77003)*
Code first (0627T)
0.00 0.00 FUD 000

● 0629T **Percutaneous injection of allogeneic cellular and/or tissue-based product, intervertebral disc, unilateral or bilateral injection, with CT guidance, lumbar; first level**
INCLUDES CT guidance (77012)

● + 0630T **each additional level (List separately in addition to code for primary procedure)**
INCLUDES CT guidance (77012)
Code first (0629T)
0.00 0.00 FUD 000

0631T

EXCLUDES *Pulse oximetry (94760-94762)*
Transcutaneous biomarker measurement (0061U)

● 0631T **Transcutaneous visible light hyperspectral imaging measurement of oxyhemoglobin, deoxyhemoglobin, and tissue oxygenation, with interpretation and report, per extremity**

0632T

● 0632T **Percutaneous transcatheter ultrasound ablation of nerves innervating the pulmonary arteries, including right heart catheterization, pulmonary artery angiography, and all imaging guidance**
INCLUDES Heart catheterization (93451, 93453, 93456, 93460)
Pulmonary artery angiography/injection (75741, 75743, 75746, 93568)
Pulmonary artery catheterization (36013-36015)
Swan-Ganz catheter insertion (93503)
EXCLUDES *Endomyocardial biopsy (93505)*

0633T-0638T

INCLUDES 3D rendering (76376-76377)
EXCLUDES *Diagnostic/interventional CT (76497)*
Limited/localized follow-up CT (76380)

● 0633T **Computed tomography, breast, including 3D rendering, when performed, unilateral; without contrast material**
● 0634T **with contrast material(s)**
● 0635T **without contrast, followed by contrast material(s)**
● 0636T **Computed tomography, breast, including 3D rendering, when performed, bilateral; without contrast material(s)**
● 0637T **with contrast material(s)**
● 0638T **without contrast, followed by contrast material(s)**

0639T

EXCLUDES *Ultrasound guidance (76998-76999)*

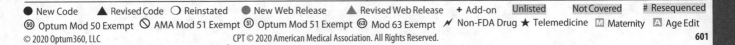

● 0639T **Wireless skin sensor thermal anisotropy measurement(s) and assessment of flow in cerebrospinal fluid shunt, including ultrasound guidance, when performed**

Appendix A — Modifiers

CPT Modifiers

A modifier is a two-position alpha or numeric code appended to a CPT® code to clarify the services being billed. Modifiers provide a means by which a service can be altered without changing the procedure code. They add more information, such as the anatomical site, to the code. In addition, they help to eliminate the appearance of duplicate billing and unbundling. Modifiers are used to increase accuracy in reimbursement, coding consistency, editing, and to capture payment data.

22 **Increased Procedural Services:** When the work required to provide a service is substantially greater than typically required, it may be identified by adding modifier 22 to the usual procedure code. Documentation must support the substantial additional work and the reason for the additional work (ie, increased intensity, time, technical difficulty of procedure, severity of patient's condition, physical and mental effort required).
Note: This modifier should not be appended to an E/M service.

23 **Unusual Anesthesia:** Occasionally, a procedure, which usually requires either no anesthesia or local anesthesia, because of unusual circumstances must be done under general anesthesia. This circumstance may be reported by adding modifier 23 to the procedure code of the basic service.

24 **Unrelated Evaluation and Management Service by the Same Physician or Other Qualified Health Care Professional During a Postoperative Period:** The physician or other qualified health care professional may need to indicate that an evaluation and management service was performed during a postoperative period for a reason(s) unrelated to the original procedure. This circumstance may be reported by adding modifier 24 to the appropriate level of E/M service.

25 **Significant, Separately Identifiable Evaluation and Management Service by the Same Physician or Other Qualified Health Care Professional on the Same Day of the Procedure or Other Service:** It may be necessary to indicate that on the day a procedure or service identified by a CPT code was performed, the patient's condition required a significant, separately identifiable E/M service above and beyond the other service provided or beyond the usual preoperative and postoperative care associated with the procedure that was performed. A significant, separately identifiable E/M service is defined or substantiated by documentation that satisfies the relevant criteria for the respective E/M service to be reported (see Evaluation and Management Services Guidelines for instructions on determining level of E/M service). The E/M service may be prompted by the symptom or condition for which the procedure and/or service was provided. As such, different diagnoses are not required for reporting of the E/M services on the same date. This circumstance may be reported by adding modifier 25 to the appropriate level of E/M service.
Note: This modifier is not used to report an E/M service that resulted in a decision to perform surgery. See modifier 57. For significant, separately identifiable non-E/M services, see modifier 59.

26 **Professional Component:** Certain procedures are a combination of a physician or other qualified health care professional component and a technical component. When the physician or other qualified health care professional component is reported separately, the service may be identified by adding modifier 26 to the usual procedure number.

32 **Mandated Services:** Services related to *mandated* consultation and/or related services (eg, third party payer, governmental, legislative or regulatory requirement) may be identified by adding modifier 32 to the basic procedure.

33 **Preventive Services:** When the primary purpose of the service is the delivery of an evidence based service in accordance with a US Preventive Services Task Force A or B rating in effect and other preventive services identified in preventive services mandates (legislative or regulatory), the service may be identified by adding 33 to the procedure. For separately reported services specifically identified as preventive, the modifier should not be used.

47 **Anesthesia by Surgeon:** Regional or general anesthesia provided by the surgeon may be reported by adding modifier 47 to the basic service. (This does not include local anesthesia.)
Note: Modifier 47 would not be used as a modifier for the anesthesia procedures.

50 **Bilateral Procedure:** Unless otherwise identified in the listings, bilateral procedures that are performed at the same session should be identified by adding modifier 50 to the appropriate 5 digit code.
Note: This modifier should not be appended to designated "add-on" codes (see Appendix F).

51 **Multiple Procedures:** When multiple procedures, other than E/M services, Physical Medicine and Rehabilitation services or provision of supplies (eg, vaccines), are performed at the same session by the same individual, the primary procedure or service may be reported as listed. The additional procedure(s) or service(s) may be identified by appending modifier 51 to the additional procedure or service code(s).
Note: This modifier should not be appended to designated "add-on" codes (see Appendix F).

52 **Reduced Services:** Under certain circumstances a service or procedure is partially reduced or eliminated at the discretion of the physician or other qualified health care professional. Under these circumstances the service provided can be identified by its usual procedure number and the addition of modifier 52, signifying that the service is reduced. This provides a means of reporting reduced services without disturbing the identification of the basic service.
Note: For hospital outpatient reporting of a previously scheduled procedure/service that is partially reduced or cancelled as a result of extenuating circumstances or those that threaten the well-being of the patient prior to or after administration of anesthesia, see modifiers 73 and 74 (see modifiers approved for ASC hospital outpatient use).

53 **Discontinued Procedure:** Under certain circumstances, the physician or other qualified health care professional may elect to terminate a surgical or diagnostic procedure. Due to extenuating circumstances or those that threaten the well being of the patient, it may be necessary to indicate that a surgical or diagnostic procedure was started but discontinued. This circumstance may be reported by adding modifier 53 to the code reported by the physician for the discontinued procedure.
Note: This modifier is not used to report the elective cancellation of a procedure prior to the patient's anesthesia induction and/or surgical preparation in the operating suite. For outpatient hospital/ambulatory surgery center (ASC) reporting of a previously scheduled procedure/service that is partially reduced or cancelled as a result of extenuating circumstances or those that threaten the well being of the patient prior to or after administration of anesthesia, see modifiers 73 and 74 (see modifiers approved for ASC hospital outpatient use).

54 **Surgical Care Only:** When 1 physician or other qualified health care professional performs a surgical procedure and another provides preoperative and/or postoperative management, surgical services may be identified by adding modifier 54 to the usual procedure number.

55 **Postoperative Management Only:** When 1 physician or other qualified health care professional performed the postoperative management and another performed the surgical procedure, the postoperative component may be identified by adding modifier 55 to the usual procedure number.

56 **Preoperative Management Only:** When 1 physician or other qualified health care professional performed the preoperative care and evaluation and another performed the surgical procedure, the preoperative component may be identified by adding modifier 56 to the usual procedure number.

57 **Decision for Surgery:** An evaluation and management service that resulted in the initial decision to perform the surgery may be identified by adding modifier 57 to the appropriate level of E/M service.

58 Staged or Related Procedure or Service by the Same Physician or Other Qualified Health Care Professional During the Postoperative Period: It may be necessary to indicate that the performance of a procedure or service during the postoperative period was (a) planned or anticipated (staged); (b) more extensive than the original procedure; or (c) for therapy following a surgical procedure. This circumstance may be reported by adding modifier 58 to the staged or related procedure.
Note: For treatment of a problem that requires a return to the operating/procedure room (eg, unanticipated clinical condition), see modifier 78.

59 Distinct Procedural Service: Under certain circumstances, it may be necessary to indicate that a procedure or service was distinct or independent from other non-E/M services performed on the same day. Modifier 59 is used to identify procedures/services, other than E/M services, that are not normally reported together but are appropriate under the circumstances. Documentation must support a different session, different procedure or surgery, different site or organ system, separate incision/excision, separate lesion, or separate injury (or area of injury in extensive injuries) not ordinarily encountered or performed on the same day by the same individual. However, when another already established modifier is appropriate it should be used rather than modifier 59. Only if no more descriptive modifier is available, and the use of modifier 59 best explains the circumstances, should modifier 59 be used.
Note: Modifier 59 should not be appended to an E/M service. To report a separate and distinct E/M service with a non-E/M service performed on the same date, see modifier 25.

62 Two Surgeons: When 2 surgeons work together as primary surgeons performing distinct part(s) of a procedure, each surgeon should report his/her distinct operative work by adding modifier 62 to the procedure code and any associated add-on code(s) for that procedure as long as both surgeons continue to work together as primary surgeons. Each surgeon should report the co-surgery once using the same procedure code. If additional procedure(s) (including add-on procedure[s]) are performed during the same surgical session, separate code(s) may also be reported with modifier 62 added.
Note: If a co-surgeon acts as an assistant in the performance of additional procedure(s), other than those reported with the modifier 62, during the same surgical session, those services may be reported using separate procedure code(s) with modifier 80 or modifier 82 added, as appropriate.

63 Procedure Performed on Infants less than 4 kg: Procedures performed on neonates and infants up to a present body weight of 4 kg may involve significantly increased complexity and physician or other qualified health care professional work commonly associated with these patients. This circumstance may be reported by adding modifier 63 to the procedure number.
Note: Unless otherwise designated, this modifier may only be appended to procedures/services listed in the 20100-69990 code series and 92920, 92928, 92953, 92960, 92986, 92987, 92990, 92997, 92998, 93312, 93313, 93314, 93315, 93316, 93317, 93318, 93452, 93505, 93530, 93531, 93532, 93533, 93561, 93562, 93563, 93564, 93568, 93580, 93582, 93590, 93591, 93592, 93615, 93616 from the Medicine/Cardiovascular section.

Modifier 63 should not be appended to any CPT codes listed in the Evaluation and Management Services, Anesthesia, Radiology, Pathology/Laboratory, or Medicine sections (other than those identified above from the Medicine/Cardiovascular section).

66 Surgical Team: Under some circumstances, highly complex procedures (requiring the concomitant services of several physicians or other qualified health care professionals, often of different specialties, plus other highly skilled, specially trained personnel, various types of complex equipment) are carried out under the "surgical team" concept. Such circumstances may be identified by each participating individual with the addition of modifier 66 to the basic procedure number used for reporting services.

76 Repeat Procedure or Service by Same Physician or Other Qualified Health Care Professional: It may be necessary to indicate that a procedure or service was repeated by the same physician or other qualified health care professional subsequent to the original procedure or service. This circumstance may be reported by adding modifier 76 to the repeated procedure or service.
Note: This modifier should not be appended to an E/M service.

77 Repeat Procedure by Another Physician or Other Qualified Health Care Professional: It may be necessary to indicate that a basic procedure or service was repeated by another physician or other qualified health care professional subsequent to the original procedure or service. This circumstance may be reported by adding modifier 77 to the repeated procedure or service.
Note: This modifier should not be appended to an E/M service.

78 Unplanned Return to the Operating/Procedure Room by the Same Physician or Other Qualified Health Care Professional Following Initial Procedure for a Related Procedure During the Postoperative Period: It may be necessary to indicate that another procedure was performed during the postoperative period of the initial procedure (unplanned procedure following initial procedure). When this procedure is related to the first, and requires the use of an operating/procedure room, it may be reported by adding modifier 78 to the related procedure. (For repeat procedures, see modifier 76.)

79 Unrelated Procedure or Service by the Same Physician or Other Qualified Health Care Professional During the Postoperative Period: The individual may need to indicate that the performance of a procedure or service during the postoperative period was unrelated to the original procedure. This circumstance may be reported by using modifier 79. (For repeat procedures on the same day, see modifier 76.)

80 Assistant Surgeon: Surgical assistant services may be identified by adding modifier 80 to the usual procedure number(s).

81 Minimum Assistant Surgeon: Minimum surgical assistant services are identified by adding modifier 81 to the usual procedure number.

82 Assistant Surgeon (when qualified resident surgeon not available): The unavailability of a qualified resident surgeon is a prerequisite for use of modifier 82 appended to the usual procedure code number(s).

90 Reference (Outside) Laboratory: When laboratory procedures are performed by a party other than the treating or reporting physician or other qualified health care professional, the procedure may be identified by adding modifier 90 to the usual procedure number.

91 Repeat Clinical Diagnostic Laboratory Test: In the course of treatment of the patient, it may be necessary to repeat the same laboratory test on the same day to obtain subsequent (multiple) test results. Under these circumstances, the laboratory test performed can be identified by its usual procedure number and the addition of modifier 91.
Note: This modifier may not be used when tests are rerun to confirm initial results; due to testing problems with specimens or equipment; or for any other reason when a normal, one-time, reportable result is all that is required. This modifier may not be used when other code(s) describe a series of test results (eg, glucose tolerance tests, evocative/suppression testing). This modifier may only be used for laboratory test(s) performed more than once on the same day on the same patient.

92 Alternative Laboratory Platform Testing: When laboratory testing is being performed using a kit or transportable instrument that wholly or in part consists of a single use, disposable analytical chamber, the service may be identified by adding modifier 92 to the usual laboratory procedure code (HIV testing 86701-86703, and 87389). The test does not require permanent dedicated space, hence by its design may be hand carried or transported to the vicinity of the patient for immediate testing at that site, although location of the testing is not in itself determinative of the use of this modifier.

95 **Synchronous Telemedicine Service Rendered Via a Real-Time Interactive Audio and Video Telecommunications System:** Synchronous telemedicine service is defined as a **real-time** interaction between a physician or other qualified health care professional and a patient who is located at a distant site from the physician or other qualified health care professional. The totality of the communication of information exchanged between the physician or other qualified health care professional and patient during the course of the synchronous telemedicine service must be of an amount and nature that would be sufficient to meet the key components and/or requirements of the same service when rendered via a face-to-face interaction. Modifier 95 may only be appended to the services listed in Appendix F. Appendix F is the list of CPT codes for services that are typically performed face-to-face, but may be rendered via real-time (synchronous) interactive audio and video telecommunications system.

96 **Habilitative Services:** When a service or procedure that may be either habilitative or rehabilitative in nature is provided for habilitative purposes, the physician or other qualified health care professional may add modifier 96 to the service or procedure code to indicate that the service or procedure provided was a habilitative service. Habilitative services help an individual learn skills and functioning for daily living that the individual has not yet developed, and then keep and/or improve those learned skills. Habilitative services also help an individual keep, learn, or improve skills and functioning for daily living.

97 **Rehabilitative Services:** When a service or procedure that may be either habilitative or rehabilitative in nature is provided for rehabilitative purposes, the physician or other qualified health care professional may add modifier 97 to the service or procedure code to indicate that the service or procedure provided was a rehabilitative service. Rehabilitative services help an individual keep, get back, or improve skills and functioning for daily living that have been lost or impaired because the individual was sick, hurt, or disabled.

99 **Multiple Modifiers:** Under certain circumstances 2 or more modifiers may be necessary to completely delineate a service. In such situations modifier 99 should be added to the basic procedure, and other applicable modifiers may be listed as part of the description of the service.

Anesthesia Physical Status Modifiers

All anesthesia services are reported by use of the five-digit anesthesia procedure code with the appropriate physical status modifier appended.

Under certain circumstances, when other modifier(s) are appropriate, they should be reported in addition to the physical status modifier.

P1 A normal healthy patient

P2 A patient with mild systemic disease

P3 A patient with severe systemic disease

P4 A patient with severe systemic disease that is a constant threat to life

P5 A moribund patient who is not expected to survive without the operation

P6 A declared brain-dead patient whose organs are being removed for donor purposes

Modifiers Approved for Ambulatory Surgery Center (ASC) Hospital Outpatient Use

CPT Level I Modifiers

25 **Significant, Separately Identifiable Evaluation and Management Service by the Same Physician or Other Qualified Health Care Professional on the Same Day of the Procedure or Other Service:** It may be necessary to indicate that on the day a procedure or service identified by a CPT code was performed, the patient's condition required a significant, separately identifiable E/M service above and beyond the other service provided or beyond the usual preoperative and postoperative care associated with the procedure that was performed. A significant, separately identifiable E/M service is defined or substantiated by documentation that satisfies the relevant criteria for the respective E/M service to be reported (see Evaluation and Management Services Guidelines for instructions on determining level of E/M service). The E/M service may be prompted by the symptom or condition for which the procedure and/or service was provided. As such, different diagnoses are not required for reporting of the E/M services on the same date. This circumstance may be reported by adding modifier 25 to the appropriate level of E/M service.
Note: This modifier is not used to report an E/M service that resulted in a decision to perform surgery. See modifier 57. For significant, separately identifiable non-E/M services, see modifier 59.

27 **Multiple Outpatient Hospital E/M Encounters on the Same Date:** For hospital outpatient reporting purposes, utilization of hospital resources related to separate and distinct E/M encounters performed in multiple outpatient hospital settings on the same date may be reported by adding modifier 27 to each appropriate level outpatient and/or emergency department E/M code(s). This modifier provides a means of reporting circumstances involving evaluation and management services provided by a physician(s) in more than one (multiple) outpatient hospital setting(s) (eg, hospital emergency department, clinic).
Note: This modifier is not to be used for physician reporting of multiple E/M services performed by the same physician on the same date. For physician reporting of all outpatient evaluation and management services provided by the same physician on the same date and performed in multiple outpatient settings (eg, hospital emergency department, clinic), see Evaluation and Management, Emergency Department, or Preventive Medicine Services codes.

33 **Preventive Services:** When the primary purpose of the service is the delivery of an evidence based service in accordance with a US Preventive Services Task Force A or B rating in effect and other preventive services identified in preventive services mandates (legislative or regulatory), the service may be identified by adding 33 to the procedure. For separately reported services specifically identified as preventive, the modifier should not be used.

50 **Bilateral Procedure:** Unless otherwise identified in the listings, bilateral procedures that are performed at the same session should be identified by adding modifier 50 to the appropriate 5 digit code.
Note: This modifier should not be appended to designated "add-on" codes (see appendix F).

52 **Reduced Services:** Under certain circumstances a service or procedure is partially reduced or eliminated at the discretion of the physician or other qualified health care professional. Under these circumstances the service provided can be identified by its usual procedure number and the addition of modifier 52, signifying that the service is reduced. This provides a means of reporting reduced services without disturbing the identification of the basic service.
Note: For hospital outpatient reporting of a previously scheduled procedure/service that is partially reduced or cancelled as a result of extenuating circumstances or those that threaten the well-being of the patient prior to or after administration of anesthesia, see modifiers 73 and 74 (see modifiers approved for ASC hospital outpatient use).

58 **Staged or Related Procedure or Service by the Same Physician or Other Qualified Health Care Professional During the Postoperative Period:** It may be necessary to indicate that the performance of a procedure or service during the postoperative period was (a) planned or anticipated (staged); (b) more extensive than the original procedure; or (c) for therapy following a surgical procedure. This circumstance may be reported by adding modifier 58 to the staged or related procedure.
Note: For treatment of a problem that requires a return to the operating or procedure room (eg, unanticipated clinical condition), see modifier 78.

59 **Distinct Procedural Service:** Under certain circumstances, it may be necessary to indicate that a procedure or service was distinct or independent from other non-E/M services performed on the same day. Modifier 59 is used to identify procedures/services, other than E/M services, that are not normally reported together but are appropriate under the circumstances. Documentation must support a different session, different procedure or surgery,

different site or organ system, separate incision/excision, separate lesion, or separate injury (or area of injury in extensive injuries) not ordinarily encountered or performed on the same day by the same individual. However, when another already established modifier is appropriate it should be used rather than modifier 59. Only if no more descriptive modifier is available, and the use of modifier 59 best explains the circumstances, should modifier 59 be used.
Note: Modifier 59 should not be appended to an E/M service. To report a separate and distinct E/M service with a non-E/M service performed on the same date, see modifier 25.

73 **Discontinued Out-Patient Hospital/Ambulatory Surgery Center (ASC) Procedure Prior to the Administration of Anesthesia:** Due to extenuating circumstances or those that threaten the well being of the patient, the physician may cancel a surgical or diagnostic procedure subsequent to the patient's surgical preparation (including sedation when provided, and being taken to the room where the procedure is to be performed), but prior to the administration of anesthesia (local, regional block(s) or general). Under these circumstances, the intended service that is prepared for but cancelled can be reported by its usual procedure number and the addition of modifier 73.
Note: The elective cancellation of a service prior to the administration of anesthesia and/or surgical preparation of the patient should not be reported. For physician reporting of a discontinued procedure, see modifier 53.

74 **Discontinued Out-Patient Hospital/Ambulatory Surgery Center (ASC) Procedure After Administration of Anesthesia:** Due to extenuating circumstances or those that threaten the well being of the patient, the physician may terminate a surgical or diagnostic procedure after the administration of anesthesia (local, regional block(s), general) or after the procedure was started (incision made, intubation started, scope inserted, etc.). Under these circumstances, the procedure started but terminated can be reported by its usual procedure number and the addition of modifier 74.
Note: The elective cancellation of a service prior to the administration of anesthesia and/or surgical preparation of the patient should not be reported. For physician reporting of a discontinued procedure, see modifier 53.

76 **Repeat Procedure or Service by Same Physician or Other Qualified Health Care Professional:** It may be necessary to indicate that a procedure or service was repeated by the same physician or other qualified health care professional subsequent to the original procedure or service. This circumstance may be reported by adding modifier 76 to the repeated procedure or service.
Note: This modifier should not be appended to an E/M service.

77 **Repeat Procedure by Another Physician or Other Qualified Health Care Professional:** It may be necessary to indicate that a basic procedure or service was repeated by another physician or other qualified health care professional subsequent to the original procedure or service. This circumstance may be reported by adding modifier 77 to the repeated procedure or service.
Note: This modifier should not be appended to an E/M service.

78 **Unplanned Return to the Operating/Procedure Room by the Same Physician or Other Qualified Health Care Professional Following Initial Procedure for a Related Procedure During the Postoperative Period:** It may be necessary to indicate that another procedure was performed during the postoperative period of the initial procedure (unplanned procedure following initial procedure). When this procedure is related to the first, and requires the use of an operating/procedure room, it may be reported by adding modifier 78 to the related procedure. (For repeat procedures, see modifier 76.)

79 **Unrelated Procedure or Service by the Same Physician During the Postoperative Period:** The individual may need to indicate that the performance of a procedure or service during the postoperative period was unrelated to the original procedure. This circumstance may be reported by using modifier 79. (For repeat procedures on the same day, see modifier 76.)

91 **Repeat Clinical Diagnostic Laboratory Test:** In the course of treatment of the patient, it may be necessary to repeat the same laboratory test on the same day to obtain subsequent (multiple) test results. Under these circumstances, the laboratory test performed can be identified by its usual procedure number and the addition of modifier 91.
Note: This modifier may not be used when tests are rerun to confirm initial results; due to testing problems with specimens or equipment; or for any other reason when a normal, one-time, reportable result is all that is required. This modifier may not be used when other code(s) describe a series of test results (eg, glucose tolerance tests, evocative/suppression testing). This modifier may only be used for laboratory test(s) performed more than once on the same day on the same patient.

Level II (HCPCS/National) Modifiers

The HCPCS Level II modifiers included here are those most commonly used when coding procedures. See your 2021 HCPCS Level II book for a complete listing.

Anatomical Modifiers

E1 Upper left, eyelid
E2 Lower left, eyelid
E3 Upper right, eyelid
E4 Lower right, eyelid
FA Left hand, thumb
F1 Left hand, second digit
F2 Left hand, third digit
F3 Left hand, fourth digit
F4 Left hand, fifth digit
F5 Right hand, thumb
F6 Right hand, second digit
F7 Right hand, third digit
F8 Right hand, fourth digit
F9 Right hand, fifth digit
LT Left side (used to identify procedures performed on the left side of the body)
RT Right side (used to identify procedures performed on the right side of the body)
TA Left foot, great toe
T1 Left foot, second digit
T2 Left foot, third digit
T3 Left foot, fourth digit
T4 Left foot, fifth digit
T5 Right foot, great toe
T6 Right foot, second digit
T7 Right foot, third digit
T8 Right foot, fourth digit
T9 Right foot, fifth digit

Anesthesia Modifiers

AA Anesthesia services performed personally by anesthesiologist
AD Medical supervision by a physician: more than four concurrent anesthesia procedures
G8 Monitored anesthesia care (MAC) for deep complex, complicated, or markedly invasive surgical procedure
G9 Monitored anesthesia care for patient who has history of severe cardiopulmonary condition
QK Medical direction of two, three, or four concurrent anesthesia procedures involving qualified individuals
QS Monitored anesthesiology care service
QX CRNA service: with medical direction by a physician
QY Medical direction of one certified registered nurse anesthetist (CRNA) by an anesthesiologist
QZ CRNA service: without medical direction by a physician

Coronary Artery Modifiers

LC Left circumflex coronary artery

LD Left anterior descending coronary artery

LM Left main coronary artery

RC Right coronary artery

RI Ramus intermedius coronary artery

Other Modifiers

CT Computed tomography services furnished using equipment that does not meet each of the attributes of the national electrical manufacturers association (NEMA) XR-29-2013 standard

EA Erythropoetic stimulating agent (ESA) administered to treat anemia due to anticancer chemotherapy

EB Erythropoetic stimulating agent (ESA) administered to treat anemia due to anticancer radiotherapy

EC Erythropoetic stimulating agent (ESA) administered to treat anemia not due to anticancer radiotherapy or anticancer chemotherapy

FP Service provided as part of family planning program

FX X-ray taken using film

G7 Pregnancy resulted from rape or incest or pregnancy certified by physician as life threatening

GA Waiver of liability statement issued as required by payer policy, individual case

GG Performance and payment of a screening mammogram and diagnostic mammogram on the same patient, same day

GH Diagnostic mammogram converted from screening mammogram on same day

GQ Via asynchronous telecommunications system

GT Via interactive audio and video telecommunication systems

GU Waiver of liability statement issued as required by payer policy, routine notice

GX Notice of liability issued, voluntary under payer policy

GY Item or service statutorily excluded, does not meet the definition of any Medicare benefit or, for non-Medicare insurers, is not a contract benefit

GZ Item or service expected to be denied as not reasonable and necessary

PI Positron emission tomography (PET) or PET/computed tomography (CT) to inform the initial treatment strategy of tumors that are biopsy proven or strongly suspected of being cancerous based on other diagnostic testing

PS Positron emission tomography (PET) or PET/computed tomography (CT) to inform the subsequent treatment strategy of cancerous tumors when the beneficiary's treating physician determines that the PET study is needed to inform subsequent antitumor strategy

PT Colorectal cancer screening test; converted to diagnostic test or other procedure

Q7 One Class A finding

Q8 Two Class B findings

Q9 One Class B and two Class C findings

QC Single channel monitoring

QM Ambulance service provided under arrangement by a provider of services

QN Ambulance service furnished directly by a provider of services

QW CLIA waived test

TC Technical component; under certain circumstances, a charge may be made for the technical component alone; under those circumstances the technical component charge is identified by adding modifier TC to the usual procedure number; technical component charges are institutional charges and not billed separately by physicians; however, portable x-ray suppliers only bill for technical component and should utilize modifier TC; the charge data from portable x-ray suppliers will then be used to build customary and prevailing profiles

* **XE** Separate encounter, a service that is distinct because it occurred during a separate encounter

* **XP** Separate practitioner, a service that is distinct because it was performed by a different practitioner

* **XS** Separate structure, a service that is distinct because it was performed on a separate organ/structure

* **XU** Unusual nonoverlapping service, the use of a service that is distinct because it does not overlap usual components of the main service

* CMS instituted additional HCPCS modifiers to define explicit subsets of modifier 59 Distinct Procedural Service.

Category II Modifiers

1P Performance Measure Exclusion Modifier due to Medical Reasons

Reasons include:

- Not indicated (absence of organ/limb, already received/performed, other)
- Contraindicated (patient allergic history, potential adverse drug interaction, other)
- Other medical reasons

2P Performance Measure Exclusion Modifier due to Patient Reasons

Reasons include:

- Patient declined
- Economic, social, or religious reasons
- Other patient reasons

3P Performance Measure Exclusion Modifier due to System Reasons

Reasons include:

- Resources to perform the services not available
- Insurance coverage/payor-related limitations
- Other reasons attributable to health care delivery system

Modifier 8P is intended to be used as a "reporting modifier" to allow the reporting of circumstances when an action described in a measure's numerator is not performed and the reason is not otherwise specified.

8P Performance measure reporting modifier-action not performed, reason not otherwise specified

Appendix B — New, Revised, and Deleted Codes

New Codes

30468 Repair of nasal valve collapse with subcutaneous/submucosal lateral wall implant(s)

32408 Core needle biopsy, lung or mediastinum, percutaneous, including imaging guidance, when performed

33741 Transcatheter atrial septostomy (TAS) for congenital cardiac anomalies to create effective atrial flow, including all imaging guidance by the proceduralist, when performed, any method (eg, Rashkind, Sang-Park, balloon, cutting balloon, blade)

33745 Transcatheter intracardiac shunt (TIS) creation by stent placement for congenital cardiac anomalies to establish effective intracardiac flow, including all imaging guidance by the proceduralist, when performed, left and right heart diagnostic cardiac catherization for congenital cardiac anomalies, and target zone angioplasty, when performed (eg, atrial septum, Fontan fenestration, right ventricular outflow tract, Mustard/Senning/Warden baffles); initial intracardiac shunt

33746 each additional intracardiac shunt location (List separately in addition to code for primary procedure)

33995 Insertion of ventricular assist device, percutaneous, including radiological supervision and interpretation; right heart, venous access only

33997 Removal of percutaneous right heart ventricular assist device, venous cannula, at separate and distinct session from insertion

55880 Ablation of malignant prostate tissue, transrectal, with high intensity–focused ultrasound (HIFU), including ultrasound guidance

57465 Computer-aided mapping of cervix uteri during colposcopy, including optical dynamic spectral imaging and algorithmic quantification of the acetowhitening effect (List separately in addition to code for primary procedure)

69705 Nasopharyngoscopy, surgical, with dilation of eustachian tube (ie, balloon dilation); unilateral

69706 bilateral

71271 Computed tomography, thorax, low dose for lung cancer screening, without contrast material(s)

76145 Medical physics dose evaluation for radiation exposure that exceeds institutional review threshold, including report

80143 Acetaminophen

80151 Amiodarone

80161 -10,11-epoxide

80167 Felbamate

80179 Salicylate

80181 Flecainide

80189 Itraconazole

80193 Leflunomide

80204 Methotrexate

80210 Rufinamide

81168 CCND1/IGH (t(11;14)) (eg, mantle cell lymphoma) translocation analysis, major breakpoint, qualitative and quantitative, if performed

81191 NTRK1 (neurotrophic receptor tyrosine kinase 1) (eg, solid tumors) translocation analysis

81192 NTRK2 (neurotrophic receptor tyrosine kinase 2) (eg, solid tumors) translocation analysis

81193 NTRK3 (neurotrophic receptor tyrosine kinase 3) (eg, solid tumors) translocation analysis

81194 NTRK (neurotrophic-tropomyosin receptor tyrosine kinase 1, 2, and 3) (eg, solid tumors) translocation analysis

81278 IGH@/BCL2 (t(14;18)) (eg, follicular lymphoma) translocation analysis, major breakpoint region (MBR) and minor cluster region (mcr) breakpoints, qualitative or quantitative

81279 JAK2 (Janus kinase 2) (eg, myeloproliferative disorder) targeted sequence analysis (eg, exons 12 and 13)

81338 MPL (MPL proto-oncogene, thrombopoietin receptor) (eg, myeloproliferative disorder) gene analysis; common variants (eg, W515A, W515K, W515L, W515R)

81339 sequence analysis, exon 10

81347 SF3B1 (splicing factor [3b] subunit B1) (eg, myelodysplastic syndrome/acute myeloid leukemia) gene analysis, common variants (eg, A672T, E622D, L833F, R625C, R625L)

81348 SRSF2 (serine and arginine-rich splicing factor 2) (eg, myelodysplastic syndrome, acute myeloid leukemia) gene analysis, common variants (eg, P95H, P95L)

81351 TP53 (tumor protein 53) (eg, Li-Fraumeni syndrome) gene analysis; full gene sequence

81352 targeted sequence analysis (eg, 4 oncology)

81353 known familial variant

81357 U2AF1 (U2 small nuclear RNA auxiliary factor 1) (eg, myelodysplastic syndrome, acute myeloid leukemia) gene analysis, common variants (eg, S34F, S34Y, Q157R, Q157P)

81360 ZRSR2 (zinc finger CCCH-type, RNA binding motif and serine/arginine-rich 2) (eg, myelodysplastic syndrome, acute myeloid leukemia) gene analysis, common variant(s) (eg, E65fs, E122fs, R448fs)

81419 Epilepsy genomic sequence analysis panel, must include analyses for ALDH7A1, CACNA1A, CDKL5, CHD2, GABRG2, GRIN2A, KCNQ2, MECP2, PCDH19, POLG, PRRT2, SCN1A, SCN1B, SCN2A, SCN8A, SLC2A1, SLC9A6, STXBP1, SYNGAP1, TCF4, TPP1, TSC1, TSC2, and ZEB2

81513 Infectious disease, bacterial vaginosis, quantitative real-time amplification of RNA markers for Atopobium vaginae, Gardnerella vaginalis, and Lactobacillus species, utilizing vaginal-fluid specimens, algorithm reported as a positive or negative result for bacterial vaginosis

81514 Infectious disease, bacterial vaginosis and vaginitis, quantitative real-time amplification of DNA markers for Gardnerella vaginalis, Atopobium vaginae, Megasphaera type 1, Bacterial Vaginosis Associated Bacteria-2 (BVAB-2), and Lactobacillus species (L. crispatus and L. jensenii), utilizing vaginal-fluid specimens, algorithm reported as a positive or negative for high likelihood of bacterial vaginosis, includes separate detection of Trichomonas vaginalis and/or Candida species (C. albicans, C. tropicalis, C. parapsilosis, C. dubliniensis), Candida glabrata, Candida krusei, when reported

81529 Oncology (cutaneous melanoma), mRNA, gene expression profiling by real-time RT-PCR of 31 genes (28 content and 3 housekeeping), utilizing formalin-fixed paraffin-embedded tissue, algorithm reported as recurrence risk, including likelihood of sentinel lymph node metastasis

81546 Oncology (thyroid), mRNA, gene expression analysis of 10,196 genes, utilizing fine needle aspirate, algorithm reported as a categorical result (eg, benign or suspicious)

81554 Pulmonary disease (idiopathic pulmonary fibrosis [IPF]), mRNA, gene expression analysis of 190 genes, utilizing transbronchial biopsies, diagnostic algorithm reported as categorical result (eg, positive or negative for high probability of usual interstitial pneumonia [UIP])

82077 Alcohol (ethanol); any specimen except urine and breath, immunoassay (eg, IA, EIA, ELISA, RIA, EMIT, FPIA) and enzymatic methods (eg, alcohol dehydrogenase)

82681 Estradiol; free, direct measurement (eg, equilibrium dialysis)

86328 Immunoassay for infectious agent antibody(ies), qualitative or semiquantitative, single-step method (eg, reagent strip); severe acute respiratory syndrome coronavirus 2 (SARS-CoV-2) (Coronavirus disease [COVID-19])

86769 Antibody; severe acute respiratory syndrome coronavirus 2 (SARS-CoV-2) (Coronavirus disease [COVID-19])

87635 Infectious agent detection by nucleic acid (DNA or RNA); severe acute respiratory syndrome coronavirus 2 (SARS-CoV-2) (Coronavirus disease [COVID-19]), amplified probe technique

90377 Rabies immune globulin, heat- and solvent/detergent-treated (RIg-HT S/D), human, for intramuscular and/or subcutaneous use

92229 Imaging of retina for detection or monitoring of disease; point-of-care automated analysis and report, unilateral or bilateral

92517 Vestibular evoked myogenic potential (VEMP) testing, with interpretation and report; cervical (cVEMP)

92518 ocular (oVEMP)

92519 cervical (cVEMP) and ocular (oVEMP)

92650 Auditory evoked potentials; screening of auditory potential with broadband stimuli, automated analysis

92651 for hearing status determination, broadband stimuli, with interpretation and report

92652 for threshold estimation at multiple frequencies, with interpretation and report

92653 neurodiagnostic, with interpretation and report

93241 External electrocardiographic recording for more than 48 hours up to 7 days by continuous rhythm recording and storage; includes recording, scanning analysis with report, review and interpretation

93242 recording (includes connection and initial recording)

93243 scanning analysis with report

93244 review and interpretation

93245 External electrocardiographic recording for more than 7 days up to 15 days by continuous rhythm recording and storage; includes recording, scanning analysis with report, review and interpretation

93246 recording (includes connection and initial recording)

93247 scanning analysis with report

93248 review and interpretation

94619 Exercise test for bronchospasm, including pre- and post-spirometry and pulse oximetry; without electrocardiographic recording(s)

99417 Prolonged office or other outpatient evaluation and management service(s) beyond the minimum required time of the primary procedure which has been selected using total time, requiring total time with or without direct patient contact beyond the usual service, on the date of the primary service, each 15 minutes of total time (List separately in addition to codes 99205, 99215 for office or other outpatient Evaluation and Management services)

99439 Chronic care management services with the following required elements: multiple (two or more) chronic conditions expected to last at least 12 months, or until the death of the patient, chronic conditions place the patient at significant risk of death, acute exacerbation/decompensation, or functional decline, comprehensive care plan established, implemented, revised, or monitored; each additional 20 minutes of clinical staff time directed by a physician or other qualified health care professional, per calendar month (List separately in addition to code for primary procedure)

0139U Neurology (autism spectrum disorder [ASD]), quantitative measurements of 6 central carbon metabolites (ie, α-ketoglutarate, alanine, lactate, phenylalanine, pyruvate, and succinate), LC-MS/MS, plasma, algorithmic analysis with result reported as negative or positive (with metabolic subtypes of ASD)

0140U Infectious disease (fungi), fungal pathogen identification, DNA (15 fungal targets), blood culture, amplified probe technique, each target reported as detected or not detected

0141U Infectious disease (bacteria and fungi), gram-positive organism identification and drug resistance element detection, DNA (20 gram-positive bacterial targets, 4 resistance genes, 1 pan gram-negative bacterial target, 1 pan Candida target), blood culture, amplified probe technique, each target reported as detected or not detected

0142U Infectious disease (bacteria and fungi), gram-negative bacterial identification and drug resistance element detection, DNA (21 gram-negative bacterial targets, 6 resistance genes, 1 pan gram-positive bacterial target, 1 pan Candida target), amplified probe technique, each target reported as detected or not detected

0143U Drug assay, definitive, 120 or more drugs or metabolites, urine, quantitative liquid chromatography with tandem mass spectrometry (LC-MS/MS) using multiple reaction monitoring (MRM), with drug or metabolite description, comments including sample validation, per date of service

0144U Drug assay, definitive, 160 or more drugs or metabolites, urine, quantitative liquid chromatography with tandem mass spectrometry (LC-MS/MS) using multiple reaction monitoring (MRM), with drug or metabolite description, comments including sample validation, per date of service

0145U Drug assay, definitive, 65 or more drugs or metabolites, urine, quantitative liquid chromatography with tandem mass spectrometry (LC-MS/MS) using multiple reaction monitoring (MRM), with drug or metabolite description, comments including sample validation, per date of service

0146U Drug assay, definitive, 80 or more drugs or metabolites, urine, by quantitative liquid chromatography with tandem mass spectrometry (LC-MS/MS) using multiple reaction monitoring (MRM), with drug or metabolite description, comments including sample validation, per date of service

0147U Drug assay, definitive, 85 or more drugs or metabolites, urine, quantitative liquid chromatography with tandem mass spectrometry (LC-MS/MS) using multiple reaction monitoring (MRM), with drug or metabolite description, comments including sample validation, per date of service

0148U Drug assay, definitive, 100 or more drugs or metabolites, urine, quantitative liquid chromatography with tandem mass spectrometry (LC-MS/MS) using multiple reaction monitoring (MRM), with drug or metabolite description, comments including sample validation, per date of service

0149U Drug assay, definitive, 60 or more drugs or metabolites, urine, quantitative liquid chromatography with tandem mass spectrometry (LC-MS/MS) using multiple reaction monitoring (MRM), with drug or metabolite description, comments including sample validation, per date of service

0150U Drug assay, definitive, 120 or more drugs or metabolites, urine, quantitative liquid chromatography with tandem mass spectrometry (LC-MS/MS) using multiple reaction monitoring (MRM), with drug or metabolite description, comments including sample validation, per date of service

0151U Infectious disease (bacterial or viral respiratory tract infection), pathogen specific nucleic acid (DNA or RNA), 33 targets, real-time semi-quantitative PCR, bronchoalveolar lavage, sputum, or endotracheal aspirate, detection of 33 organismal and antibiotic resistance genes with limited semi-quantitative results

0153U Oncology (breast), mRNA, gene expression profiling by next-generation sequencing of 101 genes, utilizing formalin-fixed paraffin-embedded tissue, algorithm reported as a triple negative breast cancer clinical subtype(s) with information on immune cell involvement

0156U Copy number (eg, intellectual disability, dysmorphology), sequence analysis

0157U APC (APC regulator of WNT signaling pathway) (eg, familial adenomatosis polyposis [FAP]) mRNA sequence analysis (List separately in addition to code for primary procedure)

0158U MLH1 (mutL homolog 1) (eg, hereditary non-polyposis colorectal cancer, Lynch syndrome) mRNA sequence analysis (List separately in addition to code for primary procedure)

0159U MSH2 (mutS homolog 2) (eg, hereditary colon cancer, Lynch syndrome) mRNA sequence analysis (List separately in addition to code for primary procedure)

0160U MSH6 (mutS homolog 6) (eg, hereditary colon cancer, Lynch syndrome) mRNA sequence analysis (List separately in addition to code for primary procedure)

0161U PMS2 (PMS1 homolog 2, mismatch repair system component) (eg, hereditary non-polyposis colorectal cancer, Lynch syndrome) mRNA sequence analysis (List separately in addition to code for primary procedure)

0162U Hereditary colon cancer (Lynch syndrome), targeted mRNA sequence analysis panel (MLH1, MSH2, MSH6, PMS2) (List separately in addition to code for primary procedure)

0163U Oncology (colorectal) screening, biochemical enzyme-linked immunosorbent assay (ELISA) of 3 plasma or serum proteins (teratocarcinoma derived growth factor-1 [TDGF-1, Cripto-1], carcinoembryonic antigen [CEA], extracellular matrix protein [ECM]), with demographic data (age, gender, CRC-screening compliance) using a proprietary algorithm and reported as likelihood of CRC or advanced adenomas

0164U Gastroenterology (irritable bowel syndrome [IBS]), immunoassay for anti-CdtB and anti-vinculin antibodies, utilizing plasma, algorithm for elevated or not elevated qualitative results

0166U Liver disease, 10 biochemical assays (α2-macroglobulin, haptoglobin, apolipoprotein A1, bilirubin, GGT, ALT, AST, triglycerides, cholesterol, fasting glucose) and biometric and demographic data, utilizing serum, algorithm reported as scores for fibrosis, necroinflammatory activity, and steatosis with a summary interpretation

0167U Gonadotropin, chorionic (hCG), immunoassay with direct optical observation, blood

0168U Fetal aneuploidy (trisomy 21, 18, and 13) DNA sequence analysis of selected regions using maternal plasma without fetal fraction cutoff, algorithm reported as a risk score for each trisomy

0169U NUDT15 (nudix hydrolase 15) and TPMT (thiopurine S-methyltransferase) (eg, drug metabolism) gene analysis, common variants

0170U Neurology (autism spectrum disorder [ASD]), RNA, next-generation sequencing, saliva, algorithmic analysis, and results reported as predictive probability of ASD diagnosis

0171U Targeted genomic sequence analysis panel, acute myeloid leukemia, myelodysplastic syndrome, and myeloproliferative neoplasms, DNA analysis, 23 genes, interrogation for sequence variants, rearrangements and minimal residual disease, reported as presence/absence

0172U Oncology (solid tumor as indicated by the label), somatic mutation analysis of BRCA1 (BRCA1, DNA repair associated), BRCA2 (BRCA2, DNA repair associated) and analysis of homologous recombination deficiency pathways, DNA, formalin-fixed paraffin-embedded tissue, algorithm quantifying tumor genomic instability score

0173U Psychiatry (ie, depression, anxiety), genomic analysis panel, includes variant analysis of 14 genes

0174U Oncology (solid tumor), mass spectrometric 30 protein targets, formalin-fixed paraffin-embedded tissue, prognostic and predictive algorithm reported as likely, unlikely, or uncertain benefit of 39 chemotherapy and targeted therapeutic oncology agents

0175U Psychiatry (eg, depression, anxiety), genomic analysis panel, variant analysis of 15 genes

0176U Cytolethal distending toxin B (CdtB) and vinculin IgG antibodies by immunoassay (ie, ELISA)

0177U Oncology (breast cancer), DNA, PIK3CA (phosphatidylinositol-4,5-bisphosphate 3-kinase catalytic subunit alpha) gene analysis of 11 gene variants utilizing plasma, reported as PIK3CA gene mutation status

0178U Peanut allergen-specific quantitative assessment of multiple epitopes using enzyme-linked immunosorbent assay (ELISA), blood, report of minimum eliciting exposure for a clinical reaction

0179U Oncology (non-small cell lung cancer), cell-free DNA, targeted sequence analysis of 23 genes (single nucleotide variations, insertions and deletions, fusions without prior knowledge of partner/breakpoint, copy number variations), with report of significant mutation(s)

0180U Red cell antigen (ABO blood group) genotyping (ABO), gene analysis Sanger/chain termination/conventional sequencing, ABO (ABO, alpha 1-3-N-acetylgalactosaminyltransferase and alpha 1-3-galactosyltransferase) gene, including subtyping, 7 exons

0181U Red cell antigen (Colton blood group) genotyping (CO), gene analysis, AQP1 (aquaporin 1 [Colton blood group]) exon 1

0182U Red cell antigen (Cromer blood group) genotyping (CROM), gene analysis, CD55 (CD55 molecule [Cromer blood group]) exons 1-10

0183U Red cell antigen (Diego blood group) genotyping (DI), gene analysis, SLC4A1 (solute carrier family 4 member 1 [Diego blood group]) exon 19

0184U Red cell antigen (Dombrock blood group) genotyping (DO), gene analysis, ART4 (ADP-ribosyltransferase 4 [Dombrock blood group]) exon 2

0185U Red cell antigen (H blood group) genotyping (FUT1), gene analysis, FUT1 (fucosyltransferase 1 [H blood group]) exon 4

0186U Red cell antigen (H blood group) genotyping (FUT2), gene analysis, FUT2 (fucosyltransferase 2) exon 2

0187U Red cell antigen (Duffy blood group) genotyping (FY), gene analysis, ACKR1 (atypical chemokine receptor 1 [Duffy blood group]) exons 1-2

0188U Red cell antigen (Gerbich blood group) genotyping (GE), gene analysis, GYPC (glycophorin C [Gerbich blood group]) exons 1-4

0189U Red cell antigen (MNS blood group) genotyping (GYPA), gene analysis, GYPA (glycophorin A [MNS blood group]) introns 1, 5, exon 2

0190U Red cell antigen (MNS blood group) genotyping (GYPB), gene analysis, GYPB (glycophorin B [MNS blood group]) introns 1, 5, pseudoexon 3

0191U Red cell antigen (Indian blood group) genotyping (IN), gene analysis, CD44 (CD44 molecule [Indian blood group]) exons 2, 3, 6

0192U Red cell antigen (Kidd blood group) genotyping (JK), gene analysis, SLC14A1 (solute carrier family 14 member 1 [Kidd blood group]) gene promoter, exon 9

0193U Red cell antigen (JR blood group) genotyping (JR), gene analysis, ABCG2 (ATP binding cassette subfamily G member 2 [Junior blood group]) exons 2-26

0194U Red cell antigen (Kell blood group) genotyping (KEL), gene analysis, KEL (Kell metallo-endopeptidase [Kell blood group]) exon 8

0195U KLF1 (Kruppel-like factor 1), targeted sequencing (ie, exon 13)

0196U Red cell antigen (Lutheran blood group) genotyping (LU), gene analysis, BCAM (basal cell adhesion molecule [Lutheran blood group]) exon 3

0197U Red cell antigen (Landsteiner-Wiener blood group) genotyping (LW), gene analysis, ICAM4 (intercellular adhesion molecule 4 [Landsteiner-Wiener blood group]) exon 1

0198U Red cell antigen (RH blood group) genotyping (RHD and RHCE), gene analysis Sanger/chain termination/conventional sequencing, RHD (Rh blood group D antigen) exons 1-10 and RHCE (Rh blood group CcEe antigens) exon 5

0199U Red cell antigen (Scianna blood group) genotyping (SC), gene analysis, ERMAP (erythroblast membrane associated protein [Scianna blood group]) exons 4, 12

0200U Red cell antigen (Kx blood group) genotyping (XK), gene analysis, XK (X-linked Kx blood group) exons 1-3

0201U Red cell antigen (Yt blood group) genotyping (YT), gene analysis, ACHE (acetylcholinesterase [Cartwright blood group]) exon 2

0202U Infectious disease (bacterial or viral respiratory tract infection), pathogen-specific nucleic acid (DNA or RNA), 22 targets including severe acute respiratory syndrome coronavirus 2 (SARS-CoV-2), qualitative RT-PCR, nasopharyngeal swab, each pathogen reported as detected or not detected

0203U Autoimmune (inflammatory bowel disease), mRNA, gene expression profiling by quantitative RT-PCR, 17 genes (15 target and 2 reference genes), whole blood, reported as a continuous risk score and classification of inflammatory bowel disease aggressiveness

0204U Oncology (thyroid), mRNA, gene expression analysis of 593 genes (including BRAF, RAS, RET, PAX8, and NTRK) for sequence variants and rearrangements, utilizing fine needle aspirate, reported as detected or not detected

0205U Ophthalmology (age-related macular degeneration), analysis of 3 gene variants (2 CFH gene, 1 ARMS2 gene), using PCR and MALDI-TOF, buccal swab, reported as positive or negative for neovascular age-related macular-degeneration risk associated with zinc supplements

0206U Neurology (Alzheimer disease); cell aggregation using morphometric imaging and protein kinase C-epsilon (PKCe) concentration in response to amylospheroid treatment by ELISA, cultured skin fibroblasts, each reported as positive or negative for Alzheimer disease

0207U quantitative imaging of phosphorylated ERK1 and ERK2 in response to bradykinin treatment by in situ immunofluorescence, using cultured skin fibroblasts, reported as a probability index for Alzheimer disease (List separately in addition to code for primary procedure)

0208U Oncology (medullary thyroid carcinoma), mRNA, gene expression analysis of 108 genes, utilizing fine needle aspirate, algorithm reported as positive or negative for medullary thyroid carcinoma

0209U Cytogenomic constitutional (genome-wide) analysis, interrogation of genomic regions for copy number, structural changes and areas of homozygosity for chromosomal abnormalities

0210U Syphilis test, non-treponemal antibody, immunoassay, quantitative (RPR)

0211U Oncology (pan-tumor), DNA and RNA by next-generation sequencing, utilizing formalin-fixed paraffin-embedded tissue, interpretative report for single nucleotide variants, copy number alterations, tumor mutational burden, and microsatellite instability, with therapy association

0212U Rare diseases (constitutional/heritable disorders), whole genome and mitochondrial DNA sequence analysis, including small sequence changes, deletions, duplications, short tandem repeat gene expansions, and variants in non-uniquely mappable regions, blood or saliva, identification and categorization of genetic variants, proband

0213U Rare diseases (constitutional/heritable disorders), whole genome and mitochondrial DNA sequence analysis, including small sequence changes, deletions, duplications, short tandem repeat gene expansions, and variants in non-uniquely mappable regions, blood or saliva, identification and categorization of genetic variants, each comparator genome (eg, parent, sibling)

0214U Rare diseases (constitutional/heritable disorders), whole exome and mitochondrial DNA sequence analysis, including small sequence changes, deletions, duplications, short tandem repeat gene expansions, and variants in non-uniquely mappable regions, blood or saliva, identification and categorization of genetic variants, proband

0215U Rare diseases (constitutional/heritable disorders), whole exome and mitochondrial DNA sequence analysis, including small sequence changes, deletions, duplications, short tandem repeat gene expansions, and variants in non-uniquely mappable regions, blood or saliva, identification and categorization of genetic variants, each comparator exome (eg, parent, sibling)

0216U Neurology (inherited ataxias), genomic DNA sequence analysis of 12 common genes including small sequence changes, deletions, duplications, short tandem repeat gene expansions, and variants in non-uniquely mappable regions, blood or saliva, identification and categorization of genetic variants

0217U Neurology (inherited ataxias), genomic DNA sequence analysis of 51 genes including small sequence changes, deletions, duplications, short tandem repeat gene expansions, and variants in non-uniquely mappable regions, blood or saliva, identification and categorization of genetic variants

0218U Neurology (muscular dystrophy), DMD gene sequence analysis, including small sequence changes, deletions, duplications, and variants in non-uniquely mappable regions, blood or saliva, identification and characterization of genetic variants

0219U Infectious agent (human immunodeficiency virus), targeted viral next-generation sequence analysis (ie, protease [PR], reverse transcriptase [RT], integrase [INT]) algorithm reported as prediction of antiviral drug susceptibility

0220U Oncology (breast cancer), image analysis with artificial intelligence assessment of 12 histologic and immunohistochemical features, reported as a recurrence score

0221U Red cell antigen (ABO blood group) genotyping (ABO), gene analysis, next-generation sequencing, ABO (ABO, alpha 1-3-N-acetylgalactosaminyltransferase and alpha 1-3-galactosyltransferase) gene

0222U Red cell antigen (RH blood group) genotyping (RHD and RHCE), gene analysis, next-generation sequencing, RH proximal promoter, exons 1-10, portions of introns 2-3

0594T Osteotomy, humerus, with insertion of an externally controlled intramedullary lengthening device, including intraoperative imaging, initial and subsequent alignment assessments, computations of adjustment schedules, and management of the intramedullary lengthening device

0596T Temporary female intraurethral valve-pump (ie, voiding prosthesis); initial insertion, including urethral measurement

0597T replacement

0598T Noncontact real-time fluorescence wound imaging, for bacterial presence, location, and load, per session; first anatomic site (eg, lower extremity)

0599T each additional anatomic site (eg, upper extremity) (List separately in addition to code for primary procedure)

0600T Ablation, irreversible electroporation; 1 or more tumors per organ, including imaging guidance, when performed, percutaneous

0601T 1 or more tumors per organ, including fluoroscopic and ultrasound guidance, when performed, open

0602T Glomerular filtration rate (GFR) measurement(s), transdermal, including sensor placement and administration of a single dose of fluorescent pyrazine agent

0603T Glomerular filtration rate (GFR) monitoring, transdermal, including sensor placement and administration of more than one dose of fluorescent pyrazine agent, each 24 hours

0604T Optical coherence tomography (OCT) of retina, remote, patient-initiated image capture and transmission to a remote surveillance center, unilateral or bilateral; initial device provision, set-up and patient education on use of equipment

0605T remote surveillance center technical support, data analyses and reports, with a minimum of 8 daily recordings, each 30 days

0606T review, interpretation and report by the prescribing physician or other qualified health care professional of remote surveillance center data analyses, each 30 days

0607T Remote monitoring of an external continuous pulmonary fluid monitoring system, including measurement of radiofrequency-derived pulmonary fluid levels, heart rate, respiration rate, activity, posture, and cardiovascular rhythm (eg, ECG data), transmitted to a remote 24-hour attended surveillance center; set-up and patient education on use of equipment

0608T analysis of data received and transmission of reports to the physician or other qualified health care professional

0609T Magnetic resonance spectroscopy, determination and localization of discogenic pain (cervical, thoracic, or lumbar); acquisition of single voxel data, per disc, on biomarkers (ie, lactic acid, carbohydrate, alanine, laal, propionic acid, proteoglycan, and collagen) in at least 3 discs

0610T transmission of biomarker data for software analysis

0611T postprocessing for algorithmic analysis of biomarker data for determination of relative chemical differences between discs

0612T interpretation and report

0613T Percutaneous transcatheter implantation of interatrial septal shunt device, including right and left heart catheterization, intracardiac echocardiography, and imaging guidance by the proceduralist, when performed

0614T Removal and replacement of substernal implantable defibrillator pulse generator

0615T Eye-movement analysis without spatial calibration, with interpretation and report

0616T Insertion of iris prosthesis, including suture fixation and repair or removal of iris, when performed; without removal of crystalline lens or intraocular lens, without insertion of intraocular lens

0617T with removal of crystalline lens and insertion of intraocular lens

0618T with secondary intraocular lens placement or intraocular lens exchange

0619T Cystourethroscopy with transurethral anterior prostate commissurotomy and drug delivery, including transrectal ultrasound and fluoroscopy, when performed

0620T Endovascular venous arterialization, tibial or peroneal vein, with transcatheter placement of intravascular stent graft(s) and closure by any method, including percutaneous or open vascular access, ultrasound guidance for vascular access when performed, all catheterization(s) and intraprocedural roadmapping and imaging guidance necessary to complete the intervention, all associated radiological supervision and interpretation, when performed

0621T Trabeculostomy ab interno by laser;

0622T with use of ophthalmic endoscope

0623T Automated quantification and characterization of coronary atherosclerotic plaque to assess severity of coronary disease, using data from coronary computed tomographic angiography; data preparation and transmission, computerized analysis of data, with review of computerized analysis output to reconcile discordant data, interpretation and report

0624T data preparation and transmission

0625T computerized analysis of data from coronary computed tomographic angiography

0626T review of computerized analysis output to reconcile discordant data, interpretation and report

0627T Percutaneous injection of allogeneic cellular and/or tissue-based product, intervertebral disc, unilateral or bilateral injection, with fluoroscopic guidance, lumbar; first level

0628T each additional level (List separately in addition to code for primary procedure)

0629T Percutaneous injection of allogeneic cellular and/or tissue-based product, intervertebral disc, unilateral or bilateral injection, with CT guidance, lumbar; first level

0630T each additional level (List separately in addition to code for primary procedure)

0631T Transcutaneous visible light hyperspectral imaging measurement of oxyhemoglobin, deoxyhemoglobin, and tissue oxygenation, with interpretation and report, per extremity

0632T Percutaneous transcatheter ultrasound ablation of nerves innervating the pulmonary arteries, including right heart catheterization, pulmonary artery angiography, and all imaging guidance

0633T Computed tomography, breast, including 3D rendering, when performed, unilateral; without contrast material

0634T with contrast material(s)

0635T without contrast, followed by contrast material(s)

0636T Computed tomography, breast, including 3D rendering, when performed, bilateral; without contrast material(s)

0637T with contrast material(s)

0638T without contrast, followed by contrast material(s)

0639T Wireless skin sensor thermal anisotropy measurement(s) and assessment of flow in cerebrospinal fluid shunt, including ultrasound guidance, when performed

0014M Liver disease, analysis of 3 biomarkers (hyaluronic acid [HA], procollagen III amino terminal peptide [PIIINP], tissue inhibitor of metalloproteinase 1 [TIMP-1]), using immunoassays, utilizing serum, prognostic algorithm reported as a risk score and risk of liver fibrosis and liver-related clinical events within 5 years

0015M Adrenal cortical tumor, biochemical assay of 25 steroid markers, utilizing 24-hour urine specimen and clinical parameters, prognostic algorithm reported as a clinical risk and integrated clinical steroid risk for adrenal cortical carcinoma, adenoma, or other adrenal malignancy

0016M Oncology (bladder), mRNA, microarray gene expression profiling of 209 genes, utilizing formalin-fixed paraffin-embedded tissue, algorithm reported as molecular subtype (luminal, luminal infiltrated, basal, basal claudin-low, neuroendocrine-like)

Revised Codes

11970 Replacement of tissue expander with permanent ~~prosthesis~~ implant

11971 Removal of tissue expander~~(s)~~ without insertion of ~~prosthesis~~ implant

19318 Breast ~~R~~ reduction ~~mammaplasty~~

19325 ~~Mammaplasty, augmentation~~ Breast augmentation with implant~~; with prosthetic implant~~

19328 Removal of intact ~~mammary~~ breast implant

19330 Removal of ~~mammary~~ ruptured breast implant ~~material,~~ including implant contents (eg, saline, silicone gel)

19340 ~~Immediate i~~Insertion of breast implant ~~prosthesis following mastopexy, mastectomy or in reconstruction~~ on same day of mastectomy (ie, immediate)

19342 ~~Delayed i~~Insertion or replacement of breast ~~prosthesis following mastopexy, mastectomy or in reconstruction~~ implant on separate day from mastectomy

19357 ~~Breast reconstruction, immediate or delayed, with tissue expander~~ Tissue expander placement in breast reconstruction, including subsequent expansion(s)

19361 Breast reconstruction; with latissimus dorsi flap~~, without prosthetic implant~~

19364 ~~Breast reconstruction~~ with free flap (eg, fTRAM, DIEP, SIEA, GAP flap)

19367 ~~Breast reconstruction~~ with single-pedicled transverse rectus abdominis myocutaneous (TRAM) flap ~~(TRAM), single pedicle, including closure of donor site;~~

19368 with single-pedicled transverse rectus abdominis myocutaneous (TRAM) flap, requiring separate microvascular anastomosis (supercharging)

19369 with bipedicled transverse rectus abdominis myocutaneous (TRAM) flap ~~Breast reconstruction with transverse rectus abdominis myocutaneous flap (TRAM), double pedicle, including closure of donor site~~

19370 ~~Open periprosthetic~~ Revision of peri-implant capsule, breast, including capsulotomy, capsulorrhaphy, ~~breast~~ and/or partial capsulectomy

19371 Peri~~prosthetic~~-implant capsulectomy, breast, complete, including removal of all intracapsular contents

19380 Revision of reconstructed breast (eg, significant removal of tissue, re-advancement and/or re-inset of flaps in autologous reconstruction or significant capsular revision combined with soft tissue excision in implant-based reconstruction)

29822 Arthroscopy, shoulder, surgical; debridement, limited, 1 or 2 discrete structures (eg, humeral bone, humeral articular cartilage, glenoid bone, glenoid articular cartilage, biceps tendon, biceps anchor complex, labrum, articular capsule, articular side of the rotator cuff, bursal side of the rotator cuff, subacromial bursa, foreign body[ies])

29823 debridement, extensive, 3 or more discrete structures (eg, humeral bone, humeral articular cartilage, glenoid bone, glenoid articular cartilage, biceps tendon, biceps anchor complex, labrum, articular capsule, articular side of the rotator cuff, bursal side of the rotator cuff, subacromial bursa, foreign body[ies])

33990 Insertion of ventricular assist device, percutaneous, including radiological supervision and interpretation; left heart, arterial access only

33991 left heart, both arterial and venous access, with transseptal puncture

33992 Removal of percutaneous left heart ventricular assist device, arterial or arterial and venous cannula(s), at separate and distinct session from insertion

33993 Repositioning of percutaneous right or left heart ventricular assist device with imaging guidance at separate and distinct session from insertion

64455 Injection(s), anesthetic agent(s) and/or steroid; plantar common digital nerve(s) (eg, Morton's neuroma)

64479 transforaminal epidural, with imaging guidance (fluoroscopy or CT), cervical or thoracic, single level

64480 transforaminal epidural, with imaging guidance (fluoroscopy or CT), cervical or thoracic, each additional level (List separately in addition to code for primary procedure)

64483 transforaminal epidural, with imaging guidance (fluoroscopy or CT), lumbar or sacral, single level

64484 transforaminal epidural, with imaging guidance (fluoroscopy or CT), lumbar or sacral, each additional level (List separately in addition to code for primary procedure)

71250 Computed tomography, thorax, diagnostic; without contrast material

71260 with contrast material(s)

71270 without contrast material, followed by contrast material(s) and further sections

74425 Urography, antegrade ~~(pyelostogram, nephrostogram, loopogram)~~, radiological supervision and interpretation

76513 [Ophthalmic ultrasound, diagnostic;] anterior segment ultrasound, immersion (water bath) B-scan or high resolution biomicroscopy, unilateral or bilateral

78130 Red cell survival study~~;~~

80415 estradiol response

81401 Molecular pathology procedure, Level 2 (eg, 2-10 SNPs, 1 methylated variant, or 1 somatic variant [typically using nonsequencing target variant analysis], or detection of a dynamic mutation disorder/triplet repeat) ~~CCND1/IGH (BCL1/IgH, t(11;14)) (eg, mantle cell lymphoma) translocation analysis, major breakpoint, qualitative, and quantitative, if performed ETV6/NTRK3 (t(12;15)) (eg, congenital/infantile fibrosarcoma), translocation analysis, qualitative, and quantitative, if performed~~

81402 Molecular pathology procedure, Level 3 (eg, >10 SNPs, 2-10 methylated variants, or 2-10 somatic variants [typically using non-sequencing target variant analysis], immunoglobulin and T-cell receptor gene rearrangements, duplication/deletion variants of 1 exon, loss of heterozygosity [LOH], uniparental disomy [UPD]) ~~IGH@/BCL2 (t(14;18)) (eg, follicular lymphoma), translocation analysis; major breakpoint region (MBR) and minor cluster region (mcr) breakpoints, qualitative or quantitative MPL (myeloproliferative leukemia virus oncogene, thrombopoietin receptor, TPOR) (eg, myeloproliferative disorder), common variants (eg, W515A, W515K, W515L, W515R)~~

81403 Molecular pathology procedure, Level 4 (eg, analysis of single exon by DNA sequence analysis, analysis of >10 amplicons using multiplex PCR in 2 or more independent reactions, mutation scanning or duplication/deletion variants of 2-5 exons) ~~JAK2 (Janus kinase 2) (eg, myeloproliferative disorder), exon 12 sequence and exon 13 sequence, if performed MPL (myeloproliferative leukemia virus oncogene, thrombopoietin receptor, TPOR) (eg, myeloproliferative disorder), exon 10 sequence~~

81404 Molecular pathology procedure, Level 5 (eg, analysis of 2-5 exons by DNA sequence analysis, mutation scanning or duplication/deletion variants of 6-10 exons, or characterization of a dynamic mutation disorder/triplet repeat by Southern blot analysis) ~~TP53 (tumor protein 53) (eg, tumor samples), targeted sequence analysis of 2-5 exons~~

81405 Molecular pathology procedure, Level 6 (eg, analysis of 6-10 exons by DNA sequence analysis, mutation scanning or duplication/deletion variants of 11-25 exons, regionally targeted cytogenomic array analysis) ~~TP53 (tumor protein 53) (eg, Li-Fraumeni syndrome, tumor samples), full gene sequence or targeted sequence analysis of >5 exons~~

82075 Alcohol (ethanol)~~, breath~~; breath

82670 Estradiol; total

86318 Immunoassay for infectious agent antibody(ies), qualitative or semiquantitative, single-step method (eg, reagent strip);

0154U Oncology (urothelial cancer), RNA, analysis by real-time RT-PCR of the FGFR3 (fibroblast growth factor receptor 3) gene analysis (ie, p.R248C [c.742C>T], p.S249C [c.746C>G], p.G370C [c.1108G>T], p.Y373C [c.1118A>G], FGFR3-TACC3v1, and FGFR3-TACC3v3), utilizing formalin-fixed paraffin-embedded urothelial cancer tumor tissue, reported as FGFR gene alteration status

0155U Oncology (breast cancer), DNA, *PIK3CA (phosphatidylinositol-4,5-bisphosphate 3-kinase, catalytic subunit alpha)* (eg, breast cancer) gene analysis (ie, p.C420R, p.E542K, p.E545A, p.E545D [g.1635G>T only], p.E545G, p.E545K, p.Q546E, p.Q546R, p.H1047L, p.H1047R, p.H1047Y[UL]), utilizing formalin-fixed paraffin-embedded breast tumor tissue, reported as PIK3CA gene mutation status

0165U Peanut allergen-specific ~~IgE and~~ quantitative assessment of 64 multiple epitopes using enzyme-linked immunosorbent assay (ELISA), blood, individual epitope results and ~~interpretation~~ probability of peanut allergy

92227 ~~Remote imaging~~ Imaging of retina for detection or monitoring of ~~retinal~~ disease ~~(eg, retinopathy in a patient with diabetes) with analysis and report under physician supervision, unilateral or bilateral~~ ; with remote clinical staff review and report, unilateral or bilateral

92228 ~~Remote imaging for monitoring and management of active retinal disease (eg, diabetic retinopathy)~~ with remote physician ~~review~~ or other qualified health care professional interpretation and report, unilateral or bilateral

94617 Exercise test for bronchospasm, including pre- and post-spirometry~~, electrocardiographic recording(s),~~ and pulse oximetry; with electrocardiographic recording(s)

95070 Inhalation bronchial challenge testing (not including necessary pulmonary function tests)~~;~~ , with histamine, methacholine, or similar compounds

99202 Office or other outpatient visit for the evaluation and management of a new patient, which requires ~~these 3 key components:~~ a medically appropriate history and/or examination and straightforward medical decision making. ~~An expanded problem focused history; An expanded problem focused examination; Straightforward medical decision making. Counseling and/or coordination of care with other physicians, other qualified health care professionals~~ When using time for code selection, ~~or agencies are provided consistent with the nature~~ 15-29 minutes of ~~the problem(s) and the patient's and/or family's needs~~ total time is spent on the date of the encounter. ~~Usually, the presenting problem(s) are of low to moderate severity. Typically, 20 minutes are spent face-to-face with the patient and/or family.~~

99203 Office or other outpatient visit for the evaluation and management of a new patient, which requires ~~these 3 key components:~~ a medically appropriate history and/or examination and low level of medical decision making. ~~A detailed history; A detailed examination; Medical decision making of low complexity. Counseling and/or coordination of care with other physicians, other qualified health care professionals~~ When using time for code selection, ~~or agencies are provided consistent with the nature~~ 30-44 minutes of ~~the problem(s) and the patient's and/or family's needs~~ total time is spent on the date of the encounter. ~~Usually, the presenting problem(s) are of moderate severity. Typically, 30 minutes are spent face-to-face with the patient and/or family.~~

99204 Office or other outpatient visit for the evaluation and management of a new patient, which requires ~~these 3 key components:~~ a medically appropriate history and/or examination and moderate level of medical decision making. ~~A comprehensive history; A comprehensive examination; Medical decision making of moderate complexity. Counseling and/or coordination of care with other physicians, other qualified health care professionals~~ When using time for code selection, ~~or agencies are provided consistent with the nature~~ 45-59 minutes of ~~the problem(s) and the patient's~~

~~and/or family's needs~~ total time is spent on the date of the encounter. ~~Usually, the presenting problem(s) are of moderate to high severity. Typically, 45 minutes are spent face-to-face with the patient and/or family.~~

99205 Office or other outpatient visit for the evaluation and management of a new patient, which requires ~~these 3 key components:~~ a medically appropriate history and/or examination and high level of medical decision making. ~~A comprehensive history; A comprehensive examination; Medical decision making of high complexity. Counseling and/or coordination of care with other physicians, other qualified health care professionals~~ When using time for code selection, ~~or agencies are provided consistent with the nature~~ 60-74 minutes ~~of the problem(s) and the patient's and/or family's needs~~ total time is spent on the date of the encounter. ~~Usually, the presenting problem(s) are of moderate to high severity. Typically, 60 minutes are spent face-to-face with the patient and/or family~~

99211 Office or other outpatient visit for the evaluation and management of an established patient, that may not require the presence of a physician or other qualified health care professional. Usually, the presenting problem(s) are minimal. ~~Typically, 5 minutes are spent performing or supervising these services~~

99212 Office or other outpatient visit for the evaluation and management of an established patient, which requires ~~at least 2 of these 3 key components:~~ medically appropriate history and/or examination and straightforward medical decision making. ~~A problem focused history; A problem focused examination; Straightforward medical decision making. Counseling and/or coordination of care with other physicians, other qualified health care professionals~~ When using time for code selection, ~~or agencies are provided consistent with the nature~~ 10-19 minutes ~~of the problem(s) and the patient's and/or family's needs~~ total time is spent on the date of the encounter. ~~Usually, the presenting problem(s) are self limited or minor. Typically, 10 minutes are spent face-to-face with the patient and/or family.~~

99213 Office or other outpatient visit for the evaluation and management of an established patient, which requires ~~at least 2 of these 3 key components:~~ medically appropriate history and/or examination and low level of medical decision making. ~~An expanded problem focused history; An expanded problem focused examination; Medical decision making of low complexity. Counseling and coordination of care with other physicians, other qualified health care professionals~~ When using time for code selection, ~~or agencies are provided consistent with the nature~~ 20-29 minutes ~~of the problem(s) and the patient's and/or family's needs~~ total time is spent on the date of the encounter. ~~Usually, the presenting problem(s) are of low to moderate severity. Typically, 15 minutes are spent face-to-face with the patient and/or family.~~

99214 Office or other outpatient visit for the evaluation and management of an established patient, which requires ~~at least 2 of these 3 key components:~~ medically appropriate history and/or examination and moderate level of medical decision making. ~~A detailed history; A detailed examination; Medical decision making of moderate complexity. Counseling and/or coordination of care with other physicians, other qualified health care professionals~~ When using time for code selection, ~~or agencies are provided consistent with the nature~~ 30-39 minutes ~~of the problem(s) and the patient's and/or family's needs~~ total time is spent on the date of the encounter. ~~Usually, the presenting problem(s) are of moderate to high severity. Typically, 25 minutes are spent face-to-face with the patient and/or family.~~

99215 Office or other outpatient visit for the evaluation and management of an established patient, which requires ~~at least 2 of these 3 key components:~~ medically appropriate history and/or examination and high level of medical decision making. ~~A comprehensive history; A comprehensive examination; Medical decision making of high complexity. Counseling and/or coordination of care with other physicians, other qualified health care professionals~~ When using time for code selection, ~~or agencies are provided consistent with the nature~~ 40-54 minutes ~~of the problem(s) and the patient's and/or family's needs~~ total time is spent on the date of the encounter. ~~Usually, the presenting problem(s) are of moderate to high severity. Typically, 40 minutes are spent face-to-face with the patient and/or family.~~

99354 Prolonged ~~evaluation and management or psychotherapy~~ service(s) ~~(beyond the typical service time of the primary procedure)~~ in the ~~office or other~~ outpatient setting requiring direct patient contact beyond the time of the usual service; first hour (List separately in addition to code for ~~office or other~~ outpatient Evaluation and Management or psychotherapy service, except with office or other outpatient services [99202, 99203, 99204, 99205, 99212, 99213, 99214, 99215])

99355 each additional 30 minutes (List separately in addition to code for prolonged service)

99356 Prolonged service in the inpatient or observation setting, requiring unit/floor time beyond the usual service; first hour (List separately in addition to code for inpatient or observation Evaluation and Management service)

99415 Prolonged clinical staff service (the service beyond the highest time in the range of total ~~typical service~~ time of the service) during an evaluation and management service in the office or outpatient setting, direct patient contact with physician supervision; first hour (List separately in addition to code for outpatient Evaluation and Management service)

99416 each additional 30 minutes (List separately in addition to code for prolonged service)

99487 Complex chronic care management services, with the following required elements: multiple (two or more) chronic conditions expected to last at least 12 months, or until the death of the patient, chronic conditions place the patient at significant risk of death, acute exacerbation/decompensation, or functional decline, ~~establishment or substantial revision of a comprehensive care plan~~comprehensive care plan established, implemented, revised, or monitored, moderate or high complexity medical decision making; ~~60 minutes of clinical staff time directed by a physician or other qualified health care professional, per calendar month.~~ first 60 minutes of clinical staff time directed by a physician or other qualified health care professional, per calendar month.

99489 each additional 30 minutes of clinical staff time directed by a physician or other qualified health care professional, per calendar month (List separately in addition to code for primary procedure)

99490 Chronic care management services, ~~at least 20 minutes of clinical staff time directed by a physician or other qualified health care professional, per calendar month,~~ with the following required elements: multiple (two or more) chronic conditions expected to last at least 12 months, or until the death of the patient, ~~;~~ chronic conditions place the patient at significant risk of death, acute exacerbation/decompensation, or functional decline, ~~;~~ comprehensive care plan established, implemented, revised, or monitored; first 20 minutes of clinical staff time directed by a physician or other qualified health care professional, per calendar month.

3170F ~~Flow~~ Baseline flow cytometry studies performed at time of diagnosis or prior to initiating treatment (HEM)[1]

0577T Electrophysiologic~~al~~ evaluation of implantable cardioverter-defibrillator system with substernal electrode (includes defibrillation threshold evaluation, induction of arrhythmia, evaluation of sensing for arrhythmia termination, and programming or reprogramming of sensing or therapeutic parameters)

Deleted Codes

0006U	0124U	0125U	0126U	0127U	0128U	0058T
0085T	0111T	0126T	0228T	0229T	0230T	0231T
0295T	0296T	0297T	0298T	0381T	0382T	0383T
0384T	0385T	0386T	0396T	0400T	0401T	0405T
0595T	19324	19366	32405	49220	57112	58293
61870	62163	63180	63182	69605	76970	78135
81545	92585	92586	92992	92993	94250	94400
94750	94770	95071	99201			

Resequenced Icon Added

33995	33997	80161	80167	80176	80179	80181
80189	80193	80204	80210	81168	81191	81192

Appendix B — New, Revised, and Deleted Codes

81193	81194	81278	81279	81338	81339	81347
81348	81351	81352	81353	81357	81419	81546
81595	81500	81503	81504	81540	81595	81596
82681	86328	87811	92517	92518	92519	92650
92651	92652	92653	93241	93242	93243	93244
93245	93246	93247	93248	94619	99417	99439
0614T	0620T	0623T	0624T	0625T	0626T	

Web Release New and Revised Codes

Codes indicated as "Web Release" codes indicate CPT codes that are in *Current Procedural Coding Expert* for the current year, but will not be in the AMA CPT book until the following year. This can also include those codes designated by the AMA as new or revised for 2021 but that actually appeared in the 2020 Optum360 book. These codes will have the appropriate new or revised icon appended to match the CPT code book, however. See the complete list that follows:

New codes, deleted codes, and revisions to codes in the 2021 *Current Procedural Coding Expert* that will not appear in the CPT code book until 2022

These codes are indicated with the following icons: ● ▲ These icons will be green in the body of the book.

New Codes

86408 Neutralizing antibody, severe acute respiratory syndrome coronavirus 2 (SARS-CoV-2) (Coronavirus disease [COVID-19]); screen

86409 titer

86413 Severe acute respiratory syndrome coronavirus 2 (SARS-CoV-2) (Coronavirus disease [COVID-19]) antibody, quantitative

87636 Infectious agent detection by nucleic acid (DNA or RNA); severe acute respiratory syndrome coronavirus 2 (SARS-CoV-2) (Coronavirus disease [COVID-19]) and influenza virus types A and B, multiplex amplified probe technique

87637 severe acute respiratory syndrome coronavirus 2 (SARS-CoV-2) (Coronavirus disease [COVID-19]), influenza virus types A and B, and respiratory syncytial virus, multiplex amplified probe technique

87811 Infectious agent antigen detection by immunoassay with direct optical (ie, visual) observation; severe acute respiratory syndrome coronavirus 2 (SARS-CoV-2) (Coronavirus disease [COVID-19])

99072 Additional supplies, materials, and clinical staff time over and above those usually included in an office visit or other nonfacility service(s), when performed during a Public Health Emergency, as defined by law, due to respiratory-transmitted infectious disease

0223U Infectious disease (bacterial or viral respiratory tract infection), pathogen-specific nucleic acid (DNA or RNA), 22 targets including severe acute respiratory syndrome coronavirus 2 (SARS-CoV-2), qualitative RT-PCR, nasopharyngeal swab, each pathogen reported as detected or not detected

0224U Antibody, severe acute respiratory syndrome coronavirus 2 (SARS-CoV-2) (Coronavirus disease [COVID-19]), includes titer(s), when performed

0225U Infectious disease (bacterial or viral respiratory tract infection) pathogen-specific DNA and RNA, 21 targets, including severe acute respiratory syndrome coronavirus 2 (SARS-CoV-2), amplified probe technique, including multiplex reverse transcription for RNA targets, each analyte reported as detected or not detected

0226U Surrogate viral neutralization test (sVNT), severe acute respiratory syndrome coronavirus 2 (SARS-CoV-2) (Coronavirus disease [COVID-19]), ELISA, plasma, serum

0227U Drug assay, presumptive, 30 or more drugs or metabolites, urine, liquid chromatography with tandem mass spectrometry (LC-MS/MS) using multiple reaction monitoring (MRM), with drug or metabolite description, includes sample validation

0228U Oncology (prostate), multianalyte molecular profile by photometric detection of macromolecules adsorbed on nanosponge array slides with machine learning, utilizing first morning voided urine, algorithm reported as likelihood of prostate cancer

0229U *BCAT1 (Branched chain amino acid transaminase 1)* or *IKZF1 (IKAROS family zinc finger 1)* (eg, colorectal cancer) promoter methylation analysis

0230U *AR (androgen receptor)* (eg, spinal and bulbar muscular atrophy, Kennedy disease, X chromosome inactivation), full sequence analysis, including small sequence changes in exonic and intronic regions, deletions, duplications, short tandem repeat (STR) expansions, mobile element insertions, and variants in non-uniquely mappable regions

0231U *CACNA1A (calcium voltage-gated channel subunit alpha 1A)* (eg, spinocerebellar ataxia), full gene analysis, including small sequence changes in exonic and intronic regions, deletions, duplications, short tandem repeat (STR) gene expansions, mobile element insertions, and variants in non-uniquely mappable regions

0232U *CSTB (cystatin B)* (eg, progressive myoclonic epilepsy type 1A, Unverricht-Lundborg disease), full gene analysis, including small sequence changes in exonic and intronic regions, deletions, duplications, short tandem repeat (STR) expansions, mobile element insertions, and variants in non-uniquely mappable regions

0233U *FXN (frataxin)* (eg, Friedreich ataxia), gene analysis, including small sequence changes in exonic and intronic regions, deletions, duplications, short tandem repeat (STR) expansions, mobile element insertions, and variants in non-uniquely mappable regions

0234U *MECP2 (methyl CpG binding protein 2)* (eg, Rett syndrome), full gene analysis, including small sequence changes in exonic and intronic regions, deletions, duplications, mobile element insertions, and variants in non-uniquely mappable regions

0235U *PTEN (phosphatase and tensin homolog)* (eg, Cowden syndrome, PTEN hamartoma tumor syndrome), full gene analysis, including small sequence changes in exonic and intronic regions, deletions, duplications, mobile element insertions, and variants in non-uniquely mappable regions

0236U *SMN1 (survival of motor neuron 1, telomeric)* and *SMN2 (survival of motor neuron 2, centromeric)* (eg, spinal muscular atrophy) full gene analysis, including small sequence changes in exonic and intronic regions, duplications and deletions, and mobile element insertions

0237U Cardiac ion channelopathies (eg, Brugada syndrome, long QT syndrome, short QT syndrome, catecholaminergic polymorphic ventricular tachycardia), genomic sequence analysis panel including *ANK2, CASQ2, CAV3, KCNE1, KCNE2, KCNH2, KCNJ2, KCNQ1, RYR2,* and *SCN5A,* including small sequence changes in exonic and intronic regions, deletions, duplications, mobile element insertions, and variants in non-uniquely mappable regions

0238U Oncology (Lynch syndrome), genomic DNA sequence analysis of *MLH1, MSH2, MSH6, PMS2,* and *EPCAM,* including small sequence changes in exonic and intronic regions, deletions, duplications, mobile element insertions, and variants in non-uniquely mappable regions

0239U Targeted genomic sequence analysis panel, solid organ neoplasm, cell-free DNA, analysis of 311 or more genes, interrogation for sequence variants, including substitutions, insertions, deletions, select rearrangements, and copy number variations

0240U Infectious disease (viral respiratory tract infection), pathogen-specific RNA, 3 targets (severe acute respiratory syndrome coronavirus 2 [SARS-CoV-2], influenza A, influenza B), upper respiratory specimen, each pathogen reported as detected or not detected

0241U Infectious disease (viral respiratory tract infection), pathogen-specific RNA, 4 targets (severe acute respiratory syndrome coronavirus 2 [SARS-CoV-2], influenza A, influenza B, respiratory syncytial virus [RSV]), upper respiratory specimen, each pathogen reported as detected or not detected

Revised Codes

87301 Infectious agent antigen detection by immunoassay technique, (eg, enzyme immunoassay [EIA], enzyme-linked immunosorbent assay [ELISA], <u>fluorescence immunoassay [FIA],</u> immunochemiluminometric assay [IMCA]) qualitative or semiquantitative, ~~multiple-step method~~; adenovirus enteric types 40/41

87305 Aspergillus

87320 Chlamydia trachomatis

87324 Clostridium difficile toxin(s)
87327 Cryptococcus neoformans
87328 cryptosporidium
87329 giardia
87332 cytomegalovirus
87335 Escherichia coli 0157
87336 Entamoeba histolytica dispar group
87337 Entamoeba histolytica group
87338 Helicobacter pylori, stool
87339 Helicobacter pylori
87340 hepatitis B surface antigen (HBsAg)
87341 hepatitis B surface antigen (HBsAg) neutralization
87350 hepatitis Be antigen (HBeAg)
87380 hepatitis, delta agent
87385 Histoplasma capsulatum
87389 HIV-1 antigen(s), with HIV-1 and HIV-2 antibodies, single result
87390 HIV-1
87391 HIV-2
87400 Influenza, A or B, each
87420 respiratory syncytial virus
87425 rotavirus
87426 severe acute respiratory syndrome coronavirus (eg, SARS-CoV, SARS-CoV-2 [COVID-19])
87427 Shiga-like toxin
87430 Streptococcus, group A
87449 not otherwise specified, each organism
87451 polyvalent for multiple organisms, each polyvalent antiserum
87802 Infectious agent antigen detection by immunoassay with direct optical (ie, visual) observation; Streptococcus, group B
87803 Clostridium difficile toxin A
87806 HIV-1 antigen(s), with HIV-1 and HIV-2 antibodies
87804 Influenza
87807 respiratory syncytial virus
87808 Trichomonas vaginalis
87809 adenovirus
87810 Chlamydia trachomatis
87850 Neisseria gonorrhoeae
87880 Streptococcus, group A
87899 not otherwise specified
0152U Infectious disease (bacteria, fungi, parasites, and DNA viruses), microbial cell-free DNA, ~~PCR and~~ plasma, untargeted next-generation sequencing, ~~plasma, detection of >1,000 potential microbial organisms for~~ report for significant positive pathogens

Deleted Codes

87450 Infectious agent antigen detection by immunoassay technique, (eg, enzyme immunoassay [EIA], enzyme-linked immunosorbent assay [ELISA], immunochemiluminometric assay [IMCA]), qualitative or semiquantitative; single step method, not otherwise specified, each organism

Appendix C — Evaluation and Management Extended Guidelines

This appendix provides an overview of evaluation and management (E/M) services, tables that identify the documentation elements associated with each code, the 2021 changes to some E/M services, and the federal documentation guidelines with emphasis on the 1997 exam guidelines. The new 2021 guidelines affect codes 99202–99215 only. The 1997 version identifies both general multi-system physical examinations and single-system examinations, but providers may also use the original 1995 version of the E/M guidelines; both are currently supported by the Centers for Medicare and Medicaid Services (CMS) for audit purposes when reporting 99217–99499.

The levels of E/M services define the wide variations in skill, effort, and time and are required for preventing and/or diagnosing and treating illness or injury, and promoting optimal health. These codes are intended to represent physician work, and because much of this work involves the amount of training, experience, expertise, and knowledge that a provider may employ when treating a given patient, the true indications of the level of this work may be difficult to recognize without some explanation.

Providers

The AMA advises coders that while a particular service or procedure may be assigned to a specific section, the service or procedure itself is not limited to use only by that specialty group (see paragraphs 2 and 3 under "Instructions for Use of the CPT® Codebook" on page xiv of the AMA CPT Book). Additionally, the procedures and services listed throughout the book are for use by any qualified physician or other qualified health care professional or entity (e.g., hospitals, laboratories, or home health agencies).

The use of the phrase "physician or other qualified health care professional" (OQHCP) was adopted to identify a health care provider other than a physician. This type of provider is further described in CPT as an individual "qualified by education, training, licensure/regulation (when applicable), and facility privileging (when applicable)." State licensure guidelines determine the scope of practice and an OQHCP must practice within these guidelines, even if more restrictive than the CPT guidelines. The OQHCP may report services independently or under incident-to guidelines. The professionals within this definition are separate from "clinical staff" and are able to practice independently. CPT defines clinical staff as "a person who works under the supervision of a physician or OQHCP and who is allowed, by law, regulation, and facility policy to perform or assist in the performance of a specified professional service, but who does not individually report that professional service." Keep in mind that there may be other policies or guidance that can affect who may report a specific service.

Types of E/M Services

When approaching E/M, the first choice that a provider must make is what type of code to use. The following tables outline the E/M codes for different levels of care for:

- Office or other outpatient services—new patient
- Office or other outpatient services—established patient
- Hospital observation services—initial care, subsequent, and discharge
- Hospital inpatient services—initial care, subsequent, and discharge
- Observation or inpatient care (including admission and discharge services)
- Consultations—office or other outpatient
- Consultations—inpatient
- Emergency department services
- Critical care
- Nursing facility—initial services
- Nursing facility—subsequent services
- Nursing facility—discharge and annual assessment
- Domiciliary, rest home, or custodial care—new patient
- Domiciliary, rest home, or custodial care—established patient
- Home services—new patient
- Home services—established patient
- Newborn care services
- Neonatal and pediatric interfacility transport
- Neonatal and pediatric critical care—inpatient
- Neonate and infant intensive care services—initial and continuing

The specifics of the code components that determine code selection are listed in the table and discussed in the next section. Before a level of service is decided upon, the correct type of service is identified.

A new patient is a patient who has not received any face-to-face professional services from the physician or OQHCP within the past three years. An established patient is a patient who has received face-to-face professional services from the physician or OQHCP within the past three years. In the case of group practices, if a physician or OQHCP of the exact same specialty or subspecialty has seen the patient within three years, the patient is considered established.

If a physician or OQHCP is on call or covering for another physician or OQHCP, the patient's encounter is classified as it would have been by the physician or OQHCP who is not available. Thus, a locum tenens physician or OQHCP who sees a patient on behalf of the patient's attending physician or OQHCP may not bill a new patient code unless the attending physician or OQHCP has not seen the patient for any problem within three years.

Office or other outpatient services are E/M services provided in the physician or OQHCP office, the outpatient area, or other ambulatory facility. Until the patient is admitted to a health care facility, he/she is considered to be an outpatient. Hospital observation services are E/M services provided to patients who are designated or admitted as "observation status" in a hospital.

Codes 99218-99220 are used to indicate initial observation care. These codes include the initiation of the observation status, supervision of patient care including writing orders, and the performance of periodic reassessments. These codes are used only by the provider "admitting" the patient for observation.

Codes 99234-99236 are used to indicate evaluation and management services to a patient who is admitted to and discharged from observation status or hospital inpatient on the same day. If the patient is admitted as an inpatient from observation on the same day, use the appropriate level of Initial Hospital Care (99221-99223).

Code 99217 indicates discharge from observation status. It includes the final physical examination of the patient, instructions, and preparation of the discharge records. It should not be used when admission and discharge are on the same date of service. As mentioned above, report codes 99234-99236 to appropriately describe same day observation services.

If a patient is in observation longer than one day, subsequent observation care codes 99224-99226 should be reported. If the patient is discharged on the second day, observation discharge code 99217 should be reported. If the patient status is changed to inpatient on a subsequent date, the appropriate inpatient code, 99221-99233, should be reported.

Initial hospital care is defined as E/M services provided during the first hospital inpatient encounter with the patient by the admitting provider. (If a physician other than the admitting physician performs the initial inpatient encounter, refer to consultations or subsequent hospital care in the CPT book.) Subsequent hospital care includes all follow-up encounters with the patient by all physicians or OQHCP. As there may only be one admitting physician, HCPCS Level II modifier AI Principal physician of record, should be appended to the initial hospital care code by the attending physician or OQHCP.

A consultation is the provision of a physician or OQHCP's opinion or advice about a patient for a specific problem at the request of another physician or other appropriate source. CPT also states that a consultation may be performed when a physician or OQHCP is determining whether to accept the transfer of patient care at the request of another physician or appropriate source. An office or other outpatient consultation is a consultation provided in the consultant's office, in the emergency department, or in an outpatient or other ambulatory facility including hospital observation services, home services, domiciliary, rest home, or custodial care. An inpatient consultation is a consultation provided in the hospital or partial hospital nursing facility setting. Report only one inpatient consultation by a consultant for each admission to the hospital or nursing facility.

If a consultant participates in the patient's management after the opinion or advice is provided, use codes for subsequent hospital or observation care or for office or other outpatient services (established patient), as appropriate.

Under CMS guidelines, the inpatient and office/outpatient consultation codes contained in the CPT manual are not covered services.

All outpatient consultation services will be reported for Medicare using the appropriate new or established evaluation and management (E/M) codes. Inpatient consultation services for the initial encounter should be reported by the physician providing the service using initial hospital care codes 99221–99223, and subsequent inpatient care codes 99231–99233.

Codes 99439, 99487, 99489, 99490, and 99491 are used to report evaluation and management services for chronic care management. These codes represent management and support services provided by clinical staff, under the direction of a physician or OQHCP, to patients residing at home or in a domiciliary, rest home, or assisted living facility. The qualified provider oversees the management and/or coordination of services for all medical conditions, psychosocial needs, and activities of daily living. These codes are reported only once per calendar month and have specific time-based thresholds.

Codes 99497-99498 are used to report the discussion and explanation of advanced directives by a physician or OQHCP. These codes represent a face-to-face service between the provider and a patient, family member, or surrogate. These codes are time-based codes and, since no active management of the problem(s) is undertaken during this time, may be reported on the same day as another E/M service.

Certain codes that CPT considers appropriate telehealth services are identified with the ★ icon and reported with modifier 95 Synchronous telemedicine service rendered via a real-time interactive audio and video telecommunications system. Medicare recognizes certain CPT and HCPCS Level II G codes as telehealth services reported with modifier GT. Check with individual payers for telehealth modifier guidance.

Revised E/M Services—Codes 99202 OCG: I.C.1.g.1.b; I.C.1.d
99215

These revised codes are used to report office or other outpatient services for a new (99202–99205) or established (99212–99215) patient.

A medically appropriate history and physical examination, as determined by the treating provider, should be documented. The level of history and physical examination are no longer used when determining the level of service. Codes should be selected based upon the CPT 2021 Medical Decision Making (MDM) table or time as documented in the patient record.

The 2021 Medical Decision Making table requires two of three levels of the three elements be met or exceeded to determine the level of code reported. The three elements are

- Number and complexity of problems addressed at the encounter
- Amount and/or complexity of data to be reviewed and analyzed
- Risk of complications and/or morbidity or mortality of patient management

Instructions and examples of each element are given in the table to enable accurate selection of the level of MDM and E/M service from 99202–99215 to be reported.

Alternatively time alone may be used to select the appropriate level of service. Total time for reporting these services includes face-to-face and non-face-to-face time personally spent by the physician or other qualified health care professional on the date of the encounter. The revised E/M codes 99202–99205 and 99212–99215 include specific time ranges used to select the appropriate code. Report new code 99417 for prolonged services when the time for code 99205 or 99215 is exceeded. Report 99417 for each minimum of 15 minutes additional prolonged services.

Code 99211 was revised but is still used to report the E/M service that does not require the presence of the physician or other qualified health care professional. The time element has also been removed from the code description.

The Centers for Medicare and Medicaid Services (CMS) recognizes these changes and will adopt the code description changes and use of time or the MDM table for codes 99202–99215 beginning January 1, 2021.

E/M Code	History	Exam	Medical Decision Making	Time Spent Face-to-Face (avg.)
99202	Medically appropriate	Medically appropriate	Straightforward	15–29 min.
99203	Medically appropriate	Medically appropriate	Low	30–44 min.
99204	Medically appropriate	Medically appropriate	Moderate	45–59 min.
99205	Medically appropriate	Medically appropriate	High	60–74 min.

Office or Other Outpatient Services—Established Patient[1]

E/M Code	History	Exam	Medical Decision Making	Time Spent Face-to-Face (avg.)
99211	—	—	Physician supervision, but presence not required	—
99212	Medically appropriate	Medically appropriate	Straightforward	10–19 min.
99213	Medically appropriate	Medically appropriate	Low	20–29 min.
99214	Medically appropriate	Medically appropriate	Moderate	30–39 min.
99215	Medically appropriate	Medically appropriate	High	40–54 min.

1 Includes follow-up, periodic reevaluation, and evaluation and management of new problems.

Hospital Observation Services

E/M Code	History[1]	Exam[1]	Medical Decision Making[1]	Problem Severity	Coordination of Care; Counseling	Time Spent Bedside and on Unit/Floor (avg.)
99217	Observation care discharge day management					
99218	Detailed or comprehensive	Detailed or comprehensive	Straightforward or low complexity	Low	Consistent with problem(s) and patient's needs	30 min.
99219	Comprehensive	Comprehensive	Moderate complexity	Moderate	Consistent with problem(s) and patient's needs	50 min.
99220	Comprehensive	Comprehensive	High complexity	High	Consistent with problem(s) and patient's needs	70 min.

1 Key component. All three components (history, exam, and medical decision making) are crucial for selecting the correct code.

Subsequent Hospital Observation Services[1]

E/M Code[2]	History[3]	Exam[3]	Medical Decision Making[3]	Problem Severity	Coordination of Care; Counseling	Time Spent Bedside and on Unit/Floor (avg.)
99224	Problem-focused interval	Problem-focused	Straightforward or low complexity	Stable, recovering, or improving	Consistent with problem(s) and patient's needs	15 min.
99225	Expanded problem-focused interval	Expanded problem-focused	Moderate complexity	Inadequate response to treatment; minor complications	Consistent with problem(s) and patient's needs	25 min.
99226	Detailed interval	Detailed	High complexity	Unstable; significant new problem or significant complication	Consistent with problem(s) and patient's needs	35 min.

1 All subsequent levels of service include reviewing the medical record, diagnostic studies, and changes in the patient's status, such as history, physical condition, and response to treatment since the last assessment.
2 These codes are resequenced in CPT and are printed following codes 99217-99220.
3 Key component. For subsequent care, at least two of the three components (history, exam, and medical decision making) are needed to select the correct code.

Hospital Inpatient Services—Initial Care[1]

E/M Code	History[2]	Exam[2]	Medical Decision Making[2]	Problem Severity	Coordination of Care; Counseling	Time Spent Bedside and on Unit/Floor (avg.)
99221	Detailed or comprehensive	Detailed or comprehensive	Straightforward or low complexity	Low	Consistent with problem(s) and patient's needs	30 min.
99222	Comprehensive	Comprehensive	Moderate complexity	Moderate	Consistent with problem(s) and patient's needs	50 min.
99223	Comprehensive	Comprehensive	High complexity	High	Consistent with problem(s) and patient's needs	70 min.

1 The admitting physician should append modifier AI, Principal physician of record, for Medicare patients

2 Key component. For initial care, all three components (history, exam, and medical decision making) are crucial for selecting the correct code.

Hospital Inpatient Services—Subsequent Care[1]

E/M Code	History[2]	Exam[2]	Medical Decision Making[2]	Problem Severity	Coordination of Care; Counseling	Time Spent Bedside and on Unit/Floor (avg.)
99231	Problem-focused interval	Problem-focused	Straightforward or low complexity	Stable, recovering or Improving	Consistent with problem(s) and patient's needs	15 min.
99232	Expanded problem-focused interval	Expanded problem-focused	Moderate complexity	Inadequate response to treatment; minor complications	Consistent with problem(s) and patient's needs	25 min.
99233	Detailed interval	Detailed	High complexity	Unstable; significant new problem or significant complication	Consistent with problem(s) and patient's needs	35 min.
99238	Hospital discharge day management					30 min. or less
99239	Hospital discharge day management					> 30 min.

1 All subsequent levels of service include reviewing the medical record, diagnostic studies, and changes in the patient's status, such as history, physical condition, and response to treatment since the last assessment.

2 Key component. For subsequent care, at least two of the three components (history, exam, and medical decision making) are needed to select the correct code.

Observation or Inpatient Care Services (Including Admission and Discharge Services)

E/M Code	History[1]	Exam[1]	Medical Decision Making[1]	Problem Severity	Coordination of Care; Counseling	Time
99234	Detailed or comprehensive	Detailed or comprehensive	Straightforward or low complexity	Low	Consistent with problem(s) and patient's needs	40 min.
99235	Comprehensive	Comprehensive	Moderate	Moderate	Consistent with problem(s) and patient's needs	50 min.
99236	Comprehensive	Comprehensive	High	High	Consistent with problem(s) and patient's needs	55 min.

1 Key component. All three components (history, exam, and medical decision making) are crucial for selecting the correct code.

Consultations—Office or Other Outpatient

E/M Code	History[1]	Exam[1]	Medical Decision Making[1]	Problem Severity	Coordination of Care; Counseling	Time Spent Face-to-Face (avg.)
99241	Problem-focused	Problem-focused	Straightforward	Minor or self-limited	Consistent with problem(s) and patient's needs	15 min.
99242	Expanded problem-focused	Expanded problem-focused	Straightforward	Low	Consistent with problem(s) and patient's needs	30 min.
99243	Detailed	Detailed	Low complexity	Moderate	Consistent with problem(s) and patient's needs	40 min.
99244	Comprehensive	Comprehensive	Moderate complexity	Moderate to high	Consistent with problem(s) and patient's needs	60 min.
99245	Comprehensive	Comprehensive	High complexity	Moderate to high	Consistent with problem(s) and patient's needs	80 min.

1 Key component. For office or other outpatient consultations, all three components (history, exam, and medical decision making) are crucial for selecting the correct code.

Consultations—Inpatient[1]

E/M Code	History[2]	Exam[2]	Medical Decision Making[2]	Problem Severity	Coordination of Care; Counseling	Time Spent Bedside and on Unit/Floor (avg.)
99251	Problem-focused	Problem-focused	Straightforward	Minor or self-limited	Consistent with problem(s) and patient's needs	20 min.
99252	Expanded problem-focused	Expanded problem-focused	Straightforward	Low	Consistent with problem(s) and patient's needs	40 min.
99253	Detailed	Detailed	Low complexity	Moderate	Consistent with problem(s) and patient's needs	55 min.
99254	Comprehensive	Comprehensive	Moderate complexity	Moderate to high	Consistent with problem(s) and patient's needs	80 min.
99255	Comprehensive	Comprehensive	High complexity	Moderate to high	Consistent with problem(s) and patient's needs	110 min.

1 These codes are used for hospital inpatients, residents of nursing facilities or patients in a partial hospital setting.
2 Key component. For initial inpatient consultations, all three components (history, exam, and medical decision making) are crucial for selecting the correct code.

Emergency Department Services, New or Established Patient

E/M Code	History[1]	Exam[1]	Medical Decision Making[1]	Problem Severity[3]	Coordination of Care; Counseling	Time Spent[2] Face-to-Face (avg.)
99281	Problem-focused	Problem-focused	Straightforward	Minor or self-limited	Consistent with problem(s) and patient's needs	N/A
99282	Expanded problem-focused	Expanded problem-focused	Low complexity	Low to moderate	Consistent with problem(s) and patient's needs	N/A
99283	Expanded problem-focused	Expanded problem-focused	Moderate complexity	Moderate	Consistent with problem(s) and patient's needs	N/A
99284	Detailed	Detailed	Moderate complexity	High; requires urgent evaluation	Consistent with problem(s) and patient's needs	N/A
99285	Comprehensive	Comprehensive	High complexity	High; poses immediate/significant threat to life or physiologic function	Consistent with problem(s) and patient's needs	N/A
99288[4]			High complexity			N/A

1 Key component. For emergency department services, all three components (history, exam, and medical decision making) are crucial for selecting the correct code and must be adequately documented in the medical record to substantiate the level of service reported.

2 Typical times have not been established for this category of services.

3 NOTE: The severity of the patient's problem, while taken into consideration when evaluating and treating the patient, does not automatically determine the level of E/M service unless the medical record documentation reflects the severity of the patient's illness, injury, or condition in the details of the history, physical examination, and medical decision making process. Federal auditors will "downcode" the level of E/M service despite the nature of the patient's problem when the documentation does not support the E/M code reported.

4 Code 99288 is used to report two-way communication with emergency medical services personnel in the field.

Critical Care

E/M Code	Patient Status	Physician Attendance	Time[1]
99291	Critically ill or critically injured	Constant	First 30–74 minutes
99292	Critically ill or critically injured	Constant	Each additional 30 minutes beyond the first 74 minutes

1 Per the guidelines for time in *CPT 2016 page xv*, "A unit of time is attained when the mid-point is passed. For example, an hour is attained when 31 minutes have elapsed (more than midway between zero and 60 minutes)."

Nursing Facility Services—Initial Nursing Facility Care[1]

E/M Code	History[1]	Exam[1]	Medical Decision Making[1]	Problem Severity	Coordination of Care; Counseling
99304	Detailed or comprehensive	Detailed or comprehensive	Straightforward or low complexity	Low	25 min.
99305	Comprehensive	Comprehensive	Moderate complexity	Moderate	35 min.
99306	Comprehensive	Comprehensive	High complexity	High	45 min.

1 These services must be performed by the physician. See CPT Corrections Document – CPT 2013 page 3 or guidelines CPT 2016 page 26.

2 Key component. For new patients, all three components (history, exam, and medical decision making) are crucial for selecting the correct code.

Nursing Facility Services—Subsequent Nursing Facility Care

E/M Code	History[1]	Exam[1]	Medical Decision Making[2]	Problem Severity	Coordination of Care; Counseling
99307	Problem-focused interval	Problem-focused	Straightforward	Stable, recovering or improving	10 min.
99308	Expanded problem-focused interval	Expanded problem-focused	Low complexity	Responding inadequately or has developed a minor complication	15 min.
99309	Detailed interval	Detailed	Moderate complexity	Significant complication or a significant new problem	25 min.
99310	Comprehensive interval	Comprehensive	High complexity	Developed a significant new problem requiring immediate attention	35 min.

1 Key component. For established patients, at least two of the three components (history, exam, and medical decision making) are needed for selecting the correct code.

Nursing Facility Discharge and Annual Assessment

E/M Code	History[1]	Exam[1]	Medical Decision Making[1]	Problem Severity	Time Spent Bedside and on Unit/Floor (avg.)
99315	Nursing facility discharge day management				30 min. or less
99316	Nursing facility discharge day management				more than 30 min.
99318	Detailed interval	Comprehensive	Low to moderate complexity	Stable, recovering or improving	30 min.

1 Key component. For annual nursing facility assessment, all three components (history, exam, and medical decision making) are crucial for selecting the correct code.

Domiciliary, Rest Home (e.g., Boarding Home) or Custodial Care Services—New Patient

E/M Code	History[1]	Exam[1]	Medical Decision Making[1]	Problem Severity	Coordination of Care; Counseling	Time Spent Face-to-Face (avg.)
99324	Problem-focused	Problem-focused	Straightforward	Low	Consistent with problem(s) and patient's needs	20 min.
99325	Expanded problem-focused	Expanded problem-focused	Low complexity	Moderate	Consistent with problem(s) and patient's needs	30 min.
99326	Detailed	Detailed	Moderate complexity	Moderate to high	Consistent with problem(s) and patient's needs	45 min.
99327	Comprehensive	Comprehensive	Moderate complexity	High	Consistent with problem(s) and patient's needs	60 min.
99328	Comprehensive	Comprehensive	High complexity	Unstable or developed a new problem requiring immediate physician attention	Consistent with problem(s) and patient's needs	75 min.

1 Key component. For new patients, all three components (history, exam, and medical decision making) are crucial for selecting the correct code and must be adequately documented in the medical record to substantiate the level of service reported.

Domiciliary, Rest Home (e.g., Boarding Home) or Custodial Care Services— Established Patient

E/M Code	History[1]	Exam[1]	Medical Decision Making[1]	Problem Severity	Coordination of Care; Counseling	Time Spent Face-to-Face (avg.)
99334	Problem-focused interval	Problem-focused	Straightforward	Minor or self-limited	Consistent with problem(s) and patient's needs	15 min.
99335	Expanded problem-focused interval	Expanded problem-focused	Low complexity	Low to moderate	Consistent with problem(s) and patient's needs	25 min.
99336	Detailed interval	Detailed	Moderate complexity	Moderate to high	Consistent with problem(s) and patient's needs	40 min.
99337	Comprehensive interval	Comprehensive	Moderate to high complexity	Moderate to high	Consistent with problem(s) and patient's needs	60 min.

1 Key component. For established patients, at least two of the three components (history, exam, and medical decision making) are needed for selecting the correct code.

Domiciliary, Rest Home (e.g., Assisted Living Facility), or Home Care Plan Oversight Services

E/M Code	Intent of Service	Presence of Patient	Time
99339	Individual physician supervision of a patient (patient not present) in home, domiciliary or rest home (e.g., assisted living facility) requiring complex and multidisciplinary care modalities involving regular physician development and/or revision of care plans, review of subsequent reports of patient status, review of related laboratory and other studies, communication (including telephone calls) for purposes of assessment or care decisions with health care professional(s), family member(s), surrogate decision maker(s) (e.g., legal guardian) and/or key caregiver(s) involved in patient's care, integration of new information into the medical treatment plan and/or adjustment of medical therapy, within a calendar month	Patient not present	15–29 min.
99340	Same as 99339	Patient not present	30 min. or more

Home Services—New Patient

E/M Code	History[1]	Exam[1]	Medical Decision Making[1]	Problem Severity	Coordination of Care; Counseling	Time Spent Face-to-Face (avg.)
99341	Problem-focused	Problem-focused	Straightforward complexity	Low	Consistent with problem(s) and patient's needs	20 min.
99342	Expanded problem-focused	Expanded problem-focused	Low complexity	Moderate	Consistent with problem(s) and patient's needs	30 min.
99343	Detailed	Detailed	Moderate complexity	Moderate to high	Consistent with problem(s) and patient's needs	45 min.
99344	Comprehensive	Comprehensive	Moderate complexity	High	Consistent with problem(s) and patient's needs	60 min.
99345	Comprehensive	Comprehensive	High complexity	Usually the patient has developed a significant new problem requiring immediate physician attention	Consistent with problem(s) and patient's needs	75 min.

1 Key component. For new patients, all three components (history, exam, and medical decision making) are crucial for selecting the correct code and must be adequately documented in the medical record to substantiate the level of service reported.

Home Services—Established Patient

E/M Code	History[1]	Exam[1]	Medical Decision Making[1]	Problem Severity	Coordination of Care; Counseling	Time Spent Face-to-Face (avg.)
99347	Problem-focused interval	Problem-focused	Straightforward	Minor or self-limited	Consistent with problem(s) and patient's needs	15 min.
99348	Expanded problem-focused interval	Expanded problem-focused	Low complexity	Low to moderate	Consistent with problem(s) and patient's needs	25 min.
99349	Detailed interval	Detailed	Moderate complexity	Moderate to high	Consistent with problem(s) and patient's needs	40 min.
99350	Comprehensive interval	Comprehensive	Moderate to high complexity	Moderate to high Usually the patient has developed a significant new problem requiring immediate physician attention	Consistent with problem(s) and patient's needs	60 min.

1 Key component. For established patients, at least two of the three components (history, exam, and medical decision making) are needed for selecting the correct code.

Newborn Care Services

E/M Code	Patient Status	Type of Visit
99460	Normal newborn	Inpatient initial inpatient hospital or birthing center per day
99461	Normal newborn	Inpatient initial treatment not in hospital or birthing center per day
99462	Normal newborn	Inpatient subsequent per day
99463	Normal newborn	Inpatient initial inpatient and discharge in hospital or birthing center per day
99464	Unstable newborn	Attendance at delivery
99465	High-risk newborn at delivery	Resuscitation, ventilation, and cardiac treatment

Neonatal and Pediatric Interfacility Transportation

E/M Code	Patient Status	Type of Visit
99466	Critically ill or injured infant or young child, to 24 months	Face-to-face transportation from one facility to another, initial 30-74 minutes
99467	Critically ill or injured infant or young child, to 24 months	Face-to-face transportation from one facility to another, each additional 30 minutes
99485[1]	Critically ill or injured infant or young child, to 24 months	Supervision of patient transport from one facility to another, initial 30 minutes
99486[1]	Critically ill or injured infant or young child, to 24 months	Supervision of patient transport from one facility to another, each additional 30 minutes

1 These codes are resequenced in CPT and are printed following codes 99466-99467.

Inpatient Neonatal and Pediatric Critical Care

E/M Code	Patient Status	Type of Visit
99468[1]	Critically ill neonate, aged 28 days or less	Inpatient initial per day
99469[2]	Critically ill neonate, aged 28 days or less	Inpatient subsequent per day
99471	Critically ill infant or young child, aged 29 days to 24 months	Inpatient initial per day
99472	Critically ill infant or young child, aged 29 days to 24 months	Inpatient subsequent per day
99475	Critically ill infant or young child, 2 to 5 years[3]	Inpatient initial per day
99476	Critically ill infant or young child, 2 to 5 years	Inpatient subsequent per day

1 Codes 99468, 99471, and 99475 may be reported only once per admission.
2 Codes 99469, 99472, and 99476 may be reported only once per day and by only one provider.
3 See 99291-99292 for patients 6 years of age and older.

Neonate and Infant Initial and Continuing Intensive Care Services

E/M Code	Patient Status	Type of Visit
99477	Neonate, aged 28 days or less	Inpatient initial per day
99478	Infant with present body weight of less than 1500 grams, no longer critically ill	Inpatient subsequent per day
99479	Infant with present body weight of 1500-2500 grams, no longer critically ill	Inpatient subsequent per day
99480	Infant with present body weight of 2501-5000 grams, no longer critically ill	Inpatient subsequent per day

Levels of E/M Services Codes 99217–99499

Confusion may be experienced when first approaching E/M codes 99217–99499 due to the way that each description of a code component or element seems to have another layer of description beneath. The three key components—history, exam, and decision making—are each comprised of elements that combine to create varying levels of that component.

For example, an expanded problem-focused history includes the chief complaint, a brief history of the present illness, and a system review focusing on the patient's problems. The level of exam is not made up of different elements but rather distinguished by the extent of exam across body areas or organ systems.

The single largest source of confusion are the "labels" or names applied to the varying degrees of history, exam, and decision-making. Terms such as expanded problem-focused, detailed, and comprehensive are somewhat meaningless unless they are defined. The lack of definition in CPT guidelines relative to these terms is precisely what caused the first set of federal guidelines to be developed in 1995 and again in 1997.

Documentation Guidelines for Evaluation and Management Services

Both versions of the federal guidelines go well beyond CPT guidelines in defining specific code requirements. The current version of the CPT guidelines does not explain the number of history of present illness (HPI) elements or the specific number of organ systems or body areas to be examined as they are in the federal guidelines. Adherence to some version of the guidelines is required when billing E/M to federal payers, but at this time, the CPT guidelines do not incorporate this level of detail into the code definitions. Although that could be interpreted to mean that non-governmental payers have a lesser documentation standard, it is best to adopt one set of the federal versions for all payer types for both consistency and ease of use.

The 1997 guidelines supply a great amount of detail relative to history and exam and will give the provider clear direction to follow when documenting elements. With that stated, the 1995 guidelines are equally valid and place a lesser documentation burden on the provider in regard to the physical exam.

The 1995 guidelines ask only for a notation of "normal" on systems with normal findings. The only narrative required is for abnormal findings. The 1997 version calls for much greater detail, or an "elemental" or "bullet-point" approach to organ systems, although a notation of normal is sufficient when addressing the elements within a system. The 1997 version works well in a template or electronic health record (EHR) format for recording E/M services.

The 1997 version did produce the single system specialty exam guidelines. When reviewing the complete guidelines listed below, note the differences between exam requirements in the 1995 and 1997 versions.

A Comparison of 1995 and 1997 Exam Guidelines

There are four types of exams indicated in the levels of E/M codes. Although the descriptors or labels are the same under 1995 and 1997 guidelines, the degree of detail required is different. The remaining content on this topic references the 1997 general multi-system specialty examination, at the end of this chapter.

The levels under each set of guidelines are:

1995 Exam Guidelines:

Problem focused:	One body area or system
Expanded problem focused:	Two to seven body areas or organ systems
Detailed:	Two to seven body areas or organ systems
Comprehensive:	Eight or more organ systems or a complete single-system examination

1997 Exam Guidelines:

Problem-focused:	Perform and document examination of one to five bullet point elements in one or more organ systems/body areas from the general multi-system examination
OR	
	Perform or document examination of one to five bullet point elements from one of the 10 single-organ-system examinations, shaded or unshaded boxes
Expanded problem-focused:	Perform and document examination of at least six bullet point elements in one or more organ systems from the general multi-system examination
OR	
	Perform and document examination of at least six bullet point elements from one of the 10 single-organ-system examinations, shaded or unshaded boxes
Detailed:	Perform and document examination of at least six organ systems or body areas, including at least two bullet point elements for each organ system or body area from the general multi-system examination
OR	
	Perform and document examination of at least 12 bullet point elements in two or more organ systems or body areas from the general multisystem examination
OR	
	Perform and document examination of at least 12 bullet elements from one of the single-organ-system examinations, shaded or unshaded boxes
Comprehensive:	Perform and document examination of at least nine organ systems or body areas, with all bullet elements for each organ system or body area (unless specific instructions are expected to limit examination content with at least two bullet elements for each organ system or body area) from the general multi-system examination
OR	
	Perform and document examination of all bullet point elements from one of the 10 single-organ system examinations with documentation of every element in shaded boxes and at least one element in each unshaded box from the single-organ-system examination.

The Documentation Guidelines

The following guidelines were developed jointly by the American Medical Association (AMA) and the Centers for Medicare and Medicaid Services (CMS). Their mutual goal was to provide physicians and claims reviewers with advice about preparing or reviewing documentation for Evaluation and Management (E/M) services.

I. Introduction

What is Documentation and Why Is It Important?

Medical record documentation is required to record pertinent facts, findings, and observations about an individual's health history, including past and present illnesses, examinations, tests, treatments, and outcomes. The medical record chronologically documents the care of the patient and is an important element contributing to high quality care. The medical record facilitates:

- The ability of the physician and other health care professionals to evaluate and plan the patient's immediate treatment and to monitor his/her health care over time
- Communication and continuity of care among physicians and other health care professionals involved in the patient's care
- Accurate and timely claims review and payment
- Appropriate utilization review and quality of care evaluations
- Collection of data that may be useful for research and education

An appropriately documented medical record can reduce many of the problems associated with claims processing and may serve as a legal document to verify the care provided, if necessary.

What Do Payers Want and Why?

Because payers have a contractual obligation to enrollees, they may require reasonable documentation that services are consistent with the insurance coverage provided. They may request information to validate:

- The site of service
- The medical necessity and appropriateness of the diagnostic and/or therapeutic services provided
- Services provided have been accurately reported

II. General Principles of Medical Record Documentation

The principles of documentation listed below are applicable to all types of medical and surgical services in all settings. For Evaluation and Management (E/M) services, the nature and amount of physician work and documentation varies by type of service, place of service, and the patient's status. The general principles listed below may be modified to account for these variable circumstances in providing E/M services.

- The medical record should be complete and legible
- The documentation of each patient encounter should include:
  - A reason for the encounter and relevant history, physical examination findings, and prior diagnostic test results
  - Assessment, clinical impression, or diagnosis
  - Plan for care
  - Date and legible identity of the practitioner
- If not documented, the rationale for ordering diagnostic and other ancillary services should be easily inferred
- Past and present diagnoses should be accessible to the treating and/or consulting physician
- Appropriate health risk factors should be identified
- The patient's progress, response to, and changes in treatment and revision of diagnosis should be documented
- The CPT and ICD-9-CM codes reported on the health insurance claim form or billing statement should be supported by the documentation in the medical record

III. *Documentation of E/M Services 1995 and 1997*

The following information provides definitions and documentation guidelines for the three key components of E/M services and for visits that consist predominately of counseling or coordination of care. The three key components—history, examination, and medical decision making—appear in the descriptors for office and other outpatient services, hospital observation services, hospital inpatient services, consultations, emergency department services, nursing facility services, domiciliary care services, and home services. While some of the text of the CPT guidelines has been repeated in this document, the reader should refer to CMS or CPT for the complete descriptors for E/M services and instructions for selecting a level of service. Documentation guidelines are identified by the symbol DG.

The descriptors for the levels of E/M services recognize seven components that are used in defining the levels of E/M services. These components are:

- History
- Examination
- Medical decision making
- Counseling
- Coordination of care
- Nature of presenting problem
- Time

The first three of these components (i.e., history, examination, and medical decision making) are the key components in selecting the level of E/M services. In the case of visits that consist predominately of counseling or coordination of care, time is the key or controlling factor to qualify for a particular level of E/M service.

Because the level of E/M service is dependent on two or three key components, performance and documentation of one component (e.g., examination) at the highest level does not necessarily mean that the encounter in its entirety qualifies for the highest level of E/M service.

These Documentation Guidelines for E/M services reflect the needs of the typical adult population. For certain groups of patients, the recorded information may vary slightly from that described here. Specifically, the medical records of infants, children, adolescents, and pregnant women may have additional or modified information, as appropriate, recorded in each history and examination area.

As an example, newborn records may include under history of the present illness (HPI) the details of the mother's pregnancy and the infant's status at birth; social history will focus on family structure; and family history will focus on congenital anomalies and hereditary disorders in the family. In addition, the content of a pediatric examination will vary with the age and development of the child. Although not specifically defined in these documentation guidelines, these patient group variations on history and examination are appropriate.

A. *Documentation of History*

The levels of E/M services are based on four types of history (Problem Focused, Expanded Problem Focused, Detailed, and Comprehensive). Each type of history includes some or all of the following elements:

- Chief complaint (CC)
- History of present illness (HPI)
- Review of systems (ROS)
- Past, family, and/or social history (PFSH)

The extent of history of present illness, review of systems, and past, family, and/or social history that is obtained and documented is dependent upon clinical judgment and the nature of the presenting problem.

The chart below shows the progression of the elements required for each type of history. To qualify for a given type of history all three elements in the table must be met. (A chief complaint is indicated at all levels.)

- DG: The CC, ROS, and PFSH may be listed as separate elements of history or they may be included in the description of the history of present illness

- DG: A ROS and/or a PFSH obtained during an earlier encounter does not need to be re-recorded if there is evidence that the physician reviewed and updated the previous information. This may occur when a physician updates his/her own record or in an institutional setting or group practice where many physicians use a common record. The review and update may be documented by:
  - Describing any new ROS and/or PFSH information or noting there has been no change in the information
  - Noting the date and location of the earlier ROS and/or PFSH

- DG: The ROS and/or PFSH may be recorded by ancillary staff or on a form completed by the patient. To document that the physician reviewed the information, there must be a notation supplementing or confirming the information recorded by others

- DG: If the physician is unable to obtain a history from the patient or other source, the record should describe the patient's condition or other circumstance that precludes obtaining a history

Definitions and specific documentation guidelines for each of the elements of history are listed below.

Chief Complaint (CC)

The CC is a concise statement describing the symptom, problem, condition, diagnosis, physician recommended return, or other factor that is the reason for the encounter, usually stated in the patient's words.

- DG: The medical record should clearly reflect the chief complaint

History of Present Illness (HPI)

The HPI is a chronological description of the development of the patient's present illness from the first sign and/or symptom or from the previous encounter to the present. It includes the following elements:

- Location
- Quality
- Severity
- Duration
- Timing
- Context
- Modifying factors
- Associated signs and symptoms

Brief and extended HPIs are distinguished by the amount of detail needed to accurately characterize the clinical problem.

A brief HPI consists of one to three elements of the HPI.

- DG: The medical record should describe one to three elements of the present illness (HPI)

An extended HPI consists of at least four elements of the HPI or the status of at least three chronic or inactive conditions.

- DG: The medical record should describe at least four elements of the present illness (HPI) or the status of at least three chronic or inactive conditions

Beginning with services performed on or after September 10, 2013, CMS has stated that physicians and OQHCP will be able to use the 1997 guidelines for an extended history of present illness (HPI) in combination with other elements from the 1995 documentation guidelines to document a particular level of evaluation and management service.

History of Present Illness	Review of systems (ROS)	PFSH	Type of History
Brief	N/A	N/A	Problem-focused
Brief	Problem Pertinent	N/A	Expanded Problem-Focused
Extended	Extended	Pertinent	Detailed
Extended	Complete	Complete	Comprehensive

Review of Systems (ROS)

A ROS is an inventory of body systems obtained through a series of questions seeking to identify signs and/or symptoms that the patient may be experiencing or has experienced. For purposes of ROS, the following systems are recognized:

- Constitutional symptoms (e.g., fever, weight loss)
- Eyes
- Ears, nose, mouth, throat
- Cardiovascular
- Respiratory
- Gastrointestinal
- Genitourinary
- Musculoskeletal
- Integumentary (skin and/or breast)
- Neurological
- Psychiatric
- Endocrine
- Hematologic/lymphatic
- Allergic/immunologic

A problem pertinent ROS inquires about the system directly related to the problem identified in the HPI.

- DG: The patient's positive responses and pertinent negatives for the system related to the problem should be documented

An extended ROS inquires about the system directly related to the problem identified in the HPI and a limited number of additional systems.

- DG: The patient's positive responses and pertinent negatives for two to nine systems should be documented

A complete ROS inquires about the system directly related to the problem identified in the HPI plus all additional body systems.

- DG: At least 10 organ systems must be reviewed. Those systems with positive or pertinent negative responses must be individually documented. For the remaining systems, a notation indicating all other systems are negative is permissible. In the absence of such a notation, at least 10 systems must be individually documented

Past, Family, and/or Social History (PFSH)

The PFSH consists of a review of three areas:

- Past history (the patient's past experiences with illnesses, operations, injuries, and treatment)
- Family history (a review of medical events in the patient's family, including diseases that may be hereditary or place the patient at risk)
- Social history (an age appropriate review of past and current activities)

For certain categories of E/M services that include only an interval history, it is not necessary to record information about the PFSH. Those categories are subsequent hospital care, follow-up inpatient consultations, and subsequent nursing facility care.

A pertinent PFSH is a review of the history area directly related to the problem identified in the HPI.

- DG: At least one specific item from any of the three history areas must be documented for a pertinent PFSH

A complete PFSH is a review of two or all three of the PFSH history areas, depending on the category of the E/M service. A review of all three history areas is required for services that by their nature include a comprehensive assessment or reassessment of the patient. A review of two of the three history areas is sufficient for other services.

- DG: A least one specific item from two of the three history areas must be documented for a complete PFSH for the following categories of E/M services: office or other outpatient services, established patient; emergency department; domiciliary care, established patient; and home care, established patient

- DG: At least one specific item from each of the three history areas must be documented for a complete PFSH for the following categories of E/M services: office or other outpatient services, new patient; hospital observation services; hospital inpatient services, initial care; consultations; comprehensive nursing facility assessments; domiciliary care, new patient; and home care, new patient

B. *Documentation of Examination 1997 Guidelines*

The levels of E/M services are based on four types of examination:

- Problem Focused: A limited examination of the affected body area or organ system
- Expanded Problem Focused: A limited examination of the affected body area or organ system and any other symptomatic or related body area or organ system
- Detailed: An extended examination of the affected body area or organ system and any other symptomatic or related body area or organ system
- Comprehensive: A general multi-system examination or complete examination of a single organ system and other symptomatic or related body area or organ system

These types of examinations have been defined for general multi-system and the following single organ systems:

- Cardiovascular
- Ears, nose, mouth, and throat
- Eyes
- Genitourinary (Female)
- Genitourinary (Male)
- Hematologic/lymphatic/immunologic
- Musculoskeletal
- Neurological
- Psychiatric
- Respiratory
- Skin

Any physician regardless of specialty may perform a general multi-system examination or any of the single organ system examinations. The type (general multi-system or single organ system) and content of examination are selected by the examining physician and are based upon clinical judgment, the patient's history, and the nature of the presenting problem.

The content and documentation requirements for each type and level of examination are summarized below and described in detail in a table found later on in this document. In the table, organ systems and body areas recognized by CPT for purposes of describing examinations are shown in the left column. The content, or individual elements, of the examination pertaining to that body area or organ system are identified by bullets (•) in the right column.

Parenthetical examples "(e.g., ...)," have been used for clarification and to provide guidance regarding documentation. Documentation for each element must satisfy any numeric requirements (such as "Measurement of any three of the following seven...") included in the description of the element. Elements with multiple components but with no specific numeric requirement (such as "Examination of liver and spleen") require documentation of at least one component. It is possible for a given examination to be expanded beyond what is defined here. When that occurs, findings related to the additional systems and/or areas should be documented.

•	DG:	Specific abnormal and relevant negative findings from the examination of the affected or symptomatic body area or organ system should be documented. A notation of "abnormal" without elaboration is insufficient
•	DG:	Abnormal or unexpected findings from the examination of any asymptomatic body area or organ system should be described
•	DG:	A brief statement or notation indicating "negative" or "normal" is sufficient to document normal findings related to an unaffected areas or asymptomatic organ system

General Multi-System Examinations

General multi-system examinations are described in detail later in this document. To qualify for a given level of multi-system examination, the following content and documentation requirements should be met:

- Problem Focused Examination: It should include performance and documentation of one to five elements identified by a bullet (•) in one or more organ systems or body areas
- Expanded Problem Focused Examination: It should include performance and documentation of at least six elements identified by a bullet (•) in one or more organ systems or body areas
- Detailed Examination: It should include at least six organ systems or body areas. For each system/area selected, performance and documentation of at least two elements identified by a bullet (•) is expected. Alternatively, a detailed examination may include performance and documentation of at least 12 elements identified by a bullet (•) in two or more organ systems or body areas
- Comprehensive Examination: It should include at least nine organ systems or body areas. For each system/area selected, all elements of the examination identified by a bullet (•) should be performed, unless specific directions limit the content of the examination. For each area/system, documentation of at least two elements identified by a bullet (•) is expected

Single Organ System Examinations

The single organ system examinations recognized by CMS include eyes; ears, nose, mouth, and throat; cardiovascular; respiratory; genitourinary (male and female); musculoskeletal; neurologic; hematologic, lymphatic, and immunologic; skin; and psychiatric. Note that for each specific single organ examination type, the performance and documentation of the stated number of elements, identified by a bullet (•) should be included, whether in a box with a shaded or unshaded border. The following content and documentation requirements must be met to qualify for a given level:

- Problem Focused Examination: one to five elements
- Expanded Problem Focused Examination: at least six elements
- Detailed Examination: at least 12 elements (other than eye and psychiatric examinations)
- Comprehensive Examination: all elements (Documentation of every element in a box with a shaded border and at least one element in a box with an unshaded border is expected)

Content and Documentation Requirements

General Multisystem Examination 1997

System/Body Area	Elements of Examination
Constitutional	• Measurement of any three of the following seven vital signs: 1) sitting or standing blood pressure, 2) supine blood pressure, 3) pulse rate and regularity, 4) respiration, 5) temperature, 6) height, 7) weight (May be measured and recorded by ancillary staff). • General appearance of patient (e.g., development, nutrition, body habitus, deformities attention to grooming)
Eyes	• Inspection of conjunctivae and lids • Examination of pupils and irises (e.g., reaction to light and accommodation, size and symmetry) • Ophthalmoscopic examination of optic discs (e.g., size, C/D ratio, appearance) and posterior segments (e.g., vessel changes, exudates, hemorrhages)
Ears, nose, mouth, and throat	• External inspection of ears and nose (e.g., overall appearance, scars, lesions, masses) • Otoscopic examination of external auditory canals and tympanic membranes • Assessment of hearing (e.g., whispered voice, finger rub, tuning fork) • Inspection of nasal mucosa, septum and turbinates • Inspection of lips, teeth and gums • Examination of oropharynx: oral mucosa, salivary glands, hard and soft palates, tongue, tonsils and posterior pharynx
Neck	• Examination of neck (e.g., masses, overall appearance, symmetry, tracheal position, crepitus) • Examination of thyroid (e.g., enlargement, tenderness, mass)
Respiratory	• Assessment of respiratory effort (e.g., intercostal retractions, use of accessory muscles, diaphragmatic movement) • Percussion of chest (e.g., dullness, flatness, hyperresonance) • Palpation of chest (e.g., tactile fremitus) • Auscultation of lungs (e.g., breath sounds, adventitious sounds, rubs)
Cardiovascular	• Palpation of heart (e.g., location, size, thrills) • Auscultation of heart with notation of abnormal sounds and murmurs • Examination of: — carotid arteries (e.g., pulse amplitude, bruits) — abdominal aorta (e.g., size, bruits) — femoral arteries (e.g., pulse amplitude, bruits) — pedal pulses (e.g., pulse amplitude) — extremities for edema and/or varicosities
Chest (Breasts)	• Inspection of breasts (e.g., symmetry, nipple discharge) • Palpation of breasts and axillae (e.g., masses or lumps, tenderness)
Gastrointestinal (Abdomen)	• Examination of abdomen with notation of presence of masses or tenderness • Examination of liver and spleen • Examination for presence or absence of hernia • Examination (when indicated) of anus, perineum and rectum, including sphincter tone, presence of hemorrhoids, rectal masses • Obtain stool sample for occult blood test when indicated

System/Body Area	Elements of Examination
Genitourinary	**Male:** • Examination of the scrotal contents (e.g., hydrocele, spermatocele, tenderness of cord, testicular mass) • Examination of the penis • Digital rectal examination of prostate gland (e.g., size, symmetry, nodularity tenderness) **Female**: • Pelvic examination (with or without specimen collection for smears and cultures), including: — examination of external genitalia (e.g., general appearance, hair distribution, lesions) and vagina (e.g., general appearance, estrogen effect, discharge, lesions, pelvic support, cystocele, rectocele) — examination of urethra (e.g., masses, tenderness, scarring) — examination of bladder (e.g., fullness, masses, tenderness) • Cervix (e.g., general appearance, lesions, discharge) • Uterus (e.g., size, contour, position, mobility, tenderness, consistency, descent or support) • Adnexa/parametria (e.g., masses, tenderness)
Lymphatic	Palpation of lymph nodes in **two or more** areas: • Neck • Groin • Axillae • Other
Musculoskeletal	• Examination of gait and station *(if circled, add to total at bottom of column to the left) • Inspection and/or palpation of digits and nails (e.g., clubbing, cyanosis, inflammatory conditions, petechiae, ischemia, infections, nodes) *(if circled, add to total at bottom of column to the left) Examination of joints, bones and muscles of **one or more of the following six** areas: 1) head and neck; 2) spine, ribs, and pelvis; 3) right upper extremity; 4) left upper extremity; 5) right lower extremity; and 6) left lower extremity. The examination of a given area includes: • Inspection and/or palpation with notation of presence of any misalignment, asymmetry, crepitation, defects, tenderness, masses, effusions • Assessment of range of motion with notation of any pain, crepitation or contracture • Assessment of stability with notation of any dislocation (luxation), subluxation, or laxity • Assessment of muscle strength and tone (e.g., flaccid, cog wheel, spastic) with notation of any atrophy or abnormal movements
Skin	• Inspection of skin and subcutaneous tissue (e.g., rashes, lesions, ulcers) • Palpation of skin and subcutaneous tissue (e.g., induration, subcutaneous nodules, tightening)
Neurologic	• Test cranial nerves with notation of any deficits • Examination of deep tendon reflexes with notation of pathological reflexes (e.g., Babinski) • Examination of sensation (e.g., by touch, pin, vibration, proprioception)
Psychiatric	• Description of patient's judgment and insight • Brief assessment of mental status including: — Orientation to time, place and person — Recent and remote memory — Mood and affect (e.g., depression, anxiety, agitation)

Content and Documentation Requirements

Level of exam	Perform and document
Problem focused	**One to five** elements identified by a bullet
Expanded problem focused	**At least six** elements identified by a bullet
Detailed	**At least 12** elements identified by a bullet, whether in a box with a shaded or unshaded border
Comprehensive	Performance of **all** elements identified by a bullet; whether in a box or with a shaded or unshaded box. Documentation of every element in each with a shaded border and at least one element in a box with an unshaded border is expected

Number of Diagnoses or Management Options	Amount and/or Complexity of Data to be Reviewed	Risk of Complications and/or Morbidity or Mortality	Type of Decision Making
Minimal	Minimal or None	Minimal	Straightforward
Limited	Limited	Low	Low Complexity
Multiple	Moderate	Moderate	Moderate Complexity
Extensive	Extensive	High	High Complexity

C. *Documentation of the Complexity of Medical Decision Making 1995 and 1997*

The levels of E/M services recognize four types of medical decision-making (straightforward, low complexity, moderate complexity, and high complexity). Medical decision-making refers to the complexity of establishing a diagnosis and/or selecting a management option as measured by:

- The number of possible diagnoses and/or the number of management options that must be considered
- The amount and/or complexity of medical records, diagnostic tests, and/or other information that must be obtained, reviewed, and analyzed
- The risk of significant complications, morbidity, and/or mortality, as well as comorbidities, associated with the patient's presenting problem, the diagnostic procedure, and/or the possible management options

The following chart shows the progression of the elements required for each level of medical decision-making. To qualify for a given type of decision-making, two of the three elements in the table must be either met or exceeded.

Each of the elements of medical decision-making is described below.

Number of Diagnoses or Management Options

The number of possible diagnoses and/or the number of management options that must be considered is based on the number and types of problems addressed during the encounter, the complexity of establishing a diagnosis, and the management decisions that are made by the physician.

Generally, decision making with respect to a diagnosed problem is easier than that for an identified but undiagnosed problem. The number and type of diagnostic tests employed may be an indicator of the number of possible diagnoses. Problems that are improving or resolving are less complex than those that are worsening or failing to change as expected. The need to seek advice from others is another indicator of complexity of diagnostic or management problems.

- DG: For each encounter, an assessment, clinical impression, or diagnosis should be documented. It may be explicitly stated or implied in documented decisions regarding management plans and/or further evaluation
  - For a presenting problem with an established diagnosis, the record should reflect whether the problem is: a) improved, well controlled, resolving, or resolved; or b) inadequately controlled, worsening, or failing to change as expected
  - For a presenting problem without an established diagnosis, the assessment or clinical impression may be stated in the form of a differential diagnosis or as a "possible," "probable," or "rule-out" (R/O) diagnosis
- DG: The initiation of, or changes in, treatment should be documented. Treatment includes a wide range of management options including patient instructions, nursing instructions, therapies, and medications
- DG: If referrals are made, consultations requested, or advice sought, the record should indicate to whom or where the referral or consultation is made or from whom the advice is requested

Amount and/or Complexity of Data to be Reviewed

The amount and complexity of data to be reviewed is based on the types of diagnostic testing ordered or reviewed. A decision to obtain and review old medical records and/or obtain history from sources other than the patient increases the amount and complexity of data to be reviewed.

Discussion of contradictory or unexpected test results with the physician who performed or interpreted the test is an indication of the complexity of data being reviewed. On occasion, the physician who ordered a test may personally review the image, tracing, or specimen to supplement information from the physician who prepared the test report or interpretation; this is another indication of the complexity of data being reviewed.

- DG: If a diagnostic service (test or procedure) is ordered, planned, scheduled, or performed at the time of the E/M encounter, the type of service (e.g., lab or x-ray) should be documented
- DG: The review of lab, radiology, and/or other diagnostic tests should be documented. A simple notation such as WBC elevated" or "chest x-ray unremarkable" is acceptable. Alternatively, the review may be documented by initialing and dating the report containing the test results
- DG: A decision to obtain old records or a decision to obtain additional history from the family, caretaker, or other source to supplement that obtained from the patient should be documented
- DG: Relevant findings from the review of old records and/or the receipt of additional history from the family, caretaker, or other source to supplement that obtained from the patient should be documented. If there is no relevant information beyond that already obtained, that fact should be documented. A notation of "old records reviewed" or "additional history obtained from family" without elaboration is insufficient
- DG: The results of discussion of laboratory, radiology, or other diagnostic tests with the physician who performed or interpreted the study should be documented
- DG: The direct visualization and independent interpretation of an image, tracing, or specimen previously or subsequently interpreted by another physician should be documented

Risk of Significant Complications, Morbidity, and/or Mortality

The risk of significant complications, morbidity, and/or mortality is based on the risks associated with the presenting problem, the diagnostic procedure, and the possible management options.

- DG: Comorbidities/underlying disease or other factors that increase the complexity of medical decision making by increasing the risk of complications, morbidity, and/or mortality should be documented
- DG: If a surgical or invasive diagnostic procedure is ordered, planned, or scheduled at the time of the E/M encounter, the type of procedure (e.g., laparoscopy) should be documented
- DG: If a surgical or invasive diagnostic procedure is performed at the time of the E/M encounter, the specific procedure should be documented
- DG: The referral for or decision to perform a surgical or invasive diagnostic procedure on an urgent basis should be documented or implied

The following Table of Risk may be used to help determine whether the risk of significant complications, morbidity, and/or mortality is minimal, low, moderate, or high. Because the determination of risk is complex and not readily quantifiable, the table includes common clinical examples rather than absolute measures of risk. The assessment of risk of the presenting problem is based on the risk related to the disease process anticipated between the present encounter and the next one. The assessment of risk of selecting diagnostic procedures and management options is based on the risk during and immediately following any procedures or treatment. The highest level of risk in any one category (presenting problem, diagnostic procedure, or management options) determines the overall risk.

Table of Risk

Level of Risk	Presenting Problem(s)	Diagnostic Procedure(s) Ordered	Management Options Selected
Minimal	One self-limited or minor problem (e.g., cold, insect bite, tinea corporis)	Laboratory test requiring venipuncture Chest x-rays EKG/EEG Urinalysis Ultrasound (e.g., echocardiography) KOH prep	Rest Gargles Elastic bandages Superficial dressings
Low	Two or more self-limited or minor problems One stable chronic illness (e.g., well controlled hypertension, non-insulin dependent diabetes, cataract, BPH) Acute, uncomplicated illness or injury (e.g., cystitis, allergic rhinitis, simple sprain)	Physiologic tests not under stress (e.g., pulmonary function tests) Non-cardiovascular imaging studies with contrast (e.g., barium enema) Superficial needle biopsies Clinical laboratory tests requiring arterial puncture Skin biopsies	Over-the-counter drugs Minor surgery with no identified risk factors Physical therapy Occupational therapy IV fluids without additives
Moderate	One or more chronic illnesses with mild exacerbation, progression or side effects of treatment Two or more stable chronic illnesses Undiagnosed new problem with uncertain prognosis (e.g., lump in breast) Acute illness with systemic symptoms (e.g., pyelonephritis, pneumonitis, colitis) Acute complicated injury (e.g., head injury with brief loss of consciousness)	Physiologic tests not under stress (e.g., cardiac stress test, fetal contraction stress test) Diagnostic endoscopies with no identified risk factors Deep needle or incisional biopsy Cardiovascular imaging studies with contrast and no identified risk factors (e.g., arteriogram, cardiac catheterization) Obtain fluid from body cavity (e.g., lumbar puncture, thoracentesis, culdocentesis)	Minor surgery with identified risk factors Effective major surgery (open, percutaneous or endoscopic) with no identified risk factors Prescription drug management Therapeutic nuclear medicine IV fluids with additives Closed treatment of fracture or dislocation without manipulation
High	One or more chronic illnesses with severe exacerbation, progression or side effects of treatment Acute/chronic illnesses that may pose a threat to life or bodily function (e.g., multiple trauma, acute MI, pulmonary embolus, severe respiratory distress, progressive severe rheumatoid arthritis, psychiatric illness with potential threat to self or others, peritonitis, acute renal failure An abrupt change in neurologic status (e.g., seizure, TIA, weakness or sensory loss)	Cardiovascular imaging studies with contrast with identified risk factors Cardiac electrophysiological tests Diagnostic endoscopies with identified risk factors Discography	Elective major surgery (open, percutaneous or endoscopic) with identified risk factors Emergency major surgery (open, percutaneous or endoscopic) Parenteral controlled substances Drug therapy requiring intensive monitoring for toxicity Decision not to resuscitate or to de-escalate care because of poor prognosis

D. Documentation of an Encounter Dominated by Counseling or Coordination of Care

In the case where counseling and/or coordination of care dominates (more than 50 percent) the physician/patient and/or family encounter (face-to-face time in the office or other outpatient setting or floor-unit time in the hospital or nursing facility), time is considered the key or controlling factor to qualify for a particular level of E/M service.

- DG: If the physician elects to report the level of service based on counseling and/or coordination of care, the total length of time of the encounter (face-to-face or floor time, as appropriate) should be documented and the record should describe the counseling and/or activities to coordinate care

Appendix D — Crosswalk of Deleted Codes

The deleted code crosswalk is meant to be used as a reference tool to find active codes that could be used in place of the deleted code. This will not always be an exact match. Please review the code descriptions and guidelines before selecting a code.

Code	Cross reference
0058T	To report, see 89398
0085T	To report, see 84999
0111T	To report, see 82726
0126T	To report, see 93998
0228T	To report, see 64999
0229T	To report, see 64999
0230T	To report, see 64999
0231T	To report, see 64999
0295T	To report, see [93241, 93242, 93243, 93244, 93245, 93246, 93247, 93248]
0296T	To report, see [93241, 93242, 93243, 93244, 93245, 93246, 93247, 93248]
0297T	To report, see [93241, 93242, 93243, 93244, 93245, 93246, 93247, 93248]
0298T	To report, see [93241, 93242, 93243, 93244, 93245, 93246, 93247, 93248]
0381T	To report, see 95999
0382T	To report, see 95999
0383T	To report, see 95999
0384T	To report, see 95999
0385T	To report, see 95999
0386T	To report, see 95999
0396T	To report, see 27599
0400T	To report, see 96999
0401T	To report, see 96999
0405T	To report, see 99499
19324	To report, see 15771-15772
32405	To report, see 32408
87450	To report, see 87301-87451, 87802-87899 [87806, 87811]
92585	To report, see 92652-92653
92586	To report, see 92650-92651
99201	To report, see 99202

Appendix E — Resequenced Codes

This appendix contains a list of codes that are not in numeric order in the book. AMA resequenced some code numbers to relocate codes in the same category but not in numeric sequence. In addition to the list of resequenced codes, the page number where the code may be found is provided for ease of use.

Code	Page	Reference
10004	13	See code following 10021.
10005	13	See code following 10021.
10006	13	See code following 10021.
10007	13	See code following 10021.
10008	13	See code following 10021.
10009	13	See code following 10021.
10010	13	See code following 10021.
10011	13	See code following 10021.
10012	13	See code following 10021.
11045	15	See code following 11042.
11046	15	See code following 11043.
15769	28	See code following 15770.
20560	40	See code following 20553.
20561	40	See code before 20555.
21552	51	See code following 21555.
21554	51	See code following 21556.
22858	61	See code following 22856.
22859	60	See code following 22854.
23071	63	See code following 23075.
23073	63	See code following 23076.
24071	66	See code following 24075.
24073	66	See code following 24076.
25071	70	See code following 25075.
25073	70	See code following 25076.
26111	76	See code following 26115.
26113	76	See code following 26116.
27043	82	See code following 27047.
27045	82	See code following 27048.
27059	83	See code following 27049.
27329	88	See code following 27360.
27337	87	See code following 27327.
27339	87	See code before 27330.
27632	93	See code following 27618.
27634	93	See code following 27619.
28039	97	See code following 28043.
28041	97	See code following 28045.
28295	100	See code following 28296.
29914	107	See code following 29863.
29915	107	See code following 29863.
29916	107	See code before 29866.
31253	112	See code following 31255.
31257	112	See code following 31255.
31259	112	See code following 31255.
31551	116	See code following 31580.
31552	116	See code following 31580.
31553	116	See code following 31580.
31554	116	See code following 31580.
31572	116	See code following 31578.

Code	Page	Reference
31573	116	See code following 31578.
31574	116	See code following 31578.
31651	118	See code following 31647.
32994	124	See code following 32998.
33221	127	See code following 33213.
33227	128	See code following 33233.
33228	128	See code following 33233.
33229	128	See code before 33234.
33230	129	See code following 33240.
33231	129	See code before 33241.
33262	129	See code following 33241.
33263	130	See code following 33241.
33264	130	See code before 33243.
33270	130	See code following 33249.
33271	130	See code following 33249.
33272	130	See code following 33249.
33273	131	See code following 33249.
33274	131	See code following 33249.
33275	131	See code following 33249.
33440	134	See code following 33410.
33962	145	See code following 33959.
33963	146	See code following 33959.
33964	146	See code following 33959.
33965	146	See code following 33959.
33966	146	See code following 33959.
33969	146	See code following 33959.
33984	146	See code following 33959.
33985	146	See code following 33959.
33986	146	See code following 33959.
33987	146	See code following 33959.
33988	146	See code following 33959.
33989	146	See code following 33959.
33995	148	See code following 33983.
33997	148	See code following 33992.
34717	150	See code following 34708.
34718	151	See code following 34709.
34812	151	See code following 34713.
34820	151	See code following 34714.
34833	152	See code following 34714.
34834	152	See code following 34714.
36465	164	See code following 36471.
36466	164	See code following 36471.
36482	165	See code following 36479.
36483	165	See code following 36479.
36572	167	See code following 36569.
36573	167	See code following 36569.
37246	174	See code following 37235.
37247	175	See code following 37235.

Code	Page	Reference
37248	175	See code following 37235.
37249	175	See code following 37235.
38243	179	See code following 38241.
43210	195	See code following 43259.
43211	192	See code following 43217.
43212	192	See code following 43217.
43213	192	See code following 43220.
43214	192	See code following 43220.
43233	195	See code following 43249.
43266	195	See code following 43255.
43270	195	See code following 43257.
43274	197	See code following numeric code 43270.
43275	197	See code following numeric code 43270.
43276	197	See code following numeric code 43270.
43277	197	See code following numeric code 43270.
43278	197	See code following numeric code 43270.
44381	208	See code following 44382.
44401	208	See code following 44392.
45346	212	See code following 45338.
45388	213	See code following 45382.
45390	214	See code following 45392.
45398	214	See code following 45393.
45399	215	See code before 45990.
46220	216	See code before 46230.
46320	216	See code following 46230.
46945	215	See code following 46221.
46946	216	See code following resequenced code 46945.
46947	218	See code following 46761.
46948	216	See code before resequenced code 46220.
50430	235	See code following 50396.
50431	236	See code following 50396.
50432	236	See code following 50396.
50433	236	See code following 50396.
50434	236	See code following 50396.
50435	236	See code following 50396.
50436	235	See code following 50391.
50437	235	See code following 50391.
51797	242	See code following 51729.
52356	246	See code following 52353.
58674	264	See code before 58541.
62328	289	See code following 62270.
62329	289	See code following 62272.
64461	300	See code following 64484.

Code	Page	Reference
64462	300	See code following 64484.
64463	300	See code following 64484.
64624	302	See code following 64610.
64625	302	See code before 64611.
64633	303	See code following 64620.
64634	303	See code following 64620.
64635	303	See code following 64620.
64636	303	See code before 64630.
66987	314	See code following 66982.
66988	314	See code following 66984.
67810	319	See code following 67715.
77085	352	See code following 77081.
77086	352	See code before 77084.
77295	353	See code before 77300.
77385	364	See code following 77417.
77386	354	See code following 77417.
77387	354	See code following 77417.
77424	354	See code following 77417.
77425	354	See code following 77417.
78429	359	See code following 78459.
78430	359	See code following 78491.
78431	359	See code following 78492.
78432	359	See code following 78492.
78433	359	See code following 78492.
78434	359	See code following 78492.
78804	361	See code following 78802.
78830	361	See code following numeric code 78804.
78831	361	See code following numeric code 78804.
78832	361	See code following numeric code 78804.
78835	361	See code following numeric code 78804.
80081	363	See code following 80055.
80161	366	See code following 80157.
80164	367	See code following 80201.
80165	367	See code following 80201.
80167	366	See code following 80169.
80171	366	See code before 80170.
80176	366	See code following 80177.
80179	367	See code before 80195.
80181	366	See code following resequenced code 80167.
80189	366	See code following resequenced code 80230.
80193	366	See code before 80177.
80204	367	See code following 80178.
80210	367	See code following 80194.
80230	366	See code following 80173.
80235	366	See code before 80175.
80280	367	See code following 80202.
80285	367	See code before 80203.
80305	364	See code before 80143.
80306	364	See code before 80143.
80307	364	See code before 80143.

Code	Page	Reference
80320	364	See code before 80143.
80321	364	See code before 80143.
80322	364	See code before 80143.
80323	364	See code before 80143.
80324	364	See code before 80143.
80325	364	See code before 80143.
80326	364	See code before 80143.
80327	364	See code before 80143.
80328	364	See code before 80143.
80329	364	See code before 80143.
80330	364	See code before 80143.
80331	364	See code before 80143.
80332	364	See code before 80143.
80333	365	See code before 80143.
80334	365	See code before 80143.
80335	365	See code before 80143.
80336	365	See code before 80143.
80337	365	See code before 80143.
80338	365	See code before 80143.
80339	365	See code before 80143.
80340	365	See code before 80145.
80341	365	See code before 80143.
80342	365	See code before 80143.
80343	365	See code before 80143.
80344	365	See code before 80143.
80345	365	See code before 80143.
80346	365	See code before 80143.
80347	365	See code before 80143.
80348	365	See code before 80143.
80349	365	See code before 80143.
80350	365	See code before 80143.
80351	365	See code before 80143.
80352	365	See code before 80143.
80353	365	See code before 80143.
80354	365	See code before 80143.
80355	365	See code before 80143.
80356	365	See code before 80143.
80357	365	See code before 80143.
80358	365	See code before 80143.
80359	365	See code before 80143.
80360	365	See code before 80143.
80361	365	See code before 80143.
80362	365	See code before 80143.
80363	365	See code before 80143.
80364	365	See code before 80143.
80365	365	See code before 80143.
80366	365	See code before 80143.
80367	365	See code before 80143.
80368	365	See code before 80143.
80369	365	See code before 80143.
80370	365	See code before 80143.
80371	366	See code before 80143.
80372	366	See code before 80143.
80373	366	See code before 80143.

Code	Page	Reference
80374	366	See code before 80143.
80375	366	See code before 80143.
80376	366	See code before 80143.
80377	366	See code before 80143.
81105	375	See code before 81260.
81106	375	See code before 81260.
81107	375	See code before 81260.
81108	375	See code before 81260.
81109	375	See code before 81260.
81110	375	See code before 81260.
81111	375	See code before 81260.
81112	375	See code before 81260.
81120	375	See code before 81260.
81121	375	See code before 81260.
81161	373	See code following numeric code 81231.
81162	371	See code following resequenced code 81210.
81163	371	See code following resequenced code 81210.
81164	371	See code before 81212.
81165	372	See code following 81212.
81166	372	See code following 81212.
81167	372	See code following 81216.
81168	372	See code before 81218.
81173	370	See code following resequenced code 81204.
81174	370	See code following resequenced code 81204.
81184	372	See code following resequenced code 81233.
81185	372	See code following resequenced code 81233.
81186	372	See code following resequenced code 81233.
81187	372	See code following resequenced code 81268.
81188	373	See code following resequenced code 81266.
81189	373	See code following resequenced code 81266.
81190	373	See code following resequenced code 81266.
81191	377	See code following numeric code 81312.
81192	377	See code following numeric code 81312.
81193	377	See code following numeric code 81312.
81194	377	See code following numeric code 81312.
81200	370	See code before 81175.
81201	370	See code following numeric code 81174.
81202	370	See code following numeric code 81174.
81203	370	See code following numeric code 81174.

Code	Page	Reference
81204	370	See code following numeric code 81174.
81205	371	See code following numeric code 81210.
81206	371	See code following numeric code 81210.
81207	371	See code following numeric code 81210.
81208	371	See code following numeric code 81210.
81209	371	See code following numeric code 81210.
81210	371	See code following numeric code 81210.
81219	372	See code before 81218.
81227	373	See code before 81225.
81230	373	See code following numeric code 81227.
81231	373	See code following numeric code 81227.
81233	372	See code following 81217.
81234	373	See code following numeric code 81231.
81238	373	See code following 81241.
81239	373	See code before 81232.
81245	374	See code following 81242.
81246	374	See code following 81242.
81250	374	See code before 81247.
81257	374	See code following 81254.
81258	374	See code following 81254.
81259	374	See code following 81254.
81261	375	See code before 81260.
81262	375	See code before 81260.
81263	375	See code before 81260.
81264	375	See code before 81260.
81265	372	See code following resequenced code 81187.
81266	372	See code following resequenced code 81187.
81267	372	See code following 81224.
81268	372	See code following 81224.
81269	374	See code following resequenced code 81259.
81271	375	See code following numeric code 81259.
81274	375	See code following resequenced code 81271.
81277	373	See code following 81229.
81278	375	See code following resequenced code 81263.
81279	375	See code following 81270.
81283	375	See code following resequenced code 81121.
81284	374	See code following numeric code 81246.
81285	374	See code following numeric code 81246.
81286	374	See code following numeric code 81246.
81287	376	See code following resequenced code 81304.
81288	376	See code following resequenced code 81292.
81289	374	See code following numeric code 81246.
81291	377	See code before 81305.
81292	376	See code before numeric code 81291.
81293	376	See code before numeric code 81291.
81294	376	See code before numeric code 81291.
81295	376	See code before numeric code 81291.
81301	376	See code following resequenced code 81287.
81302	376	See code following 81290.
81303	376	See code following 81290.
81304	376	See code following 81290.
81306	377	See code following resequenced code 81194.
81307	377	See code before 81313.
81308	377	See code before 81313.
81309	377	See code following 81314.
81312	377	See code before resequenced code 81307.
81320	377	See code before 81315.
81324	377	See code following 81316.
81325	377	See code following 81316.
81326	377	See code following 81316.
81332	378	See code following 81327.
81334	378	See code following numeric code 81326.
81336	378	See code following 81329.
81337	378	See code following 81329.
81338	376	See code following resequenced code 81294.
81339	376	See code before resequenced code 81295.
81343	377	See code following numeric code 81320.
81344	378	See code following numeric code 81332.
81345	378	See code following numeric code 81332.
81347	378	See code before 81328.
81348	378	See code following numeric code 81312.
81351	378	See code before 81335.
81352	378	See code before 81335.
81353	378	See code before 81335.
81357	379	See code before 81350.
81361	374	See code following 81254.
81362	374	See code following 81254.
81363	374	See code following 81254.
81364	374	See code following 81254.
81419	391	See code following 81414.
81443	391	See code following 81422.
81448	392	See code following 81438.
81479	391	See code following 81408.
81500	394	See code following 81538.
81503	394	See code before 81539.
81504	395	See code following resequenced code 81546.
81522	394	See code following 81518.
81540	395	See code before 81552.
81546	395	See code following 81551.
81595	393	See code following 81490.
81596	394	See code following 81514.
82042	396	See code following 82045.
82652	397	See code following 82306.
82681	400	See code following 82670.
83992	365	See code following resequenced code 80365.
86152	415	See code following 86147.
86153	415	See code before 86148.
86328	416	See code following 86318.
86408	417	See code following 86382.
86409	417	See code following 86382.
86413	417	See code following resequenced code 86409.
87623	428	See code following 87539.
87624	428	See code following 87539.
87625	428	See code before 87540.
87806	430	See code following 87803.
87811	430	See code following 87807.
87906	430	See code following 87901.
87910	430	See code following 87900.
87912	430	See code before 87902.
88177	432	See code following 88173.
88341	436	See code following 88342.
88350	436	See code following 88346.
88364	437	See code following 88365.
88373	437	See code following 88367.
88374	437	See code following 88367.
88377	437	See code following 88369.
90619	457	See code following 90734.
90620	457	See code following 90734.
90621	457	See code following 90734.
90625	457	See code following 90723.
90630	455	See code following 90654.
90644	457	See code following 90732.
90672	455	See code following 90660.
90673	455	See code before 90662.
90674	455	See code following 90661.
90694	456	See code following 90689.
90750	458	See code following 90736.
90756	455	See code following 90661.
92517	470	See code following 92549.
92518	470	See code following 92549.
92519	470	See code following 92549.
92558	471	See code before 92587.

Code	Page	Reference
92597	472	See code following 92604.
92618	472	See code following 92605.
92650	471	See code following 92584.
92651	471	See code following 92584.
92652	471	See code following 92584.
92653	471	See code following 92584.
92920	475	See code following 92998.
92921	475	See code following 92998.
92924	475	See code following 92998.
92925	475	See code following 92998.
92928	475	See code following 92998.
92929	475	See code following 92998.
92933	475	See code following 92998.
92934	476	See code following 92998.
92937	476	See code following 92998.
92938	476	See code following 92998.
92941	476	See code following 92998.
92943	476	See code following 92998.
92944	476	See code following 92998.
92973	476	See code following 92998.
92974	476	See code following 92998.
92975	476	See code following 92998.
92977	476	See code following 92998.
92978	476	See code following 92998.
92979	476	See code following 92998.
93241	478	See code following 93227.
93242	478	See code following 93227.
93243	478	See code following 93227.
93244	478	See code following 93227.
93245	478	See code following 93227.
93246	478	See code following 93227.
93247	478	See code following 93227.
93248	478	See code following 93227.
93260	480	See code following 93284.
93261	480	See code following 93289.
93264	479	See code before 93279.
93356	483	See code following 93351.
94619	496	See code following 94617.
95249	499	See code following 95250.
95700	508	See code following 95967.
95705	508	See code following 95967.
95706	508	See code following 95967.
95707	508	See code following 95967.
95708	508	See code following 95967.
95709	508	See code following 95967.
95710	508	See code following 95967.
95711	508	See code following 95967.
95712	508	See code following 95967.
95713	508	See code following 95967.
95714	508	See code following 95967.
95715	508	See code following 95967.
95716	508	See code following 95967.
95717	508	See code following 95967.
95718	508	See code following 95967.
95719	508	See code following 95967.
95720	509	See code following 95967.
95721	509	See code following 95967.
95722	509	See code following 95967.
95723	509	See code following 95967.
95724	509	See code following 95967.
95725	509	See code following 95967.
95726	509	See code following 95967.
95782	501	See code following 95811.
95783	501	See code following 95811.
95800	501	See code following 95806.
95801	501	See code following 95806.
95829	502	See code following 95830.
95836	503	See code following 95830.
95885	504	See code following 95872.
95886	504	See code following 95872.
95887	504	See code before 95873.
95938	506	See code following 95926.
95939	506	See code following 95929.
95940	505	See code following 95913.
95941	505	See code following 95913.
95943	506	See code following 95924.
95983	510	See code following 95977.
95984	510	See code following 95977.
96125	513	See code following 96105.
96127	513	See code following 96113.
96164	514	See code following 96159.
96165	514	See code following 96159.
96167	514	See code following 96159.
96168	514	See code following 96159.
96170	514	See code following 96159.
96171	514	See code following 96159.
97151	511	See code following 96040.
97152	511	See code following 96040.
97153	512	See code following 96040.
97154	512	See code following 96040.
97155	512	See code following 96040.
97156	512	See code following 96040.
97157	512	See code following 96040.
97158	512	See code following 96040.
97161	521	See code before 97010.
97162	522	See code before 97010.
97163	522	See code before 97010.
97164	522	See code before 97010.
97165	522	See code before 97010.
97166	522	See code before 97010.
97167	523	See code before 97010.
97168	523	See code before 97010.
97169	523	See code before 97010.
97170	523	See code before 97010.
97171	523	See code before 97010.
97172	523	See code before 97010.
99091	557	See code following resequenced code 99454.
99177	531	See code following 99174.
99224	544	See code following 99220.
99225	544	See code following 99220.
99226	544	See code following 99220.
99415	553	See code following 99359.
99416	554	See code following 99359.
99417	554	See code following resequenced code 99416.
99421	556	See code following 99443.
99422	556	See code following 99443.
99423	556	See code following 99443.
99439	561	See code following resequenced code 99490.
99451	557	See code following 99449.
99452	557	See code following 99449.
99453	557	See code following 99449.
99454	557	See code following 99449.
99457	558	See code before 99450.
99458	558	See code before 99450.
99473	558	See code before 99450.
99474	558	See code before 99450.
99484	563	See code following 99498.
99485	559	See code following 99467.
99486	559	See code following 99467.
99490	561	See code before 99487.
99491	561	See code before 99487.
2033F	569	See code following 2026F.
3051F	570	See code following 3044F.
3052F	570	See code before 3046F.
0253T	582	See code before 0198T.
0376T	582	See code following 0191T.
0464T	585	See code following 0333T.
0488T	587	See code following 0403T.
0510T	585	See code following 0335T.
0511T	585	See code following 0335T.
0512T	581	See code following 0102T.
0513T	581	See code following 0102T.
0523T	593	See code before 0505T.
0563T	583	See code following 0207T.
0614T	598	See code following 0580T.
0620T	593	See code following 0505T.
0623T	593	See code following 0504T.
0624T	596	See code following 0504T.
0625T	593	See code following 0504T.
0626T	593	See code following 0504T.

Appendix F — Add-on Codes, Optum Modifier 50 Exempt, Modifier 51 Exempt, Optum Modifier 51 Exempt, Modifier 63 Exempt, and Modifier 95 Telemedicine Services

Codes specified as add-on, exempt from modifiers 50, 51 and 63, and modifier 95 (telemedicine services) are listed. The lists are designed to be read left to right rather than vertically.

Add-on Codes

0054T	0055T	0076T	0095T	0098T	0163T	0164T
0165T	0174T	0214T	0215T	0217T	0218T	0222T
0290T	0376T	0397T	0437T	0439T	0443T	0450T
0466T	0471T	0480T	0492T	0496T	0513T	0514T
0523T	0560T	0562T	0570T	0599T	0628T	0630T
0071U	0072U	0073U	0074U	0075U	0076U	0130U
0131U	0132U	0133U	0134U	0135U	0136U	0137U
0138U	0157U	0158U	0159U	0160U	0161U	0162U
0207U	01953	01968	01969	10004	10006	10008
10010	10012	10036	11001	11008	11045	11046
11047	11103	11105	11107	11201	11732	11922
13102	13122	13133	13153	14302	15003	15005
15101	15111	15116	15121	15131	15136	15151
15152	15156	15157	15201	15221	15241	15261
15272	15274	15276	15278	15772	15774	15777
15787	15847	16036	17003	17312	17314	17315
19001	19082	19084	19086	19126	19282	19284
19286	19288	19294	19297	20700	20701	20702
20703	20704	20705	20930	20931	20932	20933
20934	20936	20937	20938	20939	20985	22103
22116	22208	22216	22226	22328	22512	22515
22527	22534	22552	22585	22614	22632	22634
22840	22841	22842	22843	22844	22845	22846
22847	22848	22853	22854	22858	22859	22868
22870	26125	26861	26863	27358	27692	29826
31627	31632	31633	31637	31649	31651	31654
32501	32506	32507	32667	32668	32674	33141
33225	33257	33258	33259	33367	33368	33369
33419	33508	33517	33518	33519	33521	33522
33523	33530	33572	33746	33768	33866	33884
33924	33929	33987	34709	34711	34713	34714
34715	34716	34717	34808	34812	34813	34820
34833	34834	35306	35390	35400	35500	35572
35600	35681	35682	35683	35685	35686	35697
35700	36218	36227	36228	36248	36474	36476
36479	36483	36907	36908	36909	37185	37186
37222	37223	37232	37233	37234	37235	37237
37239	37247	37249	37252	37253	38102	38746
38747	38900	43273	43283	43338	43635	44015
44121	44128	44139	44203	44213	44701	44955
47001	47542	47543	47544	47550	48400	49326
49327	49412	49435	49568	49905	50606	50705
50706	51797	52442	56606	57267	57465	58110
58611	59525	60512	61316	61517	61611	61641
61642	61651	61781	61782	61783	61797	61799
61800	61864	61868	62148	62160	63035	63043
63044	63048	63057	63066	63076	63078	63082
63086	63088	63091	63103	63295	63308	63621
64421	64462	64480	64484	64491	64492	64494
64495	64634	64636	64643	64645	64727	64778
64783	64787	64832	64837	64859	64872	64874
64876	64901	64902	64913	65757	66990	67225
67320	67331	67332	67334	67335	67340	69990
74248	74301	74713	75565	75774	76125	76802
76810	76812	76814	76937	76979	76983	77001
77002	77003	77063	77293	78020	78434	78496
78730	78835	81266	81416	81426	81536	82952
86826	87187	87503	87904	88155	88177	88185
88311	88314	88332	88334	88341	88350	88364
88369	88373	88388	90461	90472	90474	90785
90833	90836	90838	90840	90863	90913	91013
92547	92608	92618	92621	92627	92921	92925
92929	92934	92938	92944	92973	92974	92978
92979	92998	93320	93321	93325	93352	93356
93462	93463	93464	93563	93564	93565	93566
93567	93568	93571	93572	93592	93609	93613
93621	93622	93623	93655	93657	93662	94645
94729	94781	95079	95873	95874	95885	95886
95887	95940	95941	95962	95967	95984	96113
96121	96131	96133	96137	96139	96159	96165
96168	96171	96361	96366	96367	96368	96370
96371	96375	96376	96411	96415	96417	96423
96570	96571	96934	96935	96936	97130	97546
97598	97811	97814	99100	99116	99135	99140
99153	99157	99292	99354	99355	99356	99357
99359	99415	99416	99417	99439	99458	99467
99486	99489	99494	99498	99602	99607	

Optum Modifier 50 Exempt Codes

0214T	0215T	0217T	0218T	15777	20939	34713
34714	34715	34716	34717	34812	34820	34833
34834	35572	36227	36228	49568	63035	63043
63044	64421	64462	64480	64484	64491	64492
64494	64495	64634	64636			

AMA Modifier 51 Exempt Codes

20697	20974	20975	44500	61107	93600	93602
93603	93610	93612	93615	93616	93618	94610
95905	99151	99152				

Optum Modifier 51 Exempt Codes

22585	22614	22632	69990	90281	90283	90284
90287	90288	90291	90296	90371	90375	90376
90377	90378	90384	90385	90386	90389	90393
90396	90399	90476	90477	90581	90585	90586
90587	90619	90620	90621	90625	90630	90632
90633	90634	90636	90644	90647	90648	90649
90650	90651	90653	90654	90655	90656	90657
90658	90660	90661	90662	90664	90666	90667
90668	90670	90672	90673	90674	90675	90676
90680	90681	90682	90685	90686	90687	90688
90689	90690	90691	90694	90696	90697	90698
90700	90702	90707	90710	90713	90714	90715
90716	90717	90723	90732	90733	90734	90736
90738	90739	90740	90743	90744	90746	90747
90748	90749	90750	90756	97010	97012	97014
97016	97018	97022	97024	97026	97028	97032
97033	97034	97035	97036	97110	97112	97113
97116	97124	97129	97130	97140	97150	97161
97162	97163	97164	97165	97166	97167	97168
97169	97170	97171	97172	97530	97533	97535
97537	97542	97545	97546	97597	97598	97602
97605	97606	97607	97608	97610	97750	97755
97760	97761	97763	99050	99051	99053	99056
99058	99060					

Modifier 63 Exempt Codes

30540	30545	31520	33470	33502	33503	33505
33506	33610	33611	33619	33647	33670	33690
33694	33730	33732	33735	33736	33750	33755
33762	33778	33786	33922	33946	33947	33948
33949	36415	36420	36450	36456	36460	36510
36660	39503	43313	43314	43520	43831	44055
44126	44127	44128	46070	46705	46715	46716

46730	46735	46740	46742	46744	47700	47701
49215	49491	49492	49495	49496	49600	49605
49606	49610	49611	53025	54000	54150	54160
63700	63702	63704	63706	65820		

Telemedicine Services Codes

The codes on the following list may be used to report telemedicine services when modifier 95 Synchronous Telemedicine Service Rendered via a Real-Time Interactive Audio and Visual Telecommunications System, is appended.

90791	90792	90832	90833	90834	90836	90837
90838	90845	90846	90847	90863	90951	90952
90954	90955	90957	90958	90960	90961	92227
92228	93228	93229	93268	93270	93271	93272
96040	96116	97802	97803	97804	98960	98961
98962	99202	99203	99204	99205	99212	99213
99214	99215	99231	99232	99233	*99241	*99242
*99243	*99244	*99245	*99251	*99252	*99253	*99254
*99255	99307	99308	99309	99310	99354	99355
99406	99407	99408	99409	99417	99495	99496

* Consultations are noncovered by Medicare

Appendix G — Medicare Internet-only Manuals (IOMs)

The Centers for Medicare and Medicaid Services restructured its paper-based manual system as a web-based system on October 1, 2003. Called the online CMS manual system, it combines all of the various program instructions into internet-only manuals (IOMs), which are used by all CMS programs and contractors. In many instances, the references from the online manuals in appendix G contain a mention of the old paper manuals from which the current information was obtained when the manuals were converted. This information is shown in the header of the text, in the following format, when applicable, as A3-3101, HO-210, and B3-2049.

Effective with implementation of the IOMs, the former method of publishing program memoranda (PMs) to communicate program instructions was replaced by the following four templates:

- One-time notification
- Manual revisions
- Business requirements
- Confidential requirements

The web-based system has been organized by functional area (e.g., eligibility, entitlement, claims processing, benefit policy, program integrity) in an effort to eliminate redundancy within the manuals, simplify updating, and make CMS program instructions available more quickly. The web-based system contains the functional areas included below:

Pub. 100	Introduction
Pub. 100-01	Medicare General Information, Eligibility and Entitlement Manual
Pub. 100-02	Medicare Benefit Policy Manual
Pub. 100-03	Medicare National Coverage Determinations (NCD) Manual
Pub. 100-04	Medicare Claims Processing Manual
Pub. 100-05	Medicare Secondary Payer Manual
Pub. 100-06	Medicare Financial Management Manual
Pub. 100-07	State Operations Manual
Pub. 100-08	Medicare Program Integrity Manual
Pub. 100-09	Medicare Contractor Beneficiary and Provider Communications Manual
Pub. 100-10	Quality Improvement Organization Manual
Pub. 100-11	Programs of All-Inclusive Care for the Elderly (PACE) Manual
Pub. 100-12	State Medicaid Manual (under development)
Pub. 100-13	Medicaid State Children's Health Insurance Program (under development)
Pub. 100-14	Medicare ESRD Network Organizations Manual
Pub. 100-15	Medicaid Integrity Program (MIP)
Pub. 100-16	Medicare Managed Care Manual
Pub. 100-17	CMS/Business Partners Systems Security Manual
Pub. 100-18	Medicare Prescription Drug Benefit Manual
Pub. 100-19	Demonstrations
Pub. 100-20	One-Time Notification
Pub. 100-21	Reserved
Pub. 100-22	Medicare Quality Reporting Incentive Programs Manual
Pub. 100-24	State Buy-In Manual
Pub. 100-25	Information Security Acceptable Risk Safeguards Manual

A brief description of the Medicare manuals primarily used for *CPC Expert* follows:

The ***National Coverage Determinations Manual*** (NCD), is organized according to categories such as diagnostic services, supplies, and medical procedures. The table of contents lists each category and subject within that category. Revision transmittals identify any new or background material, recap the changes, and provide an effective date for the change. The manual contains four sections and is organized in accordance with CPT category sequence and contains a list of HCPCS codes related to coverage determinations, where appropriate.

The ***Medicare Benefit Policy Manual*** contains Medicare general coverage instructions that are not national coverage determinations. As a general rule, in the past these instructions have been found in chapter II of the ***Medicare Carriers Manual,*** the ***Medicare Intermediary Manual***, other provider manuals, and program memoranda.

The ***Medicare Claims Processing Manual*** contains instructions for processing claims for contractors and providers.

The ***Medicare Program Integrity Manual*** communicates the priorities and standards for the Medicare integrity programs.

Medicare IOM References

A printed version of the Medicare IOM references will no longer be published in Optum360's *Current Procedural Coding* product. Complete versions of all the manuals can be found online at https://www.cms.gov/Regulations-and-Guidance/Guidance/Manuals/Internet-Only-Manuals-IOMs.

Appendix H — Quality Payment Program

In 2015, Congress passed the Medicare Access and CHIP Reauthorization Act (MACRA), which included sweeping changes for practitioners who provide services reimbursed under the Medicare physician fee schedule (MPFS). The act focused on repealing the faulty Medicare sustainable growth rate, focusing on quality of patient outcomes, and controlling Medicare spending.

A MACRA final rule in October 2016 established the Quality Payment Program (QPP) that was effective January 1, 2017.

The QPP has two tracks:

- The merit-based incentive payment system (MIPS)
- Alternative payment models (APMs)

MIPS uses the existing quality and value reporting, Medicare meaningful use (MU), and value-based modifier (VBM) programs to define certain performance categories that determine an overall score. Eligible clinicians (ECs) can obtain a composite performance score (CPS) of up to 100 points from these weighted performance categories. This performance score then defines the payment adjustments in the second calendar year after the year the score is obtained. For instance, the score obtained for the 2019 performance year is linked to payment for Medicare Part B services in 2021.

The performance categories, along with the weights used to determine the overall score, are:

- Quality
- Advancing care information (previously called meaningful use)
- Clinical practice improvement activities (CPIA)
- Resource use

ECs may also choose to participate in APMs. These payment models, created in conjunction with the clinician community, provide additional incentives to those clinicians in the APM who provide high-quality care as cost-efficiently as possible. APMs can be created around specific clinical conditions, a care episode, or a patient population type. An APM can also be described as a new way of paying the healthcare provider for the care rendered to Medicare patients.

Advanced APMs are a subset of APMs; practices participating in an advanced APM can earn even more incentives because the ECs take on risk related to their patients' outcomes. For calendar years 2019 through 2024, clinicians participating in advanced APMs have the potential to earn an additional 5 percent incentive payment; furthermore, they are exempt from having to participate in MIPS as long as they have sufficiently participated in the advanced APM.

Eligible clinicians have flexible options for submitting data to the MIPS and an option to join advanced APMs. Under the QPP, providers can receive increased payment by providing high-quality care and by controlling costs. ECs who successfully report determined criteria—defined by the pathway chosen—receive a larger payment depending on how successful they are at meeting performance thresholds. Those who do not participate or who do not fulfill the defined requirements receive a negative penalty; failure to participate in a track in 2021 results in 9 percent payment reduction in 2022.

ECs can receive incentives under the QPP. Once the performance threshold is established, ALL ECs who score above that threshold are eligible to receive a positive payment adjustment. Keep in mind that the key requirement is that an EC **submit data** to avoid the negative payment adjustment and receive the incentives. CMS has redesigned the scoring so that clinicians are able to know how well they are doing in the program, as benchmarks are known in advance of participating.

Proposed 2021 Changes

A number of revisions have been proposed for 2021. As noted earlier, in 2021, the maximum negative payment for payment adjustment is negative 9 percent. The positive payment, not including additional positive payments adjustments for exceptional performance, is also up to a 9 percent adjustment. CMS is proposing additions, revisions, and deletions to many of the current reporting measures. Other proposals affecting the MIPS program for 2021 include:

- In the MIPS performance category, CMS proposes to reduce the Quality performance category weight from 45 percent to 40 percent and to increase the Cost performance category weight from 15 percent to 20 percent. This is in accordance with CMS's effort to equalize weighting between the Quality and Cost performance categories by 2022 as indicated in MACRA.
- New specialty sets would be added for Speech Language Pathology, Audiology, Clinical Social Work, Chiropractic Medicine, Pulmonology, Nutrition/Dietician, and Endocrinology.
- CMS proposes adding telehealth services to existing total per capital cost (TPCC) and episode-based cost measures.
- In the Improvement Activities performance category, CMS recommends modification of two existing activities. Additional criteria for nomination of new improvement activity includes linking to existing and related MIPS quality and cost measures.

Within the advanced alternative payment models (APMs), CMS has proposed MIPS quality reporting options for APM participants. Previously, CMS has tried to streamline APM participation in MIPS; however, the agency feels that allowing MIPS quality measures to be reported by the APMs would offer flexibility and improve meaningful measurement.

Appendix I — Medically Unlikely Edits (MUEs)

The Centers for Medicare & Medicaid Services (CMS) began to publish many of the edits used in the medically unlikely edits (MUE) program for the first time effective October 2008. What follows below is a list of the published CPT codes that have MUEs assigned to them and the number of units allowed with each code. CMS publishes the updates on a quarterly basis. Not all MUEs will be published, however. MUEs intended to detect and discourage any questionable payments will not be published as the agency feels the efficacy of these edits would be compromised. CMS added another component to the MUEs—the MUE Adjudication Indicator (MAI). The appropriate MAI can be found in parentheses following the MUE in this table and specify the maximum units of service (UOS) for a CPT/HCPCS code for the service. The MAI designates whether the UOS edit is applied to the line or claim.

The three MAIs are defined as follows:

MAI 1 (Line Edit) This MAI will continue to be adjudicated as the line edit on the claim and is auto-adjudicated by the contractor.

MAI 2 (Date of Service Edit, Policy) This MAI is considered to be the "absolute date of service edit" and is based on policy. The total unit of services (UOS) for that CPT code and that date of service (DOS) are combined for this edit. Medicare contractors are required to review all claims for the same patient, same date of service, and same provider.

MAI 3 (Date of Service Edit: Clinical) This MAI is also a date-of-service edit but is based upon clinical standards. The review takes current and previously submitted claims for the same patient, same date of service, and same provider into account. When medical necessity is clearly documented, the edit may be bypassed or the claim resubmitted.

The quarterly updates are published on the CMS website at https://www.cms.gov/Medicare/Coding/NationalCorrectCodInitEd/MUE. The following was updated on 10/01/2020.

Professional

CPT	MUE
0001U	1(2)
0002M	1(3)
0002U	1(2)
0003M	1(3)
0003U	1(2)
0004M	1(2)
0005U	1(2)
0006M	1(2)
0007M	1(2)
0007U	1(2)
0008U	1(3)
0009U	2(3)
0010U	2(3)
0011M	1(2)
0011U	1(2)
0012M	1(2)
0012U	1(2)
0013M	1(2)
0013U	1(3)
0014M	1(2)
0014U	1(3)
0016U	1(3)
0017U	1(3)
0018U	1(1)
0019U	1(3)
0021U	1(2)
0022U	2(3)
0023U	1(2)
0024U	1(2)
0025U	1(2)
0026U	1(3)
0027U	1(2)
0029U	1(2)
0030U	1(2)
0031U	1(2)
0032U	1(2)
0033U	1(2)
0034U	1(2)
0035U	1(2)
0036U	1(3)
0037U	1(3)
0038U	1(2)
0039U	1(2)
0040U	1(2)
0041U	1(2)
0042T	1(3)
0042U	1(2)
0043U	1(2)
0044U	1(2)
0045U	1(3)
0046U	1(3)
0047U	1(3)
0048U	1(3)
0049U	1(3)
0050U	1(3)
0051U	1(2)
0052U	1(2)
0053U	1(3)
0054T	1(3)
0054U	1(2)
0055T	1(3)
0055U	1(2)
0056U	1(3)
0058T	1(2)
0058U	1(2)
0059U	1(2)
0060U	1(2)
0061U	2(3)
0062U	1(2)
0063U	1(2)
0064U	2(3)
0065U	2(3)
0066U	1(3)
0067U	2(3)
0068U	1(3)
0069U	1(3)
0070U	1(2)
0071T	1(2)
0071U	1(2)
0072T	1(2)
0072U	1(2)
0073U	1(2)
0074U	1(2)
0075T	1(2)
0075U	1(2)
0076T	1(2)
0076U	1(2)
0077U	2(2)
0078U	1(2)
0079U	0(3)
0080U	1(2)
0082U	1(2)
0083U	1(3)
0084U	1(2)
0085T	0(3)
0086U	1(3)
0087U	1(2)
0088U	1(2)
0089U	1(2)
0090U	1(2)
0091U	1(2)
0092U	1(2)
0093U	1(2)
0094U	1(2)
0095T	1(3)
0095U	1(2)
0096U	1(2)
0097U	1(2)
0098T	2(3)
0098U	1(2)
0099U	1(2)
0100T	1(2)
0100U	1(2)
0101T	1(3)
0101U	1(2)
0102T	2(2)
0102U	1(2)
0103U	1(2)
0105U	1(2)
0106T	4(2)
0106U	1(2)
0107T	4(2)
0107U	1(3)
0108T	4(2)
0108U	1(2)
0109T	4(2)
0109U	1(3)
0110T	4(2)
0110U	1(2)
0111T	1(3)
0111U	1(2)
0112U	1(3)
0113U	1(2)
0114U	1(2)
0115U	1(3)
0116U	1(2)
0117U	1(2)
0118U	1(2)
0119U	1(2)
0120U	1(2)
0121U	1(2)
0122U	1(2)
0123U	1(2)
0126T	1(3)
0129U	1(2)
0130U	1(2)
0131U	1(2)
0132U	1(2)
0133U	1(2)
0134U	1(2)
0135U	1(2)
0136U	1(2)
0137U	1(2)
0138U	1(2)
0139U	1(2)
0140U	1(2)
0141U	1(2)
0142U	1(2)
0143U	1(2)
0144U	1(2)
0145U	1(2)
0146U	1(2)
0147U	1(2)
0148U	1(2)
0149U	1(2)
0150U	1(2)
0151U	1(2)
0152U	1(2)
0153U	1(2)
0154U	1(2)
0155U	1(2)
0156U	1(2)
0157U	1(2)
0158U	1(2)
0159U	1(2)
0160U	1(2)
0161U	1(2)
0162U	1(2)
0163T	1(3)
0163U	0(3)
0164T	4(2)
0164U	1(2)
0165T	4(2)
0165U	1(2)
0166U	1(2)
0167U	1(2)
0168U	1(2)
0169U	1(2)
0170U	1(2)
0171U	1(2)
0172U	1(2)
0173U	1(2)
0174T	1(3)
0174U	1(2)
0175T	1(3)
0175U	1(2)
0176U	1(3)
0177U	1(2)
0178U	1(2)
0179U	1(2)
0184T	1(3)
0191T	2(2)
0198T	2(2)
01996	1(2)
0200T	1(2)
0201T	1(2)
0202T	1(3)
0202U	1(3)
0207T	2(2)
0208T	1(3)
0209T	1(3)
0210T	1(3)
0211T	1(3)
0212T	1(3)
0213T	1(2)
0214T	1(2)
0215T	1(2)
0216T	1(2)
0217T	1(2)
0218T	1(2)
0219T	1(2)
0220T	1(2)
0221T	1(2)
0222T	1(3)
0223U	1(3)
0224U	3(3)
0228T	1(2)
0229T	2(3)
0230T	1(2)
0231T	2(3)
0232T	1(3)
0234T	2(2)
0235T	2(3)
0236T	1(2)
0237T	2(3)
0238T	2(3)
0253T	1(3)
0263T	1(3)
0264T	1(3)
0265T	1(3)
0266T	1(2)
0267T	1(3)
0268T	1(3)
0269T	1(2)
0270T	1(3)
0271T	1(3)
0272T	1(3)
0273T	1(3)
0274T	1(2)
0275T	1(2)
0278T	1(3)
0290T	1(3)
0295T	1(2)
0296T	1(2)
0297T	1(2)
0298T	1(2)
0308T	1(3)
0312T	1(3)
0313T	1(3)
0314T	1(3)
0315T	1(3)
0316T	1(3)
0317T	1(3)
0329T	1(2)
0330T	1(2)
0331T	1(3)
0332T	1(3)
0333T	1(2)
0335T	2(2)
0338T	1(2)
0339T	1(2)
0342T	1(3)
0345T	1(2)
0347T	1(3)
0348T	1(3)
0349T	1(3)
0350T	1(3)
0351T	5(3)
0352T	5(3)
0353T	2(3)
0354T	2(3)
0355T	1(2)
0356T	4(2)
0358T	1(2)
0362T	8(3)
0373T	24(3)
0376T	2(3)
0378T	1(2)
0379T	1(2)
0381T	1(2)
0382T	1(2)
0383T	1(2)
0384T	1(2)
0385T	1(2)
0386T	1(2)
0394T	2(3)
0395T	2(3)
0396T	2(2)
0397T	1(3)
0398T	1(3)
0400T	1(2)
0401T	1(2)
0402T	2(2)
0403T	1(2)
0404T	1(2)
0405T	1(2)
0408T	1(3)
0409T	1(3)
0410T	1(3)
0411T	1(3)
0412T	1(2)
0413T	1(3)
0414T	1(2)
0415T	1(3)
0416T	1(3)
0417T	1(3)
0418T	1(3)
0419T	1(2)
0420T	1(2)
0421T	1(2)
0422T	1(3)
0423T	1(3)
0424T	1(3)
0425T	1(3)
0426T	1(3)
0427T	1(3)
0428T	1(2)
0429T	1(2)
0430T	1(2)
0431T	1(2)
0432T	1(3)
0433T	1(3)
0434T	1(3)
0435T	1(3)
0436T	1(3)
0437T	1(3)
0439T	1(3)
0440T	3(3)
0441T	3(3)
0442T	3(3)
0443T	1(2)
0444T	1(2)
0445T	1(2)
0446T	1(3)
0447T	1(3)
0448T	1(3)
0449T	1(2)
0450T	1(3)
0451T	1(3)
0452T	1(3)
0453T	1(3)

CPT	MUE
0454T	3(3)
0455T	1(3)
0456T	1(3)
0457T	1(3)
0458T	3(3)
0459T	1(3)
0460T	3(3)
0461T	1(3)
0462T	1(2)
0463T	1(2)
0464T	1(2)
0465T	1(3)
0466T	1(3)
0467T	1(3)
0468T	1(3)
0469T	1(2)
0470T	1(2)
0471T	2(1)
0472T	1(2)
0473T	1(2)
0474T	2(2)
0475T	1(3)
0476T	1(3)
0477T	1(3)
0478T	1(3)
0479T	1(2)
0480T	4(1)
0481T	1(3)
0483T	1(2)
0484T	1(2)
0485T	1(2)
0486T	1(2)
0487T	1(3)
0488T	1(2)
0489T	1(2)
0490T	1(2)
0491T	1(2)
0492T	4(3)
0493T	1(3)
0494T	1(2)
0495T	1(2)
0496T	4(3)
0497T	1(3)
0498T	1(2)
0499T	1(2)
0500T	1(3)
0501T	1(2)
0502T	1(2)
0503T	1(2)
0504T	1(2)
0505T	1(3)
0506T	1(2)
0507T	1(2)
0508T	1(3)
0509T	1(2)
0510T	1(2)
0511T	1(2)
0512T	1(2)
0513T	2(3)
0514T	2(2)
0515T	1(3)
0516T	1(3)
0517T	1(3)
0518T	1(3)
0519T	1(3)

CPT	MUE
0520T	1(3)
0521T	1(3)
0522T	1(3)
0523T	1(3)
0524T	3(3)
0525T	1(3)
0526T	1(3)
0527T	1(3)
0528T	1(3)
0529T	1(3)
0530T	1(3)
0531T	1(3)
0532T	1(3)
0533T	1(2)
0534T	1(2)
0535T	1(2)
0536T	1(2)
0537T	1(2)
0538T	1(3)
0539T	1(3)
0540T	1(3)
0541T	1(3)
0542T	1(3)
0543T	1(2)
0544T	1(2)
0545T	1(2)
0546T	2(2)
0547T	1(2)
0548T	1(2)
0549T	1(2)
0550T	2(3)
0551T	1(2)
0552T	1(3)
0553T	2(2)
0554T	1(2)
0555T	1(2)
0556T	1(2)
0557T	1(2)
0558T	1(2)
0559T	1(2)
0560T	1(3)
0561T	1(2)
0562T	1(3)
0563T	1(2)
0564T	1(2)
0565T	1(2)
0566T	1(2)
0567T	1(2)
0568T	1(2)
0569T	1(2)
0570T	1(3)
0571T	1(2)
0572T	1(2)
0573T	1(2)
0574T	1(2)
0575T	1(2)
0576T	1(2)
0577T	1(2)
0578T	1(2)
0579T	1(2)
0580T	1(2)
0581T	0(3)
0582T	0(3)
0583T	2(2)
0584T	1(2)

CPT	MUE
0585T	1(2)
0586T	1(2)
0587T	1(2)
0588T	1(2)
0589T	1(2)
0590T	1(2)
0591T	1(2)
0592T	1(2)
0593T	1(2)
10004	3(3)
10005	1(2)
10006	3(3)
10007	1(2)
10008	2(3)
10009	1(2)
10010	3(3)
10011	1(2)
10012	3(3)
10021	1(2)
10030	2(3)
10035	1(2)
10036	2(3)
10040	1(2)
10060	1(2)
10061	1(2)
10080	1(3)
10081	1(3)
10120	3(3)
10121	2(3)
10140	2(3)
10160	3(3)
10180	2(3)
11000	1(2)
11001	1(3)
11004	1(2)
11005	1(2)
11006	1(2)
11008	1(2)
11010	2(3)
11011	2(3)
11012	2(3)
11042	1(2)
11043	1(2)
11044	1(2)
11045	12(3)
11046	10(3)
11047	10(3)
11055	1(2)
11056	1(2)
11057	1(2)
11102	1(2)
11103	6(3)
11104	1(2)
11105	3(3)
11106	1(2)
11107	2(3)
11200	1(2)
11201	1(3)
11300	5(3)
11301	6(3)
11302	4(3)
11303	3(3)
11305	4(3)
11306	4(3)
11307	3(3)

CPT	MUE
11308	2(3)
11310	4(3)
11311	4(3)
11312	3(3)
11313	3(3)
11400	3(3)
11401	3(3)
11402	3(3)
11403	2(3)
11404	2(3)
11406	2(3)
11420	3(3)
11421	3(3)
11422	3(3)
11423	2(3)
11424	2(3)
11426	2(3)
11440	4(3)
11441	3(3)
11442	3(3)
11443	2(3)
11444	2(3)
11446	2(3)
11450	1(2)
11451	1(2)
11462	1(2)
11463	1(2)
11470	3(2)
11471	2(3)
11600	2(3)
11601	2(3)
11602	3(3)
11603	2(3)
11604	2(3)
11606	2(3)
11620	2(3)
11621	2(3)
11622	2(3)
11623	2(3)
11624	2(3)
11626	2(3)
11640	2(3)
11641	2(3)
11642	3(3)
11643	2(3)
11644	2(3)
11646	2(3)
11719	1(2)
11720	1(2)
11721	1(2)
11730	1(2)
11732	4(3)
11740	2(3)
11750	6(3)
11755	2(3)
11760	4(3)
11762	2(3)
11765	4(3)
11770	1(3)
11771	1(3)
11772	1(3)
11900	1(2)
11901	1(2)
11920	1(2)
11921	1(2)

CPT	MUE
11922	1(3)
11950	1(2)
11951	1(2)
11952	1(2)
11954	1(3)
11960	2(3)
11970	2(3)
11971	2(3)
11976	1(2)
11980	1(2)
11981	1(3)
11982	1(3)
11983	1(3)
12001	1(2)
12002	1(2)
12004	1(2)
12005	1(2)
12006	1(2)
12007	1(2)
12011	1(2)
12013	1(2)
12014	1(2)
12015	1(2)
12016	1(2)
12017	1(2)
12018	1(2)
12020	2(3)
12021	3(3)
12031	1(2)
12032	1(2)
12034	1(2)
12035	1(2)
12036	1(2)
12037	1(2)
12041	1(2)
12042	1(2)
12044	1(2)
12045	1(2)
12046	1(2)
12047	1(2)
12051	1(2)
12052	1(2)
12053	1(2)
12054	1(2)
12055	1(2)
12056	1(2)
12057	1(2)
13100	1(2)
13101	1(2)
13102	9(3)
13120	1(2)
13121	1(2)
13122	9(3)
13131	1(2)
13132	1(2)
13133	7(3)
13151	1(2)
13152	1(2)
13153	2(3)
13160	2(3)
14000	2(3)
14001	2(3)
14020	2(3)
14021	2(3)
14040	2(3)

CPT	MUE
14041	3(3)
14060	2(3)
14061	2(3)
14301	2(3)
14302	8(3)
14350	2(3)
15002	1(2)
15003	60(3)
15004	1(2)
15005	19(3)
15040	1(2)
15050	1(3)
15100	1(2)
15101	40(3)
15110	1(2)
15111	5(3)
15115	1(2)
15116	2(3)
15120	1(2)
15121	8(3)
15130	1(2)
15131	2(3)
15135	1(2)
15136	1(3)
15150	1(2)
15151	1(2)
15152	5(3)
15155	1(2)
15156	1(2)
15157	1(3)
15200	1(2)
15201	7(3)
15220	1(2)
15221	9(3)
15240	1(2)
15241	9(3)
15260	1(2)
15261	6(3)
15271	1(2)
15272	3(3)
15273	1(2)
15274	60(3)
15275	1(2)
15276	3(2)
15277	1(2)
15278	15(3)
15570	2(3)
15572	2(3)
15574	2(3)
15576	2(3)
15600	2(3)
15610	2(3)
15620	2(3)
15630	2(3)
15650	1(3)
15730	1(3)
15731	1(3)
15733	2(3)
15734	4(3)
15736	2(3)
15738	3(3)
15740	2(3)
15750	2(3)
15756	2(3)
15757	2(3)

CPT	MUE
15758	2(3)
15760	2(3)
15769	1(3)
15770	2(3)
15771	1(2)
15772	9(3)
15773	1(2)
15774	3(3)
15775	1(2)
15776	1(2)
15777	1(3)
15780	1(2)
15781	1(3)
15782	1(3)
15783	1(3)
15786	1(2)
15787	2(3)
15788	1(2)
15789	1(2)
15792	1(3)
15793	1(3)
15819	1(2)
15820	1(2)
15821	1(2)
15822	1(2)
15823	1(2)
15824	1(2)
15825	1(2)
15826	1(2)
15828	1(2)
15829	1(2)
15830	1(2)
15832	1(2)
15833	1(2)
15834	1(2)
15835	1(3)
15836	1(2)
15837	2(3)
15838	1(2)
15839	2(3)
15840	1(3)
15841	2(3)
15842	2(3)
15845	2(3)
15847	1(2)
15850	0(3)
15851	1(2)
15852	1(3)
15860	1(3)
15876	1(2)
15877	1(2)
15878	1(2)
15879	1(2)
15920	1(3)
15922	1(3)
15931	1(3)
15933	1(3)
15934	1(3)
15935	1(3)
15936	1(3)
15937	1(3)
15940	2(3)
15941	2(3)
15944	2(3)
15945	2(3)

CPT	MUE
15946	2(3)
15950	2(3)
15951	2(3)
15952	2(3)
15953	2(3)
15956	2(3)
15958	2(3)
15999	1(3)
16000	1(2)
16020	1(3)
16025	1(3)
16030	1(3)
16035	1(2)
16036	8(3)
17000	1(2)
17003	13(2)
17004	1(2)
17106	1(2)
17107	1(2)
17108	1(2)
17110	1(2)
17111	1(2)
17250	4(3)
17260	7(3)
17261	7(3)
17262	6(3)
17263	3(3)
17264	3(3)
17266	2(3)
17270	6(3)
17271	4(3)
17272	5(3)
17273	4(3)
17274	2(3)
17276	2(3)
17280	6(3)
17281	5(3)
17282	4(3)
17283	4(3)
17284	2(3)
17286	2(3)
17311	4(3)
17312	6(3)
17313	3(3)
17314	4(3)
17315	15(3)
17340	1(2)
17360	1(2)
17380	1(3)
17999	1(3)
19000	2(3)
19001	5(3)
19020	2(3)
19030	1(2)
19081	1(2)
19082	2(3)
19083	1(2)
19084	2(3)
19085	1(2)
19086	2(3)
19100	4(3)
19101	3(3)
19105	2(3)
19110	1(3)
19112	2(3)

CPT	MUE
19120	1(2)
19125	1(2)
19126	3(3)
19281	1(2)
19282	2(3)
19283	1(2)
19284	2(3)
19285	1(2)
19286	2(3)
19287	1(2)
19288	2(3)
19294	2(3)
19296	1(3)
19297	2(3)
19298	1(2)
19300	1(2)
19301	1(2)
19302	1(2)
19303	1(2)
19305	1(2)
19306	1(2)
19307	1(2)
19316	1(2)
19318	1(2)
19324	1(2)
19325	1(2)
19328	1(2)
19330	1(2)
19340	1(2)
19342	1(2)
19350	1(2)
19355	1(2)
19357	1(2)
19361	1(2)
19364	1(2)
19366	1(2)
19367	1(2)
19368	1(2)
19369	1(2)
19370	1(2)
19371	1(2)
19380	1(2)
19396	1(2)
19499	1(3)
20100	2(3)
20101	2(3)
20102	3(3)
20103	3(3)
20150	2(3)
20200	2(3)
20205	3(3)
20206	3(3)
20220	3(3)
20225	2(3)
20240	4(3)
20245	3(3)
20250	1(3)
20251	2(3)
20500	2(3)
20501	2(3)
20520	2(3)
20525	4(3)
20526	1(2)
20527	2(3)
20550	5(3)

CPT	MUE
20551	5(3)
20552	1(2)
20553	1(2)
20555	1(3)
20560	1(2)
20561	1(2)
20600	6(3)
20604	4(3)
20605	2(3)
20606	2(3)
20610	2(3)
20611	2(3)
20612	2(3)
20615	1(3)
20650	4(3)
20660	1(2)
20661	1(2)
20662	1(2)
20663	1(2)
20664	1(2)
20665	1(2)
20670	3(3)
20680	3(3)
20690	2(3)
20692	2(3)
20693	2(3)
20694	2(3)
20696	2(3)
20697	4(3)
20700	1(3)
20701	1(3)
20702	1(3)
20703	1(3)
20704	1(3)
20705	1(3)
20802	1(2)
20805	1(2)
20808	1(2)
20816	3(3)
20822	3(3)
20824	1(2)
20827	1(2)
20838	1(2)
20900	2(3)
20902	2(3)
20910	1(3)
20912	1(3)
20920	1(3)
20922	1(3)
20924	2(3)
20930	0(3)
20931	1(2)
20932	1(3)
20933	1(3)
20934	1(3)
20936	0(3)
20937	1(2)
20938	1(2)
20939	1(3)
20950	2(3)
20955	1(3)
20956	1(3)
20957	1(3)
20962	1(3)
20969	2(3)

CPT	MUE
20970	1(3)
20972	2(3)
20973	1(2)
20974	1(3)
20975	1(3)
20979	1(3)
20982	1(2)
20983	1(2)
20985	2(3)
20999	1(3)
21010	1(2)
21011	4(3)
21012	3(3)
21013	2(3)
21014	2(3)
21015	1(3)
21016	2(3)
21025	2(3)
21026	2(3)
21029	1(3)
21030	1(3)
21031	2(3)
21032	1(3)
21034	1(3)
21040	2(3)
21044	1(3)
21045	1(3)
21046	2(3)
21047	2(3)
21048	2(3)
21049	1(3)
21050	1(2)
21060	1(2)
21070	1(2)
21073	1(2)
21076	1(2)
21077	1(2)
21079	1(2)
21080	1(2)
21081	1(2)
21082	1(2)
21083	1(2)
21084	1(2)
21085	1(3)
21086	1(2)
21087	1(2)
21088	1(2)
21089	1(3)
21100	1(2)
21110	2(3)
21116	1(2)
21120	1(2)
21121	1(2)
21122	1(2)
21123	1(2)
21125	2(2)
21127	2(3)
21137	1(2)
21138	1(2)
21139	1(2)
21141	1(2)
21142	1(2)
21143	1(2)
21145	1(2)
21146	1(2)

CPT	MUE
21147	1(2)
21150	1(2)
21151	1(2)
21154	1(2)
21155	1(2)
21159	1(2)
21160	1(2)
21172	1(3)
21175	1(2)
21179	1(2)
21180	1(2)
21181	1(3)
21182	1(2)
21183	1(2)
21184	1(2)
21188	1(2)
21193	1(2)
21194	1(2)
21195	1(2)
21196	1(2)
21198	1(3)
21199	1(2)
21206	1(3)
21208	1(3)
21209	1(3)
21210	2(3)
21215	2(3)
21230	2(3)
21235	2(3)
21240	1(2)
21242	1(2)
21243	1(2)
21244	1(2)
21245	2(2)
21246	2(2)
21247	1(2)
21248	2(3)
21249	2(3)
21255	1(2)
21256	1(2)
21260	1(2)
21261	1(2)
21263	1(2)
21267	1(2)
21268	1(2)
21270	1(2)
21275	1(2)
21280	1(2)
21282	1(2)
21295	1(2)
21296	1(2)
21299	1(3)
21310	1(2)
21315	1(2)
21320	1(2)
21325	1(2)
21330	1(2)
21335	1(2)
21336	1(2)
21337	1(2)
21338	1(2)
21339	1(2)
21340	1(2)
21343	1(2)
21344	1(2)

CPT	MUE
21345	1(2)
21346	1(2)
21347	1(2)
21348	1(2)
21355	1(2)
21356	1(2)
21360	1(2)
21365	1(2)
21366	1(2)
21385	1(2)
21386	1(2)
21387	1(2)
21390	1(2)
21395	1(2)
21400	1(2)
21401	1(2)
21406	1(2)
21407	1(2)
21408	1(2)
21421	1(2)
21422	1(2)
21423	1(2)
21431	1(2)
21432	1(2)
21433	1(2)
21435	1(2)
21436	1(2)
21440	2(2)
21445	2(2)
21450	1(2)
21451	1(2)
21452	1(2)
21453	1(2)
21454	1(2)
21461	1(2)
21462	1(2)
21465	1(2)
21470	1(2)
21480	1(2)
21485	1(2)
21490	1(2)
21497	1(2)
21499	1(3)
21501	3(3)
21502	1(3)
21510	1(3)
21550	2(3)
21552	2(3)
21554	2(3)
21555	2(3)
21556	2(3)
21557	1(3)
21558	1(3)
21600	5(3)
21601	2(3)
21602	1(3)
21603	1(3)
21610	1(3)
21615	1(2)
21616	1(2)
21620	1(2)
21627	1(2)
21630	1(2)
21632	1(2)
21685	1(2)

CPT	MUE
21700	1(2)
21705	1(2)
21720	1(3)
21725	1(3)
21740	1(2)
21742	1(2)
21743	1(2)
21750	1(2)
21811	1(2)
21812	1(2)
21813	1(2)
21820	1(2)
21825	1(2)
21899	1(3)
21920	2(3)
21925	2(3)
21930	5(3)
21931	3(3)
21932	2(3)
21933	2(3)
21935	1(3)
21936	1(3)
22010	2(3)
22015	2(3)
22100	1(2)
22101	1(2)
22102	1(2)
22103	3(3)
22110	1(2)
22112	1(2)
22114	1(2)
22116	3(3)
22206	1(2)
22207	1(2)
22208	5(3)
22210	1(2)
22212	1(2)
22214	1(2)
22216	6(3)
22220	1(2)
22222	1(2)
22224	1(2)
22226	4(3)
22310	1(2)
22315	1(2)
22318	1(2)
22319	1(2)
22325	1(2)
22326	1(2)
22327	1(2)
22328	6(3)
22505	1(2)
22510	1(2)
22511	1(2)
22512	3(3)
22513	1(2)
22514	1(2)
22515	4(3)
22526	0(3)
22527	0(3)
22532	1(2)
22533	1(2)
22534	3(3)
22548	1(2)
22551	1(2)

CPT	MUE
22552	5(3)
22554	1(2)
22556	1(2)
22558	1(2)
22585	5(3)
22586	1(2)
22590	1(2)
22595	1(2)
22600	1(2)
22610	1(2)
22612	1(2)
22614	13(3)
22630	1(2)
22632	4(2)
22633	1(2)
22634	4(2)
22800	1(2)
22802	1(2)
22804	1(2)
22808	1(2)
22810	1(2)
22812	1(2)
22818	1(2)
22819	1(2)
22830	1(2)
22840	1(3)
22841	0(3)
22842	1(3)
22843	1(3)
22844	1(3)
22845	1(3)
22846	1(3)
22847	1(3)
22848	1(2)
22849	1(2)
22850	1(2)
22852	1(2)
22853	4(3)
22854	4(3)
22855	1(2)
22856	1(2)
22857	1(2)
22858	1(2)
22859	4(3)
22861	1(2)
22862	1(2)
22864	1(2)
22865	1(2)
22867	1(2)
22868	1(2)
22869	1(2)
22870	1(2)
22899	1(3)
22900	3(3)
22901	2(3)
22902	4(3)
22903	3(3)
22904	1(3)
22905	1(3)
22999	1(3)
23000	1(2)
23020	1(2)
23030	2(3)
23031	1(3)
23035	1(3)

CPT	MUE
23040	1(2)
23044	1(3)
23065	2(3)
23066	2(3)
23071	2(3)
23073	2(3)
23075	2(3)
23076	2(3)
23077	1(3)
23078	1(3)
23100	1(2)
23101	1(3)
23105	1(2)
23106	1(2)
23107	1(2)
23120	1(2)
23125	1(2)
23130	1(2)
23140	1(3)
23145	1(3)
23146	1(3)
23150	1(3)
23155	1(3)
23156	1(3)
23170	1(3)
23172	1(3)
23174	1(3)
23180	1(3)
23182	1(3)
23184	1(3)
23190	1(3)
23195	1(2)
23200	1(3)
23210	1(3)
23220	1(3)
23330	2(3)
23333	1(3)
23334	1(2)
23335	1(2)
23350	1(2)
23395	1(2)
23397	1(3)
23400	1(2)
23405	2(3)
23406	1(3)
23410	1(2)
23412	1(2)
23415	1(2)
23420	1(2)
23430	1(2)
23440	1(2)
23450	1(2)
23455	1(2)
23460	1(2)
23462	1(2)
23465	1(2)
23466	1(2)
23470	1(2)
23472	1(2)
23473	1(2)
23474	1(2)
23480	1(2)
23485	1(2)
23490	1(2)
23491	1(2)

CPT	MUE
23500	1(2)
23505	1(2)
23515	1(2)
23520	1(2)
23525	1(2)
23530	1(2)
23532	1(2)
23540	1(2)
23545	1(2)
23550	1(2)
23552	1(2)
23570	1(2)
23575	1(2)
23585	1(2)
23600	1(2)
23605	1(2)
23615	1(2)
23616	1(2)
23620	1(2)
23625	1(2)
23630	1(2)
23650	1(2)
23655	1(2)
23660	1(2)
23665	1(2)
23670	1(2)
23675	1(2)
23680	1(2)
23700	1(2)
23800	1(2)
23802	1(2)
23900	1(2)
23920	1(2)
23921	1(2)
23929	1(3)
23930	2(3)
23931	2(3)
23935	2(3)
24000	1(2)
24006	1(2)
24065	2(3)
24066	2(3)
24071	2(3)
24073	2(3)
24075	5(3)
24076	4(3)
24077	1(3)
24079	1(3)
24100	1(2)
24101	1(2)
24102	1(2)
24105	1(2)
24110	1(3)
24115	1(3)
24116	1(3)
24120	1(3)
24125	1(3)
24126	1(3)
24130	1(2)
24134	1(3)
24136	1(3)
24138	1(3)
24140	1(3)
24145	1(3)
24147	1(2)

CPT	MUE
24149	1(2)
24150	1(3)
24152	1(3)
24155	1(2)
24160	1(2)
24164	1(2)
24200	3(3)
24201	3(3)
24220	1(2)
24300	1(2)
24301	2(3)
24305	4(3)
24310	2(3)
24320	2(3)
24330	1(3)
24331	1(3)
24332	1(2)
24340	1(2)
24341	2(3)
24342	2(3)
24343	1(2)
24344	1(2)
24345	1(2)
24346	1(2)
24357	1(3)
24358	1(3)
24359	2(3)
24360	1(2)
24361	1(2)
24362	1(2)
24363	1(2)
24365	1(2)
24366	1(2)
24370	1(2)
24371	1(2)
24400	1(3)
24410	1(2)
24420	1(2)
24430	1(3)
24435	1(3)
24470	1(2)
24495	1(2)
24498	1(2)
24500	1(2)
24505	1(2)
24515	1(2)
24516	1(2)
24530	1(2)
24535	1(2)
24538	1(2)
24545	1(2)
24546	1(2)
24560	1(3)
24565	1(3)
24566	1(3)
24575	1(3)
24576	1(3)
24577	1(3)
24579	1(3)
24582	1(3)
24586	1(3)
24587	1(2)
24600	1(2)
24605	1(2)
24615	1(2)

CPT	MUE
24620	1(2)
24635	1(2)
24640	1(2)
24650	1(2)
24655	1(2)
24665	1(2)
24666	1(2)
24670	1(2)
24675	1(2)
24685	1(2)
24800	1(2)
24802	1(2)
24900	1(2)
24920	1(2)
24925	1(2)
24930	1(2)
24931	1(2)
24935	1(2)
24940	1(2)
24999	1(3)
25000	2(3)
25001	1(3)
25020	1(2)
25023	1(2)
25024	1(2)
25025	1(2)
25028	4(3)
25031	2(3)
25035	2(3)
25040	1(3)
25065	2(3)
25066	2(3)
25071	3(3)
25073	2(3)
25075	6(3)
25076	3(3)
25077	1(3)
25078	1(3)
25085	1(2)
25100	1(2)
25101	1(2)
25105	1(2)
25107	1(2)
25109	4(3)
25110	2(3)
25111	1(3)
25112	1(3)
25115	1(3)
25116	1(3)
25118	5(3)
25119	1(2)
25120	1(3)
25125	1(3)
25126	1(3)
25130	1(3)
25135	1(3)
25136	1(3)
25145	1(3)
25150	1(3)
25151	1(3)
25170	1(3)
25210	2(3)
25215	1(2)
25230	1(2)
25240	1(2)

CPT	MUE
25246	1(2)
25248	3(3)
25250	1(2)
25251	1(2)
25259	1(2)
25260	9(3)
25263	4(3)
25265	4(3)
25270	8(3)
25272	4(3)
25274	4(3)
25275	2(3)
25280	9(3)
25290	10(3)
25295	9(3)
25300	1(2)
25301	1(2)
25310	5(3)
25312	4(3)
25315	1(3)
25316	1(3)
25320	1(2)
25332	1(2)
25335	1(2)
25337	1(2)
25350	1(3)
25355	1(3)
25360	1(3)
25365	1(3)
25370	1(2)
25375	1(2)
25390	1(2)
25391	1(2)
25392	1(2)
25393	1(2)
25394	1(3)
25400	1(2)
25405	1(2)
25415	1(2)
25420	1(2)
25425	1(2)
25426	1(2)
25430	1(3)
25431	1(3)
25440	1(2)
25441	1(2)
25442	1(2)
25443	1(2)
25444	1(2)
25445	1(2)
25446	1(2)
25447	4(3)
25449	1(2)
25450	1(2)
25455	1(2)
25490	1(2)
25491	1(2)
25492	1(2)
25500	1(2)
25505	1(2)
25515	1(2)
25520	1(2)
25525	1(2)
25526	1(2)
25530	1(2)

CPT	MUE
25535	1(2)
25545	1(2)
25560	1(2)
25565	1(2)
25574	1(2)
25575	1(2)
25600	1(2)
25605	1(2)
25606	1(2)
25607	1(2)
25608	1(2)
25609	1(2)
25622	1(2)
25624	1(2)
25628	1(2)
25630	1(3)
25635	1(3)
25645	1(3)
25650	1(2)
25651	1(2)
25652	1(2)
25660	1(2)
25670	1(2)
25671	1(2)
25675	1(2)
25676	1(2)
25680	1(2)
25685	1(2)
25690	1(2)
25695	1(2)
25800	1(2)
25805	1(2)
25810	1(2)
25820	1(2)
25825	1(2)
25830	1(2)
25900	1(2)
25905	1(2)
25907	1(2)
25909	1(2)
25915	1(2)
25920	1(2)
25922	1(2)
25924	1(2)
25927	1(2)
25929	1(2)
25931	1(2)
25999	1(3)
26010	2(3)
26011	3(3)
26020	4(3)
26025	1(2)
26030	1(2)
26034	2(3)
26035	1(3)
26037	1(3)
26040	1(2)
26045	1(2)
26055	5(3)
26060	5(3)
26070	2(3)
26075	3(3)
26080	3(3)
26100	1(3)
26105	2(3)

CPT	MUE
26110	2(3)
26111	4(3)
26113	3(3)
26115	4(3)
26116	2(3)
26117	2(3)
26118	1(3)
26121	1(2)
26123	1(2)
26125	4(3)
26130	1(3)
26135	4(3)
26140	2(3)
26145	6(3)
26160	4(3)
26170	4(3)
26180	4(3)
26185	1(3)
26200	2(3)
26205	1(3)
26210	2(3)
26215	2(3)
26230	2(3)
26235	2(3)
26236	2(3)
26250	2(3)
26260	1(3)
26262	1(3)
26320	4(3)
26340	4(3)
26341	2(3)
26350	6(3)
26352	2(3)
26356	4(3)
26357	2(3)
26358	2(3)
26370	3(3)
26372	1(3)
26373	2(3)
26390	2(3)
26392	2(3)
26410	4(3)
26412	3(3)
26415	2(3)
26416	2(3)
26418	4(3)
26420	3(3)
26426	4(3)
26428	2(3)
26432	2(3)
26433	2(3)
26434	2(3)
26437	4(3)
26440	6(3)
26442	5(3)
26445	5(3)
26449	5(3)
26450	6(3)
26455	6(3)
26460	4(3)
26471	4(3)
26474	4(3)
26476	4(3)
26477	2(3)
26478	6(3)

CPT	MUE
26479	4(3)
26480	4(3)
26483	4(3)
26485	4(3)
26489	2(3)
26490	3(3)
26492	2(3)
26494	1(3)
26496	1(3)
26497	2(3)
26498	1(3)
26499	2(3)
26500	3(3)
26502	2(3)
26508	1(2)
26510	4(3)
26516	1(2)
26517	1(2)
26518	1(2)
26520	4(3)
26525	4(3)
26530	4(3)
26531	4(3)
26535	3(3)
26536	4(3)
26540	4(3)
26541	4(3)
26542	4(3)
26545	4(3)
26546	2(3)
26548	3(3)
26550	1(2)
26551	1(2)
26553	1(3)
26554	1(3)
26555	2(3)
26556	2(3)
26560	2(3)
26561	2(3)
26562	2(3)
26565	2(3)
26567	3(3)
26568	2(3)
26580	1(2)
26587	2(3)
26590	2(3)
26591	4(3)
26593	8(3)
26596	1(3)
26600	2(3)
26605	3(3)
26607	2(3)
26608	4(3)
26615	3(3)
26641	1(2)
26645	1(2)
26650	1(2)
26665	1(2)
26670	2(3)
26675	1(3)
26676	2(3)
26685	3(3)
26686	3(3)
26700	2(3)
26705	3(3)

CPT	MUE
26706	2(3)
26715	3(3)
26720	4(3)
26725	3(3)
26727	3(3)
26735	4(3)
26740	3(3)
26742	3(3)
26746	3(3)
26750	3(3)
26755	2(3)
26756	2(3)
26765	3(3)
26770	3(3)
26775	2(3)
26776	4(3)
26785	3(3)
26820	1(2)
26841	1(2)
26842	1(2)
26843	2(3)
26844	2(3)
26850	5(3)
26852	2(3)
26860	1(2)
26861	4(3)
26862	1(2)
26863	2(3)
26910	4(3)
26951	8(3)
26952	4(3)
26989	1(3)
26990	2(3)
26991	1(3)
26992	2(3)
27000	1(3)
27001	1(3)
27003	1(2)
27005	1(2)
27006	1(2)
27025	1(3)
27027	1(2)
27030	1(2)
27033	1(2)
27035	1(2)
27036	1(2)
27040	2(3)
27041	3(3)
27043	2(3)
27045	3(3)
27047	2(3)
27048	2(3)
27049	1(3)
27050	1(2)
27052	1(2)
27054	1(2)
27057	1(2)
27059	1(3)
27060	1(2)
27062	1(2)
27065	1(3)
27066	1(3)
27067	1(3)
27070	1(3)
27071	1(3)

CPT	MUE
27075	1(3)
27076	1(2)
27077	1(2)
27078	1(2)
27080	1(2)
27086	1(3)
27087	1(3)
27090	1(2)
27091	1(2)
27093	1(2)
27095	1(2)
27096	1(2)
27097	1(3)
27098	1(2)
27100	1(2)
27105	1(3)
27110	1(2)
27111	1(2)
27120	1(2)
27122	1(2)
27125	1(2)
27130	1(2)
27132	1(2)
27134	1(2)
27137	1(2)
27138	1(2)
27140	1(2)
27146	1(3)
27147	1(3)
27151	1(3)
27156	1(2)
27158	1(2)
27161	1(2)
27165	1(2)
27170	1(2)
27175	1(2)
27176	1(2)
27177	1(2)
27178	1(2)
27179	1(2)
27181	1(2)
27185	1(2)
27187	1(2)
27197	1(2)
27198	1(2)
27200	1(2)
27202	1(2)
27215	0(3)
27216	0(3)
27217	0(3)
27218	0(3)
27220	1(2)
27222	1(2)
27226	1(2)
27227	1(2)
27228	1(2)
27230	1(2)
27232	1(2)
27235	1(2)
27236	1(2)
27238	1(2)
27240	1(2)
27244	1(2)
27245	1(2)
27246	1(2)

CPT	MUE
27248	1(2)
27250	1(2)
27252	1(2)
27253	1(2)
27254	1(2)
27256	1(2)
27257	1(2)
27258	1(2)
27259	1(2)
27265	1(2)
27266	1(2)
27267	1(2)
27268	1(2)
27269	1(2)
27275	2(2)
27279	1(2)
27280	1(2)
27282	1(2)
27284	1(2)
27286	1(2)
27290	1(2)
27295	1(2)
27299	1(3)
27301	3(3)
27303	2(3)
27305	1(2)
27306	1(2)
27307	1(2)
27310	1(2)
27323	2(3)
27324	3(3)
27325	1(2)
27326	1(2)
27327	5(3)
27328	3(3)
27329	1(3)
27330	1(2)
27331	1(2)
27332	1(2)
27333	1(2)
27334	1(2)
27335	1(2)
27337	3(3)
27339	4(3)
27340	1(2)
27345	1(2)
27347	1(2)
27350	1(2)
27355	1(3)
27356	1(3)
27357	1(3)
27358	1(3)
27360	2(3)
27364	1(3)
27365	1(3)
27369	1(2)
27372	2(3)
27380	1(2)
27381	1(2)
27385	2(3)
27386	2(3)
27390	1(2)
27391	1(2)
27392	1(2)
27393	1(2)

CPT	MUE
27394	1(2)
27395	1(2)
27396	1(2)
27397	1(2)
27400	1(2)
27403	1(3)
27405	2(2)
27407	2(2)
27409	1(2)
27412	1(2)
27415	1(2)
27416	1(2)
27418	1(2)
27420	1(2)
27422	1(2)
27424	1(2)
27425	1(2)
27427	1(2)
27428	1(2)
27429	1(2)
27430	1(2)
27435	1(2)
27437	1(2)
27438	1(2)
27440	1(2)
27441	1(2)
27442	1(2)
27443	1(2)
27445	1(2)
27446	1(2)
27447	1(2)
27448	1(3)
27450	1(3)
27454	1(2)
27455	1(3)
27457	1(3)
27465	1(2)
27466	1(2)
27468	1(2)
27470	1(2)
27472	1(2)
27475	1(2)
27477	1(2)
27479	1(2)
27485	1(2)
27486	1(2)
27487	1(2)
27488	1(2)
27495	1(2)
27496	1(2)
27497	1(2)
27498	1(2)
27499	1(2)
27500	1(2)
27501	1(2)
27502	1(2)
27503	1(2)
27506	1(2)
27507	1(2)
27508	1(2)
27509	1(2)
27510	1(2)
27511	1(2)
27513	1(2)
27514	1(2)

CPT	MUE
27516	1(2)
27517	1(2)
27519	1(2)
27520	1(2)
27524	1(2)
27530	1(2)
27532	1(2)
27535	1(2)
27536	1(2)
27538	1(2)
27540	1(2)
27550	1(2)
27552	1(2)
27556	1(2)
27557	1(2)
27558	1(2)
27560	1(2)
27562	1(2)
27566	1(2)
27570	1(2)
27580	1(2)
27590	1(2)
27591	1(2)
27592	1(2)
27594	1(2)
27596	1(2)
27598	1(2)
27599	1(3)
27600	1(2)
27601	1(2)
27602	1(2)
27603	2(3)
27604	2(3)
27605	1(2)
27606	1(2)
27607	2(3)
27610	1(2)
27612	1(2)
27613	3(3)
27614	3(3)
27615	1(3)
27616	1(3)
27618	3(3)
27619	2(3)
27620	1(2)
27625	1(2)
27626	1(2)
27630	2(3)
27632	3(3)
27634	2(3)
27635	1(3)
27637	1(3)
27638	1(3)
27640	1(3)
27641	1(3)
27645	1(3)
27646	1(3)
27647	1(3)
27648	1(2)
27650	1(2)
27652	1(2)
27654	1(2)
27656	1(3)
27658	2(3)
27659	2(3)

CPT	MUE
27664	2(3)
27665	2(3)
27675	1(2)
27676	1(2)
27680	2(3)
27681	1(2)
27685	2(3)
27686	3(3)
27687	1(2)
27690	2(3)
27691	2(3)
27692	4(3)
27695	1(2)
27696	1(2)
27698	2(2)
27700	1(2)
27702	1(2)
27703	1(2)
27704	1(2)
27705	1(3)
27707	1(3)
27709	1(3)
27712	1(2)
27715	1(2)
27720	1(2)
27722	1(2)
27724	1(2)
27725	1(2)
27726	1(2)
27727	1(2)
27730	1(2)
27732	1(2)
27734	1(2)
27740	1(2)
27742	1(2)
27745	1(2)
27750	1(2)
27752	1(2)
27756	1(2)
27758	1(2)
27759	1(2)
27760	1(2)
27762	1(2)
27766	1(2)
27767	1(2)
27768	1(2)
27769	1(2)
27780	1(2)
27781	1(2)
27784	1(2)
27786	1(2)
27788	1(2)
27792	1(2)
27808	1(2)
27810	1(2)
27814	1(2)
27816	1(2)
27818	1(2)
27822	1(2)
27823	1(2)
27824	1(2)
27825	1(2)
27826	1(2)
27827	1(2)
27828	1(2)

CPT	MUE
27829	1(2)
27830	1(2)
27831	1(2)
27832	1(2)
27840	1(2)
27842	1(2)
27846	1(2)
27848	1(2)
27860	1(2)
27870	1(2)
27871	1(3)
27880	1(2)
27881	1(2)
27882	1(2)
27884	1(2)
27886	1(2)
27888	1(2)
27889	1(2)
27892	1(2)
27893	1(2)
27894	1(2)
27899	1(3)
28001	2(3)
28002	3(3)
28003	2(3)
28005	3(3)
28008	2(3)
28010	4(3)
28011	4(3)
28020	2(3)
28022	3(3)
28024	4(3)
28035	1(2)
28039	2(3)
28041	2(3)
28043	4(3)
28045	4(3)
28046	1(3)
28047	1(3)
28050	2(3)
28052	2(3)
28054	2(3)
28055	1(3)
28060	1(2)
28062	1(2)
28070	2(3)
28072	4(3)
28080	3(3)
28086	2(3)
28088	2(3)
28090	2(3)
28092	2(3)
28100	1(3)
28102	1(3)
28103	1(3)
28104	2(3)
28106	1(3)
28107	1(3)
28108	2(3)
28110	1(2)
28111	1(2)
28112	4(3)
28113	1(2)
28114	1(2)
28116	1(2)

CPT	MUE
28118	1(2)
28119	1(2)
28120	2(3)
28122	4(3)
28124	4(3)
28126	4(3)
28130	1(2)
28140	3(3)
28150	4(3)
28153	4(3)
28160	5(3)
28171	1(3)
28173	2(3)
28175	2(3)
28190	3(3)
28192	2(3)
28193	2(3)
28200	4(3)
28202	2(3)
28208	4(3)
28210	2(3)
28220	1(2)
28222	1(2)
28225	1(2)
28226	1(2)
28230	1(2)
28232	6(3)
28234	6(3)
28238	1(2)
28240	1(2)
28250	1(2)
28260	1(2)
28261	1(3)
28262	1(2)
28264	1(2)
28270	6(3)
28272	6(3)
28280	1(2)
28285	4(3)
28286	1(2)
28288	4(3)
28289	1(2)
28291	1(2)
28292	1(2)
28295	1(2)
28296	1(2)
28297	1(2)
28298	1(2)
28299	1(2)
28300	1(2)
28302	1(2)
28304	1(3)
28305	1(3)
28306	1(2)
28307	1(2)
28308	4(3)
28309	1(2)
28310	1(2)
28312	4(3)
28313	4(3)
28315	1(2)
28320	1(2)
28322	2(3)
28340	2(3)
28341	2(3)

CPT	MUE
28344	1(2)
28345	2(3)
28360	1(2)
28400	1(2)
28405	1(2)
28406	1(2)
28415	1(2)
28420	1(2)
28430	1(2)
28435	1(2)
28436	1(2)
28445	1(2)
28446	1(2)
28450	2(3)
28455	3(3)
28456	2(3)
28465	3(3)
28470	2(3)
28475	5(3)
28476	4(3)
28485	5(3)
28490	1(2)
28495	1(2)
28496	1(2)
28505	1(2)
28510	4(3)
28515	4(3)
28525	4(3)
28530	1(2)
28531	1(2)
28540	1(3)
28545	1(3)
28546	1(3)
28555	1(3)
28570	1(2)
28575	1(2)
28576	1(2)
28585	1(3)
28600	2(3)
28605	2(3)
28606	3(3)
28615	5(3)
28630	2(3)
28635	2(3)
28636	4(3)
28645	4(3)
28660	4(3)
28665	3(3)
28666	4(3)
28675	3(3)
28705	1(2)
28715	1(2)
28725	1(2)
28730	1(2)
28735	1(2)
28737	1(2)
28740	1(2)
28750	1(2)
28755	1(2)
28760	1(2)
28800	1(2)
28805	1(2)
28810	5(3)
28820	6(3)
28825	8(2)

CPT	MUE	CPT	MUE	CPT	MUE	CPT	MUE	CPT	MUE	CPT	MUE	CPT	MUE	CPT	MUE
28890	1(2)	29825	1(2)	30000	1(3)	31201	1(2)	31545	1(2)	31661	1(2)	32556	2(3)	33130	1(3)
28899	1(3)	29826	1(2)	30020	1(3)	31205	1(2)	31546	1(2)	31717	1(3)	32557	2(3)	33140	1(2)
29000	1(3)	29827	1(2)	30100	2(3)	31225	1(2)	31551	1(2)	31720	1(3)	32560	1(3)	33141	1(2)
29010	1(3)	29828	1(2)	30110	1(2)	31230	1(2)	31552	1(2)	31725	1(3)	32561	1(2)	33202	1(2)
29015	1(3)	29830	1(2)	30115	1(2)	31231	1(2)	31553	1(2)	31730	1(3)	32562	1(2)	33203	1(2)
29035	1(3)	29834	1(2)	30117	2(3)	31233	1(2)	31554	1(2)	31750	1(2)	32601	1(3)	33206	1(3)
29040	1(3)	29835	1(2)	30118	1(3)	31235	1(2)	31560	1(2)	31755	1(2)	32604	1(3)	33207	1(3)
29044	1(3)	29836	1(2)	30120	1(2)	31237	1(2)	31561	1(2)	31760	1(2)	32606	1(3)	33208	1(3)
29046	1(3)	29837	1(2)	30124	2(3)	31238	1(3)	31570	1(2)	31766	1(2)	32607	1(3)	33210	1(3)
29049	1(3)	29838	1(2)	30125	1(3)	31239	1(2)	31571	1(2)	31770	2(3)	32608	1(3)	33211	1(3)
29055	1(3)	29840	1(2)	30130	1(2)	31240	1(2)	31572	1(2)	31775	1(3)	32609	1(3)	33212	1(3)
29058	1(3)	29843	1(2)	30140	1(2)	31241	1(2)	31573	1(2)	31780	1(2)	32650	1(2)	33213	1(3)
29065	1(3)	29844	1(2)	30150	1(2)	31253	1(2)	31574	1(2)	31781	1(2)	32651	1(2)	33214	1(3)
29075	1(3)	29845	1(2)	30160	1(2)	31254	1(2)	31575	1(3)	31785	1(3)	32652	1(2)	33215	2(3)
29085	1(3)	29846	1(2)	30200	1(2)	31255	1(2)	31576	1(3)	31786	1(3)	32653	1(3)	33216	1(3)
29086	2(3)	29847	1(2)	30210	1(3)	31256	1(2)	31577	1(3)	31800	1(3)	32654	1(3)	33217	1(3)
29105	1(2)	29848	1(2)	30220	1(2)	31257	1(2)	31578	1(3)	31805	1(3)	32655	1(3)	33218	1(3)
29125	1(2)	29850	1(2)	30300	1(3)	31259	1(2)	31579	1(2)	31820	1(2)	32656	1(2)	33220	1(3)
29126	1(2)	29851	1(2)	30310	1(3)	31267	1(2)	31580	1(2)	31825	1(2)	32658	1(3)	33221	1(3)
29130	3(3)	29855	1(2)	30320	1(3)	31276	1(2)	31584	1(2)	31830	1(2)	32659	1(2)	33222	1(3)
29131	2(3)	29856	1(2)	30400	1(2)	31287	1(2)	31587	1(2)	31899	1(3)	32661	1(3)	33223	1(3)
29200	1(2)	29860	1(2)	30410	1(2)	31288	1(2)	31590	1(2)	32035	1(2)	32662	1(3)	33224	1(3)
29240	1(2)	29861	1(2)	30420	1(2)	31290	1(2)	31591	1(2)	32036	1(3)	32663	1(3)	33225	1(3)
29260	1(3)	29862	1(2)	30430	1(2)	31291	1(2)	31592	1(2)	32096	1(3)	32664	1(2)	33226	1(3)
29280	2(3)	29863	1(2)	30435	1(2)	31292	1(2)	31599	1(3)	32097	1(3)	32665	1(2)	33227	1(3)
29305	1(3)	29866	1(2)	30450	1(2)	31293	1(2)	31600	1(2)	32098	1(2)	32666	1(3)	33228	1(3)
29325	1(3)	29867	1(2)	30460	1(2)	31294	1(2)	31601	1(2)	32100	1(3)	32667	3(3)	33229	1(3)
29345	1(3)	29868	1(3)	30462	1(2)	31295	1(2)	31603	1(2)	32110	1(3)	32668	2(3)	33230	1(3)
29355	1(3)	29870	1(2)	30465	1(2)	31296	1(2)	31605	1(2)	32120	1(3)	32669	2(3)	33231	1(3)
29358	1(3)	29871	1(2)	30520	1(2)	31297	1(2)	31610	1(2)	32124	1(3)	32670	1(2)	33233	1(2)
29365	1(3)	29873	1(2)	30540	1(2)	31298	1(2)	31611	1(2)	32140	1(3)	32671	1(2)	33234	1(2)
29405	1(3)	29874	1(2)	30545	1(2)	31299	1(3)	31612	1(3)	32141	1(3)	32672	1(3)	33235	1(2)
29425	1(3)	29875	1(2)	30560	1(2)	31300	1(2)	31613	1(2)	32150	1(3)	32673	1(2)	33236	1(2)
29435	1(3)	29876	1(2)	30580	2(3)	31360	1(2)	31614	1(2)	32151	1(3)	32674	1(2)	33237	1(2)
29440	1(2)	29877	1(2)	30600	1(3)	31365	1(2)	31615	1(3)	32160	1(3)	32701	1(2)	33238	1(2)
29445	1(3)	29879	1(2)	30620	1(2)	31367	1(2)	31622	1(3)	32200	2(3)	32800	1(3)	33240	1(3)
29450	1(3)	29880	1(2)	30630	1(2)	31368	1(2)	31623	1(3)	32215	1(2)	32810	1(3)	33241	1(2)
29505	1(2)	29881	1(2)	30801	1(2)	31370	1(2)	31624	1(3)	32220	1(2)	32815	1(3)	33243	1(2)
29515	1(2)	29882	1(2)	30802	1(2)	31375	1(2)	31625	1(2)	32225	1(2)	32820	1(2)	33244	1(2)
29520	1(2)	29883	1(2)	30901	1(3)	31380	1(2)	31626	1(2)	32310	1(3)	32850	1(2)	33249	1(3)
29530	1(2)	29884	1(2)	30903	1(3)	31382	1(2)	31627	1(3)	32320	1(3)	32851	1(2)	33250	1(2)
29540	1(2)	29885	1(2)	30905	1(2)	31390	1(2)	31628	1(2)	32400	2(3)	32852	1(2)	33251	1(2)
29550	1(2)	29886	1(2)	30906	1(3)	31395	1(2)	31629	1(2)	32405	2(3)	32853	1(2)	33254	1(2)
29580	1(2)	29887	1(2)	30915	1(3)	31400	1(3)	31630	1(3)	32440	1(2)	32854	1(2)	33255	1(2)
29581	1(2)	29888	1(2)	30920	1(3)	31420	1(2)	31631	1(2)	32442	1(2)	32855	1(2)	33256	1(2)
29584	1(2)	29889	1(2)	30930	1(2)	31500	2(3)	31632	2(3)	32445	1(2)	32856	1(2)	33257	1(2)
29700	2(3)	29891	1(2)	30999	1(3)	31502	1(3)	31633	2(3)	32480	1(2)	32900	1(2)	33258	1(2)
29705	1(3)	29892	1(2)	31000	1(2)	31505	1(3)	31634	1(3)	32482	1(2)	32905	1(2)	33259	1(2)
29710	1(2)	29893	1(2)	31002	1(2)	31510	1(2)	31635	1(3)	32484	2(3)	32906	1(2)	33261	1(2)
29720	1(2)	29894	1(2)	31020	1(2)	31511	1(3)	31636	1(2)	32486	1(3)	32940	1(3)	33262	1(3)
29730	1(3)	29895	1(2)	31030	1(2)	31512	1(3)	31637	2(3)	32488	1(2)	32960	1(2)	33263	1(3)
29740	1(3)	29897	1(2)	31032	1(2)	31513	1(3)	31638	1(3)	32491	1(2)	32994	1(2)	33264	1(3)
29750	1(3)	29898	1(2)	31040	1(2)	31515	1(3)	31640	1(3)	32501	1(3)	32997	1(2)	33265	1(2)
29799	1(3)	29899	1(2)	31050	1(2)	31520	1(3)	31641	1(3)	32503	1(2)	32998	1(2)	33266	1(2)
29800	1(2)	29900	2(3)	31051	1(2)	31525	1(3)	31643	1(2)	32504	1(2)	32999	1(3)	33270	1(3)
29804	1(2)	29901	2(3)	31070	1(2)	31526	1(3)	31645	1(2)	32505	1(2)	33016	1(3)	33271	1(3)
29805	1(2)	29902	2(3)	31075	1(2)	31527	1(2)	31646	2(3)	32506	3(3)	33017	1(3)	33272	1(3)
29806	1(2)	29904	1(2)	31080	1(2)	31528	1(2)	31647	1(2)	32507	2(3)	33018	1(3)	33273	1(3)
29807	1(2)	29905	1(2)	31081	1(2)	31529	1(3)	31648	1(2)	32540	1(3)	33019	1(3)	33274	1(3)
29819	1(2)	29906	1(2)	31084	1(2)	31530	1(3)	31649	2(3)	32550	2(3)	33020	1(3)	33275	1(3)
29820	1(2)	29907	1(2)	31085	1(2)	31531	1(3)	31651	3(3)	32551	2(3)	33025	1(2)	33285	1(3)
29821	1(2)	29914	1(2)	31086	1(2)	31535	1(3)	31652	1(2)	32552	2(2)	33030	1(2)	33286	1(3)
29822	1(2)	29915	1(2)	31087	1(2)	31536	1(3)	31653	1(2)	32553	1(2)	33031	1(2)	33289	1(3)
29823	1(2)	29916	1(2)	31090	1(2)	31540	1(3)	31654	1(3)	32554	2(3)	33050	1(2)	33300	1(3)
29824	1(2)	29999	1(3)	31200	1(2)	31541	1(3)	31660	1(2)	32555	2(3)	33120	1(3)	33305	1(3)

CPT	MUE
33310	1(2)
33315	1(2)
33320	1(3)
33321	1(3)
33322	1(3)
33330	1(3)
33335	1(3)
33340	1(2)
33361	1(2)
33362	1(2)
33363	1(2)
33364	1(2)
33365	1(2)
33366	1(3)
33367	1(2)
33368	1(2)
33369	1(2)
33390	1(2)
33391	1(2)
33404	1(2)
33405	1(2)
33406	1(2)
33410	1(2)
33411	1(2)
33412	1(2)
33413	1(2)
33414	1(2)
33415	1(2)
33416	1(2)
33417	1(2)
33418	1(3)
33419	1(2)
33420	1(2)
33422	1(2)
33425	1(2)
33426	1(2)
33427	1(2)
33430	1(2)
33440	1(2)
33460	1(2)
33463	1(2)
33464	1(2)
33465	1(2)
33468	1(2)
33470	1(2)
33471	1(2)
33474	1(2)
33475	1(2)
33476	1(2)
33477	1(2)
33478	1(2)
33496	1(3)
33500	1(3)
33501	1(3)
33502	1(3)
33503	1(3)
33504	1(3)
33505	1(3)
33506	1(3)
33507	1(3)
33508	1(2)
33510	1(2)
33511	1(2)
33512	1(2)
33513	1(2)

CPT	MUE
33514	1(2)
33516	1(2)
33517	1(2)
33518	1(2)
33519	1(2)
33521	1(2)
33522	1(2)
33523	1(2)
33530	1(2)
33533	1(2)
33534	1(2)
33535	1(2)
33536	1(2)
33542	1(2)
33545	1(2)
33548	1(2)
33572	3(2)
33600	1(3)
33602	1(3)
33606	1(2)
33608	1(2)
33610	1(2)
33611	1(2)
33612	1(2)
33615	1(2)
33617	1(2)
33619	1(2)
33620	1(2)
33621	1(3)
33622	1(2)
33641	1(2)
33645	1(2)
33647	1(2)
33660	1(2)
33665	1(2)
33670	1(2)
33675	1(2)
33676	1(2)
33677	1(2)
33681	1(2)
33684	1(2)
33688	1(2)
33690	1(2)
33692	1(2)
33694	1(2)
33697	1(2)
33702	1(2)
33710	1(2)
33720	1(2)
33722	1(3)
33724	1(2)
33726	1(2)
33730	1(2)
33732	1(2)
33735	1(2)
33736	1(2)
33737	1(2)
33750	1(3)
33755	1(2)
33762	1(2)
33764	1(3)
33766	1(2)
33767	1(2)
33768	1(2)
33770	1(2)

CPT	MUE
33771	1(2)
33774	1(2)
33775	1(2)
33776	1(2)
33777	1(2)
33778	1(2)
33779	1(2)
33780	1(2)
33781	1(2)
33782	1(2)
33783	1(2)
33786	1(2)
33788	1(2)
33800	1(2)
33802	1(3)
33803	1(3)
33813	1(2)
33814	1(2)
33820	1(2)
33822	1(2)
33824	1(2)
33840	1(2)
33845	1(2)
33851	1(2)
33852	1(2)
33853	1(2)
33858	1(2)
33859	1(2)
33863	1(2)
33864	1(2)
33866	1(2)
33871	1(2)
33875	1(2)
33877	1(2)
33880	1(2)
33881	1(2)
33883	1(2)
33884	2(3)
33886	1(2)
33889	1(2)
33891	1(2)
33910	1(3)
33915	1(3)
33916	1(3)
33917	1(2)
33920	1(2)
33922	1(2)
33924	1(2)
33925	1(2)
33926	1(2)
33927	1(3)
33928	1(3)
33929	1(3)
33930	1(2)
33933	1(2)
33935	1(2)
33940	1(2)
33944	1(2)
33945	1(2)
33946	1(2)
33947	1(2)
33948	1(2)
33949	1(2)
33951	1(3)
33952	1(3)

CPT	MUE
33953	1(3)
33954	1(3)
33955	1(3)
33956	1(3)
33957	1(3)
33958	1(3)
33959	1(3)
33962	1(3)
33963	1(3)
33964	1(3)
33965	1(3)
33966	1(3)
33967	1(3)
33968	1(3)
33969	1(3)
33970	1(3)
33971	1(3)
33973	1(3)
33974	1(3)
33975	1(3)
33976	1(3)
33977	1(3)
33978	1(3)
33979	1(3)
33980	1(3)
33981	1(3)
33982	1(3)
33983	1(3)
33984	1(3)
33985	1(3)
33986	1(3)
33987	1(3)
33988	1(3)
33989	1(3)
33990	1(3)
33991	1(3)
33992	1(2)
33993	1(3)
33999	1(3)
34001	1(3)
34051	1(3)
34101	1(3)
34111	2(3)
34151	1(3)
34201	1(3)
34203	1(2)
34401	1(3)
34421	1(3)
34451	1(3)
34471	1(2)
34490	1(2)
34501	1(2)
34502	1(2)
34510	2(3)
34520	1(3)
34530	1(2)
34701	1(2)
34702	1(2)
34703	1(2)
34704	1(2)
34705	1(2)
34706	1(2)
34707	1(2)
34708	1(2)
34709	3(3)

CPT	MUE
34710	1(2)
34711	2(3)
34712	1(2)
34713	1(2)
34714	1(2)
34715	1(2)
34716	1(2)
34717	2(2)
34718	2(2)
34808	1(3)
34812	1(2)
34813	1(2)
34820	1(2)
34830	1(2)
34831	1(2)
34832	1(2)
34833	1(2)
34834	1(2)
34839	1(2)
34841	1(2)
34842	1(2)
34843	1(2)
34844	1(2)
34845	1(2)
34846	1(2)
34847	1(2)
34848	1(2)
35001	1(2)
35002	1(2)
35005	1(2)
35011	1(2)
35013	1(2)
35021	1(2)
35022	1(2)
35045	1(3)
35081	1(2)
35082	1(2)
35091	1(2)
35092	1(2)
35102	1(2)
35103	1(2)
35111	1(2)
35112	1(2)
35121	1(3)
35122	1(3)
35131	1(2)
35132	1(2)
35141	1(2)
35142	1(2)
35151	1(2)
35152	1(2)
35180	2(3)
35182	2(3)
35184	2(3)
35188	2(3)
35189	1(3)
35190	2(3)
35201	2(3)
35206	2(3)
35207	3(3)
35211	3(3)
35216	2(3)
35221	3(3)
35226	3(3)
35231	2(3)

CPT	MUE
35236	2(3)
35241	2(3)
35246	2(3)
35251	2(3)
35256	2(3)
35261	1(3)
35266	2(3)
35271	2(3)
35276	2(3)
35281	2(3)
35286	2(3)
35301	2(3)
35302	1(2)
35303	1(2)
35304	1(2)
35305	1(2)
35306	2(3)
35311	1(2)
35321	1(2)
35331	1(2)
35341	3(3)
35351	1(3)
35355	1(2)
35361	1(2)
35363	1(2)
35371	1(2)
35372	1(2)
35390	1(3)
35400	1(3)
35500	2(3)
35501	1(3)
35506	1(3)
35508	1(3)
35509	1(3)
35510	1(3)
35511	1(3)
35512	1(3)
35515	1(3)
35516	1(3)
35518	1(3)
35521	1(3)
35522	1(3)
35523	1(3)
35525	1(3)
35526	1(3)
35531	1(3)
35533	1(3)
35535	1(3)
35536	1(3)
35537	1(3)
35538	1(3)
35539	1(3)
35540	1(3)
35556	1(3)
35558	1(3)
35560	1(3)
35563	1(3)
35565	1(3)
35566	1(3)
35570	1(3)
35571	1(3)
35572	2(3)
35583	1(2)
35585	2(3)
35587	1(3)

CPT	MUE
35600	2(3)
35601	1(3)
35606	1(3)
35612	1(3)
35616	1(3)
35621	1(3)
35623	1(3)
35626	3(3)
35631	4(3)
35632	1(3)
35633	1(3)
35634	1(3)
35636	1(3)
35637	1(3)
35638	1(3)
35642	1(3)
35645	1(3)
35646	1(3)
35647	1(3)
35650	1(3)
35654	1(3)
35656	1(3)
35661	1(3)
35663	1(3)
35665	1(3)
35666	2(3)
35671	2(3)
35681	1(3)
35682	1(2)
35683	1(2)
35685	2(3)
35686	1(3)
35691	1(3)
35693	1(3)
35694	1(3)
35695	1(3)
35697	2(3)
35700	2(3)
35701	1(2)
35702	2(2)
35703	2(2)
35800	2(3)
35820	2(3)
35840	2(3)
35860	2(3)
35870	1(3)
35875	2(3)
35876	2(3)
35879	2(3)
35881	1(3)
35883	1(3)
35884	1(3)
35901	1(3)
35903	2(3)
35905	1(3)
35907	1(3)
36000	4(3)
36002	2(3)
36005	2(3)
36010	2(3)
36011	4(3)
36012	4(3)
36013	2(3)
36014	2(3)
36015	4(3)

CPT	MUE
36100	2(3)
36140	3(3)
36160	2(3)
36200	2(3)
36215	6(3)
36216	4(3)
36217	2(3)
36218	6(3)
36221	1(3)
36222	1(3)
36223	1(3)
36224	1(3)
36225	1(3)
36226	1(3)
36227	2(2)
36228	4(3)
36245	6(3)
36246	4(3)
36247	3(3)
36248	6(3)
36251	1(3)
36252	1(3)
36253	1(3)
36254	1(3)
36260	1(2)
36261	1(2)
36262	1(2)
36299	1(3)
36400	1(3)
36405	1(3)
36406	1(3)
36410	3(3)
36415	2(3)
36416	0(3)
36420	2(3)
36425	2(3)
36430	1(2)
36440	1(3)
36450	1(3)
36455	1(3)
36456	1(3)
36460	2(3)
36465	1(2)
36466	1(2)
36468	2(3)
36470	1(2)
36471	1(2)
36473	1(3)
36474	1(3)
36475	1(3)
36476	2(3)
36478	1(3)
36479	2(3)
36481	1(3)
36482	1(3)
36483	2(3)
36500	4(3)
36510	1(3)
36511	1(3)
36512	1(3)
36513	1(3)
36514	1(3)
36516	1(3)
36522	1(3)
36555	2(3)

CPT	MUE
36556	2(3)
36557	2(3)
36558	2(3)
36560	2(3)
36561	2(3)
36563	1(3)
36565	1(3)
36566	1(3)
36568	2(3)
36569	2(3)
36570	2(3)
36571	2(3)
36572	1(3)
36573	1(3)
36575	2(3)
36576	2(3)
36578	2(3)
36580	2(3)
36581	2(3)
36582	2(3)
36583	2(3)
36584	2(3)
36585	2(3)
36589	2(3)
36590	2(3)
36591	2(3)
36592	1(3)
36593	2(3)
36595	2(3)
36596	2(3)
36597	2(3)
36598	2(3)
36600	4(3)
36620	3(3)
36625	2(3)
36640	1(3)
36660	1(3)
36680	1(3)
36800	1(3)
36810	1(3)
36815	1(3)
36818	1(3)
36819	1(3)
36820	1(3)
36821	2(3)
36823	1(3)
36825	1(3)
36830	2(3)
36831	1(3)
36832	2(3)
36833	1(3)
36835	1(3)
36838	1(3)
36860	2(3)
36861	2(3)
36901	1(3)
36902	1(3)
36903	1(3)
36904	1(3)
36905	1(3)
36906	1(3)
36907	1(3)
36908	1(3)
36909	1(3)
37140	1(2)

CPT	MUE
37145	1(3)
37160	1(3)
37180	1(2)
37181	1(2)
37182	1(2)
37183	1(2)
37184	1(2)
37185	2(3)
37186	2(3)
37187	1(3)
37188	1(3)
37191	1(3)
37192	1(3)
37193	1(3)
37195	1(3)
37197	2(3)
37200	2(3)
37211	1(2)
37212	1(2)
37213	1(2)
37214	1(2)
37215	1(2)
37216	0(3)
37217	1(2)
37218	1(2)
37220	1(2)
37221	1(2)
37222	2(2)
37223	2(2)
37224	1(2)
37225	1(2)
37226	1(2)
37227	1(2)
37228	1(2)
37229	1(2)
37230	1(2)
37231	1(2)
37232	2(3)
37233	2(3)
37234	2(3)
37235	2(3)
37236	1(2)
37237	2(3)
37238	1(2)
37239	2(3)
37241	2(3)
37242	2(3)
37243	1(3)
37244	2(3)
37246	1(2)
37247	2(3)
37248	1(2)
37249	3(3)
37252	1(2)
37253	5(3)
37500	1(3)
37501	1(3)
37565	1(2)
37600	1(3)
37605	1(3)
37606	1(3)
37607	1(3)
37609	1(2)
37615	2(3)
37616	1(3)

CPT	MUE
37617	3(3)
37618	2(3)
37619	1(2)
37650	1(2)
37660	1(2)
37700	1(2)
37718	1(2)
37722	1(2)
37735	1(2)
37760	1(2)
37761	1(2)
37765	1(2)
37766	1(2)
37780	1(2)
37785	1(2)
37788	1(2)
37790	1(2)
37799	1(3)
38100	1(2)
38101	1(3)
38102	1(2)
38115	1(3)
38120	1(2)
38129	1(3)
38200	1(3)
38204	0(3)
38205	1(3)
38206	1(3)
38207	0(3)
38208	0(3)
38209	0(3)
38210	0(3)
38211	0(3)
38212	0(3)
38213	0(3)
38214	0(3)
38215	0(3)
38220	1(3)
38221	1(3)
38222	1(2)
38230	1(2)
38232	1(2)
38240	1(3)
38241	1(2)
38242	1(2)
38243	1(3)
38300	1(3)
38305	1(3)
38308	1(3)
38380	1(2)
38381	1(2)
38382	1(2)
38500	2(3)
38505	2(3)
38510	1(2)
38520	1(2)
38525	1(2)
38530	1(2)
38531	1(2)
38542	1(2)
38550	1(3)
38555	1(3)
38562	1(2)
38564	1(2)
38570	1(2)

CPT	MUE
38571	1(2)
38572	1(2)
38573	1(2)
38589	1(3)
38700	1(2)
38720	1(2)
38724	1(2)
38740	1(2)
38745	1(2)
38746	1(2)
38747	1(2)
38760	1(2)
38765	1(2)
38770	1(2)
38780	1(2)
38790	1(2)
38792	1(3)
38794	1(2)
38900	1(3)
38999	1(3)
39000	1(2)
39010	1(2)
39200	1(2)
39220	1(2)
39401	1(3)
39402	1(3)
39499	1(3)
39501	1(3)
39503	1(2)
39540	1(2)
39541	1(2)
39545	1(2)
39560	1(3)
39561	1(3)
39599	1(3)
40490	2(3)
40500	2(3)
40510	2(3)
40520	2(3)
40525	2(3)
40527	2(3)
40530	2(3)
40650	2(3)
40652	2(3)
40654	2(3)
40700	1(2)
40701	1(2)
40702	1(2)
40720	1(2)
40761	1(2)
40799	1(3)
40800	2(3)
40801	2(3)
40804	1(3)
40805	2(3)
40806	2(2)
40808	2(3)
40810	2(3)
40812	2(3)
40814	4(3)
40816	2(3)
40818	2(3)
40819	2(2)
40820	2(3)
40830	2(3)

CPT	MUE
40831	2(3)
40840	1(2)
40842	1(2)
40843	1(2)
40844	1(2)
40845	1(3)
40899	1(3)
41000	1(3)
41005	1(3)
41006	2(3)
41007	2(3)
41008	2(3)
41009	2(3)
41010	1(2)
41015	2(3)
41016	1(3)
41017	2(3)
41018	2(3)
41019	1(2)
41100	2(3)
41105	2(3)
41108	2(3)
41110	2(3)
41112	2(3)
41113	2(3)
41114	2(3)
41115	1(2)
41116	2(3)
41120	1(2)
41130	1(2)
41135	1(2)
41140	1(2)
41145	1(2)
41150	1(2)
41153	1(2)
41155	1(2)
41250	2(3)
41251	2(3)
41252	2(3)
41510	1(2)
41512	1(2)
41520	1(3)
41530	1(3)
41599	1(3)
41800	2(3)
41805	1(3)
41806	1(3)
41820	4(2)
41821	2(3)
41822	1(2)
41823	1(2)
41825	2(3)
41826	2(3)
41827	2(3)
41828	4(2)
41830	2(3)
41850	2(3)
41870	2(3)
41872	4(2)
41874	4(2)
41899	1(3)
42000	1(3)
42100	2(3)
42104	2(3)
42106	2(3)

CPT	MUE
42107	2(3)
42120	1(2)
42140	1(2)
42145	1(2)
42160	1(3)
42180	1(3)
42182	1(3)
42200	1(2)
42205	1(2)
42210	1(2)
42215	1(2)
42220	1(2)
42225	1(2)
42226	1(2)
42227	1(2)
42235	1(2)
42260	1(3)
42280	1(2)
42281	1(2)
42299	1(3)
42300	2(3)
42305	2(3)
42310	2(3)
42320	2(3)
42330	1(3)
42335	2(2)
42340	1(2)
42400	2(3)
42405	2(3)
42408	1(3)
42409	1(3)
42410	1(2)
42415	1(2)
42420	1(2)
42425	1(2)
42426	1(2)
42440	1(2)
42450	1(3)
42500	2(3)
42505	2(3)
42507	1(2)
42509	1(2)
42510	1(2)
42550	2(3)
42600	1(3)
42650	2(3)
42660	2(3)
42665	2(3)
42699	1(3)
42700	2(3)
42720	1(3)
42725	1(3)
42800	3(3)
42804	1(3)
42806	1(3)
42808	2(3)
42809	1(3)
42810	1(3)
42815	1(3)
42820	1(2)
42821	1(2)
42825	1(2)
42826	1(2)
42830	1(2)
42831	1(2)

CPT	MUE
42835	1(2)
42836	1(2)
42842	1(3)
42844	1(3)
42845	1(3)
42860	1(3)
42870	1(3)
42890	1(2)
42892	1(3)
42894	1(3)
42900	1(3)
42950	1(2)
42953	1(3)
42955	1(2)
42960	1(3)
42961	1(3)
42962	1(3)
42970	1(3)
42971	1(3)
42972	1(3)
42999	1(3)
43020	1(2)
43030	1(2)
43045	1(2)
43100	1(3)
43101	1(3)
43107	1(2)
43108	1(2)
43112	1(2)
43113	1(2)
43116	1(2)
43117	1(2)
43118	1(2)
43121	1(2)
43122	1(2)
43123	1(2)
43124	1(2)
43130	1(3)
43135	1(3)
43180	1(2)
43191	1(3)
43192	1(3)
43193	1(3)
43194	1(3)
43195	1(3)
43196	1(3)
43197	1(3)
43198	1(3)
43200	1(3)
43201	1(2)
43202	1(2)
43204	1(2)
43205	1(2)
43206	1(2)
43210	1(2)
43211	1(3)
43212	1(3)
43213	1(2)
43214	1(3)
43215	1(3)
43216	1(2)
43217	1(2)
43220	1(3)
43226	1(3)
43227	1(3)

CPT	MUE
43229	1(3)
43231	1(2)
43232	1(2)
43233	1(3)
43235	1(3)
43236	1(2)
43237	1(2)
43238	1(2)
43239	1(2)
43240	1(2)
43241	1(3)
43242	1(2)
43243	1(2)
43244	1(2)
43245	1(2)
43246	1(2)
43247	1(2)
43248	1(3)
43249	1(3)
43250	1(2)
43251	1(2)
43252	1(2)
43253	1(3)
43254	1(3)
43255	2(3)
43257	1(2)
43259	1(2)
43260	1(3)
43261	1(2)
43262	2(2)
43263	1(2)
43264	1(2)
43265	1(2)
43266	1(3)
43270	1(3)
43273	1(2)
43274	2(3)
43275	1(3)
43276	2(3)
43277	3(3)
43278	1(3)
43279	1(2)
43280	1(2)
43281	1(2)
43282	1(2)
43283	1(2)
43284	1(2)
43285	1(2)
43286	1(2)
43287	1(2)
43288	1(2)
43289	1(3)
43300	1(2)
43305	1(2)
43310	1(2)
43312	1(2)
43313	1(2)
43314	1(2)
43320	1(2)
43325	1(2)
43327	1(2)
43328	1(2)
43330	1(2)
43331	1(2)
43332	1(2)

CPT	MUE
43333	1(2)
43334	1(2)
43335	1(2)
43336	1(2)
43337	1(2)
43338	1(2)
43340	1(2)
43341	1(2)
43351	1(2)
43352	1(2)
43360	1(2)
43361	1(2)
43400	1(2)
43405	1(2)
43410	1(3)
43415	1(3)
43420	1(3)
43425	1(3)
43450	1(3)
43453	1(3)
43460	1(3)
43496	1(3)
43499	1(3)
43500	1(2)
43501	1(3)
43502	1(2)
43510	1(2)
43520	1(2)
43605	1(2)
43610	2(3)
43611	2(3)
43620	1(2)
43621	1(2)
43622	1(2)
43631	1(2)
43632	1(2)
43633	1(2)
43634	1(2)
43635	1(2)
43640	1(2)
43641	1(2)
43644	1(2)
43645	1(2)
43647	1(2)
43648	1(2)
43651	1(2)
43652	1(2)
43653	1(2)
43659	1(3)
43752	2(3)
43753	1(3)
43754	1(3)
43755	1(3)
43756	1(2)
43757	1(2)
43761	2(3)
43762	2(3)
43763	2(3)
43770	1(2)
43771	1(2)
43772	1(2)
43773	1(2)
43774	1(2)
43775	1(2)
43800	1(2)

CPT	MUE
43810	1(2)
43820	1(2)
43825	1(2)
43830	1(2)
43831	1(2)
43832	1(2)
43840	2(3)
43842	0(3)
43843	1(2)
43845	1(2)
43846	1(2)
43847	1(2)
43848	1(2)
43850	1(2)
43855	1(2)
43860	1(2)
43865	1(2)
43870	1(2)
43880	1(3)
43881	1(3)
43882	1(3)
43886	1(2)
43887	1(2)
43888	1(2)
43999	1(3)
44005	1(2)
44010	1(2)
44015	1(2)
44020	2(3)
44021	1(3)
44025	1(3)
44050	1(2)
44055	1(2)
44100	1(2)
44110	1(2)
44111	1(2)
44120	1(2)
44121	2(3)
44125	1(2)
44126	1(2)
44127	1(2)
44128	2(3)
44130	2(3)
44132	1(2)
44133	1(2)
44135	1(2)
44136	1(2)
44137	1(2)
44139	1(2)
44140	2(3)
44141	1(3)
44143	1(2)
44144	1(3)
44145	1(2)
44146	1(2)
44147	1(3)
44150	1(2)
44151	1(2)
44155	1(2)
44156	1(2)
44157	1(2)
44158	1(2)
44160	1(2)
44180	1(2)
44186	1(2)

CPT	MUE
44187	1(3)
44188	1(3)
44202	1(2)
44203	2(3)
44204	2(3)
44205	1(2)
44206	1(2)
44207	1(2)
44208	1(2)
44210	1(2)
44211	1(2)
44212	1(2)
44213	1(2)
44227	1(3)
44238	1(3)
44300	1(3)
44310	2(3)
44312	1(2)
44314	1(2)
44316	1(2)
44320	1(2)
44322	1(2)
44340	1(2)
44345	1(2)
44346	1(2)
44360	1(3)
44361	1(2)
44363	1(3)
44364	1(2)
44365	1(2)
44366	1(3)
44369	1(2)
44370	1(2)
44372	1(2)
44373	1(2)
44376	1(3)
44377	1(2)
44378	1(3)
44379	1(2)
44380	1(3)
44381	1(3)
44382	1(2)
44384	1(3)
44385	1(3)
44386	1(2)
44388	1(3)
44389	1(2)
44390	1(3)
44391	1(3)
44392	1(2)
44394	1(2)
44401	1(2)
44402	1(3)
44403	1(3)
44404	1(3)
44405	1(3)
44406	1(3)
44407	1(2)
44408	1(3)
44500	1(3)
44602	1(2)
44603	1(2)
44604	1(2)
44605	1(2)
44615	3(3)

CPT	MUE
44620	2(3)
44625	1(3)
44626	1(3)
44640	2(3)
44650	2(3)
44660	1(3)
44661	1(3)
44680	1(3)
44700	1(2)
44701	1(2)
44705	1(3)
44715	1(2)
44720	2(3)
44721	2(3)
44799	1(3)
44800	1(3)
44820	1(3)
44850	1(3)
44899	1(3)
44900	1(2)
44950	1(2)
44955	1(2)
44960	1(2)
44970	1(2)
44979	1(3)
45000	1(3)
45005	1(3)
45020	1(3)
45100	2(3)
45108	1(2)
45110	1(2)
45111	1(2)
45112	1(2)
45113	1(2)
45114	1(2)
45116	1(2)
45119	1(2)
45120	1(2)
45121	1(2)
45123	1(2)
45126	1(2)
45130	1(2)
45135	1(2)
45136	1(2)
45150	1(2)
45160	1(3)
45171	2(3)
45172	2(3)
45190	1(3)
45300	1(3)
45303	1(3)
45305	1(2)
45307	1(3)
45308	1(2)
45309	1(2)
45315	1(2)
45317	1(3)
45320	1(2)
45321	1(2)
45327	1(2)
45330	1(3)
45331	1(2)
45332	1(3)
45333	1(2)
45334	1(3)

CPT	MUE
45335	1(2)
45337	1(2)
45338	1(2)
45340	1(2)
45341	1(2)
45342	1(2)
45346	1(2)
45347	1(3)
45349	1(3)
45350	1(2)
45378	1(3)
45379	1(3)
45380	1(2)
45381	1(2)
45382	1(3)
45384	1(2)
45385	1(2)
45386	1(2)
45388	1(2)
45389	1(3)
45390	1(3)
45391	1(2)
45392	1(2)
45393	1(3)
45395	1(2)
45397	1(2)
45398	1(2)
45399	1(3)
45400	1(2)
45402	1(2)
45499	1(3)
45500	1(2)
45505	1(2)
45520	1(2)
45540	1(2)
45541	1(2)
45550	1(2)
45560	1(2)
45562	1(2)
45563	1(2)
45800	1(3)
45805	1(3)
45820	1(3)
45825	1(3)
45900	1(2)
45905	1(2)
45910	1(2)
45915	1(2)
45990	1(2)
45999	1(3)
46020	2(3)
46030	1(3)
46040	2(3)
46045	2(3)
46050	2(3)
46060	2(3)
46070	1(2)
46080	1(2)
46083	2(3)
46200	1(3)
46220	1(2)
46221	1(2)
46230	1(2)
46250	1(2)
46255	1(2)

CPT	MUE
46257	1(2)
46258	1(2)
46260	1(2)
46261	1(2)
46262	1(2)
46270	1(3)
46275	1(3)
46280	1(2)
46285	1(3)
46288	1(3)
46320	2(3)
46500	1(2)
46505	1(2)
46600	1(3)
46601	1(3)
46604	1(2)
46606	1(2)
46607	1(2)
46608	1(3)
46610	1(2)
46611	1(2)
46612	1(2)
46614	1(3)
46615	1(2)
46700	1(2)
46705	1(2)
46706	1(3)
46707	1(3)
46710	1(3)
46712	1(3)
46715	1(2)
46716	1(2)
46730	1(2)
46735	1(2)
46740	1(2)
46742	1(2)
46744	1(2)
46746	1(2)
46748	1(2)
46750	1(2)
46751	1(2)
46753	1(2)
46754	1(3)
46760	1(2)
46761	1(2)
46900	1(2)
46910	1(2)
46916	1(2)
46917	1(2)
46922	1(2)
46924	1(2)
46930	1(2)
46940	1(2)
46942	1(3)
46945	1(2)
46946	1(2)
46947	1(2)
46948	1(2)
46999	1(3)
47000	3(3)
47001	3(3)
47010	1(3)
47015	1(2)
47100	3(3)
47120	2(3)

CPT	MUE
47122	1(2)
47125	1(2)
47130	1(2)
47133	1(2)
47135	1(2)
47140	1(2)
47141	1(2)
47142	1(2)
47143	1(2)
47144	1(2)
47145	1(2)
47146	2(3)
47147	1(3)
47300	2(3)
47350	1(3)
47360	1(3)
47361	1(3)
47362	1(3)
47370	1(2)
47371	1(2)
47379	1(3)
47380	1(2)
47381	1(2)
47382	1(2)
47383	1(2)
47399	1(3)
47400	1(3)
47420	1(2)
47425	1(2)
47460	1(2)
47480	1(2)
47490	1(2)
47531	2(3)
47532	1(3)
47533	1(3)
47534	2(3)
47535	1(3)
47536	2(3)
47537	1(3)
47538	2(3)
47539	2(3)
47540	2(3)
47541	1(3)
47542	2(3)
47543	1(3)
47544	1(3)
47550	1(3)
47552	1(3)
47553	1(2)
47554	1(3)
47555	1(2)
47556	1(2)
47562	1(2)
47563	1(2)
47564	1(2)
47570	1(2)
47579	1(3)
47600	1(2)
47605	1(2)
47610	1(2)
47612	1(2)
47620	1(2)
47700	1(2)
47701	1(2)
47711	1(2)

CPT	MUE
47712	1(2)
47715	1(2)
47720	1(2)
47721	1(2)
47740	1(2)
47741	1(2)
47760	1(2)
47765	1(2)
47780	1(2)
47785	1(2)
47800	1(2)
47801	1(3)
47802	1(2)
47900	1(2)
47999	1(3)
48000	1(2)
48001	1(2)
48020	1(3)
48100	1(3)
48102	1(3)
48105	1(2)
48120	1(3)
48140	1(2)
48145	1(2)
48146	1(2)
48148	1(2)
48150	1(2)
48152	1(2)
48153	1(2)
48154	1(2)
48155	1(2)
48160	0(3)
48400	1(3)
48500	1(3)
48510	1(3)
48520	1(3)
48540	1(3)
48545	1(3)
48547	1(2)
48548	1(2)
48550	1(2)
48551	1(2)
48552	2(3)
48554	1(2)
48556	1(2)
48999	1(3)
49000	1(2)
49002	1(3)
49010	1(3)
49013	1(2)
49014	1(3)
49020	2(3)
49040	2(3)
49060	2(3)
49062	1(3)
49082	1(3)
49083	2(3)
49084	1(3)
49180	2(3)
49185	2(3)
49203	1(2)
49204	1(2)
49205	1(2)
49215	1(2)
49220	1(2)

CPT	MUE	CPT	MUE	CPT	MUE	CPT	MUE	CPT	MUE	CPT	MUE	CPT	MUE	CPT	MUE
49250	1(2)	49585	1(2)	50389	1(3)	50728	1(3)	51610	1(3)	52310	1(3)	53444	1(3)	54316	1(2)
49255	1(2)	49587	1(2)	50390	2(3)	50740	1(2)	51700	1(3)	52315	2(3)	53445	1(2)	54318	1(2)
49320	1(3)	49590	1(2)	50391	1(3)	50750	1(2)	51701	2(3)	52317	1(3)	53446	1(2)	54322	1(2)
49321	1(2)	49600	1(2)	50396	1(3)	50760	1(2)	51702	2(3)	52318	1(3)	53447	1(2)	54324	1(2)
49322	1(2)	49605	1(2)	50400	1(2)	50770	1(2)	51703	2(3)	52320	1(2)	53448	1(2)	54326	1(2)
49323	1(2)	49606	1(2)	50405	1(2)	50780	1(2)	51705	1(3)	52325	1(3)	53449	1(2)	54328	1(2)
49324	1(2)	49610	1(2)	50430	2(3)	50782	1(2)	51710	1(3)	52327	1(2)	53450	1(2)	54332	1(2)
49325	1(2)	49611	1(2)	50431	2(3)	50783	1(2)	51715	1(2)	52330	1(2)	53460	1(2)	54336	1(2)
49326	1(2)	49650	1(2)	50432	2(3)	50785	1(2)	51720	1(3)	52332	1(2)	53500	1(2)	54340	1(2)
49327	1(2)	49651	1(2)	50433	2(3)	50800	1(2)	51725	1(3)	52334	1(2)	53502	1(3)	54344	1(2)
49329	1(3)	49652	2(3)	50434	2(3)	50810	1(3)	51726	1(3)	52341	1(2)	53505	1(3)	54348	1(2)
49400	1(3)	49653	2(3)	50435	2(3)	50815	1(2)	51727	1(3)	52342	1(2)	53510	1(3)	54352	1(2)
49402	1(3)	49654	1(3)	50436	1(3)	50820	1(2)	51728	1(3)	52343	1(2)	53515	1(3)	54360	1(2)
49405	2(3)	49655	1(3)	50437	1(3)	50825	1(3)	51729	1(3)	52344	1(2)	53520	1(3)	54380	1(2)
49406	2(3)	49656	1(3)	50500	1(3)	50830	1(3)	51736	1(3)	52345	1(2)	53600	1(3)	54385	1(2)
49407	1(3)	49657	1(3)	50520	1(3)	50840	1(2)	51741	1(3)	52346	1(2)	53601	1(3)	54390	1(2)
49411	1(2)	49659	1(3)	50525	1(3)	50845	1(2)	51784	1(3)	52351	1(3)	53605	1(3)	54400	1(2)
49412	1(2)	49900	1(3)	50526	1(3)	50860	1(2)	51785	1(3)	52352	1(2)	53620	1(2)	54401	1(2)
49418	1(3)	49904	1(3)	50540	1(2)	50900	1(3)	51792	1(3)	52353	1(2)	53621	1(3)	54405	1(2)
49419	1(2)	49905	1(3)	50541	1(2)	50920	2(3)	51797	1(3)	52354	1(3)	53660	1(2)	54406	1(2)
49421	1(2)	49906	1(3)	50542	1(2)	50930	2(3)	51798	1(3)	52355	1(3)	53661	1(3)	54408	1(2)
49422	1(2)	49999	1(3)	50543	1(2)	50940	1(2)	51800	1(2)	52356	1(2)	53665	1(3)	54410	1(2)
49423	2(3)	50010	1(2)	50544	1(2)	50945	1(2)	51820	1(2)	52400	1(2)	53850	1(2)	54411	1(2)
49424	3(3)	50020	1(3)	50545	1(2)	50947	1(2)	51840	1(2)	52402	1(2)	53852	1(2)	54415	1(2)
49425	1(2)	50040	1(2)	50546	1(2)	50948	1(2)	51841	1(2)	52441	1(2)	53854	1(2)	54416	1(2)
49426	1(3)	50045	1(2)	50547	1(2)	50949	1(3)	51845	1(2)	52442	6(3)	53855	1(2)	54417	1(2)
49427	1(3)	50060	1(2)	50548	1(2)	50951	1(3)	51860	1(3)	52450	1(2)	53860	1(2)	54420	1(2)
49428	1(2)	50065	1(2)	50549	1(3)	50953	1(3)	51865	1(3)	52500	1(2)	53899	1(3)	54430	1(2)
49429	1(2)	50070	1(2)	50551	1(3)	50955	1(2)	51880	1(2)	52601	1(2)	54000	1(2)	54435	1(2)
49435	1(2)	50075	1(2)	50553	1(3)	50957	1(2)	51900	1(3)	52630	1(2)	54001	1(2)	54437	1(2)
49436	1(2)	50080	1(2)	50555	1(2)	50961	1(2)	51920	1(3)	52640	1(2)	54015	1(3)	54438	1(2)
49440	1(3)	50081	1(2)	50557	1(2)	50970	1(3)	51925	1(2)	52647	1(2)	54050	1(2)	54440	1(2)
49441	1(3)	50100	1(2)	50561	1(2)	50972	1(3)	51940	1(2)	52648	1(2)	54055	1(2)	54450	1(2)
49442	1(3)	50120	1(2)	50562	1(3)	50974	1(2)	51960	1(2)	52649	1(2)	54056	1(2)	54500	1(3)
49446	1(2)	50125	1(2)	50570	1(3)	50976	1(2)	51980	1(2)	52700	1(3)	54057	1(2)	54505	1(3)
49450	1(3)	50130	1(2)	50572	1(3)	50980	1(2)	51990	1(2)	53000	1(2)	54060	1(2)	54512	1(3)
49451	1(3)	50135	1(2)	50574	1(2)	51020	1(2)	51992	1(2)	53010	1(2)	54065	1(2)	54520	1(2)
49452	1(3)	50200	1(3)	50575	1(2)	51030	1(2)	51999	1(3)	53020	1(2)	54100	2(3)	54522	1(2)
49460	1(3)	50205	1(3)	50576	1(2)	51040	1(3)	52000	1(3)	53025	1(2)	54105	2(3)	54530	1(2)
49465	1(3)	50220	1(2)	50580	1(2)	51045	2(3)	52001	1(3)	53040	1(3)	54110	1(2)	54535	1(2)
49491	1(2)	50225	1(2)	50590	1(2)	51050	1(3)	52005	2(3)	53060	1(3)	54111	1(2)	54550	1(2)
49492	1(2)	50230	1(2)	50592	1(2)	51060	1(3)	52007	1(2)	53080	1(3)	54112	1(3)	54560	1(2)
49495	1(2)	50234	1(2)	50593	1(2)	51065	1(3)	52010	1(2)	53085	1(3)	54115	1(3)	54600	1(2)
49496	1(2)	50236	1(2)	50600	1(3)	51080	1(3)	52204	1(2)	53200	1(3)	54120	1(2)	54620	1(2)
49500	1(2)	50240	1(2)	50605	1(3)	51100	1(3)	52214	1(2)	53210	1(2)	54125	1(2)	54640	1(2)
49501	1(2)	50250	1(3)	50606	1(3)	51101	1(3)	52224	1(2)	53215	1(2)	54130	1(2)	54650	1(2)
49505	1(2)	50280	1(2)	50610	1(2)	51102	1(3)	52234	1(2)	53220	1(3)	54135	1(2)	54660	1(2)
49507	1(2)	50290	1(3)	50620	1(2)	51500	1(2)	52235	1(2)	53230	1(3)	54150	1(2)	54670	1(3)
49520	1(2)	50300	1(2)	50630	1(2)	51520	1(2)	52240	1(2)	53235	1(3)	54160	1(2)	54680	1(2)
49521	1(2)	50320	1(2)	50650	1(2)	51525	1(2)	52250	1(2)	53240	1(3)	54161	1(2)	54690	1(2)
49525	1(2)	50323	1(2)	50660	1(3)	51530	1(2)	52260	1(2)	53250	1(3)	54162	1(2)	54692	1(2)
49540	1(2)	50325	1(2)	50684	1(3)	51535	1(2)	52265	1(2)	53260	1(2)	54163	1(2)	54699	1(3)
49550	1(2)	50327	2(3)	50686	2(3)	51550	1(2)	52270	1(2)	53265	1(3)	54164	1(2)	54700	1(3)
49553	1(2)	50328	1(3)	50688	2(3)	51555	1(2)	52275	1(2)	53270	1(2)	54200	1(2)	54800	1(2)
49555	1(2)	50329	1(3)	50690	2(3)	51565	1(2)	52276	1(2)	53275	1(2)	54205	1(2)	54830	1(2)
49557	1(2)	50340	1(2)	50693	2(3)	51570	1(2)	52277	1(2)	53400	1(2)	54220	1(3)	54840	1(2)
49560	2(3)	50360	1(2)	50694	2(3)	51575	1(2)	52281	1(2)	53405	1(2)	54230	1(3)	54860	1(2)
49561	1(3)	50365	1(2)	50695	2(3)	51580	1(2)	52282	1(2)	53410	1(2)	54231	1(3)	54861	1(2)
49565	2(3)	50370	1(2)	50700	1(2)	51585	1(2)	52283	1(2)	53415	1(2)	54235	1(3)	54865	1(3)
49566	2(3)	50380	1(2)	50705	2(3)	51590	1(2)	52285	1(2)	53420	1(2)	54240	1(2)	54900	1(2)
49568	2(3)	50382	1(3)	50706	2(3)	51595	1(2)	52287	1(2)	53425	1(2)	54250	1(2)	54901	1(2)
49570	1(3)	50384	1(3)	50715	1(2)	51596	1(2)	52290	1(2)	53430	1(2)	54300	1(2)	55000	1(3)
49572	1(3)	50385	1(3)	50722	1(2)	51597	1(2)	52300	1(2)	53431	1(2)	54304	1(2)	55040	1(2)
49580	1(2)	50386	1(3)	50725	1(3)	51600	1(3)	52301	1(2)	53440	1(2)	54308	1(2)	55041	1(2)
49582	1(2)	50387	1(3)	50727	1(3)	51605	1(3)	52305	1(2)	53442	1(2)	54312	1(2)	55060	1(2)

CPT	MUE
55100	2(3)
55110	1(2)
55120	1(3)
55150	1(2)
55175	1(2)
55180	1(2)
55200	1(2)
55250	1(2)
55300	1(2)
55400	1(2)
55500	1(2)
55520	1(2)
55530	1(2)
55535	1(2)
55540	1(2)
55550	1(2)
55559	1(3)
55600	1(2)
55605	1(2)
55650	1(2)
55680	1(3)
55700	1(2)
55705	1(2)
55706	1(2)
55720	1(3)
55725	1(3)
55801	1(2)
55810	1(2)
55812	1(2)
55815	1(2)
55821	1(2)
55831	1(2)
55840	1(2)
55842	1(2)
55845	1(2)
55860	1(2)
55862	1(2)
55865	1(2)
55866	1(2)
55870	1(2)
55873	1(2)
55874	1(2)
55875	1(2)
55876	1(2)
55899	1(3)
55920	1(2)
55970	1(2)
55980	1(2)
56405	2(3)
56420	1(3)
56440	1(3)
56441	1(2)
56442	1(2)
56501	1(2)
56515	1(2)
56605	1(2)
56606	6(3)
56620	1(2)
56625	1(2)
56630	1(2)
56631	1(2)
56632	1(2)
56633	1(2)
56634	1(2)
56637	1(2)

CPT	MUE
56640	1(2)
56700	1(2)
56740	1(3)
56800	1(2)
56805	1(2)
56810	1(2)
56820	1(2)
56821	1(2)
57000	1(3)
57010	1(3)
57020	1(3)
57022	1(3)
57023	1(3)
57061	1(2)
57065	1(2)
57100	2(3)
57105	2(3)
57106	1(2)
57107	1(2)
57109	1(2)
57110	1(2)
57111	1(2)
57112	1(2)
57120	1(2)
57130	1(2)
57135	2(3)
57150	1(3)
57155	1(3)
57156	1(3)
57160	1(2)
57170	1(2)
57180	1(3)
57200	1(3)
57210	1(3)
57220	1(2)
57230	1(2)
57240	1(2)
57250	1(2)
57260	1(2)
57265	1(2)
57267	2(3)
57268	1(2)
57270	1(2)
57280	1(2)
57282	1(2)
57283	1(2)
57284	1(2)
57285	1(2)
57287	1(2)
57288	1(2)
57289	1(2)
57291	1(2)
57292	1(2)
57295	1(2)
57296	1(2)
57300	1(3)
57305	1(3)
57307	1(3)
57308	1(3)
57310	1(3)
57311	1(3)
57320	1(3)
57330	1(3)
57335	1(2)
57400	1(2)

CPT	MUE
57410	1(2)
57415	1(3)
57420	1(3)
57421	1(3)
57423	1(2)
57425	1(2)
57426	1(2)
57452	1(3)
57454	1(3)
57455	1(3)
57456	1(3)
57460	1(3)
57461	1(3)
57500	1(3)
57505	1(3)
57510	1(3)
57511	1(3)
57513	1(3)
57520	1(3)
57522	1(3)
57530	1(3)
57531	1(2)
57540	1(2)
57545	1(3)
57550	1(3)
57555	1(2)
57556	1(2)
57558	1(3)
57700	1(3)
57720	1(3)
57800	1(3)
58100	1(3)
58110	1(3)
58120	1(3)
58140	1(3)
58145	1(3)
58146	1(3)
58150	1(3)
58152	1(2)
58180	1(3)
58200	1(2)
58210	1(2)
58240	1(2)
58260	1(3)
58262	1(3)
58263	1(2)
58267	1(2)
58270	1(2)
58275	1(2)
58280	1(2)
58285	1(3)
58290	1(3)
58291	1(2)
58292	1(2)
58293	1(2)
58294	1(2)
58300	0(3)
58301	1(3)
58321	1(2)
58322	1(2)
58323	1(3)
58340	1(3)
58345	1(3)
58346	1(2)
58350	1(2)

CPT	MUE
58353	1(3)
58356	1(3)
58400	1(3)
58410	1(2)
58520	1(2)
58540	1(3)
58541	1(3)
58542	1(2)
58543	1(3)
58544	1(2)
58545	1(2)
58546	1(2)
58548	1(2)
58550	1(3)
58552	1(3)
58553	1(3)
58554	1(2)
58555	1(3)
58558	1(3)
58559	1(3)
58560	1(3)
58561	1(3)
58562	1(3)
58563	1(3)
58565	1(2)
58570	1(3)
58571	1(2)
58572	1(3)
58573	1(2)
58575	1(2)
58578	1(3)
58579	1(3)
58600	1(2)
58605	1(2)
58611	1(2)
58615	1(2)
58660	1(2)
58661	1(2)
58662	1(2)
58670	1(2)
58671	1(2)
58672	1(2)
58673	1(2)
58674	1(2)
58679	1(3)
58700	1(2)
58720	1(2)
58740	1(2)
58750	1(2)
58752	1(2)
58760	1(2)
58770	1(2)
58800	1(2)
58805	1(2)
58820	1(3)
58822	1(3)
58825	1(2)
58900	1(2)
58920	1(2)
58925	1(3)
58940	1(2)
58943	1(2)
58950	1(2)
58951	1(2)
58952	1(2)

CPT	MUE
58953	1(2)
58954	1(2)
58956	1(2)
58957	1(2)
58958	1(2)
58960	1(2)
58970	1(3)
58974	1(3)
58976	2(3)
58999	1(3)
59000	2(3)
59001	2(3)
59012	2(3)
59015	2(3)
59020	2(3)
59025	2(3)
59030	2(3)
59050	2(3)
59051	2(3)
59070	2(3)
59072	2(3)
59074	2(3)
59076	2(3)
59100	1(2)
59120	1(3)
59121	1(3)
59130	1(3)
59135	1(3)
59136	1(3)
59140	1(2)
59150	1(3)
59151	1(3)
59160	1(2)
59200	1(3)
59300	1(2)
59320	1(2)
59325	1(2)
59350	1(2)
59400	1(2)
59409	2(3)
59410	1(2)
59412	1(3)
59414	1(3)
59425	1(2)
59426	1(2)
59430	1(2)
59510	1(2)
59514	1(3)
59515	1(2)
59525	1(2)
59610	1(2)
59612	2(3)
59614	1(2)
59618	1(2)
59620	1(2)
59622	1(2)
59812	1(2)
59820	1(2)
59821	1(2)
59830	1(2)
59840	1(2)
59841	1(2)
59850	1(2)
59851	1(2)
59852	1(2)

CPT	MUE
59855	1(2)
59856	1(2)
59857	1(2)
59866	1(2)
59870	1(2)
59871	1(2)
59897	1(3)
59898	1(3)
59899	1(3)
60000	1(3)
60100	3(3)
60200	2(3)
60210	1(2)
60212	1(2)
60220	1(3)
60225	1(2)
60240	1(2)
60252	1(2)
60254	1(2)
60260	1(2)
60270	1(2)
60271	1(2)
60280	1(3)
60281	1(3)
60300	2(3)
60500	1(2)
60502	1(3)
60505	1(3)
60512	1(3)
60520	1(2)
60521	1(2)
60522	1(2)
60540	1(2)
60545	1(2)
60600	1(3)
60605	1(3)
60650	1(2)
60659	1(3)
60699	1(3)
61000	1(2)
61001	1(2)
61020	2(3)
61026	2(3)
61050	1(3)
61055	1(3)
61070	2(3)
61105	1(3)
61107	1(3)
61108	1(3)
61120	1(3)
61140	1(3)
61150	1(3)
61151	1(3)
61154	1(3)
61156	1(3)
61210	1(3)
61215	1(3)
61250	1(3)
61253	1(3)
61304	1(3)
61305	1(3)
61312	2(3)
61313	2(3)
61314	2(3)
61315	1(3)

CPT	MUE
61316	1(3)
61320	2(3)
61321	1(3)
61322	1(3)
61323	1(3)
61330	1(2)
61333	1(2)
61340	1(2)
61343	1(2)
61345	1(3)
61450	1(3)
61458	1(2)
61460	1(2)
61500	1(3)
61501	1(3)
61510	1(3)
61512	1(3)
61514	2(3)
61516	1(3)
61517	1(3)
61518	1(3)
61519	1(3)
61520	1(3)
61521	1(3)
61522	1(3)
61524	2(3)
61526	1(3)
61530	1(3)
61531	1(2)
61533	2(3)
61534	1(3)
61535	2(3)
61536	1(3)
61537	1(3)
61538	1(2)
61539	1(3)
61540	1(3)
61541	1(2)
61543	1(2)
61544	1(3)
61545	1(2)
61546	1(2)
61548	1(2)
61550	1(2)
61552	1(2)
61556	1(3)
61557	1(2)
61558	1(3)
61559	1(3)
61563	2(3)
61564	1(2)
61566	1(3)
61567	1(2)
61570	1(3)
61571	1(3)
61575	1(2)
61576	1(2)
61580	1(2)
61581	1(2)
61582	1(2)
61583	1(2)
61584	1(2)
61585	1(2)
61586	1(3)
61590	1(2)

CPT	MUE
61591	1(2)
61592	1(2)
61595	1(2)
61596	1(2)
61597	1(2)
61598	1(3)
61600	1(3)
61601	1(3)
61605	1(3)
61606	1(3)
61607	1(3)
61608	1(3)
61611	1(3)
61613	1(3)
61615	1(3)
61616	1(3)
61618	2(3)
61619	2(3)
61623	2(3)
61624	2(3)
61626	2(3)
61630	1(3)
61635	2(3)
61640	0(3)
61641	0(3)
61642	0(3)
61645	1(3)
61650	1(2)
61651	2(2)
61680	1(3)
61682	1(3)
61684	1(3)
61686	1(3)
61690	1(3)
61692	1(3)
61697	2(3)
61698	1(3)
61700	2(3)
61702	1(3)
61703	1(3)
61705	1(3)
61708	1(3)
61710	1(3)
61711	1(3)
61720	1(3)
61735	1(3)
61750	2(3)
61751	2(3)
61760	1(2)
61770	1(2)
61781	1(3)
61782	1(3)
61783	1(3)
61790	1(2)
61791	1(2)
61796	1(2)
61797	4(3)
61798	1(2)
61799	4(3)
61800	1(2)
61850	1(3)
61860	1(3)
61863	1(2)
61864	1(3)
61867	1(2)

CPT	MUE	CPT	MUE	CPT	MUE	CPT	MUE	CPT	MUE	CPT	MUE	CPT	MUE	CPT	MUE
61868	2(3)	62323	1(3)	63185	1(2)	63746	1(2)	64620	5(3)	64822	1(2)	65273	1(3)	66500	1(2)
61870	1(3)	62324	1(3)	63190	1(2)	64400	4(3)	64624	2(2)	64823	1(2)	65275	1(3)	66505	1(2)
61880	1(2)	62325	1(3)	63191	1(2)	64405	1(3)	64625	2(2)	64831	1(2)	65280	1(3)	66600	1(2)
61885	1(3)	62326	1(3)	63194	1(2)	64408	1(3)	64630	1(3)	64832	3(3)	65285	1(3)	66605	1(2)
61886	1(3)	62327	1(3)	63195	1(2)	64415	1(3)	64632	1(2)	64834	1(2)	65286	1(3)	66625	1(2)
61888	1(3)	62328	2(3)	63196	1(2)	64416	1(2)	64633	1(2)	64835	1(2)	65290	1(3)	66630	1(2)
62000	1(3)	62329	1(3)	63197	1(2)	64417	1(3)	64634	4(3)	64836	1(2)	65400	1(3)	66635	1(2)
62005	1(3)	62350	1(3)	63198	1(2)	64418	1(3)	64635	1(2)	64837	2(3)	65410	1(3)	66680	1(2)
62010	1(3)	62351	1(3)	63199	1(2)	64420	2(2)	64636	4(2)	64840	1(2)	65420	1(2)	66682	1(2)
62100	1(3)	62355	1(3)	63200	1(2)	64421	3(3)	64640	5(3)	64856	2(3)	65426	1(2)	66700	1(2)
62115	1(2)	62360	1(2)	63250	1(3)	64425	1(3)	64642	1(2)	64857	2(3)	65430	1(2)	66710	1(2)
62117	1(2)	62361	1(2)	63251	1(3)	64430	1(3)	64643	3(2)	64858	1(2)	65435	1(2)	66711	1(2)
62120	1(2)	62362	1(2)	63252	1(3)	64435	1(3)	64644	1(2)	64859	2(3)	65436	1(2)	66720	1(2)
62121	1(2)	62365	1(2)	63265	1(3)	64445	1(3)	64645	3(2)	64861	1(2)	65450	1(3)	66740	1(2)
62140	1(3)	62367	1(3)	63266	1(3)	64446	1(2)	64646	1(2)	64862	1(2)	65600	1(2)	66761	1(2)
62141	1(3)	62368	1(3)	63267	1(3)	64447	1(3)	64647	1(2)	64864	2(3)	65710	1(2)	66762	1(2)
62142	2(3)	62369	1(3)	63268	1(3)	64448	1(2)	64650	1(2)	64865	1(3)	65730	1(2)	66770	1(3)
62143	2(3)	62370	1(3)	63270	1(3)	64449	1(2)	64653	1(2)	64866	1(3)	65750	1(2)	66820	1(2)
62145	2(3)	62380	2(3)	63271	1(3)	64450	10(3)	64680	1(2)	64868	1(3)	65755	1(2)	66821	1(2)
62146	2(3)	63001	1(2)	63272	1(3)	64451	2(2)	64681	1(2)	64872	1(3)	65756	1(2)	66825	1(2)
62147	1(3)	63003	1(2)	63273	1(3)	64454	2(2)	64702	2(3)	64874	1(3)	65757	1(3)	66830	1(2)
62148	1(3)	63005	1(2)	63275	1(3)	64455	1(2)	64704	4(3)	64876	1(3)	65760	0(3)	66840	1(2)
62160	1(3)	63011	1(2)	63276	1(3)	64461	1(2)	64708	3(3)	64885	1(3)	65765	0(3)	66850	1(2)
62161	1(3)	63012	1(2)	63277	1(3)	64462	1(2)	64712	1(2)	64886	1(3)	65767	0(3)	66852	1(2)
62162	1(3)	63015	1(2)	63278	1(3)	64463	1(3)	64713	1(2)	64890	2(3)	65770	1(2)	66920	1(2)
62163	1(3)	63016	1(2)	63280	1(3)	64479	1(2)	64714	1(2)	64891	2(3)	65771	0(3)	66930	1(2)
62164	1(3)	63017	1(2)	63281	1(3)	64480	4(3)	64716	2(3)	64892	2(3)	65772	1(2)	66940	1(2)
62165	1(2)	63020	1(2)	63282	1(3)	64483	1(2)	64718	1(2)	64893	2(3)	65775	1(2)	66982	1(2)
62180	1(3)	63030	1(2)	63283	1(3)	64484	4(3)	64719	1(2)	64895	2(3)	65778	1(2)	66983	1(2)
62190	1(3)	63035	4(3)	63285	1(3)	64486	1(3)	64721	1(2)	64896	2(3)	65779	1(2)	66984	1(2)
62192	1(3)	63040	1(2)	63286	1(3)	64487	1(2)	64722	4(3)	64897	2(3)	65780	1(2)	66985	1(2)
62194	1(3)	63042	1(2)	63287	1(3)	64488	1(3)	64726	2(3)	64898	2(3)	65781	1(2)	66986	1(2)
62200	1(2)	63043	4(3)	63290	1(3)	64489	1(2)	64727	2(3)	64901	2(3)	65782	1(2)	66987	2(2)
62201	1(2)	63044	4(2)	63295	1(2)	64490	1(2)	64732	1(2)	64902	1(3)	65785	1(2)	66988	2(2)
62220	1(3)	63045	1(2)	63300	1(2)	64491	1(2)	64734	1(2)	64905	1(3)	65800	1(2)	66990	1(3)
62223	1(3)	63046	1(2)	63301	1(2)	64492	1(2)	64736	1(2)	64907	1(3)	65810	1(2)	66999	1(3)
62225	2(3)	63047	1(2)	63302	1(2)	64493	1(2)	64738	1(2)	64910	3(3)	65815	1(3)	67005	1(2)
62230	2(3)	63048	5(3)	63303	1(2)	64494	1(2)	64740	1(2)	64911	2(3)	65820	1(2)	67010	1(2)
62252	2(3)	63050	1(2)	63304	1(2)	64495	1(2)	64742	1(2)	64912	3(3)	65850	1(2)	67015	1(2)
62256	1(3)	63051	1(2)	63305	1(2)	64505	1(3)	64744	1(2)	64913	3(3)	65855	1(2)	67025	1(2)
62258	1(3)	63055	1(2)	63306	1(2)	64510	1(3)	64746	1(2)	64999	1(3)	65860	1(2)	67027	1(2)
62263	1(2)	63056	1(2)	63307	1(2)	64517	1(3)	64755	1(2)	65091	1(2)	65865	1(2)	67028	1(3)
62264	1(2)	63057	3(3)	63308	3(3)	64520	1(3)	64760	1(2)	65093	1(2)	65870	1(2)	67030	1(2)
62267	2(3)	63064	1(2)	63600	2(3)	64530	1(3)	64763	1(2)	65101	1(2)	65875	1(2)	67031	1(2)
62268	1(3)	63066	1(3)	63610	1(3)	64553	1(3)	64766	1(2)	65103	1(2)	65880	1(2)	67036	1(2)
62269	2(3)	63075	1(2)	63620	1(2)	64555	2(3)	64771	2(3)	65105	1(2)	65900	1(3)	67039	1(2)
62270	2(3)	63076	3(3)	63621	2(2)	64561	1(3)	64772	2(3)	65110	1(2)	65920	1(2)	67040	1(2)
62272	1(3)	63077	1(2)	63650	2(3)	64566	1(3)	64774	2(3)	65112	1(2)	65930	1(3)	67041	1(2)
62273	2(3)	63078	3(3)	63655	1(3)	64568	1(3)	64776	1(2)	65114	1(2)	66020	1(3)	67042	1(2)
62280	1(3)	63081	1(2)	63661	1(2)	64569	1(3)	64778	1(3)	65125	1(2)	66030	1(3)	67043	1(2)
62281	1(3)	63082	6(2)	63662	1(2)	64570	1(3)	64782	2(2)	65130	1(2)	66130	1(3)	67101	1(2)
62282	1(3)	63085	1(2)	63663	1(3)	64575	2(3)	64783	2(3)	65135	1(2)	66150	1(2)	67105	1(2)
62284	1(3)	63086	2(3)	63664	1(3)	64580	2(3)	64784	3(3)	65140	1(2)	66155	1(2)	67107	1(2)
62287	1(2)	63087	1(2)	63685	1(3)	64581	2(3)	64786	1(3)	65150	1(2)	66160	1(2)	67108	1(2)
62290	5(2)	63088	3(3)	63688	1(3)	64585	2(3)	64787	4(3)	65155	1(2)	66170	1(2)	67110	1(2)
62291	4(3)	63090	1(2)	63700	1(3)	64590	1(3)	64788	5(3)	65175	1(2)	66172	1(2)	67113	1(2)
62292	1(2)	63091	3(3)	63702	1(3)	64595	1(3)	64790	1(3)	65205	1(3)	66174	1(2)	67115	1(2)
62294	1(3)	63101	1(2)	63704	1(3)	64600	2(3)	64792	2(3)	65210	1(3)	66175	1(2)	67120	1(2)
62302	1(3)	63102	1(2)	63706	1(3)	64605	1(2)	64795	2(3)	65220	1(3)	66179	1(2)	67121	1(2)
62303	1(3)	63103	3(3)	63707	1(3)	64610	1(2)	64802	1(2)	65222	1(3)	66180	1(2)	67141	1(2)
62304	1(3)	63170	1(3)	63709	1(3)	64611	1(2)	64804	1(2)	65235	1(3)	66183	1(3)	67145	1(2)
62305	1(3)	63172	1(3)	63710	1(3)	64612	1(2)	64809	1(2)	65260	1(3)	66184	1(2)	67208	1(2)
62320	1(3)	63173	1(3)	63740	1(3)	64615	1(2)	64818	1(2)	65265	1(3)	66185	1(2)	67210	1(2)
62321	1(3)	63180	1(2)	63741	1(3)	64616	1(2)	64820	4(3)	65270	1(3)	66225	1(2)	67218	1(2)
62322	1(3)	63182	1(2)	63744	1(3)	64617	1(2)	64821	1(2)	65272	1(3)	66250	1(2)	67220	1(2)

CPT	MUE	CPT	MUE	CPT	MUE	CPT	MUE	CPT	MUE	CPT	MUE	CPT	MUE	CPT	MUE
67221	1(2)	67909	1(2)	68840	1(2)	69666	1(2)	70470	2(3)	72127	1(3)	73225	2(3)	74270	1(3)
67225	1(2)	67911	2(3)	68850	1(3)	69667	1(2)	70480	1(3)	72128	1(3)	73501	2(3)	74280	1(3)
67227	1(2)	67912	1(2)	68899	1(3)	69670	1(2)	70481	1(3)	72129	1(3)	73502	2(3)	74283	1(3)
67228	1(2)	67914	2(3)	69000	1(3)	69676	1(2)	70482	1(3)	72130	1(3)	73503	2(3)	74290	1(3)
67229	1(2)	67915	2(3)	69005	1(3)	69700	1(3)	70486	1(3)	72131	1(3)	73521	2(3)	74300	1(3)
67250	1(2)	67916	2(3)	69020	1(3)	69710	0(3)	70487	1(3)	72132	1(3)	73522	2(3)	74301	1(3)
67255	1(2)	67917	2(3)	69090	0(3)	69711	1(2)	70488	1(3)	72133	1(3)	73523	2(3)	74328	1(3)
67299	1(3)	67921	2(3)	69100	3(3)	69714	1(2)	70490	1(3)	72141	1(3)	73525	2(2)	74329	1(3)
67311	1(2)	67922	2(3)	69105	1(3)	69715	1(3)	70491	1(3)	72142	1(3)	73551	2(3)	74330	1(3)
67312	1(2)	67923	2(3)	69110	1(2)	69717	1(2)	70492	1(3)	72146	1(3)	73552	2(3)	74340	1(3)
67314	1(2)	67924	2(3)	69120	1(3)	69718	1(2)	70496	2(3)	72147	1(3)	73560	4(3)	74355	1(3)
67316	1(2)	67930	2(3)	69140	1(2)	69720	1(2)	70498	2(3)	72148	1(3)	73562	3(3)	74360	1(3)
67318	1(2)	67935	2(3)	69145	1(3)	69725	1(2)	70540	1(3)	72149	1(3)	73564	4(3)	74363	2(3)
67320	2(3)	67938	2(3)	69150	1(3)	69740	1(2)	70542	1(3)	72156	1(3)	73565	1(3)	74400	1(3)
67331	1(2)	67950	2(2)	69155	1(3)	69745	1(2)	70543	1(3)	72157	1(3)	73580	2(2)	74410	1(3)
67332	1(2)	67961	2(3)	69200	1(2)	69799	1(3)	70544	2(3)	72158	1(3)	73590	3(3)	74415	1(3)
67334	1(2)	67966	2(3)	69205	1(3)	69801	1(3)	70545	1(3)	72159	1(3)	73592	2(3)	74420	2(3)
67335	1(2)	67971	1(2)	69209	1(2)	69805	1(3)	70546	1(3)	72170	2(3)	73600	2(3)	74425	2(3)
67340	2(2)	67973	1(2)	69210	1(2)	69806	1(3)	70547	1(3)	72190	1(3)	73610	3(3)	74430	1(3)
67343	1(2)	67974	1(2)	69220	1(2)	69905	1(2)	70548	1(3)	72191	1(3)	73615	2(2)	74440	1(2)
67345	1(3)	67975	1(2)	69222	1(2)	69910	1(2)	70549	1(3)	72192	1(3)	73620	2(3)	74445	1(2)
67346	1(3)	67999	1(3)	69300	1(2)	69915	1(3)	70551	2(3)	72193	1(3)	73630	3(3)	74450	1(3)
67399	1(3)	68020	1(3)	69310	1(2)	69930	1(2)	70552	2(3)	72194	1(3)	73650	2(3)	74455	1(3)
67400	1(2)	68040	1(2)	69320	1(2)	69949	1(3)	70553	2(3)	72195	1(3)	73660	2(3)	74470	2(2)
67405	1(2)	68100	1(3)	69399	1(3)	69950	1(2)	70554	1(3)	72196	1(3)	73700	2(3)	74485	2(3)
67412	1(2)	68110	1(3)	69420	1(2)	69955	1(2)	70555	1(3)	72197	1(3)	73701	2(3)	74710	1(3)
67413	1(2)	68115	1(3)	69421	1(2)	69960	1(2)	70557	1(3)	72198	1(3)	73702	2(3)	74712	1(3)
67414	1(2)	68130	1(3)	69424	1(2)	69970	1(3)	70558	1(3)	72200	2(3)	73706	2(3)	74713	2(3)
67415	1(3)	68135	1(3)	69433	1(2)	69979	1(3)	70559	1(3)	72202	1(3)	73718	2(3)	74740	1(3)
67420	1(2)	68200	1(3)	69436	1(2)	69990	1(3)	71045	4(3)	72220	1(3)	73719	2(3)	74742	2(2)
67430	1(2)	68320	1(2)	69440	1(2)	70010	1(3)	71046	2(3)	72240	1(2)	73720	2(3)	74775	1(2)
67440	1(2)	68325	1(2)	69450	1(2)	70015	1(3)	71047	1(3)	72255	1(2)	73721	3(3)	75557	1(3)
67445	1(2)	68326	1(2)	69501	1(3)	70030	2(2)	71048	1(3)	72265	1(2)	73722	2(3)	75559	1(3)
67450	1(2)	68328	1(2)	69502	1(2)	70100	2(3)	71100	2(3)	72270	1(2)	73723	2(3)	75561	1(3)
67500	1(3)	68330	1(3)	69505	1(2)	70110	2(3)	71101	2(3)	72275	1(3)	73725	2(3)	75563	1(3)
67505	1(3)	68335	1(3)	69511	1(2)	70120	1(3)	71110	1(3)	72285	4(3)	74018	3(3)	75565	1(3)
67515	1(3)	68340	1(3)	69530	1(2)	70130	1(3)	71111	1(3)	72295	5(3)	74019	2(3)	75571	1(3)
67550	1(2)	68360	1(3)	69535	1(2)	70134	1(3)	71120	1(3)	73000	2(3)	74021	2(3)	75572	1(3)
67560	1(2)	68362	1(3)	69540	1(3)	70140	2(3)	71130	1(3)	73010	2(3)	74022	2(3)	75573	1(3)
67570	1(2)	68371	1(3)	69550	1(3)	70150	1(3)	71250	2(3)	73020	2(3)	74150	1(3)	75574	1(3)
67599	1(3)	68399	1(3)	69552	1(2)	70160	1(3)	71260	2(3)	73030	4(3)	74160	1(3)	75600	1(3)
67700	2(3)	68400	1(2)	69554	1(2)	70170	2(2)	71270	1(3)	73040	2(2)	74170	1(3)	75605	1(3)
67710	1(2)	68420	1(2)	69601	1(2)	70190	1(2)	71275	1(3)	73050	1(3)	74174	1(3)	75625	1(3)
67715	1(3)	68440	2(3)	69602	1(2)	70200	2(3)	71550	1(3)	73060	2(3)	74175	1(3)	75630	1(3)
67800	1(2)	68500	1(2)	69603	1(2)	70210	1(3)	71551	1(3)	73070	2(3)	74176	2(3)	75635	1(3)
67801	1(2)	68505	1(2)	69604	1(2)	70220	1(3)	71552	1(3)	73080	2(3)	74177	2(3)	75705	20(3)
67805	1(2)	68510	1(2)	69605	1(2)	70240	1(2)	71555	1(3)	73085	2(2)	74178	1(3)	75710	2(3)
67808	1(2)	68520	1(2)	69610	1(2)	70250	2(3)	72020	4(3)	73090	2(3)	74181	1(3)	75716	1(3)
67810	2(3)	68525	1(2)	69620	1(2)	70260	1(3)	72040	3(3)	73092	2(3)	74182	1(3)	75726	3(3)
67820	1(2)	68530	1(2)	69631	1(2)	70300	1(3)	72050	1(3)	73100	2(3)	74183	1(3)	75731	1(3)
67825	1(2)	68540	1(2)	69632	1(3)	70310	1(3)	72052	1(3)	73110	3(3)	74185	1(3)	75733	1(3)
67830	1(2)	68550	1(2)	69633	1(2)	70320	1(3)	72070	1(3)	73115	2(2)	74190	1(3)	75736	2(3)
67835	1(2)	68700	1(2)	69635	1(3)	70328	1(3)	72072	1(3)	73120	2(3)	74210	1(3)	75741	1(3)
67840	3(3)	68705	2(3)	69636	1(3)	70330	1(3)	72074	1(3)	73130	3(3)	74220	1(3)	75743	1(3)
67850	3(3)	68720	1(2)	69637	1(3)	70332	2(3)	72080	1(3)	73140	3(3)	74221	1(3)	75746	1(3)
67875	1(2)	68745	1(2)	69641	1(2)	70336	1(3)	72081	1(3)	73200	2(3)	74230	1(3)	75756	2(3)
67880	1(2)	68750	1(2)	69642	1(2)	70350	1(3)	72082	1(3)	73201	2(3)	74235	1(3)	75774	7(3)
67882	1(2)	68760	4(2)	69643	1(2)	70355	1(3)	72083	1(3)	73202	2(3)	74240	2(3)	75801	1(3)
67900	1(2)	68761	4(2)	69644	1(2)	70360	2(3)	72084	1(3)	73206	2(3)	74246	1(3)	75803	1(3)
67901	1(2)	68770	1(3)	69645	1(2)	70370	1(3)	72100	2(3)	73218	2(3)	74248	1(2)	75805	1(2)
67902	1(2)	68801	4(2)	69646	1(2)	70371	1(2)	72110	1(3)	73219	2(3)	74250	1(3)	75807	1(2)
67903	1(2)	68810	1(2)	69650	1(2)	70380	2(3)	72114	1(3)	73220	2(3)	74251	1(3)	75809	1(3)
67904	1(2)	68811	1(2)	69660	1(2)	70390	2(3)	72120	1(3)	73221	2(3)	74261	1(2)	75810	1(3)
67906	1(2)	68815	1(2)	69661	1(2)	70450	3(3)	72125	1(3)	73222	2(3)	74262	1(2)	75820	2(3)
67908	1(2)	68816	1(2)	69662	1(2)	70460	1(3)	72126	1(3)	73223	2(3)	74263	0(3)	75822	1(3)

CPT	MUE
75825	1(3)
75827	1(3)
75831	1(3)
75833	1(3)
75840	1(3)
75842	1(3)
75860	2(3)
75870	1(3)
75872	1(3)
75880	1(3)
75885	1(3)
75887	1(3)
75889	1(3)
75891	1(3)
75893	2(3)
75894	2(3)
75898	2(3)
75901	1(3)
75902	2(3)
75956	1(2)
75957	1(2)
75958	2(3)
75959	1(2)
75970	1(3)
75984	2(3)
75989	2(3)
76000	3(3)
76010	2(3)
76080	3(3)
76098	3(3)
76100	2(3)
76101	1(3)
76102	1(3)
76120	1(3)
76125	1(3)
76140	0(3)
76376	2(3)
76377	2(3)
76380	2(3)
76390	0(3)
76391	1(3)
76496	1(3)
76497	1(3)
76498	1(3)
76499	1(3)
76506	1(2)
76510	2(2)
76511	2(2)
76512	2(2)
76513	2(2)
76514	1(2)
76516	1(2)
76519	2(2)
76529	2(2)
76536	1(3)
76604	1(3)
76641	2(2)
76642	2(2)
76700	1(3)
76705	2(3)
76706	1(2)
76770	1(3)
76775	2(3)
76776	2(3)
76800	1(3)

CPT	MUE
76801	1(2)
76802	2(3)
76805	1(2)
76810	2(3)
76811	1(2)
76812	2(3)
76813	1(2)
76814	2(3)
76815	1(2)
76816	2(3)
76817	1(3)
76818	2(3)
76819	2(3)
76820	3(3)
76821	2(3)
76825	2(3)
76826	2(3)
76827	2(3)
76828	2(3)
76830	1(3)
76831	1(3)
76856	1(3)
76857	1(3)
76870	1(2)
76872	1(3)
76873	1(2)
76881	2(3)
76882	2(3)
76885	1(2)
76886	1(2)
76932	1(2)
76936	1(3)
76937	2(3)
76940	1(3)
76941	3(3)
76942	1(3)
76945	1(3)
76946	1(3)
76948	1(2)
76965	2(3)
76970	2(3)
76975	1(3)
76977	1(2)
76978	1(2)
76979	3(3)
76981	1(3)
76982	1(2)
76983	2(3)
76998	1(3)
76999	1(3)
77001	2(3)
77002	1(3)
77003	1(3)
77011	1(3)
77012	1(3)
77013	1(3)
77014	2(3)
77021	1(3)
77022	1(3)
77046	1(2)
77047	1(2)
77048	1(2)
77049	1(2)
77053	2(2)
77054	2(2)

CPT	MUE
77061	1(2)
77062	1(2)
77063	1(2)
77065	1(2)
77066	1(2)
77067	1(2)
77071	1(3)
77072	1(2)
77073	1(2)
77074	1(2)
77075	1(2)
77076	1(2)
77077	1(2)
77078	1(2)
77080	1(2)
77081	1(2)
77084	1(2)
77085	1(2)
77086	1(2)
77261	1(3)
77262	1(3)
77263	1(3)
77280	2(3)
77285	1(3)
77290	1(3)
77293	1(3)
77295	1(3)
77299	1(3)
77300	10(3)
77301	1(3)
77306	1(3)
77307	1(3)
77316	1(3)
77317	1(3)
77318	1(3)
77321	1(2)
77331	3(3)
77332	4(3)
77333	2(3)
77334	10(3)
77336	1(2)
77338	1(3)
77370	1(3)
77371	1(2)
77372	1(2)
77373	1(3)
77385	1(3)
77386	1(3)
77387	1(3)
77399	1(3)
77401	1(2)
77402	2(3)
77407	2(3)
77412	2(3)
77417	1(2)
77423	1(3)
77424	1(2)
77425	1(3)
77427	1(2)
77431	1(2)
77432	1(2)
77435	1(2)
77469	1(2)
77470	1(2)
77499	1(3)

CPT	MUE
77520	1(3)
77522	1(3)
77523	1(3)
77525	1(3)
77600	1(3)
77605	1(3)
77610	1(3)
77615	1(3)
77620	1(3)
77750	1(3)
77761	1(3)
77762	1(3)
77763	1(3)
77767	2(3)
77768	2(3)
77770	2(3)
77771	2(3)
77772	2(3)
77778	1(3)
77789	2(3)
77790	1(3)
77799	1(3)
78012	1(3)
78013	1(3)
78014	1(2)
78015	1(3)
78016	1(3)
78018	1(2)
78020	1(3)
78070	1(2)
78071	1(3)
78072	1(3)
78075	1(2)
78099	1(3)
78102	1(2)
78103	1(2)
78104	1(2)
78110	1(2)
78111	1(2)
78120	1(2)
78121	1(2)
78122	1(2)
78130	1(2)
78135	1(3)
78140	1(3)
78185	1(2)
78191	1(2)
78195	1(2)
78199	1(3)
78201	1(3)
78202	1(3)
78215	1(3)
78216	1(3)
78226	1(3)
78227	1(3)
78230	1(3)
78231	1(3)
78232	1(3)
78258	1(2)
78261	1(2)
78262	1(2)
78264	1(2)
78265	1(2)
78266	1(2)
78267	1(2)

CPT	MUE
78268	1(2)
78278	2(3)
78282	1(2)
78290	1(3)
78291	1(3)
78299	1(3)
78300	1(2)
78305	1(2)
78306	1(2)
78315	1(2)
78350	0(3)
78351	0(3)
78399	1(3)
78414	1(2)
78428	1(3)
78429	1(2)
78430	1(2)
78431	1(2)
78432	1(2)
78433	1(2)
78434	1(2)
78445	1(3)
78451	1(2)
78452	1(2)
78453	1(2)
78454	1(2)
78456	1(3)
78457	1(2)
78458	1(2)
78459	1(3)
78466	1(3)
78468	1(3)
78469	1(3)
78472	1(2)
78473	1(2)
78481	1(2)
78483	1(2)
78491	1(3)
78492	1(2)
78494	1(3)
78496	1(3)
78499	1(3)
78579	1(3)
78580	1(3)
78582	1(3)
78597	1(3)
78598	1(3)
78599	1(3)
78600	1(3)
78601	1(3)
78605	1(3)
78606	1(3)
78608	1(3)
78609	0(3)
78610	1(3)
78630	1(3)
78635	1(3)
78645	1(3)
78650	1(3)
78660	1(2)
78699	1(3)
78700	1(3)
78701	1(3)
78707	1(2)
78708	1(2)

CPT	MUE
78709	1(2)
78725	1(3)
78730	1(2)
78740	1(2)
78761	1(2)
78799	1(3)
78800	1(2)
78801	1(2)
78802	1(2)
78803	1(2)
78804	1(2)
78808	1(2)
78811	1(2)
78812	1(2)
78813	1(2)
78814	1(2)
78815	1(2)
78816	1(2)
78830	1(2)
78831	1(2)
78832	1(2)
78835	4(3)
78999	1(3)
79005	1(3)
79101	1(3)
79200	1(3)
79300	1(3)
79403	1(3)
79440	1(3)
79445	1(3)
79999	1(3)
80047	2(3)
80048	2(3)
80050	0(3)
80051	2(3)
80053	1(3)
80055	1(3)
80061	1(3)
80069	1(3)
80074	1(2)
80076	1(3)
80081	1(2)
80145	1(3)
80150	2(3)
80155	1(3)
80156	2(3)
80157	2(3)
80158	1(3)
80159	2(3)
80162	2(3)
80163	1(3)
80164	2(3)
80165	1(3)
80168	2(3)
80169	1(3)
80170	2(3)
80171	1(3)
80173	2(3)
80175	1(3)
80176	1(3)
80177	1(3)
80178	2(3)
80180	1(3)
80183	1(3)
80184	2(3)

CPT	MUE
80185	2(3)
80186	2(3)
80187	1(3)
80188	2(3)
80190	2(3)
80192	2(3)
80194	2(3)
80195	2(3)
80197	2(3)
80198	2(3)
80199	1(3)
80200	2(3)
80201	2(3)
80202	2(3)
80203	1(3)
80230	1(3)
80235	1(3)
80280	1(3)
80285	1(3)
80299	3(3)
80305	1(2)
80306	1(2)
80307	1(2)
80320	1(3)
80321	1(3)
80322	1(3)
80323	1(3)
80324	1(3)
80325	1(3)
80326	1(3)
80327	1(3)
80328	1(3)
80329	1(3)
80330	1(3)
80331	1(3)
80332	1(3)
80333	1(3)
80334	1(3)
80335	1(3)
80336	1(3)
80337	1(3)
80338	1(3)
80339	1(3)
80340	1(3)
80341	1(3)
80342	1(3)
80343	1(3)
80344	1(3)
80345	1(3)
80346	1(3)
80347	1(3)
80348	1(3)
80349	1(3)
80350	1(3)
80351	1(3)
80352	1(3)
80353	1(3)
80354	1(3)
80355	1(3)
80356	1(3)
80357	1(3)
80358	1(3)
80359	1(3)
80360	1(3)
80361	1(3)

CPT	MUE
80362	1(3)
80363	1(3)
80364	1(3)
80365	1(3)
80366	1(3)
80367	1(3)
80368	1(3)
80369	1(3)
80370	1(3)
80371	1(3)
80372	1(3)
80373	1(3)
80374	1(3)
80375	1(3)
80376	1(3)
80377	1(3)
80400	1(3)
80402	1(3)
80406	1(3)
80408	1(3)
80410	1(3)
80412	1(3)
80414	1(3)
80415	1(3)
80416	1(3)
80417	1(3)
80418	1(3)
80420	1(2)
80422	1(3)
80424	1(3)
80426	1(3)
80428	1(3)
80430	1(3)
80432	1(3)
80434	1(3)
80435	1(3)
80436	1(3)
80438	1(3)
80439	1(3)
80500	1(3)
80502	1(3)
81000	2(3)
81001	2(3)
81002	2(3)
81003	2(3)
81005	2(3)
81007	1(3)
81015	2(3)
81020	1(3)
81025	1(3)
81050	2(3)
81099	1(3)
81105	1(2)
81106	1(2)
81107	1(2)
81108	1(2)
81109	1(2)
81110	1(2)
81111	1(2)
81112	1(2)
81120	1(3)
81121	1(3)
81161	1(3)
81162	1(2)
81163	1(2)

CPT	MUE	CPT	MUE	CPT	MUE	CPT	MUE	CPT	MUE	CPT	MUE	CPT	MUE	CPT	MUE
81164	1(2)	81243	1(3)	81313	1(3)	81414	1(2)	82013	1(3)	82378	1(3)	82728	1(3)	83080	2(3)
81165	1(2)	81244	1(3)	81314	1(3)	81415	1(2)	82016	1(3)	82379	1(3)	82731	1(3)	83088	1(3)
81166	1(2)	81245	1(3)	81315	1(3)	81416	2(3)	82017	1(3)	82380	1(3)	82735	1(3)	83090	2(3)
81167	1(2)	81246	1(3)	81316	1(2)	81417	1(3)	82024	4(3)	82382	1(2)	82746	1(2)	83150	1(3)
81170	1(2)	81247	1(2)	81317	1(2)	81420	1(2)	82030	1(3)	82383	1(3)	82747	1(2)	83491	1(3)
81171	1(2)	81248	1(2)	81318	1(3)	81422	1(2)	82040	1(3)	82384	2(3)	82757	1(2)	83497	1(3)
81172	1(2)	81249	1(2)	81319	1(2)	81425	1(2)	82042	2(3)	82387	1(3)	82759	1(3)	83498	2(3)
81173	1(2)	81250	1(3)	81320	1(3)	81426	2(3)	82043	1(3)	82390	1(2)	82760	1(3)	83500	1(3)
81174	1(2)	81251	1(3)	81321	1(3)	81427	1(3)	82044	1(3)	82397	3(3)	82775	1(3)	83505	1(3)
81175	1(3)	81252	1(3)	81322	1(3)	81430	1(2)	82045	1(3)	82415	1(3)	82776	1(2)	83516	4(3)
81176	1(3)	81253	1(3)	81323	1(3)	81431	1(2)	82075	2(3)	82435	1(3)	82777	1(3)	83518	1(3)
81177	1(2)	81254	1(3)	81324	1(3)	81432	1(2)	82085	1(3)	82436	1(3)	82784	6(3)	83519	5(3)
81178	1(2)	81255	1(3)	81325	1(3)	81433	1(2)	82088	2(3)	82438	1(3)	82785	1(3)	83520	9(3)
81179	1(2)	81256	1(2)	81326	1(3)	81434	1(2)	82103	1(3)	82441	1(2)	82787	4(3)	83525	4(3)
81180	1(2)	81257	1(2)	81327	1(2)	81435	1(2)	82104	1(2)	82465	1(3)	82800	1(3)	83527	1(3)
81181	1(2)	81258	1(2)	81328	1(2)	81436	1(2)	82105	1(3)	82480	2(3)	82803	2(3)	83528	1(3)
81182	1(2)	81259	1(2)	81329	1(2)	81437	1(2)	82106	2(3)	82482	1(3)	82805	2(3)	83540	2(3)
81183	1(2)	81260	1(3)	81330	1(3)	81438	1(2)	82107	1(3)	82485	1(3)	82810	2(3)	83550	1(3)
81184	1(2)	81261	1(3)	81331	1(3)	81439	1(2)	82108	1(3)	82495	1(2)	82820	1(3)	83570	1(3)
81185	1(2)	81262	1(3)	81332	1(3)	81440	1(2)	82120	1(3)	82507	1(3)	82930	1(3)	83582	1(3)
81186	1(2)	81263	1(3)	81333	1(2)	81442	1(2)	82127	1(3)	82523	1(3)	82938	1(3)	83586	1(3)
81187	1(2)	81264	1(3)	81334	1(3)	81443	1(2)	82128	2(3)	82525	2(3)	82941	1(3)	83593	1(3)
81188	1(2)	81265	1(3)	81335	1(2)	81445	1(2)	82131	2(3)	82528	1(3)	82943	1(3)	83605	1(3)
81189	1(2)	81266	2(3)	81336	1(2)	81448	1(2)	82135	1(3)	82530	4(3)	82945	4(3)	83615	2(3)
81190	1(2)	81267	1(3)	81337	1(2)	81450	1(2)	82136	2(3)	82533	5(3)	82946	1(2)	83625	1(3)
81200	1(2)	81268	4(3)	81340	1(3)	81455	1(2)	82139	2(3)	82540	1(3)	82947	5(3)	83630	1(3)
81201	1(2)	81269	1(2)	81341	1(3)	81460	1(2)	82140	2(3)	82542	6(3)	82948	2(3)	83631	1(3)
81202	1(3)	81270	1(2)	81342	1(3)	81465	1(2)	82143	2(3)	82550	3(3)	82950	3(3)	83632	1(3)
81203	1(3)	81271	1(2)	81343	1(2)	81470	1(2)	82150	2(3)	82552	3(3)	82951	1(2)	83633	1(3)
81204	1(2)	81272	1(3)	81344	1(2)	81471	1(2)	82154	1(3)	82553	3(3)	82952	3(3)	83655	2(3)
81205	1(3)	81273	1(3)	81345	1(3)	81479	3(3)	82157	1(3)	82554	1(3)	82955	1(2)	83661	3(3)
81206	1(3)	81274	1(2)	81346	1(2)	81490	1(2)	82160	1(3)	82565	2(3)	82960	1(2)	83662	4(3)
81207	1(3)	81275	1(3)	81350	1(3)	81493	1(2)	82163	1(3)	82570	3(3)	82962	2(3)	83663	3(3)
81208	1(3)	81276	1(3)	81355	1(3)	81500	1(2)	82164	1(3)	82575	1(3)	82963	1(3)	83664	3(3)
81209	1(3)	81277	1(2)	81361	1(2)	81503	1(2)	82172	2(3)	82585	1(2)	82965	1(3)	83670	1(3)
81210	1(3)	81283	1(2)	81362	1(2)	81504	1(2)	82175	2(3)	82595	1(3)	82977	1(3)	83690	2(3)
81212	1(2)	81284	1(2)	81363	1(2)	81506	1(2)	82180	1(2)	82600	1(3)	82978	1(3)	83695	1(3)
81215	1(2)	81285	1(2)	81364	1(2)	81507	1(2)	82190	2(3)	82607	1(2)	82979	1(3)	83698	1(3)
81216	1(2)	81286	1(2)	81370	1(2)	81508	1(2)	82232	2(3)	82608	1(2)	82985	1(3)	83700	1(2)
81217	1(2)	81287	1(3)	81371	1(2)	81509	1(2)	82239	1(3)	82610	1(3)	83001	1(3)	83701	1(3)
81218	1(3)	81288	1(3)	81372	1(2)	81510	1(2)	82240	1(3)	82615	1(3)	83002	1(3)	83704	1(3)
81219	1(3)	81289	1(2)	81373	2(2)	81511	1(2)	82247	2(3)	82626	1(3)	83003	5(3)	83718	1(3)
81220	1(3)	81290	1(3)	81374	1(3)	81512	1(2)	82248	2(3)	82627	1(3)	83006	1(2)	83719	1(3)
81221	1(3)	81291	1(3)	81375	1(2)	81518	1(2)	82252	1(3)	82633	1(3)	83009	1(3)	83721	1(3)
81222	1(3)	81292	1(2)	81376	5(3)	81519	1(2)	82261	1(3)	82634	1(3)	83010	1(3)	83722	1(2)
81223	1(2)	81293	1(3)	81377	2(3)	81520	1(2)	82270	1(3)	82638	1(3)	83012	1(2)	83727	1(3)
81224	1(3)	81294	1(3)	81378	1(2)	81521	1(2)	82271	1(3)	82642	1(2)	83013	1(3)	83735	4(3)
81225	1(3)	81295	1(2)	81379	1(2)	81522	1(2)	82272	1(3)	82652	1(2)	83014	1(2)	83775	1(3)
81226	1(3)	81296	1(3)	81380	2(2)	81525	1(2)	82274	1(3)	82656	1(3)	83015	1(2)	83785	1(3)
81227	1(3)	81297	1(3)	81381	3(3)	81528	1(2)	82286	1(3)	82657	2(3)	83018	4(3)	83789	4(3)
81228	1(3)	81298	1(2)	81382	6(3)	81535	1(2)	82300	1(3)	82658	2(3)	83020	2(3)	83825	2(3)
81229	1(3)	81299	1(3)	81383	2(3)	81536	11(3)	82306	1(2)	82664	2(3)	83021	2(3)	83835	2(3)
81230	1(2)	81300	1(3)	81400	2(3)	81538	1(2)	82308	1(3)	82668	1(3)	83026	1(3)	83857	1(3)
81231	1(2)	81301	1(3)	81401	2(3)	81539	1(2)	82310	2(3)	82670	2(3)	83030	1(3)	83861	2(2)
81232	1(2)	81302	1(3)	81402	1(3)	81540	1(2)	82330	2(3)	82671	1(3)	83033	1(3)	83864	1(2)
81233	1(3)	81303	1(3)	81403	4(3)	81541	1(2)	82331	1(3)	82672	1(3)	83036	1(2)	83872	2(3)
81234	1(2)	81304	1(3)	81404	5(3)	81542	1(2)	82340	1(3)	82677	1(3)	83037	1(2)	83873	1(3)
81235	1(3)	81305	1(3)	81405	2(3)	81545	1(2)	82355	2(3)	82679	1(3)	83045	1(3)	83874	2(3)
81236	1(3)	81306	1(2)	81406	2(3)	81551	1(2)	82360	2(3)	82693	2(3)	83050	1(3)	83876	1(3)
81237	1(3)	81307	1(2)	81407	1(3)	81552	1(2)	82365	2(3)	82696	1(3)	83051	1(3)	83880	1(3)
81238	1(2)	81308	1(2)	81408	2(3)	81595	1(2)	82370	2(3)	82705	1(3)	83060	1(3)	83883	4(3)
81239	1(2)	81309	1(2)	81410	1(2)	81596	1(2)	82373	1(3)	82710	1(3)	83065	1(2)	83885	2(3)
81240	1(2)	81310	1(3)	81411	1(2)	81599	1(3)	82374	1(3)	82715	3(3)	83068	1(2)	83915	1(3)
81241	1(2)	81311	1(3)	81412	1(2)	82009	1(3)	82375	1(3)	82725	1(3)	83069	1(3)	83916	2(3)
81242	1(3)	81312	1(2)	81413	1(2)	82010	1(3)	82376	1(3)	82726	1(3)	83070	1(2)	83918	2(3)

CPT	MUE
83919	1(3)
83921	2(3)
83930	2(3)
83935	2(3)
83937	1(3)
83945	2(3)
83950	1(2)
83951	1(2)
83970	2(3)
83986	2(3)
83987	1(3)
83992	2(3)
83993	1(3)
84030	1(2)
84035	1(2)
84060	1(3)
84066	1(3)
84075	2(3)
84078	1(2)
84080	1(3)
84081	1(3)
84085	1(2)
84087	1(3)
84100	2(3)
84105	1(3)
84106	1(2)
84110	1(3)
84112	1(3)
84119	1(2)
84120	1(3)
84126	1(3)
84132	2(3)
84133	2(3)
84134	1(3)
84135	1(3)
84138	1(3)
84140	1(3)
84143	2(3)
84144	1(3)
84145	1(3)
84146	3(3)
84150	2(3)
84152	1(2)
84153	1(2)
84154	1(2)
84155	1(3)
84156	1(3)
84157	2(3)
84160	2(3)
84163	1(3)
84165	1(2)
84166	2(3)
84181	3(3)
84182	6(3)
84202	1(2)
84203	1(2)
84206	1(2)
84207	1(2)
84210	1(3)
84220	1(3)
84228	1(3)
84233	1(3)
84234	1(3)
84235	1(3)
84238	3(3)

CPT	MUE
84244	2(3)
84252	1(2)
84255	2(3)
84260	1(3)
84270	1(3)
84275	1(3)
84285	1(3)
84295	1(3)
84300	2(3)
84302	1(3)
84305	1(3)
84307	1(3)
84311	2(3)
84315	1(3)
84375	1(3)
84376	1(3)
84377	1(3)
84378	2(3)
84379	1(3)
84392	1(3)
84402	1(3)
84403	2(3)
84410	1(2)
84425	1(2)
84430	1(3)
84431	1(3)
84432	1(2)
84436	1(2)
84437	1(2)
84439	1(2)
84442	1(2)
84443	4(2)
84445	1(2)
84446	1(2)
84449	1(3)
84450	1(3)
84460	1(3)
84466	1(3)
84478	1(3)
84479	1(2)
84480	1(2)
84481	1(2)
84482	1(2)
84484	2(3)
84485	1(3)
84488	1(3)
84490	1(2)
84510	1(3)
84512	1(3)
84520	1(3)
84525	1(3)
84540	2(3)
84545	1(3)
84550	1(3)
84560	2(3)
84577	1(3)
84578	1(3)
84580	1(3)
84583	1(3)
84585	1(2)
84586	1(2)
84588	1(3)
84590	1(2)
84591	1(3)
84597	1(3)

CPT	MUE
84600	2(3)
84620	1(2)
84630	2(3)
84681	1(3)
84702	2(3)
84703	1(3)
84704	1(3)
84830	1(2)
84999	1(3)
85002	1(3)
85004	1(3)
85007	1(3)
85008	1(3)
85009	1(3)
85013	1(3)
85014	2(3)
85018	2(3)
85025	2(3)
85027	2(3)
85032	1(3)
85041	1(3)
85044	1(2)
85045	1(2)
85046	1(2)
85048	2(3)
85049	2(3)
85055	1(3)
85060	1(3)
85097	2(3)
85130	1(3)
85170	1(3)
85175	1(3)
85210	2(3)
85220	2(3)
85230	2(3)
85240	2(3)
85244	1(3)
85245	2(3)
85246	2(3)
85247	2(3)
85250	2(3)
85260	2(3)
85270	2(3)
85280	2(3)
85290	2(3)
85291	1(3)
85292	1(3)
85293	1(3)
85300	2(3)
85301	1(3)
85302	1(3)
85303	2(3)
85305	2(3)
85306	2(3)
85307	2(3)
85335	2(3)
85337	1(3)
85345	1(3)
85347	3(3)
85348	1(3)
85360	1(3)
85362	2(3)
85366	1(3)
85370	1(3)
85378	1(3)

CPT	MUE
85379	2(3)
85380	1(3)
85384	2(3)
85385	1(3)
85390	3(3)
85396	1(2)
85397	2(3)
85400	1(3)
85410	1(3)
85415	2(3)
85420	2(3)
85421	1(3)
85441	1(2)
85445	1(2)
85460	1(3)
85461	1(2)
85475	1(3)
85520	1(3)
85525	2(3)
85530	1(3)
85536	1(2)
85540	1(2)
85547	1(2)
85549	1(3)
85555	1(2)
85557	1(2)
85576	7(3)
85597	1(3)
85598	1(3)
85610	4(3)
85611	2(3)
85612	1(3)
85613	3(3)
85635	1(3)
85651	1(2)
85652	1(2)
85660	2(3)
85670	2(3)
85675	1(3)
85705	1(3)
85730	4(3)
85732	4(3)
85810	2(3)
85999	1(3)
86000	6(3)
86001	20(3)
86005	2(3)
86008	20(3)
86021	1(2)
86022	1(2)
86023	3(3)
86038	1(3)
86039	1(3)
86060	1(3)
86063	1(3)
86077	1(2)
86078	1(3)
86079	1(3)
86140	1(2)
86141	1(2)
86146	3(3)
86147	4(3)
86148	3(3)
86152	1(3)
86153	1(3)

CPT	MUE
86155	1(3)
86156	1(2)
86157	1(2)
86160	4(3)
86161	2(3)
86162	1(2)
86171	2(3)
86200	1(3)
86215	1(3)
86225	1(3)
86226	1(3)
86235	10(3)
86255	5(3)
86256	9(3)
86277	1(3)
86280	1(3)
86294	1(3)
86300	2(3)
86301	1(2)
86304	1(2)
86305	1(2)
86308	1(2)
86309	1(2)
86310	1(2)
86316	2(3)
86317	6(3)
86318	2(3)
86320	1(2)
86325	2(3)
86327	1(3)
86328	3(3)
86329	3(3)
86331	12(3)
86332	1(3)
86334	2(2)
86335	2(3)
86336	1(3)
86337	1(2)
86340	1(2)
86341	1(3)
86343	1(3)
86344	1(2)
86352	1(3)
86353	7(3)
86355	1(2)
86356	7(3)
86357	1(2)
86359	1(2)
86360	1(2)
86361	1(2)
86367	1(3)
86376	2(3)
86382	3(3)
86384	1(3)
86386	1(2)
86403	2(3)
86406	2(3)
86430	2(3)
86431	2(3)
86480	1(3)
86481	1(3)
86485	1(2)
86486	2(3)
86490	1(2)
86510	1(2)

CPT	MUE
86580	1(2)
86590	1(3)
86592	2(3)
86593	2(3)
86602	3(3)
86603	2(3)
86609	14(3)
86611	4(3)
86612	2(3)
86615	6(3)
86617	2(3)
86618	2(3)
86619	2(3)
86622	2(3)
86625	1(3)
86628	3(3)
86631	6(3)
86632	3(3)
86635	4(3)
86638	6(3)
86641	2(3)
86644	2(3)
86645	1(3)
86648	2(3)
86651	2(3)
86652	2(3)
86653	2(3)
86654	2(3)
86658	12(3)
86663	2(3)
86664	2(3)
86665	2(3)
86666	4(3)
86668	2(3)
86671	3(3)
86674	3(3)
86677	3(3)
86682	2(3)
86684	2(3)
86687	1(3)
86688	1(3)
86689	2(3)
86692	2(3)
86694	2(3)
86695	2(3)
86696	2(3)
86698	3(3)
86701	1(3)
86702	2(3)
86703	1(2)
86704	1(2)
86705	1(2)
86706	2(3)
86707	1(3)
86708	1(2)
86709	1(2)
86710	4(3)
86711	2(3)
86713	3(3)
86717	8(3)
86720	2(3)
86723	2(3)
86727	2(3)
86732	2(3)
86735	2(3)

CPT	MUE
86738	2(3)
86741	2(3)
86744	2(3)
86747	2(3)
86750	4(3)
86753	3(3)
86756	2(3)
86757	6(3)
86759	2(3)
86762	2(3)
86765	2(3)
86768	5(3)
86769	3(3)
86771	2(3)
86774	2(3)
86777	2(3)
86778	2(3)
86780	2(3)
86784	1(3)
86787	2(3)
86788	2(3)
86789	2(3)
86790	4(3)
86793	2(3)
86794	1(3)
86800	1(3)
86803	1(3)
86804	1(2)
86805	2(3)
86806	2(3)
86807	2(3)
86808	1(3)
86812	1(2)
86813	1(2)
86816	1(2)
86817	1(2)
86821	1(3)
86825	1(3)
86826	2(3)
86828	1(3)
86829	1(3)
86830	2(3)
86831	2(3)
86832	2(3)
86833	1(3)
86834	1(3)
86835	1(3)
86849	1(3)
86850	3(3)
86860	2(3)
86870	2(3)
86880	4(3)
86885	2(3)
86886	3(3)
86890	1(3)
86891	1(3)
86900	1(3)
86901	1(3)
86902	6(3)
86904	2(3)
86905	8(3)
86906	1(2)
86910	0(3)
86911	0(3)
86920	9(3)

CPT	MUE
86921	2(3)
86922	5(3)
86923	10(3)
86927	2(3)
86930	0(3)
86931	1(3)
86932	1(3)
86940	1(3)
86941	1(3)
86945	2(3)
86950	1(3)
86960	1(3)
86965	1(3)
86970	1(3)
86971	1(3)
86972	1(3)
86975	1(3)
86976	1(3)
86977	1(3)
86978	1(3)
86985	1(3)
86999	1(3)
87003	1(3)
87015	3(3)
87040	2(3)
87045	3(3)
87046	6(3)
87070	3(3)
87071	2(3)
87073	2(3)
87075	6(3)
87076	2(3)
87077	4(3)
87081	2(3)
87084	1(3)
87086	3(3)
87088	3(3)
87101	2(3)
87102	4(3)
87103	2(3)
87106	3(3)
87107	4(3)
87109	2(3)
87110	2(3)
87116	2(3)
87118	3(3)
87140	3(3)
87143	2(3)
87149	4(3)
87150	12(3)
87152	1(3)
87153	3(3)
87158	1(3)
87164	2(3)
87166	2(3)
87168	2(3)
87169	2(3)
87172	1(3)
87176	2(3)
87177	3(3)
87181	12(3)
87184	8(3)
87185	4(3)
87186	12(3)
87187	3(3)

CPT	MUE	CPT	MUE	CPT	MUE	CPT	MUE	CPT	MUE	CPT	MUE	CPT	MUE	CPT	MUE
87188	6(3)	87471	1(3)	87590	1(3)	88112	6(3)	88307	8(3)	89255	1(3)	90621	1(2)	90746	1(2)
87190	9(3)	87472	1(3)	87591	3(3)	88120	2(3)	88309	3(3)	89257	1(3)	90625	1(2)	90747	1(2)
87197	1(3)	87475	1(3)	87592	1(3)	88121	2(3)	88311	4(3)	89258	1(2)	90630	1(2)	90748	0(3)
87205	3(3)	87476	1(3)	87623	1(2)	88125	1(3)	88312	9(3)	89259	1(2)	90632	1(2)	90749	1(3)
87206	6(3)	87480	1(3)	87624	1(3)	88130	1(2)	88313	8(3)	89260	1(2)	90633	1(2)	90750	1(2)
87207	3(3)	87481	5(3)	87625	1(3)	88140	1(2)	88314	6(3)	89261	1(2)	90634	1(2)	90756	1(2)
87209	4(3)	87482	1(3)	87631	1(3)	88141	1(3)	88319	11(3)	89264	1(3)	90636	1(2)	90785	3(3)
87210	4(3)	87483	1(2)	87632	1(3)	88142	1(3)	88321	1(2)	89268	1(2)	90644	1(2)	90791	1(3)
87220	3(3)	87485	1(3)	87633	1(3)	88143	1(3)	88323	1(2)	89272	1(2)	90647	1(2)	90792	1(3)
87230	2(3)	87486	1(3)	87634	1(3)	88147	1(3)	88325	1(2)	89280	1(2)	90648	1(2)	90832	2(3)
87250	1(3)	87487	1(3)	87635	2(3)	88148	1(3)	88329	2(3)	89281	1(2)	90649	1(2)	90833	2(3)
87252	2(3)	87490	1(3)	87640	1(3)	88150	1(3)	88331	11(3)	89290	1(2)	90650	1(2)	90834	2(3)
87253	2(3)	87491	3(3)	87641	1(3)	88152	1(3)	88332	13(3)	89291	1(2)	90651	1(2)	90836	2(3)
87254	7(3)	87492	1(3)	87650	1(3)	88153	1(3)	88333	4(3)	89300	1(2)	90653	1(2)	90837	2(3)
87255	2(3)	87493	2(3)	87651	1(3)	88155	1(3)	88334	5(3)	89310	1(2)	90654	1(2)	90838	2(3)
87260	1(3)	87495	1(3)	87652	1(3)	88160	4(3)	88341	13(3)	89320	1(2)	90655	1(2)	90839	1(2)
87265	1(3)	87496	1(3)	87653	1(3)	88161	4(3)	88342	4(3)	89321	1(2)	90656	1(2)	90840	3(3)
87267	1(3)	87497	2(3)	87660	1(3)	88162	3(3)	88344	6(3)	89322	1(2)	90657	1(2)	90845	1(2)
87269	1(3)	87498	1(3)	87661	1(3)	88164	1(3)	88346	2(3)	89325	1(2)	90658	1(2)	90846	1(3)
87270	1(3)	87500	1(3)	87662	2(3)	88165	1(3)	88348	1(3)	89329	1(2)	90660	1(2)	90847	1(3)
87271	1(3)	87501	1(3)	87797	3(3)	88166	1(3)	88350	8(3)	89330	1(2)	90661	1(2)	90849	1(3)
87272	1(3)	87502	1(3)	87798	13(3)	88167	1(3)	88355	1(3)	89331	1(2)	90662	1(2)	90853	1(3)
87273	1(3)	87503	1(3)	87799	3(3)	88172	5(3)	88356	3(3)	89335	1(3)	90664	1(2)	90863	1(3)
87274	1(3)	87505	1(2)	87800	2(3)	88173	5(3)	88358	2(3)	89337	1(2)	90666	1(2)	90865	1(3)
87275	1(3)	87506	1(2)	87801	3(3)	88174	1(3)	88360	6(3)	89342	1(2)	90667	1(2)	90867	1(2)
87276	1(3)	87507	1(2)	87802	2(3)	88175	1(3)	88361	6(3)	89343	1(2)	90668	1(2)	90868	1(3)
87278	1(3)	87510	1(3)	87803	3(3)	88177	6(3)	88362	1(3)	89344	1(2)	90670	1(2)	90869	1(3)
87279	1(3)	87511	1(3)	87804	3(3)	88182	2(3)	88363	2(3)	89346	1(2)	90672	1(2)	90870	2(3)
87280	1(3)	87512	1(3)	87806	1(2)	88184	2(3)	88364	3(3)	89352	1(2)	90673	1(2)	90875	1(3)
87281	1(3)	87516	1(3)	87807	2(3)	88185	35(3)	88365	4(3)	89353	1(3)	90674	1(2)	90876	0(3)
87283	1(3)	87517	1(3)	87808	1(3)	88187	2(3)	88366	2(3)	89354	1(3)	90675	1(2)	90880	1(3)
87285	1(3)	87520	1(3)	87809	2(3)	88188	2(3)	88367	3(3)	89356	2(3)	90676	1(2)	90882	0(3)
87290	1(3)	87521	1(3)	87810	2(3)	88189	2(3)	88368	3(3)	89398	1(3)	90680	1(2)	90885	0(3)
87299	1(3)	87522	1(3)	87850	1(3)	88199	1(3)	88369	3(3)	90281	0(3)	90681	1(2)	90887	0(3)
87300	2(3)	87525	1(3)	87880	2(3)	88230	2(3)	88371	1(3)	90283	0(3)	90682	1(2)	90889	0(3)
87301	1(3)	87526	1(3)	87899	4(3)	88233	2(3)	88372	1(3)	90284	0(3)	90685	1(2)	90899	1(3)
87305	1(3)	87527	1(3)	87900	1(2)	88235	2(3)	88373	3(3)	90287	0(3)	90686	1(2)	90901	1(3)
87320	1(3)	87528	1(3)	87901	1(2)	88237	4(3)	88374	5(3)	90288	0(3)	90687	1(2)	90912	1(2)
87324	2(3)	87529	2(3)	87902	1(2)	88239	3(3)	88375	1(3)	90291	0(3)	90688	1(2)	90913	3(3)
87327	1(3)	87530	2(3)	87903	1(2)	88240	1(3)	88377	5(3)	90296	1(2)	90689	1(2)	90935	1(3)
87328	2(3)	87531	1(3)	87904	14(3)	88241	3(3)	88380	1(3)	90371	10(3)	90690	1(2)	90937	1(3)
87329	2(3)	87532	1(3)	87905	2(3)	88245	1(2)	88381	1(3)	90375	20(3)	90691	1(2)	90940	1(3)
87332	1(3)	87533	1(3)	87906	2(3)	88248	1(2)	88387	2(3)	90376	20(3)	90694	1(2)	90945	1(3)
87335	1(3)	87534	1(3)	87910	1(3)	88249	1(2)	88388	1(3)	90378	4(3)	90696	1(2)	90947	1(3)
87336	1(3)	87535	1(3)	87912	1(3)	88261	2(3)	88399	1(3)	90384	0(3)	90697	1(2)	90951	1(2)
87337	1(3)	87536	1(3)	87999	1(3)	88262	2(3)	88720	1(3)	90385	1(2)	90698	1(2)	90952	1(2)
87338	1(3)	87537	1(3)	88000	0(3)	88263	1(3)	88738	1(3)	90386	0(3)	90700	1(2)	90953	1(2)
87339	1(3)	87538	1(3)	88005	0(3)	88264	1(3)	88740	1(2)	90389	0(3)	90702	1(2)	90954	1(2)
87340	1(2)	87539	1(3)	88007	0(3)	88267	2(3)	88741	1(2)	90393	1(2)	90707	1(2)	90955	1(2)
87341	1(2)	87540	1(3)	88012	0(3)	88269	2(3)	88749	1(3)	90396	1(2)	90710	1(2)	90956	1(2)
87350	1(2)	87541	1(3)	88014	0(3)	88271	16(3)	89049	1(3)	90399	0(3)	90713	1(2)	90957	1(2)
87380	1(2)	87542	1(3)	88016	0(3)	88272	12(3)	89050	2(3)	90460	9(3)	90714	1(2)	90958	1(2)
87385	2(3)	87550	1(3)	88020	0(3)	88273	3(3)	89051	2(3)	90461	8(3)	90715	1(2)	90959	1(2)
87389	1(3)	87551	2(3)	88025	0(3)	88274	5(3)	89055	2(3)	90471	1(2)	90716	1(2)	90960	1(2)
87390	1(3)	87552	1(3)	88027	0(3)	88275	12(3)	89060	2(3)	90472	8(3)	90717	1(2)	90961	1(2)
87391	1(3)	87555	1(3)	88028	0(3)	88280	1(3)	89125	2(3)	90473	1(2)	90723	0(3)	90962	1(2)
87400	2(3)	87556	1(3)	88029	0(3)	88283	5(3)	89160	1(3)	90474	1(3)	90732	1(2)	90963	1(2)
87420	1(3)	87557	1(3)	88036	0(3)	88285	10(3)	89190	1(3)	90476	1(2)	90733	1(2)	90964	1(2)
87425	1(3)	87560	1(3)	88037	0(3)	88289	1(3)	89220	2(3)	90477	1(2)	90734	1(2)	90965	1(2)
87426	3(3)	87561	1(3)	88040	0(3)	88291	1(3)	89230	1(2)	90581	1(2)	90736	1(2)	90966	1(2)
87427	2(3)	87562	1(3)	88045	0(3)	88299	1(3)	89240	1(3)	90585	1(2)	90738	1(2)	90967	1(2)
87430	1(3)	87563	3(3)	88099	0(3)	88300	4(3)	89250	1(2)	90586	1(2)	90739	1(2)	90968	1(2)
87449	3(3)	87580	1(3)	88104	5(3)	88302	4(3)	89251	1(2)	90587	1(2)	90740	1(2)	90969	1(2)
87450	2(3)	87581	1(3)	88106	5(3)	88304	5(3)	89253	1(3)	90619	1(2)	90743	1(2)	90970	1(2)
87451	2(3)	87582	1(3)	88108	6(3)	88305	16(3)	89254	1(3)	90620	1(2)	90744	1(2)	90989	1(2)

CPT	MUE
90993	1(3)
90997	1(3)
90999	1(3)
91010	1(2)
91013	1(3)
91020	1(2)
91022	1(2)
91030	1(2)
91034	1(2)
91035	1(2)
91037	1(2)
91038	1(2)
91040	1(2)
91065	2(2)
91110	1(2)
91111	1(2)
91112	1(3)
91117	1(2)
91120	1(2)
91122	1(2)
91132	1(3)
91133	1(3)
91200	1(2)
91299	1(3)
92002	1(2)
92004	1(2)
92012	1(3)
92014	1(3)
92015	0(3)
92018	1(2)
92019	1(2)
92020	1(2)
92025	1(2)
92060	1(2)
92065	1(2)
92071	2(2)
92072	1(2)
92081	1(2)
92082	1(2)
92083	1(2)
92100	1(2)
92132	1(2)
92133	1(2)
92134	1(2)
92136	2(2)
92145	1(2)
92201	1(2)
92202	1(2)
92227	1(2)
92228	1(2)
92230	2(2)
92235	1(2)
92240	1(2)
92242	1(2)
92250	1(2)
92260	1(2)
92265	1(2)
92270	1(2)
92273	1(2)
92274	1(2)
92283	1(2)
92284	1(2)
92285	1(2)
92286	1(2)
92287	1(2)

CPT	MUE
92310	0(3)
92311	1(2)
92312	1(2)
92313	1(3)
92314	0(3)
92315	1(2)
92316	1(2)
92317	1(3)
92325	1(3)
92326	2(2)
92340	0(3)
92341	0(3)
92342	0(3)
92352	0(3)
92353	0(3)
92354	0(3)
92355	0(3)
92358	0(3)
92370	0(3)
92371	0(3)
92499	1(3)
92502	1(3)
92504	1(3)
92507	1(3)
92508	1(3)
92511	1(3)
92512	1(2)
92516	1(3)
92520	1(2)
92521	1(2)
92522	1(2)
92523	1(2)
92524	1(2)
92526	1(2)
92531	0(3)
92532	0(3)
92533	0(3)
92534	0(3)
92537	1(2)
92538	1(2)
92540	1(3)
92541	1(3)
92542	1(3)
92544	1(3)
92545	1(3)
92546	1(3)
92547	1(3)
92548	1(3)
92549	1(3)
92550	1(2)
92551	0(3)
92552	1(2)
92553	1(2)
92555	1(2)
92556	1(2)
92557	1(2)
92558	0(3)
92559	0(3)
92560	0(3)
92561	1(2)
92562	1(2)
92563	1(2)
92564	1(2)
92565	1(2)
92567	1(2)

CPT	MUE
92568	1(2)
92570	1(2)
92571	1(2)
92572	1(2)
92575	1(2)
92576	1(2)
92577	1(2)
92579	1(2)
92582	1(2)
92583	1(2)
92584	1(2)
92585	1(2)
92586	1(2)
92587	1(2)
92588	1(2)
92590	0(3)
92591	0(3)
92592	0(3)
92593	0(3)
92594	0(3)
92595	0(3)
92596	1(2)
92597	1(3)
92601	1(3)
92602	1(3)
92603	1(3)
92604	1(3)
92605	0(3)
92606	0(3)
92607	1(3)
92608	4(3)
92609	1(3)
92610	1(2)
92611	1(3)
92612	1(3)
92613	1(2)
92614	1(3)
92615	1(2)
92616	1(3)
92617	1(2)
92618	1(3)
92620	1(2)
92621	2(3)
92625	1(2)
92626	1(2)
92627	6(3)
92630	0(3)
92633	0(3)
92640	1(3)
92700	1(3)
92920	3(3)
92921	6(2)
92924	2(3)
92925	6(2)
92928	3(3)
92929	6(2)
92933	2(3)
92934	6(2)
92937	2(3)
92938	6(3)
92941	1(3)
92943	2(3)
92944	3(3)
92950	2(3)
92953	2(3)

CPT	MUE
92960	2(3)
92961	1(3)
92970	1(3)
92971	1(3)
92973	2(3)
92974	1(3)
92975	1(3)
92977	1(3)
92978	1(3)
92979	2(3)
92986	1(2)
92987	1(2)
92990	1(2)
92992	1(2)
92993	1(2)
92997	1(2)
92998	2(3)
93000	3(3)
93005	3(3)
93010	5(3)
93015	1(3)
93016	1(3)
93017	1(3)
93018	1(3)
93024	1(3)
93025	1(2)
93040	3(3)
93041	2(3)
93042	3(3)
93050	1(3)
93224	1(2)
93225	1(2)
93226	1(2)
93227	1(2)
93228	1(2)
93229	1(2)
93260	1(2)
93261	1(3)
93264	1(2)
93268	1(2)
93270	1(2)
93271	1(2)
93272	1(2)
93278	1(3)
93279	1(3)
93280	1(3)
93281	1(3)
93282	1(3)
93283	1(3)
93284	1(3)
93285	1(3)
93286	2(3)
93287	2(3)
93288	1(3)
93289	1(3)
93290	1(3)
93291	1(3)
93292	1(3)
93293	1(2)
93294	1(2)
93295	1(2)
93296	1(2)
93297	1(2)
93298	1(2)
93303	1(3)

CPT	MUE
93304	1(3)
93306	1(3)
93307	1(3)
93308	1(3)
93312	1(3)
93313	1(3)
93314	1(3)
93315	1(3)
93316	1(3)
93317	1(3)
93318	1(3)
93320	2(3)
93321	1(3)
93325	2(3)
93350	1(2)
93351	1(2)
93352	1(3)
93355	1(3)
93356	1(3)
93451	1(3)
93452	1(3)
93453	1(3)
93454	1(3)
93455	1(3)
93456	1(3)
93457	1(3)
93458	1(3)
93459	1(3)
93460	1(3)
93461	1(3)
93462	1(3)
93463	1(3)
93464	1(3)
93503	2(3)
93505	1(2)
93530	1(3)
93531	1(3)
93532	1(3)
93533	1(3)
93561	1(3)
93562	1(3)
93563	1(3)
93564	1(3)
93565	1(3)
93566	1(3)
93567	1(3)
93568	1(3)
93571	1(3)
93572	2(3)
93580	1(3)
93581	1(3)
93582	1(2)
93583	1(2)
93590	1(2)
93591	1(2)
93592	2(3)
93600	1(3)
93602	1(3)
93603	1(3)
93609	1(3)
93610	1(3)
93612	1(3)
93613	1(3)
93615	1(3)
93616	1(3)

CPT	MUE
93618	1(3)
93619	1(3)
93620	1(3)
93621	1(3)
93622	1(3)
93623	1(3)
93624	1(3)
93631	1(3)
93640	1(3)
93641	1(2)
93642	1(3)
93644	1(3)
93650	1(2)
93653	1(3)
93654	1(3)
93655	2(3)
93656	1(3)
93657	2(3)
93660	1(3)
93662	1(3)
93668	1(3)
93701	1(2)
93702	1(2)
93724	1(3)
93740	0(3)
93745	1(2)
93750	4(3)
93770	0(3)
93784	1(2)
93786	1(2)
93788	1(2)
93790	1(2)
93792	1(2)
93793	1(2)
93797	2(2)
93798	2(2)
93799	1(3)
93880	1(3)
93882	1(3)
93886	1(3)
93888	1(3)
93890	1(3)
93892	1(3)
93893	1(3)
93895	1(3)
93922	2(2)
93923	2(2)
93924	1(2)
93925	1(3)
93926	1(3)
93930	1(3)
93931	1(3)
93970	1(3)
93971	1(3)
93975	1(3)
93976	1(3)
93978	1(3)
93979	1(3)
93980	1(3)
93981	1(3)
93985	1(3)
93986	1(3)
93990	2(3)
93998	1(3)
94002	1(2)

CPT	MUE
94003	1(2)
94004	1(2)
94005	1(3)
94010	1(3)
94011	1(3)
94012	1(3)
94013	1(3)
94014	1(2)
94015	1(2)
94016	1(2)
94060	1(3)
94070	1(2)
94150	0(3)
94200	1(3)
94250	1(3)
94375	1(3)
94400	1(3)
94450	1(3)
94452	1(2)
94453	1(2)
94610	2(3)
94617	1(3)
94618	1(3)
94621	1(3)
94640	4(3)
94642	1(3)
94644	1(2)
94645	2(3)
94660	1(2)
94662	1(2)
94664	1(3)
94667	1(2)
94668	2(3)
94669	2(3)
94680	1(3)
94681	1(3)
94690	1(3)
94726	1(3)
94727	1(3)
94728	1(3)
94729	1(3)
94750	1(3)
94760	1(3)
94761	1(2)
94762	1(2)
94770	1(3)
94772	1(2)
94774	1(2)
94775	1(2)
94776	1(2)
94777	1(2)
94780	1(2)
94781	2(3)
94799	1(3)
95004	80(3)
95012	2(3)
95017	27(3)
95018	19(3)
95024	40(3)
95027	90(3)
95028	30(3)
95044	80(3)
95052	20(3)
95056	1(2)
95060	1(2)

CPT	MUE
95065	1(3)
95070	1(3)
95071	1(2)
95076	1(2)
95079	2(3)
95115	1(2)
95117	1(2)
95120	0(3)
95125	0(3)
95130	0(3)
95131	0(3)
95132	0(3)
95133	0(3)
95134	0(3)
95144	30(3)
95145	10(3)
95146	10(3)
95147	10(3)
95148	10(3)
95149	10(3)
95165	30(3)
95170	10(3)
95180	6(3)
95199	1(3)
95249	1(2)
95250	1(2)
95251	1(2)
95700	1(2)
95705	1(2)
95706	1(2)
95707	1(2)
95708	4(3)
95709	4(3)
95710	4(3)
95711	1(2)
95712	1(2)
95713	1(2)
95714	4(3)
95715	4(3)
95716	4(3)
95717	1(2)
95718	1(2)
95719	1(2)
95720	1(2)
95721	1(2)
95722	1(2)
95723	1(2)
95724	1(2)
95725	1(2)
95726	1(2)
95782	1(2)
95783	1(2)
95800	1(2)
95801	1(2)
95803	1(2)
95805	1(2)
95806	1(2)
95807	1(2)
95808	1(2)
95810	1(2)
95811	1(2)
95812	1(3)
95813	1(3)
95816	1(3)
95819	1(3)

CPT	MUE	CPT	MUE	CPT	MUE	CPT	MUE	CPT	MUE	CPT	MUE	CPT	MUE	CPT	MUE
95822	1(3)	95981	1(3)	96413	1(3)	97154	12(3)	99002	0(3)	99235	1(3)	99378	0(3)	99477	1(2)
95824	1(3)	95982	1(3)	96415	8(3)	97155	24(3)	99024	1(3)	99236	1(3)	99379	0(3)	99478	1(2)
95829	1(3)	95983	1(2)	96416	1(3)	97156	16(3)	99026	0(3)	99238	1(3)	99380	0(3)	99479	1(2)
95830	1(3)	95984	11(3)	96417	3(3)	97157	16(3)	99027	0(3)	99239	1(3)	99381	0(3)	99480	1(2)
95836	1(2)	95990	1(3)	96420	1(3)	97158	16(3)	99050	0(3)	99241	0(3)	99382	0(3)	99483	1(2)
95851	3(3)	95991	1(3)	96422	2(3)	97161	1(2)	99051	0(3)	99242	0(3)	99383	0(3)	99484	1(2)
95852	1(3)	95992	1(2)	96423	1(3)	97162	1(2)	99053	0(3)	99243	0(3)	99384	0(3)	99485	1(3)
95857	1(2)	95999	1(3)	96425	1(3)	97163	1(2)	99056	0(3)	99244	0(3)	99385	0(3)	99486	4(1)
95860	1(3)	96000	1(2)	96440	1(3)	97164	1(2)	99058	0(3)	99245	0(3)	99386	0(3)	99487	1(2)
95861	1(3)	96001	1(2)	96446	1(3)	97165	1(2)	99060	0(3)	99251	0(3)	99387	0(3)	99489	10(3)
95863	1(3)	96002	1(3)	96450	1(3)	97166	1(2)	99070	0(3)	99252	0(3)	99391	0(3)	99490	1(2)
95864	1(3)	96003	1(3)	96521	2(3)	97167	1(2)	99071	0(3)	99253	0(3)	99392	0(3)	99491	1(2)
95865	1(3)	96004	1(2)	96522	1(3)	97168	1(2)	99075	0(3)	99254	0(3)	99393	0(3)	99492	1(2)
95866	1(3)	96020	1(2)	96523	1(3)	97169	0(3)	99078	0(3)	99255	0(3)	99394	0(3)	99493	1(2)
95867	1(3)	96040	4(3)	96542	1(3)	97170	0(3)	99080	0(3)	99281	1(3)	99395	0(3)	99494	2(3)
95868	1(3)	96105	3(3)	96549	1(3)	97171	0(3)	99082	1(3)	99282	1(3)	99396	0(3)	99495	1(2)
95869	1(3)	96110	3(3)	96567	1(3)	97172	0(3)	99091	1(2)	99283	1(3)	99397	0(3)	99496	1(2)
95870	4(3)	96112	1(2)	96570	1(2)	97530	6(3)	99100	1(3)	99284	1(3)	99401	0(3)	99497	1(2)
95872	4(3)	96113	6(3)	96571	2(3)	97533	4(3)	99116	0(3)	99285	1(3)	99402	0(3)	99498	3(3)
95873	1(2)	96116	1(2)	96573	1(2)	97535	8(3)	99135	0(3)	99288	0(3)	99403	0(3)	99499	1(3)
95874	1(2)	96121	3(3)	96574	1(2)	97537	6(3)	99140	0(3)	99291	1(2)	99404	0(3)	99500	0(3)
95875	2(3)	96125	2(3)	96900	1(3)	97542	8(3)	99151	1(3)	99292	8(3)	99406	1(2)	99501	0(3)
95885	4(2)	96127	2(3)	96902	0(3)	97545	1(2)	99152	2(3)	99304	1(2)	99407	1(2)	99502	0(3)
95886	4(2)	96130	1(2)	96904	1(2)	97546	2(3)	99153	9(3)	99305	1(2)	99408	0(3)	99503	0(3)
95887	1(2)	96131	7(3)	96910	1(3)	97597	1(3)	99155	1(3)	99306	1(2)	99409	0(3)	99504	0(3)
95905	2(3)	96132	1(2)	96912	1(3)	97598	8(3)	99156	1(3)	99307	1(2)	99411	0(3)	99505	0(3)
95907	1(2)	96133	7(3)	96913	1(3)	97602	0(3)	99157	6(3)	99308	1(2)	99412	0(3)	99506	0(3)
95908	1(2)	96136	1(2)	96920	1(2)	97605	1(3)	99170	1(3)	99309	1(2)	99415	1(2)	99507	0(3)
95909	1(2)	96137	11(3)	96921	1(2)	97606	1(3)	99172	0(3)	99310	1(2)	99416	3(3)	99509	0(3)
95910	1(2)	96138	1(2)	96922	1(2)	97607	1(3)	99173	0(3)	99315	1(2)	99421	1(2)	99510	0(3)
95911	1(2)	96139	11(3)	96931	1(2)	97608	1(3)	99174	0(3)	99316	1(2)	99422	1(2)	99511	0(3)
95912	1(2)	96146	1(2)	96932	1(2)	97610	1(2)	99175	1(3)	99318	1(2)	99423	1(2)	99512	0(3)
95913	1(2)	96156	1(3)	96933	1(2)	97750	8(3)	99177	1(2)	99324	1(2)	99429	0(3)	99600	0(3)
95921	1(3)	96158	1(2)	96934	2(3)	97755	8(3)	99183	1(3)	99325	1(2)	99441	1(2)	99601	0(3)
95922	1(3)	96159	4(3)	96935	2(3)	97760	6(3)	99184	1(2)	99326	1(2)	99442	1(2)	99602	0(3)
95923	1(3)	96160	3(3)	96936	2(3)	97761	6(3)	99188	1(2)	99327	1(2)	99443	1(2)	99605	0(2)
95924	1(3)	96161	1(3)	96999	1(3)	97763	6(3)	99190	1(3)	99328	1(2)	99446	1(2)	99606	0(3)
95925	1(3)	96164	1(2)	97010	0(3)	97799	1(3)	99191	1(3)	99334	1(3)	99447	1(2)	99607	0(3)
95926	1(3)	96165	6(3)	97012	1(3)	97802	8(3)	99192	1(3)	99335	1(3)	99448	1(2)	A0021	0(3)
95927	1(3)	96167	1(2)	97014	0(3)	97803	8(3)	99195	2(3)	99336	1(3)	99449	1(2)	A0080	0(3)
95928	1(3)	96168	6(3)	97016	1(3)	97804	6(3)	99199	1(3)	99337	1(3)	99450	0(3)	A0090	0(3)
95929	1(3)	96170	1(3)	97018	1(3)	97810	1(2)	99201	1(2)	99339	0(3)	99451	1(2)	A0100	0(3)
95930	1(3)	96171	1(3)	97022	1(3)	97811	2(3)	99202	1(2)	99340	0(3)	99452	1(2)	A0110	0(3)
95933	1(3)	96360	1(3)	97024	1(3)	97813	1(2)	99203	1(2)	99341	1(2)	99453	1(2)	A0120	0(3)
95937	4(3)	96361	8(3)	97026	1(3)	97814	2(3)	99204	1(2)	99342	1(2)	99454	1(2)	A0130	0(3)
95938	1(3)	96365	1(3)	97028	1(3)	98925	1(2)	99205	1(2)	99343	1(2)	99455	1(3)	A0140	0(3)
95939	1(3)	96366	8(3)	97032	4(3)	98926	1(2)	99211	1(3)	99344	1(2)	99456	1(3)	A0160	0(3)
95940	32(3)	96367	4(3)	97033	4(3)	98927	1(2)	99212	2(3)	99345	1(2)	99457	1(2)	A0170	0(3)
95941	0(3)	96368	1(2)	97034	2(3)	98928	1(2)	99213	2(3)	99347	1(3)	99458	3(3)	A0180	0(3)
95943	1(3)	96369	1(2)	97035	2(3)	98929	1(2)	99214	2(3)	99348	1(3)	99460	1(2)	A0190	0(3)
95954	1(3)	96370	3(3)	97036	3(3)	98940	1(2)	99215	1(3)	99349	1(3)	99461	1(2)	A0200	0(3)
95955	1(3)	96371	1(3)	97039	1(3)	98941	1(2)	99217	1(2)	99350	1(3)	99462	1(2)	A0210	0(3)
95957	1(3)	96372	4(3)	97110	6(3)	98942	1(2)	99218	1(2)	99354	1(2)	99463	1(2)	A0225	0(3)
95958	1(3)	96373	2(3)	97112	4(3)	98943	0(3)	99219	1(2)	99355	4(3)	99464	1(2)	A0380	0(3)
95961	1(2)	96374	1(3)	97113	6(3)	98960	0(3)	99220	1(2)	99356	1(2)	99465	1(2)	A0382	0(3)
95962	5(3)	96375	6(3)	97116	4(3)	98961	0(3)	99221	1(3)	99357	4(3)	99466	1(2)	A0384	0(3)
95965	1(3)	96376	0(3)	97124	4(3)	98962	0(3)	99222	1(3)	99358	1(2)	99467	4(3)	A0390	0(3)
95966	1(3)	96377	1(3)	97129	1(2)	98966	1(2)	99223	1(3)	99359	2(3)	99468	1(2)	A0392	0(3)
95967	3(3)	96379	1(3)	97130	7(3)	98967	1(2)	99224	1(2)	99360	1(3)	99469	1(2)	A0394	0(3)
95970	1(3)	96401	3(3)	97139	1(3)	98968	1(2)	99225	1(2)	99366	0(3)	99471	1(2)	A0396	0(3)
95971	1(3)	96402	2(3)	97140	6(3)	98970	1(2)	99226	1(2)	99367	0(3)	99472	1(2)	A0398	0(3)
95972	1(3)	96405	1(2)	97150	1(3)	98971	1(2)	99231	1(3)	99368	0(3)	99473	1(2)	A0420	0(3)
95976	1(3)	96406	1(2)	97151	8(3)	98972	1(2)	99232	1(3)	99374	0(3)	99474	1(2)	A0422	0(3)
95977	1(3)	96409	1(3)	97152	8(3)	99000	0(3)	99233	1(3)	99375	0(3)	99475	1(2)	A0424	0(3)
95980	1(3)	96411	3(3)	97153	32(3)	99001	0(3)	99234	1(3)	99377	0(3)	99476	1(2)	A0425	250(1)

CPT	MUE
A0426	2(3)
A0427	2(3)
A0428	2(3)
A0429	2(3)
A0430	1(3)
A0431	1(3)
A0432	1(3)
A0433	1(3)
A0434	2(3)
A0435	999(3)
A0436	300(3)
A0888	0(3)
A0998	0(3)
A0999	1(3)
A4206	0(3)
A4207	0(3)
A4208	0(3)
A4209	0(3)
A4210	0(3)
A4211	0(3)
A4212	0(3)
A4213	0(3)
A4215	0(3)
A4216	0(3)
A4217	0(3)
A4218	0(3)
A4220	1(3)
A4221	0(3)
A4222	0(3)
A4223	0(3)
A4224	0(3)
A4225	0(3)
A4226	0(3)
A4230	0(3)
A4231	0(3)
A4232	0(3)
A4233	0(3)
A4234	0(3)
A4235	0(3)
A4236	0(3)
A4244	0(3)
A4245	0(3)
A4246	0(3)
A4247	0(3)
A4248	0(3)
A4250	0(3)
A4252	0(3)
A4253	0(3)
A4255	0(3)
A4256	0(3)
A4257	0(3)
A4258	0(3)
A4259	0(3)
A4261	0(3)
A4262	0(3)
A4263	0(3)
A4264	0(3)
A4265	0(3)
A4266	0(3)
A4267	0(3)
A4268	0(3)
A4269	0(3)
A4270	0(3)
A4280	0(3)
A4281	0(3)

CPT	MUE
A4282	0(3)
A4283	0(3)
A4284	0(3)
A4285	0(3)
A4286	0(3)
A4290	2(3)
A4300	0(3)
A4301	1(2)
A4305	0(3)
A4306	0(3)
A4310	0(3)
A4311	0(3)
A4312	0(3)
A4313	0(3)
A4314	0(3)
A4315	0(3)
A4316	0(3)
A4320	0(3)
A4321	1(3)
A4322	0(3)
A4326	0(3)
A4327	0(3)
A4328	0(3)
A4330	0(3)
A4331	1(3)
A4332	2(3)
A4333	1(3)
A4334	1(3)
A4335	0(3)
A4336	1(3)
A4337	0(3)
A4338	0(3)
A4340	0(3)
A4344	0(3)
A4346	0(3)
A4349	1(3)
A4351	0(3)
A4352	0(3)
A4353	1(3)
A4354	0(3)
A4355	0(3)
A4356	0(3)
A4357	0(3)
A4358	0(3)
A4360	1(3)
A4361	0(3)
A4362	0(3)
A4363	1(3)
A4364	0(3)
A4366	1(3)
A4367	0(3)
A4368	1(3)
A4369	1(3)
A4371	1(3)
A4372	1(3)
A4373	1(3)
A4375	2(3)
A4376	2(3)
A4377	2(3)
A4378	2(3)
A4379	2(3)
A4380	2(3)
A4381	2(3)
A4382	2(3)
A4383	2(3)

CPT	MUE
A4384	2(3)
A4385	2(3)
A4387	1(3)
A4388	1(3)
A4389	2(3)
A4390	1(3)
A4391	1(3)
A4392	2(3)
A4393	1(3)
A4394	1(3)
A4395	3(3)
A4396	2(3)
A4397	0(3)
A4398	0(3)
A4399	0(3)
A4400	0(3)
A4402	0(3)
A4404	0(3)
A4405	1(3)
A4406	1(3)
A4407	2(3)
A4408	1(3)
A4409	1(3)
A4410	2(3)
A4411	1(3)
A4412	1(3)
A4413	2(3)
A4414	1(3)
A4415	1(3)
A4416	2(3)
A4417	2(3)
A4418	2(3)
A4419	2(3)
A4420	1(3)
A4422	7(3)
A4423	2(3)
A4424	1(3)
A4425	1(3)
A4426	2(3)
A4427	1(3)
A4428	1(3)
A4429	2(3)
A4430	1(3)
A4431	1(3)
A4432	2(3)
A4433	1(3)
A4434	1(3)
A4435	2(3)
A4450	0(3)
A4452	0(3)
A4455	0(3)
A4458	0(3)
A4459	0(3)
A4461	2(3)
A4463	0(3)
A4465	0(3)
A4467	0(3)
A4470	0(3)
A4480	0(3)
A4481	0(3)
A4483	0(3)
A4490	0(3)
A4495	0(3)
A4500	0(3)
A4510	0(3)

CPT	MUE
A4520	0(3)
A4550	0(3)
A4553	0(3)
A4554	0(3)
A4555	0(3)
A4556	0(3)
A4557	0(3)
A4558	0(3)
A4559	0(3)
A4561	1(3)
A4562	1(3)
A4563	1(2)
A4565	2(3)
A4566	0(3)
A4570	0(3)
A4575	0(3)
A4580	0(3)
A4590	0(3)
A4595	0(3)
A4600	0(3)
A4601	0(3)
A4602	0(3)
A4604	0(3)
A4605	0(3)
A4606	0(3)
A4608	0(3)
A4611	0(3)
A4612	0(3)
A4613	0(3)
A4614	0(3)
A4615	0(3)
A4616	0(3)
A4617	0(3)
A4618	1(3)
A4619	0(3)
A4620	0(3)
A4623	0(3)
A4624	0(3)
A4625	30(3)
A4626	0(3)
A4627	0(3)
A4628	0(3)
A4629	0(3)
A4630	0(3)
A4633	0(3)
A4634	0(3)
A4635	0(3)
A4636	0(3)
A4637	0(3)
A4638	0(3)
A4639	0(3)
A4640	0(3)
A4642	1(3)
A4648	5(3)
A4649	1(3)
A4650	3(3)
A4651	0(3)
A4652	0(3)
A4653	0(3)
A4657	0(3)
A4660	0(3)
A4663	0(3)
A4670	0(3)
A4671	0(3)
A4672	0(3)

CPT	MUE
A4673	0(3)
A4674	0(3)
A4680	0(3)
A4690	0(3)
A4706	0(3)
A4707	0(3)
A4708	0(3)
A4709	0(3)
A4714	0(3)
A4719	0(3)
A4720	0(3)
A4721	0(3)
A4722	0(3)
A4723	0(3)
A4724	0(3)
A4725	0(3)
A4726	0(3)
A4728	0(3)
A4730	0(3)
A4736	0(3)
A4737	0(3)
A4740	0(3)
A4750	0(3)
A4755	0(3)
A4760	0(3)
A4765	0(3)
A4766	0(3)
A4770	0(3)
A4771	0(3)
A4772	0(3)
A4773	0(3)
A4774	0(3)
A4802	0(3)
A4860	0(3)
A4870	0(3)
A4890	0(3)
A4911	0(3)
A4913	0(3)
A4918	0(3)
A4927	0(3)
A4928	0(3)
A4929	0(3)
A4930	0(3)
A4931	0(3)
A4932	0(3)
A5051	0(3)
A5052	0(3)
A5053	0(3)
A5054	0(3)
A5055	0(3)
A5056	90(3)
A5057	90(3)
A5061	0(3)
A5062	0(3)
A5063	0(3)
A5071	0(3)
A5072	0(3)
A5073	0(3)
A5081	0(3)
A5082	0(3)
A5083	5(3)
A5093	0(3)
A5102	0(3)
A5105	0(3)
A5112	0(3)

CPT	MUE
A5113	0(3)
A5114	0(3)
A5120	150(3)
A5121	0(3)
A5122	0(3)
A5126	0(3)
A5131	0(3)
A5200	2(3)
A5500	0(3)
A5501	0(3)
A5503	0(3)
A5504	0(3)
A5505	0(3)
A5506	0(3)
A5507	0(3)
A5508	0(3)
A5510	0(3)
A5512	0(3)
A5513	0(3)
A5514	0(3)
A6000	0(3)
A6010	0(3)
A6011	0(3)
A6021	0(3)
A6022	0(3)
A6023	0(3)
A6024	0(3)
A6025	0(3)
A6154	0(3)
A6196	0(3)
A6197	0(3)
A6198	0(3)
A6199	0(3)
A6203	0(3)
A6204	0(3)
A6205	0(3)
A6206	0(3)
A6207	0(3)
A6208	0(3)
A6209	0(3)
A6210	0(3)
A6211	0(3)
A6212	0(3)
A6213	0(3)
A6214	0(3)
A6215	0(3)
A6216	0(3)
A6217	0(3)
A6218	0(3)
A6219	0(3)
A6220	0(3)
A6221	0(3)
A6222	0(3)
A6223	0(3)
A6224	0(3)
A6228	0(3)
A6229	0(3)
A6230	0(3)
A6231	0(3)
A6232	0(3)
A6233	0(3)
A6234	0(3)
A6235	0(3)
A6236	0(3)
A6237	0(3)

CPT	MUE
A6238	0(3)
A6239	0(3)
A6240	0(3)
A6241	0(3)
A6242	0(3)
A6243	0(3)
A6244	0(3)
A6245	0(3)
A6246	0(3)
A6247	0(3)
A6248	0(3)
A6250	0(3)
A6251	0(3)
A6252	0(3)
A6253	0(3)
A6254	0(3)
A6255	0(3)
A6256	0(3)
A6257	0(3)
A6258	0(3)
A6259	0(3)
A6260	0(3)
A6261	0(3)
A6262	0(3)
A6266	0(3)
A6402	0(3)
A6403	0(3)
A6404	0(3)
A6407	0(3)
A6410	2(3)
A6411	0(3)
A6412	0(3)
A6413	0(3)
A6441	0(3)
A6442	0(3)
A6443	0(3)
A6444	0(3)
A6445	0(3)
A6446	0(3)
A6447	0(3)
A6448	0(3)
A6449	0(3)
A6450	0(3)
A6451	0(3)
A6452	0(3)
A6453	0(3)
A6454	0(3)
A6455	0(3)
A6456	0(3)
A6457	0(3)
A6460	1(1)
A6461	1(1)
A6501	0(3)
A6502	0(3)
A6503	0(3)
A6504	0(3)
A6505	0(3)
A6506	0(3)
A6507	0(3)
A6508	0(3)
A6509	0(3)
A6510	0(3)
A6511	0(3)
A6513	0(3)
A6530	0(3)

CPT	MUE
A6531	0(3)
A6532	0(3)
A6533	0(3)
A6534	0(3)
A6535	0(3)
A6536	0(3)
A6537	0(3)
A6538	0(3)
A6539	0(3)
A6540	0(3)
A6541	0(3)
A6544	0(3)
A6545	0(3)
A6549	0(3)
A6550	0(3)
A7000	0(3)
A7001	0(3)
A7002	0(3)
A7003	0(3)
A7004	0(3)
A7005	0(3)
A7006	0(3)
A7007	0(3)
A7008	0(3)
A7009	0(3)
A7010	0(3)
A7012	0(3)
A7013	0(3)
A7014	0(3)
A7015	0(3)
A7016	0(3)
A7017	0(3)
A7018	0(3)
A7020	0(3)
A7025	0(3)
A7026	0(3)
A7027	0(3)
A7028	0(3)
A7029	0(3)
A7030	0(3)
A7031	0(3)
A7032	0(3)
A7033	0(3)
A7034	0(3)
A7035	0(3)
A7036	0(3)
A7037	0(3)
A7038	0(3)
A7039	0(3)
A7040	2(3)
A7041	2(3)
A7044	0(3)
A7045	0(3)
A7046	0(3)
A7047	0(3)
A7048	2(3)
A7501	0(3)
A7502	0(3)
A7503	0(3)
A7504	0(3)
A7505	0(3)
A7506	0(3)
A7507	0(3)
A7508	0(3)
A7509	0(3)

CPT	MUE
A7520	0(3)
A7521	0(3)
A7522	0(3)
A7523	0(3)
A7524	0(3)
A7525	0(3)
A7526	0(3)
A7527	0(3)
A8000	0(3)
A8001	0(3)
A8002	0(3)
A8003	0(3)
A8004	0(3)
A9152	0(3)
A9153	0(3)
A9155	1(3)
A9180	0(3)
A9270	0(3)
A9272	0(3)
A9273	0(3)
A9274	0(3)
A9275	0(3)
A9276	0(3)
A9277	0(3)
A9278	0(3)
A9279	0(3)
A9280	0(3)
A9281	0(3)
A9282	0(3)
A9283	0(3)
A9284	0(3)
A9285	0(3)
A9286	0(3)
A9300	0(3)
A9500	3(3)
A9501	1(3)
A9502	3(3)
A9503	1(3)
A9504	1(3)
A9505	4(3)
A9507	1(3)
A9508	2(3)
A9509	5(3)
A9510	1(3)
A9512	30(3)
A9513	200(3)
A9515	1(3)
A9516	4(3)
A9517	200(3)
A9520	1(3)
A9521	2(3)
A9524	10(3)
A9526	2(3)
A9527	195(3)
A9528	10(3)
A9529	10(3)
A9530	200(3)
A9531	100(3)
A9532	10(3)
A9536	1(3)
A9537	1(3)
A9538	1(3)
A9539	2(3)
A9540	2(3)
A9541	1(3)

CPT	MUE
A9542	1(3)
A9543	1(3)
A9546	1(3)
A9547	2(3)
A9548	2(3)
A9550	1(3)
A9551	1(3)
A9552	1(3)
A9553	1(3)
A9554	1(3)
A9555	2(3)
A9556	10(3)
A9557	2(3)
A9558	7(3)
A9559	1(3)
A9560	2(3)
A9561	1(3)
A9562	2(3)
A9563	10(3)
A9564	20(3)
A9566	1(3)
A9567	2(3)
A9568	0(3)
A9569	1(3)
A9570	1(3)
A9571	1(3)
A9572	1(3)
A9575	300(3)
A9576	40(3)
A9577	50(3)
A9578	50(3)
A9579	100(3)
A9580	1(3)
A9581	20(3)
A9582	1(3)
A9583	18(3)
A9584	1(3)
A9585	300(3)
A9586	1(3)
A9587	54(3)
A9588	10(3)
A9589	1(3)
A9590	675(3)
A9600	7(3)
A9604	1(3)
A9606	224(3)
A9698	2(3)
A9700	2(3)
A9900	1(3)
A9901	0(3)
A9999	1(3)
B4034	0(3)
B4035	0(3)
B4036	0(3)
B4081	0(3)
B4082	0(3)
B4083	0(3)
B4087	0(3)
B4088	0(3)
B4100	0(3)
B4102	0(3)
B4103	0(3)
B4104	0(3)
B4149	0(3)
B4150	0(3)

CPT	MUE
B4152	0(3)
B4153	0(3)
B4154	0(3)
B4155	0(3)
B4157	0(3)
B4158	0(3)
B4159	0(3)
B4160	0(3)
B4161	0(3)
B4162	0(3)
B4164	0(3)
B4168	0(3)
B4172	0(3)
B4176	0(3)
B4178	0(3)
B4180	0(3)
B4185	0(3)
B4189	0(3)
B4193	0(3)
B4197	0(3)
B4199	0(3)
B4216	0(3)
B4220	0(3)
B4222	0(3)
B4224	0(3)
B5000	0(3)
B5100	0(3)
B5200	0(3)
B9002	0(3)
B9004	0(3)
B9006	0(3)
B9998	0(3)
B9999	0(3)
C1713	20(3)
C1714	4(3)
C1715	45(3)
C1716	4(3)
C1717	10(3)
C1719	99(3)
C1721	1(3)
C1722	1(3)
C1724	5(3)
C1725	9(3)
C1726	5(3)
C1727	4(3)
C1728	5(3)
C1729	6(3)
C1730	4(3)
C1731	2(3)
C1732	3(3)
C1733	3(3)
C1734	2(3)
C1749	1(3)
C1750	2(3)
C1751	3(3)
C1752	2(3)
C1753	2(3)
C1754	2(3)
C1755	2(3)
C1756	2(3)
C1757	6(3)
C1758	2(3)
C1759	2(3)
C1760	4(3)
C1762	4(3)

CPT	MUE
C1763	4(3)
C1764	1(3)
C1765	4(3)
C1766	4(3)
C1767	2(3)
C1768	3(3)
C1769	9(3)
C1770	3(3)
C1771	1(3)
C1772	1(3)
C1773	3(3)
C1776	10(3)
C1777	2(3)
C1778	4(3)
C1779	2(3)
C1780	2(3)
C1781	4(3)
C1782	1(3)
C1783	2(3)
C1784	2(3)
C1785	1(3)
C1786	1(3)
C1787	2(3)
C1788	2(3)
C1789	2(3)
C1813	1(3)
C1814	2(3)
C1815	1(3)
C1816	2(3)
C1817	1(3)
C1818	2(3)
C1819	4(3)
C1820	2(3)
C1821	4(3)
C1822	1(3)
C1823	1(3)
C1824	1(2)
C1830	2(3)
C1839	2(2)
C1840	1(3)
C1841	1(2)
C1842	1(2)
C1874	5(3)
C1875	4(3)
C1876	5(3)
C1877	5(3)
C1878	2(3)
C1880	2(3)
C1881	2(3)
C1882	1(3)
C1883	4(3)
C1884	4(3)
C1885	2(3)
C1886	1(3)
C1887	7(3)
C1888	2(3)
C1889	1(3)
C1890	1(3)
C1891	1(3)
C1892	6(3)
C1893	6(3)
C1894	6(3)
C1895	2(3)
C1896	2(3)
C1897	2(3)

CPT	MUE
C1898	2(3)
C1899	2(3)
C1900	1(3)
C1982	1(3)
C2596	1(3)
C2613	2(3)
C2614	3(3)
C2615	2(3)
C2616	1(3)
C2617	4(3)
C2618	4(3)
C2619	1(3)
C2620	1(3)
C2621	1(3)
C2622	1(3)
C2623	2(3)
C2624	1(3)
C2625	4(3)
C2626	1(3)
C2627	2(3)
C2628	4(3)
C2629	4(3)
C2630	3(3)
C2631	1(3)
C2634	24(3)
C2635	124(3)
C2636	690(3)
C2637	0(3)
C2638	150(3)
C2639	150(3)
C2640	150(3)
C2641	150(3)
C2642	120(3)
C2643	120(3)
C2644	500(1)
C2645	4608(3)
C5271	1(2)
C5272	3(2)
C5273	1(2)
C5274	35(3)
C5275	1(2)
C5276	3(2)
C5277	1(2)
C5278	15(3)
C8900	1(3)
C8901	1(3)
C8902	1(3)
C8903	1(3)
C8905	1(3)
C8906	1(3)
C8908	1(3)
C8909	1(3)
C8910	1(3)
C8911	1(3)
C8912	1(3)
C8913	1(3)
C8914	1(3)
C8918	1(3)
C8919	1(3)
C8920	1(3)
C8921	1(3)
C8922	1(3)
C8923	1(3)
C8924	1(3)
C8925	1(3)

CPT	MUE
C8926	1(3)
C8927	1(3)
C8928	1(2)
C8929	1(3)
C8930	1(2)
C8931	1(3)
C8932	1(3)
C8933	1(3)
C8934	2(3)
C8935	2(3)
C8936	2(3)
C8937	2(2)
C8957	2(3)
C9046	160(3)
C9047	22(3)
C9055	400(3)
C9113	10(3)
C9132	5500(3)
C9248	25(3)
C9250	1(3)
C9254	400(3)
C9257	5(3)
C9285	2(3)
C9290	266(3)
C9293	700(3)
C9352	3(3)
C9353	4(3)
C9354	300(3)
C9355	3(3)
C9356	125(3)
C9358	800(3)
C9359	30(3)
C9360	300(3)
C9361	10(3)
C9362	60(3)
C9363	500(3)
C9364	600(3)
C9460	1(3)
C9462	600(3)
C9482	150(3)
C9488	20(3)
C9600	3(3)
C9601	2(3)
C9602	2(3)
C9603	2(3)
C9604	2(3)
C9605	2(3)
C9606	1(3)
C9607	1(2)
C9608	2(3)
C9725	1(3)
C9726	2(3)
C9727	1(2)
C9728	1(2)
C9733	1(3)
C9734	1(3)
C9738	1(3)
C9739	1(2)
C9740	1(2)
C9745	2(2)
C9747	1(2)
C9749	1(2)
C9751	1(3)
C9752	1(2)
C9753	3(3)

CPT	MUE
C9756	1(3)
C9757	2(2)
C9758	1(2)
C9803	2(3)
D0150	1(3)
D0240	1(3)
D0250	2(3)
D0270	1(3)
D0272	1(3)
D0274	1(3)
D0277	1(3)
D0412	0(3)
D0416	1(3)
D0431	1(3)
D0460	1(2)
D0484	1(2)
D0485	1(2)
D0601	1(2)
D0602	1(2)
D0603	1(2)
D1510	2(2)
D1516	1(2)
D1517	1(2)
D1520	2(2)
D1526	1(2)
D1527	1(2)
D1551	1(2)
D1552	1(2)
D1553	2(2)
D1575	4(2)
D4260	4(2)
D4263	4(2)
D4264	3(3)
D4270	4(3)
D4273	1(2)
D4277	1(2)
D4278	3(3)
D4355	1(2)
D4381	12(3)
D5282	0(3)
D5283	0(3)
D5876	0(3)
D5911	1(3)
D5912	1(2)
D5983	1(3)
D5984	1(3)
D5985	1(3)
D7111	20(3)
D7140	32(2)
D7210	32(2)
D7220	6(3)
D7230	6(3)
D7240	6(3)
D7241	6(3)
D7250	32(2)
D7260	1(3)
D7261	1(3)
D7283	4(3)
D7288	2(3)
D7321	4(2)
D9110	1(3)
D9130	0(3)
D9230	1(3)
D9248	1(3)
D9613	0(3)

CPT	MUE
D9930	1(2)
D9944	0(3)
D9945	0(3)
D9946	0(3)
D9950	1(3)
D9951	1(3)
D9952	1(3)
D9961	0(3)
D9990	0(3)
E0100	0(3)
E0105	0(3)
E0110	0(3)
E0111	0(3)
E0112	0(3)
E0113	0(3)
E0114	0(3)
E0116	0(3)
E0117	0(3)
E0118	0(3)
E0130	0(3)
E0135	0(3)
E0140	0(3)
E0141	0(3)
E0143	0(3)
E0144	0(3)
E0147	0(3)
E0148	0(3)
E0149	0(3)
E0153	0(3)
E0154	0(3)
E0155	0(3)
E0156	0(3)
E0157	0(3)
E0158	0(3)
E0159	2(2)
E0160	0(3)
E0161	0(3)
E0162	0(3)
E0163	0(3)
E0165	0(3)
E0167	0(3)
E0168	0(3)
E0170	0(3)
E0171	0(3)
E0172	0(3)
E0175	0(3)
E0181	0(3)
E0182	0(3)
E0184	0(3)
E0185	0(3)
E0186	0(3)
E0187	0(3)
E0188	0(3)
E0189	0(3)
E0190	0(3)
E0191	0(3)
E0193	0(3)
E0194	0(3)
E0196	0(3)
E0197	0(3)
E0198	0(3)
E0199	0(3)
E0200	0(3)
E0202	0(3)
E0203	0(3)

CPT	MUE
E0205	0(3)
E0210	0(3)
E0215	0(3)
E0217	0(3)
E0218	0(3)
E0221	0(3)
E0225	0(3)
E0231	0(3)
E0232	0(3)
E0235	0(3)
E0236	0(3)
E0239	0(3)
E0240	0(3)
E0241	0(3)
E0242	0(3)
E0243	0(3)
E0244	0(3)
E0245	0(3)
E0246	0(3)
E0247	0(3)
E0248	0(3)
E0249	0(3)
E0250	0(3)
E0251	0(3)
E0255	0(3)
E0256	0(3)
E0260	0(3)
E0261	0(3)
E0265	0(3)
E0266	0(3)
E0270	0(3)
E0271	0(3)
E0272	0(3)
E0273	0(3)
E0274	0(3)
E0275	0(3)
E0276	0(3)
E0277	0(3)
E0280	0(3)
E0290	0(3)
E0291	0(3)
E0292	0(3)
E0293	0(3)
E0294	0(3)
E0295	0(3)
E0296	0(3)
E0297	0(3)
E0300	0(3)
E0301	0(3)
E0302	0(3)
E0303	0(3)
E0304	0(3)
E0305	0(3)
E0310	0(3)
E0315	0(3)
E0316	0(3)
E0325	0(3)
E0326	0(3)
E0328	0(3)
E0329	0(3)
E0350	0(3)
E0352	0(3)
E0370	0(3)
E0371	0(3)
E0372	0(3)

CPT	MUE
E0373	0(3)
E0424	0(3)
E0425	0(3)
E0430	0(3)
E0431	0(3)
E0433	0(3)
E0434	0(3)
E0435	0(3)
E0439	0(3)
E0440	0(3)
E0441	0(3)
E0442	0(3)
E0443	0(3)
E0444	0(3)
E0445	0(3)
E0446	0(3)
E0447	0(3)
E0455	0(3)
E0457	0(3)
E0459	0(3)
E0462	0(3)
E0465	0(3)
E0466	0(3)
E0467	0(3)
E0470	0(3)
E0471	0(3)
E0472	0(3)
E0480	0(3)
E0481	0(3)
E0482	0(3)
E0483	0(3)
E0484	0(3)
E0485	0(3)
E0486	0(3)
E0487	0(3)
E0500	0(3)
E0550	0(3)
E0555	0(3)
E0560	0(3)
E0561	0(3)
E0562	0(3)
E0565	0(3)
E0570	0(3)
E0572	0(3)
E0574	0(3)
E0575	0(3)
E0580	0(3)
E0585	0(3)
E0600	0(3)
E0601	0(3)
E0602	0(3)
E0603	0(3)
E0604	0(3)
E0605	0(3)
E0606	0(3)
E0607	0(3)
E0610	0(3)
E0615	0(3)
E0616	1(2)
E0617	0(3)
E0618	0(3)
E0619	0(3)
E0620	0(3)
E0621	0(3)
E0625	0(3)

CPT	MUE
E0627	0(3)
E0629	0(3)
E0630	0(3)
E0635	0(3)
E0636	0(3)
E0637	0(3)
E0638	0(3)
E0639	0(3)
E0640	0(3)
E0641	0(3)
E0642	0(3)
E0650	0(3)
E0651	0(3)
E0652	0(3)
E0655	0(3)
E0656	0(3)
E0657	0(3)
E0660	0(3)
E0665	0(3)
E0666	0(3)
E0667	0(3)
E0668	0(3)
E0669	0(3)
E0670	0(3)
E0671	0(3)
E0672	0(3)
E0673	0(3)
E0675	0(3)
E0676	1(3)
E0691	0(3)
E0692	0(3)
E0693	0(3)
E0694	0(3)
E0700	0(3)
E0705	0(3)
E0710	0(3)
E0720	0(3)
E0730	0(3)
E0731	0(3)
E0740	0(3)
E0744	0(3)
E0745	0(3)
E0746	1(3)
E0747	0(3)
E0748	0(3)
E0749	1(3)
E0755	0(3)
E0760	0(3)
E0761	0(3)
E0762	0(3)
E0764	0(3)
E0765	0(3)
E0766	0(3)
E0769	0(3)
E0770	1(3)
E0776	0(3)
E0779	0(3)
E0780	0(3)
E0781	1(2)
E0782	1(2)
E0783	1(2)
E0784	0(3)
E0785	1(2)
E0786	1(2)
E0787	0(3)

CPT	MUE
E0791	0(3)
E0830	0(3)
E0840	0(3)
E0849	0(3)
E0850	0(3)
E0855	0(3)
E0856	0(3)
E0860	0(3)
E0870	0(3)
E0880	0(3)
E0890	0(3)
E0900	0(3)
E0910	0(3)
E0911	0(3)
E0912	0(3)
E0920	0(3)
E0930	0(3)
E0935	0(3)
E0936	0(3)
E0940	0(3)
E0941	0(3)
E0942	0(3)
E0944	0(3)
E0945	0(3)
E0946	0(3)
E0947	0(3)
E0948	0(3)
E0950	0(3)
E0951	0(3)
E0952	0(3)
E0953	0(3)
E0954	0(3)
E0955	0(3)
E0956	0(3)
E0957	0(3)
E0958	0(3)
E0959	0(3)
E0960	0(3)
E0961	0(3)
E0966	0(3)
E0967	0(3)
E0968	0(3)
E0969	0(3)
E0970	0(3)
E0971	0(3)
E0973	0(3)
E0974	0(3)
E0978	0(3)
E0980	0(3)
E0981	0(3)
E0982	0(3)
E0983	0(3)
E0984	0(3)
E0985	0(3)
E0986	0(3)
E0988	0(3)
E0990	0(3)
E0992	0(3)
E0994	0(3)
E0995	0(3)
E1002	0(3)
E1003	0(3)
E1004	0(3)
E1005	0(3)
E1006	0(3)

CPT	MUE
E1007	0(3)
E1008	0(3)
E1009	0(3)
E1010	0(3)
E1011	0(3)
E1012	0(3)
E1014	0(3)
E1015	0(3)
E1016	0(3)
E1017	0(3)
E1018	0(3)
E1020	0(3)
E1028	0(3)
E1029	0(3)
E1030	0(3)
E1031	0(3)
E1035	0(3)
E1036	0(3)
E1037	0(3)
E1038	0(3)
E1039	0(3)
E1050	0(3)
E1060	0(3)
E1070	0(3)
E1083	0(3)
E1084	0(3)
E1085	0(3)
E1086	0(3)
E1087	0(3)
E1088	0(3)
E1089	0(3)
E1090	0(3)
E1092	0(3)
E1093	0(3)
E1100	0(3)
E1110	0(3)
E1130	0(3)
E1140	0(3)
E1150	0(3)
E1160	0(3)
E1161	0(3)
E1170	0(3)
E1171	0(3)
E1172	0(3)
E1180	0(3)
E1190	0(3)
E1195	0(3)
E1200	0(3)
E1220	0(3)
E1221	0(3)
E1222	0(3)
E1223	0(3)
E1224	0(3)
E1225	0(3)
E1226	0(3)
E1227	0(3)
E1228	0(3)
E1229	0(3)
E1230	0(3)
E1231	0(3)
E1232	0(3)
E1233	0(3)
E1234	0(3)
E1235	0(3)
E1236	0(3)

CPT	MUE
E1237	0(3)
E1238	0(3)
E1239	0(3)
E1240	0(3)
E1250	0(3)
E1260	0(3)
E1270	0(3)
E1280	0(3)
E1285	0(3)
E1290	0(3)
E1295	0(3)
E1296	0(3)
E1297	0(3)
E1298	0(3)
E1300	0(3)
E1310	0(3)
E1352	0(3)
E1353	0(3)
E1354	0(3)
E1355	0(3)
E1356	0(3)
E1357	0(3)
E1358	0(3)
E1372	0(3)
E1390	0(3)
E1391	0(3)
E1392	0(3)
E1399	1(3)
E1405	0(3)
E1406	0(3)
E1500	0(3)
E1510	0(3)
E1520	0(3)
E1530	0(3)
E1540	0(3)
E1550	0(3)
E1560	0(3)
E1570	0(3)
E1575	0(3)
E1580	0(3)
E1590	0(3)
E1592	0(3)
E1594	0(3)
E1600	0(3)
E1610	0(3)
E1615	0(3)
E1620	0(3)
E1625	0(3)
E1630	0(3)
E1632	0(3)
E1634	0(3)
E1635	0(3)
E1636	0(3)
E1637	0(3)
E1639	0(3)
E1699	0(3)
E1700	0(3)
E1701	0(3)
E1702	0(3)
E1800	0(3)
E1801	0(3)
E1802	0(3)
E1805	0(3)
E1806	0(3)
E1810	0(3)

CPT	MUE
E1811	0(3)
E1812	0(3)
E1815	0(3)
E1816	0(3)
E1818	0(3)
E1820	0(3)
E1821	0(3)
E1825	0(3)
E1830	0(3)
E1831	0(3)
E1840	0(3)
E1841	0(3)
E1902	0(3)
E2000	0(3)
E2100	0(3)
E2101	0(3)
E2120	0(3)
E2201	0(3)
E2202	0(3)
E2203	0(3)
E2204	0(3)
E2205	0(3)
E2206	0(3)
E2207	0(3)
E2208	0(3)
E2209	0(3)
E2210	0(3)
E2211	0(3)
E2212	0(3)
E2213	0(3)
E2214	0(3)
E2215	0(3)
E2216	0(3)
E2217	0(3)
E2218	0(3)
E2219	0(3)
E2220	0(3)
E2221	0(3)
E2222	0(3)
E2224	0(3)
E2225	0(3)
E2226	0(3)
E2227	0(3)
E2228	0(3)
E2230	0(3)
E2231	0(3)
E2291	1(2)
E2292	1(2)
E2293	1(2)
E2294	1(2)
E2295	0(3)
E2300	0(3)
E2301	0(3)
E2310	0(3)
E2311	0(3)
E2312	0(3)
E2313	0(3)
E2321	0(3)
E2322	0(3)
E2323	0(3)
E2324	0(3)
E2325	0(3)
E2326	0(3)
E2327	0(3)
E2328	0(3)

CPT	MUE
E2329	0(3)
E2330	0(3)
E2331	0(3)
E2340	0(3)
E2341	0(3)
E2342	0(3)
E2343	0(3)
E2351	0(3)
E2358	0(3)
E2359	0(3)
E2360	0(3)
E2361	0(3)
E2362	0(3)
E2363	0(3)
E2364	0(3)
E2365	0(3)
E2366	0(3)
E2367	0(3)
E2368	0(3)
E2369	0(3)
E2370	0(3)
E2371	0(3)
E2372	0(3)
E2373	0(3)
E2374	0(3)
E2375	0(3)
E2376	0(3)
E2377	0(3)
E2378	0(3)
E2381	0(3)
E2382	0(3)
E2383	0(3)
E2384	0(3)
E2385	0(3)
E2386	0(3)
E2387	0(3)
E2388	0(3)
E2389	0(3)
E2390	0(3)
E2391	0(3)
E2392	0(3)
E2394	0(3)
E2395	0(3)
E2396	0(3)
E2397	0(3)
E2398	0(3)
E2402	0(3)
E2500	0(3)
E2502	0(3)
E2504	0(3)
E2506	0(3)
E2508	0(3)
E2510	0(3)
E2511	0(3)
E2512	0(3)
E2599	0(3)
E2601	0(3)
E2602	0(3)
E2603	0(3)
E2604	0(3)
E2605	0(3)
E2606	0(3)
E2607	0(3)
E2608	0(3)
E2609	0(3)

CPT	MUE
E2610	0(3)
E2611	0(3)
E2612	0(3)
E2613	0(3)
E2614	0(3)
E2615	0(3)
E2616	0(3)
E2617	0(3)
E2619	0(3)
E2620	0(3)
E2621	0(3)
E2622	0(3)
E2623	0(3)
E2624	0(3)
E2625	0(3)
E2626	0(3)
E2627	0(3)
E2628	0(3)
E2629	0(3)
E2630	0(3)
E2631	0(3)
E2632	0(3)
E2633	0(3)
E8000	0(3)
E8001	0(3)
E8002	0(3)
G0008	1(2)
G0009	1(2)
G0010	1(3)
G0027	1(2)
G0068	16(3)
G0069	16(3)
G0070	16(3)
G0071	1(3)
G0076	1(3)
G0077	1(3)
G0078	1(3)
G0079	1(3)
G0080	1(3)
G0081	1(3)
G0082	1(3)
G0083	1(3)
G0084	1(3)
G0085	1(3)
G0086	1(3)
G0087	1(3)
G0101	1(2)
G0102	1(2)
G0103	1(2)
G0104	1(2)
G0105	1(2)
G0106	1(2)
G0108	6(3)
G0109	12(3)
G0117	1(2)
G0118	1(2)
G0120	1(2)
G0121	1(2)
G0122	0(3)
G0123	1(3)
G0124	1(3)
G0127	1(2)
G0128	1(3)
G0130	1(2)
G0141	1(3)

CPT	MUE
G0143	1(3)
G0144	1(3)
G0145	1(3)
G0147	1(3)
G0148	1(3)
G0166	2(3)
G0168	2(3)
G0175	1(3)
G0177	0(3)
G0179	1(2)
G0180	1(2)
G0181	1(2)
G0182	1(2)
G0186	1(2)
G0219	0(3)
G0235	1(3)
G0237	8(3)
G0238	8(3)
G0239	1(3)
G0245	1(2)
G0246	1(2)
G0247	1(2)
G0248	1(2)
G0249	3(3)
G0250	1(2)
G0252	0(3)
G0255	0(3)
G0257	0(3)
G0259	2(3)
G0260	2(3)
G0268	1(2)
G0269	0(3)
G0270	8(3)
G0271	4(3)
G0276	1(3)
G0277	5(3)
G0278	1(2)
G0279	1(2)
G0281	1(3)
G0282	0(3)
G0283	1(3)
G0288	1(2)
G0289	1(2)
G0293	1(2)
G0294	1(2)
G0295	0(3)
G0296	1(2)
G0297	1(2)
G0302	1(2)
G0303	1(2)
G0304	1(2)
G0305	1(2)
G0306	1(3)
G0307	1(3)
G0328	1(2)
G0329	1(3)
G0333	0(3)
G0337	1(2)
G0339	1(2)
G0340	1(3)
G0341	1(2)
G0342	1(2)
G0343	1(2)
G0372	1(2)
G0378	0(3)

CPT	MUE
G0379	0(3)
G0380	0(3)
G0381	0(3)
G0382	0(3)
G0383	0(3)
G0384	0(3)
G0390	0(3)
G0396	1(2)
G0397	1(2)
G0398	1(2)
G0399	1(2)
G0400	1(2)
G0402	1(2)
G0403	1(2)
G0404	1(2)
G0405	1(2)
G0406	1(3)
G0407	1(3)
G0408	1(3)
G0410	4(3)
G0411	4(3)
G0412	1(2)
G0413	1(2)
G0414	1(2)
G0415	1(2)
G0416	1(2)
G0420	2(3)
G0421	2(3)
G0422	6(2)
G0423	6(2)
G0424	2(2)
G0425	1(3)
G0426	1(3)
G0427	1(3)
G0428	0(3)
G0429	1(2)
G0432	1(2)
G0433	1(2)
G0435	1(2)
G0438	1(2)
G0439	1(2)
G0442	1(2)
G0443	1(2)
G0444	1(2)
G0445	1(2)
G0446	1(3)
G0447	4(3)
G0448	1(3)
G0451	1(3)
G0452	6(3)
G0453	40(3)
G0454	1(2)
G0455	1(2)
G0458	1(3)
G0459	1(3)
G0460	1(3)
G0463	0(3)
G0466	1(2)
G0467	1(3)
G0468	1(2)
G0469	1(2)
G0470	1(3)
G0471	2(3)
G0472	1(2)
G0473	1(3)

CPT	MUE
G0475	1(2)
G0476	1(2)
G0480	1(2)
G0481	1(2)
G0482	1(2)
G0483	1(2)
G0490	1(3)
G0491	1(3)
G0492	1(3)
G0493	1(3)
G0494	1(3)
G0495	1(3)
G0496	1(3)
G0498	1(2)
G0499	1(2)
G0500	1(3)
G0501	0(3)
G0506	1(2)
G0508	1(2)
G0509	1(2)
G0511	1(2)
G0512	1(2)
G0513	1(2)
G0514	1(1)
G0516	1(2)
G0517	1(2)
G0518	1(2)
G0659	1(2)
G2000	1(3)
G2001	1(3)
G2002	1(3)
G2003	1(3)
G2004	1(3)
G2005	1(3)
G2006	1(3)
G2007	1(3)
G2008	1(3)
G2009	1(3)
G2010	1(3)
G2011	1(2)
G2012	1(3)
G2013	1(3)
G2014	1(3)
G2015	1(3)
G2023	2(3)
G2024	2(3)
G2058	2(3)
G2061	1(2)
G2062	1(2)
G2063	1(2)
G2064	1(2)
G2065	1(2)
G2066	1(2)
G2067	1(2)
G2068	1(2)
G2069	1(2)
G2070	1(2)
G2071	1(2)
G2072	1(2)
G2073	1(2)
G2074	1(2)
G2075	1(2)
G2076	1(2)
G2078	3(3)
G2079	3(3)

CPT	MUE
G2081	1(2)
G2082	1(2)
G2083	1(2)
G2086	1(3)
G2087	2(3)
G6001	2(3)
G6002	2(3)
G6003	2(3)
G6004	2(3)
G6005	2(3)
G6006	2(3)
G6007	2(3)
G6008	2(3)
G6009	2(3)
G6010	2(3)
G6011	2(3)
G6012	2(3)
G6013	2(3)
G6014	2(3)
G6015	2(3)
G6016	2(3)
G6017	2(3)
G9143	1(2)
G9147	0(3)
G9148	1(3)
G9149	1(3)
G9150	1(3)
G9151	1(3)
G9152	1(3)
G9153	1(3)
G9156	1(2)
G9157	1(2)
G9187	1(3)
G9480	1(3)
G9481	1(3)
G9482	1(3)
G9483	1(3)
G9484	1(3)
G9485	1(3)
G9486	1(3)
G9487	1(3)
G9488	1(3)
G9489	1(3)
G9490	1(3)
G9678	1(2)
G9685	1(3)
G9978	1(3)
G9979	1(3)
G9980	1(3)
G9981	1(3)
G9982	1(3)
G9983	1(3)
G9984	1(3)
G9985	1(3)
G9986	1(3)
G9987	1(3)
J0120	1(3)
J0121	200(3)
J0122	300(3)
J0129	100(3)
J0130	4(3)
J0131	400(3)
J0132	12(3)
J0133	1200(3)
J0135	8(3)

CPT	MUE
J0153	180(3)
J0171	20(3)
J0178	4(2)
J0179	12(2)
J0180	140(3)
J0185	130(3)
J0190	0(3)
J0200	0(3)
J0202	12(3)
J0205	0(3)
J0207	4(3)
J0210	4(3)
J0215	30(3)
J0220	1(3)
J0221	250(3)
J0222	300(3)
J0223	756(3)
J0256	1600(3)
J0257	1400(3)
J0270	32(3)
J0275	1(3)
J0278	15(3)
J0280	7(3)
J0282	5(3)
J0285	5(3)
J0287	50(3)
J0288	0(3)
J0289	50(3)
J0290	24(3)
J0291	500(3)
J0295	12(3)
J0300	8(3)
J0330	10(3)
J0348	200(3)
J0350	0(3)
J0360	2(3)
J0364	6(3)
J0365	0(3)
J0380	1(3)
J0390	0(3)
J0395	0(3)
J0400	39(3)
J0401	400(3)
J0456	4(3)
J0461	200(3)
J0470	2(3)
J0475	8(3)
J0476	2(3)
J0480	1(3)
J0485	1500(3)
J0490	160(3)
J0500	4(3)
J0515	3(3)
J0517	30(3)
J0520	0(3)
J0558	24(3)
J0561	24(3)
J0565	200(3)
J0567	300(3)
J0570	4(3)
J0571	0(3)
J0572	0(3)
J0573	0(3)
J0574	0(3)
J0575	0(3)

CPT	MUE
J0583	250(3)
J0584	90(3)
J0585	600(3)
J0586	300(3)
J0587	300(3)
J0588	600(3)
J0592	6(3)
J0593	300(3)
J0594	320(3)
J0595	8(3)
J0596	840(3)
J0597	250(3)
J0598	100(3)
J0599	900(3)
J0600	3(3)
J0606	150(3)
J0610	15(3)
J0620	1(3)
J0630	1(3)
J0636	100(3)
J0637	20(3)
J0638	300(3)
J0640	24(3)
J0641	600(3)
J0642	600(3)
J0670	10(3)
J0690	12(3)
J0691	300(3)
J0692	12(3)
J0694	8(3)
J0695	60(3)
J0696	16(3)
J0697	4(3)
J0698	10(3)
J0702	18(3)
J0706	1(3)
J0710	0(3)
J0712	120(3)
J0713	12(3)
J0714	4(3)
J0715	0(3)
J0716	4(3)
J0717	400(3)
J0720	15(3)
J0725	10(3)
J0735	50(3)
J0740	2(3)
J0743	16(3)
J0744	6(3)
J0745	2(3)
J0770	5(3)
J0775	180(3)
J0780	4(3)
J0795	100(3)
J0800	3(3)
J0834	3(3)
J0840	6(3)
J0841	20(3)
J0850	9(3)
J0875	300(3)
J0878	1500(3)
J0881	500(3)
J0882	300(3)
J0883	1125(3)
J0884	1125(3)

CPT	MUE
J0885	60(3)
J0887	360(3)
J0888	360(3)
J0890	0(3)
J0894	100(3)
J0895	12(3)
J0897	120(3)
J0945	4(3)
J1000	1(3)
J1020	8(3)
J1030	8(3)
J1040	4(3)
J1050	1000(3)
J1071	400(3)
J1094	0(3)
J1095	1034(2)
J1096	4(3)
J1097	4(3)
J1100	120(3)
J1110	3(3)
J1120	2(3)
J1130	300(3)
J1160	2(3)
J1162	1(3)
J1165	50(3)
J1170	350(3)
J1180	0(3)
J1190	8(3)
J1200	8(3)
J1205	4(3)
J1212	1(3)
J1230	3(3)
J1240	6(3)
J1245	6(3)
J1250	2(3)
J1260	2(3)
J1265	20(3)
J1267	150(3)
J1270	8(3)
J1290	30(3)
J1300	120(3)
J1301	60(3)
J1303	360(3)
J1320	0(3)
J1322	150(3)
J1324	108(3)
J1325	1(3)
J1327	1(3)
J1330	1(3)
J1335	2(3)
J1364	2(3)
J1380	4(3)
J1410	4(3)
J1428	450(3)
J1430	10(3)
J1435	1(3)
J1436	0(3)
J1438	2(3)
J1439	750(3)
J1442	1500(3)
J1443	272(3)
J1444	272(3)
J1447	960(3)
J1450	4(3)
J1451	1(3)

CPT	MUE
J1452	0(3)
J1453	150(3)
J1454	1(3)
J1455	18(3)
J1457	0(3)
J1458	100(3)
J1459	300(3)
J1460	10(2)
J1555	480(3)
J1556	300(3)
J1557	300(3)
J1559	300(3)
J1560	1(2)
J1561	300(3)
J1562	0(3)
J1566	300(3)
J1568	300(3)
J1569	300(3)
J1570	4(3)
J1571	20(3)
J1572	300(3)
J1573	130(3)
J1575	650(3)
J1580	9(3)
J1595	1(3)
J1599	300(3)
J1600	2(3)
J1602	300(3)
J1610	2(3)
J1620	0(3)
J1626	30(3)
J1627	100(3)
J1628	100(3)
J1630	5(3)
J1631	9(3)
J1640	672(3)
J1642	100(3)
J1644	40(3)
J1645	10(3)
J1650	30(3)
J1652	20(3)
J1655	0(3)
J1670	1(3)
J1675	0(3)
J1700	0(3)
J1710	0(3)
J1720	10(3)
J1726	28(3)
J1729	25(3)
J1730	0(3)
J1740	3(3)
J1741	8(3)
J1742	2(3)
J1743	66(3)
J1744	30(3)
J1745	150(3)
J1746	200(3)
J1750	45(3)
J1756	500(3)
J1786	680(3)
J1790	2(3)
J1800	6(3)
J1810	0(3)
J1815	8(3)
J1817	0(3)

CPT	MUE
J1826	1(3)
J1830	1(3)
J1833	372(3)
J1835	0(3)
J1840	3(3)
J1850	4(3)
J1885	8(3)
J1890	0(3)
J1930	120(3)
J1931	377(3)
J1940	6(3)
J1943	675(3)
J1944	1064(3)
J1945	0(3)
J1950	12(3)
J1953	300(3)
J1955	11(3)
J1956	4(3)
J1960	0(3)
J1980	2(3)
J1990	0(3)
J2001	60(3)
J2010	10(3)
J2020	6(3)
J2060	4(3)
J2062	10(3)
J2150	8(3)
J2170	8(3)
J2175	4(3)
J2180	0(3)
J2182	300(3)
J2185	30(3)
J2186	600(3)
J2210	1(3)
J2212	240(3)
J2248	150(3)
J2250	22(3)
J2260	4(3)
J2265	400(3)
J2270	9(3)
J2274	250(3)
J2278	1000(3)
J2280	4(3)
J2300	4(3)
J2310	4(3)
J2315	380(3)
J2320	4(3)
J2323	300(3)
J2325	0(3)
J2326	120(3)
J2350	600(3)
J2353	60(3)
J2354	60(3)
J2355	2(3)
J2357	90(3)
J2358	405(3)
J2360	2(3)
J2370	2(3)
J2400	4(3)
J2405	64(3)
J2407	120(3)
J2410	2(3)
J2425	125(3)
J2426	819(3)
J2430	3(3)

CPT	MUE
J2440	4(3)
J2460	0(3)
J2469	10(3)
J2501	2(3)
J2502	60(3)
J2503	2(3)
J2504	15(3)
J2505	1(3)
J2507	8(3)
J2510	4(3)
J2513	1(3)
J2515	1(3)
J2540	75(3)
J2543	16(3)
J2545	1(3)
J2547	600(3)
J2550	3(3)
J2560	1(3)
J2562	48(3)
J2590	3(3)
J2597	45(3)
J2650	0(3)
J2670	0(3)
J2675	1(3)
J2680	4(3)
J2690	4(3)
J2700	48(3)
J2704	80(3)
J2710	2(3)
J2720	5(3)
J2724	3500(3)
J2725	0(3)
J2730	2(3)
J2760	2(3)
J2765	10(3)
J2770	6(3)
J2778	10(2)
J2780	16(3)
J2783	60(3)
J2785	4(3)
J2786	500(3)
J2787	2(3)
J2788	1(3)
J2790	1(3)
J2791	15(3)
J2792	450(3)
J2793	320(3)
J2794	100(3)
J2795	200(3)
J2796	150(3)
J2797	333(3)
J2798	240(3)
J2800	3(3)
J2805	3(3)
J2810	5(3)
J2820	15(3)
J2840	160(3)
J2850	16(3)
J2860	170(3)
J2910	0(3)
J2916	20(3)
J2920	25(3)
J2930	25(3)
J2940	0(3)
J2941	8(3)

CPT	MUE
J2950	0(3)
J2993	2(3)
J2995	0(3)
J2997	8(3)
J3000	2(3)
J3010	100(3)
J3030	1(3)
J3031	675(3)
J3060	760(3)
J3070	3(3)
J3090	200(3)
J3095	150(3)
J3101	50(3)
J3105	2(3)
J3110	2(3)
J3111	210(3)
J3121	400(3)
J3145	750(3)
J3230	2(3)
J3240	1(3)
J3243	150(3)
J3245	100(3)
J3246	1(3)
J3250	2(3)
J3260	8(3)
J3262	800(3)
J3265	0(3)
J3280	0(3)
J3285	1(3)
J3300	160(3)
J3301	16(3)
J3302	0(3)
J3303	24(3)
J3304	64(2)
J3305	0(3)
J3310	0(3)
J3315	6(3)
J3316	6(3)
J3320	0(3)
J3350	0(3)
J3355	1(3)
J3357	90(3)
J3358	520(3)
J3360	6(3)
J3364	0(3)
J3365	0(3)
J3370	12(3)
J3380	300(3)
J3385	80(3)
J3396	150(3)
J3397	600(3)
J3398	150(2)
J3400	0(3)
J3410	8(3)
J3411	4(3)
J3415	6(3)
J3420	1(3)
J3430	25(3)
J3465	40(3)
J3470	3(3)
J3471	999(2)
J3472	2(3)
J3473	450(3)
J3475	20(3)
J3480	40(3)

CPT	MUE
J3485	160(3)
J3486	4(3)
J3489	5(3)
J3520	0(3)
J3530	0(3)
J3535	0(3)
J3570	0(3)
J7030	5(3)
J7040	6(3)
J7042	6(3)
J7050	10(3)
J7060	10(3)
J7070	4(3)
J7100	2(3)
J7110	2(3)
J7120	4(3)
J7121	4(3)
J7131	500(3)
J7169	180(3)
J7170	1800(3)
J7175	9000(1)
J7177	10500(3)
J7178	7700(1)
J7179	7500(1)
J7180	6000(1)
J7181	3850(1)
J7182	22000(1)
J7183	7500(1)
J7185	22000(1)
J7186	7500(1)
J7187	7500(1)
J7188	22000(1)
J7189	13000(1)
J7190	22000(1)
J7191	0(3)
J7192	22000(1)
J7193	4000(1)
J7194	9000(1)
J7195	6000(1)
J7196	175(3)
J7197	6300(1)
J7198	6000(1)
J7200	20000(1)
J7201	9000(1)
J7202	11550(1)
J7203	12000(1)
J7205	9750(1)
J7207	22500(1)
J7208	12000(1)
J7209	7500(1)
J7210	22000(1)
J7211	22000(1)
J7296	0(3)
J7297	0(3)
J7298	0(3)
J7300	0(3)
J7301	0(3)
J7303	0(3)
J7304	0(3)
J7306	0(3)
J7307	0(3)
J7308	3(3)
J7309	1(3)
J7310	0(3)
J7311	118(2)

CPT	MUE
J7312	14(2)
J7313	38(2)
J7314	36(2)
J7315	2(3)
J7316	3(3)
J7318	120(3)
J7320	50(3)
J7321	2(2)
J7322	48(3)
J7323	2(2)
J7324	2(2)
J7325	96(3)
J7326	2(2)
J7327	2(2)
J7328	336(3)
J7329	50(2)
J7330	1(3)
J7331	40(3)
J7332	40(3)
J7336	1120(3)
J7340	1(3)
J7342	10(3)
J7345	200(3)
J7401	270(2)
J7500	0(3)
J7501	1(3)
J7502	0(3)
J7503	0(3)
J7504	15(3)
J7505	1(3)
J7507	0(3)
J7508	0(3)
J7509	0(3)
J7510	0(3)
J7511	9(3)
J7512	0(3)
J7513	0(3)
J7515	0(3)
J7516	1(3)
J7517	0(3)
J7518	0(3)
J7520	0(3)
J7525	2(3)
J7527	0(3)
J7599	1(3)
J7604	0(3)
J7605	2(3)
J7606	2(3)
J7607	0(3)
J7608	3(3)
J7609	0(3)
J7610	0(3)
J7611	10(3)
J7612	10(3)
J7613	10(3)
J7614	10(3)
J7615	0(3)
J7620	6(3)
J7622	0(3)
J7624	0(3)
J7626	2(3)
J7627	0(3)
J7628	0(3)
J7629	0(3)
J7631	4(3)

CPT	MUE
J7632	0(3)
J7633	0(3)
J7634	0(3)
J7635	0(3)
J7636	0(3)
J7637	0(3)
J7638	0(3)
J7639	3(3)
J7640	0(3)
J7641	0(3)
J7642	0(3)
J7643	0(3)
J7644	3(3)
J7645	0(3)
J7647	0(3)
J7648	0(3)
J7649	0(3)
J7650	0(3)
J7657	0(3)
J7658	0(3)
J7659	0(3)
J7660	0(3)
J7665	0(3)
J7667	0(3)
J7668	0(3)
J7669	0(3)
J7670	0(3)
J7674	100(3)
J7676	0(3)
J7677	175(3)
J7680	0(3)
J7681	0(3)
J7682	2(3)
J7683	0(3)
J7684	0(3)
J7685	0(3)
J7686	1(3)
J7699	1(3)
J7799	2(3)
J7999	2(3)
J8498	0(3)
J8499	0(3)
J8501	0(3)
J8510	0(3)
J8515	0(3)
J8520	0(3)
J8521	0(3)
J8530	0(3)
J8540	0(3)
J8560	0(3)
J8562	0(3)
J8565	0(3)
J8597	0(3)
J8600	0(3)
J8610	0(3)
J8650	0(3)
J8655	1(3)
J8670	0(3)
J8700	0(3)
J8705	0(3)
J8999	0(3)
J9000	20(3)
J9015	1(3)
J9017	30(3)
J9019	60(3)

CPT	MUE
J9020	0(3)
J9022	168(3)
J9023	140(3)
J9025	300(3)
J9027	100(3)
J9030	50(3)
J9032	300(3)
J9033	300(3)
J9034	360(3)
J9035	170(3)
J9036	360(3)
J9039	210(3)
J9040	4(3)
J9041	35(3)
J9042	200(3)
J9043	60(3)
J9044	35(3)
J9045	22(3)
J9047	160(3)
J9050	6(3)
J9055	120(3)
J9057	60(3)
J9060	24(3)
J9065	100(3)
J9070	55(3)
J9098	5(3)
J9100	120(3)
J9118	750(3)
J9119	350(3)
J9120	5(3)
J9130	24(3)
J9145	240(3)
J9150	12(3)
J9151	12(3)
J9153	132(3)
J9155	240(3)
J9160	7(3)
J9165	0(3)
J9171	240(3)
J9173	150(3)
J9175	10(3)
J9176	3000(3)
J9178	150(3)
J9179	50(3)
J9181	100(3)
J9185	2(3)
J9190	20(3)
J9200	5(3)
J9201	20(3)
J9202	3(3)
J9203	180(3)
J9204	160(3)
J9205	215(3)
J9206	42(3)
J9207	90(3)
J9208	15(3)
J9209	55(3)
J9210	1500(3)
J9211	6(3)
J9212	0(3)
J9213	12(3)
J9214	100(3)
J9215	0(3)
J9216	2(3)
J9217	6(3)

CPT	MUE	CPT	MUE	CPT	MUE	CPT	MUE	CPT	MUE	CPT	MUE	CPT	MUE	CPT	MUE
J9218	1(3)	K0012	0(3)	K0815	0(3)	L0140	0(3)	L0830	0(3)	L1833	0(3)	L2192	0(3)	L2810	0(3)
J9219	1(3)	K0013	0(3)	K0816	0(3)	L0150	0(3)	L0859	0(3)	L1834	0(3)	L2200	0(3)	L2820	0(3)
J9225	1(3)	K0014	0(3)	K0820	0(3)	L0160	0(3)	L0861	0(3)	L1836	0(3)	L2210	0(3)	L2830	0(3)
J9226	1(3)	K0015	0(3)	K0821	0(3)	L0170	0(3)	L0970	0(3)	L1840	0(3)	L2220	0(3)	L2840	0(3)
J9228	1100(3)	K0017	0(3)	K0822	0(3)	L0172	0(3)	L0972	0(3)	L1843	0(3)	L2230	0(3)	L2850	0(3)
J9229	27(3)	K0018	0(3)	K0823	0(3)	L0174	0(3)	L0974	0(3)	L1844	0(3)	L2232	0(3)	L2861	0(3)
J9230	5(3)	K0019	0(3)	K0824	0(3)	L0180	0(3)	L0976	0(3)	L1845	0(3)	L2240	0(3)	L2999	0(3)
J9245	9(3)	K0020	0(3)	K0825	0(3)	L0190	0(3)	L0978	0(3)	L1846	0(3)	L2250	0(3)	L3000	0(3)
J9250	25(3)	K0037	0(3)	K0826	0(3)	L0200	0(3)	L0980	0(3)	L1847	0(3)	L2260	0(3)	L3001	0(3)
J9260	20(3)	K0038	0(3)	K0827	0(3)	L0220	0(3)	L0982	0(3)	L1848	0(3)	L2265	0(3)	L3002	0(3)
J9261	80(3)	K0039	0(3)	K0828	0(3)	L0450	0(3)	L0984	0(3)	L1850	0(3)	L2270	0(3)	L3003	0(3)
J9262	700(3)	K0040	0(3)	K0829	0(3)	L0452	0(3)	L0999	0(3)	L1851	0(3)	L2275	0(3)	L3010	0(3)
J9263	700(3)	K0041	0(3)	K0830	0(3)	L0454	0(3)	L1000	0(3)	L1852	0(3)	L2280	0(3)	L3020	0(3)
J9264	600(3)	K0042	0(3)	K0831	0(3)	L0455	0(3)	L1001	0(3)	L1860	0(3)	L2300	0(3)	L3030	0(3)
J9266	2(3)	K0043	0(3)	K0835	0(3)	L0456	0(3)	L1005	0(3)	L1900	0(3)	L2310	0(3)	L3031	0(3)
J9267	750(3)	K0044	0(3)	K0836	0(3)	L0457	0(3)	L1010	0(3)	L1902	0(3)	L2320	0(3)	L3040	0(3)
J9268	1(3)	K0045	0(3)	K0837	0(3)	L0458	0(3)	L1020	0(3)	L1904	0(3)	L2330	0(3)	L3050	0(3)
J9270	0(3)	K0046	0(3)	K0838	0(3)	L0460	0(3)	L1025	0(3)	L1906	0(3)	L2335	0(3)	L3060	0(3)
J9271	400(3)	K0047	0(3)	K0839	0(3)	L0462	0(3)	L1030	0(3)	L1907	0(3)	L2340	0(3)	L3070	0(3)
J9280	12(3)	K0050	0(3)	K0840	0(3)	L0464	0(3)	L1040	0(3)	L1910	0(3)	L2350	0(3)	L3080	0(3)
J9285	200(3)	K0051	0(3)	K0841	0(3)	L0466	0(3)	L1050	0(3)	L1920	0(3)	L2360	0(3)	L3090	0(3)
J9293	8(3)	K0052	0(3)	K0842	0(3)	L0467	0(3)	L1060	0(3)	L1930	0(3)	L2370	0(3)	L3100	0(3)
J9295	800(3)	K0053	0(3)	K0843	0(3)	L0468	0(3)	L1070	0(3)	L1932	0(3)	L2375	0(3)	L3140	0(3)
J9299	480(3)	K0056	0(3)	K0848	0(3)	L0469	0(3)	L1080	0(3)	L1940	0(3)	L2380	0(3)	L3150	0(3)
J9301	100(3)	K0065	0(3)	K0849	0(3)	L0470	0(3)	L1085	0(3)	L1945	0(3)	L2385	0(3)	L3160	0(3)
J9302	200(3)	K0069	0(3)	K0850	0(3)	L0472	0(3)	L1090	0(3)	L1950	0(3)	L2387	0(3)	L3170	0(3)
J9303	90(3)	K0070	0(3)	K0851	0(3)	L0480	0(3)	L1100	0(3)	L1951	0(3)	L2390	0(3)	L3201	0(3)
J9305	150(3)	K0071	0(3)	K0852	0(3)	L0482	0(3)	L1110	0(3)	L1960	0(3)	L2395	0(3)	L3202	0(3)
J9306	840(3)	K0072	0(3)	K0853	0(3)	L0484	0(3)	L1120	0(3)	L1970	0(3)	L2397	0(3)	L3203	0(3)
J9307	60(3)	K0073	0(3)	K0854	0(3)	L0486	0(3)	L1200	0(3)	L1971	0(3)	L2405	0(3)	L3204	0(3)
J9308	280(3)	K0077	0(3)	K0855	0(3)	L0488	0(3)	L1210	0(3)	L1980	0(3)	L2415	0(3)	L3206	0(3)
J9309	280(3)	K0098	0(3)	K0856	0(3)	L0490	0(3)	L1220	0(3)	L1990	0(3)	L2425	0(3)	L3207	0(3)
J9311	160(3)	K0105	0(3)	K0857	0(3)	L0491	0(3)	L1230	0(3)	L2000	0(3)	L2430	0(3)	L3208	0(3)
J9312	150(3)	K0108	0(3)	K0858	0(3)	L0492	0(3)	L1240	0(3)	L2005	0(3)	L2492	0(3)	L3209	0(3)
J9313	600(3)	K0195	0(3)	K0859	0(3)	L0621	0(3)	L1250	0(3)	L2006	0(3)	L2500	0(3)	L3211	0(3)
J9315	40(3)	K0455	0(3)	K0860	0(3)	L0622	0(3)	L1260	0(3)	L2010	0(3)	L2510	0(3)	L3212	0(3)
J9320	4(3)	K0462	0(3)	K0861	0(3)	L0623	0(3)	L1270	0(3)	L2020	0(3)	L2520	0(3)	L3213	0(3)
J9325	400(3)	K0553	0(3)	K0862	0(3)	L0624	0(3)	L1280	0(3)	L2030	0(3)	L2525	0(3)	L3214	0(3)
J9328	400(3)	K0554	0(3)	K0863	0(3)	L0625	0(3)	L1290	0(3)	L2034	0(3)	L2526	0(3)	L3215	0(3)
J9330	50(3)	K0602	0(3)	K0864	0(3)	L0626	0(3)	L1300	0(3)	L2035	0(3)	L2530	0(3)	L3216	0(3)
J9340	4(3)	K0604	0(3)	K0868	0(3)	L0627	0(3)	L1310	0(3)	L2036	0(3)	L2540	0(3)	L3217	0(3)
J9351	120(3)	K0605	0(3)	K0869	0(3)	L0628	0(3)	L1499	1(3)	L2037	0(3)	L2550	0(3)	L3219	0(3)
J9352	40(3)	K0606	0(3)	K0870	0(3)	L0629	0(3)	L1600	0(3)	L2038	0(3)	L2570	0(3)	L3221	0(3)
J9354	600(3)	K0607	0(3)	K0871	0(3)	L0630	0(3)	L1610	0(3)	L2040	0(3)	L2580	0(3)	L3222	0(3)
J9355	105(3)	K0608	0(3)	K0877	0(3)	L0631	0(3)	L1620	0(3)	L2050	0(3)	L2600	0(3)	L3224	0(3)
J9356	60(3)	K0609	0(3)	K0878	0(3)	L0632	0(3)	L1630	0(3)	L2060	0(3)	L2610	0(3)	L3225	0(3)
J9357	4(3)	K0669	0(3)	K0879	0(3)	L0633	0(3)	L1640	0(3)	L2070	0(3)	L2620	0(3)	L3230	0(3)
J9360	40(3)	K0672	0(3)	K0880	0(3)	L0634	0(3)	L1650	0(3)	L2080	0(3)	L2622	0(3)	L3250	0(3)
J9370	4(3)	K0730	0(3)	K0884	0(3)	L0635	0(3)	L1652	0(3)	L2090	0(3)	L2624	0(3)	L3251	0(3)
J9371	5(3)	K0733	0(3)	K0885	0(3)	L0636	0(3)	L1660	0(3)	L2106	0(3)	L2627	0(3)	L3252	0(3)
J9390	36(3)	K0738	0(3)	K0886	0(3)	L0637	0(3)	L1680	0(3)	L2108	0(3)	L2628	0(3)	L3253	0(3)
J9395	20(3)	K0740	0(3)	K0890	0(3)	L0638	0(3)	L1685	0(3)	L2112	0(3)	L2630	0(3)	L3254	0(3)
J9400	500(3)	K0743	0(3)	K0891	0(3)	L0639	0(3)	L1686	0(3)	L2114	0(3)	L2640	0(3)	L3255	0(3)
J9600	4(3)	K0744	0(3)	K0898	1(2)	L0640	0(3)	L1690	0(3)	L2116	0(3)	L2650	0(3)	L3257	0(3)
K0001	0(3)	K0745	0(3)	K0899	0(3)	L0641	0(3)	L1700	0(3)	L2126	0(3)	L2660	0(3)	L3260	0(3)
K0002	0(3)	K0746	0(3)	K0900	0(3)	L0642	0(3)	L1710	0(3)	L2128	0(3)	L2670	0(3)	L3265	0(3)
K0003	0(3)	K0800	0(3)	K1001	0(3)	L0643	0(3)	L1720	0(3)	L2132	0(3)	L2680	0(3)	L3300	0(3)
K0004	0(3)	K0801	0(3)	K1002	0(3)	L0648	0(3)	L1730	0(3)	L2134	0(3)	L2750	0(3)	L3310	0(3)
K0005	0(3)	K0802	0(3)	K1003	0(3)	L0649	0(3)	L1755	0(3)	L2136	0(3)	L2755	0(3)	L3320	0(3)
K0006	0(3)	K0806	0(3)	K1004	0(3)	L0650	0(3)	L1810	0(3)	L2180	0(3)	L2760	0(3)	L3330	0(3)
K0007	0(3)	K0807	0(3)	K1005	0(3)	L0651	0(3)	L1812	0(3)	L2182	0(3)	L2768	0(3)	L3332	0(3)
K0008	0(3)	K0808	0(3)	L0112	0(3)	L0700	0(3)	L1820	0(3)	L2184	0(3)	L2780	0(3)	L3334	0(3)
K0009	0(3)	K0812	0(3)	L0113	0(3)	L0710	0(3)	L1830	0(3)	L2186	0(3)	L2785	0(3)	L3340	0(3)
K0010	0(3)	K0813	0(3)	L0120	0(3)	L0810	0(3)	L1831	0(3)	L2188	0(3)	L2795	0(3)	L3350	0(3)
K0011	0(3)	K0814	0(3)	L0130	0(3)	L0820	0(3)	L1832	0(3)	L2190	0(3)	L2800	0(3)	L3360	0(3)

CPT	MUE
L3370	0(3)
L3380	0(3)
L3390	0(3)
L3400	0(3)
L3410	0(3)
L3420	0(3)
L3430	0(3)
L3440	0(3)
L3450	0(3)
L3455	0(3)
L3460	0(3)
L3465	0(3)
L3470	0(3)
L3480	0(3)
L3485	0(3)
L3500	0(3)
L3510	0(3)
L3520	0(3)
L3530	0(3)
L3540	0(3)
L3550	0(3)
L3560	0(3)
L3570	0(3)
L3580	0(3)
L3590	0(3)
L3595	0(3)
L3600	0(3)
L3610	0(3)
L3620	0(3)
L3630	0(3)
L3640	0(3)
L3649	0(3)
L3650	0(3)
L3660	0(3)
L3670	0(3)
L3671	0(3)
L3674	0(3)
L3675	0(3)
L3677	0(3)
L3678	0(3)
L3702	0(3)
L3710	0(3)
L3720	0(3)
L3730	0(3)
L3740	0(3)
L3760	0(3)
L3761	0(3)
L3762	0(3)
L3763	0(3)
L3764	0(3)
L3765	0(3)
L3766	0(3)
L3806	0(3)
L3807	0(3)
L3808	0(3)
L3809	0(3)
L3891	0(3)
L3900	0(3)
L3901	0(3)
L3904	0(3)
L3905	0(3)
L3906	0(3)
L3908	0(3)
L3912	0(3)
L3913	0(3)

CPT	MUE
L3915	0(3)
L3916	0(3)
L3917	0(3)
L3918	0(3)
L3919	0(3)
L3921	0(3)
L3923	0(3)
L3924	0(3)
L3925	0(3)
L3927	0(3)
L3929	0(3)
L3930	0(3)
L3931	0(3)
L3933	0(3)
L3935	0(3)
L3956	0(3)
L3960	0(3)
L3961	0(3)
L3962	0(3)
L3967	0(3)
L3971	0(3)
L3973	0(3)
L3975	0(3)
L3976	0(3)
L3977	0(3)
L3978	0(3)
L3980	0(3)
L3981	0(3)
L3982	0(3)
L3984	0(3)
L3995	0(3)
L3999	0(3)
L4000	0(3)
L4002	0(3)
L4010	0(3)
L4020	0(3)
L4030	0(3)
L4040	0(3)
L4045	0(3)
L4050	0(3)
L4055	0(3)
L4060	0(3)
L4070	0(3)
L4080	0(3)
L4090	0(3)
L4100	0(3)
L4110	0(3)
L4130	0(3)
L4205	0(3)
L4210	0(3)
L4350	0(3)
L4360	0(3)
L4361	0(3)
L4370	0(3)
L4386	0(3)
L4387	0(3)
L4392	0(3)
L4394	0(3)
L4396	0(3)
L4397	0(3)
L4398	0(3)
L4631	0(3)
L5000	0(3)
L5010	0(3)
L5020	0(3)

CPT	MUE
L5050	0(3)
L5060	0(3)
L5100	0(3)
L5105	0(3)
L5150	0(3)
L5160	0(3)
L5200	0(3)
L5210	0(3)
L5220	0(3)
L5230	0(3)
L5250	0(3)
L5270	0(3)
L5280	0(3)
L5301	0(3)
L5312	0(3)
L5321	0(3)
L5331	0(3)
L5341	0(3)
L5400	0(3)
L5410	0(3)
L5420	0(3)
L5430	0(3)
L5450	0(3)
L5460	0(3)
L5500	0(3)
L5505	0(3)
L5510	0(3)
L5520	0(3)
L5530	0(3)
L5535	0(3)
L5540	0(3)
L5560	0(3)
L5570	0(3)
L5580	0(3)
L5585	0(3)
L5590	0(3)
L5595	0(3)
L5600	0(3)
L5610	0(3)
L5611	0(3)
L5613	0(3)
L5614	0(3)
L5616	0(3)
L5617	0(3)
L5618	0(3)
L5620	0(3)
L5622	0(3)
L5624	0(3)
L5626	0(3)
L5628	0(3)
L5629	0(3)
L5630	0(3)
L5631	0(3)
L5632	0(3)
L5634	0(3)
L5636	0(3)
L5637	0(3)
L5638	0(3)
L5639	0(3)
L5640	0(3)
L5642	0(3)
L5643	0(3)
L5644	0(3)
L5645	0(3)
L5646	0(3)

CPT	MUE
L5647	0(3)
L5648	0(3)
L5649	0(3)
L5650	0(3)
L5651	0(3)
L5652	0(3)
L5653	0(3)
L5654	0(3)
L5655	0(3)
L5656	0(3)
L5658	0(3)
L5661	0(3)
L5665	0(3)
L5666	0(3)
L5668	0(3)
L5670	0(3)
L5671	0(3)
L5672	0(3)
L5673	0(3)
L5676	0(3)
L5677	0(3)
L5678	0(3)
L5679	0(3)
L5680	0(3)
L5681	0(3)
L5682	0(3)
L5683	0(3)
L5684	0(3)
L5685	0(3)
L5686	0(3)
L5688	0(3)
L5690	0(3)
L5692	0(3)
L5694	0(3)
L5695	0(3)
L5696	0(3)
L5697	0(3)
L5698	0(3)
L5699	0(3)
L5700	0(3)
L5701	0(3)
L5702	0(3)
L5703	0(3)
L5704	0(3)
L5705	0(3)
L5706	0(3)
L5707	0(3)
L5710	0(3)
L5711	0(3)
L5712	0(3)
L5714	0(3)
L5716	0(3)
L5718	0(3)
L5722	0(3)
L5724	0(3)
L5726	0(3)
L5728	0(3)
L5780	0(3)
L5781	0(3)
L5782	0(3)
L5785	0(3)
L5790	0(3)
L5795	0(3)
L5810	0(3)
L5811	0(3)

CPT	MUE
L5812	0(3)
L5814	0(3)
L5816	0(3)
L5818	0(3)
L5822	0(3)
L5824	0(3)
L5826	0(3)
L5828	0(3)
L5830	0(3)
L5840	0(3)
L5845	0(3)
L5848	0(3)
L5850	0(3)
L5855	0(3)
L5856	0(3)
L5857	0(3)
L5858	0(3)
L5859	0(3)
L5910	0(3)
L5920	0(3)
L5925	0(3)
L5930	0(3)
L5940	0(3)
L5950	0(3)
L5960	0(3)
L5961	0(3)
L5962	0(3)
L5964	0(3)
L5966	0(3)
L5968	0(3)
L5969	0(3)
L5970	0(3)
L5971	0(3)
L5972	0(3)
L5973	0(3)
L5974	0(3)
L5975	0(3)
L5976	0(3)
L5978	0(3)
L5979	0(3)
L5980	0(3)
L5981	0(3)
L5982	0(3)
L5984	0(3)
L5985	0(3)
L5986	0(3)
L5987	0(3)
L5988	0(3)
L5990	0(3)
L5999	0(3)
L6000	0(3)
L6010	0(3)
L6020	0(3)
L6026	0(3)
L6050	0(3)
L6055	0(3)
L6100	0(3)
L6110	0(3)
L6120	0(3)
L6130	0(3)
L6200	0(3)
L6205	0(3)
L6250	0(3)
L6300	0(3)
L6310	0(3)

CPT	MUE
L6320	0(3)
L6350	0(3)
L6360	0(3)
L6370	0(3)
L6380	0(3)
L6382	0(3)
L6384	0(3)
L6386	0(3)
L6388	0(3)
L6400	0(3)
L6450	0(3)
L6500	0(3)
L6550	0(3)
L6570	0(3)
L6580	0(3)
L6582	0(3)
L6584	0(3)
L6586	0(3)
L6588	0(3)
L6590	0(3)
L6600	0(3)
L6605	0(3)
L6610	0(3)
L6611	0(3)
L6615	0(3)
L6616	0(3)
L6620	0(3)
L6621	0(3)
L6623	0(3)
L6624	0(3)
L6625	0(3)
L6628	0(3)
L6629	0(3)
L6630	0(3)
L6632	0(3)
L6635	0(3)
L6637	0(3)
L6638	0(3)
L6640	0(3)
L6641	0(3)
L6642	0(3)
L6645	0(3)
L6646	0(3)
L6647	0(3)
L6648	0(3)
L6650	0(3)
L6655	0(3)
L6660	0(3)
L6665	0(3)
L6670	0(3)
L6672	0(3)
L6675	0(3)
L6676	0(3)
L6677	0(3)
L6680	0(3)
L6682	0(3)
L6684	0(3)
L6686	0(3)
L6687	0(3)
L6688	0(3)
L6689	0(3)
L6690	0(3)
L6691	0(3)
L6692	0(3)
L6693	0(3)

CPT	MUE
L6694	0(3)
L6695	0(3)
L6696	0(3)
L6697	0(3)
L6698	0(3)
L6703	0(3)
L6704	0(3)
L6706	0(3)
L6707	0(3)
L6708	0(3)
L6709	0(3)
L6711	0(3)
L6712	0(3)
L6713	0(3)
L6714	0(3)
L6715	0(3)
L6721	0(3)
L6722	0(3)
L6805	0(3)
L6810	0(3)
L6880	0(3)
L6881	0(3)
L6882	0(3)
L6883	0(3)
L6884	0(3)
L6885	0(3)
L6890	0(3)
L6895	0(3)
L6900	0(3)
L6905	0(3)
L6910	0(3)
L6915	0(3)
L6920	0(3)
L6925	0(3)
L6930	0(3)
L6935	0(3)
L6940	0(3)
L6945	0(3)
L6950	0(3)
L6955	0(3)
L6960	0(3)
L6965	0(3)
L6970	0(3)
L6975	0(3)
L7007	0(3)
L7008	0(3)
L7009	0(3)
L7040	0(3)
L7045	0(3)
L7170	0(3)
L7180	0(3)
L7181	0(3)
L7185	0(3)
L7186	0(3)
L7190	0(3)
L7191	0(3)
L7259	0(3)
L7360	0(3)
L7362	0(3)
L7364	0(3)
L7366	0(3)
L7367	0(3)
L7368	0(3)
L7400	0(3)
L7401	0(3)

CPT	MUE
L7402	0(3)
L7403	0(3)
L7404	0(3)
L7405	0(3)
L7499	0(3)
L7510	4(3)
L7600	0(3)
L7700	0(3)
L7900	0(3)
L7902	0(3)
L8000	0(3)
L8001	0(3)
L8002	0(3)
L8010	0(3)
L8015	0(3)
L8020	0(3)
L8030	0(3)
L8031	0(3)
L8032	0(3)
L8033	0(3)
L8035	0(3)
L8039	0(3)
L8040	0(3)
L8041	0(3)
L8042	0(3)
L8043	0(3)
L8044	0(3)
L8045	0(3)
L8046	0(3)
L8047	0(3)
L8048	1(3)
L8049	0(3)
L8300	0(3)
L8310	0(3)
L8320	0(3)
L8330	0(3)
L8400	0(3)
L8410	0(3)
L8415	0(3)
L8417	0(3)
L8420	0(3)
L8430	0(3)
L8435	0(3)
L8440	0(3)
L8460	0(3)
L8465	0(3)
L8470	0(3)
L8480	0(3)
L8485	0(3)
L8499	1(3)
L8500	0(3)
L8501	0(3)
L8505	0(3)
L8507	0(3)
L8509	1(3)
L8510	0(3)
L8511	1(3)
L8512	1(3)
L8513	1(3)
L8514	1(3)
L8515	1(3)
L8600	2(3)
L8603	4(3)
L8604	3(3)
L8605	4(3)

CPT	MUE
L8606	5(3)
L8607	20(3)
L8609	1(3)
L8610	1(3)
L8612	1(3)
L8613	1(3)
L8614	1(3)
L8615	2(3)
L8616	2(3)
L8617	2(3)
L8618	2(3)
L8619	2(3)
L8621	360(3)
L8622	2(3)
L8625	1(3)
L8627	2(2)
L8628	2(2)
L8629	2(2)
L8631	1(3)
L8641	4(3)
L8642	2(3)
L8658	2(3)
L8659	2(3)
L8670	2(3)
L8679	1(3)
L8681	1(3)
L8682	2(3)
L8683	1(3)
L8684	1(3)
L8685	1(3)
L8686	2(3)
L8687	1(3)
L8688	1(3)
L8689	1(3)
L8690	2(2)
L8691	1(3)
L8692	0(3)
L8693	1(3)
L8694	1(3)
L8695	1(3)
L8696	1(3)
L8701	0(3)
L8702	0(3)
M0075	0(3)
M0076	0(3)
M0100	0(3)
M0300	0(3)
M0301	0(3)
P2028	1(2)
P2029	1(2)
P2031	0(3)
P2033	1(2)
P2038	1(2)
P3000	1(3)
P3001	1(3)
P7001	0(3)
P9010	2(3)
P9011	2(3)

CPT	MUE
P9012	8(3)
P9016	3(3)
P9017	2(3)
P9019	2(3)
P9020	2(3)
P9021	3(3)
P9022	2(3)
P9023	2(3)
P9031	12(3)
P9032	12(3)
P9033	12(3)
P9034	2(3)
P9035	2(3)
P9036	2(3)
P9037	2(3)
P9038	2(3)
P9039	2(3)
P9040	3(3)
P9041	5(3)
P9043	5(3)
P9044	10(3)
P9045	20(3)
P9046	25(3)
P9047	20(3)
P9048	1(3)
P9050	1(3)
P9051	2(3)
P9052	2(3)
P9053	2(3)
P9054	2(3)
P9055	2(3)
P9056	2(3)
P9057	2(3)
P9058	2(3)
P9059	2(3)
P9060	2(3)
P9070	2(3)
P9071	2(3)
P9073	2(3)
P9099	1(3)
P9100	2(3)
P9603	300(3)
P9604	2(3)
P9612	1(3)
P9615	1(3)
Q0035	1(3)
Q0081	1(3)
Q0083	1(3)
Q0084	1(3)
Q0085	1(3)
Q0091	1(3)
Q0111	2(3)
Q0112	3(3)
Q0113	1(3)
Q0114	1(3)
Q0115	1(3)
Q0138	510(3)
Q0139	510(3)

CPT	MUE
Q0144	0(3)
Q0161	0(3)
Q0162	0(3)
Q0163	0(3)
Q0164	0(3)
Q0166	0(3)
Q0167	0(3)
Q0169	0(3)
Q0173	0(3)
Q0174	0(3)
Q0175	0(3)
Q0177	0(3)
Q0180	0(3)
Q0181	0(3)
Q0477	1(1)
Q0478	1(3)
Q0479	1(3)
Q0480	1(3)
Q0481	1(2)
Q0482	1(3)
Q0483	1(3)
Q0484	1(3)
Q0485	1(3)
Q0486	1(3)
Q0487	1(3)
Q0488	1(3)
Q0489	1(3)
Q0490	1(3)
Q0491	1(3)
Q0492	1(3)
Q0493	1(3)
Q0494	1(3)
Q0495	1(3)
Q0496	1(3)
Q0497	2(3)
Q0498	1(3)
Q0499	1(3)
Q0501	1(3)
Q0502	1(3)
Q0503	3(3)
Q0504	1(3)
Q0506	8(3)
Q0507	1(3)
Q0508	4(3)
Q0509	2(3)
Q0510	0(3)
Q0511	0(3)
Q0512	0(3)
Q0513	0(3)
Q0514	0(3)
Q0515	0(3)
Q1004	2(2)
Q1005	2(2)
Q2004	1(3)
Q2009	100(3)
Q2017	12(3)
Q2026	30(3)
Q2028	1470(3)

CPT	MUE
Q2034	1(2)
Q2035	1(2)
Q2036	1(2)
Q2037	1(2)
Q2038	1(2)
Q2039	1(2)
Q2043	1(2)
Q2049	10(3)
Q2050	14(3)
Q2052	1(3)
Q3014	1(3)
Q3027	30(3)
Q3028	0(3)
Q3031	1(3)
Q4001	1(3)
Q4002	1(3)
Q4003	2(3)
Q4004	2(3)
Q4012	2(3)
Q4013	2(3)
Q4014	2(3)
Q4018	2(3)
Q4021	2(3)
Q4025	1(3)
Q4026	1(3)
Q4027	1(3)
Q4028	1(3)
Q4030	2(3)
Q4037	2(3)
Q4042	2(3)
Q4046	2(3)
Q4050	2(3)
Q4051	2(3)
Q4074	3(3)
Q4081	100(3)
Q5101	1500(3)
Q5103	150(3)
Q5104	150(3)
Q5105	100(3)
Q5106	60(3)
Q5107	170(3)
Q5108	12(3)
Q5109	150(3)
Q5110	1500(3)
Q5111	12(3)
Q5112	120(3)
Q5113	120(3)
Q5114	120(3)
Q5115	120(3)
Q5116	120(3)
Q5117	120(3)
Q5118	230(3)
Q9950	5(3)
Q9951	0(3)
Q9953	10(3)
Q9954	18(3)
Q9955	0(3)
Q9956	9(3)

CPT	MUE
Q9957	3(3)
Q9958	300(3)
Q9959	0(3)
Q9960	250(3)
Q9961	200(3)
Q9962	150(3)
Q9963	240(3)
Q9964	0(3)
Q9966	250(3)
Q9967	300(3)
Q9969	3(3)
Q9982	1(3)
Q9983	1(3)
Q9991	1(2)
Q9992	1(2)
R0070	2(3)
R0075	2(3)
R0076	1(3)
U0001	2(3)
U0002	2(3)
U0003	2(3)
U0004	2(3)
V2020	0(3)
V2025	0(3)
V2100	0(3)
V2101	0(3)
V2102	0(3)
V2103	0(3)
V2104	0(3)
V2105	0(3)
V2106	0(3)
V2107	0(3)
V2108	0(3)
V2109	0(3)
V2110	0(3)
V2111	0(3)
V2112	0(3)
V2113	0(3)
V2114	0(3)
V2115	0(3)
V2118	0(3)
V2121	0(3)
V2199	2(3)
V2200	0(3)
V2201	0(3)
V2202	0(3)
V2203	0(3)
V2204	0(3)
V2205	0(3)
V2206	0(3)
V2207	0(3)
V2208	0(3)
V2209	0(3)
V2210	0(3)
V2211	0(3)
V2212	0(3)
V2213	0(3)
V2214	0(3)

CPT	MUE
V2215	0(3)
V2218	0(3)
V2219	0(3)
V2220	0(3)
V2221	0(3)
V2299	0(3)
V2300	0(3)
V2301	0(3)
V2302	0(3)
V2303	0(3)
V2304	0(3)
V2305	0(3)
V2306	0(3)
V2307	0(3)
V2308	0(3)
V2309	0(3)
V2310	0(3)
V2311	0(3)
V2312	0(3)
V2313	0(3)
V2314	0(3)
V2315	0(3)
V2318	0(3)
V2319	0(3)
V2320	0(3)
V2321	0(3)
V2399	0(3)
V2410	0(3)
V2430	0(3)
V2499	2(3)
V2500	0(3)
V2501	0(3)
V2502	0(3)
V2503	0(3)
V2510	0(3)
V2511	0(3)
V2512	0(3)
V2513	0(3)
V2520	2(3)
V2521	2(3)
V2522	2(3)
V2523	2(3)
V2530	0(3)
V2531	0(3)
V2599	2(3)
V2600	0(2)
V2610	0(2)
V2615	0(2)
V2623	0(3)
V2624	0(3)
V2625	0(3)
V2626	0(3)
V2627	0(3)
V2628	0(3)
V2629	0(3)
V2630	2(2)
V2631	2(2)
V2632	2(2)

CPT	MUE
V2700	0(3)
V2702	0(3)
V2710	0(3)
V2715	0(3)
V2718	0(3)
V2730	0(3)
V2744	0(3)
V2745	0(3)
V2750	0(3)
V2755	0(3)
V2756	0(3)
V2760	0(3)
V2761	0(2)
V2762	0(3)
V2770	0(3)
V2780	0(3)
V2781	0(2)
V2782	0(3)
V2783	0(3)
V2784	0(3)
V2785	2(2)
V2786	0(3)
V2787	0(3)
V2788	0(3)
V2790	1(3)
V2797	0(3)
V5008	0(3)
V5010	0(3)
V5011	0(3)
V5014	0(3)
V5020	0(3)
V5030	0(3)
V5040	0(3)
V5050	0(3)
V5060	0(3)
V5070	0(3)
V5080	0(3)
V5090	0(3)
V5095	0(3)
V5100	0(3)
V5110	0(3)
V5120	0(3)
V5130	0(3)
V5140	0(3)
V5150	0(3)
V5160	0(3)
V5171	0(3)
V5172	0(3)
V5181	0(3)
V5190	0(3)
V5200	0(3)
V5211	0(3)
V5212	0(3)
V5213	0(3)
V5214	0(3)
V5215	0(3)
V5221	0(3)
V5230	0(3)

CPT	MUE
V5240	0(3)
V5241	0(3)
V5242	0(3)
V5243	0(3)
V5244	0(3)
V5245	0(3)
V5246	0(3)
V5247	0(3)
V5248	0(3)
V5249	0(3)
V5250	0(3)
V5251	0(3)
V5252	0(3)
V5253	0(3)
V5254	0(3)
V5255	0(3)
V5256	0(3)
V5257	0(3)
V5258	0(3)
V5259	0(3)
V5260	0(3)
V5261	0(3)
V5262	0(3)
V5263	0(3)
V5264	0(3)
V5265	0(3)
V5266	0(3)
V5267	0(3)
V5268	0(3)
V5269	0(3)
V5270	0(3)
V5271	0(3)
V5272	0(3)
V5273	0(3)
V5274	0(3)
V5275	0(3)
V5281	0(3)
V5282	0(3)
V5283	0(3)
V5284	0(3)
V5285	0(3)
V5286	0(3)
V5287	0(3)
V5288	0(3)
V5289	0(3)
V5290	0(3)
V5298	0(3)
V5299	1(3)
V5336	0(3)
V5362	0(3)
V5363	0(3)
V5364	0(3)

OPPS

CPT	MUE
0001U	1(2)
0002M	1(3)
0002U	1(2)
0003M	1(3)
0003U	1(2)
0004M	1(2)
0005U	1(2)
0006M	1(2)
0007M	1(2)
0007U	1(2)
0008U	1(3)
0009U	2(3)
0010U	2(3)
0011M	1(2)
0011U	1(2)
0012M	1(2)
0012U	1(2)
0013M	1(2)
0013U	1(3)
0014M	1(2)
0014U	1(3)
0016U	1(3)
0017U	1(3)
0018U	1(1)
0019U	1(3)
0021U	1(2)
0022U	2(3)
0023U	1(2)
0024U	1(2)
0025U	1(2)
0026U	1(3)
0027U	1(2)
0029U	1(2)
0030U	1(2)
0031U	1(2)
0032U	1(2)
0033U	1(2)
0034U	1(2)
0035U	1(2)
0036U	1(3)
0037U	1(3)
0038U	1(2)
0039U	1(2)
0040U	1(2)
0041U	1(2)
0042T	1(3)
0042U	1(2)
0043U	1(2)
0044U	1(2)
0045U	1(3)
0046U	1(3)
0047U	1(3)
0048U	1(3)
0049U	1(3)
0050U	1(3)
0051U	1(2)
0052U	1(2)
0053U	1(3)
0054T	1(3)
0054U	1(2)
0055T	1(3)
0055U	1(2)
0056U	1(3)
0058T	1(2)

CPT	MUE
0058U	1(2)
0059U	1(2)
0060U	1(2)
0061U	2(3)
0062U	1(2)
0063U	1(2)
0064U	2(3)
0065U	2(3)
0066U	1(3)
0067U	2(3)
0068U	1(3)
0069U	1(3)
0070U	1(2)
0071T	1(2)
0071U	1(2)
0072T	1(2)
0072U	1(2)
0073U	1(2)
0074U	1(2)
0075T	1(2)
0075U	1(2)
0076T	1(2)
0076U	1(2)
0077U	2(2)
0078U	1(2)
0079U	0(3)
0080U	1(2)
0082U	1(2)
0083U	1(3)
0084U	1(2)
0085T	0(3)
0086U	1(3)
0087U	1(2)
0088U	1(2)
0089U	1(2)
0090U	1(2)
0091U	1(2)
0092U	1(2)
0093U	1(2)
0094U	1(2)
0095T	1(3)
0095U	1(2)
0096U	1(2)
0097U	1(2)
0098T	2(3)
0098U	1(2)
0099U	1(2)
0100T	1(2)
0100U	1(2)
0101T	1(3)
0101U	1(2)
0102T	2(2)
0102U	1(2)
0103U	1(2)
0105U	1(2)
0106T	4(2)
0106U	1(2)
0107T	4(2)
0107U	1(3)
0108T	4(2)
0108U	1(2)
0109T	4(2)
0109U	1(3)
0110T	4(2)

CPT	MUE
0110U	1(2)
0111T	1(3)
0111U	1(2)
0112U	1(3)
0113U	1(2)
0114U	1(2)
0115U	1(3)
0116U	1(2)
0117U	1(2)
0118U	1(2)
0119U	1(2)
0120U	1(2)
0121U	1(2)
0122U	1(2)
0123U	1(2)
0126T	1(3)
0129U	1(2)
0130U	1(2)
0131U	1(2)
0132U	1(2)
0133U	1(2)
0134U	1(2)
0135U	1(2)
0136U	1(2)
0137U	1(2)
0138U	1(2)
0139U	1(2)
0140U	1(2)
0141U	1(2)
0142U	1(2)
0143U	1(2)
0144U	1(2)
0145U	1(2)
0146U	1(2)
0147U	1(2)
0148U	1(2)
0149U	1(2)
0150U	1(2)
0151U	1(2)
0152U	1(2)
0153U	1(2)
0154U	1(2)
0155U	1(2)
0156U	1(2)
0157U	1(2)
0158U	1(2)
0159U	1(2)
0160U	1(2)
0161U	1(2)
0162U	1(2)
0163T	1(3)
0163U	0(3)
0164T	4(2)
0164U	1(2)
0165T	4(2)
0165U	1(2)
0166U	1(2)
0167U	1(2)
0168U	1(2)
0169U	1(2)
0170U	1(2)
0171U	1(2)
0172U	1(2)
0173U	1(2)

CPT	MUE
0174T	1(3)
0174U	1(2)
0175T	1(3)
0175U	1(2)
0176U	1(3)
0177U	1(2)
0178U	1(2)
0179U	1(2)
0184T	1(3)
0191T	2(2)
0198T	2(2)
0199T	1(2)
0200T	1(2)
0201T	1(2)
0202T	1(3)
0202U	1(3)
0207T	2(2)
0208T	1(3)
0209T	1(3)
0210T	1(3)
0211T	1(3)
0212T	1(3)
0213T	1(2)
0214T	1(2)
0215T	1(2)
0216T	1(2)
0217T	1(2)
0218T	1(2)
0219T	1(2)
0220T	1(2)
0221T	1(2)
0222T	1(3)
0223U	1(3)
0224U	3(3)
0228T	1(2)
0229T	2(3)
0230T	1(2)
0231T	2(3)
0232T	1(3)
0234T	2(2)
0235T	2(3)
0236T	1(2)
0237T	2(3)
0238T	2(3)
0253T	1(3)
0263T	1(3)
0264T	1(3)
0265T	1(3)
0266T	1(2)
0267T	1(3)
0268T	1(3)
0269T	1(2)
0270T	1(3)
0271T	1(3)
0272T	1(3)
0273T	1(3)
0274T	1(2)
0275T	1(2)
0278T	1(3)
0290T	1(3)
0295T	1(2)
0296T	1(2)
0297T	1(2)
0298T	1(2)

CPT	MUE
0308T	1(3)
0312T	1(3)
0313T	1(3)
0314T	1(3)
0315T	1(3)
0316T	1(3)
0317T	1(3)
0329T	0(3)
0330T	1(2)
0331T	1(3)
0332T	1(3)
0333T	0(3)
0335T	2(2)
0338T	1(2)
0339T	1(2)
0342T	1(3)
0345T	1(2)
0347T	1(3)
0348T	1(3)
0349T	1(3)
0350T	1(3)
0351T	5(3)
0352T	5(3)
0353T	2(3)
0354T	2(3)
0355T	1(2)
0356T	4(2)
0358T	1(2)
0362T	8(3)
0373T	24(3)
0376T	2(3)
0378T	1(2)
0379T	1(2)
0381T	1(2)
0382T	1(2)
0383T	1(2)
0384T	1(2)
0385T	1(2)
0386T	1(2)
0394T	2(3)
0395T	2(3)
0396T	2(2)
0397T	1(3)
0398T	1(3)
0400T	1(2)
0401T	1(2)
0402T	2(2)
0403T	0(3)
0404T	1(2)
0405T	1(2)
0408T	1(3)
0409T	1(3)
0410T	1(3)
0411T	1(3)
0412T	1(2)
0413T	1(3)
0414T	1(2)
0415T	1(3)
0416T	1(3)
0417T	1(3)
0418T	1(3)
0419T	1(2)
0420T	1(2)
0421T	1(2)

CPT	MUE
0422T	1(3)
0423T	1(3)
0424T	1(3)
0425T	1(3)
0426T	1(3)
0427T	1(3)
0428T	1(2)
0429T	1(2)
0430T	1(2)
0431T	1(2)
0432T	1(3)
0433T	1(3)
0434T	1(3)
0435T	1(3)
0436T	1(3)
0437T	1(3)
0439T	1(3)
0440T	3(3)
0441T	3(3)
0442T	3(3)
0443T	1(2)
0444T	1(2)
0445T	1(2)
0446T	1(3)
0447T	1(3)
0448T	1(3)
0449T	1(2)
0450T	1(3)
0451T	1(3)
0452T	1(3)
0453T	1(3)
0454T	3(3)
0455T	1(3)
0456T	1(3)
0457T	1(3)
0458T	3(3)
0459T	1(3)
0460T	3(3)
0461T	1(3)
0462T	1(2)
0463T	1(2)
0464T	1(2)
0465T	1(3)
0466T	1(3)
0467T	1(3)
0468T	1(3)
0469T	1(2)
0470T	1(2)
0471T	2(1)
0472T	1(2)
0473T	1(2)
0474T	0(3)
0475T	1(3)
0476T	1(3)
0477T	1(3)
0478T	1(3)
0479T	1(2)
0480T	4(1)
0481T	1(3)
0483T	1(2)
0484T	1(2)
0485T	1(2)
0486T	1(2)
0487T	1(3)

CPT	MUE
0488T	1(2)
0489T	1(2)
0490T	1(2)
0491T	1(2)
0492T	4(3)
0493T	1(3)
0494T	1(2)
0495T	1(2)
0496T	4(3)
0497T	1(3)
0498T	1(2)
0499T	1(2)
0500T	1(3)
0501T	1(2)
0502T	1(2)
0503T	1(2)
0504T	1(2)
0505T	1(3)
0506T	1(2)
0507T	1(2)
0508T	1(3)
0509T	1(2)
0510T	1(2)
0511T	1(2)
0512T	1(2)
0513T	2(3)
0514T	2(2)
0515T	1(3)
0516T	1(3)
0517T	1(3)
0518T	1(3)
0519T	1(3)
0520T	1(3)
0521T	1(3)
0522T	1(3)
0523T	1(3)
0524T	3(3)
0525T	1(3)
0526T	1(3)
0527T	1(3)
0528T	1(3)
0529T	1(3)
0530T	1(3)
0531T	1(3)
0532T	1(3)
0533T	1(2)
0534T	1(2)
0535T	1(2)
0536T	1(2)
0537T	1(2)
0538T	1(3)
0539T	1(3)
0540T	1(3)
0541T	1(3)
0542T	1(3)
0543T	1(2)
0544T	1(2)
0545T	1(2)
0546T	2(2)
0547T	1(2)
0548T	1(2)
0549T	1(2)
0550T	2(3)
0551T	1(2)

CPT	MUE
0552T	0(3)
0553T	0(3)
0554T	0(3)
0555T	1(2)
0556T	1(2)
0557T	0(3)
0558T	1(2)
0559T	1(2)
0560T	1(3)
0561T	1(2)
0562T	1(3)
0563T	1(2)
0564T	1(2)
0565T	1(2)
0566T	1(2)
0567T	1(2)
0568T	1(2)
0569T	1(2)
0570T	1(3)
0571T	1(2)
0572T	1(2)
0573T	1(2)
0574T	1(2)
0575T	1(2)
0576T	1(2)
0577T	1(2)
0578T	1(2)
0579T	1(2)
0580T	1(2)
0581T	0(3)
0582T	0(3)
0583T	2(2)
0584T	1(2)
0585T	1(2)
0586T	1(2)
0587T	1(2)
0588T	1(2)
0589T	1(2)
0590T	1(2)
0591T	1(2)
0592T	1(2)
0593T	1(2)
10004	3(3)
10005	1(2)
10006	3(3)
10007	1(2)
10008	2(3)
10009	1(2)
10010	3(3)
10011	1(2)
10012	3(3)
10021	1(2)
10030	2(3)
10035	1(2)
10036	3(3)
10040	1(2)
10060	1(2)
10061	1(2)
10080	1(3)
10081	1(3)
10120	3(3)
10121	2(3)
10140	2(3)
10160	3(3)

CPT	MUE
10180	2(3)
11000	1(2)
11001	1(3)
11004	1(2)
11005	1(2)
11006	1(2)
11008	1(2)
11010	2(3)
11011	2(3)
11012	2(3)
11042	1(2)
11043	1(2)
11044	1(2)
11045	12(3)
11046	4(3)
11047	4(3)
11055	1(2)
11056	1(2)
11057	1(2)
11102	1(2)
11103	6(3)
11104	1(2)
11105	3(3)
11106	1(2)
11107	2(3)
11200	1(2)
11201	1(3)
11300	5(3)
11301	6(3)
11302	4(3)
11303	3(3)
11305	4(3)
11306	4(3)
11307	3(3)
11308	2(3)
11310	4(3)
11311	4(3)
11312	3(3)
11313	3(3)
11400	3(3)
11401	3(3)
11402	3(3)
11403	2(3)
11404	2(3)
11406	2(3)
11420	3(3)
11421	3(3)
11422	3(3)
11423	2(3)
11424	2(3)
11426	2(3)
11440	4(3)
11441	3(3)
11442	3(3)
11443	2(3)
11444	2(3)
11446	2(3)
11450	1(2)
11451	1(2)
11462	1(2)
11463	1(2)
11470	3(2)
11471	2(3)
11600	2(3)
11601	2(3)
11602	3(3)
11603	2(3)
11604	2(3)
11606	2(3)
11620	2(3)
11621	2(3)
11622	2(3)
11623	2(3)
11624	2(3)
11626	2(3)
11640	2(3)
11641	2(3)
11642	3(3)
11643	2(3)
11644	2(3)
11646	2(3)
11719	1(2)
11720	1(2)
11721	1(2)
11730	1(2)
11732	4(3)
11740	2(3)
11750	6(3)
11755	2(3)
11760	4(3)
11762	2(3)
11765	4(3)
11770	1(3)
11771	1(3)
11772	1(3)
11900	1(2)
11901	1(2)
11920	1(2)
11921	1(2)
11922	1(3)
11950	1(2)
11951	1(2)
11952	1(2)
11954	1(3)
11960	2(3)
11970	2(3)
11971	2(3)
11976	1(2)
11980	1(2)
11981	1(3)
11982	1(3)
11983	1(3)
12001	1(2)
12002	1(2)
12004	1(2)
12005	1(2)
12006	1(2)
12007	1(2)
12011	1(2)
12013	1(2)
12014	1(2)
12015	1(2)
12016	1(2)
12017	1(2)
12018	1(2)
12020	2(3)
12021	3(3)
12031	1(2)
12032	1(2)
12034	1(2)
12035	1(2)
12036	1(2)
12037	1(2)
12041	1(2)
12042	1(2)
12044	1(2)
12045	1(2)
12046	1(2)
12047	1(2)
12051	1(2)
12052	1(2)
12053	1(2)
12054	1(2)
12055	1(2)
12056	1(2)
12057	1(2)
13100	1(2)
13101	1(2)
13102	9(3)
13120	1(2)
13121	1(2)
13122	9(3)
13131	1(2)
13132	1(2)
13133	7(3)
13151	1(2)
13152	1(2)
13153	2(3)
13160	2(3)
14000	2(3)
14001	2(3)
14020	2(3)
14021	2(3)
14040	2(3)
14041	3(3)
14060	2(3)
14061	2(3)
14301	2(3)
14302	8(3)
14350	2(3)
15002	1(2)
15003	9(3)
15004	1(2)
15005	2(3)
15040	1(2)
15050	1(3)
15100	1(2)
15101	9(3)
15110	1(2)
15111	2(3)
15115	1(2)
15116	2(3)
15120	1(2)
15121	5(3)
15130	1(2)
15131	2(3)
15135	1(2)
15136	1(3)
15150	1(2)
15151	1(2)
15152	2(3)
15155	1(2)
15156	1(2)
15157	1(3)
15200	1(2)
15201	7(3)
15220	1(2)
15221	9(3)
15240	1(2)
15241	9(3)
15260	1(2)
15261	6(3)
15271	1(2)
15272	3(3)
15273	1(2)
15274	6(3)
15275	1(2)
15276	3(2)
15277	1(2)
15278	3(3)
15570	2(3)
15572	2(3)
15574	2(3)
15576	2(3)
15600	2(3)
15610	2(3)
15620	2(3)
15630	2(3)
15650	1(3)
15730	1(3)
15731	1(3)
15733	2(3)
15734	4(3)
15736	2(3)
15738	3(3)
15740	2(3)
15750	2(3)
15756	2(3)
15757	2(3)
15758	2(3)
15760	2(3)
15769	1(3)
15770	2(3)
15771	1(2)
15772	9(3)
15773	1(2)
15774	3(3)
15775	1(2)
15776	1(2)
15777	1(3)
15780	1(2)
15781	1(3)
15782	1(3)
15783	1(3)
15786	1(2)
15787	2(3)
15788	1(2)
15789	1(2)
15792	1(3)
15793	1(3)
15819	1(2)
15820	1(2)
15821	1(2)
15822	1(2)
15823	1(2)
15824	1(2)
15825	1(2)
15826	1(2)
15828	1(2)
15829	1(2)
15830	1(2)
15832	1(2)
15833	1(2)
15834	1(2)
15835	1(3)
15836	1(2)
15837	2(3)
15838	1(2)
15839	2(3)
15840	1(3)
15841	2(3)
15842	2(3)
15845	2(3)
15847	1(2)
15850	1(2)
15851	1(2)
15852	1(3)
15860	1(3)
15876	1(2)
15877	1(2)
15878	1(2)
15879	1(2)
15920	1(3)
15922	1(3)
15931	1(3)
15933	1(3)
15934	1(3)
15935	1(3)
15936	1(3)
15937	1(3)
15940	2(3)
15941	2(3)
15944	2(3)
15945	2(3)
15946	2(3)
15950	2(3)
15951	2(3)
15952	2(3)
15953	2(3)
15956	2(3)
15958	2(3)
15999	1(3)
16000	1(2)
16020	1(3)
16025	1(3)
16030	1(3)
16035	1(2)
16036	2(3)
17000	1(2)
17003	13(2)
17004	1(2)
17106	1(2)
17107	1(2)
17108	1(2)
17110	1(2)
17111	1(2)
17250	4(3)
17260	7(3)
17261	7(3)
17262	6(3)
17263	3(3)
17264	3(3)
17266	2(3)
17270	6(3)
17271	4(3)
17272	5(3)
17273	4(3)
17274	2(3)
17276	2(3)
17280	6(3)
17281	5(3)
17282	4(3)
17283	4(3)
17284	2(3)
17286	2(3)
17311	4(3)
17312	6(3)
17313	3(3)
17314	4(3)
17315	15(3)
17340	1(2)
17360	1(2)
17380	1(3)
17999	1(3)
19000	2(3)
19001	5(3)
19020	2(3)
19030	1(2)
19081	1(2)
19082	2(3)
19083	1(2)
19084	2(3)
19085	1(2)
19086	2(3)
19100	4(3)
19101	3(3)
19105	2(3)
19110	1(3)
19112	2(3)
19120	1(2)
19125	1(2)
19126	3(3)
19281	1(2)
19282	2(3)
19283	1(2)
19284	2(3)
19285	1(2)
19286	2(3)
19287	1(2)
19288	2(3)
19294	2(3)
19296	1(3)
19297	2(3)
19298	1(2)
19300	1(2)
19301	1(2)
19302	1(2)
19303	1(2)
19305	1(2)
19306	1(2)
19307	1(2)
19316	1(2)
19318	1(2)
19324	1(2)
19325	1(2)
19328	1(2)
19330	1(2)
19340	1(2)
19342	1(2)
19350	1(2)
19355	1(2)
19357	1(2)
19361	1(2)
19364	1(2)
19366	1(2)
19367	1(2)
19368	1(2)
19369	1(2)
19370	1(2)
19371	1(2)
19380	1(2)
19396	1(2)
19499	1(3)
20100	2(3)
20101	2(3)
20102	3(3)
20103	3(3)
20150	2(3)
20200	2(3)
20205	3(3)
20206	3(3)
20220	3(3)
20225	2(3)
20240	4(3)
20245	3(3)
20250	1(3)
20251	2(3)
20500	2(3)
20501	2(3)
20520	2(3)
20525	4(3)
20526	1(2)
20527	2(3)
20550	5(3)
20551	5(3)
20552	1(2)
20553	1(2)
20555	1(3)
20560	1(2)
20561	1(2)
20600	6(3)
20604	4(3)
20605	2(3)
20606	2(3)
20610	2(3)
20611	2(3)
20612	2(3)
20615	1(3)
20650	4(3)
20660	1(2)
20661	1(2)
20662	1(2)
20663	1(2)
20664	1(2)
20665	1(2)
20670	3(3)
20680	3(3)
20690	2(3)
20692	2(3)
20693	2(3)
20694	2(3)
20696	2(3)
20697	4(3)
20700	1(3)
20701	1(3)
20702	1(3)
20703	1(3)
20704	1(3)
20705	1(3)
20802	1(2)
20805	1(2)
20808	1(2)
20816	3(3)
20822	3(3)
20824	1(2)
20827	1(2)
20838	1(2)
20900	2(3)
20902	2(3)
20910	1(3)
20912	1(3)
20920	1(3)
20922	1(3)
20924	2(3)
20930	1(3)
20931	1(2)
20932	1(3)
20933	1(3)
20934	1(3)
20936	1(3)
20937	1(2)
20938	1(2)
20939	1(3)
20950	2(3)
20955	1(3)
20956	1(3)
20957	1(3)
20962	1(3)
20969	2(3)
20970	1(3)
20972	2(3)
20973	1(2)
20974	1(3)
20975	1(3)
20979	1(3)
20982	1(2)
20983	1(2)
20985	2(3)
20999	1(3)
21010	1(2)
21011	4(3)
21012	3(3)
21013	2(3)
21014	2(3)
21015	1(3)
21016	2(3)
21025	2(3)
21026	2(3)
21029	1(3)
21030	1(3)
21031	2(3)
21032	1(3)
21034	1(3)
21040	2(3)
21044	1(3)
21045	1(3)
21046	2(3)
21047	2(3)
21048	2(3)
21049	1(3)

CPT	MUE	CPT	MUE	CPT	MUE	CPT	MUE	CPT	MUE	CPT	MUE	CPT	MUE	CPT	MUE
21050	1(2)	21243	1(2)	21452	1(2)	22116	3(3)	22846	1(3)	23195	1(2)	23900	1(2)	24365	1(2)
21060	1(2)	21244	1(2)	21453	1(2)	22206	1(2)	22847	1(3)	23200	1(3)	23920	1(2)	24366	1(2)
21070	1(2)	21245	2(2)	21454	1(2)	22207	1(2)	22848	1(2)	23210	1(3)	23921	1(2)	24370	1(2)
21073	1(2)	21246	2(2)	21461	1(2)	22208	5(3)	22849	1(2)	23220	1(3)	23929	1(3)	24371	1(2)
21076	1(2)	21247	1(2)	21462	1(2)	22210	1(2)	22850	1(2)	23330	2(3)	23930	2(3)	24400	1(3)
21077	1(2)	21248	2(3)	21465	1(2)	22212	1(2)	22852	1(2)	23333	1(3)	23931	2(3)	24410	1(2)
21079	1(2)	21249	2(3)	21470	1(2)	22214	1(2)	22853	4(3)	23334	1(2)	23935	2(3)	24420	1(2)
21080	1(2)	21255	1(2)	21480	1(2)	22216	6(3)	22854	4(3)	23335	1(2)	24000	1(2)	24430	1(3)
21081	1(2)	21256	1(2)	21485	1(2)	22220	1(2)	22855	1(2)	23350	1(2)	24006	1(2)	24435	1(3)
21082	1(2)	21260	1(2)	21490	1(2)	22222	1(2)	22856	1(2)	23395	1(2)	24065	2(3)	24470	1(2)
21083	1(2)	21261	1(2)	21497	1(2)	22224	1(2)	22857	1(2)	23397	1(3)	24066	2(3)	24495	1(2)
21084	1(2)	21263	1(2)	21499	1(3)	22226	4(3)	22858	1(2)	23400	1(2)	24071	2(3)	24498	1(2)
21085	1(3)	21267	1(2)	21501	3(3)	22310	1(2)	22859	4(3)	23405	2(3)	24073	2(3)	24500	1(2)
21086	1(2)	21268	1(2)	21502	1(3)	22315	1(2)	22861	1(2)	23406	1(3)	24075	5(3)	24505	1(2)
21087	1(2)	21270	1(2)	21510	1(3)	22318	1(2)	22862	1(2)	23410	1(2)	24076	4(3)	24515	1(2)
21088	1(2)	21275	1(2)	21550	2(3)	22319	1(2)	22864	1(2)	23412	1(2)	24077	1(3)	24516	1(2)
21089	1(3)	21280	1(2)	21552	2(3)	22325	1(2)	22865	1(2)	23415	1(2)	24079	1(3)	24530	1(2)
21100	1(2)	21282	1(2)	21554	2(3)	22326	1(2)	22867	1(2)	23420	1(2)	24100	1(2)	24535	1(2)
21110	2(3)	21295	1(2)	21555	2(3)	22327	1(2)	22868	1(2)	23430	1(2)	24101	1(2)	24538	1(2)
21116	1(2)	21296	1(2)	21556	2(3)	22328	6(3)	22869	1(2)	23440	1(2)	24102	1(2)	24545	1(2)
21120	1(2)	21299	1(3)	21557	1(3)	22505	1(2)	22870	1(2)	23450	1(2)	24105	1(2)	24546	1(2)
21121	1(2)	21310	1(2)	21558	1(3)	22510	1(2)	22899	1(3)	23455	1(2)	24110	1(3)	24560	1(3)
21122	1(2)	21315	1(2)	21600	5(3)	22511	1(2)	22900	3(3)	23460	1(2)	24115	1(3)	24565	1(3)
21123	1(2)	21320	1(2)	21601	2(3)	22512	3(3)	22901	2(3)	23462	1(2)	24116	1(3)	24566	1(3)
21125	2(2)	21325	1(2)	21602	1(3)	22513	1(2)	22902	4(3)	23465	1(2)	24120	1(3)	24575	1(3)
21127	2(3)	21330	1(2)	21603	1(3)	22514	1(2)	22903	3(3)	23466	1(2)	24125	1(3)	24576	1(3)
21137	1(2)	21335	1(2)	21610	1(3)	22515	4(3)	22904	1(3)	23470	1(2)	24126	1(3)	24577	1(3)
21138	1(2)	21336	1(2)	21615	1(2)	22526	0(3)	22905	1(3)	23472	1(2)	24130	1(2)	24579	1(3)
21139	1(2)	21337	1(2)	21616	1(2)	22527	0(3)	22999	1(3)	23473	1(2)	24134	1(3)	24582	1(3)
21141	1(2)	21338	1(2)	21620	1(2)	22532	1(2)	23000	1(2)	23474	1(2)	24136	1(3)	24586	1(3)
21142	1(2)	21339	1(2)	21627	1(2)	22533	1(2)	23020	1(2)	23480	1(2)	24138	1(3)	24587	1(2)
21143	1(2)	21340	1(2)	21630	1(2)	22534	3(3)	23030	2(3)	23485	1(2)	24140	1(3)	24600	1(2)
21145	1(2)	21343	1(2)	21632	1(2)	22548	1(2)	23031	1(3)	23490	1(2)	24145	1(3)	24605	1(2)
21146	1(2)	21344	1(2)	21685	1(2)	22551	1(2)	23035	1(3)	23491	1(2)	24147	1(2)	24615	1(2)
21147	1(2)	21345	1(2)	21700	1(2)	22552	5(3)	23040	1(2)	23500	1(2)	24149	1(2)	24620	1(2)
21150	1(2)	21346	1(2)	21705	1(2)	22554	1(2)	23044	1(3)	23505	1(2)	24150	1(3)	24635	1(2)
21151	1(2)	21347	1(2)	21720	1(3)	22556	1(2)	23065	2(3)	23515	1(2)	24152	1(3)	24640	1(2)
21154	1(2)	21348	1(2)	21725	1(3)	22558	1(2)	23066	2(3)	23520	1(2)	24155	1(2)	24650	1(2)
21155	1(2)	21355	1(2)	21740	1(2)	22585	5(3)	23071	2(3)	23525	1(2)	24160	1(2)	24655	1(2)
21159	1(2)	21356	1(2)	21742	1(2)	22586	1(2)	23073	2(3)	23530	1(2)	24164	1(2)	24665	1(2)
21160	1(2)	21360	1(2)	21743	1(2)	22590	1(2)	23075	2(3)	23532	1(2)	24200	3(3)	24666	1(2)
21172	1(3)	21365	1(2)	21750	1(2)	22595	1(2)	23076	2(3)	23540	1(2)	24201	3(3)	24670	1(2)
21175	1(2)	21366	1(2)	21811	1(2)	22600	1(2)	23077	1(3)	23545	1(2)	24220	1(2)	24675	1(2)
21179	1(2)	21385	1(2)	21812	1(2)	22610	1(2)	23078	1(3)	23550	1(2)	24300	1(2)	24685	1(2)
21180	1(2)	21386	1(2)	21813	1(2)	22612	1(2)	23100	1(2)	23552	1(2)	24301	2(3)	24800	1(2)
21181	1(3)	21387	1(2)	21820	1(2)	22614	13(3)	23101	1(3)	23570	1(2)	24305	4(3)	24802	1(2)
21182	1(2)	21390	1(2)	21825	1(2)	22630	1(2)	23105	1(2)	23575	1(2)	24310	2(3)	24900	1(2)
21183	1(2)	21395	1(2)	21899	1(3)	22632	4(2)	23106	1(2)	23585	1(2)	24320	2(3)	24920	1(2)
21184	1(2)	21400	1(2)	21920	2(3)	22633	1(2)	23107	1(2)	23600	1(2)	24330	1(3)	24925	1(2)
21188	1(2)	21401	1(2)	21925	2(3)	22634	4(2)	23120	1(2)	23605	1(2)	24331	1(3)	24930	1(2)
21193	1(2)	21406	1(2)	21930	5(3)	22800	1(2)	23125	1(2)	23615	1(2)	24332	1(2)	24931	1(2)
21194	1(2)	21407	1(2)	21931	3(3)	22802	1(2)	23130	1(2)	23616	1(2)	24340	1(2)	24935	1(2)
21195	1(2)	21408	1(2)	21932	2(3)	22804	1(2)	23140	1(3)	23620	1(2)	24341	2(3)	24940	1(2)
21196	1(2)	21421	1(2)	21933	2(3)	22808	1(2)	23145	1(3)	23625	1(2)	24342	2(3)	24999	1(3)
21198	1(3)	21422	1(2)	21935	1(3)	22810	1(2)	23146	1(3)	23630	1(2)	24343	1(2)	25000	2(3)
21199	1(2)	21423	1(2)	21936	1(3)	22812	1(2)	23150	1(3)	23650	1(2)	24344	1(2)	25001	1(3)
21206	1(3)	21431	1(2)	22010	2(3)	22818	1(2)	23155	1(3)	23655	1(2)	24345	1(2)	25020	1(2)
21208	1(3)	21432	1(2)	22015	2(3)	22819	1(2)	23156	1(3)	23660	1(2)	24346	1(2)	25023	1(2)
21209	1(3)	21433	1(2)	22100	1(2)	22830	1(2)	23170	1(3)	23665	1(2)	24357	1(3)	25024	1(2)
21210	2(3)	21435	1(2)	22101	1(2)	22840	1(3)	23172	1(3)	23670	1(2)	24358	1(3)	25025	1(2)
21215	2(3)	21436	1(2)	22102	1(2)	22841	0(3)	23174	1(3)	23675	1(2)	24359	2(3)	25028	4(3)
21230	2(3)	21440	2(2)	22103	3(3)	22842	1(3)	23180	1(3)	23680	1(2)	24360	1(2)	25031	2(3)
21235	2(3)	21445	2(2)	22110	1(2)	22843	1(3)	23182	1(3)	23700	1(2)	24361	1(2)	25035	2(3)
21240	1(2)	21450	1(2)	22112	1(2)	22844	1(3)	23184	1(3)	23800	1(2)	24362	1(2)	25040	1(3)
21242	1(2)	21451	1(2)	22114	1(2)	22845	1(3)	23190	1(3)	23802	1(2)	24363	1(2)	25065	2(3)

CPT	MUE	CPT	MUE	CPT	MUE	CPT	MUE	CPT	MUE	CPT	MUE	CPT	MUE	CPT	MUE
25066	2(3)	25390	1(2)	25805	1(2)	26350	6(3)	26550	1(2)	26989	1(3)	27158	1(2)	27325	1(2)
25071	3(3)	25391	1(2)	25810	1(2)	26352	2(3)	26551	1(2)	26990	2(3)	27161	1(2)	27326	1(2)
25073	2(3)	25392	1(2)	25820	1(2)	26356	4(3)	26553	1(3)	26991	1(3)	27165	1(2)	27327	5(3)
25075	6(3)	25393	1(2)	25825	1(2)	26357	2(3)	26554	1(3)	26992	2(3)	27170	1(2)	27328	3(3)
25076	3(3)	25394	1(3)	25830	1(2)	26358	2(3)	26555	2(3)	27000	1(3)	27175	1(2)	27329	1(3)
25077	1(3)	25400	1(2)	25900	1(2)	26370	3(3)	26556	2(3)	27001	1(3)	27176	1(2)	27330	1(2)
25078	1(3)	25405	1(2)	25905	1(2)	26372	1(3)	26560	2(3)	27003	1(2)	27177	1(2)	27331	1(2)
25085	1(2)	25415	1(2)	25907	1(2)	26373	2(3)	26561	2(3)	27005	1(2)	27178	1(2)	27332	1(2)
25100	1(2)	25420	1(2)	25909	1(2)	26390	2(3)	26562	2(3)	27006	1(2)	27179	1(2)	27333	1(2)
25101	1(2)	25425	1(2)	25915	1(2)	26392	2(3)	26565	2(3)	27025	1(3)	27181	1(2)	27334	1(2)
25105	1(2)	25426	1(2)	25920	1(2)	26410	4(3)	26567	3(3)	27027	1(2)	27185	1(2)	27335	1(2)
25107	1(2)	25430	1(3)	25922	1(2)	26412	3(3)	26568	2(3)	27030	1(2)	27187	1(2)	27337	3(3)
25109	4(3)	25431	1(3)	25924	1(2)	26415	2(3)	26580	1(2)	27033	1(2)	27197	1(2)	27339	4(3)
25110	2(3)	25440	1(2)	25927	1(2)	26416	2(3)	26587	2(3)	27035	1(2)	27198	1(2)	27340	1(2)
25111	1(3)	25441	1(2)	25929	1(2)	26418	4(3)	26590	2(3)	27036	1(2)	27200	1(2)	27345	1(2)
25112	1(3)	25442	1(2)	25931	1(2)	26420	3(3)	26591	4(3)	27040	2(3)	27202	1(2)	27347	1(2)
25115	1(3)	25443	1(2)	25999	1(3)	26426	4(3)	26593	8(3)	27041	3(3)	27215	0(3)	27350	1(2)
25116	1(3)	25444	1(2)	26010	2(3)	26428	2(3)	26596	1(3)	27043	2(3)	27216	0(3)	27355	1(3)
25118	5(3)	25445	1(2)	26011	3(3)	26432	2(3)	26600	2(3)	27045	3(3)	27217	0(3)	27356	1(3)
25119	1(2)	25446	1(2)	26020	4(3)	26433	2(3)	26605	3(3)	27047	2(3)	27218	0(3)	27357	1(3)
25120	1(3)	25447	4(3)	26025	1(2)	26434	2(3)	26607	2(3)	27048	2(3)	27220	1(2)	27358	1(3)
25125	1(3)	25449	1(2)	26030	1(2)	26437	4(3)	26608	4(3)	27049	1(3)	27222	1(2)	27360	2(3)
25126	1(3)	25450	1(2)	26034	2(3)	26440	6(3)	26615	3(3)	27050	1(2)	27226	1(2)	27364	1(3)
25130	1(3)	25455	1(2)	26035	1(3)	26442	5(3)	26641	1(2)	27052	1(2)	27227	1(2)	27365	1(3)
25135	1(3)	25490	1(2)	26037	1(3)	26445	5(3)	26645	1(2)	27054	1(2)	27228	1(2)	27369	1(2)
25136	1(3)	25491	1(2)	26040	1(2)	26449	5(3)	26650	1(2)	27057	1(2)	27230	1(2)	27372	2(3)
25145	1(3)	25492	1(2)	26045	1(2)	26450	6(3)	26665	1(2)	27059	1(3)	27232	1(2)	27380	1(2)
25150	1(3)	25500	1(2)	26055	5(3)	26455	6(3)	26670	2(3)	27060	1(2)	27235	1(2)	27381	1(2)
25151	1(3)	25505	1(2)	26060	5(3)	26460	4(3)	26675	1(3)	27062	1(2)	27236	1(2)	27385	2(3)
25170	1(3)	25515	1(2)	26070	2(3)	26471	4(3)	26676	2(3)	27065	1(3)	27238	1(2)	27386	2(3)
25210	2(3)	25520	1(2)	26075	3(3)	26474	4(3)	26685	3(3)	27066	1(3)	27240	1(2)	27390	1(2)
25215	1(2)	25525	1(2)	26080	3(3)	26476	4(3)	26686	3(3)	27067	1(3)	27244	1(2)	27391	1(2)
25230	1(2)	25526	1(2)	26100	1(3)	26477	2(3)	26700	2(3)	27070	1(3)	27245	1(2)	27392	1(2)
25240	1(2)	25530	1(2)	26105	2(3)	26478	6(3)	26705	3(3)	27071	1(3)	27246	1(2)	27393	1(2)
25246	1(2)	25535	1(2)	26110	2(3)	26479	4(3)	26706	2(3)	27075	1(3)	27248	1(2)	27394	1(2)
25248	3(3)	25545	1(2)	26111	4(3)	26480	4(3)	26715	3(3)	27076	1(2)	27250	1(2)	27395	1(2)
25250	1(2)	25560	1(2)	26113	3(3)	26483	4(3)	26720	4(3)	27077	1(2)	27252	1(2)	27396	1(2)
25251	1(2)	25565	1(2)	26115	4(3)	26485	4(3)	26725	3(3)	27078	1(2)	27253	1(2)	27397	1(2)
25259	1(2)	25574	1(2)	26116	2(3)	26489	2(3)	26727	3(3)	27080	1(2)	27254	1(2)	27400	1(2)
25260	7(3)	25575	1(2)	26117	2(3)	26490	3(3)	26735	4(3)	27086	1(3)	27256	1(2)	27403	1(3)
25263	4(3)	25600	1(2)	26118	1(3)	26492	2(3)	26740	3(3)	27087	1(3)	27257	1(2)	27405	2(2)
25265	4(3)	25605	1(2)	26121	1(2)	26494	1(3)	26742	3(3)	27090	1(2)	27258	1(2)	27407	2(2)
25270	8(3)	25606	1(2)	26123	1(2)	26496	1(3)	26746	3(3)	27091	1(2)	27259	1(2)	27409	1(2)
25272	4(3)	25607	1(2)	26125	4(3)	26497	2(3)	26750	3(3)	27093	1(2)	27265	1(2)	27412	1(2)
25274	4(3)	25608	1(2)	26130	1(3)	26498	1(3)	26755	2(3)	27095	1(2)	27266	1(2)	27415	1(2)
25275	2(3)	25609	1(2)	26135	4(3)	26499	2(3)	26756	2(3)	27096	1(2)	27267	1(2)	27416	1(2)
25280	9(3)	25622	1(2)	26140	2(3)	26500	3(3)	26765	3(3)	27097	1(3)	27268	1(2)	27418	1(2)
25290	10(3)	25624	1(2)	26145	6(3)	26502	2(3)	26770	3(3)	27098	1(2)	27269	1(2)	27420	1(2)
25295	9(3)	25628	1(2)	26160	4(3)	26508	1(2)	26775	2(3)	27100	1(2)	27275	2(2)	27422	1(2)
25300	1(2)	25630	1(3)	26170	4(3)	26510	4(3)	26776	4(3)	27105	1(3)	27279	1(2)	27424	1(2)
25301	1(2)	25635	1(3)	26180	4(3)	26516	1(2)	26785	3(3)	27110	1(2)	27280	1(2)	27425	1(2)
25310	5(3)	25645	1(3)	26185	1(3)	26517	1(2)	26820	1(2)	27111	1(2)	27282	1(2)	27427	1(2)
25312	4(3)	25650	1(2)	26200	2(3)	26518	1(2)	26841	1(2)	27120	1(2)	27284	1(2)	27428	1(2)
25315	1(3)	25651	1(2)	26205	1(3)	26520	4(3)	26842	1(2)	27122	1(2)	27286	1(2)	27429	1(2)
25316	1(3)	25652	1(2)	26210	2(3)	26525	4(3)	26843	2(3)	27125	1(2)	27290	1(2)	27430	1(2)
25320	1(2)	25660	1(2)	26215	2(3)	26530	4(3)	26844	2(3)	27130	1(2)	27295	1(2)	27435	1(2)
25332	1(2)	25670	1(2)	26230	2(3)	26531	4(3)	26850	5(3)	27132	1(2)	27299	1(3)	27437	1(2)
25335	1(2)	25671	1(2)	26235	2(3)	26535	3(3)	26852	2(3)	27134	1(2)	27301	3(3)	27438	1(2)
25337	1(2)	25675	1(2)	26236	2(3)	26536	4(3)	26860	1(2)	27137	1(2)	27303	2(3)	27440	1(2)
25350	1(3)	25676	1(2)	26250	2(3)	26540	4(3)	26861	4(3)	27138	1(2)	27305	1(2)	27441	1(2)
25355	1(3)	25680	1(2)	26260	1(3)	26541	4(3)	26862	1(2)	27140	1(2)	27306	1(2)	27442	1(2)
25360	1(3)	25685	1(2)	26262	1(3)	26542	4(3)	26863	2(3)	27146	1(3)	27307	1(2)	27443	1(2)
25365	1(3)	25690	1(2)	26320	4(3)	26545	4(3)	26910	4(3)	27147	1(3)	27310	1(2)	27445	1(2)
25370	1(2)	25695	1(2)	26340	4(3)	26546	2(3)	26951	8(3)	27151	1(3)	27323	2(3)	27446	1(2)
25375	1(2)	25800	1(2)	26341	2(3)	26548	3(3)	26952	4(3)	27156	1(2)	27324	3(3)	27447	1(2)

CPT	MUE
27448	1(3)
27450	1(3)
27454	1(2)
27455	1(3)
27457	1(3)
27465	1(2)
27466	1(2)
27468	1(2)
27470	1(2)
27472	1(2)
27475	1(2)
27477	1(2)
27479	1(2)
27485	1(2)
27486	1(2)
27487	1(2)
27488	1(2)
27495	1(2)
27496	1(2)
27497	1(2)
27498	1(2)
27499	1(2)
27500	1(2)
27501	1(2)
27502	1(2)
27503	1(2)
27506	1(2)
27507	1(2)
27508	1(2)
27509	1(2)
27510	1(2)
27511	1(2)
27513	1(2)
27514	1(2)
27516	1(2)
27517	1(2)
27519	1(2)
27520	1(2)
27524	1(2)
27530	1(2)
27532	1(2)
27535	1(2)
27536	1(2)
27538	1(2)
27540	1(2)
27550	1(2)
27552	1(2)
27556	1(2)
27557	1(2)
27558	1(2)
27560	1(2)
27562	1(2)
27566	1(2)
27570	1(2)
27580	1(2)
27590	1(2)
27591	1(2)
27592	1(2)
27594	1(2)
27596	1(2)
27598	1(2)
27599	1(3)
27600	1(2)
27601	1(2)
27602	1(2)

CPT	MUE
27603	2(3)
27604	2(3)
27605	1(2)
27606	1(2)
27607	2(3)
27610	1(2)
27612	1(2)
27613	3(3)
27614	3(3)
27615	1(3)
27616	1(3)
27618	3(3)
27619	2(3)
27620	1(2)
27625	1(2)
27626	1(2)
27630	2(3)
27632	3(3)
27634	2(3)
27635	1(3)
27637	1(3)
27638	1(3)
27640	1(3)
27641	1(3)
27645	1(3)
27646	1(3)
27647	1(3)
27648	1(2)
27650	1(2)
27652	1(2)
27654	1(2)
27656	1(3)
27658	2(3)
27659	2(3)
27664	2(3)
27665	2(3)
27675	1(2)
27676	1(2)
27680	2(3)
27681	1(2)
27685	2(3)
27686	3(3)
27687	1(2)
27690	2(3)
27691	2(3)
27692	4(3)
27695	1(2)
27696	1(2)
27698	2(2)
27700	1(2)
27702	1(2)
27703	1(2)
27704	1(2)
27705	1(3)
27707	1(3)
27709	1(3)
27712	1(2)
27715	1(2)
27720	1(2)
27722	1(2)
27724	1(2)
27725	1(2)
27726	1(2)
27727	1(2)
27730	1(2)

CPT	MUE
27732	1(2)
27734	1(2)
27740	1(2)
27742	1(2)
27745	1(2)
27750	1(2)
27752	1(2)
27756	1(2)
27758	1(2)
27759	1(2)
27760	1(2)
27762	1(2)
27766	1(2)
27767	1(2)
27768	1(2)
27769	1(2)
27780	1(2)
27781	1(2)
27784	1(2)
27786	1(2)
27788	1(2)
27792	1(2)
27808	1(2)
27810	1(2)
27814	1(2)
27816	1(2)
27818	1(2)
27822	1(2)
27823	1(2)
27824	1(2)
27825	1(2)
27826	1(2)
27827	1(2)
27828	1(2)
27829	1(2)
27830	1(2)
27831	1(2)
27832	1(2)
27840	1(2)
27842	1(2)
27846	1(2)
27848	1(2)
27860	1(2)
27870	1(2)
27871	1(3)
27880	1(2)
27881	1(2)
27882	1(2)
27884	1(2)
27886	1(2)
27888	1(2)
27889	1(2)
27892	1(2)
27893	1(2)
27894	1(2)
27899	1(3)
28001	2(3)
28002	3(3)
28003	2(3)
28005	3(3)
28008	2(3)
28010	4(3)
28011	4(3)
28020	2(3)
28022	3(3)

CPT	MUE
28024	4(3)
28035	1(2)
28039	2(3)
28041	2(3)
28043	4(3)
28045	4(3)
28046	1(3)
28047	1(3)
28050	2(3)
28052	2(3)
28054	2(3)
28055	1(3)
28060	1(2)
28062	1(2)
28070	2(3)
28072	4(3)
28080	3(3)
28086	2(3)
28088	2(3)
28090	2(3)
28092	2(3)
28100	1(3)
28102	1(3)
28103	1(3)
28104	2(3)
28106	1(3)
28107	1(3)
28108	2(3)
28110	1(2)
28111	1(2)
28112	4(3)
28113	1(2)
28114	1(2)
28116	1(2)
28118	1(2)
28119	1(2)
28120	2(3)
28122	4(3)
28124	4(3)
28126	4(3)
28130	1(2)
28140	3(3)
28150	4(3)
28153	4(3)
28160	5(3)
28171	1(3)
28173	2(3)
28175	2(3)
28190	3(3)
28192	2(3)
28193	2(3)
28200	4(3)
28202	2(3)
28208	4(3)
28210	2(3)
28220	1(2)
28222	1(2)
28225	1(2)
28226	1(2)
28230	1(2)
28232	6(3)
28234	6(3)
28238	1(2)
28240	1(2)
28250	1(2)

CPT	MUE
28260	1(2)
28261	1(3)
28262	1(2)
28264	1(2)
28270	6(3)
28272	6(3)
28280	1(2)
28285	4(3)
28286	1(2)
28288	4(3)
28289	1(2)
28291	1(2)
28292	1(2)
28295	1(2)
28296	1(2)
28297	1(2)
28298	1(2)
28299	1(2)
28300	1(2)
28302	1(2)
28304	1(3)
28305	1(3)
28306	1(2)
28307	1(2)
28308	4(3)
28309	1(2)
28310	1(2)
28312	4(3)
28313	4(3)
28315	1(2)
28320	1(2)
28322	2(3)
28340	2(3)
28341	2(3)
28344	1(2)
28345	2(3)
28360	1(2)
28400	1(2)
28405	1(2)
28406	1(2)
28415	1(2)
28420	1(2)
28430	1(2)
28435	1(2)
28436	1(2)
28445	1(2)
28446	1(2)
28450	2(3)
28455	3(3)
28456	2(3)
28465	3(3)
28470	2(3)
28475	5(3)
28476	4(3)
28485	5(3)
28490	1(2)
28495	1(2)
28496	1(2)
28505	1(2)
28510	4(3)
28515	4(3)
28525	4(3)
28530	1(2)
28531	1(2)
28540	1(3)

CPT	MUE
28545	1(3)
28546	1(3)
28555	1(3)
28570	1(2)
28575	1(2)
28576	1(2)
28585	1(3)
28600	2(3)
28605	2(3)
28606	3(3)
28615	5(3)
28630	2(3)
28635	2(3)
28636	4(3)
28645	4(3)
28660	4(3)
28665	3(3)
28666	4(3)
28675	3(3)
28705	1(2)
28715	1(2)
28725	1(2)
28730	1(2)
28735	1(2)
28737	1(2)
28740	1(2)
28750	1(2)
28755	1(2)
28760	1(2)
28800	1(2)
28805	1(2)
28810	5(3)
28820	6(3)
28825	8(2)
28890	1(2)
28899	1(3)
29000	1(3)
29010	1(3)
29015	1(3)
29035	1(3)
29040	1(3)
29044	1(3)
29046	1(3)
29049	1(3)
29055	1(3)
29058	1(3)
29065	1(3)
29075	1(3)
29085	1(3)
29086	2(3)
29105	1(2)
29125	1(2)
29126	1(2)
29130	3(3)
29131	2(3)
29200	1(2)
29240	1(2)
29260	1(3)
29280	2(3)
29305	1(3)
29325	1(3)
29345	1(3)
29355	1(3)
29358	1(3)
29365	1(3)

CPT	MUE
29405	1(3)
29425	1(3)
29435	1(3)
29440	1(2)
29445	1(3)
29450	1(3)
29505	1(2)
29515	1(2)
29520	1(2)
29530	1(2)
29540	1(2)
29550	1(2)
29580	1(2)
29581	1(2)
29584	1(2)
29700	2(3)
29705	1(3)
29710	1(2)
29720	1(2)
29730	1(3)
29740	1(3)
29750	1(3)
29799	1(3)
29800	1(2)
29804	1(2)
29805	1(2)
29806	1(2)
29807	1(2)
29819	1(2)
29820	1(2)
29821	1(2)
29822	1(2)
29823	1(2)
29824	1(2)
29825	1(2)
29826	1(2)
29827	1(2)
29828	1(2)
29830	1(2)
29834	1(2)
29835	1(2)
29836	1(2)
29837	1(2)
29838	1(2)
29840	1(2)
29843	1(2)
29844	1(2)
29845	1(2)
29846	1(2)
29847	1(2)
29848	1(2)
29850	1(2)
29851	1(2)
29855	1(2)
29856	1(2)
29860	1(2)
29861	1(2)
29862	1(2)
29863	1(2)
29866	1(2)
29867	1(2)
29868	1(3)
29870	1(2)
29871	1(2)
29873	1(2)

CPT	MUE
29874	1(2)
29875	1(2)
29876	1(2)
29877	1(2)
29879	1(2)
29880	1(2)
29881	1(2)
29882	1(2)
29883	1(2)
29884	1(2)
29885	1(2)
29886	1(2)
29887	1(2)
29888	1(2)
29889	1(2)
29891	1(2)
29892	1(2)
29893	1(2)
29894	1(2)
29895	1(2)
29897	1(2)
29898	1(2)
29899	1(2)
29900	2(3)
29901	2(3)
29902	2(3)
29904	1(2)
29905	1(2)
29906	1(2)
29907	1(2)
29914	1(2)
29915	1(2)
29916	1(2)
29999	1(3)
30000	1(3)
30020	1(3)
30100	2(3)
30110	1(2)
30115	1(2)
30117	2(3)
30118	1(3)
30120	1(2)
30124	2(3)
30125	1(3)
30130	1(2)
30140	1(2)
30150	1(2)
30160	1(2)
30200	1(2)
30210	1(3)
30220	1(2)
30300	1(3)
30310	1(3)
30320	1(3)
30400	1(2)
30410	1(2)
30420	1(2)
30430	1(2)
30435	1(2)
30450	1(2)
30460	1(2)
30462	1(2)
30465	1(2)
30520	1(2)
30540	1(2)

CPT	MUE
30545	1(2)
30560	1(2)
30580	2(3)
30600	1(3)
30620	1(2)
30630	1(2)
30801	1(2)
30802	1(2)
30901	1(3)
30903	1(3)
30905	1(2)
30906	1(3)
30915	1(3)
30920	1(3)
30930	1(2)
30999	1(3)
31000	1(2)
31002	1(2)
31020	1(2)
31030	1(2)
31032	1(2)
31040	1(2)
31050	1(2)
31051	1(2)
31070	1(2)
31075	1(2)
31080	1(2)
31081	1(2)
31084	1(2)
31085	1(2)
31086	1(2)
31087	1(2)
31090	1(2)
31200	1(2)
31201	1(2)
31205	1(2)
31225	1(2)
31230	1(2)
31231	1(2)
31233	1(2)
31235	1(2)
31237	1(2)
31238	1(3)
31239	1(2)
31240	1(2)
31241	1(2)
31253	1(2)
31254	1(2)
31255	1(2)
31256	1(2)
31257	1(2)
31259	1(2)
31267	1(2)
31276	1(2)
31287	1(2)
31288	1(2)
31290	1(2)
31291	1(2)
31292	1(2)
31293	1(2)
31294	1(2)
31295	1(2)
31296	1(2)
31297	1(2)
31298	1(2)

CPT	MUE
31299	1(3)
31300	1(2)
31360	1(2)
31365	1(2)
31367	1(2)
31368	1(2)
31370	1(2)
31375	1(2)
31380	1(2)
31382	1(2)
31390	1(2)
31395	1(2)
31400	1(3)
31420	1(2)
31500	2(3)
31502	1(3)
31505	1(3)
31510	1(2)
31511	1(3)
31512	1(3)
31513	1(3)
31515	1(3)
31520	1(3)
31525	1(3)
31526	1(3)
31527	1(2)
31528	1(2)
31529	1(3)
31530	1(3)
31531	1(3)
31535	1(3)
31536	1(3)
31540	1(3)
31541	1(3)
31545	1(2)
31546	1(2)
31551	1(2)
31552	1(2)
31553	1(2)
31554	1(2)
31560	1(2)
31561	1(2)
31570	1(2)
31571	1(2)
31572	1(2)
31573	1(2)
31574	1(2)
31575	1(3)
31576	1(3)
31577	1(3)
31578	1(3)
31579	1(2)
31580	1(2)
31584	1(2)
31587	1(2)
31590	1(2)
31591	1(2)
31592	1(2)
31599	1(3)
31600	1(2)
31601	1(2)
31603	1(2)
31605	1(2)
31610	1(2)
31611	1(2)

CPT	MUE
31612	1(3)
31613	1(2)
31614	1(2)
31615	1(3)
31622	1(3)
31623	1(3)
31624	1(3)
31625	1(2)
31626	1(2)
31627	1(3)
31628	1(2)
31629	1(2)
31630	1(3)
31631	1(2)
31632	2(3)
31633	2(3)
31634	1(3)
31635	1(3)
31636	1(2)
31637	2(3)
31638	1(3)
31640	1(3)
31641	1(3)
31643	1(2)
31645	1(2)
31646	2(3)
31647	1(2)
31648	1(2)
31649	2(3)
31651	3(3)
31652	1(2)
31653	1(2)
31654	1(3)
31660	1(2)
31661	1(2)
31717	1(3)
31720	3(3)
31725	1(3)
31730	1(3)
31750	1(2)
31755	1(2)
31760	1(2)
31766	1(2)
31770	2(3)
31775	1(3)
31780	1(2)
31781	1(2)
31785	1(3)
31786	1(3)
31800	1(3)
31805	1(3)
31820	1(2)
31825	1(2)
31830	1(2)
31899	1(3)
32035	1(2)
32036	1(3)
32096	1(3)
32097	1(3)
32098	1(2)
32100	1(3)
32110	1(3)
32120	1(3)
32124	1(3)
32140	1(3)

CPT	MUE
32141	1(3)
32150	1(3)
32151	1(3)
32160	1(3)
32200	2(3)
32215	1(2)
32220	1(2)
32225	1(2)
32310	1(3)
32320	1(3)
32400	2(3)
32405	2(3)
32440	1(2)
32442	1(2)
32445	1(2)
32480	1(2)
32482	1(2)
32484	2(3)
32486	1(3)
32488	1(2)
32491	1(2)
32501	1(3)
32503	1(2)
32504	1(2)
32505	1(2)
32506	3(3)
32507	2(3)
32540	1(3)
32550	2(3)
32551	2(3)
32552	2(2)
32553	1(2)
32554	2(3)
32555	2(3)
32556	2(3)
32557	2(3)
32560	1(3)
32561	1(2)
32562	1(2)
32601	1(3)
32604	1(3)
32606	1(3)
32607	1(3)
32608	1(3)
32609	1(3)
32650	1(2)
32651	1(2)
32652	1(2)
32653	1(3)
32654	1(3)
32655	1(3)
32656	1(2)
32658	1(3)
32659	1(2)
32661	1(3)
32662	1(3)
32663	1(3)
32664	1(2)
32665	1(2)
32666	1(3)
32667	3(3)
32668	2(3)
32669	2(3)
32670	1(2)
32671	1(2)

CPT	MUE
32672	1(3)
32673	1(2)
32674	1(2)
32701	1(2)
32800	1(3)
32810	1(3)
32815	1(3)
32820	1(2)
32850	1(2)
32851	1(2)
32852	1(2)
32853	1(2)
32854	1(2)
32855	1(2)
32856	1(2)
32900	1(2)
32905	1(2)
32906	1(2)
32940	1(3)
32960	1(2)
32994	1(2)
32997	1(2)
32998	1(2)
32999	1(3)
33016	1(3)
33017	1(3)
33018	1(3)
33019	1(3)
33020	1(3)
33025	1(2)
33030	1(2)
33031	1(2)
33050	1(2)
33120	1(3)
33130	1(3)
33140	1(2)
33141	1(2)
33202	1(2)
33203	1(2)
33206	1(3)
33207	1(3)
33208	1(3)
33210	1(3)
33211	1(3)
33212	1(3)
33213	1(3)
33214	1(3)
33215	2(3)
33216	1(3)
33217	1(3)
33218	1(3)
33220	1(3)
33221	1(3)
33222	1(3)
33223	1(3)
33224	1(3)
33225	1(3)
33226	1(3)
33227	1(3)
33228	1(3)
33229	1(3)
33230	1(3)
33231	1(3)
33233	1(2)
33234	1(2)

CPT	MUE
33235	1(2)
33236	1(2)
33237	1(2)
33238	1(2)
33240	1(3)
33241	1(2)
33243	1(2)
33244	1(2)
33249	1(3)
33250	1(2)
33251	1(2)
33254	1(2)
33255	1(2)
33256	1(2)
33257	1(2)
33258	1(2)
33259	1(2)
33261	1(2)
33262	1(3)
33263	1(3)
33264	1(3)
33265	1(2)
33266	1(2)
33270	1(3)
33271	1(3)
33272	1(3)
33273	1(3)
33274	1(3)
33275	1(3)
33285	1(3)
33286	1(3)
33289	1(3)
33300	1(3)
33305	1(3)
33310	1(2)
33315	1(2)
33320	1(3)
33321	1(3)
33322	1(3)
33330	1(3)
33335	1(3)
33340	1(2)
33361	1(2)
33362	1(2)
33363	1(2)
33364	1(2)
33365	1(2)
33366	1(3)
33367	1(2)
33368	1(2)
33369	1(2)
33390	1(2)
33391	1(2)
33404	1(2)
33405	1(2)
33406	1(2)
33410	1(2)
33411	1(2)
33412	1(2)
33413	1(2)
33414	1(2)
33415	1(2)
33416	1(2)
33417	1(2)
33418	1(3)

CPT	MUE
33419	1(2)
33420	1(2)
33422	1(2)
33425	1(2)
33426	1(2)
33427	1(2)
33430	1(2)
33440	1(2)
33460	1(2)
33463	1(2)
33464	1(2)
33465	1(2)
33468	1(2)
33470	1(2)
33471	1(2)
33474	1(2)
33475	1(2)
33476	1(2)
33477	1(2)
33478	1(2)
33496	1(3)
33500	1(3)
33501	1(3)
33502	1(3)
33503	1(3)
33504	1(3)
33505	1(3)
33506	1(3)
33507	1(3)
33508	1(2)
33510	1(2)
33511	1(2)
33512	1(2)
33513	1(2)
33514	1(2)
33516	1(2)
33517	1(2)
33518	1(2)
33519	1(2)
33521	1(2)
33522	1(2)
33523	1(2)
33530	1(2)
33533	1(2)
33534	1(2)
33535	1(2)
33536	1(2)
33542	1(2)
33545	1(2)
33548	1(2)
33572	3(2)
33600	1(3)
33602	1(3)
33606	1(2)
33608	1(2)
33610	1(2)
33611	1(2)
33612	1(2)
33615	1(2)
33617	1(2)
33619	1(2)
33620	1(2)
33621	1(3)
33622	1(2)
33641	1(2)

CPT	MUE
33645	1(2)
33647	1(2)
33660	1(2)
33665	1(2)
33670	1(2)
33675	1(2)
33676	1(2)
33677	1(2)
33681	1(2)
33684	1(2)
33688	1(2)
33690	1(2)
33692	1(2)
33694	1(2)
33697	1(2)
33702	1(2)
33710	1(2)
33720	1(2)
33722	1(3)
33724	1(2)
33726	1(2)
33730	1(2)
33732	1(2)
33735	1(2)
33736	1(2)
33737	1(2)
33750	1(3)
33755	1(2)
33762	1(2)
33764	1(3)
33766	1(2)
33767	1(2)
33768	1(2)
33770	1(2)
33771	1(2)
33774	1(2)
33775	1(2)
33776	1(2)
33777	1(2)
33778	1(2)
33779	1(2)
33780	1(2)
33781	1(2)
33782	1(2)
33783	1(2)
33786	1(2)
33788	1(2)
33800	1(2)
33802	1(3)
33803	1(3)
33813	1(2)
33814	1(2)
33820	1(2)
33822	1(2)
33824	1(2)
33840	1(2)
33845	1(2)
33851	1(2)
33852	1(2)
33853	1(2)
33858	1(2)
33859	1(2)
33863	1(2)
33864	1(2)
33866	1(2)

CPT	MUE
33871	1(2)
33875	1(2)
33877	1(2)
33880	1(2)
33881	1(2)
33883	1(2)
33884	2(3)
33886	1(2)
33889	1(2)
33891	1(2)
33910	1(3)
33915	1(3)
33916	1(3)
33917	1(2)
33920	1(2)
33922	1(2)
33924	1(2)
33925	1(2)
33926	1(2)
33927	1(3)
33928	1(3)
33929	1(3)
33930	1(2)
33933	1(2)
33935	1(2)
33940	1(2)
33944	1(2)
33945	1(2)
33946	1(2)
33947	1(2)
33948	1(2)
33949	1(2)
33951	1(3)
33952	1(3)
33953	1(3)
33954	1(3)
33955	1(3)
33956	1(3)
33957	1(3)
33958	1(3)
33959	1(3)
33962	1(3)
33963	1(3)
33964	1(3)
33965	1(3)
33966	1(3)
33967	1(3)
33968	1(3)
33969	1(3)
33970	1(3)
33971	1(3)
33973	1(3)
33974	1(3)
33975	1(3)
33976	1(3)
33977	1(3)
33978	1(3)
33979	1(3)
33980	1(3)
33981	1(3)
33982	1(3)
33983	1(3)
33984	1(3)
33985	1(3)
33986	1(3)

CPT	MUE
33987	1(3)
33988	1(3)
33989	1(3)
33990	1(3)
33991	1(3)
33992	1(2)
33993	1(3)
33999	1(3)
34001	1(3)
34051	1(3)
34101	1(3)
34111	2(3)
34151	1(3)
34201	1(3)
34203	1(2)
34401	1(3)
34421	1(3)
34451	1(3)
34471	1(2)
34490	1(2)
34501	1(2)
34502	1(2)
34510	2(3)
34520	1(3)
34530	1(2)
34701	1(2)
34702	1(2)
34703	1(2)
34704	1(2)
34705	1(2)
34706	1(2)
34707	1(2)
34708	1(2)
34709	3(3)
34710	1(2)
34711	2(3)
34712	1(2)
34713	1(2)
34714	1(2)
34715	1(2)
34716	1(2)
34717	2(2)
34718	2(2)
34808	1(3)
34812	1(2)
34813	1(2)
34820	1(2)
34830	1(2)
34831	1(2)
34832	1(2)
34833	1(2)
34834	1(2)
34839	1(2)
34841	1(2)
34842	1(2)
34843	1(2)
34844	1(2)
34845	1(2)
34846	1(2)
34847	1(2)
34848	1(2)
35001	1(2)
35002	1(2)
35005	1(2)
35011	1(2)

CPT	MUE
35013	1(2)
35021	1(2)
35022	1(2)
35045	1(3)
35081	1(2)
35082	1(2)
35091	1(2)
35092	1(2)
35102	1(2)
35103	1(2)
35111	1(2)
35112	1(2)
35121	1(3)
35122	1(3)
35131	1(2)
35132	1(2)
35141	1(2)
35142	1(2)
35151	1(2)
35152	1(2)
35180	2(3)
35182	2(3)
35184	2(3)
35188	2(3)
35189	1(3)
35190	2(3)
35201	2(3)
35206	2(3)
35207	3(3)
35211	3(3)
35216	2(3)
35221	3(3)
35226	3(3)
35231	2(3)
35236	2(3)
35241	2(3)
35246	2(3)
35251	2(3)
35256	2(3)
35261	1(3)
35266	2(3)
35271	2(3)
35276	2(3)
35281	2(3)
35286	2(3)
35301	2(3)
35302	1(2)
35303	1(2)
35304	1(2)
35305	1(2)
35306	2(3)
35311	1(2)
35321	1(2)
35331	1(2)
35341	3(3)
35351	1(3)
35355	1(2)
35361	1(2)
35363	1(2)
35371	1(2)
35372	1(2)
35390	1(3)
35400	1(3)
35500	2(3)
35501	1(3)

CPT	MUE
35506	1(3)
35508	1(3)
35509	1(3)
35510	1(3)
35511	1(3)
35512	1(3)
35515	1(3)
35516	1(3)
35518	1(3)
35521	1(3)
35522	1(3)
35523	1(3)
35525	1(3)
35526	1(3)
35531	1(3)
35533	1(3)
35535	1(3)
35536	1(3)
35537	1(3)
35538	1(3)
35539	1(3)
35540	1(3)
35556	1(3)
35558	1(3)
35560	1(3)
35563	1(3)
35565	1(3)
35566	1(3)
35570	1(3)
35571	1(3)
35572	2(3)
35583	1(2)
35585	2(3)
35587	1(3)
35600	2(3)
35601	1(3)
35606	1(3)
35612	1(3)
35616	1(3)
35621	1(3)
35623	1(3)
35626	3(3)
35631	4(3)
35632	1(3)
35633	1(3)
35634	1(3)
35636	1(3)
35637	1(3)
35638	1(3)
35642	1(3)
35645	1(3)
35646	1(3)
35647	1(3)
35650	1(3)
35654	1(3)
35656	1(3)
35661	1(3)
35663	1(3)
35665	1(3)
35666	2(3)
35671	2(3)
35681	1(3)
35682	1(2)
35683	1(2)
35685	2(3)

CPT	MUE
35686	1(3)
35691	1(3)
35693	1(3)
35694	1(3)
35695	1(3)
35697	2(3)
35700	2(3)
35701	1(2)
35702	2(2)
35703	2(2)
35800	2(3)
35820	2(3)
35840	2(3)
35860	2(3)
35870	1(3)
35875	2(3)
35876	2(3)
35879	2(3)
35881	1(3)
35883	1(3)
35884	1(3)
35901	1(3)
35903	2(3)
35905	1(3)
35907	1(3)
36000	4(3)
36002	2(3)
36005	2(3)
36010	2(3)
36011	4(3)
36012	4(3)
36013	2(3)
36014	2(3)
36015	4(3)
36100	2(3)
36140	3(3)
36160	2(3)
36200	2(3)
36215	2(3)
36216	2(3)
36217	2(3)
36218	2(3)
36221	1(3)
36222	1(3)
36223	1(3)
36224	1(3)
36225	1(3)
36226	1(3)
36227	2(2)
36228	2(3)
36245	3(3)
36246	4(3)
36247	2(3)
36248	2(3)
36251	1(3)
36252	1(3)
36253	1(3)
36254	1(3)
36260	1(2)
36261	1(2)
36262	1(2)
36299	1(3)
36400	1(3)
36405	1(3)
36406	1(3)

CPT	MUE
36410	3(3)
36415	2(3)
36416	6(3)
36420	2(3)
36425	2(3)
36430	1(2)
36440	1(3)
36450	1(3)
36455	1(3)
36456	1(3)
36460	2(3)
36465	1(2)
36466	1(2)
36468	2(3)
36470	1(2)
36471	1(2)
36473	1(3)
36474	1(3)
36475	1(3)
36476	2(3)
36478	1(3)
36479	2(3)
36481	1(3)
36482	1(3)
36483	2(3)
36500	4(3)
36510	1(3)
36511	1(3)
36512	1(3)
36513	1(3)
36514	1(3)
36516	1(3)
36522	1(3)
36555	2(3)
36556	2(3)
36557	2(3)
36558	2(3)
36560	2(3)
36561	2(3)
36563	1(3)
36565	1(3)
36566	1(3)
36568	2(3)
36569	2(3)
36570	2(3)
36571	2(3)
36572	1(3)
36573	1(3)
36575	2(3)
36576	2(3)
36578	2(3)
36580	2(3)
36581	2(3)
36582	2(3)
36583	2(3)
36584	2(3)
36585	2(3)
36589	2(3)
36590	2(3)
36591	2(3)
36592	1(3)
36593	2(3)
36595	2(3)
36596	2(3)
36597	2(3)

CPT	MUE
36598	2(3)
36600	4(3)
36620	3(3)
36625	2(3)
36640	1(3)
36660	1(3)
36680	1(3)
36800	1(3)
36810	1(3)
36815	1(3)
36818	1(3)
36819	1(3)
36820	1(3)
36821	2(3)
36823	1(3)
36825	1(3)
36830	2(3)
36831	1(3)
36832	2(3)
36833	1(3)
36835	1(3)
36838	1(3)
36860	2(3)
36861	2(3)
36901	1(3)
36902	1(3)
36903	1(3)
36904	1(3)
36905	1(3)
36906	1(3)
36907	1(3)
36908	1(3)
36909	1(3)
37140	1(2)
37145	1(3)
37160	1(3)
37180	1(2)
37181	1(2)
37182	1(2)
37183	1(2)
37184	1(2)
37185	2(3)
37186	2(3)
37187	1(3)
37188	1(3)
37191	1(3)
37192	1(3)
37193	1(3)
37195	1(3)
37197	2(3)
37200	2(3)
37211	1(2)
37212	1(2)
37213	1(2)
37214	1(2)
37215	1(2)
37216	0(3)
37217	1(2)
37218	1(2)
37220	1(2)
37221	1(2)
37222	2(2)
37223	2(2)
37224	1(2)
37225	1(2)

CPT	MUE
37226	1(2)
37227	1(2)
37228	1(2)
37229	1(2)
37230	1(2)
37231	1(2)
37232	2(3)
37233	2(3)
37234	2(3)
37235	2(3)
37236	1(2)
37237	2(3)
37238	1(2)
37239	2(3)
37241	2(3)
37242	2(3)
37243	1(3)
37244	2(3)
37246	1(2)
37247	2(3)
37248	1(2)
37249	3(3)
37252	1(2)
37253	5(3)
37500	1(3)
37501	1(3)
37565	1(2)
37600	1(3)
37605	1(3)
37606	1(3)
37607	1(3)
37609	1(2)
37615	2(3)
37616	1(3)
37617	3(3)
37618	2(3)
37619	1(2)
37650	1(2)
37660	1(2)
37700	1(2)
37718	1(2)
37722	1(2)
37735	1(2)
37760	1(2)
37761	1(2)
37765	1(2)
37766	1(2)
37780	1(2)
37785	1(2)
37788	1(2)
37790	1(2)
37799	1(3)
38100	1(2)
38101	1(3)
38102	1(2)
38115	1(3)
38120	1(2)
38129	1(3)
38200	1(3)
38204	1(2)
38205	1(3)
38206	1(3)
38207	1(3)
38208	1(3)
38209	1(3)

CPT	MUE
38210	1(3)
38211	1(3)
38212	1(3)
38213	1(3)
38214	1(3)
38215	1(3)
38220	1(3)
38221	1(3)
38222	1(2)
38230	1(2)
38232	1(2)
38240	1(3)
38241	1(2)
38242	1(2)
38243	1(3)
38300	1(3)
38305	1(3)
38308	1(3)
38380	1(2)
38381	1(2)
38382	1(2)
38500	2(3)
38505	2(3)
38510	1(2)
38520	1(2)
38525	1(2)
38530	1(2)
38531	1(2)
38542	1(2)
38550	1(3)
38555	1(3)
38562	1(2)
38564	1(2)
38570	1(2)
38571	1(2)
38572	1(2)
38573	1(2)
38589	1(3)
38700	1(2)
38720	1(2)
38724	1(2)
38740	1(2)
38745	1(2)
38746	1(2)
38747	1(2)
38760	1(2)
38765	1(2)
38770	1(2)
38780	1(2)
38790	1(2)
38792	1(3)
38794	1(2)
38900	1(3)
38999	1(3)
39000	1(2)
39010	1(2)
39200	1(2)
39220	1(2)
39401	1(3)
39402	1(3)
39499	1(3)
39501	1(3)
39503	1(2)
39540	1(2)
39541	1(2)

CPT	MUE
39545	1(2)
39560	1(3)
39561	1(3)
39599	1(3)
40490	2(3)
40500	2(3)
40510	2(3)
40520	2(3)
40525	2(3)
40527	2(3)
40530	2(3)
40650	2(3)
40652	2(3)
40654	2(3)
40700	1(2)
40701	1(2)
40702	1(2)
40720	1(2)
40761	1(2)
40799	1(3)
40800	2(3)
40801	2(3)
40804	1(3)
40805	2(3)
40806	2(2)
40808	2(3)
40810	2(3)
40812	2(3)
40814	4(3)
40816	2(3)
40818	2(3)
40819	2(2)
40820	2(3)
40830	2(3)
40831	2(3)
40840	1(2)
40842	1(2)
40843	1(2)
40844	1(2)
40845	1(3)
40899	1(3)
41000	1(3)
41005	1(3)
41006	2(3)
41007	2(3)
41008	2(3)
41009	2(3)
41010	1(2)
41015	2(3)
41016	1(3)
41017	2(3)
41018	2(3)
41019	1(2)
41100	2(3)
41105	2(3)
41108	2(3)
41110	2(3)
41112	2(3)
41113	2(3)
41114	2(3)
41115	1(2)
41116	2(3)
41120	1(2)
41130	1(2)
41135	1(2)

CPT	MUE
41140	1(2)
41145	1(2)
41150	1(2)
41153	1(2)
41155	1(2)
41250	2(3)
41251	2(3)
41252	2(3)
41510	1(2)
41512	1(2)
41520	1(3)
41530	1(3)
41599	1(3)
41800	2(3)
41805	1(3)
41806	1(3)
41820	4(2)
41821	2(3)
41822	1(2)
41823	1(2)
41825	2(3)
41826	2(3)
41827	2(3)
41828	4(2)
41830	2(3)
41850	2(3)
41870	2(3)
41872	4(2)
41874	4(2)
41899	1(3)
42000	1(3)
42100	2(3)
42104	2(3)
42106	2(3)
42107	2(3)
42120	1(2)
42140	1(2)
42145	1(2)
42160	1(3)
42180	1(3)
42182	1(3)
42200	1(2)
42205	1(2)
42210	1(2)
42215	1(2)
42220	1(2)
42225	1(2)
42226	1(2)
42227	1(2)
42235	1(2)
42260	1(3)
42280	1(2)
42281	1(2)
42299	1(3)
42300	2(3)
42305	2(3)
42310	2(3)
42320	2(3)
42330	1(3)
42335	2(2)
42340	1(2)
42400	2(3)
42405	2(3)
42408	1(3)
42409	1(3)

CPT	MUE
42410	1(2)
42415	1(2)
42420	1(2)
42425	1(2)
42426	1(2)
42440	1(2)
42450	1(3)
42500	2(3)
42505	2(3)
42507	1(2)
42509	1(2)
42510	1(2)
42550	2(3)
42600	1(3)
42650	2(3)
42660	2(3)
42665	2(3)
42699	1(3)
42700	2(3)
42720	1(3)
42725	1(3)
42800	3(3)
42804	1(3)
42806	1(3)
42808	2(3)
42809	1(3)
42810	1(3)
42815	1(3)
42820	1(2)
42821	1(2)
42825	1(2)
42826	1(2)
42830	1(2)
42831	1(2)
42835	1(2)
42836	1(2)
42842	1(3)
42844	1(3)
42845	1(3)
42860	1(3)
42870	1(3)
42890	1(2)
42892	1(3)
42894	1(3)
42900	1(3)
42950	1(2)
42953	1(3)
42955	1(2)
42960	1(3)
42961	1(3)
42962	1(3)
42970	1(3)
42971	1(3)
42972	1(3)
42999	1(3)
43020	1(2)
43030	1(2)
43045	1(2)
43100	1(3)
43101	1(3)
43107	1(2)
43108	1(2)
43112	1(2)
43113	1(2)
43116	1(2)

CPT	MUE
43117	1(2)
43118	1(2)
43121	1(2)
43122	1(2)
43123	1(2)
43124	1(2)
43130	1(3)
43135	1(3)
43180	1(2)
43191	1(3)
43192	1(3)
43193	1(3)
43194	1(3)
43195	1(3)
43196	1(3)
43197	1(3)
43198	1(3)
43200	1(3)
43201	1(2)
43202	1(2)
43204	1(2)
43205	1(2)
43206	1(2)
43210	1(2)
43211	1(3)
43212	1(3)
43213	1(2)
43214	1(3)
43215	1(3)
43216	1(2)
43217	1(2)
43220	1(3)
43226	1(3)
43227	1(3)
43229	1(3)
43231	1(2)
43232	1(2)
43233	1(3)
43235	1(3)
43236	1(2)
43237	1(2)
43238	1(2)
43239	1(2)
43240	1(2)
43241	1(3)
43242	1(2)
43243	1(2)
43244	1(2)
43245	1(2)
43246	1(2)
43247	1(2)
43248	1(3)
43249	1(3)
43250	1(2)
43251	1(2)
43252	1(2)
43253	1(3)
43254	1(3)
43255	2(3)
43257	1(2)
43259	1(2)
43260	1(3)
43261	1(2)
43262	2(2)
43263	1(2)

CPT	MUE
43264	1(2)
43265	1(2)
43266	1(3)
43270	1(3)
43273	1(2)
43274	2(3)
43275	1(3)
43276	2(3)
43277	3(3)
43278	1(3)
43279	1(2)
43280	1(2)
43281	1(2)
43282	1(2)
43283	1(2)
43284	1(2)
43285	1(2)
43286	1(2)
43287	1(2)
43288	1(2)
43289	1(3)
43300	1(2)
43305	1(2)
43310	1(2)
43312	1(2)
43313	1(2)
43314	1(2)
43320	1(2)
43325	1(2)
43327	1(2)
43328	1(2)
43330	1(2)
43331	1(2)
43332	1(2)
43333	1(2)
43334	1(2)
43335	1(2)
43336	1(2)
43337	1(2)
43338	1(2)
43340	1(2)
43341	1(2)
43351	1(2)
43352	1(2)
43360	1(2)
43361	1(2)
43400	1(2)
43405	1(2)
43410	1(3)
43415	1(3)
43420	1(3)
43425	1(3)
43450	1(3)
43453	1(3)
43460	1(3)
43496	1(3)
43499	1(3)
43500	1(2)
43501	1(3)
43502	1(2)
43510	1(2)
43520	1(2)
43605	1(2)
43610	2(3)
43611	2(3)

CPT	MUE
43620	1(2)
43621	1(2)
43622	1(2)
43631	1(2)
43632	1(2)
43633	1(2)
43634	1(2)
43635	1(2)
43640	1(2)
43641	1(2)
43644	1(2)
43645	1(2)
43647	1(2)
43648	1(2)
43651	1(2)
43652	1(2)
43653	1(2)
43659	1(3)
43752	2(3)
43753	1(3)
43754	1(3)
43755	1(3)
43756	1(2)
43757	1(2)
43761	2(3)
43762	2(3)
43763	2(3)
43770	1(2)
43771	1(2)
43772	1(2)
43773	1(2)
43774	1(2)
43775	1(2)
43800	1(2)
43810	1(2)
43820	1(2)
43825	1(2)
43830	1(2)
43831	1(2)
43832	1(2)
43840	2(3)
43842	0(3)
43843	1(2)
43845	1(2)
43846	1(2)
43847	1(2)
43848	1(2)
43850	1(2)
43855	1(2)
43860	1(2)
43865	1(2)
43870	1(2)
43880	1(3)
43881	1(3)
43882	1(3)
43886	1(2)
43887	1(2)
43888	1(2)
43999	1(3)
44005	1(2)
44010	1(2)
44015	1(2)
44020	2(3)
44021	1(3)
44025	1(3)

CPT	MUE
44050	1(2)
44055	1(2)
44100	1(2)
44110	1(2)
44111	1(2)
44120	1(2)
44121	2(3)
44125	1(2)
44126	1(2)
44127	1(2)
44128	2(3)
44130	2(3)
44132	1(2)
44133	1(2)
44135	1(2)
44136	1(2)
44137	1(2)
44139	1(2)
44140	2(3)
44141	1(3)
44143	1(2)
44144	1(3)
44145	1(2)
44146	1(2)
44147	1(3)
44150	1(2)
44151	1(2)
44155	1(2)
44156	1(2)
44157	1(2)
44158	1(2)
44160	1(2)
44180	1(2)
44186	1(2)
44187	1(3)
44188	1(3)
44202	1(2)
44203	2(3)
44204	2(3)
44205	1(2)
44206	1(2)
44207	1(2)
44208	1(2)
44210	1(2)
44211	1(2)
44212	1(2)
44213	1(2)
44227	1(3)
44238	1(3)
44300	1(3)
44310	2(3)
44312	1(2)
44314	1(2)
44316	1(2)
44320	1(2)
44322	1(2)
44340	1(2)
44345	1(2)
44346	1(2)
44360	1(3)
44361	1(2)
44363	1(3)
44364	1(2)
44365	1(2)
44366	1(3)

CPT	MUE	CPT	MUE	CPT	MUE	CPT	MUE	CPT	MUE	CPT	MUE	CPT	MUE	CPT	MUE
44369	1(2)	45111	1(2)	45500	1(2)	46716	1(2)	47490	1(2)	48160	0(3)	49440	1(3)	50081	1(2)
44370	1(2)	45112	1(2)	45505	1(2)	46730	1(2)	47531	2(3)	48400	1(3)	49441	1(3)	50100	1(2)
44372	1(2)	45113	1(2)	45520	1(2)	46735	1(2)	47532	1(3)	48500	1(3)	49442	1(3)	50120	1(2)
44373	1(2)	45114	1(2)	45540	1(2)	46740	1(2)	47533	1(3)	48510	1(3)	49446	1(2)	50125	1(2)
44376	1(3)	45116	1(2)	45541	1(2)	46742	1(2)	47534	2(3)	48520	1(3)	49450	1(3)	50130	1(2)
44377	1(2)	45119	1(2)	45550	1(2)	46744	1(2)	47535	1(3)	48540	1(3)	49451	1(3)	50135	1(2)
44378	1(3)	45120	1(2)	45560	1(2)	46746	1(2)	47536	2(3)	48545	1(3)	49452	1(3)	50200	1(3)
44379	1(2)	45121	1(2)	45562	1(2)	46748	1(2)	47537	1(3)	48547	1(2)	49460	1(3)	50205	1(3)
44380	1(3)	45123	1(2)	45563	1(2)	46750	1(2)	47538	2(3)	48548	1(2)	49465	1(3)	50220	1(2)
44381	1(3)	45126	1(2)	45800	1(3)	46751	1(2)	47539	2(3)	48550	1(2)	49491	1(2)	50225	1(2)
44382	1(2)	45130	1(2)	45805	1(3)	46753	1(2)	47540	2(3)	48551	1(2)	49492	1(2)	50230	1(2)
44384	1(3)	45135	1(2)	45820	1(3)	46754	1(3)	47541	1(3)	48552	2(3)	49495	1(2)	50234	1(2)
44385	1(3)	45136	1(2)	45825	1(3)	46760	1(2)	47542	2(3)	48554	1(2)	49496	1(2)	50236	1(2)
44386	1(2)	45150	1(2)	45900	1(2)	46761	1(2)	47543	1(3)	48556	1(2)	49500	1(2)	50240	1(2)
44388	1(3)	45160	1(3)	45905	1(2)	46900	1(2)	47544	1(3)	48999	1(3)	49501	1(2)	50250	1(3)
44389	1(2)	45171	2(3)	45910	1(2)	46910	1(2)	47550	1(3)	49000	1(2)	49505	1(2)	50280	1(2)
44390	1(3)	45172	2(3)	45915	1(2)	46916	1(2)	47552	1(3)	49002	1(3)	49507	1(2)	50290	1(3)
44391	1(3)	45190	1(3)	45990	1(2)	46917	1(2)	47553	1(2)	49010	1(3)	49520	1(2)	50300	1(2)
44392	1(2)	45300	1(3)	45999	1(3)	46922	1(2)	47554	1(3)	49013	1(2)	49521	1(2)	50320	1(2)
44394	1(2)	45303	1(3)	46020	2(3)	46924	1(2)	47555	1(2)	49014	1(3)	49525	1(2)	50323	1(2)
44401	1(2)	45305	1(2)	46030	1(3)	46930	1(2)	47556	1(2)	49020	2(3)	49540	1(2)	50325	1(2)
44402	1(3)	45307	1(3)	46040	2(3)	46940	1(2)	47562	1(2)	49040	2(3)	49550	1(2)	50327	2(3)
44403	1(3)	45308	1(2)	46045	2(3)	46942	1(3)	47563	1(2)	49060	2(3)	49553	1(2)	50328	1(3)
44404	1(3)	45309	1(2)	46050	2(3)	46945	1(2)	47564	1(2)	49062	1(3)	49555	1(2)	50329	1(3)
44405	1(3)	45315	1(2)	46060	2(3)	46946	1(2)	47570	1(2)	49082	1(3)	49557	1(2)	50340	1(2)
44406	1(3)	45317	1(3)	46070	1(2)	46947	1(2)	47579	1(3)	49083	2(3)	49560	2(3)	50360	1(2)
44407	1(2)	45320	1(2)	46080	1(2)	46948	1(2)	47600	1(2)	49084	1(3)	49561	1(3)	50365	1(2)
44408	1(3)	45321	1(2)	46083	2(3)	46999	1(3)	47605	1(2)	49180	2(3)	49565	2(3)	50370	1(2)
44500	1(3)	45327	1(2)	46200	1(3)	47000	3(3)	47610	1(2)	49185	2(3)	49566	2(3)	50380	1(2)
44602	1(2)	45330	1(3)	46220	1(2)	47001	3(3)	47612	1(2)	49203	1(2)	49568	2(3)	50382	1(3)
44603	1(2)	45331	1(2)	46221	1(2)	47010	1(3)	47620	1(2)	49204	1(2)	49570	1(3)	50384	1(3)
44604	1(2)	45332	1(3)	46230	1(2)	47015	1(2)	47700	1(2)	49205	1(2)	49572	1(3)	50385	1(3)
44605	1(2)	45333	1(2)	46250	1(2)	47100	3(3)	47701	1(2)	49215	1(2)	49580	1(2)	50386	1(3)
44615	3(3)	45334	1(3)	46255	1(2)	47120	2(3)	47711	1(2)	49220	1(2)	49582	1(2)	50387	1(3)
44620	2(3)	45335	1(2)	46257	1(2)	47122	1(2)	47712	1(2)	49250	1(2)	49585	1(2)	50389	1(3)
44625	1(3)	45337	1(2)	46258	1(2)	47125	1(2)	47715	1(2)	49255	1(2)	49587	1(2)	50390	2(3)
44626	1(3)	45338	1(2)	46260	1(2)	47130	1(2)	47720	1(2)	49320	1(3)	49590	1(2)	50391	1(3)
44640	2(3)	45340	1(2)	46261	1(2)	47133	1(2)	47721	1(2)	49321	1(2)	49600	1(2)	50396	1(3)
44650	2(3)	45341	1(2)	46262	1(2)	47135	1(2)	47740	1(2)	49322	1(2)	49605	1(2)	50400	1(2)
44660	1(3)	45342	1(2)	46270	1(3)	47140	1(2)	47741	1(2)	49323	1(2)	49606	1(2)	50405	1(2)
44661	1(3)	45346	1(2)	46275	1(3)	47141	1(2)	47760	1(2)	49324	1(2)	49610	1(2)	50430	2(3)
44680	1(3)	45347	1(3)	46280	1(2)	47142	1(2)	47765	1(2)	49325	1(2)	49611	1(2)	50431	2(3)
44700	1(2)	45349	1(3)	46285	1(3)	47143	1(2)	47780	1(2)	49326	1(2)	49650	1(2)	50432	2(3)
44701	1(2)	45350	1(2)	46288	1(3)	47144	1(2)	47785	1(2)	49327	1(2)	49651	1(2)	50433	2(3)
44705	1(3)	45378	1(3)	46320	2(3)	47145	1(2)	47800	1(2)	49329	1(3)	49652	2(3)	50434	2(3)
44715	1(2)	45379	1(3)	46500	1(2)	47146	2(3)	47801	1(3)	49400	1(3)	49653	2(3)	50435	2(3)
44720	2(3)	45380	1(2)	46505	1(2)	47147	1(3)	47802	1(2)	49402	1(3)	49654	1(3)	50436	1(3)
44721	2(3)	45381	1(2)	46600	1(3)	47300	2(3)	47900	1(2)	49405	2(3)	49655	1(3)	50437	1(3)
44799	1(3)	45382	1(3)	46601	1(3)	47350	1(3)	47999	1(3)	49406	2(3)	49656	1(3)	50500	1(3)
44800	1(3)	45384	1(2)	46604	1(2)	47360	1(3)	48000	1(2)	49407	1(3)	49657	1(3)	50520	1(3)
44820	1(3)	45385	1(2)	46606	1(2)	47361	1(3)	48001	1(2)	49411	1(2)	49659	1(3)	50525	1(3)
44850	1(3)	45386	1(2)	46607	1(2)	47362	1(3)	48020	1(3)	49412	1(2)	49900	1(3)	50526	1(3)
44899	1(3)	45388	1(2)	46608	1(3)	47370	1(2)	48100	1(3)	49418	1(3)	49904	1(3)	50540	1(2)
44900	1(2)	45389	1(3)	46610	1(2)	47371	1(2)	48102	1(3)	49419	1(2)	49905	1(3)	50541	1(2)
44950	1(2)	45390	1(3)	46611	1(2)	47379	1(3)	48105	1(2)	49421	1(2)	49906	1(3)	50542	1(2)
44955	1(2)	45391	1(2)	46612	1(2)	47380	1(2)	48120	1(3)	49422	1(2)	49999	1(3)	50543	1(2)
44960	1(2)	45392	1(2)	46614	1(3)	47381	1(2)	48140	1(2)	49423	2(3)	50010	1(2)	50544	1(2)
44970	1(2)	45393	1(3)	46615	1(2)	47382	1(2)	48145	1(2)	49424	3(3)	50020	1(3)	50545	1(2)
44979	1(3)	45395	1(2)	46700	1(2)	47383	1(2)	48146	1(2)	49425	1(2)	50040	1(2)	50546	1(2)
45000	1(3)	45397	1(2)	46705	1(2)	47399	1(3)	48148	1(2)	49426	1(3)	50045	1(2)	50547	1(2)
45005	1(3)	45398	1(2)	46706	1(3)	47400	1(3)	48150	1(2)	49427	1(3)	50060	1(2)	50548	1(2)
45020	1(3)	45399	1(3)	46707	1(3)	47420	1(2)	48152	1(2)	49428	1(2)	50065	1(2)	50549	1(3)
45100	2(3)	45400	1(2)	46710	1(3)	47425	1(2)	48153	1(2)	49429	1(2)	50070	1(2)	50551	1(3)
45108	1(2)	45402	1(2)	46712	1(3)	47460	1(2)	48154	1(2)	49435	1(2)	50075	1(2)	50553	1(3)
45110	1(2)	45499	1(3)	46715	1(2)	47480	1(2)	48155	1(2)	49436	1(2)	50080	1(2)	50555	1(2)

CPT	MUE
50557	1(2)
50561	1(2)
50562	1(3)
50570	1(3)
50572	1(3)
50574	1(2)
50575	1(2)
50576	1(2)
50580	1(2)
50590	1(2)
50592	1(2)
50593	1(2)
50600	1(3)
50605	1(3)
50606	1(3)
50610	1(2)
50620	1(2)
50630	1(2)
50650	1(2)
50660	1(3)
50684	1(3)
50686	2(3)
50688	2(3)
50690	2(3)
50693	2(3)
50694	2(3)
50695	2(3)
50700	1(2)
50705	2(3)
50706	2(3)
50715	1(2)
50722	1(2)
50725	1(3)
50727	1(3)
50728	1(3)
50740	1(2)
50750	1(2)
50760	1(2)
50770	1(2)
50780	1(2)
50782	1(2)
50783	1(2)
50785	1(2)
50800	1(2)
50810	1(3)
50815	1(2)
50820	1(2)
50825	1(3)
50830	1(3)
50840	1(2)
50845	1(2)
50860	1(2)
50900	1(3)
50920	2(3)
50930	2(3)
50940	1(2)
50945	1(2)
50947	1(2)
50948	1(2)
50949	1(3)
50951	1(3)
50953	1(3)
50955	1(2)
50957	1(2)
50961	1(2)

CPT	MUE
50970	1(3)
50972	1(3)
50974	1(2)
50976	1(2)
50980	1(2)
51020	1(2)
51030	1(2)
51040	1(3)
51045	2(3)
51050	1(3)
51060	1(3)
51065	1(3)
51080	1(3)
51100	1(3)
51101	1(3)
51102	1(3)
51500	1(2)
51520	1(2)
51525	1(2)
51530	1(2)
51535	1(2)
51550	1(2)
51555	1(2)
51565	1(2)
51570	1(2)
51575	1(2)
51580	1(2)
51585	1(2)
51590	1(2)
51595	1(2)
51596	1(2)
51597	1(2)
51600	1(3)
51605	1(3)
51610	1(3)
51700	1(3)
51701	2(3)
51702	2(3)
51703	2(3)
51705	2(3)
51710	1(3)
51715	1(2)
51720	1(3)
51725	1(3)
51726	1(3)
51727	1(3)
51728	1(3)
51729	1(3)
51736	1(3)
51741	1(3)
51784	1(3)
51785	1(3)
51792	1(3)
51797	1(3)
51798	1(3)
51800	1(2)
51820	1(2)
51840	1(2)
51841	1(2)
51845	1(2)
51860	1(3)
51865	1(3)
51880	1(2)
51900	1(3)
51920	1(3)

CPT	MUE
51925	1(2)
51940	1(2)
51960	1(2)
51980	1(2)
51990	1(2)
51992	1(2)
51999	1(3)
52000	1(3)
52001	1(3)
52005	2(3)
52007	1(2)
52010	1(2)
52204	1(2)
52214	1(2)
52224	1(2)
52234	1(2)
52235	1(2)
52240	1(2)
52250	1(2)
52260	1(2)
52265	1(2)
52270	1(2)
52275	1(2)
52276	1(2)
52277	1(2)
52281	1(2)
52282	1(2)
52283	1(2)
52285	1(2)
52287	1(2)
52290	1(2)
52300	1(2)
52301	1(2)
52305	1(2)
52310	1(3)
52315	2(3)
52317	1(3)
52318	1(3)
52320	1(2)
52325	1(3)
52327	1(2)
52330	1(2)
52332	1(2)
52334	1(2)
52341	1(2)
52342	1(2)
52343	1(2)
52344	1(2)
52345	1(2)
52346	1(2)
52351	1(3)
52352	1(2)
52353	1(2)
52354	1(3)
52355	1(3)
52356	1(2)
52400	1(2)
52402	1(2)
52441	1(2)
52442	6(3)
52450	1(2)
52500	1(2)
52601	1(2)
52630	1(2)
52640	1(2)

CPT	MUE
52647	1(2)
52648	1(2)
52649	1(2)
52700	1(3)
53000	1(2)
53010	1(2)
53020	1(2)
53025	1(2)
53040	1(3)
53060	1(3)
53080	1(3)
53085	1(3)
53200	1(3)
53210	1(2)
53215	1(2)
53220	1(3)
53230	1(3)
53235	1(3)
53240	1(3)
53250	1(3)
53260	1(2)
53265	1(3)
53270	1(2)
53275	1(2)
53400	1(2)
53405	1(2)
53410	1(2)
53415	1(2)
53420	1(2)
53425	1(2)
53430	1(2)
53431	1(2)
53440	1(2)
53442	1(2)
53444	1(3)
53445	1(2)
53446	1(2)
53447	1(2)
53448	1(2)
53449	1(2)
53450	1(2)
53460	1(2)
53500	1(2)
53502	1(3)
53505	1(3)
53510	1(3)
53515	1(3)
53520	1(3)
53600	1(3)
53601	1(3)
53605	1(3)
53620	1(2)
53621	1(3)
53660	1(2)
53661	1(3)
53665	1(3)
53850	1(2)
53852	1(2)
53854	1(2)
53855	1(2)
53860	1(2)
53899	1(3)
54000	1(2)
54001	1(2)
54015	1(3)

CPT	MUE
54050	1(2)
54055	1(2)
54056	1(2)
54057	1(2)
54060	1(2)
54065	1(2)
54100	2(3)
54105	2(3)
54110	1(2)
54111	1(2)
54112	1(3)
54115	1(3)
54120	1(2)
54125	1(2)
54130	1(2)
54135	1(2)
54150	1(2)
54160	1(2)
54161	1(2)
54162	1(2)
54163	1(2)
54164	1(2)
54200	1(2)
54205	1(2)
54220	1(3)
54230	1(3)
54231	1(3)
54235	1(3)
54240	1(2)
54250	1(2)
54300	1(2)
54304	1(2)
54308	1(2)
54312	1(2)
54316	1(2)
54318	1(2)
54322	1(2)
54324	1(2)
54326	1(2)
54328	1(2)
54332	1(2)
54336	1(2)
54340	1(2)
54344	1(2)
54348	1(2)
54352	1(2)
54360	1(2)
54380	1(2)
54385	1(2)
54390	1(2)
54400	1(2)
54401	1(2)
54405	1(2)
54406	1(2)
54408	1(2)
54410	1(2)
54411	1(2)
54415	1(2)
54416	1(2)
54417	1(2)
54420	1(2)
54430	1(2)
54435	1(2)
54437	1(2)
54438	1(2)

CPT	MUE
54440	1(2)
54450	1(2)
54500	1(3)
54505	1(3)
54512	1(3)
54520	1(2)
54522	1(2)
54530	1(2)
54535	1(2)
54550	1(2)
54560	1(2)
54600	1(2)
54620	1(2)
54640	1(2)
54650	1(2)
54660	1(2)
54670	1(3)
54680	1(2)
54690	1(2)
54692	1(2)
54699	1(3)
54700	1(3)
54800	1(2)
54830	1(2)
54840	1(2)
54860	1(2)
54861	1(2)
54865	1(3)
54900	1(2)
54901	1(2)
55000	1(3)
55040	1(2)
55041	1(2)
55060	1(2)
55100	2(3)
55110	1(2)
55120	1(3)
55150	1(2)
55175	1(2)
55180	1(2)
55200	1(2)
55250	1(2)
55300	1(2)
55400	1(2)
55500	1(2)
55520	1(2)
55530	1(2)
55535	1(2)
55540	1(2)
55550	1(2)
55559	1(3)
55600	1(2)
55605	1(2)
55650	1(2)
55680	1(3)
55700	1(2)
55705	1(2)
55706	1(2)
55720	1(3)
55725	1(3)
55801	1(2)
55810	1(2)
55812	1(2)
55815	1(2)
55821	1(2)

CPT	MUE
55831	1(2)
55840	1(2)
55842	1(2)
55845	1(2)
55860	1(2)
55862	1(2)
55865	1(2)
55866	1(2)
55870	1(2)
55873	1(2)
55874	1(2)
55875	1(2)
55876	1(2)
55899	1(3)
55920	1(2)
55970	1(2)
55980	1(2)
56405	2(3)
56420	1(3)
56440	1(3)
56441	1(2)
56442	1(2)
56501	1(2)
56515	1(2)
56605	1(2)
56606	6(3)
56620	1(2)
56625	1(2)
56630	1(2)
56631	1(2)
56632	1(2)
56633	1(2)
56634	1(2)
56637	1(2)
56640	1(2)
56700	1(2)
56740	1(3)
56800	1(2)
56805	1(2)
56810	1(2)
56820	1(2)
56821	1(2)
57000	1(3)
57010	1(3)
57020	1(3)
57022	1(3)
57023	1(3)
57061	1(2)
57065	1(2)
57100	2(3)
57105	2(3)
57106	1(2)
57107	1(2)
57109	1(2)
57110	1(2)
57111	1(2)
57112	1(2)
57120	1(2)
57130	1(2)
57135	2(3)
57150	1(3)
57155	1(3)
57156	1(3)
57160	1(2)
57170	1(2)

CPT	MUE
57180	1(3)
57200	1(3)
57210	1(3)
57220	1(2)
57230	1(2)
57240	1(2)
57250	1(2)
57260	1(2)
57265	1(2)
57267	2(3)
57268	1(2)
57270	1(2)
57280	1(2)
57282	1(2)
57283	1(2)
57284	1(2)
57285	1(2)
57287	1(2)
57288	1(2)
57289	1(2)
57291	1(2)
57292	1(2)
57295	1(2)
57296	1(2)
57300	1(3)
57305	1(3)
57307	1(3)
57308	1(3)
57310	1(3)
57311	1(3)
57320	1(3)
57330	1(3)
57335	1(2)
57400	1(2)
57410	1(2)
57415	1(3)
57420	1(3)
57421	1(3)
57423	1(2)
57425	1(2)
57426	1(2)
57452	1(3)
57454	1(3)
57455	1(3)
57456	1(3)
57460	1(3)
57461	1(3)
57500	1(3)
57505	1(3)
57510	1(3)
57511	1(3)
57513	1(3)
57520	1(3)
57522	1(3)
57530	1(3)
57531	1(2)
57540	1(2)
57545	1(3)
57550	1(3)
57555	1(2)
57556	1(2)
57558	1(3)
57700	1(3)
57720	1(3)
57800	1(3)

CPT	MUE
58100	1(3)
58110	1(3)
58120	1(3)
58140	1(3)
58145	1(3)
58146	1(3)
58150	1(3)
58152	1(2)
58180	1(3)
58200	1(2)
58210	1(2)
58240	1(2)
58260	1(3)
58262	1(3)
58263	1(2)
58267	1(2)
58270	1(2)
58275	1(2)
58280	1(2)
58285	1(3)
58290	1(3)
58291	1(2)
58292	1(2)
58293	1(2)
58294	1(2)
58300	0(3)
58301	1(3)
58321	1(2)
58322	1(2)
58323	1(3)
58340	1(3)
58345	1(3)
58346	1(2)
58350	1(2)
58353	1(3)
58356	1(3)
58400	1(3)
58410	1(2)
58520	1(2)
58540	1(3)
58541	1(3)
58542	1(2)
58543	1(3)
58544	1(2)
58545	1(2)
58546	1(2)
58548	1(2)
58550	1(3)
58552	1(3)
58553	1(3)
58554	1(2)
58555	1(3)
58558	1(3)
58559	1(3)
58560	1(3)
58561	1(3)
58562	1(3)
58563	1(3)
58565	1(2)
58570	1(3)
58571	1(2)
58572	1(3)
58573	1(2)
58575	1(2)
58578	1(3)

CPT	MUE
58579	1(3)
58600	1(2)
58605	1(2)
58611	1(2)
58615	1(2)
58660	1(2)
58661	1(2)
58662	1(2)
58670	1(2)
58671	1(2)
58672	1(2)
58673	1(2)
58674	1(2)
58679	1(3)
58700	1(2)
58720	1(2)
58740	1(2)
58750	1(2)
58752	1(2)
58760	1(2)
58770	1(2)
58800	1(2)
58805	1(2)
58820	1(3)
58822	1(3)
58825	1(2)
58900	1(2)
58920	1(2)
58925	1(3)
58940	1(2)
58943	1(2)
58950	1(2)
58951	1(2)
58952	1(2)
58953	1(2)
58954	1(2)
58956	1(2)
58957	1(2)
58958	1(2)
58960	1(2)
58970	1(3)
58974	1(3)
58976	2(3)
58999	1(3)
59000	2(3)
59001	2(3)
59012	2(3)
59015	2(3)
59020	2(3)
59025	2(3)
59030	2(3)
59050	2(3)
59051	2(3)
59070	2(3)
59072	2(3)
59074	2(3)
59076	2(3)
59100	1(2)
59120	1(3)
59121	1(3)
59130	1(3)
59135	1(3)
59136	1(3)
59140	1(2)
59150	1(3)

CPT	MUE
59151	1(3)
59160	1(2)
59200	1(3)
59300	1(2)
59320	1(2)
59325	1(2)
59350	1(2)
59400	1(2)
59409	2(3)
59410	1(2)
59412	1(3)
59414	1(3)
59425	1(2)
59426	1(2)
59430	1(2)
59510	1(2)
59514	1(3)
59515	1(2)
59525	1(2)
59610	1(2)
59612	2(3)
59614	1(2)
59618	1(2)
59620	1(2)
59622	1(2)
59812	1(2)
59820	1(2)
59821	1(2)
59830	1(2)
59840	1(2)
59841	1(2)
59850	1(2)
59851	1(2)
59852	1(2)
59855	1(2)
59856	1(2)
59857	1(2)
59866	1(2)
59870	1(2)
59871	1(2)
59897	1(3)
59898	1(3)
59899	1(3)
60000	1(3)
60100	3(3)
60200	2(3)
60210	1(2)
60212	1(2)
60220	1(3)
60225	1(2)
60240	1(2)
60252	1(2)
60254	1(2)
60260	1(2)
60270	1(2)
60271	1(2)
60280	1(3)
60281	1(3)
60300	2(3)
60500	1(2)
60502	1(3)
60505	1(3)
60512	1(3)
60520	1(2)
60521	1(2)

CPT	MUE
60522	1(2)
60540	1(2)
60545	1(2)
60600	1(3)
60605	1(3)
60650	1(2)
60659	1(3)
60699	1(3)
61000	1(2)
61001	1(2)
61020	2(3)
61026	2(3)
61050	1(3)
61055	1(3)
61070	2(3)
61105	1(3)
61107	1(3)
61108	1(3)
61120	1(3)
61140	1(3)
61150	1(3)
61151	1(3)
61154	1(3)
61156	1(3)
61210	1(3)
61215	1(3)
61250	1(3)
61253	1(3)
61304	1(3)
61305	1(3)
61312	2(3)
61313	2(3)
61314	2(3)
61315	1(3)
61316	1(3)
61320	2(3)
61321	1(3)
61322	1(3)
61323	1(3)
61330	1(2)
61333	1(2)
61340	1(2)
61343	1(2)
61345	1(3)
61450	1(3)
61458	1(2)
61460	1(2)
61500	1(3)
61501	1(3)
61510	1(3)
61512	1(3)
61514	2(3)
61516	1(3)
61517	1(3)
61518	1(3)
61519	1(3)
61520	1(3)
61521	1(3)
61522	1(3)
61524	2(3)
61526	1(3)
61530	1(3)
61531	1(2)
61533	2(3)
61534	1(3)

CPT	MUE
61535	2(3)
61536	1(3)
61537	1(3)
61538	1(2)
61539	1(3)
61540	1(3)
61541	1(2)
61543	1(2)
61544	1(3)
61545	1(2)
61546	1(2)
61548	1(2)
61550	1(2)
61552	1(2)
61556	1(3)
61557	1(2)
61558	1(3)
61559	1(3)
61563	2(3)
61564	1(2)
61566	1(3)
61567	1(2)
61570	1(3)
61571	1(3)
61575	1(2)
61576	1(2)
61580	1(2)
61581	1(2)
61582	1(2)
61583	1(2)
61584	1(2)
61585	1(2)
61586	1(3)
61590	1(2)
61591	1(2)
61592	1(2)
61595	1(2)
61596	1(2)
61597	1(2)
61598	1(3)
61600	1(3)
61601	1(3)
61605	1(3)
61606	1(3)
61607	1(3)
61608	1(3)
61611	1(3)
61613	1(3)
61615	1(3)
61616	1(3)
61618	2(3)
61619	2(3)
61623	2(3)
61624	2(3)
61626	2(3)
61630	1(3)
61635	2(3)
61640	0(3)
61641	0(3)
61642	0(3)
61645	1(3)
61650	1(2)
61651	2(2)
61680	1(3)
61682	1(3)

CPT	MUE
61684	1(3)
61686	1(3)
61690	1(3)
61692	1(3)
61697	2(3)
61698	1(3)
61700	2(3)
61702	1(3)
61703	1(3)
61705	1(3)
61708	1(3)
61710	1(3)
61711	1(3)
61720	1(3)
61735	1(3)
61750	2(3)
61751	2(3)
61760	1(2)
61770	1(2)
61781	1(3)
61782	1(3)
61783	1(3)
61790	1(2)
61791	1(2)
61796	1(2)
61797	4(3)
61798	1(2)
61799	4(3)
61800	1(2)
61850	1(3)
61860	1(3)
61863	1(2)
61864	1(3)
61867	1(2)
61868	2(3)
61870	1(3)
61880	1(2)
61885	1(3)
61886	1(3)
61888	1(3)
62000	1(3)
62005	1(3)
62010	1(3)
62100	1(3)
62115	1(2)
62117	1(2)
62120	1(2)
62121	1(2)
62140	1(3)
62141	1(3)
62142	2(3)
62143	2(3)
62145	2(3)
62146	2(3)
62147	1(3)
62148	1(3)
62160	1(3)
62161	1(3)
62162	1(3)
62163	1(3)
62164	1(3)
62165	1(2)
62180	1(3)
62190	1(3)
62192	1(3)

CPT	MUE
62194	1(3)
62200	1(2)
62201	1(2)
62220	1(3)
62223	1(3)
62225	2(3)
62230	2(3)
62252	2(3)
62256	1(3)
62258	1(3)
62263	1(2)
62264	1(2)
62267	2(3)
62268	1(3)
62269	2(3)
62270	2(3)
62272	2(3)
62273	2(3)
62280	1(3)
62281	1(3)
62282	1(3)
62284	1(3)
62287	1(2)
62290	5(2)
62291	4(3)
62292	1(2)
62294	1(3)
62302	1(3)
62303	1(3)
62304	1(3)
62305	1(3)
62320	1(3)
62321	1(3)
62322	1(3)
62323	1(3)
62324	1(3)
62325	1(3)
62326	1(3)
62327	1(3)
62328	2(3)
62329	1(3)
62350	1(3)
62351	1(3)
62355	1(3)
62360	1(2)
62361	1(2)
62362	1(2)
62365	1(2)
62367	1(3)
62368	1(3)
62369	1(3)
62370	1(3)
62380	2(3)
63001	1(2)
63003	1(2)
63005	1(2)
63011	1(2)
63012	1(2)
63015	1(2)
63016	1(2)
63017	1(2)
63020	1(2)
63030	1(2)
63035	4(3)
63040	1(2)

CPT	MUE
63042	1(2)
63043	4(3)
63044	4(2)
63045	1(2)
63046	1(2)
63047	1(2)
63048	5(3)
63050	1(2)
63051	1(2)
63055	1(2)
63056	1(2)
63057	3(3)
63064	1(2)
63066	1(3)
63075	1(2)
63076	3(3)
63077	1(2)
63078	3(3)
63081	1(2)
63082	6(2)
63085	1(2)
63086	2(3)
63087	1(2)
63088	3(3)
63090	1(2)
63091	3(3)
63101	1(2)
63102	1(2)
63103	3(3)
63170	1(3)
63172	1(3)
63173	1(3)
63180	1(2)
63182	1(2)
63185	1(2)
63190	1(2)
63191	1(2)
63194	1(2)
63195	1(2)
63196	1(2)
63197	1(2)
63198	1(2)
63199	1(2)
63200	1(2)
63250	1(3)
63251	1(3)
63252	1(3)
63265	1(3)
63266	1(3)
63267	1(3)
63268	1(3)
63270	1(3)
63271	1(3)
63272	1(3)
63273	1(3)
63275	1(3)
63276	1(3)
63277	1(3)
63278	1(3)
63280	1(3)
63281	1(3)
63282	1(3)
63283	1(3)
63285	1(3)
63286	1(3)

CPT	MUE
63287	1(3)
63290	1(3)
63295	1(2)
63300	1(2)
63301	1(2)
63302	1(2)
63303	1(2)
63304	1(2)
63305	1(2)
63306	1(2)
63307	1(2)
63308	3(3)
63600	2(3)
63610	1(3)
63620	1(2)
63621	2(2)
63650	2(3)
63655	1(3)
63661	1(2)
63662	1(2)
63663	1(3)
63664	1(3)
63685	1(3)
63688	1(3)
63700	1(3)
63702	1(3)
63704	1(3)
63706	1(3)
63707	1(3)
63709	1(3)
63710	1(3)
63740	1(3)
63741	1(3)
63744	1(3)
63746	1(2)
64400	4(3)
64405	1(3)
64408	1(3)
64415	1(3)
64416	1(2)
64417	1(3)
64418	1(3)
64420	2(2)
64421	3(3)
64425	1(3)
64430	1(3)
64435	1(3)
64445	1(3)
64446	1(2)
64447	1(3)
64448	1(2)
64449	1(2)
64450	10(3)
64451	2(2)
64454	2(2)
64455	1(2)
64461	1(2)
64462	1(2)
64463	1(3)
64479	1(2)
64480	4(3)
64483	1(2)
64484	4(3)
64486	1(3)
64487	1(2)

CPT	MUE
64488	1(3)
64489	1(2)
64490	1(2)
64491	1(2)
64492	1(2)
64493	1(2)
64494	1(2)
64495	1(2)
64505	1(3)
64510	1(3)
64517	1(3)
64520	1(3)
64530	1(3)
64553	1(3)
64555	2(3)
64561	1(3)
64566	1(3)
64568	1(3)
64569	1(3)
64570	1(3)
64575	2(3)
64580	2(3)
64581	2(3)
64585	2(3)
64590	1(3)
64595	1(3)
64600	2(3)
64605	1(2)
64610	1(2)
64611	1(2)
64612	1(2)
64615	1(2)
64616	1(2)
64617	1(2)
64620	5(3)
64624	2(2)
64625	2(2)
64630	1(3)
64632	1(2)
64633	1(2)
64634	4(3)
64635	1(2)
64636	4(2)
64640	5(3)
64642	1(2)
64643	3(2)
64644	1(2)
64645	3(2)
64646	1(2)
64647	1(2)
64650	1(2)
64653	1(2)
64680	1(2)
64681	1(2)
64702	2(3)
64704	4(3)
64708	3(3)
64712	1(2)
64713	1(2)
64714	1(2)
64716	2(3)
64718	1(2)
64719	1(2)
64721	1(2)
64722	4(3)

CPT	MUE
64726	2(3)
64727	2(3)
64732	1(2)
64734	1(2)
64736	1(2)
64738	1(2)
64740	1(2)
64742	1(2)
64744	1(2)
64746	1(2)
64755	1(2)
64760	1(2)
64763	1(2)
64766	1(2)
64771	2(3)
64772	2(3)
64774	2(3)
64776	1(2)
64778	1(3)
64782	2(2)
64783	2(3)
64784	3(3)
64786	1(3)
64787	4(3)
64788	5(3)
64790	1(3)
64792	2(3)
64795	2(3)
64802	1(2)
64804	1(2)
64809	1(2)
64818	1(2)
64820	4(3)
64821	1(2)
64822	1(2)
64823	1(2)
64831	1(2)
64832	3(3)
64834	1(2)
64835	1(2)
64836	1(2)
64837	2(3)
64840	1(2)
64856	2(3)
64857	2(3)
64858	1(2)
64859	2(3)
64861	1(2)
64862	1(2)
64864	2(3)
64865	1(3)
64866	1(3)
64868	1(3)
64872	1(3)
64874	1(3)
64876	1(3)
64885	1(3)
64886	1(3)
64890	2(3)
64891	2(3)
64892	2(3)
64893	2(3)
64895	2(3)
64896	2(3)
64897	2(3)

CPT	MUE
64898	2(3)
64901	2(3)
64902	1(3)
64905	1(3)
64907	1(3)
64910	3(3)
64911	2(3)
64912	3(3)
64913	3(3)
64999	1(3)
65091	1(2)
65093	1(2)
65101	1(2)
65103	1(2)
65105	1(2)
65110	1(2)
65112	1(2)
65114	1(2)
65125	1(2)
65130	1(2)
65135	1(2)
65140	1(2)
65150	1(2)
65155	1(2)
65175	1(2)
65205	1(3)
65210	1(3)
65220	1(3)
65222	1(3)
65235	1(3)
65260	1(3)
65265	1(3)
65270	1(3)
65272	1(3)
65273	1(3)
65275	1(3)
65280	1(3)
65285	1(3)
65286	1(3)
65290	1(3)
65400	1(3)
65410	1(3)
65420	1(2)
65426	1(2)
65430	1(2)
65435	1(2)
65436	1(2)
65450	1(3)
65600	1(2)
65710	1(2)
65730	1(2)
65750	1(2)
65755	1(2)
65756	1(2)
65757	1(3)
65760	0(3)
65765	0(3)
65767	0(3)
65770	1(2)
65771	0(3)
65772	1(2)
65775	1(2)
65778	1(2)
65779	1(2)
65780	1(2)

CPT	MUE
65781	1(2)
65782	1(2)
65785	1(2)
65800	1(2)
65810	1(2)
65815	1(3)
65820	1(2)
65850	1(2)
65855	1(2)
65860	1(2)
65865	1(2)
65870	1(2)
65875	1(2)
65880	1(2)
65900	1(3)
65920	1(2)
65930	1(3)
66020	1(3)
66030	1(3)
66130	1(3)
66150	1(2)
66155	1(2)
66160	1(2)
66170	1(2)
66172	1(2)
66174	1(2)
66175	1(2)
66179	1(2)
66180	1(2)
66183	1(3)
66184	1(2)
66185	1(2)
66225	1(2)
66250	1(2)
66500	1(2)
66505	1(2)
66600	1(2)
66605	1(2)
66625	1(2)
66630	1(2)
66635	1(2)
66680	1(2)
66682	1(2)
66700	1(2)
66710	1(2)
66711	1(2)
66720	1(2)
66740	1(2)
66761	1(2)
66762	1(2)
66770	1(3)
66820	1(2)
66821	1(2)
66825	1(2)
66830	1(2)
66840	1(2)
66850	1(2)
66852	1(2)
66920	1(2)
66930	1(2)
66940	1(2)
66982	1(2)
66983	1(2)
66984	1(2)
66985	1(2)

CPT	MUE
66986	1(2)
66987	2(2)
66988	2(2)
66990	1(3)
66999	1(3)
67005	1(2)
67010	1(2)
67015	1(2)
67025	1(2)
67027	1(2)
67028	1(3)
67030	1(2)
67031	1(2)
67036	1(2)
67039	1(2)
67040	1(2)
67041	1(2)
67042	1(2)
67043	1(2)
67101	1(2)
67105	1(2)
67107	1(2)
67108	1(2)
67110	1(2)
67113	1(2)
67115	1(2)
67120	1(2)
67121	1(2)
67141	1(2)
67145	1(2)
67208	1(2)
67210	1(2)
67218	1(2)
67220	1(2)
67221	1(2)
67225	1(2)
67227	1(2)
67228	1(2)
67229	1(2)
67250	1(2)
67255	1(2)
67299	1(3)
67311	1(2)
67312	1(2)
67314	1(2)
67316	1(2)
67318	1(2)
67320	2(3)
67331	1(2)
67332	1(2)
67334	1(2)
67335	1(2)
67340	2(2)
67343	1(2)
67345	1(3)
67346	1(3)
67399	1(3)
67400	1(2)
67405	1(2)
67412	1(2)
67413	1(2)
67414	1(2)
67415	1(3)
67420	1(2)
67430	1(2)

CPT	MUE
67440	1(2)
67445	1(2)
67450	1(2)
67500	1(3)
67505	1(3)
67515	1(3)
67550	1(2)
67560	1(2)
67570	1(2)
67599	1(3)
67700	2(3)
67710	1(2)
67715	1(3)
67800	1(2)
67801	1(2)
67805	1(2)
67808	1(2)
67810	2(3)
67820	1(2)
67825	1(2)
67830	1(2)
67835	1(2)
67840	3(3)
67850	3(3)
67875	1(2)
67880	1(2)
67882	1(2)
67900	1(2)
67901	1(2)
67902	1(2)
67903	1(2)
67904	1(2)
67906	1(2)
67908	1(2)
67909	1(2)
67911	2(3)
67912	1(2)
67914	2(3)
67915	2(3)
67916	2(3)
67917	2(3)
67921	2(3)
67922	2(3)
67923	2(3)
67924	2(3)
67930	2(3)
67935	2(3)
67938	2(3)
67950	2(2)
67961	2(3)
67966	2(3)
67971	1(2)
67973	1(2)
67974	1(2)
67975	1(2)
67999	1(3)
68020	1(3)
68040	1(3)
68100	1(3)
68110	1(3)
68115	1(3)
68130	1(3)
68135	1(3)
68200	1(3)
68320	1(2)

CPT	MUE
68325	1(2)
68326	1(2)
68328	1(2)
68330	1(3)
68335	1(3)
68340	1(3)
68360	1(3)
68362	1(3)
68371	1(3)
68399	1(3)
68400	1(2)
68420	1(2)
68440	2(3)
68500	1(2)
68505	1(2)
68510	1(2)
68520	1(2)
68525	1(2)
68530	1(2)
68540	1(2)
68550	1(2)
68700	1(2)
68705	2(3)
68720	1(2)
68745	1(2)
68750	1(2)
68760	4(2)
68761	4(2)
68770	1(3)
68801	4(2)
68810	1(2)
68811	1(2)
68815	1(2)
68816	1(2)
68840	1(2)
68850	1(3)
68899	1(3)
69000	1(3)
69005	1(3)
69020	1(3)
69090	0(3)
69100	3(3)
69105	1(3)
69110	1(2)
69120	1(3)
69140	1(2)
69145	1(3)
69150	1(3)
69155	1(3)
69200	1(2)
69205	1(3)
69209	1(2)
69210	1(2)
69220	1(2)
69222	1(2)
69300	1(2)
69310	1(2)
69320	1(2)
69399	1(3)
69420	1(2)
69421	1(2)
69424	1(2)
69433	1(2)
69436	1(2)
69440	1(2)

CPT	MUE
69450	1(2)
69501	1(3)
69502	1(2)
69505	1(2)
69511	1(2)
69530	1(2)
69535	1(2)
69540	1(3)
69550	1(3)
69552	1(2)
69554	1(2)
69601	1(2)
69602	1(2)
69603	1(2)
69604	1(2)
69605	1(2)
69610	1(2)
69620	1(2)
69631	1(2)
69632	1(3)
69633	1(2)
69635	1(3)
69636	1(3)
69637	1(3)
69641	1(2)
69642	1(2)
69643	1(2)
69644	1(2)
69645	1(2)
69646	1(2)
69650	1(2)
69660	1(2)
69661	1(2)
69662	1(2)
69666	1(2)
69667	1(2)
69670	1(2)
69676	1(2)
69700	1(3)
69710	0(3)
69711	1(2)
69714	1(2)
69715	1(3)
69717	1(2)
69718	1(2)
69720	1(2)
69725	1(2)
69740	1(2)
69745	1(2)
69799	1(3)
69801	1(3)
69805	1(3)
69806	1(3)
69905	1(2)
69910	1(2)
69915	1(3)
69930	1(2)
69949	1(3)
69950	1(2)
69955	1(2)
69960	1(2)
69970	1(3)
69979	1(3)
69990	1(3)
70010	1(3)

CPT	MUE
70015	1(3)
70030	2(2)
70100	2(3)
70110	2(3)
70120	1(3)
70130	1(3)
70134	1(3)
70140	2(3)
70150	1(3)
70160	1(3)
70170	2(2)
70190	1(2)
70200	2(3)
70210	1(3)
70220	1(3)
70240	1(2)
70250	2(3)
70260	1(3)
70300	1(3)
70310	1(3)
70320	1(3)
70328	1(3)
70330	1(3)
70332	2(3)
70336	1(3)
70350	1(3)
70355	1(3)
70360	2(3)
70370	1(3)
70371	1(2)
70380	2(3)
70390	2(3)
70450	3(3)
70460	1(3)
70470	2(3)
70480	1(3)
70481	1(3)
70482	1(3)
70486	1(3)
70487	1(3)
70488	1(3)
70490	1(3)
70491	1(3)
70492	1(3)
70496	2(3)
70498	2(3)
70540	1(3)
70542	1(3)
70543	1(3)
70544	2(3)
70545	1(3)
70546	1(3)
70547	1(3)
70548	1(3)
70549	1(3)
70551	2(3)
70552	2(3)
70553	2(3)
70554	1(3)
70555	1(3)
70557	1(3)
70558	1(3)
70559	1(3)
71045	4(3)
71046	3(3)

CPT	MUE
71047	2(3)
71048	1(3)
71100	2(3)
71101	2(3)
71110	1(3)
71111	1(3)
71120	1(3)
71130	1(3)
71250	2(3)
71260	2(3)
71270	1(3)
71275	1(3)
71550	1(3)
71551	1(3)
71552	1(3)
71555	1(3)
72020	4(3)
72040	3(3)
72050	1(3)
72052	1(3)
72070	1(3)
72072	1(3)
72074	1(3)
72080	1(3)
72081	1(3)
72082	1(3)
72083	1(3)
72084	1(3)
72100	2(3)
72110	1(3)
72114	1(3)
72120	1(3)
72125	1(3)
72126	1(3)
72127	1(3)
72128	1(3)
72129	1(3)
72130	1(3)
72131	1(3)
72132	1(3)
72133	1(3)
72141	1(3)
72142	1(3)
72146	1(3)
72147	1(3)
72148	1(3)
72149	1(3)
72156	1(3)
72157	1(3)
72158	1(3)
72159	1(3)
72170	2(3)
72190	1(3)
72191	1(3)
72192	1(3)
72193	1(3)
72194	1(3)
72195	1(3)
72196	1(3)
72197	1(3)
72198	1(3)
72200	2(3)
72202	1(3)
72220	1(3)
72240	1(2)

CPT	MUE
72255	1(2)
72265	1(2)
72270	1(2)
72275	1(3)
72285	4(3)
72295	5(3)
73000	2(3)
73010	2(3)
73020	2(3)
73030	4(3)
73040	2(2)
73050	1(3)
73060	2(3)
73070	2(3)
73080	2(3)
73085	2(2)
73090	2(3)
73092	2(3)
73100	2(3)
73110	3(3)
73115	2(2)
73120	2(3)
73130	3(3)
73140	3(3)
73200	2(3)
73201	2(3)
73202	2(3)
73206	2(3)
73218	2(3)
73219	2(3)
73220	2(3)
73221	2(3)
73222	2(3)
73223	2(3)
73225	2(3)
73501	2(3)
73502	2(3)
73503	2(3)
73521	2(3)
73522	2(3)
73523	2(3)
73525	2(2)
73551	2(3)
73552	2(3)
73560	4(3)
73562	3(3)
73564	4(3)
73565	1(3)
73580	2(2)
73590	3(3)
73592	2(3)
73600	2(3)
73610	3(3)
73615	2(2)
73620	2(3)
73630	3(3)
73650	2(3)
73660	2(3)
73700	2(3)
73701	2(3)
73702	2(3)
73706	2(3)
73718	2(3)
73719	2(3)
73720	2(3)

CPT	MUE
73721	3(3)
73722	2(3)
73723	2(3)
73725	2(3)
74018	3(3)
74019	2(3)
74021	2(3)
74022	2(3)
74150	1(3)
74160	1(3)
74170	1(3)
74174	1(3)
74175	1(3)
74176	2(3)
74177	2(3)
74178	1(3)
74181	1(3)
74182	1(3)
74183	1(3)
74185	1(3)
74190	1(3)
74210	1(3)
74220	1(3)
74221	1(3)
74230	1(3)
74235	1(3)
74240	2(3)
74246	1(3)
74248	1(2)
74250	1(3)
74251	1(3)
74261	1(2)
74262	1(2)
74263	0(3)
74270	1(3)
74280	1(3)
74283	1(3)
74290	1(3)
74300	1(3)
74301	1(3)
74328	1(3)
74329	1(3)
74330	1(3)
74340	1(3)
74355	1(3)
74360	1(3)
74363	2(3)
74400	1(3)
74410	1(3)
74415	1(3)
74420	2(3)
74425	2(3)
74430	1(3)
74440	1(2)
74445	1(2)
74450	1(3)
74455	1(3)
74470	2(2)
74485	2(3)
74710	1(3)
74712	1(3)
74713	2(3)
74740	1(3)
74742	2(2)
74775	1(2)

CPT	MUE
75557	1(3)
75559	1(3)
75561	1(3)
75563	1(3)
75565	1(3)
75571	1(3)
75572	1(3)
75573	1(3)
75574	1(3)
75600	1(3)
75605	1(3)
75625	1(3)
75630	1(3)
75635	1(3)
75705	20(3)
75710	2(3)
75716	1(3)
75726	3(3)
75731	1(3)
75733	1(3)
75736	2(3)
75741	1(3)
75743	1(3)
75746	1(3)
75756	2(3)
75774	7(3)
75801	1(3)
75803	1(3)
75805	1(2)
75807	1(2)
75809	1(3)
75810	1(3)
75820	2(3)
75822	1(3)
75825	1(3)
75827	1(3)
75831	1(3)
75833	1(3)
75840	1(3)
75842	1(3)
75860	2(3)
75870	1(3)
75872	1(3)
75880	1(3)
75885	1(3)
75887	1(3)
75889	1(3)
75891	1(3)
75893	2(3)
75894	2(3)
75898	2(3)
75901	1(3)
75902	2(3)
75956	1(2)
75957	1(2)
75958	2(3)
75959	1(2)
75970	1(3)
75984	2(3)
75989	2(3)
76000	3(3)
76010	2(3)
76080	3(3)
76098	3(3)
76100	2(3)

CPT	MUE
76101	1(3)
76102	1(3)
76120	1(3)
76125	1(3)
76140	0(3)
76376	2(3)
76377	2(3)
76380	2(3)
76390	0(3)
76391	1(3)
76496	1(3)
76497	1(3)
76498	1(3)
76499	1(3)
76506	1(2)
76510	2(2)
76511	2(2)
76512	2(2)
76513	2(2)
76514	1(2)
76516	1(2)
76519	1(3)
76529	2(2)
76536	1(3)
76604	1(3)
76641	2(2)
76642	2(2)
76700	1(3)
76705	2(3)
76706	1(2)
76770	1(3)
76775	2(3)
76776	2(3)
76800	1(3)
76801	1(2)
76802	2(3)
76805	1(2)
76810	2(3)
76811	1(2)
76812	2(3)
76813	1(2)
76814	2(3)
76815	1(2)
76816	2(3)
76817	1(3)
76818	2(3)
76819	2(3)
76820	3(3)
76821	2(3)
76825	2(3)
76826	2(3)
76827	2(3)
76828	2(3)
76830	1(3)
76831	1(3)
76856	1(3)
76857	1(3)
76870	1(2)
76872	1(3)
76873	1(2)
76881	2(3)
76882	2(3)
76885	1(2)
76886	1(2)
76932	1(2)

CPT	MUE
76936	1(3)
76937	2(3)
76940	1(3)
76941	3(3)
76942	1(3)
76945	1(3)
76946	1(3)
76948	1(2)
76965	2(3)
76970	2(3)
76975	1(3)
76977	1(2)
76978	1(2)
76979	3(3)
76981	1(3)
76982	1(2)
76983	2(3)
76998	1(3)
76999	1(3)
77001	2(3)
77002	1(3)
77003	1(3)
77011	1(3)
77012	1(3)
77013	1(3)
77014	2(3)
77021	1(3)
77022	1(3)
77046	1(2)
77047	1(2)
77048	1(2)
77049	1(2)
77053	2(2)
77054	2(2)
77061	1(2)
77062	1(2)
77063	1(2)
77065	1(2)
77066	1(2)
77067	1(2)
77071	1(3)
77072	1(2)
77073	1(2)
77074	1(2)
77075	1(2)
77076	1(2)
77077	1(2)
77078	1(2)
77080	1(2)
77081	1(2)
77084	1(2)
77085	1(2)
77086	1(2)
77261	1(3)
77262	1(3)
77263	1(3)
77280	2(3)
77285	1(3)
77290	1(3)
77293	1(3)
77295	1(3)
77299	1(3)
77300	10(3)
77301	1(3)
77306	1(3)

CPT	MUE
77307	1(3)
77316	1(3)
77317	1(3)
77318	1(3)
77321	1(2)
77331	3(3)
77332	4(3)
77333	2(3)
77334	10(3)
77336	1(2)
77338	1(3)
77370	1(3)
77371	1(2)
77372	1(2)
77373	1(3)
77385	2(3)
77386	2(3)
77387	2(3)
77399	1(3)
77401	1(2)
77402	2(3)
77407	2(3)
77412	2(3)
77417	1(2)
77423	1(3)
77424	1(2)
77425	1(3)
77427	1(2)
77431	1(2)
77432	1(2)
77435	1(2)
77469	1(2)
77470	1(2)
77499	1(3)
77520	2(3)
77522	2(3)
77523	2(3)
77525	2(3)
77600	1(3)
77605	1(3)
77610	1(3)
77615	1(3)
77620	1(3)
77750	1(3)
77761	1(3)
77762	1(3)
77763	1(3)
77767	2(3)
77768	2(3)
77770	2(3)
77771	2(3)
77772	2(3)
77778	1(3)
77789	2(3)
77790	1(3)
77799	1(3)
78012	1(3)
78013	1(3)
78014	1(2)
78015	1(3)
78016	1(3)
78018	1(2)
78020	1(3)
78070	1(2)
78071	1(3)

CPT	MUE
78072	1(3)
78075	1(2)
78099	1(3)
78102	1(2)
78103	1(2)
78104	1(2)
78110	1(2)
78111	1(2)
78120	1(2)
78121	1(2)
78122	1(2)
78130	1(2)
78135	1(3)
78140	1(3)
78185	1(2)
78191	1(2)
78195	1(2)
78199	1(3)
78201	1(3)
78202	1(3)
78215	1(3)
78216	1(3)
78226	1(3)
78227	1(3)
78230	1(3)
78231	1(3)
78232	1(3)
78258	1(2)
78261	1(2)
78262	1(2)
78264	1(2)
78265	1(2)
78266	1(2)
78267	1(2)
78268	1(2)
78278	2(3)
78282	1(2)
78290	1(3)
78291	1(3)
78299	1(3)
78300	1(2)
78305	1(2)
78306	1(2)
78315	1(2)
78350	0(3)
78351	0(3)
78399	1(3)
78414	1(2)
78428	1(3)
78429	1(2)
78430	1(2)
78431	1(2)
78432	1(2)
78433	1(2)
78434	1(2)
78445	1(3)
78451	1(2)
78452	1(2)
78453	1(2)
78454	1(2)
78456	1(3)
78457	1(2)
78458	1(2)
78459	1(3)
78466	1(3)

CPT	MUE
78468	1(3)
78469	1(3)
78472	1(2)
78473	1(2)
78481	1(2)
78483	1(2)
78491	1(3)
78492	1(2)
78494	1(3)
78496	1(3)
78499	1(3)
78579	1(3)
78580	1(3)
78582	1(3)
78597	1(3)
78598	1(3)
78599	1(3)
78600	1(3)
78601	1(3)
78605	1(3)
78606	1(3)
78608	1(3)
78609	0(3)
78610	1(3)
78630	1(3)
78635	1(3)
78645	1(3)
78650	1(3)
78660	1(2)
78699	1(3)
78700	1(3)
78701	1(3)
78707	1(2)
78708	1(2)
78709	1(2)
78725	1(3)
78730	1(2)
78740	1(2)
78761	1(2)
78799	1(3)
78800	1(2)
78801	1(2)
78802	1(2)
78803	1(2)
78804	1(2)
78808	1(2)
78811	1(2)
78812	1(2)
78813	1(2)
78814	1(2)
78815	1(2)
78816	1(2)
78830	1(2)
78831	1(2)
78832	1(2)
78835	4(3)
78999	1(3)
79005	1(3)
79101	1(3)
79200	1(3)
79300	1(3)
79403	1(3)
79440	1(3)
79445	1(3)
79999	1(3)

CPT	MUE
80047	2(3)
80048	2(3)
80050	0(3)
80051	4(3)
80053	1(3)
80055	1(3)
80061	1(3)
80069	1(3)
80074	1(2)
80076	1(3)
80081	1(2)
80145	1(3)
80150	2(3)
80155	1(3)
80156	2(3)
80157	2(3)
80158	2(3)
80159	2(3)
80162	2(3)
80163	1(3)
80164	2(3)
80165	1(3)
80168	2(3)
80169	2(3)
80170	2(3)
80171	1(3)
80173	2(3)
80175	1(3)
80176	1(3)
80177	1(3)
80178	2(3)
80180	1(3)
80183	1(3)
80184	2(3)
80185	2(3)
80186	2(3)
80187	1(3)
80188	2(3)
80190	2(3)
80192	2(3)
80194	2(3)
80195	2(3)
80197	2(3)
80198	2(3)
80199	1(3)
80200	2(3)
80201	2(3)
80202	2(3)
80203	1(3)
80230	1(3)
80235	1(3)
80280	1(3)
80285	1(3)
80299	3(3)
80305	1(2)
80306	1(2)
80307	1(2)
80320	2(3)
80321	1(3)
80322	1(3)
80323	1(3)
80324	1(3)
80325	1(3)
80326	1(3)
80327	1(3)

CPT	MUE
80328	1(3)
80329	2(3)
80330	1(3)
80331	1(3)
80332	1(3)
80333	1(3)
80334	1(3)
80335	1(3)
80336	1(3)
80337	1(3)
80338	1(3)
80339	2(3)
80340	1(3)
80341	1(3)
80342	1(3)
80343	1(3)
80344	1(3)
80345	2(3)
80346	1(3)
80347	1(3)
80348	1(3)
80349	1(3)
80350	1(3)
80351	1(3)
80352	1(3)
80353	1(3)
80354	1(3)
80355	1(3)
80356	1(3)
80357	1(3)
80358	1(3)
80359	1(3)
80360	1(3)
80361	2(3)
80362	1(3)
80363	1(3)
80364	1(3)
80365	2(3)
80366	1(3)
80367	1(3)
80368	1(3)
80369	1(3)
80370	1(3)
80371	1(3)
80372	1(3)
80373	1(3)
80374	1(3)
80375	1(3)
80376	1(3)
80377	1(3)
80400	1(3)
80402	1(3)
80406	1(3)
80408	1(3)
80410	1(3)
80412	1(3)
80414	1(3)
80415	1(3)
80416	1(3)
80417	1(3)
80418	1(3)
80420	1(2)
80422	1(3)
80424	1(3)
80426	1(3)

CPT	MUE
80428	1(3)
80430	1(3)
80432	1(3)
80434	1(3)
80435	1(3)
80436	1(3)
80438	1(3)
80439	1(3)
80500	1(3)
80502	1(3)
81000	2(3)
81001	2(3)
81002	2(3)
81003	2(3)
81005	2(3)
81007	1(3)
81015	2(3)
81020	1(3)
81025	1(3)
81050	2(3)
81099	1(3)
81105	1(2)
81106	1(2)
81107	1(2)
81108	1(2)
81109	1(2)
81110	1(2)
81111	1(2)
81112	1(2)
81120	1(3)
81121	1(3)
81161	1(3)
81162	1(2)
81163	1(2)
81164	1(2)
81165	1(2)
81166	1(2)
81167	1(2)
81170	1(2)
81171	1(2)
81172	1(2)
81173	1(2)
81174	1(2)
81175	1(3)
81176	1(3)
81177	1(2)
81178	1(2)
81179	1(2)
81180	1(2)
81181	1(2)
81182	1(2)
81183	1(2)
81184	1(2)
81185	1(2)
81186	1(2)
81187	1(2)
81188	1(2)
81189	1(2)
81190	1(2)
81200	1(2)
81201	1(2)
81202	1(3)
81203	1(3)
81204	1(2)
81205	1(3)

CPT	MUE
81206	1(3)
81207	1(3)
81208	1(3)
81209	1(3)
81210	1(3)
81212	1(2)
81215	1(2)
81216	1(2)
81217	1(2)
81218	1(3)
81219	1(3)
81220	1(3)
81221	1(3)
81222	1(3)
81223	1(2)
81224	1(3)
81225	1(3)
81226	1(3)
81227	1(3)
81228	1(3)
81229	1(3)
81230	1(2)
81231	1(2)
81232	1(2)
81233	1(3)
81234	1(2)
81235	1(3)
81236	1(3)
81237	1(3)
81238	1(2)
81239	1(2)
81240	1(2)
81241	1(2)
81242	1(3)
81243	1(3)
81244	1(3)
81245	1(3)
81246	1(3)
81247	1(2)
81248	1(2)
81249	1(2)
81250	1(3)
81251	1(3)
81252	1(3)
81253	1(3)
81254	1(3)
81255	1(3)
81256	1(2)
81257	1(2)
81258	1(2)
81259	1(2)
81260	1(3)
81261	1(3)
81262	1(3)
81263	1(3)
81264	1(3)
81265	1(3)
81266	2(3)
81267	1(3)
81268	4(3)
81269	1(2)
81270	1(2)
81271	1(2)
81272	1(3)
81273	1(3)

CPT	MUE
81274	1(2)
81275	1(3)
81276	1(3)
81277	1(2)
81283	1(2)
81284	1(2)
81285	1(2)
81286	1(2)
81287	1(3)
81288	1(3)
81289	1(2)
81290	1(3)
81291	1(3)
81292	1(2)
81293	1(3)
81294	1(3)
81295	1(2)
81296	1(3)
81297	1(3)
81298	1(2)
81299	1(3)
81300	1(3)
81301	1(3)
81302	1(3)
81303	1(3)
81304	1(3)
81305	1(3)
81306	1(2)
81307	1(2)
81308	1(2)
81309	1(2)
81310	1(3)
81311	1(3)
81312	1(2)
81313	1(3)
81314	1(3)
81315	1(3)
81316	1(2)
81317	1(2)
81318	1(3)
81319	1(2)
81320	1(3)
81321	1(3)
81322	1(3)
81323	1(3)
81324	1(3)
81325	1(3)
81326	1(3)
81327	1(2)
81328	1(2)
81329	1(2)
81330	1(3)
81331	1(3)
81332	1(3)
81333	1(2)
81334	1(3)
81335	1(2)
81336	1(2)
81337	1(2)
81340	1(3)
81341	1(3)
81342	1(3)
81343	1(2)
81344	1(2)
81345	1(3)

CPT	MUE	CPT	MUE	CPT	MUE	CPT	MUE	CPT	MUE	CPT	MUE	CPT	MUE	CPT	MUE
81346	1(2)	81490	1(2)	82160	1(3)	82565	2(3)	82965	1(3)	83670	1(3)	84135	1(3)	84449	1(3)
81350	1(3)	81493	1(2)	82163	1(3)	82570	3(3)	82977	1(3)	83690	2(3)	84138	1(3)	84450	1(3)
81355	1(3)	81500	1(2)	82164	1(3)	82575	1(3)	82978	1(3)	83695	1(3)	84140	1(3)	84460	1(3)
81361	1(2)	81503	1(2)	82172	2(3)	82585	1(2)	82979	1(3)	83698	1(3)	84143	2(3)	84466	1(3)
81362	1(2)	81504	1(2)	82175	2(3)	82595	1(3)	82985	1(3)	83700	1(2)	84144	1(3)	84478	1(3)
81363	1(2)	81506	1(2)	82180	1(2)	82600	1(3)	83001	1(3)	83701	1(3)	84145	1(3)	84479	1(2)
81364	1(2)	81507	1(2)	82190	2(3)	82607	1(2)	83002	1(3)	83704	1(3)	84146	3(3)	84480	1(2)
81370	1(2)	81508	1(2)	82232	2(3)	82608	1(2)	83003	5(3)	83718	1(3)	84150	2(3)	84481	1(2)
81371	1(2)	81509	1(2)	82239	1(3)	82610	1(3)	83006	1(2)	83719	1(3)	84152	1(2)	84482	1(2)
81372	1(2)	81510	1(2)	82240	1(3)	82615	1(3)	83009	1(3)	83721	1(3)	84153	1(2)	84484	4(3)
81373	2(2)	81511	1(2)	82247	2(3)	82626	1(3)	83010	1(3)	83722	1(2)	84154	1(2)	84485	1(3)
81374	1(3)	81512	1(2)	82248	2(3)	82627	1(3)	83012	1(2)	83727	1(3)	84155	1(3)	84488	1(3)
81375	1(2)	81518	1(2)	82252	1(3)	82633	1(3)	83013	1(3)	83735	4(3)	84156	1(3)	84490	1(2)
81376	5(3)	81519	1(2)	82261	1(3)	82634	1(3)	83014	1(2)	83775	1(3)	84157	2(3)	84510	1(3)
81377	2(3)	81520	1(2)	82270	1(3)	82638	1(3)	83015	1(2)	83785	1(3)	84160	2(3)	84512	3(3)
81378	1(2)	81521	1(2)	82271	3(3)	82642	1(2)	83018	4(3)	83789	4(3)	84163	1(3)	84520	2(3)
81379	1(2)	81522	1(2)	82272	1(3)	82652	1(2)	83020	2(3)	83825	2(3)	84165	1(2)	84525	1(3)
81380	2(2)	81525	1(2)	82274	1(3)	82656	1(3)	83021	2(3)	83835	2(3)	84166	2(3)	84540	2(3)
81381	3(3)	81528	1(2)	82286	1(3)	82657	2(3)	83026	1(3)	83857	1(3)	84181	3(3)	84545	1(3)
81382	6(3)	81535	1(2)	82300	1(3)	82658	2(3)	83030	1(3)	83861	2(2)	84182	6(3)	84550	1(3)
81383	2(3)	81536	11(3)	82306	1(2)	82664	2(3)	83033	1(3)	83864	1(2)	84202	1(2)	84560	2(3)
81400	2(3)	81538	1(2)	82308	1(3)	82668	1(3)	83036	1(2)	83872	2(3)	84203	1(2)	84577	1(3)
81401	3(3)	81539	1(2)	82310	4(3)	82670	2(3)	83037	1(2)	83873	1(3)	84206	1(2)	84578	1(3)
81402	1(3)	81540	1(2)	82330	4(3)	82671	1(3)	83045	1(3)	83874	4(3)	84207	1(2)	84580	1(3)
81403	3(3)	81541	1(2)	82331	1(3)	82672	1(3)	83050	2(3)	83876	1(3)	84210	1(3)	84583	1(3)
81404	3(3)	81542	1(2)	82340	1(3)	82677	1(3)	83051	1(3)	83880	1(3)	84220	1(3)	84585	1(2)
81405	2(3)	81545	1(2)	82355	2(3)	82679	1(3)	83060	1(3)	83883	4(3)	84228	1(3)	84586	1(2)
81406	3(3)	81551	1(2)	82360	2(3)	82693	2(3)	83065	1(2)	83885	2(3)	84233	1(3)	84588	1(3)
81407	1(3)	81552	1(2)	82365	2(3)	82696	1(3)	83068	1(2)	83915	1(3)	84234	1(3)	84590	1(2)
81408	1(3)	81595	1(2)	82370	2(3)	82705	1(3)	83069	1(3)	83916	2(3)	84235	1(3)	84591	1(3)
81410	1(2)	81596	1(2)	82373	1(3)	82710	1(3)	83070	1(2)	83918	2(3)	84238	3(3)	84597	1(3)
81411	1(2)	81599	1(3)	82374	2(3)	82715	3(3)	83080	2(3)	83919	1(3)	84244	2(3)	84600	2(3)
81412	1(2)	82009	3(3)	82375	4(3)	82725	1(3)	83088	1(3)	83921	2(3)	84252	1(2)	84620	1(2)
81413	1(2)	82010	3(3)	82376	2(3)	82726	1(3)	83090	2(3)	83930	2(3)	84255	2(3)	84630	2(3)
81414	1(2)	82013	1(3)	82378	1(3)	82728	1(3)	83150	1(3)	83935	2(3)	84260	1(3)	84681	1(3)
81415	1(2)	82016	1(3)	82379	1(3)	82731	1(3)	83491	1(3)	83937	1(3)	84270	1(3)	84702	2(3)
81416	2(3)	82017	1(3)	82380	1(3)	82735	1(3)	83497	1(3)	83945	2(3)	84275	1(3)	84703	1(3)
81417	1(3)	82024	4(3)	82382	1(2)	82746	1(2)	83498	2(3)	83950	1(2)	84285	1(3)	84704	1(3)
81420	1(2)	82030	1(3)	82383	1(3)	82747	1(2)	83500	1(3)	83951	1(2)	84295	2(3)	84830	1(2)
81422	1(2)	82040	1(3)	82384	2(3)	82757	1(2)	83505	1(3)	83970	4(3)	84300	2(3)	84999	1(3)
81425	1(2)	82042	2(3)	82387	1(3)	82759	1(3)	83516	5(3)	83986	2(3)	84302	1(3)	85002	1(3)
81426	2(3)	82043	1(3)	82390	1(2)	82760	1(3)	83518	1(3)	83987	1(3)	84305	1(3)	85004	2(3)
81427	1(3)	82044	1(3)	82397	4(3)	82775	1(3)	83519	5(3)	83992	2(3)	84307	1(3)	85007	1(3)
81430	1(2)	82045	1(3)	82415	1(3)	82776	1(2)	83520	9(3)	83993	1(3)	84311	2(3)	85008	1(3)
81431	1(2)	82075	2(3)	82435	2(3)	82777	1(3)	83525	4(3)	84030	1(2)	84315	1(3)	85009	1(3)
81432	1(2)	82085	1(3)	82436	1(3)	82784	6(3)	83527	1(3)	84035	1(2)	84375	1(3)	85013	1(3)
81433	1(2)	82088	2(3)	82438	1(3)	82785	1(3)	83528	1(3)	84060	1(3)	84376	1(3)	85014	4(3)
81434	1(2)	82103	1(3)	82441	1(2)	82787	4(3)	83540	2(3)	84066	1(3)	84377	1(3)	85018	4(3)
81435	1(2)	82104	1(2)	82465	1(3)	82800	2(3)	83550	1(3)	84075	2(3)	84378	2(3)	85025	4(3)
81436	1(2)	82105	1(3)	82480	2(3)	82805	3(3)	83570	1(3)	84078	1(2)	84379	1(3)	85027	4(3)
81437	1(2)	82106	2(3)	82482	1(3)	82810	4(3)	83582	1(3)	84080	1(3)	84392	1(3)	85032	2(3)
81438	1(2)	82107	1(3)	82485	1(3)	82820	1(3)	83586	1(3)	84081	1(3)	84402	1(3)	85041	1(3)
81439	1(2)	82108	1(3)	82495	1(2)	82930	1(3)	83593	1(3)	84085	1(2)	84403	2(3)	85044	1(2)
81440	1(2)	82120	1(3)	82507	1(3)	82938	1(3)	83605	2(3)	84087	1(3)	84410	1(2)	85045	1(2)
81442	1(2)	82127	1(3)	82523	1(3)	82941	1(3)	83615	3(3)	84100	2(3)	84425	1(2)	85046	1(2)
81443	1(2)	82128	2(3)	82525	2(3)	82943	1(3)	83625	1(3)	84105	1(3)	84430	1(3)	85048	2(3)
81445	1(2)	82131	2(3)	82528	1(3)	82945	4(3)	83630	1(3)	84106	1(2)	84431	1(3)	85049	2(3)
81448	1(2)	82135	1(3)	82530	4(3)	82946	1(2)	83631	1(3)	84110	1(3)	84432	1(2)	85055	1(3)
81450	1(2)	82136	2(3)	82533	5(3)	82947	5(3)	83632	1(3)	84112	1(3)	84436	1(2)	85060	1(3)
81455	1(2)	82139	2(3)	82540	1(3)	82950	3(3)	83633	1(3)	84119	1(2)	84437	1(2)	85097	2(3)
81460	1(2)	82140	2(3)	82542	6(3)	82951	1(2)	83655	2(3)	84120	1(3)	84439	1(2)	85130	1(3)
81465	1(2)	82143	2(3)	82550	3(3)	82952	3(3)	83661	3(3)	84126	1(3)	84442	1(2)	85170	1(3)
81470	1(2)	82150	4(3)	82552	3(3)	82955	1(2)	83662	4(3)	84132	3(3)	84443	4(2)	85175	1(3)
81471	1(2)	82154	1(3)	82553	3(3)	82960	1(2)	83663	3(3)	84133	2(3)	84445	1(2)	85210	2(3)
81479	3(3)	82157	1(3)	82554	2(3)	82963	1(3)	83664	3(3)	84134	1(3)	84446	1(2)	85220	2(3)

CPT	MUE	CPT	MUE	CPT	MUE	CPT	MUE	CPT	MUE	CPT	MUE	CPT	MUE	CPT	MUE
85230	2(3)	85651	1(2)	86334	2(2)	86671	3(3)	86816	1(2)	87110	2(3)	87338	1(3)	87537	1(3)
85240	2(3)	85652	1(2)	86335	2(3)	86674	3(3)	86817	1(2)	87118	3(3)	87339	1(3)	87538	1(3)
85244	1(3)	85660	2(3)	86336	1(3)	86677	3(3)	86821	1(3)	87140	3(3)	87340	1(2)	87539	1(3)
85245	2(3)	85670	2(3)	86337	1(2)	86682	2(3)	86825	1(3)	87143	2(3)	87341	1(2)	87540	1(3)
85246	2(3)	85675	1(3)	86340	1(2)	86684	2(3)	86826	8(3)	87149	11(3)	87350	1(2)	87541	1(3)
85247	2(3)	85705	1(3)	86341	1(3)	86687	1(3)	86828	2(3)	87150	12(3)	87380	1(2)	87542	1(3)
85250	2(3)	85730	4(3)	86343	1(3)	86688	1(3)	86829	2(3)	87152	1(3)	87385	2(3)	87550	1(3)
85260	2(3)	85732	4(3)	86344	1(2)	86689	2(3)	86830	2(3)	87153	3(3)	87389	1(3)	87551	2(3)
85270	2(3)	85810	2(3)	86352	1(3)	86692	2(3)	86831	2(3)	87164	2(3)	87390	1(3)	87552	1(3)
85280	2(3)	85999	1(3)	86353	7(3)	86694	2(3)	86832	2(3)	87166	2(3)	87391	1(3)	87555	1(3)
85290	2(3)	86000	6(3)	86355	1(2)	86695	2(3)	86833	1(3)	87168	2(3)	87400	2(3)	87556	1(3)
85291	1(3)	86001	20(3)	86356	7(3)	86696	2(3)	86834	1(3)	87169	2(3)	87420	1(3)	87557	1(3)
85292	1(3)	86005	6(3)	86357	1(2)	86698	3(3)	86835	1(3)	87172	1(3)	87425	1(3)	87560	1(3)
85293	1(3)	86008	20(3)	86359	1(2)	86701	1(3)	86849	1(3)	87176	3(3)	87426	3(3)	87561	1(3)
85300	2(3)	86021	1(2)	86360	1(2)	86702	2(3)	86850	3(3)	87177	3(3)	87427	2(3)	87562	1(3)
85301	1(3)	86022	1(2)	86361	1(2)	86703	1(2)	86860	2(3)	87181	12(3)	87430	1(3)	87563	3(3)
85302	1(3)	86023	3(3)	86367	2(3)	86704	1(2)	86870	6(3)	87184	8(3)	87449	3(3)	87580	1(3)
85303	2(3)	86038	1(3)	86376	2(3)	86705	1(2)	86880	4(3)	87185	4(3)	87450	2(3)	87581	1(3)
85305	2(3)	86039	1(3)	86382	3(3)	86706	2(3)	86885	3(3)	87186	12(3)	87451	2(3)	87582	1(3)
85306	2(3)	86060	1(3)	86384	1(3)	86707	1(3)	86886	3(3)	87187	3(3)	87471	1(3)	87590	1(3)
85307	2(3)	86063	1(3)	86386	1(2)	86708	1(2)	86890	2(3)	87188	14(3)	87472	1(3)	87591	3(3)
85335	2(3)	86077	1(2)	86403	3(3)	86709	1(2)	86891	2(3)	87190	10(3)	87475	1(3)	87592	1(3)
85337	1(3)	86078	1(3)	86406	2(3)	86710	4(3)	86900	3(3)	87197	1(3)	87476	1(3)	87623	1(2)
85345	1(3)	86079	1(3)	86430	2(3)	86711	2(3)	86901	3(3)	87206	6(3)	87480	1(3)	87624	1(3)
85347	9(3)	86140	1(2)	86431	2(3)	86713	3(3)	86902	40(3)	87207	3(3)	87481	6(3)	87625	1(3)
85348	4(3)	86141	1(2)	86480	1(3)	86717	8(3)	86905	28(3)	87209	4(3)	87482	1(3)	87631	1(3)
85360	1(3)	86146	3(3)	86481	1(3)	86720	2(3)	86906	1(2)	87210	4(3)	87483	1(2)	87632	1(3)
85362	2(3)	86147	4(3)	86485	1(2)	86723	2(3)	86910	0(3)	87220	3(3)	87485	1(3)	87633	1(3)
85366	1(3)	86148	3(3)	86486	2(3)	86727	2(3)	86911	0(3)	87230	2(3)	87486	1(3)	87634	1(3)
85370	1(3)	86152	1(3)	86490	1(2)	86732	2(3)	86920	19(3)	87250	1(3)	87487	1(3)	87635	2(3)
85378	2(3)	86153	1(3)	86510	1(2)	86735	2(3)	86922	10(3)	87252	4(3)	87490	1(3)	87640	1(3)
85379	2(3)	86155	1(3)	86580	1(2)	86738	2(3)	86923	10(3)	87253	3(3)	87491	3(3)	87641	1(3)
85380	2(3)	86156	1(2)	86590	1(3)	86741	2(3)	86930	3(3)	87254	10(3)	87492	1(3)	87650	1(3)
85384	2(3)	86157	1(2)	86592	2(3)	86744	2(3)	86931	4(3)	87255	2(3)	87493	2(3)	87651	1(3)
85385	1(3)	86160	4(3)	86593	2(3)	86747	2(3)	86940	3(3)	87260	1(3)	87495	1(3)	87652	1(3)
85390	3(3)	86161	2(3)	86602	3(3)	86750	4(3)	86941	3(3)	87265	1(3)	87496	1(3)	87653	1(3)
85396	1(2)	86162	1(2)	86603	2(3)	86753	3(3)	86945	5(3)	87267	1(3)	87497	2(3)	87660	1(3)
85397	2(3)	86171	2(3)	86609	14(3)	86756	2(3)	86950	1(3)	87269	1(3)	87498	1(3)	87661	1(3)
85400	1(3)	86200	1(3)	86611	4(3)	86757	6(3)	86960	3(3)	87270	1(3)	87500	1(3)	87662	2(3)
85410	1(3)	86215	1(3)	86612	2(3)	86759	2(3)	86965	4(3)	87271	1(3)	87501	1(3)	87797	3(3)
85415	2(3)	86225	1(3)	86615	6(3)	86762	2(3)	86971	6(3)	87272	1(3)	87502	1(3)	87798	21(3)
85420	2(3)	86226	1(3)	86617	2(3)	86765	2(3)	86972	2(3)	87273	1(3)	87503	1(3)	87799	3(3)
85421	1(3)	86235	10(3)	86618	2(3)	86768	5(3)	86975	2(3)	87274	1(3)	87505	1(2)	87800	2(3)
85441	1(2)	86255	5(3)	86619	2(3)	86769	3(3)	86976	2(3)	87275	1(3)	87506	1(2)	87801	3(3)
85445	1(2)	86256	9(3)	86622	2(3)	86771	2(3)	86977	2(3)	87276	1(3)	87507	1(2)	87802	2(3)
85460	1(3)	86277	1(3)	86625	1(3)	86774	2(3)	86999	1(3)	87278	1(3)	87510	1(3)	87803	3(3)
85461	1(2)	86280	1(3)	86628	3(3)	86777	2(3)	87003	1(3)	87279	1(3)	87511	1(3)	87804	3(3)
85475	1(3)	86294	1(3)	86631	6(3)	86778	2(3)	87015	3(3)	87280	1(3)	87512	1(3)	87806	1(2)
85520	3(3)	86300	2(3)	86632	3(3)	86780	2(3)	87045	3(3)	87281	1(3)	87516	1(3)	87807	2(3)
85525	2(3)	86301	1(2)	86635	4(3)	86784	1(3)	87046	6(3)	87283	1(3)	87517	1(3)	87808	1(3)
85530	1(3)	86304	1(2)	86638	6(3)	86787	2(3)	87071	2(3)	87285	1(3)	87520	1(3)	87809	2(3)
85536	1(2)	86305	1(2)	86641	2(3)	86788	2(3)	87073	2(3)	87290	1(3)	87521	1(3)	87810	2(3)
85540	1(2)	86308	1(2)	86644	2(3)	86789	2(3)	87075	6(3)	87299	1(3)	87522	1(3)	87850	1(3)
85547	1(2)	86309	1(2)	86645	1(3)	86790	4(3)	87076	4(3)	87300	2(3)	87525	1(3)	87880	2(3)
85549	1(3)	86310	1(2)	86648	2(3)	86793	2(3)	87077	6(3)	87301	1(3)	87526	1(3)	87899	6(3)
85555	1(2)	86316	2(3)	86651	2(3)	86794	1(3)	87081	4(3)	87305	1(3)	87527	1(3)	87900	1(2)
85557	1(2)	86317	6(3)	86652	2(3)	86800	1(3)	87084	1(3)	87320	1(3)	87528	1(3)	87901	1(2)
85576	7(3)	86318	2(3)	86653	2(3)	86803	1(3)	87086	3(3)	87324	2(3)	87529	2(3)	87902	1(2)
85597	1(3)	86320	1(2)	86654	2(3)	86804	1(2)	87088	3(3)	87327	1(3)	87530	2(3)	87903	1(2)
85598	1(3)	86325	2(3)	86658	12(3)	86805	12(3)	87101	3(3)	87328	2(3)	87531	1(3)	87904	14(3)
85610	4(3)	86327	1(3)	86663	2(3)	86806	2(3)	87102	4(3)	87329	2(3)	87532	1(3)	87905	2(3)
85611	2(3)	86328	3(3)	86664	2(3)	86807	2(3)	87103	2(3)	87332	1(3)	87533	1(3)	87906	2(3)
85612	1(3)	86329	3(3)	86665	2(3)	86808	1(3)	87106	4(3)	87335	1(3)	87534	1(3)	87910	1(3)
85613	3(3)	86331	12(3)	86666	4(3)	86812	1(2)	87107	4(3)	87336	1(3)	87535	1(3)	87912	1(3)
85635	1(3)	86332	1(3)	86668	2(3)	86813	1(2)	87109	2(3)	87337	1(3)	87536	1(3)	87999	1(3)

CPT	MUE
88000	0(3)
88005	0(3)
88007	0(3)
88012	0(3)
88014	0(3)
88016	0(3)
88020	0(3)
88025	0(3)
88027	0(3)
88028	0(3)
88029	0(3)
88036	0(3)
88037	0(3)
88040	0(3)
88045	0(3)
88099	0(3)
88104	5(3)
88106	5(3)
88108	6(3)
88112	6(3)
88120	2(3)
88121	2(3)
88125	1(3)
88130	1(2)
88140	1(2)
88141	1(3)
88142	1(3)
88143	1(3)
88147	1(3)
88148	1(3)
88150	1(3)
88152	1(3)
88153	1(3)
88155	1(3)
88160	4(3)
88161	4(3)
88162	3(3)
88164	1(3)
88165	1(3)
88166	1(3)
88167	1(3)
88172	7(3)
88173	7(3)
88174	1(3)
88175	1(3)
88177	6(3)
88182	2(3)
88184	2(3)
88185	35(3)
88187	2(3)
88188	2(3)
88189	2(3)
88199	1(3)
88230	2(3)
88233	2(3)
88235	2(3)
88237	4(3)
88239	3(3)
88240	3(3)
88241	3(3)
88245	1(2)
88248	1(2)
88249	1(2)
88261	2(3)
88262	2(3)

CPT	MUE
88263	1(3)
88264	1(3)
88267	2(3)
88269	2(3)
88271	16(3)
88272	12(3)
88273	3(3)
88274	5(3)
88275	12(3)
88280	1(3)
88283	5(3)
88285	10(3)
88289	1(3)
88291	0(3)
88299	1(3)
88300	4(3)
88302	4(3)
88304	5(3)
88305	16(3)
88307	8(3)
88309	3(3)
88311	4(3)
88312	9(3)
88313	8(3)
88314	6(3)
88319	11(3)
88321	1(2)
88323	1(2)
88325	1(2)
88329	2(3)
88331	11(3)
88332	13(3)
88333	4(3)
88334	5(3)
88341	13(3)
88342	4(3)
88344	6(3)
88346	2(3)
88348	1(3)
88350	8(3)
88355	1(3)
88356	3(3)
88358	2(3)
88360	6(3)
88361	6(3)
88362	1(3)
88363	2(3)
88364	3(3)
88365	4(3)
88366	2(3)
88367	3(3)
88368	3(3)
88369	3(3)
88371	1(3)
88372	1(3)
88373	3(3)
88374	5(3)
88375	1(3)
88377	5(3)
88380	1(3)
88381	1(3)
88387	2(3)
88388	1(3)
88399	1(3)
88720	1(3)

CPT	MUE
88738	1(3)
88740	1(2)
88741	1(2)
88749	1(3)
89049	1(3)
89050	2(3)
89051	2(3)
89055	2(3)
89060	2(3)
89125	2(3)
89160	1(3)
89190	1(3)
89220	2(3)
89230	1(2)
89240	1(3)
89250	1(2)
89251	1(2)
89253	1(3)
89254	1(3)
89255	1(3)
89257	1(3)
89258	1(2)
89259	1(2)
89260	1(2)
89261	1(2)
89264	1(3)
89268	1(2)
89272	1(2)
89280	1(2)
89281	1(2)
89290	1(2)
89291	1(2)
89300	1(2)
89310	1(2)
89320	1(2)
89321	1(2)
89322	1(2)
89325	1(2)
89329	1(2)
89330	1(2)
89331	1(2)
89335	1(3)
89337	1(2)
89342	1(2)
89343	1(2)
89344	1(2)
89346	1(2)
89352	1(2)
89353	1(3)
89354	1(3)
89356	2(3)
89398	1(3)
90281	0(3)
90283	0(3)
90284	0(3)
90287	0(3)
90288	0(3)
90291	0(3)
90296	1(2)
90371	10(3)
90375	20(3)
90376	20(3)
90378	4(3)
90384	0(3)
90385	1(2)

CPT	MUE
90386	0(3)
90389	0(3)
90393	1(2)
90396	1(2)
90399	0(3)
90460	9(3)
90461	8(3)
90471	1(2)
90472	8(3)
90473	1(2)
90474	1(3)
90476	1(2)
90477	1(2)
90581	1(2)
90585	1(2)
90586	1(2)
90587	1(2)
90619	1(2)
90620	1(2)
90621	1(2)
90625	1(2)
90630	1(2)
90632	1(2)
90633	1(2)
90634	1(2)
90636	1(2)
90644	1(2)
90647	1(2)
90648	1(2)
90649	1(2)
90650	1(2)
90651	1(2)
90653	1(2)
90654	1(2)
90655	1(2)
90656	1(2)
90657	1(2)
90658	1(2)
90660	1(2)
90661	1(2)
90662	1(2)
90664	1(2)
90666	1(2)
90667	1(2)
90668	1(2)
90670	1(2)
90672	1(2)
90673	1(2)
90674	1(2)
90675	1(2)
90676	1(2)
90680	1(2)
90681	1(2)
90682	1(2)
90685	1(2)
90686	1(2)
90687	1(2)
90688	1(2)
90689	1(2)
90690	1(2)
90691	1(2)
90694	1(2)
90696	1(2)
90697	1(2)
90698	1(2)

CPT	MUE
90700	1(2)
90702	1(2)
90707	1(2)
90710	1(2)
90713	1(2)
90714	1(2)
90715	1(2)
90716	1(2)
90717	1(2)
90723	0(3)
90732	1(2)
90733	1(2)
90734	1(2)
90736	1(2)
90738	1(2)
90739	1(2)
90740	1(2)
90743	1(2)
90744	1(2)
90746	1(2)
90747	1(2)
90748	0(3)
90749	1(3)
90750	1(2)
90756	1(2)
90785	3(3)
90791	1(3)
90792	2(3)
90832	3(3)
90833	3(3)
90834	3(3)
90836	3(3)
90837	3(3)
90838	3(3)
90839	1(2)
90840	4(3)
90845	1(2)
90846	2(3)
90847	2(3)
90849	2(3)
90853	4(3)
90863	1(3)
90865	1(3)
90867	1(2)
90868	1(3)
90869	1(3)
90870	2(3)
90875	1(3)
90876	0(3)
90880	1(3)
90882	0(3)
90885	1(3)
90887	1(3)
90889	1(3)
90899	1(3)
90901	1(3)
90912	1(2)
90913	3(3)
90935	1(3)
90937	1(3)
90940	1(3)
90945	1(3)
90947	1(3)
90951	1(2)
90952	1(2)

CPT	MUE
90953	1(2)
90954	1(2)
90955	1(2)
90956	1(2)
90957	1(2)
90958	1(2)
90959	1(2)
90960	1(2)
90961	1(2)
90962	1(2)
90963	1(2)
90964	1(2)
90965	1(2)
90966	1(2)
90967	1(2)
90968	1(2)
90969	1(2)
90970	1(2)
90989	1(2)
90993	1(3)
90997	1(3)
90999	1(3)
91010	1(2)
91013	1(3)
91020	1(2)
91022	1(2)
91030	1(2)
91034	1(2)
91035	1(2)
91037	1(2)
91038	1(2)
91040	1(2)
91065	2(2)
91110	1(2)
91111	1(2)
91112	1(3)
91117	1(2)
91120	1(2)
91122	1(2)
91132	1(3)
91133	1(3)
91200	1(2)
91299	1(3)
92002	1(2)
92004	1(2)
92012	1(3)
92014	1(3)
92015	0(3)
92018	1(2)
92019	1(2)
92020	1(2)
92025	1(2)
92060	1(2)
92065	1(2)
92071	2(2)
92072	1(2)
92081	1(2)
92082	1(2)
92083	1(2)
92100	1(2)
92132	1(2)
92133	1(2)
92134	1(2)
92136	1(3)
92145	1(2)

CPT	MUE
92201	1(2)
92202	1(2)
92227	1(2)
92228	1(2)
92230	2(2)
92235	1(2)
92240	1(2)
92242	1(2)
92250	1(2)
92260	1(2)
92265	1(2)
92270	1(2)
92273	1(2)
92274	1(2)
92283	1(2)
92284	1(2)
92285	1(2)
92286	1(2)
92287	1(2)
92310	0(3)
92311	1(2)
92312	1(2)
92313	1(3)
92314	0(3)
92315	1(2)
92316	1(2)
92317	1(3)
92325	1(3)
92326	2(2)
92340	0(3)
92341	0(3)
92342	0(3)
92352	1(3)
92353	1(3)
92354	1(3)
92355	1(3)
92358	1(3)
92370	0(3)
92371	1(3)
92499	1(3)
92502	1(3)
92504	1(3)
92507	1(3)
92508	1(3)
92511	1(3)
92512	1(2)
92516	1(3)
92520	1(2)
92521	1(2)
92522	1(2)
92523	1(2)
92524	1(2)
92526	1(2)
92531	1(3)
92532	1(3)
92533	4(2)
92534	1(3)
92537	1(2)
92538	1(2)
92540	1(3)
92541	1(3)
92542	1(3)
92544	1(3)
92545	1(3)
92546	1(3)

CPT	MUE
92547	1(3)
92548	1(3)
92549	1(3)
92550	1(2)
92551	0(3)
92552	1(2)
92553	1(2)
92555	1(2)
92556	1(2)
92557	1(2)
92558	0(3)
92559	0(3)
92560	0(3)
92561	1(2)
92562	1(2)
92563	1(2)
92564	1(2)
92565	1(2)
92567	1(2)
92568	1(2)
92570	1(2)
92571	1(2)
92572	1(2)
92575	1(2)
92576	1(2)
92577	1(2)
92579	1(2)
92582	1(2)
92583	1(2)
92584	1(2)
92585	1(2)
92586	1(2)
92587	1(2)
92588	1(2)
92590	0(3)
92591	0(3)
92592	0(3)
92593	0(3)
92594	0(3)
92595	0(3)
92596	1(2)
92597	1(3)
92601	1(3)
92602	1(3)
92603	1(3)
92604	1(3)
92605	1(2)
92606	1(2)
92607	1(3)
92608	4(3)
92609	1(3)
92610	1(2)
92611	1(3)
92612	1(3)
92613	1(2)
92614	1(3)
92615	1(2)
92616	1(3)
92617	1(2)
92618	1(3)
92620	1(2)
92621	4(3)
92625	1(2)
92626	1(2)
92627	6(3)

CPT	MUE
92630	0(3)
92633	0(3)
92640	1(3)
92700	1(3)
92920	3(3)
92921	6(2)
92924	2(3)
92925	6(2)
92928	3(3)
92929	6(2)
92933	2(3)
92934	6(2)
92937	2(3)
92938	6(3)
92941	1(3)
92943	2(3)
92944	3(3)
92950	2(3)
92953	2(3)
92960	2(3)
92961	1(3)
92970	1(3)
92971	1(3)
92973	2(3)
92974	1(3)
92975	1(3)
92977	1(3)
92978	1(3)
92979	2(3)
92986	1(2)
92987	1(2)
92990	1(2)
92992	1(2)
92993	1(2)
92997	1(2)
92998	2(3)
93000	3(3)
93005	5(3)
93010	5(3)
93015	1(3)
93016	1(3)
93017	1(3)
93018	1(3)
93024	1(3)
93025	1(2)
93040	3(3)
93041	3(3)
93042	3(3)
93050	1(3)
93224	1(2)
93225	1(2)
93226	1(2)
93227	1(2)
93228	1(2)
93229	1(2)
93260	1(2)
93261	1(3)
93264	1(2)
93268	1(2)
93270	1(2)
93271	1(2)
93272	1(2)
93278	1(3)
93279	1(3)
93280	1(3)

CPT	MUE
93281	1(3)
93282	1(3)
93283	1(3)
93284	1(3)
93285	1(3)
93286	2(3)
93287	2(3)
93288	1(3)
93289	1(3)
93290	1(3)
93291	1(3)
93292	1(3)
93293	1(2)
93294	1(2)
93295	1(2)
93296	1(2)
93297	1(2)
93298	1(2)
93303	1(3)
93304	1(3)
93306	1(3)
93307	1(3)
93308	1(3)
93312	1(3)
93313	1(3)
93314	1(3)
93315	1(3)
93316	1(3)
93317	1(3)
93318	1(3)
93320	2(3)
93321	1(3)
93325	2(3)
93350	1(2)
93351	1(2)
93352	1(3)
93355	1(3)
93356	1(3)
93451	1(3)
93452	1(3)
93453	1(3)
93454	1(3)
93455	1(3)
93456	1(3)
93457	1(3)
93458	1(3)
93459	1(3)
93460	1(3)
93461	1(3)
93462	1(3)
93463	1(3)
93464	1(3)
93503	2(3)
93505	1(2)
93530	1(3)
93531	1(3)
93532	1(3)
93533	1(3)
93561	1(3)
93562	1(3)
93563	1(3)
93564	1(3)
93565	1(3)
93566	1(3)
93567	1(3)

CPT	MUE
93568	1(3)
93571	1(3)
93572	2(3)
93580	1(3)
93581	1(3)
93582	1(2)
93583	1(2)
93590	1(2)
93591	1(2)
93592	2(3)
93600	1(3)
93602	1(3)
93603	1(3)
93609	1(3)
93610	1(3)
93612	1(3)
93613	1(3)
93615	1(3)
93616	1(3)
93618	1(3)
93619	1(3)
93620	1(3)
93621	1(3)
93622	1(3)
93623	1(3)
93624	1(3)
93631	1(3)
93640	1(3)
93641	1(2)
93642	1(3)
93644	1(3)
93650	1(2)
93653	1(3)
93654	1(3)
93655	2(3)
93656	1(3)
93657	2(3)
93660	1(3)
93662	1(3)
93668	1(3)
93701	1(2)
93702	1(2)
93724	1(3)
93740	1(3)
93745	1(2)
93750	1(3)
93770	1(3)
93784	1(2)
93786	1(2)
93788	1(2)
93790	1(2)
93792	1(2)
93793	1(2)
93797	2(2)
93798	2(2)
93799	1(3)
93880	1(3)
93882	1(3)
93886	1(3)
93888	1(3)
93890	1(3)
93892	1(3)
93893	1(3)
93895	1(3)
93922	2(2)

CPT	MUE
93923	2(2)
93924	1(2)
93925	1(3)
93926	1(3)
93930	1(3)
93931	1(3)
93970	1(3)
93971	1(3)
93975	1(3)
93976	1(3)
93978	1(3)
93979	1(3)
93980	1(3)
93981	1(3)
93985	1(3)
93986	1(3)
93990	2(3)
93998	1(3)
94002	1(2)
94003	1(2)
94004	1(2)
94005	1(3)
94010	1(3)
94011	1(3)
94012	1(3)
94013	1(3)
94014	1(2)
94015	1(2)
94016	1(2)
94060	1(3)
94070	1(2)
94150	2(3)
94200	1(3)
94250	1(3)
94375	1(3)
94400	1(3)
94450	1(3)
94452	1(2)
94453	1(2)
94610	2(3)
94617	1(3)
94618	1(3)
94621	1(3)
94640	1(3)
94642	1(3)
94644	1(2)
94645	4(3)
94660	1(2)
94662	1(2)
94664	1(3)
94667	1(2)
94668	5(3)
94669	4(3)
94680	1(3)
94681	1(3)
94690	1(3)
94726	1(3)
94727	1(3)
94728	1(3)
94729	1(3)
94750	1(3)
94760	1(3)
94761	1(2)
94762	1(2)
94770	1(3)

CPT	MUE
94772	1(2)
94774	1(2)
94775	1(2)
94776	1(2)
94777	1(2)
94780	1(2)
94781	2(3)
94799	1(3)
95004	80(3)
95012	2(3)
95017	27(3)
95018	19(3)
95024	40(3)
95027	90(3)
95028	30(3)
95044	80(3)
95052	20(3)
95056	1(2)
95060	1(2)
95065	1(3)
95070	1(3)
95071	1(2)
95076	1(2)
95079	2(3)
95115	1(2)
95117	1(2)
95120	0(3)
95125	0(3)
95130	0(3)
95131	0(3)
95132	0(3)
95133	0(3)
95134	0(3)
95144	30(3)
95145	10(3)
95146	10(3)
95147	10(3)
95148	10(3)
95149	10(3)
95165	30(3)
95170	10(3)
95180	8(3)
95199	1(3)
95249	1(2)
95250	1(2)
95251	1(2)
95700	1(2)
95705	1(2)
95706	1(2)
95707	1(2)
95708	4(3)
95709	4(3)
95710	4(3)
95711	1(2)
95712	1(2)
95713	1(2)
95714	4(3)
95715	4(3)
95716	4(3)
95717	1(2)
95718	1(2)
95719	1(2)
95720	1(2)
95721	1(2)
95722	1(2)

CPT	MUE
95723	1(2)
95724	1(2)
95725	1(2)
95726	1(2)
95782	1(2)
95783	1(2)
95800	1(2)
95801	1(2)
95803	1(2)
95805	1(2)
95806	1(2)
95807	1(2)
95808	1(2)
95810	1(2)
95811	1(2)
95812	1(3)
95813	1(3)
95816	1(3)
95819	1(3)
95822	1(3)
95824	1(3)
95829	1(3)
95830	1(3)
95836	1(2)
95851	3(3)
95852	1(3)
95857	1(2)
95860	1(3)
95861	1(3)
95863	1(3)
95864	1(3)
95865	1(3)
95866	1(3)
95867	1(3)
95868	1(3)
95869	1(3)
95870	4(3)
95872	4(3)
95873	1(2)
95874	1(2)
95875	2(3)
95885	4(2)
95886	4(2)
95887	1(2)
95905	2(3)
95907	1(2)
95908	1(2)
95909	1(2)
95910	1(2)
95911	1(2)
95912	1(2)
95913	1(2)
95921	1(3)
95922	1(3)
95923	1(3)
95924	1(3)
95925	1(3)
95926	1(3)
95927	1(3)
95928	1(3)
95929	1(3)
95930	1(3)
95933	1(3)
95937	4(3)
95938	1(3)

CPT	MUE
95939	1(3)
95940	20(3)
95941	8(3)
95943	1(3)
95954	1(3)
95955	1(3)
95957	1(3)
95958	1(3)
95961	1(2)
95962	3(3)
95965	1(3)
95966	1(3)
95967	3(3)
95970	1(3)
95971	1(3)
95972	1(3)
95976	1(3)
95977	1(3)
95980	1(3)
95981	1(3)
95982	1(3)
95983	1(2)
95984	11(3)
95990	1(3)
95991	1(3)
95992	1(2)
95999	1(3)
96000	1(2)
96001	1(2)
96002	1(3)
96003	1(3)
96004	1(2)
96020	1(2)
96040	4(3)
96105	3(3)
96110	3(3)
96112	1(2)
96113	6(3)
96116	1(2)
96121	3(3)
96125	2(3)
96127	2(3)
96130	1(2)
96131	7(3)
96132	1(2)
96133	7(3)
96136	1(2)
96137	11(3)
96138	1(2)
96139	11(3)
96146	1(2)
96156	1(3)
96158	1(2)
96159	4(3)
96160	3(3)
96161	1(3)
96164	1(2)
96165	6(3)
96167	1(2)
96168	6(3)
96170	1(3)
96171	1(3)
96360	2(3)
96361	24(3)
96365	2(3)

CPT	MUE
96366	24(3)
96367	4(3)
96368	1(2)
96369	1(2)
96370	3(3)
96371	1(3)
96372	5(3)
96373	3(3)
96374	1(3)
96375	6(3)
96376	10(3)
96377	1(3)
96379	2(3)
96401	4(3)
96402	2(3)
96405	1(2)
96406	1(2)
96409	1(3)
96411	3(3)
96413	1(3)
96415	8(3)
96416	1(3)
96417	3(3)
96420	2(3)
96422	2(3)
96423	2(3)
96425	1(3)
96440	1(3)
96446	1(3)
96450	1(3)
96521	2(3)
96522	1(3)
96523	2(3)
96542	1(3)
96549	1(3)
96567	1(3)
96570	1(2)
96571	2(3)
96573	1(2)
96574	1(2)
96900	1(3)
96902	1(3)
96904	1(2)
96910	1(3)
96912	1(3)
96913	1(3)
96920	1(2)
96921	1(2)
96922	1(2)
96931	1(2)
96932	1(2)
96933	1(2)
96934	2(3)
96935	2(3)
96936	2(3)
96999	1(3)
97010	1(3)
97012	1(3)
97014	0(3)
97016	1(3)
97018	1(3)
97022	1(3)
97024	1(3)
97026	1(3)
97028	1(3)

CPT	MUE	CPT	MUE	CPT	MUE	CPT	MUE	CPT	MUE	CPT	MUE	CPT	MUE	CPT	MUE
97032	4(3)	98926	1(2)	99211	2(3)	99344	1(2)	99456	1(3)	A0160	0(3)	A4252	0(3)	A4367	1(3)
97033	4(3)	98927	1(2)	99212	2(3)	99345	1(2)	99457	1(2)	A0170	0(3)	A4253	0(3)	A4368	1(3)
97034	2(3)	98928	1(2)	99213	2(3)	99347	1(3)	99458	3(3)	A0180	0(3)	A4255	0(3)	A4369	1(3)
97035	2(3)	98929	1(2)	99214	2(3)	99348	1(3)	99460	1(2)	A0190	0(3)	A4256	1(3)	A4371	1(3)
97036	3(3)	98940	1(2)	99215	2(3)	99349	1(3)	99461	1(2)	A0200	0(3)	A4257	0(3)	A4372	1(3)
97039	1(3)	98941	1(2)	99217	1(2)	99350	1(3)	99462	1(2)	A0210	0(3)	A4258	0(3)	A4373	1(3)
97110	8(3)	98942	1(2)	99218	1(2)	99354	1(2)	99463	1(2)	A0225	0(3)	A4259	0(3)	A4375	2(3)
97112	6(3)	98943	0(3)	99219	1(2)	99355	4(3)	99464	1(2)	A0380	0(3)	A4261	0(3)	A4376	2(3)
97113	6(3)	98960	0(3)	99220	1(2)	99356	1(2)	99465	1(2)	A0382	0(3)	A4262	4(2)	A4377	2(3)
97116	4(3)	98961	0(3)	99221	0(3)	99357	1(3)	99466	1(2)	A0384	0(3)	A4263	4(2)	A4378	2(3)
97124	4(3)	98962	0(3)	99222	0(3)	99358	1(2)	99467	4(3)	A0390	0(3)	A4264	0(3)	A4379	2(3)
97129	1(2)	98966	1(2)	99223	0(3)	99359	1(3)	99468	1(2)	A0392	0(3)	A4265	1(3)	A4380	2(3)
97130	7(3)	98967	1(2)	99224	1(2)	99360	1(3)	99469	1(2)	A0394	0(3)	A4266	0(3)	A4381	2(3)
97139	1(3)	98968	1(2)	99225	1(2)	99366	2(3)	99471	1(2)	A0396	0(3)	A4267	0(3)	A4382	2(3)
97140	6(3)	98970	1(2)	99226	1(2)	99367	1(3)	99472	1(2)	A0398	0(3)	A4268	0(3)	A4383	2(3)
97150	2(3)	98971	1(2)	99231	0(3)	99368	2(3)	99473	1(2)	A0420	0(3)	A4269	0(3)	A4384	2(3)
97151	8(3)	98972	1(2)	99232	0(3)	99374	1(2)	99474	1(2)	A0422	0(3)	A4270	3(3)	A4385	2(3)
97152	8(3)	99000	0(3)	99233	0(3)	99375	0(3)	99475	1(2)	A0424	0(3)	A4280	1(3)	A4387	1(3)
97153	32(3)	99001	0(3)	99234	1(3)	99377	1(2)	99476	1(2)	A0425	250(1)	A4281	0(3)	A4388	1(3)
97154	12(3)	99002	1(3)	99235	1(3)	99378	0(3)	99477	1(2)	A0426	2(3)	A4282	0(3)	A4389	2(3)
97155	24(3)	99024	1(3)	99236	1(3)	99379	1(2)	99478	1(2)	A0427	2(3)	A4283	0(3)	A4390	1(3)
97156	16(3)	99026	0(3)	99238	0(3)	99380	1(2)	99479	1(2)	A0428	2(3)	A4284	0(3)	A4391	1(3)
97157	16(3)	99027	0(3)	99239	0(3)	99381	0(3)	99480	1(2)	A0429	2(3)	A4285	0(3)	A4392	2(3)
97158	16(3)	99050	1(3)	99241	0(3)	99382	0(3)	99483	1(2)	A0430	1(3)	A4286	0(3)	A4393	1(3)
97161	1(2)	99051	1(3)	99242	0(3)	99383	0(3)	99484	1(2)	A0431	1(3)	A4290	2(3)	A4394	1(3)
97162	1(2)	99053	1(3)	99243	0(3)	99384	0(3)	99485	1(3)	A0432	1(3)	A4300	4(3)	A4395	3(3)
97163	1(2)	99056	1(3)	99244	0(3)	99385	0(3)	99486	4(1)	A0433	1(3)	A4301	1(2)	A4396	2(3)
97164	1(2)	99058	1(3)	99245	0(3)	99386	0(3)	99487	1(2)	A0434	2(3)	A4305	2(3)	A4397	1(3)
97165	1(2)	99060	1(3)	99251	0(3)	99387	0(3)	99489	4(3)	A0435	999(3)	A4306	2(3)	A4398	2(3)
97166	1(2)	99070	1(3)	99252	0(3)	99391	0(3)	99490	1(2)	A0436	300(3)	A4310	2(3)	A4399	1(3)
97167	1(2)	99071	1(3)	99253	0(3)	99392	0(3)	99491	1(2)	A0888	0(3)	A4311	2(3)	A4400	1(3)
97168	1(2)	99075	0(3)	99254	0(3)	99393	0(3)	99492	1(2)	A0998	0(3)	A4312	1(3)	A4402	1(3)
97169	0(3)	99078	3(3)	99255	0(3)	99394	0(3)	99493	1(2)	A0999	1(3)	A4313	1(3)	A4404	1(3)
97170	0(3)	99080	1(3)	99281	2(3)	99395	0(3)	99494	2(3)	A4206	1(3)	A4314	2(3)	A4405	1(3)
97171	0(3)	99082	1(3)	99282	2(3)	99396	0(3)	99495	1(2)	A4207	1(3)	A4315	2(3)	A4406	1(3)
97172	0(3)	99091	1(2)	99283	2(3)	99397	0(3)	99496	1(2)	A4208	4(3)	A4316	1(3)	A4407	2(3)
97530	6(3)	99100	1(3)	99284	2(3)	99401	0(3)	99497	1(2)	A4209	6(3)	A4320	2(3)	A4408	1(3)
97533	4(3)	99116	1(3)	99285	2(3)	99402	0(3)	99498	3(3)	A4210	0(3)	A4321	1(3)	A4409	1(3)
97535	8(3)	99135	1(3)	99288	1(3)	99403	0(3)	99499	1(3)	A4211	1(3)	A4322	2(3)	A4410	2(3)
97537	8(3)	99140	2(3)	99291	1(2)	99404	0(3)	99500	0(3)	A4212	2(3)	A4326	1(3)	A4411	1(3)
97542	8(3)	99151	1(3)	99292	8(3)	99406	1(2)	99501	0(3)	A4213	5(3)	A4327	2(3)	A4412	1(3)
97545	1(2)	99152	2(3)	99304	1(2)	99407	1(2)	99502	0(3)	A4215	9(3)	A4328	1(3)	A4413	2(3)
97546	2(3)	99153	12(3)	99305	1(2)	99408	0(3)	99503	0(3)	A4216	25(3)	A4330	1(3)	A4414	1(3)
97597	1(3)	99155	1(3)	99306	1(2)	99409	0(3)	99504	0(3)	A4217	4(3)	A4331	3(3)	A4415	1(3)
97598	8(3)	99156	1(3)	99307	1(2)	99411	0(3)	99505	0(3)	A4218	20(3)	A4332	2(3)	A4416	2(3)
97602	1(3)	99157	6(3)	99308	1(2)	99412	0(3)	99506	0(3)	A4220	1(3)	A4335	1(3)	A4417	2(3)
97605	1(3)	99170	1(3)	99309	1(2)	99415	1(2)	99507	0(3)	A4221	1(3)	A4336	1(3)	A4418	2(3)
97606	1(3)	99172	0(3)	99310	1(2)	99416	3(3)	99509	0(3)	A4222	2(3)	A4337	2(3)	A4419	2(3)
97607	1(3)	99173	0(3)	99315	1(2)	99421	1(2)	99510	0(3)	A4223	1(3)	A4338	3(3)	A4420	1(3)
97608	1(3)	99174	0(3)	99316	1(2)	99422	1(2)	99511	0(3)	A4224	1(2)	A4340	2(3)	A4423	2(3)
97610	1(2)	99175	1(3)	99318	1(2)	99423	1(2)	99512	0(3)	A4225	1(3)	A4344	2(3)	A4424	1(3)
97750	8(3)	99177	1(2)	99324	1(2)	99429	0(3)	99600	0(3)	A4226	0(3)	A4346	2(3)	A4425	1(3)
97755	8(3)	99183	1(3)	99325	1(2)	99441	1(2)	99601	0(3)	A4230	1(3)	A4351	2(3)	A4426	2(3)
97760	6(3)	99184	1(2)	99326	1(2)	99442	1(2)	99602	0(3)	A4231	1(3)	A4352	2(3)	A4427	1(3)
97761	6(3)	99188	1(2)	99327	1(2)	99443	1(2)	99605	0(2)	A4232	0(3)	A4353	3(3)	A4428	1(3)
97763	6(3)	99190	1(3)	99328	1(2)	99446	1(2)	99606	0(3)	A4233	0(3)	A4354	2(3)	A4429	2(3)
97799	1(3)	99191	1(3)	99334	1(3)	99447	1(2)	99607	0(3)	A4234	0(3)	A4355	2(3)	A4430	1(3)
97802	8(3)	99192	1(3)	99335	1(3)	99448	1(2)	A0021	0(3)	A4235	1(3)	A4356	2(3)	A4431	1(3)
97803	8(3)	99195	2(3)	99336	1(3)	99449	1(2)	A0080	0(3)	A4236	0(3)	A4357	2(3)	A4432	2(3)
97804	6(3)	99199	1(3)	99337	1(3)	99450	0(3)	A0090	0(3)	A4244	1(3)	A4360	1(3)	A4433	1(3)
97810	1(2)	99201	1(2)	99339	1(2)	99451	1(2)	A0100	0(3)	A4245	1(3)	A4361	1(3)	A4434	1(3)
97811	2(3)	99202	1(2)	99340	1(2)	99452	1(2)	A0110	0(3)	A4246	1(3)	A4362	2(3)	A4435	2(3)
97813	1(2)	99203	1(2)	99341	1(2)	99453	1(2)	A0120	0(3)	A4247	1(3)	A4363	0(3)	A4450	20(3)
97814	2(3)	99204	1(2)	99342	1(2)	99454	1(2)	A0130	0(3)	A4248	10(3)	A4364	2(3)	A4452	4(3)
98925	1(2)	99205	1(2)	99343	1(2)	99455	1(3)	A0140	0(3)	A4250	0(3)	A4366	1(3)	A4455	1(3)

CPT	MUE
A4458	1(3)
A4459	1(3)
A4461	2(3)
A4463	2(3)
A4465	1(3)
A4467	0(3)
A4470	1(3)
A4480	1(3)
A4481	2(3)
A4483	1(3)
A4490	0(3)
A4495	0(3)
A4500	0(3)
A4510	0(3)
A4520	0(3)
A4550	3(3)
A4553	0(3)
A4554	0(3)
A4555	0(3)
A4556	2(3)
A4557	2(3)
A4558	1(3)
A4559	1(3)
A4561	1(3)
A4562	1(3)
A4563	1(2)
A4565	2(3)
A4566	0(3)
A4570	0(3)
A4575	0(3)
A4580	0(3)
A4590	0(3)
A4595	2(3)
A4600	0(3)
A4601	0(3)
A4602	1(3)
A4604	1(3)
A4605	1(3)
A4606	1(3)
A4608	1(3)
A4611	0(3)
A4612	0(3)
A4613	0(3)
A4614	1(2)
A4615	2(3)
A4616	1(3)
A4617	1(3)
A4618	1(3)
A4619	1(3)
A4620	1(3)
A4623	10(3)
A4624	2(3)
A4625	30(3)
A4626	1(3)
A4627	0(3)
A4628	1(3)
A4629	1(3)
A4630	0(3)
A4633	0(3)
A4634	1(3)
A4635	0(3)
A4636	0(3)
A4637	0(3)
A4638	0(3)
A4639	0(3)

CPT	MUE
A4640	0(3)
A4642	1(3)
A4648	3(3)
A4650	3(3)
A4651	2(3)
A4652	2(3)
A4653	0(3)
A4657	0(3)
A4660	0(3)
A4663	0(3)
A4670	0(3)
A4671	0(3)
A4672	0(3)
A4673	0(3)
A4674	0(3)
A4680	0(3)
A4690	0(3)
A4706	0(3)
A4707	0(3)
A4708	0(3)
A4709	0(3)
A4714	0(3)
A4719	0(3)
A4720	0(3)
A4721	0(3)
A4722	0(3)
A4723	0(3)
A4724	0(3)
A4725	0(3)
A4726	0(3)
A4728	0(3)
A4730	0(3)
A4736	0(3)
A4737	0(3)
A4740	0(3)
A4750	0(3)
A4755	0(3)
A4760	0(3)
A4765	0(3)
A4766	0(3)
A4770	0(3)
A4771	0(3)
A4772	0(3)
A4773	0(3)
A4774	0(3)
A4802	0(3)
A4860	0(3)
A4870	0(3)
A4890	0(3)
A4911	0(3)
A4913	0(3)
A4918	0(3)
A4927	0(3)
A4928	0(3)
A4929	0(3)
A4930	0(3)
A4931	0(3)
A4932	0(3)
A5051	1(3)
A5052	1(3)
A5053	2(3)
A5054	1(3)
A5055	1(3)
A5056	90(3)
A5057	90(3)

CPT	MUE
A5061	2(3)
A5062	1(3)
A5063	1(3)
A5071	2(3)
A5072	1(3)
A5073	1(3)
A5081	2(3)
A5082	1(3)
A5083	5(3)
A5093	2(3)
A5102	1(3)
A5105	1(3)
A5112	2(3)
A5113	0(3)
A5114	0(3)
A5120	150(3)
A5121	1(3)
A5122	1(3)
A5126	2(3)
A5131	1(3)
A5200	2(3)
A5500	0(3)
A5501	0(3)
A5503	0(3)
A5504	0(3)
A5505	0(3)
A5506	0(3)
A5507	0(3)
A5508	0(3)
A5510	0(3)
A5512	0(3)
A5513	0(3)
A5514	0(3)
A6000	0(3)
A6010	3(3)
A6011	20(3)
A6024	1(3)
A6025	4(3)
A6154	1(3)
A6205	1(3)
A6221	9(3)
A6228	2(3)
A6230	1(3)
A6236	1(3)
A6238	3(3)
A6239	1(3)
A6240	2(3)
A6241	1(3)
A6244	1(3)
A6246	3(3)
A6247	2(3)
A6250	1(3)
A6256	3(3)
A6259	3(3)
A6261	3(3)
A6262	3(3)
A6404	2(3)
A6407	4(3)
A6410	2(3)
A6411	2(3)
A6412	2(3)
A6413	0(3)
A6441	8(3)
A6442	8(3)
A6443	8(3)

CPT	MUE
A6444	4(3)
A6445	8(3)
A6446	14(3)
A6447	6(3)
A6448	24(3)
A6449	12(3)
A6450	8(3)
A6451	8(3)
A6452	22(3)
A6453	6(3)
A6454	25(3)
A6455	4(3)
A6456	20(3)
A6457	12(3)
A6460	1(1)
A6461	1(1)
A6501	1(3)
A6502	1(3)
A6503	1(3)
A6504	2(3)
A6505	2(3)
A6506	2(3)
A6507	2(3)
A6508	2(3)
A6509	1(3)
A6510	1(3)
A6511	1(3)
A6513	1(3)
A6530	0(3)
A6531	2(3)
A6532	2(3)
A6533	0(3)
A6534	0(3)
A6535	0(3)
A6536	0(3)
A6537	0(3)
A6538	0(3)
A6539	0(3)
A6540	0(3)
A6541	0(3)
A6544	0(3)
A6545	2(3)
A6549	0(3)
A6550	1(3)
A7000	0(3)
A7001	0(3)
A7002	0(3)
A7003	0(3)
A7004	0(3)
A7005	0(3)
A7006	0(3)
A7007	0(3)
A7008	0(3)
A7009	0(3)
A7010	0(3)
A7012	0(3)
A7013	0(3)
A7014	0(3)
A7015	0(3)
A7016	0(3)
A7017	0(3)
A7018	0(3)
A7020	0(3)
A7025	0(3)
A7026	0(3)

CPT	MUE
A7027	0(3)
A7028	0(3)
A7029	0(3)
A7030	0(3)
A7031	0(3)
A7032	0(3)
A7033	0(3)
A7034	0(3)
A7035	0(3)
A7036	0(3)
A7037	0(3)
A7038	0(3)
A7039	0(3)
A7040	2(3)
A7041	2(3)
A7044	0(3)
A7045	0(3)
A7046	0(3)
A7047	1(3)
A7048	2(3)
A7501	1(3)
A7502	1(3)
A7503	1(3)
A7504	180(3)
A7505	1(3)
A7506	0(3)
A7507	200(3)
A7508	0(3)
A7509	0(3)
A7520	1(3)
A7521	1(3)
A7522	0(3)
A7523	0(3)
A7524	1(3)
A7525	0(3)
A7526	0(3)
A7527	1(3)
A8000	0(3)
A8001	0(3)
A8002	0(3)
A8003	0(3)
A8004	0(3)
A9152	0(3)
A9153	0(3)
A9155	1(3)
A9180	0(3)
A9270	0(3)
A9272	0(3)
A9273	0(3)
A9274	0(3)
A9275	0(3)
A9276	0(3)
A9277	0(3)
A9278	0(3)
A9279	0(3)
A9280	0(3)
A9281	0(3)
A9282	0(3)
A9283	0(3)
A9284	0(3)
A9285	0(3)
A9286	0(3)
A9300	0(3)
A9500	3(3)
A9501	1(3)

CPT	MUE
A9502	3(3)
A9503	1(3)
A9504	1(3)
A9505	4(3)
A9507	1(3)
A9508	2(3)
A9509	5(3)
A9510	1(3)
A9512	30(3)
A9513	200(3)
A9515	1(3)
A9516	4(3)
A9517	200(3)
A9520	1(3)
A9521	2(3)
A9524	10(3)
A9526	2(3)
A9527	195(3)
A9528	10(3)
A9529	10(3)
A9530	200(3)
A9531	100(3)
A9532	10(3)
A9536	1(3)
A9537	1(3)
A9538	1(3)
A9539	2(3)
A9540	2(3)
A9541	1(3)
A9542	1(3)
A9543	1(3)
A9546	1(3)
A9547	2(3)
A9548	2(3)
A9550	1(3)
A9551	1(3)
A9552	1(3)
A9553	1(3)
A9554	1(3)
A9555	2(3)
A9556	10(3)
A9557	2(3)
A9558	7(3)
A9559	1(3)
A9560	2(3)
A9561	1(3)
A9562	2(3)
A9563	10(3)
A9564	0(3)
A9566	1(3)
A9567	2(3)
A9568	0(3)
A9569	1(3)
A9570	1(3)
A9571	1(3)
A9572	1(3)
A9575	300(3)
A9576	100(3)
A9577	50(3)
A9578	50(3)
A9579	100(3)
A9580	1(3)
A9581	20(3)
A9582	1(3)
A9583	18(3)

CPT	MUE
A9584	1(3)
A9585	300(3)
A9586	1(3)
A9587	54(3)
A9588	10(3)
A9589	1(3)
A9590	675(3)
A9600	7(3)
A9604	1(3)
A9606	224(3)
A9698	3(3)
A9700	2(3)
A9900	0(3)
A9901	0(3)
A9999	0(3)
B4034	0(3)
B4035	0(3)
B4036	0(3)
B4081	0(3)
B4082	0(3)
B4083	0(3)
B4087	0(3)
B4088	0(3)
B4100	0(3)
B4102	0(3)
B4103	0(3)
B4104	0(3)
B4149	0(3)
B4150	0(3)
B4152	0(3)
B4153	0(3)
B4154	0(3)
B4155	0(3)
B4157	0(3)
B4158	0(3)
B4159	0(3)
B4160	0(3)
B4161	0(3)
B4162	0(3)
B4164	0(3)
B4168	0(3)
B4172	0(3)
B4176	0(3)
B4178	0(3)
B4180	0(3)
B4185	0(3)
B4189	0(3)
B4193	0(3)
B4197	0(3)
B4199	0(3)
B4216	0(3)
B4220	0(3)
B4222	0(3)
B4224	0(3)
B5000	0(3)
B5100	0(3)
B5200	0(3)
B9002	0(3)
B9004	0(3)
B9006	0(3)
B9998	0(3)
B9999	0(3)
C1713	20(3)
C1714	4(3)
C1715	45(3)

CPT	MUE
C1716	4(3)
C1717	10(3)
C1719	99(3)
C1721	1(3)
C1722	1(3)
C1724	5(3)
C1725	9(3)
C1726	5(3)
C1727	4(3)
C1728	5(3)
C1729	6(3)
C1730	4(3)
C1731	2(3)
C1732	3(3)
C1733	3(3)
C1734	2(3)
C1749	1(3)
C1750	2(3)
C1751	3(3)
C1752	2(3)
C1753	2(3)
C1754	2(3)
C1755	2(3)
C1756	2(3)
C1757	6(3)
C1758	2(3)
C1759	2(3)
C1760	4(3)
C1762	4(3)
C1763	4(3)
C1764	1(3)
C1765	4(3)
C1766	4(3)
C1767	2(3)
C1768	3(3)
C1769	9(3)
C1770	3(3)
C1771	1(3)
C1772	1(3)
C1773	3(3)
C1776	10(3)
C1777	2(3)
C1778	4(3)
C1779	2(3)
C1780	2(3)
C1781	4(3)
C1782	1(3)
C1783	2(3)
C1784	2(3)
C1785	1(3)
C1786	1(3)
C1787	2(3)
C1788	2(3)
C1789	2(3)
C1813	1(3)
C1814	2(3)
C1815	1(3)
C1816	2(3)
C1817	1(3)
C1818	2(3)
C1819	4(3)
C1820	2(3)
C1821	4(3)
C1822	1(3)
C1823	1(3)

CPT	MUE
C1824	1(2)
C1830	2(3)
C1839	2(2)
C1840	1(3)
C1841	1(2)
C1842	0(3)
C1874	5(3)
C1875	4(3)
C1876	5(3)
C1877	5(3)
C1878	2(3)
C1880	2(3)
C1881	2(3)
C1882	1(3)
C1883	4(3)
C1884	4(3)
C1885	2(3)
C1886	1(3)
C1887	7(3)
C1888	2(3)
C1889	2(3)
C1890	1(3)
C1891	1(3)
C1892	6(3)
C1893	6(3)
C1894	6(3)
C1895	2(3)
C1896	2(3)
C1897	2(3)
C1898	2(3)
C1899	2(3)
C1900	1(3)
C1982	1(3)
C2596	1(3)
C2613	2(3)
C2614	3(3)
C2615	2(3)
C2616	1(3)
C2617	4(3)
C2618	4(3)
C2619	1(3)
C2620	1(3)
C2621	1(3)
C2622	1(3)
C2623	4(3)
C2624	1(3)
C2625	4(3)
C2626	1(3)
C2627	2(3)
C2628	4(3)
C2629	4(3)
C2630	3(3)
C2631	1(3)
C2634	24(3)
C2635	124(3)
C2636	690(3)
C2637	0(3)
C2638	150(3)
C2639	150(3)
C2640	150(3)
C2641	150(3)
C2642	120(3)
C2643	120(3)
C2644	0(3)
C2645	4608(3)

CPT	MUE
C5271	1(2)
C5272	3(2)
C5273	1(2)
C5274	35(3)
C5275	1(2)
C5276	3(2)
C5277	1(2)
C5278	15(3)
C8900	1(3)
C8901	1(3)
C8902	1(3)
C8903	1(3)
C8905	1(3)
C8906	1(3)
C8908	1(3)
C8909	1(3)
C8910	1(3)
C8911	1(3)
C8912	1(3)
C8913	1(3)
C8914	1(3)
C8918	1(3)
C8919	1(3)
C8920	1(3)
C8921	1(3)
C8922	1(3)
C8923	1(3)
C8924	1(3)
C8925	1(3)
C8926	1(3)
C8927	1(3)
C8928	1(2)
C8929	1(3)
C8930	1(2)
C8931	1(3)
C8932	1(3)
C8933	1(3)
C8934	2(3)
C8935	2(3)
C8936	2(3)
C8937	2(2)
C8957	2(3)
C9046	160(3)
C9047	22(3)
C9055	400(3)
C9113	10(3)
C9132	5500(3)
C9248	25(3)
C9250	5(3)
C9254	400(3)
C9257	8000(3)
C9285	2(3)
C9290	266(3)
C9293	700(3)
C9352	3(3)
C9353	4(3)
C9354	300(3)
C9355	3(3)
C9356	125(3)
C9358	800(3)
C9359	30(3)
C9360	300(3)
C9361	10(3)
C9362	60(3)
C9363	500(3)

CPT	MUE
C9364	600(3)
C9460	100(3)
C9462	600(3)
C9482	300(3)
C9488	40(3)
C9600	3(3)
C9601	2(3)
C9602	2(3)
C9603	2(3)
C9604	2(3)
C9605	2(3)
C9606	1(3)
C9607	1(2)
C9608	2(3)
C9725	1(3)
C9726	2(3)
C9727	1(2)
C9728	1(2)
C9733	1(3)
C9734	1(3)
C9738	1(3)
C9739	1(2)
C9740	1(2)
C9745	1(2)
C9747	1(2)
C9749	1(2)
C9751	1(3)
C9752	1(2)
C9753	3(3)
C9756	1(3)
C9757	2(2)
C9758	1(2)
C9803	2(3)
C9898	1(3)
D0150	1(3)
D0240	1(3)
D0250	2(3)
D0270	1(3)
D0272	1(3)
D0274	1(3)
D0277	1(3)
D0412	0(3)
D0416	1(3)
D0431	1(3)
D0460	1(2)
D0484	1(2)
D0485	1(2)
D0601	0(3)
D0602	0(3)
D0603	0(3)
D1510	2(2)
D1516	1(2)
D1517	1(2)
D1520	2(2)
D1526	1(2)
D1527	1(2)
D1551	1(2)
D1552	1(2)
D1553	2(2)
D1575	4(2)
D1999	0(3)
D4260	4(2)
D4263	4(2)
D4264	3(3)
D4270	4(3)

CPT	MUE
D4273	1(2)
D4277	0(3)
D4278	0(3)
D4355	1(2)
D4381	12(3)
D5282	0(3)
D5283	0(3)
D5876	0(3)
D5911	1(3)
D5912	1(2)
D5951	0(3)
D5983	1(3)
D5984	1(3)
D5985	1(3)
D6052	0(3)
D7111	20(3)
D7140	32(2)
D7210	32(2)
D7220	6(3)
D7230	6(3)
D7240	6(3)
D7241	6(3)
D7250	32(2)
D7260	1(3)
D7261	1(3)
D7283	4(3)
D7288	2(3)
D7321	4(2)
D9110	1(3)
D9130	0(3)
D9230	1(3)
D9248	1(3)
D9613	0(3)
D9930	1(2)
D9944	2(2)
D9945	2(2)
D9946	2(2)
D9950	1(3)
D9951	1(3)
D9952	1(3)
D9961	0(3)
D9990	0(3)
E0100	0(3)
E0105	0(3)
E0110	0(3)
E0111	0(3)
E0112	0(3)
E0113	0(3)
E0114	0(3)
E0116	0(3)
E0117	0(3)
E0118	0(3)
E0130	0(3)
E0135	0(3)
E0140	0(3)
E0141	0(3)
E0143	0(3)
E0144	0(3)
E0147	0(3)
E0148	0(3)
E0149	0(3)
E0153	0(3)
E0154	0(3)
E0155	0(3)
E0156	0(3)

CPT	MUE
E0157	0(3)
E0158	0(3)
E0159	0(3)
E0160	0(3)
E0161	0(3)
E0162	0(3)
E0163	0(3)
E0165	0(3)
E0167	0(3)
E0168	0(3)
E0170	0(3)
E0171	0(3)
E0172	0(3)
E0175	0(3)
E0181	0(3)
E0182	0(3)
E0184	0(3)
E0185	0(3)
E0186	0(3)
E0187	0(3)
E0188	0(3)
E0189	0(3)
E0190	0(3)
E0191	0(3)
E0193	0(3)
E0194	0(3)
E0196	0(3)
E0197	0(3)
E0198	0(3)
E0199	0(3)
E0200	0(3)
E0202	0(3)
E0203	0(3)
E0205	0(3)
E0210	0(3)
E0215	0(3)
E0217	0(3)
E0218	0(3)
E0221	0(3)
E0225	0(3)
E0231	0(3)
E0232	0(3)
E0235	0(3)
E0236	0(3)
E0239	0(3)
E0240	0(3)
E0241	0(3)
E0242	0(3)
E0243	0(3)
E0244	0(3)
E0245	0(3)
E0246	0(3)
E0247	0(3)
E0248	0(3)
E0249	0(3)
E0250	0(3)
E0251	0(3)
E0255	0(3)
E0256	0(3)
E0260	0(3)
E0261	0(3)
E0265	0(3)
E0266	0(3)
E0270	0(3)
E0271	0(3)

CPT	MUE
E0272	0(3)
E0273	0(3)
E0274	0(3)
E0275	0(3)
E0276	0(3)
E0277	0(3)
E0280	0(3)
E0290	0(3)
E0291	0(3)
E0292	0(3)
E0293	0(3)
E0294	0(3)
E0295	0(3)
E0296	0(3)
E0297	0(3)
E0300	0(3)
E0301	0(3)
E0302	0(3)
E0303	0(3)
E0304	0(3)
E0305	0(3)
E0310	0(3)
E0315	0(3)
E0316	0(3)
E0325	0(3)
E0326	0(3)
E0328	0(3)
E0329	0(3)
E0350	0(3)
E0352	0(3)
E0370	0(3)
E0371	0(3)
E0372	0(3)
E0373	0(3)
E0424	0(3)
E0425	0(3)
E0430	0(3)
E0431	0(3)
E0433	0(3)
E0434	0(3)
E0435	0(3)
E0439	0(3)
E0440	0(3)
E0441	0(3)
E0442	0(3)
E0443	0(3)
E0444	0(3)
E0445	0(3)
E0446	0(3)
E0447	0(3)
E0455	0(3)
E0457	0(3)
E0459	0(3)
E0462	0(3)
E0465	0(3)
E0466	0(3)
E0467	0(3)
E0470	0(3)
E0471	0(3)
E0472	0(3)
E0480	0(3)
E0481	0(3)
E0482	0(3)
E0483	0(3)
E0484	0(3)

CPT	MUE
E0485	0(3)
E0486	0(3)
E0487	0(3)
E0500	0(3)
E0550	0(3)
E0555	0(3)
E0560	0(3)
E0561	0(3)
E0562	0(3)
E0565	0(3)
E0570	0(3)
E0572	0(3)
E0574	0(3)
E0575	0(3)
E0580	0(3)
E0585	0(3)
E0600	0(3)
E0601	0(3)
E0602	0(3)
E0603	0(3)
E0604	0(3)
E0605	0(3)
E0606	0(3)
E0607	0(3)
E0610	0(3)
E0615	0(3)
E0616	1(2)
E0617	0(3)
E0618	0(3)
E0619	0(3)
E0620	0(3)
E0621	0(3)
E0625	0(3)
E0627	0(3)
E0629	0(3)
E0630	0(3)
E0635	0(3)
E0636	0(3)
E0637	0(3)
E0638	0(3)
E0639	0(3)
E0640	0(3)
E0641	0(3)
E0642	0(3)
E0650	0(3)
E0651	0(3)
E0652	0(3)
E0655	0(3)
E0656	0(3)
E0657	0(3)
E0660	0(3)
E0665	0(3)
E0666	0(3)
E0667	0(3)
E0668	0(3)
E0669	0(3)
E0670	0(3)
E0671	0(3)
E0672	0(3)
E0673	0(3)
E0675	0(3)
E0676	1(3)
E0691	0(3)
E0692	0(3)
E0693	0(3)

CPT	MUE
E0694	0(3)
E0700	0(3)
E0705	1(2)
E0710	0(3)
E0720	0(3)
E0730	0(3)
E0731	0(3)
E0740	0(3)
E0744	0(3)
E0745	0(3)
E0746	1(3)
E0747	0(3)
E0748	0(3)
E0749	1(3)
E0755	0(3)
E0760	0(3)
E0761	0(3)
E0762	1(3)
E0764	0(3)
E0765	0(3)
E0766	0(3)
E0769	0(3)
E0770	1(3)
E0776	0(3)
E0779	0(3)
E0780	0(3)
E0781	0(3)
E0782	1(2)
E0783	1(2)
E0784	0(3)
E0785	1(2)
E0786	1(2)
E0787	0(3)
E0791	0(3)
E0830	0(3)
E0840	0(3)
E0849	0(3)
E0850	0(3)
E0855	0(3)
E0856	0(3)
E0860	0(3)
E0870	0(3)
E0880	0(3)
E0890	0(3)
E0900	0(3)
E0910	0(3)
E0911	0(3)
E0912	0(3)
E0920	0(3)
E0930	0(3)
E0935	0(3)
E0936	0(3)
E0940	0(3)
E0941	0(3)
E0942	0(3)
E0944	0(3)
E0945	0(3)
E0946	0(3)
E0947	0(3)
E0948	0(3)
E0950	0(3)
E0951	0(3)
E0952	0(3)
E0953	0(3)
E0954	0(3)

CPT	MUE
E0955	0(3)
E0956	0(3)
E0957	0(3)
E0958	0(3)
E0959	2(2)
E0960	0(3)
E0961	2(2)
E0966	1(2)
E0967	0(3)
E0968	0(3)
E0969	0(3)
E0970	0(3)
E0971	2(3)
E0973	2(2)
E0974	2(2)
E0978	1(3)
E0980	0(3)
E0981	0(3)
E0982	0(3)
E0983	0(3)
E0984	0(3)
E0985	0(3)
E0986	0(3)
E0988	0(3)
E0990	2(2)
E0992	1(2)
E0994	0(3)
E0995	2(2)
E1002	0(3)
E1003	0(3)
E1004	0(3)
E1005	0(3)
E1006	0(3)
E1007	0(3)
E1008	0(3)
E1009	0(3)
E1010	0(3)
E1011	0(3)
E1012	0(3)
E1014	0(3)
E1015	0(3)
E1016	0(3)
E1017	0(3)
E1018	0(3)
E1020	0(3)
E1028	0(3)
E1029	0(3)
E1030	0(3)
E1031	0(3)
E1035	0(3)
E1036	0(3)
E1037	0(3)
E1038	0(3)
E1039	0(3)
E1050	0(3)
E1060	0(3)
E1070	0(3)
E1083	0(3)
E1084	0(3)
E1085	0(3)
E1086	0(3)
E1087	0(3)
E1088	0(3)
E1089	0(3)
E1090	0(3)

CPT	MUE
E1092	0(3)
E1093	0(3)
E1100	0(3)
E1110	0(3)
E1130	0(3)
E1140	0(3)
E1150	0(3)
E1160	0(3)
E1161	0(3)
E1170	0(3)
E1171	0(3)
E1172	0(3)
E1180	0(3)
E1190	0(3)
E1195	0(3)
E1200	0(3)
E1220	0(3)
E1221	0(3)
E1222	0(3)
E1223	0(3)
E1224	0(3)
E1225	0(3)
E1226	1(2)
E1227	0(3)
E1228	0(3)
E1229	0(3)
E1230	0(3)
E1231	0(3)
E1232	0(3)
E1233	0(3)
E1234	0(3)
E1235	0(3)
E1236	0(3)
E1237	0(3)
E1238	0(3)
E1239	0(3)
E1240	0(3)
E1250	0(3)
E1260	0(3)
E1270	0(3)
E1280	0(3)
E1285	0(3)
E1290	0(3)
E1295	0(3)
E1296	0(3)
E1297	0(3)
E1298	0(3)
E1300	0(3)
E1310	0(3)
E1352	0(3)
E1353	0(3)
E1354	0(3)
E1355	0(3)
E1356	0(3)
E1357	0(3)
E1358	0(3)
E1372	0(3)
E1390	0(3)
E1391	0(3)
E1392	0(3)
E1399	0(3)
E1405	0(3)
E1406	0(3)
E1500	0(3)
E1510	0(3)

CPT	MUE
E1520	0(3)
E1530	0(3)
E1540	0(3)
E1550	0(3)
E1560	0(3)
E1570	0(3)
E1575	0(3)
E1580	0(3)
E1590	0(3)
E1592	0(3)
E1594	0(3)
E1600	0(3)
E1610	0(3)
E1615	0(3)
E1620	0(3)
E1625	0(3)
E1630	0(3)
E1632	0(3)
E1634	0(3)
E1635	0(3)
E1636	0(3)
E1637	0(3)
E1639	0(3)
E1699	1(3)
E1700	0(3)
E1701	0(3)
E1702	0(3)
E1800	0(3)
E1801	0(3)
E1802	0(3)
E1805	0(3)
E1806	0(3)
E1810	0(3)
E1811	0(3)
E1812	0(3)
E1815	0(3)
E1816	0(3)
E1818	0(3)
E1820	0(3)
E1821	0(3)
E1825	0(3)
E1830	0(3)
E1831	0(3)
E1840	0(3)
E1841	0(3)
E1902	0(3)
E2000	0(3)
E2100	0(3)
E2101	0(3)
E2120	0(3)
E2201	0(3)
E2202	0(3)
E2203	0(3)
E2204	0(3)
E2205	0(3)
E2206	0(3)
E2207	0(3)
E2208	0(3)
E2209	0(3)
E2210	0(3)
E2211	0(3)
E2212	0(3)
E2213	0(3)
E2214	0(3)
E2215	0(3)

CPT	MUE
E2216	0(3)
E2217	0(3)
E2218	0(3)
E2219	0(3)
E2220	0(3)
E2221	0(3)
E2222	0(3)
E2224	0(3)
E2225	0(3)
E2226	0(3)
E2227	0(3)
E2228	0(3)
E2230	0(3)
E2231	0(3)
E2291	1(2)
E2292	1(2)
E2293	1(2)
E2294	1(2)
E2295	0(3)
E2300	0(3)
E2301	0(3)
E2310	0(3)
E2311	0(3)
E2312	0(3)
E2313	0(3)
E2321	0(3)
E2322	0(3)
E2323	0(3)
E2324	0(3)
E2325	0(3)
E2326	0(3)
E2327	0(3)
E2328	0(3)
E2329	0(3)
E2330	0(3)
E2331	0(3)
E2340	0(3)
E2341	0(3)
E2342	0(3)
E2343	0(3)
E2351	0(3)
E2358	0(3)
E2359	0(3)
E2360	0(3)
E2361	0(3)
E2362	0(3)
E2363	0(3)
E2364	0(3)
E2365	0(3)
E2366	0(3)
E2367	0(3)
E2368	0(3)
E2369	0(3)
E2370	0(3)
E2371	0(3)
E2372	0(3)
E2373	0(3)
E2374	0(3)
E2375	0(3)
E2376	0(3)
E2377	0(3)
E2378	0(3)
E2381	0(3)
E2382	0(3)
E2383	0(3)

CPT	MUE
E2384	0(3)
E2385	0(3)
E2386	0(3)
E2387	0(3)
E2388	0(3)
E2389	0(3)
E2390	0(3)
E2391	0(3)
E2392	0(3)
E2394	0(3)
E2395	0(3)
E2396	0(3)
E2397	0(3)
E2398	0(3)
E2402	0(3)
E2500	0(3)
E2502	0(3)
E2504	0(3)
E2506	0(3)
E2508	0(3)
E2510	0(3)
E2511	0(3)
E2512	0(3)
E2599	0(3)
E2601	0(3)
E2602	0(3)
E2603	0(3)
E2604	0(3)
E2605	0(3)
E2606	0(3)
E2607	0(3)
E2608	0(3)
E2609	0(3)
E2610	1(3)
E2611	0(3)
E2612	0(3)
E2613	0(3)
E2614	0(3)
E2615	0(3)
E2616	0(3)
E2617	0(3)
E2619	0(3)
E2620	0(3)
E2621	0(3)
E2622	0(3)
E2623	0(3)
E2624	0(3)
E2625	0(3)
E2626	0(3)
E2627	0(3)
E2628	0(3)
E2629	0(3)
E2630	0(3)
E2631	0(3)
E2632	0(3)
E2633	0(3)
E8000	0(3)
E8001	0(3)
E8002	0(3)
G0008	1(2)
G0009	1(2)
G0010	1(3)
G0027	1(2)
G0068	16(3)
G0069	16(3)

CPT	MUE
G0070	16(3)
G0071	1(3)
G0076	1(3)
G0077	1(3)
G0078	1(3)
G0079	1(3)
G0080	1(3)
G0081	1(3)
G0082	1(3)
G0083	1(3)
G0084	1(3)
G0085	1(3)
G0086	1(3)
G0087	1(3)
G0101	1(2)
G0102	1(2)
G0103	1(2)
G0104	1(2)
G0105	1(2)
G0106	1(2)
G0108	8(3)
G0109	12(3)
G0117	1(2)
G0118	1(2)
G0120	1(2)
G0121	1(2)
G0122	0(3)
G0123	1(3)
G0124	1(3)
G0127	1(2)
G0128	1(3)
G0129	6(3)
G0130	1(2)
G0141	1(3)
G0143	1(3)
G0144	1(3)
G0145	1(3)
G0147	1(3)
G0148	1(3)
G0166	2(3)
G0168	2(3)
G0175	1(3)
G0176	5(3)
G0177	5(3)
G0179	1(2)
G0180	1(2)
G0181	1(2)
G0182	1(2)
G0186	1(2)
G0219	0(3)
G0235	1(3)
G0237	8(3)
G0238	8(3)
G0239	2(3)
G0245	1(2)
G0246	1(2)
G0247	1(2)
G0248	1(2)
G0249	3(3)
G0250	1(2)
G0252	0(3)
G0255	0(3)
G0257	1(3)
G0259	2(3)
G0260	2(3)

CPT	MUE
G0268	1(2)
G0269	2(3)
G0270	8(3)
G0271	4(3)
G0276	1(3)
G0277	5(3)
G0278	1(2)
G0279	1(2)
G0281	1(3)
G0282	0(3)
G0283	1(3)
G0288	1(2)
G0289	1(2)
G0293	1(2)
G0294	1(2)
G0295	0(3)
G0296	1(2)
G0297	1(2)
G0302	1(2)
G0303	1(2)
G0304	1(2)
G0305	1(2)
G0306	4(3)
G0307	4(3)
G0328	1(2)
G0329	1(3)
G0333	0(3)
G0337	1(2)
G0339	1(2)
G0340	1(3)
G0341	1(2)
G0342	1(2)
G0343	1(2)
G0372	1(2)
G0379	1(2)
G0380	2(3)
G0381	2(3)
G0382	2(3)
G0383	2(3)
G0384	2(3)
G0390	1(2)
G0396	1(2)
G0397	1(2)
G0398	1(2)
G0399	1(2)
G0400	1(2)
G0402	1(2)
G0403	1(2)
G0404	1(2)
G0405	1(2)
G0406	1(3)
G0407	1(3)
G0408	1(3)
G0410	6(3)
G0411	6(3)
G0412	1(2)
G0413	1(2)
G0414	1(2)
G0415	1(2)
G0416	1(2)
G0420	2(3)
G0421	2(3)
G0422	6(2)
G0423	6(2)
G0424	2(2)

CPT	MUE
G0425	1(3)
G0426	1(3)
G0427	1(3)
G0428	0(3)
G0429	1(2)
G0432	1(2)
G0433	1(2)
G0435	1(2)
G0438	1(2)
G0439	1(2)
G0442	1(2)
G0443	1(2)
G0444	1(2)
G0445	1(2)
G0446	1(3)
G0447	4(3)
G0448	1(3)
G0451	1(3)
G0452	1(3)
G0453	10(3)
G0454	1(2)
G0455	1(2)
G0458	1(3)
G0459	1(3)
G0460	1(3)
G0463	4(3)
G0466	1(2)
G0467	1(3)
G0468	1(2)
G0469	1(2)
G0470	1(3)
G0471	2(3)
G0472	1(2)
G0473	1(3)
G0475	1(2)
G0476	1(2)
G0480	1(2)
G0481	1(2)
G0482	1(2)
G0483	1(2)
G0490	1(3)
G0491	1(3)
G0492	1(3)
G0493	1(3)
G0494	1(3)
G0495	1(3)
G0496	1(3)
G0498	1(2)
G0499	1(2)
G0500	1(3)
G0501	1(3)
G0506	1(2)
G0508	1(2)
G0509	1(2)
G0511	1(2)
G0512	1(2)
G0513	1(2)
G0514	1(1)
G0516	1(2)
G0517	1(2)
G0518	1(2)
G0659	1(2)
G2000	1(3)
G2001	1(3)
G2002	1(3)

CPT	MUE
G2003	1(3)
G2004	1(3)
G2005	1(3)
G2006	1(3)
G2007	1(3)
G2008	1(3)
G2009	1(3)
G2010	1(3)
G2011	1(2)
G2012	1(3)
G2013	1(3)
G2014	1(3)
G2015	1(3)
G2023	2(3)
G2024	2(3)
G2058	2(3)
G2061	1(2)
G2062	1(2)
G2063	1(2)
G2064	1(2)
G2065	1(2)
G2066	1(2)
G2067	1(2)
G2068	1(2)
G2069	1(2)
G2070	1(2)
G2071	1(2)
G2072	1(2)
G2073	1(2)
G2074	1(2)
G2075	1(2)
G2076	1(2)
G2078	3(3)
G2079	3(3)
G2081	1(2)
G2082	1(2)
G2083	1(2)
G2086	1(3)
G2087	2(3)
G6001	2(3)
G6002	2(3)
G6003	2(3)
G6004	2(3)
G6005	2(3)
G6006	2(3)
G6007	2(3)
G6008	2(3)
G6009	2(3)
G6010	2(3)
G6011	2(3)
G6012	2(3)
G6013	2(3)
G6014	2(3)
G6015	2(3)
G6016	2(3)
G6017	2(3)
G9143	1(2)
G9147	0(3)
G9148	0(3)
G9149	0(3)
G9150	0(3)
G9151	0(3)
G9152	0(3)
G9153	0(3)
G9156	1(2)

CPT	MUE
G9157	1(2)
G9187	0(3)
G9480	1(3)
G9481	2(3)
G9482	2(3)
G9483	2(3)
G9484	2(3)
G9485	2(3)
G9486	2(3)
G9487	2(3)
G9488	2(3)
G9489	2(3)
G9490	2(3)
G9678	1(2)
G9685	1(3)
G9978	2(3)
G9979	2(3)
G9980	2(3)
G9981	2(3)
G9982	2(3)
G9983	2(3)
G9984	2(3)
G9985	2(3)
G9986	2(3)
G9987	2(3)
J0120	1(3)
J0121	200(3)
J0122	300(3)
J0129	100(3)
J0130	6(3)
J0131	400(3)
J0132	300(3)
J0133	1200(3)
J0135	8(3)
J0153	180(3)
J0171	120(3)
J0178	4(2)
J0179	12(2)
J0180	140(3)
J0185	130(3)
J0190	0(3)
J0200	0(3)
J0202	12(3)
J0205	0(3)
J0207	4(3)
J0210	16(3)
J0215	0(3)
J0220	20(3)
J0221	300(3)
J0222	300(3)
J0223	756(3)
J0256	1600(3)
J0257	1400(3)
J0270	32(3)
J0275	1(3)
J0278	15(3)
J0280	10(3)
J0282	70(3)
J0285	5(3)
J0287	60(3)
J0288	0(3)
J0289	115(3)
J0290	24(3)
J0291	500(3)
J0295	12(3)

CPT	MUE
J0300	8(3)
J0330	50(3)
J0348	200(3)
J0350	0(3)
J0360	6(3)
J0364	6(3)
J0365	0(3)
J0380	1(3)
J0390	0(3)
J0395	0(3)
J0400	120(3)
J0401	400(3)
J0456	4(3)
J0461	800(3)
J0470	2(3)
J0475	8(3)
J0476	2(3)
J0480	1(3)
J0485	1500(3)
J0490	160(3)
J0500	4(3)
J0515	6(3)
J0517	30(3)
J0520	0(3)
J0558	24(3)
J0561	24(3)
J0565	200(3)
J0567	300(3)
J0570	4(3)
J0571	0(3)
J0572	0(3)
J0573	0(3)
J0574	0(3)
J0575	0(3)
J0583	1250(3)
J0584	90(3)
J0585	600(3)
J0586	300(3)
J0587	300(3)
J0588	600(3)
J0592	12(3)
J0593	300(3)
J0594	320(3)
J0595	12(3)
J0596	840(3)
J0597	250(3)
J0598	100(3)
J0599	900(3)
J0600	3(3)
J0606	150(3)
J0610	15(3)
J0620	1(3)
J0630	8(3)
J0636	100(3)
J0637	20(3)
J0638	300(3)
J0640	24(3)
J0641	1200(3)
J0642	1200(3)
J0670	10(3)
J0690	16(3)
J0691	300(3)
J0692	12(3)
J0694	12(3)
J0695	60(3)

CPT	MUE
J0696	16(3)
J0697	12(3)
J0698	12(3)
J0702	20(3)
J0706	16(3)
J0710	0(3)
J0712	180(3)
J0713	12(3)
J0714	12(3)
J0715	0(3)
J0716	4(1)
J0717	400(3)
J0720	15(3)
J0725	10(3)
J0735	50(3)
J0740	2(3)
J0743	16(3)
J0744	8(3)
J0745	8(3)
J0770	5(3)
J0775	180(3)
J0780	10(3)
J0795	100(3)
J0800	3(3)
J0834	3(3)
J0840	18(3)
J0841	24(3)
J0850	9(3)
J0875	300(3)
J0878	1500(3)
J0881	500(3)
J0882	300(3)
J0883	1250(3)
J0884	1250(3)
J0885	60(3)
J0887	360(3)
J0888	360(3)
J0890	0(3)
J0894	100(3)
J0895	12(3)
J0897	120(3)
J0945	4(3)
J1000	1(3)
J1020	8(3)
J1030	8(3)
J1040	4(3)
J1050	1000(3)
J1071	400(3)
J1094	0(3)
J1095	1034(2)
J1096	4(3)
J1097	4(3)
J1100	120(3)
J1110	3(3)
J1120	2(3)
J1130	300(3)
J1160	3(3)
J1162	10(3)
J1165	50(3)
J1170	50(3)
J1180	0(3)
J1190	8(3)
J1200	8(3)
J1205	4(3)
J1212	1(3)

CPT	MUE
J1230	5(3)
J1240	6(3)
J1245	6(3)
J1250	4(3)
J1260	2(3)
J1265	100(3)
J1267	150(3)
J1270	16(3)
J1290	60(3)
J1300	120(3)
J1301	60(3)
J1303	360(3)
J1320	0(3)
J1322	150(3)
J1324	0(3)
J1325	18(3)
J1327	99(3)
J1330	0(3)
J1335	2(3)
J1364	8(3)
J1380	4(3)
J1410	4(3)
J1428	450(3)
J1430	10(3)
J1435	0(3)
J1436	0(3)
J1438	2(3)
J1439	750(3)
J1442	1500(3)
J1443	0(3)
J1444	272(3)
J1447	960(3)
J1450	4(3)
J1451	200(3)
J1452	0(3)
J1453	150(3)
J1454	1(3)
J1455	18(3)
J1457	0(3)
J1458	100(3)
J1459	300(3)
J1460	10(2)
J1555	480(3)
J1556	300(3)
J1557	300(3)
J1559	300(3)
J1560	1(2)
J1561	300(3)
J1562	0(3)
J1566	300(3)
J1568	300(3)
J1569	300(3)
J1570	4(3)
J1571	20(3)
J1572	300(3)
J1573	130(3)
J1575	650(3)
J1580	9(3)
J1595	2(3)
J1599	300(3)
J1600	0(3)
J1602	300(3)
J1610	3(3)
J1620	0(3)
J1626	30(3)

CPT	MUE
J1627	100(3)
J1628	100(3)
J1630	7(3)
J1631	9(3)
J1640	672(3)
J1642	150(3)
J1644	50(3)
J1645	10(3)
J1650	30(3)
J1652	20(3)
J1655	0(3)
J1670	2(3)
J1675	0(3)
J1700	0(3)
J1710	0(3)
J1720	10(3)
J1726	28(3)
J1729	25(3)
J1730	0(3)
J1740	3(3)
J1741	32(3)
J1742	4(3)
J1743	66(3)
J1744	90(3)
J1745	150(3)
J1746	200(3)
J1750	45(3)
J1756	500(3)
J1786	680(3)
J1790	2(3)
J1800	12(3)
J1810	0(3)
J1815	200(3)
J1817	0(3)
J1826	1(3)
J1830	1(3)
J1833	1116(3)
J1835	0(3)
J1840	3(3)
J1850	14(3)
J1885	8(3)
J1890	0(3)
J1930	120(3)
J1931	609(3)
J1940	10(3)
J1943	675(3)
J1944	1064(3)
J1945	0(3)
J1950	12(3)
J1953	300(3)
J1955	11(3)
J1956	4(3)
J1960	0(3)
J1980	8(3)
J1990	0(3)
J2001	400(3)
J2010	10(3)
J2020	6(3)
J2060	10(3)
J2062	10(3)
J2150	8(3)
J2170	8(3)
J2175	6(3)
J2180	0(3)
J2182	300(3)

CPT	MUE
J2185	60(3)
J2186	600(3)
J2210	5(3)
J2212	240(3)
J2248	300(3)
J2250	30(3)
J2260	16(3)
J2265	400(3)
J2270	15(3)
J2274	100(3)
J2278	1000(3)
J2280	8(3)
J2300	10(3)
J2310	10(3)
J2315	380(3)
J2320	4(3)
J2323	300(3)
J2325	34(3)
J2326	120(3)
J2350	600(3)
J2353	60(3)
J2354	60(3)
J2355	2(3)
J2357	90(3)
J2358	405(3)
J2360	3(3)
J2370	30(3)
J2400	4(3)
J2405	64(3)
J2407	120(3)
J2410	2(3)
J2425	125(3)
J2426	819(3)
J2430	3(3)
J2440	4(3)
J2460	0(3)
J2469	10(3)
J2501	25(3)
J2502	60(3)
J2503	2(3)
J2504	15(3)
J2505	1(3)
J2507	8(3)
J2510	4(3)
J2513	1(3)
J2515	8(3)
J2540	75(3)
J2543	20(3)
J2545	1(3)
J2547	600(3)
J2550	3(3)
J2560	16(3)
J2562	48(3)
J2590	15(3)
J2597	45(3)
J2650	0(3)
J2670	0(3)
J2675	1(3)
J2680	4(3)
J2690	4(3)
J2700	48(3)
J2704	400(3)
J2710	10(3)
J2720	10(3)
J2724	3500(3)

CPT	MUE
J2725	0(3)
J2730	2(3)
J2760	2(3)
J2765	18(3)
J2770	7(3)
J2778	10(2)
J2780	16(3)
J2783	60(3)
J2785	4(3)
J2786	500(3)
J2787	2(3)
J2788	1(3)
J2790	3(3)
J2791	15(3)
J2792	450(3)
J2793	320(3)
J2794	100(3)
J2795	2400(3)
J2796	150(3)
J2797	333(3)
J2798	240(3)
J2800	3(3)
J2805	3(3)
J2810	20(3)
J2820	10(3)
J2840	160(3)
J2850	48(3)
J2860	170(3)
J2910	0(3)
J2916	20(3)
J2920	25(3)
J2930	25(3)
J2940	0(3)
J2941	8(3)
J2950	0(3)
J2993	2(3)
J2995	0(3)
J2997	100(3)
J3000	2(3)
J3010	100(3)
J3030	2(3)
J3031	675(3)
J3060	760(3)
J3070	3(3)
J3090	200(3)
J3095	150(3)
J3101	50(3)
J3105	4(3)
J3110	2(3)
J3111	210(3)
J3121	400(3)
J3145	750(3)
J3230	6(3)
J3240	1(3)
J3243	200(3)
J3245	100(3)
J3246	100(3)
J3250	4(3)
J3260	12(3)
J3262	800(3)
J3265	0(3)
J3280	0(3)
J3285	9(3)
J3300	160(3)
J3301	16(3)

CPT	MUE
J3302	0(3)
J3303	24(3)
J3304	64(2)
J3305	0(3)
J3310	0(3)
J3315	6(3)
J3316	6(3)
J3320	0(3)
J3350	0(3)
J3355	0(3)
J3357	90(3)
J3358	520(3)
J3360	6(3)
J3364	0(3)
J3365	0(3)
J3370	12(3)
J3380	300(3)
J3385	80(3)
J3396	150(3)
J3397	600(3)
J3398	150(2)
J3400	0(3)
J3410	16(3)
J3411	8(3)
J3415	6(3)
J3420	1(3)
J3430	50(3)
J3465	120(3)
J3470	3(3)
J3471	999(2)
J3472	2(3)
J3473	450(3)
J3475	80(3)
J3480	200(3)
J3485	160(3)
J3486	4(3)
J3489	5(3)
J3520	0(3)
J3530	0(3)
J3535	0(3)
J3570	0(3)
J7030	20(3)
J7040	12(3)
J7042	12(3)
J7050	20(3)
J7060	10(3)
J7070	7(3)
J7100	2(3)
J7110	3(3)
J7120	20(3)
J7121	5(3)
J7131	500(3)
J7169	180(3)
J7170	1800(3)
J7175	9000(1)
J7177	10500(3)
J7178	7700(1)
J7179	9600(1)
J7180	6000(1)
J7181	3850(1)
J7182	22000(1)
J7183	9600(1)
J7185	22000(1)
J7186	9600(1)
J7187	9600(1)

CPT	MUE
J7188	22000(1)
J7189	26000(1)
J7190	22000(1)
J7191	0(3)
J7192	22000(1)
J7193	20000(1)
J7194	9000(1)
J7195	20000(1)
J7196	175(3)
J7197	6300(1)
J7198	30000(1)
J7200	20000(1)
J7201	9000(1)
J7202	11550(1)
J7203	12000(1)
J7205	9750(1)
J7207	22500(1)
J7208	18000(1)
J7209	7500(1)
J7210	22000(1)
J7211	22000(1)
J7296	0(3)
J7297	0(3)
J7298	0(3)
J7300	0(3)
J7301	0(3)
J7303	0(3)
J7304	0(3)
J7306	0(3)
J7307	0(3)
J7308	3(3)
J7309	0(3)
J7310	0(3)
J7311	118(2)
J7312	14(2)
J7313	38(2)
J7314	36(2)
J7315	2(3)
J7316	3(3)
J7318	120(3)
J7320	50(3)
J7321	2(2)
J7322	48(3)
J7323	2(2)
J7324	2(2)
J7325	96(3)
J7326	2(2)
J7327	2(2)
J7328	336(3)
J7329	0(3)
J7330	1(3)
J7331	40(3)
J7332	40(3)
J7336	1120(3)
J7340	1(3)
J7342	10(3)
J7345	200(3)
J7401	270(2)
J7500	15(3)
J7501	8(3)
J7502	60(3)
J7503	120(3)
J7504	15(3)
J7505	1(3)
J7507	40(3)

CPT	MUE
J7508	300(3)
J7509	60(3)
J7510	60(3)
J7511	9(3)
J7512	300(3)
J7513	0(3)
J7515	90(3)
J7516	4(3)
J7517	16(3)
J7518	12(3)
J7520	40(3)
J7525	2(3)
J7527	20(3)
J7599	1(3)
J7604	0(3)
J7605	0(3)
J7606	0(3)
J7607	0(3)
J7608	0(3)
J7609	0(3)
J7610	0(3)
J7611	0(3)
J7612	0(3)
J7613	0(3)
J7614	0(3)
J7615	0(3)
J7620	0(3)
J7622	0(3)
J7624	0(3)
J7626	0(3)
J7627	0(3)
J7628	0(3)
J7629	0(3)
J7631	0(3)
J7632	0(3)
J7633	0(3)
J7634	0(3)
J7635	0(3)
J7636	0(3)
J7637	0(3)
J7638	0(3)
J7639	0(3)
J7640	0(3)
J7641	0(3)
J7642	0(3)
J7643	0(3)
J7644	0(3)
J7645	0(3)
J7647	0(3)
J7648	0(3)
J7649	0(3)
J7650	0(3)
J7657	0(3)
J7658	0(3)
J7659	0(3)
J7660	0(3)
J7665	0(3)
J7667	0(3)
J7668	0(3)
J7669	0(3)
J7670	0(3)
J7674	100(3)
J7676	0(3)
J7677	175(3)
J7680	0(3)

CPT	MUE
J7681	0(3)
J7682	0(3)
J7683	0(3)
J7684	0(3)
J7685	0(3)
J7686	0(3)
J7699	0(3)
J7799	2(3)
J7999	6(3)
J8498	1(3)
J8499	0(3)
J8501	57(3)
J8510	5(3)
J8515	0(3)
J8520	50(3)
J8521	15(3)
J8530	60(3)
J8540	48(3)
J8560	6(3)
J8562	12(3)
J8565	0(3)
J8597	4(3)
J8600	40(3)
J8610	20(3)
J8650	0(3)
J8655	1(3)
J8670	180(3)
J8700	120(3)
J8705	22(3)
J8999	2(3)
J9000	20(3)
J9015	1(3)
J9017	30(3)
J9019	60(3)
J9020	0(3)
J9022	168(3)
J9023	140(3)
J9025	300(3)
J9027	100(3)
J9030	50(3)
J9032	300(3)
J9033	300(3)
J9034	360(3)
J9035	170(3)
J9036	360(3)
J9039	210(3)
J9040	4(3)
J9041	35(3)
J9042	200(3)
J9043	60(3)
J9044	35(3)
J9045	22(3)
J9047	160(3)
J9050	6(3)
J9055	120(3)
J9057	60(3)
J9060	24(3)
J9065	100(3)
J9070	55(3)
J9098	5(3)
J9100	120(3)
J9118	750(3)
J9119	350(3)
J9120	5(3)
J9130	24(3)

CPT	MUE
J9145	240(3)
J9150	12(3)
J9151	12(3)
J9153	132(3)
J9155	240(3)
J9160	0(3)
J9165	0(3)
J9171	240(3)
J9173	150(3)
J9175	10(3)
J9176	3000(3)
J9178	150(3)
J9179	50(3)
J9181	100(3)
J9185	2(3)
J9190	20(3)
J9200	20(3)
J9201	20(3)
J9202	3(3)
J9203	180(3)
J9204	160(3)
J9205	215(3)
J9206	42(3)
J9207	90(3)
J9208	15(3)
J9209	55(3)
J9210	1500(3)
J9211	6(3)
J9212	0(3)
J9213	12(3)
J9214	100(3)
J9215	0(3)
J9216	0(3)
J9217	6(3)
J9218	1(3)
J9219	0(3)
J9225	1(3)
J9226	1(3)
J9228	1100(3)
J9229	27(3)
J9230	5(3)
J9245	11(3)
J9250	50(3)
J9260	20(3)
J9261	80(3)
J9262	700(3)
J9263	700(3)
J9264	600(3)
J9266	2(3)
J9267	750(3)
J9268	1(3)
J9270	0(3)
J9271	400(3)
J9280	12(3)
J9285	200(3)
J9293	8(3)
J9295	800(3)
J9299	480(3)
J9301	100(3)
J9302	200(3)
J9303	90(3)
J9305	150(3)
J9306	840(3)
J9307	80(3)
J9308	280(3)

CPT	MUE
J9309	280(3)
J9311	160(3)
J9312	150(3)
J9313	600(3)
J9315	40(3)
J9320	4(3)
J9325	400(3)
J9328	400(3)
J9330	50(3)
J9340	4(3)
J9351	120(3)
J9352	40(3)
J9354	600(3)
J9355	105(3)
J9356	60(3)
J9357	4(3)
J9360	40(3)
J9370	4(3)
J9371	5(3)
J9390	36(3)
J9395	20(3)
J9400	500(3)
J9600	4(3)
K0001	0(3)
K0002	0(3)
K0003	0(3)
K0004	0(3)
K0005	0(3)
K0006	0(3)
K0007	0(3)
K0008	0(3)
K0009	0(3)
K0010	0(3)
K0011	0(3)
K0012	0(3)
K0013	0(3)
K0014	0(3)
K0015	0(3)
K0017	0(3)
K0018	0(3)
K0019	0(3)
K0020	0(3)
K0037	0(3)
K0038	0(3)
K0039	0(3)
K0040	0(3)
K0041	0(3)
K0042	0(3)
K0043	0(3)
K0044	0(3)
K0045	0(3)
K0046	0(3)
K0047	0(3)
K0050	0(3)
K0051	0(3)
K0052	0(3)
K0053	0(3)
K0056	0(3)
K0065	0(3)
K0069	0(3)
K0070	0(3)
K0071	0(3)
K0072	0(3)
K0073	0(3)
K0077	0(3)

CPT	MUE
K0098	0(3)
K0105	0(3)
K0108	0(3)
K0195	0(3)
K0455	0(3)
K0462	0(3)
K0552	0(3)
K0553	0(3)
K0554	0(3)
K0601	0(3)
K0602	0(3)
K0603	0(3)
K0604	0(3)
K0605	0(3)
K0606	0(3)
K0607	0(3)
K0608	0(3)
K0609	0(3)
K0669	0(3)
K0672	4(3)
K0730	0(3)
K0733	0(3)
K0738	0(3)
K0740	0(3)
K0743	0(3)
K0800	0(3)
K0801	0(3)
K0802	0(3)
K0806	0(3)
K0807	0(3)
K0808	0(3)
K0812	0(3)
K0813	0(3)
K0814	0(3)
K0815	0(3)
K0816	0(3)
K0820	0(3)
K0821	0(3)
K0822	0(3)
K0823	0(3)
K0824	0(3)
K0825	0(3)
K0826	0(3)
K0827	0(3)
K0828	0(3)
K0829	0(3)
K0830	0(3)
K0831	0(3)
K0835	0(3)
K0836	0(3)
K0837	0(3)
K0838	0(3)
K0839	0(3)
K0840	0(3)
K0841	0(3)
K0842	0(3)
K0843	0(3)
K0848	0(3)
K0849	0(3)
K0850	0(3)
K0851	0(3)
K0852	0(3)
K0853	0(3)
K0854	0(3)
K0855	0(3)

CPT	MUE
K0856	0(3)
K0857	0(3)
K0858	0(3)
K0859	0(3)
K0860	0(3)
K0861	0(3)
K0862	0(3)
K0863	0(3)
K0864	0(3)
K0868	0(3)
K0869	0(3)
K0870	0(3)
K0871	0(3)
K0877	0(3)
K0878	0(3)
K0879	0(3)
K0880	0(3)
K0884	0(3)
K0885	0(3)
K0886	0(3)
K0890	0(3)
K0891	0(3)
K0898	1(2)
K0899	0(3)
K0900	0(3)
K1001	0(3)
K1002	0(3)
K1003	0(3)
K1004	0(3)
K1005	0(3)
L0112	1(2)
L0113	1(2)
L0120	1(2)
L0130	1(2)
L0140	1(2)
L0150	1(2)
L0160	1(2)
L0170	1(2)
L0172	1(2)
L0174	1(2)
L0180	1(2)
L0190	1(2)
L0200	1(2)
L0220	1(3)
L0450	1(2)
L0452	1(2)
L0454	1(2)
L0455	1(2)
L0456	1(2)
L0457	1(2)
L0458	1(2)
L0460	1(2)
L0462	1(2)
L0464	1(2)
L0466	1(2)
L0467	1(2)
L0468	1(2)
L0469	1(2)
L0470	1(2)
L0472	1(2)
L0480	1(2)
L0482	1(2)
L0484	1(2)
L0486	1(2)
L0488	1(2)

CPT	MUE
L0490	1(2)
L0491	1(2)
L0492	1(2)
L0621	1(2)
L0622	1(2)
L0623	1(2)
L0624	1(2)
L0625	1(2)
L0626	1(2)
L0627	1(2)
L0628	1(2)
L0629	1(2)
L0630	1(2)
L0631	1(2)
L0632	1(2)
L0633	1(2)
L0634	1(2)
L0635	1(2)
L0636	1(2)
L0637	1(2)
L0638	1(2)
L0639	1(2)
L0640	1(2)
L0641	1(2)
L0642	1(2)
L0643	1(2)
L0648	1(2)
L0649	1(2)
L0650	1(2)
L0651	1(2)
L0700	1(2)
L0710	1(2)
L0810	1(2)
L0820	1(2)
L0830	1(2)
L0859	1(2)
L0861	1(2)
L0970	1(2)
L0972	1(2)
L0974	1(2)
L0976	1(2)
L0978	2(3)
L0980	1(2)
L0982	1(3)
L0984	3(3)
L0999	1(3)
L1000	1(2)
L1001	1(2)
L1005	1(2)
L1010	2(2)
L1020	2(3)
L1025	1(3)
L1030	1(3)
L1040	1(3)
L1050	1(3)
L1060	1(3)
L1070	2(2)
L1080	2(2)
L1085	1(2)
L1090	1(3)
L1100	2(2)
L1110	2(2)
L1120	3(3)
L1200	1(2)
L1210	2(3)

CPT	MUE
L1220	1(3)
L1230	1(2)
L1240	1(3)
L1250	2(3)
L1260	1(3)
L1270	3(3)
L1280	2(3)
L1290	2(3)
L1300	1(2)
L1310	1(2)
L1499	1(3)
L1600	1(2)
L1610	1(2)
L1620	1(2)
L1630	1(2)
L1640	1(2)
L1650	1(2)
L1652	1(2)
L1660	1(2)
L1680	1(2)
L1685	1(2)
L1686	1(3)
L1690	1(2)
L1700	1(2)
L1710	1(2)
L1720	2(2)
L1730	1(2)
L1755	2(2)
L1810	2(2)
L1812	2(2)
L1820	2(2)
L1830	2(2)
L1831	2(2)
L1832	2(2)
L1833	2(2)
L1834	2(2)
L1836	2(2)
L1840	2(2)
L1843	2(2)
L1844	2(2)
L1845	2(2)
L1846	2(2)
L1847	2(2)
L1848	2(2)
L1850	2(2)
L1851	2(2)
L1852	2(2)
L1860	2(2)
L1900	2(2)
L1902	2(2)
L1904	2(2)
L1906	2(2)
L1907	2(2)
L1910	2(2)
L1920	2(2)
L1930	2(2)
L1932	2(2)
L1940	2(2)
L1945	2(2)
L1950	2(2)
L1951	2(2)
L1960	2(2)
L1970	2(2)
L1971	2(2)
L1980	2(2)

CPT	MUE
L1990	2(2)
L2000	2(2)
L2005	2(2)
L2006	0(3)
L2010	2(2)
L2020	2(2)
L2030	2(2)
L2034	2(2)
L2035	2(2)
L2036	2(2)
L2037	2(2)
L2038	2(2)
L2040	1(2)
L2050	1(2)
L2060	1(2)
L2070	1(2)
L2080	1(2)
L2090	1(2)
L2106	2(2)
L2108	2(2)
L2112	2(2)
L2114	2(2)
L2116	2(2)
L2126	2(2)
L2128	2(2)
L2132	2(2)
L2134	2(2)
L2136	2(2)
L2180	2(2)
L2182	4(2)
L2184	4(2)
L2186	4(2)
L2188	2(2)
L2190	2(2)
L2192	2(2)
L2200	4(2)
L2210	4(2)
L2220	4(2)
L2230	2(2)
L2232	2(2)
L2240	2(2)
L2250	2(2)
L2260	2(2)
L2265	2(2)
L2270	2(3)
L2275	2(3)
L2280	2(2)
L2300	1(2)
L2310	1(2)
L2320	2(3)
L2330	2(3)
L2335	2(2)
L2340	2(2)
L2350	2(2)
L2360	2(2)
L2370	2(2)
L2375	2(2)
L2380	2(3)
L2385	4(2)
L2387	4(2)
L2390	4(2)
L2395	4(2)
L2397	4(3)
L2405	4(2)
L2415	4(2)

CPT	MUE
L2425	4(2)
L2430	4(2)
L2492	4(2)
L2500	2(2)
L2510	2(2)
L2520	2(2)
L2525	2(2)
L2526	2(2)
L2530	2(2)
L2540	2(2)
L2550	2(2)
L2570	2(2)
L2580	2(2)
L2600	2(2)
L2610	2(2)
L2620	2(2)
L2622	2(2)
L2624	2(2)
L2627	1(3)
L2628	1(3)
L2630	1(2)
L2640	1(2)
L2650	2(3)
L2660	1(3)
L2670	2(3)
L2680	2(3)
L2750	8(3)
L2755	8(3)
L2760	8(2)
L2768	4(2)
L2780	8(3)
L2785	4(2)
L2795	2(2)
L2800	2(2)
L2810	4(2)
L2820	2(3)
L2830	2(3)
L2861	0(3)
L2999	2(3)
L3000	2(3)
L3001	2(3)
L3002	2(3)
L3003	2(3)
L3010	2(3)
L3020	2(3)
L3030	2(3)
L3031	2(3)
L3040	2(3)
L3050	2(3)
L3060	2(3)
L3070	2(3)
L3080	2(3)
L3090	2(3)
L3100	2(2)
L3140	1(2)
L3150	1(2)
L3160	2(2)
L3170	2(2)
L3201	1(3)
L3202	1(3)
L3203	1(3)
L3204	1(3)
L3206	1(3)
L3207	1(3)
L3208	1(3)

CPT	MUE
L3209	1(3)
L3211	1(3)
L3212	1(3)
L3213	1(3)
L3214	1(3)
L3215	0(3)
L3216	0(3)
L3217	0(3)
L3219	0(3)
L3221	0(3)
L3222	0(3)
L3224	2(2)
L3225	2(2)
L3230	2(2)
L3250	2(2)
L3251	2(2)
L3252	2(2)
L3253	2(2)
L3254	1(3)
L3255	1(3)
L3257	1(3)
L3260	0(3)
L3265	1(3)
L3300	4(3)
L3310	4(3)
L3330	2(2)
L3332	2(2)
L3334	4(3)
L3340	2(2)
L3350	2(2)
L3360	2(2)
L3370	2(2)
L3380	2(2)
L3390	2(2)
L3400	2(2)
L3410	2(2)
L3420	2(2)
L3430	2(2)
L3440	2(2)
L3450	2(2)
L3455	2(2)
L3460	2(2)
L3465	2(2)
L3470	2(2)
L3480	2(2)
L3485	2(2)
L3500	2(2)
L3510	2(2)
L3520	2(2)
L3530	2(2)
L3540	2(2)
L3550	2(2)
L3560	2(2)
L3570	2(2)
L3580	2(2)
L3590	2(2)
L3595	2(2)
L3600	2(2)
L3610	2(2)
L3620	2(2)
L3630	2(2)
L3640	1(2)
L3649	2(3)
L3650	1(2)
L3660	1(2)

CPT	MUE
L3670	1(3)
L3671	1(3)
L3674	1(3)
L3675	1(2)
L3677	1(2)
L3678	1(2)
L3702	2(2)
L3710	2(2)
L3720	2(2)
L3730	2(2)
L3740	2(2)
L3760	2(2)
L3761	2(2)
L3762	2(2)
L3763	2(2)
L3764	2(2)
L3765	2(2)
L3766	2(2)
L3806	2(2)
L3807	2(2)
L3808	2(2)
L3809	2(2)
L3891	0(3)
L3900	2(2)
L3901	2(2)
L3904	2(2)
L3905	2(2)
L3906	2(2)
L3908	2(2)
L3912	2(3)
L3913	2(2)
L3915	2(2)
L3916	2(3)
L3917	2(2)
L3918	2(2)
L3919	2(2)
L3921	2(2)
L3923	2(2)
L3924	2(2)
L3925	4(3)
L3927	4(3)
L3929	2(2)
L3930	2(2)
L3931	2(2)
L3933	3(3)
L3935	3(3)
L3956	4(3)
L3960	1(3)
L3961	1(3)
L3962	1(3)
L3967	1(3)
L3971	1(3)
L3973	1(3)
L3975	1(3)
L3976	1(3)
L3977	1(3)
L3978	1(3)
L3980	2(2)
L3981	2(2)
L3982	2(2)
L3984	2(2)
L3999	2(3)
L4000	1(2)
L4002	4(3)
L4010	2(2)

CPT	MUE
L4020	2(2)
L4030	2(2)
L4040	2(2)
L4045	2(2)
L4050	2(2)
L4055	2(2)
L4060	2(2)
L4070	2(3)
L4080	2(2)
L4090	4(2)
L4100	2(2)
L4110	4(2)
L4130	2(2)
L4205	8(3)
L4210	4(3)
L4350	2(2)
L4360	2(2)
L4361	2(2)
L4370	2(2)
L4386	2(2)
L4387	2(2)
L4392	2(3)
L4394	2(3)
L4396	2(2)
L4397	2(2)
L4398	2(2)
L4631	2(2)
L5000	2(3)
L5010	2(2)
L5020	2(2)
L5050	2(2)
L5060	2(2)
L5100	2(2)
L5105	2(2)
L5150	2(2)
L5160	2(2)
L5200	2(2)
L5210	2(2)
L5220	2(2)
L5230	2(2)
L5250	2(2)
L5270	2(2)
L5280	2(2)
L5301	2(2)
L5312	2(2)
L5321	2(2)
L5331	2(2)
L5341	2(2)
L5400	2(2)
L5410	2(2)
L5420	2(2)
L5430	2(2)
L5450	2(2)
L5460	2(2)
L5500	2(2)
L5505	2(2)
L5510	2(2)
L5520	2(2)
L5530	2(2)
L5535	2(2)
L5540	2(2)
L5560	2(2)
L5570	2(2)
L5580	2(2)
L5585	2(2)

CPT	MUE
L5590	2(2)
L5595	2(2)
L5600	2(2)
L5610	2(2)
L5611	2(2)
L5613	2(2)
L5614	2(2)
L5616	2(2)
L5617	2(3)
L5618	4(3)
L5620	4(3)
L5622	4(3)
L5624	4(3)
L5626	4(3)
L5628	2(3)
L5629	2(2)
L5630	2(2)
L5631	2(2)
L5632	2(2)
L5634	2(2)
L5636	2(2)
L5637	2(2)
L5638	2(2)
L5639	2(2)
L5640	2(2)
L5642	2(2)
L5643	2(2)
L5644	2(2)
L5645	2(2)
L5646	2(2)
L5647	2(2)
L5648	2(2)
L5649	2(2)
L5650	2(2)
L5651	2(2)
L5652	2(2)
L5653	2(2)
L5654	2(2)
L5655	2(2)
L5656	2(2)
L5658	2(2)
L5661	2(2)
L5665	2(2)
L5666	2(2)
L5668	2(2)
L5670	2(2)
L5671	2(2)
L5672	2(2)
L5673	4(3)
L5676	2(2)
L5677	2(2)
L5678	2(2)
L5679	4(3)
L5680	2(2)
L5681	2(2)
L5682	2(2)
L5683	2(2)
L5684	2(3)
L5685	4(3)
L5686	2(2)
L5688	2(3)
L5690	2(3)
L5692	2(2)
L5694	2(2)
L5695	2(3)

CPT	MUE	CPT	MUE	CPT	MUE	CPT	MUE	CPT	MUE	CPT	MUE	CPT	MUE	CPT	MUE
L5696	2(2)	L5974	2(2)	L6635	2(2)	L6935	2(2)	L8330	2(3)	L8691	1(3)	P9604	2(3)	Q0514	1(2)
L5697	2(2)	L5975	2(2)	L6637	2(2)	L6940	2(2)	L8400	12(3)	L8692	0(3)	P9612	1(3)	Q0515	0(3)
L5698	2(2)	L5976	2(2)	L6638	2(2)	L6945	2(2)	L8410	12(3)	L8693	1(3)	P9615	1(3)	Q1004	0(3)
L5699	2(3)	L5978	2(2)	L6640	2(2)	L6950	2(2)	L8415	6(3)	L8694	1(3)	Q0035	1(3)	Q1005	0(3)
L5700	2(2)	L5979	2(2)	L6641	2(3)	L6955	2(2)	L8417	12(3)	L8695	1(3)	Q0081	2(3)	Q2004	1(3)
L5701	2(2)	L5980	2(2)	L6642	2(3)	L6960	2(2)	L8420	14(3)	L8696	1(3)	Q0083	2(3)	Q2009	100(3)
L5702	2(2)	L5981	2(2)	L6645	2(2)	L6965	2(2)	L8430	12(3)	L8701	1(3)	Q0084	2(3)	Q2017	12(3)
L5703	2(2)	L5982	2(2)	L6646	2(2)	L6970	2(2)	L8435	12(3)	L8702	1(3)	Q0085	2(3)	Q2026	30(3)
L5704	2(2)	L5984	2(2)	L6647	2(2)	L6975	2(2)	L8440	4(3)	M0075	0(3)	Q0091	1(3)	Q2028	1470(3)
L5705	2(2)	L5985	2(2)	L6648	2(2)	L7007	2(2)	L8460	4(3)	M0076	0(3)	Q0092	2(3)	Q2034	1(2)
L5706	2(2)	L5986	2(2)	L6650	2(2)	L7008	2(2)	L8465	4(3)	M0100	0(3)	Q0111	2(3)	Q2035	1(2)
L5707	2(2)	L5987	2(2)	L6655	4(3)	L7009	2(2)	L8470	14(3)	M0300	0(3)	Q0112	3(3)	Q2036	1(2)
L5710	2(2)	L5988	2(2)	L6660	4(3)	L7040	2(2)	L8480	12(3)	M0301	0(3)	Q0113	1(3)	Q2037	1(2)
L5711	2(2)	L5990	2(2)	L6665	4(3)	L7045	2(2)	L8485	12(3)	P2028	1(2)	Q0114	1(3)	Q2038	1(2)
L5712	2(2)	L5999	2(3)	L6670	2(2)	L7170	2(2)	L8499	1(3)	P2029	1(2)	Q0115	1(3)	Q2039	1(2)
L5714	2(2)	L6000	2(2)	L6672	2(2)	L7180	2(2)	L8500	1(2)	P2031	0(3)	Q0138	510(3)	Q2043	1(2)
L5716	2(2)	L6010	2(2)	L6675	2(2)	L7181	2(2)	L8501	2(3)	P2033	1(2)	Q0139	510(3)	Q2049	10(3)
L5718	2(2)	L6020	2(2)	L6676	2(2)	L7185	2(2)	L8507	3(3)	P2038	1(2)	Q0144	0(3)	Q2050	20(3)
L5722	2(2)	L6026	2(2)	L6677	2(2)	L7186	2(2)	L8509	1(3)	P3000	1(3)	Q0161	66(3)	Q2052	0(3)
L5724	2(2)	L6050	2(2)	L6680	4(3)	L7190	2(2)	L8510	1(2)	P3001	1(3)	Q0162	24(3)	Q3014	2(3)
L5726	2(2)	L6055	2(2)	L6682	4(3)	L7191	2(2)	L8511	1(3)	P7001	0(3)	Q0163	6(3)	Q3027	30(3)
L5728	2(2)	L6100	2(2)	L6684	4(3)	L7259	2(2)	L8512	1(3)	P9010	4(3)	Q0164	8(3)	Q3028	0(3)
L5780	2(2)	L6110	2(2)	L6686	2(2)	L7360	1(3)	L8513	1(3)	P9011	4(3)	Q0166	2(3)	Q3031	1(3)
L5781	2(2)	L6120	2(2)	L6687	2(2)	L7362	1(2)	L8514	1(3)	P9012	12(3)	Q0167	108(3)	Q4001	1(3)
L5782	2(2)	L6130	2(2)	L6688	2(2)	L7364	1(3)	L8515	1(3)	P9016	12(3)	Q0169	12(3)	Q4002	1(3)
L5785	2(2)	L6200	2(2)	L6689	2(2)	L7366	1(2)	L8600	2(3)	P9017	24(3)	Q0173	5(3)	Q4003	2(3)
L5790	2(2)	L6205	2(2)	L6690	2(2)	L7367	2(3)	L8603	4(3)	P9019	12(3)	Q0174	0(3)	Q4004	2(3)
L5795	2(2)	L6250	2(2)	L6691	2(3)	L7368	1(2)	L8604	3(3)	P9020	5(3)	Q0175	6(3)	Q4012	2(3)
L5810	2(2)	L6300	2(2)	L6692	2(3)	L7400	2(2)	L8605	4(3)	P9021	8(3)	Q0177	16(3)	Q4013	2(3)
L5811	2(2)	L6310	2(2)	L6693	2(2)	L7401	2(2)	L8606	5(3)	P9022	12(3)	Q0180	1(3)	Q4014	2(3)
L5812	2(2)	L6320	2(2)	L6694	2(3)	L7402	2(2)	L8607	20(3)	P9023	15(3)	Q0181	2(3)	Q4018	2(3)
L5814	2(2)	L6350	2(2)	L6695	2(3)	L7403	2(2)	L8609	1(3)	P9031	12(3)	Q0477	1(1)	Q4021	2(3)
L5816	2(2)	L6360	2(2)	L6696	2(2)	L7404	2(2)	L8610	2(3)	P9032	12(3)	Q0478	1(3)	Q4025	1(3)
L5818	2(2)	L6370	2(2)	L6697	2(2)	L7405	2(2)	L8612	1(3)	P9033	12(3)	Q0479	1(3)	Q4026	1(3)
L5822	2(2)	L6380	2(2)	L6698	2(2)	L7499	2(3)	L8613	2(3)	P9034	4(3)	Q0480	1(3)	Q4027	1(3)
L5824	2(2)	L6382	2(2)	L6703	2(2)	L7510	4(3)	L8614	2(3)	P9035	4(3)	Q0481	1(2)	Q4028	1(3)
L5826	2(2)	L6384	2(2)	L6704	2(2)	L7600	0(3)	L8615	2(3)	P9036	4(3)	Q0482	1(3)	Q4030	2(3)
L5828	2(2)	L6386	2(2)	L6706	2(2)	L7700	2(1)	L8616	2(3)	P9037	4(3)	Q0483	1(3)	Q4037	2(3)
L5830	2(2)	L6388	2(2)	L6707	2(2)	L7900	0(3)	L8617	2(3)	P9038	4(3)	Q0484	1(3)	Q4042	2(3)
L5840	2(2)	L6400	2(2)	L6708	2(2)	L7902	0(3)	L8618	2(3)	P9039	2(3)	Q0485	1(3)	Q4046	2(3)
L5845	2(2)	L6450	2(2)	L6709	2(2)	L8000	6(3)	L8619	2(3)	P9040	8(3)	Q0486	1(3)	Q4050	2(3)
L5848	2(2)	L6500	2(2)	L6711	2(2)	L8001	4(3)	L8621	360(3)	P9041	100(3)	Q0487	1(3)	Q4051	2(3)
L5850	2(2)	L6550	2(2)	L6712	2(2)	L8002	4(3)	L8622	2(3)	P9043	10(3)	Q0488	1(3)	Q4074	0(3)
L5855	2(2)	L6570	2(2)	L6713	2(2)	L8010	4(3)	L8625	1(3)	P9044	20(3)	Q0489	1(3)	Q4081	400(3)
L5856	2(2)	L6580	2(2)	L6714	2(2)	L8015	4(3)	L8627	2(2)	P9045	20(3)	Q0490	1(3)	Q5101	1500(3)
L5857	2(2)	L6582	2(2)	L6715	5(3)	L8020	4(3)	L8628	2(2)	P9046	40(3)	Q0491	1(3)	Q5103	150(3)
L5858	2(2)	L6584	2(2)	L6721	2(2)	L8030	2(3)	L8629	2(2)	P9047	20(3)	Q0492	1(3)	Q5104	150(3)
L5859	2(2)	L6586	2(2)	L6722	2(2)	L8031	2(3)	L8631	2(3)	P9048	2(3)	Q0493	1(3)	Q5105	400(3)
L5910	2(2)	L6588	2(2)	L6805	2(2)	L8032	2(2)	L8641	4(3)	P9050	1(3)	Q0494	1(3)	Q5106	60(3)
L5920	2(2)	L6590	2(2)	L6810	2(3)	L8033	0(3)	L8642	2(3)	P9051	4(3)	Q0495	1(3)	Q5107	170(3)
L5925	2(3)	L6600	2(2)	L6880	2(2)	L8035	2(3)	L8658	3(3)	P9052	3(3)	Q0497	2(3)	Q5108	12(3)
L5930	2(2)	L6605	2(2)	L6881	2(2)	L8039	2(3)	L8659	4(3)	P9053	3(3)	Q0498	1(3)	Q5109	150(3)
L5940	2(2)	L6610	2(2)	L6882	2(2)	L8040	1(2)	L8670	3(3)	P9054	2(3)	Q0499	1(3)	Q5110	1500(3)
L5950	2(2)	L6611	2(3)	L6883	2(2)	L8041	1(2)	L8679	3(3)	P9055	2(3)	Q0501	1(3)	Q5111	12(3)
L5960	2(2)	L6615	2(2)	L6884	2(2)	L8042	2(2)	L8680	0(3)	P9056	3(3)	Q0502	1(3)	Q5112	120(3)
L5961	1(3)	L6616	2(2)	L6885	2(2)	L8043	1(2)	L8681	1(3)	P9057	4(3)	Q0503	3(3)	Q5113	120(3)
L5962	2(2)	L6620	2(2)	L6890	2(3)	L8044	1(2)	L8682	2(3)	P9058	4(3)	Q0504	1(3)	Q5114	120(3)
L5964	2(2)	L6621	2(2)	L6895	2(3)	L8045	2(2)	L8683	1(3)	P9059	15(3)	Q0506	8(3)	Q5115	120(3)
L5966	2(2)	L6623	2(2)	L6900	2(2)	L8046	1(3)	L8684	1(3)	P9060	4(3)	Q0507	1(3)	Q5116	120(3)
L5968	2(2)	L6624	2(2)	L6905	2(2)	L8047	1(2)	L8685	0(3)	P9070	15(3)	Q0508	24(3)	Q5117	120(3)
L5969	0(3)	L6625	2(2)	L6910	2(2)	L8048	1(3)	L8686	0(3)	P9071	15(3)	Q0509	2(3)	Q5118	230(3)
L5970	2(2)	L6628	2(2)	L6915	2(2)	L8049	6(3)	L8687	0(3)	P9073	4(3)	Q0510	1(2)	Q9950	5(3)
L5971	2(2)	L6629	2(2)	L6920	2(2)	L8300	1(3)	L8688	0(3)	P9099	1(3)	Q0511	1(2)	Q9951	0(3)
L5972	2(2)	L6630	2(2)	L6925	2(2)	L8310	1(3)	L8689	1(3)	P9100	12(3)	Q0512	4(3)	Q9953	10(3)
L5973	2(3)	L6632	4(3)	L6930	2(2)	L8320	2(3)	L8690	2(2)	P9603	100(3)	Q0513	1(2)	Q9954	18(3)

CPT	MUE
Q9955	0(3)
Q9956	9(3)
Q9957	3(3)
Q9958	600(3)
Q9959	0(3)
Q9960	250(3)
Q9961	200(3)
Q9962	200(3)
Q9963	240(3)
Q9964	0(3)
Q9966	250(3)
Q9967	300(3)
Q9969	3(3)
Q9982	1(3)
Q9983	1(3)
Q9991	1(2)
Q9992	1(2)
R0070	2(3)
R0075	2(3)
R0076	1(3)
U0001	2(3)
U0002	2(3)
U0003	2(3)
U0004	2(3)
V2020	1(3)
V2025	0(3)
V2100	2(3)
V2101	2(3)
V2102	2(3)

CPT	MUE
V2103	2(3)
V2104	2(3)
V2105	2(3)
V2106	2(3)
V2107	2(3)
V2108	2(3)
V2109	2(3)
V2110	2(3)
V2111	2(3)
V2112	2(3)
V2113	2(3)
V2114	2(3)
V2115	2(3)
V2118	2(3)
V2121	2(3)
V2199	2(3)
V2200	2(3)
V2201	2(3)
V2202	2(3)
V2203	2(3)
V2204	2(3)
V2205	2(3)
V2206	2(3)
V2207	2(3)
V2208	2(3)
V2209	2(3)
V2210	2(3)
V2211	2(3)
V2212	2(3)

CPT	MUE
V2213	2(3)
V2214	2(3)
V2215	2(3)
V2218	2(3)
V2219	2(3)
V2220	2(3)
V2221	2(3)
V2299	2(3)
V2300	2(3)
V2301	2(3)
V2302	2(3)
V2303	2(3)
V2304	2(3)
V2305	2(3)
V2306	2(3)
V2307	2(3)
V2308	2(3)
V2309	2(3)
V2310	2(3)
V2311	2(3)
V2312	2(3)
V2313	2(3)
V2314	2(3)
V2315	2(3)
V2318	2(3)
V2319	2(3)
V2320	2(3)
V2321	2(3)
V2399	2(3)

CPT	MUE
V2410	2(3)
V2430	2(3)
V2499	2(3)
V2500	2(3)
V2501	2(3)
V2502	2(3)
V2503	2(3)
V2510	2(3)
V2511	2(3)
V2512	2(3)
V2513	2(3)
V2520	2(3)
V2521	2(3)
V2522	2(3)
V2523	2(3)
V2530	2(3)
V2531	2(3)
V2599	2(3)
V2600	0(2)
V2610	0(2)
V2615	0(2)
V2623	2(2)
V2624	2(2)
V2625	2(2)
V2626	2(2)
V2627	2(2)
V2628	2(3)
V2629	2(2)
V2630	2(2)

CPT	MUE
V2631	2(2)
V2632	2(2)
V2700	2(3)
V2702	0(3)
V2710	2(3)
V2715	4(3)
V2718	2(3)
V2730	2(3)
V2744	2(3)
V2745	2(3)
V2750	2(3)
V2755	2(3)
V2756	0(3)
V2760	0(3)
V2761	0(2)
V2762	0(3)
V2770	2(3)
V2780	2(3)
V2781	0(2)
V2782	2(3)
V2783	2(3)
V2784	2(3)
V2785	2(2)
V2786	0(3)
V2787	0(3)
V2788	0(3)
V2790	1(3)
V2797	0(3)
V5008	0(3)

CPT	MUE
V5010	0(3)
V5011	0(3)
V5014	0(3)
V5020	0(3)
V5030	0(3)
V5040	0(3)
V5050	0(3)
V5060	0(3)
V5070	0(3)
V5080	0(3)
V5090	0(3)
V5095	0(3)
V5100	0(3)
V5110	0(3)
V5120	0(3)
V5130	0(3)
V5140	0(3)
V5150	0(3)
V5160	0(3)
V5171	0(3)
V5172	0(3)
V5181	0(3)
V5190	0(3)
V5200	0(3)
V5211	0(3)
V5212	0(3)
V5213	0(3)
V5214	0(3)
V5215	0(3)

CPT	MUE
V5221	0(3)
V5230	0(3)
V5240	0(3)
V5241	0(3)
V5242	0(3)
V5243	0(3)
V5244	0(3)
V5245	0(3)
V5246	0(3)
V5247	0(3)
V5248	0(3)
V5249	0(3)
V5250	0(3)
V5251	0(3)
V5252	0(3)
V5253	0(3)
V5254	0(3)
V5255	0(3)
V5256	0(3)
V5257	0(3)
V5258	0(3)
V5259	0(3)
V5260	0(3)
V5261	0(3)
V5262	0(3)
V5263	0(3)
V5264	0(3)
V5265	0(3)
V5266	0(3)

CPT	MUE
V5267	0(3)
V5268	0(3)
V5269	0(3)
V5270	0(3)
V5271	0(3)
V5272	0(3)
V5273	0(3)
V5274	0(3)
V5275	0(3)
V5281	0(3)
V5282	0(3)
V5283	0(3)
V5284	0(3)
V5285	0(3)
V5286	0(3)
V5287	0(3)
V5288	0(3)
V5289	0(3)
V5290	0(3)
V5298	0(3)
V5299	1(3)
V5336	0(3)
V5362	0(3)
V5363	0(3)
V5364	0(3)

Appendix J — Inpatient-Only Procedures

Inpatient Only Procedures—This appendix identifies services with the status indicator C. Medicare will not pay an OPPS hospital or ASC when they are performed on a Medicare patient as an outpatient. Physicians should refer to this list when scheduling Medicare patients for surgical procedures. CMS updates this list quarterly. The following was updated 10/01/2020.

00176	Anesth pharyngeal surgery
00192	Anesth facial bone surgery
00211	Anesth cran surg hematoma
00214	Anesth skull drainage
00215	Anesth skull repair/fract
00474	Anesth surgery of rib
00524	Anesth chest drainage
00540	Anesth chest surgery
00542	Anesthesia removal pleura
00546	Anesth lung chest wall surg
00560	Anesth heart surg w/o pump
00561	Anesth heart surg <1 yr
00562	Anesth hrt surg w/pmp age 1+
00567	Anesth CABG w/pump
00580	Anesth heart/lung transplnt
00604	Anesth sitting procedure
00632	Anesth removal of nerves
0075T	Perq stent/chest vert art
0076T	S&i stent/chest vert art
00792	Anesth hemorr/excise liver
00794	Anesth pancreas removal
00796	Anesth for liver transplant
00844	Anesth pelvis surgery
00846	Anesth hysterectomy
00848	Anesth pelvic organ surg
00864	Anesth removal of bladder
00866	Anesth removal of adrenal
00868	Anesth kidney transplant
00882	Anesth major vein ligation
00904	Anesth perineal surgery
00908	Anesth removal of prostate
00932	Anesth amputation of penis
00934	Anesth penis nodes removal
00936	Anesth penis nodes removal
0095T	Rmvl artific disc addl crvcl
0098T	Rev artific disc addl
01140	Anesth amputation at pelvis
01150	Anesth pelvic tumor surgery
01212	Anesth hip disarticulation
01232	Anesth amputation of femur
01234	Anesth radical femur surg
01272	Anesth femoral artery surg
01274	Anesth femoral embolectomy
01404	Anesth amputation at knee
01442	Anesth knee artery surg
01444	Anesth knee artery repair
01486	Anesth ankle replacement
01502	Anesth lwr leg embolectomy
01634	Anesth shoulder joint amput
01636	Anesth forequarter amput
01638	Anesth shoulder replacement
0163T	Lumb artif diskectomy addl
0164T	Remove lumb artif disc addl
01652	Anesth shoulder vessel surg
01654	Anesth shoulder vessel surg
01656	Anesth arm-leg vessel surg
0165T	Revise lumb artif disc addl
01756	Anesth radical humerus surg
01990	Support for organ donor
0202T	Post vert arthrplst 1 lumbar
0219T	Plmt post facet implt cerv
0220T	Plmt post facet implt thor
0235T	Trluml perip athrc visceral
0345T	Transcath mtral vlve repair
0451T	Insj/rplcmt aortic ventr sys
0452T	Insj/rplcmt dev vasc seal
0455T	Remvl aortic ventr cmpl sys
0456T	Remvl aortic dev vasc seal
0459T	Relocaj rplcmt aortic ventr
0461T	Repos aortic contrpulsj dev
0483T	Tmvi percutaneous approach
0484T	Tmvi transthoracic exposure
0494T	Prep & cannulj cdvr don lung
0495T	Mntr cdvr don lng 1st 2 hrs
0496T	Mntr cdvr don lng ea addl hr
0543T	Ta mv rpr w/artif chord tend
0544T	Tcat mv annulus rcnstj
0545T	Tcat tv annulus rcnstj
0569T	Ttvr perq appr 1st prosth
0570T	Ttvr perq ea addl prosth
0584T	Perq islet cell transplant
0585T	Laps islet cell transplant
0586T	Open islet cell transplant
11004	Debride genitalia & perineum
11005	Debride abdom wall
11006	Debride genit/per/abdom wall
11008	Remove mesh from abd wall
15756	Free myo/skin flap microvasc
15757	Free skin flap microvasc
15758	Free fascial flap microvasc
16036	Escharotomy addl incision
19305	Mast radical
19306	Mast rad urban type
19361	Breast reconstr w/lat flap
19364	Breast reconstruction
19367	Breast reconstruction
19368	Breast reconstruction
19369	Breast reconstruction
20661	Application of head brace
20664	Application of halo
20802	Replantation arm complete
20805	Replant forearm complete
20808	Replantation hand complete
20816	Replantation digit complete
20824	Replantation thumb complete
20827	Replantation thumb complete
20838	Replantation foot complete
20955	Fibula bone graft microvasc
20956	Iliac bone graft microvasc
20957	Mt bone graft microvasc
20962	Other bone graft microvasc
20969	Bone/skin graft microvasc
20970	Bone/skin graft iliac crest
21045	Extensive jaw surgery
21141	Lefort i-1 piece w/o graft
21142	Lefort i-2 piece w/o graft
21143	Lefort i-3/> piece w/o graft
21145	Lefort i-1 piece w/ graft
21146	Lefort i-2 piece w/ graft
21147	Lefort i-3/> piece w/ graft
21151	Lefort ii w/bone grafts
21154	Lefort iii w/o lefort i
21155	Lefort iii w/ lefort i
21159	Lefort iii w/fhdw/o lefort i
21160	Lefort iii w/fhd w/ lefort i
21179	Reconstruct entire forehead
21180	Reconstruct entire forehead
21182	Reconstruct cranial bone
21183	Reconstruct cranial bone
21184	Reconstruct cranial bone
21188	Reconstruction of midface
21194	Reconst lwr jaw w/graft
21196	Reconst lwr jaw w/fixation
21247	Reconstruct lower jaw bone
21255	Reconstruct lower jaw bone
21268	Revise eye sockets
21343	Open tx dprsd front sinus fx
21344	Open tx compl front sinus fx
21347	Opn tx nasomax fx multple
21348	Opn tx nasomax fx w/graft
21366	Opn tx complx malar w/grft
21422	Treat mouth roof fracture
21423	Treat mouth roof fracture
21431	Treat craniofacial fracture
21432	Treat craniofacial fracture
21433	Treat craniofacial fracture
21435	Treat craniofacial fracture
21436	Treat craniofacial fracture
21510	Drainage of bone lesion
21602	Exc ch wal tum w/o lymphadec
21603	Exc ch wal tum w/lymphadec
21615	Removal of rib
21616	Removal of rib and nerves
21620	Partial removal of sternum
21627	Sternal debridement
21630	Extensive sternum surgery
21632	Extensive sternum surgery
21705	Revision of neck muscle/rib
21740	Reconstruction of sternum

Appendix J — Inpatient-Only Procedures

21750	Repair of sternum separation
21825	Treat sternum fracture
22010	I&d p-spine c/t/cerv-thor
22015	I&d abscess p-spine l/s/ls
22110	Remove part of neck vertebra
22112	Remove part thorax vertebra
22114	Remove part lumbar vertebra
22116	Remove extra spine segment
22206	Incis spine 3 column thorac
22207	Incis spine 3 column lumbar
22208	Incis spine 3 column adl seg
22210	Incis 1 vertebral seg cerv
22212	Incis 1 vertebral seg thorac
22214	Incis 1 vertebral seg lumbar
22216	Incis addl spine segment
22220	Incis w/discectomy cervical
22222	Incis w/discectomy thoracic
22224	Incis w/discectomy lumbar
22226	Revise extra spine segment
22318	Treat odontoid fx w/o graft
22319	Treat odontoid fx w/graft
22325	Treat spine fracture
22326	Treat neck spine fracture
22327	Treat thorax spine fracture
22328	Treat each add spine fx
22532	Lat thorax spine fusion
22533	Lat lumbar spine fusion
22534	Lat thor/lumb addl seg
22548	Neck spine fusion
22556	Thorax spine fusion
22558	Lumbar spine fusion
22586	Prescrl fuse w/ instr l5-s1
22590	Spine & skull spinal fusion
22595	Neck spinal fusion
22600	Neck spine fusion
22610	Thorax spine fusion
22630	Lumbar spine fusion
22632	Spine fusion extra segment
22800	Post fusion </6 vert seg
22802	Post fusion 7-12 vert seg
22804	Post fusion 13/> vert seg
22808	Ant fusion 2-3 vert seg
22810	Ant fusion 4-7 vert seg
22812	Ant fusion 8/> vert seg
22818	Kyphectomy 1-2 segments
22819	Kyphectomy 3 or more
22830	Exploration of spinal fusion
22841	Insert spine fixation device
22843	Insert spine fixation device
22844	Insert spine fixation device
22846	Insert spine fixation device
22847	Insert spine fixation device
22848	Insert pelv fixation device
22849	Reinsert spinal fixation
22850	Remove spine fixation device
22852	Remove spine fixation device
22855	Remove spine fixation device
22857	Lumbar artif diskectomy
22861	Revise cerv artific disc
22862	Revise lumbar artif disc
22864	Remove cerv artif disc
22865	Remove lumb artif disc
23200	Resect clavicle tumor
23210	Resect scapula tumor
23220	Resect prox humerus tumor
23335	Shoulder prosthesis removal
23472	Reconstruct shoulder joint
23474	Revis reconst shoulder joint
23900	Amputation of arm & girdle
23920	Amputation at shoulder joint
24900	Amputation of upper arm
24920	Amputation of upper arm
24930	Amputation follow-up surgery
24931	Amputate upper arm & implant
24940	Revision of upper arm
25900	Amputation of forearm
25905	Amputation of forearm
25915	Amputation of forearm
25920	Amputate hand at wrist
25924	Amputation follow-up surgery
25927	Amputation of hand
26551	Great toe-hand transfer
26553	Single transfer toe-hand
26554	Double transfer toe-hand
26556	Toe joint transfer
26992	Drainage of bone lesion
27005	Incision of hip tendon
27025	Incision of hip/thigh fascia
27030	Drainage of hip joint
27036	Excision of hip joint/muscle
27054	Removal of hip joint lining
27070	Part remove hip bone super
27071	Part removal hip bone deep
27075	Resect hip tumor
27076	Resect hip tum incl acetabul
27077	Resect hip tum w/innom bone
27078	Rsect hip tum incl femur
27090	Removal of hip prosthesis
27091	Removal of hip prosthesis
27120	Reconstruction of hip socket
27122	Reconstruction of hip socket
27125	Partial hip replacement
27132	Total hip arthroplasty
27134	Revise hip joint replacement
27137	Revise hip joint replacement
27138	Revise hip joint replacement
27140	Transplant femur ridge
27146	Incision of hip bone
27147	Revision of hip bone
27151	Incision of hip bones
27156	Revision of hip bones
27158	Revision of pelvis
27161	Incision of neck of femur
27165	Incision/fixation of femur
27170	Repair/graft femur head/neck
27175	Treat slipped epiphysis
27176	Treat slipped epiphysis
27177	Treat slipped epiphysis
27178	Treat slipped epiphysis
27181	Treat slipped epiphysis
27185	Revision of femur epiphysis
27187	Reinforce hip bones
27222	Treat hip socket fracture
27226	Treat hip wall fracture
27227	Treat hip fracture(s)
27228	Treat hip fracture(s)
27232	Treat thigh fracture
27236	Treat thigh fracture
27240	Treat thigh fracture
27244	Treat thigh fracture
27245	Treat thigh fracture
27248	Treat thigh fracture
27253	Treat hip dislocation
27254	Treat hip dislocation
27258	Treat hip dislocation
27259	Treat hip dislocation
27268	Cltx thigh fx w/mnpj
27269	Optx thigh fx
27280	Fusion of sacroiliac joint
27282	Fusion of pubic bones
27284	Fusion of hip joint
27286	Fusion of hip joint
27290	Amputation of leg at hip
27295	Amputation of leg at hip
27303	Drainage of bone lesion
27365	Resect femur/knee tumor
27445	Revision of knee joint
27448	Incision of thigh
27450	Incision of thigh
27454	Realignment of thigh bone
27455	Realignment of knee
27457	Realignment of knee
27465	Shortening of thigh bone
27466	Lengthening of thigh bone
27468	Shorten/lengthen thighs
27470	Repair of thigh
27472	Repair/graft of thigh
27486	Revise/replace knee joint
27487	Revise/replace knee joint
27488	Removal of knee prosthesis
27495	Reinforce thigh
27506	Treatment of thigh fracture
27507	Treatment of thigh fracture
27511	Treatment of thigh fracture
27513	Treatment of thigh fracture
27514	Treatment of thigh fracture
27519	Treat thigh fx growth plate
27535	Treat knee fracture
27536	Treat knee fracture
27540	Treat knee fracture
27556	Treat knee dislocation
27557	Treat knee dislocation
27558	Treat knee dislocation
27580	Fusion of knee
27590	Amputate leg at thigh
27591	Amputate leg at thigh
27592	Amputate leg at thigh

27596 Amputation follow-up surgery
27598 Amputate lower leg at knee
27645 Resect tibia tumor
27646 Resect fibula tumor
27702 Reconstruct ankle joint
27703 Reconstruction ankle joint
27712 Realignment of lower leg
27715 Revision of lower leg
27724 Repair/graft of tibia
27725 Repair of lower leg
27727 Repair of lower leg
27880 Amputation of lower leg
27881 Amputation of lower leg
27882 Amputation of lower leg
27886 Amputation follow-up surgery
27888 Amputation of foot at ankle
28800 Amputation of midfoot
31225 Removal of upper jaw
31230 Removal of upper jaw
31290 Nasal/sinus endoscopy surg
31291 Nasal/sinus endoscopy surg
31360 Removal of larynx
31365 Removal of larynx
31367 Partial removal of larynx
31368 Partial removal of larynx
31370 Partial removal of larynx
31375 Partial removal of larynx
31380 Partial removal of larynx
31382 Partial removal of larynx
31390 Removal of larynx & pharynx
31395 Reconstruct larynx & pharynx
31725 Clearance of airways
31760 Repair of windpipe
31766 Reconstruction of windpipe
31770 Repair/graft of bronchus
31775 Reconstruct bronchus
31780 Reconstruct windpipe
31781 Reconstruct windpipe
31786 Remove windpipe lesion
31800 Repair of windpipe injury
31805 Repair of windpipe injury
32035 Thoracostomy w/rib resection
32036 Thoracostomy w/flap drainage
32096 Open wedge/bx lung infiltr
32097 Open wedge/bx lung nodule
32098 Open biopsy of lung pleura
32100 Exploration of chest
32110 Explore/repair chest
32120 Re-exploration of chest
32124 Explore chest free adhesions
32140 Removal of lung lesion(s)
32141 Remove/treat lung lesions
32150 Removal of lung lesion(s)
32151 Remove lung foreign body
32160 Open chest heart massage
32200 Drain open lung lesion
32215 Treat chest lining
32220 Release of lung
32225 Partial release of lung
32310 Removal of chest lining
32320 Free/remove chest lining
32440 Remove lung pneumonectomy
32442 Sleeve pneumonectomy
32445 Removal of lung extrapleural
32480 Partial removal of lung
32482 Bilobectomy
32484 Segmentectomy
32486 Sleeve lobectomy
32488 Completion pneumonectomy
32491 Lung volume reduction
32501 Repair bronchus add-on
32503 Resect apical lung tumor
32504 Resect apical lung tum/chest
32505 Wedge resect of lung initial
32506 Wedge resect of lung add-on
32507 Wedge resect of lung diag
32540 Removal of lung lesion
32650 Thoracoscopy w/pleurodesis
32651 Thoracoscopy remove cortex
32652 Thoracoscopy rem totl cortex
32653 Thoracoscopy remov fb/fibrin
32654 Thoracoscopy contrl bleeding
32655 Thoracoscopy resect bullae
32656 Thoracoscopy w/pleurectomy
32658 Thoracoscopy w/sac fb remove
32659 Thoracoscopy w/sac drainage
32661 Thoracoscopy w/pericard exc
32662 Thoracoscopy w/mediast exc
32663 Thoracoscopy w/lobectomy
32664 Thoracoscopy w/ th nrv exc
32665 Thoracoscop w/esoph musc exc
32666 Thoracoscopy w/wedge resect
32667 Thoracoscopy w/w resect addl
32668 Thoracoscopy w/w resect diag
32669 Thoracoscopy remove segment
32670 Thoracoscopy bilobectomy
32671 Thoracoscopy pneumonectomy
32672 Thoracoscopy for lvrs
32673 Thoracoscopy w/thymus resect
32674 Thoracoscopy lymph node exc
32800 Repair lung hernia
32810 Close chest after drainage
32815 Close bronchial fistula
32820 Reconstruct injured chest
32850 Donor pneumonectomy
32851 Lung transplant single
32852 Lung transplant with bypass
32853 Lung transplant double
32854 Lung transplant with bypass
32855 Prepare donor lung single
32856 Prepare donor lung double
32900 Removal of rib(s)
32905 Revise & repair chest wall
32906 Revise & repair chest wall
32940 Revision of lung
32997 Total lung lavage
33017 Prcrd drg 6yr+ w/o cgen car
33018 Prcrd drg 0-5yr or w/anomly
33019 Perq prcrd drg insj cath ct
33020 Incision of heart sac
33025 Incision of heart sac
33030 Partial removal of heart sac
33031 Partial removal of heart sac
33050 Resect heart sac lesion
33120 Removal of heart lesion
33130 Removal of heart lesion
33140 Heart revascularize (tmr)
33141 Heart tmr w/other procedure
33202 Insert epicard eltrd open
33203 Insert epicard eltrd endo
33236 Remove electrode/thoracotomy
33237 Remove electrode/thoracotomy
33238 Remove electrode/thoracotomy
33243 Remove eltrd/thoracotomy
33250 Ablate heart dysrhythm focus
33251 Ablate heart dysrhythm focus
33254 Ablate atria lmtd
33255 Ablate atria w/o bypass ext
33256 Ablate atria w/bypass exten
33257 Ablate atria lmtd add-on
33258 Ablate atria x10sv add-on
33259 Ablate atria w/bypass add-on
33261 Ablate heart dysrhythm focus
33265 Ablate atria lmtd endo
33266 Ablate atria x10sv endo
33300 Repair of heart wound
33305 Repair of heart wound
33310 Exploratory heart surgery
33315 Exploratory heart surgery
33320 Repair major blood vessel(s)
33321 Repair major vessel
33322 Repair major blood vessel(s)
33330 Insert major vessel graft
33335 Insert major vessel graft
33340 Perq clsr tcat l atr apndge
33361 Replace aortic valve perq
33362 Replace aortic valve open
33363 Replace aortic valve open
33364 Replace aortic valve open
33365 Replace aortic valve open
33366 Trcath replace aortic valve
33367 Replace aortic valve w/byp
33368 Replace aortic valve w/byp
33369 Replace aortic valve w/byp
33390 Valvuloplasty aortic valve
33391 Valvuloplasty aortic valve
33404 Prepare heart-aorta conduit
33405 Replacement of aortic valve
33406 Replacement of aortic valve
33410 Replacement of aortic valve
33411 Replacement of aortic valve
33412 Replacement of aortic valve
33413 Replacement of aortic valve
33414 Repair of aortic valve
33415 Revision subvalvular tissue
33416 Revise ventricle muscle
33417 Repair of aortic valve

Appendix J — Inpatient-Only Procedures

33418	Repair tcat mitral valve
33420	Revision of mitral valve
33422	Revision of mitral valve
33425	Repair of mitral valve
33426	Repair of mitral valve
33427	Repair of mitral valve
33430	Replacement of mitral valve
33440	Rplcmt a-valve tlcj autol pv
33460	Revision of tricuspid valve
33463	Valvuloplasty tricuspid
33464	Valvuloplasty tricuspid
33465	Replace tricuspid valve
33468	Revision of tricuspid valve
33470	Revision of pulmonary valve
33471	Valvotomy pulmonary valve
33474	Revision of pulmonary valve
33475	Replacement pulmonary valve
33476	Revision of heart chamber
33477	Implant tcat pulm vlv perq
33478	Revision of heart chamber
33496	Repair prosth valve clot
33500	Repair heart vessel fistula
33501	Repair heart vessel fistula
33502	Coronary artery correction
33503	Coronary artery graft
33504	Coronary artery graft
33505	Repair artery w/tunnel
33506	Repair artery translocation
33507	Repair art intramural
33510	Cabg vein single
33511	Cabg vein two
33512	Cabg vein three
33513	Cabg vein four
33514	Cabg vein five
33516	Cabg vein six or more
33517	Cabg artery-vein single
33518	Cabg artery-vein two
33519	Cabg artery-vein three
33521	Cabg artery-vein four
33522	Cabg artery-vein five
33523	Cabg art-vein six or more
33530	Coronary artery bypass/reop
33533	Cabg arterial single
33534	Cabg arterial two
33535	Cabg arterial three
33536	Cabg arterial four or more
33542	Removal of heart lesion
33545	Repair of heart damage
33548	Restore/remodel ventricle
33572	Open coronary endarterectomy
33600	Closure of valve
33602	Closure of valve
33606	Anastomosis/artery-aorta
33608	Repair anomaly w/conduit
33610	Repair by enlargement
33611	Repair double ventricle
33612	Repair double ventricle
33615	Repair modified fontan
33617	Repair single ventricle
33619	Repair single ventricle
33620	Apply r&l pulm art bands
33621	Transthor cath for stent
33622	Redo compl cardiac anomaly
33641	Repair heart septum defect
33645	Revision of heart veins
33647	Repair heart septum defects
33660	Repair of heart defects
33665	Repair of heart defects
33670	Repair of heart chambers
33675	Close mult vsd
33676	Close mult vsd w/resection
33677	Cl mult vsd w/rem pul band
33681	Repair heart septum defect
33684	Repair heart septum defect
33688	Repair heart septum defect
33690	Reinforce pulmonary artery
33692	Repair of heart defects
33694	Repair of heart defects
33697	Repair of heart defects
33702	Repair of heart defects
33710	Repair of heart defects
33720	Repair of heart defect
33722	Repair of heart defect
33724	Repair venous anomaly
33726	Repair pul venous stenosis
33730	Repair heart-vein defect(s)
33732	Repair heart-vein defect
33735	Revision of heart chamber
33736	Revision of heart chamber
33737	Revision of heart chamber
33750	Major vessel shunt
33755	Major vessel shunt
33762	Major vessel shunt
33764	Major vessel shunt & graft
33766	Major vessel shunt
33767	Major vessel shunt
33768	Cavopulmonary shunting
33770	Repair great vessels defect
33771	Repair great vessels defect
33774	Repair great vessels defect
33775	Repair great vessels defect
33776	Repair great vessels defect
33777	Repair great vessels defect
33778	Repair great vessels defect
33779	Repair great vessels defect
33780	Repair great vessels defect
33781	Repair great vessels defect
33782	Nikaidoh proc
33783	Nikaidoh proc w/ostia implt
33786	Repair arterial trunk
33788	Revision of pulmonary artery
33800	Aortic suspension
33802	Repair vessel defect
33803	Repair vessel defect
33813	Repair septal defect
33814	Repair septal defect
33820	Revise major vessel
33822	Revise major vessel
33824	Revise major vessel
33840	Remove aorta constriction
33845	Remove aorta constriction
33851	Remove aorta constriction
33852	Repair septal defect
33853	Repair septal defect
33858	As-aort grf f/aortic dsj
33859	As-aort grf f/ds oth/thn dsj
33863	Ascending aortic graft
33864	Ascending aortic graft
33871	Transvrs a-arch grf hypthrm
33875	Thoracic aortic graft
33877	Thoracoabdominal graft
33880	Endovasc taa repr incl subcl
33881	Endovasc taa repr w/o subcl
33883	Insert endovasc prosth taa
33884	Endovasc prosth taa add-on
33886	Endovasc prosth delayed
33889	Artery transpose/endovas taa
33891	Car-car bp grft/endovas taa
33910	Remove lung artery emboli
33915	Remove lung artery emboli
33916	Surgery of great vessel
33917	Repair pulmonary artery
33920	Repair pulmonary atresia
33922	Transect pulmonary artery
33924	Remove pulmonary shunt
33925	Rpr pul art unifocal w/o cpb
33926	Repr pul art unifocal w/cpb
33927	Impltj tot rplcmt hrt sys
33928	Rmvl & rplcmt tot hrt sys
33929	Rmvl rplcmt hrt sys f/trnspl
33930	Removal of donor heart/lung
33933	Prepare donor heart/lung
33935	Transplantation heart/lung
33940	Removal of donor heart
33944	Prepare donor heart
33945	Transplantation of heart
33946	Ecmo/ecls initiation venous
33947	Ecmo/ecls initiation artery
33948	Ecmo/ecls daily mgmt-venous
33949	Ecmo/ecls daily mgmt artery
33951	Ecmo/ecls insj prph cannula
33952	Ecmo/ecls insj prph cannula
33953	Ecmo/ecls insj prph cannula
33954	Ecmo/ecls insj prph cannula
33955	Ecmo/ecls insj ctr cannula
33956	Ecmo/ecls insj ctr cannula
33957	Ecmo/ecls repos perph cnula
33958	Ecmo/ecls repos perph cnula
33959	Ecmo/ecls repos perph cnula
33962	Ecmo/ecls repos perph cnula
33963	Ecmo/ecls repos perph cnula
33964	Ecmo/ecls repos perph cnula
33965	Ecmo/ecls rmvl perph cannula
33966	Ecmo/ecls rmvl prph cannula
33967	Insert i-aort percut device
33968	Remove aortic assist device
33969	Ecmo/ecls rmvl perph cannula

33970 Aortic circulation assist
33971 Aortic circulation assist
33973 Insert balloon device
33974 Remove intra-aortic balloon
33975 Implant ventricular device
33976 Implant ventricular device
33977 Remove ventricular device
33978 Remove ventricular device
33979 Insert intracorporeal device
33980 Remove intracorporeal device
33981 Replace vad pump ext
33982 Replace vad intra w/o bp
33983 Replace vad intra w/bp
33984 Ecmo/ecls rmvl prph cannula
33985 Ecmo/ecls rmvl ctr cannula
33986 Ecmo/ecls rmvl ctr cannula
33987 Artery expos/graft artery
33988 Insertion of left heart vent
33989 Removal of left heart vent
33990 Insert vad artery access
33991 Insert vad art&vein access
33992 Remove vad different session
33993 Reposition vad diff session
34001 Removal of artery clot
34051 Removal of artery clot
34151 Removal of artery clot
34401 Removal of vein clot
34451 Removal of vein clot
34502 Reconstruct vena cava
34701 Evasc rpr a-ao ndgft
34702 Evasc rpr a-ao ndgft rpt
34703 Evasc rpr a-unilac ndgft
34704 Evasc rpr a-unilac ndgft rpt
34705 Evac rpr a-biiliac ndgft
34706 Evasc rpr a-biiliac rpt
34707 Evasc rpr ilio-iliac ndgft
34708 Evasc rpr ilio-iliac rpt
34709 Plmt xtn prosth evasc rpr
34710 Dlyd plmt xtn prosth 1st vsl
34711 Dlyd plmt xtn prosth ea addl
34712 Tcat dlvr enhncd fixj dev
34717 Evasc rpr a-iliac ndgft
34718 Evasc rpr n/a a-iliac ndgft
34808 Endovas iliac a device addon
34812 Xpose for endoprosth femorl
34813 Femoral endovas graft add-on
34820 Xpose for endoprosth iliac
34830 Open aortic tube prosth repr
34831 Open aortoiliac prosth repr
34832 Open aortofemor prosth repr
34833 Xpose for endoprosth iliac
34834 Xpose endoprosth brachial
34841 Endovasc visc aorta 1 graft
34842 Endovasc visc aorta 2 graft
34843 Endovasc visc aorta 3 graft
34844 Endovasc visc aorta 4 graft
34845 Visc & infraren abd 1 prosth
34846 Visc & infraren abd 2 prosth
34847 Visc & infraren abd 3 prosth
34848 Visc & infraren abd 4+ prost
35001 Repair defect of artery
35002 Repair artery rupture neck
35005 Repair defect of artery
35013 Repair artery rupture arm
35021 Repair defect of artery
35022 Repair artery rupture chest
35081 Repair defect of artery
35082 Repair artery rupture aorta
35091 Repair defect of artery
35092 Repair artery rupture aorta
35102 Repair defect of artery
35103 Repair artery rupture aorta
35111 Repair defect of artery
35112 Repair artery rupture spleen
35121 Repair defect of artery
35122 Repair artery rupture belly
35131 Repair defect of artery
35132 Repair artery rupture groin
35141 Repair defect of artery
35142 Repair artery rupture thigh
35151 Repair defect of artery
35152 Repair ruptd popliteal art
35182 Repair blood vessel lesion
35189 Repair blood vessel lesion
35211 Repair blood vessel lesion
35216 Repair blood vessel lesion
35221 Repair blood vessel lesion
35241 Repair blood vessel lesion
35246 Repair blood vessel lesion
35251 Repair blood vessel lesion
35271 Repair blood vessel lesion
35276 Repair blood vessel lesion
35281 Repair blood vessel lesion
35301 Rechanneling of artery
35302 Rechanneling of artery
35303 Rechanneling of artery
35304 Rechanneling of artery
35305 Rechanneling of artery
35306 Rechanneling of artery
35311 Rechanneling of artery
35331 Rechanneling of artery
35341 Rechanneling of artery
35351 Rechanneling of artery
35355 Rechanneling of artery
35361 Rechanneling of artery
35363 Rechanneling of artery
35371 Rechanneling of artery
35372 Rechanneling of artery
35390 Reoperation carotid add-on
35400 Angioscopy
35501 Art byp grft ipsilat carotid
35506 Art byp grft subclav-carotid
35508 Art byp grft carotid-vertbrl
35509 Art byp grft contral carotid
35510 Art byp grft carotid-brchial
35511 Art byp grft subclav-subclav
35512 Art byp grft subclav-brchial
35515 Art byp grft subclav-vertbrl
35516 Art byp grft subclav-axilary
35518 Art byp grft axillary-axilry
35521 Art byp grft axill-femoral
35522 Art byp grft axill-brachial
35523 Art byp grft brchl-ulnr-rdl
35525 Art byp grft brachial-brchl
35526 Art byp grft aor/carot/innom
35531 Art byp grft aorcel/aormesen
35533 Art byp grft axill/fem/fem
35535 Art byp grft hepatorenal
35536 Art byp grft splenorenal
35537 Art byp grft aortoiliac
35538 Art byp grft aortobi-iliac
35539 Art byp grft aortofemoral
35540 Art byp grft aortbifemoral
35556 Art byp grft fem-popliteal
35558 Art byp grft fem-femoral
35560 Art byp grft aortorenal
35563 Art byp grft ilioiliac
35565 Art byp grft iliofemoral
35566 Art byp fem-ant-post tib/prl
35570 Art byp tibial-tib/peroneal
35571 Art byp pop-tibl-prl-other
35583 Vein byp grft fem-popliteal
35585 Vein byp fem-tibial peroneal
35587 Vein byp pop-tibl peroneal
35600 Harvest art for cabg add-on
35601 Art byp common ipsi carotid
35606 Art byp carotid-subclavian
35612 Art byp subclav-subclavian
35616 Art byp subclav-axillary
35621 Art byp axillary-femoral
35623 Art byp axillary-pop-tibial
35626 Art byp aorsubcl/carot/innom
35631 Art byp aor-celiac-msn-renal
35632 Art byp ilio-celiac
35633 Art byp ilio-mesenteric
35634 Art byp iliorenal
35636 Art byp spenorenal
35637 Art byp aortoiliac
35638 Art byp aortobi-iliac
35642 Art byp carotid-vertebral
35645 Art byp subclav-vertebrl
35646 Art byp aortobifemoral
35647 Art byp aortofemoral
35650 Art byp axillary-axillary
35654 Art byp axill-fem-femoral
35656 Art byp femoral-popliteal
35661 Art byp femoral-femoral
35663 Art byp ilioiliac
35665 Art byp iliofemoral
35666 Art byp fem-ant-post tib/prl
35671 Art byp pop-tibl-prl-other
35681 Composite byp grft pros&vein
35682 Composite byp grft 2 veins
35683 Composite byp grft 3/> segmt
35691 Art trnsposj vertbrl carotid
35693 Art trnsposj subclavian
35694 Art trnsposj subclav carotid

35695	Art trnsposj carotid subclav
35697	Reimplant artery each
35700	Reoperation bypass graft
35701	Exploration carotid artery
35702	Expl n/flwd surg uxtr art
35703	Expl n/flwd surg lxtr art
35721	Exploration femoral artery
35800	Explore neck vessels
35820	Explore chest vessels
35840	Explore abdominal vessels
35870	Repair vessel graft defect
35901	Excision graft neck
35905	Excision graft thorax
35907	Excision graft abdomen
36660	Insertion catheter artery
36823	Insertion of cannula(s)
37140	Revision of circulation
37145	Revision of circulation
37160	Revision of circulation
37180	Revision of circulation
37181	Splice spleen/kidney veins
37182	Insert hepatic shunt (tips)
37215	Transcath stent cca w/eps
37217	Stent placemt retro carotid
37218	Stent placemt ante carotid
37616	Ligation of chest artery
37617	Ligation of abdomen artery
37618	Ligation of extremity artery
37660	Revision of major vein
37788	Revascularization penis
38100	Removal of spleen total
38101	Removal of spleen partial
38102	Removal of spleen total
38115	Repair of ruptured spleen
38380	Thoracic duct procedure
38381	Thoracic duct procedure
38382	Thoracic duct procedure
38562	Removal pelvic lymph nodes
38564	Removal abdomen lymph nodes
38724	Removal of lymph nodes neck
38746	Remove thoracic lymph nodes
38747	Remove abdominal lymph nodes
38765	Remove groin lymph nodes
38770	Remove pelvis lymph nodes
38780	Remove abdomen lymph nodes
39000	Exploration of chest
39010	Exploration of chest
39200	Resect mediastinal cyst
39220	Resect mediastinal tumor
39499	Chest procedure
39501	Repair diaphragm laceration
39503	Repair of diaphragm hernia
39540	Repair of diaphragm hernia
39541	Repair of diaphragm hernia
39545	Revision of diaphragm
39560	Resect diaphragm simple
39561	Resect diaphragm complex
39599	Diaphragm surgery procedure
41130	Partial removal of tongue
41135	Tongue and neck surgery
41140	Removal of tongue
41145	Tongue removal neck surgery
41150	Tongue mouth jaw surgery
41153	Tongue mouth neck surgery
41155	Tongue jaw & neck surgery
42426	Excise parotid gland/lesion
42845	Extensive surgery of throat
42894	Revision of pharyngeal walls
42953	Repair throat esophagus
42961	Control throat bleeding
42971	Control nose/throat bleeding
43045	Incision of esophagus
43100	Excision of esophagus lesion
43101	Excision of esophagus lesion
43107	Removal of esophagus
43108	Removal of esophagus
43112	Removal of esophagus
43113	Removal of esophagus
43116	Partial removal of esophagus
43117	Partial removal of esophagus
43118	Partial removal of esophagus
43121	Partial removal of esophagus
43122	Partial removal of esophagus
43123	Partial removal of esophagus
43124	Removal of esophagus
43135	Removal of esophagus pouch
43279	Lap myotomy heller
43283	Lap esoph lengthening
43286	Esphg tot w/laps moblj
43287	Esphg dstl 2/3 w/laps moblj
43288	Esphg thrsc moblj
43300	Repair of esophagus
43305	Repair esophagus and fistula
43310	Repair of esophagus
43312	Repair esophagus and fistula
43313	Esophagoplasty congenital
43314	Tracheo-esophagoplasty cong
43320	Fuse esophagus & stomach
43325	Revise esophagus & stomach
43327	Esoph fundoplasty lap
43328	Esoph fundoplasty thor
43330	Esophagomyotomy abdominal
43331	Esophagomyotomy thoracic
43332	Transab esoph hiat hern rpr
43333	Transab esoph hiat hern rpr
43334	Transthor diaphrag hern rpr
43335	Transthor diaphrag hern rpr
43336	Thorabd diaphr hern repair
43337	Thorabd diaphr hern repair
43338	Esoph lengthening
43340	Fuse esophagus & intestine
43341	Fuse esophagus & intestine
43351	Surgical opening esophagus
43352	Surgical opening esophagus
43360	Gastrointestinal repair
43361	Gastrointestinal repair
43400	Ligate esophagus veins
43405	Ligate/staple esophagus
43410	Repair esophagus wound
43415	Repair esophagus wound
43425	Repair esophagus opening
43460	Pressure treatment esophagus
43496	Free jejunum flap microvasc
43500	Surgical opening of stomach
43501	Surgical repair of stomach
43502	Surgical repair of stomach
43520	Incision of pyloric muscle
43605	Biopsy of stomach
43610	Excision of stomach lesion
43611	Excision of stomach lesion
43620	Removal of stomach
43621	Removal of stomach
43622	Removal of stomach
43631	Removal of stomach partial
43632	Removal of stomach partial
43633	Removal of stomach partial
43634	Removal of stomach partial
43635	Removal of stomach partial
43640	Vagotomy & pylorus repair
43641	Vagotomy & pylorus repair
43644	Lap gastric bypass/roux-en-y
43645	Lap gastr bypass incl smll i
43771	Lap revise gastr adj device
43775	Lap sleeve gastrectomy
43800	Reconstruction of pylorus
43810	Fusion of stomach and bowel
43820	Fusion of stomach and bowel
43825	Fusion of stomach and bowel
43832	Place gastrostomy tube
43840	Repair of stomach lesion
43843	Gastroplasty w/o v-band
43845	Gastroplasty duodenal switch
43846	Gastric bypass for obesity
43847	Gastric bypass incl small i
43848	Revision gastroplasty
43850	Revise stomach-bowel fusion
43855	Revise stomach-bowel fusion
43860	Revise stomach-bowel fusion
43865	Revise stomach-bowel fusion
43880	Repair stomach-bowel fistula
43881	Impl/redo electrd antrum
43882	Revise/remove electrd antrum
44005	Freeing of bowel adhesion
44010	Incision of small bowel
44015	Insert needle cath bowel
44020	Explore small intestine
44021	Decompress small bowel
44025	Incision of large bowel
44050	Reduce bowel obstruction
44055	Correct malrotation of bowel
44110	Excise intestine lesion(s)
44111	Excision of bowel lesion(s)
44120	Removal of small intestine
44121	Removal of small intestine
44125	Removal of small intestine
44126	Enterectomy w/o taper cong
44127	Enterectomy w/taper cong

44128 Enterectomy cong add-on
44130 Bowel to bowel fusion
44132 Enterectomy cadaver donor
44133 Enterectomy live donor
44135 Intestine transplnt cadaver
44136 Intestine transplant live
44137 Remove intestinal allograft
44139 Mobilization of colon
44140 Partial removal of colon
44141 Partial removal of colon
44143 Partial removal of colon
44144 Partial removal of colon
44145 Partial removal of colon
44146 Partial removal of colon
44147 Partial removal of colon
44150 Removal of colon
44151 Removal of colon/ileostomy
44155 Removal of colon/ileostomy
44156 Removal of colon/ileostomy
44157 Colectomy w/ileoanal anast
44158 Colectomy w/neo-rectum pouch
44160 Removal of colon
44187 Lap ileo/jejuno-stomy
44188 Lap colostomy
44202 Lap enterectomy
44203 Lap resect s/intestine addl
44204 Laparo partial colectomy
44205 Lap colectomy part w/ileum
44206 Lap part colectomy w/stoma
44207 L colectomy/coloproctostomy
44208 L colectomy/coloproctostomy
44210 Laparo total proctocolectomy
44211 Lap colectomy w/proctectomy
44212 Laparo total proctocolectomy
44213 Lap mobil splenic fl add-on
44227 Lap close enterostomy
44300 Open bowel to skin
44310 Ileostomy/jejunostomy
44314 Revision of ileostomy
44316 Devise bowel pouch
44320 Colostomy
44322 Colostomy with biopsies
44345 Revision of colostomy
44346 Revision of colostomy
44602 Suture small intestine
44603 Suture small intestine
44604 Suture large intestine
44605 Repair of bowel lesion
44615 Intestinal strictureplasty
44620 Repair bowel opening
44625 Repair bowel opening
44626 Repair bowel opening
44640 Repair bowel-skin fistula
44650 Repair bowel fistula
44660 Repair bowel-bladder fistula
44661 Repair bowel-bladder fistula
44680 Surgical revision intestine
44700 Suspend bowel w/prosthesis
44715 Prepare donor intestine
44720 Prep donor intestine/venous
44721 Prep donor intestine/artery
44800 Excision of bowel pouch
44820 Excision of mesentery lesion
44850 Repair of mesentery
44899 Bowel surgery procedure
44900 Drain appendix abscess open
44960 Appendectomy
45110 Removal of rectum
45111 Partial removal of rectum
45112 Removal of rectum
45113 Partial proctectomy
45114 Partial removal of rectum
45116 Partial removal of rectum
45119 Remove rectum w/reservoir
45120 Removal of rectum
45121 Removal of rectum and colon
45123 Partial proctectomy
45126 Pelvic exenteration
45130 Excision of rectal prolapse
45135 Excision of rectal prolapse
45136 Excise ileoanal reservior
45395 Lap removal of rectum
45397 Lap remove rectum w/pouch
45400 Laparoscopic proc
45402 Lap proctopexy w/sig resect
45540 Correct rectal prolapse
45550 Repair rectum/remove sigmoid
45562 Exploration/repair of rectum
45563 Exploration/repair of rectum
45800 Repair rect/bladder fistula
45805 Repair fistula w/colostomy
45820 Repair rectourethral fistula
45825 Repair fistula w/colostomy
46705 Repair of anal stricture
46710 Repr per/vag pouch sngl proc
46712 Repr per/vag pouch dbl proc
46715 Rep perf anoper fistu
46716 Rep perf anoper/vestib fistu
46730 Construction of absent anus
46735 Construction of absent anus
46740 Construction of absent anus
46742 Repair of imperforated anus
46744 Repair of cloacal anomaly
46746 Repair of cloacal anomaly
46748 Repair of cloacal anomaly
46751 Repair of anal sphincter
47010 Open drainage liver lesion
47015 Inject/aspirate liver cyst
47100 Wedge biopsy of liver
47120 Partial removal of liver
47122 Extensive removal of liver
47125 Partial removal of liver
47130 Partial removal of liver
47133 Removal of donor liver
47135 Transplantation of liver
47140 Partial removal donor liver
47141 Partial removal donor liver
47142 Partial removal donor liver
47143 Prep donor liver whole
47144 Prep donor liver 3-segment
47145 Prep donor liver lobe split
47146 Prep donor liver/venous
47147 Prep donor liver/arterial
47300 Surgery for liver lesion
47350 Repair liver wound
47360 Repair liver wound
47361 Repair liver wound
47362 Repair liver wound
47380 Open ablate liver tumor rf
47381 Open ablate liver tumor cryo
47400 Incision of liver duct
47420 Incision of bile duct
47425 Incision of bile duct
47460 Incise bile duct sphincter
47480 Incision of gallbladder
47550 Bile duct endoscopy add-on
47570 Laparo cholecystoenterostomy
47600 Removal of gallbladder
47605 Removal of gallbladder
47610 Removal of gallbladder
47612 Removal of gallbladder
47620 Removal of gallbladder
47700 Exploration of bile ducts
47701 Bile duct revision
47711 Excision of bile duct tumor
47712 Excision of bile duct tumor
47715 Excision of bile duct cyst
47720 Fuse gallbladder & bowel
47721 Fuse upper gi structures
47740 Fuse gallbladder & bowel
47741 Fuse gallbladder & bowel
47760 Fuse bile ducts and bowel
47765 Fuse liver ducts & bowel
47780 Fuse bile ducts and bowel
47785 Fuse bile ducts and bowel
47800 Reconstruction of bile ducts
47801 Placement bile duct support
47802 Fuse liver duct & intestine
47900 Suture bile duct injury
48000 Drainage of abdomen
48001 Placement of drain pancreas
48020 Removal of pancreatic stone
48100 Biopsy of pancreas open
48105 Resect/debride pancreas
48120 Removal of pancreas lesion
48140 Partial removal of pancreas
48145 Partial removal of pancreas
48146 Pancreatectomy
48148 Removal of pancreatic duct
48150 Partial removal of pancreas
48152 Pancreatectomy
48153 Pancreatectomy
48154 Pancreatectomy
48155 Removal of pancreas
48400 Injection intraop add-on
48500 Surgery of pancreatic cyst
48510 Drain pancreatic pseudocyst

48520	Fuse pancreas cyst and bowel
48540	Fuse pancreas cyst and bowel
48545	Pancreatorrhaphy
48547	Duodenal exclusion
48548	Fuse pancreas and bowel
48551	Prep donor pancreas
48552	Prep donor pancreas/venous
48554	Transpl allograft pancreas
48556	Removal allograft pancreas
49000	Exploration of abdomen
49002	Reopening of abdomen
49010	Exploration behind abdomen
49013	Prpertl pel pack hemrrg trma
49014	Reexploration pelvic wound
49020	Drainage abdom abscess open
49040	Drain open abdom abscess
49060	Drain open retroperi abscess
49062	Drain to peritoneal cavity
49203	Exc abd tum 5 cm or less
49204	Exc abd tum over 5 cm
49205	Exc abd tum over 10 cm
49215	Excise sacral spine tumor
49220	Multiple surgery abdomen
49255	Removal of omentum
49412	Ins device for rt guide open
49425	Insert abdomen-venous drain
49428	Ligation of shunt
49605	Repair umbilical lesion
49606	Repair umbilical lesion
49610	Repair umbilical lesion
49611	Repair umbilical lesion
49900	Repair of abdominal wall
49904	Omental flap extra-abdom
49905	Omental flap intra-abdom
49906	Free omental flap microvasc
50010	Exploration of kidney
50040	Drainage of kidney
50045	Exploration of kidney
50060	Removal of kidney stone
50065	Incision of kidney
50070	Incision of kidney
50075	Removal of kidney stone
50100	Revise kidney blood vessels
50120	Exploration of kidney
50125	Explore and drain kidney
50130	Removal of kidney stone
50135	Exploration of kidney
50205	Renal biopsy open
50220	Remove kidney open
50225	Removal kidney open complex
50230	Removal kidney open radical
50234	Removal of kidney & ureter
50236	Removal of kidney & ureter
50240	Partial removal of kidney
50250	Cryoablate renal mass open
50280	Removal of kidney lesion
50290	Removal of kidney lesion
50300	Remove cadaver donor kidney
50320	Remove kidney living donor
50323	Prep cadaver renal allograft
50325	Prep donor renal graft
50327	Prep renal graft/venous
50328	Prep renal graft/arterial
50329	Prep renal graft/ureteral
50340	Removal of kidney
50360	Transplantation of kidney
50365	Transplantation of kidney
50370	Remove transplanted kidney
50380	Reimplantation of kidney
50400	Revision of kidney/ureter
50405	Revision of kidney/ureter
50500	Repair of kidney wound
50520	Close kidney-skin fistula
50525	Close nephrovisceral fistula
50526	Close nephrovisceral fistula
50540	Revision of horseshoe kidney
50545	Laparo radical nephrectomy
50546	Laparoscopic nephrectomy
50547	Laparo removal donor kidney
50548	Laparo remove w/ureter
50600	Exploration of ureter
50605	Insert ureteral support
50610	Removal of ureter stone
50620	Removal of ureter stone
50630	Removal of ureter stone
50650	Removal of ureter
50660	Removal of ureter
50700	Revision of ureter
50715	Release of ureter
50722	Release of ureter
50725	Release/revise ureter
50728	Revise ureter
50740	Fusion of ureter & kidney
50750	Fusion of ureter & kidney
50760	Fusion of ureters
50770	Splicing of ureters
50780	Reimplant ureter in bladder
50782	Reimplant ureter in bladder
50783	Reimplant ureter in bladder
50785	Reimplant ureter in bladder
50800	Implant ureter in bowel
50810	Fusion of ureter & bowel
50815	Urine shunt to intestine
50820	Construct bowel bladder
50825	Construct bowel bladder
50830	Revise urine flow
50840	Replace ureter by bowel
50845	Appendico-vesicostomy
50860	Transplant ureter to skin
50900	Repair of ureter
50920	Closure ureter/skin fistula
50930	Closure ureter/bowel fistula
50940	Release of ureter
51525	Removal of bladder lesion
51530	Removal of bladder lesion
51550	Partial removal of bladder
51555	Partial removal of bladder
51565	Revise bladder & ureter(s)
51570	Removal of bladder
51575	Removal of bladder & nodes
51580	Remove bladder/revise tract
51585	Removal of bladder & nodes
51590	Remove bladder/revise tract
51595	Remove bladder/revise tract
51596	Remove bladder/create pouch
51597	Removal of pelvic structures
51800	Revision of bladder/urethra
51820	Revision of urinary tract
51840	Attach bladder/urethra
51841	Attach bladder/urethra
51865	Repair of bladder wound
51900	Repair bladder/vagina lesion
51920	Close bladder-uterus fistula
51925	Hysterectomy/bladder repair
51940	Correction of bladder defect
51960	Revision of bladder & bowel
51980	Construct bladder opening
53415	Reconstruction of urethra
53448	Remov/replc ur sphinctr comp
54125	Removal of penis
54130	Remove penis & nodes
54135	Remove penis & nodes
54390	Repair penis and bladder
54430	Revision of penis
54438	Replantation of penis
55605	Incise sperm duct pouch
55650	Remove sperm duct pouch
55801	Removal of prostate
55810	Extensive prostate surgery
55812	Extensive prostate surgery
55815	Extensive prostate surgery
55821	Removal of prostate
55831	Removal of prostate
55840	Extensive prostate surgery
55842	Extensive prostate surgery
55845	Extensive prostate surgery
55862	Extensive prostate surgery
55865	Extensive prostate surgery
56630	Extensive vulva surgery
56631	Extensive vulva surgery
56632	Extensive vulva surgery
56633	Extensive vulva surgery
56634	Extensive vulva surgery
56637	Extensive vulva surgery
56640	Extensive vulva surgery
57110	Remove vagina wall complete
57111	Remove vagina tissue compl
57112	Vaginectomy w/nodes compl
57270	Repair of bowel pouch
57280	Suspension of vagina
57296	Revise vag graft open abd
57305	Repair rectum-vagina fistula
57307	Fistula repair & colostomy
57308	Fistula repair transperine
57311	Repair urethrovaginal lesion
57531	Removal of cervix radical
57540	Removal of residual cervix

57545 Remove cervix/repair pelvis
58140 Myomectomy abdom method
58146 Myomectomy abdom complex
58150 Total hysterectomy
58152 Total hysterectomy
58180 Partial hysterectomy
58200 Extensive hysterectomy
58210 Extensive hysterectomy
58240 Removal of pelvis contents
58267 Vag hyst w/urinary repair
58275 Hysterectomy/revise vagina
58280 Hysterectomy/revise vagina
58285 Extensive hysterectomy
58293 Vag hyst w/uro repair compl
58400 Suspension of uterus
58410 Suspension of uterus
58520 Repair of ruptured uterus
58540 Revision of uterus
58548 Lap radical hyst
58575 Laps tot hyst resj mal
58605 Division of fallopian tube
58611 Ligate oviduct(s) add-on
58700 Removal of fallopian tube
58720 Removal of ovary/tube(s)
58740 Adhesiolysis tube ovary
58750 Repair oviduct
58752 Revise ovarian tube(s)
58760 Fimbrioplasty
58822 Drain ovary abscess percut
58825 Transposition ovary(s)
58940 Removal of ovary(s)
58943 Removal of ovary(s)
58950 Resect ovarian malignancy
58951 Resect ovarian malignancy
58952 Resect ovarian malignancy
58953 Tah rad dissect for debulk
58954 Tah rad debulk/lymph remove
58956 Bso omentectomy w/tah
58957 Resect recurrent gyn mal
58958 Resect recur gyn mal w/lym
58960 Exploration of abdomen
59120 Treat ectopic pregnancy
59121 Treat ectopic pregnancy
59130 Treat ectopic pregnancy
59135 Treat ectopic pregnancy
59136 Treat ectopic pregnancy
59140 Treat ectopic pregnancy
59325 Revision of cervix
59350 Repair of uterus
59514 Cesarean delivery only
59525 Remove uterus after cesarean
59620 Attempted vbac delivery only
59830 Treat uterus infection
59850 Abortion
59851 Abortion
59852 Abortion
59855 Abortion
59856 Abortion
59857 Abortion
60254 Extensive thyroid surgery
60270 Removal of thyroid
60505 Explore parathyroid glands
60521 Removal of thymus gland
60522 Removal of thymus gland
60540 Explore adrenal gland
60545 Explore adrenal gland
60600 Remove carotid body lesion
60605 Remove carotid body lesion
60650 Laparoscopy adrenalectomy
61105 Twist drill hole
61107 Drill skull for implantation
61108 Drill skull for drainage
61120 Burr hole for puncture
61140 Pierce skull for biopsy
61150 Pierce skull for drainage
61151 Pierce skull for drainage
61154 Pierce skull & remove clot
61156 Pierce skull for drainage
61210 Pierce skull implant device
61250 Pierce skull & explore
61253 Pierce skull & explore
61304 Open skull for exploration
61305 Open skull for exploration
61312 Open skull for drainage
61313 Open skull for drainage
61314 Open skull for drainage
61315 Open skull for drainage
61316 Implt cran bone flap to abdo
61320 Open skull for drainage
61321 Open skull for drainage
61322 Decompressive craniotomy
61323 Decompressive lobectomy
61333 Explore orbit/remove lesion
61340 Subtemporal decompression
61343 Incise skull (press relief)
61345 Relieve cranial pressure
61450 Incise skull for surgery
61458 Incise skull for brain wound
61460 Incise skull for surgery
61500 Removal of skull lesion
61501 Remove infected skull bone
61510 Removal of brain lesion
61512 Remove brain lining lesion
61514 Removal of brain abscess
61516 Removal of brain lesion
61517 Implt brain chemotx add-on
61518 Removal of brain lesion
61519 Remove brain lining lesion
61520 Removal of brain lesion
61521 Removal of brain lesion
61522 Removal of brain abscess
61524 Removal of brain lesion
61526 Removal of brain lesion
61530 Removal of brain lesion
61531 Implant brain electrodes
61533 Implant brain electrodes
61534 Removal of brain lesion
61535 Remove brain electrodes
61536 Removal of brain lesion
61537 Removal of brain tissue
61538 Removal of brain tissue
61539 Removal of brain tissue
61540 Removal of brain tissue
61541 Incision of brain tissue
61543 Removal of brain tissue
61544 Remove & treat brain lesion
61545 Excision of brain tumor
61546 Removal of pituitary gland
61548 Removal of pituitary gland
61550 Release of skull seams
61552 Release of skull seams
61556 Incise skull/sutures
61557 Incise skull/sutures
61558 Excision of skull/sutures
61559 Excision of skull/sutures
61563 Excision of skull tumor
61564 Excision of skull tumor
61566 Removal of brain tissue
61567 Incision of brain tissue
61570 Remove foreign body brain
61571 Incise skull for brain wound
61575 Skull base/brainstem surgery
61576 Skull base/brainstem surgery
61580 Craniofacial approach skull
61581 Craniofacial approach skull
61582 Craniofacial approach skull
61583 Craniofacial approach skull
61584 Orbitocranial approach/skull
61585 Orbitocranial approach/skull
61586 Resect nasopharynx skull
61590 Infratemporal approach/skull
61591 Infratemporal approach/skull
61592 Orbitocranial approach/skull
61595 Transtemporal approach/skull
61596 Transcochlear approach/skull
61597 Transcondylar approach/skull
61598 Transpetrosal approach/skull
61600 Resect/excise cranial lesion
61601 Resect/excise cranial lesion
61605 Resect/excise cranial lesion
61606 Resect/excise cranial lesion
61607 Resect/excise cranial lesion
61608 Resect/excise cranial lesion
61611 Transect artery sinus
61613 Remove aneurysm sinus
61615 Resect/excise lesion skull
61616 Resect/excise lesion skull
61618 Repair dura
61619 Repair dura
61624 Transcath occlusion cns
61630 Intracranial angioplasty
61635 Intracran angioplsty w/stent
61645 Perq art m-thrombect &/nfs
61650 Evasc prlng admn rx agnt 1st
61651 Evasc prlng admn rx agnt add
61680 Intracranial vessel surgery
61682 Intracranial vessel surgery

Appendix J — Inpatient-Only Procedures

61684	Intracranial vessel surgery
61686	Intracranial vessel surgery
61690	Intracranial vessel surgery
61692	Intracranial vessel surgery
61697	Brain aneurysm repr complx
61698	Brain aneurysm repr complx
61700	Brain aneurysm repr simple
61702	Inner skull vessel surgery
61703	Clamp neck artery
61705	Revise circulation to head
61708	Revise circulation to head
61710	Revise circulation to head
61711	Fusion of skull arteries
61735	Incise skull/brain surgery
61750	Incise skull/brain biopsy
61751	Brain biopsy w/ct/mr guide
61760	Implant brain electrodes
61850	Implant neuroelectrodes
61860	Implant neuroelectrodes
61863	Implant neuroelectrode
61864	Implant neuroelectrde addl
61867	Implant neuroelectrode
61868	Implant neuroelectrde addl
61870	Implant neuroelectrodes
62005	Treat skull fracture
62010	Treatment of head injury
62100	Repair brain fluid leakage
62115	Reduction of skull defect
62117	Reduction of skull defect
62120	Repair skull cavity lesion
62121	Incise skull repair
62140	Repair of skull defect
62141	Repair of skull defect
62142	Remove skull plate/flap
62143	Replace skull plate/flap
62145	Repair of skull & brain
62146	Repair of skull with graft
62147	Repair of skull with graft
62148	Retr bone flap to fix skull
62161	Dissect brain w/scope
62162	Remove colloid cyst w/scope
62163	Zneuroendoscopy w/fb removal
62164	Remove brain tumor w/scope
62165	Remove pituit tumor w/scope
62180	Establish brain cavity shunt
62190	Establish brain cavity shunt
62192	Establish brain cavity shunt
62200	Establish brain cavity shunt
62201	Brain cavity shunt w/scope
62220	Establish brain cavity shunt
62223	Establish brain cavity shunt
62256	Remove brain cavity shunt
62258	Replace brain cavity shunt
63050	Cervical laminoplsty 2/> seg
63051	C-laminoplasty w/graft/plate
63077	Spine disk surgery thorax
63078	Spine disk surgery thorax
63081	Remove vert body dcmprn crvl
63082	Remove vertebral body add-on
63085	Remove vert body dcmprn thrc
63086	Remove vertebral body add-on
63087	Remov vertbr dcmprn thrclmbr
63088	Remove vertebral body add-on
63090	Remove vert body dcmprn lmbr
63091	Remove vertebral body add-on
63101	Remove vert body dcmprn thrc
63102	Remove vert body dcmprn lmbr
63103	Remove vertebral body add-on
63170	Incise spinal cord tract(s)
63172	Drainage of spinal cyst
63173	Drainage of spinal cyst
63180	Revise spinal cord ligaments
63182	Revise spinal cord ligaments
63185	Incise spine nrv half segmnt
63190	Incise spine nrv >2 segmnts
63191	Incise spine accessory nerve
63194	Incise spine & cord cervical
63195	Incise spine & cord thoracic
63196	Incise spine&cord 2 trx crvl
63197	Incise spine&cord 2 trx thrc
63198	Incise spin&cord 2 stgs crvl
63199	Incise spin&cord 2 stgs thrc
63200	Release spinal cord lumbar
63250	Revise spinal cord vsls crvl
63251	Revise spinal cord vsls thrc
63252	Revise spine cord vsl thrlmb
63270	Excise intrspinl lesion crvl
63271	Excise intrspinl lesion thrc
63272	Excise intrspinl lesion lmbr
63273	Excise intrspinl lesion scrl
63275	Bx/exc xdrl spine lesn crvl
63276	Bx/exc xdrl spine lesn thrc
63277	Bx/exc xdrl spine lesn lmbr
63278	Bx/exc xdrl spine lesn scrl
63280	Bx/exc idrl spine lesn crvl
63281	Bx/exc idrl spine lesn thrc
63282	Bx/exc idrl spine lesn lmbr
63283	Bx/exc idrl spine lesn scrl
63285	Bx/exc idrl imed lesn cervl
63286	Bx/exc idrl imed lesn thrc
63287	Bx/exc idrl imed lesn thrlmb
63290	Bx/exc xdrl/idrl lsn any lvl
63295	Repair laminectomy defect
63300	Remove vert xdrl body crvcl
63301	Remove vert xdrl body thrc
63302	Remove vert xdrl body thrlmb
63303	Remov vert xdrl bdy lmbr/sac
63304	Remove vert idrl body crvcl
63305	Remove vert idrl body thrc
63306	Remov vert idrl bdy thrclmbr
63307	Remov vert idrl bdy lmbr/sac
63308	Remove vertebral body add-on
63700	Repair of spinal herniation
63702	Repair of spinal herniation
63704	Repair of spinal herniation
63706	Repair of spinal herniation
63707	Repair spinal fluid leakage
63709	Repair spinal fluid leakage
63710	Graft repair of spine defect
63740	Install spinal shunt
64755	Incision of stomach nerves
64760	Incision of vagus nerve
64809	Remove sympathetic nerves
64818	Remove sympathetic nerves
64866	Fusion of facial/other nerve
64868	Fusion of facial/other nerve
65273	Repair of eye wound
69155	Extensive ear/neck surgery
69535	Remove part of temporal bone
69554	Remove ear lesion
69950	Incise inner ear nerve
75956	Xray endovasc thor ao repr
75957	Xray endovasc thor ao repr
75958	Xray place prox ext thor ao
75959	Xray place dist ext thor ao
92941	Prq card revasc mi 1 vsl
92970	Cardioassist internal
92971	Cardioassist external
92975	Dissolve clot heart vessel
92992	Revision of heart chamber
92993	Revision of heart chamber
93583	Perq transcath septal reduxn
99184	Hypothermia ill neonate
99190	Special pump services
99191	Special pump services
99192	Special pump services
99356	Prolonged service inpatient
99357	Prolonged service inpatient
99462	Sbsq nb em per day hosp
99468	Neonate crit care initial
99469	Neonate crit care subsq
99471	Ped critical care initial
99472	Ped critical care subsq
99475	Ped crit care age 2-5 init
99476	Ped crit care age 2-5 subsq
99477	Init day hosp neonate care
99478	Ic lbw inf < 1500 gm subsq
99479	Ic lbw inf 1500-2500 g subsq
99480	Ic inf pbw 2501-5000 g subsq
C9606	PC H rev ac tot/subtot occl 1 ves
G0341	Percutaneous islet celltrans
G0342	Laparoscopy islet cell trans
G0343	Laparotomy islet cell transp
G0412	Open tx iliac spine uni/bil
G0414	Pelvic ring fx treat int fix
G0415	Open tx post pelvic fxcture

Appendix K — Place of Service and Type of Service

Place-of-Service Codes for Professional Claims

Listed below are place of service codes and descriptions. These codes should be used on professional claims to specify the entity where service(s) were rendered. Check with individual payers (e.g., Medicare, Medicaid, other private insurance) for reimbursement policies regarding these codes. To comment on a code(s) or description(s), please send your request to posinfo@cms.gov.

01	Pharmacy	A facility or location where drugs and other medically related items and services are sold, dispensed, or otherwise provided directly to patients.
02	Telehealth	The location where health services and health related services are provided or received through telecommunication technology.
03	School	A facility whose primary purpose is education.
04	Homeless shelter	A facility or location whose primary purpose is to provide temporary housing to homeless individuals (e.g., emergency shelters, individual or family shelters).
05	Indian Health Service freestanding facility	A facility or location, owned and operated by the Indian Health Service, which provides diagnostic, therapeutic (surgical and non-surgical), and rehabilitation services to American Indians and Alaska natives who do not require hospitalization.
06	Indian Health Service provider-based facility	A facility or location, owned and operated by the Indian Health Service, which provides diagnostic, therapeutic (surgical and nonsurgical), and rehabilitation services rendered by, or under the supervision of, physicians to American Indians and Alaska natives admitted as inpatients or outpatients.
07	Tribal 638 freestanding facility	A facility or location owned and operated by a federally recognized American Indian or Alaska native tribe or tribal organization under a 638 agreement, which provides diagnostic, therapeutic (surgical and nonsurgical), and rehabilitation services to tribal members who do not require hospitalization.
08	Tribal 638 provider-based Facility	A facility or location owned and operated by a federally recognized American Indian or Alaska native tribe or tribal organization under a 638 agreement, which provides diagnostic, therapeutic (surgical and nonsurgical), and rehabilitation services to tribal members admitted as inpatients or outpatients.
09	Prison/correctional facility	A prison, jail, reformatory, work farm, detention center, or any other similar facility maintained by either federal, state or local authorities for the purpose of confinement or rehabilitation of adult or juvenile criminal offenders.
10	Unassigned	N/A
11	Office	Location, other than a hospital, skilled nursing facility (SNF), military treatment facility, community health center, State or local public health clinic, or intermediate care facility (ICF), where the health professional routinely provides health examinations, diagnosis, and treatment of illness or injury on an ambulatory basis.
12	Home	Location, other than a hospital or other facility, where the patient receives care in a private residence.
13	Assisted living facility	Congregate residential facility with self-contained living units providing assessment of each resident's needs and on-site support 24 hours a day, 7 days a week, with the capacity to deliver or arrange for services including some health care and other services.
14	Group home	A residence, with shared living areas, where clients receive supervision and other services such as social and/or behavioral services, custodial service, and minimal services (e.g., medication administration).
15	Mobile unit	A facility/unit that moves from place-to-place equipped to provide preventive, screening, diagnostic, and/or treatment services.
16	Temporary lodging	A short-term accommodation such as a hotel, campground, hostel, cruise ship or resort where the patient receives care, and which is not identified by any other POS code.
17	Walk-in retail health clinic	A walk-in health clinic, other than an office, urgent care facility, pharmacy, or independent clinic and not described by any other place of service code, that is located within a retail operation and provides preventive and primary care services on an ambulatory basis.
18	Place of employment/ worksite	A location, not described by any other POS code, owned or operated by a public or private entity where the patient is employed, and where a health professional provides on-going or episodic occupational medical, therapeutic or rehabilitative services to the individual.
19	Off campus-outpatient hospital	A portion of an off-campus hospital provider based department which provides diagnostic, therapeutic (both surgical and nonsurgical), and rehabilitation services to sick or injured persons who do not require hospitalization or institutionalization.
20	Urgent care facility	Location, distinct from a hospital emergency room, an office, or a clinic, whose purpose is to diagnose and treat illness or injury for unscheduled, ambulatory patients seeking immediate medical attention.

21	Inpatient hospital	A facility, other than psychiatric, which primarily provides diagnostic, therapeutic (both surgical and nonsurgical), and rehabilitation services by, or under, the supervision of physicians to patients admitted for a variety of medical conditions.
22	On campus-outpatient hospital	A portion of a hospital's main campus which provides diagnostic, therapeutic (both surgical and nonsurgical), and rehabilitation services to sick or injured persons who do not require hospitalization or institutionalization.
23	Emergency room—hospital	A portion of a hospital where emergency diagnosis and treatment of illness or injury is provided.
24	Ambulatory surgical center	A freestanding facility, other than a physician's office, where surgical and diagnostic services are provided on an ambulatory basis.
25	Birthing center	A facility, other than a hospital's maternity facilities or a physician's office, which provides a setting for labor, delivery, and immediate post-partum care as well as immediate care of new born infants.
26	Military treatment facility	A medical facility operated by one or more of the uniformed services. Military treatment facility (MTF) also refers to certain former U.S. Public Health Service (USPHS) facilities now designated as uniformed service treatment facilities (USTF).
27-30	Unassigned	N/A
31	Skilled nursing facility	A facility which primarily provides inpatient skilled nursing care and related services to patients who require medical, nursing, or rehabilitative services but does not provide the level of care or treatment available in a hospital.
32	Nursing facility	A facility which primarily provides to residents skilled nursing care and related services for the rehabilitation of injured, disabled, or sick persons, or, on a regular basis, health-related care services above the level of custodial care to individuals other than those with intellectual disabilities.
33	Custodial care facility	A facility which provides room, board, and other personal assistance services, generally on a long-term basis, and which does not include a medical component.
34	Hospice	A facility, other than a patient's home, in which palliative and supportive care for terminally ill patients and their families is provided.
35-40	Unassigned	N/A
41	Ambulance—land	A land vehicle specifically designed, equipped and staffed for lifesaving and transporting the sick or injured.
42	Ambulance—air or water	An air or water vehicle specifically designed, equipped and staffed for lifesaving and transporting the sick or injured.
43-48	Unassigned	N/A
49	Independent clinic	A location, not part of a hospital and not described by any other place-of-service code, that is organized and operated to provide preventive, diagnostic, therapeutic, rehabilitative, or palliative services to outpatients only.
50	Federally qualified health center	A facility located in a medically underserved area that provides Medicare beneficiaries with preventive primary medical care under the general direction of a physician.
51	Inpatient psychiatric facility	A facility that provides inpatient psychiatric services for the diagnosis and treatment of mental illness on a 24-hour basis, by or under the supervision of a physician.
52	Psychiatric facility-partial hospitalization	A facility for the diagnosis and treatment of mental illness that provides a planned therapeutic program for patients who do not require full time hospitalization, but who need broader programs than are possible from outpatient visits to a hospital-based or hospital-affiliated facility.
53	Community mental health center	A facility that provides the following services: outpatient services, including specialized outpatient services for children, the elderly, individuals who are chronically ill, and residents of the CMHC's mental health services area who have been discharged from inpatient treatment at a mental health facility; 24 hour a day emergency care services; day treatment, other partial hospitalization services, or psychosocial rehabilitation services; screening for patients being considered for admission to state mental health facilities to determine the appropriateness of such admission; and consultation and education services.
54	Intermediate care facility/individuals with intellectual disabilities	A facility which primarily provides health-related care and services above the level of custodial care to individuals with Intellectual Disabilities but does not provide the level of care or treatment available in a hospital or SNF.
55	Residential substance abuse treatment facility	A facility which provides treatment for substance (alcohol and drug) abuse to live-in residents who do not require acute medical care. Services include individual and group therapy and counseling, family counseling, laboratory tests, drugs and supplies, psychological testing, and room and board.
56	Psychiatric residential treatment center	A facility or distinct part of a facility for psychiatric care which provides a total 24-hour therapeutically planned and professionally staffed group living and learning environment.
57	Non-residential substance abuse treatment facility	A location which provides treatment for substance (alcohol and drug) abuse on an ambulatory basis. Services include individual and group therapy and counseling, family counseling, laboratory tests, drugs and supplies, and psychological testing.

58	Non-residential opioid treatment facility	A location that provides treatment for opioid use disorder on an ambulatory basis. Services include methadone and other forms of medication assisted treatment (MAT).
59	Unassigned	N/A
60	Mass immunization center	A location where providers administer pneumococcal pneumonia and influenza virus vaccinations and submit these services as electronic media claims, paper claims, or using the roster billing method. This generally takes place in a mass immunization setting, such as, a public health center, pharmacy, or mall but may include a physician office setting.
61	Comprehensive inpatient rehabilitation facility	A facility that provides comprehensive rehabilitation services under the supervision of a physician to inpatients with physical disabilities. Services include physical therapy, occupational therapy, speech pathology, social or psychological services, and orthotics and prosthetics services.
62	Comprehensive outpatient rehabilitation facility	A facility that provides comprehensive rehabilitation services under the supervision of a physician to outpatients with physical disabilities. Services include physical therapy, occupational therapy, and speech pathology services.
63-64	Unassigned	N/A
65	End-stage renal disease treatment facility	A facility other than a hospital, which provides dialysis treatment, maintenance, and/or training to patients or caregivers on an ambulatory or home-care basis.
66-70	Unassigned	N/A
71	Public health clinic	A facility maintained by either state or local health departments that provides ambulatory primary medical care under the general direction of a physician.
72	Rural health clinic	A certified facility which is located in a rural medically underserved area that provides ambulatory primary medical care under the general direction of a physician.
73-80	Unassigned	N/A
81	Independent laboratory	A laboratory certified to perform diagnostic and/or clinical tests independent of an institution or a physician's office.
82-98	Unassigned	N/A
99	Other place of service	Other place of service not identified above.

Type of Service

Common Working File Type of Service (TOS) Indicators

For submitting a claim to the Common Working File (CWF), use the following table to assign the proper TOS. Some procedures may have more than one applicable TOS. CWF will reject codes with incorrect TOS designations. CWF will produce alerts on codes with incorrect TOS designations.

The only exceptions to this annual update are:

- Surgical services billed for dates of service through December 31, 2007, containing the ASC facility service modifier SG must be reported as TOS F. Effective for services on or after January 1, 2008, the SG modifier is no longer applicable for Medicare services. ASC providers should discontinue applying the SG modifier on ASC facility claims. The indicator F does not appear in the TOS table because its use depends upon claims submitted with POS 24 (ASC facility) from an ASC (specialty 49). This became effective for dates of service January 1, 2008, or after.
- Surgical services billed with an assistant-at-surgery modifier (80-82, AS) must be reported with TOS 8. The 8 indicator does not appear on the TOS table because its use is dependent upon the use of the appropriate modifier. (See Pub. 100-4 *Medicare Claims Processing Manual,* chapter 12, "Physician/Practitioner Billing," for instructions on when assistant-at-surgery is allowable.)
- TOS H appears in the list of descriptors. However, it does not appear in the table. In CWF, "H" is used only as an indicator for hospice. The contractor should not submit TOS H to CWF at this time.
- For outpatient services, when a transfusion medicine code appears on a claim that also contains a blood product, the service is paid under reasonable charge at 80 percent; coinsurance and deductible apply. When transfusion medicine codes are paid under the clinical laboratory fee schedule they are paid at 100 percent; coinsurance and deductible do not apply.

Note: For injection codes with more than one possible TOS designation, use the following guidelines when assigning the TOS:

When the choice is L or 1:

- Use TOS L when the drug is used related to ESRD; or
- Use TOS 1 when the drug is not related to ESRD and is administered in the office.

When the choice is G or 1:

- Use TOS G when the drug is an immunosuppressive drug; or
- Use TOS 1 when the drug is used for other than immunosuppression.

When the choice is P or 1:

- Use TOS P if the drug is administered through durable medical equipment (DME); or
- Use TOS 1 if the drug is administered in the office.

The place of service or diagnosis may be considered when determining the appropriate TOS. The descriptors for each of the TOS codes listed in the annual HCPCS update are:

0	Whole blood
1	Medical care
2	Surgery
3	Consultation
4	Diagnostic radiology
5	Diagnostic laboratory
6	Therapeutic radiology
7	Anesthesia
8	Assistant at surgery
9	Other medical items or services
A	Used DME
B	High risk screening mammography
C	Low risk screening mammography
D	Ambulance
E	Enteral/parenteral nutrients/supplies
F	Ambulatory surgical center (facility usage for surgical services)
G	Immunosuppressive drugs
H	Hospice
J	Diabetic shoes
K	Hearing items and services
L	ESRD supplies
M	Monthly capitation payment for dialysis
N	Kidney donor
P	Lump sum purchase of DME, prosthetics, orthotics
Q	Vision items or services

R	Rental of DME
S	Surgical dressings or other medical supplies
U	Occupational therapy
V	Pneumococcal/flu vaccine
W	Physical therapy

Appendix L — Multianalyte Assays with Algorithmic Analyses

The following tables contain the Administrative Codes for Multianalyte Assays with Algorithmic Analyses (MAAA), category I codes for MAAA and the most current list of Proprietary Laboratory Analysis (PLA) codes.

The following is a list of MAAA procedures that are usually exclusive to one single clinical laboratory or manufacturer. These tests use the results from several different assays, including molecular pathology assays, fluorescent in situ hybridization assays, and nonnucleic acid-based assays (e.g., proteins, polypeptides, lipids, and carbohydrates) to perform an algorithmic analysis that is reported as a numeric score or probability. Although the laboratory report may list results of individual component tests of the MAAAs, these assays are not separately reportable.

The following list includes the proprietary name and clinical laboratory/manufacturer, an alphanumeric code, and the code descriptor.

The format for the code descriptor usually includes:

- Type of disease (e.g., oncology, autoimmune, tissue rejection)
- Chemical(s) analyzed (e.g., DNA, RNA, protein, antibody)
- Number of markers (e.g., number of genes, number of proteins)
- Methodology(s) (e.g., microarray, real-time [RT]-PCR, in situ hybridization [ISH], enzyme linked immunosorbent assays [ELISA])
- Number of functional domains (when indicated)
- Type of specimen (e.g., blood, fresh tissue, formalin-fixed paraffin embedded)
- Type of algorithm result (e.g., prognostic, diagnostic)
- Report (e.g., probability index, risk score)

MAAA procedures with a Category I code are noted on the following list and can also be found in code range 81500–81599 in the pathology and laboratory chapter. If a specific MAAA test does not have a Category I code, it is denoted with a four-digit number and the letter M. Use code 81599 if an MAAA test is not included on the following list or in the Category I codes. The codes on the list are exclusive to the assays identified by proprietary name. Report code 81599 also when an analysis is performed that may possibly fall within a specific descriptor but the proprietary name is not included in the list. The list does not contain all MAAA procedures.

Proprietary Name/Clinical Laboratory/Manufacturer	Code	Descriptor
Administrative Codes for Multianalyte Assays with Algorithmic Analyses (MAAA)		
	0001M (0001M has been deleted. To report, see 81596.)	
ASH FibroSURE™, BioPredictive S.A.S	0002M	Liver disease, ten biochemical assays (ALT, A2-macroglobulin, apolipoprotein A-1, total bilirubin, GGT, haptoglobin, AST, glucose, total cholesterol and triglycerides) utilizing serum, prognostic algorithm reported as quantitative scores for fibrosis, steatosis and alcoholic steatohepatitis (ASH)
NASH FibroSURE™, BioPredictive S.A.S	0003M	Liver disease, ten biochemical assays (ALT, A2-macroglobulin, apolipoprotein A-1, total bilirubin, GGT, haptoglobin, AST, glucose, total cholesterol and triglycerides) utilizing serum, prognostic algorithm reported as quantitative scores for fibrosis, steatosis and nonalcoholic steatohepatitis (NASH)
ScoliScore™ Transgenomic	0004M	Scoliosis, DNA analysis of 53 single nucleotide polymorphisms (SNPs), using saliva, prognostic algorithm reported as a risk score
HeproDX™, GoPath Laboratories, LLC	0006M	Oncology (hepatic), mRNA expression levels of 161 genes, utilizing fresh hepatocellular carcinoma tumor tissue, with alpha-fetoprotein level, algorithm reported as a risk classifier
NETest (Wren Laboratories, LLC)	0007M	Oncology (gastrointestinal neuroendocrine tumors), real-time PCR expression analysis of 51 genes, utilizing whole peripheral blood, algorithm reported as a nomogram of tumor disease index
	(0009M has been deleted)	
NeoLAB™ Prostate Liquid Biopsy, NeoGenomics Laboratories	0011M	Oncology, prostate cancer, mRNA expression assay of 12 genes (10 content and 2 housekeeping), RT-PCR test utilizing blood plasma and urine, algorithms to predict high-grade prostate cancer risk
Cxbladder™ Detect, Pacific Edge Diagnostics USA, Ltd.	0012M	Oncology (urothelial), mRNA, gene expression profiling by real-time quantitative PCR of five genes (*MDK, HOXA13, CDC2 [CDK1], IGFBP5*, and *CXCR2*), utilizing urine, algorithm reported as a risk score for having urothelial carcinoma
Cxbladder™ Monitor, Pacific Edge Diagnostics USA, Ltd.	0013M	Oncology (urothelial), mRNA, gene expression profiling by real-time quantitative PCR of five genes (*MDK, HOXA13, CDC2 [CDK1], IGFBP5*, and *CXCR2*), utilizing urine, algorithm reported as a risk score for having recurrent urothelial carcinoma
Enhanced Liver Fibrosis™ (ELF™) Test, Siemens Healthcare Diagnostics Inc/Siemens Healthcare Laboratory LLC	● 0014M	Liver disease, analysis of 3 biomarkers (hyaluronic acid [HA], procollagen III amino terminal peptide [PIIINP], tissue inhibitor of metalloproteinase 1 [TIMP-1]), using immunoassays, utilizing serum, prognostic algorithm reported as a risk score and risk of liver fibrosis and liver-related clinical events within 5 years
Adrenal Mass Panel, 24 Hour, Urine, Mayo Clinic Laboratories (MCL), Mayo Clinic	● 0015M	Adrenal cortical tumor, biochemical assay of 25 steroid markers, utilizing 24-hour urine specimen and clinical parameters, prognostic algorithm reported as a clinical risk and integrated clinical steroid risk for adrenal cortical carcinoma, adenoma, or other adrenal malignancy

Proprietary Name/Clinical Laboratory/Manufacturer	Code	Descriptor
Decipher Bladder TURBT®, Decipher Biosciences, Inc	● 0016M	Oncology (bladder), mRNA, microarray gene expression profiling of 209 genes, utilizing formalin fixed paraffin-embedded tissue, algorithm reported as molecular subtype (luminal, luminal infiltrated, basal, basal claudin-low, neuroendocrine-like)
Category I Codes for Multianalyte Assays with Algorithmic Analyses (MAAA)		
Vectra® DA, Crescendo Bioscience, Inc	81490	Autoimmune (rheumatoid arthritis), analysis of 12 biomarkers using immunoassays, utilizing serum, prognostic algorithm reported as a disease activity score (Do not report 81490 with 86140)
AlloMap®, CareDx, Inc	# 81595	Cardiology (heart transplant), mRNA, gene expression profiling by real-time quantitative PCR of 20 genes (11 content and 9 housekeeping), utilizing subfraction of peripheral blood, algorithm reported as a rejection risk score
Corus® CAD, CardioDx, Inc	81493	Coronary artery disease, mRNA, gene expression profiling by real-time RT-PCR of 23 genes, utilizing whole peripheral blood, algorithm reported as a risk score
PreDx Diabetes Risk Score™, Tethys Clinical Laboratory	81506	Endocrinology (type 2 diabetes), biochemical assays of seven analytes (glucose, HbA1c, insulin, hs-CRP, adiponectin, ferritin, interleukin 2-receptor alpha), utilizing serum or plasma, algorithm reporting a risk score
Harmony™ Prenatal Test, Ariosa Diagnostics	81507	Fetal aneuploidy (trisomy 21, 18, and 13) DNA sequence analysis of selected regions using maternal plasma, algorithm reported as a risk score for each trisomy
No proprietary name and clinical laboratory or manufacturer. Maternal serum screening procedures are performed by many labs and are not exclusive to a single facility.	81508	Fetal congenital abnormalities, biochemical assays of two proteins (PAPP-A, hCG [any form]), utilizing maternal serum, algorithm reported as a risk score
	81509	Fetal congenital abnormalities, biochemical assays of three proteins (PAPP-A, hCG [any form], DIA), utilizing maternal serum, algorithm reported as a risk score
	81510	Fetal congenital abnormalities, biochemical assays of three analytes (AFP, uE3, hCG [any form]), utilizing maternal serum, algorithm reported as a risk score
	81511	Fetal congenital abnormalities, biochemical assays of four analytes (AFP, uE3, hCG [any form], DIA) utilizing maternal serum, algorithm reported as a risk score (may include additional results from previous biochemical testing)
	81512	Fetal congenital abnormalities, biochemical assays of five analytes (AFP, uE3, total hCG, hyperglycosylated hCG, DIA) utilizing maternal serum, algorithm reported as a risk score
Aptima® BV Assay, Hologic, Inc	● 81513	Infectious disease, bacterial vaginosis, quantitative real-time amplification of RNA markers for Atopobium vaginae, Gardnerella vaginalis, and Lactobacillus species, utilizing vaginal-fluid specimens, algorithm reported as a positive or negative result for bacterial vaginosis
BD MAX™ Vaginal Panel, Becton Dickson and Company	● 81514	Infectious disease, bacterial vaginosis and vaginitis, quantitative real-time amplification of DNA markers for Gardnerella vaginalis, Atopobium vaginae, Megasphaera type 1, Bacterial Vaginosis Associated Bacteria-2 (BVAB-2), and Lactobacillus species (L. crispatus and L. jensenii), utilizing vaginal-fluid specimens, algorithm reported as a positive or negative for high likelihood of bacterial vaginosis, includes separate detection of Trichomonas vaginalis and/or Candida species (C. albicans, C. tropicalis, C. parapsilosis, C. dubliniensis), Candida glabrata, Candida krusei, when reported
HCV FibroSURE™, FibroTest™, BioPredictive S.A.S.	# 81596	Infectious disease, chronic hepatitis C virus (HCV) infection, six biochemical assays (ALT, A2-macroglobulin, apolipoprotein A-1, total bilirubin, GGT, and haptoglobin) utilizing serum, prognostic algorithm reported as scores for fibrosis and necroinflammatory activity in liver
Breast Cancer Index, Biotheranostics, Inc	81518	Oncology (breast), mRNA, gene expression profiling by real-time RT-PCR of 11 genes (7 content and 4 housekeeping), utilizing formalin-fixed paraffin-embedded tissue, algorithms reported as percentage risk for metastatic recurrence and likelihood of benefit from extended endocrine therapy
EndoPredict®, Myriad Genetic Laboratories, Inc	# 81522	Oncology (breast), mRNA, gene expression profiling by RT-PCR of 12 genes (8 content and 4 housekeeping), utilizing formalin-fixed paraffin-embedded tissue, algorithm reported as recurrence risk score
Oncotype DX® Genomic Health	81519	Oncology (breast), mRNA, gene expression profiling by real-time RT-PCR of 21 genes, utilizing formalin-fixed paraffin embedded tissue, algorithm reported as recurrence score
Prosigna® Breast Cancer Assay, NanoString Technologies, Inc	81520	Oncology (breast), mRNA gene expression profiling by hybrid capture of 58 genes (50 content and 8 housekeeping), utilizing formalin-fixed paraffin-embedded tissue, algorithm reported as a recurrence risk score
MammaPrint®, Agendia, Inc	81521	Oncology (breast), mRNA, microarray gene expression profiling of 70 content genes and 465 housekeeping genes, utilizing fresh frozen or formalin-fixed paraffin-embedded tissue, algorithm reported as index related to risk of distant metastasis
Oncotype DX® Colon Cancer Assay, Genomic Health	81525	Oncology (colon), mRNA, gene expression profiling by real-time RT-PCR of 12 genes (7 content and 5 housekeeping), utilizing formalin-fixed paraffin-embedded tissue, algorithm reported as a recurrence score

Proprietary Name/Clinical Laboratory/Manufacturer	Code	Descriptor
Cologuard™, Exact Sciences, Inc	81528	Oncology (colorectal) screening, quantitative real-time target and signal amplification of 10 DNA markers (*KRAS* mutations, promoter methylation of *NDRG4* and *BMP3*) and fecal hemoglobin, utilizing stool, algorithm reported as a positive or negative result
Decision Dx® Melanoma, Castle Biosciences, Inc	● 81529	Oncology (cutaneous melanoma), mRNA, gene expression profiling by real-time RT-PCR of 31 genes (28 content and 3 housekeeping), utilizing formalin-fixed paraffin-embedded tissue, algorithm reported as recurrence risk, including likelihood of sentinel lymph node metastasis
ChemoFX®, Helomics, Corp.	81535	Oncology (gynecologic), live tumor cell culture and chemotherapeutic response by DAPI stain and morphology, predictive algorithm reported as a drug response score; first single drug or drug combination
ChemoFX®, Helomics, Corp.	+ 81536	Oncology (gynecologic), live tumor cell culture and chemotherapeutic response by DAPI stain and morphology, predictive algorithm reported as a drug response score; each additional single drug or drug combination (List separately in addition to code for primary procedure)
VeriStrat, Biodesix, Inc	81538	Oncology (lung), mass spectrometric 8-protein signature, including amyloid A, utilizing serum, prognostic and predictive algorithm reported as good versus poor overall survival
Risk of Ovarian Malignancy Algorithm (ROMA)™, Fujirebio Diagnostics	# 81500	Oncology (ovarian), biochemical assays of two proteins (CA-125 and HE4), utilizing serum, with menopausal status, algorithm reported as a risk score
OVA1™, Vermillion, Inc	# 81503	Oncology (ovarian), biochemical assays of five proteins (CA-125, apolipoprotein A1, beta-2 microglobulin, transferrin, and pre-albumin), utilizing serum, algorithm reported as a risk score
4Kscore test, OPKO Health Inc	81539	Oncology (high-grade prostate cancer), biochemical assay of four proteins (Total PSA, Free PSA, Intact PSA, and human kallikrein-2 [hK2]), utilizing plasma or serum, prognostic algorithm reported as a probability score
Prolaris®, Myriad Genetic Laboratories, Inc	81541	Oncology (prostate), mRNA gene expression profiling by real-time RT-PCR of 46 genes (31 content and 15 housekeeping), utilizing formalin-fixed paraffin-embedded tissue, algorithm reported as a disease-specific mortality risk score
Decipher® Prostate, Decipher® Biosciences	81542	Oncology (prostate), mRNA, microarray gene expression profiling of 22 content genes, utilizing formalin-fixed paraffin-embedded tissue, algorithm reported as metastasis risk score
	(81545 has been deleted)	
ConfirmMDx® for Prostate Cancer, MDxHealth, Inc	81551	Oncology (prostate), promoter methylation profiling by real-time PCR of 3 genes (*GSTP1, APC, RASSF1*), utilizing formalin-fixed paraffin-embedded tissue, algorithm reported as a likelihood of prostate cancer detection on repeat biopsy
Afirma® Genomic Sequencing Classifier, Veracyte, Inc	# ● 81546	Oncology (thyroid), mRNA, gene expression analysis of 10,196 genes, utilizing fine needle aspirate, algorithm reported as a categorical result (eg, benign or suspicious)
Tissue of Origin Test, Kit-FFPE, Cancer Genetics, Inc	# 81504	Oncology (tissue of origin), microarray gene expression profiling of >2000 genes, utilizing formalin-fixed paraffin-embedded tissue, algorithm reported as tissue similarity scores
CancerTYPE ID, bioTheranostics, Inc	# 81540	Oncology (tumor of unknown origin), mRNA, gene expression profiling by real-time RT-PCR of 92 genes (87 content and 5 housekeeping) to classify tumor into main cancer type and subtype, utilizing formalin-fixed paraffin-embedded tissue, algorithm reported as a probability of a predicted main cancer type and subtype
DecisionDx®-UM test, Castle Biosciences, Inc	81552	Oncology (uveal melanoma), mRNA, gene expression profiling by real-time RT-PCR of 15 genes (12 content and 3 housekeeping), utilizing fine needle aspirate or formalin-fixed paraffin-embedded tissue, algorithm reported as risk of metastasis
Envisia® Genomic Classifier, Veracyte, Inc	● 81554	Pulmonary disease (idiopathic pulmonary fibrosis [IPF]), mRNA, gene expression analysis of 190 genes, utilizing transbronchial biopsies, diagnostic algorithm reported as categorical result (eg, positive or negative for high probability of usual interstitial pneumonia [UIP])
Proprietary Laboratory Analyses (PLA)		
PreciseType® HEA Test, Immucor, Inc	0001U	Red blood cell antigen typing, DNA, human erythrocyte antigen gene analysis of 35 antigens from 11 blood groups, utilizing whole blood, common RBC alleles reported
PolypDX™, Atlantic Diagnostic Laboratories, LLC, Metabolomic Technologies, Inc	0002U	Oncology (colorectal), quantitative assessment of three urine metabolites (ascorbic acid, succinic acid and carnitine) by liquid chromatography with tandem mass spectrometry (LC-MS/MS) using multiple reaction monitoring acquisition, algorithm reported as likelihood of adenomatous polyps
Overa (OVA1 Next Generation), Aspira Labs, Inc, Vermillion, Inc	0003U	Oncology (ovarian) biochemical assays of five proteins (apolipoprotein A-1, CA 125 II, follicle stimulating hormone, human epididymis protein 4, transferrin), utilizing serum, algorithm reported as a likelihood score
	(0004U has been deleted)	

Proprietary Name/Clinical Laboratory/Manufacturer	Code	Descriptor
ExosomeDx®, Prostate (IntelliScore), Exosome Diagnostics, Inc, Exosome Diagnostics, Inc	0005U	Oncology (prostate) gene expression profile by real-time RT-PCR of 3 genes *ERG, PCA3,* and *SPDEF*), urine, algorithm reported as risk score
	(0006U has been deleted)	
ToxProtect, Genotox Laboratories Ltd	0007U	Drug test(s), presumptive, with definitive confirmation of positive results, any number of drug classes, urine, includes specimen verification including DNA authentication in comparison to buccal DNA, per date of service.
AmHPR® H. pylori Antibiotic Resistance Panel, American Molecular Laboratories, Inc	0008U	Helicobacter pylori detection and antibiotic resistance, DNA, 16S and 23S rRNA, gyrA, pbp1,rdxA and rpoB, next generation sequencing, formalin-fixed paraffin-embedded or fresh tissue or fecal sample, predictive, reported as positive or negative for resistance to clarithromycin, fluoroquinolones, metronidazole, amoxicillin, tetracycline, and rifabutin
DEPArray™HER2, PacificDx	0009U	Oncology (breast cancer), *ERBB2* (HER2) copy number by FISH, tumor cells from formalin-fixed paraffin-embedded tissue isolated using image-based dielectrophoresis (DEP) sorting, reported as *ERBB2* gene amplified or non-amplified
Bacterial Typing by Whole Genome Sequencing, Mayo Clinic	0010U	Infectious disease (bacterial), strain typing by whole genome sequencing, phylogenetic-based report of strain relatedness, per submitted isolate
Cordant CORE™, Cordant Health Solutions	0011U	Prescription drug monitoring, evaluation of drugs present by LC-MS/MS, using oral fluid, reported as a comparison to an estimated steady-state range, per date of service including all drug compounds and metabolites
MatePair Targeted Rearrangements, Congenital, Mayo Clinic	0012U	Germline disorders, gene rearrangement detection by whole genome next-generation sequencing, DNA, whole blood, report of specific gene rearrangement(s)
MatePair Targeted Rearrangements, Oncology, Mayo Clinic	0013U	Oncology (solid organ neoplasia), gene rearrangement detection by whole genome next-generation sequencing, DNA, fresh or frozen tissue or cells, report of specific gene rearrangement(s)
MatePair Targeted Rearrangements, Hematologic, Mayo Clinic	0014U	Hematology (hematolymphoid neoplasia), gene rearrangement detection by whole genome next-generation sequencing, DNA, whole blood or bone marrow, report of specific gene rearrangement(s)
	(0015U has been deleted)	
BCR-ABL1 major and minor breakpoint fusion transcripts, University of Iowa, Department of Pathology, Asuragen	0016U	Oncology (hematolymphoid neoplasia), RNA, *BCR/ABL1* major and minor breakpoint fusion transcripts, quantitative PCR amplification, blood or bone marrow, report of fusion not detected or detected with quantitation
JAK2 Mutation, University of Iowa, Department of Pathology	0017U	Oncology (hematolymphoid neoplasia), *JAK2* mutation, DNA, PCR amplification of exons 12-14 and sequence analysis, blood or bone marrow, report of JAK2 mutation not detected or detected
ThyraMIR™, Interpace Diagnostics	0018U	Oncology (thyroid), microRNA profiling by RT-PCR of 10 microRNA sequences, utilizing fine needle aspirate, algorithm reported as a positive or negative result for moderate to high risk of malignancy
OncoTarget/OncoTreat, Columbia University Department of Pathology and Cell Biology, Darwin Health	0019U	Oncology, RNA, gene expression by whole transcriptome sequencing, formalin-fixed paraffin embedded tissue or fresh frozen tissue, predictive algorithm reported as potential targets for therapeutic agents
	(0020U has been deleted)	
Apifiny®, Armune BioScience, Inc	0021U	Oncology (prostate), detection of 8 autoantibodies (ARF 6, NKX3-1, 5'-UTR-BMI1, CEP 164, 3'-UTR-Ropporin, Desmocollin, AURKAIP-1, CSNK2A2), multiplexed immunoassay and flow cytometry serum, algorithm reported as risk score
Oncomine™ Dx Target Test, Thermo Fisher Scientific	0022U	Targeted genomic sequence analysis panel, non-small cell lung neoplasia, DNA and RNA analysis, 23 genes, interrogation for sequence variants and rearrangements, reported as presence/absence of variants and associated therapy(ies) to consider
LeukoStrat® CDx *FLT3* Mutation Assay, LabPMM LLC, an Invivoscribe Technologies, Inc Company, Invivoscribe Technologies, Inc	0023U	Oncology (acute myelogenous leukemia), DNA, genotyping of internal tandem duplication, p.D835, p.I836, using mononuclear cells, reported as detection or non-detection of *FLT3* mutation and indication for or against the use of midostaurin
GlycA, Laboratory Corporation of America, Laboratory Corporation of America	0024U	Glycosylated acute phase proteins (GlycA), nuclear magnetic resonance spectroscopy, quantitative
UrSure Tenofovir Quantification Test, Synergy Medical Laboratories, UrSure Inc	0025U	Tenofovir, by liquid chromatography with tandem mass spectrometry (LC-MS/MS), urine, quantitative
Thyroseq Genomic Classifier, CBLPath, Inc, University of Pittsburgh Medical Center	0026U	Oncology (thyroid), DNA and mRNA of 112 genes, next-generation sequencing, fine needle aspirate of thyroid nodule, algorithmic analysis reported as a categorical result ("Positive, high probability of malignancy" or "Negative, low probability of malignancy")
JAK2 Exons 12 to 15 Sequencing, Mayo Clinic, Mayo Clinic	0027U	*JAK2 (Janus kinase 2)* (eg, myeloproliferative disorder) gene analysis, targeted sequence analysis exons 12-15
	(0028U has been deleted)	
Focused Pharmacogenomics Panel, Mayo Clinic, Mayo Clinic	0029U	Drug metabolism (adverse drug reactions and drug response), targeted sequence analysis (ie, *CYP1A2, CYP2C19, CYP2C9, CYP2D6, CYP3A4, CYP3A5, CYP4F2, SLCO1B1, VKORC1* and rs12777823)

Proprietary Name/Clinical Laboratory/Manufacturer	Code	Descriptor
Warfarin Response Genotype, Mayo Clinic, Mayo Clinic	0030U	Drug metabolism (warfarin drug response), targeted sequence analysis (i.e., *CYP2C9, CYP4F2, VKORC1,* rs12777823)
Cytochrome P450 1A2 Genotype, Mayo Clinic, Mayo Clinic	0031U	*CYP1A2 (cytochrome P450 family 1, subfamily A, member 2)* (eg, drug metabolism) gene analysis, common variants (ie, *1F, *1K, *6, *7)
Catechol-O- Methyltransferase *(COMT)* Genotype, Mayo Clinic, Mayo Clinic	0032U	*COMT (catechol-O-methyltransferase)* (eg, drug metabolism) gene analysis, c.472G>A (rs4680) variant
Serotonin Receptor Genotype *(HTR2A* and *HTR2C)*, Mayo Clinic, Mayo Clinic	0033U	*HTR2A (5-hydroxytryptamine receptor 2A), HTR2C (5-hydroxytryptamine receptor 2C) (eg, citalopram metabolism) gene analysis, common variants* (i.e., *HTR2A* rs7997012 [c.614-2211T>C], *HTR2C* rs3813929 [c.- 759C>T] and rs1414334 [c.551-3008C>G])
Thiopurine Methyltransferase *(TPMT)* and Nudix Hydrolase *(NUDT15)* Genotyping, Mayo Clinic, Mayo Clinic	0034U	*TPMT (thiopurine S-methyltransferase), NUDT15 (nudix hydroxylase 15)* (eg, thiopurine metabolism) gene analysis, common variants (i.e., *TPMT* *2, *3A, *3B, *3C, *4, *5, *6, *8, *12; *NUDT15* *3, *4, *5)
Real-time quaking induced conversion for prion detection (RT QuIC), National Prion Disease Pathology Surveillance Center	0035U	Neurology (prion disease), cerebrospinal fluid, detection of prion protein by quaking induced conformational conversion, qualitative
EXaCT-1 Whole Exome Testing, Lab of Oncology-Molecular Detection, Weill Cornell Medicine-Clinical Genomics Laboratory	0036U	Exome (ie, somatic mutations), paired formalin-fixed paraffin-embedded tumor tissue and normal specimen, sequence analyses
FoundationOne CDx™ (F1CDx), Foundation Medicine, Inc, Foundation Medicine, Inc	0037U	Targeted genomic sequence analysis, solid organ neoplasm, DNA analysis of 324 genes, interrogation for sequence variants, gene copy number amplifications, gene rearrangements, microsatellite instability and tumor mutational burden
Sensieva ™ Droplet 25OH Vitamin D2/D3 Microvolume LC/MS Assay, InSource Diagnostics, InSource Diagnostics	0038U	Vitamin D, 25 hydroxy D2 and D3, by LC- MS/MS, serum microsample, quantitative
Anti-dsDNA, High Salt/Avidity, University of Washington, Department of Laboratory Medicine, Bio-Rad	0039U	Deoxyribonucleic acid (DNA) antibody, double stranded, high avidity
MRDx BCR-ABL Test, MolecularMD, MolecularMD	0040U	*BCR/ABL1 (t(9;22))* (eg, chronic myelogenous leukemia) translocation analysis, major breakpoint, quantitative
Lyme ImmunoBlot IgM, IGeneX Inc, ID-FISH Technology Inc (ASR) (Lyme ImmunoBlot IgM Strips Only)	0041U	Borrelia burgdorferi, antibody detection of 5 recombinant protein groups, by immunoblot, IgM
Lyme ImmunoBlot IgG, IGeneX Inc, ID-FISH Technology Inc (ASR) (Lyme ImmunoBlot IgG Strips Only)	0042U	Borrelia burgdorferi, antibody detection of 12 recombinant protein groups, by immunoblot, IgG
Tick-Borne Relapsing Fever (TBRF) Borrelia ImmunoBlots IgM Test, IGeneX Inc, ID-FISH Technology Inc (Provides TBRF ImmunoBlot IgM Strips)	0043U	Tick-borne relapsing fever Borrelia group, antibody detection to 4 recombinant protein groups, by immunoblot, IgM
Tick-Borne Relapsing Fever (TBRF) Borrelia ImmunoBlots IgG Test, IGeneX Inc, ID-FISH Technology Inc (Provides TBRF ImmunoBlot IgG Strips)	0044U	Tick-borne relapsing fever Borrelia group, antibody detection to 4 recombinant protein groups, by immunoblot, IgG
The Oncotype DX® Breast DCIS Score™ Test, Genomic Health, Inc, Genomic Health, Inc	0045U	Oncology (breast ductal carcinoma in situ), mRNA, gene expression profiling by real- time RT-PCR of 12 genes (7 content and 5 housekeeping), utilizing formalin-fixed paraffin-embedded tissue, algorithm reported as recurrence score
FLT3 ITD MRD by NGS, LabPMM LLC, an Invivoscribe Technologies, Inc Company	0046U	*FLT3 (fms-related tyrosine kinase 3)* (eg, acute myeloid leukemia) internal tandem duplication (ITD) variants, quantitative
Oncotype DX Genomic Prostate Score, Genomic Health, Inc, Genomic Health, Inc	0047U	Oncology (prostate), mRNA, gene expression profiling by real-time RT-PCR of 17 genes (12 content and 5 housekeeping), utilizing formalin-fixed paraffin-embedded tissue, algorithm reported as a risk score
MSK-IMPACT (Integrated Mutation Profiling of Actionable Cancer Targets), Memorial Sloan Kettering Cancer Center	0048U	Oncology (solid organ neoplasia), DNA, targeted sequencing of protein-coding exons of 468 cancer-associated genes, including interrogation for somatic mutations and microsatellite instability, matched with normal specimens, utilizing formalin-fixed paraffin-embedded tumor tissue, report of clinically significant mutation(s)
NPM1 MRD by NGS, LabPMM LLC, an Invivoscribe Technologies, Inc Company	0049U	*NPM1 (nucleophosmin)* (eg, acute myeloid leukemia) gene analysis, quantitative
MyAML NGS Panel, LabPMM LLC, an Invivoscribe Technologies, Inc Company	0050U	Targeted genomic sequence analysis panel, acute myelogenous leukemia, DNA analysis, 194 genes, interrogation for sequence variants, copy number variants or rearrangements
UCompliDx, Elite Medical Laboratory Solutions, LLC, Elite Medical Laboratory Solutions, LLC (LDT)	0051U	Prescription drug monitoring, evaluation of drugs present by LC-MS/MS, urine, 31 drug panel, reported as quantitative results, detected or not detected, per date of service
VAP Cholesterol Test, VAP Diagnostics Laboratory, Inc, VAP Diagnostics Laboratory, Inc	0052U	Lipoprotein, blood, high resolution fractionation and quantitation of lipoproteins, including all five major lipoprotein classes and subclasses of HDL, LDL, and VLDL by vertical auto profile ultracentrifugation

Appendix L — Multianalyte Assays with Algorithmic Analyses

Proprietary Name/Clinical Laboratory/Manufacturer	Code	Descriptor
Prostate Cancer Risk Panel, Mayo Clinic, Laboratory Developed Test	0053U	Oncology (prostate cancer), FISH analysis of 4 genes (*ASAP1, HDAC9, CHD1 and PTEN*), needle biopsy specimen, algorithm reported as probability of higher tumor grade
AssuranceRx Micro Serum, Firstox Laboratories, LLC, Firstox Laboratories, LLC	0054U	Prescription drug monitoring, 14 or more classes of drugs and substances, definitive tandem mass spectrometry with chromatography, capillary blood, quantitative report with therapeutic and toxic ranges, including steady-state range for the prescribed dose when detected, per date of service
myTAIHEART, TAI Diagnostics, Inc, TAI Diagnostics, Inc	0055U	Cardiology (heart transplant), cell-free DNA, PCR assay of 96 DNA target sequences (94 single nucleotide polymorphism targets and two control targets), plasma
MatePair Acute Myeloid Leukemia Panel, Mayo Clinic, Laboratory Developed Test	0056U	Hematology (acute myelogenous leukemia), DNA, whole genome next-generation sequencing to detect gene rearrangement(s), blood or bone marrow, report of specific gene rearrangement(s)
	(0057U has been deleted)	
Merkel SmT Oncoprotein Antibody Titer, University of Washington, Department of Laboratory Medicine	0058U	Oncology (Merkel cell carcinoma), detection of antibodies to the Merkel cell polyoma virus oncoprotein (small T antigen), serum, quantitative
Merkel Virus VP1 Capsid Antibody, University of Washington, Department of Laboratory Medicine	0059U	Oncology (Merkel cell carcinoma), detection of antibodies to the Merkel cell polyoma virus capsid protein (VP1), serum, reported as positive or negative
Twins Zygosity PLA, Natera, Inc, Natera, Inc	0060U	Twin zygosity, genomic-targeted sequence analysis of chromosome 2, using circulating cell-free fetal DNA in maternal blood
Transcutaneous multispectral measurement of tissue oxygenation and hemoglobin using spatial frequency domain imaging (SFDI), Modulated Imaging, Inc, Modulated Imaging, Inc	0061U	Transcutaneous measurement of five biomarkers (tissue oxygenation [StO2], oxyhemoglobin [ctHbO2], deoxyhemoglobin [ctHbR], papillary and reticular dermal hemoglobin concentrations [ctHb1 and ctHb2]), using spatial frequency domain imaging (SFDI) and multi-spectral analysis
SLE-key® Rule Out, Veracis Inc, Veracis Inc	0062U	Autoimmune (systemic lupus erythematosus), IgG and IgM analysis of 80 biomarkers, utilizing serum, algorithm reported with a risk score
NPDX ASD ADM Panel I, Stemina Biomarker Discovery, Inc, Stemina Biomarker Discovery, Inc d/b/a NeuroPointDX	0063U	Neurology (autism), 32 amines by LC-MS/MS, using plasma, algorithm reported as metabolic signature associated with autism spectrum disorder
BioPlex 2200 Syphilis Total & RPR Assay, Bio-Rad Laboratories, Bio-Rad Laboratories	0064U	Antibody, Treponema pallidum, total and rapid plasma reagin (RPR), immunoassay, qualitative
BioPlex 2200 RPR Assay, Bio-Rad Laboratories, Bio-Rad Laboratories	0065U	Syphilis test, non-treponemal antibody, immunoassay, qualitative (RPR)
PartoSure™ Test, Parsagen Diagnostics, Inc, Parsagen Diagnostics, Inc, a QIAGEN Company	0066U	Placental alpha-micro globulin-1 (PAMG-1), immunoassay with direct optical observation, cervico-vaginal fluid, each specimen
BBDRisk Dx™, Silbiotech, Inc, Silbiotech, Inc	0067U	Oncology (breast), immunohistochemistry, protein expression profiling of 4 biomarkers (matrix metalloproteinase-1 [MMP-1], carcinoembryonic antigen-related cell adhesion molecule 6 [CEACAM6], hyaluronoglucosaminidase [HYAL1], highly expressed in cancer protein [HEC1]), formalin-fixed paraffin-embedded precancerous breast tissue, algorithm reported as carcinoma risk score
MYCODART Dual Amplification Real Time PCR Panel for 6 Candida species, RealTime Laboratories, Inc/MycoDART, Inc, RealTime Laboratories, Inc	0068U	Candida species panel *(C. albicans, C. glabrata, C. parapsilosis, C. kruseii, C tropicalis, and C. auris)*, amplified probe technique with qualitative report of the presence or absence of each species
miR-31*now*™, GoPath Laboratories, GoPath Laboratories	0069U	Oncology (colorectal), microRNA, RT-PCR expression profiling of miR-31-3p, formalin-fixed paraffin-embedded tissue, algorithm reported as an expression score
CYP2D6 Common Variants and Copy Number, Mayo Clinic, Laboratory Developed Test	0070U	*CYP2D6 (cytochrome P450, family 2, subfamily D, polypeptide 6)* (eg, drug metabolism) gene analysis, common and select rare variants (ie, *2, *3, *4, *4N, *5, *6, *7, *8, *9, *10, *11, *12, *13, *14A, *14B, *15, *17, *29, *35, *36, *41, *57, *61, *63, *68, *83, *xN)
CYP2D6 Full Gene Sequencing, Mayo Clinic, Laboratory Developed Test	+ 0071U	*CYP2D6 (cytochrome P450, family 2, subfamily D, polypeptide 6)* (eg, drug metabolism) gene analysis, full gene sequence (List separately in addition to code for primary procedure)
CYP2D6-2D7 Hybrid Gene Targeted Sequence Analysis, Mayo Clinic, Laboratory Developed Test	+ 0072U	*CYP2D6 (cytochrome P450, family 2, subfamily D, polypeptide 6)* (eg, drug metabolism) gene analysis, targeted sequence analysis (ie, CYP2D6-2D7 hybrid gene) (List separately in addition to code for primary procedure)
CYP2D7-2D6 Hybrid Gene Targeted Sequence Analysis, Mayo Clinic, Laboratory Developed Test	+ 0073U	*CYP2D6 (cytochrome P450, family 2, subfamily D, polypeptide 6)* (eg, drug metabolism) gene analysis, targeted sequence analysis (ie, CYP2D7-2D6 hybrid gene) (List separately in addition to code for primary procedure)
CYP2D6 trans-duplication/multiplication non-duplicated gene targeted sequence analysis, Mayo Clinic, Laboratory Developed Test	+ 0074U	*CYP2D6 (cytochrome P450, family 2, subfamily D, polypeptide 6)* (eg, drug metabolism) gene analysis, targeted sequence analysis (ie, non-duplicated gene when duplication/multiplication is trans) (List separately in addition to code for primary procedure)
CYP2D6 5′ gene duplication/multiplication targeted sequence analysis, Mayo Clinic, Laboratory Developed Test	+ 0075U	*CYP2D6 (cytochrome P450, family 2, subfamily D, polypeptide 6)* (eg, drug metabolism) gene analysis, targeted sequence analysis (ie, 5′ gene duplication/multiplication) (List separately in addition to code for primary procedure)

Proprietary Name/Clinical Laboratory/Manufacturer	Code	Descriptor
CYP2D6 3' gene duplication/multiplication targeted sequence analysis, Mayo Clinic, Laboratory Developed Test	+ 0076U	*CYP2D6 (cytochrome P450, family 2, subfamily D, polypeptide 6)* (eg, drug metabolism) gene analysis, targeted sequence analysis (ie, 3' gene duplication/multiplication) (List separately in addition to code for primary procedure)
M-Protein Detection and Isotyping by MALDI-TOF Mass Spectrometry, Mayo Clinic, Laboratory Developed Test	0077U	Immunoglobulin paraprotein (M-protein), qualitative, immunoprecipitation and mass spectrometry, blood or urine, including isotype
INFINITI® Neural Response Panel, PersonalizeDx Labs, AutoGenomics Inc	0078U	Pain management (opioid-use disorder) genotyping panel, 16 common variants (ie, *ABCB1, COMT, DAT1, DBH, DOR, DRD1, DRD2, DRD4, GABA, GAL, HTR2A, HTTLPR, MTHFR, MUOR, OPRK1, OPRM1*), buccal swab or other germline tissue sample, algorithm reported as positive or negative risk of opioid-use disorder
ToxLok™, InSource Diagnostics, InSource Diagnostics	0079U	Comparative DNA analysis using multiple selected single-nucleotide polymorphisms (SNPs), urine and buccal DNA, for specimen identity verification
BDX-XL2, Biodesix®, Inc, Biodesix®, Inc	0080U	Oncology (lung), mass spectrometric analysis of galectin-3-binding protein and scavenger receptor cysteine-rich type 1 protein M130, with five clinical risk factors (age, smoking status, nodule diameter, nodule-spiculation status and nodule location), utilizing plasma, algorithm reported as a categorical probability of malignancy
	(0081U has been deleted. To report, use 81552)	
NextGen Precision™ Testing, Precision Diagnostics, Precision Diagnostics LBN Precision Toxicology, LLC	0082U	Drug test(s), definitive, 90 or more drugs or substances, definitive chromatography with mass spectrometry, and presumptive, any number of drug classes, by instrument chemistry analyzer (utilizing immunoassay), urine, report of presence or absence of each drug, drug metabolite or substance with description and severity of significant interactions per date of service
Onco4D™, Animated Dynamics, Inc, Animated Dynamics, Inc	0083U	Oncology, response to chemotherapy drugs using motility contrast tomography, fresh or frozen tissue, reported as likelihood of sensitivity or resistance to drugs or drug combinations
BLOODchip®, ID CORE XT™, Grifols Diagnostic Solutions Inc	0084U	Red blood cell antigen typing, DNA, genotyping of 10 blood groups with phenotype prediction of 37 red blood cell antigens
	(0085U has been deleted)	
Accelerate PhenoTest™ BC kit, Accelerate Diagnostics, Inc	0086U	Infectious disease (bacterial and fungal), organism identification, blood culture, using rRNA FISH, 6 or more organism targets, reported as positive or negative with phenotypic minimum inhibitory concentration (MIC)-based antimicrobial susceptibility
Molecular Microscope® MMDx—Heart, Kashi Clinical Laboratories	0087U	Cardiology (heart transplant), mRNA gene expression profiling by microarray of 1283 genes, transplant biopsy tissue, allograft rejection and injury algorithm reported as a probability score
Molecular Microscope® MMDx—Kidney, Kashi Clinical Laboratories	0088U	Transplantation medicine (kidney allograft rejection), microarray gene expression profiling of 1494 genes, utilizing transplant biopsy tissue, algorithm reported as a probability score for rejection
Pigmented Lesion Assay (PLA), DermTech	0089U	Oncology (melanoma), gene expression profiling by RTqPCR, *PRAME* and *LINC00518*, superficial collection using adhesive patch(es)
myPath® Melanoma, Myriad Genetic Laboratories	0090U	Oncology (cutaneous melanoma), mRNA gene expression profiling by RT-PCR of 23 genes (14 content and 9 housekeeping), utilizing formalin-fixed paraffin-embedded tissue, algorithm reported as a categorical result (ie, benign, indeterminate, malignant)
FirstSight^{CRC}, CellMax Life	0091U	Oncology (colorectal) screening, cell enumeration of circulating tumor cells, utilizing whole blood, algorithm, for the presence of adenoma or cancer, reported as a positive or negative result
REVEAL Lung Nodule Characterization, MagArray, Inc	0092U	Oncology (lung), three protein biomarkers, immunoassay using magnetic nanosensor technology, plasma, algorithm reported as risk score for likelihood of malignancy
ComplyRX, Claro Labs	0093U	Prescription drug monitoring, evaluation of 65 common drugs by LC-MS/MS, urine, each drug reported detected or not detected
RCIGM Rapid Whole Genome Sequencing, Rady Children's Institute for Genomic Medicine (RCIGM)	0094U	Genome (eg, unexplained constitutional or heritable disorder or syndrome), rapid sequence analysis
Esophageal String Test™ (EST), Cambridge Biomedical, Inc	0095U	Inflammation (eosinophilic esophagitis), ELISA analysis of eotaxin-3 *(CCL26 [C-C motif chemokine ligand 26])* and major basic protein *(PRG2 [proteoglycan 2, pro eosinophil major basic protein])*, specimen obtained by swallowed nylon string, algorithm reported as predictive probability index for active eosinophilic esophagitis
HPV, High-Risk, Male Urine, Molecular Testing Labs	0096U	Human papillomavirus (HPV), high-risk types (ie, 16, 18, 31, 33, 35, 39, 45, 51, 52, 56, 58, 59, 66, 68), male urine

Proprietary Name/Clinical Laboratory/Manufacturer	Code	Descriptor
BioFire® FilmArray® Gastrointestinal (GI) Panel, BioFire® Diagnostics	0097U	Gastrointestinal pathogen, multiplex reverse transcription and multiplex amplified probe technique, multiple types or subtypes, 22 targets (Campylobacter [C. jejuni/C. coli/C. upsaliensis], Clostridium difficile [C. difficile] toxin A/B, Plesiomonas shigelloides, Salmonella, Vibrio [V. parahaemolyticus/V. vulnificus/V. cholerae], including specific identification of Vibrio cholerae, Yersinia enterocolitica, Enteroaggregative Escherichia coli [EAEC], Enteropathogenic Escherichia coli [EPEC], Enterotoxigenic Escherichia coli [ETEC] lt/st, Shiga-like toxin-producing Escherichia coli [STEC] stx1/stx2 [including specific identification of the E. coli O157 serogroup within STEC], Shigella/Enteroinvasive Escherichia coli [EIEC], Cryptosporidium, Cyclospora cayetanensis, Entamoeba histolytica, Giardia lamblia [also known as G. intestinalis and G. duodenalis], adenovirus F 40/41, astrovirus, norovirus GI/GII, rotavirus A, sapovirus [Genogroups I, II, IV, and V])
BioFire® FilmArray® Respiratory Panel (RP) EZ, BioFire® Diagnostics	0098U	Respiratory pathogen, multiplex reverse transcription and multiplex amplified probe technique, multiple types or subtypes, 14 targets (adenovirus, coronavirus, human metapneumovirus, influenza A, influenza A subtype H1, influenza A subtype H3, influenza A subtype H1-2009, influenza B, parainfluenza virus, human rhinovirus/enterovirus, respiratory syncytial virus, Bordetella pertussis, Chlamydophila pneumoniae, Mycoplasma pneumoniae)
BioFire® FilmArray® Respiratory Panel (RP), BioFire® Diagnostics	0099U	Respiratory pathogen, multiplex reverse transcription and multiplex amplified probe technique, multiple types or subtypes, 20 targets (adenovirus, coronavirus 229E, coronavirus HKU1, coronavirus, coronavirus OC43, human metapneumovirus, influenza A, influenza A subtype, influenza A subtype H3, influenza A subtype H1-2009, influenza, parainfluenza virus, parainfluenza virus 2, parainfluenza virus 3, parainfluenza virus 4, human rhinovirus/enterovirus, respiratory syncytial virus, Bordetella pertussis, Chlamydophila pneumonia, Mycoplasma pneumoniae)
BioFire® FilmArray® Respiratory Panel 2 (RP2), BioFire® Diagnostics	0100U	Respiratory pathogen, multiplex reverse transcription and multiplex amplified probe technique, multiple types or subtypes, 21 targets (adenovirus, coronavirus 229E, coronavirus HKU1, coronavirus NL63, coronavirus OC43, human metapneumovirus, human rhinovirus/enterovirus, influenza A, including subtypes H1, H1-2009, and H3, influenza B, parainfluenza virus 1, parainfluenza virus 2, parainfluenza virus 3, parainfluenza virus 4, respiratory syncytial virus, Bordetella parapertussis [IS1001], Bordetella pertussis [ptxP], Chlamydia pneumoniae, Mycoplasma pneumoniae)
ColoNext®, Ambry Genetics®, Ambry Genetics®	0101U	Hereditary colon cancer disorders (eg, Lynch syndrome, *PTEN* hamartoma syndrome, Cowden syndrome, familial adenomatosis polyposis), genomic sequence analysis panel utilizing a combination of NGS, Sanger, MLPA, and array CGH, with MRNA analytics to resolve variants of unknown significance when indicated (15 genes [sequencing and deletion/duplication], *EPCAM* and *GREM1* [deletion/duplication only])
BreastNext®, Ambry Genetics®, Ambry Genetics®	0102U	Hereditary breast cancer-related disorders (eg, hereditary breast cancer, hereditary ovarian cancer, hereditary endometrial cancer), genomic sequence analysis panel utilizing a combination of NGS, Sanger, MLPA, and array CGH, with MRNA analytics to resolve variants of unknown significance when indicated (17 genes [sequencing and deletion/duplication])
OvaNext®, Ambry Genetics®, Ambry Genetics®	0103U	Hereditary ovarian cancer (eg, hereditary ovarian cancer, hereditary endometrial cancer), genomic sequence analysis panel utilizing a combination of NGS, Sanger, MLPA, and array CGH, with MRNA analytics to resolve variants of unknown significance when indicated (24 genes [sequencing and deletion/duplication], *EPCAM* [deletion/duplication only])
	(0104U has been deleted)	
KidneyIntelXT™, RenalytixAI, RenalytixAI	0105U	Nephrology (chronic kidney disease), multiplex electrochemiluminescent immunoassay (ECLIA) of tumor necrosis factor receptor 1A, receptor superfamily 2 *(TNFR1, TNFR2)*, and kidney injury molecule-1 (KIM-1) combined with longitudinal clinical data, including *APOL1* genotype if available, and plasma (isolated fresh or frozen), algorithm reported as probability score for rapid kidney function decline (RKFD)
13C-Spirulina Gastric Emptying Breath Test (GEBT), Cairn Diagnostics d/b/a Advanced Breath Diagnostics, LLC, Cairn Diagnostics d/b/a Advanced Breath Diagnostics, LLC	0106U	Gastric emptying, serial collection of 7 timed breath specimens, non-radioisotope carbon-13(^{13}C) spirulina substrate, analysis of each specimen by gas isotope ratio mass spectrometry, reported as rate of $^{13}CO_2$ excretion
Singulex Clarity C.diff toxins A/B Assay, Singulex	0107U	Clostridium difficile toxin(s) antigen detection by immunoassay technique, stool, qualitative, multiple-step method
TissueCypher® Barrett's Esophagus Assay, Cernostics, Cernostics	0108U	Gastroenterology (Barrett's esophagus), whole slide-digital imaging, including morphometric analysis, computer-assisted quantitative immunolabeling of 9 protein biomarkers (p16, AMACR, p53, CD68, COX-2, CD45RO, HIF1a, HER-2, K20) and morphology, formalin-fixed paraffin-embedded tissue, algorithm reported as risk of progression to high-grade dysplasia or cancer
MYCODART Dual Amplification Real Time PCR Panel for 4 Aspergillus species, RealTime Laboratories, Inc/MycoDART, Inc	0109U	Infectious disease (Aspergillus species), real-time PCR for detection of DNA from 4 species *(A. fumigatus, A. terreus, A. niger,* and *A. flavus)*, blood, lavage fluid, or tissue, qualitative reporting of presence or absence of each species

Proprietary Name/Clinical Laboratory/Manufacturer	Code	Descriptor
Oral OncolyticAssuranceRX, Firstox Laboratories, LLC, Firstox Laboratories, LLC	0110U	Prescription drug monitoring, one or more oral oncology drug(s) and substances, definitive tandem mass spectrometry with chromatography, serum or plasma from capillary blood or venous blood, quantitative report with steady-state range for the prescribed drug(s) when detected
Praxis(™) Extended RAS Panel, Illumina, Illumina	0111U	Oncology (colon cancer), targeted *KRAS* (codons 12, 13, and 61) and *NRAS* (codons 12, 13, and 61) gene analysis utilizing formalin-fixed paraffin-embedded tissue
MicroGenDX qPCR & NGS For Infection, MicroGenDX, MicroGenDX	0112U	Infectious agent detection and identification, targeted sequence analysis (16S and 18S rRNA genes) with drug-resistance gene
MiPS (Mi-Prostate Score), MLabs, MLabs	0113U	Oncology (prostate), measurement of *PCA3* and *TMPRSS2-ERG* in urine and PSA in serum following prostatic massage, by RNA amplification and fluorescence-based detection, algorithm reported as risk score
EsoGuard™, Lucid Diagnostics, Lucid Diagnostics	0114U	Gastroenterology (Barrett's esophagus), *VIM* and *CCNA1* methylation analysis, esophageal cells, algorithm reported as likelihood for Barrett's esophagus
ePlex Respiratory Pathogen (RP) Panel, GenMark Diagnostics, Inc, GenMark Diagnostics, Inc	0115U	Respiratory infectious agent detection by nucleic acid (DNA and RNA), 18 viral types and subtypes and 2 bacterial targets, amplified probe technique, including multiplex reverse transcription for RNA targets, each analyte reported as detected or not detected
Snapshot Oral Fluid Compliance, Ethos Laboratories	0116U	Prescription drug monitoring, enzyme immunoassay of 35 or more drugs confirmed with LC-MS/MS, oral fluid, algorithm results reported as a patient-compliance measurement with risk of drug to drug interactions for prescribed medications
Foundation PI℠, Ethos Laboratories	0117U	Pain management, analysis of 11 endogenous analytes (methylmalonic acid, xanthurenic acid, homocysteine, pyroglutamic acid, vanilmandelate, 5-hydroxyindoleacetic acid, hydroxymethylglutarate, ethylmalonate, 3-hydroxypropyl mercapturic acid (3-HPMA), quinolinic acid, kynurenic acid), LC-MS/MS, urine, algorithm reported as a pain-index score with likelihood of atypical biochemical function associated with pain
Viracor TRAC™ dd-cfDNA, Viracor Eurofins, Viracor Eurofins	0118U	Transplantation medicine, quantification of donor-derived cell-free DNA using whole genome next-generation sequencing, plasma, reported as percentage of donor-derived cell-free DNA in the total cell-free DNA
MI-HEART Ceramides, Plasma, Mayo Clinic, Laboratory Developed Test	0119U	Cardiology, ceramides by liquid chromatography-tandem mass spectrometry, plasma, quantitative report with risk score for major cardiovascular events
Lymph3Cx Lymphoma Molecular Subtyping Assay, Mayo Clinic, Laboratory Developed Test	0120U	Oncology (B-cell lymphoma classification), mRNA, gene expression profiling by fluorescent probe hybridization of 58 genes (45 content and 13 housekeeping genes), formalin-fixed paraffin-embedded tissue, algorithm reported as likelihood for primary mediastinal B-cell lymphoma (PMBCL) and diffuse large B-cell lymphoma (DLBCL) with cell of origin subtyping in the latter
Flow Adhesion of Whole Blood on VCAM-1 (FAB-V), Functional Fluidics, Functional Fluidics	0121U	Sickle cell disease, microfluidic flow adhesion (VCAM-1), whole blood
Flow Adhesion of Whole Blood to P-SELECTIN (WB-PSEL), Functional Fluidics, Functional Fluidics	0122U	Sickle cell disease, microfluidic flow adhesion (P-Selectin), whole blood
Mechanical Fragility, RBC by shear stress profiling and spectral analysis, Functional Fluidics, Functional Fluidics	0123U	Mechanical fragility, RBC, shear stress and spectral analysis profiling
	(0124U has been deleted)	
	(0125U has been deleted)	
	(0126U has been deleted)	
	(0127U has been deleted)	
	(0128U has been deleted)	
BRCAplus, Ambry Genetics	0129U	Hereditary breast cancer-related disorders (eg, hereditary breast cancer, hereditary ovarian cancer, hereditary endometrial cancer), genomic sequence analysis and deletion/duplication analysis panel *(ATM, BRCA1, BRCA2, CDH1, CHEK2, PALB2, PTEN,* and *TP53)*
+RNAinsight™ for ColoNext®, Ambry Genetics	+ 0130U	Hereditary colon cancer disorders (eg, Lynch syndrome, PTEN hamartoma syndrome, Cowden syndrome, familial adenomatosis polyposis), targeted mRNA sequence analysis panel *(APC, CDH1, CHEK2, MLH1, MSH2, MSH6, MUTYH, PMS2, PTEN,* and *TP53)* (List separately in addition to code for primary procedure)
+RNAinsight™ for BreastNext®, Ambry Genetics	+ 0131U	Hereditary breast cancer-related disorders (eg, hereditary breast cancer, hereditary ovarian cancer, hereditary endometrial cancer), targeted mRNA sequence analysis panel (13 genes) (List separately in addition to code for primary procedure)
+RNAinsight™ for OvaNext®, Ambry Genetics	+ 0132U	Hereditary ovarian cancer-related disorders (eg, hereditary breast cancer, hereditary ovarian cancer, hereditary endometrial cancer), targeted mRNA sequence analysis panel (17 genes) (List separately in addition to code for primary procedure)
+RNAinsight™ for ProstateNext®, Ambry Genetics	+ 0133U	Hereditary prostate cancer-related disorders, targeted mRNA sequence analysis panel (11 genes) (List separately in addition to code for primary procedure)

Proprietary Name/Clinical Laboratory/Manufacturer	Code	Descriptor
+RNAinsight™ for CancerNext®, Ambry Genetics	+ 0134U	Hereditary pan cancer (eg, hereditary breast and ovarian cancer, hereditary endometrial cancer, hereditary colorectal cancer), targeted mRNA sequence analysis panel (18 genes) (List separately in addition to code for primary procedure)
+RNAinsight™ for GYNPlus®, Ambry Genetics	+ 0135U	Hereditary gynecological cancer (eg, hereditary breast and ovarian cancer, hereditary endometrial cancer, hereditary colorectal cancer), targeted mRNA sequence analysis panel (12 genes) (List separately in addition to code for primary procedure)
+RNAinsight™ for *ATM*, Ambry Genetics	+ 0136U	*ATM (ataxia telangiectasia mutated)* (eg, ataxia telangiectasia) mRNA sequence analysis (List separately in addition to code for primary procedure)
+RNAinsight™ for *PALB2*, Ambry Genetics	+ 0137U	*PALB2 (partner and localizer of BRCA2)* (eg, breast and pancreatic cancer) mRNA sequence analysis (List separately in addition to code for primary procedure)
+RNAinsight™ for *BRCA1/2*, Ambry Genetics	+ 0138U	*BRCA1 (BRCA1, DNA repair associated), BRCA2 (BRCA2, DNA repair associated)* (eg, hereditary breast and ovarian cancer) mRNA sequence analysis (List separately in addition to code for primary procedure)
NPDX ASD Energy Metabolism, Stemina Biomarker Discovery, Inc, Stemina Biomarker Discovery, Inc	● 0139U	Neurology (autism spectrum disorder [ASD]), quantitative measurements of 6 central carbon metabolites (ie, α-ketoglutarate, alanine, lactate, phenylalanine, pyruvate, and succinate), LC-MS/MS, plasma, algorithmic analysis with result reported as negative or positive (with metabolic subtypes of ASD)
ePlex® BCID Fungal Pathogens Panel, GenMark Diagnostics, Inc, GenMark Diagnostics, Inc	● 0140U	Infectious disease (fungi), fungal pathogen identification, DNA (15 fungal targets), blood culture, amplified probe technique, each target reported as detected or not detected
ePlex® BCID Gram-Positive Panel, GenMark Diagnostics, Inc, GenMark Diagnostics, Inc	● 0141U	Infectious disease (bacteria and fungi), gram-positive organism identification and drug resistance element detection, DNA (20 gram-positive bacterial targets, 4 resistance genes, 1 pan gram-negative bacterial target, 1 pan Candida target), blood culture, amplified probe technique, each target reported as detected or not detected
ePlex® BCID Gram-Negative Panel, GenMark Diagnostics, Inc, GenMark Diagnostics, Inc	● 0142U	Infectious disease (bacteria and fungi), gram-negative bacterial identification and drug resistance element detection, DNA (21 gram-negative bacterial targets, 6 resistance genes, 1 pan gram-positive bacterial target, 1 pan Candida target), amplified probe technique, each target reported as detected or not detected
CareViewRx, Newstar Medical Laboratories, LLC, Newstar Medical Laboratories, LLC PsychViewRx Plus analysis by Newstar Medical Laboratories, LLC. To report, see (~0150U)	● 0143U	Drug assay, definitive, 120 or more drugs or metabolites, urine, quantitative liquid chromatography with tandem mass spectrometry (LC-MS/MS) using multiple reaction monitoring (MRM), with drug or metabolite description, comments including sample validation, per date of service
CareViewRx Plus, Newstar Medical Laboratories, LLC, Newstar Medical Laboratories, LLC	● 0144U	Drug assay, definitive, 160 or more drugs or metabolites, urine, quantitative liquid chromatography with tandem mass spectrometry (LC-MS/MS) using multiple reaction monitoring (MRM), with drug or metabolite description, comments including sample validation, per date of service
PainViewRx, Newstar Medical Laboratories, LLC, Newstar Medical Laboratories, LLC	● 0145U	Drug assay, definitive, 65 or more drugs or metabolites, urine, quantitative liquid chromatography with tandem mass spectrometry (LC-MS/MS) using multiple reaction monitoring (MRM), with drug or metabolite description, comments including sample validation, per date of service
PainViewRx Plus, Newstar Medical Laboratories, LLC, Newstar Medical Laboratories, LLC	● 0146U	Drug assay, definitive, 80 or more drugs or metabolites, urine, by quantitative liquid chromatography with tandem mass spectrometry (LC-MS/MS) using multiple reaction monitoring (MRM), with drug or metabolite description, comments including sample validation, per date of service
RiskViewRx, Newstar Medical Laboratories, LLC, Newstar Medical Laboratories, LLC	● 0147U	Drug assay, definitive, 85 or more drugs or metabolites, urine, quantitative liquid chromatography with tandem mass spectrometry (LC-MS/MS) using multiple reaction monitoring (MRM), with drug or metabolite description, comments including sample validation, per date of service
RiskViewRx Plus, Newstar Medical Laboratories, LLC, Newstar Medical Laboratories, LLC	● 0148U	Drug assay, definitive, 100 or more drugs or metabolites, urine, quantitative liquid chromatography with tandem mass spectrometry (LC-MS/MS) using multiple reaction monitoring (MRM), with drug or metabolite description, comments including sample validation, per date of service
PsychViewRx, Newstar Medical Laboratories, LLC, Newstar Medical Laboratories, LLC	● 0149U	Drug assay, definitive, 60 or more drugs or metabolites, urine, quantitative liquid chromatography with tandem mass spectrometry (LC-MS/MS) using multiple reaction monitoring (MRM), with drug or metabolite description, comments including sample validation, per date of service
PsychViewRx Plus, Newstar Medical Laboratories, LLC, Newstar Medical Laboratories, LLC CareViewRx analysis by Newstar Medical Laboratories, LLC. To report, see (~0143U)	● 0150U	Drug assay, definitive, 120 or more drugs or metabolites, urine, quantitative liquid chromatography with tandem mass spectrometry (LC-MS/MS) using multiple reaction monitoring (MRM), with drug or metabolite description, comments including sample validation, per date of service
BioFire® FilmArray® Pneumonia Panel, BioFire® Diagnostics, BioFire® Diagnostics	● 0151U	Infectious disease (bacterial or viral respiratory tract infection), pathogen specific nucleic acid (DNA or RNA), 33 targets, real-time semi-quantitative PCR, bronchoalveolar lavage, sputum, or endotracheal aspirate, detection of 33 organismal and antibiotic resistance genes with limited semi-quantitative results

Proprietary Name/Clinical Laboratory/Manufacturer	Code	Descriptor
Karius® Test, Karius Inc, Karius Inc	● 0152U	Infectious disease (bacteria, fungi, parasites, and DNA viruses), microbial cell-free DNA, plasma, untargeted next-generation sequencing, report for significant positive pathogens
Insight TNBCtype™, Insight Molecular Labs	● 0153U	Oncology (breast), mRNA, gene expression profiling by next-generation sequencing of 101 genes, utilizing formalin-fixed paraffin-embedded tissue, algorithm reported as a triple negative breast cancer clinical subtype(s) with information on immune cell involvement
therascreen® *FGFR* RGQ RT-PCR Kit, QIAGEN, QIAGEN GmbH	● 0154U	Oncology (urothelial cancer), RNA, analysis by real-time RT-PCR of the *FGFR3 (fibroblast growth factor receptor3)* gene analysis (ie, p.R248C [c.742C>T], p.S249C [c.746C>G], p.G370C [c.1108G>T], p.Y373C [c.1118A>G], FGFR3-TACC3v1, and FGFR3-TACC3v3) utilizing formalin-fixed paraffin-embedded urothelial cancer tumor tissue, reported as *FGFR* gene alteration status
therascreen *PIK3CA* RGQ PCR Kit, QIAGEN, QIAGEN GmbH	● 0155U	Oncology (breast cancer), DNA, *PIK3CA (phosphatidylinositol-4,5-bisphosphate 3-kinase, catalytic subunit alpha)* (eg, breast cancer) gene analysis (ie, p.C420R, p.E542K, p.E545A, p.E545D [g.1635G>T only], p.E545G, p.E545K, p.Q546E, p.Q546R, p.H1047L, p.H1047R, p.H1047Y), utilizing formalin-fixed paraffin-embedded breast tumor tissue, reported as *PIK3CA* gene mutation status
SMASH™, New York Genome Center, Marvel Genomics™	● 0156U	Copy number (eg, intellectual disability, dysmorphology), sequence analysis
CustomNext + RNA: *APC*, Ambry Genetics®, Ambry Genetics®	+● 0157U	*APC (APC regulator of WNT signaling pathway)* (eg, familial adenomatosis polyposis [FAP]) mRNA sequence analysis (List separately in addition to code for primary procedure)
CustomNext + RNA: *MLH1*, Ambry Genetics®, Ambry Genetics®	+● 0158U	*MLH1 (mutL homolog 1)* (eg, hereditary non-polyposis colorectal cancer, Lynch syndrome) mRNA sequence analysis (List separately in addition to code for primary procedure)
CustomNext + RNA: *MSH2*, Ambry Genetics®, Ambry Genetics®	+● 0159U	*MSH2 (mutS homolog 2)* (eg, hereditary colon cancer, Lynch syndrome) mRNA sequence analysis (List separately in addition to code for primary procedure)
CustomNext + RNA: *MSH6*, Ambry Genetics®, Ambry Genetics®	+● 0160U	*MSH6 (mutS homolog 6)* (eg, hereditary colon cancer, Lynch syndrome) mRNA sequence analysis (List separately in addition to code for primary procedure)
CustomNext + RNA: *PMS2*, Ambry Genetics®, Ambry Genetics®	+● 0161U	*PMS2 (PMS1 homolog 2, mismatch repair system component)* (eg, hereditary non-polyposis colorectal cancer, Lynch syndrome) mRNA sequence analysis (List separately in addition to code for primary procedure)
CustomNext + RNA: Lynch *(MLH1, MSH2, MSH6, PMS2)*, Ambry Genetics®, Ambry Genetics®	+● 0162U	Hereditary colon cancer (Lynch syndrome), targeted mRNA sequence analysis panel *(MLH1, MSH2, MSH6, PMS2)* (List separately in addition to code for primary procedure)
BeScreened™-CRC, Beacon Biomedical Inc, Beacon Biomedical Inc	● 0163U	Oncology (colorectal) screening, biochemical enzyme-linked immunosorbent assay (ELISA) of 3 plasma or serum proteins (teratocarcinoma derived growth factor-1 [TDGF-1, Cripto-1], carcinoembryonic antigen [CEA], extracellular matrix protein [ECM]), with demographic data (age, gender, CRC-screening compliance) using a proprietary algorithm and reported as likelihood of CRC or advanced adenomas
ibs-smart™, Gemelli Biotech, Gemelli Biotech	● 0164U	Gastroenterology (irritable bowel syndrome [IBS]), immunoassay for anti-CdtB and anti-vinculin antibodies, utilizing plasma, algorithm for elevated or not elevated qualitative results
VeriMAP™ Peanut Dx—Bead-based Epitope Assay, AllerGenis™ Clinical Laboratory, AllerGenis™ LLC	▲ 0165U	Peanut allergen-specific quantitative assessment of multiple epitopes using enzyme-linked immunosorbent assay (ELISA), blood, individual epitope results and interpretation probability of peanut allergy
LiverFASt™, Fibronostics, Fibronostics	● 0166U	Liver disease, 10 biochemical assays (a2-macroglobulin, haptoglobin, apolipoprotein A1, bilirubin, GGT, ALT, AST, triglycerides, cholesterol, fasting glucose) and biometric and demographic data, utilizing serum, algorithm reported as scores for fibrosis, necroinflammatory activity, and steatosis with a summary interpretation
ADEXUSDx hCG Test, NOWDiagnostics, NOWDiagnostics	● 0167U	Gonadotropin, chorionic (hCG), immunoassay with direct optical observation, blood
Vanadis® NIPT, PerkinElmer, Inc, PerkinElmer Genomics	● 0168U	Fetal aneuploidy (trisomy 21, 18, and 13) DNA sequence analysis of selected regions using maternal plasma without fetal fraction cutoff, algorithm reported as a risk score for each trisomy
NT *(NUDT15* and *TPMT)* genotyping panel, RPRD Diagnostics	● 0169U	*NUDT15 (nudix hydrolase 15)* and *TPMT (thiopurine S-methyltransferase)* (eg, drug metabolism) gene analysis, common variants
Clarifi™, Quadrant Biosciences, Inc, Quadrant Biosciences, Inc	● 0170U	Neurology (autism spectrum disorder [ASD]), RNA, next-generation sequencing, saliva, algorithmic analysis, and results reported as predictive probability of ASD diagnosis
MyMRD® NGS Panel, Laboratory for Personalized Molecular Medicine, Laboratory for Personalized Molecular Medicine	● 0171U	Targeted genomic sequence analysis panel, acute myeloid leukemia, myelodysplastic syndrome, and myeloproliferative neoplasms, DNA analysis, 23 genes, interrogation for sequence variants, rearrangements and minimal residual disease, reported as presence/absence

Appendix L — Multianalyte Assays with Algorithmic Analyses

Proprietary Name/Clinical Laboratory/Manufacturer	Code	Descriptor
myChoice® CDx, Myriad Genetics Laboratories, Inc, Myriad Genetics Laboratories, Inc	● 0172U	Oncology (solid tumor as indicated by the label), somatic mutation analysis of *BRCA1 (BRCA1, DNA repair associated), BRCA2 (BRCA2, DNA repair associated)* and analysis of homologous recombination deficiency pathways, DNA, formalin-fixed paraffin-embedded tissue, algorithm quantifying tumor genomic instability score
Psych HealthPGx Panel, RPRD Diagnostics, RPRD Diagnostics	● 0173U	Psychiatry (ie, depression, anxiety), genomic analysis panel, includes variant analysis of 14 genes
LC-MS/MS Targeted Proteomic Assay, OncoOmicDx Laboratory, LDT	● 0174U	Oncology (solid tumor), mass spectrometric 30 protein targets, formalin-fixed paraffin-embedded tissue, prognostic and predictive algorithm reported as likely, unlikely, or uncertain benefit of 39 chemotherapy and targeted therapeutic oncology agents
Genomind® Professional PGx Express™ CORE, Genomind, Inc, Genomind, Inc	● 0175U	Psychiatry (eg, depression, anxiety), genomic analysis panel, variant analysis of 15 genes
IB*Schek*®, Commonwealth Diagnostics International, Inc, Commonwealth Diagnostics International, Inc	● 0176U	Cytolethal distending toxin B (CdtB) and vinculin IgG antibodies by immunoassay (ie, ELISA)
therascreen® *PIK3CA* RGQ PCR Kit, QIAGEN, QIAGEN GmbH	● 0177U	Oncology (breast cancer), DNA, *PIK3CA (phosphatidylinositol-4,5-bisphosphate 3-kinase catalytic subunit alpha)* gene analysis of 11 gene variants utilizing plasma, reported as PIK3CA gene mutation status
VeriMAP™ Peanut Sensitivity - Bead Based Epitope Assay, AllerGenis™ Clinical Laboratory, AllerGenis™ LLC	● 0178U	Peanut allergen-specific quantitative assessment of multiple epitopes using enzyme-linked immunosorbent assay (ELISA), blood, report of minimum eliciting exposure for a clinical reaction
Resolution ctDx Lung™, Resolution Bioscience, Resolution Bioscience, Inc	● 0179U	Oncology (non-small cell lung cancer), cell-free DNA, targeted sequence analysis of 23 genes (single nucleotide variations, insertions and deletions, fusions without prior knowledge of partner/breakpoint, copy number variations), with report of significant mutation(s)
Navigator ABO Sequencing, Grifols Immunohematology Center, Grifols Immunohematology Center	● 0180U	Red cell antigen (ABO blood group) genotyping *(ABO), gene analysis Sanger/chain termination/conventional sequencing, ABO (ABO, alpha 1-3-N-acetylgalactosaminyltransferase and alpha 1-3-galactosyltransferase)* gene, including subtyping, 7 exons
Navigator CO Sequencing, Grifols Immunohematology Center, Grifols Immunohematology Center	● 0181U	Red cell antigen (Colton blood group) genotyping (CO), gene analysis, *AQP1 (aquaporin 1 [Colton blood group])* exon 1
Navigator CROM Sequencing, Grifols Immunohematology Center, Grifols Immunohematology Center	● 0182U	Red cell antigen (Cromer blood group) genotyping (CROM), gene analysis, *CD55 (CD55 molecule [Cromer blood group])* exons 1-10
Navigator DI Sequencing, Grifols Immunohematology Center, Grifols Immunohematology Center	● 0183U	Red cell antigen (Diego blood group) genotyping (DI), gene analysis, *SLC4A1 (solute carrier family 4 member 1 [Diego blood group])* exon 19
Navigator DO Sequencing, Grifols Immunohematology Center, Grifols Immunohematology Center	● 0184U	Red cell antigen (Dombrock blood group) genotyping (DO), gene analysis, *ART4 (ADP-ribosyltransferase 4 [Dombrock blood group])* exon 2
Navigator FUT1 Sequencing, Grifols Immunohematology Center, Grifols Immunohematology Center	● 0185U	Red cell antigen (H blood group) genotyping (FUT1), gene analysis, *FUT1 (fucosyltransferase 1 [H blood group])* exon 4
Navigator FUT2 Sequencing, Grifols Immunohematology Center, Grifols Immunohematology Center	● 0186U	Red cell antigen (H blood group) genotyping (FUT2), gene analysis, *FUT2 (fucosyltransferase 2)* exon 2
Navigator FY Sequencing, Grifols Immunohematology Center, Grifols Immunohematology Center	● 0187U	Red cell antigen (Duffy blood group) genotyping (FY), gene analysis, *ACKR1 (atypical chemokine receptor 1 [Duffy blood group])* exons 1-2
Navigator GE Sequencing, Grifols Immunohematology Center, Grifols Immunohematology Center	● 0188U	Red cell antigen (Gerbich blood group) genotyping (GE), gene analysis, *GYPC (glycophorin C [Gerbich blood group])* exons 1-4
Navigator GYPA Sequencing, Grifols Immunohematology Center, Grifols Immunohematology Center	● 0189U	Red cell antigen (MNS blood group) genotyping (GYPA), gene analysis, *GYPA (glycophorin A [MNS blood group])* introns 1, 5, exon 2
Navigator GYPB Sequencing, Grifols Immunohematology Center, Grifols Immunohematology Center	● 0190U	Red cell antigen (MNS blood group) genotyping (GYPB), gene analysis, *GYPB (glycophorin B [MNS blood group])* introns 1, 5, pseudoexon 3
Navigator IN Sequencing, Grifols Immunohematology Center, Grifols Immunohematology Center	● 0191U	Red cell antigen (Indian blood group) genotyping (IN), gene analysis, *CD44 (CD44 molecule [Indian blood group])* exons 2, 3, 6
Navigator JK Sequencing, Grifols Immunohematology Center, Grifols Immunohematology Center	● 0192U	Red cell antigen (Kidd blood group) genotyping (JK), gene analysis, *SLC14A1 (solute carrier family 14 member 1 [Kidd blood group])* gene promoter, exon 9
Navigator JR Sequencing, Grifols Immunohematology Center, Grifols Immunohematology Center	● 0193U	Red cell antigen (JR blood group) genotyping (JR), gene analysis, *ABCG2 (ATP binding cassette subfamily G member 2 [Junior blood group])* exons 2-26
Navigator KEL Sequencing, Grifols Immunohematology Center, Grifols Immunohematology Center	● 0194U	Red cell antigen (Kell blood group) genotyping (KEL), gene analysis, *KEL (Kell metallo-endopeptidase [Kell blood group])* exon 8
Navigator KLF1 Sequencing, Grifols Immunohematology Center, Grifols Immunohematology Center	● 0195U	*KLF1 (Kruppel-like factor 1),* targeted sequencing (ie, exon 13)
Navigator LU Sequencing, Grifols Immunohematology Center, Grifols Immunohematology Center	● 0196U	Red cell antigen (Lutheran blood group) genotyping (LU), gene analysis, *BCAM (basal cell adhesion molecule [Lutheran blood group])* exon 3
Navigator LW Sequencing, Grifols Immunohematology Center, Grifols Immunohematology Center	● 0197U	Red cell antigen (Landsteiner-Wiener blood group) genotyping (LW), gene analysis, *ICAM4 (intercellular adhesion molecule 4 [Landsteiner-Wiener blood group])* exon 1

Proprietary Name/Clinical Laboratory/Manufacturer	Code	Descriptor
Navigator RHD/CE Sequencing, Grifols Immunohematology Center, Grifols Immunohematology Center	● 0198U	Red cell antigen (RH blood group) genotyping (RHD and RHCE), gene analysis Sanger/chain termination/conventional sequencing, *RHD (Rh blood group D antigen)* exons 1-10 and *RHCE (Rh blood group CcEe antigens)* exon 5
Navigator SC Sequencing, Grifols Immunohematology Center, Grifols Immunohematology Center	● 0199U	Red cell antigen (Scianna blood group) genotyping (SC), gene analysis, *ERMAP (erythroblast membrane associated protein [Scianna blood group])* exons 4, 12
Navigator XK Sequencing, Grifols Immunohematology Center, Grifols Immunohematology Center	● 0200U	Red cell antigen (Kx blood group) genotyping (XK), gene analysis, *XK (X-linked Kx blood group)* exons 1-3
Navigator YT Sequencing, Grifols Immunohematology Center, Grifols Immunohematology Center	● 0201U	Red cell antigen (Yt blood group) genotyping (YT), gene analysis, *ACHE (acetylcholinesterase [Cartwright blood group])* exon 2
BioFire® Respiratory Panel 2.1 (RP2.1), BioFire® Diagnostics, BioFire® Diagnostics, LLC QIAstat-Dx Respiratory SARS CoV-2 Panel, QIAGEN Sciences, QIAGEN GmbH. To report, see (~0223U)	● 0202U	Infectious disease (bacterial or viral respiratory tract infection), pathogen-specific nucleic acid (DNA or RNA), 22 targets including severe acute respiratory syndrome coronavirus 2 (SARS-CoV-2), qualitative RT-PCR, nasopharyngeal swab, each pathogen reported as detected or not detected
PredictSURE IBD™ Test, KSL Diagnostics, PredictImmune Ltd	● 0203U	Autoimmune (inflammatory bowel disease), mRNA, gene expression profiling by quantitative RT-PCR, 17 genes (15 target and 2 reference genes), whole blood, reported as a continuous risk score and classification of inflammatory bowel disease aggressiveness
Afirma Xpression Atlas, Veracyte, Inc, Veracyte, Inc	● 0204U	Oncology (thyroid), mRNA, gene expression analysis of 593 genes (including *BRAF, RAS, RET, PAX8,* and *NTRK*) for sequence variants and rearrangements, utilizing fine needle aspirate, reported as detected or not detected
Vita Risk®, Arctic Medical Laboratories, Arctic Medical Laboratories	● 0205U	Ophthalmology (age-related macular degeneration), analysis of 3 gene variants (2 *CFH* gene, 1 *ARMS2* gene), using PCR and MALDI-TOF, buccal swab, reported as positive or negative for neovascular age-related macular-degeneration risk associated with zinc supplements
DISCERN™, NeuroDiagnostics, NeuroDiagnostics	● 0206U	Neurology (Alzheimer disease); cell aggregation using morphometric imaging and protein kinase C-epsilon (PKCe) concentration in response to amylospheroid treatment by ELISA, cultured skin fibroblasts, each reported as positive or negative for Alzheimer disease
DISCERN™, NeuroDiagnostics, NeuroDiagnostics	+● 0207U	Neurology (Alzheimer disease); quantitative imaging of phosphorylated *ERK1* and *ERK2* in response to bradykinin treatment by in situ immunofluorescence, using cultured skin fibroblasts, reported as a probability index for Alzheimer disease (List separately in addition to code for primary procedure)
Afirma Medullary Thyroid Carcinoma (MTC) Classifier, Veracyte, Inc, Veracyte, Inc	● 0208U	Oncology (medullary thyroid carcinoma), mRNA, gene expression analysis of 108 genes, utilizing fine needle aspirate, algorithm reported as positive or negative for medullary thyroid carcinoma
CNGnome™, PerkinElmer Genomics, PerkinElmer Genomics	● 0209U	Cytogenomic constitutional (genome-wide) analysis, interrogation of genomic regions for copy number, structural changes and areas of homozygosity for chromosomal abnormalities
BioPlex 2200 RPR Assay - Quantitative, Bio-Rad Laboratories, Bio-Rad Laboratories	● 0210U	Syphilis test, non-treponemal antibody, immunoassay, quantitative (RPR)
MI Cancer Seek™ - NGS Analysis, Caris MPI d/b/a Caris Life Sciences, Caris MPI d/b/a Caris Life Sciences	● 0211U	Oncology (pan-tumor), DNA and RNA by next-generation sequencing, utilizing formalin-fixed paraffin-embedded tissue, interpretative report for single nucleotide variants, copy number alterations, tumor mutational burden, and microsatellite instability, with therapy association
Genomic Unity® Whole Genome Analysis—Proband, Variantyx Inc, Variantyx Inc	● 0212U	Rare diseases (constitutional/heritable disorders), whole genome and mitochondrial DNA sequence analysis, including small sequence changes, deletions, duplications, short tandem repeat gene expansions, and variants in non-uniquely mappable regions, blood or saliva, identification and categorization of genetic variants, proband
Genomic Unity® Whole Genome Analysis - Comparator, Variantyx Inc, Variantyx Inc	● 0213U	Rare diseases (constitutional/heritable disorders), whole genome and mitochondrial DNA sequence analysis, including small sequence changes, deletions, duplications, short tandem repeat gene expansions, and variants in non-uniquely mappable regions, blood or saliva, identification and categorization of genetic variants, each comparator genome (eg, parent, sibling)
Genomic Unity® Exome Plus Analysis - Proband, Variantyx Inc, Variantyx Inc	● 0214U	Rare diseases (constitutional/heritable disorders), whole exome and mitochondrial DNA sequence analysis, including small sequence changes, deletions, duplications, short tandem repeat gene expansions, and variants in non-uniquely mappable regions, blood or saliva, identification and categorization of genetic variants, proband
Genomic Unity® Exome Plus Analysis - Comparator, Variantyx Inc, Variantyx Inc	● 0215U	Rare diseases (constitutional/heritable disorders), whole exome and mitochondrial DNA sequence analysis, including small sequence changes, deletions, duplications, short tandem repeat gene expansions, and variants in non-uniquely mappable regions, blood or saliva, identification and categorization of genetic variants, each comparator exome (eg, parent, sibling)
Genomic Unity® Ataxia Repeat Expansion and Sequence Analysis, Variantyx Inc, Variantyx Inc	● 0216U	Neurology (inherited ataxias), genomic DNA sequence analysis of 12 common genes including small sequence changes, deletions, duplications, short tandem repeat gene expansions, and variants in non-uniquely mappable regions, blood or saliva, identification and categorization of genetic variants

Proprietary Name/Clinical Laboratory/Manufacturer	Code	Descriptor
Genomic Unity® Comprehensive Ataxia Repeat Expansion and Sequence Analysis, Variantyx Inc, Variantyx Inc	● 0217U	Neurology (inherited ataxias), genomic DNA sequence analysis of 51 genes including small sequence changes, deletions, duplications, short tandem repeat gene expansions, and variants in non-uniquely mappable regions, blood or saliva, identification and categorization of genetic variants
Genomic Unity® DMD Analysis, Variantyx Inc, Variantyx Inc	● 0218U	Neurology (muscular dystrophy), *DMD* gene sequence analysis, including small sequence changes, deletions, duplications, and variants in non-uniquely mappable regions, blood or saliva, identification and characterization of genetic variants
Sentosa® SQ HIV-1 Genotyping Assay, Vela Diagnostics USA, Inc, Vela Operations Singapore Pte Ltd	● 0219U	Infectious agent (human immunodeficiency virus), targeted viral next-generation sequence analysis (ie, protease [PR], reverse transcriptase [RT], integrase [INT]), algorithm reported as prediction of antiviral drug susceptibility
PreciseDx™ Breast Cancer Test, PreciseDx, PreciseDx	● 0220U	Oncology (breast cancer), image analysis with artificial intelligence assessment of 12 histologic and immunohistochemical features, reported as a recurrence score
Navigator ABO Blood Group NGS, Grifols Immunohematology Center, Grifols Immunohematology Center	● 0221U	Red cell antigen (ABO blood group) genotyping (ABO), gene analysis, next-generation sequencing, *ABO (ABO, alpha 1-3-N-acetylgalactosaminyltransferase and alpha 1-3-galactosyltransferase)* gene
Navigator Rh Blood Group NGS, Grifols Immunohematology Center, Grifols Immunohematology Center	● 0222U	Red cell antigen (RH blood group) genotyping (RHD and RHCE), gene analysis, next-generation sequencing, RH proximal promoter, exons 1-10, portions of introns 2-3
QIAstat-Dx Respiratory SARS CoV-2 Panel, QIAGEN Sciences, QIAGEN GmbH BioFire® Respiratory Panel 2.1 (RP2.1), BioFire® Diagnostics, BioFire® Diagnostics, LLC. To report, see (~0202U)	● 0223U	Infectious disease (bacterial or viral respiratory tract infection), pathogen-specific nucleic acid (DNA or RNA), 22 targets including severe acute respiratory syndrome coronavirus 2 (SARS-CoV-2), qualitative RT-PCR, nasopharyngeal swab, each pathogen reported as detected or not detected
COVID-19 Antibody Test, Mt Sinai, Mount Sinai Laboratory	● 0224U	Antibody, severe acute respiratory syndrome coronavirus 2 (SARS-CoV-2) (Coronavirus disease [COVID-19]), includes titer(s), when performed
ePlex® Respiratory Pathogen Panel 2, GenMark Dx, GenMark Diagnostics, Inc	● 0225U	Infectious disease (bacterial or viral respiratory tract infection) pathogen-specific DNA and RNA, 21 targets, including severe acute respiratory syndrome coronavirus 2 (SARS-CoV-2), amplified probe technique, including multiplex reverse transcription for RNA targets, each analyte reported as detected or not detected
Tru-Immune™, Ethos Laboratories, GenScript® USA Inc	● 0226U	Surrogate viral neutralization test (sVNT), severe acute respiratory syndrome coronavirus 2 (SARS-CoV-2) (Coronavirus disease [COVID-19]), ELISA, plasma, serum
Comprehensive Screen, Aspenti Health	● 0227U	Drug assay, presumptive, 30 or more drugs or metabolites, urine, liquid chromatography with tandem mass spectrometry (LC-MS/MS) using multiple reaction monitoring (MRM), with drug or metabolite description, includes sample validation
PanGIA Prostate, Genetics Institute of America, Entopsis, LLC	● 0228U	Oncology (prostate), multianalyte molecular profile by photometric detection of macromolecules adsorbed on nanosponge array slides with machine learning, utilizing first morning voided urine, algorithm reported as likelihood of prostate cancer
Colvera®, Clinical Genomic Pathology Inc	● 0229U	*BCAT1 (Branched chain amino acid transaminase 1) or IKZF1 (IKAROS family zinc finger 1)* (eg, colorectal cancer) promoter methylation analysis
Genomic Unity® AR Analysis, Variantyx Inc, Variantyx Inc	● 0230U	*AR (androgen receptor)* (eg, spinal and bulbar muscular atrophy, Kennedy disease, X chromosome inactivation), full sequence analysis, including small sequence changes in exonic and intronic regions, deletions, duplications, short tandem repeat (STR) expansions, mobile element insertions, and variants in non-uniquely mappable regions
Genomic Unity® CACNA1A Analysis, Variantyx Inc, Variantyx Inc	● 0231U	*CACNA1A (calcium voltage-gated channel subunit alpha 1A)* (eg, spinocerebellar ataxia), full gene analysis, including small sequence changes in exonic and intronic regions, deletions, duplications, short tandem repeat (STR) gene expansions, mobile element insertions, and variants in non-uniquely mappable regions
Genomic Unity® CSTB Analysis, Variantyx Inc, Variantyx Inc	● 0232U	*CSTB (cystatin B)* (eg, progressive myoclonic epilepsy type 1A, Unverricht-Lundborg disease), full gene analysis, including small sequence changes in exonic and intronic regions, deletions, duplications, short tandem repeat (STR) expansions, mobile element insertions, and variants in non-uniquely mappable regions
Genomic Unity® FXN Analysis, Variantyx Inc, Variantyx Inc	● 0233U	*FXN (frataxin)* (eg, Friedreich ataxia), gene analysis, including small sequence changes in exonic and intronic regions, deletions, duplications, short tandem repeat (STR) expansions, mobile element insertions, and variants in non-uniquely mappable regions
Genomic Unity® MECP2 Analysis, Variantyx Inc, Variantyx Inc	● 0234U	*MECP2 (methyl CpG binding protein 2)* (eg, Rett syndrome), full gene analysis, including small sequence changes in exonic and intronic regions, deletions, duplications, mobile element insertions, and variants in non-uniquely mappable regions

Proprietary Name/Clinical Laboratory/Manufacturer	Code	Descriptor
Genomic Unity® PTEN Analysis, Variantyx Inc, Variantyx Inc	● 0235U	*PTEN (phosphatase and tensin homolog)* (eg, Cowden syndrome, PTEN hamartoma tumor syndrome), full gene analysis, including small sequence changes in exonic and intronic regions, deletions, duplications, mobile element insertions, and variants in non-uniquely mappable regions
Genomic Unity® SMN1/2 Analysis, Variantyx Inc, Variantyx Inc	● 0236U	*SMN1 (survival of motor neuron 1, telomeric)* and *SMN2 (survival of motor neuron 2, centromeric)* (eg, spinal muscular atrophy) full gene analysis, including small sequence changes in exonic and intronic regions, duplications and deletions, and mobile element insertions
Genomic Unity® Cardiac Ion Channelopathies Analysis, Variantyx Inc, Variantyx Inc	● 0237U	Cardiac ion channelopathies (eg, Brugada syndrome, long QT syndrome, short QT syndrome, catecholaminergic polymorphic ventricular tachycardia), genomic sequence analysis panel including *ANK2, CASQ2, CAV3, KCNE1, KCNE2, KCNH2, KCNJ2, KCNQ1, RYR2,* and *SCN5A,* including small sequence changes in exonic and intronic regions, deletions, duplications, mobile element insertions, and variants in non-uniquely mappable regions
Genomic Unity® Lynch Syndrome Analysis, Variantyx Inc, Variantyx Inc	● 0238U	Oncology (Lynch syndrome), genomic DNA sequence analysis of *MLH1, MSH2, MSH6, PMS2,* and *EPCAM,* including small sequence changes in exonic and intronic regions, deletions, duplications, mobile element insertions, and variants in non-uniquely mappable regions
FoundationOne® Liquid CDx, FOUNDATION MEDICINE, INC, FOUNDATION MEDICINE, INC	● 0239U	Targeted genomic sequence analysis panel, solid organ neoplasm, cell-free DNA, analysis of 311 or more genes, interrogation for sequence variants, including substitutions, insertions, deletions, select rearrangements, and copy number variations
Xpert® Xpress SARS-CoV-2/Flu/RSV (SARS-CoV-2 & Flu targets only), Cepheid	● 0240U	Infectious disease (viral respiratory tract infection), pathogen-specific RNA, 3 targets (severe acute respiratory syndrome coronavirus 2 [SARS-CoV-2], influenza A, influenza B), upper respiratory specimen, each pathogen reported as detected or not detected
Xpert® Xpress SARS-CoV-2/Flu/RSV (all targets), Cepheid	● 0241U	Infectious disease (viral respiratory tract infection), pathogen-specific RNA, 4 targets (severe acute respiratory syndrome coronavirus 2 [SARS-CoV-2], influenza A, influenza B, respiratory syncytial virus [RSV]), upper respiratory specimen, each pathogen reported as detected or not detected

Appendix M — Glossary

-centesis. Puncture, as with a needle, trocar, or aspirator; often done for withdrawing fluid from a cavity.

-ectomy. Excision, removal.

-orrhaphy. Suturing.

-ostomy. Indicates a surgically created artificial opening.

-otomy. Making an incision or opening.

-plasty. Indicates surgically formed or molded.

abdominal lymphadenectomy. Surgical removal of the abdominal lymph nodes grouping, with or without para-aortic and vena cava nodes.

ablation. Removal or destruction of a body part or tissue or its function. Ablation may be performed by surgical means, hormones, drugs, radiofrequency, heat, chemical application, or other methods.

abnormal alleles. Form of gene that includes disease-related variations.

absorbable sutures. Strands prepared from collagen or a synthetic polymer and capable of being absorbed by tissue over time. Examples include surgical gut and collagen sutures; or synthetics like polydioxanone (PDS), polyglactin 910 (Vicryl), poliglecaprone 25 (Monocryl), polyglyconate (Maxon), and polyglycolic acid (Dexon).

acetabuloplasty. Surgical repair or reconstruction of the large cup-shaped socket in the hipbone (acetabulum) with which the head of the femur articulates.

Achilles tendon. Tendon attached to the back of the heel bone (calcaneus) that flexes the foot downward.

acromioclavicular joint. Junction between the clavicle and the scapula. The acromion is the projection from the back of the scapula that forms the highest point of the shoulder and connects with the clavicle. Trauma or injury to the acromioclavicular joint is often referred to as a dislocation of the shoulder. This is not correct, however, as a dislocation of the shoulder is a disruption of the glenohumeral joint.

acromionectomy. Surgical treatment for acromioclavicular arthritis in which the distal portion of the acromion process is removed.

acromioplasty. Repair of the part of the shoulder blade that connects to the deltoid muscles and clavicle.

actigraphy. Science of monitoring activity levels, particularly during sleep. In most cases, the patient wears a wristband that records motion while sleeping. The data are recorded, analyzed, and interpreted to study sleep/wake patterns and circadian rhythms.

air conduction. Transportation of sound from the air, through the external auditory canal, to the tympanic membrane and ossicular chain. Air conduction hearing is tested by presenting an acoustic stimulus through earphones or a loudspeaker to the ear.

air puff device. Instrument that measures intraocular pressure by evaluating the force of a reflected amount of air blown against the cornea.

alleles. Form of gene usually arising from a mutation responsible for a hereditary variation.

allogeneic collection. Collection of blood or blood components from one person for the use of another. Allogeneic collection was formerly termed homologous collection.

allograft. Graft from one individual to another of the same species.

amniocentesis. Surgical puncture through the abdominal wall, with a specialized needle and under ultrasonic guidance, into the interior of the pregnant uterus and directly into the amniotic sac to collect fluid for diagnostic analysis or therapeutic reduction of fluid levels.

anastomosis. Surgically created connection between ducts, blood vessels, or bowel segments to allow flow from one to the other.

anesthesia time. Time period factored into anesthesia procedures beginning with the anesthesiologist preparing the patient for surgery and ending when the patient is turned over to the recovery department.

Angelman syndrome. Early childhood emergence of a pattern of interrupted development, stiff, jerky gait, absence or impairment of speech, excessive laughter, and seizures.

angioplasty. Reconstruction or repair of a diseased or damaged blood vessel.

annuloplasty. Surgical plication of weakened tissue of the heart, to improve its muscular function. Annuli are thick, fibrous rings and one is found surrounding each of the cardiac chambers. The atrial and ventricular muscle fibers attach to the annuli. In annuloplasty, weakened annuli may be surgically plicated, or tucked, to improve muscular functions.

anorectal anometry. Measurement of pressure generated by anal sphincter to diagnose incontinence.

anterior chamber lenses. Lenses inserted into the anterior chamber following intracapsular cataract extraction.

applanation tonometer. Instrument that measures intraocular pressure by recording the force required to flatten an area of the cornea.

appropriateness of care. Proper setting of medical care that best meets the patient's care or diagnosis, as defined by a health care plan or other legal entity.

aqueous humor. Fluid within the anterior and posterior chambers of the eye that is continually replenished as it diffuses out into the blood. When the flow of aqueous is blocked, a build-up of fluid in the eye causes increased intraocular pressure and leads to glaucoma and blindness.

arteriogram. Radiograph of arteries.

arteriovenous fistula. Connecting passage between an artery and a vein.

arteriovenous malformation. Connecting passage between an artery and a vein.

arthrotomy. Surgical incision into a joint that may include exploration, drainage, or removal of a foreign body.

ASA. 1) Acetylsalicylic acid. Synonym(s): aspirin. 2) American Society of Anesthesiologists. National organization for anesthesiology that maintains and publishes the guidelines and relative values for anesthesia coding.

aspirate. To withdraw fluid or air from a body cavity by suction.

assay. Chemical analysis of a substance to establish the presence and strength of its components. A therapeutic drug assay is used to determine if a drug is within the expected therapeutic range for a patient.

atrial septal defect. Cardiac anomaly consisting of a patent opening in the atrial septum due to a fusion failure, classified as ostium secundum type, ostium primum defect, or endocardial cushion defect.

attended surveillance. Ability of a technician at a remote surveillance center or location to respond immediately to patient transmissions regarding rhythm or device alerts as they are produced and received at the remote location. These transmissions may originate from wearable or implanted therapy or monitoring devices.

auricle. External ear, which is a single elastic cartilage covered in skin and normal adnexal features (hair follicles, sweat glands, and sebaceous glands), shaped to channel sound waves into the acoustic meatus.

autogenous transplant. Tissue, such as bone, that is harvested from the patient and used for transplantation back into the same patient.

autograft. Any tissue harvested from one anatomical site of a person and grafted to another anatomical site of the same person. Most commonly, blood vessels, skin, tendons, fascia, and bone are used as autografts.

autologous. Tissue, cells, or structure obtained from the same individual.

AVF. Arteriovenous fistula.

AVM. Arteriovenous malformation. Clusters of abnormal blood vessels that grow in the brain comprised of a blood vessel "nidus" or nest through which arteries and veins connect directly without going through the capillaries. As time passes, the nidus may enlarge resulting in the formation of a mass that may bleed. AVMs are more prone to bleeding in patients ages 10 to 55. Once older than age 55, the possibility of bleeding is reduced dramatically.

backbench preparation. Procedures performed on a donor organ following procurement to prepare the organ for transplant into the recipient. Excess fat and other tissue may be removed, the organ may be perfused, and vital arteries may be sized, repaired, or modified to fit the patient. These procedures are done on a back table in the operating room before transplantation can begin.

Bartholin's gland. Mucous-producing gland found in the vestibular bulbs on either side of the vaginal orifice and connected to the mucosal membrane at the opening by a duct.

Bartholin's gland abscess. Pocket of pus and surrounding cellulitis caused by infection of the Bartholin's gland and causing localized swelling and pain in the posterior labia majora that may extend into the lower vagina.

basic value. Relative weighted value based upon the usual anesthesia services and the relative work or cost of the specific anesthesia service assigned to each anesthesia-specific procedure code.

Berman locator. Small, sensitive tool used to detect the location of a metallic foreign body in the eye.

bifurcated. Having two branches or divisions, such as the left pulmonary veins that split off from the left atrium to carry oxygenated blood away from the heart.

Billroth's operation. Anastomosis of the stomach to the duodenum or jejunum.

bioprosthetic heart valve. Replacement cardiac valve made of biological tissue. Allograft, xenograft or engineered tissue.

biopsy. Tissue or fluid removed for diagnostic purposes through analysis of the cells in the biopsy material.

Blalock-Hanlon procedure. Atrial septectomy procedure to allow free mixing of the blood from the right and left atria.

Blalock-Taussig procedure. Anastomosis of the left subclavian artery to the left pulmonary artery or the right subclavian artery to the right pulmonary artery in order to shunt some of the blood flow from the systemic to the pulmonary circulation.

blepharochalasis. Loss of elasticity and relaxation of skin of the eyelid, thickened or indurated skin on the eyelid associated with recurrent episodes of edema, and intracellular atrophy.

blepharoplasty. Plastic surgery of the eyelids to remove excess fat and redundant skin weighting down the lid. The eyelid is pulled tight and sutured to support sagging muscles.

blepharoptosis. Droop or displacement of the upper eyelid, caused by paralysis, muscle problems, or outside mechanical forces.

blepharorrhaphy. Suture of a portion or all of the opposing eyelids to shorten the palpebral fissure or close it entirely.

bone conduction. Transportation of sound through the bones of the skull to the inner ear.

bone mass measurement. Radiologic or radioisotopic procedure or other procedure approved by the FDA for identifying bone mass, detecting bone loss, or determining bone quality. The procedure includes a physician's interpretation of the results. Qualifying individuals must be an estrogen-deficient woman at clinical risk for osteoporosis with vertebral abnormalities.

brachytherapy. Form of radiation therapy in which radioactive pellets or seeds are implanted directly into the tissue being treated to deliver their dose of radiation in a more directed fashion. Brachytherapy provides radiation to the prescribed body area while minimizing exposure to normal tissue.

breakpoint. Point at which a chromosome breaks.

Bristow procedure. Anterior capsulorrhaphy prevents chronic separation of the shoulder. In this procedure, the bone block is affixed to the anterior glenoid rim with a screw.

buccal mucosa. Tissue from the mucous membrane on the inside of the cheek.

bundle of His. Bundle of modified cardiac fibers that begins at the atrioventricular node and passes through the right atrioventricular fibrous ring to the interventricular septum, where it divides into two branches. Bundle of His recordings are taken for intracardiac electrograms.

Caldwell-Luc operation. Intraoral antrostomy approach into the maxillary sinus for the removal of tooth roots or tissue, or for packing the sinus to reduce zygomatic fractures by creating a window above the teeth in the canine fossa area.

canthorrhaphy. Suturing of the palpebral fissure, the juncture between the eyelids, at either end of the eye.

canthotomy. Horizontal incision at the canthus (junction of upper and lower eyelids) to divide the outer canthus and enlarge lid margin separation.

cardio-. Relating to the heart.

cardiopulmonary bypass. Venous blood is diverted to a heart-lung machine, which mechanically pumps and oxygenates the blood temporarily so the heart can be bypassed while an open procedure on the heart or coronary arteries is performed. During bypass, the lungs are deflated and immobile.

cardioverter-defibrillator. Device that uses both low energy cardioversion or defibrillating shocks and antitachycardia pacing to treat ventricular tachycardia or ventricular fibrillation.

care plan oversight services. Physician's ongoing review and revision of a patient's care plan involving complex or multidisciplinary care modalities.

case management services. Physician case management is a process of involving direct patient care as well as coordinating and controlling access to the patient or initiating and/or supervising other necessary health care services.

cataract extraction. Surgical removal of the cataract or cloudy lens. Anterior chamber lenses are inserted in conjunction with intracapsular cataract extraction and posterior chamber lenses are inserted in conjunction with extracapsular cataract extraction.

catheter. Flexible tube inserted into an area of the body for introducing or withdrawing fluid.

Centers for Medicare and Medicaid Services. Federal agency that oversees the administration of the public health programs such as Medicare, Medicaid, and State Children's Insurance Program.

certified nurse midwife. Registered nurse who has successfully completed a program of study and clinical experience or has been certified by a recognized organization for the care of pregnant or delivering patients.

CFR. Code of Federal Regulations.

CGMS. Continuous glucose monitoring system.

CHAMPUS. Civilian Health and Medical Program of the Uniformed Services. See Tricare.

CHAMPVA. Civilian Health and Medical Program of the Department of Veterans Affairs.

chemodenervation. Chemical destruction of nerves. A substance, for example, Botox, is used to temporarily inhibit the transfer of chemicals at the presynaptic membrane, blocking the neuromuscular junctions.

chemoembolization. Administration of chemotherapeutic agents directly to a tumor in combination with the percutaneous administration of an occlusive substance into a vessel to deprive the tumor of its blood supply. This ensures a prolonged level of therapy directed at the tumor. Chemoembolization is primarily being used for cancers of the liver and endocrine system.

chemosurgery. Application of chemical agents to destroy tissue, originally referring to the in situ chemical fixation of premalignant or malignant lesions to facilitate surgical excision.

Chiari osteotomy. Top of the femur is altered to correct a dislocated hip caused by congenital conditions or cerebral palsy. Plate and screws are often used.

chimera. Organ or anatomic structure consisting of tissues of diverse genetic constitution.

choanal atresia. Congenital, membranous, or bony closure of one or both posterior nostrils due to failure of the embryonic bucconasal membrane to rupture and open up the nasal passageway.

chondromalacia. Condition in which the articular cartilage softens, seen in various body sites but most often in the patella, and may be congenital or acquired.

chorionic villus sampling. Aspiration of a placental sample through a catheter, under ultrasonic guidance. The specialized needle is placed transvaginally through the cervix or transabdominally into the uterine cavity.

chronic pain management services. Distinct services frequently performed by anesthesiologists who have additional training in pain management procedures. Pain management services include initial and subsequent evaluation and management (E/M) services, trigger point injections, spine and spinal cord injections, and nerve blocks.

cineplastic amputation. Amputation in which muscles and tendons of the remaining portion of the extremity are arranged so that they may be utilized for motor functions. Following this type of amputation, a specially constructed prosthetic device allows the individual to execute more complex movements because the muscles and tendons are able to communicate independent movements to the device.

circadian. Relating to a cyclic, 24-hour period.

CLIA. Clinical Laboratory Improvement Amendments. Requirements set in 1988, CLIA imposes varying levels of federal regulations on clinical procedures. Few laboratories, including those in physician offices, are exempt. Adopted by Medicare and Medicaid, CLIA regulations redefine laboratory testing in regard to laboratory certification and accreditation, proficiency testing, quality assurance, personnel standards, and program administration.

clinical social worker. Individual who possesses a master's or doctor's degree in social work and, after obtaining the degree, has performed at least two years of supervised clinical social work. A clinical social worker must be licensed by the state or, in the case of states without licensure, must completed at least two years or 3,000 hours of post-master's degree supervised clinical social work practice under the supervision of a master's level social worker.

clinical staff. Someone who works for, or under, the direction of a physician or qualified health care professional and does not bill services separately. The person may be licensed or regulated to help the physician perform specific duties.

clonal. Originating from one cell.

CMS. Centers for Medicare and Medicaid Services. Federal agency that administers the public health programs.

CO_2 laser. Carbon dioxide laser that emits an invisible beam and vaporizes water-rich tissue. The vapor is suctioned from the site.

codons. Series of three adjoining bases in one polynucleotide chain of a DNA or RNA molecule that provides the codes for a specific amino acid.

cognitive. Being aware by drawing from knowledge, such as judgment, reason, perception, and memory.

colostomy. Artificial surgical opening anywhere along the length of the colon to the skin surface for the diversion of feces.

commissurotomy. Surgical division or disruption of any two parts that are joined to form a commissure in order to increase the opening. The procedure most often refers to opening the adherent leaflet bands of fibrous tissue in a stenosed mitral valve.

common variants. Nucleotide sequence differences associated with abnormal gene function. Tests are usually performed in a single series of laboratory testing (in a single, typically multiplex, assay arrangement or using more than one assay to include all variants to be examined). Variants are representative of a mutation that mainly causes a single disease, such as cystic fibrosis. Other uncommon variants could provide additional information. Tests may be performed based on society recommendations and guidelines.

community mental health center. Facility providing outpatient mental health day treatment, assessments, and education as appropriate to community members.

component code. In the National Correct Coding Initiative (NCCI), the column II code that cannot be charged to Medicare when the column I code is reported.

comprehensive code. In the National Correct Coding Initiative (NCCI), the column I code that is reported to Medicare and precludes reporting column II codes.

computerized corneal topography. Digital imaging and analysis by computer of the shape of the corneal.

conjunctiva. Mucous membrane lining of the eyelids and covering of the exposed, anterior sclera.

conjunctivodacryocystostomy. Surgical connection of the lacrimal sac directly to the conjunctival sac.

conjunctivorhinostomy. Correction of an obstruction of the lacrimal canal achieved by suturing the posterior flaps and removing any lacrimal obstruction, preserving the conjunctiva.

constitutional. Cells containing genetic code that may be passed down to future generations. May also be referred to as germline.

consultation. Advice or opinion regarding diagnosis and treatment or determination to accept transfer of care of a patient rendered by a medical professional at the request of the primary care provider.

continuous positive airway pressure device. Pressurized device used to maintain the patient's airway for spontaneous or mechanically aided breathing. Often used for patients with mild to moderate sleep apnea.

core needle biopsy. Large-bore biopsy needle inserted into a mass and a core of tissue is removed for diagnostic study.

corpectomy. Removal of the body of a bone, such as a vertebra.

costochondral. Pertaining to the ribs and the scapula.

COTD. Cardiac output thermodilution. Cardiac output measured by thermodilution method that requires heart catheterization and then injection of a thermal indicator, usually iced saline. A computer calculates the cardiac output using an equation that incorporates body temperature, injectate volume and temperature, time, and other calculated ratios over a denominator of the integral of the change in blood temperature during the cold injection, reflected by the area of the inscribed curve.

CPT. 1) Chest physical therapy. 2) Cold pressor test. 3) Current Procedural Terminology.

craniosynostosis. Congenital condition in which one or more of the cranial sutures fuse prematurely, creating a deformed or aberrant head shape.

craterization. Excision of a portion of bone creating a crater-like depression to facilitate drainage from infected areas of bone.

cricoid. Circular cartilage around the trachea.

CRNA. Certified registered nurse anesthetist. Nurse trained and specializing in the administration of anesthesia.

cryolathe. Tool used for reshaping a button of corneal tissue.

cryosurgery. Application of intense cold, usually produced using liquid nitrogen, to locally freeze diseased or unwanted tissue and induce tissue necrosis without causing harm to adjacent tissue.

CT. Computed tomography.

cutdown. Small, incised opening in the skin to expose a blood vessel, especially over a vein (venous cutdown) to allow venipuncture and permit a needle or cannula to be inserted for the withdrawal of blood or administration of fluids.

cyclophotocoagulation. Procedure done to prevent vision loss from glaucoma in which a neodymium: YAG laser is used to burn and destroy a portion of the ciliary body in order to decrease the amount of aqueous humor being produced in the eye. This procedure is only done when creating a drain for aqueous humor to reduce intraocular pressure would not be successful. Destroying portions of the ciliary body reduces the amount of fluid present in the eye.

cytogenetic studies. Procedures in CPT that are related to the branch of genetics that studies cellular (cyto) structure and function as it relates to heredity (genetics). White blood cells, specifically T-lymphocytes, are the most commonly used specimen for chromosome analysis.

cytogenomic. Chromosomic evaluation using molecular methods.

dacryocystotome. Instrument used for incising the lacrimal duct strictures.

DBS. Deep brain stimulation. Treatment for disabling neurological symptoms associated with diseases including Parkinson's. DBS requires three components: the implanted electrode, extension, and neurostimulator. Electrical impulses are sent from the neurostimulator to the implant to block tremors.

debride. To remove all foreign objects and devitalized or infected tissue from a burn or wound to prevent infection and promote healing.

definitive drug testing. Drug tests used to further analyze or confirm the presence or absence of specific drugs or classes of drugs used by the patient. These tests are able to provide more conclusive information regarding the concentration of the drug and their metabolites. May be used for medical, workplace, or legal purposes.

definitive identification. Identification of microorganisms using additional tests to specify the genus or species (e.g., slide cultures or biochemical panels).

dentoalveolar structure. Area of alveolar bone surrounding the teeth and adjacent tissue.

Department of Health and Human Services. Cabinet department that oversees the operating divisions of the federal government responsible for health and welfare. HHS oversees the Centers for Medicare and Medicaid Services, Food and Drug Administration, Public Health Service, and other such entities.

Department of Justice. Attorneys from the DOJ and the United States Attorney's Office have, under the memorandum of understanding, the same direct access to contractor data and records as the OIG and the Federal Bureau of Investigation (FBI). DOJ is responsible for prosecution of fraud and civil or criminal cases presented.

dermis. Skin layer found under the epidermis that contains a papillary upper layer and the deep reticular layer of collagen, vascular bed, and nerves.

dermis graft. Skin graft that has been separated from the epidermal tissue and the underlying subcutaneous fat, used primarily as a substitute for fascia grafts in plastic surgery.

desensitization. 1) Administration of extracts of allergens periodically to build immunity in the patient. 2) Application of medication to decrease the symptoms, usually pain, associated with a dental condition or disease.

destruction. Ablation or eradication of a structure or tissue.

diabetes outpatient self-management training services. Educational and training services furnished by a certified provider in an outpatient setting. The physician managing the individual's diabetic condition must certify that the services are needed under a comprehensive plan of care and provide the patient with the skills and knowledge necessary for therapeutic program compliance (including skills related to the self-administration of injectable drugs). The provider must meet applicable standards established by the National Diabetes Advisory or be recognized by an organization that represents individuals with diabetes as meeting standards for furnishing the services.

diagnostic procedures. Procedure performed on a patient to obtain information to assess the medical condition of the patient or to identify a disease and to determine the nature and severity of an illness or injury.

dialysis. Artificial filtering of the blood to remove contaminating waste elements and restore normal balance.

diaphragm. 1) Muscular wall separating the thorax and its structures from the abdomen. 2) Flexible disk inserted into the vagina and against the cervix as a method of birth control.

diaphysectomy. Surgical removal of a portion of the shaft of a long bone, often done to facilitate drainage from infected bone.

diathermy. Applying heat to body tissues by various methods for therapeutic treatment or surgical purposes to coagulate and seal tissue.

dilation. Artificial increase in the diameter of an opening or lumen made by medication or by instrumentation.

dissect. Cut apart or separate tissue for surgical purposes or for visual or microscopic study.

DNA. Deoxyribonucleic acid. Chemical containing the genetic information necessary to produce and propagate living organisms. Molecules are comprised of two twisting paired strands, called a double helix.

DNA marker. Specific gene sequence within a chromosome indicating the inheritance of a certain trait.

dorsal. Pertaining to the back or posterior aspect.

drugs and biologicals. Drugs and biologicals included - or approved for inclusion - in the United States Pharmacopoeia, the National Formulary, the United States Homeopathic Pharmacopoeia, in New Drugs or Accepted Dental Remedies, or approved by the pharmacy and drug therapeutics committee of the medical staff of the hospital. Also included are medically accepted and FDA approved drugs used in an anticancer chemotherapeutic regimen. The carrier determines medical acceptance based on supportive clinical evidence.

dual-lead device. Implantable cardiac device (pacemaker or implantable cardioverter-defibrillator [ICD]) in which pacing and sensing components are placed in only two chambers of the heart.

duplex scan. Noninvasive vascular diagnostic technique that uses ultrasonic scanning to identify the pattern and direction of blood flow within arteries or veins displayed in real time images. Duplex scanning combines B-mode two-dimensional pictures of the vessel structure with spectra and/or color flow Doppler mapping or imaging of the blood as it moves through the vessels.

duplication/deletion (DUP/DEL). Term used in molecular testing which examines genomic regions to determine if there are extra chromosomes (duplication) or missing chromosomes (deletions). Normal gene dosage is two copies per cell except for the sex chromosomes which have one per cell.

DuToit staple capsulorrhaphy. Reattachment of the capsule of the shoulder and glenoid labrum to the glenoid lip using staples to anchor the avulsed capsule and glenoid labrum.

Dx. Diagnosis.

DXA. Dual energy x-ray absorptiometry. Radiological technique for bone density measurement using a two-dimensional projection system in which two x-ray beams with different levels of energy are pulsed alternately and the results are given in two scores, reported as standard deviations from peak bone mass density.

dynamic mutation. Unstable or changing polynucleotides resulting in repeats related to genes that can undergo disease-producing increases or decreases in the repeats that differ within tissues or over generations.

ECMO. Extracorporeal membrane oxygenation.

ectropion. Drooping of the lower eyelid away from the eye or outward turning or eversion of the edge of the eyelid, exposing the palpebral conjunctiva and causing irritation.

Eden-Hybinette procedure. Anterior shoulder repair using an anterior bone block to augment the bony anterior glenoid lip.

EDTA. Drug used to inhibit damage to the cornea by collagenase. EDTA is especially effective in alkali burns as it neutralizes soluble alkali, including lye.

effusion. Escape of fluid from within a body cavity.

electrocardiographic rhythm derived. Analysis of data obtained from readings of the heart's electrical activation, including heart rate and rhythm, variability of heart rate, ST analysis, and T-wave alternans. Other data may also be assessed when warranted.

electrocautery. Division or cutting of tissue using high-frequency electrical current to produce heat, which destroys cells.

electrode array. Electronic device containing more than one contact whose function can be adjusted during programming services. Electrodes are specialized for a particular electrochemical reaction that acts as a medium between a body surface and another instrument.

electromyography. Test that measures muscle response to nerve stimulation determining if muscle weakness is present and if it is related to the muscles themselves or a problem with the nerves that supply the muscles.

electrooculogram (EOG). Record of electrical activity associated with eye movements.

electrophysiologic studies. Electrical stimulation and monitoring to diagnose heart conduction abnormalities that predispose patients to bradyarrhythmias and to determine a patient's chance for developing ventricular and supraventricular tachyarrhythmias.

embolization. Placement of a clotting agent, such as a coil, plastic particles, gel, foam, etc., into an area of hemorrhage to stop the bleeding or to block blood flow to a problem area, such as an aneurysm or a tumor.

emergency. Serious medical condition or symptom (including severe pain) resulting from injury, sickness, or mental illness that arises suddenly and requires immediate care and treatment, generally received within 24 hours of onset, to avoid jeopardy to the life, limb, or health of a covered person.

empyema. Accumulation of pus within the respiratory, or pleural, cavity.

EMTALA. Emergency Medical Treatment and Active Labor Act.

end-stage renal disease. Chronic, advanced kidney disease requiring renal dialysis or a kidney transplant to prevent imminent death.

endarterectomy. Removal of the thickened, endothelial lining of a diseased or damaged artery.

endomicroscopy. Diagnostic technology that allows for the examination of tissue at the cellular level during endoscopy. The technology decreases the need for biopsy with histological examination for some types of lesions.

endovascular embolization. Procedure whereby vessels are occluded by a variety of therapeutic substances for the treatment of abnormal blood vessels by inhibiting the flow of blood to a tumor, arteriovenous malformations, lymphatic malformation, and to prevent or stop hemorrhage.

entropion. Inversion of the eyelid, turning the edge in toward the eyeball and causing irritation from contact of the lashes with the surface of the eye.

enucleation. Removal of a growth or organ cleanly so as to extract it in one piece.

epidermis. Outermost, nonvascular layer of skin that contains four to five differentiated layers depending on its body location: stratum corneum, lucidum, granulosum, spinosum, and basale.

epiphysiodesis. Surgical fusion of an epiphysis performed to prematurely stop further bone growth.

escharotomy. Surgical incision into the scab or crust resulting from a severe burn in order to relieve constriction and allow blood flow to the distal unburned tissue.

established patient. 1) Patient who has received professional services in a face-to-face setting within the last three years from the same physician/qualified health care professional or another physician/qualified health care professional of the exact same specialty and subspecialty who belongs to the same group practice. 2) For OPPS hospitals, patient who has been registered as an inpatient or outpatient in a hospital's provider-based clinic or emergency department within the past three years.

evacuation. Removal or purging of waste material.

evaluation and management codes. Assessment and management of a patient's health care.

evaluation and management service components. Key components of history, examination, and medical decision making that are key to selecting the correct E/M codes. Other non-key components include counseling, coordination of care, nature of presenting problem, and time.

event recorder. Portable, ambulatory heart monitor worn by the patient that makes electrocardiographic recordings of the length and frequency of aberrant cardiac rhythm to help diagnose heart conditions and to assess pacemaker functioning or programming.

exenteration. Surgical removal of the entire contents of a body cavity, such as the pelvis or orbit.

exon. One of multiple nucleic acid sequences used to encode information for a gene polypeptide or protein. Exons are separated from other exons by non-protein-coding sequences known as introns.

extended care services. Items and services provided to an inpatient of a skilled nursing facility, including nursing care, physical or occupational therapy, speech pathology, drugs and supplies, and medical social services.

external electrical capacitor device. External electrical stimulation device designed to promote bone healing. This device may also promote neural regeneration, revascularization, epiphyseal growth, and ligament maturation.

external pulsating electromagnetic field. External stimulation device designed to promote bone healing. This device may also promote neural regeneration, revascularization, epiphyseal growth, and ligament maturation.

extracorporeal. Located or taking place outside the body.

Eyre-Brook capsulorrhaphy. Reattachment of the capsule of the shoulder and glenoid labrum to the glenoid lip.

False Claims Act. Governs civil actions for filing false claims. Liability under this act pertains to any person who knowingly presents or causes to be presented a false or fraudulent claim to the government for payment or approval.

fascia. Fibrous sheet or band of tissue that envelops organs, muscles, and groupings of muscles.

fasciectomy. Excision of fascia or strips of fascial tissue.

fasciotomy. Incision or transection of fascial tissue.

fat graft. Graft composed of fatty tissue completely freed from surrounding tissue that is used primarily to fill in depressions.

FDA. Food and Drug Administration. Federal agency responsible for protecting public health by substantiating the safety, efficacy, and security of human and veterinary drugs, biological products, medical devices, national food supply, cosmetics, and items that give off radiation.

filtered speech test. Test most commonly used to identify central auditory dysfunction in which the patient is presented monosyllabic words that are low pass filtered, allowing only the parts of each word below a certain pitch to be presented. A score is given on the number of correct responses. This may be a subset of a standard battery of tests provided during a single encounter.

fissure. Deep furrow, groove, or cleft in tissue structures.

fistulization. Creation of a communication between two structures that were not previously connected.

flexor digitorum profundus tendon. Tendon originating in the proximal forearm and extending to the index finger and wrist. A thickened FDP sheath, usually caused by age, illness, or injury, can fill the carpal canal and lead to impingement of the median nerve.

fluoroscopy. Radiology technique that allows visual examination of part of the body or a function of an organ using a device that projects an x-ray image on a fluorescent screen.

focal length. Distance between the object in focus and the lens.

focused medical review. Process of targeting and directing medical review efforts on Medicare claims where the greatest risk of inappropriate program payment exists. The goal is to reduce the number of noncovered claims or unnecessary services. CMS analyzes national data such as internal billing, utilization, and payment data and provides its findings to the FI. Local medical review policies are developed identifying aberrances, abuse, and overutilized services. Providers are responsible for knowing national Medicare coverage and billing guidelines and local medical review policies, and for determining whether the services provided to Medicare beneficiaries are covered by Medicare.

fragile X syndrome. Intellectual disabilities, enlarged testes, big jaw, high forehead, and long ears in males. In females, fragile X presents with mild intellectual disabilities and heterozygous sexual structures. In some families, males have shown no symptoms but carry the gene.

free flap. Tissue that is completely detached from the donor site and transplanted to the recipient site, receiving its blood supply from capillary ingrowth at the recipient site.

free microvascular flap. Tissue that is completely detached from the donor site following careful dissection and preservation of the blood vessels, then attached to the recipient site with the transferred blood vessels anastomosed to the vessels in the recipient bed.

fulguration. Destruction of living tissue by using sparks from a high-frequency electric current.

gas tamponade. Absorbable gas may be injected to force the retina against the choroid. Common gases include room air, short-acting sulfahexafluoride, intermediate-acting perfluoroethane, or long-acting perfluorooctane.

Gaucher disease. Genetic metabolic disorder in which fat deposits may accumulate in the spleen, liver, lungs, bone marrow, and brain.

gene. Basic unit of heredity that contains nucleic acid. Genes are arranged in different and unique sequences or strings that determine the gene's function. Human genes usually include multiple protein coding regions such as exons separated by introns which are nonprotein coding sections.

genome. Complete set of DNA of an organism. Each cell in the human body is comprised of a complete copy of the approximately three billion DNA base pairs that constitute the human genome.

habilitative services. Procedures or services provided to assist a patient in learning, keeping, and improving new skills needed to perform daily living activities. Habilitative services assist patients in acquiring a skill for the first time.

HCPCS. Healthcare Common Procedure Coding System.

HCPCS Level I. Healthcare Common Procedure Coding System Level I. Numeric coding system used by physicians, facility outpatient departments, and ambulatory surgery centers (ASC) to code ambulatory, laboratory, radiology, and other diagnostic services for Medicare billing. This coding system contains only the American Medical Association's Physicians' Current Procedural Terminology (CPT) codes. The AMA updates codes annually.

HCPCS Level II. Healthcare Common Procedure Coding System Level II. National coding system, developed by CMS, that contains alphanumeric codes for physician and nonphysician services not included in the CPT coding system. HCPCS Level II covers such things as ambulance services, durable medical equipment, and orthotic and prosthetic devices.

HCPCS modifiers. Two-character code (AA-ZZ) that identifies circumstances that alter or enhance the description of a service or supply. They are recognized by carriers nationally and are updated annually by CMS.

Hct. Hematocrit.

health care provider. Entity that administers diagnostic and therapeutic services.

hemilaminectomy. Excision of a portion of the vertebral lamina.

hemodialysis. Cleansing of wastes and contaminating elements from the blood by virtue of different diffusion rates through a semipermeable membrane, which separates blood from a filtration solution that diffuses other elements out of the blood. The blood is slowly filtered extracorporeally through special dialysis equipment and returned to the body. Synonym(s): renal dialysis.

hemodialysis. Cleansing of wastes and contaminating elements from the blood by virtue of different diffusion rates through a semipermeable membrane, which separates blood from a filtration solution that diffuses other elements out of the blood.

hemoperitoneum. Effusion of blood into the peritoneal cavity, the space between the continuous membrane lining the abdominopelvic walls and encasing the visceral organs.

heterograft. Surgical graft of tissue from one animal species to a different animal species. A common type of heterograft is porcine (pig) tissue, used for temporary wound closure.

heterotopic transplant. Tissue transplanted from a different anatomical site for usage as is natural for that tissue, for example, buccal mucosa to a conjunctival site.

HGNC. HUGO gene nomenclature committee.

HGVS. Human genome variation society.

Hickman catheter. Central venous catheter used for long-term delivery of medications, such as antibiotics, nutritional substances, or chemotherapeutic agents.

HLA. Human leukocyte antigen.

home health services. Services furnished to patients in their homes under the care of physicians. These services include part-time or intermittent skilled nursing care, physical therapy, medical social services, medical supplies, and some rehabilitation equipment. Home health supplies and services must be prescribed by a physician, and the beneficiary must be confined at home in order for Medicare to pay the benefits in full.

homograft. Graft from one individual to another of the same species.

hospice care. Items and services provided to a terminally ill individual by a hospice program under a written plan established and periodically reviewed by the individual's attending physician and by the medical director: Nursing care provided by or under the supervision of a registered professional nurse; Physical or occupational therapy or speech-language pathology services; Medical social services under the direction of a physician; Services of a home health aide who has successfully completed a training program; Medical supplies (including drugs and biologicals) and the use of medical appliances; Physicians' services; Short-term inpatient care (including both respite care and procedures necessary for pain control and acute and chronic symptom management) in an inpatient facility on an intermittent basis and not consecutively over longer than five days; Counseling (including dietary counseling) with respect to care of the terminally ill individual and adjustment to his death; Any item or service which is specified in the plan and for which payment may be made.

hospital. Institution that provides, under the supervision of physicians, diagnostic, therapeutic, and rehabilitation services for medical diagnosis, treatment, and care of patients. Hospitals receiving federal funds must maintain clinical records on all patients, provide 24-hour nursing services, and have a discharge planning process in place. The term "hospital" also includes religious nonmedical health care institutions and facilities of 50 beds or less located in rural areas.

HUGO. Human genome organization

IA. Intra-arterial.

ICD. Implantable cardioverter defibrillator.

ICD-10-CM. International Classification of Diseases, 10th Revision, Clinical Modification. Clinical modification of the alphanumeric classification of diseases used by the World Health Organization, already in use in much of the world, and used for mortality reporting in the United States. The implementation date for ICD-10-CM diagnostic coding system to replace ICD-9-CM in the United States was October 1, 2015.

ICD-10-PCS. International Classification of Diseases, 10th Revision, Procedure Coding System. Beginning October 1, 2015, inpatient hospital services and surgical procedures must be coded using ICD-10-PCS codes, replacing ICD-9-CM, Volume 3 for procedures.

ICM. Implantable cardiovascular monitor.

ileostomy. Artificial surgical opening that brings the end of the ileum out through the abdominal wall to the skin surface for the diversion of feces through a stoma.

iliopsoas tendon. Fibrous tissue that connects muscle to bone in the pelvic region, common to the iliacus and psoas major.

ILR. Implantable loop recorder.

IM. 1) Infectious mononucleosis. 2) Internal medicine. 3) Intramuscular.

immunotherapy. Therapeutic use of serum or gamma globulin.

implant. Material or device inserted or placed within the body for therapeutic, reconstructive, or diagnostic purposes.

implantable cardiovascular monitor. Implantable electronic device that stores cardiovascular physiologic data such as intracardiac pressure waveforms collected from internal sensors or data such as weight and blood pressure collected from external sensors. The information stored in these devices is used as an aid in managing patients with heart failure and other cardiac conditions that are non-rhythm related. The data may be transmitted via local telemetry or remotely to a surveillance technician or an internet-based file server.

implantable cardioverter-defibrillator. Implantable electronic cardiac device used to control rhythm abnormalities such as tachycardia, fibrillation, or bradycardia by producing high- or low-energy stimulation and pacemaker functions. It may also have the capability to provide the functions of an implantable loop recorder or implantable cardiovascular monitor.

implantable loop recorder. Implantable electronic cardiac device that constantly monitors and records electrocardiographic rhythm. It may be triggered by the patient when a symptomatic episode occurs or activated automatically by rapid or slow heart rates. This may be the sole purpose of the device or it may be a component of another cardiac device, such as a pacemaker or implantable cardioverter-defibrillator. The data can be transmitted via local telemetry or remotely to a surveillance technician or an internet-based file server.

implantable venous access device. Catheter implanted for continuous access to the venous system for long-term parenteral feeding or for the administration of fluids or medications.

IMRT. Intensity modulated radiation therapy. External beam radiation therapy delivery using computer planning to specify the target dose and to modulate the radiation intensity, usually as a treatment for a malignancy. The delivery system approaches the patient from multiple angles, minimizing damage to normal tissue.

in situ. Located in the natural position or contained within the origin site, not spread into neighboring tissue.

incontinence. Inability to control urination or defecation.

infundibulectomy. Excision of the anterosuperior portion of the right ventricle of the heart.

internal direct current stimulator. Electrostimulation device placed directly into the surgical site designed to promote bone regeneration by encouraging cellular healing response in bone and ligaments.

interrogation device evaluation. Assessment of an implantable cardiac device (pacemaker, cardioverter-defibrillator, cardiovascular monitor, or loop recorder) in which collected data about the patient's heart rate and rhythm, battery and pulse generator function, and any leads or sensors present, are retrieved and evaluated. Determinations regarding device programming and appropriate treatment settings are made based on the findings. CPT provides required components for evaluation of the various types of devices.

intramedullary implants. Nail, rod, or pin placed into the intramedullary canal at the fracture site. Intramedullary implants not only provide a method of aligning the fracture, they also act as a splint and may reduce fracture pain. Implants may be rigid or flexible. Rigid implants are preferred for prophylactic treatment of diseased bone, while flexible implants are preferred for traumatic injuries.

intraocular lens. Artificial lens implanted into the eye to replace a damaged natural lens or cataract.

intravenous. Within a vein or veins.

introducer. Instrument, such as a catheter, needle, or tube, through which another instrument or device is introduced into the body.

intron. Nonprotein section of a gene that separates exons in human genes. Contains vital sequences that allow splicing of exons to produce a functional protein from a gene. Sometimes referred to as intervening sequences (IVS).

IP. 1) Interphalangeal. 2) Intraperitoneal.

irrigation. To wash out or cleanse a body cavity, wound, or tissue with water or other fluid.

Kayser-Fleischer ring. Condition found in Wilson's disease in which deposits of copper cause a pigmented ring around the cornea's outer border in the deep epithelial layers.

keratoprosthesis. Surgical procedure in which the physician creates a new anterior chamber with a plastic optical implant to replace a severely damaged cornea that cannot be repaired.

keratotomy. Surgical incision of the cornea.

krypton laser. Laser light energy that uses ionized krypton by electric current as the active source, has a radiation beam between the visible yellow-red spectrum, and is effective in photocoagulation of retinal bleeding, macular lesions, and vessel aberrations of the choroid.

lacrimal. Tear-producing gland or ducts that provides lubrication and flushing of the eyes and nasal cavities.

lacrimal punctum. Opening of the lacrimal papilla of the eyelid through which tears flow to the canaliculi to the lacrimal sac.

lacrimotome. Knife for cutting the lacrimal sac or duct.

lacrimotomy. Incision of the lacrimal sac or duct.

laparotomy. Incision through the flank or abdomen for therapeutic or diagnostic purposes.

laryngoscopy. Examination of the hypopharynx, larynx, and tongue base with an endoscope.

larynx. Musculocartilaginous structure between the trachea and the pharynx that functions as the valve preventing food and other particles from entering the respiratory tract, as well as the voice mechanism. Also called the voicebox, the larynx is composed of three single cartilages: cricoid, epiglottis, and thyroid; and three paired cartilages: arytenoid, corniculate, and cuneiform.

laser surgery. Use of concentrated, sharply defined light beams to cut, cauterize, coagulate, seal, or vaporize tissue.

LEEP. Loop electrode excision procedure. Biopsy specimen or cone shaped wedge of cervical tissue is removed using a hot cautery wire loop with an electrical current running through it.

levonorgestrel. Drug inhibiting ovulation and preventing sperm from penetrating cervical mucus. It is delivered subcutaneously in polysiloxone capsules. The capsules can be effective for up to five years, and provide a cumulative pregnancy rate of less than 2 percent. The capsules are not biodegradable, and therefore must be removed. Removal is more difficult than insertion of levonorgestrel capsules because fibrosis develops around the capsules. Normal hormonal activity and a return to fertility begins immediately upon removal.

ligament. Band or sheet of fibrous tissue that connects the articular surfaces of bones or supports visceral organs.

ligation. Tying off a blood vessel or duct with a suture or a soft, thin wire.

lymphadenectomy. Dissection of lymph nodes free from the vessels and removal for examination by frozen section in a separate procedure to detect early-stage metastases.

lysis. Destruction, breakdown, dissolution, or decomposition of cells or substances by a specific catalyzing agent.

Magnuson-Stack procedure. Treatment for recurrent anterior dislocation of the shoulder that involves tightening and realigning the subscapularis tendon.

maintenance of wakefulness test. Attended study determining the patient's ability to stay awake.

Manchester operation. Preservation of the uterus following prolapse by amputating the vaginal portion of the cervix, shortening the cardinal ligaments, and performing a colpoperineorrhaphy posteriorly.

mapping. Multidimensional depiction of a tachycardia that identifies its site of origin and its electrical conduction pathway after tachycardia has been induced. The recording is made from multiple catheter sites within the heart, obtaining electrograms simultaneously or sequentially.

marsupialization. Creation of a pouch in surgical treatment of a cyst in which one wall is resected and the remaining cut edges are sutured to adjacent tissue creating an open pouch of the previously enclosed cyst.

mastectomy. Surgical removal of one or both breasts.

McDonald procedure. Polyester tape is placed around the cervix with a running stitch to assist in the prevention of pre-term delivery. Tape is removed at term for vaginal delivery.

MCP. Metacarpophalangeal.

medial. Middle or midline.

mediastinotomy. Incision into the mediastinum for purposes of exploration, foreign body removal, drainage, or biopsy.

medical review. Review by a Medicare administrative contractor, carrier, and/or quality improvement organization (QIO) of services and items provided by physicians, other health care practitioners, and providers of health care services under Medicare. The review determines if the items and services are reasonable and necessary and meet Medicare coverage requirements, whether the quality meets professionally recognized standards of health care, and whether the services are medically appropriate in an inpatient, outpatient, or other setting as supported by documentation.

Medicare contractor. Medicare Part A fiscal intermediary, Medicare Part B carrier, Medicare administrative contractor (MAC), or a durable medical equipment Medicare administrative contractor (DME MAC).

Medicare physician fee schedule. List of payments Medicare allows by procedure or service. Payments may vary through geographic adjustments. The MPFS is based on the resource-based relative value scale (RBRVS). A national total relative value unit (RVU) is given to each procedure (HCPCS Level I CPT, Level II national codes). Each total RVU has three components: physician work, practice expense, and malpractice insurance.

meibomian gland. Sebaceous gland located in the tarsal plates along the eyelid margins that produces the lipid components found in tears.

metabolite. Chemical compound resulting from the natural process of metabolism. In drug testing, the metabolite of the drug may endure in a higher concentration or for a longer duration than the initial "parent" drug.

methylation. Mechanism used to regulate genes and protect DNA from some types of cleavage.

microarray. Small surface onto which multiple specific nucleic acid sequences can be attached to be used for analysis. Microarray may also be known as a gene chip or DNA chip. Tests can be run on the sequences for any variants that may be present.

mitral valve. Valve with two cusps that is between the left atrium and left ventricle of the heart.

moderate sedation. Medically controlled state of depressed consciousness, with or without analgesia, while maintaining the patient's airway, protective reflexes, and ability to respond to stimulation or verbal commands.

Mohs micrographic surgery. Special technique used to treat complex or ill-defined skin cancer and requires a single physician to provide two distinct services. The first service is surgical and involves the destruction of the lesion by a combination of chemosurgery and excision. The second service is that of a pathologist and includes mapping, color coding of specimens, microscopic examination of specimens, and complete histopathologic preparation.

monitored anesthesia care. Sedation, with or without analgesia, used to achieve a medically controlled state of depressed consciousness while maintaining the patient's airway, protective reflexes, and ability to respond to stimulation or verbal commands. In dental conscious sedation, the patient is rendered free of fear, apprehension, and anxiety through the use of pharmacological agents.

monoclonal. Relating to a single clone of cells.

mosaicplasty. Multiple, small grafts composed of bone and cartilage placed to treat osteochondral defects of the knee. The grafts are cylindrical in shape and are placed in corresponding size holes made to the desired depth to fill the defect and allow for a more naturally shaped reconstruction.

multiple sleep latency test (MSLT). Attended study to determine the tendency of the patient to fall asleep.

multiple-lead device. Implantable cardiac device (pacemaker or implantable cardioverter-defibrillator [ICD]) in which pacing and sensing components are placed in at least three chambers of the heart.

Mustard procedure. Corrective measure for transposition of great vessels involves an intra-atrial baffle made of pericardial tissue or synthetic material. The baffle is secured between pulmonary veins and mitral valve and between mitral and tricuspid valves. The baffle directs systemic venous flow into the left ventricle and lungs and pulmonary venous flow into the right ventricle and aorta.

mutation. Alteration in gene function that results in changes to a gene or chromosome. Can cause deficits or disease that can be inherited, can have beneficial effects, or result in no noticeable change.

mutation scanning. Process normally used on multiple polymerase chain reaction (PCR) amplicons to determine DNA sequence variants by differences in characteristics compared to normal. Specific DNA variants can then be studied further.

myotomy. Surgical cutting of a muscle to gain access to underlying tissues or for therapeutic reasons.

myringotomy. Incision in the eardrum done to prevent spontaneous rupture precipitated by fluid pressure build-up behind the tympanic membrane and to prevent stagnant infection and erosion of the ossicles.

nasal polyp. Fleshy outgrowth projecting from the mucous membrane of the nose or nasal sinus cavity that may obstruct ventilation or affect the sense of smell.

nasal sinus. Air-filled cavities in the cranial bones lined with mucous membrane and continuous with the nasal cavity, draining fluids through the nose.

nasogastric tube. Long, hollow, cylindrical catheter made of soft rubber or plastic that is inserted through the nose down into the stomach, and is used for feeding, instilling medication, or withdrawing gastric contents.

nasolacrimal punctum. Opening of the lacrimal duct near the nose.

nasopharynx. Membranous passage above the level of the soft palate.

Nd:YAG laser. Laser light energy that uses an yttrium, aluminum, and garnet crystal doped with neodymium ions as the active source, has a radiation beam nearing the infrared spectrum, and is effective in photocoagulation, photoablation, cataract extraction, and lysis of vitreous strands.

nebulizer. Latin for mist, a device that converts liquid into a fine spray and is commonly used to deliver medicine to the upper respiratory, bronchial, and lung areas.

nerve conduction study. Diagnostic test performed to assess muscle or nerve damage. Nerves are stimulated with electric shocks along the course of the muscle. Sensors are utilized to measure and record nerve functions, including conduction and velocity.

neurectomy. Excision of all or a portion of a nerve.

neuromuscular junction. Nerve synapse at the meeting point between the terminal end of a nerve (motor neuron) and a muscle fiber.

neuropsychological testing. Evaluation of a patient's behavioral abilities wherein a physician or other health care professional administers a series of tests in thinking, reasoning, and judgment.

new patient. Patient who is receiving face-to-face care from a provider/qualified health care professional or another physician/qualified health care professional of the exact same specialty and subspecialty who belongs to the same group practice for the first time in three years. For OPPS hospitals, a patient who has not been registered as an inpatient or outpatient, including off-campus provider based clinic or emergency department, within the past three years.

Niemann-Pick syndrome. Accumulation of phospholipid in histiocytes in the bone marrow, liver, lymph nodes, and spleen, cerebral involvement, and red macular spots similar to Tay-Sachs disease. Most commonly found in Jewish infants.

Nissen fundoplasty. Surgical repair technique that involves the fundus of the stomach being wrapped around the lower end of the esophagus to treat reflux esophagitis.

nonabsorbable sutures. Strands of natural or synthetic material that resist absorption into living tissue and are removed once healing is under way. Nonabsorbable sutures are commonly used to close skin wounds and repair tendons or collagenous tissue.

obturator. Prosthesis used to close an acquired or congenital opening in the palate that aids in speech and chewing.

obturator nerve. Lumbar plexus nerve with anterior and posterior divisions that innervate the adductor muscles (e.g., adductor longus, adductor brevis) of the leg and the skin over the medial area of the thigh or a sacral plexus nerve with anterior and posterior divisions that innervate the superior gemellus muscles.

occult blood test. Chemical or microscopic test to determine the presence of blood in a specimen.

ocular implant. Implant inside muscular cone.

oophorectomy. Surgical removal of all or part of one or both ovaries, either as open procedure or laparoscopically. Menstruation and childbearing ability continues when one ovary is removed.

orthosis. Derived from a Greek word meaning "to make straight," it is an artificial appliance that supports, aligns, or corrects an anatomical deformity or improves the use of a moveable body part. Unlike a prosthesis, an orthotic device is always functional in nature.

osteo-. Having to do with bone.

osteogenesis stimulator. Device used to stimulate the growth of bone by electrical impulses or ultrasound.

osteotomy. Surgical cutting of a bone.

ostomy. Artificial (surgical) opening in the body used for drainage or for delivery of medications or nutrients.

pacemaker. Implantable cardiac device that controls the heart's rhythm and maintains regular beats by artificial electric discharges. This device consists of the pulse generator with a battery and the electrodes, or leads, which are placed in single or dual chambers of the heart, usually transvenously.

palmaris longus tendon. Tendon located in the hand that flexes the wrist joint.

paracentesis. Surgical puncture of a body cavity with a specialized needle or hollow tubing to aspirate fluid for diagnostic or therapeutic reasons.

paratenon graft. Graft composed of the fatty tissue found between a tendon and its sheath.

passive mobilization. Pressure, movement, or pulling of a limb or body part utilizing an apparatus or device.

pedicle flap. Full-thickness skin and subcutaneous tissue for grafting that remains partially attached to the donor site by a pedicle or stem in which the blood vessels supplying the flap remain intact.

Pemberton osteotomy. Osteotomy is performed to position triradiate cartilage as a hinge for rotating the acetabular roof in cases of dysplasia of the hip in children.

penetrance. Being formed by, or pertaining to, a single clone.

percutaneous intradiscal electrothermal annuloplasty. Procedure corrects tears in the vertebral annulus by applying heat to the collagen disc walls percutaneously through a catheter. The heat contracts and thickens the wall, which may contract and close any annular tears.

percutaneous skeletal fixation. Treatment that is neither open nor closed and the injury site is not directly visualized. Fixation devices (pins, screws) are placed through the skin to stabilize the dislocation using x-ray guidance.

pericardium. Thin and slippery case in which the heart lies that is lined with fluid so that the heart is free to pulse and move as it beats.

peripheral arterial tonometry (PAT). Pulsatile volume changes in a digit are measured to determine activity in the sympathetic nervous system for respiratory analysis.

peritoneal. Space between the lining of the abdominal wall, or parietal peritoneum, and the surface layer of the abdominal organs, or visceral peritoneum. It contains a thin, watery fluid that keeps the peritoneal surfaces moist.

peritoneal dialysis. Dialysis that filters waste from blood inside the body using the peritoneum, the natural lining of the abdomen, as the semipermeable membrane across which ultrafiltration is accomplished. A special catheter is inserted into the abdomen and a dialysis solution is drained into the abdomen. This solution extracts fluids and wastes, which are then discarded when the fluid is drained. Various forms of peritoneal dialysis include CAPD, CCPD, and NIDP.

peritoneal effusion. Persistent escape of fluid within the peritoneal cavity.

pessary. Device placed in the vagina to support and reposition a prolapsing or retropositioned uterus, rectum, or vagina.

phacoemulsification. Cataract extraction in which the lens is fragmented by ultrasonic vibrations and simultaneously irrigated and aspirated.

phenotype. Physical expression of a trait or characteristic as determined by an individual's genetic makeup or genotype.

photocoagulation. Application of an intense laser beam of light to disrupt tissue and condense protein material to a residual mass, used especially for treating ocular conditions.

physical status modifiers. Alphanumeric modifier used to identify the patient's health status as it affects the work related to providing the anesthesia service.

physical therapy modality. Therapeutic agent or regimen applied or used to provide appropriate treatment of the musculoskeletal system.

physician. Legally authorized practitioners including a doctor of medicine or osteopathy, a doctor of dental surgery or of dental medicine, a doctor of podiatric medicine, a doctor of optometry, and a chiropractor only with respect to treatment by means of manual manipulation of the spine (to correct a subluxation).

PICC. Peripherally inserted central catheter. PICC is inserted into one of the large veins of the arm and threaded through the vein until the tip sits in a large vein just above the heart.

PKR. Photorefractive therapy. Procedure involving the removal of the surface layer of the cornea (epithelium) by gentle scraping and use of a computer-controlled excimer laser to reshape the stroma.

pleurodesis. Injection of a sclerosing agent into the pleural space for creating adhesions between the parietal and the visceral pleura to treat a collapsed lung caused by air trapped in the pleural cavity, or severe cases of pleural effusion.

plication. Surgical technique involving folding, tucking, or pleating to reduce the size of a hollow structure or organ.

polyclonal. Containing one or more cells.

polymorphism. Genetic variation in the same species that does not harm the gene function or create disease.

polypeptide. Chain of amino acids held together by covalent bonds. Proteins are made up of amino acids.

polysomnography. Test involving monitoring of respiratory, cardiac, muscle, brain, and ocular function during sleep.

Potts-Smith-Gibson procedure. Side-to-side anastomosis of the aorta and left pulmonary artery creating a shunt that enlarges as the child grows.

Prader-Willi syndrome. Rounded face, almond-shaped eyes, strabismus, low forehead, hypogonadism, hypotonia, intellectual disabilities, and an insatiable appetite.

presumptive drug testing. Drug screening tests to identify the presence or absence of drugs in a patient's system. Tests are usually able to identify low concentrations of the drug. These tests may be used for medical, workplace, or legal purposes.

presumptive identification. Identification of microorganisms using media growth, colony morphology, gram stains, or up to three specific tests (e.g., catalase, indole, oxidase, urease).

professional component. Portion of a charge for health care services that represents the physician's (or other practitioner's) work in providing the service, including interpretation and report of the procedure. This component of the service usually is charged for and billed separately from the inpatient hospital charges.

profunda. Denotes a part of a structure that is deeper from the surface of the body than the rest of the structure.

prolonged physician services. Extended pre- or post-service care provided to a patient whose condition requires services beyond the usual.

prostate. Male gland surrounding the bladder neck and urethra that secretes a substance into the seminal fluid.

prosthetic. Device that replaces all or part of an internal body organ or body part, or that replaces part of the function of a permanently inoperable or malfunctioning internal body organ or body part.

provider of services. Institution, individual, or organization that provides health care.

proximal. Located closest to a specified reference point, usually the midline or trunk.

psychiatric hospital. Specialized institution that provides, under the supervision of physicians, services for the diagnosis and treatment of mentally ill persons.

pterygium. Benign, wedge-shaped, conjunctival thickening that advances from the inner corner of the eye toward the cornea.

pterygomaxillary fossa. Wide depression on the external surface of the maxilla above and to the side of the canine tooth socket.

pulmonary artery banding. Surgical constriction of the pulmonary artery to prevent irreversible pulmonary vascular obstructive changes and overflow into the left ventricle.

Putti-Platt procedure. Realignment of the subscapularis tendon to treat recurrent anterior dislocation, thereby partially eliminating external rotation. The anterior capsule is also tightened and reinforced.

pyloroplasty. Enlargement and reconstruction of the lower portion of the stomach opening into the duodenum performed after vagotomy to speed gastric emptying and treat duodenal ulcers.

qualified health care professional. Educated, licensed or certified, and regulated professional operating under a specified scope of practice to provide patient services that are separate and distinct from other clinical staff. Services may be billed independently or under the facility's services.

RAC. Recovery audit contractor. National program using CMS-affiliated contractors to review claims prior to payment as well as for payments on claims already processed, including overpayments and underpayments.

radiation therapy simulation. Radiation therapy simulation. Procedure by which the specific body area to be treated with radiation is defined and marked. A CT scan is performed to define the body contours and these images are used to create a plan customized treatment for the patient, targeting the area to be treated while sparing adjacent tissue. The center of the area to be treated is marked and an immobilization device (e.g., cradle, mold) is created to make sure the patient is in the same position each time for treatment. Complexity of treatment depends on the number of treatment areas and the use of tools to isolate the area of treatment.

radioactive substances. Materials used in the diagnosis and treatment of disease that emit high-speed particles and energy-containing rays.

radiology services. Services that include diagnostic and therapeutic radiology, nuclear medicine, CT scan procedures, magnetic resonance imaging services, ultrasound, and other imaging procedures.

radiotherapy afterloading. Part of the radiation therapy process in which the chemotherapy agent is actually instilled into the tumor area subsequent to surgery and placement of an expandable catheter into the void remaining after tumor excision. The specialized catheter remains in place and the patient may come in for multiple treatments with radioisotope placed to treat the margin of tissue surrounding the excision. After the radiotherapy is completed, the patient returns to have the catheter emptied and removed. This is a new therapy in breast cancer treatment.

Rashkind procedure. Transvenous balloon atrial septectomy or septostomy performed by cardiac catheterization. A balloon catheter is inserted into the heart either to create or enlarge an opening in the interatrial septal wall.

rehabilitation services. Therapy services provided primarily for assisting in a rehabilitation program of evaluation and service including cardiac rehabilitation, medical social services, occupational therapy, physical therapy, respiratory therapy, skilled nursing, speech therapy, psychiatric rehabilitation, and alcohol and substance abuse rehabilitation.

respiratory airflow (ventilation). Assessment of air movement during inhalation and exhalation as measured by nasal pressure sensors and thermistor.

respiratory analysis. Assessment of components of respiration obtained by other methods such as airflow or peripheral arterial tone.

respiratory effort. Measurement of diaphragm and/or intercostal muscle for airflow using transducers to estimate thoracic and abdominal motion.

respiratory movement. Measurement of chest and abdomen movement during respiration.

ribbons. In oncology, small plastic tubes containing radioactive sources for interstitial placement that may be cut into specific lengths tailored to the size of the area receiving ionizing radiation treatment.

Ridell sinusotomy. Frontal sinus tissue is destroyed to eliminate tumors.

RNA. Ribonucleic acid.

rural health clinic. Clinic in an area where there is a shortage of health services staffed by a nurse practitioner, physician assistant, or certified nurse midwife under physician direction that provides routine diagnostic services, including clinical laboratory services, drugs, and biologicals and that has prompt access to additional diagnostic services from facilities meeting federal requirements.

Salter osteotomy. Innominate bone of the hip is cut, removed, and repositioned to repair a congenital dislocation, subluxation, or deformity.

saucerization. Creation of a shallow, saucer-like depression in the bone to facilitate drainage of infected areas.

Schiotz tonometer. Instrument that measures intraocular pressure by recording the depth of an indentation on the cornea by a plunger of known weight.

screening mammography. Radiologic images taken of the female breast for the early detection of breast cancer.

screening pap smear. Diagnostic laboratory test consisting of a routine exfoliative cytology test (Papanicolaou test) provided to a woman for the early detection of cervical or vaginal cancer. The exam includes a clinical breast examination and a physician's interpretation of the results.

seeds. Small (1 mm or less) sources of radioactive material that are permanently placed directly into tumors.

Senning procedure. Flaps of intra-atrial septum and right atrial wall are used to create two interatrial channels to divert the systemic and pulmonary venous circulation.

sensitivity tests. Number of methods of applying selective suspected allergens to the skin or mucous.

sensorineural conduction. Transportation of sound from the cochlea to the acoustic nerve and central auditory pathway to the brain.

sentinel lymph node. First node to which lymph drainage and metastasis from a cancer can occur.

separate procedures. Services commonly carried out as a fundamental part of a total service and, as such, do not usually warrant separate identification. These services are identified in CPT with the parenthetical phrase (separate procedure) at the end of the description and are payable only when performed alone.

septectomy. 1) Surgical removal of all or part of the nasal septum. 2) Submucosal resection of the nasal septum.

Shirodkar procedure. Treatment of an incompetent cervical os by placing nonabsorbent suture material in purse-string sutures as a cerclage to support the cervix.

short tandem repeat (STR). Short sequences of a DNA pattern that are repeated. Can be used as genetic markers for human identity testing.

sialodochoplasty. Surgical repair of a salivary gland duct.

single-lead device. Implantable cardiac device (pacemaker or implantable cardioverter-defibrillator [ICD]) in which pacing and sensing components are placed in only one chamber of the heart.

single-nucleotide polymorphism (SNP). Single nucleotide (A, T, C, or G that is different in a DNA sequence. This difference occurs at a significant frequency in the population.

sinus of Valsalva. Any of three sinuses corresponding to the individual cusps of the aortic valve, located in the most proximal part of the aorta just above the cusps. These structures are contained within the pericardium and appear as distinct but subtle outpouchings or dilations of the aortic wall between each of the semilunar cusps of the valve.

sleep apnea. Intermittent cessation of breathing during sleep that may cause hypoxemia and pulmonary arterial hypertension.

sleep latency. Time period between lying down in bed and the onset of sleep.

sleep staging. Determination of the separate levels of sleep according to physiological measurements.

somatic. 1) Pertaining to the body or trunk. 2) In genetics acquired or occurring after birth.

SPECT. Single photon emission computerized tomography. SPECT images are taken after the injection of a radionuclide using a special camera containing a detector crystal, usually sodium iodide. Images are captured as the gamma radiation from the radionuclide scintillates or gives off its energy in a flash of light when coming in contact with the crystal. This type of imaging is reported for the anatomical area and purpose such as detecting liver function or myocardial perfusion after an ischemic event.

speculoscopy. Viewing the cervix utilizing a magnifier and a special wavelength of light, allowing detection of abnormalities that may not be discovered on a routine Pap smear.

speech-language pathology services. Speech, language, and related function assessment and rehabilitation service furnished by a qualified speech-language pathologist. Audiology services include hearing and balance assessment services furnished by a qualified audiologist. A qualified speech pathologist and audiologist must have a master's or doctoral degree in their respective fields and be licensed to serve in the state. Speech pathologists and audiologists practicing in states without licensure must complete 350 hours of supervised clinical work and perform at least nine months of supervised full-time service after earning their degrees.

sphincteroplasty. Surgical repair done to correct, augment, or improve the muscular function of a sphincter, such as the anus or intestines.

spirometry. Measurement of the lungs' breathing capacity.

splint. Brace or support. 1) dynamic splint: brace that permits movement of an anatomical structure such as a hand, wrist, foot, or other part of the body after surgery or injury. 2) static splint: brace that prevents movement and maintains support and position for an anatomical structure after surgery or injury.

stent. Tube to provide support in a body cavity or lumen.

stereotactic radiosurgery. Delivery of externally-generated ionizing radiation to specific targets for destruction or inactivation. Most often utilized in the treatment of brain or spinal tumors, high-resolution stereotactic imaging is used to identify the target and then deliver the treatment. Computer-assisted planning may also be employed. Simple and complex cranial lesions and spinal lesions are typically treated in a single planning and treatment session, although a maximum of five sessions may be required. No incision is made for stereotactic radiosurgery procedures.

stereotaxis. Three-dimensional method for precisely locating structures.

Stoffel rhizotomy. Nerve roots are sectioned to relieve pain or spastic paralysis.

strabismus. Misalignment of the eyes due to an imbalance in extraocular muscles.

surgical package. Normal, uncomplicated performance of specific surgical services, with the assumption that, on average, all surgical procedures of a given type are similar with respect to skill level, duration, and length of normal follow-up care.

symblepharopterygium. Adhesion in which the eyelid is adhered to the eyeball by a band that resembles a pterygium.

sympathectomy. Surgical interruption or transection of a sympathetic nervous system pathway.

tarso-. 1) Relating to the foot. 2) Relating to the margin of the eyelid.

tarsocheiloplasty. Plastic operation upon the edge of the eyelid for the treatment of trichiasis.

tarsorrhaphy. Suture of a portion or all of the opposing eyelids together for the purpose of shortening the palpebral fissure or closing it entirely.

technical component. Portion of a health care service that identifies the provision of the equipment, supplies, technical personnel, and costs attendant to the performance of the procedure other than the professional services.

tendon. Fibrous tissue that connects muscle to bone, consisting primarily of collagen and containing little vasculature.

tendon allograft. Allografts are tissues obtained from another individual of the same species. Tendon allografts are usually obtained from cadavers and frozen or freeze dried for later use in soft tissue repairs where the physician elects not to obtain an autogenous graft (a graft obtained from the individual on whom the surgery is being performed).

tendon suture material. Tendons are composed of fibrous tissue consisting primarily of collagen and containing few cells or blood vessels. This tissue heals more slowly than tissues with more vascularization. Because of this, tendons are usually repaired with nonabsorbable suture material. Examples include surgical silk, surgical cotton, linen, stainless steel, surgical nylon, polyester fiber, polybutester (Novafil), polyethylene (Dermalene), and polypropylene (Prolene, Surilene).

tendon transplant. Replacement of a tendon with another tendon.

tenon's capsule. Connective tissue that forms the capsule enclosing the posterior eyeball, extending from the conjunctival fornix and continuous with the muscular fascia of the eye.

tenonectomy. Excision of a portion of a tendon to make it shorter.

tenotomy. Cutting into a tendon.

TENS. Transcutaneous electrical nerve stimulator. TENS is applied by placing electrode pads over the area to be stimulated and connecting the electrodes to a transmitter box, which sends a current through the skin to sensory nerve fibers to help decrease pain in that nerve distribution.

tensilon. Edrophonium chloride. Agent used for evaluation and treatment of myasthenia gravis.

terminally ill. Individual whose medical prognosis for life expectancy is six months or less.

tetralogy of Fallot. Specific combination of congenital cardiac defects: obstruction of the right ventricular outflow tract with pulmonary stenosis, interventricular septal defect, malposition of the aorta, overriding the interventricular septum and receiving blood from both the venous and arterial systems, and enlargement of the right ventricle.

therapeutic services. Services performed for treatment of a specific diagnosis. These services include performance of the procedure, various incidental elements, and normal, related follow-up care.

thoracentesis. Surgical puncture of the chest cavity with a specialized needle or hollow tubing to aspirate fluid from within the pleural space for diagnostic or therapeutic reasons.

thoracic lymphadenectomy. Procedure to cut out the lymph nodes near the lungs, around the heart, and behind the trachea.

thoracostomy. Creation of an opening in the chest wall for drainage.

thyroglossal duct. Embryonic duct at the front of the neck, which becomes the pyramidal lobe of the thyroid gland with obliteration of the remaining duct, but may form a cyst or sinus in adulthood if it persists.

total disc arthroplasty with artificial disc. Removal of an intravertebral disc and its replacement with an implant. The implant is an artificial disc consisting of two metal plates with a weight-bearing surface of polyethylene between the plates. The plates are anchored to the vertebral immediately above and below the affected disc.

total shoulder replacement. Prosthetic replacement of the entire shoulder joint, including the humeral head and the glenoid fossa.

trabeculae carneae cordis. Bands of muscular tissue that line the walls of the ventricles in the heart.

trabeculectomy. Surgical incision between the anterior portion of the eye and the canal of Schlemm to drain the aqueous humor.

tracheostomy. Formation of a tracheal opening on the neck surface with tube insertion to allow for respiration in cases of obstruction or decreased patency. A tracheostomy may be planned or performed on an emergency basis for temporary or long-term use.

tracheotomy. Formation of a tracheal opening on the neck surface with tube insertion to allow for respiration in cases of obstruction or decreased patency. A tracheotomy may be planned or performed on an emergency basis for temporary or long-term use.

traction. Drawing out or holding tension on an area by applying a direct therapeutic pulling force.

transcranial magnetic stimulation. Application of electromagnetic energy to the brain through a coil placed on the scalp. The procedure stimulates cortical neurons and is intended to activate and normalize their processes.

transcription. Process by which messenger RNA is synthesized from a DNA template resulting in the transfer of genetic information from the DNA molecule to the messenger RNA.

translocation. Disconnection of all or part of a chromosome that reattaches to another position in the DNA sequence of the same or another chromosome. Often results in a reciprocal exchange of DNA sequences between two differently numbered chromosomes. May or may not result in a clinically significant loss of DNA.

trephine. 1) Specialized round saw for cutting circular holes in bone, especially the skull. 2) Instrument that removes small disc-shaped buttons of corneal tissue for transplanting.

tricuspid atresia. Congenital absence of the valve that may occur with other defects, such as atrial septal defect, pulmonary atresia, and transposition of great vessels.

turbinates. Scroll or shell-shaped elevations from the wall of the nasal cavity, the inferior turbinate being a separate bone, while the superior and middle turbinates are of the ethmoid bone.

tympanic membrane. Thin, sensitive membrane across the entrance to the middle ear that vibrates in response to sound waves, allowing the waves to be transmitted via the ossicular chain to the internal ear.

tympanoplasty. Surgical repair of the structures of the middle ear, including the eardrum and the three small bones, or ossicles.

unlisted procedure. Procedural descriptions used when the overall procedure and outcome of the procedure are not adequately described by an existing procedure code. Such codes are used as a last resort and only when there is not a more appropriate procedure code.

ureterorrhaphy. Surgical repair using sutures to close an open wound or injury of the ureter.

vagotomy. Division of the vagus nerves, interrupting impulses resulting in lower gastric acid production and hastening gastric emptying. Used in the treatment of chronic gastric, pyloric, and duodenal ulcers that can cause severe pain and difficulties in eating and sleeping.

variant. Nucleotide deviation from the normal sequence of a region. Variations are usually either substitutions or deletions. Substitution variations are the result of one nucleotide taking the place of another. A deletion occurs when one or more nucleotides are left out. In some cases, several in a reasonably close proximity on the same chromosome in a DNA strand. These variations result in amino acid changes in the protein made by the gene. However, the term variant does not itself imply a functional change. Intron variations are usually described in one of two ways: 1) the changed nucleotide is defined by a plus or a minus sign indicating the position relative to the first or last nucleotide to the intron, or 2) the second variant description is indicated relative to the last nucleotide of the preceding exon or first nucleotide of the following exon.

vascular family. Group of vessels (family) that branch from the aorta or vena cava. At each branching, the vascular order increases by one. The first order vessel is the primary branch off the aorta or vena cava. The second order vessel branches from the first order, the third order branches from the second order, and any further branching is beyond the third order. For example, for the inferior vena cava, the common iliac artery is a first order vessel. The internal and external iliac arteries are second order vessels, as they each originate from the first order common iliac artery. The external iliac artery extends directly from the common iliac artery and the internal iliac artery bifurcates from the common iliac artery. A third order vessel from the external iliac artery is the inferior epigastric artery and a third order vessel from the internal iliac artery is the obturator artery. Note orders are not always identical bilaterally (e.g., the left common carotid artery is a first order and the right common carotid is a second order. Synonym(s): vascular origins and distributions.

vasectomy. Surgical procedure involving the removal of all or part of the vas deferens, usually performed for sterilization or in conjunction with a prostatectomy.

vena cava interruption. Procedure that places a filter device, called an umbrella or sieve, within the large vein returning deoxygenated blood to the heart to prevent pulmonary embolism caused by clots.

ventricular assist device. Temporary measure used to support the heart by substituting for left and/or right heart function. The device replaces the work of the left and/or right ventricle when a patient has a damaged or weakened heart. A left ventricular assist device (VAD) helps the heart pump blood through the rest of the body. A right VAD helps the heart pump blood to the lungs to become oxygenated again. Catheters are inserted to circulate the blood through external tubing to a pump machine located outside of the body and back to the correct artery.

ventricular septal defect. Congenital cardiac anomaly resulting in a continual opening in the septum between the ventricles that, in severe cases, causes oxygenated blood to flow back into the lungs, resulting in pulmonary hypertension.

vertebral interspace. Non-bony space between two adjacent vertebral bodies that contains the cushioning intervertebral disk.

volar. Palm of the hand (palmar) or sole of the foot (plantar).

Waterston procedure. Type of aortopulmonary shunting done to increase pulmonary blood flow. The ascending aorta is anastomosed to the right pulmonary artery.

Wharton's ducts. Salivary ducts below the mandible.

wick catheter. Device used to monitor interstitial fluid pressure, and sometimes used intraoperatively during fasciotomy procedures to evaluate the effectiveness of the decompression.

wound closure. Closure or repair of a wound created surgically or due to trauma (e.g., laceration). The closure technique depends on the type, site, and depth of the defect. Consideration is also given to cosmetic and functional outcome. A single layer closure involves approximation of the edges of the wound. The second type of closure involves closing the one or more deeper layers of tissue prior to skin closure. The most complex type of closure may include techniques such as debridement or undermining, which involves manipulation of tissue around the wound to allow the skin to cover the wound. The AMA CPT® book defines these as Simple, Intermediate and Complex repair.

xenograft. Tissue that is nonhuman and harvested from one species and grafted to another. Pigskin is the most common xenograft for human skin and is applied to a wound as a temporary closure until a permanent option is performed.

z-plasty. Plastic surgery technique used primarily to release tension or elongate contractured scar tissue in which a Z-shaped incision is made with the middle line of the Z crossing the area of greatest tension. The triangular flaps are then rotated so that they cross the incision line in the opposite direction, creating a reversed Z.

ZPIC. Zone Program Integrity Contractor. CMS contractor that replaced the existing Program Safeguard Contractors (PSC). Contractors are responsible for ensuring the integrity of all Medicare-related claims under Parts A and B (hospital, skilled nursing, home health, provider, and durable medical equipment claims), Part C (Medicare Advantage health plans), Part D (prescription drug plans), and coordination of Medicare-Medicaid data matches (Medi-Medi).

Appendix N — Listing of Sensory, Motor, and Mixed Nerves

This list contains the sensory, motor, and mixed nerves assigned to each nerve conduction study to improve coding accuracy. Each nerve makes up one single unit of service.

Motor Nerves Assigned to Codes 95907-95913

I. Upper extremity, cervical plexus, and brachial plexus motor nerves
  - A. Axillary motor nerve to the deltoid
  - B. Long thoracic motor nerve to the serratus anterior
  - C. Median nerve
    1. Median motor nerve to the abductor pollicis brevis
    2. Median motor nerve, anterior interosseous branch, to the flexor pollicis longus
    3. Median motor nerve, anterior interosseous branch, to the pronator quadratus
    4. Median motor nerve to the first lumbrical
    5. Median motor nerve to the second lumbrical
  - D. Musculocutaneous motor nerve to the biceps brachii
  - E. Radial nerve
    1. Radial motor nerve to the extensor carpi ulnaris
    2. Radial motor nerve to the extensor digitorum communis
    3. Radial motor nerve to the extensor indicis proprius
    4. Radial motor nerve to the brachioradialis
  - F. Suprascapular nerve
    1. Suprascapular motor nerve to the supraspinatus
    2. Suprascapular motor nerve to the infraspinatus
  - G. Thoracodorsal motor nerve to the latissimus dorsi
  - H. Ulnar nerve
    1. Ulnar motor nerve to the abductor digiti minimi
    2. Ulnar motor nerve to the palmar interosseous
    3. Ulnar motor nerve to the first dorsal interosseous
    4. Ulnar motor nerve to the flexor carpi ulnaris
  - I. Other

II. Lower extremity motor nerves
  - A. Femoral motor nerve to the quadriceps
    1. Femoral motor nerve to vastus medialis
    2. Femoral motor nerve to vastus lateralis
    3. Femoral motor nerve to vastus intermedius
    4. Femoral motor nerve to rectus femoris
  - B. Ilioinguinal motor nerve
  - C. Peroneal (fibular) nerve
    1. Peroneal motor nerve to the extensor digitorum brevis
    2. Peroneal motor nerve to the peroneus brevis
    3. Peroneal motor nerve to the peroneus longus
    4. Peroneal motor nerve to the tibialis anterior
  - D. Plantar motor nerve
  - E. Sciatic nerve
  - F. Tibial nerve
    1. Tibial motor nerve, inferior calcaneal branch, to the abductor digiti minimi
    2. Tibial motor nerve, medial plantar branch, to the abductor hallucis
    3. Tibial motor nerve, lateral plantar branch, to the flexor digiti minimi brevis
  - G. Other

III. Cranial nerves and trunk
  - A. Cranial nerve VII (facial motor nerve)
    1. Facial nerve to the frontalis
    2. Facial nerve to the nasalis
    3. Facial nerve to the orbicularis oculi
    4. Facial nerve to the orbicularis oris
  - B. Cranial nerve XI (spinal accessory motor nerve)
  - C. Cranial nerve XII (hypoglossal motor nerve)
  - D. Intercostal motor nerve
  - E. Phrenic motor nerve to the diaphragm
  - F. Recurrent laryngeal nerve
  - G. Other

IV. Nerve Roots
  - A. Cervical nerve root stimulation
    1. Cervical level 5 (C5)
    2. Cervical level 6 (C6)
    3. Cervical level 7 (C7)
    4. Cervical level 8 (C8)
  - B. Thoracic nerve root stimulation
    1. Thoracic level 1 (T1)
    2. Thoracic level 2 (T2)
    3. Thoracic level 3 (T3)
    4. Thoracic level 4 (T4)
    5. Thoracic level 5 (T5)
    6. Thoracic level 6 (T6)
    7. Thoracic level 7 (T7)
    8. Thoracic level 8 (T8)
    9. Thoracic level 9 (T9)
    10. Thoracic level 10 (T10)
    11. Thoracic level 11 (T11)
    12. Thoracic level 12 (T12)
  - C. Lumbar nerve root stimulation
    1. Lumbar level 1 (L1)
    2. Lumbar level 2 (L2)
    3. Lumbar level 3 (L3)
    4. Lumbar level 4 (L4)
    5. Lumbar level 5 (L5)
  - D. Sacral nerve root stimulation
    1. Sacral level 1 (S1)
    2. Sacral level 2 (S2)
    3. Sacral level 3 (S3)
    4. Sacral level 4 (S4)

Sensory and Mixed Nerves Assigned to Codes 95907–95913

I. Upper extremity sensory and mixed nerves
  A. Lateral antebrachial cutaneous sensory nerve
  B. Medial antebrachial cutaneous sensory nerve
  C. Medial brachial cutaneous sensory nerve
  D. Median nerve
    1. Median sensory nerve to the first digit
    2. Median sensory nerve to the second digit
    3. Median sensory nerve to the third digit
    4. Median sensory nerve to the fourth digit
    5. Median palmar cutaneous sensory nerve
    6. Median palmar mixed nerve
  E. Posterior antebrachial cutaneous sensory nerve
  F. Radial sensory nerve
    1. Radial sensory nerve to the base of the thumb
    2. Radial sensory nerve to digit 1
  G. Ulnar nerve
    1. Ulnar dorsal cutaneous sensory nerve
    2. Ulnar sensory nerve to the fourth digit
    3. Ulnar sensory nerve to the fifth digit
    4. Ulnar palmar mixed nerve
  H. Intercostal sensory nerve
  I. Other

II. Lower extremity sensory and mixed nerves
  A. Lateral femoral cutaneous sensory nerve
  B. Medical calcaneal sensory nerve
  C. Medial femoral cutaneous sensory nerve
  D. Peroneal nerve
    1. Deep peroneal sensory nerve
    2. Superficial peroneal sensory nerve, medial dorsal cutaneous branch
    3. Superficial peroneal sensory nerve, intermediate dorsal cutaneous branch
  E. Posterior femoral cutaneous sensory nerve
  F. Saphenous nerve
    1. Saphenous sensory nerve (distal technique)
    2. Saphenous sensory nerve (proximal technique)
  G. Sural nerve
    1. Sural sensory nerve, lateral dorsal cutaneous branch
    2. Sural sensory nerve
  H. Tibial sensory nerve (digital nerve to toe 1)
  I. Tibial sensory nerve (medial plantar nerve)
  J. Tibial sensory nerve (lateral plantar nerve)
  K. Other

III. Head and trunk sensory nerves
  A. Dorsal nerve of the penis
  B. Greater auricular nerve
  C. Ophthalmic branch of the trigeminal nerve
  D. Pudendal sensory nerve
  E. Suprascapular sensory nerves
  F. Other

In the following table, the reasonable maximum number of studies per diagnostic category is listed that allows for a physician or other qualified health care professional to obtain a diagnosis for 90 percent of patients with that same final diagnosis. The numbers denote the suggested number of studies, although the decision is up to the provider.

Type of Study/Maximum Number of Studies

Indication	Limbs Studied by Needle EMG (95860–95864, 95867–95870, 95885–95887)	Nerve Conduction Studies (Total nerves studied, 95907-95913)	Neuromuscular Junction Testing (Repetitive Stimulation 95937)
Carpal Tunnel (Unilateral)	1	7	—
Carpal Tunnel (Bilateral)	2	10	—
Radiculopathy	2	7	—
Mononeuropathy	1	8	—
Polyneuropathy/Mononeuropathy Multiplex	3	10	—
Myopathy	2	4	2
Motor Neuronopathy (e.g., ALS)	4	6	2
Plexopathy	2	12	—
Neuromuscular Junction	2	4	3
Tarsal Tunnel Syndrome (Unilateral)	1	8	—
Tarsal Tunnel Syndrome (Bilateral)	2	11	—
Weakness, Fatigue, Cramps, or Twitching (Focal)	2	7	2
Weakness, Fatigue, Cramps, or Twitching (General)	4	8	2
Pain, Numbness, or Tingling (Unilateral)	1	9	—
Pain, Numbness, or Tingling (Bilateral)	2	12	—

Appendix O — Vascular Families

This table assumes that the starting point is aortic catheterization. This categorization would not be accurate if, for instance, a femoral or carotid artery were catheterized with the blood's flow. The names of the arteries appearing in bold face type in the following table indicate those arteries that are most often the subject of arteriographic procedures.

Arterial Vascular Family

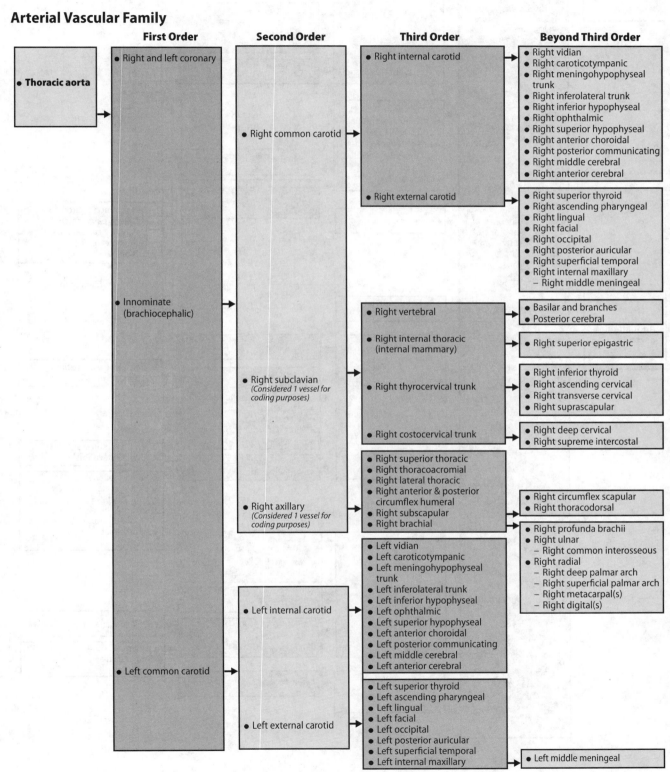

(Columns: First Order → Second Order → Third Order → Beyond Third Order)

- **Thoracic aorta**
  - First Order: Right and left coronary
  - First Order: Innominate (brachiocephalic)
    - Second Order: Right common carotid
      - Third Order: Right internal carotid
        - Beyond Third Order:
          - Right vidian
          - Right caroticotympanic
          - Right meningohypophyseal trunk
          - Right inferolateral trunk
          - Right inferior hypophyseal
          - Right ophthalmic
          - Right superior hypophyseal
          - Right anterior choroidal
          - Right posterior communicating
          - Right middle cerebral
          - Right anterior cerebral
      - Third Order: Right external carotid
        - Beyond Third Order:
          - Right superior thyroid
          - Right ascending pharyngeal
          - Right lingual
          - Right facial
          - Right occipital
          - Right posterior auricular
          - Right superficial temporal
          - Right internal maxillary
            - Right middle meningeal
    - Second Order: Right subclavian *(Considered 1 vessel for coding purposes)*
      - Third Order: Right vertebral
        - Beyond Third Order:
          - Basilar and branches
          - Posterior cerebral
      - Third Order: Right internal thoracic (internal mammary)
        - Beyond Third Order:
          - Right superior epigastric
      - Third Order: Right thyrocervical trunk
        - Beyond Third Order:
          - Right inferior thyroid
          - Right ascending cervical
          - Right transverse cervical
          - Right suprascapular
      - Third Order: Right costocervical trunk
        - Beyond Third Order:
          - Right deep cervical
          - Right supreme intercostal
    - Second Order: Right axillary *(Considered 1 vessel for coding purposes)*
      - Third Order:
        - Right superior thoracic
        - Right thoracoacromial
        - Right lateral thoracic
        - Right anterior & posterior circumflex humeral
        - Right subscapular
          - Beyond Third Order:
            - Right circumflex scapular
            - Right thoracodorsal
        - Right brachial
          - Beyond Third Order:
            - Right profunda brachii
            - Right ulnar
              - Right common interosseous
            - Right radial
              - Right deep palmar arch
              - Right superficial palmar arch
              - Right metacarpal(s)
              - Right digital(s)
  - First Order: Left common carotid
    - Second Order: Left internal carotid
      - Third Order:
        - Left vidian
        - Left caroticotympanic
        - Left meningohypophyseal trunk
        - Left inferolateral trunk
        - Left inferior hypophyseal
        - Left ophthalmic
        - Left superior hypophyseal
        - Left anterior choroidal
        - Left posterior communicating
        - Left middle cerebral
        - Left anterior cerebral
    - Second Order: Left external carotid
      - Third Order:
        - Left superior thyroid
        - Left ascending pharyngeal
        - Left lingual
        - Left facial
        - Left occipital
        - Left posterior auricular
        - Left superficial temporal
        - Left internal maxillary
          - Beyond Third Order:
            - Left middle meningeal

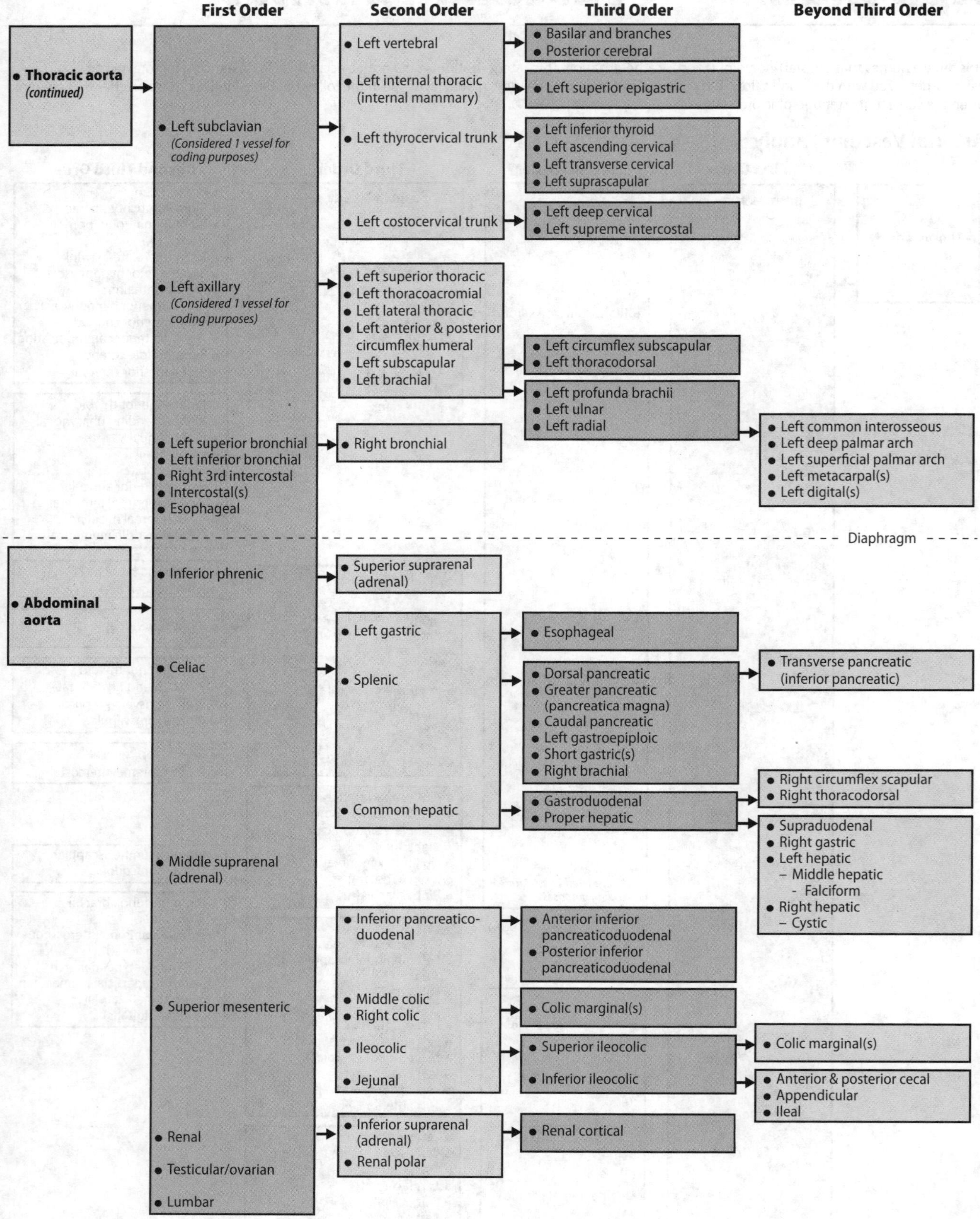
First Order
Second Order
Third Order
Beyond Third Order
• Thoracic aorta (continued)
• Left subclavian (Considered 1 vessel for coding purposes)
• Left vertebral
• Basilar and branches
• Posterior cerebral
• Left internal thoracic (internal mammary)
• Left superior epigastric
• Left thyrocervical trunk
• Left inferior thyroid
• Left ascending cervical
• Left transverse cervical
• Left suprascapular
• Left costocervical trunk
• Left deep cervical
• Left supreme intercostal
• Left axillary (Considered 1 vessel for coding purposes)
• Left superior thoracic
• Left thoracoacromial
• Left lateral thoracic
• Left anterior & posterior circumflex humeral
• Left subscapular
• Left brachial
• Left circumflex subscapular
• Left thoracodorsal
• Left profunda brachii
• Left ulnar
• Left radial
• Left common interosseous
• Left deep palmar arch
• Left superficial palmar arch
• Left metacarpal(s)
• Left digital(s)
• Left superior bronchial
• Left inferior bronchial
• Right 3rd intercostal
• Intercostal(s)
• Esophageal
• Right bronchial
Diaphragm
• Abdominal aorta
• Inferior phrenic
• Superior suprarenal (adrenal)
• Celiac
• Left gastric
• Esophageal
• Splenic
• Dorsal pancreatic
• Greater pancreatic (pancreatica magna)
• Caudal pancreatic
• Left gastroepiploic
• Short gastric(s)
• Right brachial
• Transverse pancreatic (inferior pancreatic)
• Right circumflex scapular
• Right thoracodorsal
• Common hepatic
• Gastroduodenal
• Proper hepatic
• Supraduodenal
• Right gastric
• Left hepatic
– Middle hepatic
- Falciform
• Right hepatic
– Cystic
• Middle suprarenal (adrenal)
• Superior mesenteric
• Inferior pancreatico-duodenal
• Anterior inferior pancreaticoduodenal
• Posterior inferior pancreaticoduodenal
• Middle colic
• Right colic
• Colic marginal(s)
• Ileocolic
• Superior ileocolic
• Inferior ileocolic
• Colic marginal(s)
• Anterior & posterior cecal
• Appendicular
• Ileal
• Jejunal
• Renal
• Inferior suprarenal (adrenal)
• Renal polar
• Renal cortical
• Testicular/ovarian
• Lumbar

First Order	Second Order	Third Order	Beyond Third Order

- **Abdominal aorta** *(continued)*
  - Inferior mesenteric (First Order)
    - Left colic, Sigmoid, Superior rectal (Second Order)
      - Ascending left colic, Ascending left colic (Third Order)
        - Colic marginal(s) (Beyond Third Order)
  - Middle (median) sacral (First Order)
  - Common iliac (First Order)
    - Internal iliac (Second Order)
      - Posterior division (Third Order)
        - Iliolumbar
        - Lateral sacral
        - Superior gluteal
      - Anterior division (Third Order)
        - Obturator
        - Umbilical
          - Superior vesical
        - Uterine
        - Vaginal
        - Inferior vesical
        - Middle rectal
          - Prostate
        - Internal pudendal
          - Inferior rectal
        - Inferior gluteal
    - External iliac *(Considered 1 vessel for coding purposes)* (Second Order)
      - Deep circumflex iliac, Inferior epigastric (Third Order)
        - Cremasteric
    - Common femoral *(Considered 1 vessel for coding purposes)* (Second Order)
      - Profunda femoris, Deep external pudendal, Superficial external pudendal, Superficial femoral *(Considered 1 vessel for coding purposes)*, Popliteal *(Considered 1 vessel for coding purposes)* (Third Order)
        - Medial femoral circumflex
        - Lateral femoral circumflex
        - Geniculate
        - Anterior tibial
        - Posterior tibial
        - Peroneal
        - Pedal arch
        - Digital(s)

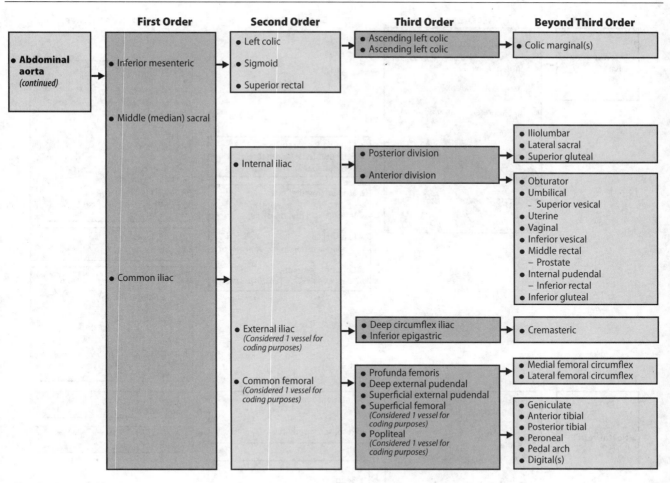

Venous Vascular Family

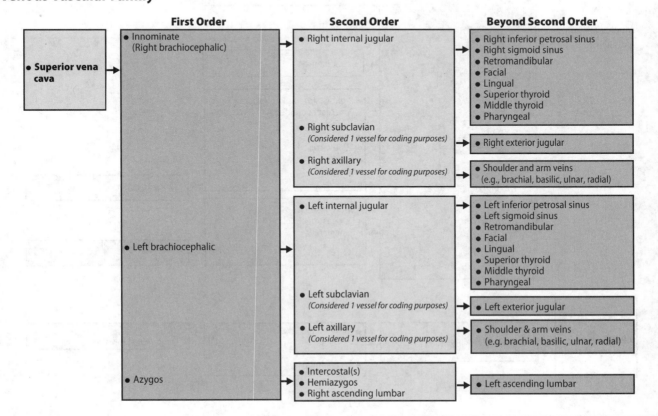

First Order	Second Order	Beyond Second Order

- **Superior vena cava**
  - Innominate (Right brachiocephalic) (First Order)
    - Right internal jugular (Second Order)
      - Right inferior petrosal sinus
      - Right sigmoid sinus
      - Retromandibular
      - Facial
      - Lingual
      - Superior thyroid
      - Middle thyroid
      - Pharyngeal
    - Right subclavian *(Considered 1 vessel for coding purposes)* (Second Order)
      - Right exterior jugular
    - Right axillary *(Considered 1 vessel for coding purposes)* (Second Order)
      - Shoulder and arm veins (e.g., brachial, basilic, ulnar, radial)
  - Left brachiocephalic (First Order)
    - Left internal jugular (Second Order)
      - Left inferior petrosal sinus
      - Left sigmoid sinus
      - Retromandibular
      - Facial
      - Lingual
      - Superior thyroid
      - Middle thyroid
      - Pharyngeal
    - Left subclavian *(Considered 1 vessel for coding purposes)* (Second Order)
      - Left exterior jugular
    - Left axillary *(Considered 1 vessel for coding purposes)* (Second Order)
      - Shoulder & arm veins (e.g. brachial, basilic, ulnar, radial)
  - Azygos (First Order)
    - Intercostal(s), Hemiazygos, Right ascending lumbar (Second Order)
      - Left ascending lumbar

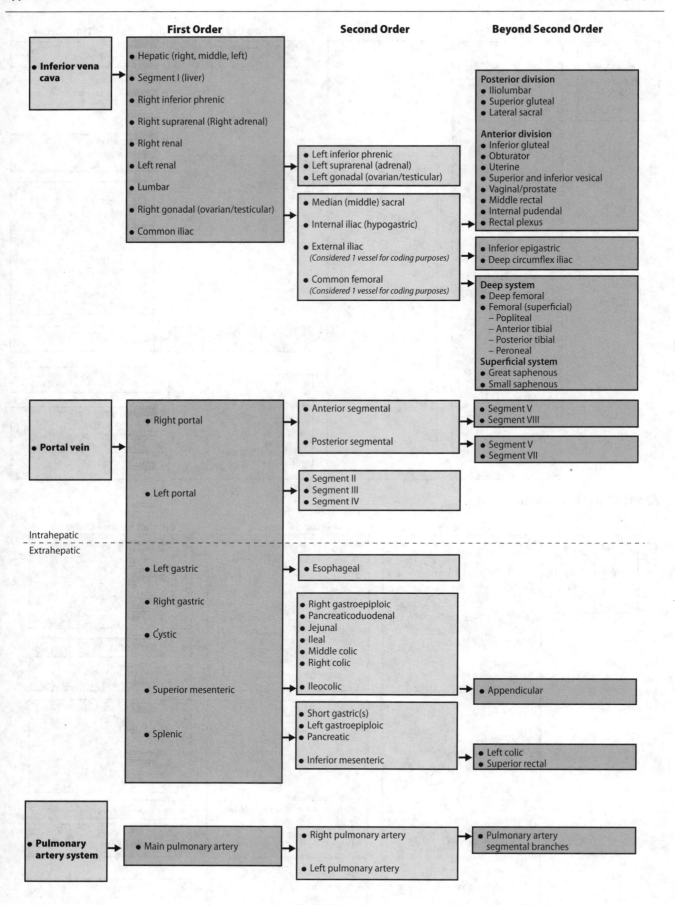

First Order | **Second Order** | **Beyond Second Order**

- **Inferior vena cava** →
  - Hepatic (right, middle, left)
  - Segment I (liver)
  - Right inferior phrenic
  - Right suprarenal (Right adrenal)
  - Right renal
  - Left renal →
    - Left inferior phrenic
    - Left suprarenal (adrenal)
    - Left gonadal (ovarian/testicular)
  - Lumbar
  - Right gonadal (ovarian/testicular)
  - Common iliac →
    - Median (middle) sacral
    - Internal iliac (hypogastric) →
      - Posterior division
        - Iliolumbar
        - Superior gluteal
        - Lateral sacral
      - Anterior division
        - Inferior gluteal
        - Obturator
        - Uterine
        - Superior and inferior vesical
        - Vaginal/prostate
        - Middle rectal
        - Internal pudendal
        - Rectal plexus
    - External iliac *(Considered 1 vessel for coding purposes)* →
      - Inferior epigastric
      - Deep circumflex iliac
    - Common femoral *(Considered 1 vessel for coding purposes)* →
      - Deep system
        - Deep femoral
        - Femoral (superficial)
          - Popliteal
          - Anterior tibial
          - Posterior tibial
          - Peroneal
      - Superficial system
        - Great saphenous
        - Small saphenous

- **Portal vein** →
  - Intrahepatic
    - Right portal →
      - Anterior segmental →
        - Segment V
        - Segment VIII
      - Posterior segmental →
        - Segment V
        - Segment VII
    - Left portal →
      - Segment II
      - Segment III
      - Segment IV
  - Extrahepatic
    - Left gastric →
      - Esophageal
    - Right gastric
    - Cystic
    - Superior mesenteric →
      - Right gastroepiploic
      - Pancreaticoduodenal
      - Jejunal
      - Ileal
      - Middle colic
      - Right colic
      - Ileocolic →
        - Appendicular
    - Splenic →
      - Short gastric(s)
      - Left gastroepiploic
      - Pancreatic
      - Inferior mesenteric →
        - Left colic
        - Superior rectal

- **Pulmonary artery system** →
  - Main pulmonary artery →
    - Right pulmonary artery →
      - Pulmonary artery segmental branches
    - Left pulmonary artery

Appendix P — Interventional Radiology Illustrations

Internal Carotid and Vertebral Arterial Anatomy

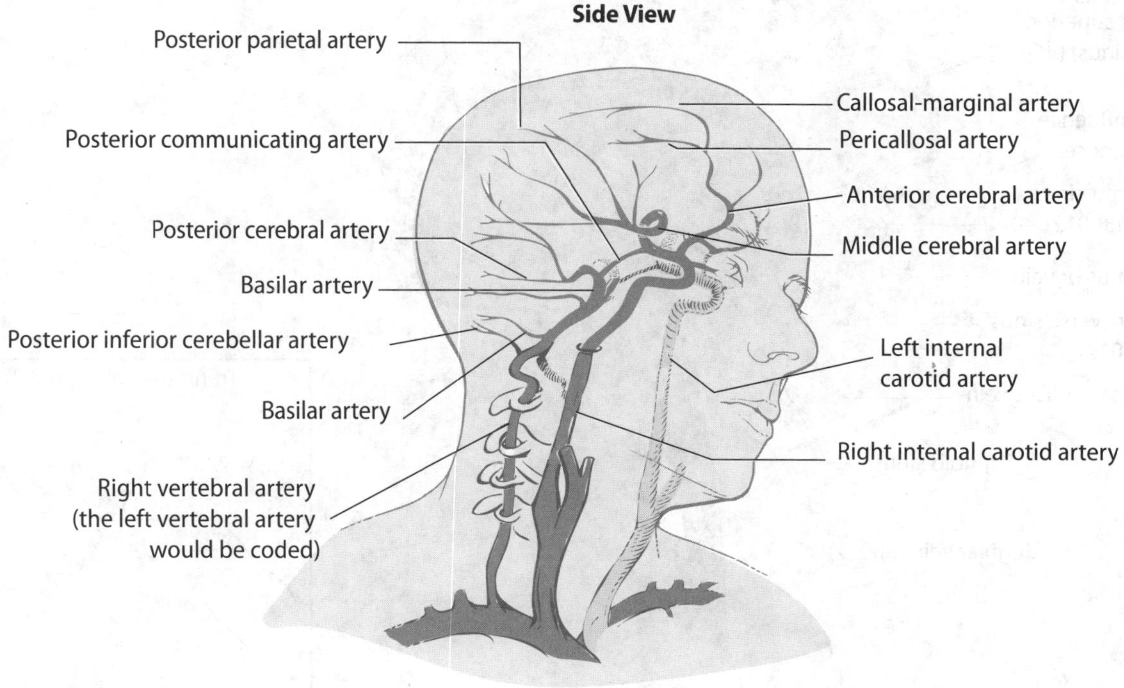

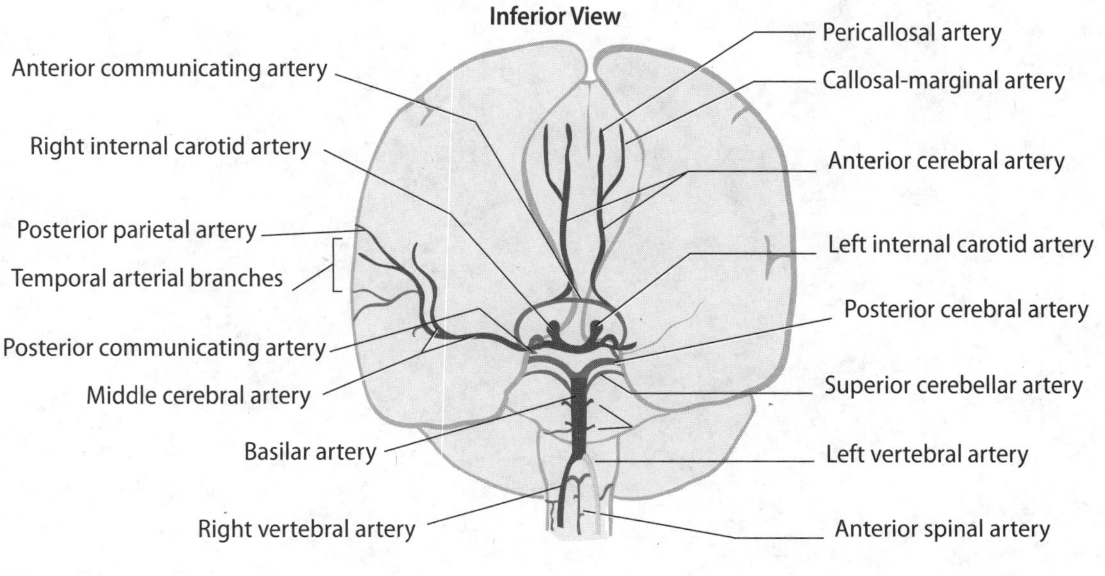

Appendix P — Interventional Radiology Illustrations

Cerebral Venous Anatomy

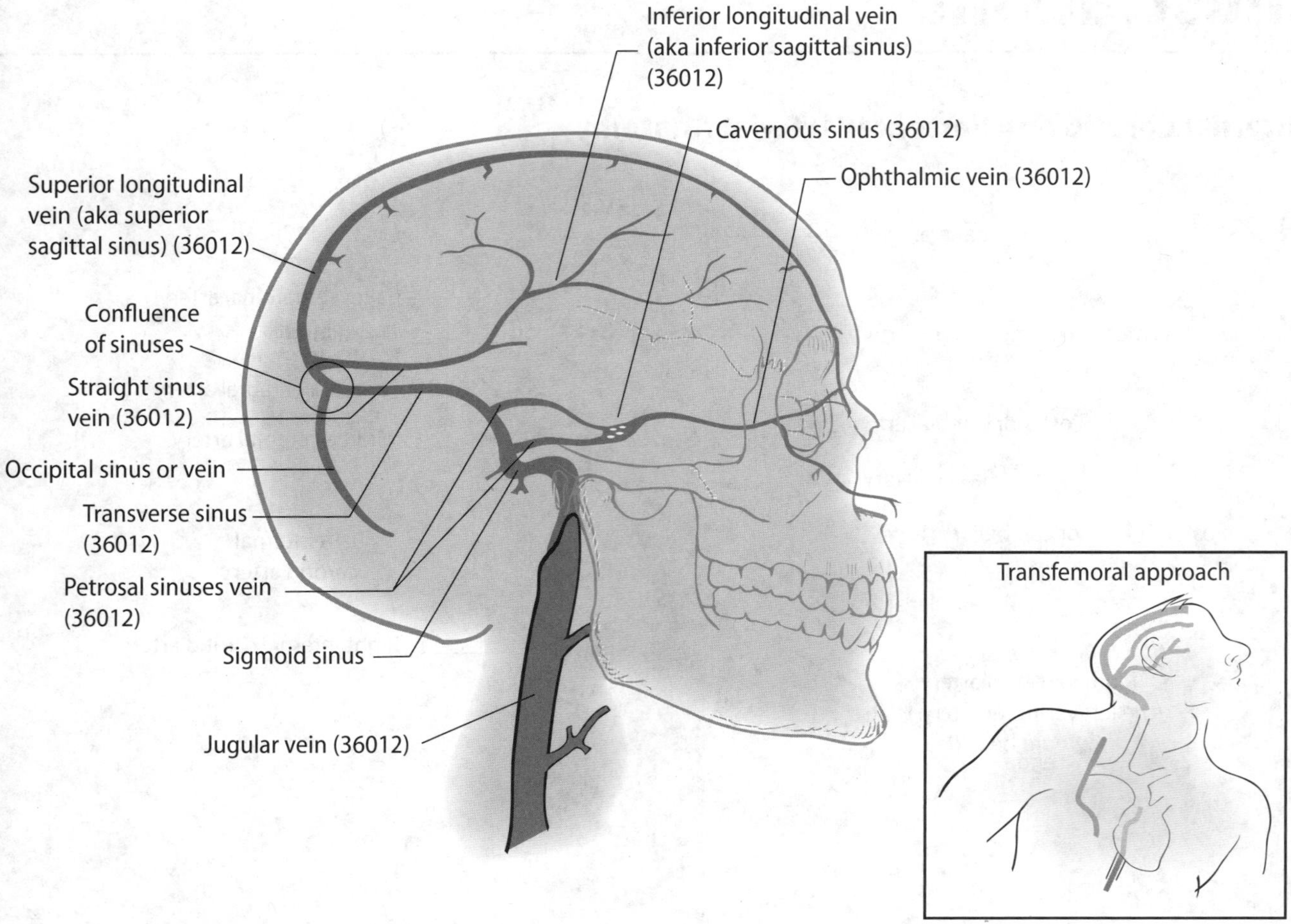

Normal Aortic Arch and Branch Anatomy—Transfemoral Approach

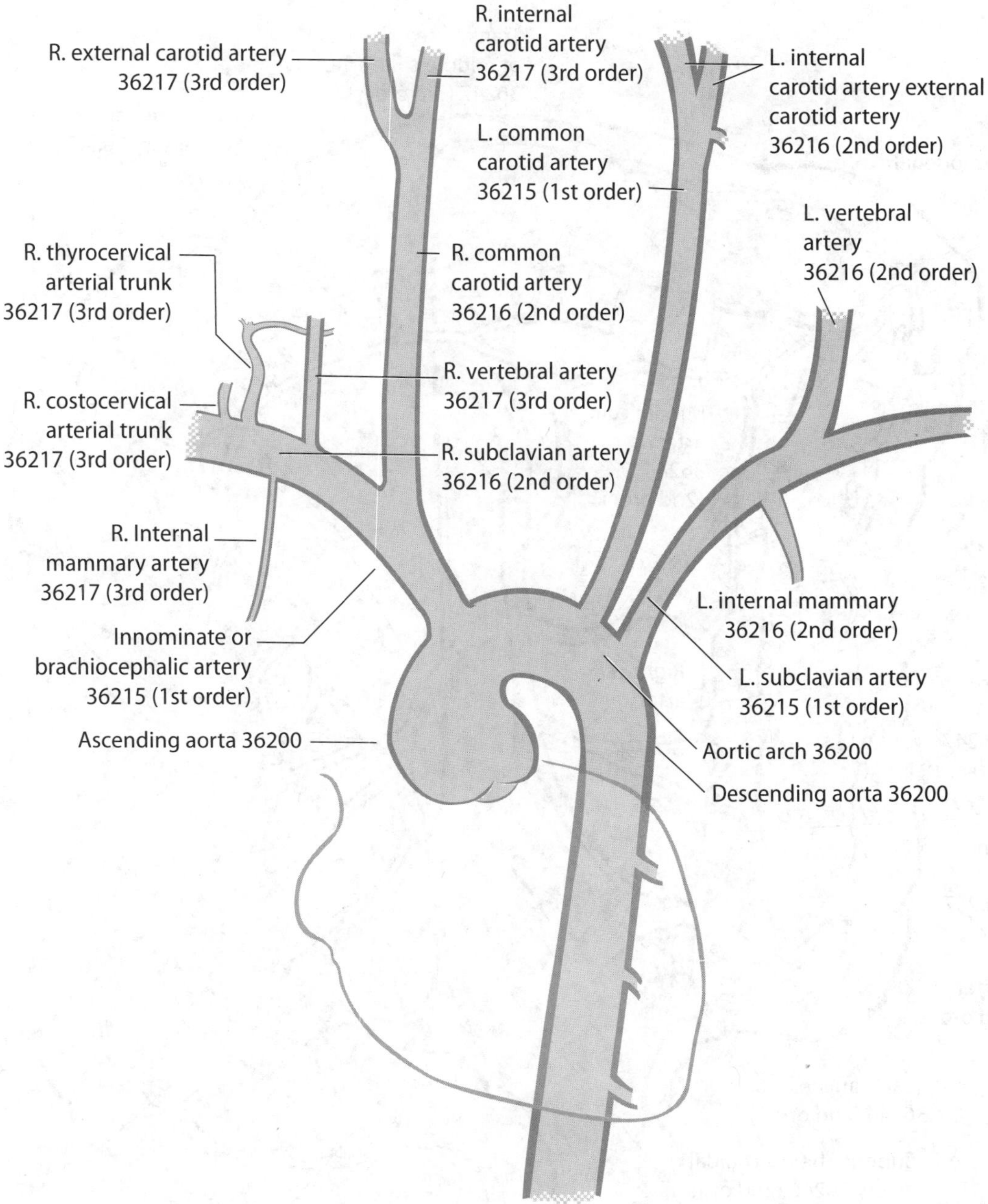
R. external carotid artery 36217 (3rd order)
R. internal carotid artery 36217 (3rd order)
L. internal carotid artery external carotid artery 36216 (2nd order)
L. common carotid artery 36215 (1st order)
L. vertebral artery 36216 (2nd order)
R. thyrocervical arterial trunk 36217 (3rd order)
R. common carotid artery 36216 (2nd order)
R. vertebral artery 36217 (3rd order)
R. costocervical arterial trunk 36217 (3rd order)
R. subclavian artery 36216 (2nd order)
R. Internal mammary artery 36217 (3rd order)
L. internal mammary 36216 (2nd order)
Innominate or brachiocephalic artery 36215 (1st order)
L. subclavian artery 36215 (1st order)
Ascending aorta 36200
Aortic arch 36200
Descending aorta 36200

Superior and Inferior Mesenteric Arteries and Branches

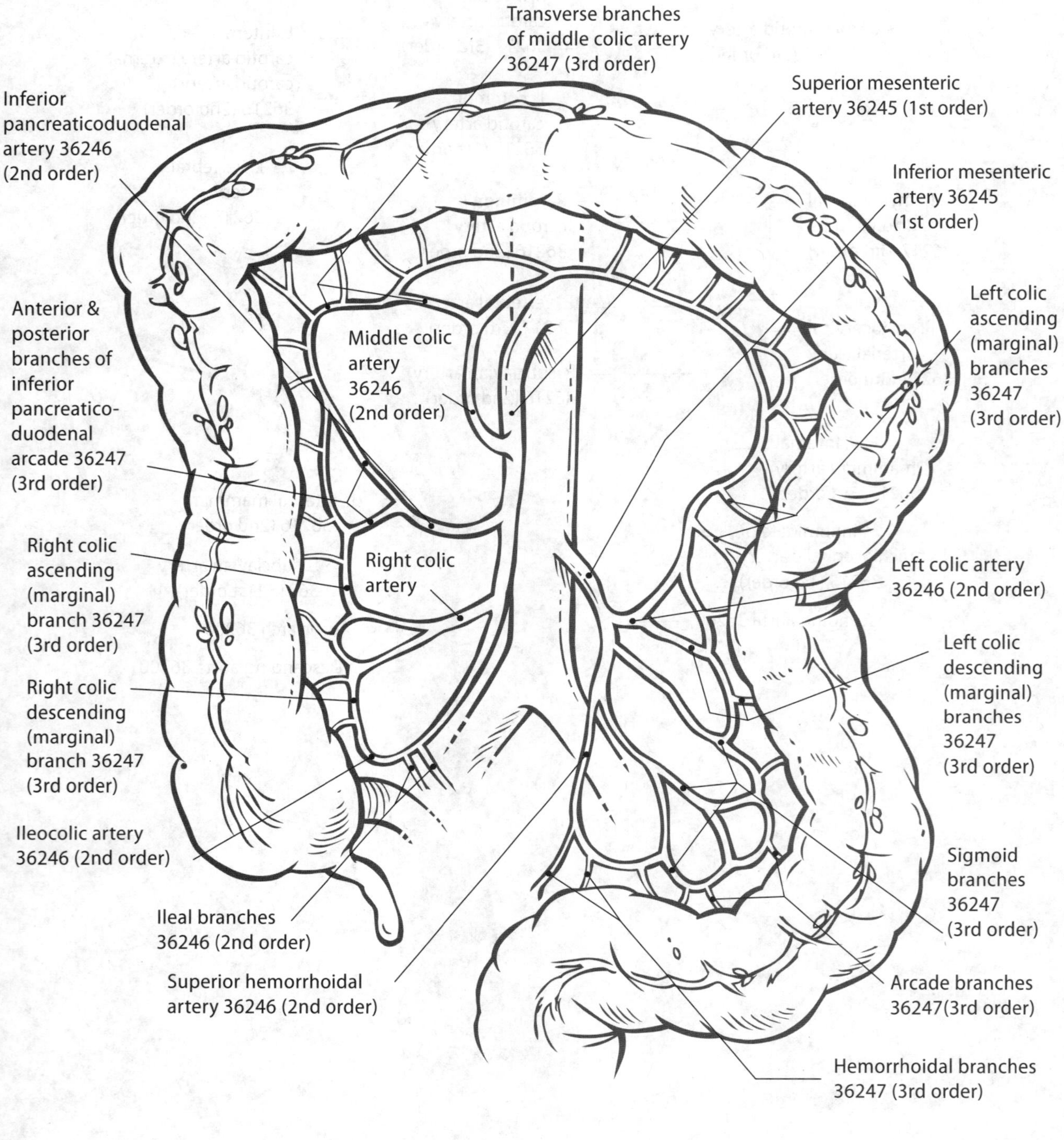
Transverse branches of middle colic artery 36247 (3rd order)
Superior mesenteric artery 36245 (1st order)
Inferior pancreaticoduodenal artery 36246 (2nd order)
Inferior mesenteric artery 36245 (1st order)
Anterior & posterior branches of inferior pancreatico-duodenal arcade 36247 (3rd order)
Middle colic artery 36246 (2nd order)
Left colic ascending (marginal) branches 36247 (3rd order)
Right colic ascending (marginal) branch 36247 (3rd order)
Right colic artery
Left colic artery 36246 (2nd order)
Right colic descending (marginal) branch 36247 (3rd order)
Left colic descending (marginal) branches 36247 (3rd order)
Ileocolic artery 36246 (2nd order)
Sigmoid branches 36247 (3rd order)
Ileal branches 36246 (2nd order)
Superior hemorrhoidal artery 36246 (2nd order)
Arcade branches 36247(3rd order)
Hemorrhoidal branches 36247 (3rd order)

Renal Artery Anatomy—Femoral Approach

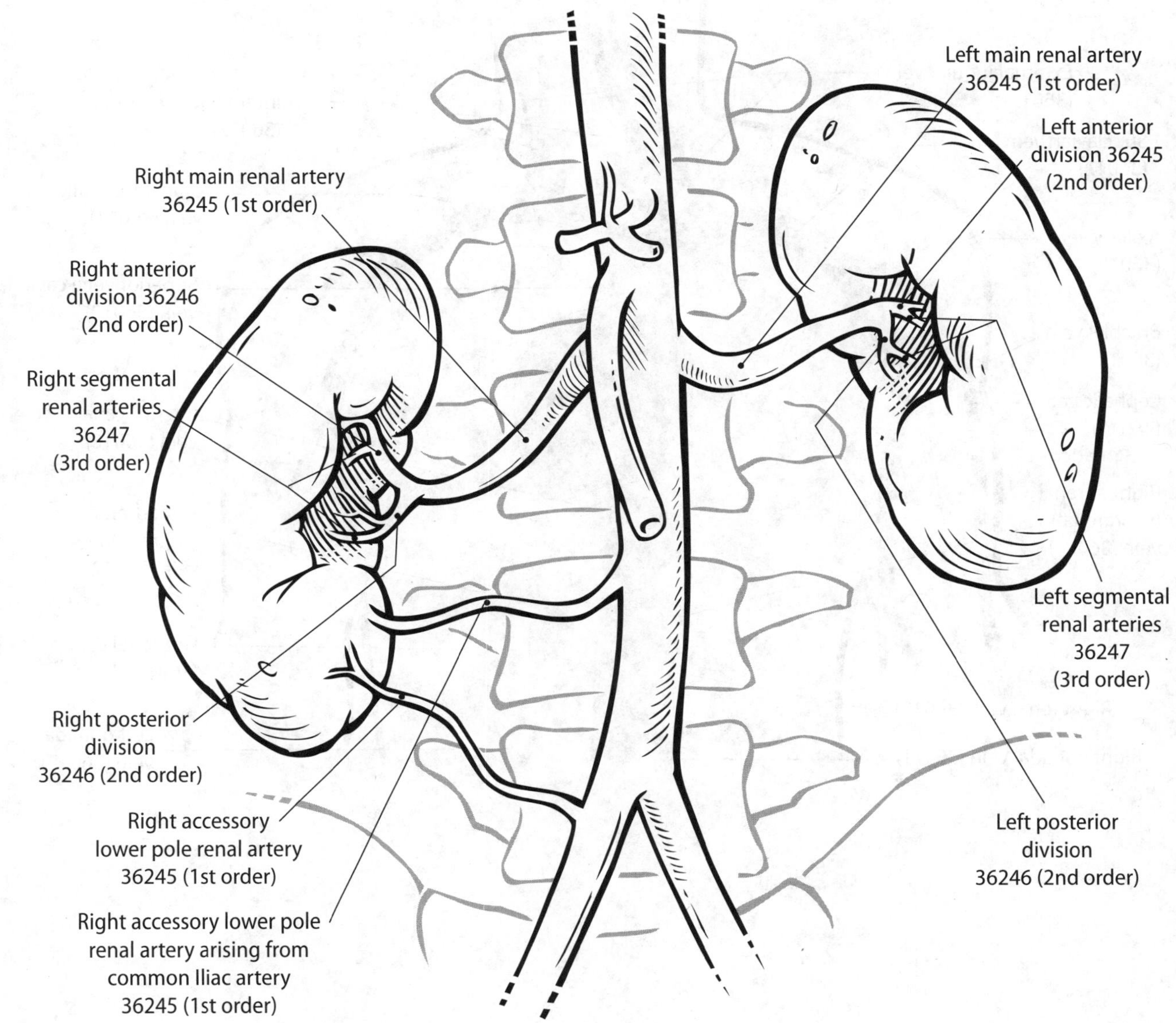
Left main renal artery
36245 (1st order)
Left anterior
division 36245
(2nd order)
Right main renal artery
36245 (1st order)
Right anterior
division 36246
(2nd order)
Right segmental
renal arteries
36247
(3rd order)
Left segmental
renal arteries
36247
(3rd order)
Right posterior
division
36246 (2nd order)
Right accessory
lower pole renal artery
36245 (1st order)
Left posterior
division
36246 (2nd order)
Right accessory lower pole
renal artery arising from
common Iliac artery
36245 (1st order)

Central Venous Anatomy

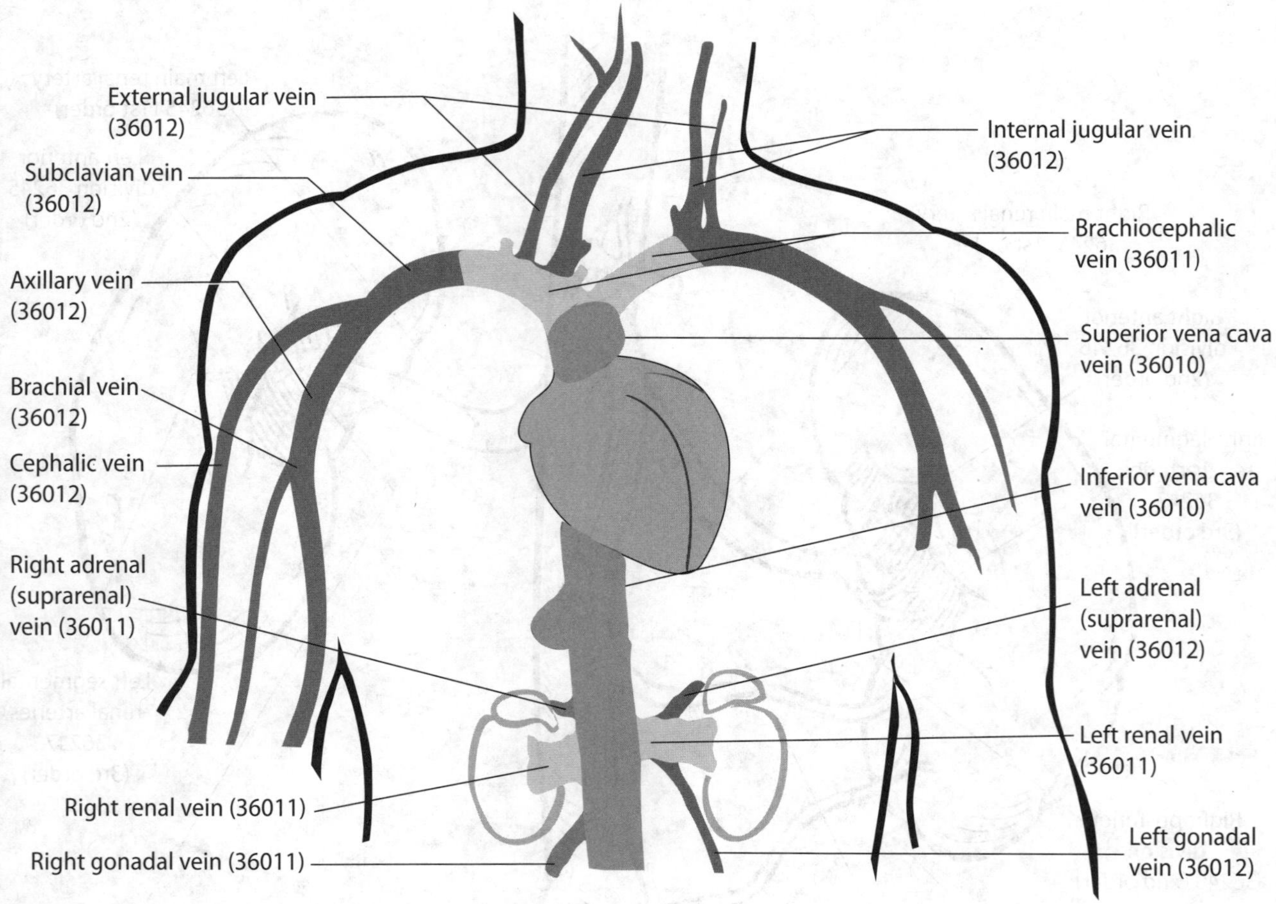
External jugular vein (36012)
Subclavian vein (36012)
Axillary vein (36012)
Brachial vein (36012)
Cephalic vein (36012)
Right adrenal (suprarenal) vein (36011)
Right renal vein (36011)
Right gonadal vein (36011)
Internal jugular vein (36012)
Brachiocephalic vein (36011)
Superior vena cava vein (36010)
Inferior vena cava vein (36010)
Left adrenal (suprarenal) vein (36012)
Left renal vein (36011)
Left gonadal vein (36012)

Portal System (Arterial)

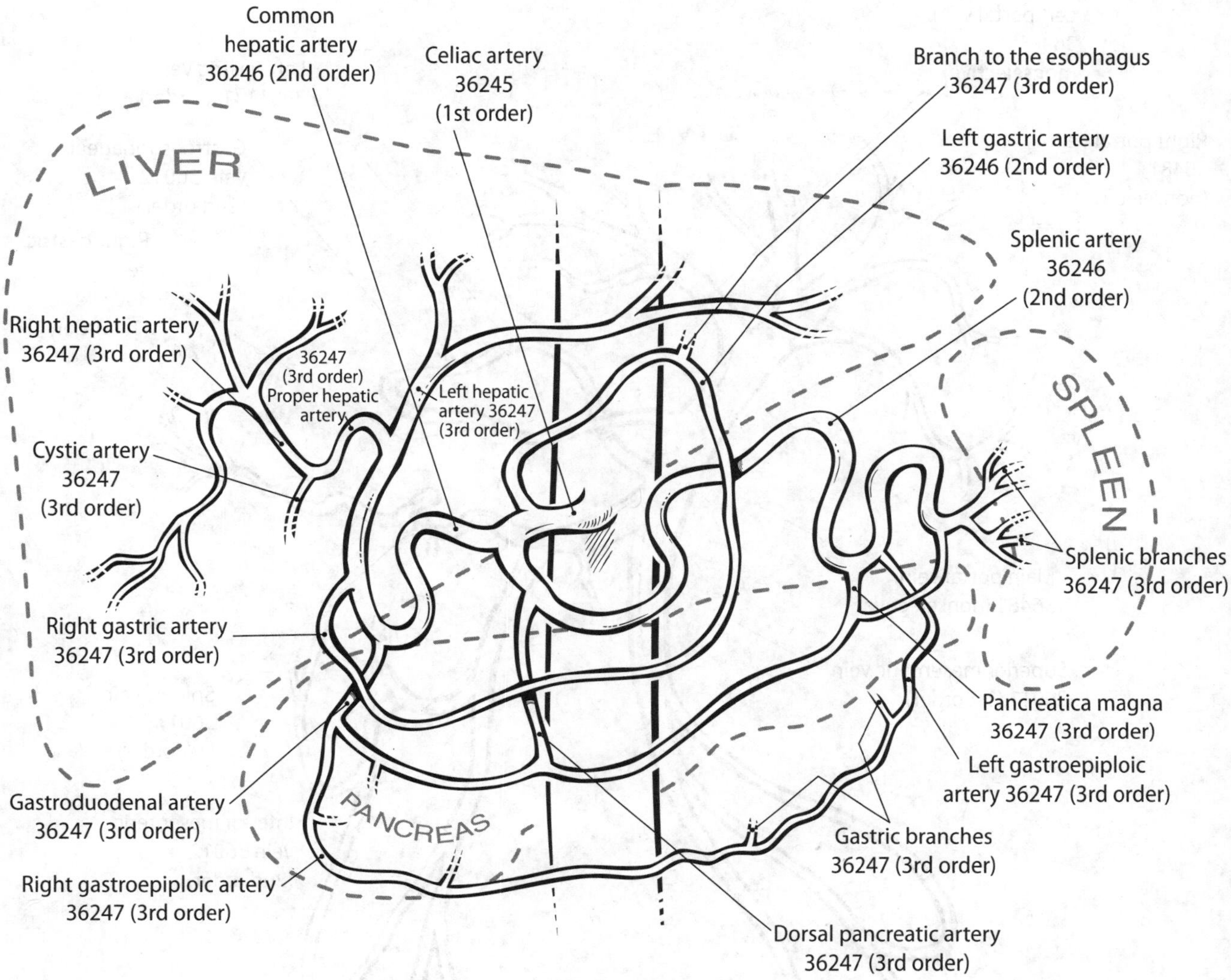
Common hepatic artery 36246 (2nd order)
Celiac artery 36245 (1st order)
Branch to the esophagus 36247 (3rd order)
Left gastric artery 36246 (2nd order)
LIVER
Splenic artery 36246 (2nd order)
Right hepatic artery 36247 (3rd order)
36247 (3rd order) Proper hepatic artery
Left hepatic artery 36247 (3rd order)
SPLEEN
Cystic artery 36247 (3rd order)
Splenic branches 36247 (3rd order)
Right gastric artery 36247 (3rd order)
Pancreatica magna 36247 (3rd order)
Left gastroepiploic artery 36247 (3rd order)
Gastroduodenal artery 36247 (3rd order)
PANCREAS
Gastric branches 36247 (3rd order)
Right gastroepiploic artery 36247 (3rd order)
Dorsal pancreatic artery 36247 (3rd order)

Portal System (Venous)

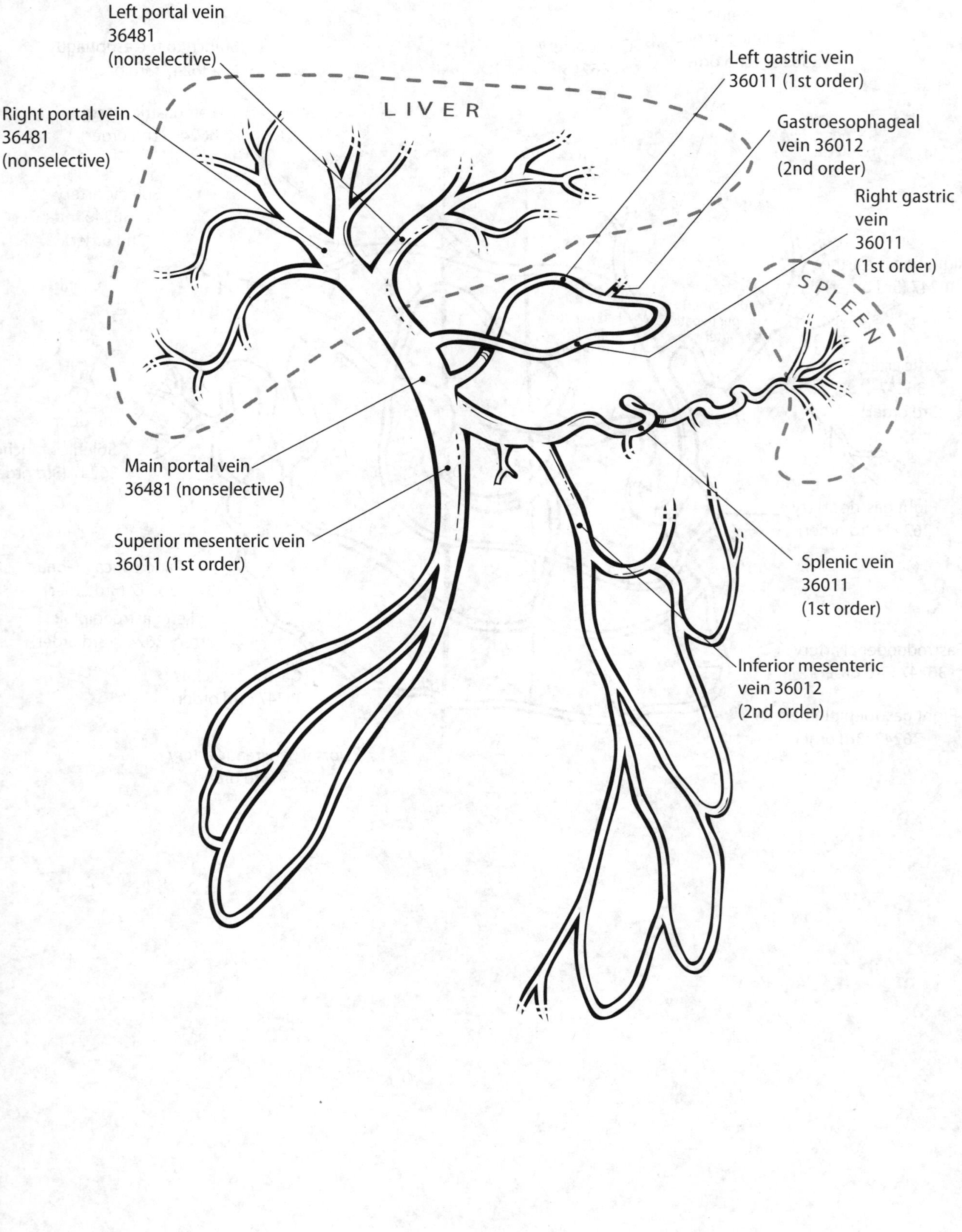
Left portal vein
36481
(nonselective)
Right portal vein
36481
(nonselective)
LIVER
Left gastric vein
36011 (1st order)
Gastroesophageal
vein 36012
(2nd order)
Right gastric
vein
36011
(1st order)
SPLEEN
Main portal vein
36481 (nonselective)
Superior mesenteric vein
36011 (1st order)
Splenic vein
36011
(1st order)
Inferior mesenteric
vein 36012
(2nd order)

Pulmonary Artery Angiography

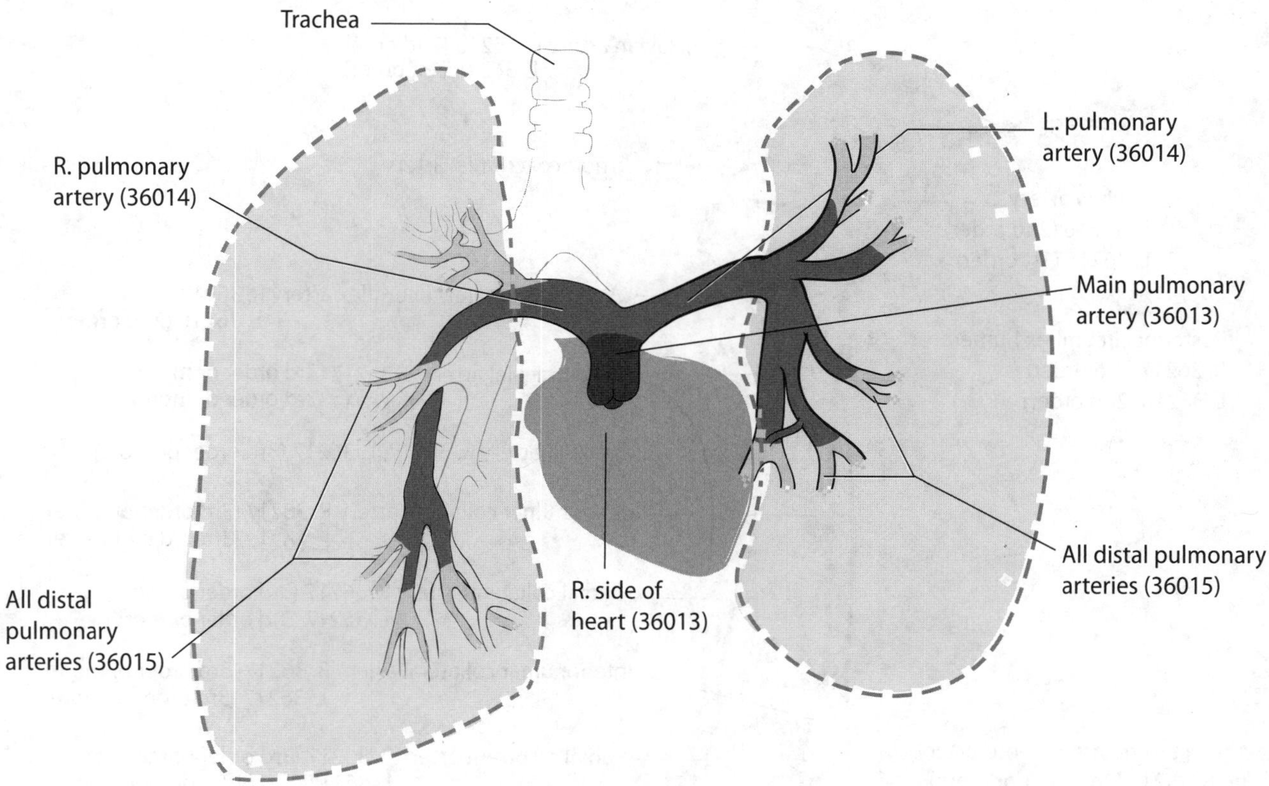

Upper Extremity Arterial Anatomy—Transfemoral or Contralateral Approach

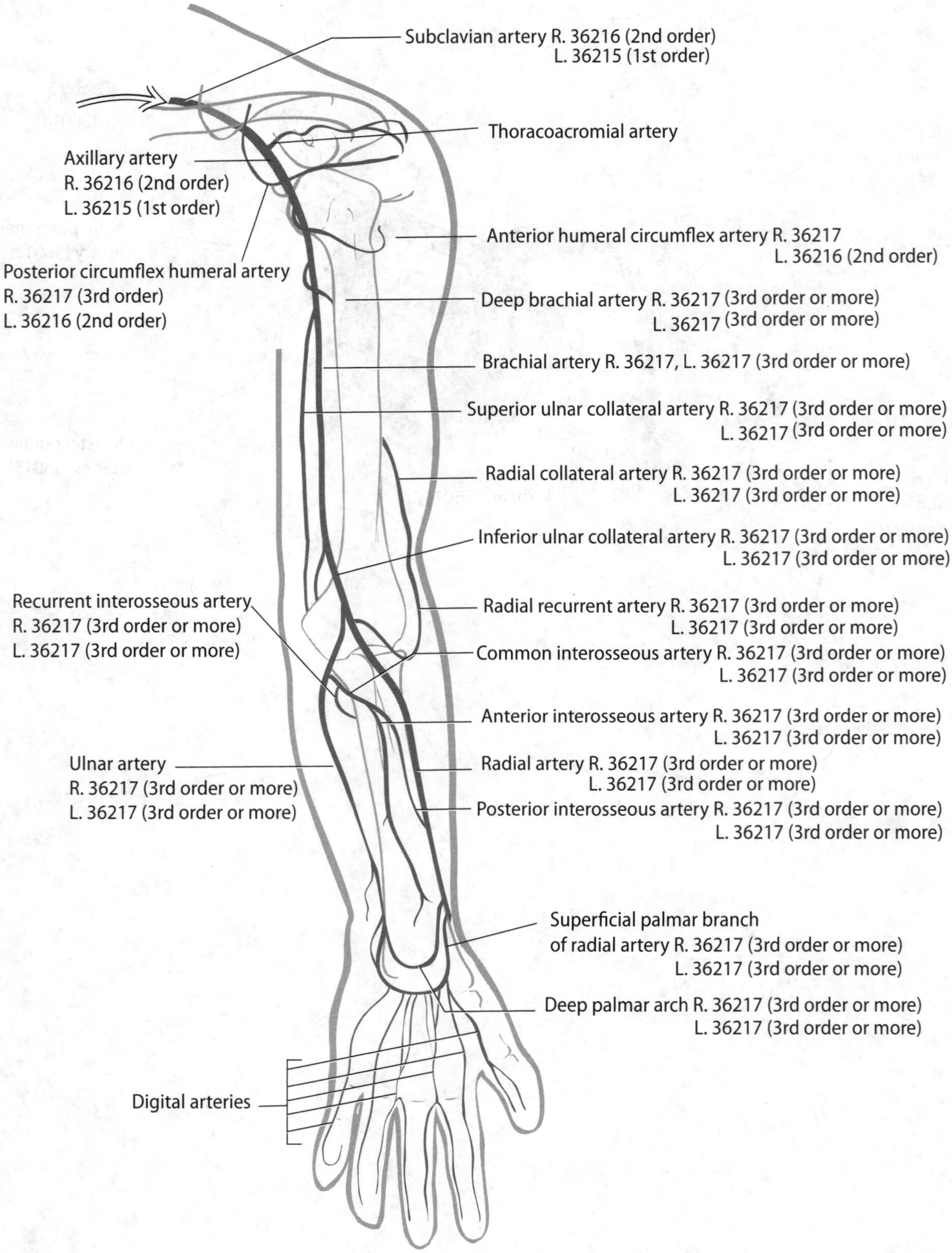

Subclavian artery R. 36216 (2nd order)
L. 36215 (1st order)

Axillary artery
R. 36216 (2nd order)
L. 36215 (1st order)

Thoracoacromial artery

Posterior circumflex humeral artery
R. 36217 (3rd order)
L. 36216 (2nd order)

Anterior humeral circumflex artery R. 36217
L. 36216 (2nd order)

Deep brachial artery R. 36217 (3rd order or more)
L. 36217 (3rd order or more)

Brachial artery R. 36217, L. 36217 (3rd order or more)

Superior ulnar collateral artery R. 36217 (3rd order or more)
L. 36217 (3rd order or more)

Radial collateral artery R. 36217 (3rd order or more)
L. 36217 (3rd order or more)

Inferior ulnar collateral artery R. 36217 (3rd order or more)
L. 36217 (3rd order or more)

Recurrent interosseous artery
R. 36217 (3rd order or more)
L. 36217 (3rd order or more)

Radial recurrent artery R. 36217 (3rd order or more)
L. 36217 (3rd order or more)

Common interosseous artery R. 36217 (3rd order or more)
L. 36217 (3rd order or more)

Anterior interosseous artery R. 36217 (3rd order or more)
L. 36217 (3rd order or more)

Ulnar artery
R. 36217 (3rd order or more)
L. 36217 (3rd order or more)

Radial artery R. 36217 (3rd order or more)
L. 36217 (3rd order or more)

Posterior interosseous artery R. 36217 (3rd order or more)
L. 36217 (3rd order or more)

Superficial palmar branch
of radial artery R. 36217 (3rd order or more)
L. 36217 (3rd order or more)

Deep palmar arch R. 36217 (3rd order or more)
L. 36217 (3rd order or more)

Digital arteries

Lower Extremity Arterial Anatomy—Contralateral, Axillary or Brachial Approach

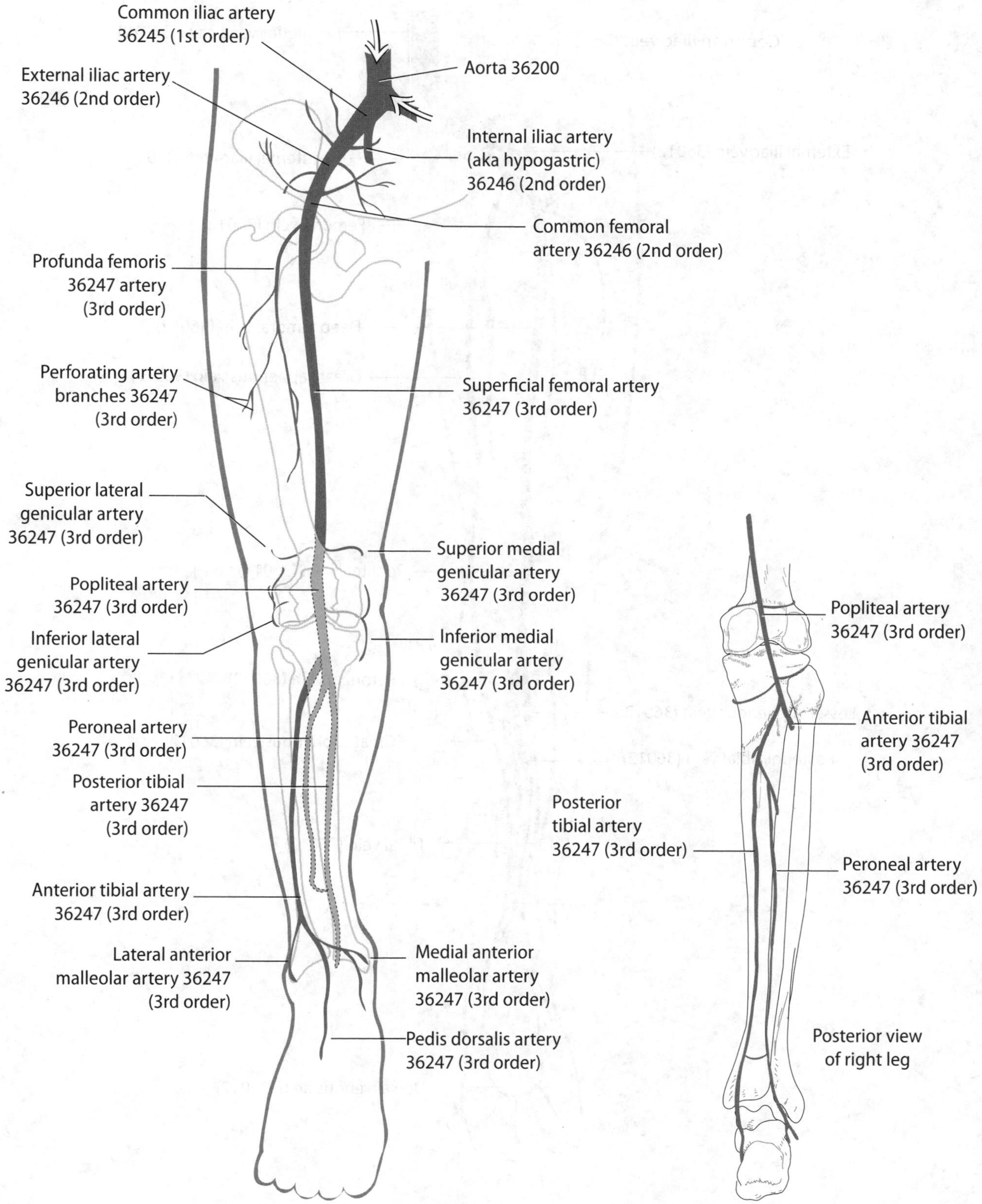
Common iliac artery 36245 (1st order)
Aorta 36200
External iliac artery 36246 (2nd order)
Internal iliac artery (aka hypogastric) 36246 (2nd order)
Common femoral artery 36246 (2nd order)
Profunda femoris 36247 artery (3rd order)
Perforating artery branches 36247 (3rd order)
Superficial femoral artery 36247 (3rd order)
Superior lateral genicular artery 36247 (3rd order)
Superior medial genicular artery 36247 (3rd order)
Popliteal artery 36247 (3rd order)
Inferior lateral genicular artery 36247 (3rd order)
Inferior medial genicular artery 36247 (3rd order)
Peroneal artery 36247 (3rd order)
Posterior tibial artery 36247 (3rd order)
Anterior tibial artery 36247 (3rd order)
Lateral anterior malleolar artery 36247 (3rd order)
Medial anterior malleolar artery 36247 (3rd order)
Pedis dorsalis artery 36247 (3rd order)
Popliteal artery 36247 (3rd order)
Anterior tibial artery 36247 (3rd order)
Posterior tibial artery 36247 (3rd order)
Peroneal artery 36247 (3rd order)
Posterior view of right leg

Lower Extremity Venous Anatomy

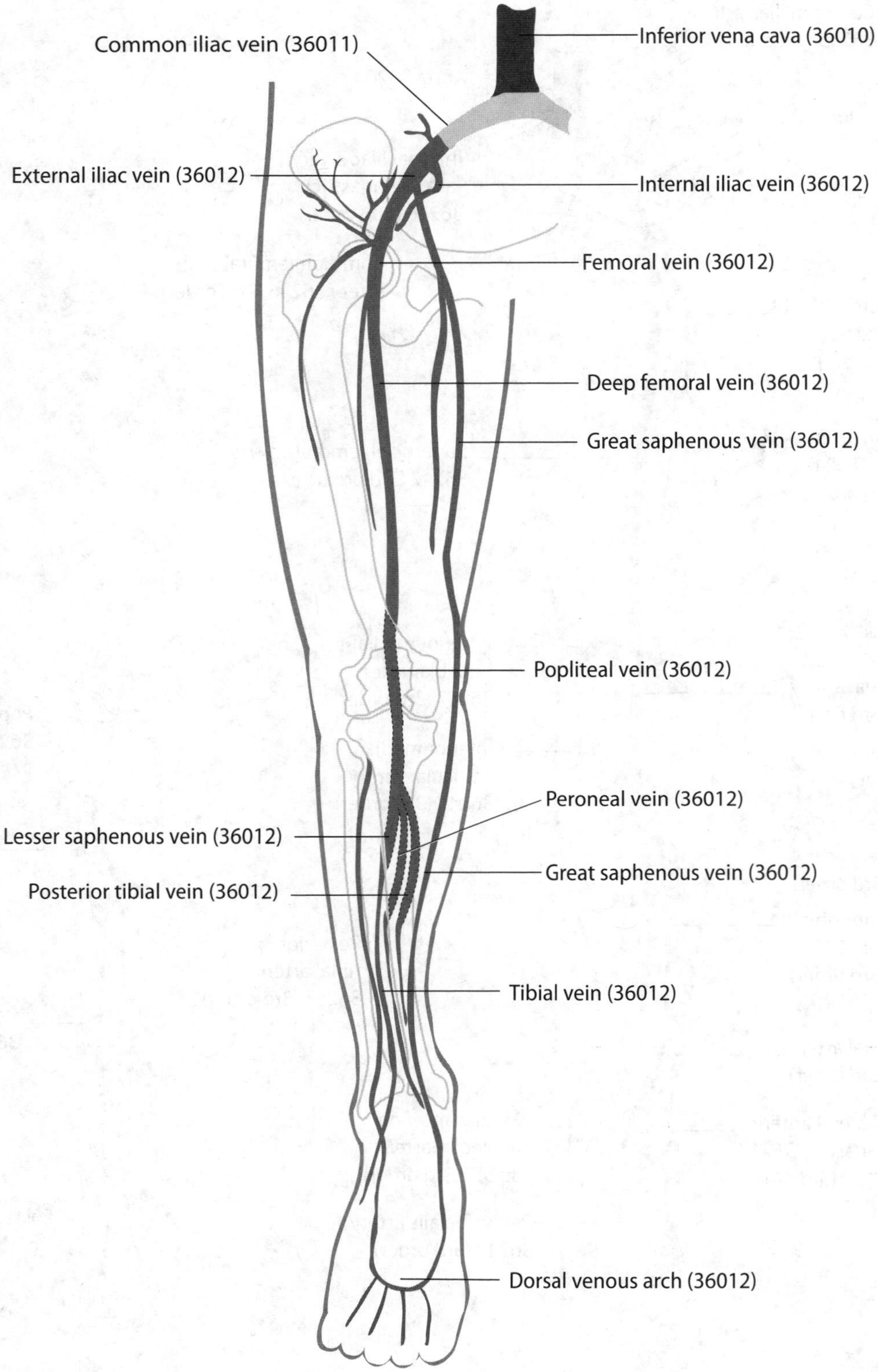
Common iliac vein (36011)
Inferior vena cava (36010)
External iliac vein (36012)
Internal iliac vein (36012)
Femoral vein (36012)
Deep femoral vein (36012)
Great saphenous vein (36012)
Popliteal vein (36012)
Peroneal vein (36012)
Lesser saphenous vein (36012)
Great saphenous vein (36012)
Posterior tibial vein (36012)
Tibial vein (36012)
Dorsal venous arch (36012)

Coronary Arteries Anterior View

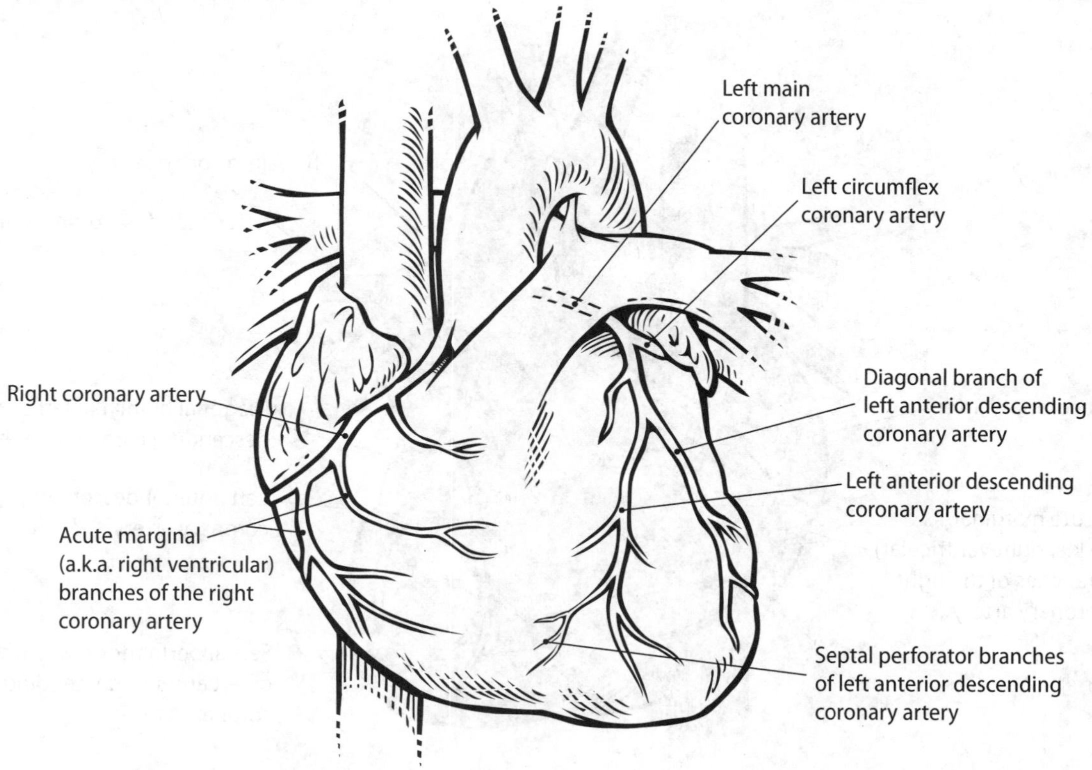

Left Heart Catheterization

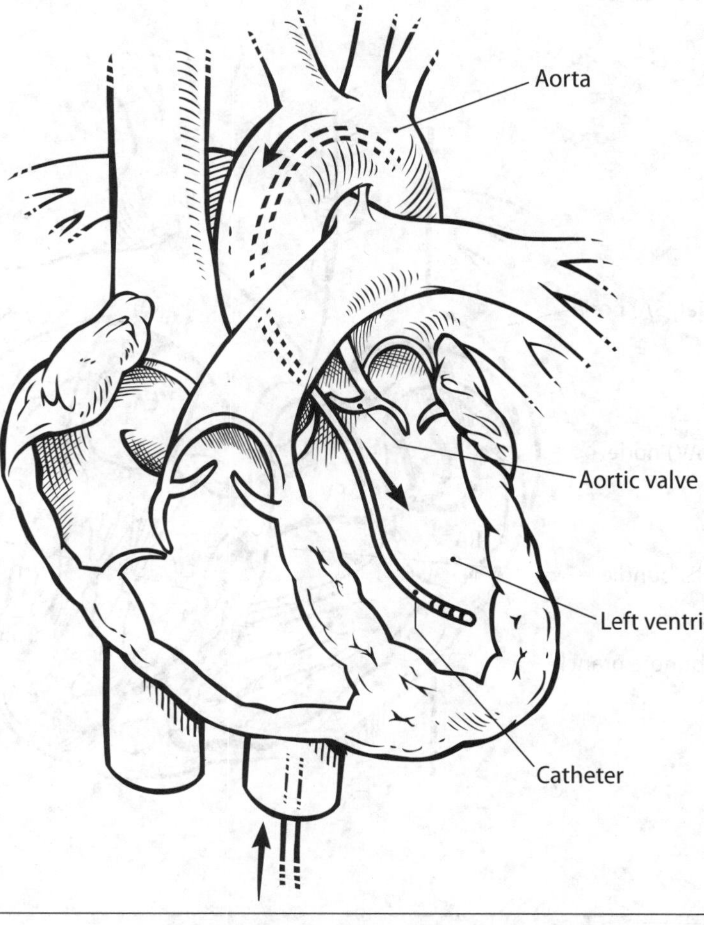

Right Heart Catheterization

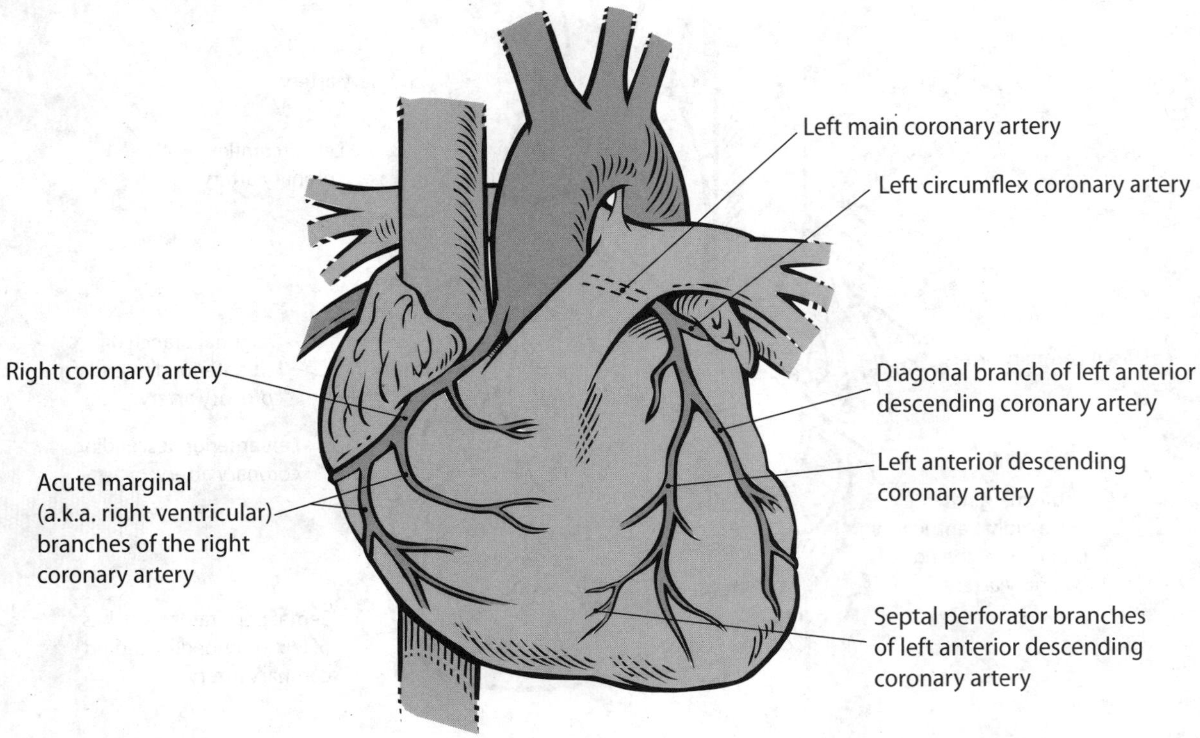

Heart Conduction System

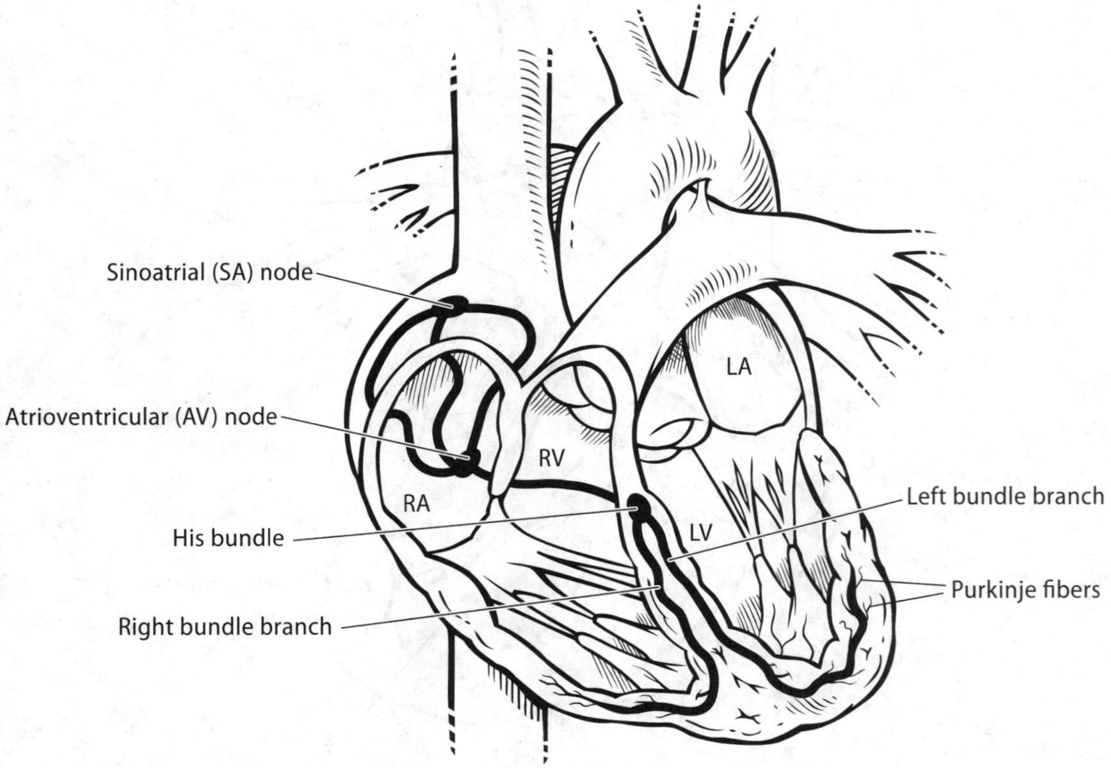